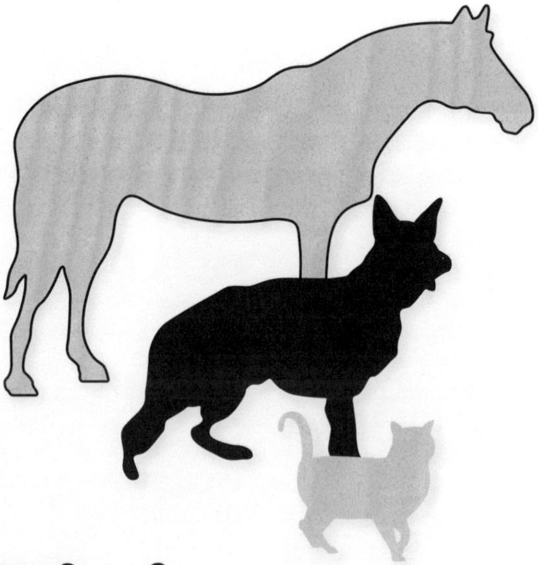

Chinese Herbal Formulas for Veterinarians

中獸醫方劑學

John K. Chen, Ph.D., Pharm.D., O.M.D., L.Ac.
Tina T. Chen, M.S., L.Ac.
Signe Beebe, D.V.M.
Michael Salewski, D.V.M.

中獸醫方劑學

Chinese Herbal Formulas for Veterinarians

Authors
John K. Chen, Ph.D., Pharm.D., O.M.D., L.Ac.
Tina T. Chen, M.S., L.Ac.
Signe Beebe, D.V.M.
Michael Salewski, D.V.M.

Co-authors
Eric K. Chen, Ph.D., O.M.D., L.Ac., J.D.
Victor Meng-Chau Jang, L.Ac.
Delicia Liu, L.Ac.
Minh T. Nguyen, L.Ac.
Shenying Tang, L.Ac.

Editors
Minh T. Nguyen, L.Ac.
Timothy Rogers, M.S.A.O.M., D.V.M.
Lily Huang, L.Ac.

International Standard Book Number (ISBN)-10: 0-9740635-9-2
International Standard Book Number (ISBN)-13: 978-0-9740635-9-1
Standard Address Number (SAN): 255-3376
Library of Congress Control Number (LCCN): 2011933459

Art of Medicine Press, Inc.
P.O. Box 90878
City of Industry, CA 91715-0878

Website: www.aompress.com
Email: editor@aompress.com

Abbreviated Table of Contents

Table of Contents

Table of Contents

Table of Contents

Table of Contents

Table of Contents

Table of Contents

Table of Contents

Table of Contents

Table of Contents

Table of Contents

Table of Contents

Preface

Chinese Herbal Formulas for Veterinarians is intended to be used with *Chinese Medical Herbology and Pharmacology*. The former text provides insight on how Chinese herbal formulas are used specifically in veterinary medicine, while the latter text provides indepth understanding of how each individual herb functions within these formulas.

In referencing between these two texts, it is important to note that the nomenclature for some herbs has been changed since the publication of ***Chinese Medical Herbology and Pharmacology*** in 2004. Most changes correspond to the 2005 edition of 中华人民共和国药典 *Zhong Hua Ren Min Gong He Guo Yao Dian* (Pharmacopoeia of the People's Republic of China), which is the official pharmacopoeia in China, as well as our primary reference. Changes have been made to:

- correctly pronounce the *pinyin* name, from *Huang Bai* (Cortex Phellodendri) to *Huang Bo* (Cortex Phellodendri Chinensis)
- precisely describe the processing method, from *Zhi Gan Cao* (Radix Glycyrrhizae Praeparata) to *Zhi Gan Cao* (Radix et Rhizoma Glycyrrhizae Praeparata cum Melle)
- be more specific: *Kun Bu* (Thallus Laminariae seu Eckloniae) is separated into *Hai Dai* (Thallus Laminariae) and *Kun Bu* (Thallus Eckloniae)
- be more inclusive: from *Shan Ci Gu* (Pseudobulbus Cremastrae) to *Shan Ci Gu* (Pseudobulbus Cremastrae seu Pleiones)
- adapt to the current rules and regulations, from *Xi Xin* (Herba Asari) to *Xi Xin* (Radix et Rhizoma Asari). Note: The aerial parts of asarum contain aristolochic acid, and have been banned by many countries around the world. As a result, the root and rhizome of asarum are now used, as they are believed to have little or no aristolochic acid.[1]
- and lastly, to humbly correct our previous errors, such as replacing the incorrect *Mu Fang Ji* (Radix Couulus Trilobus) with *Mu Fang Ji* (Radix Cocculi Trilobi).

Chinese Medical Herbology and Pharmacology	*Chinese Herbal Formulas for Veterinarians*
Ba Yue Zha (Fructus Akebiae)	*Yu Zhi Zi* (Fructus Akebiae)
Bai Dou Kou (Fructus Amomi Rotundus)	*Dou Kou* (Fructus Amomi Rotundus)
Bai Dou Kou Ke (Pericarpium Amomi Rotundus)	*Dou Kou Ke* (Pericarpium Amomi Rotundus)
Bai Hua She (Bungarus Parvus)	*Jin Qian Bai Hua She* (Bungarus Parvus)
Bai Hua She She Cao (Herba Oldenlandia)	*Bai Hua She She Cao* (Herba Hedyotis)
Bai Ji Li (Fructus Tribuli)	*Ji Li* (Fructus Tribuli)
Bai Qian (Rhizoma Cynanchi Stauntonii)	*Bai Qian* (Rhizoma et Radix Cynanchi Stauntonii)
Bai Wei (Radix Cynanchi Atrati)	*Bai Wei* (Radix et Rhizoma Cynanchi Atrati)
Bei Mu (Bulbus Fritillaria)	*Bei Mu* (Bulbus Fritillariae)
Bei Wu Jia Pi (Cortex Periploca Sepium Radicis)	*Xiang Jia Pi* (Cortex Periplocae)
Bi Ba (Fructus Piperis Longi)	*Bi Bo* (Fructus Piperis Longi)
Bi Xie (Rhizoma Dioscoreae Hypoglaucae)	*Fen Bi Xie* (Rhizoma Dioscoreae Hypoglaucae)
Bian Dou (Semen Lablab Album)	*Bai Bian Dou* (Semen Lablab Album)
Can Sha (Excrementum Bombycis Mori)	*Can Sha* (Faeces Bombycis)
Chi Fu Ling (Poria Rubrae)	*Chi Fu Ling* (Poria Rubra)
Chi Shao (Radix Paeoniae Rubrae)	*Chi Shao* (Radix Paeoniae Rubra)
Chong Wei Zi (Semen Leonuri)	*Chong Wei Zi* (Fructus Leonuri)
Chuan Xiong (Rhizoma Ligustici Chuanxiong)	*Chuan Xiong* (Rhizoma Chuanxiong)
Chun Gen Pi (Cortex Ailanthi)	*Chun Pi* (Cortex Ailanthi)
Ci Wu Jia (Radix et Caulis Acanthopanacis Senticosi)	*Ci Wu Jia* (Radix et Rhizoma seu Caulis Acanthopanacis Senticosi)
Da Hui Xiang (Fructus Anisi Stellati)	*Ba Jiao Hui Xiang* (Fructus Anisi Stellati)
Da Ji (Herba seu Radix Cirsii Japonici)	*Da Ji* (Herba Cirsii Japonici)

Chinese Medical Herbology and Pharmacology	*Chinese Herbal Formulas for Veterinarians*
Dai Zhe Shi (Haematitum)	*Zhe Shi* (Haematitum)
Dan Shen (Radix Salviae Miltiorrhizae)	*Dan Shen* (Radix et Rhizoma Salviae Miltiorrhizae)
Dang Gui (Radicis Angelicae Sinensis)	*Dang Gui* (Radix Angelicae Sinensis)
Dang Gui Shen (Corpus Radicis Angelicae Sinensis)	*Dang Gui Shen* (Corpus Radix Angelicae Sinensis)
Dang Gui Tou (Caput Radicis Angelicae Sinensis)	*Dang Gui Tou* (Caput Radix Angelicae Sinensis)
Dang Gui Wei (Extremitas Radicis Angelicae Sinensis)	*Dang Gui Wei* (Extremitas Radix Angelicae Sinensis)
Di Bie Chong (Eupolyphaga)	*Tu Bie Chong* (Eupolyphaga seu Steleophaga)
Duan Shi Gao (Gypsum Fibrosum Preparata)	*Duan Shi Gao* (Gypsum Fibrosum Praeparatum)
Fen Fang Ji (Radix Stephaniae Tetandrae)	*Fang Ji* (Radix Stephaniae Tetrandrae)
Fu Xiao Mai (Semen Tritici Aestivi Levis)	*Fu Xiao Mai* (Fructus Tritici Levis)
Gan Cao (Radix Glycyrrhizae)	*Gan Cao* (Radix et Rhizoma Glycyrrhizae)
Gan Song (Radix seu Rhizoma Nardostachys)	*Gan Song* (Radix et Rhizoma Nardostachydis)
Gan Sui (Radix Euphorbiae Kansui)	*Gan Sui* (Radix Kansui)
Gao Ben (Rhizoma Ligustici)	*Gao Ben* (Rhizoma et Radix Ligustici)
Ge Gen (Radix Puerariae)	*Ge Gen* (Radix Puerariae Lobatae)
Gu Zhi Hua (Semen Oroxyli)	*Mu Hu Die* (Semen Oroxyli)
Gua Lou Ren (Semen Trichosanthis)	*Gua Lou Zi* (Semen Trichosanthis)
Gua Lou Shi (Fructus Trichosanthis)	*Gua Lou* (Fructus Trichosanthis)
Guan Bai Fu (Rhizoma Aconitum Coreanum)	*Guan Bai Fu* (Radix Aconiti Coreani)
Guan Ye Lian Qiao (Herba Hypericum)	*Guan Ye Jin Si Tao* (Herba Hyperici Perforati)
Guan Zhong (Rhizoma Dryopteridis)	*Mian Ma Guan Zhong* (Rhizoma Dryopteridis Crassirhizomatis)
Hai Ge Fen (Concha Meretricis seu Cyclinae)	*Ge Qiao* (Concha Meretricis seu Cyclinae)
Hai Jin Sha (Herba Lygodii)	*Hai Jin Sha* (Spora Lygodii)
Han Fang Ji (Radix Stephaniae Tetandrae)	*Fang Ji* (Radix Stephaniae Tetrandrae)
Han Lian Cao (Herba Ecliptae)	*Mo Han Lian* (Herba Ecliptae)
Hei Cha (Folium Camelliae Nigrum)	*Hei Cha* (Folium Camelliae Nigrum)
Hei Dou (Semen Glycine Max)	*Hei Dou* (Semen Sojae)
Hong Dou Kou (Fructus Alphiniae Galangae)	*Hong Dou Kou* (Fructus Galangae)
Hong Teng (Caulis Sargentodoxae)	*Da Xue Teng* (Caulis Sargentodoxae)
Hu Jiao (Fructus Piper)	*Hu Jiao* (Fructus Piperis)
Hu Zhang (Rhizoma Polygoni Cuspidati)	*Hu Zhang* (Rhizoma et Radix Polygoni Cuspidati)
Huai Niu Xi (Radix Achyranthis Bidentatae)	*Niu Xi* (Radix Achyranthis Bidentatae)
Huang Bai (Cortex Phellodendri)	*Huang Bo* (Cortex Phellodendri Chinensis)
Huang Teng (Caulis Fibraurea)	*Huang Teng* (Caulis Fibraureae)
Huo Xiang (Herba Agastache)	*Huo Xiang* (Herba Agastaches)
Huo Xiang Ye (Folium Agastache)	*Huo Xiang Ye* (Folium Agastaches)
Jin Bo (Native Gold)	*Jin Bo* (gold foil)
Jin Yin Hua (Flos Lonicerae)	*Jin Yin Hua* (Flos Lonicerae Japonicae)
Jing Jie Sui (Flos Schizonepetae)	*Jing Jie Sui* (Spica Schizonepetae)
Jing Sui (Flos Schizonepetae)	*Jing Jie Sui* (Spica Schizonepetae)
Ju He (Semen Citri Rubrum)	*Ju He* (Semen Citri Reticulatae)
Ju Luo (Fibra Citri Rubrum)	*Ju Luo* (Vascular Citri Reticulatae)

Preface

Chinese Medical Herbology and Pharmacology	*Chinese Herbal Formulas for Veterinarians*
Ju Ye (Folium Citri Rubrum)	*Ju Ye* (Folium Citri Reticulatae)
Ku Shen Gen (Radix Sophorae Flavescentis)	*Ku Shen* (Radix Sophorae Flavescentis)
Kun Bu (Thallus Laminariae seu Eckloniae)	*Kun Bu* (Thallus Eckloniae)
Long Dan Cao (Radix Gentianae)	*Long Dan* (Radix et Rhizoma Gentianae)
Lu Cha (Folium Camellia Sinensis)	*Cha Ye* (Folium Camelliae)
Lu Feng Fang (Nidus Vespae)	*Feng Fang* (Nidus Vespae)
Lu Han Cao (Herba Pyrolae)	*Lu Xian Cao* (Herba Pyrolae)
Lu Jiao Jiao (Gelatinum Cornu Cervi)	*Lu Jiao Jiao* (Colla Cornus Cervi)
Lu Jiao Shuang (Cornu Cervi Degelatinatium)	*Lu Jiao Shuang* (Cornu Cervi Degelatinatum)
Ma Huang Gen (Radix Ephedrae)	*Ma Huang Gen* (Radix et Rhizoma Ephedrae)
Mai Men Dong (Radix Ophiopogonis)	*Mai Dong* (Radix Ophiopogonis)
Mi Jiao (Cornu Elapnurus)	*Mi Lu Jiao* (Cornu Elaphuri)
Mi Rong (Cornu Elapnurus Parvum)	*Mi Lu Rong* (Cornu Elaphuri Pantotrichum)
Ming Fan (Alumen)	*Bai Fan* (Alumen)
Mu Fang Ji (Radix Couulus Trilobus)	*Mu Fang Ji* (Radix Cocculi Trilobi)
Niu Xi (Radix Cyathulae seu Achyranthis)	*Niu Xi* (Radix Achyranthis Bidentatae)
Pao Jiang (Rhizoma Zingiberis Preparatum)	*Pao Jiang* (Rhizoma Zingiberis Praeparatum)
Qian Cao (Radix Rubiae)	*Qian Cao* (Radix et Rhizoma Rubiae)
Qian Jin Zi (Semen Euphorbiae Lathyridis)	*Qian Jin Zi* (Semen Euphorbiae)
Ren Dong Cao (Herba Lonicerae)	*Ren Dong Cao* (Herba Lonicerae Japonicae)
Ren Dong Teng (Caulis Lonicerae)	*Ren Dong Teng* (Caulis Lonicerae Japonicae)
Ren Gong Niu Huang (Calculus Bovis Syntheticum)	*Ren Gong Niu Huang* (Calculus Bovis Artifactus)
Ren Shen (Radix Ginseng)	*Ren Shen* (Radix et Rhizoma Ginseng)
Rui Ren (Semen Prinsepiae)	*Rui Ren* (Nux Prinsepiae)
San Qi (Radix Notoginseng)	*San Qi* (Radix et Rhizoma Notoginseng)
Sang Shen Zi (Fructus Mori)	*Sang Shen* (Fructus Mori)
Shan Ci Gu (Pseudobulbus Cremastrae)	*Shan Ci Gu* (Pseudobulbus Cremastrae seu Pleiones)
Shan Dou Gen (Radix Sophorae Tonkinensis)	*Shan Dou Gen* (Radix et Rhizoma Sophorae Tonkinensis)
Sheng Di Huang (Radix Rehmanniae)	*Di Huang* (Radix Rehmanniae)
Shi Chang Pu (Rhizoma Acori)	*Shi Chang Pu* (Rhizoma Acori Tatarinowii)
Shi Hu (Herba Dendrobii)	*Shi Hu* (Caulis Dendrobii)
Shu Di Huang (Radix Rehmanniae Preparata)	*Shu Di Huang* (Radix Rehmanniae Praeparata)
Shui Chang Pu (Rhizoma Acori Calami)	*Zang Chang Pu* (Rhizoma Acori Calami)
Su Geng (Caulis Perillae)	*Zi Su Geng* (Caulis Perillae)
Su Ye (Folium Perillae)	*Zi Su Ye* (Folium Perillae)
Su Zi (Fructus Perillae)	*Zi Su Zi* (Fructus Perillae)
Suan Zao Ren (Semen Zizyphi Spinosae)	*Suan Zao Ren* (Semen Ziziphi Spinosae)
Tian Men Dong (Radix Asparagi)	*Tian Dong* (Radix Asparagi)
Tu Bei Mu (Bulbus Bolbostemma Paniculatum)	*Tu Bei Mu* (Rhizoma Bolbostematis)
Tu Niu Xi (Radix Achyranthes Longifolia)	*Tu Niu Xi* (Radix Achyranthis Longifoliae)
Wan Nian Song (Herba Selaginellae)	*Juan Bai* (Herba Selaginellae)
Wei Ling Xian (Radix Clematidis)	*Wei Ling Xian* (Radix et Rhizoma Clematidis)
Wu Ling Zhi (Excrementum Trogopteri seu Pteromi)	*Wu Ling Zhi* (Faeces Trogopteri)

Chinese Medical Herbology and Pharmacology	*Chinese Herbal Formulas for Veterinarians*
Wu Long Cha (Folium Camellia Sinensis Fermentata)	*Wu Long Cha* (Folium Camelliae Fermentata)
Xi Xin (Herba Asari)	*Xi Xin* (Radix et Rhizoma Asari)
Xiang Ru (Herba Elsholtziae seu Moslae)	*Xiang Ru* (Herba Moslae)
Xiao Ji (Herba Cirisii)	*Xiao Ji* (Herba Cirsii)
Xing Ren (Semen Armeniacae Amarum)	*Ku Xing Ren* (Semen Armeniacae Amarum)
Xu Chang Qing (Radix Cynanchi Paniculati)	*Xu Chang Qing* (Radix et Rhizoma Cynanchi Paniculati)
Xuan Ming Fen (Matrii Sulfas Exsiccatus)	*Xuan Ming Fen* (Natrii Sulfas Exsiccatus)
Ye Jiao Teng (Caulis Polygoni Multiflori)	*Shou Wu Teng* (Caulis Polygoni Multiflori)
Ye Ming Sha (Excrementum Vespertilionis Murini)	*Ye Ming Sha* (Faeces Vespertilionis Murini)
Yi Tang (Saccharum Granorum)	*Yi Tang* (Maltosum)
Yi Zhi Ren (Fructus Alpiniae Oxyphyllae)	*Yi Zhi* (Fructus Alpiniae Oxyphyllae)
Yin Chen Hao (Herba Artemisiae Scopariae)	*Yin Chen* (Herba Artemisiae Scopariae)
Yin Guo Ye (Folium Ginkgo)	*Yin Xing Ye* (Folium Ginkgo)
Yuan Ming Fen (Matrii Sulfas Exsiccatus)	*Xuan Ming Fen* (Natrii Sulfas Exsiccatus)
Zang Hong Hua (Flos Crocus Sativus)	*Xi Hong Hua* (Stigma Croci)
Zhen Zhu Mu (Concha Margaritaferae)	*Zhen Zhu Mu* (Concha Margaritiferae)
Zhi Gan Cao (Radix Glycyrrhizae Preparata)	*Zhi Gan Cao* (Radix et Rhizoma Glycyrrhizae Praeparata cum Melle)
Zhi Ke (Fructus Aurantii)	*Zhi Qiao* (Fructus Aurantii)
Zhi Mu (Radix Anemarrhenae)	*Zhi Mu* (Rhizoma Anemarrhenae)
Zi Cao Gen (Radix Lithospermi)	*Zi Cao* (Radix Arnebiae)
Zi Wan (Radix Asteris)	*Zi Wan* (Radix et Rhizoma Asteris)
Zong Lu Pi (Fibra Stipulae Trachycarpi)	*Zong Lu* (Petiolus Trachycarpi)

[1] Wu KM, Farrelly JG, Upton R, Chen J. Complexities of the herbal nomenclature system in traditional Chinese medicine (TCM): Lessons learned from the misuse of Aristolochia-related species and the importance of the pharmaceutical name during botanical drug product development. Phytomedicine 2007;14:273-279.

Acknowledgement

We would like to thank Signe Beebe, Michael Salewski, Minh Nguyen, Timothy Rogers, and all the peer reviewers for their time, knowledge and expertise in writing and completing this text.

We would also like to thank all of our teachers, who have taught us everything we know, especially Drs. Chang Wei-Yen (Jimmy), Tan Teh-Fu (Richard), Zhang Xiao-Ping, Zhang Hua-Long, Jiao Shu-De, Sam Liang, Liu Zhi-Tong, Charlis Tsai and Tsai Wen-Qi.

Our thanks to Dan Bensky, Randall Barolet, Andrew Gamble, Giovanni Maciocia, Subhuti Dharmanada, Him-che Yeung, Nigel Wiseman and Feng Ye for establishing the credibility of traditional Chinese medicine in the western worlds.

Our thanks to the team of co-authors, Eric Chen, Victor Jang, Delicia Liu, Minh Nguyen and Shenying Tang. Without their contributions, this book would still be a work in progress.

Our utmost appreciation to a team of many fine editors, Minh Nguyen, Timothy Rogers, Thad Ekdahl, Catherine Lu, Laraine Crampton, Abba Anderson, Colleen Burke, Lily Huang, Cathy McNease, Marguerite Valance, Linda Joy Stone, and Kevin Inglis. You help to make this book a pleasure to read.

We warmly appreciate all of the other contributors and peer-reviewers, for your invaluable comments and suggestions.

Most importantly, we would like to thank our family: our father, for his vision and inspiration; our mom, for her endless love and support; and our family for reminding us to stop and smell the herbs throughout the journey of writing this book.

The publication of *Chinese Herbal Formulas for Veterinarians* would not have been possible without the help of everyone who has contributed. This book belongs to all of us.

John K. Chen
Tina T. Chen

I would like to thank Rachele Kelly and Heather Estay for their help in the research and editing of this text.

Signe Beebe

I would like to thank Signe Beebe, John Chen and Tina Chen for their invaluable work and dedication to this book. I would also like to thank my many mentors in herbal medicine including Huisheng Xie, Gary Allen, Mona Boudreaux, and Kezhuang Zhao. Finally, I would like to thank my clients and patients, whose support and spirit have made life so fulfilling.

Michael Salewski

Contributors

Authors
John K Chen, PhD, PharmD, OMD, LAc
Tina T Chen, MS, LAc
Signe Beebe, DVM
Michael Salewski, DVM

Co-Authors
Eric K Chen, PhD, OMD, LAc, JD
Victor Meng-Chau Jang, LAc
Delicia Liu, LAc
Minh T Nguyen, LAc
Shenying Tang, LAc

Editors
Minh T Nguyen, LAc
Lily Huang, LAc
Timothy Rogers, MSAOM, DVM

Associate Editors
Laraine Crampton, LAc
Thad Ekdahl, LAc
Catherine Lu, LAc

Copy Editors
Abba Anderson, LAc
Colleen Burke, LAc
Dave Karaba, LAc
Cathy McNease, DiplCH
Marguerite Valance, LAc

Draft Editors
Linda Joy Stone, LAc
Kevin Inglis, LAc

Consultants
Jize Li, LAc
Huabing Wen, LAc

Research Associates
Wei Chien
Lily Kathleen Ko, LAc
Janice Lee, LAc
Delicia Liu, LAc

Peer Reviewers
Gary Allen, DOM
Albuquerque, New Mexico, USA

Monika Bartholomé, DVM, CVT
Herne, Germany

Ihor Basko, DVM, CVA
Kapaa, Hawaii USA

Linda Boggie, DVM
Holten, The Netherlands

Mona Boudreaux, DVM, CVA, MMQ
Wonder Lake, Illinois USA

Eidín Burns, MVB
Limerick, Ireland

Bruce Ferguson, DVM, MS
Karawara, Western Australia

Barbara Fougere, BVSc, BVMS (Hons)
NSW Auustralia

Carolina Haddad, DVM
São Paulo, Brazil

Joyce Harman DVM, MRCVS
Virginia USA

Oh Soon Hock
Singapore

Carole Holland, DVM,CVA
Jupiter, Florida USA

Jean GF Joaquim, DVM, MSc, PhD
São Paulo, Brazil

Deva Khalsa, VMD,CVA, FBIH
New Zealand

Ching Ming Liu, DVM, MS, CVA
Taipei, Taiwan

Lorena Lloret, DVM, CVA, CVFT
Madrid, Spain

Deborah M Mitchell, DVM, MS
Schaumburg, Illinois USA

Carl Muller, BVSc, IVAS
Victoria, Australia

Ferdinand Niessen, DVM
Duesseldorf, Germany

Contributors

Phil Rogers, MVB, MRCVS
Dublin, Ireland

Shane Ryan, BVSc (Hons) MVS CVA
Singapore

Nancy Scanlan, DVM, MSFP, CVA
Weed, California USA

Robert G Schaeffer, Jr, DVM, PhD
St. Louis, Missouri USA

Cheryl Schwartz, DVM
Alameda, California USA

Emiel Van den Bosch
Ramsel, Belgium

Susan G Wynn, DVM, CVA, CVCH, AHG
Sandy Springs Georgia USA

Huisheng Xie, DVM, PhD, MS
Reddick, Florida USA

Kezhuang Zhao, DOM, LAc
Santa Fe, New Mexico USA

Chinese Language Consultant
Estella Huei-Mei Liu

Cover Design
Charles O Funk

Book Design
Rick Friesen
Chien-Hui Liao

Portraits
Jimmy Wei-Yen Chang, OMD, LAc

Legal Advisor
Eric K Chen, PhD, OMD, LAc, JD

Using This Book

Chinese Herbal Formulas for Veterinarians is intended to be a reference and educational text for the use of classical Chinese herbal formulas in animals. This book is adapted from ***Chinese Herbal Formulas and Applications*** by John Chen and Tina Chen, which offers a comprehensive look at the use of these formulas in humans. While this text focuses on veterinary applications of classical formulas, we retain the resource of many formulas of historical significance that may not be commonly used in veterinary medicine at this time. Other formulas that are specific to human medical conditions, and those that would never be used in veterinary medicine because of superior Western therapies, have been omitted entirely. Each chapter is prefaced with an introduction to the category of formulas that follow. These introductions have been written specifically to explain how the formulas in each chapter's category apply to common pattern imbalances found in animals. In each formula monograph, we have included the following sections: Chinese therapeutic actions, clinical manifestations, veterinary clinical applications, cautions and/or contraindications, and acupuncture treatments specific to veterinary medicine. These sections are meant to expand the practitioners' clinical skills and help assure good outcomes for patients.

Traditional Chinese veterinary medicine (TCVM) has many terms that can, on occasion, create confusion because of their similarity to Western medical terminology. This volume, like ***Chinese Herbal Formulas and Applications,*** tries to bridge this gap by providing consistent standards, such as:

- Terms that have become an accepted part of the English lexicon and are well understood by the general public, such as qi, yin, and yang, are not italicized or capitalized.
- Terms unique to the profession, understood primarily by TCVM practitioners, are given in *pinyin*, italicized and translated, but not capitalized; such as *bi zheng* (painful obstruction syndrome), *xiao ke* (wasting and thirsting syndrome), and *lin zheng* (dysuria syndrome).
- Organ names are capitalized when used in the context of traditional Chinese veterinary medicine, but <u>not</u> when referring exclusively to anatomical function. For example, *Qing Wei San* (Clear the Stomach Powder), can be used effectively to clear <u>Stomach</u> heat, a disorder of the <u>stomach</u> that commonly manifests as ulcers or gastritis in horses.
- Names and words distinct to herbal medicine are italicized, capitalized, and translated, such as *Ren Shen* (Radix et Rhizoma Ginseng) and *Bu Zhong Yi Qi Tang* (Tonify the Middle and Augment the Qi Decoction).
- Translations are omitted after the first full use of the term in one monograph or segment of a monograph, unless repetition is necessary to ensure clarity and safety in discriminating between substances or concepts.
- To avoid confusion, formulas other than the principal formula under consideration in a given monograph will be listed with their full *pinyin* and common names at each use, unless mentioned multiple times within a given paragraph.
- In the early development of TCVM, animal species were not mapped according to channel pathways, but rather were treated using collections of individual points, now referred to as "classical points." More recently, efforts have been made to use "transpositional points," that is taking human points and meridians and transferring them to animal species based on comparative anatomical locations. In monographs in which acupuncture points are suggested, transpositional points will be given, using common point nomenclature (e.g., *Jiquan* [HT 1] and *Kunlun* [BL 60]), while classical points will be listed by their *pinyin* designation (e.g., *Qian Ti Men*). In those instances where a classical point occupies the same anatomical location as a transpositional point, the transpositional point nomenclature will be used. When a classical point has the same *pinyin* name as a transpositional point, no corresponding numerical listing will be given. For example, the equine classical point *Shenshu* has the same *pinyin* name as *Shenshu* (BL 23), but is located 1 *cun* medial to *Guanyuanshu* (BL 26). In the listing of suggested treatment points, this point would be found under the classical points heading and be given simply as *Shenshu.* Practitioners unfamiliar with classical veterinary points are referred to *Xie's Veterinary Acupuncture* (Xie and Preast, Blackwell Publishing, 2007).

Using This Book

One of our objectives in writing this text is to help veterinarians interested in TCVM better integrate both Western and Chinese modalities into their clinical practice. This text includes the extensive information on pharmacologic effects, toxicology, herb-drug interactions, and research gathered by John Chen and Tina Chen in ***Chinese Medical Herbology and Pharmacology***. Moreover, this text has chapter introductions, clinical manifestations, veterinary clinical applications, formula modifications, cautions/contraindications, and practical suggestions drawn from the clinical experience of the authors and peer reviewers in small animal and equine medicine. It is hoped that texts such as this one will create greater acceptance of TCVM as a valid modality in the community and spur direct research into the actions of classic formulas in domesticated and non-domesticated animals, as well as avian species.

CHAPTER INTRODUCTIONS

The introductory section of each chapter describes traditional Chinese medical theory, therapeutic indications, and cautions specific to veterinary herbal medicine. Here, practitioners will find information on the mechanisms of pattern pathophysiology, how they manifest and are described in the context of Western veterinary medicine, and how the herbs in the chapter work to correct the imbalance, or in Western parlance, treat and/or cure the disease. The introduction should be seen as a valuable overview of theory: how pathogenic factors invade domestic animals and what environmental situations or husbandry practices lead to imbalances. Attention to this section prior to looking at specific formula monographs will be very helpful in determining which formula may be best for a specific animal.

IDENTIFICATION

Each formula is identified by four traits at the beginning of each monograph. **Chinese Characters** in both traditional and simplified forms are listed first. In cases where the traditional and simplified characters are identical, only one will be listed. ***Pinyin* Names** with Mandarin tone markings are provided to identify and provide pronunciation as accurately as possible. The **Literal Name** is the name translated directly from the *pinyin* name. **Original Source** refers to the traditional text or reference in which the formula was first documented. This is an important aspect for identification because it specifies when, where, and by whom this formula was first conceived. However, as many clinicians are using prepared formulas in tablets or granules, etc., it should be noted that these 'patent' formulas may vary slightly in ingredients, depending on which source text was used by the manufacturer. In most instances, these are minor substitutions that will not alter the intention of the formula, but clinicians should be familiar with the properties of the individual herbs in order to know how the substitutions may affect the formula's action.

COMPOSITION

The authors strive to assure the accuracy of the ingredients by giving both standardized *pinyin* and pharmaceutical names of the herbs. This nomenclature has been carried forward from ***Chinese Herbal Formulas and Applications*** to this edition, as has the conversion of herb dosages into metric units.

It should also be noted that some formulas, as originally constructed, contained species now regulated under the Convention on International Trade in Endangered Species (CITES). Obviously, there are moral and legal issues that limit or prevent the use of such species, and their inclusion in this text should not be interpreted as the authors' endorsement of their use; rather, their inclusion serves to provide a historically accurate portrayal of the original formula. In these situations, modern, non-CITES substitutions are provided in the formula monographs where appropriate.

DOSAGE / PREPARATION / ADMINISTRATION

This section describes the historical (and modern day) preparation of the formulas as decoctions. The decoction dosage form is not commonly used in veterinary medicine. The information provided in this section can be used by those veterinarians who may wish to extrapolate from the human dosage and prepare an individual formula as a decoction for their animal patients.

CHINESE THERAPEUTIC ACTIONS

These are the treatment strategies that link the therapeutic effects of the formula with the disease diagnosis .

CLINICAL MANIFESTATIONS

This section focuses on the diagnosis of the disorder and associated clinical signs. Veterinary medicine encompasses so many species and disease conditions that it would be impossible to produce a text for all. The authors decided to focus primarily on the predominant species seen in common practice: dogs, cats, and horses. However, Chinese patterns of disease and their manifestations can be extrapolated to any species, and although manifestations of poor hair coat or hoof quality may not apply to avian patients, other aspects of the clinical exam, as discussed in the **Overview**, should allow accurate assessment and treatment of any patient.

VETERINARY CLINICAL APPLICATIONS

It is extremely important that veterinarians employing this text have a complete and thorough understanding of both TCVM theory and the formulas in this text, and prescribe formulas to treat appropriate Chinese medicine patterns, with Western medical disease classification being a secondary concern. Having said this, this section summarizes the primary clinical applications of the formula in terms of biomedically-defined diseases. Please note that this is not a comprehensive list, but an account of the most commonly encountered conditions. Inclusion does not mean a formula is necessarily appropriate for use; in fact, readers will find that a specific Western disease may be listed under multiple formulas. Listing of biomedically defined diseases is designed to serve as a guide to assist practitioners in selecting the best possible herbal formula.

EXPLANATION

This section is comprised of two parts: an explanation of the etiology of the disease, and the strategy of the herbal treatment.

VETERINARY MODIFICATIONS

This section explains how the classical formulas can be modified, based on the clinical experience of the authors, to target the treatment of complications and variations of the same veterinary medical condition.

CAUTIONS / CONTRAINDICATIONS

The herbal formulas chosen for this text are very safe for use in clinical veterinary practice and have been carefully crafted with appropriate checks and balances to ensure safety and efficacy. When appropriate, cautions and/or contradictions for a specific formula are listed for individual species or as a general precaution, such as not using in pregnant animals. With appropriate diagnosis, dosage, and patient monitoring, safe and effective use of these formulas with minimal unwanted side effects should be easy to accomplish.

WESTERN SCIENCES (PHARMACOLOGICAL EFFECTS / HUMAN CLINICAL STUDIES AND RESEARCH)

An exhaustive list of the many clinical studies and research on pharmacologically active substances of herbs and formulas can be found in ***Chinese Medical Herbology and Pharmacology*** and ***Chinese Herbal Formulas and Applications***. For this text, the authors have chosen to retain those studies most pertinent to veterinary practice. While some may find the incorporation of human studies in a veterinary text disconcerting, the authors feel their inclusion is warranted for a number of reasons. Extrapolation from humans to animals frequently occurs in conventional veterinary medicine; off-label pharmaceutical use is prevalent and choosing to do the same for plant-based medicine is not so different as to ignore such valuable research. The use of Chinese herbs in animals relies heavily on information obtained from their use in humans at this point in time. There is little to no funding for

Using This Book

research on the use of Chinese herbs for veterinary use. On a more philosophical level, TCVM practitioners should understand that the Taoist theory that guides Chinese medical practice is a universal concept that applies to horses and dogs, as well as to humans. Damp-heat in the Bladder in a cat is not that much different than damp-heat in the Bladder in a human patient, and just as Western doctors and veterinarians will prescribe similar, if not identical, antibiotics for this condition, likewise TCM and TCVM practitioners will prescribe similar, if not identical, herbal formulas.

HERB-DRUG INTERACTION

Though critically important, there is little definitive information on the subject of herb-drug interaction in human medicine, let alone veterinary practice. Documented interactions between formulas and drugs are discussed in each formula monograph. Potential interactions are not included because they involve too much assumption and speculation. As TCVM becomes more integrated into daily veterinary practice, more information regarding both the safety and cautions for using formulas alongside Western medicine will become available and will be incorporated in later editions of this text.

TOXICOLOGY

In most cases, the toxicology of the herbal formulas is based on *in vitro* studies. Readers are advised to examine and understand these reports with the same attention to context, proportion, and clinical application as they would in reviewing toxicology and/or *in vitro* studies for any medicine or supplement.

SUGGESTED ACUPUNCTURE TREATMENT

The inclusion of suggested acupuncture points is unique to this book. The points listed in this section are for the same pattern of disease or clinical signs that the formula addresses, but it is by no means a comprehensive list. For the most part, transpositional point descriptions are those used as in human medicine for the pattern addressed by the formulas, as well as those recommended by the authors and reviewers of the text, based on clinical experience. Classical veterinary points are also included where appropriate. Practitioners will likely add or subtract points, based on their own experience and on the patients' specific needs and the complexity of the conditions.

RELATED FORMULAS

These formulas have composition and/or functions similar to the primary formulas. This section highlights the contrasting differences between the primary and related formula(s) without restating overlapping similarities. In select cases, the related formulas are more commonly used in veterinary medicine than the primary formula. That said, infrequently-used related formulas have been included in this text as well, as they may yet find more frequent applications as practitioners gain more experience with their use.

AUTHORS' COMMENTS

Here the authors seek to provide veterinary-specific practical insights into the use of classical herbal formulas in animals. Years of experience have been put into this section, resulting in the discussion of formula use and modification particular to conditions frequently encountered by veterinarians in the clinic or on the farm. Dietary recommendations and strategies for use alongside Western pharmaceuticals are often included to help ensure the best outcome for patients. The authors hope that as Chinese medicine is being used more widely and additional animal studies are done, future editions of this text will include even more information on how these formulas may be effectively utilized.

Using This Book

REFERENCES

Reference material is embedded in the text for ease of access via endnotes in each monograph. The key information from all of these notes has been carefully consolidated into two thorough bibliographic resources.

- The complete names of historical books (given in Chinese characters, *pinyin* names, and English names) are listed in the Bibliography of Historical Texts.
- The complete names of recent journals, articles and books are listed in the Bibliography of Contemporary References.

DISCLAIMER

Great care has been taken by the authors, editors, and other contributors to maintain the accuracy of the information contained in ***Chinese Herbal Formulas for Veterinarians***. All information has been evaluated, double-checked and cross-verified. However, in view of the potential for human, electronic, or mechanical error, neither the authors, the publisher, nor any contributors involved in the preparation or publication of this text warrant that the information contained herein is in every aspect accurate, and they are not responsible for any errors or omissions, or for the results obtained from the use of said information.

Chinese Herbal Formulas for Veterinarians is intended to be an educational guide for healthcare practitioners, as professional training and expertise are essential to the safe practice of herbal medicine, in both the selection and recommendation of formulas, and in providing effective guidance for the use and administration of herbs. We cannot anticipate all conditions under which this information may be used, nor explicit adaptations for less-commonly treated creatures or species. In view of ongoing research, changes in governmental regulation, and the constant flow of information relating to Chinese and Western medicine, the reader is urged to check with appropriate sources for all up-to-date information. In recognition of the fact that practitioners accessing information in this text will have varying levels of training and expertise, we accept no responsibility for the results obtained by the application of the information within this text. Neither the publisher, authors, editors, nor contributors can be held responsible for errors of fact or omission, or for any consequences arising from the use or misuse of the information herein.

It is our intention to continually update and improve this text to maintain and enhance its usefulness. We welcome and encourage your comments and suggestions.

Part 1

— Overview

总论

黄帝 Huǎng Dì

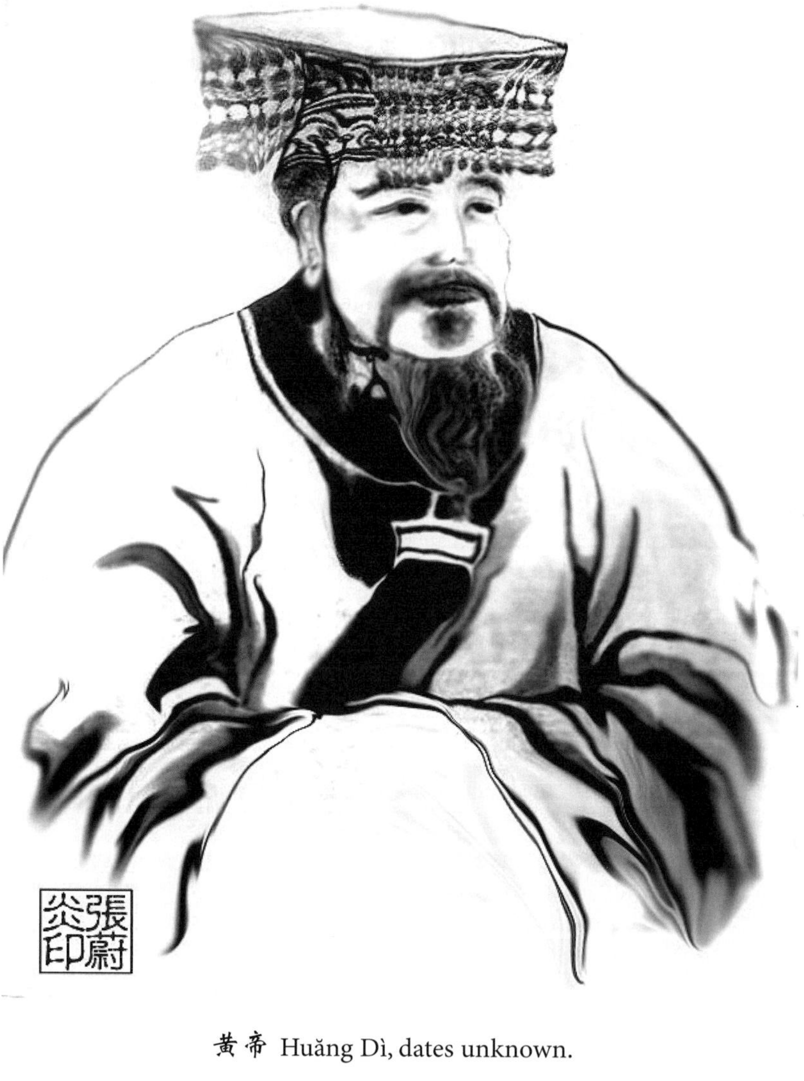

黄帝 Huǎng Dì, dates unknown.

黄帝 Huǎng Dì

Huang Di, also known as the "Yellow Emperor," was the first leader to unite all of the tribes in ancient China at the dawn of recorded civilization. Huang Di treated all citizens in his kingdoms like his own sons and daughters, and he suffered great distress when they were ill. To improve healthcare, Huang Di personally learned medicine from many of his deputies. According to legend, Huang Di inquired about all aspects of medicine: this conversation was later recorded and published as *Huang Di Nei Jing* (Yellow Emperor's Inner Classic).[a] The deputies that Huang Di consulted included 岐伯 *Qi Bo*, an authority in medicine; 桐君 *Tong Jun*, an expert in herbal medicine; 雷公 *Lei Gong*, the founder in the processing of herbs; 少俞 *Shao Yu*, an expert in acupuncture; and 伯高 *Bo Gao*, who knew pulse diagnosis in great detail. Of all the deputies, *Qi Bo* was considered the most knowledgeable, and was regarded by many as 天师 the Heavenly Physician.

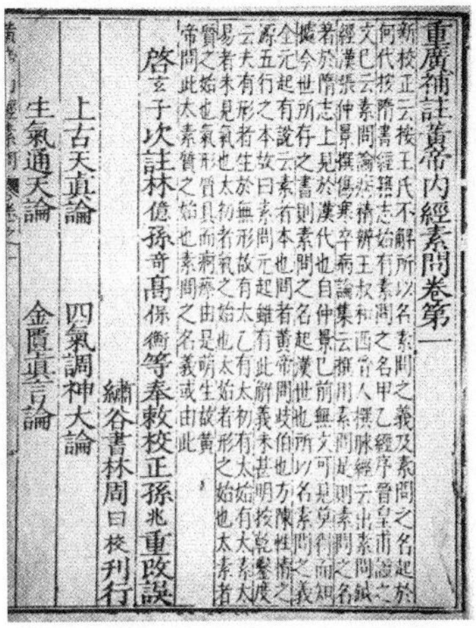

黄帝内经 *Huang Di Nei Jing* (Yellow Emperor's Inner Classic) compiled in the first or second century CE.

Huang Di Nei Jing (Yellow Emperor's Inner Classic), also abbreviated as *Nei Jing* (Inner Classic), is organized into two volumes: 素问 *Su Wen* (Basic Questions) and 灵枢 *Ling Shu* (Magic Pivot). It assembled and presented the fundamental theories of traditional Chinese medicine, including 阴阳 yin and yang, 五行 the five elements, 脏腑 the *zang fu*, and 经络 the channels and collaterals. In addition to solidifying the fundamental theories of traditional Chinese medicine, the text was crucial in shaping the study of Chinese herbal formulas. Beyond the basic concepts, the text strongly emphasized the importance of holistic medicine, that the human body is a small universe within a bigger universe represented by the environment, each having close and inseparable connections within itself and to each other. Lastly, it stressed the importance of the prevention and treatment of disease, and discouraged belief in superstition and witchcraft.

[1] This legend, however, is only folklore. In actuality, *Huang Di Nei Jing* (Yellow Emperor's Inner Classic) is believed to be a compilation of work by many physicians during the first and second century CE. They named it after *Huang Di* (Yellow Emperor) to honor his contribution to civilization in China.

Dynasties & Kingdoms	Year
Xia Dynasty 夏	**2100-1600 BCE**
Shang Dynasty 商	1600-1100 BCE
Zhou Dynasty 周	1100-221 BCE
Qin Dynasty 秦	221-207 BCE
Han Dynasty 漢	206 BCE-220
Three Kingdoms 三國	220-280
Western Jin Dynasty 西晉	265-316
Eastern Jin Dynasty 東晉	317-420
Northern and Southern Dynasties 北南朝	420-581
Sui Dynasty 隋	581-618
Tang Dynasty 唐	618-907
Five Dynasties 五代	907-960
Song Dynasty 宋	960-1279
Liao Dynasty 潦	916-1125
Jin Dynasty 金	1115-1234
Yuan Dynasty 元	1271-1368
Ming Dynasty 明	1368-1644
Qing Dynasty 清	1644-1911
Republic of China 中華民國	1912-Present Day
People's Republic of China 中華人民共和國	1949-Present Day

Table of Contents

Part I 总论 — Overview

Section 1 — Introduction

As veterinary medicine advances and becomes more specialized, domestic species, especially companion animals, are enjoying longer, healthier lives. Undoubtedly, pets have moved from the farm yard and backyard to the living room; they are viewed less as livestock and more as family members. These creatures provide valued companionship, true; but some are also prized for their competitive athleticism. This transition has created more sophisticated pet owners who are willing to explore every avenue to keep their animal companions in the best possible health. At the same time, as antibiotic resistance crops up and demand for organic foodstuffs rises, production veterinary medicine is also searching for alternatives. It is somewhat ironic that as more and more animals undergo MRI and joint replacement procedures, one of the oldest systems of medicine—Chinese medicine—is experiencing a resurgence in popularity.

Chinese Herbal Formulas for Veterinarians is a specialized adaptation of *Chinese Herbal Formulas and Applications,* the comprehensive text by doctors John K. Chen and Tina T. Chen. In this text, *Chinese Herbal Formulas for Veterinarians,* the authors have chosen many formulas likely to be used in clinical veterinary practice, and this text is intended as both a reference and educational guide. Following the Chens' lead, this book groups formulas by their Chinese energetic properties. Discussion of individual formulas provides detailed explanation as to how these properties can be used in commonly seen veterinary diseases. Recommended complementary acupuncture points are also included in the individual formula monographs when appropriate. See **Using This Book** for complete details.

Effective treatment can only follow the proper application of theory, and it is assumed that practitioners using this text have a strong foundation in traditional Chinese medicine (TCM). *The importance of this cannot be overstated.* Because Chinese medical theory relies on universal truths, as reliable and steadfast as the laws of physics, non-human species can be diagnosed and treated using the same model of disease. Proper treatment relies on correct interpretation of an individual's pattern, rather than on the allopathic label placed on the condition. For example, an aged, thin German Shepherd and an exuberant three-year-old Labrador may both present with hip dysplasia. These two animals, diagnosed as having the same affliction by Western medical standards, harbor different clinical manifestations by Chinese tenets and will be treated differently with both acupuncture and herbal formulas. For those who are new to these concepts, it is strongly recommended that you study *Traditional Chinese Veterinary Medicine* (Xie and Preast) and *Chinese Medical Herbology and Pharmacology* (Chen and Chen) before using this book in practice, in order to safely and effectively provide appropriate care.

Section 2 — History of Traditional Chinese Veterinary Medicine

As the Chinese developed the complex system of medicine we now refer to as traditional Chinese medicine, there is evidence that the medical treatment of animals progressed alongside the treatment of humans. One can imagine the value of animals in an agricultural society: they were sustenance, wealth, transportation, labor, and, in the case of horses, engines of war.

孙阳 Sun Yang and 王良 Wang Liang, considered by scholars as "the fathers of Chinese veterinary medicine," lived during the Spring and Autumn period (770-476 BCE) and established the foundation of traditional Chinese veterinary medicine. They established the principles of diagnosis in animals, theories of internal and external disorders, treatment methods, and classification of medicinal substances. During the Sui dynasty (581-618 CE), 治马牛驼骡等经 *Chi Ma Niu To Lu Ching* (Various Treatises on the Treatment of Horses, Cattle, Camels, and Donkeys) was published to provide differential diagnosis specific to these veterinary patients. During the Tang dynasty (618-907 CE), the advancement of veterinary medicine flourished. During this time, military requirements for healthy horses necessitated the development of a school of veterinary medicine. 司牧安骥集 *Si Mu An Ji Ji* (A Collection of Ways to Relieve Suffering in Horses) was published during this period. The Ming dynasty (1368-1644 CE) saw the first detailed text on equine acupuncture and herbal medicine: 元亨疗马集 *Yuan Heng Liao Ma Ji* (Horse Therapy Yuanheng Set), written by brothers Yu Ben-Yuan and Yu Ben-Heng in 1608 CE. From this time onward, many texts discussing veterinary applications of Chinese medicine were published, although all focused on agricultural species. During the Qing Dynasty (1644-1911 CE), swine disease was rampant, leading to the publication of 猪经大全 *Zhu Jing Da Quan* (A Complete Collection of Pig Diseases) in 1900 CE, which contained over sixty complete prescriptions.

In the 20th century, as Western veterinarians became interested in the traditional Chinese system, both human and veterinary texts were used to apply the different methodologies of traditional medicine - acupuncture, herbal medicine, *tuina*, and food therapy - to clinical practice. Today, the division remains much the same. Chinese veterinarians still focus primarily on agricultural species production medicine and the control of epidemic and zoonotic disease, while their Western counterparts tend to treat individual patients belonging to species that would be labeled as companions.

Section 3 — Tongue and Pulse Diagnosis

Tongue findings and pulse parameters are unique diagnostic tools in traditional Chinese medicine. When viewed within the context of the overall picture of illness, they provide insight into traditional Chinese veterinary medicine, and they aid in the selection of the appropriate herbal formula for treatment.

Tongue diagnosis in animals is similar to human tongue diagnosis in terms of tongue topography, color, body shape and moisture. However, animals do not have tongue coatings that correspond directly to the tongue coatings seen in humans. A normal dog or cat has a thin, white, moist, translucent coating that is barely perceptible. Equine tongues are usually evaluated from the side,

Section 3 — Tongue and Pulse Diagnosis

as both the coating and color of the dorsal aspect of the tongue can be influenced by plant and other material (such as creosote coating on fences). In general, most animals have tongue coating characteristics that are much more subtle and less reliable than those found in humans with a similar condition. In animals, if a significant tongue coating is present, it appears to be correlated with an increased severity of disease. That said, some animals can present with significant disease progression, but may not have a tongue coating that would be expected for that same disease state in a human. The presence or absence of a tongue coating should be interpreted judiciously. The use of a particular herbal formula should not be ruled out based on the presence or absence of tongue coating alone.

Similar to tongue findings, pulse parameters must be interpreted in light of all other physical findings, diagnostic testing, history and signalment, prior to choosing an herbal formula. Pulse evaluation and diagnosis in animals is quite different from that in humans, for obvious reasons. Most domesticated animals (dogs, cats, horses, pigs and ruminants) are quadrupeds, and there can be great variation in the overall size of these patients. The pulse is taken at the proximal femoral artery in dogs, cats and pigs, at the carotid artery in horses, and at the ventral tail artery in ruminants. Listed below are ten basic pulse images in domesticated animals, far fewer than in humans. Other pulse images do exist, but are not as commonly seen as those listed below. The pulse is not typically evaluated in avian species.

1. **Superficial or Floating** (浮脉 *fu mai*): can be easily felt with light finger pressure, but is easily obliterated by heavy pressure.
2. **Deep or Sinking** (沉脉 *chen mai*): cannot be felt with light pressure of the fingers. It can only be felt with heavy pressure.
3. **Rapid** (数脉 *shu mai*): faster speed than a normal pulse.
4. **Slow** (迟脉 *chi mai*): slower speed than a normal pulse.
5. **Deficient, Weak or Empty** (虚脉 *xu mai*): feels soft, weak and forceless, at all three levels.
6. **Excessive, Full, or Forceful Pulse** (实脉 *shi mai*): feels very forceful at all three levels (bounding pulse).
7. **Slippery or Rolling** (滑脉 *hua mai*): feels smooth and rounded and slides away from pressure when pressed.
8. **Thready, Thin, or Small** (细脉 *xi mai*): feels narrow, like a fine thread, but is very distinct and clear.
9. **Wiry or String-taut** (弦脉 *xian mai*): has decreased flexibility, feels straight and long, like pressing a violin string.
10. **Choppy** (涩脉 *se mai*): feels hesitant, rough and uneven; this type often represents pulse deficits.

These pulses are felt at three levels or depths (superficial, middle and deep) and at three positions (proximal, middle and distal) on each artery; these positions are thought to correspond to each of the internal organs in the same manner as that in human pulse evaluation at this point in time. Accurate pulse evaluation requires consistent practice. As more information accumulates on the use of tongue and pulse evaluation in animals, the information presented here can be expected to change.

Section 4 — Treatment

Traditional Chinese Veterinary Medicine commonly uses acupuncture, *tuina*, food therapy, and herbal medicine to effect change in patients. Like the underlying theoretical principles, treatment follows the balance of yin and yang; heat is treated with cold, stagnation with movement, leakage with binding, and so forth. In acute conditions, treatment often focuses on the clinical signs or manifestation(s). This is especially the case in young animals with strong constitutions that have acute bouts of diarrhea, vomiting, bleeding, or are subject to trauma or ingestion of toxins. As animals age, symptoms are often secondary to primary, or root, patterns of deficiency, and it is often more advisable to treat the underlying deficiency pattern first. In tonifying the underlying deficiency, the manifestation is tangentially attacked. For instance, if cold has invaded due to a Kidney yang deficiency, tonifying the Kidney will warm the body and disperse the cold. This makes it vitally important for practitioners to have the necessary skills to determine whether a patient has an excess or deficient pattern. Many practitioners will take a middle path, that is, treating both the root and the manifestation simultaneously, which can be very effective in *bi zheng* (painful obstruction syndrome) cases, in which patients with deficiencies of blood and/or qi are invaded by wind, cold, and dampness. Once the pattern of disease is correctly identified, treatment with the appropriate acupuncture points and herbal formulas can begin.

Section 5 — Treatment Methods

The treatment method is the bridge between any disease and its effective herbal remedy. As such, a successful treatment requires accurate diagnosis of the disease, strategic planning of treatment methods, and careful consideration of which herbal formula to prescribe. The principles of treatment methods are best delineated by Cheng Zhong-Ling in his work 医学心悟 *Yi Xue Xin Wu* (Medical Revelations) in 1732, in which the eight treatment methods are described as follows:

1. **Sweating** (汗法 *han fa*): When a pathogen enters the superficial layers of the body, sweating is often used to release these pathogens to the exterior by inducing a mild sweat in animals that sweat. In patients that do not sweat, a mild increase in panting and intolerance to heat is often observed. The herbs in such formulas are usually acrid and warming or acrid and cooling, which stimulate Lung qi and enhance its dispersing qualities and regulate the defensive layer. Common uses for this regimen would include the early stages of influenza, shipping fever, rhinopneumonitis, and *Bordatella* infections. In weak patients, sweating is combined with tonification.
2. **Vomiting** (吐法 *tu fa*): Emetic formulas are rarely used in modern clinical practice and would obviously only be used in veterinary patients with the ability to vomit. Even traditionally, vomiting was used with caution and was reserved for strong patients with acute presentations of food stagnation or toxins in the upper half of the body. Veterinarians will most likely choose modern emetics or stimulate reflux via nasogastric tube instead of herbal methods.
3. **Draining Downward or Purging** (下法 *xia fa*): Like vomiting, purging is another strong treatment method; however, it focuses on the lower half of the body to induce defecation in order to cleanse the Stomach and Intestines, remove heat, drain excess water, clear blood stasis, or unblock the Intestines. Herbs that are cold and drain downward, hot and drain downward, moisten the Intestines and drain downward, or are cathartics are generally employed for this type of treatment. Though this strong treatment is helpful for cases of constipation and many forms of colic, a wise practitioner will carefully balance draining with tonification in weak patients.
4. **Harmonizing** (和法 *he fa*): Harmonizing formulas attack and tonify simultaneously, which makes them helpful in complicated cases where a disease may present with concurrent hot and cold, or

Section 5 — Treatment Methods

deficiency and excess. These formulas are also used in cases where different parts of the body are affected, such the Stomach and Liver, or situations of *shaoyang* disorders, or for disharmonies of blood and qi.

5. **Warming** (温法 *wen fa*): Cold invasion can result from an external pathogen, but can also be generated interiorly from yang deficiency, or it can reside in the channels at the site of an old traumatic injury. Therefore, in choosing a warming formula, practitioners should take care to determine whether cold has arisen from excess or deficiency, and choose formulas that warm the correct channel, organ, or body part affected.
6. **Clearing** (清法 *qing fa*): These formulas are cooling and are used to clear heat and purge fire toxins from all three levels of the body (qi, nutritive, and organ), whether derived from excess or deficiency. Left untreated, heat will damage yin and body fluids, and this treatment method is commonly combined with tonification to combat the drying nature of heat, especially in weaker patients.
7. **Reducing** (消法 *xiao fa*): Reducing formulas eliminate stagnation and transform phlegm. This method dissolves hardenings and nodules that result from chronic disease. Rather than the stronger technique of draining downward, which expels pathogens and is usually reserved for more acute conditions, reducing is a gradual, softer treatment more suited for the dissolution of stubborn accumulations.
8. **Tonifying** (补法 *bu fa*): As the name implies, tonifying treatments replenish deficiencies of the vital substances of qi, blood, yin and yang in the *zang fu* organs. Deficient patients with concurrent excess pathogens should not be treated with tonification alone, but should have a combined treatment that addresses both the excess and deficiency so as not to draw the pathogen deeper into the interior.

These eight treatment methods are all well-documented within the history of Chinese herbal medicine. In clinical practice, it is often necessary to utilize more than one method when treating patients, as any one disease may have quite a few complications and may affect different parts of the body; moreover, patients may have different constitutions and/or underlying conditions.

Section 6 — Classification of Chinese Herbs

Individual herbs are chosen for formulas based on inherent properties that address the descriptive characteristics of the imbalances they treat. These properties are temperature, taste, direction, and channel influence. The toxicity of certain herbs and herbal combinations is also considered when constructing formulas.

Temperature: When the temperature of an herb is discussed, it is the energetic, or thermal, properties that the herb possesses that are being considered. Any herb can be placed along a continuum that runs from cold to cool to neutral to warm to hot. When treating diseases of heat invasion, cold or cool herbs will be used. As heat is yang energy, cool herbs would be yin in nature. Likewise, warming herbs would be yang and used to treat conditions where cold has accumulated. Neutral herbs walk the line between hot, cold, yang and yin, and are often used to harmonize formulas and tonify *zang* (solid organs) and *fu* (hollow organs).

Taste: There are five tastes recognized in Chinese herbal medicine: acrid, sweet, sour, bitter, and salty. These are known as the five fundamental tastes in classical herbal literature. Bland is a sixth category comprised of herbs that have little or no prominent flavor. From a conventional medicine perspective, the taste of an herb many times is associated with its biochemical components.

Section 6 — Classification of Chinese Herbs

1. ***Acrid* herbs** activate qi and blood, serve to warm and dry, and cause movement and dispersal within the body; they are particularly effective at removing pathogenic qi to the exterior by inducing sweating. Examples include *Gui Zhi* (Ramulus Cinnamomi), *Sheng Jiang* (Rhizoma Zingiberis Recens), *Bo He* (Herba Menthae), and *Ma Huang* (Herba Ephedrae).
2. ***Sweet* herbs** tonify, nourish, and harmonize. They tend to calm, cool, and moisten. Because of these properties, sweet herbs play crucial roles in treating deficiency and in balancing the other herbs in a formula. Examples include *Gan Cao* (Radix et Rhizoma Glycyrrhizae), *Ren Shen* (Radix et Rhizoma Ginseng), *Huang Qi* (Radix Astragali), and *Shu Di Huang* (Radix Rehmanniae Praeparata).
3. ***Sour* herbs** function to stabilize and bind. More specifically, they help prevent the loss of fluids from perspiration and maintain the integrity of the respiratory and gastrointestinal tracts. By drying dampness and treating phlegm, sour herbs also aid in digestion and help with problems of the urinary tract. Examples include *Wu Wei Zi* (Fructus Schisandrae Chinensis) and *Wu Mei* (Fructus Mume).
4. ***Bitter* herbs** are very effective at clearing heat toxins from the body through purging, detoxifying, cooling, drying and draining dampness, and sedating. Many have antibiotic, antiviral, and antipyretic properties, which make them useful in treating inflammation and infection. Examples are *Huang Lian* (Rhizoma Coptidis), *Da Huang* (Radix et Rhizoma Rhei), and *Long Dan* (Radix et Rhizoma Gentianae).
5. ***Salty* herbs** soften hardness, dissolve stagnation, and purge accumulation by sinking or directing qi or substances downward. They are often used to resolve masses and relieve constipation. They also help guide other herbs to the Kidney organ and channel. Examples include *Hai Zao* (Sargassum), *Kun Bu* (Thallus Ecklonia), and *Mu Li* (Concha Ostreae).
6. ***Bland* herbs** have no prominent flavor and exert a diuretic effect on the body; they are used to treat edema and dysuria. Examples include *Fu Ling* (Poria) and *Zhu Ling* (Polyporus).

Direction: describes how/where an herb will send its energy within the body. Upward-directing herbs will raise qi and go to the chest, head, and front or upper limbs. Downward-directing herbs will help purge pathogens via the stool or urine or treat the abdomen and hind limbs. They can also direct qi downward to help counteract symptoms of cough or vomiting. Outward-directing herbs disperse to the surface to induce sweating or consolidate the exterior. Inward-directing herbs penetrate interiorly and can help direct formulas to specific *zang fu*.

Channel Entered includes the primary channel affiliation of a formula or reflects guiding herbs that can direct a formula to a specific channel. Some will be used to "dredge" or clear obstruction from the channel(s).

Section 7 — Classification of Formulas

Throughout the long history of traditional Chinese medicine, many different approaches have been taken in the attempt to classify formulas. Initially, both theory and formulas were organized rather simply and were grouped into broad and very limited descriptive categories. It was not until 1682 that Wang Ang described 22 categories in his work 医方集解 *Yi Fang Ji Jie* (Analytical Collection of Medical Formulas). Wang divided formulas based on their primary action, etiology of the disease, and specific branches of medicine, such as obstetrics and gynecology. Variations of this comprehensive system are still used today in many texts, including this one.

Section 8 — Composition of Formulas

Formula construction is a complex business. Fortunately, there are hundreds of formulas put together throughout the centuries by masters of the art for treating common patterns seen in practice. However, many practitioners may choose to combine formulas or modify an existing formula in order to treat an individual animal. Knowing how and why formulas are put together is very important in these situations.

Formulas are built through a metaphorical hierarchy based on a model first described in the 黄帝内经 *Huang Di Nei Jing* (Yellow Emperor's Inner Classic) from the second century BCE and are balanced to enhance the strengths and minimize the complications of its individual components. There are four components of a formula: the chief herb (君药 *jun yao*), deputy herb (臣药 *chen yao*), assistant herb (佐药 *zuo yao*), and envoy herb (使药 *shi yao*). The *chief herb* is indispensable to the formula; its action is directed against and has the strongest effect on the principal imbalance or invasive pathogen in the disease pattern. The *deputy herb* aids the chief in its fight against the primary concern, but is also the main ingredient against any secondary issues. The *assistant herb*, like most assistants, often has multiple duties. It reinforces the chief or deputy by dealing with less important issues; it curbs any toxic properties of the chief and deputy; and, in more complex formulas, can have the *opposite* effect of the chief. This helps in cooling formulas, for instance, by having a warming assistant herb that can help keep too much cold from disrupting the whole system. An *envoy herb*, sometimes called a directing herb, focuses the action of a formula on a specific channel, organ, or region of the body and also works to harmonize the entire formula. Not every formula will employ all four components, and some will have more than one from each category. For example, diseases of a rather simple etiology may only require a chief and two deputies, while complex diseases may require multiple assistant and envoy herbs.

When formulas are modified, it is usually done with small changes to minor ingredients to fine tune the action, either by increasing the dose of an herb, adding another deputy, assistant, or envoy, or replacing one of the non-chief herbs with another without changing the overall purpose of the formula. For example, *Jiang Can* (Bombyx Batryticatus) may be added to a formula such as *Tian Ma Gou Teng Yin* (Gastrodia and Uncaria Decoction) for greater control of seizures in epilepsy cases, or *Yan Hu Suo* (Rhizoma Corydalis) can be added in higher doses to *Shao Fu Zhu Yu Tang* (Drive Out Blood Stasis in the Lower Abdomen Decoction) to improve pain management in colic cases. Additionally, formulas can be changed by altering all but the chief herb in order to change the purpose of the formula. Only practitioners very experienced in constructing formulas should attempt this method or try to construct new formulas from scratch.

Section 9 — Dosages

In general, large doses are used for acute or severe conditions and smaller doses for chronic or mild conditions. Dosage adjustments may also be needed for pediatric or geriatric patients, or for patients with weak constitutions. Dosage may also change during the course of treatment. For example, an acute case that is initially treated with a large dose may have the daily dose tapered as the condition improves. Likewise, delicate patients may start out on smaller doses and have their dose increased as they become stronger and show that they can tolerate the formula without any ill effects. Species differences need to be considered as well. Dogs and cats can often be treated with the recommended dose for humans, when adjusted for weight. Horses and other herbivores, however, often do well on 70 to 80 percent of the human dose, when adjusted for weight. A dosing guideline is included at the end of this section.

Section 10 — Dosage Forms

Throughout the centuries, many different dosage forms have been described, and as modern preparation techniques developed, more and more variations are available to practitioners. A brief discussion of various forms and their application in veterinary medicine follows.

1. **Decoction** (汤剂 *tang ji*) is one of the most commonly used forms of Chinese herbal formula administration in human practice. The general protocol for administration is to first soak the herbs in water, then cook the herbs, filter, and administer the decoction while it is warm. Decoctions can also be used topically as a soaking solution or herbal wash. This dosage form becomes a bit unwieldy in veterinary practice, as the decoction will most often have to be mixed in with food, and sometimes the volume of the decoction makes this impractical. Some owners will also balk at the time involved in preparation. Horses tend to take to this dosage form most readily and can even be fed the herbal residue in most cases. For those interested in using decoctions, *Chinese Herbal Formulas and Applications* has an excellent section on preparing decoctions.
2. **Powder** (散剂 *san ji*), made by grinding and blending the ingredients into small particles, is a common dosage form and readily available to practitioners. Powders are easily mixed into food, but although the dose can be relatively small, many animals (cats in particular) will refuse to eat powdered formulations. This issue can be avoided in finicky dogs by encapsulating the powder into capsules.
3. **Pill** (丸剂 *wan ji*) is a solid dosage form that is made by combining the herbal powder with a binding agent, such as water, honey, alcohol, vinegar, or other aqueous agents. This dosage form is available from many manufacturers and has the advantage of having a long shelf life and increased patient compliance. The biggest disadvantage to pills is that the practitioner loses the ability to modify the formula for the individual patient.
4. **Soft extract** (膏剂 *gao ji*) is prepared by cooking the herbs with water or vegetable oil to concentrate the herbs into a soft extract. This dosage form is very practical for topical use, in particular as poultices on the lower limbs of horses. They can also be used on small animals, usually for wounds or trauma, though the hair will often need to be clipped, and the paste will need to be covered with a light wrap to avoid ingestion.
5. **Pellet** (丹剂 *dan ji*) is a solid dosage form similar to a pill. They are smaller than pills and more concentrated, which can make them indispensable for treating smaller patients such as cats. Like pills, their biggest disadvantage is the inability to modify for the individual patient.
6. **Medicinal wine** or **tincture** (酒剂 *jiu ji*) uses grain-based alcohol to extract the active constituents in the herbs. Internally administered, medicinal wines can be used in veterinary practice; however, glycerine-based tinctures often provide better patient compliance. Those designed for topical use, especially liniments for *bi zheng* (painful obstruction syndrome), can be very helpful.
7. **Tea** (茶剂 *cha ji*), prepared by soaking herbs in hot water, is not very effective and is impractical for use in veterinary medicine.
8. **Distillation** (药露 *yao lu*) captures the essential oils in many fragrant and aromatic herbs. This method is used when fresh herbs are available and are uncommon in veterinary practice.
9. **Lozenge** (锭剂 *ding ji*) is a dose form not used in veterinary medicine.
10. **Moxa** (灸剂 *jiu ji*) is prepared by crushing and rolling *Ai Ye* (Folium Artemisiae Argyi) in paper to form a stick that resembles the shape of a cigar. Upon burning the moxa stick, the resultant heat and the effects of the herb are delivered to the affected area. Moxa can be very useful in veterinary medicine, though caution needs to be used on patients with long hair coats.
11. **Syrup** (糖浆剂 *tang jiang ji*) refers to the addition of cane syrup to liquid dosage forms to mask the taste of herbs. This is similar to the practice of mixing Western medicines with molasses for horses and can be effective in all species. There are commercial syrup preparations (often for cough) that can be used in veterinary patients.
12. **Tablet** (片剂 *pian ji*) is a contemporary form that is made by combining raw herbs or (more commonly) concentrated powder and pressing them into tablets. This preparation, as with tablets and pills, can greatly enhance patient and owner compliance. There are many classic formulas now available in this form.

Section 10 — Dosage Forms

13. **Capsule** (胶囊剂 *jiao nang ji*) is constructed by taking powdered herbs or concentrates and placing them into empty capsules. As discussed previously, this can enhance patient compliance, though capsules may be difficult to swallow for some small patients.
14. **Granule** or **powder** (冲服剂 *chong fu ji*) is a contemporary form that is very commonly used in veterinary practice. The process of low-heat/high-pressure extraction allows for the production of quality, concentrated powders that are quickly absorbed and require much smaller volumes per dose. This greatly enhances patient compliance and still allows for construction and modification of custom formulations for patients.
15. **Injection** (针剂 *zhen ji*) is a preparation that can be administered via intravenous, subcutaneous, or intramuscular injection. They are currently not available in the United States.

Section 11 — Veterinary Dosing Guidelines

The following table is intended to assist veterinarians in administering proper doses of Chinese herbal formulas. These recommended dosages are a guideline, which is why there is such a wide range of suggestions. Different manufacturers of the same formula may arrive at different strengths, so that the practitioner may need to adjust the dose of a given formula and may even require increasing beyond the recommended dose in the table below. Though common sense and a strong knowledge of herbal formulas guided by experience should accompany their use, the vast majority of the formulas in this text have a very wide margin of safety, and practitioners should feel comfortable in exploring dose requirements for individual patients. As discussed in the **Dosage** section, modifications may be needed, based on the constitution or age of the patient, the severity of the condition, and the progression of the treatment. As with any protocol, patients should be monitored and changes made as necessary. Dosing three times daily is often recommended for best therapeutic effect. Because this schedule can be difficult for many owners, our general recommendations are for twice daily administration. When optimal administration is possible, divide the total daily dose recommended below by three. If owners can only dose once daily, use the highest dose listed.

Special Dosing Note: Herbal formula may also be administered via rectal enema. This route of administration may be necessary in emergent cases and for those patients for which oral administration is contraindicated or not possible. Extract granular herb formulas are best suited for rectal use and are easily prepared by mixing with warm water. The dosage required to obtain an effective therapeutic effect is 3-4 times that of the recommended oral dose, and the herbal enema solution retained for a minimum of 5-10 minutes to promote maximum absorption.

Puppies, kittens, foals, and other newborns should be dosed at half of the adult dose.

Section 11 — Veterinary Dosing Guidelines

VETERINARY DOSING GUIDELINES

Animals	Weight	Powder	Extract Granules	Tablets	Pills	Tinctures
Dogs	Up to 15 kg (Up to 25 lbs)	0.5-1.5 g bid	0.5-1 g bid	½ bid	1-3 bid	2-5 drops bid
	15-30 kg (25-50 lbs)	1.5-3 g bid	1-2 g bid	½-1 bid	3-4 bid	5-10 drops bid
	30-45 kg (50-75 lbs)	3-4 g bid	2-3 g bid	1-1½ bid	4-6 bid	10-15 drops bid
	45-60 kg (75-100 lbs)	4-6 g bid	3 g bid	1½-2 bid	6-8 bid	12-20 drops bid
	60-75kg (100-125 lbs)	6-7 g bid	3-4 g bid	2 bid	8-10 bid	15-25 drops bid
Cats	Up to 6 kg (Up to10 lbs)	0.25-0.5 g bid	0.25-0.5 g bid	½ bid	1 bid	1-2 drops bid
	6-9 kg (10-15 lbs)	0.5-1 g bid	0.5 g bid	1 bid	1-2 bid	2 drops bid
	>9 kg (>15 lbs)	1-1.5 g bid	0.5-1 g bid	1 bid	2 bid	2-3 drops bid
Horses*	Minis	5-10 g bid	5-10 g bid	3-5 bid	20 bid	Tinctures in horses are not advised due to volume requirements
	Ponies	10-20 g bid	10-15 g bid	6-8 bid	40-60 bid	
	550-725 kg (900-1200 lbs)	20-30 g bid	15-20 g bid	10 bid	Impractical	
	725-900 kg (1200-1500lbs)	30-40 g bid	20-25 g bid	15 bid	Impractical	

*Ruminants, camelids, and pigs may be dosed like horses, extrapolating for like weights.

Part II

— Formula Monographs

各论

神农 Shén Nŏng

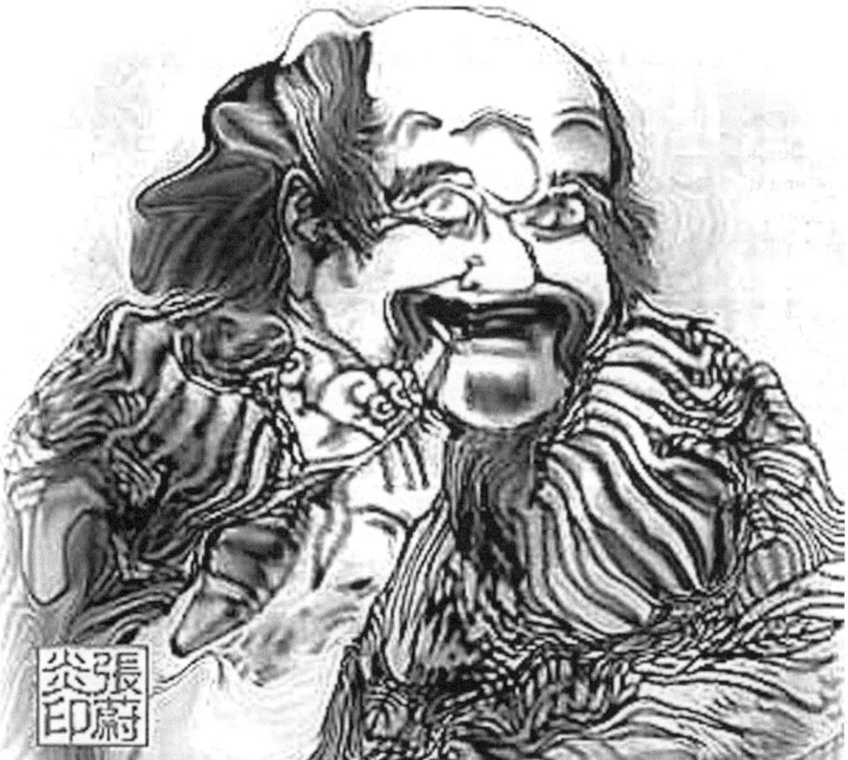

神农 Shén Nŏng, dates unknown.

神农 Shén Nǒng

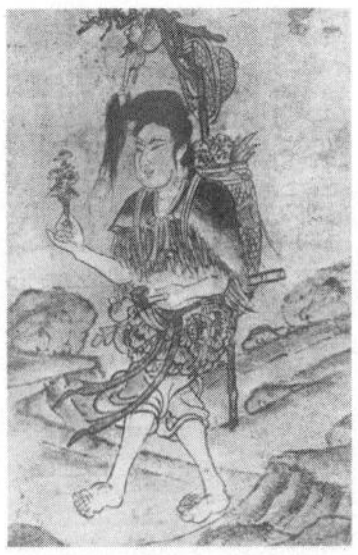

Shen Nong personally picking herbs.

According to folklore and legend, Shen Nong, also known as the "Divine Husbandman," was the person credited for converting the nomads in ancient China from seasonal wanderers into a settled, agricultural society. He taught people what plants to consume as food, when to plant seeds and harvest crops, and how to make tools. In addition, he dedicated his life to searching for herbal medicines to treat disease. He traveled all throughout ancient China, and personally collected and tasted each and every medicinal substance. After years of personal trial and error, he gained an uncommon understanding of the therapeutic effects and side effects of many medicinal substances. He reportedly ingested as many as 70 poisonous substances per day, but used *Cha Ye* (Folium Camelliae) to successfully neutralize these poisons. Unfortunately, Shen Nong died when he experimented with an extremely toxic herb called 断肠草 *Duan Chang Cao.*[a] To commemorate Shen Nong and his contributions to medicine, numerous authors and physicians compiled and published *Shen Nong Ben Cao Jing* (Divine Husbandman's Classic of the Materia Medica) in his name.

Shen Nong Ben Cao Jing (Divine Husbandman's Classic of the Materia Medica) is the first, and one of the most authoritative, texts on Chinese herbal medicine. It contains information on 365 medicinal substances (252 plants, 67 animals, and 46 minerals) including details such as taste, thermal properties, dosages, and toxicity. It also includes descriptions of how to cultivate the herbs, process the herbs, and distinguish true from false herbs. This is one of the earliest records of Chinese herbal medicine, and much of its documentations still holds true today, such as the use of *Ma Huang* (Herba Ephedrae) to treat wheezing and dyspnea, *Hai Zao* (Sargassum) to treat goiter, *Huang Lian* (Rhizoma Coptidis) to stop diarrhea, *Gua Di* (Pedicellus Cucumeris) to induce vomiting, *Lei Wan* (Omphalia) to kill parasites, *Huang Qin* (Radix Scutellariae) to reduce fever, and so on.

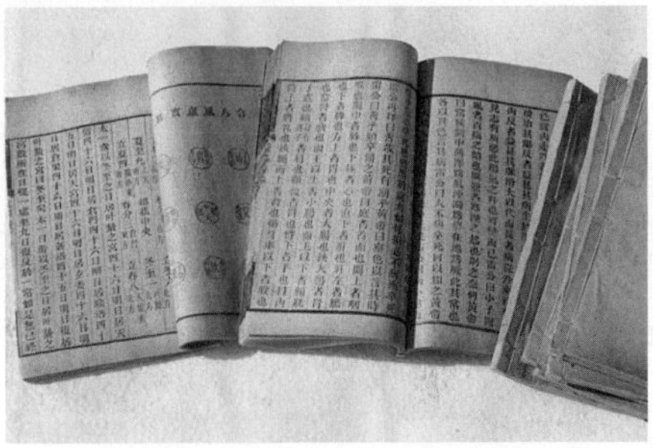

神农本草经 *Shen Nong Ben Cao Jing* (Divine Husbandman's Classic of the Materia Medica) compiled during the second century CE.

[1] 断肠草 *Duan Chang Cao*, literally "break the intestines herb," is a name given to many herbs that are toxic. Historians believe that the actual herb that poisoned and killed Shen Nong was *Gou Wen* (Herba Gelsemii Elegantis). The toxicity of this herb was later documented in great detail in *Ben Cao Gang Mu* (Materia Medica) by Li Shi-Zhen in 1596.

Dynasties & Kingdoms	Year
Xia Dynasty 夏	**2100-1600 BCE**
Shang Dynasty 商	1600-1100 BCE
Zhou Dynasty 周	1100-221 BCE
Qin Dynasty 秦	221-207 BCE
Han Dynasty 漢	206 BCE-220
Three Kingdoms 三國	220-280
Western Jin Dynasty 西晉	265-316
Eastern Jin Dynasty 東晉	317-420
Northern and Southern Dynasties 北南朝	420-581
Sui Dynasty 隋	581-618
Tang Dynasty 唐	618-907
Five Dynasties 五代	907-960
Song Dynasty 宋	960-1279
Liao Dynasty 遼	916-1125
Jin Dynasty 金	1115-1234
Yuan Dynasty 元	1271-1368
Ming Dynasty 明	1368-1644
Qing Dynasty 清	1644-1911
Republic of China 中華民國	1912-Present Day
People's Republic of China 中華人民共和國	1949-Present Day

Table of Contents

Chapter 1

— Exterior-Releasing Formulas

解表剂

张仲景 Zhāng Zhòng-Jǐng

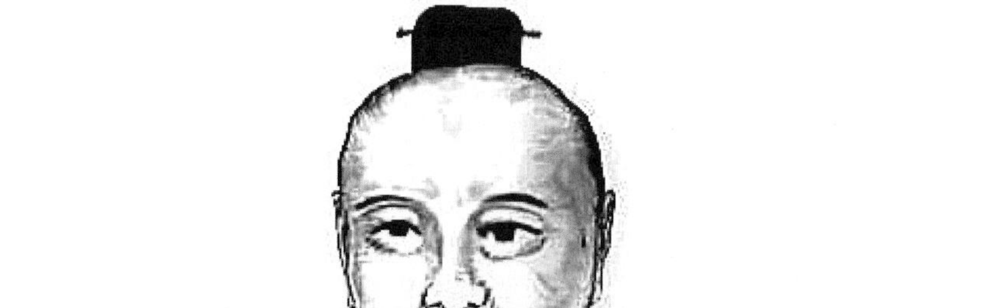

张仲景Zhāng Zhòng-Jǐng, also known as 张机Zhāng Jī, 150 – 219 CE.

张仲景 Zhāng Zhòng-Jǐng

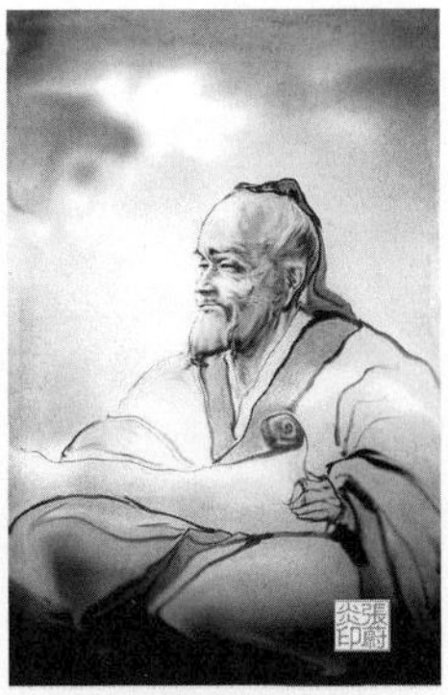

Zhang Zhong-Jing
with his manuscripts.

Zhang Zhong-Jing, also known as Zhang Ji, was born near the end of the Eastern Han dynasty. During the transition from the collapse of the Eastern Han to the beginning of the Three Kingdoms era, China was ravaged by constant civil war, and people suffered from crime, poverty, infection and death. During a ten-year period near the end of the Eastern Han, two-thirds of the population fell ill and died. Seventy percent of the fatalities were due to *shang han* (cold damage). Although Zhang was from a wealthy family of over 200 members, even his family members could not escape the common fate and many succumbed to the epidemic. Greatly affected by the loss of his family members and the devastating impact of widespread losses in the community and nation, Zhang dedicated his entire life to studying and practicing medicine.

伤寒杂病论*Shang Han Za Bing Lun* (Discussion of Cold-Induced Disorders and Miscellaneous Diseases) is the most famous work by Zhang. This original work later was divided by Wang Shu-He into two volumes: 伤寒论*Shang Han Lun* (Discussion of Cold-Induced Disorders) and 金匮要略 *Jin Gui Yao Lue* (Essentials from the Golden Cabinet).

- *Shang Han Lun* (Discussion of Cold-Induced Disorders) emphasized external disorders, and classified them according to *Liu Jing Bian Zheng* (Six Stages Differentiation).
- *Jin Gui Yao Lue* (Essentials from the Golden Cabinet) focused on internal and miscellaneous diseases, and classified them according to *Ba Gang Bian Zheng* (Eight Principle Differentiation).

Zhang's work clearly established the relationships among disease, progression, complications, treatment strategies, dosage forms, and herbal formulas. Zhang Zhong-Jing forever changed the practice of traditional Chinese medicine. Over 1,700 years after their original publication, his works are still studied as required textbooks in schools of Traditional Chinese Medicine around the world. Many of the formulas he used are still considered to be the standard herbal treatment, such as *Bai Hu Tang* (White Tiger Decoction) for fever, *Bai Tou Weng Tang* (Pulsatilla Decoction) for dysentery, *Yin Chen Hao Tang* (Artemisia Scoparia Decoction) for jaundice, and *Gua Lou Xie Bai Ban Xia Tang* (Trichosanthes Fruit, Chinese Chive, and Pinellia Decoction) for chest pain.

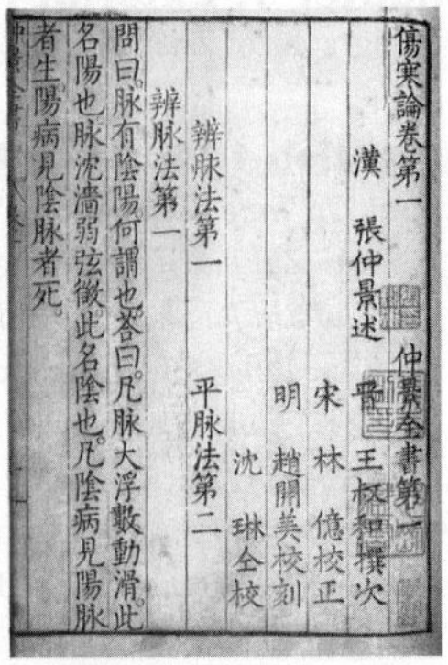

傷寒論卷第一 仲景全書第一
漢 張仲景述 晉 王叔和撰次
宋 林億校正
明 趙開美校刻
沈琳仝校
辨脈法第一 平脈法第二
辨脈法第一
問曰脈有陰陽何謂也荅曰凡脈大浮數動滑此
名陽也脈沈濇弱弦微此名陰也凡陰病見陽脈
者生陽病見陰脈者死

伤寒论*Shang Han Lun*
(Discussion of Cold-Induced
Disorders)

Because of his lasting influence, Zhang Zhong-Jing has always been remembered as 医圣the Sage of Medicine.

Dynasties & Kingdoms	Year
Xia Dynasty 夏	2100-1600 BCE
Shang Dynasty 商	1600-1100 BCE
Zhou Dynasty 周	1100-221 BCE
Qin Dynasty 秦	221-207 BCE
Han Dynasty 漢	**206 BCE-220**
Three Kingdoms 三國	220-280
Western Jin Dynasty 西晉	265-316
Eastern Jin Dynasty 東晉	317-420
Northern and Southern Dynasties 北南朝	420-581
Sui Dynasty 隋	581-618
Tang Dynasty 唐	618-907
Five Dynasties 五代	907-960
Song Dynasty 宋	960-1279
Liao Dynasty 遼	916-1125
Jin Dynasty 金	1115-1234
Yuan Dynasty 元	1271-1368
Ming Dynasty 明	1368-1644
Qing Dynasty 清	1644-1911
Republic of China 中華民國	1912-Present Day
People's Republic of China 中華人民共和國	1949-Present Day

Examples of formulas of Zhang Zhong-Jing that are in common use today include:

- *Gui Zhi Tang* (Cinnamon Twig Decoction)
- *Da Cheng Qi Tang* (Major Order the Qi Decoction)
- *Xiao Chai Hu Tang* (Minor Bupleurum Decoction)
- *Bai Hu Tang* (White Tiger Decoction)
- *Li Zhong Wan* (Regulate the Middle Pill)
- *Jin Gui Shen Qi Wan* (Kidney Qi Pill from the Golden Cabinet)
- *Mai Men Dong Tang* (Ophiopogonis Decoction)
- *Wu Mei Wan* (Mume Pill)

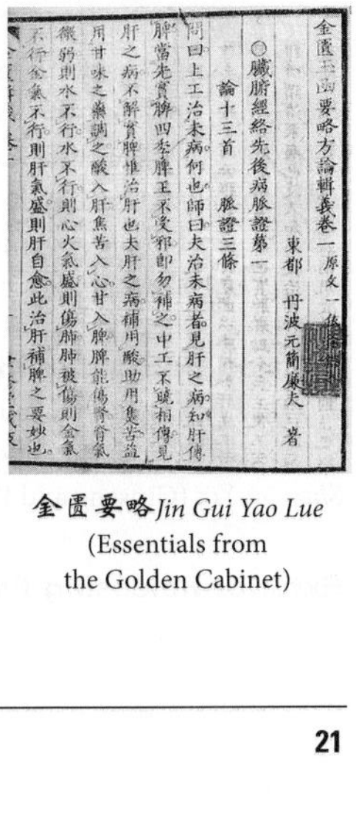

金匱玉函要略方論輯義卷一 原文一條
東都 丹波元簡廉夫 著
臟腑經絡先後病脈證第一
論十三首 脈證三條
問曰上工治未病何也師曰夫治未病者見肝之病知肝傳
脾當先實脾四季脾王不受邪即勿補之中工不曉相傳見
肝之病不解實脾惟治肝也夫肝之病補用酸助用焦苦益
用甘味之藥調之酸入肝焦苦入心甘入脾脾能傷腎腎氣
微弱則水不行水不行則心火氣盛則傷肺肺被傷則金氣
不行金氣不行則肝氣盛則肝自愈此治肝補脾之要妙也

金匱要略*Jin Gui Yao Lue*
(Essentials from
the Golden Cabinet)

Table of Contents

Chapter 1 — Overview

解表剂 — Exterior-Releasing Formulas

Definition: Exterior-releasing formulas induce sweating and release exterior factors from the skin and muscles. This method of treatment is known as *han fa* (sweating), one of the *ba fa* (eight treatment methods) described in the *Huang Di Nei Jing* (Yellow Emperor's Inner Classic) in the first or second century A.D.

The term "exterior releasing" primarily refers to the method of inducing diaphoresis or sweating. The primary focus of these formulas is to induce sweating to dispel exogenous factors from the external and superficial areas of the body, that is the skin and muscle layers. Exterior-releasing formulas are the first line of defense to keep exogenous factors from penetrating the interior of the body and causing more serious disease. Most exterior-releasing formulas are comprised of herbs that are aromatic in nature, and these herbs contain volatile oils and are scattering in nature, which is why they should not be used long term. In addition to inducing sweating, they stimulate immune function, relieve pain, and regulate body temperature.

Wind is viewed as the master pathogen in Chinese medicine, and it is considered to be the vehicle by which all exogenous factors enter the body. Wind is involved in all exterior conditions, including heat as well as cold conditions; thus most exterior-releasing formulas target either wind-cold or wind-heat syndromes. These formulas may address specific complaints (e.g. fever, cough, wheezing, nasal congestion) or specific locations of distress, such as the head, neck and throat. Alternatively, they can be used to treat disorders such as skin eruptions, abscesses and sores, edema, dysentery and the early stage of *shang han* (cold damage) or *wen bing* (warm disease). Typically, these formulas treat exterior disorders which are acute in nature. Dogs, cats, birds, and many other animals do not sweat appreciably, thus the effectiveness of exterior releasing formula can not be ascertained by the presence and quantity of sweat induced in these species. These formulas have been shown to be clinically effective in treating exterior syndromes, and opening the pores alone without inducing obvious perspiration still produces the intended therapeutic effects in non-sweating species. In horses, the ideal effect would be the induction of a mild sweat, particularly on the head and neck, or until the entire body surface feels slightly warm. An excessive, foamy sweat would be contraindicated and an indication to decrease the dose of a formula.

Exterior syndrome refers to an attack or invasion of the superficial parts of the body from outside via the mouth, nose and skin by *liu yin* (six exogenous factors). Chinese medicine categorizes these six exogenous factors according to the climatic characteristics of wind, cold, fire, dampness, dryness and summer-heat. As normal climatic factors, they are called the six qi. Once they invade the body due to abrupt or seasonal weather changes, and or because the body is too weak to compensate for these climatic changes, they are then referred to as the six exogenous factors. This category also includes early invasion of the body by infectious diseases like flu virus, or noxious epidemic pathogens (qi) such as the plague, anthrax, and other toxic infectious epidemic disease agents. The six exogenous factors can be used to describe or represent many different types of disease agents, as long as that agent produces the same effects and clinical signs in the body as one of the six exogenous factors. The clinical signs of early stage exterior syndrome include: mild fever and slight

Chapter 1 — Overview

chills without sweating, stiffness and pain of the head and neck, wheezing, and a superficial pulse. Early stage exterior syndromes are typically divided into wind-cold and wind-heat disorders.

Wind-cold disorders are characterized by fever and (more predominantly) shivering (chills), sneezing, stiff and painful neck and forequarters, clear or white secretions (ocular, nasal and sputum), a superficial pulse, moist or white greasy tongue coating, and lack of thirst. Cats with acute feline upper respiratory disease (feline URI) and feline asthma from wind-cold, as well as dogs with acute infectious tracheobronchitis (kennel cough) will often show these classic signs.

In veterinary medicine, it is often the case that wind-cold conditions have already progressed or transformed into a wind-heat condition by the time the owner brings the animal in for examination. It is only after the animal begins to become lethargic, eats poorly, develops obvious yellow oculonasal discharge, cough and/or exhibits pain and stiffness of the body and extremities, that they are determined to be ill by the owner. All of the aforementioned are clinical signs associated with wind-heat disorder. In addition, animals may also present with moderate fever; excessive thirst; coughing; swollen, sore throat; red, swollen eyes; a rapid, superficial pulse; and a red, dry tongue with a thin, white to yellow coating. When wind-heat exogenous factors become established and settle in the head and neck areas, swollen lymph nodes may be seen with ocular and nasal discharge that is thick and yellow-green. The nasal discharge can have a foul smell. Common veterinary diseases in this category include sinusitis, bacterial conjunctivitis, equine strangles, chronic canine kennel cough, feline URI and fever of unknown origin (FUO), and common equine pathogens such as rhinopneumonitis and strangles.

Animals with conditions due to exterior-interior excess can present with high fever, anorexia, lethargy, depression, sweating (in those species that sweat), a thick, yellow-green nasal discharge, thick saliva, vomiting, foul-smelling mucoid diarrhea or constipation, dark, turbid urination, red tongue with yellow, greasy coating, and a forceful rapid or wiry pulse. In general, many of the serious toxic infectious diseases seen in veterinary medicine will initially present with wind-cold or wind-heat signs that progress to the interior and are seen in this category. These include the rickettsial diseases such as Lyme disease, feline infectious peritonitis (FIP), feline leukemia (FeLV), feline immunodeficiency virus (FIV), canine distemper virus, and equine encephalomyelitis. Some fungal diseases may also fit this classification early in their development. General applications of exterior releasing formulas in veterinary medicine include acute viral and bacterial infections, asthma, coughing, edema, arthritis, fever, sinusitis, nasal discharge and selected eye disorders.

Accurate diagnosis is essential when using exterior-releasing formulas. They are not appropriate for treating interior disorders alone, fully-expressed skin rashes, or edema due to deficiency. If the pathogenic influence is present at the exterior level (skin and muscle) only, treatment should focus on releasing it from that level to ensure that the influence does not penetrate inward and cause more serious disease by attacking the *zang* (solid) and *fu* (hollow) organs. In this instance, exterior-releasing formulas are indicated. However, if it is obvious that exogenous factors have penetrated to the interior with signs of an interior disorder present, a choice must be made whether to release the exterior first or to treat both interior and exterior simultaneously. For animals that have a weak constitution, or are debilitated or geriatric, it is critical to tonify existing deficiencies and strengthen body resistance while at the same time releasing the exterior to dispel invading pathogenic factors.

SUBCATEGORIES OF ACTION

Since there is a variety of exterior factors and individual constitutional differences, exterior-releasing formulas are divided into three subcategories to reflect the nature of the disorders, the characteristics of the herbal formulas, and the constitutions of the patients.

Chapter 1 — Overview

1. **Acrid and Warm Exterior-Releasing Formulas**
   These formulas treat exterior wind-cold syndromes. Common symptoms include a dislike of cold, fever, neck and forequarter stiffness, soreness and pain of the body and the extremities, absence of thirst, no sweating (or continued presence of fever and dislike of cold after sweating), a thin, white tongue coating, and a superficial, tight or superficial, moderate pulse.
   Herbs commonly used to release exterior wind-cold include *Ma Huang* (Herba Ephedrae), *Gui Zhi* (Ramulus Cinnamomi), *Fang Feng* (Radix Saposhnikoviae), *Jing Jie* (Herba Schizonepetae), and *Zi Su Ye* (Folium Perillae). Formulas commonly used to release exterior wind-cold include *Gui Zhi Tang* (Cinnamon Twig Decoction), *Xiao Qing Long Tang* (Minor Bluegreen Dragon Decoction), and *Jiu Wei Qiang Huo Tang* (Nine-Herb Decoction with Notopterygium).

2. **Acrid and Cold Exterior-Releasing Formulas**
   These formulas treat exterior wind-heat syndromes with the following commonly seen clinical manifestations: fever, sweating, aversion to wind and cold, stiff and painful body and extremities, thirst, a painful and/or swollen throat, cough, a thin, white or thin, yellow tongue coating, and a superficial, rapid pulse.
   Herbs commonly used to release exterior wind-heat include *Bo He* (Herba Menthae), *Niu Bang Zi* (Fructus Arctii), *Sang Ye* (Folium Mori), *Ju Hua* (Flos Chrysanthemi), and *Ge Gen* (Radix Puerariae Lobatae). Formulas commonly used to release exterior wind-heat include *Sang Ju Yin* (Mulberry Leaf and Chrysanthemum Decoction), *Yin Qiao San* (Honeysuckle and Forsythia Powder), and *Ma Huang Xing Ren Gan Cao Shi Gao Tang* (Ephedra, Apricot Kernel, Licorice, and Gypsum Decoction).

3. **Supporting [the Upright] and Releasing [the Exterior] Formulas**
   These formulas are used for constitutionally deficient patients who are attacked by *liu yin* (six exogenous factors). However, this situation presents two dilemmas. First, exterior-releasing formulas induce diaphoresis to dispel exterior exogenous factors but, in the process, may damage yin and body fluids, especially in animals who already have underlying deficiencies. Second, animals who have underlying deficiencies often do not have enough *zheng* (upright) *qi* and body fluids (sweat), and are often unable to push out the exterior pathogens, even when they take exterior-releasing herbs. Therefore, in order to safely dispel exterior pathogenic factors in deficient patients, the underlying constitution of these animals must be simultaneously supported. Supporting and releasing formulas usually consist of both exterior-releasing herbs and qi- or yang-tonifying herbs to accomplish both goals.
   Herbs commonly used to support *zheng* (upright) *qi* include *Ren Shen* (Radix et Rhizoma Ginseng) and *Gan Cao* (Radix et Rhizoma Glycyrrhizae). Formulas that simultaneously support the upright and release the exterior include *Bai Du San* (Overcome Pathogenic Influences Powder) and *Shen Su Yin* (Ginseng and Perilla Leaf Decoction).

CAUTIONS / CONTRAINDICATIONS

- Correct dosage is particularly important with exterior-releasing formulas because of their acrid and diaphoretic effects. Dosage is also dictated by individual species sensitivity, propensity and ability to sweat, climate, season, and the acuteness of the disorder. Inducing a slight sweat is optimal; excessive sweating injures the qi and fluids. In general, exterior-releasing formulas should be monitored carefully so they do not contribute in any way to interior disharmony.
- Excessive panting, excessive increase in heart and respiratory rate, and hyperactivity are indications that the dosage of formula used is too high and should be lowered or discontinued.
- As a species, cats are particularly sensitive to *Ma Huang* (Herba Ephedrae). Herbal formula containing this herb should be used with caution. Begin with a single formula and using the lowest therapeutic dose before adding any additional formula.
- Horses should be monitored for dry stool. Often, concurrent administration of a warm bran mash can prevent constipation caused by fluid loss.

Chapter 1 — Overview

- Exterior-releasing formulas are generally taken as warm decoctions to induce sweating. Mild sweating over the whole body is ideal. The body may be covered with a blanket to ensure and facilitate sweating, and this is particularly effective in horses. However, profuse sweating should be avoided since it may deplete qi and yin and, in severe cases, may cause qi or yang collapse.
- Avoid exposure to wind after taking the decoction lest recurrent attacks occur.
- Avoid foods that are raw, cold, oily or greasy, as they may decrease the absorption and compromise the therapeutic effects of these formulas.
- If interior symptoms are observed along with exterior symptoms, the normal treatment plan is to treat the exterior first, and the interior condition second, or treat both interior and exterior conditions at the same time.
- Exterior-releasing formulas are contraindicated if the disease factor has progressed completely into the interior; and contraindicated in cases of ulcerated sores, deficiency-type of edema, and dehydration from vomiting or diarrhea.

PROCESSING

Many exterior-releasing formulas contain acrid herbs to induce sweating. These formulas should not be over-cooked, since the essential oils, which give these herbs their acrid, aromatic, and diaphoretic effects, evaporate very easily. Therefore, many exterior-releasing herbs are post-decocted, added at the last five to ten minutes of cooking.

PHARMACOLOGICAL EFFECTS & CLINICAL APPLICATIONS

While exterior-releasing formulas have a wide range of clinical applications, they are mainly used to treat various respiratory and infectious disorders.

1. **Cough**: Many exterior-releasing formulas have antitussive effects to suppress cough. *Ma Huang Xing Ren Gan Cao Shi Gao Tang* (Ephedra, Apricot Kernel, Licorice, and Gypsum Decoction) alleviates cough and dyspnea in cases of asthma or respiratory tract infection.[1] As an active ingredient in this formula, *Ku Xing Ren* (Semen Armeniacae Amarum) has an inhibitory effect on the respiratory center in the brain, thereby producing antitussive and antiasthmatic effects.[2]
2. **Wheezing and dyspnea**: *Xiao Qing Long Tang* (Minor Bluegreen Dragon Decoction) has been used successfully to treat wheezing and dyspnea. Several clinical studies have shown *Xiao Qing Long Tang* (Minor Bluegreen Dragon Decoction) to be effective in treating wheezing and dyspnea in patients with acute and chronic bronchial asthma.[3]
3. **Asthma**: Many exterior-releasing formulas have marked antiasthmatic effects, and may be used to treat asthma.[4,5] The proposed mechanisms of actions include: 1) stimulating the beta-adrenoceptors to achieve bronchorelaxation; and 2) inhibiting the infiltration of eosinophils into the airway.[6,7] Exemplar formulas include *Xiao Qing Long Tang* (Minor Bluegreen Dragon Decoction) and *She Gan Ma Huang Tang* (Belamcanda and Ephedra Decoction).
4. **Bronchitis**: Many exterior-releasing formulas are effective in treating bronchitis and related symptoms. *Xiao Qing Long Tang* (Minor Bluegreen Dragon Decoction) has both antibiotic and antiasthmatic effects, and is an excellent formula for treating bronchitis in both juveniles and adults.[8,9,10,11,12] *Ma Huang Xing Ren Gan Cao Shi Gao Tang* (Ephedra, Apricot Kernel, Licorice, and Gypsum Decoction) treats both acute and chronic bronchitis,[13,14] as it has antitussive effects to suppress cough,[15] bronchodilating effects to relieve wheezing and dyspnea,[16] and antiallergic effects to reduce swelling and inflammation.[17]
5. **Pneumonia**: Exterior-releasing formulas can treat both the cause and symptoms of pneumonia. For example, *Xiao Qing Long Tang* (Minor Bluegreen Dragon Decoction) and *Yin Qiao San* (Honeysuckle and Forsythia Powder) have antibiotic effects to treat infection of the lungs.[18,19] In addition, *Xiao Qing Long Tang* (Minor Bluegreen Dragon Decoction), *Yin Qiao San* (Honeysuckle and Forsythia Powder), and *Ma Huang Xing Ren Gan Cao Shi Gao Tang* (Ephedra, Apricot Kernel, Licorice, and Gypsum Decoction) address the associated symptoms of pneumonia, such as aversion to cold, fever, cough, dyspnea, chest congestion, and the presence of sputum.[20,21]

6. **Respiratory tract disorders**: Exterior-releasing formulas treat various types of respiratory tract disorders. In addition to the examples listed above, other indications include rhinitis,[22] allergic rhinitis,[23,24] nasosinusitis,[25] tonsillitis,[26,27] pharyngitis,[28,29] and many others.
7. **Nasal disorders**: Exterior wind-releasing formulas effectively treat various nasal disorders, such as sinusitis,[30] rhinitis,[31] and nasal polyps.[32] The mechanisms of action are attributed to the antiallergic effects,[33] mast cell stabilizing effects,[34] and anti-inflammatory effects that suppress inflammation of the nasal mucosa.[35] Two representative formulas that treat nasal disorders are *Cang Er Zi San* (Xanthium Powder) and *Xin Yi San* (Magnolia Flower Powder).
8. **Fever**: Many formulas in this category have antipyretic effects to treat fever. The mechanisms of the antipyretic effects vary. *Gui Zhi Tang* (Cinnamon Twig Decoction) has regulatory effects on body temperature to reduce fever.[36] *Ge Gen Tang* (Kudzu Decoction) lowers body temperature by suppressing interferon-induced interleukin-1alpha production.[37] *Yin Qiao San* (Honeysuckle and Forsythia Powder) has a broad spectrum of antibiotic effects to treat infection with fever.[38,39]
9. **Common colds and influenza**: Exterior-releasing formulas are frequently used to treat viral infections such as common colds and influenza, since these formulas are effective in treating both the cause and the symptoms. *Ge Gen Tang* (Kudzu Decoction) has antiviral effects to treat the infection, and antipyretic and anti-inflammatory effects to alleviate fever and muscle aches and pains.[40,41,42] *Xiao Qing Long Tang* (Minor Bluegreen Dragon Decoction) is useful as both a prophylaxis and a treatment for influenza virus infection, since its antiviral effects are attributed to stimulation and increased production of anti-influenza virus antibody.[43] Lastly, *Yin Qiao San* (Honeysuckle and Forsythia Powder) is one of the most frequently used formulas for common colds and influenza, since it treats both the cause and symptoms of viral infection with its antiviral, analgesic, anti-inflammatory and antipyretic activities.[44,45,46]
10. **Infectious disorders**: In addition to the infections listed above (common cold, influenza, bronchitis, pneumonia, etc.), exterior-releasing formulas are also effective in treating herpes zoster,[47] measles,[48] viral myocarditis,[49] infectious meningitis, and many other disorders.

References

1. *Jiang Su Zhong Yi Za Zhi* (Jiangsu Journal of Chinese Medicine), 1965; 11:15.
2. Life Sci, 1980; 27(8):659.
3. *Shan Dong Zhong Yi Xue Yuan Xue Bao* (Journal of Shandong University School of Chinese Medicine), 1992; 1:43.
4. *Si Chuan Zhong Yi* (Sichuan Chinese Medicine), 1998; 9:42.
5. *Shi Yong Zhong Yi Yao Za Zhi* (Journal of Practical Chinese Medicine and Medicinals), 1997; 5:14.
6. Kao ST, Lin CS, Hsieh CC, Hsieh WT, Lin JG. Effects of xiao-qing-long-tang (XQLT) on bronchoconstriction and airway eosinophil infiltration in ovalbumin-sensitized guinea pigs: in vivo and in vitro studies. Allergy. 2001 Dec; 56(12):1164-71.
7. *Zhong Yi Fang Ji Xian Dai Yan Jiu* (Modern Study of Medical Formulas in Traditional Chinese Medicine), 1997; (1):62.
8. T. Nagai, H. Yamada, In vivo anti-influenza virus activity of kampo (Japanese herbal) medicine "sho-seiryu-to" and its mode of action. Int. J. Immunopharmacol. 1994; 16, 605-613.
9. Kao ST, Lin CS, Hsieh CC, Hsieh WT, Lin JG. Effects of xiao-qing-long-tang (XQLT) on bronchoconstriction and airway eosinophil infiltration in ovalbumin-sensitized guinea pigs: in vivo and in vitro studies. Allergy. 2001 Dec; 56(12):1164-71.
10. *Zhong Yi Fang Ji Xian Dai Yan Jiu* (Modern Study of Medical Formulas in Traditional Chinese Medicine), 1997; (1):62
11. *Si Chuan Zhong Yi* (Sichuan Chinese Medicine), 1986; 12:15.
12. *Shan Xi Zhong Yi* (Shanxi Chinese Medicine), 1997; 4:174
13. *Shang Hai Zhong Yi Yao Za Zhi* (Shanghai Journal of Chinese Medicine and Herbology), 1986; 1:26
14. *Shang Hai Zhong Yi Yao Za Zhi* (Shanghai Journal of Chinese Medicine and Herbology), 1986; 1:26
15. *Zhong Cheng Yao Yan Jiu* (Research of Chinese Patent Medicine), 1987; (4):47
16. Kao ST, Yeh TJ, Hsieh CC, Shiau HB, Yeh FT, and Lin JG. The effects of Ma-Xing-Gan-Shi-Tang on respiratory resistance and airway leukocyte infiltration in asthmatic guinea pigs. Immunopharmacol Immunotoxicol. 2001 Aug; 23(3):445-58.
17. Shichijo K and Saito H. Effect of Chinese herbal medicines and disodium cromoglycate on IgE-dependent histamine release from mouse cultured mast cells. Int J Immunopharmacol. 1997 Nov-Dec; 19(11-12):677-82.
18. T. Nagai and H. Yamada, In vivo anti-influenza virus activity of kampo (Japanese herbal) medicine "sho-seiryu-to" and its mode of action. Int. J. Immunopharmacol. 1994; 16, 605-613.
19. *Zhong Cheng Yao* (Study of Chinese Patent Medicine), 1990; 12(1):22.
20. *Hu Bei Zhong Yi Za Zhi* (Hubei Journal of Chinese Medicine), 1982; 1:55.
21. *Zhong Yi Fang Ji Xian Dai Yan Jiu* (Modern Study of Medical Formulas in Traditional Chinese Medicine), 1997; (1):113.
22. *Nan Jing Zhong Yi Yao Da Xue Xue Bao* (Journal of Nanjing University of Traditional Chinese Medicine and Medicinals), 1995; (4):14.

Chapter 1 — Overview

23. *Xin Jiang Zhong Yi Yao* (Xinjiang Chinese Medicine and Herbology), 1996; 4:20.
24. *Si Chuan Zhong Yi* (Sichuan Chinese Medicine), 1991; 10:46.
25. *Zhong Yi Ming Fang Lin Chuang Xin Yong* (Contemporary Clinical Applications of Classic Chinese Formulas), 2001; 646.
26. *Hu Bei Zhong Yi Za Zhi* (Hubei Journal of Chinese Medicine), 1998; 2:41.
27. *Fu Jian Zhong Yi Yao* (Fujian Chinese Medicine and Herbology), 1999; 4(3).
28. *Jiang Xi Zhong Yi Yao* (Jiangxi Chinese Medicine and Herbology), 1989; 4:36.
29. *Fu Jian Zhong Yi Yao* (Fujian Chinese Medicine and Herbology), 1956; (2):13.
30. *Zhe Jiang Zhong Yi Za Zhi* (Zhejiang Journal of Chinese Medicine), 1989; 10:454.
31. Yang SH, Hong CY, and Yu CL. The stimulatory effects of nasal discharge from patients with perennial allergic rhinitis on normal human neutrophils are normalized after treatment with a new mixed formula of Chinese herbs. International Immunopharmacology. 2002 Nov; 2(12):1627-39.
32. *Fu Jian Zhong Yi Yao* (Fujian Chinese Medicine and Herbology), 1991; 6:17.
33. *Zhong Guo Yao Li Xue Bao* (Chinese Herbal Pharmacology Journal), 1990; 5:34.
34. Shichijo K and Saito H. Effect of Chinese herbal medicines and disodium cromoglycate on IgE-dependent histamine release from mouse cultured mast cells. Int J Immunopharmacol. 1997 Nov-Dec; 19(11-12):677-82.
35. Yang SH, Hong CY, and Yu CL. The stimulatory effects of nasal discharge from patients with perennial allergic rhinitis on normal human neutrophils are normalized after treatment with a new mixed formula of Chinese herbs. International Immunopharmacology, 2002 Nov.; 2(12):1627-39 .
36. *Zhong Yao Yao Li Yu Ying Yong* (Pharmacology and Applications of Chinese Herbs), 1987; 3(2):1.
37. Kurokawa M, Kumeda CA, Yamamura J, Kamiyama T, and Shiraki K. Antipyretic activity of cinnamyl derivatives and related compounds in influenza virus-infected mice. Eur J Pharmacol., 1998 May 1; 348(1):45-51.
38. *Zhong Cheng Yao* (Study of Chinese Patent Medicine), 1990; 12(1):22.
39. *Liao Ning Zhong Yi Za Zhi* (Liaoning Journal of Chinese Medicine), 1994; 12:548.
40. Kurokawa M, Tsurita M, Brown J, Fukuda Y, and Shiraki K. Effect of interleukin-12 level augmented by Kakkon-to, a herbal medicine, on the early stage of influenza infection in mice. Antiviral Res. 2002 Nov; 56(2):183-8.
41. Kurokawa M, Kumeda CA, Yamamura J, Kamiyama T, and Shiraki K. Antipyretic activity of cinnamyl derivatives and related compounds in influenza virus-infected mice. Eur J Pharmacol. 1998 May 1; 348(1):45-51.
42. Ozaki Y. Studies on antiinflammatory effect of Japanese Oriental medicines (kampo medicines) used to treat inflammatory diseases. Biol Pharm Bull. 1995 Apr; 1(4):559-62.
43. T. Nagai and H. Yamada, In vivo anti-influenza virus activity of kampo (Japanese herbal) medicine "sho-seiryu-to" and its mode of action. Int. J. Immunopharmacol. 1994; 16, 605-613
44. *Zhong Cheng Yao* (Study of Chinese Patent Medicine), 1990; 12(1):22.
45. *Zhong Yi Za Zhi* (Journal of Chinese Medicine), 1986; 27(3):59.
46. *Zhong Yao Tong Bao* (Journal of Chinese Herbology), 1986; 11(1):51.
47. *Xin Zhong Yi* (New Chinese Medicine), 1977; 51.
48. Huang SP. Shieh GJ. Lee L. Teng HJ. Kao ST. Lin JG. Inhibition effect of shengma-gegen-tang on measles virus in Vero cells and human peripheral blood mononuclear cells. American Journal of Chinese Medicine, 1997; 25(1):89-96.
49. *Hu Nan Zhong Yi Za Zhi* (Hunan Journal of Chinese Medicine), 1997; 4:29.

Section 1

幸温解表剂
— Acrid and Warm Exterior-Releasing Formulas

Gui Zhī Tāng (Cinnamon Twig Decoction)
桂枝湯
桂枝汤

Pinyin Name: *Gui Zhi Tang*
Literal Name: Cinnamon Twig Decoction
Alternate Names: *Kuei Chih Tang*, Cinnamon Decoction, Cassia Twig Decoction, Cinnamon Combination
Original Source: *Shang Han Lun* (Discussion of Cold-Induced Disorders) by Zhang Zhong-Jing in the Eastern Han Dynasty

COMPOSITION

Gui Zhi (Ramulus Cinnamomi)	9g
Bai Shao (Radix Paeoniae Alba)	9g
Zhi Gan Cao (Radix et Rhizoma Glycyrrhizae Praeparata cum Melle)	6g
Sheng Jiang (Rhizoma Zingiberis Recens), *qie* (sliced)	9g
Da Zao (Fructus Jujubae), *bo* (opened)	12 pieces [3 pieces]

DOSAGE / PREPARATION / ADMINISTRATION

The source text states to coarsely crush the ingredients and cook with 7 cups [1,400 mL] of water over low intensity fire until 3 cups [600 mL] of the liquid remain. Take 1 cup [200 mL] of the warm, strained decoction, followed by 1 cup [200 mL] of hot porridge, to promote and enhance the therapeutic effect of the herbs. For best results, have the patient sweat slightly all over the body but do not induce profuse sweating. Once slight sweating has been achieved, stop taking the formula. If sweating does not occur, repeat the dose one or two more times, progressively reducing the time interval between doses within half of a day.

If the patient's condition is severe, administer the dose twice daily (morning and night), and progressively add another two to three doses if no sweating has been induced within two hours after taking the formula. Today, this formula may be prepared as a decoction with the doses suggested in brackets.

CHINESE THERAPEUTIC ACTIONS

1. Releases the exterior and muscle layer
2. Regulates and harmonizes *ying* (nutritive) *qi* and *wei* (defensive) *qi*

CLINICAL MANIFESTATIONS

Exterior-deficient, wind-cold syndrome: fever, sweating or panting, aversion to wind, nasal congestion, dry heaves, absence of thirst, a thin, white tongue coating, and a superficial and moderate, or superficial and weak pulse.

Disharmony of the *ying* (nutritive) and *wei* (defensive) levels: fever and aversion to wind in constitutionally weak, chronic and debilitated animals.

VETERINARY CLINICAL APPLICATIONS

Fever, fever of unknown origin, feline upper respiratory tract disease, canine infectious tracheobronchitis, equine influenza and rhinopneumonitis infections, allergic rhinitis and sinusitis, bronchial asthma, and urinary incontinence.

EXPLANATION

Gui Zhi Tang (Cinnamon Twig Decoction), first presented in the *Shang Han Lun* (Discussion of Cold-Induced Disorders), is designed to treat *taiyang* wind syndrome.

Guì Zhī Tāng (Cinnamon Twig Decoction)

Taiyang wind syndrome refers to attack by wind-cold pathogenic factor at the body's exterior, with wind being the dominant pathogen. Unlike cold, which constricts the body, wind is dispersing and highly mobile in character. Wind usually attacks the exterior of the body and leaves after the attack, taking with it some of the body's *wei* (defensive) *qi*. This etiology can have special significance in horses as they are often body-clipped for shows and exposed to the elements.

Wei (defensive) *qi* controls the opening and closing of the skin pores; the subsequent depletion of *wei qi* impairs the body's regulation of the skin pores. The pores are left open after the wind invasion, which allows yang qi to leak out of the body, carrying body fluids with it. Hence, animals will experience sweating and aversion to wind. Some horses will develop chills that are alleviated with blanketing. Note that sweating, one of the key characteristics of this syndrome, is absent in *taiyang* cold syndrome.

Since cold is also involved in *taiyang* wind syndrome, stagnation of qi and blood and obstruction of the channels may also occur, causing neck stiffness and pain. However, the severity of the neck stiffness seen in *taiyang* wind syndrome is much less than that found in *taiyang* cold syndrome. Since the disease is at the exterior, the tongue coating is still normal. The pulse, superficial and moderate, or superficial and weak, indicates an exterior-deficiency syndrome.

Gui Zhi Tang contains only five ingredients, but it has multiple functions: disperse, tonify, release, and constrict. *Gui Zhi* (Ramulus Cinnamomi), the chief herb, releases wind-cold from the exterior and muscle layer to relieve body aches and pains. *Bai Shao* (Radix Paeoniae Alba), the deputy herb, consolidates the body's interior (e.g., yin and body fluids). Used together, *Gui Zhi* (Ramulus Cinnamomi) and *Bai Shao* (Radix Paeoniae Alba) harmonize *wei* (defensive) *qi* and *ying* (nutritive) *qi*. *Gui Zhi* (Ramulus Cinnamomi) is acrid and warm; *Bai Shao* (Radix Paeoniae Alba) is sour and cool. The former is dispersing in nature, while the latter is nourishing.

Zhi Gan Cao (Radix et Rhizoma Glycyrrhizae Praeparata cum Melle) serves as both assistant and envoy herb. As an assistant, it helps *Gui Zhi* (Ramulus Cinnamomi) relieve aches and pains and helps *Bai Shao* (Radix Paeoniae Alba) benefit yin; as an envoy, it harmonizes the formula. *Sheng Jiang* (Rhizoma Zingiberis Recens), besides helping *Gui Zhi* (Ramulus Cinnamomi) to dispel exterior wind and cold, stops nausea and relieves dry heaves. *Da Zao* (Fructus Jujubae) tonifies qi and body fluids. *Sheng Jiang* (Rhizoma Zingiberis Recens) and *Da Zao* (Fructus Jujubae) work synergistically to benefit the middle *jiao* and assist in qi production.

Lastly, this formula also treats disharmony of *ying* (nutritive) *qi* and *wei* (defensive) *qi* brought on by major illnesses, and qi or blood deficiency. Clinical manifestations in such cases include slight fever with sweating and aversion to wind.

VETERINARY MODIFICATIONS

- With more fever than signs of cold, add *Shi Gao* (Gypsum Fibrosum) and *Zhi Mu* (Rhizoma Anemarrhenae).
- For neck and shoulder pain, add *Ge Gen* (Radix Puerariae Lobatae).
- For sneezing, nasal discharge, and nasal obstruction, add *Jing Jie* (Herba Schizonepetae), *Fang Feng* (Radix Saposhnikoviae), and *Xin Yi Hua* (Flos Magnoliae).
- If accompanied by coughing and wheezing, add *Hou Po* (Cortex Magnoliae Officinalis) and *Ku Xing Ren* (Semen Armeniacae Amarum).

***Gui Zhi Tang* (Cinnamon Twig Decoction)**

Diagnosis	Clinical Signs	Treatment	Herbs
Exterior-deficient, wind-cold syndrome	• Fever and aversion to wind: exterior wind-cold with deficiency of *wei* (defensive) *qi* • Sweating (horses): disharmony of the *ying* (nutritive) and *wei* (defensive) levels • Thin, white tongue coating: exterior wind-cold • Superficial and weak pulse: exterior condition with underlying deficiency	• Releases the exterior and the muscle layer • Regulates and harmonizes *ying* (nutritive) *qi* and *wei* (defensive) *qi*	• *Gui Zhi* (Ramulus Cinnamomi) releases wind-cold from the exterior and muscle layer. • *Bai Shao* (Radix Paeoniae Alba) consolidates the interior (yin and body fluids). • *Zhi Gan Cao* (Radix et Rhizoma Glycyrrhizae Praeparata cum Melle) relieves aches and pains, benefits yin, and harmonizes the herbs. • *Sheng Jiang* (Rhizoma Zingiberis Recens) and *Da Zao* (Fructus Jujubae) benefit the middle *jiao* and tonify qi.

Guì Zhī Tāng (Cinnamon Twig Decoction)

- If there is profuse, white phlegm, remove *Bai Shao* (Radix Paeoniae Alba) and *Da Zao* (Fructus Jujubae), and add *Ban Xia* (Rhizoma Pinelliae) and *Chen Pi* (Pericarpium Citri Reticulatae).
- For animals recovering from wind-cold invasion, add *Xiao Chai Hu Tang* (Minor Bupleurum Decoction).

CAUTIONS / CONTRAINDICATIONS

- *Gui Zhi Tang* is contraindicated in *taiyang* cold syndrome, because *Gui Zhi* (Ramulus Cinnamomi) is not strong enough to dispel excess cold; moreover, the consolidating characteristic of *Bai Shao* (Radix Paeoniae Alba) may actually lead cold into the interior.
- This formula is contraindicated in patients with wind-heat syndrome, exterior cold and interior heat, absence of sweating with irritability, exterior excess conditions without sweating, or beginning stages of febrile disorders with fever, sore throat, and thirst.
- During the course of the disease, avoid foods that are raw, cold, greasy or fatty. Foods such as, meat, cheese, garlic and products that are fermented or preserved should also be avoided.
- This formula is contraindicated in patients with obvious damp-heat conditions. Ingestion of the decoction may cause vomiting or colic, since *Zhi Gan Cao* (Radix et Rhizoma Glycyrrhizae Praeparata cum Melle) and *Gui Zhi* (Ramulus Cinnamomi) are both sweet and warm herbs that can aggravate the damp-heat condition.

PHARMACOLOGICAL EFFECTS

1. **Effect on sweating regulation**: Use of *Gui Zhi Tang* in rats was associated with a bidirectional modulating effect on sweating. *Gui Zhi Tang* reduced sweating in polyhidrosis induced by aminopyrine, and promoted sweating in hypohidrosis induced by atropine.[1]
2. **Effect on temperature regulation**: *Gui Zhi Tang* has marked effects to reduce body temperature in cases of fever and normal body temperature. According to laboratory studies, oral ingestion of this formula reduced body temperature for up to five hours in rats with fever, and up to four hours in rats with normal body temperature.[2] Another study in rabbits and mice on the pharmacokinetics of this formula stated that the initial onset of action was observed 60 minutes after administration, and reached the peak effect after 120 minutes. The average reduction of temperature was 3.8°C.[3,4]
3. **Anti-inflammatory**: Intraperitoneal injection of *Gui Zhi Tang* at 7.5 g/kg demonstrated marked anti-inflammatory effect in mice with swollen feet. The onset of effect began one hour after the injection, and lasted for approximately 24 hours.[5] According to another study in mice, the anti-inflammatory effect of *Gui Zhi Tang* (25.32 g/kg) was stronger than aspirin (100 mg/kg).[6]
4. **Analgesic and sedative**: Intraperitoneal injection of *Gui Zhi Tang* in mice at doses of 7.5 g/kg and 15 g/kg showed marked analgesic and sedative effects. Though effective, delayed onset of effect up to 120 minutes was observed.[7]
5. **Antibiotic**: According to *in vitro* studies, administration of *Gui Zhi Tang* was associated with inhibitory effects against *Helicobacter pylori*, *Staphylococcus aureus*, *Salmonella typhi* and *Mycobacterium tuberculosis*.[8]
6. **Cardiovascular**: Administration of *Gui Zhi Tang* induced an increase of systolic blood pressure and stroke volume in 7 healthy adult males (age, 22.3 +/- 1.8 years old).[9]

HUMAN CLINICAL STUDIES AND RESEARCH

1. **Fever**: In one clinical study, *Gui Zhi Tang* was evaluated for its effect to reduce body temperature in subjects with fever due to infectious diseases. Out of 24 cases with high fever, the temperature was reduced to normal in 16 cases, reduced to mild fever in 4 cases, and no effect in 2 cases. Two cases were excluded from the study as the causes of fever were determined later to be other than infectious disorders.[10]
2. **Common cold**: In one study involving 42 patients with common cold in the summertime, administration of *Gui Zhi Tang* was associated with complete recovery within 2-3 packs of herbs.[11]
3. **Bronchial asthma**: One study reported 97.5% effectiveness using modified *Gui Zhi Tang* plus *Hou Po* (Cortex Magnoliae Officinalis) to treat bronchial asthma in 40 infants (29 males and 11 females, between 2-10 years of age, with 7 days to 6 months history of illness). The duration of treatment ranged from 1-5 days. Of 40 patients, the study reported recovery in 36 cases, improvement in 3 cases, and no effect in 1 case.[12]
4. **Atrioventricular block**: One study reported success using modified *Gui Zhi Tang* to treat atrioventricular block. The herbal treatment contained *Gui Zhi Tang* plus *San Qi* (Radix et Rhizoma Notoginseng) and *Huang Qi* (Radix Astragali) as the base formula, with addition of *Suan Zao Ren* (Semen Ziziphi Spinosae) for palpitations, and *Yu Jin* (Radix Curcumae) and *Gua Lou Pi* (Pericarpium Trichosanthis) for feeling of chest oppression. Of 30 patients, the study reported recovery in 28 cases and improvement in 2 cases after 14-21 days of treatment.[13]
5. **Enuresis**: One study reported great success in treating enuresis in young children using modified *Gui Zhi Tang*. The herbal treatment contained *Gui Zhi* (Ramulus Cinnamomi) 10g, *Bai Shao* (Radix Paeoniae Alba) 10g, *Sheng Jiang* (Rhizoma Zingiberis Recens) 3 slices, *Da Zao* (Fructus Jujubae) 5 pieces, *Zhi Gan Cao* (Radix et Rhizoma Glycyrrhizae Praeparata cum Melle) 6g, *Yi Zhi*

Guì Zhī Tāng (Cinnamon Twig Decoction)

(Fructus Alpiniae Oxyphyllae) 15g, *Tu Si Zi* (Semen Cuscutae) 15g, *Wu Yao* (Radix Linderae) 10g, and *Mu Gua* (Fructus Chaenomelis) 2 pieces. Of 30 infants, the study reported complete recovery in 4 cases, significant improvement in 15 cases, and moderate improvement in 11 cases. The overall effectiveness was 100%.[14] Another study reported marked effectiveness in treating enuresis in 10 of 15 children using *Gui Zhi Tang* plus *Suo Quan Wan* (Shut the Sluice Pill). The average duration of treatment was 10 packs of herbs.[15]

TOXICOLOGY

The LD_{50} of *Gui Zhi Tang* in mice is 28.125 g/kg within 72 hours via intraperitoneal injection.[16]

SUGGESTED ACUPUNCTURE TREATMENT

1. Points: *Fengmen* (BL 12), *Feishu* (BL 13), *Dazhui* (GV 14), *Lieque* (LU 7), *Fengchi* (GB 20), *Jinggu* (BL 64), *Houxi* (SI 3), *Shenmai* (BL 62), and *Housanli* (ST 36). Equine: *Dingchuan* and *Feizhishu*. Canine: *Dingchuan* and *Bitong*.
2. Technique: even method.

The acupuncture treatment for this syndrome focuses on dispelling wind from the skin and muscles, as well as harmonizing *ying* (nutritive) and *wei* (defensive) levels. *Fengmen* (BL 12) is the influential point for wind and the trachea and helps to dispel wind-cold, cough, and cervical stiffness, while *Feishu* (BL 13) is the Lung *shu* (transport) point and can relieve cough, asthmatic breathing, and clear nasal congestion. *Jinggu* (BL 64), the *yuan* (source) point of the foot *taiyang* channel, is combined with *Fengchi* (GB 20) to dispel exterior wind and relieve fever and aversion to wind. These two points may be sedated. *Houxi* (SI 3) and *Shenmai* (BL 62) relieve muscle aches and dispel exterior wind. *Housanli* (ST 36) strengthens qi of the body to help harmonize the *ying* (nutritive) and *wei* (defensive) levels.

Dingchuan is used symptomatically in both equine and canine species to relieve cough and dyspnea. *Feizhishu* is an alternate Lung *shu* (transport) point found in horses, and *Bitong* is used in dogs for the relief of nasal congestion and sinusitis.

RELATED FORMULAS

Guì Zhī Jiā Gě Gēn Tāng
(Cinnamon Twig Decoction plus Kudzu)
桂枝加葛根湯
桂枝加葛根汤
Pinyin Name: *Gui Zhi Jia Ge Gen Tang*
Literal Name: Cinnamon Twig Decoction plus Kudzu
Original Source: *Shang Han Lun* (Discussion of Cold-Induced Disorders) by Zhang Zhong-Jing in the Eastern Han Dynasty

Gui Zhi (Ramulus Cinnamomi)	6g
Bai Shao (Radix Paeoniae Alba)	6g
Zhi Gan Cao (Radix et Rhizoma Glycyrrhizae Praeparata cum Melle)	6g
Sheng Jiang (Rhizoma Zingiberis Recens), *qie* (sliced)	9g
Da Zao (Fructus Jujubae), *bo* (opened)	12 pieces [3 pieces]
Ge Gen (Radix Puerariae Lobatae)	12g

The source text states to cook the ingredients with 8 cups [1,600 mL] of water until 3 cups [600 mL] of the liquid remain. Take 1 cup [200 mL] of the warm, strained decoction and cover the body with blankets to promote mild sweating. Patients do not need to consume hot porridge after taking this formula. Please refer to *Gui Zhi Tang* (Cinnamon Twig Decoction) for additional information on administration and contraindications. Today, this formula may be prepared as a decoction with the doses suggested in brackets.

Gui Zhi Jia Ge Gen Tang (Cinnamon Twig Decoction plus Kudzu) treats *taiyang* wind syndrome with severe neck stiffness. The addition of *Ge Gen* (Radix Puerariae Lobatae) directs the formula to the head and neck and relieves muscle tension and neck stiffness. Other clinical signs include sweating with aversion to wind.

Gui Zhi Jia Ge Gen Tang (Cinnamon Twig Decoction plus Kudzu) is used to treat cervical pain and stiffness during periods of seasonal cold. This formula has proven to be successful in relieving neck pain in the absence of radiographic findings of structural abnormalities.

Guì Zhī Jiā Sháo Yào Tāng
(Cinnamon Twig Decoction plus Peony)
桂枝加芍藥湯
桂枝加芍药汤
Pinyin Name: *Gui Zhi Jia Shao Yao Tang*
Literal Name: Cinnamon Twig Decoction plus Peony
Original Source: *Shang Han Lun* (Discussion of Cold-Induced Disorders) by Zhang Zhong-Jing in the Eastern Han Dynasty

Gui Zhi (Ramulus Cinnamomi)	9g
Bai Shao (Radix Paeoniae Alba)	18g
Zhi Gan Cao (Radix et Rhizoma Glycyrrhizae Praeparata cum Melle)	6g

Guì Zhī Tāng (Cinnamon Twig Decoction)

Da Zao (Fructus Jujubae), *bo* (opened)	12 pieces [3 pieces]
Sheng Jiang (Rhizoma Zingiberis Recens), *qie* (sliced)	9g

Gui Zhi Jia Shao Yao Tang (Cinnamon Twig Decoction plus Peony) treats patients with *taiyang* syndrome who have been improperly treated with downward-draining methods. In these situations, the downward-draining methods damage Spleen qi, allowing the Liver to attack the deficient Spleen. As the exterior wind-cold condition moves into the interior, the *taiyang* syndrome is now complicated by *taiyin* syndrome. Clinically, this condition is characterized by both exterior and interior signs of aversion to cold, fever, sweating, abdominal fullness, distention and pain, and diarrhea.

Gui Zhi Jia Shao Yao Tang (Cinnamon Twig Decoction plus Peony) is a modification of *Gui Zhi Tang*. The ingredients and the doses of the two formulas are exactly the same, with the exception of *Bai Shao* (Radix Paeoniae Alba). The dose of *Bai Shao* is doubled in *Gui Zhi Jia Shao Yao Tang*, making it a formula for treating interior disharmony instead of exterior conditions. Today, *Gui Zhi Jia Shao Yao Tang* is used to treat abdominal pain and cramps, enteritis, and food poisoning.

Gui Zhi Jia Shao Yao Tang (Cinnamon Twig Decoction plus Peony) can be used to treat pancreatitis with abdominal pain and post-abdominal surgical pain with cold signs and cramping.

AUTHORS' COMMENTS

Gui Zhi Tang is not typically used as a single formula in small animal veterinary medicine; instead it is combined with single herbs or combined directly with other formula just as it is in human medicine. A notable exception to this is the use of *Gui Zhi Tang* as a single formula to treat fever of unknown origin in dogs and cats. The use of this formula has shown to decrease fever within 24-72 hours of administration, which is typically 3-6 doses. Cats appear to have a faster response time than dogs. In horses, however, this formula can be very useful on its own. Practitioners are often confronted with patients with mild to no fever, little if any changes in laboratory values, and yet who are off feed, slightly depressed, stiff, and may have slight upper respiratory signs. Many of these patients likely have a mild equine influenza/type-1 infection and can be treated successfully with *Gui Zhi Tang* alone. The ingredients are also balanced nicely for the equine gastro-intestinal system, and it is unlikely that this formula will cause any problems, if given appropriately.

Since dogs, cats, birds, and many other animals do not sweat, the effectiveness of exterior releasing formula cannot be ascertained by the presence and quantity of sweat induced in these species. These formulas have been shown to be clinically effective in treating exterior syndromes, and opening the pores alone to expel pathogens without inducing obvious sweating still produces the intended therapeutic effects in non-sweating species.

In the clinic, animals may not show all the signs, or it may be difficult to match the exact clinical signs. The key to selecting *Gui Zhi Tang* is to identify the main clinical signs: fever, aversion to wind, sweating, and a superficial pulse. Deficient animals often catch colds frequently as their *wei* (defensive) *qi* is low. Animals that are kenneled, travel, and/or compete frequently are particularly vulnerable.

Gui Zhi Tang can be used in deficient patients who show both wind-cold and wind-heat clinical signs. These mixed clinical signs may include aversion to cold, fever, aversion to wind, sweating, a sore throat, neck pain and stiffness, and other conflicting clinical signs. When it is difficult to diagnose whether the animal has wind-cold or wind-heat, many times the condition is transitioning from wind-cold to wind-heat, and then to Lung heat. In the stage between wind-cold and wind-heat, mixed clinical signs such as the ones described above will be present and the *ying* (nutritive) and *wei* (defensive) levels will be disrupted. *Gui Zhi Tang* is often combined with *Yin Qiao San* (Honeysuckle and Forsythia Powder) in a 1:1 ratio to help expel the exterior pathogenic factors of both wind-cold and wind-heat.

Gui Zhi Tang and *Yu Ping Feng San* (Jade Windscreen Powder) both treat spontaneous sweating and aversion to wind, but have completely different clinical applications.

- *Gui Zhi Tang* is an exterior-releasing formula that treats wind-cold invasion with disharmony between the *ying* (nutritive) and *wei* (defensive) levels, causing clinical signs such as fever, neck pain and stiffness, stuffy nose, and a superficial pulse. This formula is used for patients who suffer from exterior conditions.
- *Yu Ping Feng San* is an astringent formula that also treats sweating and aversion to wind. However, these clinical signs are caused by *wei* (defensive) *qi* deficiency and its inability to consolidate the exterior. Besides leakage of body fluids, other clinical signs include frequent catching of common colds, generalized weakness, and a deficient pulse. This formula is appropriate for patients who frequently suffer from exterior conditions but do not currently have one.[17]

Guì Zhī Tāng (Cinnamon Twig Decoction)

Gui Zhi Tang and *Xiao Jian Zhong Tang* (Minor Construct the Middle Decoction) contain very similar ingredients, but have drastically different applications. *Xiao Jian Zhong Tang* is comprised of *Gui Zhi Tang* plus *Yi Tang* (Maltosum). However, because of dose differences, the main functions of the two formulas differ significantly.

- *Gui Zhi Tang* is an exterior-releasing formula. It contains *Gui Zhi* (Ramulus Cinnamomi) and *Bai Shao* (Radix Paeoniae Alba) as chief and deputy herbs to release the exterior and harmonize the *ying* (nutritive) and *wei* (defensive) levels.
- *Xiao Jian Zhong Tang* is an interior-warming formula. It contains *Yi Tang* (Maltosum) as the chief herb to warm and tonify the Spleen to relieve pain. As deputy herbs, *Gui Zhi* (Ramulus Cinnamomi) warms yang qi, and *Bai Shao* (Radix Paeoniae Alba) relieves pain.
- Although both formulas contain similar ingredients, *Gui Zhi Tang* primarily expels exterior wind-cold invasion, while *Xiao Jian Zhong Tang* (Minor Construct the Middle Decoction) warms and tonifies the middle *jiao* to relieve pain.

Gui Zhi Tang can be combined with *Suo Quan Wan* (Shut the Sluice Pill) in the treatment of urinary incontinence in dogs. Usually, *Suo Quan Wan* (Shut the Sluice Pill) is not strong enough to warm the Kidney, and the addition of *Gui Zhi Tang* greatly improves long term treatment success.

The follow formulas are variations of *Gui Zhi Tang*, and are used for different indications:

- *Gui Zhi Ren Shen Tang* (Cinnamon Twig and Ginseng Decoction) has been found to be useful in treating cardiac arrhythmia that occur in heart yang deficiency. From a western perspective, this corresponds to animals with atrial fibrillation secondary to cardiomyopathy and/or congestive heart failure. In horses, a better option for atrial fibrillation is *Zhi Gan Cao Tang* (Honey-Fried Licorice Decoction), reserving *Gui Zhi Ren Shen Tang* (Cinnamon Twig and Ginseng Decoction) for those cases where *Gui Zhi Tang* alone would be chosen, but for more prominent clinical signs of anorexia or mild colic.
- *Gui Zhi Jia Long Gu Mu Li Tang* (Cinnamon Twig Decoction plus Dragon Bone and Oyster Shell) is useful in treating *shen* (spirit) disturbance in aging canines who are deficient in yin and yang, with disharmony between the *ying* (nutritive) level and *wei* (defensive) level and lack of communication between the Heart and Kidney. Because the formula aids this communication, it is especially useful in dogs that require regular cardiac monitoring and whose nervousness and anxiety interfere with obtaining valid evaluations of heart function. It can be combined with conventional medications with appropriate monitoring. Older dogs that have lost a long-time canine housemate or littermate and that the owner reports won't stop "looking" for the deceased animal will also benefit from harmonizing yin and yang. Show horses and competition dogs that have become depleted from a long season and are becoming "ring sour" or anxious can become better focused without sacrificing performance on this formula. Many of these animals will also show signs of lumbar pain commonly associated with being "cold-backed."

References

1. Fu HY, He YZ. Studies on the hidropoiesis of the decoction of gui-zhi tang in mice and rats. Zhong Xi Yi Jie He Za Zhi. 1991 Jan; 11(1): 34-6, 6.
2. *Zhong Yao Yao Li Yu Ying Yong* (Pharmacology and Applications of Chinese Herbs), 1987; 3(2):1.
3. *Zhong Cheng Yao Yan Jiu* (Research of Chinese Patent Medicine), 1983; (3):25.
4. *Zhong Yi Za Zhi* (Journal of Chinese Medicine), 1984; 8:63.
5. *Zhong Cheng Yao Yan Jiu* (Research of Chinese Patent Medicine), 1983; (3):25.
6. *Zhong Yao Yao Li Yu Ying Yong* (Pharmacology and Applications of Chinese Herbs), 1987; 3(2):1.
7. *Zhong Cheng Yao Yan Jiu* (Research of Chinese Patent Medicine), 1983; (3):25.
8. *Zhong Yao Yao Li Yu Ying Yong* (Pharmacology and Applications of Chinese Herbs), 1987; 3(3):1.
9. Xu FH, Uebaba K. Effect of Kampo formulations (traditional Chinese medicine) on circulatory parameters. Acupuncture & Electro-Therapeutics Research. 1999; 24(1):11-28.
10. *Jiang Su Yi Yao* (Jiangsu Journal of Medicine and Herbology), 1979; (1):43.
11. *Zhong Yi Ming Fang Lin Chuang Xin Yong* (Contemporary Clinical Applications of Classic Chinese Formulas), 2001; 547.
12. *Si Chuan Zhong Yi* (Sichuan Chinese Medicine), 1998; 9:42.
13. *Jiang Xi Zhong Yi Yao* (Jiangxi Chinese Medicine and Herbology), 1999; 6:56.
14. *Ji Lin Zhong Yi Yao* (Jilin Chinese Medicine and Herbology), 1998; 4:36.
15. *Shi Yong Zhong Xi Yi Jie He Za Zhi* (Practical Journal of Integrated Chinese and Western Medicines), 1992; 1:44.
16. *Zhong Cheng Yao Yan Jiu* (Research of Chinese Patent Medicine), 1983; (3):25
17. Wang MZ, et al. *Zhong Yi Xue Wen Da Ti Ku* (Questions and Answers on Traditional Chinese Medicine: Herbal Formulas).

Gĕ Gēn Tāng (Kudzu Decoction)

葛根湯
葛根汤

Pinyin Name: *Ge Gen Tang*
Literal Name: Kudzu Decoction
Alternate Names: *Ko Ken Tang*, Pueraria Decoction, Pueraria Combination
Original Source: *Shang Han Lun* (Discussion of Cold-Induced Disorders) by Zhang Zhong-Jing in the Eastern Han Dynasty

COMPOSITION

Ge Gen (Radix Puerariae Lobatae)	12g
Ma Huang (Herba Ephedrae)	9g
Gui Zhi (Ramulus Cinnamomi)	6g
Bai Shao (Radix Paeoniae Alba)	6g
Zhi Gan Cao (Radix et Rhizoma Glycyrrhizae Praeparata cum Melle)	6g
Sheng Jiang (Rhizoma Zingiberis Recens), *qie* (sliced)	9g
Da Zao (Fructus Jujubae), *bo* (opened)	12 pieces [3 pieces]

DOSAGE / PREPARATION / ADMINISTRATION

The source text states to cook *Ma Huang* (Herba Ephedrae) and *Ge Gen* (Radix Puerariae Lobatae) first with 10 cups [2,000 mL] of water until 8 cups [1,400 mL] of the liquid remain. Remove the foam from the top, add in the other ingredients, and cook until the liquid is reduced to 3 cups [600 mL]. Take 1 cup [200 mL] of the strained decoction while it is warm to promote mild sweating.

CHINESE THERAPEUTIC ACTIONS

1. Releases the exterior and muscle layer
2. Promotes generation of body fluids

CLINICAL MANIFESTATIONS

Taiyang syndrome with wind-cold invasion: severe muscle stiffness of the neck and back, aversion to cold with or without fever, aversion to wind and diarrhea.

VETERNIARY CLINICAL APPLICATIONS

Fever, upper respiratory tract infection, allergic rhinitis, chronic rhinitis, neck and shoulder stiffness and pain, periarthritis of shoulder, tendonitis or bursitis of the shoulders, cervical intervertebral disk disease, cervical spondylosis, soft tissues injuries, facial paralysis, meningitis, encephalitis and diarrhea.

EXPLANATION

Ge Gen Tang (Kudzu Decoction) treats *taiyang* syndrome with wind-cold invasion. In comparison to the clinical signs and conditions applicable to *Gui Zhi Tang* (Cinnamon Twig Decoction), the distinguishing symptom for the use of this formula is the severe stiffness and pain in the neck and back. The severe neck stiffness and pain are caused by cold constriction, and by lack of body fluids which fail to nourish the muscle layer. Other clinical signs of *taiyang* syndrome with wind-cold invasion include fever and aversion to cold and wind.

Ge Gen Tang is formulated by adding *Ge Gen* (Radix Puerariae Lobatae) and *Ma Huang* (Herba Ephedrae) to *Gui Zhi Tang* (Cinnamon Twig Decoction). *Ge Gen* (Radix Puerariae Lobatae), however, acts as the chief herb. It promotes generation of body fluids and relieves muscle stiffness. *Ma Huang* (Herba Ephedrae) and *Gui Zhi* (Ramulus Cinnamomi) release wind and cold from the exterior. Also, the sweet and acrid properties of *Gui Zhi* (Ramulus Cinnamomi) help to relieve body aches and pains. *Bai Shao* (Radix Paeoniae Alba), the deputy herb, consolidates the interior (yin and body fluids) of the body. Used together, *Gui Zhi* (Ramulus Cinnamomi) and *Bai Shao* (Radix Paeoniae Alba) harmonize qi at the *wei* (defensive) and *ying* (nutritive) levels. *Zhi Gan Cao* (Radix et Rhizoma Glycyrrhizae Praeparata cum Melle) serves as both an auxiliary and envoy herb. As an auxiliary herb, it relieves aches and pains and promotes the production of body fluids; as an envoy herb, it harmonizes the formula. *Sheng Jiang* (Rhizoma Zingiberis Recens) helps *Gui Zhi* (Ramulus Cinnamomi) to dispel exterior wind-cold. *Da Zao* (Fructus Jujubae) tonifies deficient qi and body fluids.

VETERINARY MODIFICATIONS

- For nausea and vomiting caused by reversed flow of Stomach qi, add *Ban Xia* (Rhizoma Pinelliae) and *Fu Ling* (Poria).
- If there are signs of fever and thirst, add *Zhi Mu* (Rhizoma Anemarrhenae) and *Shi Gao* (Gypsum Fibrosum).
- If accompanied by severe pain of the shoulders, add *Fu Ling* (Poria), *Bai Zhu* (Rhizoma Atractylodis Macrocephalae) and *Fu Zi* (Radix Aconiti Lateralis Praeparata).

Gě Gēn Tāng (Kudzu Decoction)

Ge Gen Tang (Kudzu Decoction)

Diagnosis	Clinical Signs	Treatment	Herbs
Taiyang syndrome with wind-cold invasion	• Neck stiffness and pain: cold constriction and lack of body fluids • Fever, aversion to cold, aversion to wind: *taiyang* syndrome with exterior wind-cold	• Releases the exterior and muscle layer • Promotes generation of body fluids	• *Ge Gen* (Radix Puerariae Lobatae) promotes generation of body fluids and relieves muscle stiffness. • *Ma Huang* (Herba Ephedrae) and *Gui Zhi* (Ramulus Cinnamomi) release wind and cold from the exterior. • *Gui Zhi* (Ramulus Cinnamomi) and *Bai Shao* (Radix Paeoniae Alba) harmonize *wei* (defensive) and *ying* (nutritive) levels. • *Zhi Gan Cao* (Radix et Rhizoma Glycyrrhizae Praeparata cum Melle) relieves aches and pains and promotes the production of body fluids. • *Sheng Jiang* (Rhizoma Zingiberis Recens) dispels exterior wind and cold. • *Da Zao* (Fructus Jujubae) tonifies deficient qi and body fluids.

- For abdominal pain and diarrhea, add *Huang Qin* (Radix Scutellariae) and *Huang Lian* (Rhizoma Coptidis).

CAUTIONS / CONTRAINDICATIONS

- *Ma Huang* (Herba Ephedrae) is extremely acrid and warm, induces diaphoresis, releases exterior wind-cold, and relieves dyspnea. It can induce profuse sweating and damage the qi and yin of the body when used at high doses. Therefore, formulas containing this herb should only be used in conditions having all of the following characteristics: wind, cold, exterior, and excess.
- *Ge Gen Tang* should be used with care in the following patients: cats and horses, geriatric and debilitated patients and individuals with generalized weakness, animals on long-term non-steroidal anti-inflammatory drugs. In geriatric animals, it is best to combine this formula with an appropriate Spleen tonic to promote qi and blood production and prevent gastrointestinal upset.
- It is contraindicated in animals with hypertension.
- The lowest therapeutic dose is advised when used to treat cats and horses. It is contraindicated in those with obvious yin deficiency. Signs of overdose include aggression, anxiety, hyperactivity, salivation, vomiting/colic, increased respiratory and heart rate and elevation of blood pressure.
- This formula is not recommended for the following syndromes: exterior wind-heat syndrome, exterior febrile conditions, transformation of wind-cold to wind-heat, interior heat, damp-heat accumulation, and qi or blood deficiency.
- This formula is not suitable for animals with the following conditions: thirst caused by deficiency of body fluids, spontaneous sweating due to *wei* (defensive) *qi* deficiency, weak pulse from deficient conditions, rapid pulse from excess conditions, and palpitations and a sensation of heaviness in the body as a result of misuse of herbs.
- This formula is contraindicated in the following conditions: animals with ulceration, abscesses and sores; *lin zheng* (dysuria syndrome); and animals with bleeding or excessive bleeding on the verge of collapse.

PHARMACOLOGICAL EFFECTS

1. **Antibacterial**: According to *in vitro* studies, *Ge Gen Tang* demonstrated an inhibitory effect against *E. coli* and *Staphylococcus aureus*, but only at high concentration.[1]
2. **Antiviral**: One study reported marked effectiveness using *Ge Gen Tang* to treat mice with early stage of influenza infection. The dose of the formula was 5.0 mg per mouse three times daily. The mechanism of this action was attributed to significant enhancement of interleukin-12 correlated with the reduction of virus yields in broncho-alveolar lavage fluid in the early phase of infection.[2]
3. **Antipyretic**: Administration of *Ge Gen Tang* effectively reduced fever in mice infected with influenza virus. The mechanism of the antipyretic effects was attributed to the suppression of interferon-induced interleukin-1-alpha production.[3]
4. **Anti-inflammatory**: Oral administration of *Ge Gen Tang* was associated with inhibition of the inflammatory processes in both the early exudative stage and the late proliferative stage. This study stated *Ge Gen Tang* was

Gě Gēn Tāng (Kudzu Decoction)

useful in treating stomatitis, tonsillitis, cold and chronic inflammatory diseases.[4]

5. **Cardiovascular**: In anesthetized dogs and cats, intravenous injection of *Ge Gen Tang* at 0.25-0.5 g/kg was associated with dilation of the blood vessels and increased blood perfusion to the brain. The duration of action was approximately one hour.[5]
6. **Immunostimulant**: Continuous administration of extract of *Ge Gen Tang* in mice was associated with a significant influence to the immune system. Increase in phagocytic activity of the immune cells was observed in mice with suppressed immune system. However, a suppression of the immune response was observed in mice with hyperactive immune system.[6,7] In another study involving 10 subjects, use of *Ge Gen Tang* daily was associated with an increase of natural killer (NK) cells.[8]

HUMAN CLINICAL STUDIES AND RESEARCH

1. **Fever**: One hundred and ten children with fever were effectively treated with modified *Ge Gen Tang*. The study reported reduction of body temperature in 66 cases (60%) after 1 dose, 43 cases (39%) after 2 doses, and 1 case (0.9%) after 3 doses. Minor modifications to the original formula were made based on the clinical manifestations of the patients.[9]
2. **Upper respiratory tract infection**: In one study, *Ge Gen Tang* demonstrated a rate of effectiveness of approximately 80% in releasing the pathogenic factor from the exterior. The main improvements were seen in runny nose, sneezing, and aversion to cold.[10]
3. **Meningitis**: Thirteen patients with infectious meningitis were treated with *Ge Gen Tang* with complete recovery in all cases. Resolution of clinical signs range from 40 hours to 15 days. No complications were reported.[11] It has also been reported that this formula is also effective in treating encephalitis, though treatment must begin within the first two days.[12]
4. **Neck and shoulder pain**: Seventy patients with neck and shoulder disorders were treated with a modified *Ge Gen Tang* with complete recovery in 9 cases, significant improvement in 30 cases, moderate improvement in 29 cases, and no improvement in 2 cases. *Ge Gen Tang* was modified by increasing the doses of *Ge Gen* (Radix Puerariae Lobatae) and *Gui Zhi* (Ramulus Cinnamomi).[13] Another study reported a 94% rate of effectiveness using modified *Ge Gen Tang* to treat 50 patients between 40-60 years of age, with neck and shoulder pain with history of illness ranging from 5 days to 10 years. The duration of treatment ranged from 30-50 days. Of 50 patients, the study reported complete recovery in 16 cases, significant improvement in 25 cases, moderate improvement in 6 cases, and no benefit in 3 cases.[14]
5. **Periarthritis of shoulder**: Forty-eight patients with periarthritis of the shoulder was treated for 10-20 days with complete recovery in 34 cases, significant improvement in 8 cases, and no benefit in 6 cases. The herbal treatment contained *Ge Gen Tang* plus *Xi Xin* (Radix et Rhizoma Asari), *Qiang Huo* (Rhizoma et Radix Notopterygii), *Fang Feng* (Radix Saposhnikoviae) and others.[15]
6. **Soft tissues injuries**: One study reported a 96.88% rate of effectiveness using modified *Ge Gen Tang* to treat soft tissues injuries in 32 patients (25 males and 7 females), between 10-55 years of age, and 1 hour to 1½ year history of illness. The herbal treatment consisted of *Ge Gen Tang*, with the dose of *Ge Gen* (Radix Puerariae Lobatae) increased to 50g. Of 32 patients, the study reported complete recovery in 19 cases, significant improvement in 12 cases, and no benefit in 1 case.[16]
7. **Facial paralysis**: Use of modified *Ge Gen Tang* was associated with varying degrees of improvement to complete recovery in all 216 patients with facial paralysis. The herbal treatment contained *Ge Gen Tang* plus *Bai Fu Zi* (Rhizoma Typhonii), *Jiang Can* (Bombyx Batryticatus), *Quan Xie* (Scorpio), and others as needed. The herbs were given in decoction daily, for 5 packs of herbs per course of treatment. The duration of treatment ranged from 5-35 packs of herbs.[17] Another study reported 97.67% effectiveness in treating 86 patients with facial paralysis. The herbal treatment contained *Ge Gen Tang* plus *Qian Zheng San* (Lead to Symmetry Powder), with addition of *Fu Ling* (Poria) and *Cang Zhu* (Rhizoma Atractylodis) for presence of dampness; and addition of *Chai Hu* (Radix Bupleuri) and *Huang Qin* (Radix Scutellariae) for fever. After 3-5 packs of herbs and induction of sweating, the herbal treatment was modified by adding *Hong Hua* (Flos Carthami), *Dang Gui* (Radix Angelicae Sinensis) and *Huang Qi* (Radix Astragali); and eliminating *Ma Huang* (Herba Ephedrae), *Gui Zhi* (Ramulus Cinnamomi), *Qiang Huo* (Rhizoma et Radix Notopterygii) and *Ge Gen* (Radix Puerariae Lobatae). Upon stabilization and during the recovery phase, the herbal treatment was switched to *Shi Quan Da Bu Tang* (All-Inclusive Great Tonifying Decoction) for consolidation and maintenance. Of 86 patients, the study reported complete recovery in 79 cases, improvement in 5 cases, and no benefit in 2 cases.[18]

HERB-DRUG INTERACTION

Acetaminophen: One study evaluated the pharmacokinetics of acetaminophen under co-administration of *Ge Gen Tang* in human volunteers. The pharmacokinetic parameters were calculated from the blood acetaminophen concentration-time curves. No significant differences were noted between the group that received only acetaminophen

Gĕ Gēn Tāng (Kudzu Decoction)

and the group that received both acetaminophen and *Ge Gen Tang.*[19]

TOXICOLOGY

Ge Gen Tang is relatively safe, even at a high dosage. No side effects or toxicities were observed following oral administration of this formula at 2.5 g/kg in mice. Furthermore, adverse reactions were not observed following oral administration of this formula to mice at a dosage equivalent to seventeen times the normal adult human dose.[20] In humans, administration of this formula in extract at 7.5 g/day was associated with mild nausea, vomiting, fatigue and constipation.[21]

SUGGESTED ACUPUNCTURE TREATMENT

1. Points: *Lieque* (LU 7), *Yingxiang* (LI 20), *Zhizheng* (SI 7), *Fengmen* (BL 12), *Fengchi* (GB 20), *Hegu* (LI 4), *Tianzhu* (BL 10), *Qiuxu* (GB 40), *Jiuwei* and *Jingjiaji.*
2. Technique: sedation in general; use even method in cases of deficiency; may also use moxibustion.

Lieque (LU 7), the *luo* (connecting) point of the Lung channel, is combined with *Yingxiang* (LI 20) to ventilate the Lung and relieve various clinical signs associated with Lung qi rising. *Zhizheng* (SI 7), the *luo* (connecting) point of the hand *taiyang* channel, is combined with *Fengmen* (BL 12) and *Fengchi* (GB 20) to expel exterior cold and relieve fever and aversion to cold. *Hegu* (LI 4) helps relieve the wind-cold factor. *Tianzhu* (BL 10) and *Qiuxu* (GB 40) relieve neck and shoulder stiffness.

As this formula is used often in animals with neck and shoulder stiffness, both *Jiuwei* and *Jingjiaji* can be very effective in this regard. Practitioners should choose points in the area of greatest stiffness/pain. In horses moxibustion is extremely helpful, while in dogs electroacupuncture is usually the method of choice. [Note: *Jiuwei* is known as the equine cervical nine points, and *Jingjiaji* is known as the cervical paravertebral points.]

AUTHORS' COMMENTS

Historically, *Ge Gen Tang* has been used for *taiyang* syndrome with wind-cold, and accompanied by stiffness of the neck and shoulders. Today, it is commonly used to treat neck and shoulder stiffness and pain associated with musculoskeletal injuries, with or without *taiyang* syndrome or wind-cold condition.

For best results, combine *Ge Gen Tang* with *Shao Yao Gan Cao Tang* (Peony and Licorice Decoction) to treat acute neck and shoulder disorders with stiffness and pain. This combination is especially useful for animals of any age with acute exacerbation of pre-existing cervical intervertebral disk disease, cervical spondylosis, elbow or shoulder dysplasia or degenerative joint disease, chronic injury, and cervical/shoulder pain in the absence of structural abnormalities during abrupt seasonal weather changes. It is also effective for performance and service animals that suffer an acute strain or sprain of the neck or joints of the front limbs. In these cases it is typical to increase the amount of *Ge Gen* (Radix Puerariae Lobatae) to further generate body fluids and relieve muscle stiffness and add herbs to move the blood and dispel wind-dampness. *Yan Huo Suo* (Rhizoma Corydalis) activates qi and blood to relieve pain and *Qiang Huo* (Rhizoma et Radix Notopterygii), which is warm and aromatic, disperses wind, cold and dampness from the exterior and opens the channels in the upper body; both are good additions. Caution should be exercised in the treatment of geriatric, debilitated and generally weak patients; the lowest therapeutic dose should be given initially and increased as needed. In these cases, it is best to combine this formula with an appropriate Spleen tonic to prevent gastrointestinal upset and to promote qi and blood production. The use of a Spleen tonic is particularly important, as many weak and geriatric animals are on long-term non-steroidal, anti-inflammatory drugs. Once the condition has stabilized and pain is under control, the formula should be discontinued and the maintenance formula re-instituted.

Ge Gen Tang can be used with *Cang Er Zi San* (Xanthium Powder) to treat chronic nasal discharge that is thick and yellow. For clear, watery nasal discharge combine with *Xin Yi San* (Magnolia Flower Powder).

References

1. *Zhong Yi Za Zhi* (Journal of Chinese Medicine), 1955; (10):36.
2. Kurokawa M, Tsurita M, Brown J, Fukuda Y, Shiraki K. Effect of interleukin-12 level augmented by Kakkon-to, a herbal medicine, on the early stage of influenza infection in mice. Antiviral Res. 2002 Nov; 56(2):183-8.
3. Kurokawa M, Kumeda CA, Yamamura J, Kamiyama T, Shiraki K. Antipyretic activity of cinnamyl derivatives and related compounds in influenza virus-infected mice. Eur J Pharmacol. 1998 May 1; 348(1):45-51.
4. Ozaki Y. Studies on antiinflammatory effect of Japanese Oriental medicines (kampo medicines) used to treat inflammatory diseases. Biol Pharm Bull. 1995 Apr; 18(4):559-62.
5. *Zhong Yao Yao Li Yu Ying Yong* (Pharmacology and Applications of Chinese Herbs), 1987; 4(4):33.
6. *Guo Wai Yi Xue* (Foreign Medicine), 1993; 15(3):23.
7. *Guo Wai Yi Xue* (Foreign Medicine), 1995; 17(3):64.
8. *Han Fang Yi Xue* (Kampo Medicine), 1985, 9(5):12.
9. *Yun Nan Zhong Yi Za Zhi* (Yunan Journal of Chinese Medicine), 1987; 8(2):35.
10. *Zhong Yi Fang Ji Xian Dai Yan Jiu* (Modern Study of Medical Formulas in Traditional Chinese Medicine), 1997; 63(6):2007.

Gě Gēn Tāng (Kudzu Decoction)

11. *Jiang Su Zhong Yi Za Zhi* (Jiangsu Journal of Chinese Medicine), 1963; (11):17.
12. *Fu Jian Zhong Yi Yao* (Fujian Chinese Medicine and Herbology), 1956; (2):13.
13. *Liao Ning Zhong Yi Za Zhi* (Liaoning Journal of Chinese Medicine), 1983; (6):34.
14. *Zhong Yi Han Shou Tong Xun* (Reports of Chinese Medicine), 1993; 3:42.
15. *Hu Bei Zhong Yi Za Zhi* (Hubei Journal of Chinese Medicine), 1995; 2:31.
16. *Zhong Yi Ming Fang Lin Chuang Xin Yong* (Contemporary Clinical Applications of Classic Chinese Formulas), 2001; 677.
17. *Hu Nan Zhong Yi Za Zhi* (Hunan Journal of Chinese Medicine), 1992; 1:43.
18. *Ji Lin Zhong Yi Yao* (Jilin Chinese Medicine and Herbology), 1995; 1:18.
19. Qi J, Toyoshima A, Honda Y, Mineshita S. Pharmacokinetic study on acetaminophen: interaction with a Chinese medicine. Journal of Medical & Dental Sciences. 1997 Mar.; 44(1):31-5.
20. *Guo Wai Yi Xue* (Foreign Medicine), 1993; 15(3):23.
21. *Guo Wai Yi Xue* (Foreign Medicine), 1989; 11(1):52.

Jiǔ Wèi Qiāng Huó Tāng (Nine-Herb Decoction with Notopterygium)

九味羌活湯
九味羌活汤

Pinyin Name: *Jiu Wei Qiang Huo Tang*
Literal Name: Nine-Herb Decoction with Notopterygium
Alternate Names: *Chiu Wei Qiang Huo Tang, Jiu Wei Chiang Huo Tang*, Nine-Flavour Chiang-hou Decoction, Notopterygium Decoction with Nine Herbs, Notopterigium Nine Herb Combination
Original Source: *Ci Shi Nan Zhi* (Hard-Won Knowledge) by Wang Hao-Gu in 1308

COMPOSITION

Qiang Huo (Rhizoma et Radix Notopterygii)	4.5g [6g]
Fang Feng (Radix Saposhnikoviae)	4.5g [6g]
Cang Zhu (Rhizoma Atractylodis)	4.5g [6g]
Xi Xin (Radix et Rhizoma Asari)	1.5g [2g]
Chuan Xiong (Rhizoma Chuanxiong)	3g
Bai Zhi (Radix Angelicae Dahuricae)	3g
Di Huang (Radix Rehmanniae)	3g
Huang Qin (Radix Scutellariae)	3g
Gan Cao (Radix et Rhizoma Glycyrrhizae)	3g

DOSAGE / PREPARATION / ADMINISTRATION

The source text states to grind the ingredients coarsely and cook the coarse powder in water to make a decoction. Today, this formula may be prepared as a decoction with the doses suggested in brackets. In addition, 3 slices of *Sheng Jiang* (Rhizoma Zingiberis Recens) and 3 stalks of *Cong Bai* (Bulbus Allii Fistulosi) can be added to enhance the effects of unblocking yang qi and releasing the exterior.

CHINESE THERAPEUTIC ACTIONS

1. Induces sweating and dispels dampness
2. Clears interior heat

CLINICAL MANIFESTATIONS

Wind, cold and dampness at the exterior and heat in the interior: aversion to cold, fever, neck pain and stiffness, soreness and pain of the body and limbs, a white tongue coating, and a superficial pulse.

VETERINARY CLINICAL APPLICATIONS

Arthritis, cervical and shoulder pain, intervertebral disk disease and spondylosis, whole body soreness and stiffness.

EXPLANATION

Jiu Wei Qiang Huo Tang (Nine-Herb Decoction with Notopterygium) treats wind, cold and dampness constricting

Jiǔ Wèi Qiāng Huó Tāng (Nine-Herb Decoction with Notopterygium)

Jiu Wei Qiang Huo Tang (Nine-Herb Decoction with Notopterygium)

Diagnosis	Clinical Signs	Treatment	Herbs
Exterior wind, cold and dampness, with interior heat	• Fever and aversion to cold: exterior wind-cold • Soreness and pain in the body and extremities: exterior wind-dampness causing qi and blood stagnation • White tongue coating and a superficial pulse: exterior condition • Thirst: interior heat	• Dispels exterior wind, cold and dampness • Clears interior heat	• *Qiang Huo* (Rhizoma et Radix Notopterygii) disperses wind, cold and dampness at the exterior. • *Fang Feng* (Radix Saposhnikoviae) dispels wind and cold. • *Cang Zhu* (Rhizoma Atractylodis) dries dampness. • *Xi Xin* (Radix et Rhizoma Asari), *Chuan Xiong* (Rhizoma Chuanxiong), and *Bai Zhi* (Radix Angelicae Dahuricae) dispel wind-cold factor, disperse dampness, and activate qi and blood flow. • *Di Huang* (Radix Rehmanniae) prevents the acrid and warm herbs from damaging body fluids. • *Huang Qin* (Radix Scutellariae) clears interior heat. • *Gan Cao* (Radix et Rhizoma Glycyrrhizae) harmonizes the herbs.

the exterior and heat forming in the interior. Aversion to cold and fever is caused by wind-cold constricting the pores and blocking the yang qi from reaching the *wei* (defensive) level. The wind, cold and dampness at the exterior block qi and blood circulation in the channels and collaterals, which results in neck pain and stiffness, body aches, and pain. Constriction at the exterior can lead to heat formation in the interior. The disease location is mainly at the exterior, as indicated by the white tongue coating and the superficial pulse. Treatment should thus focus primarily on releasing the exterior, and secondarily on clearing interior heat.

Acrid, aromatic and warm, *Qiang Huo* (Rhizoma et Radix Notopterygii) enters the *taiyang* channel and disperses wind, cold and dampness at the exterior. It releases wind-cold, dispels wind-dampness, benefits the joints, and relieves pain. *Fang Feng* (Radix Saposhnikoviae) helps dispel wind, and *Cang Zhu* (Rhizoma Atractylodis) dries dampness. *Xi Xin* (Radix et Rhizoma Asari), *Chuan Xiong* (Rhizoma Chuanxiong), and *Bai Zhi* (Radix Angelicae Dahuricae) dispel wind-cold factors, disperse dampness, activate qi and blood flow, and relieve neck pain, stiffness, and body aches. *Di Huang* (Radix Rehmanniae) prevents the acrid and warm herbs from damaging body fluids. *Huang Qin* (Radix Scutellariae) clears interior heat. *Gan Cao* (Radix et Rhizoma Glycyrrhizae) harmonizes the herbs.

VETERINARY MODIFICATIONS

- With clear or watery nasal discharge, add *Xin Yi San* (Magnolia Flower Powder).
- If accompanied by cough, add *Ku Xing Ren* (Semen Armeniacae Amarum) and *Zhi Sou San* (Stop Coughing Powder).
- If there is severe pain caused by more damp accumulation, increase the dose of *Qiang Huo* (Rhizoma et Radix Notopterygii) and *Cang Zhu* (Rhizoma Atractylodis).
- If the pain is moderate or mild because there is less damp accumulation, remove *Cang Zhu* (Rhizoma Atractylodis) and *Xi Xin* (Radix et Rhizoma Asari).
- If there is severe neck pain and stiffness, add *Yan Huo Suo* (Rhizoma Corydalis) and *Gao Ben* (Rhizoma et Radix Ligustici).
- For vomiting or thirst, add *Zhi Shi* (Fructus Aurantii Immaturus) and *Jie Geng* (Radix Platycodonis).
- To enhance the exterior-releasing functions, add *Cong Bai* (Bulbus Allii Fistulosi) and *Sheng Jiang* (Rhizoma Zingiberis Recens).

CAUTIONS / CONTRAINDICATIONS

- *Jiu Wei Qiang Huo Tang* contains many warm, acrid, and drying herbs. It should be used with caution in patients with yin, qi or body fluid deficiencies.
- This formula is contraindicated in patients with wind-heat, yin-deficient heat, or generalized weakness and deficiency with heat.

Jiǔ Wèi Qiāng Huó Tāng (Nine-Herb Decoction with Notopterygium)

PHARMACOLOGICAL EFFECTS

1. **Antipyretic**: Administration of *Jiu Wei Qiang Huo Tang* was effective in reducing body temperature in rabbits with artificially-induced fever. The antipyretic effects of the herbs started 2 hours after ingestion, and lasted for 6 hours. The reduction of body temperature was 0.7°C after 4 hours. The study also noted that the potency of the formula was similar to 0.2 mg/kg of aspirin.[1]
2. **Analgesic and anti-inflammatory**: One study reported that both water and alcohol extracts of *Jiu Wei Qiang Huo Tang* had marked analgesic and anti-inflammatory effects in mice.[2]

HUMAN CLINICAL STUDIES AND RESEARCH

Sciatica: Modified *Jiu Wei Qiang Huo Tang* was used to treat 38 patients with sciatica with an overall effectiveness rate of 94.7%.[3]

SUGGESTED ACUPUNCTURE TREATMENT

1. Points: *Fengchi* (GB 20), *Kongzui* (LU 6), *Hegu* (LI 4), *Zhigou* (TH 6), *Housanli* (ST 36), *Neiting* (ST 44), *Rangu* (KI 2). *Dashu* (BL 11), *Kunlun* (BL 60), and *Xuanzhong* (GB 39).
2. Technique: sedation.

Fengchi (GB 20), *Kongzui* (LU 6), and *Hegu* (LI 4) ventilate the Lung and dispel exterior wind, cold and dampness. *Zhigou* (TH 6) activates qi flow of the *San Jiao* channel to dissolve dampness. *Housanli* (ST 36) harmonizes the middle *jiao* and strengthens the Spleen to dispel dampness. *Neiting* (ST 44) sedates heat. *Rangu* (KI 2) cools heat in the blood. *Dashu* (BL 11), *Kunlun* (BL 60), and *Xuanzhong* (GB 39) are all helpful in treating cervical stiffness and general body aches.

AUTHORS' COMMENTS

Jiu Wei Qiang Huo Tang is a formula that can be used in all four seasons to treat conditions characterized by wind, cold and damp factors at the exterior, with heat in the interior. The main diagnostic clinical signs include fever, aversion to cold, muscle aches and pains, and slight thirst.

Jiu Wei Qiang Huo Tang is useful to treat dogs that are used for hunting or performance events and are exposed to wind, cold and dampness for prolonged periods of time. Many of these animals are fed dry food diets high in carbohydrates (grains such as corn, wheat and soybean) and already have pre-existing heat and/or dampness in the interior, which exterior constriction worsens. Similarly, many performance horses are fed diets high in concentrates and have limited time for grazing, both of which can lead to damp accumulation, stagnation, and interior heat development. When these animals are then body-clipped, which exacerbates the exposure factor, and subjected to the stresses of performance, the invasion of wind, cold and dampness easily follows. *Jiu Wei Qiang Huo Tang* is also useful in treating older animals of any species with arthritis, chronic injuries, cervical spondylosis or intervertebral disk disease, with aggravation of their disease during abrupt seasonal changes.

The difference between the use of *Jiu Wei Qiang Huo Tang* and *Ge Gen Tang* (Kudzu Decoction) is that *Ge Gen Tang* treats exterior-excess, wind-cold syndromes accompanied by stiffness and pain of the neck, while *Jiu Wei Qiang Huo Tang* dispels exterior wind, cold, and dampness and relieves muscle stiffness and pain throughout the whole body.

References

1. *Zhong Yao Tong Bao* (Journal of Chinese Herbology), 1986; 11(1):51.
2. *Zhong Cheng Yao* (Study of Chinese Patent Medicine), 1992; 14(2):25.
3. *Shang Hai Zhong Yi Yao Za Zhi* (Shanghai Journal of Chinese Medicine and Herbology), 1988; 7:23.

Xìng Sū Yǐn (Apricot Kernel and Perilla Leaf Decoction)

杏蘇飲
杏苏饮

Pinyin Name: *Xing Su Yin*
Literal Name: Apricot Kernel and Perilla Leaf Decoction
Alternate Names: *Er Ke Xing Su Yin* (Pediatric Apricot Kernel and Perilla Leaf Decoction), Apricot Seed and Perilla Pediatric Formula
Original Source: *Yi Zong Jin Jian* (Golden Mirror of the Medical Tradition) by Wu Qian in 1742

COMPOSITION

Zi Su Ye (Folium Perillae)	[3-6g]
Ku Xing Ren (Semen Armeniacae Amarum), *chao* (dry-fried)	[3-6g]
Mai Dong (Radix Ophiopogonis)	[3-6g]
Jie Geng (Radix Platycodonis)	[3-6g]
Ju Hong (Exocarpium Citri Reticulatae)	[1-3g]
Qian Hu (Radix Peucedani)	[3-6g]
Zhi Qiao (Fructus Citri Aurantii), *chao* (dry-fried) with bran	[3-6g]
Zhe Bei Mu (Bulbus Fritillariae Thunbergii)	[3-6g]
Huang Qin (Radix Scutellariae)	[3-6g]
Sang Bai Pi (Cortex Mori), *chao* (dry-fried)	[3-6g]
Gan Cao (Radix et Rhizoma Glycyrrhizae)	[1-3g]

DOSAGE / PREPARATION / ADMINISTRATION

The source text states to decoct the ingredients with *Sheng Jiang* (Rhizoma Zingiberis Recens). Note: The doses of herbs are unavailable from the source text. Suggested doses are listed above in brackets. Actual doses vary, depending on the condition and age of the patients.

CHINESE THERAPEUTIC ACTIONS

1. Dispels wind-cold
2. Ventilates the Lung and dissolves phlegm

CLINICAL MANIFESTATIONS

Wind-cold at the exterior: fever, aversion to cold, nausea, vomiting, drooling, sticky nasal discharge, sneezing, and cough.

VETERINARY CLINICAL APPLICATIONS

Upper respiratory tract infection in kittens, puppies and foals, as well as in debilitated and geriatric animals.

EXPLANATION

Xing Su Yin (Apricot Kernel and Perilla Leaf Decoction) is specifically designed to treat juvenile, geriatric and chronically debilitated animals who have wind-cold attacking the exterior. If wind travels to the upper parts of the body, animals may have neck pain and stiffness. If cold blocks the normal flow of qi, patients may experience aversion to cold, cough, nasal obstruction, and sneezing with gastrointestinal signs.

Zi Su Ye (Folium Perillae) warms the exterior and dispels wind-cold. *Ku Xing Ren* (Semen Armeniacae Amarum) redirects the reversed flow of Lung qi and relieves cough. *Mai Dong* (Radix Ophiopogonis) nourishes yin and fluids of the Lung and Stomach. *Jie Geng* (Radix Platycodonis), *Ju Hong* (Exocarpium Citri Rubrum), and *Qian Hu* (Radix Peucedani) ventilate Lung qi and relieve cough. *Zhi Qiao* (Fructus Aurantii), *Zhe Bei Mu* (Bulbus Fritillariae Thunbergii), and *Qian Hu* (Radix Peucedani) dissolve phlegm and eliminate stagnation. *Huang Qin* (Radix Scutellariae) and *Sang Bai Pi* (Cortex Mori) clear heat from the Lung and prevent the wind-cold condition from turning into Lung heat. *Gan Cao* (Radix et Rhizoma Glycyrrhizae) and *Sheng Jiang* (Rhizoma Zingiberis Recens) harmonize the formula and relieve nausea and vomiting.

VETERINARY MODIFICATIONS

- For exterior conditions caused by more wind-cold, add *Fang Feng* (Radix Saposhnikoviae) and *Jing Jie* (Herba Schizonepetae).
- When there is cough and dyspnea, add *Zi Su Zi* (Fructus Perillae) and *Ting Li Zi* (Semen Descurainiae seu Lepidii).
- For cough caused by wind-cold, add *Ding Chuan Tang* (Arrest Wheezing Decoction).
- For cough caused by phlegm, add *Er Chen Tang* (Two-Cured Decoction).

Xìng Sū Yǐn (Apricot Kernel and Perilla Leaf Decoction)

***Xing Su Yin* (Apricot Kernel and Perilla Leaf Decoction)**

Diagnosis	Clinical Signs	Treatment	Herbs
Wind-cold at the exterior	• Fever, aversion to cold, sticky nasal discharge, and sneezing: exterior wind-cold • Nausea and vomiting: wind-cold affecting Stomach qi flow • Coughing: wind-cold affecting Lung qi flow	• Dispels wind-cold • Ventilates the Lung and dissolves phlegm	• *Zi Su Ye* (Folium Perillae) warms the exterior and dispels wind-cold. • *Ku Xing Ren* (Semen Armeniacae Amarum) corrects the reversed flow of Lung qi and relieves cough. • *Mai Dong* (Radix Ophiopogonis) nourishes yin and fluids of the Lung and Stomach. • *Jie Geng* (Radix Platycodonis), *Ju Hong* (Exocarpium Citri Rubrum), and *Qian Hu* (Radix Peucedani) ventilate Lung qi and relieve cough. • *Zhi Qiao* (Fructus Aurantii), *Zhe Bei Mu* (Bulbus Fritillariae Thunbergii), and *Qian Hu* (Radix Peucedani) dissolve phlegm and eliminate stagnation. • *Huang Qin* (Radix Scutellariae) and *Sang Bai Pi* (Cortex Mori) clear heat from the Lung, and prevents the wind-cold condition from turning into Lung heat. • *Gan Cao* (Radix et Rhizoma Glycyrrhizae) and *Sheng Jiang* (Rhizoma Zingiberis Recens) harmonize the formula and relieve nausea and vomiting.

SUGGESTED ACUPUNCTURE TREATMENT

1. Points: *Lieque* (LU 7), *Hegu* (LI 4), *Fengchi* (GB 20), *Tianzhu* (BL 10), *Feishu* (BL 13), *Tiantu* (CV 22), and *Dingchuan.*
2. Technique: sedation

Lieque (LU 7) is the *Luo* connecting point and can disperse the Lung and clear wind-cold. *Fengchi* (GB 20) and *Hegu* (LI 4) ventilate the Lung and can enhance the ability of *Lieque* to expel pathogens. *Tianzhu* (BL 10) can clear wind-cold. *Tiantu* (CV 22) and *Dingchuan* can stop coughing.

AUTHORS' COMMENTS

Xing Su Yin is also known as *Er Ke Xing Su Yin* (Pediatric Apricot Kernel and Perilla Leaf Decoction). It is a gentle formula that safely treats exterior wind-cold condition in young patients because it transforms phlegm and diffuses the lung to relieve cough and contains herbs to moisten and protect Lung yin. Older animals and pets younger than one year of age are particularly susceptible to yin damage. In veterinary medicine this formula has found application in the treatment of kittens with upper respiratory disease that also exhibit gastrointestinal signs with lethargy, anorexia, drooling and vomiting. It can also be used in puppies with acute kennel cough, as well as geriatric and chronically debilitated animals due to its mild and safe nature. In foals and weanlings a common presentation for this formula is what is colloquially known as the "snots": sticky nasal discharge, and often accompanied by a cough, which is often very persistent. These cases are likely mild or early infections with rhinopneumonitis or various *Streptococcus* infections that have not developed into a more serious stage.

Xiǎo Qīng Lóng Tāng (Minor Bluegreen Dragon Decoction)

小青龍湯
小青龙汤

Pinyin Name: *Xiao Qing Long Tang*
Literal Name: Minor Bluegreen Dragon Decoction
Alternate Names: *Hsiao Ching Lung Tang, Xiao Ching Long Tang*, Minor Blue Dragon Decoction, Minor Blue Dragon Combination
Original Source: *Shang Han Lun* (Discussion of Cold-Induced Disorders) by Zhang Zhong-Jing in the Eastern Han Dynasty

COMPOSITION

Ma Huang (Herba Ephedrae)	9g
Gui Zhi (Ramulus Cinnamomi)	9g [6-9g]
Xi Xin (Radix et Rhizoma Asari)	9g [3-6g]
Gan Jiang (Rhizoma Zingiberis)	9g [3-6g]
Ban Xia (Rhizoma Pinelliae), *xi* (washed)	0.5 cup [9g]
Bai Shao (Radix Paeoniae Alba)	9g
Wu Wei Zi (Fructus Schisandrae Chinensis)	0.5 cup [3-6g]
Zhi Gan Cao (Radix et Rhizoma Glycyrrhizae Praeparata cum Melle)	9g [6g]

DOSAGE / PREPARATION / ADMINISTRATION

The source text instructions are to cook *Ma Huang* (Herba Ephedrae) with 10 cups [2,000 mL] of water until the liquid is reduced to 8 cups [1,600 mL]. Remove the foam from the top, add the other ingredients, and cook until the liquid is reduced to 3 cups [600 mL]. Take 1 cup [200 mL] of the warm, strained decoction. Today, the decoction may be prepared using the doses suggested in brackets.

CHINESE THERAPEUTIC ACTIONS

1. Releases the exterior and dispels *yin* (invisible phlegm)
2. Relieves wheezing and coughing

CLINICAL MANIFESTATIONS

Wind-cold at the exterior with water accumulation in the interior: aversion to cold and fever, absence of sweating, coughing and wheezing with profuse, clear, watery sputum, heaviness in movement and pain of the body, edema of the face and limbs, and a superficial pulse.

VETERINARY CLINICAL APPLICATIONS

Acute feline asthma, acute dyspnea from equine RAO (recurrent airway obstruction), acute allergic bronchitis, pneumonia, bronchiectasis, wheezing and dyspnea, forequarter and rear-quarter edema, cough and allergic rhinitis and sinusitis.

EXPLANATION

Xiao Qing Long Tang (Minor Bluegreen Dragon Decoction) treats conditions characterized by wind-cold invasion at the exterior and water accumulation in the interior. Individuals who have pre-existing water accumulation in the interior generally have Spleen and Lung qi deficiencies. After being attacked by wind-cold at the exterior, patients may experience dysfunctioning of the Lung and Spleen, causing more water retention, especially in the epigastrium and the chest. Water retention in the chest causes an inability to breathe properly when lying in a horizontal position.

Aversion to cold and fever are caused by the wind-cold factor at the exterior. Cough, dyspnea and wheezing are the result of reversed flow of Lung qi, which is secondary to wind-cold attack and phlegm accumulation. Profuse, watery sputum, heaviness and pain of the body, swollen face and extremities, and a white, slippery tongue coating all suggest water accumulation and the failure of the Lung to metabolize water. The superficial pulse indicates that the disease is located at the exterior.

In this syndrome, the exterior and the interior must be treated at the same time. If only exterior herbs are used, the interior water accumulation remains. If only water-regulating herbs are used to address the water accumulation, the exterior condition remains untreated, and there may be further complications as the pathogenic factors move inward.

Ma Huang (Herba Ephedrae) and *Gui Zhi* (Ramulus Cinnamomi), the chief herbs, dispel exterior wind-cold factor through diaphoresis. *Ma Huang* (Herba Ephedrae)

Xiǎo Qīng Lóng Tāng (Minor Bluegreen Dragon Decoction)

Xiao Qing Long Tang (Minor Bluegreen Dragon Decoction)

Diagnosis	Clinical Signs	Treatment	Herbs
Exterior wind-cold, interior water accumulation	• Fever, aversion: exterior-excess wind-cold condition • Profuse, clear, watery sputum and edema of the face and limbs: water accumulation • Coughing, dyspnea and wheezing: reversed flow of Lung qi • Heaviness and pain of the body: damp and phlegm accumulation	• Relieves exterior wind-cold • Dispels water accumulation and phlegm • Relieves wheezing and coughing	• *Ma Huang* (Herba Ephedrae) and *Gui Zhi* (Ramulus Cinnamomi) dispel the exterior wind-cold. • *Xi Xin* (Radix et Rhizoma Asari) releases wind-cold from the exterior and warms the Lung in the interior. • *Gan Jiang* (Rhizoma Zingiberis) warms the middle *jiao* to dispel cold. • *Ban Xia* (Rhizoma Pinelliae) eliminates phlegm, directs Stomach qi downward, and harmonizes the middle *jiao*. • *Bai Shao* (Radix Paeoniae Alba) and *Wu Wei Zi* (Fructus Schisandrae Chinensis) prevent the acrid and warm herbs from damaging qi, yin, and body fluids. • *Zhi Gan Cao* (Radix et Rhizoma Glycyrrhizae Praeparata cum Melle) tonifies qi and harmonizes the herbs.

also smoothes Lung qi flow to relieve cough, dyspnea, and wheezing. *Gui Zhi* (Ramulus Cinnamomi) warms the yang and eliminates cold. *Xi Xin* (Radix et Rhizoma Asari), acrid and hot, enters the *shaoyin* channel and warms the Lung to resolve phlegm accumulation. It also assists *Ma Huang* (Herba Ephedrae) and *Gui Zhi* (Ramulus Cinnamomi) in releasing the exterior. *Gan Jiang* (Rhizoma Zingiberis) enters the *yangming* channel to warm the yang of the middle *jiao* to dispel cold. *Ban Xia* (Rhizoma Pinelliae) eliminates phlegm, directs Stomach qi downward, and harmonizes the middle *jiao*.

If only arid and warm herbs are used in this syndrome, however, the Lung qi may become dispersed or lost, and yin may be injured. For this reason, *Wu Wei Zi* (Fructus Schisandrae Chinensis) is added to contain and prevent the leakage of Lung qi. *Bai Shao* (Radix Paeoniae Alba) nourishes yin, tonifies the blood, and prevents the acrid herbs from drying up body fluids. Both *Wu Wei Zi* (Fructus Schisandrae Chinensis) and *Bai Shao* (Radix Paeoniae Alba) are used only in small doses, as large doses might interfere with the exterior-releasing effect. *Zhi Gan Cao* (Radix et Rhizoma Glycyrrhizae Praeparata cum Melle) supplements qi and harmonizes the exterior-releasing and astringent herbs in this formula.

VETERINARY MODIFICATIONS

- With cough and dyspnea, add *Ku Xing Ren* (Semen Armeniacae Amarum) and *Hou Po* (Cortex Magnoliae Officinalis).
- With fever, add *Jie Geng* (Radix Platycodonis) and *Shi Gao* (Gypsum Fibrosum).
- With more heat, add *Shi Gao* (Gypsum Fibrosum).
- With thirst as a result of Lung heat, add *Shi Gao* (Gypsum Fibrosum) and *Huang Qin* (Radix Scutellariae).
- If the exterior clinical signs are not severe, remove *Gui Zhi* (Ramulus Cinnamomi) and use honey-fried *Ma Huang* (Herba Ephedrae) instead.

CAUTIONS / CONTRAINDICATIONS

- *Xiao Qing Long Tang* should not be taken for a prolonged period of time. It should be discontinued when the desired effects have been achieved.
- This formula is contraindicated in the following situations: heat condition with a sore throat or a rapid pulse; wind-heat or beginning stages of *wen bing* (warm diseases); yin deficiency with dry cough or thirst; phlegm-heat conditions with thick, yellow sputum; cough with streaks of blood in the sputum; and cough with thick, yellow sputum, thirst, a red tongue with yellow tongue coating, and a rapid pulse.
- Because this is a relatively strong formula, caution must be used when prescribing this formula. *Xi Xin* (Radix et Rhizoma Asari) must be prescribed carefully because it

is potentially toxic at a high dose. *Wu Wei Zi* (Fructus Schisandrae Chinensis) must not be used at a large dose to avoid retaining the pathogenic factors inside the body with its astringent effect.

- Rare cases of gastrointestinal discomfort (nausea, vomiting, and diarrhea) and skin itching have been linked to *Xiao Qing Long Tang*. These reactions were self-limiting and resolved upon the discontinuation of the formula.[1]
- Use of *Xiao Qing Long Tang* has been associated with only a few side effects, such as dry mouth, sedation and drowsiness, due mainly to the blockage of histamine H1 and muscarinic receptors in the salivary glands and the brain.[2,3]

PHARMACOLOGICAL EFFECTS

1. **Antiasthmatic**: *Xiao Qing Long Tang* has marked antiasthmatic effects, and has been used for centuries to treat bronchial asthma. There are two proposed mechanisms of the antiasthmatic effects. One, it stimulates the beta2-adrenoceptors to produce bronchorelaxation. Two, it inhibits the infiltration of eosinophils into the airway. Thus, *Xiao Qing Long Tang* is useful for both prevention and treatment of asthma.[4,5]
2. **Antiallergic**: One study reported that *Xiao Qing Long Tang* has antiallergic effects and may be useful and reasonable for controlling allergic diseases including bronchial asthma, allergic asthma and allergic rhinitis.[6] One demonstrated mechanism of the antiallergic effects was the inhibitory activity on histamine release and suppression of Th2 differentiation at the stage of antigen-presenting cells (APCs)-CD4(+)T cell interaction.[7] Another demonstrated mechanism is the inhibition of mast cell activities.[8] Lastly, it has been shown to control the allergen-induced inflammatory process by substantially inhibiting the allergen-induced synthesis of TNF-alpha.[9]
3. **Antiviral**: One study found *Xiao Qing Long Tang* to be useful for both prophylaxis and treatment of influenza virus infection in patients with allergic pulmonary inflammation, such as bronchial asthma. The mechanism of this action was attributed to the effects of the formula to augment the antiviral IgA antibody titer in the nasal and broncho-alveolar cavities, activate T-cells in Peyer's patch lymphocytic tissue, and stimulate the production of anti-influenza virus IgA antibody by nasal lymphocytes.[10] *Xiao Qing Long Tang*, however, has not shown direct action against the virus.[11] Clinically, *Xiao Qing Long Tang* can be used to prevent influenza virus infection by cross-protection of subtypes of influenza A virus and B virus. It is also useful for the treatment of influenza virus infection in elderly patients and individuals with a history of influenza virus infection, influenza vaccination, and allergic pulmonary inflammation.[12,13]
4. **Immunomodulatory**: Administration of *Xiao Qing Long Tang* has immunomodulatory effects in reducing bronchial inflammation in allergen-sensitized mice. *Xiao Qing Long Tang* suppressed airway inflammation by decreasing the number of total cells and eosinophil infiltration in the bronchoalveolar lavage fluid, and down-regulated the allergen- or mitogen-induced intrapulmonary lymphocyte response of sensitized mice as compared to those of controls.[14]
5. **Sympathomimetic**: Administration of *Xiao Qing Long Tang* was associated with increased respiratory rate, heart rate, blood pressure, systolic pressure, diastolic pressure, and decreased blood flow in dogs at all doses of 0.5, 1 and 2 g/kg via duodenal administration.[15]

HUMAN CLINICAL STUDIES AND RESEARCH

1. **Pulmonary disorders**: In a clinical study, 258 patients between 6 to 67 years of age with various pulmonary disorders for over one month characterized by cough and dyspnea were examined and treated. According to western diagnosis, 120 patients had acute pneumonia, 68 had chronic pneumonia, 60 had acute asthma, 4 had pulmonary emphysema, 4 had pleurisy, 1 had pulmonary tuberculosis and 1 had pulmonary carcinoma. Patients with the first four diagnoses were treated with herbs only, while those with the last three diagnoses were treated with both herbs and drugs. The herbal treatment was based on *Xiao Qing Long Tang*, with minor modifications when necessary. The study reported significant improvement to complete recovery within 4-6 doses in all patients except ones with tuberculosis and carcinoma.[16]
2. **Bronchitis**: Use of modified *Xiao Qing Long Tang* was effective in treating bronchitis. Of 51 patients, the study reported significant improvement in 27 cases, moderate improvement in 15 cases, and no benefit in 1 case.[17]
3. **Bronchitis in children**: Modified *Xiao Qing Long Tang* demonstrated a 96% rate of effectiveness in treating bronchitis in children. The herbal treatment contained *Xiao Qing Long Tang* plus *Chuan Bei Mu* (Bulbus Fritillariae Cirrhosae), *Jie Geng* (Radix Platycodonis), *Zi Wan* (Radix et Rhizoma Asteris) and others as the base formula. Modifications were made as follows: *Jin Yin Hua* (Flos Lonicerae Japonicae), *Zhi Zi* (Fructus Gardeniae) and *Shi Gao* (Gypsum Fibrosum) were added for heat; *Jing Jie* (Herba Schizonepetae) and *Bai Qian* (Rhizoma et Radix Cynanchi Stauntonii) were added for wind-cold; *Ku Xing Ren* (Semen Armeniacae Amarum), *Niu Bang Zi* (Fructus Arctii) and *Xuan Shen* (Radix Scrophulariae) were added for repetitive cough with a hoarse voice; and *Cang Zhu* (Rhizoma Atractylodis) and *Huo Xiang* (Herba Agastaches) were added for profuse dampness and phlegm. Of 65

Xiǎo Qīng Lóng Tāng (Minor Bluegreen Dragon Decoction)

patients, the study reported complete recovery in 57 cases, improvement in 6 cases, and no benefit in 2 cases.[18]

4. **Pneumonia**: Use of modified *Xiao Qing Long Tang* effectively treated 72 of 89 patients with pneumonia within 2 weeks. Seventeen patients who did not respond were then treated with concurrent herb and drug therapy. The herbal treatment contained *Xiao Qing Long Tang* plus *Yu Xing Cao* (Herba Houttuyniae), *Huang Qin* (Radix Scutellariae) and *Ku Xing Ren* (Semen Armeniacae Amarum) as the base formula. For presence of sticky cold phlegm, *Bai Jie Zi* (Semen Sinapis), *Zi Su Zi* (Fructus Perillae) and *Xuan Fu Hua* (Flos Inulae) were added, and *Huang Qin* (Radix Scutellariae) and *Bai Shao* (Radix Paeoniae Alba) were removed. For accumulation of hot phlegm in the Lung, *Shi Gao* (Gypsum Fibrosum) and *Chuan Bei Mu* (Bulbus Fritillariae Cirrhosae) were added, and *Gan Jiang* (Rhizoma Zingiberis), *Gui Zhi* (Ramulus Cinnamomi) and *Xi Xin* (Radix et Rhizoma Asari) were removed. For generalized deficiency and weakness, *Ren Shen* (Radix et Rhizoma Ginseng), *Bai Zhu* (Rhizoma Atractylodis Macrocephalae), *Dang Gui* (Radix Angelicae Sinensis) and *Shu Di Huang* (Radix Rehmanniae Praeparata) were added, and *Huang Qin* (Radix Scutellariae) and *Ma Huang* (Herba Ephedrae) were removed.[19]
5. **Wheezing and dyspnea**: *Xiao Qing Long Tang* has been shown in many studies to effectively treat wheezing and dyspnea. One study reported 86.7% effectiveness using this formula in liquid form three times daily for 1-3 weeks to treat 30 patients with bronchial asthma.[20] Another study with 39 patients noted that *Xiao Qing Long Tang* was effective for both acute and chronic bronchial asthma.[21] Lastly, in one study of pediatric patients with bronchial asthma, the use of modified *Xiao Qing Long Tang* was associated with 64.5% rate of effectiveness.[22]
6. **Cough**: Sixty patients with cough characterized by wind-cold were treated with modified *Xiao Qing Long Tang* with marked success within 3-6 packs of herbs. The herbal treatment included *Xiao Qing Long Tang* plus *Sha Shen* (Radix Glehniae seu Adenophorae), *Zi Wan* (Radix et Rhizoma Asteris) and others as deemed necessary. *Zhi Mu* (Rhizoma Anemarrhenae) was added for fever. *Huang Qi* (Radix Astragali) was added for qi deficiency with profuse sweating. Lower doses of *Xi Xin* (Radix et Rhizoma Asari) and *Gan Jiang* (Rhizoma Zingiberis), and addition of *Shi Gao* (Gypsum Fibrosum) and *Huang Qin* (Radix Scutellariae), were used for presence of scanty, thick, yellow sputum.[23]
7. **Rhinitis**: Fifty-three patients with a past history of rhinitis between 2 weeks to 12 years were treated with *Xiao Qing Long Tang*. Clinical presentation included sneezing, itching and irritation of the nose, and profuse, clear and watery nasal discharge. The study reported an overall rate of effectiveness of 94.3%, with complete recovery in 26 cases, moderate improvement in 24 cases, and no benefit in 3 cases.[24]
8. **Allergic rhinitis**: *Xiao Qing Long Tang* plus *Chai Hu* (Radix Bupleuri) was used to treat 386 patients with allergic rhinitis with marked effectiveness in 164 cases, moderate effect in 177 cases, and no effect in 45 cases. The overall rate of effectiveness was 88.3%.[25]

HERB-DRUG INTERACTION

- **Fluticasone**: Forty-two asthma patients were divided into three groups: one group treated with *Xiao Qing Long Tang*, one group treated with fluticasone inhalation, and one group treated with both. The study reported that concurrent administration of fluticasone and *Xiao Qing Long Tang* was associated with superior results based on pulmonary function and serum interleukin (IL)-16 levels, in comparison with the other two groups. The study concluded that the combination (of inhaled fluticasone and oral *Xiao Qing Long Tang*) could become an important therapeutical method in treating mild and severe asthma patients.[26]
- **Carbamazepine**: One study evaluated the potential herb-drug interaction between *Xiao Qing Long Tang* and carbamazepine in rats. With simultaneous oral administration, *Xiao Qing Long Tang* delayed the oral absorption of carbamazepine, but did not influence the peak plasma concentration, area under the plasma concentration-time curve, or terminal elimination half-life (T½). With 1-week pre-treatment with *Xiao Qing Long Tang*, the Tmax and the elimination rate constant for carbamazepine were significantly increased, but the protein binding was not affected.[27]

SUGGESTED ACUPUNCTURE TREATMENT

1. Points: *Pianli* (LI 6), *Hegu* (LI 4), *Feishu* (BL 13), *Lieque* (LU 7), *Jingqu* (LU 8), *Sanjiaoshu* (BL 22), and *Yinlingquan* (SP 9). Classical: *Feishu* (equine), *Dingchuan*, *Bitong* (canine)
2. Technique: sedation.

Pianli (LI 6) is the *luo* (connecting) point of the hand *yangming* channel, connecting with the hand *taiyin* channel. Therefore, *Pianli* (LI 6) is used with *Hegu* (LI 4) and *Feishu* (BL 13) to ventilate the Lung and release the exterior. *Lieque* (LU 7) and *Jingqu* (LU 8) relieve coughing and wheezing. *Sanjiaoshu* (BL 22) regulates the water pathways, and *Yinlingquan* (SP 9) eliminates water retention to strengthen the Spleen.

Feishu (equine), which, it should be noted, does not correspond to the transpositional point of *Feishu* (BL 13),

Xiǎo Qīng Lóng Tāng (Minor Bluegreen Dragon Decoction)

supports the Lung in the equine patient. *Dingchuan* helps to relieve cough, and *Bitong* relieves sinus congestion in the dog.

AUTHORS' COMMENTS

Xiao Qing Long Tang in veterinary medicine can be used to treat acute cases of feline asthma or exacerbation of chronic cases, canine allergic bronchitis and acute rhinitis-sinusitis associated with wind-cold. It has extremely strong dispersing and warming effects. Thus, accurate diagnosis is necessary before prescribing this formula. Chief diagnostic signs for selecting this formula include profuse, clear or white nasal discharge or sputum with aversion to cold, dyspnea, wheezing or cough, and a white tongue coating. There should be no clinical signs of heat. It should not be used for a prolonged period of time, since the warm herbs may change the condition from cold to heat. Animals should also be monitored closely as exterior wind-cold condition can turn into wind-heat condition rather quickly. As soon as signs of heat are evident, immediately stop the use of the formula and select a more appropriate formula. Cats as a species are especially sensitive to the effects of *Ma Huang* (Herba Ephedrae). Treatment should begin using the lowest therapeutic dose and increased as needed with close monitoring to avoid adverse effects. In the treatment of feline asthma, this formula is chosen for acute onset of wheezing and/or cough with copious clear or foamy phlegm. In acute onset of asthmatic breathing in the dog or cat it is necessary to use formulas containing *Ma Huang* (Herba Ephedrae) in order to adequately ventilate the Lung to control the clinical signs and prevent hospitalization. For cats with chronic asthma and dogs with chronic bronchitis that have Lung yin-deficiency heat and chronic cough and experience an acute asthma attack due to wind-cold, combine with *Ren Shen Ge Jie San* (Ginseng and Gecko Powder). This can occur as a result of abrupt seasonal change.

Equine RAO (recurrent airway obstruction) is a common cause of dyspnea, wheezing, and coughing in the horse. It should be noted that equine RAO cases typically fall into categories of deficiency encompassing the Lung and Kidney, and that long-term treatment will be focused on correcting these imbalances. *Xiao Qing Long Tang,* then, is used for acute exacerbations of clinical signs brought on by wind-cold invasion (e.g. abrupt weather change, viral infection) and discontinued once clinical signs resolve. Concurrent administration of formulas such as *Bai He Gu Jin Tang* (Lily Bulb Decoction to Preserve the Metal) or *Ren Shen Ge Jie San* (Ginseng and Gecko Powder) is recommended. More commonly, this formula is administered to horses with bronchitis and a wet, deep-seated cough. These patients also often have significant limb edema, which, if not resolved with the base formula, may resolve with the addition of *Fu Ling* (Poria) or combination with *Wu Ling San* (Five-Ingredient Powder with Poria). The stool should be monitored in these cases for dryness, and a mild laxative such as psyllium may be added to the feed if impaction is a concern.

References

1. *Zhong Yao Ming Fang Yao Li Yu Ying Yong* (Pharmacology and Applications of Famous Herbal Formulas), 1989; 44-45.
2. Sakaguchi M, Mase A, Iizuka A, Yuzurihara M, Ishige A, Amagaya S, Komatsu Y, Takeda H, Matsumiya T. Further pharmacological study on Sho-seiryu-to as an antiallergic. Methods Find Exp Clin Pharmacol. 1997 Dec;19(10):707-13.
3. Sakaguchi M, Iizuka A, Yuzurihara M, Ishige A, Komatsu Y, Matsumiya T, Takeda H. Pharmacological characteristics of Sho-seiryu-to, an antiallergic Kampo medicine without effects on histamine H1 receptors and muscarinic cholinergic system in the brain. Methods Find Exp Clin Pharmacol. 1996 Jan-Feb;18(1):41-7.
4. Kao ST, Lin CS, Hsieh CC, Hsieh WT, Lin JG. Effects of xiao-qing-long-tang (XQLT) on bronchoconstriction and airway eosinophil infiltration in ovalbumin-sensitized guinea pigs: in vivo and in vitro studies. Allergy. 2001 Dec; 56(12):1164-71.
5. *Zhong Yi Fang Ji Xian Dai Yan Jiu* (Modern Study of Medical Formulas in Traditional Chinese Medicine), 1997; (1):62.
6. Tanno Y, Shindoh Y, Takishima T. Modulation of human basophil growth in vitro by xiao-qing-long-tang (syo-seiryu-to), chai-pu-tang (saiboku-to), qing-fei-tang (seihai-to), baicalein and ketotifen. American Journal of Chinese Medicine. 1989; 17(1-2):45-50.
7. Ikeda Y, Kaneko A, Yamamoto M, Ishige A, Sasaki H. Possible involvement of suppression of Th2 differentiation in the antiallergic effect of Sho-seiryu-to in mice. Jpn J Pharmacol. 2002 Dec; 90(4):328-36.
8. Sakaguchi M, Mase A, Iizuka A, Yuzurihara M, Ishige A, Amagaya S, Komatsu Y, Takeda H, Matsumiya T. Further pharmacological study on Sho-seiryu-to as an antiallergic. Methods Find Exp Clin Pharmacol. 1997 Dec; 19(10):707-13.
9. Tanaka A, Ohashi Y, Kakinoki Y, Washio Y, Yamada K, Nakai Y, Nakano T, Nakai Y, Ohmoto Y. The herbal medicine shoseiryu-to inhibits allergen-induced synthesis of tumour necrosis factor alpha by peripheral blood mononuclear cells in patients with perennial allergic rhinitis. Acta Otolaryngol Suppl. 1998;538:118-25.
10. Nagai T, Yamada H. In vivo anti-influenza virus activity of kampo (Japanese herbal) medicine "sho-seiryu-to" and its mode of action. Int. J. Immunopharmacol. 1994, 16, 605-613.
11. Nagai T, Yamada H. In vivo anti-influenza virus activity of Kampo (Japanese herbal) medicine "sho-seiryu-to"--stimulation of mucosal immune system and effect on allergic pulmonary inflammation model mice. Immunopharmacol Immunotoxicol. 1998 May;20(2):267-81.
12. Yamada H, Nagai T. In vivo antiinfluenza virus activity of Kampo medicine Sho-seiryu-to through mucosal immune system. Methods Find Exp Clin Pharmacol. 1998 Apr;20(3):185-92.
13. Nagai T, Urata M, Yamada H. In vivo anti-influenza virus activity of Kampo (Japanese herbal) medicine "Sho-seiryu-to"--effects on aged mice, against subtypes of a viruses and B virus, and therapeutic effect. Immunopharmacol Immunotoxicol. 1996 May;18(2):193-208.
14. Kao ST, Wang SD, Wang JY, Yu CK, Lei HY. The effect of Chinese herbal medicine, xiao-qing-long tang (XQLT), on allergen-induced bronchial inflammation in mite-sensitized mice. Allergy. 2000 Dec;55(12):1127-33.

Xiǎo Qīng Lóng Tāng (Minor Bluegreen Dragon Decoction)

15. Amagaya S, Iizuka A, Makino B, Kubo M, Komatsu Y, Cheng FC, Ruo TI, Itoh T, Terasawa K. General pharmacological properties of Sho-seiryu-to (TJ-19) extracts. Phytomedicine. 2001 Sep;8(5):338-47.
16. *Shan Dong Zhong Yi Za Zhi* (Shandong Journal of Chinese Medicine), 1994; 13(8):342.
17. *Si Chuan Zhong Yi* (Sichuan Chinese Medicine), 1986; 12:15.
18. *Shan Xi Zhong Yi* (Shanxi Chinese Medicine), 1997; 4:174.
19. *He Bei Zhong Yi* (Hebei Chinese Medicine), 1998; 2:114.
20. *Shang Hai Zhong Yi Yao Za Zhi* (Shanghai Journal of Chinese Medicine and Herbology), 1993; 9:25.
21. *Shan Dong Zhong Yi Xue Yuan Xue Bao* (Journal of Shandong University School of Chinese Medicine), 1992; 1:43.
22. *Guo Wai Yi Xue Zhong Yi Zhong Yao Fen Ce* (Monograph of Chinese Herbology from Foreign Medicine), 1979; 1:33.
23. *He Bei Zhong Yi* (Hebei Chinese Medicine), 1999; 2:16.
24. *Nan Jing Zhong Yi Yao Da Xue Xue Bao* (Journal of Nanjing University of Traditional Chinese Medicine and Medicinals), 1995, (4):14.
25. *Xin Jiang Zhong Yi Yao* (Xinjiang Chinese Medicine and Herbology), 1996; 4:20.
26. Zhang X, Wang L, Shi Q. Effect of fluticasone inhalation combined with xiaoqinglong decoction on pulmonary function and serum interleukin-16 level in asthma patients. Zhongguo Zhong Xi Yi Jie He Za Zhi. 2003 Jun; 23(6):426-9.
27. Ohnishi N, Yonekawa Y, Nakasako S, Nagasawa K, Yokoyama T, Yoshioka M, Kuroda K. Studies on interactions between traditional herbal and Western medicines. I. Effects of Sho-seiryu-to on the pharmacokinetics of carbamazepine in rats. Biol Pharm Bull. 1999 May; 22(5):527-31.

Shè Gān Má Huáng Tāng (Belamcanda and Ephedra Decoction)

射幹麻黃湯
射干麻黄汤

Pinyin Name: *She Gan Ma Huang Tang*
Literal Name: Belamcanda and Ephedra Decoction
Alternate Name: Belamcanda and Mahuang Combination
Original Source: *Jin Gui Yao Lue* (Essentials from the Golden Cabinet) by Zhang Zhong-Jing in the Eastern Han Dynasty

COMPOSITION

Ma Huang (Herba Ephedrae)	12g [9g]
She Gan (Rhizoma Belamcandae)	9g [6-g]
Sheng Jiang (Rhizoma Zingiberis Recens)	12g [9g]
Xi Xin (Radix et Rhizoma Asari)	9g [3g]
Zi Wan (Radix et Rhizoma Asteris)	9g [6g]
Kuan Dong Hua (Flos Farfarae)	9g [6g]
Ban Xia (Rhizoma Pinelliae)	0.5 cup [9g]
Wu Wei Zi (Fructus Schisandrae Chinensis)	0.5 cup [3g]
Da Zao (Fructus Jujubae)	7 pieces [3 pieces]

DOSAGE / PREPARATION / ADMINISTRATION

The source text states to cook *Ma Huang* (Herba Ephedrae) with 12 cups [2,400 mL] of water and bring to a boil twice. Remove the foam from the top, add the other ingredients, and cook until the liquid is reduced to 3 cups [600 mL]. Take the warm, strained decoction in three equally-divided doses daily. Today, the decoction may be prepared using the doses suggested in brackets.

CHINESE THERAPEUTIC ACTIONS

1. Ventilates the Lung and dispels phlegm
2. Directs Lung qi downward and stops coughing

CLINICAL MANIFESTATIONS

Tan yin (phlegm retention) with reversed flow of Lung qi: excessive coughing, wheezing, dyspnea, profuse clear, watery sputum, rattling sounds in the throat, heaviness and pain of the body, swollen face and extremities, and may have a white, slippery tongue coating.

VETERINARY CLINICAL APPLICATIONS

Cough, acute feline asthma, acute exacerbation of equine RAO (recurrent airway obstruction), bronchitis and bronchiectasis.

Shè Gān Má Huáng Tāng (Belamcanda and Ephedra Decoction)

***She Gan Ma Huang Tang* (Belamcanda and Ephedra Decoction)**

Diagnosis	Clinical Signs	Treatment	Herbs
Tan yin (phlegm retention) with reversed flow of Lung qi	• Profuse, clear, watery sputum and rattling sounds in the throat: *tan yin* (phlegm retention) • Severe coughing and dyspnea: phlegm accumulation blocking Lung qi circulation • White, slippery tongue coating: water accumulation	• Ventilates the Lung and dispels phlegm • Redirects Lung qi downward and stops coughing	• *Ma Huang* (Herba Ephedrae) ventilates the Lung and relieves dyspnea. • *She Gan* (Rhizoma Belamcandae) dispels *tan yin* (phlegm retention). • *Sheng Jiang* (Rhizoma Zingiberis Recens), *Xi Xin* (Radix et Rhizoma Asari), *Zi Wan* (Radix et Rhizoma Asteris), *Kuan Dong Hua* (Flos Farfarae), and *Ban Xia* (Rhizoma Pinelliae) dissolve phlegm, clear the throat, and direct the rising qi downward. • *Wu Wei Zi* (Fructus Schisandrae Chinensis) contains the leakage of Lung qi and stops coughing. • *Da Zao* (Fructus Jujubae) harmonizes the middle *jiao*.

EXPLANATION

She Gan Ma Huang Tang (Belamcanda and Ephedra Decoction) is a modification of *Xiao Qing Long Tang* (Minor Bluegreen Dragon Decoction). It treats *tan yin* (phlegm retention) with reversed flow of Lung qi, and is suitable for conditions characterized by severe phlegm and water retention. Clinically, the cough and sputum are more severe in this case than that found in *Xiao Qing Long Tang* (Minor Bluegreen Dragon Decoction).

Ma Huang (Herba Ephedrae) ventilates the Lung and relieves dyspnea. *She Gan* (Rhizoma Belamcandae) dispels *tan yin* (phlegm retention). *Sheng Jiang* (Rhizoma Zingiberis Recens), *Xi Xin* (Radix et Rhizoma Asari), *Zi Wan* (Radix et Rhizoma Asteris), *Kuan Dong Hua* (Flos Farfarae), and *Ban Xia* (Rhizoma Pinelliae) dissolve phlegm, clear the throat, and redirect the rising qi. *Wu Wei Zi* (Fructus Schisandrae Chinensis) contains the leakage of Lung qi and stops coughing. *Da Zao* (Fructus Jujubae) harmonizes the middle *jiao*.

She Gan Ma Huang Tang is modified from *Xiao Qing Long Tang* (Minor Bluegreen Dragon Decoction), with the removal of *Gui Zhi* (Ramulus Cinnamomi), *Bai Shao* (Radix Paeoniae Alba), and *Gan Cao* (Radix et Rhizoma Glycyrrhizae), and the addition of *She Gan* (Rhizoma Belamcandae), *Zi Wan* (Radix et Rhizoma Asteris), *Kuan Dong Hua* (Flos Farfarae), and *Da Zao* (Fructus Jujubae). These additional herbs enable *She Gan Ma Huang Tang* to strongly dispel phlegm and direct Lung qi downward to treat cough and dyspnea.

VETERINARY MODIFICATIONS

- For Lung heat from respiratory tract infection, add *Yu Xing Cao* (Herba Houttuyniae), *Jin Yin Hua* (Flos Lonicerae Japonicae), *Lian Qiao* (Fructus Forsythiae), and *Huang Qin* (Radix Scutellariae).
- If there is high fever, add *Shi Gao* (Gypsum Fibrosum) and *Geng Mi* (Semen Oryzae).
- When there is profuse sputum, add *Gua Lou Pi* (Pericarpium Trichosanthis).

PHARMACOLOGICAL EFFECTS

1. **Antitussive**: Administration of a *She Gan Ma Huang Tang* preparation at 0.4 mL/10g was associated with marked antitussive effects in mice with artificially-induced cough.[1]
2. **Expectorant**: Administration of *She Gan Ma Huang Tang* in mice was associated with marked expectorant effects at high doses, but not at low doses.[2]
3. **Antiasthmatic**: Administration of *She Gan Ma Huang Tang* has been shown to have a relaxant effect on the bronchial smooth muscle to relieve wheezing and dyspnea.[3]

HUMAN CLINICAL STUDIES AND RESEARCH

1. **Bronchitis**: Use of modified *She Gan Ma Huang Tang* was associated with 90.75% effectiveness in treating bronchitis. The herbal treatment used *She Gan Ma Huang Tang* as the base formula, and added *Wu Gong* (Scolopendra) for spastic cough; *Shi Gao* (Gypsum Fibrosum) and *Huang Qin* (Radix Scutellariae) for fever; and *Che Qian Zi* (Semen Plantaginis) for diarrhea.[4]
2. **Bronchitis in children**: Use of modified *She Gan Ma Huang Tang* was associated with 94.7% effectiveness in

Shè Gān Má Huáng Tāng (Belamcanda and Ephedra Decoction)

treating dyspnea and bronchitis in 38 children. *She Gan Ma Huang Tang* was modified as follows: for the presence of excess heat, *Huang Qin* (Radix Scutellariae), *Yu Xing Cao* (Herba Houttuyniae), and *Shi Gao* (Gypsum Fibrosum) were added, and *Wu Wei Zi* (Fructus Schisandrae Chinensis), *Xi Xin* (Radix et Rhizoma Asari), and *Ban Xia* (Rhizoma Pinelliae) were removed; for dry cough without sputum, *Mai Dong* (Radix Ophiopogonis), *Pi Pa Ye* (Folium Eriobotryae), and *Bai Bu* (Radix Stemonae) were added; for cough with clear, watery sputum, *Zi Su Zi* (Fructus Perillae) and *Ku Xing Ren* (Semen Armeniacae Amarum) were added; for sticky, yellow sputum, *Gua Lou Pi* (Pericarpium Trichosanthis) and *Tian Zhu Huang* (Concretio Silicea Bambusae) were added, and *Xi Xin* (Radix et Rhizoma Asari), *Sheng Jiang* (Rhizoma Zingiberis Recens), and *Da Zao* (Fructus Jujubae) were removed; for wheezing with chest congestion, *Bai Jie Zi* (Semen Sinapis), *Zi Su Zi* (Fructus Perillae), and *Di Long* (Pheretima) were added; and for Spleen and Lung qi deficiencies, *Dang Shen* (Radix Codonopsis) and *Bai Zhu* (Rhizoma Atractylodis Macrocephalae) were added. Of 38 patients, the study reported complete recovery in 34 cases, improvement in 2 cases, and no benefit in 2 cases.[5]

3. **Asthma**: Use of modified *She Gan Ma Huang Tang* was effective in treating asthma. The herbal treatment contained *She Gan Ma Huang Tang* plus *Dan Nan Xing* (Arisaema cum Bile) and *Ku Xing Ren* (Semen Armeniacae Amarum) as the base formula, with addition of *Yin Yang Huo* (Herba Epimedii), *Fu Zi* (Radix Aconiti Lateralis Praeparata), and *Rou Gui* (Cortex Cinnamomi) for cold-type asthma; *Shi Gao* (Gypsum Fibrosum), *Sang Bai Pi* (Cortex Mori), and *Yu Xing Cao* (Herba Houttuyniae) for heat-type asthma; and *Bu Gu Zhi* (Fructus Psoraleae), *Zhong Ru Shi* (Stalactitum), and *Huang Qi* (Radix Astragali) during remission of asthma. *Wang Bu Liu Xing* (Semen Vaccariae) seeds were applied topically to acupuncture points on the ear. Of 100 patients, the study reported significant improvement in 35 cases, moderate improvement in 57 cases, and no benefit in 8 cases. The overall rate of effectiveness was 92%.[6]

SUGGESTED ACUPUNCTURE TREATMENT

1. Points: *Pianli* (LI 6), *Hegu* (LI 4), *Feishu* (BL 13), *Lieque* (LU 7), *Jingqu* (LU 8), *Sanjiaoshu* (BL 22), *Yinlingquan* (SP 9), *Fenglong* (ST 40), *Tiantu* (CV 22), *Qihaishu*, *Feimen*, *Feipan*, and *Dingchuan*.
2. Technique: sedation.

Pianli (LI 6), *Hegu* (LI 4), and *Feishu* (BL 13) ventilate the Lung and relieve the exterior. *Lieque* (LU 7) and *Jingqu* (LU 8) relieve coughing and wheezing. *Sanjiaoshu* (BL 22) regulates the water pathways, and *Yinlingquan* (SP 9) removes water retention to strengthen the Spleen. *Fenglong* (ST 40) dispels phlegm. *Tiantu* (CV 22) helps stop dyspnea and asthma. *Qihaishu*, *Feimen*, and *Feipan* are used in the equine patient to tonify the Lung and qi. *Dingchuan* helps to stop dyspnea and cough.

AUTHORS' COMMENTS

Xiao Qing Long Tang (Minor Bluegreen Dragon Decoction) and *She Gan Ma Huang Tang* both release exterior wind-cold and treat interior *tan yin* (phlegm retention).

- *Xiao Qing Long Tang* is indicated for severe wind-cold attack with constitutional water accumulation; it involves more severe clinical signs of profuse, watery nasal discharge and sputum. It treats internal fluid accumulation with exterior excess, wind-cold invasion. This formula focuses on exterior clinical signs in the treatment of acute feline asthma, acute dyspnea in equine RAO, acute canine and feline allergic bronchitis, or infectious equine bronchitis.
- *She Gan Ma Huang Tang* focuses less on wind-cold condition and more on phlegm stagnation causing clinical signs of cough and dyspnea with sputum. It more strongly directs Lung qi downward and relieves dyspnea. This formula contains nearly twice the amount of *Ma Huang* (Herba Ephedrae) to ventilate the Lung and relieve dyspnea as does *Xiao Qing Long Tang*. It can be used in cases of acute feline asthma with short rapid breathing, wheezing, inability to lie down and, in severe cases, cyanosis. This presentation can be seen in newly diagnosed cases or in chronic cases with acute exacerbation of the disease. This formula is especially useful in cats with severe life threatening asthma that are fed dry, kibbled food, which promotes the development and retention of phlegm. This formula relieves cough and wheezing rather than addressing exterior signs as with *Xiao Qing Long Tang*. Once the clinical signs have been controlled and the animal is stable, a formula to tonify deficiencies of the Spleen, Lung and/or Kidney should be used. The same holds true for horses with RAO; this formula would be used in cases of acute respiratory distress where fluid buildup in the lungs and trachea are obvious. *She Gan Ma Huang Tang* can also be useful for the resolution of bronchitis that persists after the original wind-cold invasion has passed when the phlegm becomes severe causing dyspnea and rattling, raspy breath sounds in the trachea. Cats and horses are particularly sensitive to the effects of *Ma Huang* (Herba Ephedrae). It is advised to use the smallest therapeutic dose of either formula to begin treatment.

References

1. *Zhong Yi Fang Ji Xian Dai Yan Jiu* (Modern Study of Medical Formulas in Traditional Chinese Medicine), 1997; 66.

Shè Gān Má Huáng Tāng (Belamcanda and Ephedra Decoction)

2. *Zhong Yi Fang Ji Xian Dai Yan Jiu* (Modern Study of Medical Formulas in Traditional Chinese Medicine), 1997; 66-67.
3. *Zhong Yi Yao Xue Bao* (Report of Chinese Medicine and Herbology), 1990; 3:36.
4. *Nan Jing Zhong Yi Xue Yuan Xue Bao* (Journal of Nanjing University of Traditional Chinese Medicine), 1993; 4:46.
5. *Shan Dong Zhong Yi Za Zhi* (Shandong Journal of Chinese Medicine), 1996; 11:499.
6. *Shi Yong Zhong Yi Yao Za Zhi* (Journal of Practical Chinese Medicine and Medicinals), 1997; 5:14.

Cāng Ěr Zǐ Sǎn (Xanthium Powder)

蒼耳子散
苍耳子散

Pinyin Name: *Cang Er Zi San*
Literal Name: Xanthium Powder
Alternate Names: *Cang Er San*, *Tsang Erh San*, Xanthium Formula
Original Source: *Ji Sheng Fang* (Formulas to Aid the Living) by Yan Yong-He in 1253

COMPOSITION

Cang Er Zi (Fructus Xanthii), *chao* (dry-fried)	7.5g
Xin Yi Hua (Flos Magnoliae)	15g
Bai Zhi (Radix Angelicae Dahuricae)	30g
Bo He (Herba Menthae)	1.5g

DOSAGE / PREPARATION / ADMINISTRATION

Sun-dry the ingredients and then grind them into a fine powder. Take 6g per dose after meals with an herbal tea made from *Cong Bai* (Bulbus Allii Fistulosi) and *Cha Ye* (Folium Camelliae).

CHINESE THERAPEUTIC ACTIONS

1. Dispels wind
2. Opens the nasal orifices

CLINICAL MANIFESTATIONS

Nasal obstruction caused by wind: thick, yellow nasal discharge, frontal and temporal pain.

VETERINARY CLINICAL APPLICAITONS

Acute or chronic sinusitis, acute or chronic allergic rhinitis.

EXPLANATION

Cang Er Zi San (Xanthium Powder) treats wind attacking the exterior. Wind invasion is characterized by clinical

***Cang Er Zi San* (Xanthium Powder)**

Diagnosis	Clinical Signs	Treatment	Herbs
Nasal obstruction due to wind	• Nasal obstruction and sinus pain: exterior wind • Runny nose with thick, yellow nasal discharge: wind condition	• Dispels wind • Opens the nasal orifices	• *Cang Er Zi* (Fructus Xanthii) and *Xin Yi Hua* (Flos Magnoliae) unblock the nasal passages. • *Bai Zhi* (Radix Angelicae Dahuricae) opens the nasal orifices, dispels wind, and discharges pus. • *Bo He* (Herba Menthae) releases wind-heat from the exterior. • *Cong Bai* (Bulbus Allii Fistulosi) and *Cha Ye* (Folium Camelliae) enhance the overall effects of the formula

Cāng Ěr Zǐ Sǎn (Xanthium Powder)

signs such as nasal discharge and sinus pain, while heat invasion is characterized by thick, yellow nasal discharge. Clinically, this formula may be used for animals suffering from acute and chronic bacterial, viral and lymphoplasmacytic rhinitis or sinusitis.

Cang Er Zi (Fructus Xanthii) and *Xin Yi Hua* (Flos Magnoliae), the two chief herbs, unblock the nasal passages and are commonly used together for their synergistic effect. *Bai Zhi* (Radix Angelicae Dahuricae) opens the nasal orifices, dispels wind, and discharges pus. *Bo He* (Herba Menthae) releases wind-heat from the exterior. *Bai Zhi* (Radix Angelicae Dahuricae) and *Bo He* (Herba Menthae) relieve sinus pain caused by wind. *Cong Bai* (Bulbus Allii Fistulosi) and *Cha Ye* (Folium Camelliae) enhance the overall effects of the formula.

CAUTIONS / CONTRAINDICATIONS

Cang Er Zi San (Xanthium Powder) contains a large amount of acrid and warm herbs and is not intended for long-term use. It can aggravate yin deficiency in animals with yin-deficient heat.

VETERINARY MODIFICATIONS

- If there is increased Lung heat, add *Shi Gao* (Gypsum Fibrosum) and *Zhi Mu* (Rhizoma Anemarrhenae).
- For copious, purulent nasal discharge, add *Jin Yin Hua* (Flos Lonicerae Japonicae), *Lian Qiao* (Fructus Forsythiae), *Ju Hua* (Flos Chrysanthemi), *Huang Qin* (Radix Scutellariae) and *Ge Gen* (Radix Puerariae Lobatae).

SUGGESTED ACUPUNCTURE TREATMENT

1. Points: *Lieque* (LU 7), *Hegu* (LI 4), *Yingxiang* (LI 20), *Bitong* (canine classical point) and *Longhui*.
2. Technique: even method or sedation.

Lieque (LU 7) opens the Lung and disperses wind, *Hegu* (LI 4) releases the exterior and relieves sinus pain, and *Yingxiang* (LI 20) opens the nasal passages. Combined with *Bitong* and *Longhui*, these points treat stuffy nose, nasal congestion, and rhinitis.

AUTHORS' COMMENTS

Cang Er Zi San can be used to treat both acute and chronic rhinitis-sinusitis. It is more suitable for chronic, deeply entrenched rhinitis-sinusitis than *Xin Yi San* (Magnolia Flower Powder), which is one of the most commonly used formulas for opening the nasal orifices. *Xin Yi San* consists mostly of warm exterior-releasing herbs and is used more for acute rhinitis problems caused by wind-cold, which is characterized by clear, watery nasal discharge.

In order to successfully treat chronic rhinitis-sinusitis in dogs and cats, *Cang Er Zi San* (Xanthium Powder) is typically combined with single herbs or another formula to enhance its heat clearing properties. It can be combined with *Sang Ju Yin* (Mulberry Leaf and Chrysanthemum Decoction) or *Yin Qiao San* (Honeysuckle and Forsythia Powder) to treat chronic sinusitis-rhinitis, or as an adjunct to chemotherapy in the treatment of nasal adenocarcinoma to control nasal discharge.

Cang Er Zi San is an exceptional formula for use in horses. Alone, it is indispensable for treating the nasal discharge from rhinopneumonitis and influenza infections. Combined with *Yu Ping Feng San* (Jade Windscreen Powder) in a 1:1 ratio, it treats the chronic, frustrating cases of "snotty nose" so common in young horses. Given along with *Sang Ju Yin* (Mulberry Leaf and Chrysanthemum Decoction), *Yin Qiao San* (Honeysuckle and Forsythia Powder), or *Pu Ji Xiao Du Yin* (Universal Benefit Decoction to Eliminate Toxin) a practitioner can treat sinus infection, pneumonia, and *Streptococcus equi* infections that are not too entrenched in the interior. Ethmoid hematomas can be treated by adding *San Qi* (Radix et Rhizoma Notoginseng) or by combining this formula with a formula like *Xue Fu Zhu Yu Tang* (Drive Out Stasis in the Mansion of Blood Decoction).

Xīn Yí Sǎn (Magnolia Flower Powder)

辛夷散

Pinyin Name: *Xin Yi San*
Literal Name: Magnolia Flower Powder
Alternate Names: *Hsin I San*, Magnolia Flower Formula
Original Source: *Ji Sheng Fang* (Formulas to Aid the Living) by Yan Yong-He in 1253

COMPOSITION

Xin Yi Hua (Flos Magnoliae)
Sheng Ma (Rhizoma Cimicifugae)
Bai Zhi (Radix Angelicae Dahuricae)
Xi Xin (Radix et Rhizoma Asari)
Fang Feng (Radix Saposhnikoviae)
Qiang Huo (Rhizoma et Radix Notopterygii)
Gao Ben (Rhizoma et Radix Ligustici)
Chuan Xiong (Rhizoma Chuanxiong)
Mu Tong (Caulis Akebiae)
Zhi Gan Cao (Radix et Rhizoma Glycyrrhizae Praeparata cum Melle)

DOSAGE / PREPARATION / ADMINISTRATION

The source text states to grind equal amounts of the ingredients into powder. Take 6g of the powder per dose with tea after meals.

CHINESE THERAPEUTIC ACTIONS

1. Releases wind-cold from the exterior
2. Opens the nasal orifices

CLINICAL MANIFESTATIONS

Nasal obstruction caused by wind-cold: profuse, clear or white nasal discharge, and sinus pain.

VETERINARY CLINICAL APPLICATIONS

Allergic rhinitis, sinus congestion and sinusitis, and acute feline rhinotracheitis.

EXPLANATION

Xin Yi San (Magnolia Flower Powder) is one of the most commonly used formulas for opening the nasal orifices. Consisting of mostly warm exterior-releasing herbs, this formula is suitable for nasal problems caused by wind-cold. As wind-cold attacks the exterior of the body, it travels upward to affect the nose. Clinical presentations

***Xin Yi San* (Magnolia Flower Powder)**

Diagnosis	Clinical Signs	Treatment	Herbs
Nasal obstruction caused by wind-cold	• Nasal obstruction and sinus pain: exterior wind • Runny nose with clear or white nasal discharge: wind-cold condition	• Releases wind-cold from the exterior • Opens the nasal orifices	• *Xin Yi Hua* (Flos Magnoliae), *Sheng Ma* (Rhizoma Cimicifugae), and *Bai Zhi* (Radix Angelicae Dahuricae) raise clear qi to the head to open the nasal orifices. • *Xi Xin* (Radix et Rhizoma Asari) warms the Lung to resolve phlegm and helps open the nasal orifices. • *Fang Feng* (Radix Saposhnikoviae) and *Qiang Huo* (Rhizoma et Radix Notopterygii) dispel wind-cold. • *Gao Ben* (Rhizoma et Radix Ligustici) and *Chuan Xiong* (Rhizoma Chuanxiong) relieve headache. • *Mu Tong* (Caulis Akebiae) opens obstruction in the nose, and drains dampness and eliminates water accumulation through urination. • *Zhi Gan Cao* (Radix et Rhizoma Glycyrrhizae Praeparata cum Melle) harmonizes the herbs.

Xīn Yí Săn (Magnolia Flower Powder)

include runny nose with clear or white nasal discharge, and sinus pain.

In this formula, the herbs of light quality – *Xin Yi Hua* (Flos Magnoliae), *Sheng Ma* (Rhizoma Cimicifugae), and *Bai Zhi* (Radix Angelicae Dahuricae) – raise clear qi to the head to open the nasal orifices. *Xin Yi Hua* (Flos Magnoliae) and *Bai Zhi* (Radix Angelicae Dahuricae) are two commonly used herbs for nasal problems. *Xi Xin* (Radix et Rhizoma Asari) warms the Lung to resolve phlegm and helps the previous two herbs open the nasal orifices. *Fang Feng* (Radix Saposhnikoviae) and *Qiang Huo* (Rhizoma et Radix Notopterygii) dispel wind-cold. *Gao Ben* (Rhizoma et Radix Ligustici) and *Chuan Xiong* (Rhizoma Chuanxiong) relieve headache. *Mu Tong* (Caulis Akebiae) opens obstruction in the nose, and drains dampness and eliminates water accumulation through urination. *Zhi Gan Cao* (Radix et Rhizoma Glycyrrhizae Praeparata cum Melle) harmonizes the formula.

VETERINARY MODIFICATIONS

- For clear nasal discharge from wind-cold invasion, add *Jing Jie* (Herba Schizonepetae) and *Qiang Huo* (Rhizoma et Radix Notopterygii).
- For abscess caused by accumulation of wind-dampness, add *Cang Zhu* (Rhizoma Atractylodis) and *Lian Qiao* (Fructus Forsythiae).
- With abscess and loss of smell, add *Pai Nong San* (Drain the Pus Powder).

HUMAN CLINICAL STUDIES AND RESEARCH

Allergic rhinitis: Perennial allergic rhinitis was effectively treated with *Xin Yi San* 9g, *Xiao Qing Long Tang* (Minor Bluegreen Dragon Decoction) 3g, and *Xiang Sha Liu Jun Zi Tang* (Six-Gentlemen Decoction with Aucklandia and Amomum) 3g. The patients were given 15g (9+3+3) of herbal extract per day in three equal doses. The mechanism of action was attributed to the suppression of nasal mucosa inflammation by normalizing stimulatory effects of allergic nasal discharge in patients with H-IgE allergic rhinitis.[1]

SUGGESTED ACUPUNCTURE TREATMENT

1. Points: *Yingxiang* (LI 20), *Bitong* (extra point), *Longhui*, *Baihui* (GV 20), *Shangxing* (GV 23), *Fengchi* (GB 20), and *Hegu* (LI 4).
2. Technique: even method or sedation.

Yingxiang (LI 20), *Bitong* (extra point) and *Longhui* together open the nasal orifices and relieve nasal congestion. *Baihui* (GV 20) and *Shangxing* (GV 23) activate yang to relieve nasal congestion. *Fengchi* (GB 20) and *Hegu* (LI 4) dispel exterior pathogens.

RELATED FORMULA

***Xīn Yí Săn* (Magnolia Flower Powder)**

辛夷散

Pinyin Name: *Xin Yi San*

Literal Name: Magnolia Flower Powder

Original Source: *Yi Fang Ji Jie* (Analytical Collection of Medical Formulas) by Wang Ang in 1682

Xin Yi Hua (Flos Magnoliae)
Sheng Ma (Rhizoma Cimicifugae)
Bai Zhi (Radix Angelicae Dahuricae)
Xi Xin (Radix et Rhizoma Asari)
Fang Feng (Radix Saposhnikoviae)
Qiang Huo (Rhizoma et Radix Notopterygii)
Gao Ben (Rhizoma et Radix Ligustici)
Chuan Xiong (Rhizoma Chuanxiong)
Mu Tong (Caulis Akebiae)
Zhi Gan Cao (Radix et Rhizoma Glycyrrhizae Praeparata cum Melle)

This formula is commonly used to treat nasal problems caused by wind-cold. Clinical presentations include stuffy nose with clear or white nasal discharge.

There are two variations of *Xin Yi San*:

- *Xin Yi San* from *Ji Sheng Fang* (Formulas to Aid the Living) contains *Qiang Huo* (Rhizoma et Radix Notopterygii), and is slightly better for treating sinus pain.
- *Xin Yi San* from *Yi Fang Ji Jie* (Analytical Collection of Medical Formulas) uses *Gan Cao* (Radix et Rhizoma Glycyrrhizae) and *Cha Ye* (Folium Camelliae), and is slightly better for reducing swelling and nasal obstruction.

AUTHORS' COMMENTS

Xin Yi San is one of the most commonly used formulas in veterinary medicine for treating nasal discharge. It is especially good for allergic rhinitis-sinusitis during seasonal changes. The key clinical signs include nasal congestion, clear, watery nasal discharge and loss of smell. Horses can have the additional symptom of head-tossing, most noticeable under saddle. This is caused by an irritating post-nasal drip subsequent to an allergic rhinitis. It should not be used in cases when heat signs are present. It can be combined with *Cang Er Zi* (Fructus Xanthii), *Ge Gen* (Radix Puerariae Lobatae) and *Ze Lan* (Herba Lycopi) for chronic or allergic type rhinitis and sinusitis.

Reference

1. Yang SH, Hong CY, Yu CL. The stimulatory effects of nasal discharge from patients with perennial allergic rhinitis on normal human neutrophils are normalized after treatment with a new mixed formula of Chinese herbs. International Immunopharmacology. 2002 Nov. 2(12):1627-39.

Qīng Bí Tāng (Clear the Nose Decoction)

清鼻湯
清鼻汤

Pinyin Name: *Qing Bi Tang*
Literal Name: Clear the Nose Decoction
Alternate Name: Pueraria Nasal Combination
Original Source: *Yan Fang* (Time-Tested Formulas) of unknown author and date

COMPOSITION

Ge Gen (Radix Puerariae Lobatae)	12g
Ma Huang (Herba Ephedrae)	6g
Sheng Jiang (Rhizoma Zingiberis Recens)	3g
Yi Yi Ren (Semen Coicis)	10g
Jie Geng (Radix Platycodonis)	9g
Xin Yi Hua (Flos Magnoliae)	8g
Shi Gao (Gypsum Fibrosum)	2g
Da Huang (Radix et Rhizoma Rhei)	3g
Chuan Xiong (Rhizoma Chuanxiong)	3g
Rou Gui (Cortex Cinnamomi)	5g
Bai Shao (Radix Paeoniae Alba)	3g
Da Zao (Fructus Jujubae)	2g
Gan Cao (Radix et Rhizoma Glycyrrhizae)	2g

DOSAGE / PREPARATION / ADMINISTRATION

Prepare the ingredients as a decoction and take while warm with meals, to avoid possible digestive discomfort.

CHINESE THERAPEUTIC ACTIONS

1. Clears nasal obstruction
2. Releases the exterior

CLINICAL MANIFESTATIONS

Nasal and/or sinus obstruction caused by damp-heat: nasal congestion, yellow, sticky nasal discharge, sneezing, decreased energy level and fatigue.

VETERINARY CLINICAL APPLICATIONS

Acute and chronic sinusitis and rhinitis with foul smelling, sticky, yellow nasal discharge.

EXPLANATION

Qing Bi Tang (Clear the Nose Decoction) specifically treats nasal and sinus obstruction caused by damp-heat, with the diagnostic symptom of yellow and sticky discharge. This syndrome may occur secondary to an acute exterior attack or a chronic condition. If the nasal obstruction is the result of an exterior condition, other clinical signs of an exterior attack may be present, such as sneezing, aversion to cold and itching of the nose and throat. If the nasal and sinus obstruction is chronic in nature, patients may experience a decreased sense of smell, decreased energy level, fatigue and other allergy clinical signs.

Ge Gen (Radix Puerariae Lobatae), *Ma Huang* (Herba Ephedrae), and *Sheng Jiang* (Rhizoma Zingiberis Recens) release exterior pathogens. *Yi Yi Ren* (Semen Coicis) and *Jie Geng* (Radix Platycodonis) drain dampness and eliminate pus. *Xin Yi Hua* (Flos Magnoliae) opens the nasal passages and unblocks nasal obstruction. *Shi Gao* (Gypsum Fibrosum) and *Da Huang* (Radix et Rhizoma Rhei), both cold in nature, clear heat and reduce swelling. *Chuan Xiong* (Rhizoma Chuanxiong) activates blood circulation and relieves sinus pain associated with nasal clinical signs. *Rou Gui* (Cortex Cinnamomi) warms the body, dispels cold, and moderates the harsh and cold properties of *Shi Gao* (Gypsum Fibrosum) and *Da Huang* (Radix et Rhizoma Rhei). *Bai Shao* (Radix Paeoniae Alba) harmonizes *ying* (nutritive) and *wei* (defensive) levels, and balances the acrid and warm herbs in this formula. *Da Zao* (Fructus Jujubae) and *Gan Cao* (Radix et Rhizoma Glycyrrhizae) harmonize the formula.

VETERINARY MODIFICATIONS

- If there is sinus pain, add *Bai Zhi* (Radix Angelicae Dahuricae) and *Yan Hu Suo* (Rhizoma Corydalis).
- For sinus infection with yellow discharge, add *Jin Yin Hua* (Flos Lonicerae Japonicae), *Lian Qiao* (Fructus Forsythiae), *Ju Hua* (Flos Chrysanthemi), *Huang Qin* (Radix Scutellariae) and *Huang Lian* (Rhizoma Coptidis).
- For blood-tinged pus, add *San Qi* (Radix et Rhizoma Notoginseng).

Qīng Bí Tāng (Clear the Nose Decoction)

***Qing Bi Tang* (Clear the Nose Decoction)**

Diagnosis	Clinical Signs	Treatment	Herbs
Nasal obstruction caused by damp-heat	• Stuffy nose with yellow, sticky discharge: accumulation of damp-heat • Decreased sense of smell: damp-heat blocking the sensory orifices • Sneezing, headache, aversion to cold, and an itching sensation in the nose and throat: exterior condition	• Clears nasal obstruction • Releases the exterior	• *Ge Gen* (Radix Puerariae Lobatae), *Ma Huang* (Herba Ephedrae), and *Sheng Jiang* (Rhizoma Zingiberis Recens) release exterior pathogens. • *Yi Yi Ren* (Semen Coicis) and *Jie Geng* (Radix Platycodonis) drain dampness and eliminate pus. • *Xin Yi Hua* (Flos Magnoliae) opens the nasal passages and unblocks nasal obstruction. • *Shi Gao* (Gypsum Fibrosum) and *Da Huang* (Radix et Rhizoma Rhei) clear heat and reduce swelling. • *Chuan Xiong* (Rhizoma Chuanxiong) activates blood circulation and unblocks stagnation. • *Rou Gui* (Cortex Cinnamomi) warms the body and moderates the effects of the harsh and cold herbs. • *Bai Shao* (Radix Paeoniae Alba) balances the acrid and warm herbs. • *Da Zao* (Fructus Jujubae) and *Gan Cao* (Radix et Rhizoma Glycyrrhizae) harmonize the formula.

CAUTIONS / CONTRAINDICATIONS

Qing Bi Tang contains *Ma Huang* (Herba Ephedrae), *Shi Gao* (Gypsum Fibrosum) and *Da Huang* (Radix et Rhizoma Rhei) and is not appropriate for long-term use. Once the acute phase of rhinitis and sinusitis has cleared, another formula that is not as dispersing, draining and cooling should be used. This formula is not typically used more than 10-14 days without modification.

SUGGESTED ACUPUNCTURE TREATMENT

1. Points: *Yingxiang* (LI 20), *Bitong* (extra point), *Longhui*, *Quchi* (LI 11), *Fengmen* (BL 12), *Hegu* (LI 4), *Sanjian* (LI 3), *Neiting* (ST 44), *Yinlingquan* (SP 9), *Fenglong* (ST 40), and *Dazhui* (GV 14).
2. Technique: sedation.

Yingxiang (LI 20), *Bitong*, and *Longhui* are the classic combination for treating nasal congestion. *Fengmen* (BL 12) and *Hegu* (LI 4) release the exterior. *Hegu* (LI 4), *Sanjian* (LI 3), *Neiting* (ST 44), *Yinlingquan* (SP 9), and *Fenglong* (ST 40) remove damp-heat. *Bitong* (extra point), *Yingxiang* (LI 20) and *Quchi* (LI 11) lead qi and blood to the nose and clear nasal obstruction. *Dazhui* (GV 14) and *Quchi* (LI 11) clear wind-heat. If there is sinus pain, add *Longhui* and *Yuyao* (extra point). For sinus infection, bleed *Erjian* (the ear apex).

AUTHORS' COMMENTS

Qing Bi Tang was formulated based on the clinical experience of past herbalists and has been refined after years of trial and error and found to be very effective in the treatment of sinusitis and rhinitis. The original source for *Qing Bi Tang* is unavailable because it has not been formally cited in any reference or textbook.

Qing Bi Tang can be combined with *Yin Qiao San* (Honeysuckle and Forsythia Powder) or *Jing Jie Lian Qiao Tang* (Schizonepeta and Forsythia Decoction) to treat severe sinusitis-rhinitis. In dogs and cats, it can be used in these combinations to treat mycotic (fungal) nasal infections and nasal adenocarcinoma with nasal discharge which develops secondary to bacterial invasion. Horses can be treated with the formula alone or in the above combinations for all matter of sinus infections, including those caused from feed material after an episode of choke and from tooth root abscesses. The nature of these conditions almost always requires long treatment intervals, and as such will require diligent patient monitoring, formula modification, and the addition of formulas to support the Spleen and Stomach.

There are three formulas that commonly treat various types of sinusitis and rhinitis:

- *Cang Er Zi San* (Xanthium Powder) is best for wind-heat condition characterized by nasal obstruction with yellow

Qīng Bí Tāng (Clear the Nose Decoction)

discharge. *Cang Er Zi San* can be used to treat both acute and chronic rhinitis-sinusitis with signs of wind-heat. It is more suitable for chronic deeply entrenched rhinitis-sinusitis than *Xin Yi San* (Magnolia Flower Powder) which is one of the most commonly used formulas for opening the nasal orifices.

- *Xin Yi San* (Magnolia Flower Powder) is most effective for wind-cold condition characterized by nasal obstruction with clear, white discharge. *Xin Yi San* consists of mostly warm exterior-releasing herbs and is used more for acute rhinitis problems such as those seen in feline upper respiratory disease, acute kennel cough, equine influenza type-1, and allergic rhinitis caused by wind-cold, which is characterized by clear, watery nasal discharge.
- *Qing Bi Tang* (Clear the Nose Decoction) targets damp-heat condition characterized by nasal obstruction with yellow, sticky nasal discharge that has a foul smell, and is not for long term use without modification. *Qing Bi Tang* (Clear the Nose Decoction) is particularly useful in the treatment of more severe rhinitis-sinusitis with damp-heat. The ability to clear damp-heat is what makes this formula more suited to treat fungal and neoplastic conditions of the nares and sinuses in addition to bacterial infections. It is not typically used alone and is combined with other formula(s) to increase both its heat and damp clearing abilities in these cases.

The treatment of chronic nasal discharge in veterinary patients can be very frustrating and challenging. The authors have used these three formulas as a sole therapy for the treatment of acute and chronic rhinitis-sinusitis due to viral, bacterial and fungal infections, allergies, infections secondary to foreign body invasion of the nasal cavity, and to help control nasal discharge secondary to neoplasia. These formulas can be safely combined with antibiotic therapy to control or resolve chronic severe infections. When using these formulas and antibiotics together, herbal medications to support the Spleen and Stomach are highly recommended to avoid gastrointestinal upset caused by the combination of cold herbs in these formulas with antibiotics, which are also cold in nature. Generally, all of the chronic rhinitis-sinusitis cases already have a variable component of Spleen deficiency and Liver qi stagnation which allowed dampness and phlegm to develop in the first place. The use of both systems of medicine together greatly improves the probability of resolving chronic infections over using one system of medicine alone.

Section 2

辛凉解表剂
— Acrid and Cold Exterior-Releasing Formulas

Sāng Jú Yǐn (Mulberry Leaf and Chrysanthemum Decoction)

桑菊飲
桑菊饮

Pinyin Name: *Sang Ju Yin*
Literal Name: Mulberry Leaf and Chrysanthemum Decoction
Alternate Names: *Sang Chu Yin*, Morus Leaves and Chrysanthemum Drink, Mulberry and Chrysanthemum Decoction, Morus and Chrysanthemum Combination
Original Source: *Wen Bing Tiao Bian* (Systematic Differentiation of Warm Disease) by Wu Ju-Tong in 1798

COMPOSITION

Sang Ye (Folium Mori)	7.5g
Ju Hua (Flos Chrysanthemi)	3g
Bo He (Herba Menthae)	2.4g
Lian Qiao (Fructus Forsythiae)	4.5g
Jie Geng (Radix Platycodonis)	6g
Ku Xing Ren (Semen Armeniacae Amarum)	6g
Lu Gen (Rhizoma Phragmitis)	6g
Gan Cao (Radix et Rhizoma Glycyrrhizae)	2.4g

DOSAGE / PREPARATION / ADMINISTRATION

Cook the ingredients with 2 cups of water until the liquid is reduced to 1 cup. Take the decoction twice daily.

CHINESE THERAPEUTIC ACTIONS

1. Dispels wind and clears heat
2. Ventilates the Lung and arrests coughing

CLINICAL MANIFESTATIONS

Early stage of wind-warmth syndrome: cough, mild fever, and slight thirst.

VETERINARY CLINICAL APPLICATIONS

Acute bronchitis, hacking dry cough, or cough with sticky, yellow mucous that is difficult to expectorate, feline upper respiratory infections, equine influenza and rhinopneumonitis.

EXPLANATION

Sang Ju Yin (Mulberry Leaf and Chrysanthemum Decoction) is a relatively mild formula that treats the early stage or a mild case of wind-warmth syndrome. Coughing, the prominent clinical sign in these animals, arises when the wind-warmth factor affects the normal Lung qi flow. Since this wind-warmth syndrome is mild in nature, the fever and thirst will be slight.

Sang Ye (Folium Mori) and *Ju Hua* (Flos Chrysanthemi) expel the wind-warmth factor and clear Lung heat. *Bo He* (Herba Menthae) helps clear the wind-warmth from the upper *jiao*. *Jie Geng* (Radix Platycodonis), with its ascending tendency, and *Ku Xing Ren* (Semen Armeniacae Amarum), with its descending tendency, regulate Lung qi to relieve cough. *Lian Qiao* (Fructus Forsythiae) clears heat and eliminates toxins in the upper *jiao*. *Lu Gen* (Rhizoma Phragmitis) clears heat and promotes the generation of body fluids to relieve thirst. *Gan Cao* (Radix et Rhizoma Glycyrrhizae) harmonizes the herbs.

In this formula, *Sang Ye* (Folium Mori) and *Ju Hua* (Flos Chrysanthemi) are used as chief herbs to gently disperse early-stage wind-warmth factor that is beginning to affect

Sāng Jú Yǐn (Mulberry Leaf and Chrysanthemum Decoction)

Sang Ju Yin (Mulberry Leaf and Chrysanthemum Decoction)

Diagnosis	Clinical Signs	Treatment	Herbs
Early stage of wind-warmth syndrome	• Mild fever: exterior wind-warmth • Slight thirst: heat consuming body fluids • Cough: wind-warmth affecting Lung qi circulation	• Dispels wind and clears heat • Ventilates the Lung and arrests cough	• *Sang Ye* (Folium Mori) and *Ju Hua* (Flos Chrysanthemi) dispel exterior wind-warmth factor and clear interior Lung heat. • *Bo He* (Herba Menthae) clears wind-warmth factor from the upper *jiao*. • *Lian Qiao* (Fructus Forsythiae) clears heat and eliminates toxins in the upper *jiao*. • *Jie Geng* (Radix Platycodonis) and *Ku Xing Ren* (Semen Armeniacae Amarum) regulate Lung qi to relieve coughing. • *Lu Gen* (Rhizoma Phragmitis) clears heat and promotes the generation of body fluids to relieve thirst. • *Gan Cao* (Radix et Rhizoma Glycyrrhizae) harmonizes the herbs.

the Lung. Although *Bo He* (Herba Menthae) is colder, and has a stronger exterior-releasing effect, it is not suitable as the chief herb for two main reasons. First, its exterior-releasing effect is too strong, and may further damage body fluids, creating heat phlegm and aggravating cough. Second, it does not clear Lung heat nor arrest the cough. Therefore, *Bo He* (Herba Menthae) is not suitable as the chief ingredient, but is used as the deputy herb to help *Sang Ye* (Folium Mori) and *Ju Hua* (Flos Chrysanthemi) release the wind-warmth factor.

VETERINARY MODIFICATIONS

- For severe cough with yellow sputum caused by Lung heat, add *Huang Qin* (Radix Scutellariae) and *Sang Bai Pi* (Cortex Mori).
- For cough with sticky sputum that is difficult to expectorate, add *Gua Lou Pi* (Pericarpium Trichosanthis), *Dong Gua Zi* (Semen Benincasae), and *Zhe Bei Mu* (Bulbus Fritillariae Thunbergii).
- For cough with blood-streaked sputum, add *Bai Mao Gen* (Rhizoma Imperatae), *Ou Jie* (Nodus Nelumbinis Rhizomatis), and *Qian Cao* (Radix et Rhizoma Rubiae).
- If there is labored breathing or dyspnea characterized by more heat and dryness in the *qi* (energy) level, add *Shi Gao* (Gypsum Fibrosum) and *Zhi Mu* (Rhizoma Anemarrhenae) to clear the Lung.
- When there is more thirst, add *Tian Hua Fen* (Radix Trichosanthis) and *Zhi Mu* (Rhizoma Anemarrhenae).

CAUTIONS / CONTRAINDICATIONS

- *Sang Ju Yin* is an acrid and cold formula that treats early wind-warmth condition. It is inappropriate for cough caused by wind-cold.
- This formula has only mild potency to treat cough caused by early wind-warmth invasion. In cases of severe cough caused by Lung heat, the use of this formula alone will not be sufficient. Modification with additional herbs and doses, or selection of another formula is necessary for proper treatment.

PHARMACOLOGICAL EFFECTS

1. **Effect on temperature regulation**: Administration of *Sang Ju Yin* was associated with reduction of body temperature in rabbits with artificially-induced fever. The formula, however, has a slow onset of action, as the effect was not observed until 4 hours later. The researchers noted that the potency of this formula is similar to that of aspirin at 2 mg/kg.[1]
2. **Anti-inflammatory**: Administration of *Sang Ju Yin* was associated with marked anti-inflammatory effects in mice with swelling and inflammation. The mechanism of action is attributed to reversal of the increased capillary permeability. The minimum effective dose for anti-inflammatory effects was 0.307 g/kg. The pharmacokinetic parameters of *Sang Ju Yin* are: 4.83 hours for half life, 3.1 hours for time to reach peak concentration, and 24.48 hours for duration of action.[2]

HUMAN CLINICAL STUDIES AND RESEARCH

1. **Upper respiratory tract infection**: Patients with upper respiratory tract infection characterized by cough, fever, sticky sputum, and a dry mouth were treated with *Sang*

Sāng Jú Yĭn (Mulberry Leaf and Chrysanthemum Decoction)

Ju Yin. Out of 375 cases, the study reported satisfactory results in 359 cases (95.5%). No side effects were reported.[3]

2. **Cough**: Eighty pediatric patients with cough were treated with *Sang Ju Yin* plus *Ma Huang* (Herba Ephedrae) and *Gan Jiang* (Rhizoma Zingiberis) with 94% effectiveness. Additional modifications were made by adding *Shi Gao* (Gypsum Fibrosum) and *Huang Qin* (Radix Scutellariae) for Lung heat; *Ge Gen* (Radix Puerariae Lobatae) and *Tian Hua Fen* (Radix Trichosanthis) for thirst; *Bai Bu* (Radix Stemonae) and *Zi Wan* (Radix et Rhizoma Asteris) for severe cough; *Bai Guo* (Semen Ginkgo) and *Di Long* (Pheretima) for wheezing; *Xi Xin* (Radix et Rhizoma Asari) and *Fu Zi* (Radix Aconiti Lateralis Praeparata) for cold; *Chuan Bei Mu* (Bulbus Fritillariae Cirrhosae) and *Gua Lou Pi* (Pericarpium Trichosanthis) for profuse phlegm; *She Gan* (Rhizoma Belamcandae) and *Niu Bang Zi* (Fructus Arctii) for redness and swelling of the throat; *Bai Mao Gen* (Rhizoma Imperatae) and *Xian He Cao* (Herba Agrimoniae) for nosebleeds; and charred *Shan Zha* (Fructus Crataegi), charred *Shen Qu* (Massa Fermentata), and charred *Mai Ya* (Fructus Hordei Germinatus) for poor appetite. Of 80 cases, the study reported complete recovery in 64 cases after 2 packs of herbs, in 11 cases after 3-5 packs of herbs, and no benefit in 5 cases.[4]

SUGGESTED ACUPUNCTURE TREATMENT

1. Points: *Quchi* (LI 11), *Hegu* (LI 4), *Dazhui* (GV 14), *Feishu* (BL 13), *Lieque* (LU 7), *Tiantu* (CV 22), *Waiguan* (TH 5), and *Dingchuan*.
2. Technique: shallow needling; sedation.

Since the hand *yangming* channel connects with the hand *taiyin* channel, needle *Quchi* (LI 11) and *Hegu* (LI 4), *he* (uniting) point and *yuan* (source) point of the hand *yangming* channel respectively, to clear Lung heat and regulate the qi flow of the Lung. *Dazhui* (GV 14) will also clear wind heat. *Feishu* (BL 13) and *Lieque* (LU 7) can disperse the Lung and consolidate the exterior. *Tiantu* (CV 22) can stop cough. *Waiguan* (TH 5) dispels exterior wind-warmth factor. *Dingchuan* stops cough and dyspnea.

AUTHORS' COMMENTS

Sang Ju Yin is one of the most essential and effective formulas for treating mild cases of cough caused by wind-warmth invasion. This formula is also effective in treating dry cough, with scanty or no sputum, during the autumn. Because this formula is mild in nature, it is necessary to modify it to increase its potency and/or address associated complications. Please see the **Veterinary Modifications** section for details.

Sang Ju Yin is suitable for young, geriatric or chronically debilitated animals. It is especially useful in kittens, puppies, and foals with upper respiratory infection that presents with mild signs of wind heat. It is also helpful for animals that are depleted from competition, breeding, or extensive travel and are showing early signs of respiratory infection. These animals are alert, playful, eating and appear normal otherwise with the exception of mild fever and cough. If these animals have yellow nasal and ocular discharge with sneezing, lethargy and poor appetite, then *Yin Qiao San* (Honeysuckle and Forsythia Powder) would be more appropriate to use. Both formulas are most effective if administered every 8 hours instead of every 12 hours. This dosing schedule used early in the treatment of upper respiratory tract infection can prevent the pathogen from invading deeper into the body.

Sang Ju Yin and *Yin Qiao San* (Honeysuckle and Forsythia Powder) are cool, acrid formulas used for the initial stages of warm febrile disorders. Both contain *Lian Qiao* (Fructus Forsythiae), *Jie Geng* (Radix Platycodonis), *Gan Cao* (Radix et Rhizoma Glycyrrhizae), *Bo He* (Herba Menthae), and *Lu Gen* (Rhizoma Phragmitis).

- *Sang Ju Yin* more effectively ventilates the Lung to arrest coughing.
- *Yin Qiao San* has stronger heat-clearing and exterior-releasing effects.

References

1. *Zhong Yao Tong Bao* (Journal of Chinese Herbology), 1986; 11(1):51.
2. *Zhong Yao Yao Li Yu Ying Yong* (Pharmacology and Applications of Chinese Herbs), 1993; (1):1.
3. *Fu Jian Zhong Yi Yao* (Fujian Chinese Medicine and Herbology), 1957; 2(6):25.
4. *Shi Yong Zhong Yi Yao Za Zhi* (Journal of Practical Chinese Medicine and Medicinals), 1999; 7:16.

Yín Qiào Sǎn (Honeysuckle and Forsythia Powder)

銀翹散
银翘散

Pinyin Name: *Yin Qiao San*
Literal Name: Honeysuckle and Forsythia Powder
Alternate Names: *Yin Jiao San*, Lonicera and Forsythia Formula
Original Source: *Wen Bing Tiao Bian* (Systematic Differentiation of Warm Disease) by Wu Ju-Tong in 1798

COMPOSITION

Jin Yin Hua (Flos Lonicerae Japonicae)	30g [15g]
Lian Qiao (Fructus Forsythiae)	30g [15g]
Jing Jie Sui (Spica Schizonepetae)	12g [4g]
Dan Dou Chi (Semen Sojae Praeparatum)	15g [5g]
Jie Geng (Radix Platycodonis)	18g [6g]
Niu Bang Zi (Fructus Arctii)	18g [6g]
Bo He (Herba Menthae)	18g [6g]
Zhu Ye (Herba Phyllostachys)	12g [4g]
Gan Cao (Radix et Rhizoma Glycyrrhizae)	15g [5g]

DOSAGE / PREPARATION / ADMINISTRATION

Grind the ingredients into powder and take 18g of the powder with a decoction made from fresh *Lu Gen* (Rhizoma Phragmitis). The decoction of *Lu Gen* (Rhizoma Phragmitis) is prepared by cooking the herb in water until its aroma fills the air. Do not overcook the herb, since a light decoction (cooking for a short period of time) enters and treats the Lung, while a heavy decoction (cooking for a long period of time) enters the middle *jiao*.

For patients with serious conditions, take the decoction three times during the day (2 hours apart) and one time at night. For patients with mild conditions, take the decoction twice during the day (3 hours apart) and one time at night. The treatment should be continued until the condition is resolved. Today, this formula may be prepared as a decoction with the doses suggested in brackets above.

CHINESE THERAPEUTIC ACTIONS

1. Releases the exterior with acrid and cold herbs
2. Clears heat and eliminates toxins

CLINICAL MANIFESTATIONS

Onset of *wen bing* (warm diseases): fever, aversion to cold, slight aversion to wind, little to no sweating, stiff and painful neck, thirst, a sore throat, cough, a red tongue and a superficial, rapid pulse.

VETERINARY CLINICAL APPLICATIONS

Fever, viral and bacterial pneumonia, acute canine infectious tracheobronchitis, feline rhinotracheitis, beginning of any febrile disease, epidemic encephalitis (early stage), as well as early onset West Nile Virus patients.

EXPLANATION

Yin Qiao San (Honeysuckle and Forsythia Powder) treats the early stage of *wen bing* (warm diseases), when heat enters through the nose and mouth and attacks the Lung. When heat attacks the *wei* (defensive) level of the skin, it produces clinical signs of fever and aversion to cold and wind. When heat invades the Lung, it produces cough. Thirst and a red tongue tip are indications of heat damaging body fluids. A red tongue and a superficial, rapid pulse are signs of heat at the exterior.

Jin Yin Hua (Flos Lonicerae Japonicae) and *Lian Qiao* (Fructus Forsythiae) are the chief herbs in this formula. Acrid, aromatic and cold, they release exterior heat and eliminate toxins. *Jing Jie Sui* (Spica Schizonepetae) and *Dan Dou Chi* (Semen Sojae Praeparatum) open the skin pores to help expel exterior factors through the induction of a mild sweat. *Jie Geng* (Radix Platycodonis) regulates Lung qi and relieves the sore throat. *Bo He* (Herba Menthae) dispels wind-heat. *Zhu Ye* (Herba Phyllostachys) clears upper *jiao* heat, while *Niu Bang Zi* (Fructus Arctii) clears heat and eliminates toxins to relieve the sore throat. *Gan Cao* (Radix et Rhizoma Glycyrrhizae) clears heat and eliminates toxins. Finally, *Lu Gen* (Rhizoma Phragmitis) clears heat and promotes the generation of body fluids to relieve thirst.

Yín Qiào Săn (Honeysuckle and Forsythia Powder)

Yin Qiao San (Honeysuckle and Forsythia Powder)

Diagnosis	Clinical Signs	Treatment	Herbs
Onset of *wen bing* (warm diseases)	• Fever, aversion to cold and wind: heat attacks the *wei* (defensive) level • Cough: heat enters the Lung through the mouth and nose • Thirst and a red tongue: body fluids damaged by heat • Red tongue and a superficial, rapid pulse: heat at the exterior	• Releases the exterior • Clears heat and eliminates toxins	• *Jin Yin Hua* (Flos Lonicerae Japonicae) and *Lian Qiao* (Fructus Forsythiae) release exterior heat and eliminate toxins. • *Jing Jie Sui* (Spica Schizonepetae) and *Dan Dou Chi* (Semen Sojae Praeparatum) open the skin pores to expel exterior factors via mild sweating. • *Jie Geng* (Radix Platycodonis) regulates Lung qi and relieves sore throat. • *Niu Bang Zi* (Fructus Arctii) clears heat and eliminates toxins. • *Bo He* (Herba Menthae) dispels exterior wind-heat. • *Zhu Ye* (Herba Phyllostachys) clears interior heat from upper *jiao*. • *Lu Gen* (Rhizoma Phragmitis) clears heat and promotes the generation of body fluids. • *Gan Cao* (Radix et Rhizoma Glycyrrhizae) clears heat and eliminates toxins.

VETERINARY MODIFICATIONS

- With irritability and thirst, add *Mai Dong* (Radix Ophiopogonis) and *Shi Gao* (Gypsum Fibrosum).
- If there is nausea and vomiting, add *Huo Xiang* (Herba Agastaches) and *Zhi Qiao* (Fructus Aurantii).
- If there is thirst, add *Tian Hua Fen* (Radix Trichosanthis) or *Lu Gen* (Rhizoma Phragmitis).
- If there is cough, add *Ku Xing Ren* (Semen Armeniacae Amarum) and *Zhe Bei Mu* (Bulbus Fritillariae Thunbergii).
- For atopic dermatitis, combine with *Xiao Feng San* (Eliminate Wind Powder) and *Zi Cao* (Radix Arnebiae).
- When there is more interior heat, add *Zhi Zi* (Fructus Gardeniae) and *Huang Qin* (Radix Scutellariae).
- When heat in the Lung has injured body fluids, add *Di Huang* (Radix Rehmanniae) and *Mai Dong* (Radix Ophiopogonis).

CAUTIONS / CONTRAINDICATIONS

- *Yin Qiao San* is contraindicated in cases of wind-cold invasion or in initial stages of damp-heat conditions.
- Wind-heat conditions can change rapidly. Optimal treatment requires close monitoring of clinical presentations and immediate adjustment of the herbal treatment.
- Avoid feeding foods that are oily, greasy, raw, cold, or sour in nature while taking this herbal formula.[1]

PHARMACOLOGICAL EFFECTS

1. **Antibiotic**: According to *in vitro* studies, *Yin Qiao San* has broad spectrum of inhibitory effects against such pathogens as *Staphylococcus aureus*, *Bacillus subtilis*, *Bacillus proteus*, *Pseudomonas aeruginosa*, and *Candida albicans*. The minimum inhibitory concentration was 110 mg/mL (equivalent to 550 mg/mL of raw herb).[2]
2. **Effect on temperature regulation**: Administration of *Yin Qiao San* was effective in reducing body temperature in rabbits with artificially-induced fever. Oral ingestion of decoction at 3.8 mL/kg (equivalent to 8.8 g/kg of dried herbs) was effective in reducing body temperature by 1°C for up to six hours. In comparison with aspirin (0.2 mg/kg), the herbal formula and the drug are approximately the same in their effect to reduce fever.[3]
3. **Anti-inflammatory**: Administration of various dosage forms of *Yin Qiao San* was effective in reducing swelling and inflammation in rats. The dosage forms tested include decoction, pills, and tea bags. It has been determined that to achieve an anti-inflammatory effect, the minimum effective dose is 1.5 g/kg. The pharmacokinetic parameters of *Yin Qiao San* are: 2.31 hours to reach peak therapeutic effect, 16.23 hours for duration of action, and 4.53 hours for half life.[4]
4. **Analgesic**: Administration of *Yin Qiao San* at doses of 50 mg/kg and 100 mg/kg via intraperitoneal injection was associated with mild analgesic effects in mice for up to one hour.[5]

Yín Qiào Săn (Honeysuckle and Forsythia Powder)

HUMAN CLINICAL STUDIES AND RESEARCH

1. **Common cold and influenza**: Three hundred patients with infectious viral infection were treated with *Yin Qiao San* with most reporting improvement after 1-2 doses.[6]
2. **High fever**: In one study, 102 children with high fever caused by infection were treated with 87.25% effectiveness using modified *Yin Qiao San*. Modifications included addition of *Shi Gao* (Gypsum Fibrosum), *Di Gu Pi* (Cortex Lycii), and *Zhi Mu* (Rhizoma Anemarrhenae) for persistent high fever; *Jiang Can* (Bombyx Batryticatus) and *Gou Teng* (Ramulus Uncariae cum Uncis) for spasms and cramps; *Ma Huang* (Herba Ephedrae), *Ku Xing Ren* (Semen Armeniacae Amarum), and *Qian Hu* (Radix Peucedani) for cough; *Chi Shao* (Radix Paeoniae Rubra), *Chan Tui* (Periostracum Cicadae), and *Ju Hua* (Flos Chrysanthemi) for red eyes; *Ban Xia* (Rhizoma Pinelliae) and *Sheng Jiang* (Rhizoma Zingiberis Recens) for nausea and vomiting; and *Yi Yi Ren* (Semen Coicis) and *Hua Shi* (Talcum) for diarrhea. After using 1-3 packs of the herbs, the study reported improvement in 89 of 102 patients.[7]
3. **Pneumonia**: One study reported recovery in all 25 children with pneumonia after they were treated with 3-5 packs of modified *Yin Qiao San* plus *Zhi Mu* (Rhizoma Anemarrhenae) and *Ku Xing Ren* (Semen Armeniacae Amarum). Additional modifications were made as needed. For irritability and thirst due to excess heat, *Tian Hua Fen* (Radix Trichosanthis) and *Huang Lian* (Rhizoma Coptidis) were added, and *Jing Jie Sui* (Spica Schizonepetae), *Bo He* (Herba Menthae) and *Niu Bang Zi* (Fructus Arctii) were removed. For severe cough with thick sputum, *Chuan Bei Mu* (Bulbus Fritillariae Cirrhosae) and *Gua Lou* (Fructus Trichosanthis) were added, and *Niu Bang Zi* (Fructus Arctii) and *Jing Jie Sui* (Spica Schizonepetae) were removed. For dry or foul-smelling stools, *Da Huang* (Radix et Rhizoma Rhei) was added, and *Jie Geng* (Radix Platycodonis) and *Bo He* (Herba Menthae) were removed. For reduced frequency and volume of urine with painful urination, *Che Qian Zi* (Semen Plantaginis) was added, and *Niu Bang Zi* (Fructus Arctii) and *Jing Jie Sui* (Spica Schizonepetae) were removed.[8]
4. **Acute upper respiratory infection**: In one report, 1150 patients with wind-heat exterior infection were treated with *Yin Qiao San* with relief of fever within an average of 2.7 days.[9]

TOXICOLOGY

The LD_{50} for *Yin Qiao San* in mice via oral ingestion was 100 g/kg in decoction, and 75 g/kg in pills.[10]

SUGGESTED ACUPUNCTURE TREATMENT

1. Points: *Dazhui* (GV 14), *Fengchi* (GB 20), *Waiguan* (TH 5), *Quchi* (LI 11), *Hegu* (LI 4), *Chize* (LU 5), *Shangyang* (LI 1), *Feishu* (BL 13), *Lieque* (LU 7), *Tiantu* (CV 22), *Yuji* (LU 10), *Shaoshang* (LU 11) and *Dingchuan*.
2. Technique: sedation.

Dazhui (GV 14) dispels heat from the exterior. *Fengchi* (GB 20) relieves exterior wind. *Waiguan* (TH 5), *Quchi* (LI 11), and *Hegu* (LI 4) dispel wind-heat and regulate the qi flow of the Lung. *Chize* (LU 5) clears Lung heat. *Shangyang* (LI 1) opens the channel and clears wind-heat. *Feishu* (BL 13) and *Lieque* (LU 7) disperse the Lung and consolidate the exterior. *Tiantu* (CV 22) stops cough. *Yuji* (LU 10) and *Shaoshang* (LU 11) sedate Lung heat and relieve sore throat. *Dingchuan* stops cough and dyspnea.

AUTHORS' COMMENTS

Yin Qiao San is the representative formula for treating the initial stage of *wen bing* (warm diseases), with chief manifestations of fever, aversion to cold, slight aversion to wind, thirst, and a superficial, rapid pulse. It is widely used in the treatment of various types of respiratory diseases and is most effective when administered immediately after clinical signs appear. Appropriate use of this formula will reduce the severity and duration of viral infections. It is best to administer *Yin Qiao San* three to four times daily instead of twice for optimal clinical results. Cattery, kennel, and stable owners have used this formula at the first sign of respiratory disease to prevent the remainder of the population in their care from becoming ill.

Yin Qiao San is also effective in the treatment of chronic rhinitis-sinusitis with nasal discharge and significant nasal-sinus tissue destruction (as evidenced upon radiographs or computerized tomography) in the dog and cat when combined with *Xue Fu Zhu Yu Tang* (Drive Out Stasis in the Mansion of Blood Decoction) or *Tong Qiao Huo Xue Tang* (Unblock the Orifices and Invigorate the Blood Decoction). They can be combined in a 3:1 or 4:1 ratio of *Yin Qiao San* to *Xue Fu Zhu Yu Tang* (Drive Out Stasis in the Mansion of Blood Decoction) or *Tong Qiao Huo Xue Tang* (Unblock the Orifices and Invigorate the Blood Decoction), depending on the case. This protocol can be used in a similar fashion in horses that develop chronic sinusitis subsequent to intranasal vaccination. This protocol may also be useful in many cases of ethmoid hematoma in patients that are not bleeding profusely, in which case herbs such as *San Qi* (Radix et Rhizoma Notoginseng) should be used initially until bleeding is controlled. The authors have also used *Yin Qiao San* in combination with *San Qi* (Radix et Rhizoma Notoginseng) and *Gui Pi Tang* (Restore the Spleen Decoction) in cases of exercise induced pulmonary hemorrhage (EIPH).

Yín Qiào Săn (Honeysuckle and Forsythia Powder)

Xue Fu Zhu Yu Tang (Drive Out Stasis in the Mansion of Blood Decoction) activates qi and blood circulation, removes blood stagnation, and relieves pain. It is used to treat qi and blood stagnation in the chest, which includes the Lung. In Chinese medicine, the nose is the sensory orifice related to the Lung, and, as such, this formula can be used to treat rhinitis-sinusitis. *Xue Fu Zhu Yu Tang* (Drive Out Stasis in the Mansion of Blood Decoction) has the unique ability to activate blood circulation and dispel blood stasis without injuring the blood, soothe the Liver, and relieve qi stagnation without consuming qi. *Tong Qiao Huo Xue Tang* (Unblock the Orifices and Invigorate the Blood Decoction) specifically activates blood circulation to the head and face and opens the sensory orifices. The use of blood-moving formulas in chronic rhinitis-sinusitis is essential because long-term tissue destruction, toxic heat, and dampness cause stagnation, which leads to blood stasis. In addition, herbal formulas that invigorate blood flow to the upper orifices help to increase delivery of antibiotics, oxygen, nutrients, immune factors, and other formulas to compromised tissue and help to drain discharge and enhance chemotherapeutic effects.

Yin Qiao San can be used in combination with *Ma Huang Xing Ren Gan Cao Shi Gao Tang* (Ephedra, Apricot Kernel, Licorice, and Gypsum Decoction) to treat pneumonia in the dog and horse. *Ma Huang Xing Ren Gan Cao Shi Gao Tang* (Ephedra, Apricot Kernel, Licorice, and Gypsum Decoction) is a strong formula that clears and ventilates the Lung to treat cough and dyspnea caused by Lung heat. When used with *Yin Qiao San* this combination can cleat heat toxins, disperse the Lung, relieve the exterior, and unblock the collaterals. In the treatment of acute bacterial pneumonia, it can be combined with *Yin Qiao San* in a ratio of 1:4. Diseases of the horse such as Eastern, Western, and Venezuelan equine encephalitis, West Nile Virus, strangles, and Rhodococcus, which all can move quickly to generate heat toxins, can be treated using a combination of *Yin Qiao San* with *Huang Lian Jie Du Tang* (Coptis Decoction to Relieve Toxicity), also in a 1:4 ratio. The latter formula is quite effective at draining heat, but it is very cold and should be used with caution in weak or debilitated animals. Additionally, when used to treat *Streptococcus equi,* abscesses that can be drained to the exterior should be opened at the onset of treatment.

It is common in the treatment of bacterial, neoplastic or mycotic pneumonia to add additional single herbs to improve the ability of *Yin Qiao San* to clear heat and toxins from the Lungs. The following herbs can be added to enhance the overall effects: *Yu Xing Cao* (Herba Houttuyniae), *Zi Hua Di Ding* (Herba Violae), *Ma Bian Cao* (Herba Verbenae), *Chuan Xin Lian* (Herba Andrographis), *Da Qing Ye* (Folium Isatidis), and *Ban Lan Gen* (Radix Isatidis). Once the acute signs (e.g., fever, nasal discharge, cough with thick, yellow phlegm, dyspnea, anorexia, lethargy) of pneumonia have been cleared, those herbal formulas administered to clear heat, eliminate toxins and ventilate the Lung should be decreased, and herbal formulas to tonify Lung qi and yin and to tonify the Spleen and Stomach should be added.

Sang Ju Yin (Mulberry Leaf and Chrysanthemum Decoction) and *Yin Qiao San* both clear heat, eliminate toxins, disperse wind-heat, and ventilate the Lung. Both are suitable for wind-heat invasion with fever and cough. The differences between the two formulas are as follows:

- *Sang Ju Yin* contains *Sang Ye* (Folium Mori), *Ju Hua* (Flos Chrysanthemi), and *Ku Xing Ren* (Semen Armeniacae Amarum). This formula ventilates the Lung and arrests cough associated with initial stages of wind-heat invasion.
- *Yin Qiao San* contains *Jin Yin Hua* (Flos Lonicerae Japonicae), *Jing Jie* (Herba Schizonepetae), *Dan Dou Chi* (Semen Sojae Praeparatum), *Niu Bang Zi* (Fructus Arctii), and *Zhu Ye* (Herba Phyllostachys). This formula eliminates toxins to treat *wen bing* (warm disease) conditions with chief manifestations of sore throat and fever.

References

1. *Zhong Yao Ming Fang Yao Li Yu Ying Yong* (Pharmacology and Applications of Famous Herbal Formulas), 1989; 55-57.
2. *Zhong Cheng Yao* (Study of Chinese Patent Medicine), 1990; 12(1):22.
3. *Zhong Yao Tong Bao* (Journal of Chinese Herbology), 1986; 11(1):51.
4. *Zhong Yi Za Zhi* (Journal of Chinese Medicine), 1986; 27(3):59.
5. *Zhong Cheng Yao* (Study of Chinese Patent Medicine), 1990; 12(1):22.
6. *Hu Bei Zhong Yi Za Zhi* (Hubei Journal of Chinese Medicine), 1983; (2):19.
7. *Liao Ning Zhong Yi Za Zhi* (Liaoning Journal of Chinese Medicine), 1994; 12:548.
8. *Hu Bei Zhong Yi Za Zhi* (Hubei Journal of Chinese Medicine), 1982; 1:55.
9. *Zhong Cheng Yao Yan Jiu* (Research of Chinese Patent Medicine), 1986; (12):39.
10. *Zhong Yi Za Zhi* (Journal of Chinese Medicine), 1986; 27(3):59.

Má Huáng Xìng Rén Gān Cǎo Shí Gāo Tāng

(Ephedra, Apricot Kernel, Licorice, and Gypsum Decoction)

麻黃杏仁甘草石膏湯

麻黄杏仁甘草石膏汤

Pinyin Name: *Ma Huang Xing Ren Gan Cao Shi Gao Tang*

Literal Name: Ephedra, Apricot Kernel, Licorice, and Gypsum Decoction

Alternate Names: *Ma Xing Gan Shi Tang, Ma Xing Shi Gan Tang, Ma Hsing Kan Shih Tang*, Ephedra, Apricot, Licorice and Gypsum Decoction; Ephedra, Apricot Kernel, Gypsum and Licorice Decoction; Ma-huang and Apricot Seed Decoction, Mahuang and Apricot Seed Combination

Original Source: *Shang Han Lun* (Discussion of Cold-Induced Disorders) by Zhang Zhong-Jing in the Eastern Han Dynasty

COMPOSITION

Ma Huang (Herba Ephedrae)	12g [5-9g]
Shi Gao (Gypsum Fibrosum), *fen sui* (pulverized)	24g [18g]
Ku Xing Ren (Semen Armeniacae Amarum)	50 kernels [9g]
Zhi Gan Cao (Radix et Rhizoma Glycyrrhizae Praeparata cum Melle)	6g

DOSAGE / PREPARATION / ADMINISTRATION

The source text states to cook *Ma Huang* (Herba Ephedrae) in 7 cups [1,400 mL] of water until it is reduced to 5 cups [1,000 mL]. Remove the foam from the top, add the other ingredients, and cook until the liquid reduces to 2 cups [400 mL]. Take 1 cup [200 mL] of the warm, strained decoction. Today, the decoction may be prepared using the doses suggested in brackets.

CHINESE THERAPEUTIC ACTIONS

1. Ventilates Lung qi
2. Clears Lung heat
3. Relieves cough and dyspnea

CLINICAL MANIFESTATIONS

Cough and dyspnea in Lung heat syndrome caused by exterior pathogenic factors: unremitting fever, thirst with a desire to drink, rhinitis, dry, painful cough with little or no mucus, dyspnea, red tongue and a slippery, rapid pulse.

VETERINARY CLINICAL APPLICATIONS

Acute feline and equine upper respiratory tract infection, acute pharyngitis, acute infectious canine tracheobronchitis, viral and bacterial pneumonia, pleuritis, cough and dyspnea, acute feline asthma, fever and nasosinusitis.

EXPLANATION

Ma Huang Xing Ren Gan Cao Shi Gao Tang (Ephedra, Apricot Kernel, Licorice, and Gypsum Decoction) is indicated for Lung heat syndrome characterized by cough and dyspnea. This syndrome can be caused by an exterior wind-heat factor directly invading the Lung, or by an exterior wind-cold factor constricting the Lung. Both situations can create stagnation in the Lung that later transforms into heat.

***Ma Huang Xing Ren Gan Cao Shi Gao Tang* (Ephedra, Apricot Kernel, Licorice, and Gypsum Decoction)**

Diagnosis	Clinical Signs	Treatment	Herbs
Cough and dyspnea in Lung heat syndrome	• Coughing and dyspnea: heat affecting Lung qi circulation • Thirst with a desire to drink: heat damaging body fluids • Unremitting fever and nasal discharge: Lung heat • Red tongue and rapid pulse: heat	• Releases exterior factors • Clears Lung heat • Corrects reversed flow of Lung qi	• *Ma Huang* (Herba Ephedrae) ventilates the Lung and directs Lung qi downward. • *Shi Gao* (Gypsum Fibrosum) clears Lung heat and restrains the warm property of *Ma Huang* (Herba Ephedrae). • *Ku Xing Ren* (Semen Armeniacae Amarum) corrects the reversed flow of Lung qi to relieve cough and dyspnea. • *Zhi Gan Cao* (Radix et Rhizoma Glycyrrhizae Praeparata cum Melle) generates body fluids and relieves thirst.

Má Huáng Xìng Rén Gān Căo Shí Gāo Tāng

(Ephedra, Apricot Kernel, Licorice, and Gypsum Decoction)

Unremitting fever and rhinitis occur as a result of heat trapped in the Lung. Coughing and dyspnea are the result of heat disrupting the proper descending flow of Lung qi. Heat damages body fluids, leading to thirst with a desire to drink. Heat also forces fluids out of the body, causing sweating in horses. However, this condition cannot be relieved by diaphoresis because it is no longer at the exterior level. If the heat damages body fluids extensively, there will be no sweating.

Ma Huang (Herba Ephedrae), the chief herb, ventilates the Lung and directs Lung qi downward. *Shi Gao* (Gypsum Fibrosum) is the deputy herb, yet its dose is double the amount of the chief herb for two key reasons: to sedate Lung heat, and to prevent the warm property of *Ma Huang* (Herba Ephedrae) from creating more heat. *Ku Xing Ren* (Semen Armeniacae Amarum) helps *Ma Huang* (Herba Ephedrae) to correct the reversed flow of Lung qi and relieve cough and dyspnea. *Zhi Gan Cao* (Radix et Rhizoma Glycyrrhizae Praeparata cum Melle) helps *Shi Gao* (Gypsum Fibrosum) generate body fluids and relieve thirst. It also harmonizes the descending, dispersing, warm, and cold properties of all of the herbs in this formula.

VETERINARY MODIFICATIONS

- When there is more cough and dyspnea, add *Sang Bai Pi* (Cortex Mori) and *Di Gu Pi* (Cortex Lycii).
- For severe cough and dyspnea, add *Xie Bai San* (Drain the White Powder).
- If there is cough with sputum, add *Jie Geng* (Radix Platycodonis).
- If there is blood in the sputum, add *Bai Mao Gen* (Rhizoma Imperatae) and *Ce Bai Ye* (Cacumen Platycladi).
- For fever, increased respiration, a thin, yellow tongue coating, and a rapid pulse, add *Zi Su Ye* (Folium Perillae), *Sang Ye* (Folium Mori), *Di Long* (Pheretima) and *Sang Bai Pi* (Cortex Mori).
- If high fever is present, add *Jin Yin Hua* (Flos Lonicerae Japonicae) and *Lian Qiao* (Fructus Forsythiae).
- If accompanied by edema of the face and lower limbs, add *Ting Li Zi* (Semen Descurainiae seu Lepidii) and *Che Qian Zi* (Semen Plantaginis).
- For thick, profuse and yellow sputum, add *Huang Qin* (Radix Scutellariae), *Gua Lou* (Fructus Trichosanthis), and *Zhe Bei Mu* (Bulbus Fritillariae Thunbergii).
- To increase heat-clearing ability and treat bacterial infection, one or more of the following can be added: *Yu Xing Cao* (Herba Houttuyniae), *Ban Lan Gen* (Radix Isatidis), *Da Qing Ye* (Folium Isatidis), *Huang Qin* (Radix Scutellariae), *Lian Qiao* (Fructus Forsythiae), *Jin Yin Hua* (Flos Lonicerae Japonicae) and *Pu Gong Ying* (Herba Taraxaci).
- For dry stool or constipation, add *Da Huang* (Radix et Rhizoma Rhei), *Mang Xiao* (Natrii Sulfas), and *Huo Ma Ren* (Fructus Cannabis).

CAUTIONS / CONTRAINDICATIONS

- *Ma Huang Xing Ren Gan Cao Shi Gao Tang* should be used with caution in the following situations: animals with Spleen and Stomach qi deficiencies; juvenile and geriatric patients; and those with general weakness or convalescing from chronic illness. When the use of this formula is necessary in such patients, it should be modified by adding *Sang Bai Pi* (Cortex Mori) and reducing the dose of *Shi Gao* (Gypsum Fibrosum).
- This formula is contraindicated for cough or dyspnea caused by wind-cold invasion or deficiency.
- According to one report, continuous use of over 10 packs of this formula in decoction has been associated with occasional incidents of poor appetite and abdominal distention.[1]
- The use of this formula in cats should be carefully monitored, as this species is sensitive to the effects of *Ma Huang* (Herba Ephedrae).

PHARMACOLOGICAL EFFECTS

1. **Antiasthmatic**: *Ma Huang Xing Ren Gan Cao Shi Gao Tang* demonstrated antiasthmatic effects to dilate the lung to treat asthma. The proposed mechanism of its antiasthmatic effects is its stimulation of beta2-adrenoceptors on bronchial smooth muscle and its anti-inflammatory ability to inhibit the neutrophil into the airway.[2] Though the individual component of *Ma Huang* (Herba Ephedrae) has effect to dilate the lung and treat cough and dyspnea, the effect is significantly less than the formula as a whole. It was pointed out that the maximum effect is achieved only when the four herbs are combined together. The stronger effect of the formula is attributed to the other three herbs, which not only help to treat the disorders, but also help to increase the extraction of ephedrine alkaloids by an additional 50%.[3]
2. **Antitussive**: Administration of *Ma Huang Xing Ren Gan Cao Shi Gao Tang* was associated with marked antitussive effects in mice and dogs with artificially-induced cough.[4]
3. **Effect on temperature regulation**: A group of rabbits with artificially-induced fever was divided into two groups to evaluate the effect of *Ma Huang Xing Ren Gan Cao Shi Gao Tang* on body temperature. Rabbits that received oral ingestion of the formula had an average of 1.27°C reduction of body temperature. Rabbits in the control

Má Huáng Xìng Rén Gān Cǎo Shí Gāo Tāng

(Ephedra, Apricot Kernel, Licorice, and Gypsum Decoction)

group that did not receive any treatment had an average of 0.93°C increase of body temperature.[5]

4. **Mast cell stabilizer**: Administration of *Ma Huang Xing Ren Gan Cao Shi Gao Tang* and *Xiao Feng San* (Eliminate Wind Powder) at 4-40 mcg/mL was found to inhibit IgE-dependent histamine released from mouse cultured mast cells.[6]

HUMAN CLINICAL STUDIES AND RESEARCH

1. **Acute bronchitis**: Use of *Ma Huang Xing Ren Gan Cao Shi Gao Tang* plus *Xiao Xian Xiong Tang* (Minor Sinking into the Chest Decoction) demonstrated a rate of effectiveness of 88% in treating acute bronchitis in 50 children. Additional modifications were made as deemed necessary. The herbs were cooked in water, and the resultant decoction (100 mL total) was taken in three to four equally-divided doses.[7]
2. **Chronic bronchitis**: Use of modified *Ma Huang Xing Ren Gan Cao Shi Gao Tang* produced good results in treating individuals with chronic bronchitis. The herbal treatment contained this formula plus *Huang Qin* (Radix Scutellariae), *Ban Xia* (Rhizoma Pinelliae) and *Yu Jin* (Radix Curcumae) as the base formula, plus *Yu Xing Cao* (Herba Houttuyniae) and *Jin Yin Hua* (Flos Lonicerae Japonicae) for presence of phlegm and heat; *Da Huang* (Radix et Rhizoma Rhei) and *Gua Lou* (Fructus Trichosanthis) for constipation; *Huang Qi* (Radix Astragali) and *Bai Zhu* (Rhizoma Atractylodis Macrocephalae) for qi deficiency; and *Tai Zi Shen* (Radix Pseudostellariae) and *Mai Dong* (Radix Ophiopogonis) for damaged yin. Of 46 cases, the study reported significant improvement in 34 cases, improvement in 8 cases, and no effect in 4 cases.[8]
3. **Pneumonia**: Use of *Ma Huang Xing Ren Gan Cao Shi Gao Tang* plus *Qing Dai* (Indigo Naturalis), *Huang Qin* (Radix Scutellariae) and others was associated with marked success in treating pneumonia in children. Modifications included addition of *Zi Su Zi* (Fructus Perillae), *Lai Fu Zi* (Semen Raphani) and *Di Long* (Pheretima) for hurried respiration with profuse sputum. The average duration of treatment was 6.2 days. Of 61 cases, the study reported complete recovery in 21 cases, near-recovery in 22 cases, improvement in 13 cases, and no effect in 5 cases.[9] According to another study, use of *Ma Huang Xing Ren Gan Cao Shi Gao Tang* plus *Ting Li Zi* (Semen Descurainiae seu Lepidii), *Da Qing Ye* (Folium Isatidis) and others was associated with 98.22% effectiveness in treating pneumonia in 56 children.[10] Lastly, 300 patients with pneumonia were treated with modified *Ma Huang Xing Ren Gan Cao Shi Gao Tang* with complete recovery in most patients within 2-3 days.[11]
4. **Upper respiratory tract infection**: Good results were reported in treating patients with upper respiratory tract infection using *Ma Huang Xing Ren Gan Cao Shi Gao Tang*. The study reported that 69.8% of patients had improvement of cough, 75.9% had reduction of sputum, and 78.3% had improvement of cough and dyspnea.[12]
5. **Cough and dyspnea**: *Ma Huang Xing Ren Gan Cao Shi Gao Tang* plus *Ting Li Zi* (Semen Descurainiae seu Lepidii) and other herbs was effective in treating all 40 children with cough and dyspnea.[13] Another study reported 93.75% effectiveness in treating bronchial cough and dyspnea in 80 children using *Ma Huang Xing Ren Gan Cao Shi Gao Tang* plus *Zao Jiao Ci* (Spina Gleditsiae), *Sang Bai Pi* (Cortex Mori) and others as needed.[14] Lastly, use of *Ma Huang Xing Ren Gan Cao Shi Gao Tang* plus *Dan Nan Xing* (Arisaema cum Bile), *Qian Hu* (Radix Peucedani) and others was successful in treating 82 children with cough and dyspnea. The duration of treatment ranged from 10 to 13 days.[15]
6. **Asthma**: Use of modified *Ma Huang Xing Ren Gan Cao Shi Gao Tang* produced marked results in treating asthma. Of 47 cases, the study reported complete recovery in 17 cases, significant improvement in 13 cases, moderate improvement in 11 cases, and no benefit in 6 cases. The average duration of herbal treatment was 34 days.[16] In another study, use of modified *Ma Huang Xing Ren Gan Cao Shi Gao Tang* in 37 patients with asthma was associated with 91.9% effectiveness. The herbal treatment contained *Ma Huang Xing Ren Gan Cao Shi Gao Tang* plus *Yu Xing Cao* (Herba Houttuyniae), *Zi Su Zi* (Fructus Perillae) and others as the base formula. Furthermore, *Lai Fu Zi* (Semen Raphani), *She Gan* (Rhizoma Belamcandae) and *Di Long* (Pheretima) were added for severe asthma; *Huang Qin* (Radix Scutellariae) and *Tian Hua Fen* (Radix Trichosanthis) for heat; *Tian Zhu Huang* (Concretio Silicea Bambusae), *Dan Nan Xing* (Arisaema cum Bile) and *Zhu Ru* (Caulis Bambusae in Taenia) for phlegm; and *Sha Shen* (Radix Glehniae seu Adenophorae), *Mai Dong* (Radix Ophiopogonis) and *Yu Zhu* (Rhizoma Polygonati Odorati) for dry cough with little or no sputum.[17]
7. **Fever**: Use of modified *Ma Huang Xing Ren Gan Cao Shi Gao Tang* in decoction was effective in treating 40 children with fever caused by infection. The herbal treatment contained this formula plus *Jin Yin Hua* (Flos Lonicerae Japonicae), *Lian Qiao* (Fructus Forsythiae), and *Huang Qin* (Radix Scutellariae) for presence of heat and toxins; *Jie Geng* (Radix Platycodonis) for cough; and *Huang Lian* (Rhizoma Coptidis) for diarrhea. The study reported normal body temperature within 12 hours in 39 of 40 children.[18] Another report pointed out that while this formula is effective in reducing fever, it does not address

Má Huáng Xìng Rén Gān Cǎo Shí Gāo Tāng

(Ephedra, Apricot Kernel, Licorice, and Gypsum Decoction)

the infection itself. Therefore, herbs with antibiotic effects should be added to increase the effectiveness of the treatment.[19]

8. **Acute pharyngitis**: One study involving 50 patients reported 94% effectiveness in treating acute pharyngitis using *Ma Huang Xing Ren Gan Cao Shi Gao Tang* plus *Ban Lan Gen* (Radix Isatidis), *Lian Qiao* (Fructus Forsythiae), and *Pu Gong Ying* (Herba Taraxaci).[20]
9. **Nasosinusitis**: In one study, 112 patients with acute nasosinusitis were treated with complete recovery in 90 patients, improvement in 19 patients, and no benefit in 3 patients. The overall rate of effectiveness was 97.4%. The herbal treatment contained *Ma Huang Xing Ren Gan Cao Shi Gao Tang* plus *Bai Zhi* (Radix Angelicae Dahuricae), *Cang Er Zi* (Fructus Xanthii), *Xin Yi Hua* (Flos Magnoliae), and others as needed. The duration of treatment ranged from 7-20 packs of herbs.[21]

SUGGESTED ACUPUNCTURE TREATMENT

1. Points: *Fengchi* (GB 20), *Dazhui* (GV 14), *Shaoshang* (LU 11), *Chize* (LU 5), *Hegu* (LI 4), *Lieque* (LU 7), *Erjian, Weijian, Dingchuan, Feizhishu* and *Feishu.*
2. Technique: sedation.

Fengchi (GB 20) releases the exterior. *Shaoshang* (LU 11) should be bled to sedate excess heat in the Lung. *Dazhui* (GV 14) is used to clear wind-heat. *Chize* (LU 5), the *he* (uniting) point of the Lung channel, relieves coughing and dyspnea. *Hegu* (LI 4) is the *yuan* (source) point of the Large Intestine channel, and *Lieque* (LU 7) is the *luo* (connecting) point of the Lung channel. Used together, *Hegu* (LI 4) and *Lieque* (LU 7) sedate Lung heat and dispel exterior factors. *Erjian* and *Weijian* are classical points that can be bled to clear heat. *Dingchuan*, another classical point can be used to stop cough. *Feizhishu* and *Feishu* are classical points that can clear Lung heat.

AUTHORS' COMMENTS

Ma Huang Xing Ren Gan Cao Shi Gao Tang is an effective formula for treating respiratory disorders in which the main diagnostic criterion is interior Lung heat. It is typically combined with other heat-clearing herbs in the treatment of Lung heat. It can be combined with *Yin Qiao San* (Honeysuckle and Forsythia Powder) to treat bronchitis and pneumonia in the dog and horse [see Authors' Comments for *Yin Qiao San* (Honeysuckle and Forsythia Powder)]. This formula addresses exogenous pathogen invasion of the Lung, which causes fever, stagnation and heat with phlegm, all factors that disrupt the Lung qi dispersing function. Pneumonia resulting from either infectious pathogens or aspiration may be treated with this formula. This formula is intended for otherwise healthy animals with normal gastrointestinal function. It is not for long-term use; once heat and phlegm have resolved, it is best to change to another formula to finish clearing heat, mildly ventilate the Lung, and tonify existing deficiencies. Combine this formula with *Ren Shen Ge Jie San* (Ginseng and Gecko Powder) for cats with chronic asthma. Similarly this combination can be used for dogs with chronic bronchitis that have Lung yin-deficient heat and chronic cough and/or that experience an acute asthma attack due to wind-heat, which typically occurs during abrupt seasonal changes.

Many modern disorders are not as simple as the clinical signs described above for this formula. For this reason, it is important to recognize when and how the patterns are different, and to modify the formula accordingly to treat the complications. Depending on each individual case, this formula can be prescribed singularly, or used as a base formula with the addition of herbs from the phlegm-eliminating, heat-clearing, cough-arresting and other categories. Its versatility is what makes it so useful.

- For cats with chronic asthma and dogs with chronic bronchitis that have Lung yin-deficiency heat and chronic cough and/or that experience an acute asthma attack due to wind-heat, combine with *Ren Shen Ge Jie San* (Ginseng and Gecko Powder).
- To treat bronchitis and pneumonia due to Lung heat in the dog and horse, combine this formula with other heat-clearing herbs or formulas, such as *Yin Qiao San* (Honeysuckle and Forsythia Powder).
- *Ma Huang Xing Ren Gan Cao Shi Gao Tang* contains a large amount of *Shi Gao* (Gypsum Fibrosum) to clear heat, restrain the effects of *Ma Huang* (Herba Ephedrae), ventilate the Lung, and direct Lung qi downward; the treatment of phlegm is secondary. If phlegm is the primary concern in the treatment of pneumonia, a formula such as *Qing Qi Hua Tan Wan* (Clear the Qi and Transform Phlegm Pill) would be more appropriate.

Ma Huang Xing Ren Gan Cao Shi Gao Tang and *Sang Ju Yin* (Mulberry Leaf and Chrysanthemum Decoction) both arrest cough, but have the following differences:

- *Ma Huang Xing Ren Gan Cao Shi Gao Tang* is a strong formula that clears and ventilates the Lung to arrest cough and dyspnea caused by Lung heat.
- *Sang Ju Yin* is a mild formula that treats the initial attack of wind-heat manifesting in cough. Patients will not show severe clinical signs, since the pathogenic factor still resides at the *wei* (defensive) level.

Má Huáng Xìng Rén Gān Căo Shí Gāo Tāng

(Ephedra, Apricot Kernel, Licorice, and Gypsum Decoction)

Ma Huang Xing Ren Gan Cao Shi Gao Tang and *Xie Bai San* (Drain the White Powder) both clear Lung heat to relieve cough and dyspnea, but have contrasting differences:

- *Ma Huang Xing Ren Gan Cao Shi Gao Tang* treats Lung heat syndrome following a wind-heat or wind-cold invasion. Besides addressing clinical signs of cough and dyspnea, this formula also treats fever, thirst with a preference to drink, and a rapid, forceful pulse. It sedates Lung heat and ventilates Lung qi and primarily treats cases of excess pathogenic factors invading the Lung.
- *Xie Bai San* is designed for juvenile and yin-deficient animals who have hidden stagnant Lung heat that leads to qi reversal and gradual body fluid depletion. Aside from cough and dyspnea, accompanying clinical signs include warm, steaming sensations on the skin, especially in the late afternoon, and a rapid, fine pulse. Because the *zang fu* organs in young animals are still tender, they are much more susceptible to damage. For this reason, the draining herbs in this formula, such as *Sang Bai Pi* (Cortex Mori), are milder in nature. *Di Gu Pi* (Cortex Lycii) clears deficiency heat, while *Geng Mi* (Semen Oryzae) and *Gan Cao* (Radix et Rhizoma Glycyrrhizae) strengthen the Spleen and Stomach (earth element) in order to promote the Lung (metal element). Together, the herbs clear heat without injuring yin, and sedate the Lung without injuring *zheng* (upright) *qi*. In short, *Xie Bai San* cools and nourishes the Lung, and is indicated for chronic cases of cough or dyspnea in yin-deficient patients.[22]

References

1. *Zhong Xi Yi Jie He Za Zhi* (Journal of Integrated Chinese and Western Medicine), 1885; (9):540.
2. Kao ST, Yeh TJ, Hsieh CC, Shiau HB, Yeh FT, Lin JG. The effects of Ma-Xing-Gan-Shi-Tang on respiratory resistance and airway leukocyte infiltration in asthmatic guinea pigs. Immunopharmacol Immunotoxicol. 2001 Aug; 23(3):445-58.
3. *Zhong Yi Yao Yan Jiu Zi Liao* (Research and Resource of Chinese Medicine and Herbology), 1986; (1):31.
4. *Zhong Cheng Yao Yan Jiu* (Research of Chinese Patent Medicine), 1987; (4):47.
5. *Zhong Cheng Yao Yan Jiu* (Research of Chinese Patent Medicine), 1984; (6):21.
6. Shichijo K, Saito H. Effect of Chinese herbal medicines and disodium cromoglycate on IgE-dependent histamine release from mouse cultured mast cells. Int J Immunopharmacol. 1997 Nov-Dec; 19 (11-12):677-82.
7. *Shang Hai Zhong Yi Yao Za Zhi* (Shanghai Journal of Chinese Medicine and Herbology), 1986; 1:26.
8. *Nan Jing Zhong Yi Yao Da Xue Xue Bao* (Journal of Nanjing University of Traditional Chinese Medicine and Medicinals), 1996; 1:59.
9. *Zhe Jiang Zhong Yi Za Zhi* (Zhejiang Journal of Chinese Medicine), 1982; 11-12:498.
10. *Hei Long Jiang Zhong Yi Yao* (Heilongjiang Chinese Medicine and Herbology), 1994; 3:38.
11. *Zhong Yi Fang Ji Xian Dai Yan Jiu* (Modern Study of Medical Formulas in Traditional Chinese Medicine), 1997; (1):113.
12. *Zhong Yi Fang Ji Xian Dai Yan Jiu* (Modern Study of Medical Formulas in Traditional Chinese Medicine), 1997; (1):113.
13. *Jiang Su Zhong Yi Za Zhi* (Jiangsu Journal of Chinese Medicine), 1965; 11:15.
14. *Jiang Su Zhong Yi* (Jiangsu Chinese Medicine), 1988; 7:11.
15. *Hu Bei Zhong Yi Za Zhi* (Hubei Journal of Chinese Medicine), 1992; 3:16.
16. *Shi Yong Zhong Yi Nei Ke Za Zhi* (Journal of Practical Chinese Internal Medicine), 1989; 4:23.
17. *Zhe Jiang Zhong Yi Xue Yuan Xue Bao* (Journal of Zhejiang University of Chinese Medicine), 1998; 3:22.
18. *Hu Bei Zhong Yi Za Zhi* (Hubei Journal of Chinese Medicine), 1987; 1:15.
19. *Hu Bei Zhong Yi Za Zhi* (Hubei Journal of Chinese Medicine), 1987; (1):15.
20. *Jiang Xi Zhong Yi Yao* (Jiangxi Chinese Medicine and Herbology), 1989; 4:36.
21. *Zhong Yi Ming Fang Lin Chuang Xin Yong* (Contemporary Clinical Applications of Classic Chinese Formulas), 2001; 646.
22. Wang MZ, et al. *Zhong Yi Xue Wen Da Ti Ku* (Questions and Answers on Traditional Chinese Medicine: Herbal Formulas).

Níng Sòu Wán (Quiet the Cough Pill)

寧嗽丸
宁嗽丸

Pinyin Name: *Ning Sou Wan*
Literal Name: Quiet the Cough Pill
Alternate Names: Cough-Stopping Pill, Fritillaria and Platycodon Formula
Original Source: *Zhong Guo Guo Yao Gu You Cheng Fang Xuan Ji* (A Selection of Traditional Prescriptions of Chinese Medicine) by the Chinese Herbal Medicine Committee of the Ministry of the Interior in 1967

COMPOSITION

Zi Su Zi (Fructus Perillae)	60g
Ku Xing Ren (Semen Armeniacae Amarum)	45g
Jie Geng (Radix Platycodonis)	60g
Ban Xia (Rhizoma Pinelliae), *zhi* (prepared)	60g
Chuan Bei Mu (Bulbus Fritillariae Cirrhosae)	60g
Ju Hong (Exocarpium Citri Reticulatae)	30g
Bo He (Herba Menthae)	45g
Fu Ling (Poria)	60g
Gu Ya (Fructus Setariae Germinatus)	30g
Sang Bai Pi (Cortex Mori)	45g
Shi Hu (Caulis Dendrobii)	60g
Zhi Gan Cao (Radix et Rhizoma Glycyrrhizae Praeparata cum Melle)	15g

DOSAGE / PREPARATION / ADMINISTRATION

First, cook *Sang Bai Pi* (Cortex Mori) and *Shi Hu* (Caulis Dendrobii) in water to obtain a decoction. Grind the rest of the ingredients into a fine powder. Mix the decoction and the powder together to form pills, which should resemble *Lu Dou* (Semen Phaseoli Radiati) in size. Take 4.5g of pills twice daily with warm water.

CHINESE THERAPEUTIC ACTIONS

1. Clears the Lung and disperses stagnation
2. Dissolves phlegm and relieves cough

CLINICAL MANIFESTATIONS

Fever, cough with phlegm, wheezing and dyspnea, sneezing, and aversion to wind.

VETERINARY CLINICAL APPLICATIONS

Cough, upper respiratory infection with cough with clear or white phlegm, feline asthma, tracheitis, cough from acute and chronic bronchitis.

EXPLANATION

Ning Sou Wan (Quiet the Cough Pill) treats cases of exterior wind-heat attacking the body, with chief complaints of cough with phlegm and fever. Since wind-heat can interfere with the normal functions of the Lung, clinical signs usually include cough, wheezing, dyspnea, nasal obstruction, nasal discharge, and stiff neck.

Many herbs in this formula have distinct effects to dispel phlegm, clear the Lung, and arrest coughing; such herbs include *Zi Su Zi* (Fructus Perillae), *Ku Xing Ren* (Semen Armeniacae Amarum), *Jie Geng* (Radix Platycodonis), *Ban Xia* (Rhizoma Pinelliae), *Chuan Bei Mu* (Bulbus Fritillariae Cirrhosae), and *Ju Hong* (Exocarpium Citri Rubrum). *Bo He* (Herba Menthae) dispels exterior wind-heat. Its cooling property also helps restrict the other warm herbs from creating heat in the body. *Fu Ling* (Poria) and *Gu Ya* (Fructus Setariae Germinatus) strengthen the Spleen, transform water, and prevent further formation of dampness and phlegm. *Sang Bai Pi* (Cortex Mori) promotes urination and drains dampness from the body. *Shi Hu* (Caulis Dendrobii) moistens the Lung, relieves cough, and prevents the phlegm-eliminating herbs from injuring yin. *Zhi Gan Cao* (Radix et Rhizoma Glycyrrhizae Praeparata cum Melle) harmonizes the entire formula.

Níng Sòu Wán (Quiet the Cough Pill)

***Ning Sou Wan* (Quiet the Cough Pill)**

Diagnosis	Clinical Signs	Treatment	Herbs
Cough due to exterior wind-heat	• Fever, and aversion to wind: exterior wind-heat condition • Nasal obstruction, nasal discharge, and sneezing: wind-heat affecting Lung qi circulation • Cough, wheezing and dyspnea: reversed flow of Lung qi • Phlegm: presence of dampness	• Clears the Lung and disperses stagnation • Dissolves phlegm and relieves cough	• *Zi Su Zi* (Fructus Perillae), *Ku Xing Ren* (Semen Armeniacae Amarum), *Jie Geng* (Radix Platycodonis), *Ban Xia* (Rhizoma Pinelliae), *Chuan Bei Mu* (Bulbus Fritillariae Cirrhosae), and *Ju Hong* (Exocarpium Citri Rubrum) dispel phlegm, clear the Lung, and arrest cough. • *Bo He* (Herba Menthae) dispels exterior wind-heat. • *Fu Ling* (Poria) and *Gu Ya* (Fructus Setariae Germinatus) strengthen the Spleen and prevent the formation of dampness and phlegm. • *Sang Bai Pi* (Cortex Mori) promotes urination and drains dampness out of the body. • *Shi Hu* (Caulis Dendrobii) moistens the Lung, relieves cough, and prevents the phlegm-eliminating herbs from injuring yin. • *Zhi Gan Cao* (Radix et Rhizoma Glycyrrhizae Praeparata cum Melle) harmonizes the herbs.

VETERINARY MODIFICATIONS

- For cough caused by upper respiratory infection, add *Hua Gai San* (Canopy Powder).
- For cough caused by Lung heat, add *Xie Bai San* (Drain the White Powder).
- For cough caused by phlegm, add *Er Chen Tang* (Two-Cured Decoction).
- If there is a dry throat and thirst, add *Mai Dong* (Radix Ophiopogonis) and *Wu Wei Zi* (Fructus Schisandrae Chinensis).

SUGGESTED ACUPUNCTURE TREATMENT

1. Points: *Quchi* (LI 11), *Hegu* (LI 4), *Tiantu* (CV 22), *Fengmen* (BL 12), *Feishu* (BL 13), *Fenglong* (ST 40), *Housanli* (ST 36), *Lieque* (LU 7), *Chize* (LU 5), and *Dingchuan*.
2. Technique: sedation.

Quchi (LI 11), *Hegu* (LI 4), *Tiantu* (CV 22), *Fengmen* (BL 12), *Feishu* (BL 13), and *Fenglong* (ST 40) dispel phlegm and arrest cough. *Lieque* (LU 7) and *Chize* (LU 5) clear Lung heat and preserve yin. *Housanli* (ST 36) strengthens the Spleen to dissolve phlegm. *Dingchuan* stops cough.

AUTHORS' COMMENTS

Ning Sou Wan can be used in veterinary medicine to quiet cough caused by wind-heat and phlegm obstructing the qi flow of the Lung. In addition to herbs which clear wind-heat and phlegm, it contains herbs which moisten and protect the Lung and strengthen the Spleen to prevent continued accumulation of dampness and phlegm. Overall, it is a balanced formula for the treatment of chronic cough and, because of its energetic neutrality, can be used in combination with other respiratory formulas solely to address the symptom of coughing. However, chronic cough will often damage the Lung, and once clinical signs have resolved, administration of a Lung tonic, such as *Bu Fei Tang* (Tonify the Lung Decoction), would be prudent. *Ning Sou Wan* can be used to treat feline asthma in cats with residual wheezing and asthmatic breathing that occur after an acute asthma attack.

Please see **Authors' Comments** for *Zhi Sou San* (Stop Coughing Powder) for a comparison of formulas to stop coughing.

Dùn Sòu Sǎn (Long-Bout Cough Powder)

頓嗽散
顿嗽散

Pinyin Name: *Dun Sou San*
Literal Name: Long-Bout Cough Powder
Alternate Name: Morus and Platycodon Formula
Original Source: *Yan Fang* (Time-Tested Formulas) of unknown author and date

COMPOSITION

Chai Hu (Radix Bupleuri)	15g
Huang Qin (Radix Scutellariae)	9g
Sang Bai Pi (Cortex Mori)	9g
Jie Geng (Radix Platycodonis)	9g
Zhi Zi (Fructus Gardeniae)	7.5g
Shi Gao (Gypsum Fibrosum)	15g
Gan Cao (Radix et Rhizoma Glycyrrhizae)	3g

CHINESE THERAPEUTIC ACTIONS

1. Arrests cough
2. Clears heat and dissolves phlegm

CLINICAL MANIFESTATIONS

Cough caused by heat: persistent or violent cough, cough with or without sputum.

VETERINARY CLINICAL APPLICATIONS

Cough, cough from upper respiratory infection or bronchitis, cough with heat and phlegm, and post-heartworm treatment in dogs.

EXPLANATION

Dun Sou San (Long-Bout Cough Powder) treats cough caused by heat. This formula uses *Chai Hu* (Radix Bupleuri) and *Huang Qin* (Radix Scutellariae) to clear heat from the chest to relieve the stifling sensation or the feeling of oppression and congestion. *Sang Bai Pi* (Cortex Mori) and *Jie Geng* (Radix Platycodonis) dissolve phlegm and relieve coughing. *Zhi Zi* (Fructus Gardeniae) clears heat from the Lung to relieve irritability. *Shi Gao* (Gypsum Fibrosum) clears heat from the Lung and lowers fever. *Gan Cao* (Radix et Rhizoma Glycyrrhizae) tonifies qi and harmonizes the formula.

SUGGESTED ACUPUNCTURE TREATMENT

1. Points: *Shanzhong* (CV 17), *Lieque* (LU 7), *Tiantu* (CV 22), *Quchi* (LI 11), *Yuji* (LU 10), *Housanli* (ST 36) and *Dingchuan*.
2. Technique: sedation.

Shanzhong (CV 17) opens the chest, while *Quchi* (LI 11) and *Yuji* (LU 10) clear heat in the Lung. *Lieque* (LU 7) and

***Dun Sou San* (Long-Bout Cough Powder)**

Diagnosis	Clinical Signs	Treatment	Herbs
Cough caused by heat	• Persistent or violent cough: heat disturbing Lung qi circulation • Cough with little sputum or no sputum: heat consuming body fluids	• Arrests cough • Clears heat and dissolves phlegm	• *Chai Hu* (Radix Bupleuri) and *Huang Qin* (Radix Scutellariae) clear heat from the chest and relieve the feeling of oppression or congestion. • *Sang Bai Pi* (Cortex Mori) and *Jie Geng* (Radix Platycodonis) dissolve phlegm and relieve coughing. • *Zhi Zi* (Fructus Gardeniae) clears heat and eliminates toxins. • *Shi Gao* (Gypsum Fibrosum) clears heat from the Lung and reduces fever. • *Gan Cao* (Radix et Rhizoma Glycyrrhizae) tonifies qi and harmonizes the herbs.

Dùn Sòu Săn (Long-Bout Cough Powder)

Tiantu (CV 22) dissolve phlegm and direct qi downward. *Housanli* (ST 36) regulates and harmonizes qi. *Dingchuan* stops cough.

AUTHORS' COMMENTS

Dun Sou San was originally developed in Japan for treating cough. Clinically, it treats cough secondary to pulmonary infections, such as viral pneumonia or bronchitis, and is useful in horses that suffer from a persistent cough after recovering from pleuropneumonia, rhinopneumonitis, and *Streptococcus equi* infections.

Dun Sou San can be used to treat coughing due to interior heat and phlegm in the Lung which has not resolved despite antibiotic therapy following treatment for canine heartworm disease. These animals may present with mild to moderate fever and have a harsh choking cough that sounds dry without mucus. These animals nearly always have a variable component of Lung qi and yin deficiencies in addition to retained heat and phlegm. This formula is comprised of seven herbs, four of which clear heat: *Shi Gao* (Gypsum Fibrosum), *Chai Hu* (Radix Bupleuri), *Huang Qin* (Radix Scutellariae) and *Zhi Zi* (Fructus Gardeniae). If significant heat and phlegm are not present and cough is due to phlegm that is hard to expectorate, use *Zhi Sou San* (Stop Coughing Powder). *Dun Sou San* is not for long-term use; once heat and phlegm have been resolved it should be discontinued. It should not be used in Spleen qi deficient animals without modification.

Please see **Authors' Comments** for *Zhi Sou San* (Stop Coughing Powder) for a comparison of formulas to stop coughing.

Zhĭ Sòu Săn (Stop Coughing Powder)

止嗽散

Pinyin Name: *Zhi Sou San*
Literal Name: Stop Coughing Powder
Alternate Names: *Chih Sou San*, Cough-Stopping Powder, Platycodon and Schizonepeta Formula, Citrus and Apricot Seed Formula
Original Source: *Yi Xue Xin Wu* (Medical Revelations) by Cheng Guo-Peng in 1732

COMPOSITION

Zi Wan (Radix et Rhizoma Asteris), *zheng* (steamed)	1,000g [9g]
Bai Qian (Rhizoma et Radix Cynanchi Stauntonii), *zheng* (steamed)	1,000g [9g]
Bai Bu (Radix Stemonae), *zheng* (steamed)	1,000g [9g]
Jie Geng (Radix Platycodonis), *chao* (dry-fried)	1,000g [9g]
Chen Pi (Pericarpium Citri Reticulatae)	500g [9g]
Jing Jie (Herba Schizonepetae)	1,000g [9g]
Gan Cao (Radix et Rhizoma Glycyrrhizae), *chao* (dry-fried)	375g [3g]

DOSAGE / PREPARATION / ADMINISTRATION

The source text instructions are to grind the ingredients into powder. Take 9g of the powder with boiled water after meals and before bedtime. This formula may be taken with a decoction of *Sheng Jiang* (Rhizoma Zingiberis Recens) if there are external wind-cold clinical signs present. Today, this formula is generally administered by giving 6g of the powdered herbs with warm, boiled water or with a decoction of *Sheng Jiang* (Rhizoma Zingiberis Recens). This formula may also be prepared as a decoction with the doses suggested in brackets above.

CHINESE THERAPEUTIC ACTIONS

1. Stops coughing and dissolves phlegm
2. Releases exterior factors and ventilates the Lung

CLINICAL MANIFESTATIONS

Wind invading the Lung: coughing, mild fever and aversion to cold.

Zhǐ Sòu Sǎn (Stop Coughing Powder)

VETERINARY CLINICAL APPLICATIONS

Cough with exterior condition, allergic bronchitis, feline upper respiratory tract infection, persistent cough secondary to infection, canine chronic bronchitis and cough following heartworm treatment.

EXPLANATION

Zhi Sou San (Stop Coughing Powder) treats persistent coughing that cannot be alleviated after the administration of exterior-releasing herbs. In this situation, the exterior clinical signs, such as fever and aversion to cold, will be mostly resolved by the exterior-releasing method, but the abnormal Lung qi flow persists.

The treatment approach for this syndrome places more emphasis on arresting the cough, and less on releasing the exterior. *Zi Wan* (Radix et Rhizoma Asteris), *Bai Qian* (Rhizoma et Radix Cynanchi Stauntonii), and *Bai Bu* (Radix Stemonae) dissolve phlegm and stop cough. These three herbs have excellent synergistic effects to treat both acute and chronic cough. *Jie Geng* (Radix Platycodonis) and *Chen Pi* (Pericarpium Citri Reticulatae) ventilate the Lung, cause the Lung qi to descend, and dissolve phlegm. *Jing Jie* (Herba Schizonepetae) expels wind and relieves exterior clinical signs. *Gan Cao* (Radix et Rhizoma Glycyrrhizae), besides harmonizing all of the herbs, works with *Jie Geng* (Radix Platycodonis) to relieve itchy throat.

VETERINARY MODIFICATIONS

- For cough caused by wind-heat, add *Sang Ye* (Folium Mori), *Ju Hua* (Flos Chrysanthemi), and *Bo He* (Herba Menthae).
- For cough with white sputum caused by a wind-cold invasion, add *Zi Su Ye* (Folium Perillae), *Fang Feng* (Radix Saposhnikoviae), and *Ku Xing Ren* (Semen Armeniacae Amarum).
- For dry cough with absence of sputum because of Lung dryness, add *Gua Lou* (Fructus Trichosanthis), *Bei Mu* (Bulbus Fritillariae), and *Zhi Mu* (Rhizoma Anemarrhenae).
- For dry cough with a sore throat, add *Sang Ye* (Folium Mori), *Sha Shen* (Radix Glehniae seu Adenophorae), and *She Gan* (Rhizoma Belamcandae).
- For cough and a greasy tongue coating caused by summer-dampness, add *Huo Xiang* (Herba Agastaches), *Pei Lan* (Herba Eupatorii), and *Xiang Ru* (Herba Moslae).
- For cough with profuse sputum, add *Ban Xia* (Rhizoma Pinelliae) and *Fu Ling* (Poria).
- For cough with profuse sputum and a stifling sensation in the chest due to phlegm-damp obstruction, add *Ban Xia* (Rhizoma Pinelliae), *Fu Ling* (Poria), and *Chen Pi* (Pericarpium Citri Reticulatae).
- For cough and fever in children, add *Jin Yin Hua* (Flos Lonicerae Japonicae), *Niu Bang Zi* (Fructus Arctii), *Huang Qin* (Radix Scutellariae), *Zi Su Zi* (Fructus Perillae), *Ku Xing Ren* (Semen Armeniacae Amarum), and *Chuan Bei Mu* (Bulbus Fritillariae Cirrhosae).
- If there is profuse, thick sputum as a result of damp accumulation, add *Ban Xia* (Rhizoma Pinelliae), *Fu Ling* (Poria), and *Sang Bai Pi* (Cortex Mori).

CAUTIONS / CONTRAINDICATIONS

- *Zhi Sou San* contains many herbs that are warm and drying in nature; thus, it is not suitable for chronic cough caused by yin deficiency, Lung heat, or phlegm heat.
- This formula should be used with extreme caution if the cough is accompanied by blood-streaked phlegm.[1]

HUMAN CLINICAL STUDIES AND RESEARCH

1. **Cough**: Modified *Zhi Sou San* demonstrated 90% effectiveness in treating cough associated with various causes and conditions. In addition to *Zhi Sou San*, modifications

***Zhi Sou San* (Stop Coughing Powder)**

Diagnosis	Clinical Signs	Treatment	Herbs
Cough due to wind invading the Lung	• Coughing: obstruction of Lung qi circulation • Fever, and aversion to cold: exterior wind	• Stops coughing and dissolves phlegm • Releases exterior factors and ventilates the Lung	• *Zi Wan* (Radix et Rhizoma Asteris), *Bai Qian* (Rhizoma et Radix Cynanchi Stauntonii) and *Bai Bu* (Radix Stemonae) dissolve phlegm and stop cough. • *Jie Geng* (Radix Platycodonis) and *Chen Pi* (Pericarpium Citri Reticulatae) ventilate the Lung, cause the Lung qi to descend, and dissolve phlegm. • *Jing Jie* (Herba Schizonepetae) expels wind and relieves exterior clinical signs. • *Gan Cao* (Radix et Rhizoma Glycyrrhizae) harmonizes the herbs.

Zhǐ Sòu Sǎn (Stop Coughing Powder)

were made as follows: for cough due to wind-cold, *Fang Feng* (Radix Saposhnikoviae), *Ku Xing Ren* (Semen Armeniacae Amarum), and *Qiang Huo* (Rhizoma et Radix Notopterygii) were added; for cough due to wind-heat, *Sang Ye* (Folium Mori) and *Ku Xing Ren* (Semen Armeniacae Amarum) were added and the dose of *Jing Jie* (Herba Schizonepetae) was reduced; for dampness and phlegm affecting the Lung, *Huang Qin* (Radix Scutellariae), *Jie Geng* (Radix Platycodonis), and *Ku Xing Ren* (Semen Armeniacae Amarum) were added, and *Jing Jie* (Herba Schizonepetae) was removed; for dryness affecting the Lung, *Sha Shen* (Radix Glehniae seu Adenophorae), *Xuan Shen* (Radix Scrophulariae), and *Zhi Mu* (Rhizoma Anemarrhenae) were added, and the doses were reduced for *Jing Jie* (Herba Schizonepetae), *Bai Qian* (Rhizoma et Radix Cynanchi Stauntonii), and *Chen Pi* (Pericarpium Citri Reticulatae).[2]

2. **Cough with exterior condition**: One study reported 94% effectiveness using modified *Zhi Sou San* to treat cough associated with an exterior condition. The herbal treatment contained *Zhi Sou San* plus *Mu Dan Pi* (Cortex Moutan) and *Dan Shen* (Radix et Rhizoma Salviae Miltiorrhizae) as the base formula. In addition, *Bai He* (Bulbus Lilii) and *Mai Dong* (Radix Ophiopogonis) were added for dry cough caused by dryness and heat damaging the Lung; *Yuan Zhi* (Radix Polygalae) and *Ban Xia* (Rhizoma Pinelliae) were added for cough with profuse, white sputum; and *Sang Bai Pi* (Cortex Mori) and *Huang Qin* (Radix Scutellariae) were added for cough with yellow sputum. Of 50 cases, the study reported complete recovery in 23 cases, improvement in 24 cases, and no benefit in 3 cases.[3]
3. **Respiratory tract infection**: Eighty patients with respiratory tract infections were divided into two groups and treated with herbs or drugs three times daily, for 3 days per course of treatment. Group one of 40 patients received *Zhi Sou San*, and group two of 40 patients received antibiotic drugs. For group one, the study reported complete recovery in 34 patients, moderate improvement in 5 patients, and no benefit in 1 case. For group two, the study reported complete recovery in 10 patients, moderate improvement in 12 patients, and no effect in 18 patients.[4]
4. **Acute bronchitis**: One hundred children with acute bronchitis were treated with complete recovery in 92 cases and improvement in 2 cases. The herbal treatment was based on *Zhi Sou San* with the addition of *Tian Zhu Huang* (Concretio Silicea Bambusae), *Gua Lou Pi* (Pericarpium Trichosanthis), *Huang Qi* (Radix Astragali), *Sang Bai Pi* (Cortex Mori), *Qian Hu* (Radix Peucedani), and *Jin Yin Hua* (Flos Lonicerae Japonicae). Most patients had complete recovery within 4-6 packs of herbs.[5] In another study, *Zhi Sou San* successfully treated 147 of 153 patients (91 males and 62 females) with bronchitis for 2-32 days. The duration of treatment was between 2 and 8 packs of herbs.[6]
5. **Chronic bronchitis**: One study reported marked effectiveness using modified *Zhi Sou San* to treat chronic bronchitis. Of 30 patients, 23 had significant improvement, 6 had improvement, and 1 had slight improvement. The herbal treatment was modified by removing *Jing Jie* (Herba Schizonepetae) and adding *Ku Xing Ren* (Semen Armeniacae Amarum) and *Dan Shen* (Radix et Rhizoma Salviae Miltiorrhizae) to *Zhi Sou San*. Furthermore, *Huang Qin* (Radix Scutellariae) and *Sang Bai Pi* (Cortex Mori) were added for hot phlegm; *Ma Huang* (Herba Ephedrae) and *Xi Xin* (Radix et Rhizoma Asari) for cold phlegm; *Sha Shen* (Radix Glehniae seu Adenophorae) and *Mai Dong* (Radix Ophiopogonis) for Lung dryness; and *Dang Shen* (Radix Codonopsis) and *Huang Qi* (Radix Astragali) for Lung and Spleen qi deficiencies.[7]
6. **Interstitial pneumonia**: Modified *Zhi Sou San* showed marked effectiveness in treating interstitial pneumonia. The base formula included *Zhi Sou San* plus *Tao Ren* (Semen Persicae) and *Ban Lan Gen* (Radix Isatidis). Other herbs were added as deemed necessary: *San Ao Tang* (Three-Unbinding Decoction) for wind-cold; *Ma Huang Xing Ren Gan Cao Shi Gao Tang* (Ephedra, Apricot Kernel, Licorice, and Gypsum Decoction), *Jin Yin Hua* (Flos Lonicerae Japonicae), and *Lian Qiao* (Fructus Forsythiae) for fever with cough; and *Ping Wei San* (Calm the Stomach Powder) for excessive dampness and phlegm. Each course of treatment was 6 days. The average duration of treatment was 1.6 courses.[8]

SUGGESTED ACUPUNCTURE TREATMENT

1. Points: *Lieque* (LU 7), *Feishu* (BL 13), *Zhaohai* (KI 6), *Hegu* (LI 4), *Waiguan* (TH 5), and *Dingchuan*.
2. Technique: sedation.

The aim of the acupuncture treatment is to stop cough, dissolve phlegm, dispel exterior factors, and ventilate the Lung. *Lieque* (LU 7), the *luo* (connecting) point of the Lung channel, and *Feishu* (BL 13), the *shu* (transport) point of the Lung, regulate Lung qi, ventilate the Lung, and stop coughing. *Zhaohai* (KI 6) has a specific function to relieve itchy throat. *Hegu* (LI 4) and *Waiguan* (TH 5) together dispel exterior factors. *Dingchuan* stops cough.

AUTHORS' COMMENTS

Zhi Sou San ventilates the Lung, expels wind, and is widely used to treat cough due to various causes. It is especially effective in treating cough with lingering exterior pathogenic factors. Key clinical signs include cough with a tickling sensation in the throat, slight aversion to wind, fever, and a thin, white tongue coating. This pattern may

Zhǐ Sòu Sǎn (Stop Coughing Powder)

be seen in canine kennel cough and in chronic feline rhinotracheitis where there is residual cough, especially if antibiotic therapy was administered, and with phlegm that is hard to expectorate. Many owners describe this type of cough as productive, with the pet "gagging but can't get anything to come up" despite repeated bouts of cough. Horses may also have a lingering cough post-infection. While *Dun Sou San* (Long-Bout Cough Powder) is appropriate if heat is still lingering in the patient, *Zhi Sou San* is more suited for those in which wind and cold were the primary pathogens. Exercise will often induce a violent, productive cough, even in those patients that appear fully recovered.

Ning Sou Wan (Quiet the Cough Pill), *Dun Sou San* (Long-Bout Cough Powder), and *Zhi Sou San* (Stop Coughing Powder) are three formulas commonly used to treat cough in veterinary medicine. Their major differences are as follows:

- *Ning Sou Wan* quiets cough caused by wind-heat and transforms phlegm. It contains *Shi Hu* (Caulis Dendrobii) which moistens the Lung, and prevents the phlegm-eliminating herbs from damaging Lung yin, as well as herbs to strengthen the Spleen to prevent continued accumulation of dampness and phlegm. It contains *Zhi Gan Cao* (Radix et Rhizoma Glycyrrhizae Praeparata cum Melle), the honey-processed form of *Gan Cao* (Radix et Rhizoma Glycyrrhizae), making this formula a better choice to tonify the Spleen, benefit qi, moisten the Lung and stop cough than the other formulas in this group. Overall, it is the most balanced formula for the treatment of chronic cough. It can also be used to treat feline asthma in cats with residual wheezing and asthmatic breathing that can often occur after an acute asthma attack has been stabilized. In effect, it is a good transition formula before the employment of tonifying maintenance formulas for the Lung and Spleen.
- *Dun Sou San* stops cough caused by heat and phlegm in the interior. Its focus is on clearing heat prior to clearing phlegm, rather than releasing the exterior. It is made up of seven herbs, four of which clear heat: (*Shi Gao* (Gypsum Fibrosum), *Chai Hu* (Radix Bupleuri), *Huang Qin* (Radix Scutellariae) and *Zhi Zi* (Fructus Gardeniae)). It is not for long-term use; once heat and phlegm have been resolved it should be discontinued. It should not be used in Spleen qi deficient animals without modification.
- *Zhi Sou San* stops cough caused by wind at the exterior and phlegm in the interior. It focuses more on resolving phlegm and restoring the normal flow of Lung qi, than on releasing the exterior.

References

1. Chen Q, *Zhong Yao Ming Fang Yao Li Yu Ying Yong* (Pharmacology and Applications of Famous Herbal Formulas), 1989; 599-600.
2. *Yun Nan Zhong Yi Zhong Yao Za Zhi* (Yunnan Journal of Traditional Chinese Medicine and Herbal Medicine), 1999; 4:15.
3. *Zhong Yi Ming Fang Lin Chuang Xin Yong* (Contemporary Clinical Applications of Classic Chinese Formulas), 2001; 136.
4. *Shi Zhen Guo Yao Yan Jiu* (Research of Shizhen Herbs), 1995; 2:37.
5. *Shi Yong Zhong Xi Yi Jie He Za Zhi* (Practical Journal of Integrated Chinese and Western Medicines), 1995; 10:634.
6. *Zhong Yi Ming Fang Lin Chuang Xin Yong* (Contemporary Clinical Applications of Classic Chinese Formulas), 2001; 138.
7. *Zhong Yuan Yi Kan* (Resource Journal of Chinese Medicine), 1994; 5:44.
8. *Shi Yong Zhong Xi Yi Jie He Za Zhi* (Practical Journal of Integrated Chinese and Western Medicines), 1995; 3:152.

Jīng Jiè Lián Qiào Tāng (Schizonepeta and Forsythia Decoction)

荊芥連翹湯
荆芥连翘汤

Pinyin Name: *Jing Jie Lian Qiao Tang*
Literal Name: Schizonepeta and Forsythia Decoction
Alternate Names: *Ching Chieh Lien Chiao Tang, Jing Jie Lian Chiao Tang*, Schizonepeta and Forsythia Combination
Original Source: *Wan Bing Hui Chun* (Restoration of Health from the Myriad Diseases) by Gong Ting-Xian in 1587

COMPOSITION

Jing Jie (Herba Schizonepetae)
Fang Feng (Radix Saposhnikoviae)
Lian Qiao (Fructus Forsythiae)
Jie Geng (Radix Platycodonis)
Huang Qin (Radix Scutellariae)
Zhi Zi (Fructus Gardeniae)
Bai Zhi (Radix Angelicae Dahuricae)
Chai Hu (Radix Bupleuri)
Zhi Qiao (Fructus Citri Aurantii)
Dang Gui (Radix Angelicae Sinensis)
Chuan Xiong (Rhizoma Chuanxiong)
Bai Shao (Radix Paeoniae Alba)
Gan Cao (Radix et Rhizoma Glycyrrhizae)

DOSAGE / PREPARATION / ADMINISTRATION

Cook all of the ingredients in water, and take the decoction after meals. Note: Exact doses of the herbs are unavailable. The source text only states to use equal amounts of all of the herbs, except for *Gan Cao* (Radix et Rhizoma Glycyrrhizae), which should be used at half the dose of the other herbs.

CHINESE THERAPEUTIC ACTIONS

1. Releases wind-heat from the exterior
2. Dispels heat, fire, and toxins

CLINICAL MANIFESTATIONS

Purulent infection of the ears and nose due to wind-heat attacking the upper *jiao*: swelling, inflammation and infection of the ears and nose, abscess and suppuration of the affected area.

VETERINARY CLINICAL APPLICATIONS

Otitis externa/media due to bacteria or yeast, rhinitis and sinusitis with purulent discharge in the dog and cat; rhinopneumonitis, sinus infection, pharyngitis, and *Streptococcus equi* in the horse.

EXPLANATION

Jing Jie Lian Qiao Tang (Schizonepeta and Forsythia Decoction) treats inflammation and swelling of the ears and nose. The disease progression begins with wind-heat attacking the upper *jiao*. As wind-heat travels upward, it directly attacks the ears and nose, leading to inflammation and swelling. As heat accumulates in the affected area, suppuration develops, leading to the formation and discharge of pus.

Clinically, wind-heat attacking the ears is characterized by swelling and pain of the inner ear, abscess and discharge of pus, deafness, and tinnitus; wind-heat attacking the nose is characterized by swelling and obstruction of the nasal passages, loss of smell, abscess, and yellow nasal discharge.

Jing Jie (Herba Schizonepetae) and *Fang Feng* (Radix Saposhnikoviae) release exterior wind. *Lian Qiao* (Fructus Forsythiae) and *Jie Geng* (Radix Platycodonis) reduce swelling and inflammation, as well as eliminate pus and toxins. *Huang Qin* (Radix Scutellariae) and *Zhi Zi* (Fructus Gardeniae) purge fire and reduce inflammation. *Bai Zhi* (Radix Angelicae Dahuricae) dispels wind and unblocks obstruction in the ears and nose. *Chai Hu* (Radix Bupleuri) dispels wind, and with *Zhi Qiao* (Fructus Aurantii), relieves the feeling of distention caused by qi stagnation. *Dang Gui* (Radix Angelicae Sinensis), *Chuan Xiong* (Rhizoma Chuanxiong), and *Bai Shao* (Radix Paeoniae Alba) tonify the blood and promote blood circulation. *Gan Cao* (Radix et Rhizoma Glycyrrhizae) harmonizes the formula.

Jīng Jiè Lián Qiào Tāng (Schizonepeta and Forsythia Decoction)

***Jing Jie Lian Qiao Tang* (Schizonepeta and Forsythia Decoction)**

Diagnosis	Clinical Signs	Treatment	Herbs
Suppuration of the ears and nose	Swelling, inflammation and infection of the ears and nose: wind-heat attacking the upper body	• Releases wind-heat from the exterior • Dispels heat, fire, and toxins	• *Jing Jie* (Herba Schizonepetae) and *Fang Feng* (Radix Saposhnikoviae) release exterior wind and relieve itching. • *Lian Qiao* (Fructus Forsythiae) and *Jie Geng* (Radix Platycodonis) reduce swelling and inflammation and eliminate pus and abscesses. • *Huang Qin* (Radix Scutellariae) and *Zhi Zi* (Fructus Gardeniae) purge fire and reduce inflammation. • *Bai Zhi* (Radix Angelicae Dahuricae) dispels wind and unblocks obstruction in the ears and nose. • *Chai Hu* (Radix Bupleuri) dispels wind. • *Zhi Qiao* (Fructus Aurantii) activates qi circulation and relieves distention. • *Dang Gui* (Radix Angelicae Sinensis), *Chuan Xiong* (Rhizoma Chuanxiong), and *Bai Shao* (Radix Paeoniae Alba) tonify the blood and promote blood circulation. • *Gan Cao* (Radix et Rhizoma Glycyrrhizae) harmonizes the herbs.

VETERINARY MODIFICATIONS

- For hypertrophic sinusitis or rhinitis, add *Xin Yi Hua* (Flos Magnoliae) and *Cang Er Zi* (Fructus Xanthii).
- If there is swelling and pain caused by wind-heat, add *Jin Yin Hua* (Flos Lonicerae Japonicae) and *Huang Lian* (Rhizoma Coptidis).
- For nasal obstruction, combine with *Qing Bi Tang* (Clear the Nose Decoction).
- If there is loss of smell, combine with *Xin Yi San* (Magnolia Flower Powder).

SUGGESTED ACUPUNCTURE TREATMENT

1. Points: *Fengmen* (BL 12), *Weizhong* (BL 40), *Xuehai* (SP 10), *Quchi* (LI 11), *Waiguan* (TH 5), *Hegu* (LI 4), *Taichong* (LR 3), *Tinggong* (SI 19), *Yifeng* (TH 17), and *Sanyinjiao* (SP 6).
2. Technique: bleeding and sedation.

Waiguan (TH 5) and *Hegu* (LI 4) release exterior wind-heat and clear the ears and nose. *Xuehai* (SP 10), *Quchi* (LI 11) and bleeding on *Weizhong* (BL 40) clear heat-toxin. *Taichong* (LR 3) regulates qi, and *Sanyinjiao* (SP 6) regulates blood. *Fengmen* (BL 12) dispels wind. *Tinggong* (SI 19) and *Yifeng* (TH 17) along with *Hegu* (LI 4) help to clear the ears of heat. *Yifeng* (TH 17) also helps disperse swelling of the face.

AUTHORS' COMMENTS

There are three common causes of suppurative otitis externa/media in the dog. One is damp-heat in the Liver and Gallbladder channels which is caused by poor diet and results from internal organ dysfunction. There are two external causes: one that develops secondary to foreign body invasion of the ear by plant material, and the other that is due to invasion of the ear by ectoparasites. This formula is appropriate to treat the latter condition. Otitis externa/media is uncommon in the horse, and this formula is not likely to be used frequently for this reason, though it can be tried if otitis is suspected as the cause of headshaking. Further, it can be used in the horse for nasal discharge and sinus infections either alone or in the combinations listed below, and as an adjunct in the treatment of strangles.

Jing Jie Lian Qiao Tang can be combined with *Cang Er Zi San* (Xanthium Powder) or *Qing Bi Tang* (Clear the Nose Decoction) to treat chronic rhinitis and sinusitis with thick, yellow discharge. The ratio of each formula will vary depending on the case, but it can be as high as 1:1.

Section 3

扶正解表剂

Supporting [the Upright] and Releasing [the Exterior] Formulas

Bài Dú Săn (Overcome Pathogenic Influences Powder)

敗毒散

败毒散

Pinyin Name: *Bai Du San*

Literal Name: Overcome Pathogenic Influences Powder

Alternate Names: *Ren Shen Bai Du San*, *Jen Shen Pai Tu San*, Ginseng Detoxifying Formula, Ginseng Antiphlogistic Powder, Ginseng Powder to Overcome Pathogenic Influences, Ginseng and Mentha Formula

Original Source: *Xiao Er Yao Zheng Zhi Jue* (Craft of Medicinal Treatment for Childhood Disease Patterns) by Qian Yi in 1119

COMPOSITION

Qiang Huo (Rhizoma et Radix Notopterygii)	30g [9g]
Du Huo (Radix Angelicae Pubescentis)	30g [9g]
Chuan Xiong (Rhizoma Chuanxiong)	30g [9g]
Zhi Qiao (Fructus Aurantii)	30g [9g]
Jie Geng (Radix Platycodonis), *chao* (dry-fried)	30g [9g]
Qian Hu (Radix Peucedani)	30g [9g]
Fu Ling (Poria)	30g [9g]
Chai Hu (Radix Bupleuri), *xi* (washed)	30g [9g]
Gan Cao (Radix et Rhizoma Glycyrrhizae)	15g [5g]
Ren Shen (Radix et Rhizoma Ginseng)	30g [9g]

DOSAGE / PREPARATION / ADMINISTRATION

The source text states to grind the ingredients into powder. Cook 6g of the powder with *Sheng Jiang* (Rhizoma Zingiberis Recens) and *Bo He* (Herba Menthae) in water to obtain a decoction. Today, this formula may be prepared as a decoction with the doses suggested in brackets above.

CHINESE THERAPEUTIC ACTIONS

1. Releases the exterior through diaphoresis
2. Dispels wind, cold, and dampness
3. Tonifies qi

CLINICAL MANIFESTATIONS

Exterior wind, cold and dampness with qi deficiency: aversion to cold, fever, neck stiffness, joint pain, body aches, nasal obstruction, cough with sputum, a pale tongue, and a superficial, soft, rapid pulse that is forceless upon pressure.

VETERINARY CLINICAL APPLICATIONS

Upper and lower respiratory tract infections, infection with fever, cough, and nasal congestion.

EXPLANATION

Bai Du San (Overcome Pathogenic Influences Powder) treats weak and deficient patients who suffer from an attack by exterior wind, cold and dampness. Aversion to cold, fever, absence of sweating, neck stiffness, joint pain, and body aches are all indications of wind, cold and dampness attacking the exterior and muscles. Wind-cold may constrict the Lung, and cause nasal obstruction and cough with sputum. A superficial, soft pulse is a sign of dampness. A pale tongue and a pulse that is forceless upon pressure indicate underlying qi deficiency.

Bài Dú Săn (Overcome Pathogenic Influences Powder)

Bai Du San (Overcome Pathogenic Influences Powder)

Diagnosis	Clinical Signs	Treatment	Herbs
Exterior wind, cold and dampness with qi deficiency	• Aversion to cold, fever, neck stiffness, joint pain, and body aches: wind, cold and dampness attacking the exterior and the muscles • Nasal obstruction, cough: wind-cold invading the Lung • Pale tongue and a forceless pulse: qi deficiency	• Releases the exterior through diaphoresis • Dispels wind, cold and dampness • Tonifies *yuan* (source) *qi*	• *Qiang Huo* (Rhizoma et Radix Notopterygii) and *Du Huo* (Radix Angelicae Pubescentis) dispel wind, cold, and dampness from the body. • *Chuan Xiong* (Rhizoma Chuanxiong) activates blood circulation and dispels exterior wind-cold. • *Zhi Qiao* (Fructus Aurantii) regulates Lung qi to relieve distention and fullness. • *Jie Geng* (Radix Platycodonis) and *Qian Hu* (Radix Peucedani) dispel phlegm and relieve coughing. • *Fu Ling* (Poria) dispels dampness and tonifies the middle *jiao*. • *Chai Hu* (Radix Bupleuri), *Bo He* (Herba Menthae) and *Sheng Jiang* (Rhizoma Zingiberis Recens) release the exterior factors. • *Gan Cao* (Radix et Rhizoma Glycyrrhizae) harmonizes the herbs. • *Ren Shen* (Radix et Rhizoma Ginseng) tonifies *yuan* (source) *qi*.

The treatment goals are to dispel wind, cold, and dampness and to tonify *yuan* (source) *qi*. *Qiang Huo* (Rhizoma et Radix Notopterygii) and *Du Huo* (Radix Angelicae Pubescentis) act as the chief herbs to dispel wind, cold, and dampness from the whole body. *Chuan Xiong* (Rhizoma Chuanxiong) activates blood circulation to relieve pain. It also dispels exterior wind and cold. *Chai Hu* (Radix Bupleuri) helps the chief herbs release the exterior. *Zhi Qiao* (Fructus Aurantii) regulates the qi flow of the Lung to relieve chest distention and fullness. *Jie Geng* (Radix Platycodonis) and *Qian Hu* (Radix Peucedani) relieve coughing and dispel phlegm. *Fu Ling* (Poria) dispels dampness through diuresis and tonifies the middle *jiao*. *Bo He* (Herba Menthae) and *Sheng Jiang* (Rhizoma Zingiberis Recens) help relieve exterior clinical signs. *Gan Cao* (Radix et Rhizoma Glycyrrhizae) harmonizes the herbs.

To help a deficient body dispel exterior factors, the interior must also be strengthened; hence, a small amount of *Ren Shen* (Radix et Rhizoma Ginseng) is used to tonify *yuan* (source) *qi*, which strengthens the body to help expel the exterior factors. Moreover, *Ren Shen* (Radix et Rhizoma Ginseng) balances and prevents the acrid and strong properties of the exterior-releasing herbs from damaging the weak body. Lastly, by tonifying qi, this herb prevents future re-infections and reduces the susceptibility of the body to exterior pathogens.

CAUTIONS / CONTRAINDICATIONS

- *Bai Du San* is a warm, acrid formula that is contraindicated in cases of exterior wind-heat invasion, interior heat, or yin deficiency with exterior invasion.
- The dose of *Ren Shen* (Radix et Rhizoma Ginseng) should be carefully adjusted according to each patient's condition. It should not constitute more than ten percent of the entire formula. *Bai Du San* was originally designed for children. In animals that do not have significant qi deficiency, the dose of *Ren Shen* (Radix et Rhizoma Ginseng) should be decreased.

HUMAN CLINICAL STUDIES AND RESEARCH

1. **Infection with fever**: In one study, 136 children with epidemic infection and fever were evaluated and treated. The ages of the children ranged from 6 months to 12 years, with length of illness between 1-7 days prior to the evaluation and herbal treatment. Out of 136 cases, 36 had been treated previously with antibiotic drugs without success, 79 were treated with herbs only, and 21 received concurrent herbal and drug treatment. The study reported complete recovery in 125 cases after 3 days. The other 11

Bài Dú Sǎn (Overcome Pathogenic Influences Powder)

cases continued to have fever and needed additional treatment.[1]

2. **Respiratory tract infection**: Use of *Bai Du San* in decoction was associated with 94% effectiveness in treating infants and young children with upper respiratory infection caused by virus. The herbal treatment contained 6g each of *Chai Hu* (Radix Bupleuri), *Qian Hu* (Radix Peucedani), *Tai Zi Shen* (Radix Pseudostellariae), *Chuan Xiong* (Rhizoma Chuanxiong), *Zhi Qiao* (Fructus Aurantii), *Fu Ling* (Poria), and *Jie Geng* (Radix Platycodonis); 5g each of *Qiang Huo* (Rhizoma et Radix Notopterygii) and *Du Huo* (Radix Angelicae Pubescentis); 3g of *Bo He* (Herba Menthae); and 3 pieces of *Sheng Jiang* (Rhizoma Zingiberis Recens). Of 37 cases, the study reported complete recovery in 17 cases, marked improvement in 18 cases, and no benefit in 2 cases.[2]

SUGGESTED ACUPUNCTURE TREATMENT

1. Points: *Fengchi* (GB 20), *Dazhui* (GV 14), *Quchi* (LI 11), *Hegu* (LI 4), *Housanli* (ST 36), and *Yinlingquan* (SP 9).
2. Technique: even method; may use moxibustion.

Fengchi (GB 20) and *Dazhui* (GV 14) dispel wind and relieve the exterior. *Quchi* (LI 11) and *Hegu* (LI 4) relieve the exterior and regulate the qi flow of the Lung. *Housanli* (ST 36) and *Yinlingquan* (SP 9) strengthen qi and eliminate dampness.

RELATED FORMULA

Rén Shēn Bài Dú Sǎn
(Ginseng Powder to Overcome Pathogenic Influences)
人參敗毒散
人参败毒散

Pinyin Name: *Ren Shen Bai Du San*

Literal Name: Ginseng Powder to Overcome Pathogenic Influences

Original Source: *Tai Ping Hui Min He Ji Ju Fang* (Imperial Grace Formulary of the Tai Ping Era) by the Imperial Medical Department in 1078-85

COMPOSITION

Chai Hu (Radix Bupleuri)
Gan Cao (Radix et Rhizoma Glycyrrhizae)
Jie Geng (Radix Platycodonis)
Ren Shen (Radix et Rhizoma Ginseng)
Chuan Xiong (Rhizoma Chuanxiong)
Fu Ling (Poria), [remove the peel]
Zhi Qiao (Fructus Aurantii), *chao* (dry-fried) with bran
Qian Hu (Radix Peucedani)
Qiang Huo (Rhizoma et Radix Notopterygii)
Du Huo (Radix Angelicae Pubescentis)

The source text states to grind equal amounts of the ingredients into powder, and cook 6g of the powder with *Sheng Jiang* (Rhizoma Zingiberis Recens) and *Bo He* (Herba Menthae) in water to obtain a decoction.

Ren Shen Bai Du San (Ginseng Powder to Overcome Pathogenic Influences) is used to treat juvenile, geriatric and debilitated animals that have wind-cold with dampness attacking a constitutionally deficient body. The types of cases requiring this formula include patients that have been hospitalized (post-surgical, chemotherapy, postpartum) and that acquire a wind-cold invasion (upper respiratory infection).

Bai Du San (Overcome Pathogenic Influences Powder) and *Ren Shen Bai Du San* (Ginseng Powder to Overcome Pathogenic Influences) are essentially the same formulas with the same indications. The minor differences between these two formulas are preparation of some of the ingredients, and the dose of *Gan Cao* (Radix et Rhizoma Glycyrrhizae). Because of their overwhelming similarities, the names "*Bai Du San*" and "*Ren Shen Bai Du San*" are sometimes used interchangeably.

References

1. *Shan Xi Yi Kan* (Shanxi Journal of Medicine), 1994; 15(8):347.
2. *Shan Xi Zhong Yi* (Shanxi Chinese Medicine), 1999; 7:297.

Shēn Sū Yǐn (Ginseng and Perilla Leaf Decoction)

參蘇飲
参苏饮

Pinyin Name: *Shen Su Yin*
Literal Name: Ginseng and Perilla Leaf Decoction
Alternate Names: Ginseng and Perilla Drink, Ginseng and Perilla Decoction, Ginseng and Perilla Combination
Original Source: *Tai Ping Hui Min He Ji Ju Fang* (Imperial Grace Formulary of the Tai Ping Era) by the Imperial Medical Department in 1078-85

COMPOSITION

Ge Gen (Radix Puerariae Lobatae)	22.5g [6g]
Zi Su Ye (Folium Perillae)	22.5g [6g]
Qian Hu (Radix Peucedani)	22.5g [6g]
Ban Xia (Rhizoma Pinelliae), *chao* (dry-fried with ginger juice)	22.5g [6g]
Jie Geng (Radix Platycodonis)	15g [4g]
Chen Pi (Pericarpium Citri Reticulatae)	15g [4g]
Zhi Qiao (Fructus Aurantii), *chao* (dry-fried) with bran	15g [4g]
Mu Xiang (Radix Aucklandiae)	15g [4g]
Ren Shen (Radix et Rhizoma Ginseng)	22.5g [6g]
Fu Ling (Poria)	22.5g [6g]
Gan Cao (Radix et Rhizoma Glycyrrhizae)	15g [4g]

DOSAGE / PREPARATION / ADMINISTRATION

Grind the ingredients coarsely and cook 12g of the powder with 7 slices of *Sheng Jiang* (Rhizoma Zingiberis Recens) and 1 piece of *Da Zao* (Fructus Jujubae) in 1.5 bowls of water until it is reduced to 60%. Take the warm, strained decoction any time during the day. This formula may also be prepared as a decoction with the doses suggested in brackets above.

CHINESE THERAPEUTIC ACTIONS

1. Tonifies qi and releases the exterior
2. Expels phlegm and stops cough

CLINICAL MANIFESTATIONS

Exterior wind-cold syndrome with interior *tan yin* (phlegm retention): aversion to cold, fever, neck stiffness and pain, nasal obstruction, coughing with profuse sputum, exercise intolerance, lethargy, shortness of breath, weak vocalization and a weak, superficial pulse.

VETERINARY CLINICAL APPLICATIONS

Bronchitis, pneumonia, and upper respiratory tract infection.

EXPLANATION

Shen Su Yin (Ginseng and Perilla Leaf Decoction) tonifies qi, dispels exterior pathogenic factors, expels phlegm, and stops cough. Clinically, patients will manifest wind-cold at the exterior (aversion to cold, fever, and nasal obstruction) and *tan yin* (phlegm retention) in the interior (coughing with profuse sputum, epigastric bloating and distention in the chest and diaphragm). In addition, patients will have qi deficiency, with clinical signs such as fatigue, lethargy, shortness of breath, and weak vocalization.

Ge Gen (Radix Puerariae Lobatae) and *Zi Su Ye* (Folium Perillae), the chief herbs, release exterior wind-cold factor. *Qian Hu* (Radix Peucedani), *Ban Xia* (Rhizoma Pinelliae), and *Jie Geng* (Radix Platycodonis) arrest cough, dissolve phlegm, and ventilate Lung qi. *Chen Pi* (Pericarpium Citri Reticulatae) and *Zhi Qiao* (Fructus Aurantii) regulate qi and expand the chest. *Mu Xiang* (Radix Aucklandiae) regulates qi, dries dampness, and unblocks stagnation. *Ren Shen* (Radix et Rhizoma Ginseng) tonifies qi, while *Fu Ling* (Poria) strengthens the Spleen and drains dampness. *Gan Cao* (Radix et Rhizoma Glycyrrhizae) harmonizes the middle *jiao* and the entire formula.

Shēn Sū Yǐn (Ginseng and Perilla Leaf Decoction)

Shen Su Yin (Ginseng and Perilla Leaf Decoction)

Diagnosis	Clinical Signs	Treatment	Herbs
Exterior wind-cold and interior *tan yin* (phlegm retention) with underlying qi deficiency	• Aversion to cold, fever, neck pain and stiffness and nasal obstruction: exterior wind-cold • Coughing with profuse sputum: interior *tan yin* (phlegm retention) • Fatigue, lethargy, shortness of breath, weak vocalization: qi deficiency	• Tonifies qi and releases the exterior • Expels phlegm and stops cough	• *Ge Gen* (Radix Puerariae Lobatae) and *Zi Su Ye* (Folium Perillae) release exterior wind-cold and regulate qi. • *Qian Hu* (Radix Peucedani), *Ban Xia* (Rhizoma Pinelliae), and *Jie Geng* (Radix Platycodonis) ventilate Lung qi, expel phlegm, and arrest cough. • *Chen Pi* (Pericarpium Citri Reticulatae) and *Zhi Qiao* (Fructus Aurantii) regulate qi and expand the chest. • *Mu Xiang* (Radix Aucklandiae) regulates qi and unblocks stagnation. • *Ren Shen* (Radix et Rhizoma Ginseng) tonifies Lung and Spleen qi. • *Fu Ling* (Poria) strengthens the Spleen and drains dampness. • *Gan Cao* (Radix et Rhizoma Glycyrrhizae) harmonizes the middle *jiao* and the entire formula.

VETERINARY MODIFICATIONS

- For cough, wheezing, and aversion to cold caused by wind-cold, add *Ma Huang* (Herba Ephedrae), *Ku Xing Ren* (Semen Armeniacae Amarum), and *Jin Fei Cao* (Herba Inulae).
- For cough, wheezing and rapid respiration caused by wind-heat, add *Zhi Mu* (Rhizoma Anemarrhenae) and *Bei Mu* (Bulbus Fritillariae).
- For cough caused by Lung cold, add *Wu Wei Zi* (Fructus Schisandrae Chinensis) and *Gan Jiang* (Rhizoma Zingiberis).
- For cough caused by Lung heat, add *Ku Xing Ren* (Semen Armeniacae Amarum), *Huang Qin* (Radix Scutellariae), and *Sang Bai Pi* (Cortex Mori).
- When there is profuse sputum, add *Gua Lou Zi* (Semen Trichosanthis).
- If there is abdominal pain (colic) and diarrhea, add *Huo Xiang* (Herba Agastaches) and *Sha Ren* (Fructus Amomi).

PHARMACOLOGICAL EFFECTS

1. **Antipyretic**: Administration of *Shen Su Yin* at 0.54g/kg in rabbits was associated with marked antipyretic effects in rabbits with artificially-induced fever.[1]
2. **Antitussive and expectorant**: Use of *Shen Su Yin* was associated with both antitussive and expectorant effects in mice.[2]

HUMAN CLINICAL STUDIES AND RESEARCH

1. **Upper respiratory tract infection**: One study reported good results using modified *Shen Su Yin* to treat 39 patients with upper respiratory tract infection arising from various causes (34 with viral infection and 5 with bacterial infection). In addition to *Shen Su Yin* as the base formula, modifications included addition of *Huang Qin* (Radix Scutellariae) and *Zhe Bei Mu* (Bulbus Fritillariae Thunbergii) for phlegm and heat obstructing the Lung; and *Gua Lou* (Fructus Trichosanthis) for constipation. Of 39 cases, the study reported recovery in 33 cases within 4-17 days, and 6 more cases in 18-20 days.[3]
2. **Infection**: Use of modified *Shen Su Yin* was associated with good results in treating 60 patients with frequent infection caused by qi deficiency. The herbal treatment included *Ren Shen* (Radix et Rhizoma Ginseng), *Fu Ling* (Poria), *Chen Pi* (Pericarpium Citri Reticulatae), *Ban Xia* (Rhizoma Pinelliae), *Zi Su Ye* (Folium Perillae), *Qian Hu* (Radix Peucedani), *Ge Gen* (Radix Puerariae Lobatae), *Jie Geng* (Radix Platycodonis), *Chai Hu* (Radix Bupleuri), *Zhi Qiao* (Fructus Aurantii), *Mu Xiang* (Radix Aucklandiae), and *Zhi Gan Cao* (Radix et Rhizoma Glycyrrhizae Praeparata cum Melle). *Bai Bu* (Radix Stemonae) and *Xian He Cao* (Herba Agrimoniae) were added for chronic and frequent cough; *Bai Qian* (Rhizoma et Radix Cynanchi Stauntonii) and *Zi Wan* (Radix et Rhizoma Asteris) were added for cough with profuse white sputum; and *Huang*

Shēn Sū Yǐn (Ginseng and Perilla Leaf Decoction)

Qi (Radix Astragali) was added for profuse sweating with weakness and fatigue. Of 60 cases, the study reported complete recovery in 38 cases within 3 packs of herbs, in 20 cases after 4-6 packs, and 2 cases after 7-10 packs.[4]

3. **Common cold**: *Shen Su Yin* was used to treat 100 geriatric patients with common cold with good results. The treatment protocol was to use this formula in suspension form, using 20g of the herbs per dose two times daily. Of cases patients, the study reported complete recovery in 49 cases, significant improvement in 33 cases, moderate improvement in 9 cases, and no benefit in 9 cases. The overall rate of effectiveness was 91%.[5]

SUGGESTED ACUPUNCTURE TREATMENT

1. Points: *Fengchi* (GB 20), *Dazhui* (GV 14), *Quchi* (LI 11), *Hegu* (LI 4), *Housanli* (ST 36), *Yinlingquan* (SP 9), *Fenglong* (ST 40), and *Neiguan* (PC 6).
2. Technique: even method; may use moxibustion.

Fengchi (GB 20) and *Dazhui* (GV 14) dispel wind and relieve the exterior. *Quchi* (LI 11) and *Hegu* (LI 4) relieve the exterior and regulate the qi flow of the Lung. *Housanli* (ST 36) and *Yinlingquan* (SP 9) strengthen qi and eliminate dampness. *Fenglong* (ST 40) dispels phlegm. *Neiguan* (PC 6) regulates qi and relieves chest congestion.

AUTHORS' COMMENTS

Shen Su Yin was originally designed to treat wind-cold invasion with pre-existing damp and phlegm accumulation in the interior. Thus, *Shen Su Yin* contains the ingredients of *Er Chen Tang* (Two-Cured Decoction) to dispel dampness and phlegm.

Shen Su Yin dispels dampness affecting the Lung, manifesting in white nasal discharge, white sputum and chest congestion. It focuses on dispelling exterior wind and cold, harmonizing *ying* (nutritive) *qi* and *wei* (defensive) *qi*, dispelling phlegm, and stopping cough. It is used for wind-cold invasion in those animals with pre-existing Lung qi deficiency. The *zheng* (upright) *qi* in these patients is weak as is the body's response to exterior pathogen invasion. The clinical signs seen may be mild to moderate, and serious disease could quickly develop in these cases. This formula is most suitable for young, geriatric and chronically ill animals that are qi deficient, and animals that have weak digestive function and damp accumulation. It is not appropriate to use in animals with heat signs.

References

1. *Zhong Yao Yao Li Yu Lin Chuang* (Pharmacology and Clinical Applications of Chinese Herbs), 1992; 8(3):6.
2. *Zhong Yao Yao Li Yu Lin Chuang* (Pharmacology and Clinical Applications of Chinese Herbs), 1992; 8(3):6.
3. *Liao Ning Zhong Yi Za Zhi* (Liaoning Journal of Chinese Medicine), 1987; 12:48.
4. *Fu Jian Zhong Yi Yao* (Fujian Chinese Medicine and Herbology), 1996; 6:49.
5. *Xin Zhong Yi* (New Chinese Medicine), 1987; 8:54.

Chapter 1 — Summary — Exterior-Releasing Formulas

SECTION 1: ACRID AND WARM EXTERIOR-RELEASING FORMULAS

Name	Similarities	Differences
Gui Zhi Tang (Cinnamon Twig Decoction)	Releases wind-cold in exterior-deficient conditions	Harmonizes *ying* (nutritive) and *wei* (defensive) levels
Ge Gen Tang (Kudzu Decoction)	Release exterior wind-cold, relieve muscle stiffness and pain	Relieves muscle stiffness and pain in the neck
Jiu Wei Qiang Huo Tang (Nine-Herb Decoction with Notopterygium)		Relieves muscle stiffness and pain throughout the body
Xing Su Yin (Apricot Kernel and Perilla Leaf Decoction)	Releases wind-cold, regulates qi circulation	Dispels wind-cold, dissolves phlegm, regulates qi circulation in the upper *jiao*
Xiao Qing Long Tang (Minor Bluegreen Dragon Decoction)	Release exterior wind-cold, eliminate interior phlegm	Relieves severe wind-cold attack
She Gan Ma Huang Tang (Belamcanda and Ephedra Decoction)		Relieves phlegm retention
Cang Er Zi San (Xanthium Powder)	Release exterior wind, open the nasal orifices	Treats nasal disorders caused by exterior wind
Xin Yi San (Magnolia Flower Powder)		Treats nasal disorders caused by wind-cold
Qing Bi Tang (Clear the Nose Decoction)		Treats nasal disorders caused by damp-heat

Gui Zhi Tang (Cinnamon Twig Decoction), containing *Gui Zhi* (Ramulus Cinnamomi) but not *Ma Huang* (Herba Ephedrae), is moderate in its exterior-releasing effects. However, because it contains *Bai Shao* (Radix Paeoniae Alba), it can harmonize the *ying* (nutritive) and *wei* (defensive) levels. It is suitable for exterior deficiency-cold syndromes.

Ge Gen Tang (Kudzu Decoction) and ***Jiu Wei Qiang Huo Tang*** (Nine-Herb Decoction with Notopterygium) both release exterior wind-cold and relieve muscle stiffness and pain.

- *Ge Gen Tang* treats exterior-excess, wind-cold syndromes accompanied by stiffness and pain of the neck.
- *Jiu Wei Qiang Huo Tang* dispels exterior wind, cold, and dampness. It relieves muscle stiffness and pain throughout the body.

Xing Su Yin (Apricot Kernel and Perilla Leaf Decoction) is designed for juvenile, geriatric and chronically debilitated animals that have wind-cold attacking the exterior parts of the body, with clinical signs such as, fever, aversion to cold, nausea, vomiting, drooling, sticky nasal discharge, sneezing, and cough.

Xiao Qing Long Tang (Minor Bluegreen Dragon Decoction) and ***She Gan Ma Huang Tang*** (Belamcanda and Ephedra Decoction) both release exterior wind-cold and treat interior phlegm retention.

- *Xiao Qing Long Tang* emphasizes releasing severe cases of wind-cold attack and dispels *yin* (invisible phlegm).
- *She Gan Ma Huang Tang* focuses on restoring the appropriate flow of Lung qi, relieving dyspnea, and eliminating *tan yin* (phlegm retention).

Chapter 1 — Summary

Cang Er Zi San (Xanthium Powder), ***Xin Yi San*** (Magnolia Flower Powder), and ***Qing Bi Tang*** (Clear the Nose Decoction) treat nasal disorders, such as sinusitis and rhinitis.

- *Cang Er Zi San* treats nasal disorders caused by wind, with clinical signs such as stuffy nose, and thick, yellow nasal discharge.
- *Xin Yi San* treats nasal disorders caused by wind-cold, with clinical signs such as stuffy nose, and profuse, clear and white nasal discharge.
- *Qing Bi Tang* treats nasal disorders that are changing from an exterior (wind-cold or wind-heat) to an interior (damp-heat) condition. Clinical manifestations include stuffy nose, yellow and sticky nasal discharge, sneezing, fatigue, itchy nose, a decreased sense of smell, and decreased energy level.

SECTION 2: ACRID AND COLD EXTERIOR-RELEASING FORMULAS

Name	Similarities	Differences
Sang Ju Yin (Mulberry Leaf and Chrysanthemum Decoction)	Release exterior wind-heat	Stronger functions to ventilate the Lung to suppress cough
Yin Qiao San (Honeysuckle and Forsythia Powder)		Stronger functions to clear heat, relieve sore throat, and release the exterior
Ma Xing Gan Shi Tang (Ephedra, Apricot Kernel, Licorice, and Gypsum Decoction)	Releases exterior wind-heat, clears Lung heat	Ventilates the Lung, clears Lung heat, and relieves cough and dyspnea.
Ning Sou Wan (Quiet the Cough Pill)	Clear Lung heat, suppress cough	Releases exterior wind-heat, clears Lung heat
Dun Sou San (Long-Bout Cough Powder)		Clears heat and dissolves phlegm
Zhi Sou San (Stop Coughing Powder)		Releases exterior wind, dissolves phlegm
Jing Jie Lian Qiao Tang (Schizonepeta and Forsythia Decoction)	Dispels wind-heat from the upper parts of the body	Dispels heat, fire, and toxins, treats ear and nose disorders

Sang Ju Yin (Mulberry Leaf and Chrysanthemum Decoction) and ***Yin Qiao San*** (Honeysuckle and Forsythia Powder) are cool, acrid formulas that release exterior wind-heat to treat the initial stages of warm febrile disorders.

- *Sang Ju Yin* has a stronger effect to ventilate the Lung to arrest cough. It treats exterior wind-heat syndrome characterized by reversed flow of Lung qi and other mild exterior wind-heat clinical signs.
- *Yin Qiao San* has stronger heat-clearing and exterior-releasing effects. It is suitable for severe wind-heat conditions or *wen bing* (warm diseases) disorders, with signs of heat and toxicity, such as fever and thirst.

Ma Huang Xing Ren Gan Cao Shi Gao Tang (Ephedra, Apricot Kernel, Licorice, and Gypsum Decoction) has strong functions to clear Lung heat and ventilate the Lung. It treats Lung heat caused by exterior pathogenic factors, with clinical signs such as unremitting fever, thirst with a desire to drink, coughing and dyspnea.

Ning Sou Wan (Quiet the Cough Pill), ***Dun Sou San*** (Long-Bout Cough Powder) and ***Zhi Sou San*** (Stop Coughing Powder) clear heat and suppress cough.

- *Ning Sou Wan* releases exterior wind-heat and clears Lung heat to relieve cough.
- *Dun Sou San* clears heat and dissolves phlegm to suppress cough.
- *Zhi Sou San* releases exterior wind and dissolves phlegm to stop cough.

Jing Jie Lian Qiao Tang (Schizonepeta and Forsythia Decoction) dispels wind-heat from the upper parts of the body to treat inflammation and swelling of the ears and nose.

Chapter 1 — Summary

SECTION 3: SUPPORTING [THE UPRIGHT] AND RELEASING [THE EXTERIOR] FORMULAS

Name	Similarities	Differences
Bai Du San (Overcome Pathogenic Influences Powder)	Release exterior wind-cold, tonify qi	Tonifies qi, dispels wind, cold and dampness
Shen Su Yin (Ginseng and Perilla Leaf Decoction)		Tonifies Lung and Spleen qi, dispels phlegm, and stops cough

Bai Du San (Overcome Pathogenic Influences Powder) and ***Shen Su Yin*** (Ginseng and Perilla Leaf Decoction) both release exterior wind-cold. They both contain *Ren Shen* (Radix et Rhizoma Ginseng) to tonify qi in animals with underlying weakness and deficiency.

- *Bai Du San* relieves dampness lodged in the channels, causing body aches, and neck and shoulder stiffness. It is better at treating wind-cold and dampness at the superficial level.
- *Shen Su Yin* focuses on dispelling dampness affecting the Lung, manifesting in white nasal discharge, white sputum, chest congestion, and a feeling of heaviness. It is stronger in regulating Lung qi and dissolving phlegm. It is better for treating invasion of wind-cold in animals that are qi deficient and that also have interior *tan yin* (phlegm retention).

Chapter 2

— Downward Draining Formulas

泻下剂

张景岳 Zhāng Jǐng-Yuè

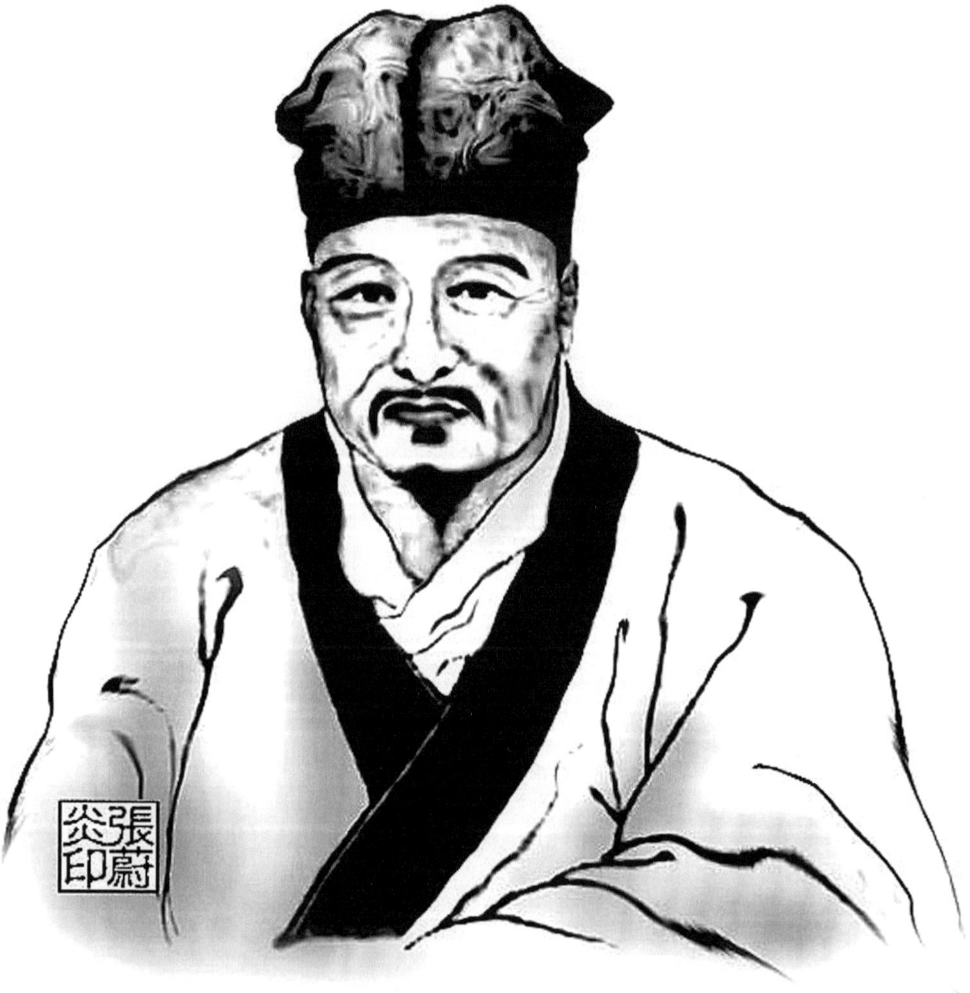

张景岳 Zhāng Jǐng-Yuè, also known as 张介宾 Zhāng Jīe-Bín, 1563 – 1640.

张景岳 Zhāng Jǐng-Yuè

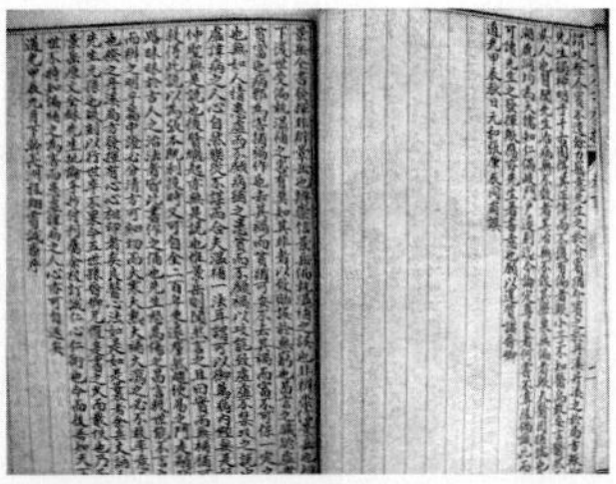

景岳全书 *Jing Yue Quan Shu* (Collected Treatises of [Zhang] Jing Yue) in 1624.

Born into a wealthy military family, Zhang Jing-Yue was intensely curious and could afford the time and money to explore many different interests. Zhang studied astrology, philosophy, music, medicine, and more. Of all topics, Zhang was most interested in and excelled in medicine. He specialized in and studied the *Huang Di Nei Jing* (Yellow Emperor's Inner Classic) for 30 years.

During the Ming dynasty when Zhang practiced medicine, many physicians over-prescribed the use of herbs that were acrid, hot and drying, and consequently injured yin and body fluids. Zhang proposed and used tonic herbs to rescue damaged yin and body fluids, and significantly influenced the practice of Traditional Chinese Medicine. Many tonic formulas he used then are still frequently prescribed today.

Zhang published many texts in his lifetime, and is best known for 景岳全书 *Jing Yue Quan Shu* (Collected Treatises of [Zhang] Jing Yue) in 1624. This comprehensive text discussed many aspects of medicine, including theory, treatment strategies, herbs, formulas, gynecology, pediatrics, and more. Because of his military background, Zhang also proposed treatment strategies based on miliary tactics, such as 八阵 *Ba Zhen* (Eight Arrays of Formulas): 补 *bu* (tonic) formulas to treat deficiency, 和 *he* (harmonizing) formulas to treat disharmony, 攻 *gong* (attack) formulas to treat excess, 散 *san* (disperse) formulas to disperse exterior conditions, 寒 *han* (cold) formulas to clear heat, 热 *re* (hot) formulas to dispel cold, 固 *gu* (stabilize) formulas to stop loss (of body fluids), and 因 *yin* (pattern-specific) formulas to treat specific disorders.

As a great compliment, Zhang Jing-Yue is remembered by many as the reincarnation of Zhang Zhong-Jing.

Exemplar formulas of Zhang Jing-Yue that are in common use today include:

- *Zhou Che Wan* (Vessel and Vehicle Pill)
- *Ji Chuan Jian* (Benefit the River [Flow] Decoction)
- *Chai Hu Shu Gan San* (Bupleurum Powder to Spread the Liver)
- *Tong Xie Yao Fang* (Important Formula for Painful Diarrhea)
- *Yu Nu Jian* (Jade Woman Decoction)
- *Zuo Gui Wan* (Restore the Left [Kidney] Pill)
- *You Gui Wan* (Restore the Right [Kidney] Pill)
- *Tai Shan Pan Shi San* (Powder that Gives the Stability of Mount Tai)

Dynasties & Kingdoms	Year
Xia Dynasty 夏	2100-1600 BCE
Shang Dynasty 商	1600-1100 BCE
Zhou Dynasty 周	1100-221 BCE
Qin Dynasty 秦	221-207 BCE
Han Dynasty 漢	206 BCE-220
Three Kingdoms 三國	220-280
Western Jin Dynasty 西晉	265-316
Eastern Jin Dynasty 東晉	317-420
Northern and Southern Dynasties 北南朝	420-581
Sui Dynasty 隋	581-618
Tang Dynasty 唐	618-907
Five Dynasties 五代	907-960
Song Dynasty 宋	960-1279
Liao Dynasty 遼	916-1125
Jin Dynasty 金	1115-1234
Yuan Dynasty 元	1271-1368
Ming Dynasty 明	**1368-1644**
Qing Dynasty 清	1644-1911
Republic of China 中華民國	1912-Present Day
People's Republic of China 中華人民共和國	1949-Present Day

Table of Contents

Chapter 2 — Overview

泻下剂 — Downward Draining Formulas

Definition: Downward draining formulas consist mostly of purgative herbs, and function to pass stools, drain excess heat, dispel accumulation and stagnation from the Stomach and Intestines, and drastically eliminate water retention and cold stagnation. This method of treatment is known as *xia fa* (draining downward), one of the *ba fa* (eight treatment methods) described in the *Huang Di Nei Jing* (Yellow Emperor's Inner Classic) in the first or second century A.D.

Downward draining formulas break up and eliminate interior accumulations of cold, heat, dampness, stool, food and water that would otherwise interfere with normal functioning of the body. Many of these formulas contain herbs with laxative (softening-lubricant) effects, while others have a cathartic (increased peristalsis) effect to break up and eliminate accumulated pathogenic factors through defecation and urination.

In general, downward draining formulas treat interior excess syndromes. Interior excess refers to a wide variety of disorders that include qi stagnation, blood stagnation, phlegm retention, food stagnation, constipation, water retention, parasitic infestation, and many others. This chapter discusses downward draining formulas that treat interior excess syndromes characterized by constipation and water retention. These disorders can occur acutely in healthy animals, or may be seen chronically in those with underlying deficiencies of qi, blood, yin, yang and body fluids. Each downward draining formula is designed for specific disease patterns and for the particular constitution of the individual animal. Except for the formulas that moisten and lubricate the Intestines, most downward draining formulas contain purgative herbs; thus they should be prescribed and monitored with great care. Treatments for those types of interior excess conditions *not* characterized by constipation are discussed in other chapters of this book.

The greatest application of these formulas in small animal veterinary medicine is in the treatment of canine and feline constipation and idiopathic feline megacolon. In the equine, impaction colic is a common presentation. In most cases, this is an acute condition that quickly resolves with treatment. However, persistent dry stool also occurs frequently in older patients, and addressing the condition at this mild stage with the appropriate formula can prevent a more serious event. Constipation in animals can develop acutely from inactivity, dietary indiscretion, attack by an external pathogenic factor, or as a secondary complication from chronic disease, pharmaceuticals, surgery, or parturition. According to Chinese medicine, constipation is generally divided into excess or deficient. Excess patterns of constipation can develop from heat (external and internal), phlegm, and stagnation, factors that obstruct the qi flow of the middle *jiao* and the descent of the Large Intestine qi, resulting in accumulation and retention of feces. Deficient patterns of constipation are due to a depletion or insufficient production of yin (body fluids and blood), causing lack of normal moistening and lubrication of stool in the Large Intestine, or insufficient qi and yang leading to weak or absent peristaltic movement. Yang-deficiency causes of constipation are not as common as constipation from other conditions. Cold constricts the normal qi flow of the Large Intestine, preventing normal evacuation of feces; the result is constipation and loose stools instead of dry. In animals with deficiency, constipation can often become chronic. The most commonly seen pattern of constipation in geriatric dogs and cats is a deficiency of yin and blood; in younger animals, particularly dogs, constipation is often seen following dietary indiscretion.

Chapter 2 — Overview

Idiopathic megacolon in the cat can be one of the more challenging presentations of constipation seen in veterinary practice. By far, the greatest factors in the development of chronic constipation in the cat, which can progress to idiopathic megacolon, are diet, obesity, and lack of regular exercise. From a Chinese medicine perspective, eating a diet low in fiber can generate heat and dampness (mucus) and lead to chronic constipation. In the cat, this commonly occurs from eating commercial pet food diet containing high levels of carbohydrates in the form of grains (corn, wheat, soybeans) without natural prey fiber. Cats have evolved as strict carnivores metabolically adapted to preferentially utilize protein and fat as energy sources; they have limited ability to properly digest diets high in carbohydrates. Cats are natural hunters and normally obtain fiber and bulk in their diet by consuming the entire animal (muscle, bone, hide, hair, feather, entrails). This natural fiber and bulk is not available to many domesticated cats, most of whom are confined indoors and have no access to regular prey such as birds and mice. Adequate fiber and bulk is required to increase the volume of stool, which in turn triggers receptors in the intestinal wall, stimulating peristalsis and decreasing the travel time of waste through the intestines. The tendency towards constipation increases if the diet consists of processed dry food. Cats that hunt obtain most of their water intake from consumption of their prey. Cats have a less sensitive response to thirst and dehydration than dogs and other omnivorous species. The amount of water consumed by domesticated cats depends on how much dry matter their food contains rather than the food's moisture content. This means that cats who eat exclusively dry foods will consume half the amount of water of those who eat canned pet food; a canned diet will increase the amount of water taken in by the cat.

Obesity in Chinese medicine coincides with retention of dampness and phlegm. Over time, dampness combines with heat and is then "cooked" to produce thick, hot phlegm, which results in thick, sticky feces that interfere with the normal descent of the flow of qi in the Lung, Stomach and Large Intestine, and the ascent of Spleen qi. Many cats become obese as a consequence of eating a dry, high-carbohydrate diet that is fed freely in many cases. In addition to diet, chronic stress can produce Liver qi stagnation, causing heat and Spleen dysfunction, which, in turn, creates dampness and phlegm. Liver qi stagnation can occur when a cat has to share a litter box with multiple feline housemates, is regularly forced to use a litter box which is dirty, too small, or that contains material that is objectionable to the cat. Submissive cats (those most picked on) in a multi-animal household may also develop Liver qi stagnation. Many cats are kept strictly indoors, and, as such, do not have the freedom to exercise normally (hunting, running, etc). Lack of regular physical activity, common in cats kept strictly indoors with no freedom to hunt and play, also contributes to sluggish bowel activity, qi and blood stagnation, weak Spleen and Lung functions. This situation also contributes to elevated body condition scores and obesity, especially when combined with a high-carbohydrate, low-fiber diet. In summary, cats that regularly consume a species-inappropriate diet, are obese, and are unable or unwilling to exercise are those most at risk for development of habitual constipation and progression to feline megacolon. Cats with habitual constipation may also have concurrent conditions such as diabetes, chronic skin disease, feline lower urinary tract disease, inflammatory bowel disease, spondylosis, and feline asthma.

In general, the treatment of constipation involves unblocking the Large Intestine by lubrication of the stool and promoting normal intestinal transportation (qi) function. Herbs that open the Lung qi to assist with its descending function are helpful because of the yin-yang relationship that exists between the Large Intestine and the Lung. This includes herbs such as *Yu Li Ren* (Semen Pruni) *Shan Zha* (Fructus Crataegi), *Lai Fu Zi* (Semen Raphani), *Jie Geng* (Radix Platycodonis), *Xing Ren Shu Pi* (Cortex Pruni Armeniacae), *Sang Bai Pi* (Cortex Mori), *Gua Lou Pi* (Pericarpium Trichosanthis) and *Sheng Ma* (Rhizoma Cimicifugae). Herbs that regulate Liver qi to prevent and relieve stagnation are also recommended, such as *Chai Hu* (Radix Bupleuri), *Bai Shao* (Radix Paeoniae Alba), and *Xiang Fu* (Rhizoma Cyperi).

Chapter 2 — Overview

SUBCATEGORIES OF ACTION

1. **Cold Purgatives**

These formulas contain purgative herbs which are bitter and cold, and are suitable for eliminating interior excess conditions with heat stagnation and accumulation of stool. There is a history of chronic constipation in the dog or cat or a diagnosis of feline megacolon. Conversely, in the horse this pattern will present as acute cases of impaction colic that occur after eating poor quality feed, eating too soon after strenuous exercise, or secondary to the accumulation of heat in hot weather. Common clinical manifestations include a palpably painful distended colon, distention, or pain. In severe cases, the animal may have a fever. The tongue coating can be thick white, sticky, and/or yellow, with a forceful, slippery-wiry pulse. These animals may constantly strain to defecate without producing any stool; or may pass loose, foul smelling fluid and small amounts of loose stool around the impacted stool. Many cats vocalize loudly and repeatedly. Cold purgatives are often combined with qi-regulating herbs, as most conditions of excess have some degree of qi stagnation present; and cold purgative formulas are combined with herbs that tonify blood and yin in constitutionally weak, chronically debilitated and geriatric animals.

Herbs commonly used to purge interior heat and excess include *Da Huang* (Radix et Rhizoma Rhei) and *Mang Xiao* (Natrii Sulfas). Formulas commonly used to purge interior heat and excess include *Da Cheng Qi Tang* (Major Order the Qi Decoction) and *Xiao Cheng Qi Tang* (Minor Order the Qi Decoction).

2. **Moist Laxatives**

These formulas treat constipation that is caused by heat and dryness in the Intestines, which damage yin, and some of the animals may have obvious increased thirst. These formulas lubricate the Intestines and promote normal bowel movements; they are comprised of sweet and nourishing seeds that contain lipids to moisten the bowel and relieve constipation. Many of these formulas contain both laxative and cold purgative herbs and are suitable for the treatment of mild to moderate constipation. This is the group of formulas typically chosen to treat animals that are weak, have chronic disease and/or are yin and blood deficient.

Representative herbs include *Huo Ma Ren* (Fructus Cannabis), *Ku Xing Ren* (Semen Armeniacae Amarum), *Tao Ren* (Semen Persicae), and *Yu Li Ren* (Semen Pruni). Representative formulas include *Ma Zi Ren Wan* (Hemp Seed Pill) and *Run Chang Wan* (Moisten the Intestines Pill).

3. **Purgative and Tonic Formulas**

These formulas treat constipation characterized by concurrent excess and deficiency in the interior. This syndrome requires the use of downward draining and tonifying methods together to ensure that the stools are moved and the qi is not damaged. These two methods cannot be used individually if both conditions are present. If only the downward draining method is employed, the qi may consequently become more deficient. If only the tonifying method is used, then the constipated stool may become more stagnant.

Downward draining herbs commonly used to drain interior excess include *Da Huang* (Radix et Rhizoma Rhei) and *Mang Xiao* (Natrii Sulfas). Tonic herbs frequently used to tonify interior deficiency include *Ren Shen* (Radix et Rhizoma Ginseng), *Dang Gui* (Radix Angelicae Sinensis), *Di Huang* (Radix Rehmanniae), and *Xuan Shen* (Radix Scrophulariae). An exemplar formula with both downward draining and tonic actions is *Zeng Ye Cheng Qi Tang* (Increase the Fluids and Order the Qi Decoction).

CAUTIONS / CONTRAINDICATIONS

- Downward draining formulas are designed to treat interior excess syndromes. If patients have both exterior and interior excess symptoms, then one should dispel the exterior factor first before eliminating the interior excess. In some cases, both exterior and interior factors may be dispelled at the same time.

Chapter 2 — Overview

- Downward draining formulas should be used with caution during pregnancy, in postpartum and nursing mothers, in geriatric or pediatric animals, or any animal with bleeding disorders, or with underlying qi, blood, and/or body fluid deficiencies. In general, for these animals, use tonic herbs either after or in conjunction with the downward draining formulas.
- Since most of the downward draining formulas have a tendency to consume Stomach qi, they should be discontinued immediately once the desired effects have been achieved.
- When properly administered these herbal formula are very effective to treat constipation both acute and chronic; animals receiving these formula should be given adequate amounts of water and have appropriate monitoring of electrolytes, especially in chronic cases when these formulas are used in conjunction with conventional laxative drugs.
- Lastly, avoid foods that are oily, greasy, or hard to digest to prevent further consumption of Stomach qi.

PROCESSING

Da Huang (Radix et Rhizoma Rhei) and *Mang Xiao* (Natrii Sulfas) are commonly used in downward draining formulas. To potentiate the downward draining effect, *Da Huang* (Radix et Rhizoma Rhei) is usually post-decocted, and *Mang Xiao* (Natrii Sulfas) is usually dissolved in the decoction immediately prior to ingestion. Cooking these two herbs in the decoction with the rest of the herbs will compromise the overall potency and effectiveness of the formulas.

PHARMACOLOGICAL EFFECTS & CLINICAL APPLICATIONS

Downward draining formulas primarily treat gastrointestinal disorders, such as constipation, intestinal obstruction, and others.

1. **Constipation**: Almost all downward draining formulas have purgative and/or laxative effects, and commonly treat constipation. Downward draining formulas have different potency and mechanisms of action, and proper selection of the formula depends on the characteristics of the constipation and the overall constitution of the patient. *Da Cheng Qi Tang* (Major Order the Qi Decoction) and *Xiao Cheng Qi Tang* (Minor Order the Qi Decoction) have potent purgative actions to treat moderate to severe constipation. Their mechanism of action involves stimulating the intestines to increase contraction and peristalsis.[1,2] *Ma Zi Ren Wan* (Hemp Seed Pill) and *Run Chang Wan* (Moisten the Intestines Pill) have moderate laxative effects to treat mild to moderate constipation. Their mechanisms of action are lubrication of the intestines and promotion of bowel movement.[3]
2. **Intestinal obstruction**: Some potent downward draining formulas, such as *Da Cheng Qi Tang* (Major Order the Qi Decoction) and *Da Xian Xiong Tang* (Major Sinking into the Chest Decoction), treat intestinal obstruction by dramatically stimulating the intestines to promote the evacuation of bowels.[4,5,6]
3. **Gastrointestinal disorders**: Downward draining formulas can treat gastrointestinal disorders, such as acute abdominal pain,[7] chronic colitis,[8] chronic gastritis,[9] peptic ulcer disease,[10] acute gastroenteritis,[11] acute appendicitis,[12] and post-surgical constipation.[13]

References

1. *Zhong Guo Zhong Xi Yi Jie He Za Zhi* (Chinese Journal of Integrative Chinese and Western Medicine), 1993; (1):33.
2. *Zhong Yi Fang Ji Xian Dai Yan Jiu* (Modern Study of Medical Formulas in Traditional Chinese Medicine), 1997; 146-147.
3. *Zhong Xi Yi Jie He Za Zhi* (Journal of Integrated Chinese and Western Medicine), 1990; (6):5.
4. *Zhong Guo Zhong Xi Yi Jie He Za Zhi* (Chinese Journal of Integrative Chinese and Western Medicine), 1993; (1):33.
5. *Zhong Guo Zhong Xi Yi Jie He Za Zhi* (Chinese Journal of Integrative Chinese and Western Medicine), 1989; 5:282.
6. *Chi Jiao Yi Sheng Za Zhi* (Journal of Barefoot Doctors), 1975; (2):26.
7. *Zhong Yi Fang Ji Xian Dai Yan Jiu* (Modern Study of Medical Formulas in Traditional Chinese Medicine), 1997; 4(1):20.
8. *Yun Nan Zhong Yi Za Zhi* (Yunan Journal of Chinese Medicine), 1993; 2:10.
9. *Hu Bei Zhong Yi Za Zhi* (Hubei Journal of Chinese Medicine), 1988; 6:8.
10. *Zhong Yi Za Zhi* (Journal of Chinese Medicine), 1985; 8:52.
11. *Zhong Yi Ming Fang Lin Chuang Xin Yong* (Contemporary Clinical Applications of Classic Chinese Formulas), 2001; 85-86.
12. *Xin Zhong Yi* (New Chinese Medicine), 1985; (11):22.
13. *Zhong Yi Za Zhi* (Journal of Chinese Medicine), 1965; 10:40.

Section 1

寒下剂
— Cold Purgatives

Dà Chéng Qì Tāng (Major Order the Qi Decoction)
大承氣湯
大承气汤

Pinyin Name: *Da Cheng Qi Tang*
Literal Name: Major Order the Qi Decoction
Alternate Names: *Ta Cheng Chi Tang, Da Cheng Chi Tang*, Major Chi-Infusing Decoction, Major Purgative Decoction, Major Rhubarb Combination
Original Source: *Shang Han Lun* (Discussion of Cold-Induced Disorders) by Zhang Zhong-Jing in the Eastern Han Dynasty

COMPOSITION

Da Huang (Radix et Rhizoma Rhei), *xi* (washed) with liquor	12g
Mang Xiao (Natrii Sulfas)	0.3 cup [6-9g]
Hou Po (Cortex Magnoliae Officinalis), *zhi* (fried with liquid)	24g [15-24g]
Zhi Shi (Fructus Aurantii Immaturus)	5 pieces [12g]

DOSAGE / PREPARATION / ADMINISTRATION

The source text instructions are to first cook *Zhi Shi* (Fructus Aurantii Immaturus) and *Hou Po* (Cortex Magnoliae Officinalis) with 10 cups [2,000 mL] of water until 5 cups [1,000 mL] of the liquid remain. Discard the residue, add *Da Huang* (Radix et Rhizoma Rhei), and cook until the liquid is further reduced to 2 cups [400 mL]. Discard the residue, add *Mang Xiao* (Natrii Sulfas), and bring the decoction to a boil 1-2 times using only low intensity fire. Take half [1 cup] of the warm decoction twice daily. Discontinue the formula once bowel movement has been induced.

Today, this formula is prepared as a decoction using the doses suggested in brackets above, with *Da Huang* (Radix et Rhizoma Rhei) post-decocted only for a short period of time and *Mang Xiao* (Natrii Sulfas) dissolved into the warm, strained decoction immediately before ingestion.

CHINESE THERAPEUTIC ACTIONS

Strongly and quickly drains heat and accumulation downward

CLINICAL MANIFESTATIONS

1. Excess *yangming fu* (hollow organ) syndrome: constipation, pain and bloating of the abdomen, abdominal pain aggravated by pressure, a feeling of hardness upon palpation, and, in severe cases, fever, trembling of the extremities, a dry, yellow, prickly or dry, black tongue coating, and a deep, slippery, and excess pulse.
2. Impacted stools accompanied by watery fluids with a foul smell, abdominal pain and bloating, solid mass of feces palpated in the colon, a dry tongue and mouth, and a slippery, excess pulse.

VETERINARY CLINICAL APPLICATIONS

Acute severe constipation, constipation or impaction secondary to dietary indiscretion, recurrent severe habitual constipation, feline megacolon, post-operative constipation, enteroparalysis, cholecystitis, hepatitis, pancreatitis, acute pancreatitis, food poisoning requiring purging of toxic substances, organophosphorus poisoning, and lead poisoning.

EXPLANATION

Da Cheng Qi Tang (Major Order the Qi Decoction) is representative of cold purgative formulas and has a wide range of functions. This formula was first presented in

Dà Chéng Qì Tāng (Major Order the Qi Decoction)

***Da Cheng Qi Tang* (Major Order the Qi Decoction)**

Diagnosis	Clinical Signs	Treatment	Herbs
Accumulation of excess heat in the Stomach and Intestines	• Constipation, pain and bloating of the abdomen, abdominal pain aggravated by pressure, and a palpably enlarged colon: accumulation of excess heat in the Stomach and Intestines • Dry mouth and tongue: heat drying up body fluids • Dry, yellow, prickly or dry, black tongue coating, and a deep, slippery, excess pulse: interior excess heat	Strongly drains heat and stool downward	• *Da Huang* (Radix et Rhizoma Rhei) clears heat and purges constipated stools. • *Mang Xiao* (Natrii Sulfas) clears heat, moistens dryness, and softens the stool. • *Hou Po* (Cortex Magnoliae Officinalis) activates qi circulation and disperses accumulation. • *Zhi Shi* (Fructus Aurantii Immaturus) relieves fullness and distention.

Shang Han Lun (Discussion of Cold-Induced Disorders) for treating *yangming fu* (hollow organs) syndrome. This syndrome arises when the wind-cold factor is not dispelled at the exterior. It then travels into the interior *zang fu* organs, where it transforms into heat, and binds with the stools.

This *yangming fu* syndrome is a condition characterized by interior excess heat. Because the heat is bound up with the stool, the stool becomes hard, causing constipation. The dry stool may disturb qi circulation, causing pain and bloating of the abdomen. Trembling of the extremities is the consequence of interior excess heat forcing body fluids out of the body. The dry mouth and tongue signify heat drying up body fluids. The tongue and pulse conditions both suggest interior excess heat.

Some animals with interior excess heat may present with different clinical manifestations. Some may actually pass watery stool rectally. The animal is actually constipated, but the owner is seeing loose watery stool with a foul odor and brings the animal in with a primary complaint of diarrhea. This is an important clinical pattern to recognize. The reason loose stool is seen is because the heat and stools are so tightly interlocked that the turbid water in the intestines has nowhere to go but to be excreted rectally as watery fluids. The fetid smell is caused by heat and stagnation. Because the stools are so hard in the large intestine, they feel like a solid mass when palpated.

All of the above conditions have the same etiology: interior heat accumulates in the Stomach and Intestines, causing consumption of yin and body fluids. The four diagnostic signs associated with the use of this formula are: *pi* (distention), *man* (fullness), *zao* (dryness), and *shi* (hardness), with a dry, yellow or black tongue coating, and a deep, slippery and excess pulse. Treatment calls for the use of drastic purgative herbs to quickly dispel heat and accumulation. Immediate action must be taken in order to preserve yin and body fluids from being consumed further.

Da Huang (Radix et Rhizoma Rhei), the chief herb, clears the Stomach and Intestines by quickly purging heat and constipated stools. *Mang Xiao* (Natrii Sulfas), the deputy herb, clears heat, moistens dryness, and softens the stools. *Da Huang* (Radix et Rhizoma Rhei) and *Mang Xiao* (Natrii Sulfas) mutually enforce each other in their actions of dispelling heat and purging constipated stools. *Hou Po* (Cortex Magnoliae Officinalis) and *Zhi Shi* (Fructus Aurantii Immaturus) regulate qi flow to relieve fullness and distention, and activate qi circulation to help dispel heat and stagnant stools.

VETERINARY MODIFICATIONS

- If there is severe thirst as a result of dryness and heat, add *Shi Gao* (Gypsum Fibrosum) and *Zhi Mu* (Rhizoma Anemarrhenae).
- When there is qi and blood stagnation, add *Chi Shao* (Radix Paeoniae Rubra) and *Tao Ren* (Semen Persicae).
- If accompanied by qi deficiency, add *Ren Shen* (Radix et Rhizoma Ginseng).
- For yin or body fluid deficiencies, add *Xuan Shen* (Radix Scrophulariae) and *Di Huang* (Radix Rehmanniae).
- For dry stools and pain, increase the dose of *Mang Xiao* (Natrii Sulfas) and add *Gua Lou Zi* (Semen Trichosanthis).
- For ascites, add *Gan Sui* (Radix Kansui) and *Yuan Hua* (Flos Genkwa).

Dà Chéng Qì Tāng (Major Order the Qi Decoction)

CAUTIONS / CONTRAINDICATIONS

- Do not use *Da Cheng Qi Tang* when the exterior syndrome is not yet resolved, or for mild to moderate cases of constipation.
- This is a drastic downward draining formula. This formula is contraindicated in pregnant animals, meconium impaction in foals, and in geriatric or convalescing patients. It is also contraindicated in animals with yin or qi deficiency, or generalized weakness.
- Discontinue this formula once the desired effects are achieved. Prolonged use may injure the qi.
- This formula is not to be used in cases of intractable constipation (obstipation) with severe colonic dilation seen in feline megacolon. It can be used to treat habitual constipation before it reaches the stage of obstipation in the management of feline megacolon and following manual relief of obstipation.

PHARMACOLOGICAL EFFECTS

1. **Gastrointestinal**: Administration of *Da Cheng Qi Tang* in guinea pigs was been associated with increased contraction and peristalsis. The mechanism of action is attributed to the stimulating effect on the smooth muscles of the intestines.[1]
2. **Digestive**: The effect of *Da Cheng Qi Tang* on the organs associated with digestion was evaluated by administering the formula to rats. The study reported that the herbs had a stimulating effect on the gastrointestinal system and increased the production of gastric acid and pancreatic enzymes. The herbs, however, had little influence on the production and release of bile acid.[2]
3. **Antibiotic**: Administration of *Da Cheng Qi Tang* was associated with an inhibitory effect *in vitro* against *Staphylococcus aureus*, *Salmonella typhi*, *Bacillus dysenteriae*, and *Bacillus paratyphosus*.[3]

HUMAN CLINICAL STUDIES AND RESEARCH

1. **Intestinal obstruction**: Sixty-six patients with intestinal obstruction were treated with *Da Cheng Qi Tang* with 100% success rate. In follow-ups, 46 patients had no recurrence within 3 years. The 20 patients who had recurrences were treated with the same formula with complete recovery.[4] In another study, individuals with intestinal obstruction were divided into two groups and treated with herbs accordingly. Group one with 78 patients (42 males, 36 females, average of 43 years of age) was treated with *Da Cheng Qi Tang* plus *Lai Fu Zi* (Semen Raphani) and *Huang Qin* (Radix Scutellariae) in decoction one time daily for up to three days with 92.3% effectiveness. Group two with 92 patients (52 males, 40 females, average of 41 years of age) was treated with *Da Cheng Qi Tang* only in decoction one time daily for up to two days with 76.1% effectiveness.[5]
2. **Enteroparalysis**: Administration of modified *Da Cheng Qi Tang* was associated with good results in treating 40 patients with enteroparalysis. Clinical results include passage of gas, bowel movement, and relief of abdominal distention and pain within 2 to 6 hours.[6]
3. **Infection of gallbladder and bile duct**: A modification of *Da Cheng Qi Tang* was used to treat 128 patients with acute infection of the gallbladder or the bile duct with complete recovery in 81 patients, moderate improvement in 33 patients, and no benefit in 14 patients. The study concluded an overall rate of effectiveness of 89%.[7]
4. **Cholecystitis**: One study reported marked improvement using modified *Da Cheng Qi Tang* to treat 75 patients with acute inflammation of the gallbladder. The herbal treatment contained *Da Cheng Qi Tang* plus *Pu Gong Ying* (Herba Taraxaci), *Jin Qian Cao* (Herba Lysimachiae) and *San Qi* (Radix et Rhizoma Notoginseng) as the base formula. Modifications included addition of *Xiang Fu* (Rhizoma Cyperi) and *Yu Jin* (Radix Curcumae) for qi stagnation; *Jin Yin Hua* (Flos Lonicerae Japonicae) and *Lian Qiao* (Fructus Forsythiae) for excess heat; and *Yin Chen* (Herba Artemisiae Scopariae) and *Zhi Zi* (Fructus Gardeniae) for damp-heat. The herbs were given in decoction two times daily. The average duration of treatment was 8.34 days. The study reported recovery in 50 of 75 patients.[8]
5. **Acute pancreatitis**: Modified *Da Cheng Qi Tang* has been shown to effectively treat acute pancreatitis. The study used *Da Cheng Qi Tang* plus *Huang Qin* (Radix Scutellariae), *Huang Bo* (Cortex Phellodendri Chinensis), and *Chai Hu* (Radix Bupleuri) as the base formula, with addition of *Jin Yin Hua* (Flos Lonicerae Japonicae) and *Lian Qiao* (Fructus Forsythiae) for excess heat in the Stomach and Intestines; *Yin Chen* (Herba Artemisiae Scopariae) and *Zhi Zi* (Fructus Gardeniae) for damp-heat jaundice; and *Ku Lian Pi* (Cortex Meliae), *Bing Lang* (Semen Arecae), and *Xi Xin* (Radix et Rhizoma Asari) for biliary ascariasis. The treatment protocol was to administer 500 mL of the decoction twice daily six hours apart. For those without constipation, *Mang Xiao* (Natrii Sulfas) and *Da Huang* (Radix et Rhizoma Rhei) were removed from the formula, and the decoction was given only one time per day. The study reported complete recovery in all 48 patients (20 males and 28 females) with an average of 8.34 days.[9]
6. **Organophosphorus poisoning**: Patients with acute organophosphorus poisoning were first treated with gastric lavage followed by administration of one dose of *Da Cheng Qi Tang* via gastric tube. Of 35 patients, the study reported complete recovery in 32 patients and fatality in 3 patients.[10]
7. **Lead poisoning**: One study reported complete recovery in all 30 patients suffering from chronic lead poisoning.

Dà Chéng Qì Tāng (Major Order the Qi Decoction)

The herbal formula used *Da Cheng Qi Tang* as the base formula, and added *Yan Hu Suo* (Rhizoma Corydalis) and *Wu Yao* (Radix Linderae) for acute and excruciating abdominal pain; *Qian Niu Zi* (Semen Pharbitidis) and *Yu Li Ren* (Semen Pruni) for chronic constipation; *Shan Zha* (Fructus Crataegi), *Lai Fu Zi* (Semen Raphani), and *Ji Nei Jin* (Endothelium Corneum Gigeriae Galli) for poor appetite; *Ren Shen* (Radix et Rhizoma Ginseng), *Huang Qi* (Radix Astragali), *Dang Gui* (Radix Angelicae Sinensis), and *Bai Shao* (Radix Paeoniae Alba) for qi and blood deficiencies.[11]

SUGGESTED ACUPUNCTURE TREATMENT

1. Points: *Hegu* (LI 4), *Quchi* (LI 11), *Dazhui* (GV 14), *Sibai* (ST 2), *Neiting* (ST 44), *Lidui* (ST 45), *Guanchong* (TH 1), *Pishu* (BL 20), *Weishu* (BL 21), *Changqiang* (GV 1), *Shangjuxu* (ST 37), *Tianshu* (ST 25), *Lieque* (LU 7), *Zhaohai* (KI 6), *Weijian*, *Jiangya* and *Erding*.
2. Technique: sedation.

Hegu (LI 4) and *Quchi* (LI 11) sedate heat and relieve pain in the *yangming* channel. *Dazhui* (GV 14), *Sibai* (ST 2), *Neiting* (ST 44), *Lidui* (ST 45), and *Guanchong* (TH 1) clear heat, move qi, and relieve pain. *Pishu* (BL 20) and *Weishu* (BL 21) tonify the Spleen and Stomach and promote motility. *Changqiang* (GV 1) opens the yang channels and regulates gastrointestinal motility. *Shangjuxu* (ST 37), the lower *he* (uniting) point of the Large Intestine, is combined with *Tianshu* (ST 25) to expel the constipated stool. *Lieque* (LU 7), the *luo* (connecting) point of the Lung channel, regulates qi flow of the Large Intestine. *Zhaohai* (KI 6) nourishes body fluids and helps clear heat. *Weijian* clears heat. *Jiangya* and *Erding* are classical equine points to relieve colic pain and promote intestinal motility.

AUTHORS' COMMENTS

Da Cheng Qi Tang is the standard downward draining formula in the treatment of excess *yangming fu* (hollow organs) syndrome. Traditionally, the four main diagnostic clinical signs are *pi* (distention), *man* (fullness), *zao* (dryness) and *shi* (hardness).

- *Pi* (distention) is the feeling of oppression, obstruction, and increased pressure in the chest and epigastrium.
- *Man* (fullness) is the feeling of bloating and fullness in the epigastric and abdominal regions.
- *Zao* (dryness) refers to the dry, compacted stool, which feels hard upon abdominal palpation.
- *Shi* (hardness) signifies an excess condition in which the dry, hard stools are interlocked with heat, causing constipation and abdominal pain that intensifies with palpation.

The potency of *Da Cheng Qi Tang* is directly dependent on the preparation of two ingredients: *Da Huang* (Radix et Rhizoma Rhei) and *Mang Xiao* (Natrii Sulfas). *Da Huang* (Radix et Rhizoma Rhei) must be post-decocted to preserve its purgative functions; otherwise, it will lose much of its purgative effect if it is cooked together with the rest of the herbs. *Mang Xiao* (Natrii Sulfas) is also kept aside during the cooking process. When the cooking process is finished and the herb residue is filtered out, *Mang Xiao* (Natrii Sulfas) should be dissolved into the warm decoction immediately before ingestion. The rationale for this preparation can also be explained from a biochemical perspective. *Da Huang* (Radix et Rhizoma Rhei) contains sennoside and emodin as the main active ingredients responsible for purgative and laxative actions. These two compounds are highly sensitive to heat, and will be deactivated with prolonged exposure if cooked for a long period of time. *Mang Xiao* (Natrii Sulfas), on the other hand, is a mineral substance that does not require extraction with cooking. If added to the decoction during the cooking process, it will simply be lost when the decoction is filtered out and the herb residues discarded. For these reasons, it is important to following the specific instructions according to the source text to ensure the efficacy of this formula. Commerical products of this formula sometimes vary greatly in efficacy, depending on how these two herbs are handled in the manufacturing process.

Da Cheng Qi Tang can be used in postpartum animals that show no signs of exterior conditions but have lower abdominal pain and hardness with retention of lochia, constipation, irritability and fever. However, this formula must be given carefully as most postpartum animals can be weak and deficient.

This formula can be used for any excess heat conditions, or for fire flaring upward accompanied by constipation or hardness of the stool, since it can purge out the excess. Three of the most effective outlets for clearing fire from the body include inducing sweating, diuresis, and purging the bowels. Since this formula helps guide heat down and out of the body, it is extremely effective in enhancing the overall effect of other heat-clearing herbs.

Da Cheng Qi Tang (Major Order the Qi Decoction), *Xiao Cheng Qi Tang* (Minor Order the Qi Decoction), and *Tiao Wei Cheng Qi Tang* (Regulate the Stomach and Order the Qi Decoction) share many similarities, but have notable differences. All three formulas contain *Da Huang* (Radix et Rhizoma Rhei) to purge stagnation and heat in the Large Intestine to treat *yangming fu* (hollow organs) syndrome.

Dà Chéng Qì Tāng (Major Order the Qi Decoction)

Common clinical signs include constipation and abdominal pain that worsens upon pressure. The differences are as follows:

- *Da Cheng Qi Tang* is the strongest of the formula to drain excess heat in the Stomach and Intestines, relieve obstruction of the abdomen, and restore the normal flow of qi, thus the name "Major Order the Qi Decoction." This also helps differentiate it from its less powerful version "Minor Order the Qi Decoction." This formula contains *Da Huang* (Radix et Rhizoma Rhei), *Mang Xiao* (Natrii Sulfas), *Zhi Shi* (Fructus Aurantii Immaturus), and *Hou Po* (Cortex Magnoliae Officinalis). The four ingredients together treat *pi* (distention), *man* (fullness), *zao* (dryness), and *shi* (hardness). The constipation is characterized by extremely hard stools. *Da Huang* (Radix et Rhizoma Rhei) and *Mang Xiao* (Natrii Sulfas) are commonly used together to treat excess constipation caused by heat. From a pharmacological standpoint, the two herbs work synergistically because *Da Huang* (Radix et Rhizoma Rhei) increases intestinal peristalsis and *Mang Xiao* (Natrii Sulfas) increases bowel fluid content in order to produce a bowel movement. From a TCM perspective, *Da Huang* (Radix et Rhizoma Rhei) has a strong purgative function to relieve stagnation; *Mang Xiao* (Natrii Sulfas) softens the stool to promote its passage. This formula is most often used in cases of habitual constipation seen with eventual progression to feline megacolon. It is not used in cases of obstipation (intractable constipation with severe colonic dilation-impaction) seen in feline megacolon. This formula is used after the relief of obstipation by enema and/or manual extraction of feces. In these cases it functions to keep the colon moving and prevent re-impaction while also resolving or stabilizing the condition to avoid surgical intervention. This formula has also been used in veterinary medicine to relieve impaction caused by dietary indiscretion in the dog (food and bone impaction, gravel, dirt, plant materials, manure, etc.) The type of materials ingested by the dog causing obstruction is only limited by the imagination. In the horse, this formula can be used in acute cases of impaction colic. Heat can accumulate from high environmental temperatures, from eating too soon after exercise while the body is still hot, and, most commonly, by feed stagnating in the colon. Practitioners will likely need to administer this formula via nasogastric tube. In foals, however, *Da Cheng Qi Tang* will likely be too strong. In these cases, if enemas will not relieve the impaction, administration of the mildest formula in the group, *Tiao Wei Cheng Qi Tang* (Regulate the Stomach and Order the Qi Decoction), is recommended. If there is abdominal pain, add *Yan Hu Suo* (Rhizoma Corydalis) and *Wu Yao* (Radix Linderae).
- *Xiao Cheng Qi Tang* treats the same disorders as *Da Cheng Qi Tang*. It is not as strong as *Da Cheng Qi Tang* to drain heat and accumulation downward, and it has a moderate action to relieve constipation characterized by moderately hard stools. It contains the same amount of *Da Huang* (Radix et Rhizoma Rhei) and decreased doses of *Zhi Shi* (Fructus Aurantii Immaturus) and *Hou Po* (Cortex Magnoliae Officinalis), and it does not contain *Mang Xiao* (Natrii Sulfas). This formula focuses more on relieving qi stagnation and signs of *pi* (distention), *man* (fullness) and *shi* (hardness), rather than dryness. This is an important consideration in the horse. Cases may respond better to *Xiao Cheng Qi Tang* where rectal palpation reveals impaction that is overly large and firm but gives to light pressure. Cases that palpate hard, almost like an enterolith, would be better served by the moistening qualities of *Da Cheng Qi Tang*.
- *Tiao Wei Cheng Qi Tang* contains *Da Huang* (Radix et Rhizoma Rhei), *Mang Xiao* (Natrii Sulfas), and *Gan Cao* (Radix et Rhizoma Glycyrrhizae), and is the mildest of the three formulas and the most commonly used formula for constipation in small animals. It softens the stools and focuses more on relief of dryness rather than treating *pi* (distention) and *man* (fullness). The use of sweet, tonifying *Zhi Gan Cao* (Radix et Rhizoma Glycyrrhizae Praeparata cum Melle) protects the Stomach yin and makes this formula the best choice to treat mild to moderate constipation in weak, geriatric and post-surgical animals. It is also a nice formula to use in postpartum mares to prevent of postpartum colic and in foals with meconium impaction. It is also used to treat painful, swollen gums

Comparison of Three "*Cheng Qi Tang* (Order the Qi Decoctions)"

Formula Names	*Pi* (Distention)	*Man* (Fullness)	*Zao* (Dryness)	*Shi* (Hardness)
Da Cheng Qi Tang (Major Order the Qi Decoction)	severe	severe	severe	severe
Xiao Cheng Qi Tang (Minor Order the Qi Decoction)	moderate	moderate		moderate
Tiao Wei Cheng Qi Tang (Regulate the Stomach and Order the Qi Decoction)			severe	severe

and gingivitis-stomatitis caused by heat in the Stomach and Large Intestine in the cat and dog.

It is important to note that all three of these formulas are purgatives and are not for long term use. They typically take effect quickly, and in general a course of treatment does not exceed 2-4 days. Once the bowel movements have normalized, the formula is modified or another formula is chosen to tonify any underlying deficiencies.

References

1. *Zhong Guo Zhong Xi Yi Jie He Za Zhi* (Chinese Journal of Integrative Chinese and Western Medicine), 1993; (1):33.
2. *Zhong Xi Yi Jie He Za Zhi* (Journal of Integrated Chinese and Western Medicine), 1985; (6):338.
3. *Zhong Yao Yao Li Yu Ying Yong* (Pharmacology and Applications of Chinese Herbs), 1988; 4(3):1.
4. *Zhong Yi Yao Xin Xi* (Information on Chinese Medicine and Herbology), 1995; (3):46.
5. *Zhong Guo Zhong Xi Yi Jie He Za Zhi* (Chinese Journal of Integrative Chinese and Western Medicine), 1989; 5:282.
6. *Zhong Guo Zhong Xi Yi Jie He Za Zhi* (Chinese Journal of Integrative Chinese and Western Medicine), 1992; 11:695.
7. *Ji Lin Zhong Yi Yao* (Jilin Chinese Medicine and Herbology), 1988; (2):12.
8. *Fu Jian Zhong Yi Yao* (Fujian Chinese Medicine and Herbology), 1992; 1:31.
9. *Liao Ning Zhong Yi Za Zhi* (Liaoning Journal of Chinese Medicine), 1985; 2:24.
10. *Shi Yong Zhong Xi Yi Jie He Za Zhi* (Practical Journal of Integrated Chinese and Western Medicines), 1993; 2:755.
11. *Jiang Xi Zhong Yi Yao* (Jiangxi Chinese Medicine and Herbology), 1993; 1:17.

Xiǎo Chéng Qì Tāng (Minor Order the Qi Decoction)

小承氣湯
小承气汤

Pinyin Name: *Xiao Cheng Qi Tang*
Literal Name: Minor Order the Qi Decoction
Alternate Names: *Hsiao Cheng Chi Tang*, Minor Qi-Infusing Decoction, Minor Purgative Decoction, Minor Rhubarb Combination
Original Source: *Shang Han Lun* (Discussion of Cold-Induced Disorders) by Zhang Zhong-Jing in the Eastern Han Dynasty

COMPOSITION

Da Huang (Radix et Rhizoma Rhei), *xi* (washed) with liquor	12g
Hou Po (Cortex Magnoliae Officinalis), *zhi* (fried with liquid)	6g
Zhi Shi (Fructus Aurantii Immaturus), *zhi* (fried with liquid)	3 large pieces [9g]

DOSAGE / PREPARATION / ADMINISTRATION

Cook the ingredients with 4 cups [800 mL] of water until reduced to 1.2 cups [240 mL]. Take the warm, strained decoction in two equally-divided doses twice daily.

CHINESE THERAPEUTIC ACTIONS

Moderate action to drain heat and accumulation downward

CLINICAL MANIFESTATIONS

1. Excess *yangming fu* (hollow organs) syndrome: constipation, pain and distention of the abdomen, a yellow, greasy tongue coating and a rapid, slippery pulse.
2. Early stage of dysentery with rectal tenesmus, and epigastric and abdominal distention and pain.

VETERINARY CLINICAL APPLICATIONS

Acute constipation, recurrent habitual constipation, feline megacolon, post-operative constipation, constipation secondary to dietary indiscretion, intestinal paralysis, absence of intestinal peristalsis, abdominal distention and pain, chronic gastritis, acute gastroenteritis and acute cholecystitis

Xiǎo Chéng Qì Tāng (Minor Order the Qì Decoction)

EXPLANATION

Xiao Cheng Qi Tang (Minor Order the Qi Decoction) treats *yangming fu* (hollow organs) syndrome of moderate severity, characterized by the presence of *pi* (distention), *man* (fullness), and *shi* (hardness). However, there is no *zao* (dryness) associated with this pattern, and thus it contains no *Mang Xiao* (Natrii Sulfas). *Da Huang* (Radix et Rhizoma Rhei), the chief herb, clears heat in the Stomach and Intestines and purges constipated stools. *Hou Po* (Cortex Magnoliae Officinalis) and *Zhi Shi* (Fructus Aurantii Immaturus) regulate qi flow to relieve fullness and distention, and activate qi circulation to help dispel heat and stagnant stools.

Xiao Cheng Qi Tang is a variation of *Da Cheng Qi Tang* (Major Order the Qi Decoction) and basically has the same purgative effect, except that it is a milder formula for *yangming fu* (hollow organs) syndrome of moderate severity. Therefore, it is not necessary to post-decoct *Da Huang* (Radix et Rhizoma Rhei), as in *Da Cheng Qi Tang* (Major Order the Qi Decoction). Instead, *Da Huang* (Radix et Rhizoma Rhei) is fully cooked to moderate its potent downward draining effects. Additionally, the doses of *Hou Po* (Cortex Magnoliae Officinalis) and *Zhi Shi* (Fructus Aurantii Immaturus) are decreased, since the condition is not as severe. Lastly, *Mang Xiao* (Natrii Sulfas) is not included in this formula since there is an absence of *zao* (dryness).

VETERINARY MODIFICATIONS

- If there is generalized weakness and qi deficiency, add *Huang Qi* (Radix Astragali) and *Ren Shen* (Radix et Rhizoma Ginseng).
- If there is generalized weakness and blood deficiency, add *Dang Gui* (Radix Angelicae Sinensis) and *Chuan Xiong* (Rhizoma Chuanxiong).
- When there is irritability and restlessness as a result of Lung deficiency, add *Mai Dong* (Radix Ophiopogonis) and *Wu Wei Zi* (Fructus Schisandrae Chinensis).

CAUTIONS / CONTRAINDICATIONS

Refer to *Da Cheng Qi Tang* (Major Order the Qi Decoction).

PHARMACOLOGICAL EFFECTS

1. **Gastrointestinal**: Administration of *Xiao Cheng Qi Tang* was associated with increased contraction and peristalsis. The mechanism of action was attributed to the stimulating effect on the smooth muscles of the intestines.[1,2]
2. **Antibiotic**: Administration of *Xiao Cheng Qi Tang* was associated with an inhibitory effect *in vitro* against *Staphylococcus aureus* and *E. coli*. Also, the inhibitory effect of the formula was determined to be stronger than the individual ingredients.[3]

HUMAN CLINICAL STUDIES AND RESEARCH

1. **Gastrointestinal disorders**: *Xiao Cheng Qi Tang* has been shown in many studies to treat various types of gastro-intestinal disorders, such as post-operative constipation, intestinal paralysis, absence of intestinal peristalsis, abdominal distention and pain, etc.[4]
2. **Post-operative constipation**: Eighty-six geriatric patients were treated with modified *Xiao Cheng Qi Tang* for prevention and treatment of post-operative constipation. The first dose of the formula was given 48 hours after the surgery, and the second dose was given 6 hours later (54 hours after the surgery) only if necessary. The study reported 100% success rate, with 53 patients showing gas or bowel movement after the first dose, and the remaining 33 patients after the second dose.[5]
3. **Chronic gastritis**: Use of modified *Xiao Cheng Qi Tang* was associated with 96.36% effectiveness in the treatment of chronic gastritis in 55 patients.[6]
4. **Acute gastroenteritis**: Modified *Xiao Cheng Qi Tang* effectively treated acute gastroenteritis in 91 patients (49 males and 42 females) between 1 and 5 years of age, with 1-3 days history of illness. The study reported immediate improvement in 16 cases, significant improvement in 42 cases, moderate improvement in 26 cases, and no benefit in 7 cases. The overall rate of effectiveness was 92.3%. The

Xiao Cheng Qi Tang **(Minor Order the Qi Decoction)**

Diagnosis	Clinical Signs	Treatment	Herbs
Accumulation of excess heat in the Stomach and Intestines	• Constipation with pain and bloating of the abdomen: accumulation of excess heat in the Stomach and Intestines • Yellow tongue coating and rapid slippery excess pulse: interior excess heat	Gently drains heat and accumulation downward	• Fully-cooked *Da Huang* (Radix et Rhizoma Rhei) gently clears heat and purges the constipated stools. • *Hou Po* (Cortex Magnoliae Officinalis) activates qi circulation and disperses accumulation. • *Zhi Shi* (Fructus Aurantii Immaturus) relieves pain and bloating.

Xiǎo Chéng Qì Tāng (Minor Order the Qi Decoction)

herbal treatment used *Xiao Cheng Qi Tang* plus charred *Shan Zha* (Fructus Crataegi) and charred *Shen Qu* (Massa Fermentata) as the base formula. *Mu Xiang* (Radix Aucklandiae) was added for abdominal pain; *Lian Qiao* (Fructus Forsythiae), and *Bo He* (Herba Menthae) were added for fever; *Sha Ren* (Fructus Amomi), *Huang Lian* (Rhizoma Coptidis), and *Ban Xia* (Rhizoma Pinelliae) were added for recurrent nausea and vomiting. The herbs were given one time daily in decoction.[7]

5. **Viral hepatitis**: Administration of modified *Xiao Cheng Qi Tang* effectively treated 39 of 40 patients with viral hepatitis. Of those who responded to the treatment, none had recurrence during the follow-up exam one year later. All patients received two courses of treatment, with 15 days per course. The herbal treatment contained *Xiao Cheng Qi Tang* plus *Gan Cao* (Radix et Rhizoma Glycyrrhizae) as the base formula. Additionally, *Cang Zhu* (Rhizoma Atractylodis) was added for dampness; and charred *Shan Zha* (Fructus Crataegi) and charred *Ji Nei Jin* (Endothelium Corneum Gigeriae Galli) were added for indigestion. Pharmaceutical drugs were added as supportive treatment when necessary.[8]

HERB-DRUG INTERACTION

Opioid-induced constipation and nausea: One study reported marked effectiveness using *Xiao Cheng Qi Tang* to relieve constipation and nausea caused by excessive use of opioid analgesics in 40 patients with terminal cancer. For constipation, the study reported complete recovery in 30 cases, improvement in 8 cases, and no benefit in 2 cases. For nausea, the study reported complete relief in 19 cases and improvement in 9 cases.[9]

SUGGESTED ACUPUNCTURE TREATMENT

1. Points: *Hegu* (LI 4), *Quchi* (LI 11), *Shangjuxu* (ST 37), *Zhigou* (TH 6), *Lieque* (LU 7), *Zhaohai* (KI 6), *Jiangya* and *Erding*.
2. Technique: sedation.

Hegu (LI 4) and *Quchi* (LI 11) sedate heat in the *yangming* channel. Combine *Shangjuxu* (ST 37), the lower *he* (uniting) point of the Large Intestine, with *Zhigou* (TH 6) to expel constipated stools. *Lieque* (LU 7), the *luo* (connecting) point of the Lung channel, regulates qi flow of the Large Intestine. *Zhaohai* (KI 6) nourishes body fluids and helps clear heat. *Jiangya* and *Erding* are the classic equine points for treating colic and improving gastrointestinal motility.

AUTHORS' COMMENTS

Please refer to *Da Cheng Qi Tang* (Major Order the Qi Decoction) for a detailed comparison with *Xiao Cheng Qi Tang* and *Tiao Wei Cheng Qi Tang* (Regulate the Stomach and Order the Qi Decoction).

References

1. *Zhong Guo Zhong Xi Yi Jie He Za Zhi* (Chinese Journal of Integrative Chinese and Western Medicine), 1993; (1):33.
2. *Zhong Yi Fang Ji Xian Dai Yan Jiu* (Modern Study of Medical Formulas in Traditional Chinese Medicine), 1997; 146-147.
3. *Zhong Yi Za Zhi* (Journal of Chinese Medicine), 1955; 10:36.
4. *Zhong Yi Ming Fang Lin Chuang Xin Yong* (Contemporary Clinical Applications of Classic Chinese Formulas), 2001; 85.
5. *Bei Jing Zhong Yi Za Zhi* (Beijing Journal of Chinese Medicine), 1991; (5):31.
6. *Hu Bei Zhong Yi Za Zhi* (Hubei Journal of Chinese Medicine), 1988; 6:8.
7. *Zhong Yi Ming Fang Lin Chuang Xin Yong* (Contemporary Clinical Applications of Classic Chinese Formulas), 2001; 85-86.
8. *Yun Nan Yi Yao* (Yunan Medicine and Herbology), 1982; 3:102.
9. *Xin Zhong Yi* (New Chinese Medicine), 1996; 2:52.

Tiáo Wèi Chéng Qì Tāng

(Regulate the Stomach and Order the Qi Decoction)

調胃承氣湯

调胃承气汤

Pinyin Name: *Tiao Wei Cheng Qi Tang*

Literal Name: Regulate the Stomach and Order the Qi Decoction

Alternate Names: *Tiao Wei Cheng Chi Tang*, Stomach-Regulating and Qi-Infusing Decoction, Stomach-Regulating and Purgative Decoction, Rhubarb and Mirabilitum Combination

Original Source: *Shang Han Lun* (Discussion of Cold-Induced Disorders) by Zhang Zhong-Jing in the Eastern Han Dynasty

COMPOSITION

Da Huang (Radix et Rhizoma Rhei), *xi* (washed) with liquor	12g
Mang Xiao (Natrii Sulfas)	0.5 cup [9-12g]
Zhi Gan Cao (Radix et Rhizoma Glycyrrhizae Praeparata cum Melle)	6g

DOSAGE / PREPARATION / ADMINISTRATION

Cook *Da Huang* (Radix et Rhizoma Rhei) and *Zhi Gan Cao* (Radix et Rhizoma Glycyrrhizae Praeparata cum Melle) in 3 cups [600 mL] of water and reduce the liquid to 1 cup [200 mL]. Filter and discard the residue, then add *Mang Xiao* (Natrii Sulfas) and bring the decoction to a boil 1-2 times using low intensity fire. Take the entire decoction while warm.

CHINESE THERAPEUTIC ACTIONS

Gently and slowly drains heat and accumulation downward

CLINICAL MANIFESTATIONS

1. *Yangming fu* (hollow organs) syndrome characterized by dryness and heat in the Stomach and Intestines: constipation, thirst, irritability, pain and bloating of the abdomen, a yellow tongue coating, and a slippery, rapid pulse.
2. Heat in the Stomach and Intestines causing hematemesis, epistaxis, swelling and pain of the gums, mouth and throat.

VETERINARY CLINICAL APPLICATIONS

Acute or chronic mild to moderate constipation in weak and geriatric patients, post-surgical constipation, painful swollen gums and gingivitis-stomatitis.

EXPLANATION

Tiao Wei Cheng Qi Tang (Regulate the Stomach and Order the Qi Decoction) treats *yangming fu* (hollow organs) syndrome characterized by dryness and heat in the Stomach and Intestines. In this condition, *zao* (dryness) and *shi* (hardness) are present, but *pi* (distension) and *man* (fullness) are absent. *Da Huang* (Radix et Rhizoma Rhei) clears heat in the Stomach and Intestines and purges constipated stools. *Mang Xiao* (Natrii Sulfas) clears heat, moistens dryness, and softens the stools. *Gan Cao* (Radix et Rhizoma Glycyrrhizae) tonifies qi and harmonizes the formula.

Tiao Wei Cheng Qi Tang, a variation of *Da Cheng Qi Tang* (Major Order the Qi Decoction), is indicated for *yangming fu* (hollow organs) syndrome characterized by mild to moderate constipation and pain and bloating

***Tiao Wei Cheng Qi Tang* (Regulate the Stomach and Order the Qi Decoction)**

Diagnosis	Clinical Signs	Treatment	Herbs
Accumulation of excess heat in the Stomach and Intestines	• Constipation with pain and bloating of the abdomen: accumulation of excess heat in the Stomach and Intestines • Thirst, irritability, fever: dryness and heat • Yellow tongue coating, rapid slippery pulse: interior excess heat	Slowly drains heat and accumulation downward	• Fully-cooked *Da Huang* (Radix et Rhizoma Rhei) slowly clears heat and purges the constipated stool. • *Mang Xiao* (Natrii Sulfas) clears heat, moistens dryness, and softens the stool. • *Gan Cao* (Radix et Rhizoma Glycyrrhizae) tonifies qi and harmonizes the formula.

Tiáo Wèi Chéng Qì Tāng
(Regulate the Stomach and Order the Qi Decoction)

of the abdomen. In this formula, *Da Huang* (Radix et Rhizoma Rhei) is fully cooked to moderate its potent downward draining effects. *Mang Xiao* (Natrii Sulfas) is used at a slightly higher dose to address dryness and heat. *Hou Po* (Cortex Magnoliae Officinalis) and *Zhi Shi* (Fructus Aurantii Immaturus) are removed, since *pi* (distention) and *man* (fullness) are absent in this condition. *Gan Cao* (Radix et Rhizoma Glycyrrhizae) is added to tonify qi and harmonize the formula. Overall, *Tiao Wei Cheng Qi Tang* has a stronger effect in treating "dry-heat" and a weaker effect in treating "fullness," in comparison to *Da Cheng Qi Tang*.

VETERINARY MODIFICATIONS

- To strengthen ability to nourish yin and blood, clear heat and cool blood, add *Di Huang* (Radix Rehmanniae).
- To nourish yin, moisten the Large Intestine and unblock the bowels, add *He Shou Wu* (Radix Polygoni Multiflori).

CAUTIONS / CONTRAINDICATIONS

Refer to *Da Cheng Qi Tang* (Major Order the Qi Decoction).

HERB-DRUG INTERACTION

Drug overdose: Use of *Tiao Wei Cheng Qi Tang* was associated with satisfactory results in treating 24 patients with overdose of illegal drugs. The herbal formula contained *Da Huang* (Radix et Rhizoma Rhei) 10g, *Gan Cao* (Radix et Rhizoma Glycyrrhizae) 10g, and *Mang Xiao* (Natrii Sulfas) 10g. The patients received gastric lavage first, followed by administration of the herbs via a gastric tube with warm water. Bowel movement was induced within 2.5 to 4.0 hours in all patients.[1]

SUGGESTED ACUPUNCTURE TREATMENT

1. Points: *Hegu* (LI 4), *Quchi* (LI 11), *Shangjuxu* (ST 37), *Tianshu* (ST 25), *Lieque* (LU 7), *Weishu* (BL 21), *Zhongwan* (CV 12), *Zhaohai* (KI 6), *Jiangya* and *Erding*.
2. Technique: sedation.

Hegu (LI 4) and *Quchi* (LI 11) sedate heat in the *yangming* channel. Combine *Shangjuxu* (ST 37), the lower *he* (uniting) point of the Large Intestine, with *Tianshu* (ST 25) to expel constipated stools. *Lieque* (LU 7), the *luo* (connecting) point of the Lung channel, regulates the qi flow of the Large Intestine. *Weishu* (BL 21) and *Zhongwan* (CV 12) are association and alarm points of the Stomach and improve motility and relieve pain. *Zhaohai* (KI 6) nourishes body fluids and helps clear heat. *Jiangya* and *Erding* are classical equine points used to relieve colic pain and improve gastrointestinal motility.

AUTHORS' COMMENTS

Tiao Wei Cheng Qi Tang is commonly used to treat constipation in small animals. It clears heat, softens the stools, and relieves dryness from excess heat in the Stomach and Large Intestine. In horses, the stomach-protecting properties of this formula make it the preferred choice in cases where stomach ulcers or phenylbutazone therapy are causing an acute episode of colic accompanied by decreased colonic motility. It is also the first choice to use in impacted foals because of its gentleness and ability to help the stomach. The use of sweet, tonifying *Zhi Gan Cao* (Radix et Rhizoma Glycyrrhizae Praeparata cum Melle) in this formula harmonizes the middle *jiao* and protects the Stomach yin while clearing heat and accumulation, and this makes the formula the best choice to treat mild to moderate constipation in weak, geriatric, post-surgical and Spleen qi deficient animals. Excess heat in the Stomach can ascend through the Stomach channel to cause swollen, painful gums and mouth; this formula can be used to treat gingivitis-stomatitis in the dog and cat. This formula is a purgative formula and is not for long-term use; once clinical signs resolve another formula should be chosen to address underlying deficiency.

Please refer to *Da Cheng Qi Tang* (Major Order the Qi Decoction) for a detailed comparison with *Xiao Cheng Qi Tang* (Minor Order the Qi Decoction) and *Tiao Wei Cheng Qi Tang*.

Reference

1. *Si Chuan Zhong Yi* (Sichuan Chinese Medicine), 1996; 1:37.

Yǐ Zì Tāng (Yi Word Decoction)

乙字湯
乙字汤

Pinyin Name: *Yi Zi Tang*
Literal Name: Yi Word Decoction
Alternate Names: *I Chi Tang*, I-Character Decoction, Cimicifuga Combination
Original Source: *Asada's Prescriptions* by Sohaku Asada

COMPOSITION

Chai Hu (Radix Bupleuri)	5g
Sheng Ma (Rhizoma Cimicifugae)	1g
Dang Gui (Radix Angelicae Sinensis)	6g
Gan Cao (Radix et Rhizoma Glycyrrhizae)	3g
Huang Qin (Radix Scutellariae)	3g
Da Huang (Radix et Rhizoma Rhei)	1g

DOSAGE / PREPARATION / ADMINISTRATION

The source text states to cook the ingredients in 1 bowl of water and reduce it to 50%. Take the warm decoction in two or three equally-divided doses daily. Today, this formula may be prepared as a decoction with higher doses of the ingredients, approximately two to three times higher.

CHINESE THERAPEUTIC ACTIONS

1. Clears heat and promotes bowel movement
2. Cools the blood and eliminates toxins
3. Raises yang qi

CLINICAL MANIFESTATIONS

Accumulation of dampness, heat and toxins in the lower *jiao*: constipation, severe pain, and perianal and vaginal itching.

VETERINARY CLINICAL APPLICATIONS

Rectal prolapse, rectal polyps with ulceration, anal fissure, anal gland infection and impaction, post-surgical constipation, perianal fistula, constipation, vaginal and perianal itching.

EXPLANATION

Yi Zi Tang (Yi Word Decoction) primarily treats perianal, anal gland and rectal infection and itching caused by accumulation of dampness, heat, and toxins in the lower *jiao*. Animals can experience constipation, severe pain, and bleeding secondary to these conditions. Because this formula is indicated for accumulation of dampness, heat, and toxins in the lower *jiao*, it can also treat vaginal itching and inflammation.

Chai Hu (Radix Bupleuri) and *Sheng Ma* (Rhizoma Cimicifugae) together have lifting functions to raise qi and restore the normal position of the rectum. *Dang Gui* (Radix Angelicae Sinensis) and *Gan Cao* (Radix et Rhizoma Glycyrrhizae) nourish the blood and replenish lost blood. Additionally, these two herbs have effects to relieve pain. *Huang Qin* (Radix Scutellariae) and *Da Huang* (Radix

***Yi Zi Tang* (Yi Word Decoction)**

Diagnosis	Clinical Signs	Treatment	Herbs
Accumulation of dampness, heat and toxins in the lower *jiao*	• Anal gland infection and/or constipation with severe pain: accumulation of dampness, heat and toxins in the lower *jiao* • Perianal fistula, anal fissure, perianal and vaginal itching: accumulation of dampness, heat and toxins in the lower *jiao*	• Clears heat and promotes bowel movement • Cools the blood and eliminates toxins • Raises yang qi	• *Chai Hu* (Radix Bupleuri) and *Sheng Ma* (Rhizoma Cimicifugae) have lifting functions to raise qi. • *Dang Gui* (Radix Angelicae Sinensis) and *Gan Cao* (Radix et Rhizoma Glycyrrhizae) nourish the blood and replenish lost blood. • *Huang Qin* (Radix Scutellariae) and *Da Huang* (Radix et Rhizoma Rhei) clear damp-heat and toxins from the Large Intestine and promote intestinal peristalsis.

Yǐ Zì Tāng (Yi Word Decoction)

et Rhizoma Rhei) clear damp-heat and toxins from the Large Intestine and promote intestinal peristalsis.

VETERINARY MODIFICATIONS

- If the constipation is severe, increase the dose of *Da Huang* (Radix et Rhizoma Rhei) and add *Zhi Shi* (Fructus Aurantii Immaturus).
- When there are dry stools, add *Yu Li Ren* (Semen Pruni) and *Huo Ma Ren* (Fructus Cannabis).
- For infection of the vulva, anal glands and perianal regions with licking and chewing add: *Long Dan* (Radix et Rhizoma Gentianae), *Ze Xie* (Rhizoma Alismatis), *Mu Tong* (Caulis Akebiae) and *Che Qian Zi* (Semen Plantaginis), *Lian Qiao* (Fructus Forsythiae), *Jin Yin Hua* (Flos Lonicerae Japonicae) and *Huang Lian* (Rhizoma Coptidis).
- With increased dampness, add *Hua Shi* (Talcum) and *Yi Yi Ren* (Semen Coicis).
- If accompanied by profuse bleeding, add charred *Di Yu* (Radix Sanguisorbae), *Di Huang* (Radix Rehmanniae), and *Huang Lian* (Rhizoma Coptidis).
- For severe rectal, perianal and anal gland pain, add *Yan Huo Suo* (Rhizoma Corydalis), *Ru Xiang* (Gummi Olibanum), *Wu Yao* (Radix Linderae), and *Xiang Fu* (Rhizoma Cyperi).
- For rectal prolapse arising from qi deficiency, add *Bu Zhong Yi Qi Tang* (Tonify the Middle and Augment the Qi Decoction).
- For rectal prolapse with excess bleeding, add *Huai Hua San* (Sophora Japonica Flower Powder) or charred *Di Yu* (Radix Sanguisorbae), *Di Huang* (Radix Rehmanniae), and *Huang Lian* (Rhizoma Coptidis).

SUGGESTED ACUPUNCTURE TREATMENT

1. Points: *Changqiang* (GV 1), *Quchi* (LI 11), *Xuehai* (SP 10), *Baihui* (GV 20) and *Gangtuo*.
2. Technique: even method and sedation.

Xuehai (SP 10) by itself nourishes blood and moistens the Intestines, and when combined with *Quchi* (LI 11), clears damp-heat, promotes bowel movement, and stops bleeding. *Changqiang* (GV 1) is located next to the affected area and thus relieves pain and reduces swelling. For animals with a prolapsed rectum, apply moxibustion on *Baihui* (GV 20). For prolapsed rectum in the horse, electroacupuncture across *Gangtuo* (lateral to the anus on both left and right) helps to prevent recurrence after rectum has been replaced.

AUTHORS' COMMENTS

In dogs, *Yi Zi Tang* has shown good efficacy in treating perianal fistula and rectal polyps with ulceration when combined with topical medical honey and golden yellow ointment. Its efficacy can be increased by the addition of herbs or formula to invigorate blood in the lower *jiao* such as *Shao Fu Zhu Yu Tang* (Drive Out Blood Stasis in the Lower Abdomen Decoction).

In horses, *Yi Zi Tang* can be used in mares after surgical repair of a rectal-vaginal tear, a prolapsed rectum, or torn rectum, where it can help to relieve pain, help prevent infection, and keep the stools soft to avoid straining during defecation. It also has application in broodmares that develop vaginitis from multiple inseminations or that develop local allergic reaction to cleansers or extenders.

Section 2

润下剂
— Moist Laxatives

Má Zǐ Rén Wán (Hemp Seed Pill)
麻子仁丸

Pinyin Name: *Ma Zi Ren Wan*
Literal Name: Hemp Seed Pill
Alternate Name: Apricot Seed and Linum Formula
Original Source: *Shang Han Lun* (Discussion of Cold-Induced Disorders) by Zhang Zhong-Jing in the Eastern Han Dynasty

COMPOSITION

Huo Ma Ren (Fructus Cannabis)	2 cups (480g) [20g]
Ku Xing Ren (Semen Armeniacae Amarum), *ao* (simmered)	1 cup (240g) [10g]
Bai Shao (Radix Paeoniae Alba)	240g [9g]
Da Huang (Radix et Rhizoma Rhei)	480g [12g]
Hou Po (Cortex Magnoliae Officinalis), *zhi* (fried with liquid)	1 *chi* (240g) [9g]
Zhi Shi (Fructus Aurantii Immaturus)	240g [9g]

Note: The source text provides the doses of some of the herbs in volume (cup) and length (*chi*). One cup is approximately 200 mL, and one *chi* is about 23 centimeters or 9 inches. To facilitate preparation, these units have been converted to weight (grams).

DOSAGE / PREPARATION / ADMINISTRATION

Grind the ingredients into powder, and mix with *Feng Mi* (Mel) to form pills. The pills should resemble *Wu Tong Zi* (Semen Firmianae), a small seed approximately 5 mm in diameter. Take 10 pills per dose, three times daily. The dose may be increased until the desired effect is achieved. Today, this formula may be prepared in pills or decoction. For pills, grind the herbs into powder and mix with honey to form pills. Take 9g of pills one to two times daily with warm water. For decoction, use the doses suggested in brackets above.

CHINESE THERAPEUTIC ACTIONS

1. Lubricates the Intestines and drains heat
2. Activates qi circulation and promotes defecation

CLINICAL MANIFESTATIONS

Dryness and heat in the Stomach and Intestines accompanied by deficiency of body fluids: mild constipation with dry, hard stools, and frequent urination, accompanied by a yellow tongue coating and a rapid pulse.

VETERINARY CLINICAL APPLICATIONS

Habitual constipation, post-surgical constipation, drug-induced constipation, and constipation in geriatric, postpartum and chronically debilitated animals.

EXPLANATION

Ma Zi Ren Wan (Hemp Seed Pill) treats dryness and heat in the Stomach and Large Intestine. Dryness and heat may consume water and body fluids in these two organs, causing dry stools, constipation, and difficult defecation. Dryness and heat in the Stomach also affects the Spleen, limiting the latter's ability to distribute water to various parts of the body. As a result, water passes out through the Urinary Bladder in the form of frequent urination.

The chief herb, *Huo Ma Ren* (Fructus Cannabis), is sweet and neutral, and enters the Spleen, Stomach, and Large Intestine to moisten dryness and lubricate the Intestines to facilitate bowel movement. The deputy herb, *Ku Xing Ren* (Semen Armeniacae Amarum), enters two organs connected by their *zang fu* relationship: the Large Intestine to moisten dryness and the Lung to regulate and guide qi

Má Zǐ Rén Wán (Hemp Seed Pill)

Ma Zi Ren Wan **(Hemp Seed Pill)**

Diagnosis	Clinical Signs	Treatment	Herbs
Dryness and heat in the Stomach and Intestines with deficiency of body fluids	• Constipation with dry, hard stools: dryness and heat consuming water and body fluids • Frequent urination: abnormal distribution of water	• Lubricates the Intestines and drains heat • Activates qi circulation and promotes defecation	• *Huo Ma Ren* (Fructus Cannabis) moistens dryness and lubricates the Intestines. • *Ku Xing Ren* (Semen Armeniacae Amarum) moistens dryness and regulates qi. • *Bai Shao* (Radix Paeoniae Alba) nourishes yin and blood. • *Da Huang* (Radix et Rhizoma Rhei) purges constipated stools and drains heat. • *Hou Po* (Cortex Magnoliae Officinalis) and *Zhi Shi* (Fructus Aurantii Immaturus) activate qi circulation. • *Feng Mi* (Mel) lubricates the Intestines and moistens dryness.

downward. *Bai Shao* (Radix Paeoniae Alba) nourishes yin and blood, preserves yin, and relieves abdominal and intestinal pain and spasms. *Da Huang* (Radix et Rhizoma Rhei) purges the constipated stool and drains heat. *Hou Po* (Cortex Magnoliae Officinalis) and *Zhi Shi* (Fructus Aurantii Immaturus) activate qi to relieve bloating and distention and to eliminate the constipated stool. *Feng Mi* (Mel) helps *Huo Ma Ren* (Fructus Cannabis) lubricate the Intestines and moisten dryness. It also moderates the harsh properties of *Da Huang* (Radix et Rhizoma Rhei).

VETERINARY MODIFICATIONS

- If constipation is severe and the stools are very hard and dry, add *Mang Xiao* (Natrii Sulfas) to soften stools.
- For habitual constipation with dry stools in geriatric patients, reduce the dose of *Da Huang* (Radix et Rhizoma Rhei) and add *Bai Zi Ren* (Semen Platycladi), *Rou Cong Rong* (Herba Cistanches), and *Dang Gui* (Radix Angelicae Sinensis).
- For post-surgical constipation, add *Huang Lian* (Rhizoma Coptidis), *Sheng Ma* (Rhizoma Cimicifugae), *Tao Ren* (Semen Persicae), and *Dang Gui* (Radix Angelicae Sinensis).
- When there is thirst and increased water intake as a result of Stomach heat, add *Shi Gao* (Gypsum Fibrosum) and *Zhi Mu* (Rhizoma Anemarrhenae).
- If there is frequent urination, add *Qian Shi* (Semen Euryales), *Sang Piao Xiao* (Ootheca Mantidis), and *Yi Zhi* (Fructus Alpiniae Oxyphyllae).

CAUTIONS / CONTRAINDICATIONS

- Though *Ma Zi Ren Wan* is classified as a moist laxative formula, it nonetheless has a moderate purgative effect since it contains *Da Huang* (Radix et Rhizoma Rhei), *Zhi Shi* (Fructus Aurantii Immaturus) and *Hou Po* (Cortex Magnoliae Officinalis) to drain downward, activate qi circulation, and purge constipated stools. Therefore, this formula should still be prescribed carefully for use in very weak or deficient patients. Moreover, it should not be taken daily over a long period of time, since this may consume qi and body fluids. Debilitated patients should be treated for underlying deficiencies with diet and/or other formulas while using *Ma Zi Ren Wan*. Once these imbalances are corrected and intestinal movement normalized *Ma Zi Ren Wan* should be discontinued.
- This formula should be used with caution during pregnancy.

PHARMACOLOGICAL EFFECTS

1. **Laxative**: According to various laboratory studies in mice, administration of *Ma Zi Ren Wan* was associated with increased bowel movement, usually within 12 hours.[1]
2. **Gastrointestinal**: Administration of *Ma Zi Ren Wan* was associated with increased intestinal peristalsis in anesthetized rabbits.[2]

HUMAN CLINICAL STUDIES AND RESEARCH

1. **Constipation**: According to one study, 557 patients with different causes and various severity of constipation were treated with *Ma Zi Ren Wan* with complete recovery in 281 patients, significant improvement in 229 patients, moderate improvement in 25 patients, and no change in 22 patients. The overall rate of effectiveness was 96%.[3]
2. **Post-surgical constipation**: Use of *Ma Zi Ren Wan* was reported to have 95.8% effectiveness in preventing post-surgical constipation. Of 500 patients, the study reported normal bowel movements (without dryness, pain or bleeding) in 479 patients. Of 21 patients who did not respond, 16 had a history of habitual constipation.[4]

Má Zǐ Rén Wán (Hemp Seed Pill)

HERB-DRUG INTERACTION

Drug-induced constipation: Constipation caused by antipsychotic drugs in 80 individuals was treated with marked success using *Ma Zi Ren Wan*. The herbs were given at 9 to 15g per dose, three times daily. For those with severe constipation, the form was switched from pills to decoction. Of 80 cases, the study reported complete recovery in 62 cases, improvement in 13 cases, and no change in 5 cases.[5]

SUGGESTED ACUPUNCTURE TREATMENT

1. Points: *Dachangshu* (BL 25), *Shangjuxu* (ST 37), *Tianshu* (ST 25), *Housanli* (ST 36), *Qiansanli* (LI 10), *Changqiang* (GV 1), *Zhigou* (TH 6), *Quchi* (LI 11), *Hegu* (LI 4), *Pishu* and *Qihaishu*.
2. Technique: even method.

Dachangshu (BL 25) regulates the qi circulation of the Large Intestine to promote fluids and lubricate the Intestines. *Shangjuxu* (ST 37), the lower *he* (uniting) point of the Large Intestine, and *Tianshu* (ST 25), the *mu* (collecting) point of the Large Intestine, activate qi circulation in the Stomach and Intestines and remove stagnation. *Housanli* (ST 36) and *Qiansanli* (LI 10) tonify qi and promote defecation. *Changqiang* (GV 1) regulates gastrointestinal motility and relieves constipation. *Zhigou* (TH 6) regulates circulation in all three *jiaos*. *Quchi* (LI 11) and *Hegu* (LI 4) clear heat in the Large Intestine. *Pishu* and *Qihaishu* are classical equine points to tonify Spleen qi.

RELATED FORMULA

***Wŭ Rén Wán* (Five-Seed Pill)**

五仁丸

Pinyin Name: *Wu Ren Wan*

Literal Name: Five-Seed Pill

Original Source: *Shi Yi De Xiao Fang* (Effective Formulas from Generations of Physicians) by Wei Yi-Lin in 1345

Tao Ren (Semen Persicae)	30g [15g]
Ku Xing Ren (Semen Armeniacae Amarum), *chao* (dry-fried)	30g [15g]
Bai Zi Ren (Semen Platycladi)	15g [9g]
Song Zi Ren (Semen Pini)	3.75g [5g]
Yu Li Ren (Semen Pruni), *chao* (dry-fried)	3g [5g]
Chen Pi (Pericarpium Citri Reticulatae), *yan* (ground) to powder	120g [15g]

Mash the five seeds into a paste. Add powdered *Chen Pi* (Pericarpium Citri Reticulatae) and blend thoroughly. Mix the powder with honey to form small pills that resemble the size of *Wu Tong Zi* (Semen Firmianae), a small seed approximately 5 mm in diameter. Take 50 pills with rice soup on an empty stomach. Today, this formula is prepared by grinding all of the ingredients into powder, mixing the powder with honey, and forming into pills. Take 12g of pills per dose with warm, boiled water on an empty stomach. This formula may also be prepared as a decoction with the doses suggested in brackets above.

Wu Ren Wan (Five-Seed Pill) is composed of five seeds rich in oil to lubricate the Intestines and facilitate bowel movement. It treats constipation and dry stool caused by severe body fluid deficiency. It may also be used for constipation in geriatric or postpartum animals with blood deficiency. Clinical manifestations include constipation, dry stool, a dry mouth, and excess thirst.

Ku Xing Ren (Semen Armeniacae Amarum), the chief herb, nourishes and treats intestinal dryness. It also directs Lung qi downward to help the functioning of the Large Intestine, as these two organs are connected by their *zang fu* relationship. *Tao Ren* (Semen Persicae), the deputy herb, helps *Ku Xing Ren* (Semen Armeniacae Amarum) moisten dryness and lubricate the bowels. *Bai Zi Ren* (Semen Platycladi) and *Yu Li Ren* (Semen Pruni), rich in oil, are moist laxatives that further lubricate the bowels and relieve dryness and heat in the Stomach and Intestines. *Song Zi Ren* (Semen Pini) moistens the five *zang* (solid) organs and treats constipation caused by deficiency. *Feng Mi* (Mel) lubricates the bowels. Finally, *Chen Pi* (Pericarpium Citri Reticulatae) regulates qi to promote circulation in the abdomen and relieve distention or bloating.

Wu Ren Wan should be taken with caution during gestation, since it contains *Tao Ren* (Semen Persicae), a blood-moving herb.

AUTHORS' COMMENTS

Ma Zi Ren Wan is one of the most commonly used formula in veterinary medicine to treat constipation characterized by heat, dryness and stagnation, and is commonly used to treat habitual and post-surgical constipation in deficient and geriatric animals. It can also be used as the base formula to treat constipation arising from heat and dryness after gastrointestinal or colon surgeries. To improve treatment efficacy in older dogs and cats, it can be combined with other formulas that tonify yin and blood.

Xiao Cheng Qi Tang (Minor Order the Qi Decoction) and *Ma Zi Ren Wan* have three ingredients in common: *Da Huang* (Radix et Rhizoma Rhei), *Zhi Shi* (Fructus Aurantii Immaturus), and *Hou Po* (Cortex Magnoliae

Má Zǐ Rén Wán (Hemp Seed Pill)

Officinalis). While *Xiao Cheng Qi Tang* (Minor Order the Qi Decoction) is classified as a cold purgative formula, *Ma Zi Ren Wan* is known as a moist laxative formula for the following reasons:

- *Xiao Cheng Qi Tang* (Minor Order the Qi Decoction) is best administered as a decoction, which is absorbed quickly to provide a more immediate and potent effect to drain and purge downwards.
- *Ma Zi Ren Wan* is administered as honey pills, which are absorbed slowly over a long period of time. Consequently, its effects are gentle, and its potency is moderate. Furthermore, *Ma Zi Ren Wan* contains additional ingredients, such as *Huo Ma Ren* (Fructus Cannabis), *Ku Xing Ren* (Semen Armeniacae Amarum), *Bai Shao* (Radix Paeoniae Alba), and *Feng Mi* (Mel). Some of these herbs are rich in oil and can lubricate the Intestines to promote the passage of stools. Others are sweet and have a moderating effect to prevent *Da Huang* (Radix et Rhizoma Rhei) from injuring *zheng* (upright) *qi*. Because the overall focus of this formula is to lubricate the Intestines and regulate bowel movement, and not to purge downwards, it is considered as a moist laxative.

References

1. *Zhong Xi Yi Jie He Za Zhi* (Journal of Integrated Chinese and Western Medicine), 1990; (6):5.
2. *Zhong Xi Yi Jie He Za Zhi* (Journal of Integrated Chinese and Western Medicine), 1990; (6):5.
3. *Hu Nan Zhong Yi Za Zhi* (Hunan Journal of Chinese Medicine), 1994; 10(4):55.
4. *Zhong Yi Za Zhi* (Journal of Chinese Medicine), 1965; 10:40.
5. *Si Chuan Zhong Yi* (Sichuan Chinese Medicine), 1996; 9:29.

Rùn Cháng Wán (Moisten the Intestines Pill)

潤腸丸

润肠丸

Pinyin Name: *Run Chang Wan*
Literal Name: Moisten the Intestines Pill
Original Source: *Pi Wei Lun* (Discussion of the Spleen and Stomach) by Li Gao in 1249

COMPOSITION

Da Huang (Radix et Rhizoma Rhei)	15g
Tao Ren (Semen Persicae), *jin* (soaked)	30g
Huo Ma Ren (Fructus Cannabis)	37.5g
Dang Gui (Radix Angelicae Sinensis)	15g
Qiang Huo (Rhizoma et Radix Notopterygii)	15g

DOSAGE / PREPARATION / ADMINISTRATION

The source text advises to separately grind *Huo Ma Ren* (Fructus Cannabis) into a paste, and pound all of the other ingredients into powder. Mix the paste and the powder with *Feng Mi* (Mel) and form into small pills that resemble the size of *Wu Tong Zi* (Semen Firmianae), a small seed approximately 5 mm in diameter. Take 50 pills with warm water on an empty stomach. Today, this formula is prepared by grinding all of the ingredients into powder and mixing with *Feng Mi* (Mel) to form into pills. Take 12g of pills per dose with warm water on an empty stomach.

CHINESE THERAPEUTIC ACTIONS

1. Lubricates the Intestines and promotes defecation
2. Tonifies and invigorates blood and dispels wind

CLINICAL MANIFESTATIONS

Constipation characterized by blood deficiency: habitual constipation, constipation in geriatric, chronically debilitated or weak animals, dry and hard stools, lack of appetite, and lethargy.

VETERINARY CLINICAL APPLICATIONS

Constipation in anemic, geriatric, and chronically ill animals.

Rùn Cháng Wán (Moisten the Intestines Pill)

***Run Chang Wan* (Moisten the Intestines Pill)**

Diagnosis	Clinical Signs	Treatment	Herbs
Constipation characterized by blood deficiency	Constipation with dry and hard stools accompanied by anemia: blood deficiency	• Lubricates the Intestines and promotes defecation • Tonifies blood circulation and dispels wind	• *Da Huang* (Radix et Rhizoma Rhei) purges the bowels and clears heat. • *Tao Ren* (Semen Persicae), *Huo Ma Ren* (Fructus Cannabis), and *Feng Mi* (Mel) moisten the Intestines and promote bowel movement. • *Dang Gui* (Radix Angelicae Sinensis) tonifies blood and yin to lubricate the bowels. • *Qiang Huo* (Rhizoma et Radix Notopterygii) expels wind and relieves pain.

EXPLANATION

Run Chang Wan (Moisten the Intestines Pill) is a moist-laxative formula that treats constipation characterized by blood deficiency and blood stasis, which can occur secondary to trauma and chronic disease, as a result of poor diet and overwork, or post-partum. It can also treat constipation that develops after an exterior wind-heat attack of the Lung in geriatric animals. This happens when wind enters the Lung and sinks to the Intestines, injuring the Spleen and Stomach function and causing constipation referred to as *feng jie* (wind bind).

Da Huang (Radix et Rhizoma Rhei) purges the bowels and clears heat. *Tao Ren* (Semen Persicae), *Huo Ma Ren* (Fructus Cannabis), and *Feng Mi* (Mel) moisten the Intestines and promote defecation. *Dang Gui* (Radix Angelicae Sinensis) tonifies blood and yin to lubricate the bowels. *Qiang Huo* (Rhizoma et Radix Notopterygii) expels wind and relieves pain in this type of constipation.

VETERINARY MODIFICATIONS

- If there is fever, add *Chai Hu* (Radix Bupleuri).
- When there is abdominal pain, add *Mu Xiang* (Radix Aucklandiae).
- For blood deficiency, increase the dose of *Dang Gui* (Radix Angelicae Sinensis) and *Tao Ren* (Semen Persicae) and add *Shu Di Huang* (Radix Rehmanniae Praeparata) and *Hong Hua* (Flos Carthami).
- For wind and dryness, add *Yu Li Ren* (Semen Pruni), *Zao Jiao Ci* (Spina Gleditsiae), and increase the dose of *Qiang Huo* (Rhizoma et Radix Notopterygii).
- If accompanied by qi deficiency, add *Ren Shen* (Radix et Rhizoma Ginseng) and *Yu Li Ren* (Semen Pruni).
- If there is qi stagnation, add *Bing Lang* (Semen Arecae) and *Mu Xiang* (Radix Aucklandiae).
- For hot phlegm accumulation, add *Gua Lou* (Fructus Trichosanthis) and *Zhu Li* (Succus Bambusae).
- When there is body fluid deficiency, add *Ren Shen* (Radix et Rhizoma Ginseng) and *Mai Dong* (Radix Ophiopogonis).

CAUTIONS / CONTRAINDICATIONS

Run Chang Wan should be used with caution during gestation.

SUGGESTED ACUPUNCTURE TREATMENT

1. Points: *Dachangshu* (BL 25), *Shangjuxu* (ST 37), *Tianshu* (ST 25), *Xuehai* (SP 10), *Sanyinjiao* (SP 6), *Taixi* (KI 3), *Geshu* (BL 17), and *Fengmen* (BL 12).
2. Technique: even method.

Dachangshu (BL 25) regulates qi circulation of the Large Intestine to help promote fluids and lubricate the Intestines. *Shangjuxu* (ST 37), the lower *he* (uniting) point of the Large Intestine, and *Tianshu* (ST 25), the *mu* (collecting) point of the Large Intestine, activate qi circulation in the Stomach and Intestines and remove stagnation. *Xuehai* (SP 10) nourishes blood and moistens the Large Intestine. *Sanyinjiao* (SP 6) and *Taixi* (KI 3) nourish yin. *Geshu* (BL 17) and *Fengmen* (BL 12) activate blood circulation and dispel wind.

RELATED FORMULA

***Rùn Cháng Wán* (Moisten the Intestines Pill)**
潤腸丸
润肠丸
Pinyin Name: *Run Chang Wan*
Literal Name: Moisten the Intestines Pill
Alternate Names: *Jun Chang Tang*, Bowel-Nourishing Decoction, Linum and Rhubarb Formula
Original Source: *Wan Bing Hui Chun* (Restoration of Health from the Myriad Diseases) by Gong Ting-Xian in 1587

Rùn Cháng Wán (Moisten the Intestines Pill)

Dang Gui (Radix Angelicae Sinensis)
Shu Di Huang (Radix Rehmanniae Praeparata)
Di Huang (Radix Rehmanniae)
Huo Ma Ren (Fructus Cannabis)
Tao Ren (Semen Persicae)
Ku Xing Ren (Semen Armeniacae Amarum)
Zhi Qiao (Fructus Aurantii)
Huang Qin (Radix Scutellariae)
Hou Po (Cortex Magnoliae Officinalis)
Da Huang (Radix et Rhizoma Rhei)
Gan Cao (Radix et Rhizoma Glycyrrhizae)

The source text states to use an equal amount for all ingredients, and half the amount for *Gan Cao* (Radix et Rhizoma Glycyrrhizae). Grind the ingredients into powder, and mix with *Feng Mi* (Mel) and form into small pills that resemble the size of *Wu Tong Zi* (Semen Firmianae), a small seed approximately 5 mm in diameter. Take 50 pills with warm water on an empty stomach. This formula treats constipation due to dryness and heat in the Stomach and Large Intestine.

AUTHORS' COMMENTS

Ma Zi Ren Wan (Hemp Seed Pill) and *Run Chang Wan* are moist-laxative formulas that gently treat mild to moderate cases of constipation. The clinical applications of *Ma Zi Ren Wan* and *Run Chang Wan* are similar: both treat constipation that results from deficiency of blood and body fluids.

- *Run Chang Wan* treats constipation characterized by blood deficiency, and is considered to be safer for use in weak or geriatric patients because it is not as dispersing as *Ma Zi Ren Wan* (Hemp Seed Pill); it may take longer to see an effect with this formula than others because of this. Adequate dosing is essential in obtaining relief from constipation.
- *Ma Zi Ren Wan* (Hemp Seed Pill) treats constipation characterized by body fluid deficiency, with stagnation, dryness and heat in the Stomach and Intestines. This formula does not contain herbs to dispel wind.

Section 3

攻补兼施剂
— Purgative and Tonic Formulas

Zēng Yè Chéng Qì Tāng
(Increase the Fluids and Order the Qi Decoction)

增液承氣湯
增液承气汤

Pinyin Name: *Zeng Ye Cheng Qi Tang*
Literal Name: Increase the Fluids and Order the Qi Decoction
Original Source: *Wen Bing Tiao Bian* (Systematic Differentiation of Warm Disease) by Wu Ju-Tong in 1798

COMPOSITION

Xuan Shen (Radix Scrophulariae)	30g
Mai Dong (Radix Ophiopogonis)	24g
Di Huang (Radix Rehmanniae)	24g
Da Huang (Radix et Rhizoma Rhei)	9g
Mang Xiao (Natrii Sulfas)	4.5g

DOSAGE / PREPARATION / ADMINISTRATION

Cook the ingredients in 8 cups of water until 2 cups of liquid remain. Take 1 cup of the decoction. If bowel movement is not induced after taking the formula, administer another cup.

CHINESE THERAPEUTIC ACTIONS

1. Nourishes yin and generates body fluids
2. Purges heat and promotes defecation

CLINICAL MANIFESTATIONS

Yangming fu (hollow organs) syndrome characterized by heat in the Stomach and Intestines damaging yin and body fluids: severe constipation that cannot be relieved by regular purgative method; dry, immobile stools; abdominal pain; increased thirst; and a dry tongue and mouth.

VETERINARY CLINICAL APPLICATIONS

Chronic renal insufficiency, diabetes mellitus, feline hyperthyroidism, chronic constipation, and feline megacolon. Any chronic disease, infection, or surgery that causes moderate to severe yin deficiency and constipation with hard, dry, immobile stool.

EXPLANATION

In *yangming fu* syndrome, heat stagnates in the Stomach and Large Intestine and causes the stools to be impacted. If the heat persists, yin and body fluids will be so severely damaged that even normal purgative methods would not be able to remove the dry, constipated stools. In such cases, two kinds of herbs must be used: sweet, cold, and moistening herbs that nourish yin and moisten dryness; and bitter and salty herbs that clear heat and drain downward. Nourishing yin and replenishing body fluids are essential steps in successfully removing the constipated stools and clearing stagnant interior heat.

Zeng Ye Cheng Qi Tang (Increase the Fluids and Order the Qi Decoction) contains *Xuan Shen* (Radix Scrophulariae), *Mai Dong* (Radix Ophiopogonis), and *Di Huang* (Radix Rehmanniae) to nourish yin and body fluids, and to moisten dryness. *Da Huang* (Radix et Rhizoma Rhei) and *Mang Xiao* (Natrii Sulfas) purge excess heat, soften hardness, and remove constipated stools.

This formula, besides treating *yangming fu* (hollow organs) syndrome, may also be used to treat chronic constipation

Zēng Yè Chéng Qì Tāng

(Increase the Fluids and Order the Qi Decoction)

***Zeng Ye Cheng Qi Tang* (Increase the Fluids and Order the Qi Decoction)**

Diagnosis	Clinical Signs	Treatment	Herbs
Yangming syndrome characterized by heat in the Stomach and Intestines damaging yin and body fluids	• Severe constipation with abdominal bloating: heat in the Stomach and Large Intestine with hard and constipated stools • Dry, immobile stools, thirst, a dry mouth and throat: damage to yin and body fluids	• Nourishes yin and generates body fluids • Purges heat and promotes defecation	• *Xuan Shen* (Radix Scrophulariae), *Mai Dong* (Radix Ophiopogonis) and *Di Huang* (Radix Rehmanniae) nourish yin and body fluids, clear heat, and moisten dryness. • *Da Huang* (Radix et Rhizoma Rhei) and *Mang Xiao* (Natrii Sulfas) purge excess heat, soften hardness, and remove constipated stools.

characterized by yin deficiency and dry heat in the Large Intestine seen in chronic disease.

VETERINARY MODIFICATIONS

- For constipation characterized by qi deficiency, add *Tai Zi Shen* (Radix Pseudostellariae) or *Xi Yang Shen* (Radix Panacis Quinquefolii).
- For bleeding hemorrhoids, add *Di Yu* (Radix Sanguisorbae) and *Huai Hua* (Flos Sophorae).
- To strengthen the ability to nourish yin and blood, clear heat, and cool the blood, increase the dose of *Di Huang* (Radix Rehmanniae).
- To nourish yin, moisten the Large Intestine, and unblock bowels, add *He Shou Wu* (Radix Polygoni Multiflori).

CAUTIONS / CONTRAINDICATIONS

Zeng Ye Cheng Qi Tang treats severe constipation characterized by heat damaging yin and body fluids. It is not suitable for mild constipation seen in postpartum animals caused by blood deficiency, or constipation caused by dryness in weak geriatric animals. For constipation in these animals remove the purgative herbs *Da Huang* (Radix et Rhizoma Rhei) and *Mang Xiao* (Natrii Sulfas); the remaining herbs make up the formula *Zeng Ye Tang* (Increase the Fluids Decoction), which is appropriate for use in these patients.

HUMAN CLINICAL STUDIES AND RESEARCH

1. **Anal fissures**: Administration of modified *Zeng Ye Cheng Qi Tang* in 31 patients with anal fissures was associated with complete recovery in 29 patients and improvement in 2 patients. The history of illness ranged from 7 days to 5 years. The herbal treatment contained the following ingredients: *Xuan Shen* (Radix Scrophulariae) 15g, *Di Huang* (Radix Rehmanniae) 15g, *Mai Dong* (Radix Ophiopogonis) 15g, post-decocted *Da Huang* (Radix et Rhizoma Rhei) 5g, and *Mang Xiao* (Natrii Sulfas) 5g. Dry-fried *Di Yu* (Radix Sanguisorbae) and dry-fried *Huai Hua* (Flos Sophorae) were added for hematochezia; and *Zhi Qiao* (Fructus Aurantii) and *Yan Hu Suo* (Rhizoma Corydalis) for severe pain. For those who experience multiple bowel movements or loose stools after herbal treatment, *Da Huang* (Radix et Rhizoma Rhei) should be reduced in dose or pre-decocted. The herbs were cooked in water, and decoction given daily, for an average of 7 packs of herbs.[1]
2. **Renal insufficiency**: Administration of *Zeng Ye Cheng Qi Tang* was shown to have beneficial effects in treating acute renal insufficiency in one study. The study entailed the administration of 200 mL of herbal solution via rectal enema two to four times daily. Of 49 patients, the study reported recovery in 41 patients, improvement in 2 patients, and fatality in 6 patients.[2]

HERB-DRUG INTERACTION

Phenothiazine-induced constipation: Use of modified *Zeng Ye Cheng Qi Tang* was beneficial in alleviating the side effects related to use of phenothiazine in 30 psychiatric patients. Phenothiazine-induced side effects include constipation, a dry mouth with a bitter taste, nausea, etc. The herbal formula contained *Xuan Shen* (Radix Scrophulariae), *Di Huang* (Radix Rehmanniae), *Mai Dong* (Radix Ophiopogonis), *Da Huang* (Radix et Rhizoma Rhei), *Zhi Shi* (Fructus Aurantii Immaturus), *Hou Po* (Cortex Magnoliae Officinalis), and *Tian Hua Fen* (Radix Trichosanthis). The herbs were given in decoction form one time daily. Patients were instructed to continue with phenothiazine and herbs concurrently for four weeks, while avoiding all other treatments. Of 30 patients, the study reported complete recovery in 14 patients, significant effect in 10 patients, moderate effect in 3 patients, and no change in 3 patients. The overall rate of effectiveness was 90%.[3]

Zēng Yè Chéng Qì Tāng

(Increase the Fluids and Order the Qi Decoction)

SUGGESTED ACUPUNCTURE TREATMENT

1. Points: *Dachangshu* (BL 25), *Shangjuxu* (ST 37), *Tianshu* (ST 25), *Daheng* (SP 15), *Changqiang* (GV 1), *Zhigou* (TH 6), *Zhaohai* (KI 6), *Yinxi* (HT 6), *Zhubin* (KI 9), and *Fuliu* (KI 7).
2. Technique: both tonification and sedation.

Dachangshu (BL 25) and *Shangjuxu* (ST 37) regulate qi and water circulation in the Stomach and Intestines. *Tianshu* (ST 25) and *Daheng* (SP 15) work together to eliminate heat and help intestinal function. *Changqiang* (GV 1) is helpful in anal and rectal dysfunction. *Zhigou* (TH 6) and *Zhaohai* (KI 6) nourish yin and promote water circulation throughout the body. *Yinxi* (HT 6), *Zhubin* (KI 9) and *Fuliu* (KI 7) increase body fluids to moisten the Intestines and clear heat.

AUTHORS' COMMENTS

Zeng Ye Cheng Qi Tang treats febrile disorders with constipation characterized by heat stagnation and yin and body fluid deficiencies. It can also be used in cases caused by high fever and acute infectious disease, both of which lead to body fluid deficiency. It can be used to treat patients with established diabetes and/or chronic renal failure that have severe constipation with dryness secondary to yin deficiency. It can also be used to treat habitual constipation in the cat to relieve colonic impaction and prevent the development of obstipation seen in feline megacolon.

References

1. *An Hui Zhong Yi Xue Yuan Xue Bao* (Journal of Anhui University School of Medicine), 1993; 4:28.
2. *Zhong Yi Za Zhi* (Journal of Chinese Medicine), 1986; 10:32.
3. *Xin Yi Xue* (New Medicine), 1997; 7:24.

Chapter 2 — Summary

— Downward Draining Formulas

Section 1: Purgatives

Name	Similarities	Differences
Da Cheng Qi Tang (Major Order the Qi Decoction)	Drain heat and accumulation downward	Strongest potency
Xiao Cheng Qi Tang (Minor Order the Qi Decoction)		Moderate to strong potency
Tiao Wei Cheng Qi Tang (Regulate the Stomach and Order the Qi Decoction)		Mild to moderate potency
Yi Zi Tang (Yi Word Decoction)	Clears heat and promotes bowel movement	Cools the blood, eliminates toxins, and raises yang qi

Da Cheng Qi Tang (Major Order the Qi Decoction), ***Xiao Cheng Qi Tang*** (Minor Order the Qi Decoction), and ***Tiao Wei Cheng Qi Tang*** (Regulate the Stomach and Order the Qi Decoction) all contain *Da Huang* (Radix et Rhizoma Rhei) to purge stagnation and heat in the Large Intestine to treat *yangming fu* (hollow organs) syndrome.

- *Da Cheng Qi Tang* is the strongest of these three formulas, and may be used to treat all four manifestations of *pi* (distention), *man* (fullness), *zao* (dryness), and *shi* (hardness). The constipation is characterized by extremely hard stools.
- *Xiao Cheng Qi Tang* has moderate to strong potency and is used to treat qi stagnation with clinical signs of *pi* (distention), *man* (fullness) and *shi* (hardness). The constipation is characterized by moderately hard stools.
- *Tiao Wei Cheng Qi Tang* is the mildest among the three formulas and mainly softens the stools in constipation characterized by *zao* (dryness) and *shi* (hardness).

Yi Zi Tang (Yi Word Decoction) clears heat and eliminates toxins from the lower *jiao* to treat constipation. In addition, it cools the blood, stops bleeding, and raises yang qi to relieve hemorrhoids.

Section 2: Moist Laxatives

Name	Similarities	Differences
Ma Zi Ren Wan (Hemp Seed Pill)	Lubricate the Intestines to relieve constipation	Drains heat and activates qi circulation
Run Chang Wan (Moisten the Intestines Pill)		Regulates blood circulation and tonifies the blood.

Ma Zi Ren Wan (Hemp Seed Pill) and ***Run Chang Wan*** (Moisten the Intestines Pill) lubricate the Intestines to relieve constipation.

- *Ma Zi Ren Wan* purges heat and activates qi circulation. It relieves constipation characterized by dry-heat in the Stomach and Large Intestine.
- *Run Chang Wan* nourishes the blood and activates blood circulation. It is used for constipation characterized by blood deficiency.

Chapter 2 — Summary

Section 3: Purgative and Tonic Formula

Name	Similarities	Differences
Zeng Ye Cheng Qi Tang (Increase the Fluids and Order the Qi Decoction)	Clears heat and promotes defecation	Nourishes yin and generates body fluids

Zeng Ye Cheng Qi Tang (Increase the Fluids and Order the Qi Decoction) has a strong nourishing and moisturizing action, and is suitable for severe constipation accompanied by severe deficiency of yin and body fluids.

Chapter 3

— Harmonizing Formulas

和解剂

吴有性 Wū Yǒu-Xìng

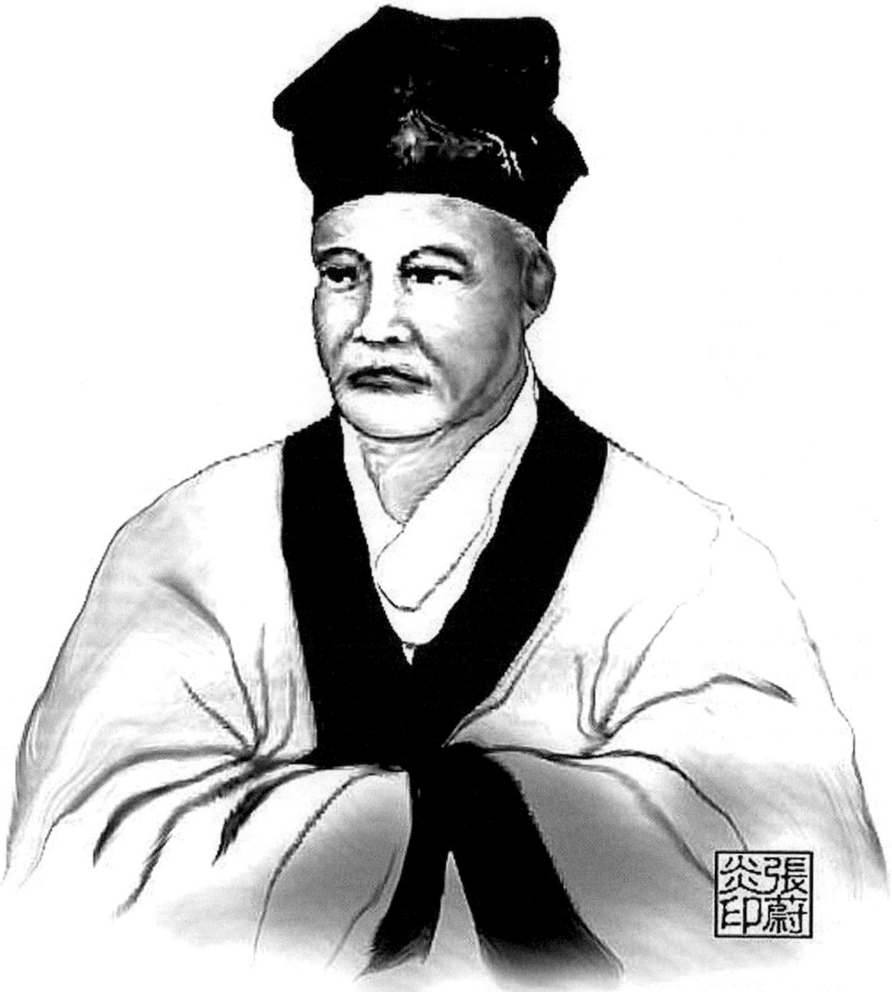

吴有性 Wū Yǒu-Xìng, also known as 吴又可 Wū Yòu-Kě, 1580's – 1660's.[1]

吴有性 Wū Yǒu-Xìng

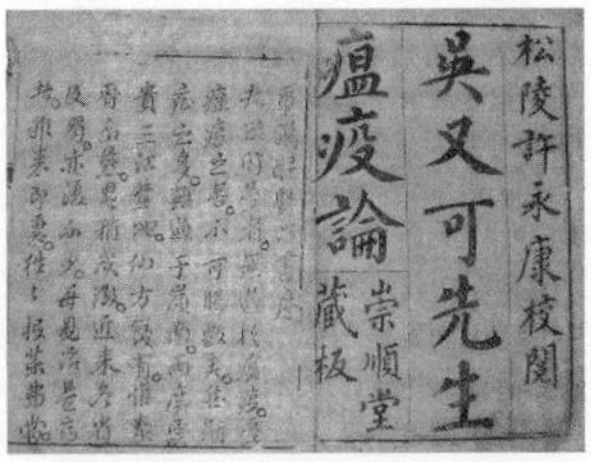

温疫论 *Wen Yi Lun* (Discussion of Epidemic Warm Disease) in 1642.

Wu You-Xing lived during the transition from the Ming dynasty to the Qing dynasty, a period dominated by war and characterized by extreme poverty and poor sanitary conditions. As a result, countless epidemics ravaged the country and killed millions of people. At the time, most physicians strictly followed the guidelines of 伤寒 *shang han* (cold damage), and achieved little or no success in treating 温疫 *wen yi* (warm epidemic). Wu observed that *wen yi* (warm epidemic) plagued everyone, starting "from one person to the entire household, from one household to the entire street, and from one street to the entire village." To better understand the patterns of this kind of disease, Wu risked his life by entering affected households and neighborhoods to personally observe and directly treat those who became ill. After years of clinical observation, Wu stated that epidemics such as *wen yi* (warm epidemic) are "***not*** caused by wind, cold, summer-heat, nor dampness, but rather by 戾气 *li qi* (perverse qi)." He further elaborated that *li qi* (perverse qi) existed in the universe, but have "no sound nor smell, and no shape nor shadow." Furthermore, he observed that *li qi* (perverse qi) may be transmitted from one person to another via "heaven [air borne]" or "earth [direct contact]," and affect weak, deficient individuals (i.e., those with low immunity).

Based on these observations, Wu You-Xing wrote *Wen Yi Lun* (Discussion of Epidemic Warm Disease) in 1642, which was published approximately 200 years before the discovery of bacteria and other micro-organisms. It accurately described the origins and transmission of epidemic disease, and the importance of the immune system in relationship to the pathogens. Wu revolutionized and significantly influenced the theory and practice of traditional Chinese medicine, changes that persist even today.

Formulas originated by Wu You-Xing include:

- *Cheng Qi Yang Ying Tang* (Order the Qi and Nourish the Nutritive Qi Decoction)
- *Da Yuan Yin* (Reach the Membrane Source Decoction)

1. Exact dates of his birth and death are unknown.

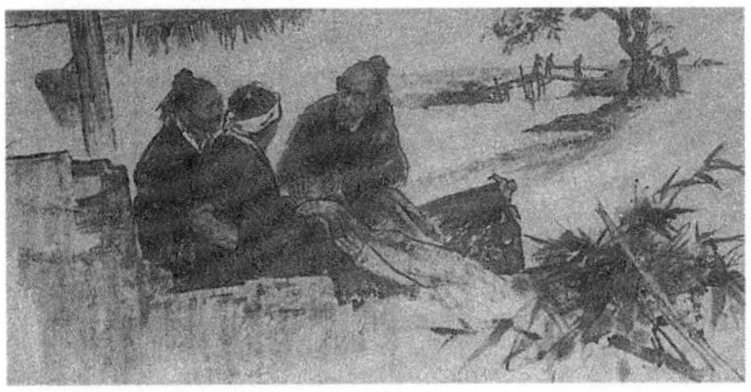

Wu personally entering the epidemic area to treat patients.

Dynasties & Kingdoms	Year
Xia Dynasty 夏	2100-1600 BCE
Shang Dynasty 商	1600-1100 BCE
Zhou Dynasty 周	1100-221 BCE
Qin Dynasty 秦	221-207 BCE
Han Dynasty 漢	206 BCE-220
Three Kingdoms 三國	220-280
Western Jin Dynasty 西晉	265-316
Eastern Jin Dynasty 東晉	317-420
Northern and Southern Dynasties 北南朝	420-581
Sui Dynasty 隋	581-618
Tang Dynasty 唐	618-907
Five Dynasties 五代	907-960
Song Dynasty 宋	960-1279
Liao Dynasty 遼	916-1125
Jin Dynasty 金	1115-1234
Yuan Dynasty 元	1271-1368
Ming Dynasty 明	**1368-1644**
Qing Dynasty 清	1644-1911
Republic of China 中華民國	1912-Present Day
People's Republic of China 中華人民共和國	1949-Present Day

Table of Contents

Chapter 3 — Overview

和解剂

— Harmonizing Formulas

Definition: Harmonizing formulas treat complicated and co-existing but contrasting illnesses that cannot be addressed by one simple treatment method. This method of treatment is known as *he fa* (harmonizing), one of the *ba fa* (eight treatment methods) described in the *Huang Di Nei Jing* (Yellow Emperor's Inner Classic) in the first or second century, A.D.

Complicated and contrasting illnesses refer to disorders that affect more than one part of the body and often have opposite characteristics. For example, these disorders can affect the exterior and interior, *ying* (nutritive) and *wei* (defensive) levels, or *qi* (energy) and *xue* (blood) levels. Moreover, the disorders can be characterized by both cold and heat, or excess and deficiency. In such complex cases, it is inappropriate to solely release the exterior, drain the interior, tonify the deficiency, or clear the excess. Instead, it is more suitable to regulate and resolve these conditions through the use of harmonizing formulas. Harmonizing formulas frequently treat three main categories of disorders: *shaoyang* (half-interior, half-exterior) syndromes, Liver and Spleen disharmony, and Intestines and Stomach disharmony.

Shaoyang syndrome is one of the six stages of disease progression described in *Shang Han Lun* (Discussion of Cold-Induced Disorders). The *shaoyang* is situated between yang and yin, or between the exterior and interior; it is characterized by pathogens residing in this layer. *Shaoyang* syndrome can be caused by exterior pathogens attacking the *taiyang* channel and invading the *shaoyang* (this is the most common situation), or by attacking the *shaoyang* level directly. Disorders in the *shaoyang* may cause qi stagnation and eventual heat formation in the Gallbladder channel (a *shaoyang* channel). Once pathogens are lodged in the *shaoyang*, they can hide for long periods of time, making these disorders difficult to resolve.

The most distinguishing characteristic of *shaoyang* syndrome is alternating fever that may be accompanied by trembling; in humans, it is characterized by alternating fever and chills. Once a pathogen enters the *shaoyang* the *zheng* (upright) *qi* will fight it; fever is seen when the *zheng qi* is stronger than the pathogen, and, conversely, trembling is seen when the pathogen dominates the *zheng qi*. It should be recognized that there are other disorders that can cause this presentation, and careful evaluation is required before prescribing a harmonizing formula. Fever and trembling (aversion to cold) are common complaints in exterior conditions, but they must be differentiated from *shaoyang* syndrome. In *taiyang* syndrome, fever and trembling present simultaneously; in *yangming* syndrome, there is high fever and absence of trembling; in *shaoyang* syndrome, there are alternating spells of fever and trembling. Other clinical signs of *shaoyang* syndrome include chest and hypochondriac fullness, and discomfort that develops from stagnation of qi along the *jueyin* (Liver) channel. A dry mouth and throat and irritability develop from excess heat in the interior. Lack of appetite, nausea, and vomiting occur from qi stagnation of the Gallbladder, which invades the Stomach and leads to reversed flow of qi. The tongue coating is thin and white because pathogenic factors have not yet transformed into internal heat, and a wiry pulse is the result of qi stagnation in the Gallbladder channel. All of the clinical signs of *shaoyang* syndrome need not be present; the presence of two or more manifestations is adequate reason to prescribe a harmonizing formula.

Chapter 3 — Overview

Shaoyang syndrome cannot be treated solely with exterior-releasing formulas as this would leave the interior pathogenic factor untreated. Similarly, this syndrome cannot be addressed by targeting the interior with heat-clearing, downward-draining, or emetic formulas, since this would leave the exterior pathogenic factor untreated, or worse, draw it into the interior. *Shaoyang* syndrome must be harmonized by addressing the exterior and interior concurrently.

In addition to *shaoyang* syndrome, there are many other applications of harmonizing formulas. An unregulated Liver may overact on the Spleen and Stomach, causing Liver and Spleen disharmony, and Stomach and Intestines disharmony. The Liver is responsible for the free flow of qi and promotes normal digestion by regulating the ascending and descending of Spleen and Stomach qi. The Spleen is in charge of the transformation and transportation of food and water. Liver and Spleen disharmony—a combination of Liver qi stagnation and impaired transportation and transformation function of the Spleen—is one of the most commonly seen disorders in veterinary medicine. Liver qi stagnation is often seen in animals that are chronically medicated, emotionally stressed (from isolation, lack of exercise, excessive confinement, boarding, grooming, and abuse) and in breeds that are constitutionally predisposed. When the Liver becomes stagnant, it can over-control the Spleen, impairing its function. Spleen qi deficiency often occurs from consumption of species-inappropriate diets made of energetically "hot" meats (lamb, venison), dampness-engendering processed carbohydrates (grains and sugars), dyes, and preservatives. Overfeeding and the feeding of cold raw or refrigerated food, chronic antibiotic use, lack of regular exercise, and/or overwork may contribute to Spleen dysfunction. Antibiotics are energetically cold and bitter and can injure the Spleen, cause Liver qi stagnation, and negatively impact the normal bacterial flora and function of the gastrointestinal tract.

Clinical signs of Liver-Spleen disharmony include: poor appetite, nausea, depression, irritability, aggression, vomiting, diarrhea, pain on defecation that decreases after the stool is passed, increased urgency to defecate, tenesmus, abdominal bloating and pain, flatulence, borborygmus, belching, and hypochondriac pain. The tongue and pulse are variable and dependent on the degree of Liver qi stagnation and Spleen qi deficiency present. A preponderance to qi stagnation results in a pulse that is wiry, and the tongue will be red to purple and may have a thicker white coating if heat is present. Qi deficiency pulses will be weaker, more slippery than wiry, and the tongue will be lighter in color, from pale pink to red and it may have a greasy coating. Chronic Liver-Spleen disharmony often progresses to damp-heat disorders involving the Liver, Gallbladder, Spleen and Stomach. Dietary therapy is often necessary for successful resolution of Liver-Spleen disharmony. Chinese food therapy and nutritional supplements are an integral part of treatment and are specifically designed to treat the individual animal and pattern of disease in the same manner as herbal medicine and acupuncture.

An accumulation of pathogenic factors, such as interlocking of heat and cold in the Stomach and Intestines, leads to disharmony between these organs. The interlocking of heat and cold interferes with the ascending and descending functions of these two organs and results in a reversal of qi flow. Stomach and Intestine disharmony develops in veterinary patients as a result of poor diet and long-term pharmaceutical therapy. These factors cause disruption of the normal ascending and descending of the middle *jiao* and also cause stagnation and heat in the Stomach (manifesting as nausea, vomiting, halitosis, epigastric distention, a thicker tongue coating that may be greasy, and a rapid pulse) and cold in the Intestines (manifesting as borborygmus, diarrhea, and a wiry pulse).

Harmonizing formulas have classically been used to treat *shaoyang* syndrome. Today, harmonizing methods can be used effectively to treat all of the above disorders.

Chapter 3 — Overview

SUBCATEGORIES OF ACTION

Harmonizing formulas are divided into three subcategories to reflect the nature of the disharmony and the characteristics of the formulas.

1. ***Shaoyang* Harmonizing Formulas**

These formulas harmonize *shaoyang* syndrome that is located half-interior and half-exterior. Common clinical manifestations include alternating spells of trembling and fever, fullness and discomfort in the chest and hypochondrium, irritability, nausea, vomiting, lack of appetite, and a dry mouth and throat.

Herbs commonly used to harmonize *shaoyang* syndromes include *Huang Qin* (Radix Scutellariae) with *Chai Hu* (Radix Bupleuri), or *Huang Qin* (Radix Scutellariae) with *Qing Hao* (Herba Artemisiae Annuae). Representative formulas that harmonize *shaoyang* are *Xiao Chai Hu Tang* (Minor Bupleurum Decoction) and *Hao Qin Qing Dan Tang* (Artemisia Annua and Scutellaria Decoction to Clear the Gallbladder).

2. **Liver and Spleen Harmonizing Formulas**

These formulas treat Liver (excess) overacting on the Spleen (deficiency). These cases usually involve Liver qi stagnation and Spleen qi deficiency. Common clinical manifestations include poor appetite, nausea, depression, irritability, aggression, vomiting, diarrhea, pain on defecation, increased urgency to defecate, tenesmus, abdominal bloating, flatulence, borborygmus, belching, and hypochondriac pain and colic. The tongue and pulse are variable, depending on the degree of Liver qi stagnation and Spleen qi deficiency. With more qi stagnation, the pulse will be wiry and the tongue will be red to purple, and, in severe cases, may have a thin, white to yellow coating depending on whether heat is present. If qi deficiency is predominant, the pulse will be weaker, more slippery than wiry, and the tongue will be lighter in color, ranging from pale pink to red, and may have a greasy, white coating.

Formulas that harmonize the Liver and Spleen are generally composed of herbs that smooth Liver qi, strengthen the Spleen, regulate qi circulation, and nourish the blood. Exemplar herbs include *Chai Hu* (Radix Bupleuri), *Zhi Qiao* (Fructus Aurantii), *Chen Pi* (Pericarpium Citri Reticulatae), *Xiang Fu* (Rhizoma Cyperi), *Dang Gui* (Radix Angelicae Sinensis), *Bai Shao* (Radix Paeoniae Alba), *Fu Ling* (Poria), and *Zhi Gan Cao* (Radix et Rhizoma Glycyrrhizae Praeparata cum Melle). Representative formulas include *Si Ni San* (Frigid Extremities Powder), *Xiao Yao San* (Rambling Powder), and *Tong Xie Yao Fang* (Important Formula for Painful Diarrhea).

3. **Intestines and Stomach Harmonizing Formulas**

These formulas treat accumulation of various pathogenic factors in the Stomach and Intestines. Such cases involve interlocking of heat and cold, which causes reversed qi flow in the Stomach and Intestines. Common clinical manifestations include; nausea, halitosis, vomiting, abdominal distention and pain, borborygmus, and diarrhea.

Two types of herbs are commonly used to harmonize the Intestines and Stomach and treat the interlocking of heat and cold: acrid and warm herbs, such as *Gan Jiang* (Rhizoma Zingiberis) and *Sheng Jiang* (Rhizoma Zingiberis Recens); and bitter and cold herbs, such as *Huang Qin* (Radix Scutellariae) and *Huang Lian* (Rhizoma Coptidis). An exemplar formula is *Ban Xia Xie Xin Tang* (Pinellia Decoction to Drain the Epigastrium).

CAUTIONS / CONTRAINDICATIONS

- In comparison to formulas from other categories, harmonizing formulas do not have drastic or potent actions. Nevertheless, harmonizing formulas eliminate pathogenic factors from the body. Incorrect diagnosis or application of harmonizing formulas may delay healing or even worsen the condition. For example, the use of harmonizing formulas for an interior condition may require an extended amount of time for healing, and using them for an exterior syndrome may worsen the condition by drawing the exterior pathogens inward.

Chapter 3 — Overview

- Harmonizing formulas should not be used in animals with alternating spells of fever and trembling accompanied by the following characteristics: fatigue, weakness, irregular diet and lifestyle, and deficiency of qi and/or blood.
- Harmonizing formulas should not be used for conditions in which the exterior pathogenic factors have not yet entered the *shaoyang*, for an interior condition that has progressed past *shaoyang*, or for *yangming* syndromes with excess heat.

PHARMACOLOGICAL EFFECTS & CLINICAL APPLICATIONS

While harmonizing formulas are divided into three subcategories based on their traditional therapeutic actions, these subcategories have contrasting pharmacological effects and clinical applications.

1. ***Shaoyang* harmonizing formulas**, as the name implies, primarily relieve "half-interior, half-exterior" *shaoyang* syndromes. In conventional medicine, internal organ diseases of a chronic nature often characterize such conditions. Clinically, *shaoyang* harmonizing formulas are most effective and most commonly used for chronic diseases affecting the liver, gallbladder, pancreas, and kidneys.
   - **Liver disorders**: *Shaoyang* harmonizing formulas have marked hepatoprotective effects and commonly treat various liver disorders, including but not limited to chronic hepatitis,[1,2,3] liver fibrosis,[4] liver cancer,[5] and alcohol-induced liver disorders (hepatitis, fatty liver, and liver cirrhosis).[6] The mechanisms of actions differ among several formulas. *Xiao Chai Hu Tang* (Minor Bupleurum Decoction) protects the liver by augmenting the natural killer (NK) activity in the liver and increasing the production of granulocyte colony-stimulating factor (G-CSF) on peripheral blood mononuclear cells.[7,8] *Si Ni San* (Frigid Extremities Powder) provides protective effects against liver injury through multiple mechanisms, such as protection of the hepatocyte membrane, enhancement of nitric oxide release, and dysfunction of liver-infiltrating cells, mainly by causing their apoptosis.[9] *Chai Hu Gui Zhi Tang* (Bupleurum and Cinnamon Twig Decoction) protects the liver by inhibiting the cell proliferation and induction of apoptosis in adjacent hepatocytes in subjects with liver lesions induced by N-nitrosomorpholine.[10]
   - **Gallbladder disorders**: Cholecystitis and cholelithiasis are two gallbladder disorders commonly addressed by formulas that harmonize *shaoyang*, such as *Xiao Chai Hu Tang* (Minor Bupleurum Decoction),[11,12] and *Hao Qin Qing Dan Tang* (Artemisia Annua and Scutellaria Decoction to Clear the Gallbladder).[13] The mechanism of this action is attributed to their cholagogic effect to increase the secretion of bile from the gallbladder and facilitate its excretion into the intestines.[14]
   - **Pancreatic disorders**: Some *shaoyang* harmonizing formulas have protective effects on the pancreas and have been used to treat various pancreatic disorders. For example, *Xiao Chai Hu Tang* (Minor Bupleurum Decoction) may be used to treat acute pancreatitis,[15] and *Chai Hu Gui Zhi Tang* (Bupleurum and Cinnamon Twig Decoction) may be used to treat chronic pancreatitis and pancreatic fibrosis.[16,17,18,19]
   - **Kidney disorders**: *Xiao Chai Hu Tang* (Minor Bupleurum Decoction) has been shown to effectively treat renal insufficiency,[20] and acute and chronic nephritis.[21] *Chai Ling Tang* (Bupleurum and Poria Decoction) has been used successfully to treat nephropathy,[22] diabetic nephropathy,[23] and steroid-dependent nephrotic syndrome.[24] The mechanisms of these nephroprotective effects have been attributed in part to the ability of the formulas to increase elimination of water,[25] and decrease serum albumin and total protein levels.[26]

2. **Liver and Spleen harmonizing formulas** treat a wide variety of disorders, including, but not limited to, liver disorders, gallbladder disorders, gastrointestinal disorders, mental disorders, and sexual and reproductive disorders.
   - **Liver disorders**: These formulas have been used effectively to treat liver disorders, such as hepatitis,[27,28] chronic hepatitis,[29] and liver cirrhosis.[30,31] The hepatoprotective effects of these formulas include enhanced protection of the hepatocyte membrane, reduced damage of liver cells, decreased liver enzymes, and increased generation of new liver cells.[32,33,34] Exemplar formulas include *Si Ni San*

Chapter 3 — Overview

(Frigid Extremities Powder), *Chai Hu Shu Gan Tang* (Bupleurum Decoction to Spread the Liver), and *Xiao Yao San* (Rambling Powder).

- **Gallbladder disorders**: Cholecystitis and cholelithiasis are two gallbladder disorders commonly addressed by these formulas, such as with *Si Ni San* (Frigid Extremities Powder),[35,36] *Chai Hu Shu Gan Tang* (Bupleurum Decoction to Spread the Liver),[37,38] and *Xiao Yao San* (Rambling Powder).[39] The mechanism has been attributed to the cholagogic effects of the formulas that increase the production and secretion of bile acids.[40]
- **Gastrointestinal disorders**: These formulas have been used to treat a wide variety of gastro-intestinal diseases, including but not limited to superficial gastritis,[41] gastritis,[42] peptic ulcer,[43] chronic ulcerative colitis,[44] enteritis,[45,46] colitis,[47] ulcerative colitis,[48] and irritable bowel syndrome.[49,50] Exemplar formulas include *Si Ni San* (Frigid Extremities Powder), *Chai Hu Shu Gan Tang* (Bupleurum Decoction to Spread the Liver), *Xiao Yao San* (Rambling Powder), and *Tong Xie Yao Fang* (Important Formula for Painful Diarrhea). The mechanisms of actions vary, depending on the disorders and the formulas.
- **Mental disorders**: Many harmonizing formulas have been used to treat various types of mental disorders. *Xiao Yao San* (Rambling Powder) has been used successfully for schizophrenia,[51] depression,[52] and neurosis.[53] *Jia Wei Xiao Yao San* (Augmented Rambling Powder) has been used effectively for affective and panic disorders.[54,55] *Chai Hu Shu Gan Tang* (Bupleurum Decoction to Spread the Liver) has been used to treat insomnia.[56] The mechanisms of actions vary, depending on the disorders and the formulas.
- **Sexual and reproductive disorders**: These formulas are effective in treating a wide variety of sexual and reproductive disorders in both men and women. *Si Ni San* (Frigid Extremities Powder) has been used effectively for impotence,[57] chronic adnexitis,[58] and infertility caused by blocked fallopian tubes.[59] *Chai Hu Shu Gan Tang* (Bupleurum Decoction to Spread the Liver) has been used successfully for orchitis,[60] male sexual dysfunction (inability to ejaculate),[61] and breast distention and pain.[62] Lastly, *Xiao Yao San* (Rambling Powder) is useful in cases of sexual dysfunction in men (impotence and inability to ejaculate),[63,64] and infertility in women.[65]

3. Unlike other harmonizing formulas that have a wide range of clinical applications, **Stomach and Intestines harmonizing formulas** target mainly gastrointestinal disorders.
   - **Gastrointestinal disorders**: The conditions these formulas treat include, but are not limited to, superficial gastritis,[66] chronic gastritis,[67] atrophic gastritis,[68] peptic ulcer disease,[69] reflux esophagitis,[70] upper gastrointestinal bleeding,[71] indigestion,[72] gastroptosis,[73] gastroenteritis,[74] irritable bowel syndrome,[75] and ulcerative colitis.[76] Exemplar formulas include *Ban Xia Xie Xin Tang* (Pinellia Decoction to Drain the Epigastrium), *Sheng Jiang Xie Xin Tang* (Fresh Ginger Decoction to Drain the Epigastrium), and *Huang Lian Tang* (Coptis Decoction).

References

1. *Xin Yao Yu Lin Chuang* (New Medicine and the Clinical Application), 1982; 4:651.
2. *Zhong Yi Fang Ji Xian Dai Yan Jiu* (Modern Study of Medical Formulas in Traditional Chinese Medicine), 1997; (1):199.
3. *Guo Wai Yi Xue Zhong Yi Zhong Yao Fen Ce* (Monograph of Chinese Herbology from Foreign Medicine), 1991; 3:168.
4. Shimizu I. Sho-saiko-to: Japanese herbal medicine for protection against hepatic fibrosis and carcinoma. Journal of Gastroenterology & Hepatology. 2000 Mar.; 15 Suppl:D84-90.
5. Oka H, Yamamoto S, Kuroki T, Harihara S, Marumo T, Kim SR, Monna T, Kobayashi K, Tango T. Prospective study of chemoprevention of hepatocellular carcinoma with Sho-saiko-to (TJ-9). Cancer. 1995 Sep 1; 76(5):743-9.
6. *Guo Wai Yi Xue Zhong Yi Zhong Yao Fen Ce* (Monograph of Chinese Herbology from Foreign Medicine), 1991; 13(6):31.
7. Kaneko M, Kawakita T, Tauchi Y, Saito Y, Suzuki A, Nomoto K. Augmentation of NK activity after oral administration of a traditional Chinese medicine, xiao-chai-hu-tang (shosaiko-to). Immunopharmacol Immunotoxicol. 1994 Feb;16(1): 41-53.
8. Yamashiki M, Asakawa M, Kayaba Y, Kosaka Y, Nishimura A.Herbal medicine "sho-saiko-to" induces in vitro granulocyte colony-stimulating factor production on peripheral blood mononuclear cells. J Clin Lab Immunol. 1992; 37(2):83-90.
9. Jiang J, Zhou C, Xu Q. Alleviating effects of Si-Ni-San, a traditional Chinese prescription, on experimental liver injury and its mechanisms. Biol Pharm Bull. 2003 Aug; 26(8):1089-94.
10. Tatsuta M, Iishi H, Baba M, Narahara H, Yano H, Sakai N.Suppression by Chai-hu-gui-zhi-tang of the development of liver lesions induced by N-nitrosomorpholine in Sprague-Dawley rats. Cancer Lett. 2000 Apr 28; 152(1):31-6.

Chapter 3 — Overview

11. *Fu Jian Zhong Yi Yao* (Fujian Chinese Medicine and Herbology), 1986; 17(3):48.
12. *Shi Yong Zhong Xi Yi Jie He Za Zhi* (Practical Journal of Integrated Chinese and Western Medicines), 1993; 4:218.
13. *Chang Chun Zhong Yi Xue Yuan Xue Bao* (Journal of Changchun University of Chinese Medicine), 1998; 1:29.
14. *Guo Wai Yi Xue* (Foreign Medicine), 1991; 13(4):46.
15. *Zhong Yi Za Zhi* (Journal of Chinese Medicine), 1982; 9:40.
16. *Guo Wai Yi Xue* (Foreign Medicine), 1992; 1:40.
17. Motoo Y, Su SB, Xie MJ, Taga H, Sawabu N. Effect of herbal medicine Saiko-keishi-to (TJ-10) on rat spontaneous chronic pancreatitis: comparison with other herbal medicines. Int J Pancreatol. 2000 Apr; 27(2):123-9.
18. Su SB, Motoo Y, Xie MJ, Sakai J, Taga H, Sawabu N. Expression of pancreatitis-associated protein (PAP) in rat spontaneous chronic pancreatitis: effect of herbal medicine Saiko-keishi-to (TJ-10). Pancreas. 1999 Oct; 19(3):239-47.
19. Su SB, Motoo Y, Xie MJ, Taga H, Sawabu N.Antifibrotic effect of the herbal medicine Saiko-keishi-to (TJ-10) on chronic pancreatitis in the WBN/Kob rat. Pancreas. 2001 Jan; 22(1):8-17.
20. *Shan Dong Zhong Yi Za Zhi* (Shandong Journal of Chinese Medicine), 1998; 8:359.
21. *Zhong Yi Fang Ji Xian Dai Yan Jiu* (Modern Study of Medical Formulas in Traditional Chinese Medicine), 1997; 190.
22. *Guo Wai Yi Xue Zhong Yi Zhong Yao Fen Ce* (Monograph of Chinese Herbology from Foreign Medicine), 1989; 11(6):18.
23. *Guo Wai Yi Xue Zhong Yi Zhong Yao Fen Ce* (Monograph of Chinese Herbology from Foreign Medicine), 1990; (5):247.
24. Yoshikawa N, Ito H, Takekoshi Y, Honda M, Awazu M, Iijima K, Nakamura H, Seino Y, Takeda N, Hattori S, Matsuda I. Standard versus long-term prednisolone with sairei-to for initial therapy in childhood steroid-responsive nephrotic syndrome: a prospective controlled study. Nippon Jinzo Gakkai Shi. 1998 Nov; 40(8):587-90.
25. Fujitsuka N, Goto K, Takeda S, Aburada M. The diuretic effect of Sairei-to is mediated by nitric oxide production in pentobarbital-anesthetized rats. J Pharmacol Sci. 2004 Feb; 94(2):185-91.
26. Li P, Fujio S. Effects of chai ling tang on proteinuria in rat models. J Tradit Chin Med. 1995 Mar; 15(1):48-52.
27. *Shan Xi Xin Zhong Yi* (New Shanxi Chinese Medicine), 1987; (5):225.
28. *Hei Long Jiang Zhong Yi Yao* (Heilongjiang Chinese Medicine and Herbology), 1987; (1):25.
29. *Zhong Yi Yao Xue Bao* (Report of Chinese Medicine and Herbology), 1992; 6:38.
30. *Liao Ning Zhong Yi Za Zhi* (Liaoning Journal of Chinese Medicine), 1996; 4:169.
31. *Ji Lin Zhong Yi Yao* (Jilin Chinese Medicine and Herbology), 1986; (5):18.
32. Jiang J, Zhou C, Xu Q. Alleviating effects of Si-Ni-San, a traditional Chinese prescription, on experimental liver injury and its mechanisms. Biol Pharm Bull. 2003 Aug; 26(8):1089-94.
33. *Zhong Cao Yao* (Chinese Herbal Medicine), 1990; 21(11):28.
34. *Zhong Cao Yao* (Chinese Herbal Medicine), 1990; 21(11):28.
35. *Hu Nan Zhong Yi Za Zhi* (Hunan Journal of Chinese Medicine), 1989; 4:39.
36. *An Hui Zhong Yi Xue Yuan Xue Bao* (Journal of Anhui University School of Medicine), 1995; 4:32.
37. *Gan Su Zhong Yi Xue Yuan Xue Bao* (Journal of Gansu University of Chinese Medicine), 1995; 2:37.
38. *Shi Yong Zhong Xi Yi Jie He Za Zhi* (Practical Journal of Integrated Chinese and Western Medicines), 1991; 4(10):618.
39. *Jiang Xi Zhong Yi Yao* (Jiangxi Chinese Medicine and Herbology), 1999; 1:27.
40. *Shi Yong Zhong Yi Nei Ke Za Zhi* (Journal of Practical Chinese Internal Medicine), 1989; 3(1):11.
41. *Zhe Jiang Zhong Yi Za Zhi* (Zhejiang Journal of Chinese Medicine), 1997; 10:439.
42. *Bei Jing Zhong Yi Yao Da Xue Xue Bao* (Journal of Beijing University of Medicine and Medicinals), 1997; 3:68.
43. *Zhe Jiang Zhong Yi Xue Yuan Xue Bao* (Journal of Zhejiang University of Chinese Medicine), 1997; 2:53.
44. *Nei Meng Gu Zhong Yi Yao* (Traditional Chinese Medicine and Medicinals of Inner Mongolia), 1998; 1:26.
45. *Hu Nan Zhong Yi Za Zhi* (Hunan Journal of Chinese Medicine), 1987; 6:12.
46. *Ha Er Bing Zhong Yi* (Haerbing Chinese Medicine), 1964; 4:25.
47. *Shan Xi Zhong Yi* (Shanxi Chinese Medicine), 1989; 11:490.
48. *Shan Dong Zhong Yi Za Zhi* (Shandong Journal of Chinese Medicine), 1996; 10:444.
49. *Si Chuan Zhong Yi* (Sichuan Chinese Medicine), 1997; 11:25.
50. *Zhe Jiang Zhong Yi Za Zhi* (Zhejiang Journal of Chinese Medicine), 1996; 11:502.
51. *Xin Zhong Yi* (New Chinese Medicine), 1983; (1):37.
52. *Bei Jing Zhong Yi* (Beijing Chinese Medicine), 1996; 2:22.
53. *Fu Jian Zhong Yi Yao* (Fujian Chinese Medicine and Herbology), 1999; 5:26.
54. Zhang LD, Zhang YL, Xu SH, Zhou G, Jin SB. Traditional Chinese medicine typing of affective disorders and treatment. American Journal of Chinese Medicine. 1994; 22(3-4):321-7.
55. Mantani N. Hisanaga A. Kogure T. Kita T. Shimada Y. Terasawa K. Four cases of panic disorder successfully treated with Kampo (Japanese herbal) medicines: Kami-shoyo-san and Hange-koboku-to. Psychiatry & Clinical Neurosciences. 56(6):617-20, 2002 Dec.
56. *Zhong Yi Ming Fang Lin Chuang Xin Yong* (Contemporary Clinical Applications of Classic Chinese Formulas), 2001, 575.
57. *Hu Bei Zhong Yi Za Zhi* (Hubei Journal of Chinese Medicine), 1986; 3:21.
58. *Chang Chun Zhong Yi Xue Yuan Xue Bao* (Journal of Changchun University of Chinese Medicine), 1995; 1:43.
59. *Zhong Yi Ming Fang Lin Chuang Xin Yong* (Contemporary Clinical Applications of Classic Chinese Formulas), 2001; 243.
60. *Shan Xi Zhong Yi* (Shanxi Chinese Medicine), 1993; 14(2):54.
61. *Zhe Jiang Zhong Yi Za Zhi* (Zhejiang Journal of Chinese Medicine), 1990; 25(6):253.
62. *Guang Xi Zhong Yi Yao* (Guangxi Chinese Medicine and Herbology), 1985; 8(2):21.
63. *Ji Lin Zhong Yi Yao* (Jilin Chinese Medicine and Herbology), 1990; 2:17.

Chapter 3 — Overview

64. *He Nan Zhong Yi* (Henan Chinese Medicine), 1997; 3:174.
65. *Xin Zhong Yi* (New Chinese Medicine), 1995; 5:38.
66. *Shan Xi Zhong Yi* (Shanxi Chinese Medicine), 1991; 12(3):128.
67. *Tian Jin Zhong Yi* (Tianjin Chinese Medicine), 1997; 1:15.
68. *Xin Zhong Yi* (New Chinese Medicine), 1988; 7:35.
69. *Hei Long Jiang Zhong Yi Yao* (Heilongjiang Chinese Medicine and Herbology), 1996; 5:27.
70. *Hei Long Jiang Zhong Yi Yao* (Heilongjiang Chinese Medicine and Herbology), 1998; 3:30.
71. *Hu Bei Zhong Yi Za Zhi* (Hubei Journal of Chinese Medicine), 1987; 3:22.
72. *Si Chuan Zhong Yi* (Sichuan Chinese Medicine), 1990; 5:11.
73. *Shang Hai Zhong Yi Yao Za Zhi* (Shanghai Journal of Chinese Medicine and Herbology), 1998; 4:30.
74. *Zhe Jiang Zhong Yi Za Zhi* (Zhejiang Journal of Chinese Medicine), 1985; 4:155.
75. *Zhong Yi Ming Fang Lin Chuang Xin Yong* (Contemporary Clinical Applications of Classic Chinese Formulas), 2001; 303.
76. *Xin Zhong Yi* (New Chinese Medicine), 1997; 6:14.

Section 1

和解少阳剂 — Shaoyang Harmonizing Formulas

Xiǎo Chái Hú Tāng (Minor Bupleurum Decoction)

小柴胡湯

小柴胡汤

Pinyin Name: *Xiao Chai Hu Tang*
Literal Name: Minor Bupleurum Decoction
Alternate Names: *Hsiao Tsai Hu Tang*, Minor Bupleurum Combination
Original Source: *Shang Han Lun* (Discussion of Cold-Induced Disorders) by Zhang Zhong-Jing in the Eastern Han Dynasty

COMPOSITION

Chai Hu (Radix Bupleuri)	24g [12g]
Huang Qin (Radix Scutellariae)	9g [9g]
Ban Xia (Rhizoma Pinelliae), *xi* (washed)	0.5 cup [9g]
Sheng Jiang (Rhizoma Zingiberis Recens), *qie* (sliced)	9g [9g]
Ren Shen (Radix et Rhizoma Ginseng)	9g [6g]
Zhi Gan Cao (Radix et Rhizoma Glycyrrhizae Praeparata cum Melle)	9g [5g]
Da Zao (Fructus Jujubae), *bo* (opened)	12 pieces [4 pieces]

DOSAGE / PREPARATION / ADMINISTRATION

The source text specifies to cook the ingredients in 12 cups [2,400 mL] of water until 6 cups [1,200 mL] of the liquid remain. Discard the residue, and cook the strained decoction again until it is reduced to 3 cups [600 mL]. Take 1 cup [200 mL] of warm decoction per dose, three times daily. Today, the decoction may be prepared using the doses suggested in brackets.

CHINESE THERAPEUTIC ACTIONS

Harmonizes *shaoyang*

CLINICAL MANIFESTATIONS

1. *Shaoyang* syndrome: intermittent fever, chest and hypochondriac discomfort, irritability, dry mouth and throat, lack of appetite, nausea, vomiting, vertigo, a dry throat, a thin, white tongue coating, and a wiry pulse.
2. Any of the following disorders with *shaoyang* characteristics: disorders involving heat in the uterus, Liver, or *chong* (thoroughfare) channel; jaundice; or any internal injury characterized by *shaoyang* syndrome.

VETERINARY CLINICAL APPLICATIONS

Hepatitis, chronic active hepatitis, hepatic cirrhosis, hepatic carcinoma, acute and chronic toxic hepatopathy, hepatic lipidosis, jaundice, cholecystitis, cholelithiasis, pancreatitis, fever of unknown origin, fever in cancer, chronic glomerulonephritis, chronic renal insufficiency, chronic urinary tract infection, upper respiratory infection, bronchitis, recurrent pneumonia, chronic gastritis, metritis, postpartum infection and postpartum fever.

EXPLANATION

Xiao Chai Hu Tang (Minor Bupleurum Decoction) is the main formula for harmonizing *shaoyang* syndrome, one of the six stages of disease progression described in *Shang Han Lun* (Discussion of Cold-Induced Disorders). The *shaoyang* is situated between yang and yin, or between the exterior and interior; therefore, intermittent fever and trembling may occur in *shaoyang* syndrome if the body is fighting both the pathogens outside and the disharmony inside.

Xiǎo Chái Hú Tāng (Minor Bupleurum Decoction)

***Xiao Chai Hu Tang* (Minor Bupleurum Decoction)**

Diagnosis	Clinical Signs	Treatment	Herbs
Shaoyang syndrome	• Intermittent fever: the location of the illness between exterior and interior • Chest and hypochondriac discomfort: qi stagnation • A dry mouth and throat, and irritability: heat in the *shaoyang* Gallbladder channel • Lack of appetite, nausea, and vomiting: Gallbladder heat invading the Stomach • Thin, white tongue coating: exterior condition • Wiry pulse: qi stagnation	Harmonizes *shaoyang*	• *Chai Hu* (Radix Bupleuri) releases the exterior, and *Huang Qin* (Radix Scutellariae) clears the interior. Together, they harmonize *shaoyang* disorders. • *Ban Xia* (Rhizoma Pinelliae) harmonizes the Stomach to relieve nausea and vomiting and disperses stagnation. • *Sheng Jiang* (Rhizoma Zingiberis Recens) harmonizes the middle *jiao*. • *Ren Shen* (Radix et Rhizoma Ginseng), *Zhi Gan Cao* (Radix et Rhizoma Glycyrrhizae Praeparata cum Melle), and *Da Zao* (Fructus Jujubae) tonify Stomach qi, nourish body fluids, and harmonize the *ying* (nutritive) and *wei* (defensive) levels.

Disorders in the *shaoyang* may cause qi stagnation and eventual heat formation in the Gallbladder channel (a *shaoyang* channel), giving rise to chest and hypochondriac discomfort, a dry mouth and throat, and irritability. Lack of appetite, nausea, and vomiting are the results of Gallbladder heat invading the Stomach. The tongue coating may be thin and white because the pathogenic factors have not yet transformed into internal heat. The wiry pulse is the result of qi stagnation in the *shaoyang* channel.

Because the disease resides between the exterior and the interior, it is not suitable to use only exterior-releasing herbs or only purgative herbs. Use of only exterior-releasing herbs will not treat the interior condition, and use of only heat-clearing or downward-draining herbs will bring the pathogens from the exterior into the interior. Therefore, the harmonizing method is the most appropriate treatment approach in this condition.

Chai Hu (Radix Bupleuri) is the main herb for treating *shaoyang* disorders. The light quality of *Chai Hu* (Radix Bupleuri) lifts and disperses stagnation, as well as releases to the exterior. *Huang Qin* (Radix Scutellariae), a bitter and cold herb that enters the Gallbladder channel, is ideal for clearing *shaoyang* heat. Together, *Chai Hu* (Radix Bupleuri) disperses the exterior while *Huang Qin* (Radix Scutellariae) clears the interior to achieve the harmonizing effect. *Ban Xia* (Rhizoma Pinelliae), besides harmonizing the Stomach to relieve nausea and vomiting, disperses stagnation in the body. *Sheng Jiang* (Rhizoma Zingiberis Recens) helps *Ban Xia* (Rhizoma Pinelliae) harmonize the middle *jiao*. It also reduces the toxicity of *Ban Xia* (Rhizoma Pinelliae). *Ren Shen* (Radix et Rhizoma Ginseng), *Zhi Gan Cao* (Radix et Rhizoma Glycyrrhizae Praeparata cum Melle), and *Da Zao* (Fructus Jujubae) tonify Stomach qi, nourish body fluids, and harmonize the *ying* (nutritive) and *wei* (defensive) levels. The combination of *Chai Hu* (Radix Bupleuri) and *Ren Shen* (Radix et Rhizoma Ginseng) also provides a mutual check and balance: *Chai Hu* (Radix Bupleuri) prevents the tonic effect of *Ren Shen* (Radix et Rhizoma Ginseng) from retaining the pathogens in the body, while *Ren Shen* (Radix et Rhizoma Ginseng) prevents the dispersing effect of *Chai Hu* (Radix Bupleuri) from damaging qi. Combined, these herbs expel the pathogens and strengthen bodily constitution.

Because the *shaoyang* stage is unstable and often short and transient, the clinical signs listed above may not be clinically present all at the same time. Therefore, as suggested in *Shang Han Lun* (Discussion of Cold-Induced Disorders), this formula can be applied even if there is only one *shaoyang* symptom present clinically.

VETERINARY MODIFICATIONS

General Clinical Signs

- If there is thirst, remove *Ban Xia* (Rhizoma Pinelliae) and add *Tian Hua Fen* (Radix Trichosanthis).
- With thirst and irritability from deficiency heat, add *Mai Dong* (Radix Ophiopogonis) and *Wu Wei Zi* (Fructus Schisandrae Chinensis).
- If there is no thirst, but a slight fever and exterior clinical signs are present, remove *Ren Shen* (Radix et Rhizoma Ginseng) and add *Gui Zhi* (Ramulus Cinnamomi).
- With irritability, add *Dan Zhu Ye* (Herba Lophatheri) and *Geng Mi* (Semen Oryzae).

Xiǎo Chái Hú Tāng (Minor Bupleurum Decoction)

- With abdominal pain, remove *Huang Qin* (Radix Scutellariae) and add *Bai Shao* (Radix Paeoniae Alba), *Yan Hu Suo* (Rhizoma Corydalis), *Xiang Fu* (Rhizoma Cyperi) and *Qing Pi* (Pericarpium Citri Reticulatae Viride).
- With more vomiting or nausea, add *Sheng Jiang* (Rhizoma Zingiberis Recens) and *Chen Pi* (Pericarpium Citri Reticulatae).
- When there is poor appetite, add *Bai Zhu* (Rhizoma Atractylodis Macrocephalae), *Chen Pi* (Pericarpium Citri Reticulatae), *Fu Ling* (Poria), and *Shan Zha* (Fructus Crataegi).

Liver and Gallbladder Disorders

- For icteric jaundice and hepatitis, add *Zhi Shi* (Fructus Aurantii Immaturus), *Yin Chen* (Herba Artemisiae Scopariae), *Bai Shao* (Radix Paeoniae Alba), and *Jin Qian Cao* (Herba Lysimachiae).
- For damp-heat jaundice, add *Yin Chen* (Herba Artemisiae Scopariae), *Zhi Zi* (Fructus Gardeniae), and *Ban Lan Gen* (Radix Isatidis).
- For jaundice with more heat, add *Zhi Zi* (Fructus Gardeniae) and *Huang Bo* (Cortex Phellodendri Chinensis).

Infectious Disorders

- For acute upper respiratory infection or kennel cough, add *Jing Jie* (Herba Schizonepetae), *Fang Feng* (Radix Saposhnikoviae), and *Ge Gen* (Radix Puerariae Lobatae).
- With wind-heat, add *Jin Yin Hua* (Flos Lonicerae Japonicae), *Lian Qiao* (Fructus Forsythiae), and *Ban Lan Gen* (Radix Isatidis).
- For acute bronchitis, add *Jie Geng* (Radix Platycodonis), *Zhi Qiao* (Fructus Aurantii), *Ku Xing Ren* (Semen Armeniacae Amarum), and *Bai Bu* (Radix Stemonae).
- For chronic bronchitis, add *Fu Ling* (Poria), *Chen Pi* (Pericarpium Citri Reticulatae), *Zi Wan* (Radix et Rhizoma Asteris), and *Kuan Dong Hua* (Flos Farfarae).
- For urinary tract infection, add *Bian Xu* (Herba Polygoni Avicularis), *Che Qian Cao* (Herba Plantaginis), and *Hai Jin Sha* (Spora Lygodii).

Parturition Disorders

- For postpartum wind invasion with increased vomiting or nausea, increase the dose of *Sheng Jiang* (Rhizoma Zingiberis Recens).
- For postpartum wind invasion with marked deficiency, increase the dose of *Ren Shen* (Radix et Rhizoma Ginseng).

CAUTIONS / CONTRAINDICATIONS

- *Xiao Chai Hu Tang* should be used with caution in patients with yin and/or blood deficiencies, in animals with upper excess and lower deficiency, and in animals with Liver fire. This formula is dry in nature, is not for long-term use, and should be discontinued once the clinical signs resolve.
- In general, there is no sweating associated with relief of clinical signs following the administration of *Xiao Chai Hu Tang* since it harmonizes, rather than releases the exterior. However, some animals may sweat prior to recovery. They should be monitored closely to prevent excessive sweating from injuring yin.
- Avoid cold and raw foods during administration.[1]

PHARMACOLOGICAL EFFECTS

1. **Hepatoprotective**: Administration of *Xiao Chai Hu Tang* was associated with preventive and beneficial effects against various types of drug- or chemical-induced liver damage. In one study, intraperitoneal injection of the formula in rats effectively controlled galactose-induced liver disorder in 65-70% of subjects by lowering the SGOT and SGPT.[2] Other studies have indicated that the formula is also effective against liver cirrhosis induced by carbon tetrachloride.[3] Yet another study reported that *Xiao Chai Hu Tang* was effective in treating liver inflammation and fibrosis.[4] One proposed mechanism of this hepatoprotective effect is the augmentation of natural killer (NK) cell activity in the liver.[5] Another proposed mechanism is a dose-dependent increase in the production of granulocyte colony-stimulating factor (G-CSF) on peripheral blood mononuclear cells.[6]
2. **Cholagogic**: Administration of *Xiao Chai Hu Tang* was associated with a marked effect of increasing the secretion of bile acid from the gallbladder and its excretion into the intestines in animals.[7]
3. **Immunostimulant**: Administration of *Xiao Chai Hu Tang* has marked effect on the immune system. In one study of mice, 100 mg/kg of the herb was associated with stimulating natural killer (NK) cells activities, while 200 mg/kg was associated with inhibition of NK cell activity.[8]
4. **Anti-inflammatory**: Intraperitoneal injection of the formula in rats at 200 mg/kg was associated with marked anti-inflammatory effects for up to 4 hours.[9] The anti-inflammatory effects were also present in rats whose adrenal glands had been surgically removed.[10]
5. **Effect on temperature regulation**: Administration of *Xiao Chai Hu Tang* was associated with effectiveness in reducing body temperature in rabbits with artificially-induced fever,[11] but it had little effect in rabbits with normal body temperature.[12]
6. **Gastrointestinal**: Administration of *Xiao Chai Hu Tang* was associated with inhibiting gastric acid production in rats. However, it had a stimulating effect on the intestines to increase peristalsis.[13]

Xiǎo Chái Hú Tāng (Minor Bupleurum Decoction)

7. **Effect on hypercholesterolemia and hyperlipidemia**: Administration of *Xiao Chai Hu Tang* and *Da Chai Hu Tang* (Major Bupleurum Decoction) was associated with beneficial effects in treating rats with cholesterol-induced hypercholesterolemia and aging-induced hyperlipidemia. Both formulas reduced total cholesterol in the liver and triglycerides in the liver and blood.[14]
8. **Antiallergic**: Administration of *Xiao Chai Hu Tang* had a dose-dependent effect to significantly inhibit histamine release to treat allergies. The proposed mechanism of this effect was attributed to the ability of *Xiao Chai Hu Tang* to inhibit IgE receptor-associated protein phosphorylation in the histamine release pathway.[15]
9. **Antiulcer**: *Xiao Chai Hu Tang* was effective in treating gastric ulcers in rats. *Xiao Chai Hu Tang* had a comparable effect to sucralfate in protecting the gastric mucosa, and had effects similar to cimetidine or atropine in inhibiting gastric acid secretions.[16] *Xiao Chai Hu Tang* also showed an antiulcer effect against both water-immersion stress-induced gastric lesions and ethanol-induced gastric injury in a dose-dependent manner.[17]
10. **Antitumor**: Administration of *Xiao Chai Hu Tang* was associated with antitumor activity, presumably because it stimulates host-mediated factors such as the phagocytic function of the reticuloendothelial system and C3 cleavage producibility, and is closely related to TNF production. It is unclear whether *Xiao Chai Hu Tang* has a direct antitumor effect.[18]
11. **Antitumor and antimetastatic**: Administration of *Xiao Chai Hu Tang* in mice with malignant melanoma was associated with slowing tumor development and the transition to malignancy, decreasing incidence of distant metastasis to brain and kidney, and, at the malignant stage, prolonging life span.[19] The mechanism of this action was attributed to the ability of *Xiao Chai Hu Tang* to inhibit the growth of malignant melanoma cells by up-regulating Fas-mediated apoptosis and arresting the cell cycle through down-regulation of cyclin dependent kinases.[20] *Xiao Chai Hu Tang* also inhibited lung carcinoma growth and metastasis, with special reference to macrophage activation.[21]
12. **Radioprotective**: Administration of *Xiao Chai Hu Tang* and/or methylprednisolone was associated with protective effects against radiation-induced damage to lung tissues. The efficacy of radioprotective effect from the mildest to the most potent were *Xiao Chai Hu Tang*, methylprednisolone, and the combination of both (more effective than either alone).[22]
13. **Bioavailability**: Oral administration of *Xiao Chai Hu Tang* before or after meals did not show any significant difference in the maximum plasma concentration or the plasma concentration-time curve. The study concluded that timing of administration (before or after meals) did not affect the blood concentration (bioavailability) of *Xiao Chai Hu Tang*.[23]

HUMAN CLINICAL STUDIES AND RESEARCH

1. **Chronic hepatitis**: In a double-blind multicenter clinical study involving 222 patients with chronic active hepatitis, use of *Xiao Chai Hu Tang* was associated with a decrease of HBeAg and an increase of Anti-HBe antibodies. No remarkable side effects were noticed.[24] In another study, two groups of patients with chronic hepatitis were treated with modified *Xiao Chai Hu Tang* with good results. In one group of 41 patients with chronic infectious hepatitis, 26 patients had significant improvement and 13 patients had moderate improvement. In another group of 21 patients with chronic active hepatitis, 10 patients had significant improvement and 8 patients had moderate improvement. The formula used contained *Chai Hu* (Radix Bupleuri) 12g, *Huang Qin* (Radix Scutellariae) 12g, *Tai Zi Shen* (Radix Pseudostellariae) 15g, *Ban Xia* (Rhizoma Pinelliae) 10g, *Gan Cao* (Radix et Rhizoma Glycyrrhizae) 6g, and dry-fried *Zhi Zi* (Fructus Gardeniae) 10g.[25] In another study, administration of *Xiao Chai Hu Tang* for 2-3 months was associated with marked symptomatic relief and improvement of liver function among 45 chronic hepatitis patients who did not respond to prednisone.[26]
2. **Viral hepatitis**: Use of *Xiao Chai Hu Tang* has been shown in many studies to effectively treat hepatitis. In one study, 307 patients with viral hepatitis were treated with 87.75% effectiveness using *Xiao Chai Hu Tang* plus *Zhi Zi* (Fructus Gardeniae) and *Hua Shi* (Talcum) as the base formula.[27] For 50 patients with chronic hepatitis B, one study reported 86.0% effectiveness using *Xiao Chai Hu Tang* plus *Zhu Ling* (Polyporus), *Huang Qi* (Radix Astragali), and *Zao Xiu* (Rhizoma Paridis) as the main herbal treatment.[28]
3. **Hepatitis C**: One study investigated the mechanism of action on the therapeutic effect of *Xiao Chai Hu Tang* to suppress liver cancer development. The study found that in hepatitis C patients, use of *Xiao Chai Hu Tang* could adjust the decreased IL-10 production and the increased IL-4 and IL-5 production of mononuclear cells, indicating that this moderate regulation of the cytokine production system may be useful in the prevention of disease progression.[29]
4. **Hepatic fibrosis and carcinoma:** *Xiao Chai Hu Tang* demonstrated chemopreventive and anti-carcinogenic effects against the development of hepatocellular carcinoma in cirrhotic patients. Evidence showed that *Xiao Chai Hu Tang* suppressed oxidative stress in hepatocytes and hepatic stellate cells, inhibited chemical hepatocarcinogenesis in animals, and acted as a biological response

modifier by suppressing the proliferation of hepatoma cells by inducing apoptosis and arresting the cell cycle. Baicalin, baicalein, and saikosaponin-a are believed to be three of the main active compounds in *Xiao Chai Hu Tang*.[30] In another study, administration of *Xiao Chai Hu Tang* inhibited collagen production, while an increase in retinoid level inhibited activation of Ito cells, leading to inhibition and prevention of liver fibrosis.[31]

5. **Hepatocellular carcinomas**: In a prospective, randomized, non-blind controlled study, 260 patients with liver cirrhosis were randomly assigned to 2 groups: patients in the trial group were given 7.5 g/day of *Xiao Chai Hu Tang* orally in addition to the conventional drugs given to the control patients. After monitoring the patients for 60 months, the study reported that the incidence of hepatocellular carcinomas was lower and the survival rate was higher for the trial group compared with the control group. The researchers concluded that *Xiao Chai Hu Tang* helped to prevent the development of hepatocellular carcinomas in patients with cirrhosis, particularly in patients without HBs antigen.[32]
6. **Cholecystitis and cholelithiasis**: One hundred patients with cholecystitis and cholelithiasis were treated with a combination of *Xiao Chai Hu Tang* and *Xiao Cheng Qi Tang* (Minor Order the Qi Decoction) with an 85% success rate of passing the stones.[33]
7. **Cholecystitis**: One study reported 98.9% effectiveness using *Xiao Chai Hu Tang* to treat cholecystitis. Of 285 patients (134 males, 151 females, average of 40.1 years of age, 2.7 years average duration of illness), 61 had acute cholecystitis and 224 had chronic cholecystitis. The treatment protocol was to administer the herbs in decoction one time daily for 15 days per course of treatment. The study reported complete recovery in 273 patients, improvement in 9 patients, and no effect in 3 patients.[34]
8. **Pancreatitis**: Fifty patients with acute pancreatitis were treated with marked improvement using acupuncture, modified *Xiao Chai Hu Tang,* and atropine. The average duration of treatment was 6.8 days, with most patients showing improvement after about 3 days.[35]
9. **Fever in cancer**: Thirty-two cancer patients with high fever were treated with good results using modified *Xiao Chai Hu Tang*. The treatment protocol was to use *Xiao Chai Hu Tang* plus *Bai Hua She She Cao* (Herba Hedyotis) and *Ban Zhi Lian* (Herba Scutellariae Barbatae) as the base formula. *Yu Ping Feng San* (Jade Windscreen Powder) and *Bie Jia* (Carapax Trionycis) were added for qi and yin deficiencies; *Yin Chen* (Herba Artemisiae Scopariae) and *Yi Yi Ren* (Semen Coicis) for damp-heat; and *Shi Gao* (Gypsum Fibrosum) and *Zhi Mu* (Rhizoma Anemarrhenae) for persistent high fever due to heat and toxins. Out of 32 patients, 17 had marked improvement, 13 had moderate improvement, and 2 had no improvement.[36]
10. **Fever**: Eighty-six patients with high fever (36 due to respiratory tract infection, 20 due to infection of the bile duct, 9 due to urinary tract infection, 4 due to postpartum infection, 2 due to toxemia, 3 due to hepatitis, 2 due to encephalitis, 2 due to influenza, 2 due to parotitis, 3 due to bacterial dysentery, and 3 due to unknown causes) were treated successfully. The study reported reduction of body temperature in 29 patients after 1-2 doses, 36 patients after 3-4 doses, and 21 patients after 4 doses.[37] According to another study, 128 patients with high fever were treated with *Xiao Chai Hu Tang* plus *Ban Lan Gen* (Radix Isatidis), *Mian Ma Guan Zhong* (Rhizoma Dryopteridis Crassirhizomatis), *Bai Wei* (Radix et Rhizoma Cynanchi Atrati) and others. *Ge Gen* (Radix Puerariae Lobatae) was added for body aches and pains; and *Mu Dan Pi* (Cortex Moutan) and *Di Huang* (Radix Rehmanniae) were added for red tongue body. Within 5 doses of herbs, the study reported normal temperature (37.2°C / 98.96°F or below) without recurrence of fever in 119 of 128 patients.[38]
11. **Nephritis**: Forty patients of acute and chronic nephritis were treated with electro-acupuncture and *Xiao Chai Hu Tang* with significant improvement. There were significant reductions of protein and cells in the urine.[39] Another study reported that the combination of *Xiao Chai Hu Tang* and *Ba Wei Di Huang Wan* (Eight-Ingredient Pill with Rehmannia) is beneficial in treating patients with chronic nephritis refractory to steroid therapy.[40]
12. **Chronic renal insufficiency**: Modified *Xiao Chai Hu Tang* was used with good results in treating 60 patients with chronic renal insufficiency. The herbal treatment included *Xiao Chai Hu Tang* plus *Dan Shen* (Radix et Rhizoma Salviae Miltiorrhizae), *Da Huang* (Radix et Rhizoma Rhei), *Yi Mu Cao* (Herba Leonuri), and other herbs as the base formula. *Tai Zi Shen* (Radix Pseudostellariae), *Di Huang* (Radix Rehmanniae), and *Gou Qi Zi* (Fructus Lycii) were added for qi and yin deficiencies with accumulation of dampness and toxins. *Fu Zi* (Radix Aconiti Lateralis Praeparata) and dry-fried *Bai Zhu* (Rhizoma Atractylodis Macrocephalae) were added for accumulation of water and dampness due to inability of Spleen and Kidney to regulate water circulation. The herbs were given for 3 months per course of treatment. Of 60 patients, the study reported significant improvement in 12 patients, moderate improvement in 24 patients, stabilization in 14 patients, and no benefit in 10 patients. The overall rate of effectiveness was 83.33%.[41]
13. **Cough**: *Xiao Chai Hu Tang* plus *Xi Xin* (Radix et Rhizoma Asari), *Gan Jiang* (Rhizoma Zingiberis), *Ku Xing Ren* (Semen Armeniacae Amarum), and others were used

to treat 52 patients with chronic cough with marked improvement in 13 patients, moderate improvement in 35 patients, and no effect in 4 patients. The overall rate of effectiveness was 92.3%.[42]

14. **Bronchial asthma**: Use of *Xiao Chai Hu Tang* was reported to have a 64.3% effectiveness rate in treating chronic bronchial asthma dependent on steroid drugs for treatment. Of 28 patients, 4 had significant improvement and 14 had moderate improvement.[43]
15. **Antral gastritis**: *Xiao Chai Hu Tang* plus *Xuan Fu Hua* (Flos Inulae), *Tao Ren* (Semen Persicae), and others were used to treat 107 patients with antral gastritis with 90.70% effectiveness. The duration of treatment ranged from 1-3 courses, with 15 packs of herbs per course of treatment.[44]
16. **Gastritis**: Thirty-six patients with gastritis due to regurgitation of bile were treated with modified *Xiao Chai Hu Tang* for 30 days with marked results. Modifications of the herbs were as follows: *Dan Shen* (Radix et Rhizoma Salviae Miltiorrhizae) was added for chronic gastritis with blood stagnation; *Huang Lian* (Rhizoma Coptidis) for accumulation of heat; *Zhi Qiao* (Fructus Aurantii) for abdominal distention and fullness; *San Qi* (Radix et Rhizoma Notoginseng), *Hai Piao Xiao* (Endoconcha Sepiae) and *Bai Fan* (Alumen) for ulceration. Most patients reported complete recovery or resolution of all clinical signs. Endoscopy also confirmed varying degrees of recovery.[45]
17. **Allergic rhinitis**: In one comparison study, patients with allergic rhinitis were treated with either herbs or drugs (antihistamine). In the herb group, *Xiao Chai Hu Tang* was used as the base formula, with the addition of *Xin Yi Hua* (Flos Magnoliae) and *Ju Hua* (Flos Chrysanthemi) for severe nose itching and sneezing; *Cang Zhu* (Rhizoma Atractylodis) and *Sheng Ma* (Rhizoma Cimicifugae) for profuse nasal discharge; *Bai Zhi* (Radix Angelicae Dahuricae) and *Bo He* (Herba Menthae) for severe sinus swelling and congestion; *Huang Qin* (Radix Scutellariae) and *Chuan Xiong* (Rhizoma Chuanxiong) for severe inflammation; *Tao Ren* (Semen Persicae) and *Ge Gen* (Radix Puerariae Lobatae) for nasal polyps; and other modifications as deemed necessary. The study reported 90.8% effectiveness for 65 patients in the herb group, and 76.9% effectiveness for 65 patients in the drug (antihistamine) group.[46]
18. **Postpartum infection**: Use of modified *Xiao Chai Hu Tang* had 96.6% effectiveness in treating 178 patients with postpartum viral infection (common cold or influenza). The herbal treatment contained *Xiao Chai Hu Tang* plus *Huang Qi* (Radix Astragali), *Yi Mu Cao* (Herba Leonuri) and *Dang Gui* (Radix Angelicae Sinensis) as the base formula. Modifications were made as needed. For dry mouth and stuffy or runny nose, *Sheng Jiang* (Rhizoma Zingiberis Recens) was removed and *Sang Ye* (Folium Mori), *Ju Hua* (Flos Chrysanthemi), *Bo He* (Herba Menthae), and *Lu Gen* (Rhizoma Phragmitis) were added. For nasal obstruction, *Zi Su Ye* (Folium Perillae) was added. For high fever without perspiration, *Qing Hao* (Herba Artemisiae Annuae) was added. For thick sticky sputum, *Zhi Mu* (Rhizoma Anemarrhenae) and *Zhe Bei Mu* (Bulbus Fritillariae Thunbergii) were added. For white foamy sputum, *Chen Pi* (Pericarpium Citri Reticulatae) and *Fu Ling* (Poria) were added. For sore throat, *Ban Lan Gen* (Radix Isatidis), *She Gan* (Rhizoma Belamcandae), and *Ma Bo* (Lasiosphaera seu Calvatia) were added. For red tongue body with little tongue coating, *Yu Zhu* (Rhizoma Polygonati Odorati) was added. After 1-2 packs of herbal treatment, the study reported complete recovery in 154 patients, improvement in 18 patients, and no effect in 6 patients.[47]
19. **Postpartum fever**: Modified *Xiao Chai Hu Tang* effectively reduced body temperature within an average of 10 hours in all 60 postpartum women with fever. The herbal treatment contained *Xiao Chai Hu Tang* plus *Dang Gui* (Radix Angelicae Sinensis), *Yi Mu Cao* (Herba Leonuri), and others as the base formula. In addition, *Jin Yin Hua* (Flos Lonicerae Japonicae) and *Jing Jie* (Herba Schizonepetae) were added for sore throat; *Tao Ren* (Semen Persicae) and *Hong Hua* (Flos Carthami) for lower abdominal pain with spotting; and *Pu Gong Ying* (Herba Taraxaci) and dry-fried *Chuan Shan Jia* (Squama Manis) for breast distention and pain.[48]

HERB-DRUG INTERACTION

- **Interferon**: Increased risk of acute pneumonitis may be associated with the use of interferon, *Xiao Chai Hu Tang*, or both in combination. Among patients with chronic hepatitis or liver cirrhosis, the frequency of drug-induced pneumonitis was 0.5% in those given only interferon-alpha, 0.7% in those given only *Xiao Chai Hu Tang*, and 4.0% in those given both interferon-alpha and *Xiao Chai Hu Tang*.[49] Many theories have been proposed on the mechanism of this interaction. One theory states that the herbs have not been shown to injure the lung tissues, but may over stimulate the neutrophils to release granulocytes, elastase and oxygen radicals, which subsequently damage lung tissue. The fibroblasts that repair the damaged tissue may increase the risk of pulmonary fibrosis.[50] Another theory states that acute pneumonitis associated with concurrent use of interferon and *Xiao Chai Hu Tang* may be due to allergic-immunological mechanisms.[51]
- **Interleukin 2**: Concurrent use of *Xiao Chai Hu Tang* and interleukin 2 showed a synergistic antitumor effect against murine renal cell carcinoma cell line in mice. The treatment protocol was to administer *Xiao Chai Hu Tang*

Xiǎo Chái Hú Tāng (Minor Bupleurum Decoction)

at 2.5 g/kg daily over 30 days, and interleukin 2 at 10(4) U/subject by subcutaneous injection every other day for a total of 8 doses. The combination of these two substances inhibited growth of the tumor and prolonged survival significantly as compared with the untreated mice.[52]

- **Lamivudine (Epivir; 3TC)**: One study reported synergistic antiviral effect when *Xiao Chai Hu Tang* is combined with antiviral drugs such as zidovudine (AZT), lamivudine (3TC) or AZT plus 3TC. Used alone, *Xiao Chai Hu Tang* moderately inhibited HIV-1 replication at a concentration of 25 mcg/mL. Used together, *Xiao Chai Hu Tang* enhanced the anti-HIV-1 activity of 3TC. The researchers suggested that the combination of *Xiao Chai Hu Tang* and 3TC has potential as a chemotherapeutic modality for HIV-1 infection.[53]
- **5-fluorouracil (5-FU)**: The combination of 5-FU and *Xiao Chai Hu Tang* had a synergistic effect for treatment of cancer in mice by increasing the life span by 56% and alleviating side effects of 5-FU.[54]
- **Drug-induced liver damage**: Administration of *Xiao Chai Hu Tang* has been shown to have beneficial effects in preventing and/or treating damage induced by drugs, such as halothane, danazol, D-galactosamine, and carbon tetrachloride.[55,56,57,58]
- **Liver enzyme inhibition**: The effect of *Xiao Chai Hu Tang* on cytochrome P450 enzymes was evaluated in 26 healthy subjects. Use of this herbal formula (2.5g twice daily for 5 days) was associated with a decreased mean activity of CYP1A2 by 16% on both day 1 and day 5 compared with the baseline (P=0.001).[59] In another study on the metabolic activity of different cytochrome P450 (CYP) isoforms, *Xiao Chai Hu Tang* was reported to be a competitive inhibitor of CYP2C9, but not CYP2D6. The study concluded that because of this inhibitory effect on liver metabolism, care should be taken with concurrent use of *Xiao Chai Hu Tang* and drugs.[60]
- **Pentobarbital**: Administration of *Xiao Chai Hu Tang* was associated with significantly shortened pentobarbital-induced sleeping time in mice. The mechanism of this interaction was attributed to the up-regulation of the mRNA expression of CYP2B, CYP3A1, CYP2E1 and CYP4A1.[61]
- **Carbamazepine**: Administration of one dose of *Xiao Chai Hu Tang* was associated with decreased peak concentration, and the time needed to reach the peak concentration, of carbamazepine in rats. However, two-week repeated treatments of *Xiao Chai Hu Tang* did not affect plasma concentration-time profile or any pharmacokinetic parameter of carbamazepine, an indication that *Xiao Chai Hu Tang* did not affect the liver metabolism of carbamazepine. The study attributed the mechanism of this interaction to decreased gastrointestinal absorption of carbamazepine due to delayed gastric emptying.[62]
- **Tolbutamide**: *Xiao Chai Hu Tang* demonstrably reduced the bioavailability of tolbutamide after oral administration in rats. The formula was found to accelerate the initial absorption rate, reduce the area under the plasma concentration-time curve, and decrease the overall bioavailability of tolbutamide.[63] The mechanism of this interaction was attributed to the inhibitory effect of *Xiao Chai Hu Tang* on the function of gastric emptying, thereby decreasing gastrointestinal absorption of tolbutamide.[64]
- **Ofloxacin**: In an open, random-crossover investigation study with seven volunteers, a single dose of ofloxacin and a one-week dose of *Xiao Chai Hu Tang* were given concurrently. Using high-performance liquid chromatography to evaluate the bioavailability of ofloxacin, it was determined that there is no significant effect on the rate or extent of bioavailability of ofloxacin when given concurrently with *Xiao Chai Hu Tang*.[65]

TOXICOLOGY

- *Xiao Chai Hu Tang* has a very low toxicology profile. In one study, rats were given up to 640 mg/kg of the extract per day continuously for 6 months. At the end of the study, the animals were examined for body weight, general behavior, water and food intake, and function of vital organs. The study concluded that no abnormality could be observed.[66]
- **Interstitial pneumonia**: Over 200 patients of interstitial pneumonia have been associated with the use of *Xiao Chai Hu Tang* in Japan. While the exact mechanism of this adverse reaction is not completely understood, it was suggested that phenolic compounds (lignans and flavonoids) present in this formula may induce apoptosis in human lung fibroblasts and peripheral blood mononuclear cells. Two phenolic compounds, baicalein and medicarpin, were found to significantly inhibit the growth and reduce the viability of lung fibroblasts. The researchers suggested that the phenolic compounds of *Xiao Chai Hu Tang* (especially baicalein and medicarpin) may have a direct effect on human lung fibroblasts and immune cells to induce apoptosis.[67] **Note:** *Xiao Chai Hu Tang* is one of the most commonly used herbal formulas in Japan. According to a study published in 1999, this formula has been administered to 1.5 million Japanese patients with chronic liver diseases.[68] In addition, there have been numerous other reports that document the safe and effective use of this formula. Thus, it is important to keep a proper perspective on the relative frequency of events, as well as risk-to-benefit analysis, in evaluating toxicology reports.

Xiǎo Chái Hú Tāng (Minor Bupleurum Decoction)

SUGGESTED ACUPUNCTURE TREATMENT

1. Points: *Yangchi* (TH 4), *Neiguan* (PC 6), *Qiuxu* (GB 40), *Ligou* (LR 5), *Housanli* (ST 36), and *Dushu* (BL 16).
2. Technique: even method.

Yangchi (TH 4), the *yuan* (source) point of the *San Jiao* channel, regulates circulation in all three *jiaos* and harmonizes the *shaoyang*. *Neiguan* (PC 6), the *luo* (connecting) point of the Pericardium channel, regulates qi circulation, removes stagnation, and directs reversed flow of Stomach qi downward. *Qiuxu* (GB 40), the *yuan* (source) point of the Gallbladder channel, sedates heat in the *shaoyang* and leads the fire downward. *Ligou* (LR 5), the *luo* (connecting) point of the Liver channel, regulates Liver qi and relieves stagnation. *Qiuxu* (GB 40) and *Ligou* (LR 5) are combined to relieve heat and stagnation associated with the Gallbladder and Liver. *Housanli* (ST 36) strengthens Spleen qi to prevent it from being attacked by the Liver and Gallbladder, and harmonizes the Stomach to relieve nausea and vomiting. *Dushu* (BL 16) is the *shu* (transport) point of *du* (governing) channel and can help to regulate *shaoyang* disorders.

RELATED FORMULA

***Chái Hú Zhǐ Jié Tāng* (Bupleurum, Bitter Orange, and Platycodon Decoction)**
柴胡枳桔湯
柴胡枳桔汤
Pinyin Name: *Chai Hu Zhi Jie Tang*
Literal Name: Bupleurum, Bitter Orange, and Platycodon Decoction
Original Source: *Chong Ding Tong Su Shang Han Lun* (Revised Popular Guide to the Discussion of Cold-Induced Disorders) by Yu Gen-Chu in the Qing Dynasty

Chai Hu (Radix Bupleuri)	3-4.5g
Zhi Qiao (Fructus Citri Aurantii)	4.5g
Ban Xia (Rhizoma Pinelliae), *zhu* (boiled) with ginger	4.5g
Sheng Jiang (Rhizoma Zingiberis Recens), fresh	3g
Huang Qin (Radix Scutellariae)	3-4.5g
Jie Geng (Radix Platycodonis)	3g
Chen Pi (Pericarpium Citri Reticulatae)	4.5g
Cha Ye (Folium Camelliae)	3g

Chai Hu Zhi Jie Tang (Bupleurum, Bitter Orange, and Platycodon Decoction) mainly harmonizes the *shaoyang*, releases the exterior, and regulates the chest and diaphragm. The main indication is *shaoyang* syndrome, with slightly greater emphasis on the exterior than the interior. Clinically, patients will show clinical signs such as intermittent fever and trembling, deafness, hypochondriac pain, a white, slippery tongue coating, and a wiry, slippery pulse. This formula can be taken with *Cha Ye* (Folium Camelliae) to enhance the overall heat-clearing and damp-dispelling effects.

In comparison to *Xiao Chai Hu Tang*, which treats *shaoyang* syndrome with equal emphasis on both the exterior and interior, *Chai Hu Zhi Jie Tang* focuses on *shaoyang* syndromes in which there are more exterior clinical signs than interior. For this reason, *Ren Shen* (Radix et Rhizoma Ginseng), *Zhi Gan Cao* (Radix et Rhizoma Glycyrrhizae Praeparata cum Melle), and *Da Zao* (Fructus Jujubae) are not used in this formula.

AUTHORS' COMMENTS

Xiao Chai Hu Tang is a formula that has diverse clinical applications. It can be used to treat febrile disorders, acute and residual infection of the respiratory system, acute and chronic disorders of the gastrointestinal system (in particular the Liver and Gallbladder), chronic urinary tract disorders, post-partum disorders, and as a preventative formula in the treatment of recurrent external pathogen invasions. A common modern application of this formula is to clear residual heat from the body following attack from exterior pathogens in animals with pre-existing chronic disease such as renal insufficiency, liver cirrhosis, cancer, nephrotic syndrome, recurrent pneumonia and chronic pyelonephritis. In chronic disease conditions, the *zheng* (upright) *qi* is weak and allows easy invasion from exterior wind-cold which then internalizes and transforms into heat in the *shaoyang*. Many of these animals will have a fever that is not alleviated with antipyretic or antibiotic drugs. Though these drugs work well to temporarily bring down body temperature, the fever tends to return as soon as the therapeutic effect is over. Even animals with strong constitutions that are used for competition may have their *zheng qi* weakened by a taxing show schedule. This allows for easy contraction of contagious disease, and, even more important for this discussion, the inability to fully eliminate the pathogen. These animals may exhibit chronic fatigue, recurrent fever, chronic cough, or recurrent mild colic post-infection.

Xiao Chai Hu Tang can also be used for fever that develops with no obvious etiology (fever of unknown origin), or fever secondary to cancer and parturition. Fever and trembling (aversion to cold) are common complaints in exterior conditions, but they must be differentiated correctly:

- In *taiyang* syndrome, fever and trembling are present simultaneously.

Xiǎo Chái Hú Tāng (Minor Bupleurum Decoction)

- In *yangming* syndrome, there is high fever and absence of trembling.
- In *shaoyang* syndrome, there can be intermittent fever and trembling.

Xiao Chai Hu Tang has also shown application in the treatment of acute and chronic immune-mediated polyarthritis in the dog. In many of these cases, the clinical signs are representative of *shaoyang* syndrome, and the use of this formula in combination with *Yi Yi Ren Tang* (Coicis Decoction), *Che Qian Zi* (Semen Plantaginis), *Lian Qiao* (Fructus Forsythiae), *Yan Hu Suo* (Rhizoma Corydalis) and *Hong Hua* (Flos Carthami) has been effective. In cases of high fever *Shi Gao* (Gypsum Fibrosum) can be added until the fever resolves.

One unique application of *Xiao Chai Hu Tang* that requires additional explanation is the treatment of an exterior condition, specifically, extensive blood loss post-partum. Loss of blood during parturition creates emptiness in the uterus and the *chong* (thoroughfare) channel. Due to this void, pathogenic factors directly and easily invade into deeper levels of the body instead of lingering at the *wei* (defensive) level. The Liver stores blood; moreover, the Liver channel travels around the genital region and traverses up the lower abdomen and is closely related to the uterus and *chong* channel. If heat enters the uterus and *chong* channel, it affects the Liver, which, in turn, affects its paired organ, the Gallbladder. This stagnant heat creates disharmony in the *shaoyang* stage, leading to intermittent fever and trembling hypochondriac discomfort, a dry mouth and throat, irritability, lack of appetite, nausea, and vomiting. *Xiao Chai Hu Tang* harmonizes the *shaoyang* and pushes the heat outward to relieve the heat trapped in the uterus and the *chong* channel.[69]

Intermittent fever and trembling is a key symptom that can be treated with *Xiao Chai Hu Tang* or *Xiao Yao San* (Rambling Powder). However, the diagnostic criteria and clinical application guidelines are very different.

- *Xiao Chai Hu Tang* treats intermittent fever and trembling caused by exterior pathogenic factors that enter the *shaoyang* level and get trapped in the half-exterior and half-interior location. *Ren Shen* (Radix et Rhizoma Ginseng), *Da Zao* (Fructus Jujubae), and *Gan Cao* (Radix et Rhizoma Glycyrrhizae) strengthen the interior to push the pathogens outward and prevent them from invading further into the body, but these herbs are ***not*** used here to tonify the deficiencies. *Sheng Jiang* (Rhizoma Zingiberis Recens) is used with *Ban Xia* (Rhizoma Pinelliae) to treat nausea and irritability caused by Gallbladder heat invading the Stomach.
- *Xiao Yao San* treats intermittent fever and trembling caused by disharmony among the Liver, Spleen, and Gallbladder accompanied by blood deficiency and Liver qi stagnation; the fever and trembling are ***not*** the result of an exterior invasion. *Dang Gui* (Radix Angelicae Sinensis), *Bai Shao* (Radix Paeoniae Alba), *Fu Ling* (Poria), and *Bai Zhu* (Rhizoma Atractylodis Macrocephalae) strengthen the Spleen to prevent the Liver from overacting. *Sheng Jiang* (Rhizoma Zingiberis Recens) warms the middle *jiao* to strengthen the Spleen.

Xiao Chai Hu Tang and *Xiao Yao San* (Rambling Powder) both use *Chai Hu* (Radix Bupleuri) as the chief herb, but with different intent and at different doses:

- *Xiao Chai Hu Tang* treats *shaoyang* syndrome in which the pathogenic heat is trapped between the exterior and interior. In this case, signs of intermittent fever and trembling are more severe. As a result, a large dose of *Chai Hu* (Radix Bupleuri) is needed to harmonize *shaoyang* and clear the heat.
- *Xiao Yao San* treats Liver qi stagnation accompanied by Spleen deficiency that manifests in emotional complaints; however, the physical clinical signs are less severe compared to that of *Xiao Chai Hu Tang*. Although *Chai Hu* (Radix Bupleuri) is also the chief herb, only a moderate dose is needed to regulate Liver qi. In this case, this herb serves more as a channel-guiding herb in this formula to address Liver qi stagnation. Using a large dose of *Chai Hu* (Radix Bupleuri) in *Xiao Yao San* is not appropriate because it shifts the effect of the formula from harmonizing to exterior-releasing. Moreover, animals with Liver qi stagnation often have underlying deficiencies, and using *Chai Hu* (Radix Bupleuri) at a large dose may exacerbate such deficiencies.

Xiao Chai Hu Tang and *Da Chai Hu Tang* (Major Bupleurum Decoction) both treat *shaoyang* disorders with intermittent fever and trembling, and hypochondriac distention and discomfort. Both formulas contain *Chai Hu* (Radix Bupleuri), *Huang Qin* (Radix Scutellariae), *Ban Xia* (Rhizoma Pinelliae), *Sheng Jiang* (Rhizoma Zingiberis Recens), and *Da Zao* (Fructus Jujubae). Despite the similarities, they have contrasting differences:

- *Xiao Chai Hu Tang* contains *Chai Hu* (Radix Bupleuri) and *Huang Qin* (Radix Scutellariae) as chief herbs to harmonize the *shaoyang*. *Ren Shen* (Radix et Rhizoma Ginseng) strengthens the interior to prevent the pathogenic factors from moving further inward. This formula treats a variety of conditions, including exterior invasion with chronic disease, and following parturition.
- *Da Chai Hu Tang* is mainly used for *yangming fu* (hollow organs) syndrome with excess heat in the body. *Da*

Xiǎo Chái Hú Tāng (Minor Bupleurum Decoction)

Huang (Radix et Rhizoma Rhei), *Zhi Shi* (Fructus Aurantii Immaturus), and *Bai Shao* (Radix Paeoniae Alba) sedate heat in the *yangming* channel. The key sign for differential diagnosis is constipation with abdominal pain.[70]

Xiao Chai Hu Tang and *Hao Qin Qing Dan Tang* (Artemisia Annua and Scutellaria Decoction to Clear the Gallbladder) both harmonize *shaoyang* and treat chief manifestations of intermittent fever and trembling, as well as chest and hypochondriac distention and pain. Their main differences are as follows:

- *Xiao Chai Hu Tang* lifts clear yang qi and pushes pathogenic factors outward. Containing *Huang Qin* (Radix Scutellariae), *Ren Shen* (Radix et Rhizoma Ginseng), *Da Zao* (Fructus Jujubae), *Gan Cao* (Radix et Rhizoma Glycyrrhizae), *Ban Xia* (Rhizoma Pinelliae), and *Sheng Jiang* (Rhizoma Zingiberis Recens), this formula harmonizes *shaoyang*, dispels pathogenic factors, and restores *zheng* (upright) *qi* to treat intermittent fever and trembling, hypochondriac pain and distention, a dry mouth and throat, a thin, white tongue coating, and a wiry pulse. This formula is better at resolving the exterior.
- *Hao Qin Qing Dan Tang* clears damp-heat in the Stomach and Gallbladder, using *Qing Hao* (Herba Artemisiae Annuae) and *Huang Qin* (Radix Scutellariae) as the two main ingredients. The formula further contains *Zhu Ru* (Caulis Bambusae in Taenia), *Ban Xia* (Rhizoma Pinelliae), *Chi Fu Ling* (Poria Rubra), *Bi Yu San* (Jasper Powder), *Chen Pi* (Pericarpium Citri Reticulatae), and *Zhi Qiao* (Fructus Aurantii) to treat damp-heat with turbid phlegm accumulation in the *shaoyang* channel. Clinical signs include intermittent fever and trembling with a greater degree of heat than cold, anorexia, nausea, bilious vomiting and a red tongue, and in severe cases the patient may present with a white to yellow greasy coating, and a slippery, rapid pulse.

References

1. *Zhong Yao Ming Fang Yao Li Yu Ying Yong* (Pharmacology and Applications of Famous Herbal Formulas), 1989; 92-96.
2. *Yao Xue Za Zhi* (Journal of Medicinals), 1984; 104(7):798.
3. *Guo Wai Yi Xue* (Foreign Medicine), 1984; (5)279.
4. Kusunose M, Qiu B, Cui T, Hamada A, Yoshioka S, Ono M, Miyamura M, Kyotani S, Nishioka Y.Effect of Sho-saiko-to extract on hepatic inflammation and fibrosis in dimethylnitrosamine induced liver injury rats. Biol Pharm Bull. 2002 Nov; 25(11):1417-21.
5. Kaneko M, Kawakita T, Tauchi Y, Saito Y, Suzuki A, Nomoto K. Augmentation of NK activity after oral administration of a traditional Chinese medicine, xiao-chai-hu-tang (shosaiko-to). Immunopharmacol Immunotoxicol. 1994 Feb; 16(1):41-53.
6. Yamashiki M, Asakawa M, Kayaba Y, Kosaka Y, Nishimura A.Herbal medicine "sho-saiko-to" induces in vitro granulocyte colony-stimulating factor production on peripheral blood mononuclear cells. J Clin Lab Immunol. 1992; 37(2):83-90.
7. *Guo Wai Yi Xue* (Foreign Medicine), 1991; 13(4):46.
8. *Guo Wai Yi Xue* (Foreign Medicine), 1991; 13(4):43.
9. *Yao Xue Za Zhi* (Journal of Medicinals), 1984; 104(5):509.
10. *Zhong Yi Fang Ji Xian Dai Yan Jiu* (Modern Study of Medical Formulas in Traditional Chinese Medicine), 1997; (1):184.
11. *Shan Xi Zhong Yi* (Shanxi Chinese Medicine), 1990; 11(8):376.
12. *Gan Su Zhong Yi Xue Yuan Xue Bao* (Journal of Gansu University of Chinese Medicine), 1991; 8(3):39.
13. *Zhong Yi Fang Ji Xian Dai Yan Jiu* (Modern Study of Medical Formulas in Traditional Chinese Medicine), 1997; (1):186.
14. Umeda M, Amagaya S, Ogihara Y. Effect of shosaikoto, daisaikoto and sannoshashinto (traditional Japanese and Chinese medicines) on experimental hyperlipidemia in rats. J Ethnopharmacol. 1989 Oct; 26(3):255-69.
15. Matsumoto T, Shibata T. The ex vivo effect of the herbal medicine sho-saiko-to on histamine release from rat mast cells. Eur Arch Otorhinolaryngol. 1998; 255(7):359-64.
16. Matsuta M, Kanita R, Tsutsui F, Yamashita A. Antiulcer properties of shosaiko-to. Nippon Yakurigaku Zasshi. 1996 Oct; 108(4):217-25.
17. Kase Y, Yuzurihara M, Iizuka S, Ishige A, Komatsu Y. The effects of hange-shashin-to on gastric function in comparison with sho-saiko-to. Biol Pharm Bull. 1997 Nov; 20(11):1155-9.
18. Ito H, Shimura K. Studies on the antitumor activity of traditional Chinese medicines. (II). The antitumor mechanism of traditional Chinese medicines. Gan To Kagaku Ryoho. 1985 Nov; 12(11):2149-54.
19. Kato M, Liu W, Yi H, Asai N, Hayakawa A, Kozaki K, Takahashi M, Nakashima I.The herbal medicine Sho-saiko-to inhibits growth and metastasis of malignant melanoma primarily developed in ret-transgenic mice. J Invest Dermatol. 1998 Oct; 111(4):640-4.
20. Liu W, Kato M, Akhand AA, Hayakawa A, Takemura M, Yoshida S, Suzuki H, Nakashima I. The herbal medicine sho-saiko-to inhibits the growth of malignant melanoma cells by upregulating Fas-mediated apoptosis and arresting cell cycle through downregulation of cyclin dependent kinases. Int J Oncol. 1998 Jun; 12(6):1321-6.
21. Ito H, Shimura K.Effects of a blended Chinese medicine, xiao-chai-hu-tang, on Lewis lung carcinoma growth and inhibition of lung metastasis, with special reference to macrophage activation. Jpn J Pharmacol. 1986 Jul; 41(3):307-14.
22. Kure F. The radioprotective effects of methylprednisolone and Sho-Saikoto on mouse lung. Nippon Igaku Hoshasen Gakkai Zasshi. 1992 Jan 25; 52(1):96-103.
23. Nishioka Y, Kyotani S, Miyamura M, Kusunose M. Influence of time of administration of a Shosaiko-to extract granule on blood concentration of its active constituents. Chem Pharm Bull (Tokyo). 1992 May; 40(5):1335-7.
24. Hirayama C, Okumura M, Tanikawa K, Yano M, Mizuta M, Ogawa N.A multicenter randomized controlled clinical trial of Shosaiko-to in chronic active hepatitis. Gastroenterol Jpn. 1989 Dec; 24(6):715-9.
25. *Hu Nan Zhong Yi Za Zhi* (Hunan Journal of Chinese Medicine), 1989; 5(3):5.
26. *Xin Yao Yu Lin Chuang* (New Medicine and the Clinical Application), 1982; 4:651.
27. *Hu Nan Zhong Yi Za Zhi* (Hunan Journal of Chinese Medicine), 1987; 3:5.
28. *Zhe Jiang Zhong Yi Xue Yuan Xue Bao* (Journal of Zhejiang University of Chinese Medicine), 1999; 3:36.
29. Yamashiki M. Nishimura A. Suzuki H. Sakaguchi S. Kosaka Y. Effects of the Japanese herbal medicine "Sho-saiko-to" (TJ-9) on in vitro interleukin-10 production by peripheral blood mononuclear cells of patients with chronic hepatitis C. Hepatology. 1997 Jun; 25(6):1390-7.
30. Shimizu I. Sho-saiko-to: Japanese herbal medicine for protection against hepatic fibrosis and carcinoma. Journal of Gastroenterology & Hepatology. 2000 Mar; 15 Suppl:D84-90.

Xiǎo Chái Hú Tāng (Minor Bupleurum Decoction)

31. Ono M, Miyamura M, Kyotani S, Saibara T, Ohnishi S, Nishioka Y. Effects of Sho-saiko-to extract on liver fibrosis in relation to the changes in hydroxyprolin—e and retinoid levels of the liver in rats. J Pharm Pharmacol. 1999 Sep; 51(9):1079-84.
32. Oka H. Yamamoto S. Kuroki T. Harihara S. Marumo T. Kim SR. Monna T. Kobayashi K. Tango T. Prospective study of chemoprevention of hepatocellular carcinoma with Sho-saiko-to (TJ-9). Cancer. 1995 Sep 1; 76(5):743-9.
33. *Fu Jian Zhong Yi Yao* (Fujian Chinese Medicine and Herbology), 1986; 17(3):48.
34. *Shi Yong Zhong Xi Yi Jie He Za Zhi* (Practical Journal of Integrated Chinese and Western Medicines), 1993; 4:218.
35. *Zhong Yi Za Zhi* (Journal of Chinese Medicine), 1982; 9:40.
36. *Shan Xi Zhong Yi* (Shanxi Chinese Medicine), 1995; 2:57.
37. *Si Chuan Zhong Yi* (Sichuan Chinese Medicine), 1986; 4(5):36.
38. *Hu Nan Zhong Yi Za Zhi* (Hunan Journal of Chinese Medicine), 1996; 2:32.
39. *Zhong Yi Fang Ji Xian Dai Yan Jiu* (Modern Study of Medical Formulas in Traditional Chinese Medicine), 1997; (1):190.
40. *Zhong Yi Fang Ji Xian Dai Yan Jiu* (Modern Study of Medical Formulas in Traditional Chinese Medicine), 1997; 190.
41. *Shan Dong Zhong Yi Za Zhi* (Shandong Journal of Chinese Medicine), 1998; 8:359.
42. *Shan Xi Zhong Yi* (Shanxi Chinese Medicine), 1995; 6:12.
43. *Guo Wai Yi Xue Zhong Yi Zhong Yao Fen Ce* (Monograph of Chinese Herbology from Foreign Medicine), 1992; 4:202.
44. *Shi Yong Zhong Xi Yi Jie He Za Zhi* (Practical Journal of Integrated Chinese and Western Medicines), 1996; 5:312.
45. *Zhong Yi Za Zhi* (Journal of Chinese Medicine), 1983; 5:41.
46. *Shi Yong Zhong Yi Za Zhi* (Journal of Practical Chinese Medicine), 1995; 2:27.
47. *Si Chuan Zhong Yi* (Sichuan Chinese Medicine), 1996; 10:41.
48. *Shi Yong Zhong Xi Yi Jie He Za Zhi* (Practical Journal of Integrated Chinese and Western Medicines), 1997; 19:1927.
49. Nakagawa A et al. Five patients of drug-induced pneumonitis due to Sho-saiko-to or interferon-alpha or both. Nihon Kyobu Shikkan Gakkai Zasshi. 1995 Dec; 33(12):1361-1366.
50. Murakami K et al. A possible mechanism of interstitial pneumonia during interferon therapy with sho-saiko-to. Nihon Kyobu Shikkan Gakkai Zasshi. 1995 Apr; 33(4):389-94
51. Ishizaki T. Sasaki F. Ameshima S. Shiozaki K. Takahashi H. Abe Y. Ito S. Kuriyama M. Nakai T. Kitagawa M. Pneumonitis during interferon and/or herbal drug therapy in patients with chronic active hepatitis. European Respiratory Journal. 1996 Dec; 9(12):2691-6.
52. Huang Y, Marumo K, Murai M.Antitumor effects and pharmacological interaction of xiao-chai-hu-tang (sho-saiko-to) and interleukin 2 in murine renal cell carcinoma. Keio J Med. 1997 Sep; 46(3):132-7.
53. Piras G. Makino M. Baba M. Sho-saiko-to, a traditional Kampo medicine, enhances the anti-HIV-1 activity of lamivudine (3TC) in vitro. Microbiology & Immunology. 1997; 41(10):835-9.
54. Ohta T, Tawara M, Tatsuka M, Abe H, Odashima S. An approach to prolongation of survival rate in tumor bearing mice using 5-fluorouracil in combination with various kinds of herb medicine. Gan To Kagaku Ryoho. 1983 Aug; 10(8):1858-65.
55. Mitsukawa H, Ikeda K. Effect of sho-saiko-to (xiao-chai-hu-tang) on hepatic injury induced by halothane in rats. Masui. 1991 May; 40(5):794-800.
56. Yaginuma T, Okamura T, Takeuchi T, Nishii O, Fujimori R.Preventive effect of traditional herbal medicine, shosaiko-to, on danazol-induced hepatic damage. Int J Gynaecol Obstet. 1989 Aug; 29(4):337-41.
57. Ohta Y, Nishida K, Sasaki E, Kongo M, Hayashi T, Nagata M, Ishiguro I. Comparative study of oral and parenteral administration of sho-saiko-to (xiao-chaihu-tang) extract on D-galactosamine-induced liver injury in rats. Am J Chin Med. 1997; 25(3-4):333-42.
58. Amagaya S, Hayakawa M, Ogihara Y, Ohta Y, Fujiwara K, Oka H, Oshio H, Kishi T. Treatment of chronic liver injury in mice by oral administration of xiao-chai-hu-tang. J Ethnopharmacol. 1989 Apr; 25(2):181-7.
59. Saruwatari J. Nakagawa K. Shindo J. Nachi S. Echizen H. Ishizaki T. The in-vivo effects of sho-saiko-to, a traditional Chinese herbal medicine, on two cytochrome P450 enzymes (1A2 and 3A) and xanthine oxidase in man. Journal of Pharmacy & Pharmacology. 2003 Nov; 55(11):1553-9.
60. Takahashi K. Uejima E. Morisaki T. Takahashi K. Kurokawa N. Azuma J. In vitro inhibitory effects of Kampo medicines on metabolic reactions catalyzed by human liver microsomes. Journal of Clinical Pharmacy & Therapeutics. 2003 Aug; 28(4):319-27.
61. Nose M, Tamura M, Ryu N, Mizukami H, Ogihara Y.Sho-saiko-to and Saiko-keisi-to, the traditional Chinese and Japanese herbal medicines, altered hepatic drug-metabolizing enzymes in mice and rats when administered orally for a long time. J Pharm Pharmacol. 2003 Oct; 55(10):1419-26.
62. Ohnishi N, Okada K, Yoshioka M, Kuroda K, Nagasawa K, Takara K, Yokoyama T.Studies on interactions between traditional herbal and western medicines. V. effects of Sho-saiko-to (Xiao-Cai-hu-Tang) on the pharmacokinetics of carbamazepine in rats. Biol Pharm Bull. 2002 Nov; 25(11):1461-6.
63. American Journal of Chinese Medicine. 1999; 27(3-4):355-63.
64. Nishimura N, Naora K, Hirano H, Iwamoto K.Effects of sho-saiko-to (xiao chai hu tang), a Chinese traditional medicine, on the gastric function and absorption of tolbutamide in rats. Yakugaku Zasshi. 2001 Feb; 121(2):153-9.
65. International Journal of Clinical Pharmacology and Therapeutics. 1994 Feb; 32(2):57-61.
66. *Yi Fang Xin Jie* (New Explanation for Medical Formulas), 1980; 42.
67. Liu ZL. Tanaka S. Horigome H. Hirano T. Oka K. Induction of apoptosis in human lung fibroblasts and peripheral lymphocytes in vitro by Shosaiko-to derived phenolic metabolites. Biological & Pharmaceutical Bulletin. 2002 Jan; 25(1):37-41.
68. Yamashiki M. Nishimura A. Huang XX. Nobori T. Sakaguchi S. Suzuki H. Effects of the Japanese herbal medicine "Sho-saiko-to" (TJ-9) on interleukin-12 production in patients with HCV-positive liver cirrhosis. Developmental Immunology. 1999; 7(1):17-22.
69. Wang MZ, et al. *Zhong Yi Xue Wen Da Ti Ku* (Questions and Answers on Traditional Chinese Medicine: Herbal Formulas).
70. Wang MZ, et al. *Zhong Yi Xue Wen Da Ti Ku* (Questions and Answers on Traditional Chinese Medicine: Herbal Formulas).

Chái Hú Guì Zhī Tāng (Bupleurum and Cinnamon Twig Decoction)

柴胡桂枝湯
柴胡桂枝汤

Pinyin Name: *Chai Hu Gui Zhi Tang*
Literal Name: Bupleurum and Cinnamon Twig Decoction
Alternate Names: *Tsai Hu Kuei Chih Tang, Cai Hu Gui Zhi Tang*, Bupleurum and Cinnamon Combination
Original Source: *Shang Han Lun* (Discussion of Cold-Induced Disorders) by Zhang Zhong-Jing in the Eastern Han Dynasty

COMPOSITION

Chai Hu (Radix Bupleuri)	12g
Huang Qin (Radix Scutellariae)	4.5g
Ren Shen (Radix et Rhizoma Ginseng)	4.5g
Ban Xia (Rhizoma Pinelliae), *xi* (washed)	0.25 cup [6-9g]
Gui Zhi (Ramulus Cinnamomi)	4.5g
Bai Shao (Radix Paeoniae Alba)	4.5g
Zhi Gan Cao (Radix et Rhizoma Glycyrrhizae Praeparata cum Melle)	3g
Sheng Jiang (Rhizoma Zingiberis Recens), *qie* (sliced)	4.5g
Da Zao (Fructus Jujubae), *bo* (opened)	6 pieces

DOSAGE / PREPARATION / ADMINISTRATION

The source text states to cook the herbs in 7 cups [1,400 mL] of water, and reduce the liquid to 3 cups [600 mL]. Take 1 cup [200 mL] of the strained decoction three times daily.

CHINESE THERAPEUTIC ACTIONS

1. Dispels pathogenic factors from *taiyang* and *shaoyang* stages
2. Harmonizes the exterior and interior

CLINICAL MANIFESTATIONS

Taiyang and *shaoyang* syndromes that appear six to seven days after the onset of illness: fever, trembling, joint pain, nausea and abdominal pain.

VETERINARY CLINICAL APPLICATIONS

Upper respiratory infection, kennel cough, fever, chronic hepatitis, liver cirrhosis, jaundice, cholecystitis, cholelithiasis, gastric or duodenal ulcers, chronic pancreatitis, nephritis, seizures and epilepsy.

EXPLANATION

Chai Hu Gui Zhi Tang (Bupleurum and Cinnamon Twig Decoction) addresses disorders characterized by *shaoyang* and *taiyang* syndromes, with *shaoyang* clinical signs predominating and *taiyang* clinical signs lingering. *Shaoyang* syndrome is characterized by distention and obstruction beneath the heart, and pain around the umbilical region or the lower abdomen. *Taiyang* syndrome is characterized by joint pain, fever and shaking.

Chai Hu Gui Zhi Tang combines two formulas: *Xiao Chai Hu Tang* (Minor Bupleurum Decoction) and *Gui Zhi Tang* (Cinnamon Twig Decoction). *Xiao Chai Hu Tang* (Minor Bupleurum Decoction) treats *shaoyang* syndrome by harmonizing the exterior and interior. *Gui Zhi Tang* (Cinnamon Twig Decoction) treats *taiyang* syndrome by releasing the exterior. Combined, *Chai Hu Gui Zhi Tang* treats both *taiyang* and *shaoyang* syndromes.

Please refer to *Xiao Chai Hu Tang* (Minor Bupleurum Decoction) and *Gui Zhi Tang* (Cinnamon Twig Decoction) for additional information on these two formulas.

***Chai Hu Gui Zhi Tang* (Bupleurum and Cinnamon Twig Decoction)**

Diagnosis	Clinical Signs	Treatment	Herbs
Taiyang and *shaoyang* syndromes	• Joint pain, fever and trembling: *taiyang* syndrome • Pain around the umbilical region or the lower abdomen: *shaoyang* syndrome	• Dispels pathogenic factors from *taiyang* and *shaoyang* stages • Harmonizes the exterior and interior	• *Gui Zhi Tang* (Cinnamon Twig Decoction) treats *taiyang* syndrome by releasing the exterior. • *Xiao Chai Hu Tang* (Minor Bupleurum Decoction) treats *shaoyang* syndrome by harmonizing the exterior and interior.

Chái Hú Guì Zhī Tāng (Bupleurum and Cinnamon Twig Decoction)

VETERINARY MODIFICATIONS

With painful joints, add *Ge Gen* (Radix Puerariae Lobatae) and *Sheng Ma* (Rhizoma Cimicifugae).

CAUTIONS / CONTRAINDICATIONS

Avoid cold, raw, oily, and greasy foods while taking *Chai Hu Gui Zhi Tang.*[1]

PHARMACOLOGICAL EFFECTS

1. **Antiulcer**: Administration of *Chai Hu Gui Zhi Tang* had a marked effect in preventing cysteamine-induced gastric ulcers in rats. The mechanism is attributed to decreased gastric acid production.[2]
2. **Immunostimulant**: Long-term administration of the formula was associated with an increase in lymphocytes in mice.[3]
3. **Anti-inflammatory**: Administration of *Chai Hu Gui Zhi Tang* was associated with marked anti-inflammatory effect in both acute and chronic inflammatory disorders in rats.[4]
4. **Analgesic**: *Chai Hu Gui Zhi Tang* was reported to be an effective treatment for trigeminal neuralgia in rats. This mechanism of action was attributed to the ability of the formula to control pain in ligatured nerves by local effect, not by general analgesic effect.[5]
5. **Protective effect on the pancreas**: According to one study in rats, administration of *Chai Hu Gui Zhi Tang* was associated with inhibiting pancreatic fibrosis by suppressing transforming growth factor beta1 (TGF-beta1) expression.[6] Another study reported that *Chai Hu Gui Zhi Tang* effectively delayed the onset of chronic pancreatitis and suppressed pancreatitis-associated protein gene expression in rats.[7,8]
6. **Hepatoprotective**: Administration of *Chai Hu Gui Zhi Tang* was associated with treating liver lesions induced by N-nitrosomorpholine in rats. The mechanism of this hepatoprotective function was attributed to inhibition of cell proliferation and induction of apoptosis in adjacent hepatocytes.[9]

HUMAN CLINICAL STUDIES AND RESEARCH

1. **Common cold and influenza**: Administration of modified *Chai Hu Gui Zhi Tang* was effective in treating common cold and influenza. Out of 2,650 patients, 2,220 were treated on an outpatient basis, and 430 were hospitalized. The study reported complete recovery in 2,405 patients, improvement in 208 patients, and no improvement in 37 patients. The overall rate effectiveness was 98.7%. The herbal treatment used *Chai Hu Gui Zhi Tang* as the base formula, and added *Ma Huang* (Herba Ephedrae) and *Xi Xin* (Radix et Rhizoma Asari) for more cold; *Qiang Huo* (Rhizoma et Radix Notopterygii) and *Fang Feng* (Radix Saposhnikoviae) for more wind; *Jin Yin Hua* (Flos Lonicerae Japonicae), *Lian Qiao* (Fructus Forsythiae), *Shi Gao* (Gypsum Fibrosum), and *Ban Lan Gen* (Radix Isatidis) for more heat; *Huo Xiang* (Herba Agastaches) and *Cang Zhu* (Rhizoma Atractylodis) for more damp; *Huang Qi* (Radix Astragali) or *Dang Shen* (Radix Codonopsis) for qi deficiency; *Fu Zi* (Radix Aconiti Lateralis Praeparata) and *Gan Jiang* (Rhizoma Zingiberis) for yang deficiency; *Mai Dong* (Radix Ophiopogonis), *Tian Hua Fen* (Radix Trichosanthis), and *Zhi Mu* (Rhizoma Anemarrhenae) for yin deficiency; and *Long Gu* (Os Draconis) and *Mu Li* (Concha Ostreae) for profuse perspiration.[10]
2. **Fever**: Administration of 5 to 8 doses of modified *Chai Hu Gui Zhi Tang* was effective in treating patients with fever due to viral infection. Out of 112 patients, the study reported complete recovery in 85 patients, improvement in 13 patients, and no effect in 14 patients.[11]
3. **Arrhythmia**: Administration of modified *Chai Hu Gui Zhi Tang* effectively treated various types of arrhythmia. Out of 24 patients, the study reported complete recovery in 16 patients, improvement in 4 patients, and no benefit in 4 patients.[12]
4. **Neurasthenia**: One study reported satisfactory result using modified *Chai Hu Gui Zhi Tang* to treat 60 patients with neurasthenia. The herbal treatment protocol was to use this formula as the base, and add *Shan Zha* (Fructus Crataegi), *Shen Qu* (Massa Fermentata), and *Mai Ya* (Fructus Hordei Germinatus) for poor appetite and epigastric fullness and distention; *Ju Hua* (Flos Chrysanthemi) and *Bai Zhi* (Radix Angelicae Dahuricae) for dizziness and headache; *He Huan Hua* (Flos Albiziae) and *Mu Li* (Concha Ostreae) for insomnia; *Bai Zi Ren* (Semen Platycladi) and *Shi Chang Pu* (Rhizoma Acori Tatarinowii) for inability to concentrate; and *Chuan Lian Zi* (Fructus Toosendan) for chest oppression and discomfort.[13]
5. **Chronic hepatitis**: According to one study, 133 patients with chronic hepatitis were treated with this formula, and the study reported a rate of effectiveness of 62.3%. Significant effect was reported in 47 patients, moderate effect in 36 patients, mild effect in 9 patients, and no effect in 28 patients. Deterioration was reported in 13 patients. .[14]
6. **Chronic pancreatitis**: Use of *Chai Hu Gui Zhi Tang* effectively treated chronic pancreatitis. Out of 21 patients who participated in the study, 10 were male, 11 were female, and the ages ranged between 15 to 84 years. The treatment protocol was to administer 7.5g of the formula daily in powdered extract for 8 weeks or more. Out of 21 patients, the study reported marked improvement in 8 patients, slight improvement in 7 patients, and no improvement in 6 patients. The overall rate effectiveness was 71%.[15]
7. **Frozen shoulder**: Administration of *Chai Hu Gui Zhi Tang* in 26 patients (2 males and 24 females) with frozen

Chái Hú Guì Zhī Tāng (Bupleurum and Cinnamon Twig Decoction)

shoulder characterized by deficiency was associated with improvement in 22 patients and no effect in 4 patients.[16]

8. **Trigeminal neuralgia**: Use of *Chai Hu Gui Zhi Tang* effectively treated patients suffering from trigeminal neuralgia. This mechanism of action was attributed to the capacity of this formula to control the manifestation of pain in ligatured nerves by local effect, not by general analgesic effect.[17]

HERB-DRUG INTERACTION

- **Benzodiazepines**: Concurrent administration of *Chai Hu Gui Zhi Tang* and anticonvulsants, such as benzodiazepines, has been found to have a synergistic effect in treating epilepsy. *Chai Hu Gui Zhi Tang* acts as a partial agonist for the GABA-A receptor, and it activates the GABA-A receptor-mediated chloride current (Icl).[18]
- **Pentobarbital**: Administration of *Chai Hu Gui Zhi Tang* was associated with significantly shortened pentobarbital-induced sleeping time in mice. The mechanism of this interaction was attributed to the up-regulation of the mRNA expression of CYP2B, CYP3A1, and CYP4A1.[19]

TOXICOLOGY

Chai Hu Gui Zhi Tang has a relatively low toxicity. Continuous administration of the formula for four weeks in rats showed no abnormalities in the liver, spleen, kidney, or adrenal glands.[20]

SUGGESTED ACUPUNCTURE TREATMENT

Please refer to *Xiao Chai Hu Tang* (Minor Bupleurum Decoction) and *Gui Zhi Tang* (Cinnamon Twig Decoction) for suggested acupuncture treatments.

AUTHORS' COMMENTS

Chai Hu Gui Zhi Tang has demonstrated useful application in the treatment of acute and chronic immune-mediated polyarthritis in the dog. In many of these cases, the clinical signs are representative of *shaoyang* syndrome, and the use of this formula in combination with *Yi Yi Ren Tang* (Coicis Decoction), *Che Qian Zi* (Semen Plantaginis), *Ge Gen* (Radix Puerariae Lobatae), *Yan Hu Suo* (Rhizoma Corydalis) and *Ji Xue Teng* (Caulis Spatholobi) has been effective. This formula has also shown efficacy in the treatment of concurrent cholangiohepatitis and chronic pancreatitis in the cat and hyperactivity and anxiety in the dog. In the comments on *Xiao Chai Hu Tang* (Minor Bupleurum Decoction), a use for that formula was given for competition animals with lingering effects of infection (fatigue, recurrent infection, etc.). *Chai Hu Gui Zhi Tang* can be used in a similar fashion but is especially useful in those animals with lingering joint pain as the predominant complaint.

Chai Hu Gui Zhi Tang can be used to treat chronic pancreatitis and chronic hepatitis in the dog and cat. It has also proven useful in treating cases of persistent infectious tracheobronchitis (kennel cough) in dogs that are unresponsive or minimally responsive to antibiotic therapy. Likewise, horses with a persistent cough that can be elicited with palpation of the trachea or throat latch can be treated with this formula. Here it helps to release pathogens that have gone slightly deeper than those treated by *Gui Zhi Tang* (Cinnamon Twig Decoction), but have not penetrated deep enough to be classified as an interior disease pattern.

References

1. *Zhong Yao Ming Fang Yao Li Yu Ying Yong* (Pharmacology and Applications of Famous Herbal Formulas), 1989; 92-96.
2. *Guo Wai Yi Xue* (Foreign Medicine), 1985; 7(6):35.
3. *Guo Wai Yi Xue* (Foreign Medicine), 1991; 13(4) 45.
4. *Yao Xue Za Zhi* (Journal of Medicinals), 1983; 103(4):466.
5. Sunagawa M, Okada M, Guo SY, Hisamitsu T. Effectiveness of Saiko-Keishi-To (TJ-10, a Kampo herbal medicine) for trigeminal neuralgia in rats. Masui. 2001 May; 50(5):486-90.
6. Su SB, Motoo Y, Xie MJ, Taga H, Sawabu N.Antifibrotic effect of the herbal medicine Saiko-keishi-to (TJ-10) on chronic pancreatitis in the WBN/Kob rat. Pancreas. 2001 Jan; 22(1):8-17.
7. Motoo Y, Su SB, Xie MJ, Taga H, Sawabu N.Effect of herbal medicine Saiko-keishi-to (TJ-10) on rat spontaneous chronic pancreatitis: comparison with other herbal medicines. Int J Pancreatol. 2000 Apr; 27(2):123-9.
8. Su SB, Motoo Y, Xie MJ, Sakai J, Taga H, Sawabu N. Expression of pancreatitis-associated protein (PAP) in rat spontaneous chronic pancreatitis: effect of herbal medicine Saiko-keishi-to (TJ-10). Pancreas. 1999 Oct; 19(3):239-47.
9. Tatsuta M, Iishi H, Baba M, Narahara H, Yano H, Sakai N.Suppression by Chai-hu-gui-zhi-tang of the development of liver lesions induced by N-nitrosomorpholine in Sprague-Dawley rats. Cancer Lett. 2000 Apr 28; 152(1):31-6.
10. *Shi Zhen Guo Yi Guo Yao* (Shizhen National Herbs and Medicine), 1998; 5:404.
11. *Shan Dong Zhong Yi Za Zhi* (Shandong Journal of Chinese Medicine), 1990; 6:17.
12. *He Nan Zhong Yi* (Henan Chinese Medicine), 1991; 4:11.
13. *Fu Jian Zhong Yi Yao* (Fujian Chinese Medicine and Herbology), 1986; 4:28.
14. *Zhong Yi Fang Ji Xian Dai Yan Jiu* (Modern Study of Medical Formulas in Traditional Chinese Medicine), 1997; (1):199.
15. *Guo Wai Yi Xue* (Foreign Medicine), 1992; 1:40.
16. *Guo Wai Yi Xue* (Foreign Medicine), 1992; 2:105-106.
17. Sunagawa M, Okada M, Guo SY, Hisamitsu T. Effectiveness of Saiko-Keishi-To (TJ-10, a Kampo herbal medicine) for trigeminal neuralgia in rats. Masui. 2001 May; 50(5):486-90.
18. Sugiyama K, Kano T, Muteki T. Intravenous anesthetics, acting on the gamma-amino butric acid (GABA)A receptor, potentiate the herbal medicine "saiko-keishi-to"-induced chloride current. Masui. 1997 Sep; 46(9):1197-203.
19. Nose M, Tamura M, Ryu N, Mizukami H, Ogihara Y.Sho-saiko-to and Saiko-keisi-to, the traditional Chinese and Japanese herbal medicines, altered hepatic drug-metabolizing enzymes in mice and rats when administered orally for a long time. J Pharm Pharmacol. 2003 Oct; 55(10):1419-26.
20. *Yao Xue Za Zhi* (Journal of Medicinals), 1980; 100(6):602.

Chái Líng Tāng (Bupleurum and Poria Decoction)

柴苓湯
柴苓汤

Pinyin Name: *Chai Ling Tang*
Literal Name: Bupleurum and Poria Decoction
Alternate Name: Bupleurum and Hoelen Combination
Original Source: *Shen Shi Zun Sheng Shu* (Master Shen's Book for Revering Life) by Shen Jin-Ao in 1773

COMPOSITION

Chai Hu (Radix Bupleuri)
Ban Xia (Rhizoma Pinelliae)
Huang Qin (Radix Scutellariae)
Ren Shen (Radix et Rhizoma Ginseng)
Gan Cao (Radix et Rhizoma Glycyrrhizae)
Bai Zhu (Rhizoma Atractylodis Macrocephalae)
Zhu Ling (Polyporus)
Fu Ling (Poria)
Ze Xie (Rhizoma Alismatis)
Gui Zhi (Ramulus Cinnamomi)

DOSAGE / PREPARATION / ADMINISTRATION

Chai Ling Tang is formulated by combining two formulas: *Xiao Chai Hu Tang* (Minor Bupleurum Decoction) and *Wu Ling San* (Five-Ingredient Powder with Poria). Please refer to these two formulas for additional information.

CHINESE THERAPEUTIC ACTIONS

1. Harmonizes the exterior and interior to relieve *shaoyang* syndrome
2. Dispels water stagnation and phlegm accumulation

CLINICAL MANIFESTATIONS

Shaoyang syndrome with water accumulation: intermittent fever, trembling, thirst, anorexia, edema, distention in the chest and hypochondriac regions, vomiting and diarrhea after drinking, and a white tongue coating.

VETERINARY CLINICAL APPLICATIONS

Liver cirrhosis and ascites, toxic hepatopathy, cholecystitis, edema, nephropathy, gastroenteritis and febrile disorders.

EXPLANATION

Chai Ling Tang (Bupleurum and Poria Decoction) treats *shaoyang* syndrome with water accumulation in the lower parts of the body. *Shaoyang* syndrome is characterized by intermittent fever, trembling, discomfort in the chest and hypochondriac regions; water accumulation is characterized by thirst, edema, and scanty urine.

Chai Ling Tang is comprised of two formulas: *Xiao Chai Hu Tang* (Minor Bupleurum Decoction) which treats *shaoyang* syndrome by harmonizing the exterior and the interior; and *Wu Ling San* (Five-Ingredient Powder with Poria) which treats water accumulation in the lower parts of the body by resolving dampness and promoting the flow of yang qi.

Please refer to *Xiao Chai Hu Tang* (Minor Bupleurum Decoction) and *Wu Ling San* (Five-Ingredient Powder with Poria) for additional information on these two formulas.

***Chai Ling Tang* (Bupleurum and Poria Decoction)**

Diagnosis	Clinical Signs	Treatment	Herbs
Shaoyang syndrome with water accumulation	• Intermittent fever and trembling and discomfort of the hypochondriac region: *shaoyang* syndrome • Thirst, edema, and scanty urine: water accumulation	• Harmonizes the exterior and interior to relieve *shaoyang* syndrome • Dispels water stagnation and phlegm accumulation	• *Xiao Chai Hu Tang* (Minor Bupleurum Decoction) treats *shaoyang* syndrome. • *Wu Ling San* (Five-Ingredient Powder with Poria) treats water accumulation.

Chái Líng Tāng (Bupleurum and Poria Decoction)

VETERINARY MODIFICATIONS

- If accompanied by irritability and a dry mouth, add *Huang Lian* (Rhizoma Coptidis) and *Mai Dong* (Radix Ophiopogonis).
- With vomiting and thirst, add *Zhi Shi* (Fructus Aurantii Immaturus) and *Zhu Ru* (Caulis Bambusae in Taenia).
- With diarrhea and a dry mouth, add *Gan Jiang* (Rhizoma Zingiberis) and *Huang Bo* (Cortex Phellodendri Chinensis).
- When the vomiting and diarrhea is due to food stagnation, add *Ping Wei San* (Calm the Stomach Powder).
- When the vomiting and diarrhea is due to deficiency and cold, add *Wu Zhu Yu Tang* (Evodia Decoction).

PHARMACOLOGICAL EFFECTS

1. **Diuretic**: Administration of *Chai Ling Tang* at 10 times the normal dose to 10-month-old rats was associated with a marked increase in water and sodium excretion in the first 24-hour period. Continuous administration for 1 month was associated with weight reduction, but no abnormal reactions.[1] The mechanism of this diuretic action was attributed to the production of nitric oxide.[2]
2. **Endocrine**: Administration of 0.01-1.0 g/kg of *Chai Ling Tang* to male Wistar rats was associated with a stimulating effect on the endocrine system, as demonstrated by an increased plasma concentration of adrenocorticotropic hormone and a decreased level of corticotropin releasing factor.[3]
3. **Nephroprotective**: Use of *Chai Ling Tang* was associated with beneficial effects in treating passive Heymann nephritis in rats, which is similar to human membranous nephropathy. The study reported that *Chai Ling Tang* significantly decreased serum albumin and total protein, and inhibited serum total cholesterol. The researchers concluded that proteinuria in passive Heymann nephritis can be significantly suppressed by *Chai Ling Tang*.[4]

HUMAN CLINICAL STUDIES AND RESEARCH

1. **Hepatitis**: Use of *Chai Ling Tang* was associated with 55.3% effectiveness in treating chronic hepatitis. Of 48 patients, the study reported significant improvement in 4 patients, moderate improvement in 13 patients, slight improvement in 9 patients, and no benefit in 22 patients.[5]
2. **Alcohol-induced liver damages**: Twenty-seven patients with various types of alcohol-induced liver disorders (13 with hepatitis, 11 with fatty liver, and 3 with liver cirrhosis) were treated with good results using *Chai Ling Tang*. The treatment protocol was to administer 3g of the powdered extract three times daily before meals for at least 3 months. All patients were instructed to avoid consumption of alcohol. The study reported improved lab values of SGOT and LDH after one month, and improved lab values of SGOT, SGPT, LDH, gamma-GPT, and total bilirubin after three months. Of 27 patients, the study reported moderate improvement in 17 patients, slight improvement in 8 patients, no effect in 1 patient, and deterioration in 1 patient. The proposed mechanism of the hepatoprotective effects was attributed to ability of this formula to reduce inflammation, regulate the production and excretion of bile, and protect liver cell membrane.[6]
3. **Nephropathy**: Thirty-nine patients with nephropathy were divided into two groups, with both groups similar in age, severity of illness, and overall condition. Group one of 21 patients received herbal treatment, and group two of 18 patients received drug treatment. Patients in group one received *Chai Ling Tang* as the base formula, with minor modifications based on the four possible patterns (Lung and Kidney qi deficiencies, Spleen and Kidney yang deficiencies, Liver and Kidney yin deficiencies, and qi and yin deficiencies). Patients in group two received 1 mg/kg of prednisone daily in the morning with meals for eight weeks, followed by a gradual reduction in dose, and eventual discontinuation. The study reported that both groups responded well to the treatments, and group one showed faster relief of proteinuria.[7]
4. **Diabetic nephropathy**: Fifteen patients with diabetic nephropathy who were treated with *Chai Ling Tang* showed the following results: moderate improvement in 10 patients, slight improvement in 3 patients, and no improvement in 2 patients.[8]
5. **Steroid-dependent nephrotic syndrome**: Administration of *Chai Ling Tang* effectively treated 4 patients with steroid-dependent relapsing nephrotic syndrome associated with the use of prednisolone and immunosuppressive agents. After treatment with *Chai Ling Tang*, the study reported that relapse was markedly suppressed in three patients but not at all in the other. Based on this information, the researchers concluded that *Chai Ling Tang* was effective for steroid-dependent nephrotic syndrome.[9] Another study reported marked improvement in 37 children with steroid-dependent nephrotic syndrome treated with *Chai Ling Tang* while taking corticosteroids. After treatment with *Chai Ling Tang*, the study reported improvement with proteinuria, reduction of prednisone dose, and relief of side effects. The study indicated that *Chai Ling Tang* may be a useful steroid substitute for patients with steroid-dependent nephrotic syndrome who fail to respond to or manifest severe toxic effect from cytotoxic agents.[10] In one multicenter, randomized, controlled clinical trial, initial 8-week prednisolone and 2-year *Chai Ling Tang* was effective in 196 children with steroid-responsive nephrotic syndrome.[11]

Cháí Líng Tāng (Bupleurum and Poria Decoction)

6. **Rheumatoid arthritis**: Administration of 9g of *Chai Ling Tang* daily for 3 months was associated with marked improvements in 17 patients with rheumatoid arthritis.[12]
7. **Systemic lupus erythematosus (SLE)**: Daily administration of *Chai Ling Tang* in powdered extract (8.1 g/day in two to three equally-divided doses) for 6 to 12 months was effective in treating 69 patients with SLE. Patients with joint pain and increased sensitivity to light showed improvement after 9-12 months. Patients with proteinuria showed improvement after 6-12 months. Patients with decreased white blood cell counts showed improvement after 3 months. Patients with decreased CD4 and CD8 counts showed improvement after 12 months. Side effects were reported in 8 of 69 patients, and included thirst, nausea, palpitations, itching, and increased SGPT (in 1 case).[13] Another report concluded long-term administration of *Chai Ling Tang* showed an inhibitory effect on SLE and was beneficial as a supportive treatment for patients with mild cases of SLE.[14]
8. **Ulcerative colitis**: Administration of *Chai Ling Tang* was effective in treating ulcerative colitis. In 3 patients, administration of this formula with 30mg of prednisolone and 4.0g of salicylazosulfapyridine effectively alleviated symptoms of ulcerative colitis. No recurrence was reported upon reduction and discontinuation of prednisolone.[15]
9. **Otitis media**: Use of *Chai Ling Tang* to treat suppurative otitis media in 35 children (with 46 affected ears) had a 78.3% rate of effectiveness.[16]
10. **Recurrent miscarriages**: Use of *Chai Ling Tang* to treat 10 of 12 women with a history of recurrent miscarriages who had shown positive antiphospholipid antibodies produced an 83.3% success rate. The 12 women had experienced a total of 27 spontaneous miscarriages in their previous pregnancies. The treatment protocol was to administer 9.0g daily of *Chai Ling Tang* before their next pregnancy. Of 12 patients, the study reported conversion of antiphospholipid antibodies from positive to negative in 9 patients, and successful pregnancy and delivery of a child in 10 patients. The study considered *Chai Ling Tang* to be an effective therapy for patients with recurrent miscarriages who were found to be positive for antiphospholipid antibodies.[17] In two other studies, use of *Chai Ling Tang* and *Dang Gui Shao Yao San* (Tangkuei and Peony Powder) helped to prevent autoimmunity-related recurrent miscarriages by correcting T helper-1/T helper-2 balance.[18,19]
11. **Anovulation in polycystic ovary syndrome**: Administration of *Chai Ling Tang* stimulated ovulation in 70.6% of anovulatory patients with polycystic ovary syndrome. Serum LH and the LH/FSH ratio significantly decreased, and serum testosterone levels did not significantly change during the treatment. The researchers concluded that *Chai Ling Tang* can be useful for the treatment of anovulation in polycystic ovary syndrome, especially because this condition does not respond well to clomiphene citrate or gonadotropin therapy.[20]

HERB-DRUG INTERACTION

- **Liver enzyme inhibition**: One study that examined the metabolic activity of different cytochrome P450 (CYP) isoforms reported *Chai Ling Tang* to be a competitive inhibitor of CYP3A4 (Ki value of 0.1 mg/mL), CYP2C9 (Ki value of 0.7-0.8 mg/mL), and CYP1A2 (inhibition > 68%), but not CYP2D6. The study concluded that because of this inhibitory effect on liver metabolism, care should be taken with concurrent use of *Chai Ling Tang* and drugs.[21]
- **Ofloxacin**: In a study with 7 volunteers in an open, random, crossover fashion, no significant effect on the rate and extent of bioavailability of ofloxacin was noted with coadministrations of *Liu Jun Zi Tang* (Six-Gentlemen Decoction), *Xiao Chai Hu Tang* (Minor Bupleurum Decoction), or *Chai Ling Tang* (Bupleurum and Poria Decoction).[22]

SUGGESTED ACUPUNCTURE TREATMENT

1. Points: *Yangchi* (TH 4), *Neiguan* (PC 6), *Qiuxu* (GB 40), *Ligou* (LR 5), *Housanli* (ST 36); and *Pangguangshu* (BL 28), *Zhongji* (CV 3), *Yinlingquan* (SP 9), *Shuifen* (CV 9), and *Waiguan* (TH 5).
2. Technique: even method for *Yangchi* (TH 4), *Neiguan* (PC 6), *Qiuxu* (GB 40), *Ligou* (LR 5), and *Housanli* (ST 36); and sedation for *Pangguangshu* (BL 28), *Zhongji* (CV 3), *Yinlingquan* (SP 9), *Shuifen* (CV 9), and *Waiguan* (TH 5).

Yangchi (TH 4), the *yuan* (source) point of the *San Jiao* channel, regulates qi circulation in all three *jiaos* and harmonizes the *shaoyang*. *Neiguan* (PC 6), the *luo* (connecting) point of the Pericardium channel, regulates qi circulation, removes stagnation, and corrects the rising qi of the Stomach. *Qiuxu* (GB 40), the *yuan* (source) point of the Gallbladder channel, sedates heat in the *shaoyang* and leads fire downward. *Ligou* (LR 5), the *luo* (connecting) point of the Liver channel, regulates Liver qi flow and relieves stagnation. Together, *Qiuxu* (GB 40) and *Ligou* (LR 5) relieve heat and stagnation in the Gallbladder and Liver. *Housanli* (ST 36) strengthens Spleen qi to prevent the Spleen from being overacted on by the Liver and Gallbladder and harmonizes the Stomach to relieve nausea and vomiting.

Pangguangshu (BL 28) and *Zhongji* (CV 3) regulate Urinary Bladder qi. When combined, *Pangguangshu* (BL 28), *Zhongji* (CV 3), and *Yinlingquan* (SP 9) dispel dampness and promote diuresis. In addition, *Shuifen* (CV 9) regulates water passages to promote urination. *Waiguan*

Chái Líng Tāng (Bupleurum and Poria Decoction)

(TH 5), which connects with the *yangwei* (linking) channel, relieves exterior pathogenic factors and regulates water within all three *jiaos*. Together, these five points regulate qi and water and induce diuresis.

AUTHORS' COMMENTS

Chai Ling Tang can be used to treat hepatotoxicity secondary to non-steroidal anti-inflammatory drugs, liver cirrhosis with ascites, and severe pancreatitis with edema in the dog.

References

1. *Guo Wai Yi Xue Zhong Yi Zhong Yao Fen Ce* (Monograph of Chinese Herbology from Foreign Medicine), 1981; 2:57.
2. Fujitsuka N, Goto K, Takeda S, Aburada M. The diuretic effect of Sairei-to is mediated by nitric oxide production in pentobarbital-anesthetized rats. J Pharmacol Sci. 2004 Feb; 94(2):185-91.
3. *Guo Wai Yi Xue Zhong Yi Zhong Yao Fen Ce* (Monograph of Chinese Herbology from Foreign Medicine), 1993; 15(2):31.
4. Li P, Fujio S. Effects of chai ling tang on proteinuria in rat models. J Tradit Chin Med. 1995 Mar; 15(1):48-52.
5. *Guo Wai Yi Xue Zhong Yi Zhong Yao Fen Ce* (Monograph of Chinese Herbology from Foreign Medicine), 1991; 3:168.
6. *Guo Wai Yi Xue Zhong Yi Zhong Yao Fen Ce* (Monograph of Chinese Herbology from Foreign Medicine), 1991; 13(6):31.
7. *Guo Wai Yi Xue Zhong Yi Zhong Yao Fen Ce* (Monograph of Chinese Herbology from Foreign Medicine), 1989; 11(6):18.
8. *Guo Wai Yi Xue Zhong Yi Zhong Yao Fen Ce* (Monograph of Chinese Herbology from Foreign Medicine), 1990; (5):247.
9. Kimura K, Nanba S, Tojo A, Matsuoka H, Sugimoto T. Effects of sairei-to on the relapse of steroid-dependent nephrotic syndrome. Am J Chin Med. 1990; 18(1-2):45-50.
10. Liu XY. Therapeutic effect of chai-ling-tang (sairei-to) on the steroid-dependent nephrotic syndrome in children. American Journal of Chinese Medicine. 1995; 23(3-4):255-60.
11. Yoshikawa N, Ito H, Takekoshi Y, Honda M, Awazu M, Iijima K, Nakamura H, Seino Y, Takeda N, Hattori S, Matsuda I. Standard versus long-term prednisolone with sairei-to for initial therapy in childhood steroid-responsive nephrotic syndrome: a prospective controlled study. Nippon Jinzo Gakkai Shi. 1998 Nov; 40(8):587-90.
12. *Guo Wai Yi Xue Zhong Yi Zhong Yao Fen Ce* (Monograph of Chinese Herbology from Foreign Medicine), 1994; 16(5):25.
13. *Guo Wai Yi Xue Zhong Yi Zhong Yao Fen Ce* (Monograph of Chinese Herbology from Foreign Medicine), 1994; 16(5):25.
14. *Guo Wai Yi Xue Zhong Yi Zhong Yao Fen Ce* (Monograph of Chinese Herbology from Foreign Medicine), 1994; 16(4):25.
15. *Guo Wai Yi Xue Zhong Yi Zhong Yao Fen Ce* (Monograph of Chinese Herbology from Foreign Medicine), 1993; 15(4):22.
16. *Guo Wai Yi Xue Zhong Yi Zhong Yao Fen Ce* (Monograph of Chinese Herbology from Foreign Medicine), 1989; (5):285.
17. Takakuwa K. Yasuda M. Hataya I. Sekizuka N. Tamura M. Arakawa M. Higashino M. Hasegawa I. Tanaka K. Treatment for patients with recurrent abortion with positive antiphospholipid antibodies using a traditional Chinese herbal medicine. Journal of Perinatal Medicine. 1996; 24(5):489-94.
18. Fujii T, Kanai T, Kozuma S, Hamai Y, Hyodo H, Yamashita T, Miki A, Unno N, Taketani Y. Theoretical basis for herbal medicines, Tokishakuyaku-san and Sairei-to, in the treatment of autoimmunity-related recurrent abortion by correcting T helper-1/T helper-2 balance. American Journal of Reproductive Immunology. 2000 Dec.; 44(6):342-6.
19. Fujii T. Herbal factors in the treatment of autoimmunity-related habitual abortion. Vitam Horm. 2002; 65:333-44.
20. Sakai A. Kondo Z. Kamei K. Izumi S. Sumi K. Induction of ovulation by Sairei-to for polycystic ovary syndrome patients. Endocrine Journal. 1999 Feb; 46(1):217-20.
21. Takahashi K. Uejima E. Morisaki T. Takahashi K. Kurokawa N. Azuma J. In vitro inhibitory effects of Kampo medicines on metabolic reactions catalyzed by human liver microsomes. Journal of Clinical Pharmacy & Therapeutics. 2003 Aug; 28(4):319-27.
22. Hasegawa T, Yamaki K, Nadai M, Muraoka I, Wang L, Takagi K, Nabeshima T. Lack of effect of Chinese medicines on bioavailability of ofloxacin in healthy volunteers. Int J Clin Pharmacol Ther. 1994 Feb; 32(2):57-61.

Hāo Qín Qīng Dǎn Tāng

(Artemisia Annua and Scutellaria Decoction to Clear the Gallbladder)

蒿芩清膽湯
蒿芩清胆汤

Pinyin Name: *Hao Qin Qing Dan Tang*

Literal Name: Artemisia Annua and Scutellaria Decoction to Clear the Gallbladder

Original Source: *Chong Ding Tong Su Shang Han Lun* (Revised Popular Guide to the Discussion of Cold-Induced Disorders) by Yu Gen-Chu in the Qing Dynasty

COMPOSITION

Qing Hao (Herba Artemisiae Annuae)	4.5-6g
Huang Qin (Radix Scutellariae)	4.5-9g
Zhu Ru (Caulis Bambusae in Taenia)	9g
Ban Xia (Rhizoma Pinelliae)	4.5g
Zhi Qiao (Fructus Aurantii)	4.5g
Chen Pi (Pericarpium Citri Reticulatae)	4.5g
Chi Fu Ling (Poria Rubra)	9g
Bi Yu San (Jasper Powder)	9g

DOSAGE / PREPARATION / ADMINISTRATION

Prepare the ingredients as a decoction. Note: *Bi Yu San* (Jasper Powder) is an herbal formula that treats the syndrome of summer-heat and dampness complicated by Liver and Gallbladder heat. It contains *Hua Shi* (Talcum) 180g, *Gan Cao* (Radix et Rhizoma Glycyrrhizae) 30g, and *Qing Dai* (Indigo Naturalis) [9g]. Please refer to *Chinese Herbal Formulas and Applications* for additional information.

CHINESE THERAPEUTIC ACTIONS

1. Clears Gallbladder heat and dispels dampness
2. Harmonizes the Stomach and dissolves phlegm

CLINICAL MANIFESTATIONS

Gallbladder damp-heat: alternating spells of fever and trembling (with fever being more prominent); dry heaves; regurgitation of yellow and sticky fluids; a red tongue, and, in severe cases, there may be a white or yellowish tongue coating; and a slippery, rapid pulse on the right and a wiry, rapid pulse on the left.

VETERINARY CLINICAL APPLICATIONS

Cholangitis, cholelithiasis, gastritis, and fever.

EXPLANATION

Hao Qin Qing Dan Tang (Artemisia Annua and Scutellaria Decoction to Clear the Gallbladder) treats damp-heat in the Gallbladder and reversed flow of Stomach qi. Damp-heat in the Gallbladder causes intermittent fever and trembling because the Gallbladder is a *shaoyang* organ, located between the exterior and the interior. Hypochondriac pain and distention arise as a result of heat in the Gallbladder and Liver channels; these channels travel through the chest and hypochondriac region. Because the wood element (Liver and Gallbladder) acts on the earth element (Spleen and Stomach), excess in the Gallbladder can negatively affect the Stomach, causing reversed flow of Stomach qi and damp obstruction, which manifest in dry heaves, nausea, and regurgitation of yellow and sticky fluids. A rapid pulse indicates heat. A slippery pulse on the right indicates damp obstruction produced by the Spleen, while a wiry pulse on the left indicates qi stagnation in the Gallbladder.

Qing Hao (Herba Artemisiae Annuae) penetrates and clears heat in the *shaoyang* level. *Huang Qin* (Radix Scutellariae) purges and sedates heat in the Gallbladder. *Zhu Ru* (Caulis Bambusae in Taenia) clears heat and resolves phlegm. *Ban Xia* (Rhizoma Pinelliae) dries dampness and eliminates phlegm. *Zhi Qiao* (Fructus Aurantii) and *Chen Pi* (Pericarpium Citri Reticulatae) activate qi flow, expand the chest, and harmonize and regulate Stomach qi. *Chi Fu Ling* (Poria Rubra) and *Hua Shi* (Talcum) drain damp-heat out of the body through urination. *Qing Dai* (Indigo Naturalis) eliminates phlegm and interior heat. *Gan Cao* (Radix et Rhizoma Glycyrrhizae) harmonizes the Stomach and the formula.

Hāo Qín Qīng Dǎn Tāng

(Artemisia Annua and Scutellaria Decoction to Clear the Gallbladder)

Hao Qin Qing Dan Tang (Artemisia Annua and Scutellaria Decoction to Clear the Gallbladder)

Diagnosis	Clinical Signs	Treatment	Herbs
Gallbladder damp-heat	• Intermittent fever and trembling: *shaoyang* level • Hypochondriac pain and distention: heat in the Gallbladder and Liver channels • Dry heaves, nausea, and regurgitation of fluids: reversed flow of Stomach qi • Red tongue body and in severe cases may have a white or yellowish tongue coating: heat condition • Slippery, rapid pulse on the right: damp obstruction • Wiry, rapid pulse on the left: qi stagnation	• Clears Gallbladder heat and dispels dampness • Harmonizes the Stomach and dissolves phlegm	• *Qing Hao* (Herba Artemisiae Annuae) penetrates and clears heat in the *shaoyang* level. • *Huang Qin* (Radix Scutellariae) purges and sedates heat in the Gallbladder. • *Zhu Ru* (Caulis Bambusae in Taenia) and *Ban Xia* (Rhizoma Pinelliae) clear heat, eliminate dampness and phlegm, and redirect Stomach qi downward. • *Zhi Qiao* (Fructus Aurantii) and *Chen Pi* (Pericarpium Citri Reticulatae) activate qi flow, expand the chest, and regulate Stomach qi. • *Chi Fu Ling* (Poria Rubra) and *Hua Shi* (Talcum) drain damp-heat out of the body through urination. • *Qing Dai* (Indigo Naturalis) eliminates phlegm and interior heat. • *Gan Cao* (Radix et Rhizoma Glycyrrhizae) harmonizes the Stomach and the formula.

VETERINARY MODIFICATIONS

- With body aches and pains, add *Sang Zhi* (Ramulus Mori), *Yi Yi Ren* (Semen Coicis), and *Si Gua Luo* (Retinervus Luffae Fructus).
- For damp-heat jaundice, remove *Ban Xia* (Rhizoma Pinelliae) and *Chen Pi* (Pericarpium Citri Reticulatae); and add *Yin Chen* (Herba Artemisiae Scopariae) and *Zhi Zi* (Fructus Gardeniae).
- With dizziness and vertigo due to phlegm accumulation, add *Tian Ma* (Rhizoma Gastrodiae).
- With insomnia and palpitations, add *Hu Po* (Succinum) and *Huang Lian* (Rhizoma Coptidis).
- For *lin zheng* (dysuria syndrome), add *Che Qian Zi* (Semen Plantaginis), *Mu Tong* (Caulis Akebiae), and *Ze Xie* (Rhizoma Alismatis).

CAUTIONS / CONTRAINDICATIONS

Avoid cold, raw or greasy foods while taking *Hao Qin Qing Dan Tang*.[1]

HUMAN CLINICAL STUDIES AND RESEARCH

1. **Cholelithiasis**: Use of modified *Hao Qin Qing Dan Tang* demonstrated a success rate of 85% in eliminating gallstones. Of 60 cases involving gallstones, the study reported elimination of all stones in 46 cases, partial elimination of stones in 5 cases, no benefit in 5 cases, and surgical intervention in 4 cases. The herbal treatment contained this formula plus *Chai Hu* (Radix Bupleuri) for Liver qi stagnation; *Da Huang* (Radix et Rhizoma Rhei) for dry stools and constipation; and *Long Dan* (Radix et Rhizoma Gentianae), *Che Qian Zi* (Semen Plantaginis), and *Yin Chen* (Herba Artemisiae Scopariae) for severe jaundice. The duration of treatment ranged from 7 to 30 days of therapy.[2]
2. **Gastritis**: Good results were reported using modified *Hao Qin Qing Dan Tang* to treat gastritis caused by regurgitation of bile. In addition to this formula, modifications included the addition of *Chuan Lian Zi* (Fructus Toosendan) and *Wu Zhu Yu* (Fructus Evodiae) for severe pain; *Xiang Fu* (Rhizoma Cyperi) and *Zi Su Geng* (Caulis Perillae) for upper abdominal distention and pain; *Huang Lian* (Rhizoma Coptidis) and *Zhe Shi* (Haematitum) for increased acidity of the stomach; and other adjustments when deemed necessary. Of 52 cases, the study reported significant improvement in 43 cases and moderate improvement in 9 cases.[3]
3. **Fever**: Use of *Hao Qin Qing Dan Tang* was associated with 95% effectiveness in treating 100 patients with fever caused by an external infection. Clinical presentations included acute onset of fever (body temperature of 38.5°C / 101.3°F or higher), elevated body temperature especially in the evening and at night with or without perspiration; chills, sore throat, a dry mouth, a bitter taste in the mouth, cough, dysuria, a red tongue body with a thin, greasy white

Hāo Qín Qīng Dǎn Tāng

(Artemisia Annua and Scutellaria Decoction to Clear the Gallbladder)

or yellow tongue coating, and a rapid pulse. The herbal treatment contained *Hao Qin Qing Dan Tang* plus *Bo He* (Herba Menthae) and *Ge Gen* (Radix Puerariae Lobatae). Of 100 cases, the study reported complete recovery in 37 cases, significant improvement in 58 cases, and no effect in 5 cases.[4] Another study reported 96.3% effectiveness using modified *Hao Qin Qing Dan Tang* to treat fever in 54 patients. Modifications included the addition of *Chai Hu* (Radix Bupleuri) for alternating spells of chills and fever; *Cang Zhu* (Rhizoma Atractylodis) and *Hou Po* (Cortex Magnoliae Officinalis) for chest fullness and distention; *Jie Geng* (Radix Platycodonis) for redness, swelling, and pain in the throat; and *Yu Jin* (Radix Curcumae) for a feeling of heaviness in the head.[5]

SUGGESTED ACUPUNCTURE TREATMENT

1. Points: *Fengchi* (GB 20), *Zhigou* (TH 6), *Yanglingquan* (GB 34), *Housanli* (ST 36), and *Fenglong* (ST 40).
2. Technique: sedation. May bleed to relieve heat.

Fengchi (GB 20) clears heat and expels wind. *Zhigou* (TH 6) regulates qi flow in the three *jiaos*. *Yanglingquan* (GB 34), the *he* (uniting) point of the Gallbladder channel, sedates the Gallbladder and Liver. *Housanli* (ST 36) harmonizes the middle *jiao* and directs Stomach qi downward. *Fenglong* (ST 40), the *luo* (connecting) point of the Stomach channel, dispels dampness and phlegm. To treat serious alternating spells of fever and chills, needle *Dazhui* (GV 14), *Zhongzhu* (TH 3), *Yemen* (TH 2), *Quchi* (LI 11), and *Hegu* (LI 4).

AUTHORS' COMMENTS

Hao Qin Qing Dan Tang is a commonly used formula for treating damp-heat with turbidity attacking the *shaoyang* level. This formula is indicated in the following conditions: jaundice with *lin zheng* (dysuria syndrome), vomiting caused by disharmony of the Liver and Stomach with turbidity in the Stomach caused by phlegm obstruction.

Xiao Chai Hu Tang (Minor Bupleurum Decoction) and *Hao Qin Qing Dan Tang* both harmonize *shaoyang* syndrome, but have important differences:

- *Xiao Chai Hu Tang* harmonizes *shaoyang* syndrome that is caused initially by wind-cold invading the *taiyang* level, which then turns into heat and moves deeper into the *shaoyang* level. The chief herb, *Chai Hu* (Radix Bupleuri), is an acrid, bitter, and cold herb that releases the exterior, lifts the clear yang, and disperses wind and heat.
- *Hao Qin Qing Dan Tang* harmonizes *shaoyang* syndrome caused by damp-heat invading the Gallbladder channel. The chief herb, *Qing Hao* (Herba Artemisiae Annuae), an acrid, bitter, and cold herb, works with the other herbs in the formula to clear damp-heat from the *shaoyang*.

References

1. *Zhong Yao Ming Fang Yao Li Yu Ying Yong* (Pharmacology and Applications of Famous Herbal Formulas), 1989; 92-96.
2. *Chang Chun Zhong Yi Xue Yuan Xue Bao* (Journal of Changchun University of Chinese Medicine), 1998; 1:29.
3. *Si Chuan Zhong Yi* (Sichuan Chinese Medicine), 1996; 6:28.
4. *Zhong Yi Ming Fang Lin Chuang Xin Yong* (Contemporary Clinical Applications of Classic Chinese Formulas), 2001; 705.
5. *Shan Xi Zhong Yi* (Shanxi Chinese Medicine), 1999; 2:81.

Section 2

调和肝脾剂
— Liver and Spleen Harmonizing Formulas

Sì Nì Săn (Frigid Extremities Powder)
四逆散

Pinyin Name: *Si Ni San*
Literal Name: Frigid Extremities Powder
Alternate Names: *Su Ni San*, Counterflow Cold Formula, Cold Limbs Powder, Bupleurum and Chih-shih Formula
Original Source: *Shang Han Lun* (Discussion of Cold-Induced Disorders) by Zhang Zhong-Jing in the Eastern Han Dynasty

COMPOSITION

Chai Hu (Radix Bupleuri)	[6g]
Zhi Shi (Fructus Aurantii Immaturus), *po* (opened) and *zhi* (fried with liquid)	[6g]
Bai Shao (Radix Paeoniae Alba)	[6g]
Zhi Gan Cao (Radix et Rhizoma Glycyrrhizae Praeparata cum Melle)	[6g]

DOSAGE / PREPARATION / ADMINISTRATION

The source text states to grind equal amounts of the ingredients into powder and sift evenly. Take one large spoonful of the powder (6-9g) with boiled water three times daily. Today, this formula may be prepared as a decoction with the doses suggested in brackets.

CHINESE THERAPEUTIC ACTIONS

1. Ventilates the pathogens outward and relieves constraint
2. Spreads Liver qi and harmonizes the Liver and Spleen

CLINICAL MANIFESTATIONS

1. *Shaoyin* syndrome with frigid extremities: cold extremities, dysuria, abdominal pain, diarrhea, and tenesmus.
2. Disharmony of the Liver and Spleen: poor appetite, nausea, hypochondriac distention, epigastric and abdominal pain, and a wiry pulse.

VETERINARY CLINICAL APPLICATIONS

Chronic hepatitis, chronic cholecystitis, liver cirrhosis, pancreatitis, acute and chronic gastritis, peptic ulcer disease, infertility and uveitis.

EXPLANATION

Si Ni San (Frigid Extremities Powder) treats *shaoyin* syndrome characterized by cold extremities. This condition begins with the progression of an exterior pathogenic factor from the *shaoyang* level into the more interior *shaoyin* level. As the disease migrates toward the interior, it blocks the circulation of Liver and Gallbladder qi to the extremities, resulting in coldness below the elbows and stifles. In other words, the cold extremities in this case result from blocked circulation of qi, and not from yang deficiency. Also, the pulse is wiry and not weak, another indication that the condition is caused by qi stagnation and not by yang deficiency.

This formula also treats disharmony of the Liver and Spleen, with clinical signs including irritability, hypochondriac discomfort and distention, and epigastric and abdominal pain. Since the flow of Liver and Gallbladder qi to the exterior is blocked, it counterflows and overacts on the Spleen and Stomach, resulting in abdominal pain, diarrhea, and lack of appetite. To treat this syndrome, qi must be lifted and extended outward; the Liver and Spleen must also be harmonized and stagnant Liver qi smoothed.

Chai Hu (Radix Bupleuri) harmonizes and spreads the Liver and relieves Liver qi stagnation. *Zhi Shi* (Fructus Aurantii Immaturus) activates qi and breaks up qi stagnation. The lifting tendency of *Chai Hu* (Radix Bupleuri), coupled with the downward-directing action of *Zhi Shi* (Fructus Aurantii Immaturus), further facilitates the flow of qi to the extremities. *Bai Shao* (Radix Paeoniae Alba) nourishes Liver blood and softens the Liver. It helps *Zhi Shi*

Sì Nì Sǎn (Frigid Extremities Powder)

***Si Ni San* (Frigid Extremities Powder)**

Diagnosis	Clinical Signs	Treatment	Herbs
Shaoyin syndrome characterized by frigid extremities	• Cold extremities: blocked qi circulation to the extremities • Poor appetite, nausea, hypochondriac discomfort and distention, and epigastric and abdominal pain: Liver and Spleen disharmony • Wiry pulse: excess condition	• Ventilates the pathogens outward and relieves constraint • Spreads Liver qi and harmonizes the Liver and Spleen	• *Chai Hu* (Radix Bupleuri) harmonizes the Liver and relieves Liver qi stagnation. • *Zhi Shi* (Fructus Aurantii Immaturus) activates qi and breaks up qi stagnation. • *Bai Shao* (Radix Paeoniae Alba) nourishes Liver blood and softens the Liver. • *Zhi Gan Cao* (Radix et Rhizoma Glycyrrhizae Praeparata cum Melle) tonifies qi and strengthens the middle *jiao*.

(Fructus Aurantii Immaturus) relieve pain in the hypochondriac area and treats other Liver qi stagnation clinical signs. *Bai Shao* (Radix Paeoniae Alba) also prevents the drying nature of *Chai Hu* (Radix Bupleuri) from damaging yin. *Zhi Gan Cao* (Radix et Rhizoma Glycyrrhizae Praeparata cum Melle) tonifies qi and strengthens the middle *jiao*. It also harmonizes the formula and relieves gastrointestinal complaints arising when the Liver overacts on the Spleen and Stomach. Combined, these herbs lift the qi, smooth Liver qi, and restore the normal functioning of the Spleen.

Si Ni San is the basic formula for treating Liver qi stagnation. The cold extremities in this case do not suggest a cold syndrome, but rather constraint and stagnation of qi. In fact, if a patient with this condition is not treated in time, interior heat is likely to result.

VETERINARY MODIFICATIONS

- With severe Liver qi stagnation, add *Xiang Fu* (Rhizoma Cyperi) and *Yu Jin* (Radix Curcumae).
- If there is dysuria, add *Fu Ling* (Poria).
- With abdominal pain due to cold, add *Fu Zi* (Radix Aconiti Lateralis Praeparata).
- With nausea and vomiting, add *Huang Lian* (Rhizoma Coptidis) and *Sheng Jiang* (Rhizoma Zingiberis Recens).
- With diarrhea with tenesmus, add *Tong Xie Yao Fang* (Important Formula for Painful Diarrhea).
- If there is Spleen deficiency, add *Dang Shen* (Radix Codonopsis) and *Bai Zhu* (Rhizoma Atractylodis Macrocephalae).
- With food stagnation or indigestion, add *Mai Ya* (Fructus Hordei Germinatus) and *Ji Nei Jin* (Endothelium Corneum Gigeriae Galli); or *Bao He Wan* (Preserve Harmony Pill).
- If there is blood stagnation, add *Dan Shen* (Radix et Rhizoma Salviae Miltiorrhizae) and *Wu Ling Zhi* (Faeces Trogopteri); or *Ge Xia Zhu Yu Tang* (Drive Out Blood Stasis Below the Diaphragm Decoction).
- For hepatic disorders, add *Yin Chen* (Herba Artemisiae Scopariae), *Jin Qian Cao* (Herba Lysimachiae), *Yu Jin* (Radix Curcumae), and *Dan Shen* (Radix et Rhizoma Salviae Miltiorrhizae).

CAUTIONS / CONTRAINDICATIONS

The presence of frigid extremities is a clinical sign that may have various causes. *Si Ni San* must ***not*** be used indiscriminately as a symptomatic treatment for frigid extremities. Instead, it should only be used for cold extremities caused by blocked qi circulation failing to warm the extremities.

PHARMACOLOGICAL EFFECTS

1. **Gastrointestinal**: Alcohol extract of *Si Ni San* demonstrated an inhibitory effect on the gastrointestinal system and decreased the production of gastric acid.[1]
2. **Cardiovascular**: Administration of 60 mL of water extract of *Si Ni San* was associated with increased blood perfusion to the brain in patients with atherosclerosis and poor peripheral blood circulation. The same treatment had little effect on normal and healthy individuals.[2]
3. **Cardiotonic**: Intravenous injection of *Si Ni San* in dogs was associated with positive inotropic effects, positive chronotropic effects, and increased blood pressure.[3]
4. **Anti-arrhythmic**: Administration of *Si Ni San* was effective against arrhythmia induced by aconitine, epinephrine, and calcium chloride in rats and rabbits.[4, 5]
5. **Hepatoprotective**: Administration of *Si Ni San* was associated with marked hepatoprotective effects against many substances, such as carbon tetrachloride (CCl4), Bacillus Calmette-Guerin (BCG), and picryl chloride (PCl-DTH). *Si Ni San* provided protective effects against liver injury through multiple mechanisms, such as protection of the hepatocyte membrane, enhancement of nitric oxide release, and dysfunction of liver-infiltrating cells, mainly by causing their apoptosis.[6]

Sì Nì Săn (Frigid Extremities Powder)

HUMAN CLINICAL STUDIES AND RESEARCH

1. **Hepatitis**: Thirty-three patients with hepatitis were treated with modified *Si Ni San* with significant improvement in 29 patients and moderate improvement in 4 patients. The herbal treatment contained *Si Ni San* plus *Yan Hu Suo* (Rhizoma Corydalis) 10g, *Hou Po* (Cortex Magnoliae Officinalis) 10g, *Yu Jin* (Radix Curcumae) 7g, and *Dan Shen* (Radix et Rhizoma Salviae Miltiorrhizae) 12g as the base formula. *Yin Chen* (Herba Artemisiae Scopariae) and *Zhi Zi* (Fructus Gardeniae) were added for jaundice; *Da Huang* (Radix et Rhizoma Rhei) was added for constipation; *Bai Zhu* (Rhizoma Atractylodis Macrocephalae), *Fu Ling* (Poria) and *Yi Yi Ren* (Semen Coicis) were added for diarrhea; *Mai Ya* (Fructus Hordei Germinatus), *Shan Zha* (Fructus Crataegi), and *Chen Pi* (Pericarpium Citri Reticulatae) were added for poor appetite; *Di Gu Pi* (Cortex Lycii) and *Qing Hao* (Herba Artemisiae Annuae) were added for low-grade fever; *Bie Jia* (Carapax Trionycis), *Mu Li* (Concha Ostreae) and *Qing Pi* (Pericarpium Citri Reticulatae Viride) were added for enlargement of the liver or spleen; and *Dang Shen* (Radix Codonopsis) was added for constant fatigue.[7]
2. **Hypochondriac pain due to hepatitis**: Administration of *Si Ni San* plus *Jin Ling Zi San* (Melia Toosendan Powder) in 65 patients with hypochondriac pain due to hepatitis was associated with complete relief in 38 patients, improvement in 16 patients, and no benefit in 11 patients.[8]
3. **Liver cirrhosis**: Use of modified *Si Ni San* to treat liver cirrhosis had beneficial effects. The herbal treatment contained *Si Ni San* plus *Huang Qi* (Radix Astragali), *Dan Shen* (Radix et Rhizoma Salviae Miltiorrhizae), *Bie Jia* (Carapax Trionycis) and others as the base formula. Strategies for modifications included the addition of *Xiang Fu* (Rhizoma Cyperi) and *Yan Hu Suo* (Rhizoma Corydalis) for Liver qi stagnation; *Yu Jin* (Radix Curcumae) and *Huang Qin* (Radix Scutellariae) for heat; *Di Huang* (Radix Rehmanniae) and *Gou Qi Zi* (Fructus Lycii) for yin deficiency; *Dang Gui* (Radix Angelicae Sinensis) and *E Zhu* (Rhizoma Curcumae) for blood stagnation; and addition of *Fu Ling* (Poria) and *Yi Yi Ren* (Semen Coicis), and elimination of *Bie Jia* (Carapax Trionycis) for Spleen deficiency.[9]
4. **Cholecystitis**: Complete recovery was reported in 78 of 84 patients with chronic cholecystitis when treated with *Si Ni San* plus *Chuan Lian Zi* (Fructus Toosendan) and *Mu Xiang* (Radix Aucklandiae) as the base formula. Modifications included the addition of *Yu Jin* (Radix Curcumae) and *Yan Hu Suo* (Rhizoma Corydalis) for qi stagnation; *Jin Qian Cao* (Herba Lysimachiae) and *Da Huang* (Radix et Rhizoma Rhei) for gallstones; and *Huang Qin* (Radix Scutellariae) and *Jin Yin Hua* (Flos Lonicerae Japonicae) for damp-heat.[10]
5. **Cholelithiasis**: Forty-two patients with gallstones were treated with complete recovery in 31 patients, improvement in 10 patients, and no effect in 1 case. The herbal treatment included *Si Ni San* plus *Yu Jin* (Radix Curcumae), *Ji Nei Jin* (Endothelium Corneum Gigeriae Galli), *Jin Qian Cao* (Herba Lysimachiae), and others.[11]
6. **Biliary ascariasis**: Use of *Si Ni San* plus *Jin Ling Zi San* (Melia Toosendan Powder) was effective in treating biliary ascariasis in 40 patients (22 males and 18 females, between 6-45 years of age). The herbal treatment included *Chai Hu* (Radix Bupleuri) 10g, *Zhi Qiao* (Fructus Aurantii) 10g, *Chuan Lian Zi* (Fructus Toosendan) 10g, *Shi Jun Zi* (Fructus Quisqualis) 10g, *Bing Lang* (Semen Arecae) 10g, *Bai Shao* (Radix Paeoniae Alba) 18g, *Gan Cao* (Radix et Rhizoma Glycyrrhizae) 6g, and *Yan Hu Suo* (Rhizoma Corydalis) 12g. The study reported complete recovery in all 40 patients, with an average of 4.2 days of treatment.[12] In another study, successful expulsion of biliary ascariasis was reported in all 51 patients after treatment for 1 to 3 days with *Si Ni San* plus *Wu Mei* (Fructus Mume) and *Ku Lian Pi* (Cortex Meliae).[13]
7. **Superficial gastritis**: Thirty-five patients with superficial gastritis were treated with good results using modified *Si Ni San*. *Zhe Bei Mu* (Bulbus Fritillariae Thunbergii), *Huang Qin* (Radix Scutellariae) and *Xiang Fu* (Rhizoma Cyperi) were added for Liver and Stomach qi stagnation. *San Leng* (Rhizoma Sparganii), *E Zhu* (Rhizoma Curcumae), *Yan Hu Suo* (Rhizoma Corydalis), *San Qi* (Radix et Rhizoma Notoginseng), and *Chuan Lian Zi* (Fructus Toosendan) were added for stagnation in the Stomach channel.[14]
8. **Gastritis**: Use of modified *Si Ni San* demonstrated 93.3% effectiveness in treating 30 patients with gastritis caused by regurgitation of bile. The herbal treatment contained *Si Ni San* plus *Pu Gong Ying* (Herba Taraxaci), *Chen Pi* (Pericarpium Citri Reticulatae), *Huang Lian* (Rhizoma Coptidis) and others as the base formula. Modifications included the addition of *Chuan Lian Zi* (Fructus Toosendan) and *Yan Hu Suo* (Rhizoma Corydalis) for upper abdominal pain; and *Da Huang* (Radix et Rhizoma Rhei) for constipation. Of 30 patients, the study reported significant improvement in 16 patients, moderate improvement in 12 patients, and no effect in 2 patients.[15]
9. **Peptic ulcer disease**: One study of 70 peptic ulcer patients reported 93% effectiveness using *Si Ni San* plus *Hou Po* (Cortex Magnoliae Officinalis), *Shi Hu* (Caulis Dendrobii), *Mai Dong* (Radix Ophiopogonis), and others as needed. The duration of treatment was 30 days. Of 70 patients, the study reported complete recovery in 63 patients, improvement in 2 patients, and no improvement in 5 patients.[16]
10. **Epigastric pain**: One study reported marked success using herbs to treat 110 patients of epigastric pain arising from various causes (such as acute or chronic gastritis, gastric

Sì Nì Săn (Frigid Extremities Powder)

ulcer, duodenal ulcer). The herbal formula included *Si Ni San* plus *Yu Jin* (Radix Curcumae), *Mai Ya* (Fructus Hordei Germinatus), *Hou Po* (Cortex Magnoliae Officinalis), and others as needed. Of 110 patients, 55 had complete recovery, 33 had significant improvement, 20 had marked improvement, and 2 had no effect.[17]

11. **Ulcerative colitis**: One study reported significant improvement in 8 of 10 patients with chronic ulcerative colitis when treated with modified *Si Ni San*. Modifications were made by adding *Bai Jiang Cao* (Herba cum Radice Patriniae), *Da Xue Teng* (Caulis Sargentodoxae), and *Yi Yi Ren* (Semen Coicis) for damp-heat; *Dang Shen* (Radix Codonopsis), *Shan Yao* (Rhizoma Dioscoreae) and dry-fried *Bai Zhu* (Rhizoma Atractylodis Macrocephalae) for Spleen deficiency; and *Si Shen Wan* (Four-Miracle Pill) for Kidney yang deficiency.[18]
12. **Infertility**: Two hundred forty-six women with infertility due to blocked fallopian tubes were treated with 72.36% effectiveness (complete resolution in 136 patients, improvement in 42 patients, and no effect in 68 patients). The herbal treatment contained as the base formula *Chai Hu* (Radix Bupleuri) 10g, *Zhi Shi* (Fructus Aurantii Immaturus) 10g, *Chi Shao* (Radix Paeoniae Rubra) 10g, *Gan Cao* (Radix et Rhizoma Glycyrrhizae) 10g, *Dan Shen* (Radix et Rhizoma Salviae Miltiorrhizae) 10g and *Chuan Shan Jia* (Squama Manis) 15g. Modifications included addition of a larger dose of *Zhi Shi* (Fructus Aurantii Immaturus) for Liver stagnation, and *Shui Zhi* (Hirudo) for blood stagnation. The herbs were given in decoction daily for 3 months per course of treatment.[19]

TOXICOLOGY

In acute toxicology studies, the LD_{50} in mice was 413 g/kg via oral ingestion of decoction and 22.4 g/kg via intravenous injection. It was also noted that intravenous injection of the formula was associated with marked changes in electrocardiogram in rats and rabbits. In chronic toxicology studies, daily administration of the formula to rats in decoction at 15 g/kg for 20 days showed no abnormalities in either liver or kidney functions. The researchers also noted that the alcohol extract of the same formula showed more toxicity in both acute and chronic toxicology studies.[20]

SUGGESTED ACUPUNCTURE TREATMENT

1. Points: *Yangchi* (TH 4), *Neiguan* (PC 6), *Gongsun* (SP 4), *Xingjian* (LR 2), *Housanli* (ST 36), and *Sanyinjiao* (SP 6).
2. Technique: sedation.

Yangchi (TH 4) regulates qi of the *shaoyang* and lifts yang qi to increase its circulation. According to the *ba hui* (eight meeting) points principle, *Neiguan* (PC 6) and *Gongsun* (SP 4) relieve chest congestion and remove stagnation. *Xingjian* (LR 2) regulates Liver qi. *Housanli* (ST 36) and *Sanyinjiao* (SP 6) tonify qi, strengthen the Spleen, and nourish yin and blood.

AUTHORS' COMMENTS

Si Ni San is the foundation of many Liver qi-regulating formulas. This formula is not typically used alone but instead is combined with other herbs or formulas to treat many conditions with Liver qi stagnation and Liver-Spleen disharmony in veterinary medicine. Understanding the principles and uses of this formula will facilitate the understanding of other Liver qi-regulating formulas that are derived from *Si Ni San,* such as *Xiao Yao San* (Rambling Powder), *Jia Wei Xiao Yao San* (Augmented Rambling Powder), and *Chai Hu Shu Gan San* (Bupleurum Powder to Spread the Liver). All four formulas can be used to treat Liver qi stagnation and Liver-Spleen disharmony. In general, *Si Ni San* lacks the blood nourishing properties of *Xiao Yao San* (Rambling Powder), the heat clearing and blood nourishing abilities of *Jia Wei Xiao Yao San* (Augmented Rambling Powder), and is less able to regulate middle *jiao* qi flow than *Chai Hu Shu Gan San* (Bupleurum Powder to Spread the Liver).

Si Ni San can be used to treat liver cirrhosis, chronic hepatitis, pancreatitis and cholangiohepatitis in the dog and cat. It can be combined with *Yan Hu Suo San* (Corydalis Powder) or *Xue Fu Zhu Yu Tang* (Drive Out Stasis in the Mansion of Blood Decoction) to improve clinical results and relieve pain.

For the treatment of uveitis in the dog, it can be combined with *Huang Qin* (Radix Scutellariae), *Zhi Zi* (Fructus Gardeniae), *Shi Jue Ming* (Concha Haliotidis), *Mi Meng Hua* (Flos Buddlejae), *Ji Li* (Fructus Tribuli), *Jue Ming Zi* (Semen Cassiae), *Chi Shao* (Radix Paeoniae Rubra), and *Long Dan* (Radix et Rhizoma Gentianae). If there is hypopyon present, add *Pu Gong Ying* (Herba Taraxaci); and with fever, add *Shi Gao* (Gypsum Fibrosum).

For post-parturition abdominal pain it can be combined with *Shi Xiao San* (Sudden Smile Powder); and for infertility due to Liver qi stagnation and Liver blood deficiency, combine with *Si Wu Tang* (Four-Substance Decoction), *Ge Xia Zhu Yu Tang* (Drive Out Blood Stasis Below the Diaphragm Decoction) and *Yi Mu Cao* (Herba Leonuri).

Si Ni San (Frigid Extremities Powder) and *Si Ni Tang* (Frigid Extremities Decoction) are two formulas with similar names that must ***not*** be confused. These two formulas

Sì Nì Sǎn (Frigid Extremities Powder)

treat different syndromes (qi stagnation vs. yang deficiency) that share similar clinical signs (e.g., cold extremities/ limbs).

- *Si Ni San*: Qi stagnation blocks and prevents yang qi from properly circulating to the extremities. Animals usually experience coldness below the stifles and elbows, not in the entire limbs as seen in animals with yang deficiency. In general, these animals also warm up faster when the extremities are exposed to heat. Other accompanying signs include abdominal discomfort and pain, and diarrhea. *Si Ni San* contains qi-regulating herbs to harmonize and smooth Liver qi flow and open channel circulation to the extremities. This condition is often seen when pathogenic factors invade from the outside and are trapped in the *shaoyang* channels concurrent with qi stagnation. When yang qi is no longer blocked by qi stagnation, the cold limbs will be resolved.
- *Si Ni Tang*: Yang deficiency with coldness manifests not only in cold extremities, but also in coldness of the whole limbs and all over the body. Comparatively speaking, this coldness is more severe and does not warm up when exposed to heat. Accompanying clinical signs include a withered *shen* (spirit), desire to sleep, intolerance of cold, preference for lying in a fetal position, vomiting, abdominal pain, diarrhea with undigested food, and a weak, fine pulse. *Si Ni Tang* contains interior-warming herbs to boost Kidney yang to warm *ming men* (life gate) fire, thus warming the limbs.[21]

Si Ni San and *Yi Guan Jian* (Linking Decoction) both treat hypochondriac pain. The difference is as follows:

- *Si Ni San* treats epigastric, abdominal, or hypochondriac pain caused by Liver qi stagnation.
- *Yi Guan Jian* treats hypochondriac pain caused by Kidney and Liver yin deficiencies.[22]

References

1. *Tian Jin Zhong Yi* (Tianjin Chinese Medicine), 1987; (5):18.
2. *Zhong Yao Yao Li Yu Ying Yong* (Pharmacology and Applications of Chinese Herbs), 1991; 7(1):29.
3. *Liao Ning Zhong Yi Za Zhi* (Liaoning Journal of Chinese Medicine), 1986; (7):40.
4. *Zhong Yao Yao Li Yu Ying Yong* (Pharmacology and Applications of Chinese Herbs), 1988; 18.
5. *Zhong Yao Yao Li Yu Ying Yong* (Pharmacology and Applications of Chinese Herbs), 1992; 8(4):37.
6. Jiang J, Zhou C, Xu Q. Alleviating effects of Si-Ni-San, a traditional Chinese prescription, on experimental liver injury and its mechanisms. Biol Pharm Bull. 2003 Aug; 26(8):1089-94.
7. *Shan Xi Xin Zhong Yi* (New Shanxi Chinese Medicine), 1987; (5):225.
8. *Zhong Yi Ming Fang Lin Chuang Xin Yong* (Contemporary Clinical Applications of Classic Chinese Formulas), 2001; 244.
9. *Liao Ning Zhong Yi Za Zhi* (Liaoning Journal of Chinese Medicine), 1996; 4:169.
10. *Hu Nan Zhong Yi Za Zhi* (Hunan Journal of Chinese Medicine), 1989; 4:39.
11. *An Hui Zhong Yi Xue Yuan Xue Bao* (Journal of Anhui University School of Medicine), 1995; 4:32.
12. *Guang Xi Zhong Yi Yao* (Guangxi Chinese Medicine and Herbology), 1985; 1:14.
13. *Fu Jian Zhong Yi Yao* (Fujian Chinese Medicine and Herbology), 1962; 2:37.
14. *Zhe Jiang Zhong Yi Za Zhi* (Zhejiang Journal of Chinese Medicine), 1997; 10:439.
15. *Bei Jing Zhong Yi Yao Da Xue Xue Bao* (Journal of Beijing University of Medicine and Medicinals), 1997; 3:68.
16. *Zhe Jiang Zhong Yi Xue Yuan Xue Bao* (Journal of Zhejiang University of Chinese Medicine), 1997; 2:53.
17. *Zhong Yi Ming Fang Lin Chuang Xin Yong* (Contemporary Clinical Applications of Classic Chinese Formulas), 2001; 245.
18. *Nei Meng Gu Zhong Yi Yao* (Traditional Chinese Medicine and Medicinals of Inner Mongolia), 1998; 1:26.
19. *Zhong Yi Ming Fang Lin Chuang Xin Yong* (Contemporary Clinical Applications of Classic Chinese Formulas), 2001; 243.
20. *Zhong Xi Yi Jie He Za Zhi* (Journal of Integrated Chinese and Western Medicine), 1988; 8(10):601.
21. Wang MZ, et al. *Zhong Yi Xue Wen Da Ti Ku* (Questions and Answers on Traditional Chinese Medicine: Herbal Formulas).
22. Wang MZ, et al. *Zhong Yi Xue Wen Da Ti Ku* (Questions and Answers on Traditional Chinese Medicine: Herbal Formulas).

Cháí Hú Shū Gān Sǎn (Bupleurum Powder to Spread the Liver)

柴胡疏肝散

Pinyin Name: *Chai Hu Shu Gan San*
Literal Name: Bupleurum Powder to Spread the Liver
Alternate Names: *Chai Hu Shu Gan Tang* (Bupleurum Decoction to Spread the Liver), Bupleurum and Cyperus Combination
Original Source: *Jing Yue Quan Shu* (Collected Treatises of [Zhang] Jing Yue) by Zhang Jie-Bin (Zhang Jing-Yue) in 1624

COMPOSITION

Chai Hu (Radix Bupleuri)	6g
Xiang Fu (Rhizoma Cyperi)	4.5g
Chen Pi (Pericarpium Citri Reticulatae), *chao* (dry-fried) with vinegar	6g
Zhi Qiao (Fructus Citri Aurantii), *chao* (dry-fried) with bran	4.5g
Bai Shao (Radix Paeoniae Alba)	4.5g
Chuan Xiong (Rhizoma Chuanxiong)	4.5g
Zhi Gan Cao (Radix et Rhizoma Glycyrrhizae Praeparata cum Melle)	1.5g

DOSAGE / PREPARATION / ADMINISTRATION

The source text states to cook the ingredients in 1.5 bowls of water until 80% of the liquid remains. Take the warm, strained decoction before meals.

CHINESE THERAPEUTIC ACTIONS

1. Regulates the Liver and promotes qi circulation
2. Harmonizes the blood and relieves pain

CLINICAL MANIFESTATIONS

Liver qi stagnation: hypochondriac pain, intermittent fever, trembling, restlessness, irritability, hyperactivity, poor digestion and abdominal pain.

VETERINARY CLINICAL APPLICATIONS

Cholecystitis, cholelithiasis, hepatitis, elevated liver enzymes, canine hyperadrenocorticism, gastritis, pancreatitis, peptic ulcer disease and mastitis.

EXPLANATION

Chai Hu Shu Gan San (Bupleurum Powder to Spread the Liver) treats Liver qi stagnation. The Liver is responsible for smoothing the qi flow in the body. If Liver qi is stagnant, pain may occur. Hypochondriac pain arises from Liver qi stagnation affecting the Liver channel, which runs through these regions of the body. The qi-smoothing function of the Liver is directly related to one's emotions. If Liver qi is stagnant, emotional disorders such as restlessness, hyperactivity and irritability occur. Liver qi stagnation may cause blood stagnation. Stagnation of Liver qi (wood element) can overact on the Spleen and Stomach (earth element), causing poor digestion and abdominal pain.

Chai Hu (Radix Bupleuri) harmonizes and spreads the Liver and relieves Liver qi stagnation. *Xiang Fu* (Rhizoma Cyperi) effectively breaks up Liver qi stagnation and relieves pain. *Chen Pi* (Pericarpium Citri Reticulatae) and

***Chai Hu Shu Gan San* (Bupleurum Powder to Spread the Liver)**

Diagnosis	Clinical Signs	Treatment	Herbs
Liver qi stagnation	• Hypochondriac pain: Liver qi stagnation along the Liver channel • Poor digestion, abdominal pain: Liver qi stagnation overacting on the Spleen and Stomach • Restlessness, hyperactivity and irritability: Liver qi stagnation affecting behavior	• Regulates the Liver and promotes qi circulation • Harmonizes the blood and relieves pain	• *Chai Hu* (Radix Bupleuri) harmonizes and spreads the Liver and relieves Liver qi stagnation. • *Xiang Fu* (Rhizoma Cyperi) breaks up Liver qi stagnation and relieves pain. • *Chen Pi* (Pericarpium Citri Reticulatae) and *Zhi Qiao* (Fructus Aurantii) activate qi circulation and break up qi stagnation. • *Bai Shao* (Radix Paeoniae Alba) nourishes Liver blood to soften the Liver. • *Chuan Xiong* (Rhizoma Chuanxiong) activates blood circulation. • *Zhi Gan Cao* (Radix et Rhizoma Glycyrrhizae Praeparata cum Melle) harmonizes the herbs and relieves pain.

Chái Hú Shū Gān Săn (Bupleurum Powder to Spread the Liver)

Zhi Qiao (Fructus Aurantii) activate qi circulation and break up qi stagnation. *Bai Shao* (Radix Paeoniae Alba) nourishes Liver blood to soften the Liver. *Chuan Xiong* (Rhizoma Chuanxiong) activates blood circulation. *Zhi Gan Cao* (Radix et Rhizoma Glycyrrhizae Praeparata cum Melle) harmonizes the herbs and relieves pain.

VETERINARY MODIFICATIONS

- With belching and acid reflux, add *Hai Piao Xiao* (Endoconcha Sepiae).
- If there is severe stomach pain, add *Yan Hu Suo* (Rhizoma Corydalis) and *Chuan Lian Zi* (Fructus Toosendan).
- For Liver qi stagnation that has turned into Liver fire, add *Zhi Zi* (Fructus Gardeniae) and *Chuan Lian Zi* (Fructus Toosendan).

CAUTIONS / CONTRAINDICATIONS

Chai Hu Shu Gan San is not recommended in patients with yin-deficient heat characterized by clinical signs such as a red tongue with no coating, a dry mouth and throat, restlessness, and insomnia. Similarly, this formula should be discontinued in those who develop these clinical signs after taking this formula.[1]

PHARMACOLOGICAL EFFECTS

1. **Cardiovascular**: Administration of *Chai Hu Shu Gan San* via intravenous injection in rabbits was associated with a marked improvement in blood circulation to various parts of the body, including the brain, heart, and liver.[2]
2. **Cholagogic**: Administration of *Chai Hu Shu Gan San* in rats was associated with increased production and release of bile acid after one hour.[3]

HUMAN CLINICAL STUDIES AND RESEARCH

1. **Cholecystitis**: One study reported complete recovery in 25 of 30 patients with chronic cholecystitis when treated with *Chai Hu Shu Gan San* plus *Qing Pi* (Pericarpium Citri Reticulatae Viride), *Yu Jin* (Radix Curcumae), *Yan Hu Suo* (Rhizoma Corydalis), *Hou Po* (Cortex Magnoliae Officinalis), *Jin Qian Cao* (Herba Lysimachiae), and *Yin Chen* (Herba Artemisiae Scopariae).[4] In another study, 132 patients with chronic cholecystitis were treated with complete recovery in 39 patients, significant improvement in 46 patients, moderate improvement in 40 patients, and no effect in 7 patients. In addition to *Chai Hu Shu Gan San*, modifications were made by adding *Yu Jin* (Radix Curcumae) and *Jin Ling Zi San* (Melia Toosendan Powder) for qi stagnation; *Jin Qian Cao* (Herba Lysimachiae), *Hu Zhang* (Rhizoma et Radix Polygoni Cuspidati), and *Huang Qin* (Radix Scutellariae) for damp-heat. Electro-acupuncture and herbal injection at acupuncture points were performed, too.[5]
2. **Cholelithiasis and bile duct infection**: One hundred and sixteen patients with gallstones and infection of the bile duct were treated with complete recovery in 27 patients, significant improvement in 68 patients, moderate improvement in 16 patients, and no benefit in 5 patients. The herbal formula was modified from *Chai Hu Shu Gan San*, with addition of *Jin Qian Cao* (Herba Lysimachiae), *Da Huang* (Radix et Rhizoma Rhei), *Yu Jin* (Radix Curcumae), *Shan Zha* (Fructus Crataegi), *Huang Qin* (Radix Scutellariae), *Qing Pi* (Pericarpium Citri Reticulatae Viride), and *Ji Nei Jin* (Endothelium Corneum Gigeriae Galli), and elimination of *Chuan Xiong* (Rhizoma Chuanxiong).[6]
3. **Hepatitis B**: Sixty patients with chronic hepatitis B were treated with good results using modified *Chai Hu Shu Gan San*. The herbal formula contained *Chai Hu* (Radix Bupleuri) 10g, dry-fried *Bai Zhu* (Rhizoma Atractylodis Macrocephalae) 10g, *Zhi Shi* (Fructus Aurantii Immaturus) 10g, *Fu Ling* (Poria) 12g, *Yu Jin* (Radix Curcumae) 12g, *Bai Jiang Cao* (Herba cum Radice Patriniae) 12g, *Dan Shen* (Radix et Rhizoma Salviae Miltiorrhizae) 20g, *Bai Hua She She Cao* (Herba Hedyotis) 15g, *Chi Shao* (Radix Paeoniae Rubra) 15g, and others as needed. The herbs were given in decoction daily 1 to 2 hours after a meal. Of 60 patients, the study reported recovery in 12 patients, improvement in 46 patients, and no improvement in 2 patients. The overall rate of effectiveness was 96%.[7]
4. **Atrophic gastritis**: Thirty-nine patients with atrophic gastritis reported good results using modified *Chai Hu Shu Gan San*. The herbal formula contained *Chai Hu* (Radix Bupleuri) 12g, *Zhi Qiao* (Fructus Aurantii) 12g, *Xiang Fu* (Rhizoma Cyperi) 12g, *Bai Shao* (Radix Paeoniae Alba) 15g, *Chuan Xiong* (Rhizoma Chuanxiong) 10g, *Gan Cao* (Radix et Rhizoma Glycyrrhizae) 6g, *Yan Hu Suo* (Rhizoma Corydalis) 10g, *Chuan Lian Zi* (Fructus Toosendan) 6g, *Mu Xiang* (Radix Aucklandiae) 6g, *Dan Shen* (Radix et Rhizoma Salviae Miltiorrhizae) 15g, *Yu Jin* (Radix Curcumae) 15g, *Ban Xia* (Rhizoma Pinelliae) 10g, *Chen Pi* (Pericarpium Citri Reticulatae) 10g, charred *Shan Zha* (Fructus Crataegi) 15g, charred *Shen Qu* (Massa Fermentata) 15g, and charred *Mai Ya* (Fructus Hordei Germinatus) 15g. The study reported complete recovery in 23 of 39 patients.[8]
5. **Peptic ulcer disease**: Use of modified *Chai Hu Shu Gan San* was associated with beneficial effects in treating gastric or duodenal ulcers. The herbal formula was modified from *Chai Hu Shu Gan San*, with the removal of *Chuan Xiong* (Rhizoma Chuanxiong), and the addition of *Bai Ji* (Rhizoma Bletillae), *Sha Ren* (Fructus Amomi), *Xuan Shen* (Radix Scrophulariae), and *Pu Gong Ying* (Herba Taraxaci). The duration of treatment ranged from 3 to 12 packs of herbs.[9]

Chái Hú Shū Gān Săn (Bupleurum Powder to Spread the Liver)

6. **Male sexual dysfunction**: Use of modified *Chai Hu Shu Gan San* was effective in treating 17 of 19 patients who were unable to ejaculate. The herbal treatment contained *Chai Hu Shu Gan San* plus *Ju He* (Semen Citri Reticulatae), *Shi Chang Pu* (Rhizoma Acori Tatarinowii), *Chuan Shan Jia* (Squama Manis), *Mu Tong* (Caulis Akebiae), *Hu Po* (Succinum), and others as needed.[10]
7. **Orchitis**: One study reported complete recovery in 32 of 37 patients with orchitis, when treated with an herbal formula that contained *Chai Hu Shu Gan San* plus *Huang Qin* (Radix Scutellariae), *Wu Yao* (Radix Linderae), *Tao Ren* (Semen Persicae), *Xiao Hui Xiang* (Fructus Foeniculi), *Ju He* (Semen Citri Reticulatae), *Bai Jiang Cao* (Herba cum Radice Patriniae), and others.[11]
8. **Breast distention and pain**: Complete relief of breast distention and pain was reported in 21 of 24 patients who were treated with modified *Chai Hu Shu Gan San*. The herbal formula contained *Chai Hu* (Radix Bupleuri) 12g, *Bai Shao* (Radix Paeoniae Alba) 12g, vinegar-fried *Chen Pi* (Pericarpium Citri Reticulatae) 10g, *Chuan Xiong* (Rhizoma Chuanxiong) 10g, *Xiang Fu* (Rhizoma Cyperi) 10g, dry-fried *Zhi Qiao* (Fructus Aurantii) 10g, *Yu Jin* (Radix Curcumae) 10g, *Tong Cao* (Medulla Tetrapanacis) 10g, *Bai Zhi* (Radix Angelicae Dahuricae) 10g, processed *Ru Xiang* (Gummi Olibanum) 10g, processed *Mo Yao* (Myrrha) 10g, *Pu Gong Ying* (Herba Taraxaci) 15g, and *Gan Cao* (Radix et Rhizoma Glycyrrhizae) 6g. The treatment protocol was to cook the herbs in water, and administer the decoction in three equally-divided doses daily, for 7 days per course of treatment.[12]
9. **Insomnia**: One study reported 96.7% effectiveness using modified *Chai Hu Shu Gan San* to treat patients with stubborn insomnia. The treatment protocol was to use this formula as the base, with the addition of *Chi Shao* (Radix Paeoniae Rubra) and *Dan Shen* (Radix et Rhizoma Salviae Miltiorrhizae) for blood stagnation; *Ju Hua* (Flos Chrysanthemi) and *Zhi Zi* (Fructus Gardeniae) for Liver excess; and *Dan Nan Xing* (Arisaema cum Bile) and *Shi Chang Pu* (Rhizoma Acori Tatarinowii) for phlegm accumulation. Of 30 patients, the study reported complete recovery in 26 patients, improvement in 3 patients, and no effect in one patient.[13]

SUGGESTED ACUPUNCTURE TREATMENT

1. Points: *Yangchi* (TH 4), *Neiguan* (PC 6), *Gongsun* (SP 4), *Xingjian* (LR 2), *Housanli* (ST 36), *Sanyinjiao* (SP 6), *Qimen* (LR 14), *Ganshu* (BL 18), *Xiaxi* (GB 43), *Zhongting* (CV 16) and *Ganshu* (equine).
2. Technique: sedation.

Yangchi (TH 4) regulates the qi flow of the *shaoyang* and raises yang qi to increase its circulation. *Neiguan* (PC 6) and *Gongsun* (SP 4) are used according to the *ba hui* (eight meeting) points principle to relieve chest congestion and remove stagnation. *Xingjian* (LR 2) regulates Liver qi. *Zusanli* (ST 36) and *Sanyinjiao* (SP 6) tonify qi, strengthen the Spleen, and nourish yin and blood. Lastly, *Qimen* (LR 14), *Ganshu* (BL 18), *Xiaxi* (GB 43), and *Zhongting* (CV 16) regulate qi circulation, smooth Liver qi, and relieve pain. *Ganshu* (equine) is a classical equine point that is effective for treating liver qi stagnation. [Note: *Ganshu* (equine) in horses is not the same as *Ganshu* (BL 18) in human, although the pinyin names are the same. *Ganshu* (equine), a classical point also known as *Ganzhishu*, is the Liver *shu* (transport) point in horses. It is located in the 13th intercostals space along a line from the shoulder to the hip joint.]

AUTHORS' COMMENTS

Chai Hu Shu Gan San is the basic formula for treating Liver qi stagnation. Many other formulas that treat Liver qi stagnation are formulated from it, modified to fit the patient's condition. It can be used to help normalize elevated liver enzymes in the absence of other abnormal laboratory values with appropriate clinical signs. It is often used to treat dogs with canine Cushing's disease (hyperadrenocorticism). Liver qi stagnation commonly disrupts the digestion, emotional balance, and qi and blood circulation of these animals. As liver qi stagnation is pervasive throughout all stages of the disease, *Chai Hu Shu Gan San* has evolved as an important formula to help effectively manage hyperadrenocorticism in these cases.

For poor appetite, belching, flatulence, loose stool and abdominal pain due to disharmony between the Stomach and Liver in the dog, add *Shen Ling Bai Zhu San* (Ginseng, Poria, and Atractylodes Macrocephala Powder). For poor digestion with irritability, restlessness and hyperactivity, combine with *Gui Pi Tang* (Restore the Spleen Decoction). For acute cholangiohepatitis in the cat, combine with *Yin Chen Hao Tang* (Artemisia Scoparia Decoction).

In the horse, Liver qi stagnation is also associated with pain in the girth area and behavioral problems, especially when being ridden and during estrus. If discomfort is the biggest problem, combining the formula with *Shao Fu Zhu Yu Tang* (Drive Out Blood Stasis in the Lower Abdomen Decoction) is helpful. If behavioral issues are more of a concern, combining with *Chai Hu Jia Long Gu Mu Li Tang* (Bupleurum plus Dragon Bone and Oyster Shell Decoction) is often very successful.

Chái Hú Shū Gān Săn (Bupleurum Powder to Spread the Liver)

Chai Hu Shu Gan San is a variation of *Si Ni San* (Frigid Extremities Powder). Although the herbs in these two formulas are similar, their doses and emphases are different.

- *Si Ni San* treats both Spleen qi deficiency and obstructed circulation of Liver and Gallbladder qi. *Chai Hu* (Radix Bupleuri) and *Zhi Shi* (Fructus Aurantii Immaturus) are the only qi-moving herbs in this formula. *Zhi Gan Cao* (Radix et Rhizoma Glycyrrhizae Praeparata cum Melle) is used at a high dose to tonify qi and strengthen the Spleen.
- *Chai Hu Shu Gan San* mainly treats Liver qi stagnation, and contains many qi- and blood-moving herbs, such as *Chai Hu* (Radix Bupleuri), *Zhi Qiao* (Fructus Aurantii), *Chen Pi* (Pericarpium Citri Reticulatae), *Chuan Xiong* (Rhizoma Chuanxiong), and *Xiang Fu* (Rhizoma Cyperi). *Zhi Gan Cao* (Radix et Rhizoma Glycyrrhizae Praeparata cum Melle) is used at a low dose for harmonizing purposes.

References

1. *Zhong Yao Ming Fang Yao Li Yu Ying Yong* (Pharmacology and Applications of Famous Herbal Formulas), 1989; 112-113.
2. *Zhong Yao Yao Li Yu Lin Chuang* (Pharmacology and Clinical Applications of Chinese Herbs), 1987; 4(4):17.
3. *Shi Yong Zhong Yi Nei Ke Za Zhi* (Journal of Practical Chinese Internal Medicine), 1989; 3(1):11.
4. *Shan Xi Zhong Yi* (Shanxi Chinese Medicine), 1990; 11(3):128.
5. *Gan Su Zhong Yi Xue Yuan Xue Bao* (Journal of Gansu University of Chinese Medicine), 1995; 2:37.
6. *Shi Yong Zhong Xi Yi Jie He Za Zhi* (Practical Journal of Integrated Chinese and Western Medicines), 1991; 4(10):618.
7. *Zhong Yi Yao Xue Bao* (Report of Chinese Medicine and Herbology), 1992; 6:38.
8. *Shan Xi Zhong Yi* (Shanxi Chinese Medicine), 1995; 16(1):28.
9. *Hei Long Jiang Zhong Yi Yao* (Heilongjiang Chinese Medicine and Herbology), 1987; 1:41.
10. *Zhe Jiang Zhong Yi Za Zhi* (Zhejiang Journal of Chinese Medicine), 1990; 25(6):253.
11. *Shan Xi Zhong Yi* (Shanxi Chinese Medicine), 1993; 14(2):54.
12. *Guang Xi Zhong Yi Yao* (Guangxi Chinese Medicine and Herbology), 1985; 8(2):21.
13. *Zhong Yi Ming Fang Lin Chuang Xin Yong* (Contemporary Clinical Applications of Classic Chinese Formulas), 2001; 575.

3 HARMONIZING FORMULAS

Shū Gān Tāng (Spread the Liver Decoction)

疏肝湯

疏肝汤

Pinyin Name: *Shu Gan Tang*
Literal Name: Spread the Liver Decoction
Alternate Name: Bupleurum and Evodia Combination
Original Source: *Wan Bing Hui Chun* (Restoration of Health from the Myriad Diseases) by Gong Ting-Xian in 1587

COMPOSITION

Chai Hu (Radix Bupleuri)	3g
Qing Pi (Pericarpium Citri Reticulatae Viride)	3g
Zhi Qiao (Fructus Aurantii)	3g
Tao Ren (Semen Persicae)	3g
Hong Hua (Flos Carthami)	1.5g
Dang Gui (Radix Angelicae Sinensis)	3g
Chuan Xiong (Rhizoma Chuanxiong)	2.1g
Bai Shao (Radix Paeoniae Alba)	2.1g
Huang Lian (Rhizoma Coptidis), *chao* (dry-fried)	6g

DOSAGE / PREPARATION / ADMINISTRATION

The source text specifies to first dry-fry *Huang Lian* (Rhizoma Coptidis) with the juice of *Wu Zhu Yu* (Fructus Evodiae). Then, grind all of the ingredients into powder and cook in water to make a decoction. Take the warm, strained decoction after meals.

Shū Gān Tāng (Spread the Liver Decoction)

CHINESE THERAPEUTIC ACTIONS

1. Regulates blood circulation and eliminates blood stasis
2. Opens the channels and collaterals and relieves pain

CLINICAL MANIFESTATIONS

Liver qi stagnation with blood stasis: hypochondriac pain and intermittent fever and trembling, poor appetite, nausea, vomiting, belching and poor digestion.

VETERINARY CLINICAL APPLICATIONS

Pain in the ribcage (hypochondrium) secondary to vehicular trauma or bite wounds, abdominal bloating, anorexia, nausea, vomiting, chronic hepatitis, chronic vomiting in the cat, recovery stage of feline hepatic lipidosis, recovery from acute pancreatitis and chronic pancreatitis.

EXPLANATION

Shu Gan Tang (Spread the Liver Decoction) treats hypochondriac pain caused by Liver qi stagnation with blood stasis. The classic text describes this condition as being characterized by pain in the hypochondrium, poor appetite, nausea, vomiting, belching and poor digestion. This condition may also develop secondary to internal or external injuries. Internal injuries include pancreatitis, and external injuries include trauma and contusion.

Because the fundamental disorder is Liver qi stagnation, *Chai Hu* (Radix Bupleuri) is used to treat the *shaoyang* syndrome and to spread Liver qi. *Qing Pi* (Pericarpium Citri Reticulatae Viride) and *Zhi Qiao* (Fructus Aurantii) regulate qi and, together with *Chai Hu* (Radix Bupleuri), relieve hypochondriac pain and fullness. Since qi and blood stagnations often occur together, blood movers are added to enhance the overall effect. *Tao Ren* (Semen Persicae) and *Hong Hua* (Flos Carthami) move the blood, eliminate blood stagnation, and relieve pain. *Dang Gui* (Radix Angelicae Sinensis) nourishes the blood and, with *Chuan Xiong* (Rhizoma Chuanxiong), moves the blood. *Dang Gui* (Radix Angelicae Sinensis) and *Bai Shao* (Radix Paeoniae Alba) soften the Liver by tonifying yin and blood. *Bai Shao* (Radix Paeoniae Alba) is one of the key herbs used to relax the muscles and relieve spasms and pain. Because Liver qi stagnation can easily turn into Liver heat and fire, *Huang Lian* (Rhizoma Coptidis) clears heat and fire. Lastly, *Wu Zhu Yu* (Fructus Evodiae) acts as a guiding herb to lead the therapeutic effect of the entire formula to the affected area.

SUGGESTED ACUPUNCTURE TREATMENT

1. Points: *Waiguan* (TH 5), *Qiuxu* (GB 40), *Qimen* (LR 14), *Xuehai* (SP 10), *Sanyinjiao* (SP 6), *Geshu* (BL 17), *Taichong* (LR 3), *Zhongwan* (CV 12) and *Ganshu* (equine).
2. Technique: sedation.

Waiguan (TH 5), *Qiuxu* (GB 40), and *Qimen* (LR 14) soothe the Liver, invigorate qi, relieve pain, and harmonize *shaoyang*; sedation on *Xuehai* (SP 10), *Sanyinjiao* (SP 6), and *Geshu* (BL 17) invigorates the blood and removes stagnation; sedation on *Taichong* (LR 3) and *Zhongwan* (CV 12) sedates Liver fire, harmonizes the Stomach, and relieves belching. *Ganshu* (equine) is a classical equine point that is effective for treating liver qi stagnation. [Note: *Ganshu* (equine) in horses is not the same as *Ganshu* (BL 18) in humans, although the pinyin names are the same.

***Shu Gan Tang* (Spread the Liver Decoction)**

Diagnosis	Clinical Signs	Treatment	Herbs
Liver qi stagnation with blood stasis	• Hypochondriac pain, poor appetite, nausea, vomiting, belching and poor digestion: Liver qi stagnation with blood stasis • Intermittent fever and trembling: *shaoyang* syndrome	• Regulates blood circulation and eliminates blood stasis • Opens the channels and collaterals and relieves pain	• *Chai Hu* (Radix Bupleuri) regulates Liver qi and spreads Liver qi stagnation. • *Qing Pi* (Pericarpium Citri Reticulatae Viride) and *Zhi Qiao* (Fructus Aurantii) regulate qi and relieve hypochondriac pain and fullness. • *Tao Ren* (Semen Persicae) and *Hong Hua* (Flos Carthami) move the blood, eliminate blood stagnation, and relieve pain. • *Dang Gui* (Radix Angelicae Sinensis) and *Chuan Xiong* (Rhizoma Chuanxiong) nourish the blood and regulate blood circulation. • *Dang Gui* (Radix Angelicae Sinensis) and *Bai Shao* (Radix Paeoniae Alba) tonify yin and blood to soften the Liver. • *Huang Lian* (Rhizoma Coptidis) clears heat and fire. • *Wu Zhu Yu* (Fructus Evodiae) guides the formula to the affected area.

Shū Gān Tāng (Spread the Liver Decoction)

Ganshu (equine), a classical point also known as *Ganzhishu*, is the Liver *shu* (transport) point in horses. It is located in the 13th intercostal space along a line from the shoulder to the hip joint.]

AUTHORS' COMMENTS

Shu Gan Tang is commonly used to treat the recovery stage of acute pancreatitis and chronic pancreatitis in the dog and cat. A course of treatment is typically 10 to 21 days. It also is effective in treating the recovery stage of hepatic lipidosis in the cat. It has application in the recovery of gastrointestinal ulceration and pain secondary to aspirin and non-steroidal anti-inflammatory drug use. It is a good choice to treat vomiting and poor appetite in the cat when Liver qi stagnation is affecting digestion. To treat ribcage pain secondary to trauma or bite wounds, it can be combined with *Xue Fu Zhu Yu Tang* (Drive Out Stasis in the Mansion of Blood Decoction). It is also applicable in horses with recurrent colic where gastric ulceration is initially suspected but endoscopic exam is normal. There are many different patent formulations on the market with variable ability to dredge the Liver, drain dampness, and move the blood.

Chai Hu Shu Gan Tang (Bupleurum Decoction to Spread the Liver) and *Shu Gan Tang* both treat Liver qi stagnation with blood stasis.

- *Chai Hu Shu Gan Tang* places more emphasis on activating qi circulation.
- *Shu Gan Tang* focuses more on invigorating blood circulation and eliminating blood stasis.

Chái Hú Qīng Gān Tāng (Bupleurum Decoction to Clear the Liver)

柴胡清肝湯

柴胡清肝汤

Pinyin Name: *Chai Hu Qing Gan Tang*
Literal Name: Bupleurum Decoction to Clear the Liver
Alternate Names: *Tsai Hu Ching Kan Tang*, Bupleurum Liver-Clearing Decoction, Bupleurum and Rehmannia Combination
Original Source: *Yi Guan Tang* (Linking Clinic)

COMPOSITION

Huang Qin (Radix Scutellariae)	3g
Huang Lian (Rhizoma Coptidis)	3g
Huang Bo (Cortex Phellodendri Chinensis)	3g
Zhi Zi (Fructus Gardeniae)	4.5g
Di Huang (Radix Rehmanniae)	4.5g
Dang Gui (Radix Angelicae Sinensis)	6g
Bai Shao (Radix Paeoniae Alba)	4.5g
Chuan Xiong (Rhizoma Chuanxiong)	3g
Chai Hu (Radix Bupleuri)	4.5g
Jie Geng (Radix Platycodonis)	3g
Niu Bang Zi (Fructus Arctii)	4.5g
Lian Qiao (Fructus Forsythiae)	6g
Tian Hua Fen (Radix Trichosanthis)	3g
Bo He (Herba Menthae)	3g
Gan Cao (Radix et Rhizoma Glycyrrhizae)	3g

DOSAGE / PREPARATION / ADMINISTRATION

Prepare the ingredients as a decoction.

CHINESE THERAPEUTIC ACTIONS

Clears heat from the Liver, Gallbladder, and *San Jiao* channels

Chái Hú Qīng Gān Tāng (Bupleurum Decoction to Clear the Liver)

CLINICAL MANIFESTATIONS

Heat in the Liver, Gallbladder, and *San Jiao* channels: fever, chills, epistaxis, itching, loss of hearing, swelling of the lymph nodes, and cellulitis.

VETERINARY CLINICAL APPLICATIONS

Lymphadenopathy with fever, puppy strangles, equine strangles and other submandibular lymphadenopathy, acute otitis media, otitis interna, systemic lupus erythematosus, food allergy dermatitis, atopy, pododermatitis, fly-bite dermatitis, cellulitis, temporal dermatitis in the cat, acute cholangiohepatitis, chronic anal sacculitis and vaginitis.

EXPLANATION

Chai Hu Qing Gan Tang (Bupleurum Decoction to Clear the Liver) clears heat in the Liver, Gallbladder, and *San Jiao* channels, characterized by clinical signs such as fever, trembling, epistaxis, loss of hearing, and swelling of the lymph nodes. Clinically, this formula is especially effective for juvenile, chronically ill and geriatric patients. Long-term use of this formula improves the physical condition of such patients and helps balance their underlying body constitution.

This formula is a modified combination of *Huang Lian Jie Du Tang* (Coptis Decoction to Relieve Toxicity) and *Si Wu Tang* (Four-Substance Decoction). *Huang Qin* (Radix Scutellariae), *Huang Lian* (Rhizoma Coptidis), *Huang Bo* (Cortex Phellodendri Chinensis), and *Zhi Zi* (Fructus Gardeniae), the four herbs in *Huang Lian Jie Du Tang* (Coptis Decoction to Relieve Toxicity), eliminate excess fire in the upper, middle, and lower *jiaos*. *Di Huang* (Radix Rehmanniae), *Dang Gui* (Radix Angelicae Sinensis), *Bai Shao* (Radix Paeoniae Alba), and *Chuan Xiong* (Rhizoma Chuanxiong), four herbs that follow the principles of *Si Wu Tang* (Four-Substance Decoction), cool the heat and moisten dryness in the blood. *Chai Hu* (Radix Bupleuri) is added as a channel-guiding herb to direct the formula to the Liver and Gallbladder. *Jie Geng* (Radix Platycodonis) clears heat from the head, eyes, throat, and chest. *Niu Bang Zi* (Fructus Arctii) and *Lian Qiao* (Fructus Forsythiae) clear heat from the Lung, benefit the throat, and dispel heat from the skin. *Tian Hua Fen* (Radix Trichosanthis) promotes the secretion of body fluids, reduces swelling, and discharges pus. *Bo He* (Herba Menthae) clears heat and relieves Liver qi stagnation. *Gan Cao* (Radix et Rhizoma Glycyrrhizae) harmonizes the formula.

***Chai Hu Qing Gan Tang* (Bupleurum Decoction to Clear the Liver)**

Diagnosis	Clinical Signs	Treatment	Herbs
Heat in the Liver, Gallbladder, and *San Jiao* channels	Fever, trembling, epistaxis, loss of hearing, dermatitis and swelling of the lymph nodes: heat in the Liver, Gallbladder, and *San Jiao* channels	Clears heat from the Liver, Gallbladder, and *San Jiao* channels	• *Huang Qin* (Radix Scutellariae), *Huang Lian* (Rhizoma Coptidis), *Huang Bo* (Cortex Phellodendri Chinensis), and *Zhi Zi* (Fructus Gardeniae) clear heat and purge fire from the entire body. • *Shu Di Huang* (Radix Rehmanniae Praeparata), *Dang Gui* (Radix Angelicae Sinensis), *Bai Shao* (Radix Paeoniae Alba), and *Chuan Xiong* (Rhizoma Chuanxiong) tonify the blood and activate blood circulation. • *Chai Hu* (Radix Bupleuri) guides the formula to the Liver and Gallbladder. • *Jie Geng* (Radix Platycodonis) clears heat from the head, eyes, throat, and chest. • *Niu Bang Zi* (Fructus Arctii) and *Lian Qiao* (Fructus Forsythiae) clear heat from the Lung, benefit the throat, and dispel heat from the skin. • *Tian Hua Fen* (Radix Trichosanthis) promotes the secretion of body fluids, reduces swelling, and discharges pus. • *Bo He* (Herba Menthae) clears heat and relieves Liver qi stagnation. • *Gan Cao* (Radix et Rhizoma Glycyrrhizae) harmonizes the formula.

Cháí Hú Qīng Gān Tāng (Bupleurum Decoction to Clear the Liver)

VETERINARY MODIFICATIONS

- For inner ear infections, combine with *Qing Bi Tang* (Clear the Nose Decoction).
- With enlarged, swollen lymph nodes, add *Xia Ku Cao* (Spica Prunellae), *Xuan Shen* (Radix Scrophulariae) and *Mu Dan Pi* (Cortex Moutan).
- For damp-heat dermatitis, add *Jia Wei Xiao Yao San* (Augmented Rambling Powder).

PHARMACOLOGICAL EFFECTS

Hepatoprotective and choleretic: Administration of *Chai Hu Qing Gan Tang* showed beneficial effects on the liver and gallbladder in rats. It had protective effects against experimental cholestasis induced by carbon tetrachloride or alpha-naphthylisothiocyanate, and a protective effect against the alterations of serum components, such as SGOT, SGPT, alkaline phosphatase and the concentration of serum bilirubin. The study concluded that *Chai Hu Qing Gan Tang* had choleretic effect to treat cholestasis and hepatoprotective effect to prevent liver parenchymal injury.[1]

SUGGESTED ACUPUNCTURE TREATMENT

1. Points: *Xingjian* (LR 2), *Quchi* (LI 11), *Neiting* (ST 44), *Zhigou* (TH 6), *Sanyinjiao* (SP 6), *Lieque* (LU 7), *Chize* (LU 5), *Taichong* (LR 3), *Waiguan* (TH 5), and *Ganshu* (BL 18).
2. Technique: sedation

Xingjian (LR 2), *Quchi* (LI 11), *Zhigou* (TH 6), and *Neiting* (ST 44) purge fire. *Sanyinjiao* (SP 6) nourishes the blood to moisten dryness. *Lieque* (LU 7) and *Chize* (LU 5) clear Lung heat. *Taichong* (LR 3), *Waiguan* (TH 5), and *Ganshu* (BL 18) soothe the Liver and disperse stagnation.

RELATED FORMULA

Chái Hú Qīng Gān Tāng
(Bupleurum Decoction to Clear the Liver)
柴胡清肝湯
柴胡清肝汤
Pinyin Name: *Chai Hu Qing Gan Tang*
Literal Name: Bupleurum Decoction to Clear the Liver
Original Source: *Wai Ke Zheng Zong* (True Lineage of External Medicine) by Chen Shi-Gong in 1617

Chai Hu (Radix Bupleuri)	4.5g
Di Huang (Radix Rehmanniae)	4.5g
Chi Shao (Radix Paeoniae Rubra)	4.5g
Niu Bang Zi (Fructus Arctii)	4.5g
Dang Gui (Radix Angelicae Sinensis)	6g
Lian Qiao (Fructus Forsythiae)	6g
Chuan Xiong (Rhizoma Chuanxiong)	3g
Huang Qin (Radix Scutellariae)	3g
Zhi Zi (Fructus Gardeniae)	3g
Tian Hua Fen (Radix Trichosanthis)	3g
Gan Cao (Radix et Rhizoma Glycyrrhizae)	3g
Fang Feng (Radix Saposhnikoviae)	3g

Cook the herbs in 2 cups of water until the liquid is reduced to 1.6 cups. Take the warm, strained decoction after meals. Note: Another source states to use *Bai Shao* (Radix Paeoniae Alba) in place of *Chi Shao* (Radix Paeoniae Rubra), and equal amounts (3g) of all of the ingredients. This formula treats Liver fire rising, causing the formation of sores and ulcers in the temple area of the head.

These two formulas have the exact same names and very similar functions, but are from different original sources.

- *Chai Hu Qing Gan Tang* from *Yi Guan Tang* (Linking Clinic) is a colder formula that strongly clears heat from the Liver, Gallbladder, and *San Jiao* channels.
- *Chai Hu Qing Gan Tang* from *Wai Ke Zheng Zong* (True Lineage of External Medicine) is not as cold, and has been used historically for early-stage sores and ulcers in the temple area of the head.

AUTHORS' COMMENTS

Chai Hu Qing Gan Tang and *Long Dan Xie Gan Tang* (Gentiana Decoction to Drain the Liver) both treat Liver-Gallbladder heat or fire.

- *Chai Hu Qing Gan Tang* also clears heat from the *san jiao* channels. It is used for less severe Liver fire patterns and thus can be given for a longer period of time. It can be combined with a tonic for the middle *jiao* to extend its use even longer. For animals that are young or weak, this formula is more appropriate.
- *Long Dan Xie Gan Tang* clears heat and in addition drains dampness; it is better for acute damp-heat and severe Liver-fire patterns and is not for long-term use without modification. It should not be used in animals with deficiency of the middle *jiao* or that are yin deficient.

Reference

1. Sasaki T, Ohta S, Kamogawa A, Shinoda M. Protective effects of various Chinese traditional medicines against experimental cholestasis. Chem Pharm Bull (Tokyo). 1990 Feb; 38(2):513-6.

Yì Gān Sǎn (Restrain the Liver Powder)

抑肝散

抑肝散

Pinyin Name: *Yi Gan San*
Literal Name: Restrain the Liver Powder
Alternate Names: *I Kan San,* Liver-Repressing Formula, Bupleurum Formula
Original Source: *Bao Ying Cuo Yao* (Synopsis of Caring for Infants) by Xue Kai in 1555

COMPOSITION

Chai Hu (Radix Bupleuri)	1.5g
Gou Teng (Ramulus Uncariae cum Uncis)	3g
Dang Gui (Radix Angelicae Sinensis)	3g
Chuan Xiong (Rhizoma Chuanxiong)	2.4g
Bai Zhu (Rhizoma Atractylodis Macrocephalae), *chao* (dry-fried)	3g
Fu Ling (Poria)	3g
Gan Cao (Radix et Rhizoma Glycyrrhizae)	1.5g

DOSAGE / PREPARATION / ADMINISTRATION

Prepare the ingredients as a decoction.

CHINESE THERAPEUTIC ACTIONS

1. Calms the Liver and clears Liver heat
2. Nourishes Liver blood and strengthens the Spleen

CLINICAL MANIFESTATIONS

Liver blood deficiency accompanied by Liver heat: fever, being easily frightened, muscle spasms and contraction, nervousness, irritability, aggression, restlessness, seizures, and intermittent fever and trembling. Animals may also vomit saliva and sputum.

VETERINARY CLINICAL APPLICATIONS

Behavioral disorders, poor digestion, aggression, irritability, restlessness and pacing at night, and epilepsy.

EXPLANATION

Yi Gan San (Restrain the Liver Powder) treats Liver blood deficiency accompanied by Liver heat. Liver heat rising leads to emotional instability, causing clinical manifestations such as irritability, excitability, nervousness, and seizures. Clinically, animals will show signs of deficiency and excess simultaneously. Liver blood deficiency is characterized by muscle spasms and contraction, being easily frightened or scared; the excess is characterized by nervousness, irritability, aggression, and restlessness at night with pacing. In addition, if the Liver overacts on the Spleen and Stomach, patients will show clinical signs such as epigastric and abdominal discomfort and bloating, lack of appetite, and vomiting of saliva and sputum.

To address the complicated situation of deficiency and excess, herbs are selected to nourish the blood, clear Liver fire, and harmonize the Liver, Spleen, and Stomach. The

***Yi Gan San* (Restrain the Liver Powder)**

Diagnosis	Clinical Signs	Treatment	Herbs
Liver blood deficiency accompanied by Liver heat rising	• Emotional instability, irritability, excitability, restlessness, nervousness, seizures: Liver heat rising • Muscle spasms and contraction, easily frightened or scared: Liver blood deficiency • Epigastric and abdominal discomfort or distention, lack of appetite, and vomiting of saliva and sputum: Liver overacting on the Spleen and Stomach	• Calms the Liver and clears Liver heat • Nourishes Liver blood and strengthens the Spleen	• *Chai Hu* (Radix Bupleuri) and *Gou Teng* (Ramulus Uncariae cum Uncis) calm the Liver and clear Liver heat. • *Dang Gui* (Radix Angelicae Sinensis) and *Chuan Xiong* (Rhizoma Chuanxiong) nourish Liver blood and soften the Liver. • *Bai Zhu* (Rhizoma Atractylodis Macrocephalae) and *Fu Ling* (Poria) strengthen the Spleen. • *Gan Cao* (Radix et Rhizoma Glycyrrhizae) harmonizes the herbs.

Yì Gān Săn (Restrain the Liver Powder)

Liver must first be calmed and Liver heat cleared. Liver blood should also be nourished and the Spleen strengthened to prevent wood from overacting on earth. This formula contains *Chai Hu* (Radix Bupleuri) and *Gou Teng* (Ramulus Uncariae cum Uncis) to calm the Liver and clear Liver heat. *Dang Gui* (Radix Angelicae Sinensis) and *Chuan Xiong* (Rhizoma Chuanxiong) nourish Liver blood and soften the Liver. *Bai Zhu* (Rhizoma Atractylodis Macrocephalae) and *Fu Ling* (Poria) strengthen the Spleen. *Gan Cao* (Radix et Rhizoma Glycyrrhizae) harmonizes the herbs.

VETERINARY MODIFICATIONS

- For both qi and blood deficiencies, add *Ren Shen* (Radix et Rhizoma Ginseng), *Huang Qi* (Radix Astragali), *Bai Shao* (Radix Paeoniae Alba), *Shu Di Huang* (Radix Rehmanniae Praeparata), and *Di Huang* (Radix Rehmanniae).
- With restless sleep, irritability and insomnia, add *Suan Zao Ren* (Semen Ziziphi Spinosae) and *Bai Zi Ren* (Semen Platycladi).
- With vomiting of sputum and saliva, add *Wen Dan Tang* (Warm the Gallbladder Decoction).
- With disturbed *shen* (spirit), add *Bai Shao* (Radix Paeoniae Alba) and *Suan Zao Ren* (Semen Ziziphi Spinosae).

PHARMACOLOGICAL EFFECTS

Antidepressive and antinociceptive: Administration of *Yi Gan San*, *Bu Zhong Yi Qi Tang* (Tonify the Middle and Augment the Qi Decoction) and *Chai Hu Jia Long Gu Mu Li Tang* (Bupleurum plus Dragon Bone and Oyster Shell Decoction) for 14 consecutive days showed both antidepressive and antinociceptive properties in mice.[1]

SUGGESTED ACUPUNCTURE TREATMENT

1. Points: *Xuehai* (SP 10), *Sanyinjiao* (SP 6), *Taichong* (LR 3), *Yanglingquan* (GB 34), *Neiguan* (PC 6), *Shenmen* (HT 7) and *Dafengmen*.
2. Technique: tonification and sedation.

This condition is characterized by Liver heat rising. The treatment priority, therefore, is to clear Liver heat and nourish Liver blood to calm the yang. *Xuehai* (SP 10) and *Sanyinjiao* (SP 6) nourish Liver blood. *Taichong* (LR 3) clears Liver heat. In addition, the combination of *Taichong* (LR 3) and *Yanglingquan* (GB 34), the *he* (uniting) point of the Gallbladder channel, clears Liver heat and relieves muscle spasms. *Neiguan* (PC 6) regulates qi and corrects the reversed flow of qi. *Shenmen* (HT 7) tranquilizes the mind and relieves insomnia. *Dafengmen* is a classical point in both the dog and horse and is used to treat *shen* (spirit) disturbances and relieve anxiety.

AUTHORS' COMMENTS

Yi Gan San was originally formulated to treat Liver blood deficiency accompanied by Liver heat. It can be used to treat behavioral disorder in dogs and horses characterized by irritability and aggression, in combination with *Tian Wang Bu Xin Dan* (Emperor of Heaven's Special Pill to Tonify the Heart) or *Yang Xin Tang* (Nourish the Heart Decoction). This formula can be given before bedtime to tranquilize the *shen* (spirit) to stop pacing and restlessness at night in older dogs and in cats with hyperthyroidism. It can be used to treat epilepsy in dogs in combination with *Ban Xia Bai Zhu Tian Ma Tang* (Pinellia, Atractylodes Macrocephala, and Gastrodia Decoction). Mares, who may show severe irritability during estrus if they are also Liver blood deficient, may be administered this formula combined with *Tao Hong Si Wu Tang* (Four-Substance Decoction with Safflower and Peach Pit). This combination has the added benefit of moving blood and can help with the ovarian pain that can accompany this syndrome.

Reference

1. Koshikawa N, Imai T, Takahashi I, Yamauchi M, Sawada S, Kansaku A. Effects of Hochu-ekki-to, Yoku-kan-san and Saiko-ka-ryukotsu-borei-to on behavioral despair and acetic acid-induced writhing in mice. Methods Find Exp Clin Pharmacol. 1998 Jan-Feb; 20(1):47-51.

Xiāo Yáo Săn (Rambling Powder)

逍遙散
逍遥散

Pinyin Name: *Xiao Yao San*
Literal Name: Rambling Powder
Alternate Names: *Hsiao Yao San*, Merry Life Powder, Bupleurum and Tang-kuei Formula, Tangkuei and Bupleurum Formula
Original Source: *Tai Ping Hui Min He Ji Ju Fang* (Imperial Grace Formulary of the Tai Ping Era) by the Imperial Medical Department in 1078-85

COMPOSITION

Chai Hu (Radix Bupleuri)	30g [9g]
Dang Gui (Radix Angelicae Sinensis), *cuo* (grated) and *chao* (dry-fried) slightly	30g [9g]
Bai Shao (Radix Paeoniae Alba)	30g [9g]
Bai Zhu (Rhizoma Atractylodis Macrocephalae)	30g [9g]
Fu Ling (Poria)	30g [9g]
Zhi Gan Cao (Radix et Rhizoma Glycyrrhizae Praeparata cum Melle)	15g [4.5g]

DOSAGE / PREPARATION / ADMINISTRATION

The source text instructs to grind the ingredients coarsely and then cook 6g of the powdered herbs with small amounts of roasted *Sheng Jiang* (Rhizoma Zingiberis Recens) and *Bo He* (Herba Menthae) in 1 large bowl of water until the liquid is reduced to 70%. Take the hot, strained decoction any time during the day. Today, this formula may be prepared as a decoction with the doses suggested in brackets, with 9g of roasted *Sheng Jiang* (Rhizoma Zingiberis Recens) and 4.5g of *Bo He* (Herba Menthae).

CHINESE THERAPEUTIC ACTIONS

1. Soothes the Liver and relieves qi stagnation
2. Strengthens the Spleen
3. Nourishes the blood

CLINICAL MANIFESTATIONS

Liver qi stagnation with blood deficiency and Spleen deficiency: bilateral hypochondriac pain, anxiety, irritability, dry eyes and mouth, lethargy, lack of appetite, pale pink tongue, and a wiry, deficient pulse.

VETERINARY CLINICAL APPLICATIONS

Behavioral disorders, lactation difficulties, ovarian cysts, infertility, benign cystic mammary hyperplasia, canine hyperadrenocorticism, feline diabetes, chronic hepatitis, liver cirrhosis, recovery from acute pancreatitis, allergic dermatitis, dandruff, poor hair coat, poor nail quality, poor athletic performance, keratoconjunctivitis sicca, cholecystitis, anorexia, chronic gastritis, gastric ulcer, duodenal ulcer, irritable bowel syndrome, and progressive retinal atrophy.

EXPLANATION

Xiao Yao San (Rambling Powder) treats Liver qi stagnation with blood deficiency and Spleen deficiency. The Liver stores blood and is responsible for dispersing and smoothing the qi flow of the body. Emotional distress, consumption of yin and blood, and malnourishment of the Liver can all cause Liver qi to become stagnant and impair the Liver's functioning. When Liver qi stagnates, it will cause clinical signs such as hypochondriac pain, irritability, aggression and elevated liver enzymes. Liver qi stagnation contributes to yin and blood deficiencies, resulting in dry eyes, dandruff, poor hair coat, and cracked and dry nails or hooves. When stagnant Liver qi overacts on a deficient Spleen, there can be poor digestion, lethargy, and lack of appetite.

Chai Hu (Radix Bupleuri) smoothes Liver qi and disperses qi stagnation. However, *Chai Hu* (Radix Bupleuri) is drying in nature, and may further damage yin and blood. Therefore, herbs that nourish yin and tonify blood must be added. *Dang Gui* (Radix Angelicae Sinensis) is sweet, and tonifies the blood and relieves pain. *Bai Shao* (Radix Paeoniae Alba) nourishes the blood to soften the Liver to relieve distention and pain. *Bai Zhu* (Rhizoma Atractylodis Macrocephalae) and *Fu Ling* (Poria) tonify the Spleen to help the generation of blood. *Zhi Gan Cao* (Radix et Rhizoma Glycyrrhizae Praeparata cum Melle) supplements qi and helps *Bai Shao* (Radix Paeoniae Alba) soften the Liver to relieve pain. Roasted *Sheng Jiang* (Rhizoma Zingiberis Recens) strongly warms and harmonizes the Stomach. A small amount of *Bo He* (Herba Menthae) helps *Chai Hu* (Radix Bupleuri) relieve Liver stagnation and clear any heat generated from qi stagnation.

Xīāo Yáo Sǎn (Rambling Powder)

***Xiao Yao San* (Rambling Powder)**

Diagnosis	Clinical Signs	Treatment	Herbs
Liver qi stagnation with blood deficiency and Spleen deficiency	• Bilateral hypochondriac pain, irritability, aggression, increased liver enzymes: Liver qi stagnation • Dry eyes, dandruff, poor hair coat, dry and cracked nails and hooves: yin and blood deficiencies • Lethargy, poor digestion and lack of appetite: Spleen deficiency	• Soothes the Liver and relieves qi stagnation • Strengthens the Spleen • Nourishes the blood	• *Chai Hu* (Radix Bupleuri) smoothes Liver qi and disperses qi stagnation. • *Dang Gui* (Radix Angelicae Sinensis) and *Bai Shao* (Radix Paeoniae Alba) tonify blood, nourish yin, and soften the Liver. • *Bai Zhu* (Rhizoma Atractylodis Macrocephalae) and *Fu Ling* (Poria) tonify the Spleen to help the generation of blood. • Roasted *Sheng Jiang* (Rhizoma Zingiberis Recens) warms and harmonizes the Stomach. • *Bo He* (Herba Menthae) helps *Chai Hu* to relieve Liver qi stagnation and clear heat. • *Zhi Gan Cao* (Radix et Rhizoma Glycyrrhizae Praeparata cum Melle) harmonizes the herbs.

VETERINARY MODIFICATIONS

- With irritability, aggression, and other signs of heat, add *Mu Dan Pi* (Cortex Moutan) and *Zhi Zi* (Fructus Gardeniae).
- With poor appetite, add *Shen Qu* (Massa Fermentata) and *Ji Nei Jin* (Endothelium Corneum Gigeriae Galli).
- If accompanied by qi deficiency, add *Huang Qi* (Radix Astragali) and *Ren Shen* (Radix et Rhizoma Ginseng).
- If accompanied by blood deficiency, add *Shu Di Huang* (Radix Rehmanniae Praeparata).
- With restlessness at night due to stress and anxiety, add *Suan Zao Ren* (Semen Ziziphi Spinosae) and *Zhen Zhu Mu* (Concha Margaritiferae).

CAUTIONS / CONTRAINDICATIONS

- *Xiao Yao San* should be used with caution during pregnancy.
- This formula should be used with caution in cases of qi stagnation with underlying Liver and Kidney yin deficiencies, characterized by clinical signs such as hypochondriac pain, chest and abdominal fullness and distention, a dry mouth and throat, a red tongue with little tongue coating, and a deep pulse.[1]
- There are two important notes on the preparation and dosing of herbs in this formula. *Sheng Jiang* (Rhizoma Zingiberis Recens) should be roasted to decrease its acrid property and exterior-releasing effect. *Bo He* (Herba Menthae) should be kept at a low dose to clear Liver qi stagnation, since a high dose may produce an undesirable exterior-releasing effect. If not prepared properly, these two herbs will act as exterior-releasing herbs and further damage yin and blood.

PHARMACOLOGICAL EFFECTS

1. **Central nervous system**: Administration of *Xiao Yao San* in mice and rats was associated with a mild inhibitory effect on the central nervous system to relieve pain and decrease the risk of seizures and epilepsy.[2]
2. **Hepatoprotective**: Administration of this formula was associated with marked hepatoprotective effect against carbon tetrachloride-induced liver damages. The formula reduced damage to liver cells, lowered liver enzymes, and promoted the generation of new liver cells.[3]
3. **Endocrine**: Administration of the formula was associated with an increase in weight of the uterus in laboratory animals. The effect was voided in animals whose ovaries had been surgically removed. The study suggested that the formula has an endocrine effect as it stimulated the ovary and increased the weight of the uterus.[4]
4. **Gastrointestinal**: Administration of the formula was associated with increased gastric acid production in mice and relaxation of the smooth muscles of the intestines in rabbits.[5]

HUMAN CLINICAL STUDIES AND RESEARCH

1. **Schizophrenia**: Fourteen cases of schizophrenia characterized by Liver qi stagnation were treated with modified *Xiao Yao San* with satisfactory results.[6]
2. **Affective psychosis**: Twenty-six cases of affective psychosis were treated with modified *Xiao Yao San* with significant improvement in 16 cases, moderate improvement in 7 cases, and no benefit in 3 cases.[7]
3. **Neurosis**: One study reported 96% effectiveness using modified *Xiao Yao San* to treat 47 patients with neurosis. The herbal treatment contained *Xiao Yao San* plus *Yuan*

Xiāo Yáo Săn (Rambling Powder)

Zhi (Radix Polygalae), *Shi Chang Pu* (Rhizoma Acori Tatarinowii) and others as the base formula. Modifications included addition of *Suan Zao Ren* (Semen Ziziphi Spinosae), *Bai Zi Ren* (Semen Platycladi) and *Shou Wu Teng* (Caulis Polygoni Multiflori) for palpitations and insomnia; *Zhe Shi* (Haematitum), *Jue Ming Zi* (Semen Cassiae) and *Di Long* (Pheretima) for Liver yang rising; *Sha Ren* (Fructus Amomi), *Shen Qu* (Massa Fermentata) and charred *Shan Zha* (Fructus Crataegi) for decreased food intake; *Gua Lou* (Fructus Trichosanthis), *Xie Bai* (Bulbus Allii Macrostemonis) and *Fo Shou* (Fructus Citri Sarcodactylis) for feeling of chest oppression; *Du Zhong* (Cortex Eucommiae), *Xu Duan* (Radix Dipsaci) and *Gou Qi Zi* (Fructus Lycii) for Kidney deficiency with low back soreness; *Huang Qi* (Radix Astragali), *Dang Shen* (Radix Codonopsis) and *Shu Di Huang* (Radix Rehmanniae Praeparata) for qi and blood deficiencies; *Dan Nan Xing* (Arisaema cum Bile), *Ban Xia* (Rhizoma Pinelliae) and *Chen Pi* (Pericarpium Citri Reticulatae) for more phlegm; and *Di Long* (Pheretima) and *Gui Zhi* (Ramulus Cinnamomi) for numbness of the fingers. Of 47 patients, the study reported complete recovery in 31 patients, improvement in 14 patients, and no improvement in 2 patients.[8]

4. **Hyperplasia of mammary glands**: One hundred and thirty-two patients with hyperplasia of mammary glands were treated with modified *Xiao Yao San* with significant improvement in 103 patients, moderate improvement in 20 patients, mild improvement in 6 patients, and no effect in 3 patients. The overall effectiveness was 97.7%. The treatment protocol was to administer 9g of herbs in pills twice daily for 20 days per course of treatment, for a total of 2 courses. The formula was modified depending on the condition of the patient. *Wang Bu Liu Xing* (Semen Vaccariae), *Ji Xue Teng* (Caulis Spatholobi), *Xiang Fu* (Rhizoma Cyperi), *Gua Lou* (Fructus Trichosanthis), and *Chi Shao* (Radix Paeoniae Rubra) were added for swelling and pain of the breast before menstruation. *Xia Ku Cao* (Spica Prunellae), *Tian Dong* (Radix Asparagi), *Ju He* (Semen Citri Reticulatae), *Zhe Bei Mu* (Bulbus Fritillariae Thunbergii), *Ru Xiang* (Gummi Olibanum), and *Mo Yao* (Myrrha) were added for swelling and pain of the breast after menstruation.[9]
5. **Breast proliferation disease**: One study reported 96.1% effectiveness in the treatment of breast proliferation disease in 51 patients using modified *Xiao Yao San* and *Er Chen Tang* (Two-Cured Decoction) for 3 months. This study demonstrated marked changes to the hormones as follows: very significant decline of saliva estradiol (P less than 0.001), significant decline of saliva progesterone (P less than 0.05), very significant decline of plasma prolactin (P less than 0.005), and insignificant changes of saliva testosterone. The researchers stated that these herbs could regulate the endocrine system to restore normal follicle function.[10]
6. **Mastadenoma**: One study reported marked success in the treatment of benign tumor of the breast in 174 women. The herbal prescription contained *Xiao Yao San* plus *San Leng* (Rhizoma Sparganii), *Gua Lou* (Fructus Trichosanthis), *Mu Li* (Concha Ostreae) and others. *Zhe Bei Mu* (Bulbus Fritillariae Thunbergii) and *Xia Ku Cao* (Spica Prunellae) were added for accumulation of heat and phlegm; *Zhi Zi* (Fructus Gardeniae) and *Zhi Mu* (Rhizoma Anemarrhenae) for restlessness and anger; *Yan Hu Suo* (Rhizoma Corydalis) and *Chuan Lian Zi* (Fructus Toosendan) for breast distention; *Huang Qi* (Radix Astragali) and *Dang Shen* (Radix Codonopsis) for qi deficiency; and *Shu Di Huang* (Radix Rehmanniae Praeparata) and *He Shou Wu* (Radix Polygoni Multiflori) for yin and blood deficiencies. Of 174 patients, the study reported recovery in 130 patients, marked improvement in 29 patients, moderate improvement in 10 patients, and no effect in 5 patients. The rate of effectiveness was 97.13%.[11]
7. **Lactation difficulties**: One study reported 93.3% effectiveness in promoting lactation among 30 postpartum women using *Xiao Yao San* plus *Tian Hua Fen* (Radix Trichosanthis), *Si Gua Luo* (Retinervus Luffae Fructus) and *Lou Lu* (Radix Rhapontici). The duration of treatment was 7 days per course of treatment.[12]
8. **Oophoritic cyst**: Use of modified *Xiao Yao San* was associated with marked effect to treat women with oophoritic cyst with pain, irregular menstruation and abnormal bleeding. The herbal treatment contained *Xiao Yao San* plus *Zao Jiao Ci* (Spina Gleditsiae), *Chuan Xiong* (Rhizoma Chuanxiong) and *Wa Leng Zi* (Concha Arcae) as the base formula, with addition of *Zhi Zi* (Fructus Gardeniae) and *Di Huang* (Radix Rehmanniae) for heat; *Rou Gui* (Cortex Cinnamomi) and *Pao Jiang* (Rhizoma Zingiberis Praeparatum) for cold; *Huang Qi* (Radix Astragali) and *Dang Shen* (Radix Codonopsis) for qi deficiency; charred *Di Huang* (Radix Rehmanniae) and charred *Huang Qin* (Radix Scutellariae) for yin deficiency; *Yu Jin* (Radix Curcumae) and *Zhi Qiao* (Fructus Aurantii) for qi and blood stagnation; and *Shu Di Huang* (Radix Rehmanniae Praeparata) and *Xu Duan* (Radix Dipsaci) for Kidney deficiency. Of 186 patients, the study reported complete recovery in 124 patients and improvement in 48 patients. The overall rate of effectiveness was 92%.[13]
9. **Orchitis**: One case of chronic orchitis was successfully treated with significant reduction of swelling and pain. The initial treatment was for 6 doses of a formula that contained *Xiao Yao San* plus *Sheng Ma* (Rhizoma Cimicifugae) 6g, *Huang Qi* (Radix Astragali) 15g, *Chen Pi* (Pericarpium Citri Reticulatae) 9g, *Ju He* (Semen Citri Reticulatae) 9g, and *Li Zhi He* (Semen Litchi) 9g. The follow-up treatment

Xiāo Yáo Sǎn (Rambling Powder)

was for another 6 doses of the same formula, with addition of *Xia Ku Cao* (Spica Prunellae) 12g.[14]

10. **Prostatitis**: Eighteen patients of chronic prostatitis were treated with modified *Xiao Yao San* with complete recovery in 16 patients and moderate improvement in 2 patients.[15]
11. **Infertility**: One study reported marked effectiveness using modified *Xiao Yao San* to treat infertility in 30 females (between 24-38 years of age). The herbal treatment contained *Xiao Yao San* plus *Yu Jin* (Radix Curcumae), *Xiang Fu* (Rhizoma Cyperi) and others as the base formula. Modifications included addition of *Fu Pen Zi* (Fructus Rubi) and *Tu Si Zi* (Semen Cuscutae) for Kidney deficiency; *Tao Ren* (Semen Persicae), *Chuan Niu Xi* (Radix Cyathulae) and *Yi Mu Cao* (Herba Leonuri) for blood stagnation; and *Chen Pi* (Pericarpium Citri Reticulatae) and *Ban Xia* (Rhizoma Pinelliae) for presence of dampness and phlegm. The herbs were given in decoction one time daily. The treatment protocol was to begin the herbal therapy for 7 days, starting on the fourth day after the end of the period, for 3 months per course of therapy, and 1-3 courses total. Of 30 patients at the end of the study, 20 were pregnant and 10 had varying degrees of improvement with menstruation.[16]
12. **Hepatitis**: Thirty patients with hepatitis B were treated with this formula with moderate improvement in 29 patients. The formula was modified slightly depending on the condition of the patient.[17]
13. **Liver cirrhosis**: Seventeen patients with liver cirrhosis were treated with modified *Xiao Yao San* with significant improvement in 6 patients, moderate improvement in 9 patients, and no improvement in 2 patients.[18]
14. **Cholecystitis**: Administration of modified *Xiao Yao San* was associated with good results in treating 168 patients with cholecystitis (32 with acute and 136 with chronic cholecystitis). Of 168 patients, the study reported significant improvement in 79 patients and moderate improvement in 89 patients. Modifications to this formula included addition of *Yu Jin* (Radix Curcumae), *Chuan Lian Zi* (Fructus Toosendan), *Qing Pi* (Pericarpium Citri Reticulatae Viride) and *Zhi Qiao* (Fructus Aurantii) for hypochondriac pain radiating to the shoulder and back; *Hong Hua* (Flos Carthami) and *Dan Shen* (Radix et Rhizoma Salviae Miltiorrhizae) for fixed, stabbing pain in the hypochondrium with dark-colored tongue; *Sha Shen* (Radix Glehniae seu Adenophorae), *Shi Hu* (Caulis Dendrobii) and *Gou Qi Zi* (Fructus Lycii) for dry mouth with red tongue; *Da Huang* (Radix et Rhizoma Rhei), *Mang Xiao* (Natrii Sulfas), *Zhi Shi* (Fructus Aurantii Immaturus), and *Zhi Zi* (Fructus Gardeniae) for fever, nausea, vomiting and constipation; and *Jin Qian Cao* (Herba Lysimachiae) and *Hai Jin Sha* (Spora Lygodii) for presence of gallstones.[19]
15. **Anorexia**: Use of modified *Xiao Yao San* was associated with 100% effectiveness in improving appetite in 50 children with anorexia. The herbal treatment contained this formula plus dry-fried *Mai Ya* (Fructus Hordei Germinatus), *Ji Nei Jin* (Endothelium Corneum Gigeriae Galli), and others as needed. The average duration of treatment was 20.5 days. Of 50 children, 30 had complete recovery and 20 had improved appetite.[20]
16. **Irritable bowel syndrome (IBS)**: Administration of modified *Xiao Yao San* for 1-2 months in 52 patients with IBS was associated with complete recovery in 34 patients and improvement in 18 patients. The herbal treatment was based on *Xiao Yao San*, with addition of *Zhi Qiao* (Fructus Aurantii), *Mu Xiang* (Radix Aucklandiae) and *Yan Hu Suo* (Rhizoma Corydalis) for severe distention and pain; *Pao Jiang* (Rhizoma Zingiberis Praeparatum) and *Rou Gui* (Cortex Cinnamomi) for feeling of coldness in the abdomen; *Huang Qin* (Radix Scutellariae) and *Huang Lian* (Rhizoma Coptidis) for burning sensations and pain in the epigastric and abdominal regions; and addition of *Sha Ren* (Fructus Amomi) and *Bai Bian Dou* (Semen Lablab Album) and elimination of *Dang Gui* (Radix Angelicae Sinensis) for diarrhea.[21]
17. **Hyperlipidemia**: The effectiveness of using *Xiao Yao San* in treating hyperlipidemia was evaluated by dividing 126 patients into two groups. Group one received *Xiao Yao San* and group two received liquid extract of *Shan Zha* (Fructus Crataegi). There were 84 patients in group one, with an average age of 53 years (ranging from 35-73). There were 42 patients in group two, with an average age of 52 years (ranging from 37-72). Both groups were treated for 15 days per course of treatment, for a total of 3 courses. At the end, the study reported that both treatments were effective in reducing total cholesterol and triglyceride levels, with *Xiao Yao San* having 90.5% and 86.9% effectiveness, and the liquid extract of *Shan Zha* (Fructus Crataegi) having 78.5% and 76.2% effectiveness, respectively. The effectiveness rate was defined as greater than 10% reduction of total cholesterol and triglyceride levels.[22]
18. **Optic nerve atrophy**: Seventy patients (136 affected eyes) with atrophy of the optic nerve were treated with modified *Xiao Yao San* with satisfactory results.[23]

TOXICOLOGY

No fatality was observed following oral ingestion of the formula up to 200 g/kg (dried herb dose) in laboratory mice.[24]

SUGGESTED ACUPUNCTURE TREATMENT

1. Points: *Ganshu* (BL 18), *Yanglingquan* (GB 34), *Ligou* (LR 5), *Pishu* (BL 20), *Housanli* (ST 36), *Sanyinjiao* (SP 6), *Qimen* (LR 14) and *Ganshu* (equine).
2. Technique: even method.

Xiāo Yáo Sǎn (Rambling Powder)

Ganshu (BL 18), *Yanglingquan* (GB 34), and *Ligou* (LR 5) remove stagnation in the Liver and regulate the blood and menstruation. *Pishu* (BL 20), *Housanli* (ST 36), and *Sanyinjiao* (SP 6) strengthen the Spleen, warm yang, and nourish qi and blood. *Qimen* (LR 14), the *mu* (collecting) point of the Liver and the intersection of the Liver, Spleen, and *yinwei* (linking) channels, harmonizes the Spleen and Liver and regulates qi and blood circulation. *Ganshu* (equine) is a classical equine point used to relieve Liver qi stagnation. [Note: *Ganshu* (equine) in horses is not the same as *Ganshu* (BL 18) in human, although the pinyin names are the same. *Ganshu* (equine), a classical point also known as *Ganzhishu*, is the Liver *shu* (transport) point in horses. It is located in the 13th intercostal space along a line from the shoulder to the hip joint.]

RELATED FORMULA

***Hēi Xiāo Yáo Sǎn* (Black Rambling Powder)**
黑逍遙散
黑逍遥散
Pinyin Name: *Hei Xiao Yao San*
Literal Name: Black Rambling Powder
Original Source: *Yi Lue Liu Shu* (Six Texts on the Essentials of Medicine)

Chai Hu (Radix Bupleuri)	1.5g
Gan Cao (Radix et Rhizoma Glycyrrhizae)	1.5g
Bai Shao (Radix Paeoniae Alba)	4.5g
Bai Zhu (Rhizoma Atractylodis Macrocephalae)	4.5g
Fu Ling (Poria)	4.5g
Dang Gui (Radix Angelicae Sinensis), *chao* (dry-fried)	9g [6g]
Di Huang (Radix Rehmanniae) or *Shu Di Huang* (Radix Rehmanniae Praeparata)	15g

The source text states to grind the ingredients coarsely and then cook 6g of the powdered herbs with one slice of *Sheng Jiang* (Rhizoma Zingiberis Recens) and a small amount of *Bo He* (Herba Menthae). Take the strained decoction while warm. Today, this formula may be prepared as a decoction using the doses suggested in brackets.

Hei Xiao Yao San (Black Rambling Powder) is formulated by adding *Di Huang* (Radix Rehmanniae) or *Shu Di Huang* (Radix Rehmanniae Praeparata) to *Xiao Yao San*. As the base, *Xiao Yao San* treats Liver qi stagnation. *Di Huang* (Radix Rehmanniae) is added if there are more heat clinical signs, and *Shu Di Huang* (Radix Rehmanniae Praeparata) is used if there is deficiency.

This formula regulates Liver qi, strengthens the Spleen, nourishes the blood, and regulates menstruation. Clinical manifestations include irregular menstruation with abdominal pain, and a wiry, deficient pulse.

AUTHORS' COMMENTS

Xiao Yao San is often used as a base formula in treating many chronic digestion and hepatic disorders. It is excellent for the treatment of gastric ulcers when combined with *Er Chen Tang* (Two-Cured Decoction) or *Yu Nu Jian* (Jade Woman Decoction) and is a wonderful follow-up herbal formula for the recovery stage of toxic hepatopathy, hepatic lipidosis and pancreatitis. It is useful for animals that have a good appetite yet remain thin and under conditioned, and it promotes consistent performance in animal athletes. It is effective for treating behavioral disorders due to Liver qi stagnation from stress, estrus, lack of regular exercise, death of a housemate, moving to a new location, excessive confinement, and frequent boarding for long periods of time. It is a relatively mild formula that can be taken long term. It has been used to treat progressive retinal atrophy in combination with *Xue Fu Zhu Yu Tang* (Drive Out Stasis in the Mansion of Blood Decoction) or *Tao Hong Si Wu Tang* (Four-Substance Decoction with Safflower and Peach Pit) to attenuate and/or slow the progression of the disease.

Chai Hu Shu Gan San (Bupleurum Powder to Spread the Liver) and *Xiao Yao San* are two of the most commonly used formulas to treat Liver qi stagnation.

- *Chai Hu Shu Gan San* focuses only on Liver qi stagnation, and is suitable for animals with more severe Liver qi stagnation.
- *Xiao Yao San* treats Liver qi stagnation with blood and Spleen deficiencies. It has a weaker qi-dispersing effect but a stronger nourishing action. Thus, it is more suitable for deficient-type patients with mild Liver qi stagnation and is appropriate for long-term use.

Si Ni San (Frigid Extremities Powder) and *Xiao Yao San* both harmonize the Liver (wood element) and Spleen (earth element) to treat such clinical signs as hypochondriac or abdominal pain. Both formulas contain *Chai Hu* (Radix Bupleuri), *Bai Shao* (Radix Paeoniae Alba), and *Gan Cao* (Radix et Rhizoma Glycyrrhizae). The differences between these two formulas are as follows:

- *Xiao Yao San* regulates Liver qi, strengthens the Spleen, and nourishes the blood. It is more suitable for combined conditions of excess (Liver qi stagnation) and deficiency (blood and Spleen qi deficiencies). Chief manifestations of *Xiao Yao San* include hypochondriac pain, dry eyes, dandruff, poor hair coat, poor nail quality, listlessness, decreased dietary intake, poor digestion, and a wiry, deficient pulse. It is also commonly used to treat emotional

Xiāo Yáo Sǎn (Rambling Powder)

disturbances. *Xiao Yao San* contains *Bai Zhu* (Rhizoma Atractylodis Macrocephalae), *Fu Ling* (Poria), *Dang Gui* (Radix Angelicae Sinensis), *Sheng Jiang* (Rhizoma Zingiberis Recens), *Bo He* (Herba Menthae), and *Zhi Gan Cao* (Radix et Rhizoma Glycyrrhizae Praeparata cum Melle) to strengthen the Spleen and nourish the blood.

- *Si Ni San* mainly treats an excess condition involving cold extremities caused by heat trapped in the body and blocking the qi from reaching the extremities. It uses *Chai Hu* (Radix Bupleuri), the chief herb, and *Zhi Shi* (Fructus Aurantii Immaturus) to break up qi stagnation to allow qi to circulate to the extremities.

Xiao Yao San and *Yi Guan Jian* (Linking Decoction) both treat hypochondriac bloating and pain, but the etiology of this condition and the focus of the formulas are quite different.

- *Xiao Yao San* addresses Liver qi stagnation accompanied by blood and Spleen deficiencies. It regulates Liver qi, spreads stagnation, strengthens the Spleen, and nourishes the blood. It is considered a harmonizing formula.
- *Yi Guan Jian* treats Liver and yin deficiencies with Liver qi stagnation. It is a tonic formula used to treat dry eyes, mouth, skin and hair coat, chronic hepatitis, seizures (epilepsy), feline hyperthyroidism and canine hyperadrenocorticism. It nourishes yin and regulates Liver qi.

References

1. *Zhong Yao Ming Fang Yao Li Yu Ying Yong* (Pharmacology and Applications of Famous Herbal Formulas), 1989; 114-115.
2. *Zhong Yao Yao Li Yu Ying Yong* (Pharmacology and Applications of Chinese Herbs), 1993; 9(2):8.
3. *Zhong Cao Yao* (Chinese Herbal Medicine), 1990; 21(11):28.
4. *Zhong Guo Yao Li Tong Xun* (Journal of Chinese Herbal Studies), 1988; (3):44.
5. *Zhong Guo Yao Li Tong Xun* (Journal of Chinese Herbal Studies), 1988; (3):44.
6. *Zhong Xi Yi Jie He Za Zhi* (Journal of Integrated Chinese and Western Medicine), 1982; (3):170.
7. *Xin Zhong Yi* (New Chinese Medicine), 1983; (1):37.
8. *Fu Jian Zhong Yi Yao* (Fujian Chinese Medicine and Herbology), 1999; 5:26.
9. *Zhong Yi Za Zhi* (Journal of Chinese Medicine), 1993; (2):86.
10. Zhang GL. Treatment of breast proliferation disease with modified xiao yao san and er chen decoction. *Zhong Xi Yi Jie He Za Zhi.* 1991 Jul; 11(7):400-2, 388.
11. *Jiang Su Zhong Yi* (Jiangsu Chinese Medicine), 1996; 8:26.
12. *An Hui Zhong Yi Lin Chuang Za Zi* (Anhui Journal of Clinical Chinese Medicine), 1995; 4:12.
13. *He Nan Zhong Yi* (Henan Chinese Medicine), 1999; 3:46.
14. *Liao Ning Zhong Yi Za Zhi* (Liaoning Journal of Chinese Medicine), 1980; (2):36.
15. *Zhong Yi Za Zhi* (Journal of Chinese Medicine), 1990; (11):20.
16. *Xin Zhong Yi* (New Chinese Medicine), 1995; 5:38.
17. *Hei Long Jiang Zhong Yi Yao* (Heilongjiang Chinese Medicine and Herbology), 1987; (1):25.
18. *Ji Lin Zhong Yi Yao* (Jilin Chinese Medicine and Herbology), 1986; (5):18.
19. *Jiang Xi Zhong Yi Yao* (Jiangxi Chinese Medicine and Herbology), 1999; 1:27.
20. *Shan Xi Zhong Yi* (Shanxi Chinese Medicine), 1995; 12:541.
21. *Si Chuan Zhong Yi* (Sichuan Chinese Medicine), 1997; 11:25.
22. *Shan Xi Yi Kan* (Shanxi Journal of Medicine), 1995; 16(3):109.
23. *Bei Jing Zhong Yi* (Beijing Chinese Medicine), 1986; (4):17.
24. *Zhong Guo Yao Li Tong Xun* (Journal of Chinese Herbal Studies), 1988; (3):44.

Jiā Wèi Xiāo Yáo Săn (Augmented Rambling Powder)

加味逍遥散
加味逍遥散

Pinyin Name: *Jia Wei Xiao Yao San*
Literal Name: Augmented Rambling Powder
Alternate Names: *Dan Zhi Xiao Yao San* (Moutan and Gardenia Rambling Powder), *Ba Wei Xiao Yao San* (Eight-Ingredient Rambling Powder), *Chia Wei Hsiao Yao San*, Modified Merry Life Powder, Bupleurum and Peony Formula
Original Source: *Nei Ke Zhai Yao* (Summary of Internal Medicine) by Wen Sheng in the mid-19th century

COMPOSITION

Chai Hu (Radix Bupleuri)	30g [9g]
Dang Gui (Radix Angelicae Sinensis), *chao* (dry-fried) slightly	30g [9g]
Bai Shao (Radix Paeoniae Alba)	30g [9g]
Bai Zhu (Rhizoma Atractylodis Macrocephalae)	30g [9g]
Fu Ling (Poria)	30g [9g]
Zhi Gan Cao (Radix et Rhizoma Glycyrrhizae Praeparata cum Melle)	15g [4.5g]
Mu Dan Pi (Cortex Moutan)	30g [9g]
Zhi Zi (Fructus Gardeniae), *chao* (dry-fried)	30g [9g]

DOSAGE / PREPARATION / ADMINISTRATION

The source text instructs to grind the ingredients into powder, and cook 9g of the powdered herbs to make a decoction. Today, this formula is usually prepared as a decoction with the doses suggested in brackets.

CHINESE THERAPEUTIC ACTIONS

1. Soothes the Liver and relieves qi stagnation
2. Strengthens the Spleen
3. Nourishes the blood
4. Sedates heat and fire

CLINICAL MANIFESTATIONS

Liver qi stagnation accompanied by interior heat and underlying blood and Spleen deficiencies: irritability, restlessness, aggression, hypochondriac pain, dandruff, poor hair coat, poor nail quality, dry eyes, lethargy, nausea, lack of appetite, poor digestion, dysuria and pollakiuria.

VETERINARY CLINICAL APPLICATIONS

Infertility, behavioral disorder with aggression and anxiety, pancreatitis, cholangiohepatitis, early stage of liver cirrhosis, elevated liver enzymes, keratoconjunctivitis sicca (KCS), uveitis, progressive retinal atrophy, dermatitis, and benign cystic mammary gland hyperplasia.

EXPLANATION

Jia Wei Xiao Yao San (Augmented Rambling Powder) treats Liver qi stagnation accompanied by interior heat and underlying blood and Spleen deficiencies. As a result of deficiency in the interior (Spleen and blood), Liver qi stagnation is unrestrained and turns into heat and fire, leading to clinical signs such as irritability, dry eyes, dry skin and hair coat, pollakiuria and dysuria.

Jia Wei Xiao Yao San is modified from *Xiao Yao San* (Rambling Powder), which resolves Liver qi stagnation, nourishes the blood, and strengthens the Spleen. The

***Jia Wei Xiao Yao San* (Augmented Rambling Powder)**

Diagnosis	Clinical Signs	Treatment	Herbs
Liver qi stagnation accompanied by interior heat and underlying blood and Spleen deficiencies	• Bilateral hypochondriac pain: Liver qi stagnation • Irritability, aggression and dysuria: interior heat • Dry eyes, poor hair coat and dandruff: yin and blood deficiencies • Lethargy and lack of appetite: Spleen deficiency	• Soothes the Liver and relieves qi stagnation • Strengthens the Spleen • Nourishes the blood • Sedates heat and fire	• *Xiao Yao San* (Rambling Powder) treats Liver qi stagnation, nourishes the blood, and strengthens the Spleen. • *Mu Dan Pi* (Cortex Moutan) and *Zhi Zi* (Fructus Gardeniae) sedate interior heat and fire.

Jiā Wèi Xiāo Yáo Sǎn (Augmented Rambling Powder)

addition of *Mu Dan Pi* (Cortex Moutan) and *Zhi Zi* (Fructus Gardeniae) sedates interior heat arising from Spleen and blood deficiencies, and from Liver qi stagnation.

VETERINARY MODIFICATIONS

- For blood deficiency, add *Chuan Xiong* (Rhizoma Chuanxiong) and *Shu Di Huang* (Radix Rehmanniae Praeparata).
- If the condition is marked by qi deficiency and fatigue, add *Huang Qi* (Radix Astragali) and *Ren Shen* (Radix et Rhizoma Ginseng).
- With *shaoyang* syndrome, combine with *Xiao Chai Hu Tang* (Minor Bupleurum Decoction).
- With yin deficiency with heat, combine with *Qing Hao Bie Jia Tang* (Artemisia Annua and Soft-Shelled Turtle Shell Decoction).

CAUTIONS / CONTRAINDICATIONS

- *Jia Wei Xiao Yao San* should be used with caution during pregnancy.
- This formula is contraindicated in animals with underlying deficiency and cold.[1]

PHARMACOLOGICAL EFFECTS

Anxiolytic: Use of *Jia Wei Xiao Yao San* showed anxiolytic effects through the neurosteroid synthesis followed by gamma-amino-butyric acid A/benzodiazepine (GABA(A)/BZP) receptor stimulations in male mice.[2]

HUMAN CLINICAL STUDIES AND RESEARCH

- **Affective disorders:** Administration of *Jia Wei Xiao Yao San* effectively treated affective disorders characterized by depressed Liver resulting in fire, mild yang deficiency and mild yin deficiency. Of 50 patients, the study reported marked improvement in 26 patients, improvement in 17 patients, and no improvement in 7 patients.[3]
- **Panic disorder**: Four patients diagnosed with panic disorder with agoraphobia, in accordance with the Diagnostic and Statistical Manual of Mental Disorders (DSM) criteria, were successfully treated with herbal medicine. Two patients were treated with *Jia Wei Xiao Yao San*, and 2 with *Ban Xia Hou Po Tang* (Pinellia and Magnolia Bark Decoction). Both formulas successfully relieved panic attacks, anticipatory anxiety and agoraphobia. The study concluded that these formulas may be useful as additional or alternative treatments for panic disorder.[4]

HERB-DRUG INTERACTION

Antipsychotic-induced Parkinsonism: Use of *Jia Wei Xiao Yao San* was associated with statistically significant reduction ($P<0.01$) in tremors caused by antipsychotic-induced Parkinsonism in 8 patients. The tremors did not worsen in any of the patients, and there were no reports of side effects.[5]

TOXICOLOGY

Use of *Jia Wei Xiao Yao San* was associated with one case of adult respiratory distress syndrome. After taking *Jia Wei Xiao Yao San* for treatment of seborrheic dermatitis, a 59-year-old female presented with a respiratory illness having clinical, radiologic and functional characteristics of adult respiratory distress syndrome, with increased number of lymphocytes, neutrophils, and eosinophils in the bronchoalveolar lavage fluid. The lymphocyte stimulation test with *Jia Wei Xiao Yao San* was positive.[6]

SUGGESTED ACUPUNCTURE TREATMENT

1. Points: *Ganshu* (BL 18), *Yanglingquan* (GB 34), *Ligou* (LR 5), *Pishu* (BL 20), *Housanli* (ST 36), *Sanyinjiao* (SP 6), *Qimen* (LR 14), *Taichong* (LR 3), and *Zhigou* (TH 6).
2. Technique: even method.

Ganshu (BL 18), *Yanglingquan* (GB 34), and *Ligou* (LR 5) remove stagnation in the Liver and regulate the blood and menstruation. *Pishu* (BL 20), *Housanli* (ST 36), and *Sanyinjiao* (SP 6) strengthen the Spleen, warm yang, and nourish qi and blood. *Qimen* (LR 14), the *mu* (collecting) point of the Liver and the intersection of the Liver, Spleen, and *yinwei* (linking) channels, harmonizes the Spleen and Liver and regulates qi and blood circulation. *Taichong* (LR 3) and *Zhigou* (TH 6) sedate heat and fire.

RELATED FORMULA

***Shí Wèi Xiāo Yáo Sǎn* (Ten-Ingredient Rambling Powder)**
十味逍遙散
十味逍遥散
Pinyin Name: *Shi Wei Xiao Yao San*
Literal Name: Ten-Ingredient Rambling Powder
Original Source: *Nei Ke Zhai Yao* (Summary of Internal Medicine) by Wen Sheng in the mid-19th century

Chai Hu (Radix Bupleuri)	30g [9g]
Dang Gui (Radix Angelicae Sinensis), *chao* (dry-fried) slightly	30g [9g]
Bai Shao (Radix Paeoniae Alba)	30g [9g]
Bai Zhu (Rhizoma Atractylodis Macrocephalae)	30g [9g]
Fu Ling (Poria)	30g [9g]
Zhi Gan Cao (Radix et Rhizoma Glycyrrhizae Praeparata cum Melle)	15g [4.5g]
Sheng Jiang (Rhizoma Zingiberis Recens)	30g [9g]
Bo He (Herba Menthae), *wei* (roasted)	15g [4.5g]
Mu Dan Pi (Cortex Moutan)	30g [9g]
Zhi Zi (Fructus Gardeniae), *chao* (dry-fried)	30g [9g]

Jiā Wèi Xiāo Yáo Săn (Augmented Rambling Powder)

The source text instructs to grind the ingredients into powder, and cook 9g of the powdered herbs to make a decoction. Today, this formula is usually prepared as a decoction with the doses suggested in brackets.

Shi Wei Xiao Yao San (Ten-Ingredient Rambling Powder) treats Liver qi stagnation accompanied by interior heat and underlying blood and Spleen deficiencies. It is formulated by combining the ingredients from both *Xiao Yao San* (Rambling Powder) and *Jia Wei Xiao Yao San* (Augmented Rambling Powder).

- In comparison with *Xiao Yao San* (Rambling Powder), this formula has stronger effect to clear heat as it contains *Mu Dan Pi* (Cortex Moutan) and *Zhi Zi* (Fructus Gardeniae).
- In contrast with *Jia Wei Xiao Yao San* (Augmented Rambling Powder), it has better effect to regulate Liver qi circulation and harmonize the Stomach since it has *Bo He* (Herba Menthae) and roasted *Sheng Jiang* (Rhizoma Zingiberis Recens).

AUTHORS' COMMENTS

Jia Wei Xiao Yao San literally means "Augmented Rambling Powder." The augmentation refers to the addition of two herbs: *Mu Dan Pi* (Cortex Moutan) and *Zhi Zi* (Fructus Gardeniae). Thus, this formula is also known as *Dan Zhi Xiao Yao San* (Moutan and Gardenia Rambling Powder). It is stronger for treating behavioral disorder characterized by aggression due to Liver heat than *Xiao Yao San.*

Jia Wei Xiao Yao San contains strong heat-clearing and qi-regulating herbs that make it unsuitable for long-term use. In cases where long-term use is required, a formula such as *Yi Guan Jian* (Linking Decoction) can be used or added to *Jia Wei Xiao Yao San* to reduce the possibility of having these strong herbs create imbalances in the body.

Jia Wei Xiao Yao San is a commonly used veterinary formula and has diverse applications:

- Combine with *Xiao Feng San* (Eliminate Wind Powder) for treatment of allergic dermatitis with pruritus.
- Combine with *Suan Zao Ren Tang* (Sour Jujube Decoction) for behavioral disorder with aggression, hyperactivity, restlessness and insomnia.
- Combine with *Xue Fu Zhu Yu Tang* (Drive Out Stasis in the Mansion of Blood Decoction) to treat keratoconjunctivitis sicca.
- Combine with *Ba Zheng San* (Eight-Herb Powder for Rectification) or *Wu Lin San* (Five-Ingredient Powder for Painful Urinary Dysfunction) for urinary tract infection.

References

1. *Zhong Yao Ming Fang Yao Li Yu Ying Yong* (Pharmacology and Applications of Famous Herbal Formulas), 1989; 115-116.
2. Mizowaki M, Toriizuka K, Hanawa T. Anxiolytic effect of Kami-Shoyo-San (TJ-24) in mice: possible mediation of neurosteroid synthesis. Life Sci. 2001 Sep 21; 69(18):2167-77.
3. Zhang LD, Zhang YL, Xu SH, Zhou G, Jin SB. Traditional Chinese medicine typing of affective disorders and treatment. American Journal of Chinese Medicine. 1994; 22(3-4):321-7.
4. Mantani N, Hisanaga A, Kogure T, Kita T, Shimada Y, Terasawa K. Four cases of panic disorder successfully treated with Kampo (Japanese herbal) medicines: Kami-shoyo-san and Hange-koboku-to. Psychiatry & Clinical Neurosciences. 2002 Dec; 56(6):617-20.
5. Ishikawa T, Funahashi T, Kudo J. Effectiveness of the Kampo kami-shoyo-san (TJ-24) for tremor of antipsychotic-induced parkinsonism. Psychiatry Clin Neurosci. 2000 Oct; 54(5):579-82.
6. Shiota Y, Wilson JG, Matsumoto H, Munemasa M, Okamura M, Hiyama J, Marukawa M, Ono T, Taniyama K, Mashiba H. Adult respiratory distress syndrome induced by a Chinese medicine, Kamisyoyo-san. Internal Medicine. 1996 Jun; 35(6):494-6.

Tōng Xiè Yào Fāng (Important Formula for Painful Diarrhea)

痛瀉要方
痛泻要方

Pinyin Name: *Tong Xie Yao Fang*
Literal Name: Important Formula for Painful Diarrhea
Alternate Names: *Bai Zhu Shao Yao San* (Atractylodes Macrocephala and Peony Powder), Important Formula for Painful Purging
Original Source: *Jing Yue Quan Shu* (Collected Treatises of [Zhang] Jing Yue) by Zhang Jie-Bin (Zhang Jing-Yue) in 1624

COMPOSITION

Bai Zhu (Rhizoma Atractylodis Macrocephalae), *chao* (dry-fried) with soil	90g [6g]
Bai Shao (Radix Paeoniae Alba), *chao* (dry-fried)	60g [6g]
Chen Pi (Pericarpium Citri Reticulatae), *chao* (dry-fried)	45g [4.5g]
Fang Feng (Radix Saposhnikoviae)	60g [3g]

DOSAGE / PREPARATION / ADMINISTRATION

The source text states that this formula may be prepared as a decoction, pills or powder. Today, this formula is usually prepared as a decoction with the doses suggested in brackets.

CHINESE THERAPEUTIC ACTIONS

1. Tonifies the Spleen and sedates the Liver
2. Dispels dampness and stops diarrhea

CLINICAL MANIFESTATIONS

Abdominal pain and diarrhea caused by Spleen deficiency and Liver excess: borborygmus, flatulence, diarrhea, tenesmus, abdominal pain which persists after defecation, a thin, white tongue coating, and a thin, wiry, pulse.

VETERINARY CLINICAL APPLICATIONS

Diarrhea, diarrhea secondary to hyperthyroidism in the cat, chronic enteritis and inflammatory bowel disease.

EXPLANATION

Tong Xie Yao Fang (Important Formula for Painful Diarrhea) treats abdominal pain and diarrhea caused by the Liver overacting on the Spleen, with abdominal pain and cramping prior to defecation that is relieved after the stool has been passed. The pain is not due to retention of food or other substances; rather, the pain is due to the Liver (excess) overacting on the Spleen (deficiency). Diarrhea is the direct reflection of digestive weakness secondary to an overactive Liver.

This formula contains *Bai Zhu* (Rhizoma Atractylodis Macrocephalae) as the chief herb to tonify the Spleen and dry dampness. *Bai Shao* (Radix Paeoniae Alba), the deputy herb, nourishes the blood and relieves pain by sedating the Liver and softening Liver qi. *Chen Pi* (Pericarpium Citri Reticulatae) regulates qi, dries dampness, awakens the Spleen and harmonizes the middle *jiao*. *Fang Feng* (Radix Saposhnikoviae) disperses Liver qi to help stop the Liver from overacting on the Spleen, and directs the effects of the formula to the Spleen and Liver.

***Tong Xie Yao Fang* (Important Formula for Painful Diarrhea)**

Diagnosis	Clinical Signs	Treatment	Herbs
Abdominal pain and diarrhea caused by Spleen deficiency and Liver excess	• Borborygmus, flatulence, diarrhea, tenesmus, abdominal pain and bloating: Liver excess overacting on Spleen deficiency • Thin, white tongue coating and a wiry, thin pulse: presence of deficient and excess conditions	• Tonifies the Spleen and sedates the Liver • Dispels dampness and stops diarrhea	• *Bai Zhu* (Rhizoma Atractylodis Macrocephalae) tonifies the Spleen and dries dampness. • *Bai Shao* (Radix Paeoniae Alba) nourishes the blood and relieves pain by sedating the Liver and softening Liver qi. • *Chen Pi* (Pericarpium Citri Reticulatae) regulates qi, dries dampness, and harmonizes the Stomach. • *Fang Feng* (Radix Saposhnikoviae) disperses Liver qi to help stop the Liver from overacting on the Spleen.

Tòng Xiè Yào Fāng (Important Formula for Painful Diarrhea)

VETERINARY MODIFICATIONS

- For chronic diarrhea, add dry-fried *Sheng Ma* (Rhizoma Cimicifugae).
- If the diarrhea is caused by acute gastroenteritis or bacterial diarrhea, add *Ge Gen Huang Qin Huang Lian Tang* (Kudzu, Coptis, and Scutellaria Decoction) and *Shan Zha* (Fructus Crataegi).
- If the diarrhea is caused by hyperthyroidism, add *Ge Gen* (Radix Puerariae Lobatae), *Mu Li* (Concha Ostreae), and *Xia Ku Cao* (Spica Prunellae), and increase the dose of *Bai Shao* (Radix Paeoniae Alba) and *Fang Feng* (Radix Saposhnikoviae).
- For diarrhea in chronic hepatic diseases, add *Ge Gen* (Radix Puerariae Lobatae), *Shan Zha* (Fructus Crataegi), *Fu Ling* (Poria), and *Yi Yi Ren* (Semen Coicis).
- With a greasy, yellow tongue coating, add *Huang Lian* (Rhizoma Coptidis).

CAUTIONS / CONTRAINDICATIONS

- *Fang Feng* (Radix Saposhnikoviae) is an important herb in this formula that serves two purposes: to disperse Liver qi stagnation and to guide the formula to the Spleen channel. However, its dose must not be arbitrarily increased, or its function will shift to an exterior-releasing emphasis.
- Avoid cold, raw, oily or greasy foods while taking *Tong Xie Yao Fang*.[1]

PHARMACOLOGICAL EFFECTS

1. **Gastrointestinal**: This formula had a marked effect on the production of gastric acid in laboratory rats. At 25g/kg and 75g/kg (dose of dried herbs), it reduced gastric acid production by 59.1% and 64.1%, respectively.[2] The use of this formula was also associated with a marked inhibitory effect on intestinal peristalsis in rabbits.[3]
2. **Antibiotic**: This formula was associated with an inhibitory effect against *Bacillus dysenteriae*, *E. coli*, and *Staphylococcus aureus*.

HUMAN CLINICAL STUDIES AND RESEARCH

1. **Diarrhea**: Use of *Tong Xie Yao Fang* was associated with recovery in 43 of 45 children with diarrhea.[4] Another study reported 93.8% effectiveness using modified *Tong Xie Yao Fang* to treat 32 patients with diarrhea.[5]
2. **Acute enteritis**: Sixty patients with acute enteritis characterized by severe pain and diarrhea were treated with *Tong Xie Yao Fang* with a 90% overall rate of effectiveness. The patients received 1-2 packs of herbs for treatment. The study reported no side effects in most patients.[6]
3. **Chronic enteritis**: Thirty-five patients with chronic enteritis were treated with modified *Tong Xie Yao Fang* with complete recovery in 28 patients, moderate improvement in 5 patients, and no effect in 2 patients. The herbal treatment contained dry-fried *Bai Shao* (Radix Paeoniae Alba) 20-30g, dry-fried *Bai Zhu* (Rhizoma Atractylodis Macrocephalae) 15g, *Chen Pi* (Pericarpium Citri Reticulatae) 6g, and *Fang Feng* (Radix Saposhnikoviae) 10g. Modification included the addition of *Sheng Ma* (Rhizoma Cimicifugae) 6g for chronic diarrhea; increased dose of *Bai Shao* (Radix Paeoniae Alba), with the addition of *Mu Gua* (Fructus Chaenomelis) 6g, and *Mu Xiang* (Radix Aucklandiae) 6g for severe abdominal pain; and *Dang Shen* (Radix Codonopsis) 10g for fatigue.[7]
4. **Chronic colitis**: Twenty patients with chronic colitis were treated with modified *Tong Xie Yao Fang* for one and a half months with marked improvement in 14 patients, moderate improvement in 4 patients, and no effect in 2 patients. The treatment included *Fang Feng* (Radix Saposhnikoviae), *Bai Zhu* (Rhizoma Atractylodis Macrocephalae), *Chen Pi* (Pericarpium Citri Reticulatae), *Bai Shao* (Radix Paeoniae Alba), *Wu Mei* (Fructus Mume), *Mu Gua* (Fructus Chaenomelis), *Dang Shen* (Radix Codonopsis), *Shan Yao* (Rhizoma Dioscoreae), and *Shan Zha* (Fructus Crataegi).[8] Another study reported 93.55% effectiveness using modified *Tong Xie Yao Fang* to treat 124 patients with chronic colitis (25 with complete recovery, 68 with significant improvement, and 23 with moderate improvement). The herbal formula contained *Yi Yi Ren* (Semen Coicis) 20g, *Che Qian Zi* (Semen Plantaginis) 20g, *Huang Qi* (Radix Astragali) 15g, *Bai Jiang Cao* (Herba cum Radice Patriniae) 15g, *Bai Zhi* (Radix Angelicae Dahuricae) 15g, dry-fried *Bai Shao* (Radix Paeoniae Alba) 12g, *Hou Po* (Cortex Magnoliae Officinalis) 12g, *Fang Feng* (Radix Saposhnikoviae) 3g, *Bai Zhu* (Rhizoma Atractylodis Macrocephalae) 10g, *Ku Shen* (Radix Sophorae Flavescentis) 10g, dry-fried *Cang Zhu* (Rhizoma Atractylodis) 10g, *Mu Xiang* (Radix Aucklandiae) 5g, *Chen Pi* (Pericarpium Citri Reticulatae) 6g, and *Chai Hu* (Radix Bupleuri) 6g. The patients were given the herbs in decoction for 2 weeks per course of treatment, with duration of 1-6 courses total.[9]
5. **Ulcerative colitis**: Thirty-five patients with ulcerative colitis were treated with modified *Tong Xie Yao Fang* for 20 days with marked improvement in 30 patients and moderate improvement in 5 patients. The formula included *Bai Zhu* (Rhizoma Atractylodis Macrocephalae), *Bai Shao* (Radix Paeoniae Alba), *Chen Pi* (Pericarpium Citri Reticulatae), *Fang Feng* (Radix Saposhnikoviae), *Sheng Ma* (Rhizoma Cimicifugae), *Qin Pi* (Cortex Fraxini), and *Chi Shi Zhi* (Halloysitum Rubrum).[10] Another study reported 93.5% effectiveness for treatment of chronic colitis using *Tong Xie Yao Fang* plus *Shan Yao* (Rhizoma Dioscoreae), *Gu Ya* (Fructus Setariae Germinatus), *Mai Ya* (Fructus Hordei Germinatus), and other herbs as deemed necessary. Modifications included the addition of *Yan Hu Suo* (Rhizoma Corydalis) and a larger dose of *Bai*

Tòng Xiè Yào Fāng (Important Formula for Painful Diarrhea)

Shao (Radix Paeoniae Alba) for severe abdominal pain; *Mu Xiang* (Radix Aucklandiae), *Zhi Qiao* (Fructus Aurantii), and *Hou Po* (Cortex Magnoliae Officinalis) for Liver qi stagnation; *Chuan Lian Zi* (Fructus Toosendan) for qi stagnation turning into fire; *Da Huang* (Radix et Rhizoma Rhei), *Bing Lang* (Semen Arecae) and *Huang Lian* (Rhizoma Coptidis) for dampness in the Intestines; *Dang Shen* (Radix Codonopsis), *Huang Qi* (Radix Astragali) and *Yi Yi Ren* (Semen Coicis) for Spleen and qi deficiency; and *Si Shen Wan* (Four-Miracle Pill) for Spleen and Kidney deficiencies. Of 32 patients, the study reported complete recovery in 21 patients, improvement in 9 patients, and no benefit in 2 patients.[11]

6. **Irritable bowel syndrome (IBS)**: *Tong Xie Yao Fang* has been shown in many studies to effectively treat IBS. Fifty patients with IBS were treated with modified *Tong Xie Yao Fang* with complete recovery in 35 patients. The average length of treatment was 28.4 days, with a range of 23 to 120 days. Fifteen patients discontinued the treatment due to various reasons, with most showing some indications of improvement.[12] Another study reported 89.9% effectiveness using *Tong Xie Yao Fang* plus *Si Shen Wan* (Four-Miracle Pill) to treat 187 patients with IBS.[13] Lastly, one study reported 93.3% effectiveness using modified *Tong Xie Yao Fang* to treat 30 patients with IBS. The herbal treatment used *Tong Xie Yao Fang* as the base, with the addition of *Sheng Ma* (Rhizoma Cimicifugae) and *Chi Shi Zhi* (Halloysitum Rubrum) for chronic diarrhea; *Bu Gu Zhi* (Fructus Psoraleae) and *Rou Gui* (Cortex Cinnamomi) for Spleen and Kidney yang deficiencies; and *Chai Hu* (Radix Bupleuri) and *Dang Gui* (Radix Angelicae Sinensis) for Liver qi stagnation with blood deficiency. Each course of treatment lasted 1 month. Of 30 patients, the study reported significant improvement in 9 patients, improvement in 19 patients, and no improvement in 2 patients.[14]

SUGGESTED ACUPUNCTURE TREATMENT

1. Points: *Ganshu* (BL 18), *Xingjian* (LR 2), *Sanyinjiao* (SP 6), *Yinlingquan* (SP 9), *Sibai* (ST 2), *Guanchong* (TH 1), *Pishu* (BL 20), *Zhongwan* (CV 12), *Housanli* (ST 36), and *Tianshu* (ST 25).
2. Technique: both tonification and sedation. Moxibustion may be used.

Ganshu (BL 18) and *Xingjian* (LR 2) together sedate the Liver and relieve pain. *Sanyinjiao* (SP 6) and *Yinlingquan* (SP 9) strengthen the Spleen and help stop diarrhea. *Sibai* (ST 2) and *Guanchong* (TH 1) encourage qi flow in the abdomen and stop pain. *Pishu* (BL 20), *Zhongwan* (CV 12), and *Housanli* (ST 36) strengthen the Spleen and Stomach. *Tianshu* (ST 25), the *mu* (collecting) point of the Large Intestine, relieves diarrhea. In patients with severe deficiency of the middle *jiao*, apply moxibustion on *Zhongwan* (CV 12) and *Housanli* (ST 36).

AUTHORS' COMMENTS

Tong Xie Yao Fang was originally called *Bai Zhu Shao Yao San* (Atractylodes Macrocephala and Peony Powder), with the understanding that this was an "important formula for painful diarrhea" and that abdominal pain may persist after defecation. *Tong Xie Yao Fang* eventually became the "official" name of this formula, however, since this name meaningfully incorporates its primary function.

Tong Xie Yao Fang is a common foundational formula for treating various types of diarrhea and inflammatory bowel disease in veterinary species. Inflammatory bowel disease due to Liver qi stagnation and Spleen qi deficiency is prevalent in dogs and cats as a result of feeding commercial diets which are species inappropriate. It is also fairly common in horses overfed concentrates and confined to a stall for long periods. The animals for which this formula is appropriate have abdominal pain and abdominal cramps manifested by a humped backed, looking at the abdomen, rolling, vocalizing while passing stool, or walking during defecation and straining to pass a relatively small amount of stool. In some cases the animal may suddenly shriek or scream and try to "run" away from their stool after it is passed. The diarrhea may be soft and pasty to watery and contain both blood and mucus and is worse when the animal is stressed. Dry food diets, which contain high amounts of dampness-engendering carbohydrates such as corn, wheat and soybean, and energetically hot meats such as lamb eventually lead to chronic Spleen qi deficiency and dampness in the dog and cat. Likewise, diets that approach and surpass 50% of concentrated feeds, especially those with a great deal of molasses, create similar patterns in the horse. In cases where the Spleen is predominantly weak and has invited the Liver to invade it, the diarrhea will not resolve until the Spleen has been sufficiently strengthened. This formula can be combined with *Dang Shen* (Radix Codonopsis), *Huang Qi* (Radix Astragali) and *Yi Yi Ren* (Semen Coicis) to further tonify the Spleen, depending on the individual case. In horses with digestive issues, combining this formula with *Shen Ling Bai Zhu San* (Ginseng, Poria, and Atractylodes Macrocephala Powder) or *Bu Zhong Yi Qi Tang* (Tonify the Middle and Augment the Qi Decoction) will be helpful.

In the treatment of lymphocytic-plasmacytic enteritis/colitis (inflammatory bowel disease), *Tong Xie Yao Fang* can be tailored to fit the individual animal's pattern of illness more closely by using the following herbs:

Tòng Xiè Yào Fāng (Important Formula for Painful Diarrhea)

- With more Liver qi stagnation, increase the dose of *Fang Feng* (Radix Saposhnikoviae) and add *Chai Hu* (Radix Bupleuri), *Qing Pi* (Pericarpium Citri Reticulatae Viride) and *Xiang Fu* (Rhizoma Cyperi).
- With watery diarrhea, add *Fu Ling* (Poria) and *Che Qian Zi* (Semen Plantaginis).
- If abdominal pain is severe, increase the dose of *Bai Shao* (Radix Paeoniae Alba) and add *Mu Gua* (Fructus Chaenomelis), *Yan Hu Suo* (Rhizoma Corydalis) and *Gan Cao* (Radix et Rhizoma Glycyrrhizae).
- With severe tenesmus, add *Mu Xiang* (Radix Aucklandiae) and *Hou Po* (Cortex Magnoliae Officinalis).
- If the stool is bloody, add *Di Yu* (Radix Sanguisorbae) and *San Qi* (Radix et Rhizoma Notoginseng).
- For increased dampness, add *Bing Lang* (Semen Arecae) and *Da Huang* (Radix et Rhizoma Rhei).

Tong Xie Yao Fang, literally meaning "important formula for painful diarrhea," treats abdominal pain and diarrhea caused by Spleen deficiency and Liver excess. Its formulation has a distinct rationale:

- *Bai Zhu* (Rhizoma Atractylodis Macrocephalae) and *Chen Pi* (Pericarpium Citri Reticulatae) strengthen the Spleen, dry dampness, and promote qi circulation. This formula does not use standard qi tonics, such as *Ren Shen* (Radix et Rhizoma Ginseng) and *Huang Qi* (Radix Astragali), because such herbs tonify qi and raise yang qi, but do not dry dampness and restore the normal transformation and transportation functions of the Spleen.
- *Fang Feng* (Radix Saposhnikoviae) is acrid, spreads Liver qi stagnation, awakens the Spleen, and dries dampness. It enters both the Liver and Spleen channels, raises yang, and stops diarrhea. When paired with *Bai Shao* (Radix Paeoniae Alba), it regulates Liver qi and relieves pain. When combined with *Bai Zhu* (Rhizoma Atractylodis Macrocephalae), it strengthens the Spleen and dispels dampness. *Chai Hu* (Radix Bupleuri), a standard Liver qi-regulating herb, is not used here because it does not strengthen the Spleen. In addition, *Chai Hu* (Radix Bupleuri) is slightly drying in nature, and may injure yin and contribute to more deficiency.[15]

Si Shen Wan (Four-Miracle Pill), *Shen Ling Bai Zhu San* (Ginseng, Poria, and Atractylodes Macrocephala Powder), and *Tong Xie Yao Fang* all treat diarrhea.

- *Si Shen Wan* warms and tonifies Spleen and Kidney yang to stop chronic diarrhea. It treats severe diarrhea that occurs in the early morning, and watery diarrhea that contains undigested food.
- *Shen Ling Bai Zhu San* treats diarrhea characterized by Spleen qi deficiency with damp accumulation, manifesting in fatigue, weakness of the limbs, and poor appetite.
- *Tong Xie Yao Fang* tonifies the Spleen and spreads Liver qi. This formula stops the type of diarrhea that accompanies stress-related abdominal pain. Animals will often have flatulence, bloating, and abdominal pain that appears relieved after stool is passed.
- Lastly, these formulas are commonly used together in clinical practices. *Tong Xie Yao Fang* can be combined with *Si Shen Wan* (Four-Miracle Pill) for the treatment of chronic diarrhea due to Kidney and Spleen yang deficiency in geriatric dogs and cats and in horses with Cushing's disease. *Tong Xie Yao Fang* may also be used with *Shen Ling Bai Zhu San* (Ginseng, Poria, and Atractylodes Macrocephala Powder) for animals with diarrhea due to predominance of Spleen qi deficiency.

References

1. *Zhong Yao Ming Fang Yao Li Yu Ying Yong* (Pharmacology and Applications of Famous Herbal Formulas), 1989; 119-120.
2. *Zhong Yao Yao Li Yu Lin Chuang* (Pharmacology and Clinical Applications of Chinese Herbs), 1992; 8:20.
3. *Hu Nan Zhong Yi Xue Yuan Xue Bao* (Journal of Hunan University of Traditional Chinese Medicine), 1987; 7:42.
4. *Yun Nan Zhong Yi Za Zhi* (Yunan Journal of Chinese Medicine), 1986; 4:24.
5. *Gan Su Zhong Yi* (Gansu Chinese Medicine), 1996; 6:21.
6. *Ha Er Bing Zhong Yi* (Haerbing Chinese Medicine), 1964; 4:25.
7. *Hu Nan Zhong Yi Za Zhi* (Hunan Journal of Chinese Medicine), 1987; 6:12.
8. *Zhong Guo Gang Chang Za Zhi* (Chinese Journal of Anus and Intestines), 1987; 4:27.
9. *Shan Xi Zhong Yi* (Shanxi Chinese Medicine), 1989; 11:490.
10. *Hu Nan Zhong Yi Za Zhi* (Hunan Journal of Chinese Medicine), 1988; 6:36.
11. *Shan Dong Zhong Yi Za Zhi* (Shandong Journal of Chinese Medicine), 1996; 10:444.
12. *Shi Yong Zhong Yi Nei Ke Za Zhi* (Journal of Practical Chinese Internal Medicine), 1991; 4:90.
13. *Hei Long Jiang Zhong Yi Yao* (Heilongjiang Chinese Medicine and Herbology), 1986; 6:23.
14. *Zhe Jiang Zhong Yi Za Zhi* (Zhejiang Journal of Chinese Medicine), 1996; 11:502.
15. Wang MZ, et al. *Zhong Yi Xue Wen Da Ti Ku* (Questions and Answers on Traditional Chinese Medicine: Herbal Formulas).

Section 3

调和肠胃剂

— Intestines and Stomach Harmonizing Formulas

Bàn Xià Xiè Xīn Tāng (Pinellia Decoction to Drain the Epigastrium)

半夏瀉心湯
半夏泻心汤

Pinyin Name: *Ban Xia Xie Xin Tang*

Literal Name: Pinellia Decoction to Drain the Epigastrium

Alternate Names: *Pan Hsia Hsieh Hsin Tang, Ban Xia Xieh Xin Tang*, Pinellia Heart-Draining Decoction, Pinellia Combination

Original Source: *Shang Han Lun* (Discussion of Cold-Induced Disorders) by Zhang Zhong-Jing in the Eastern Han Dynasty

COMPOSITION

Ban Xia (Rhizoma Pinelliae), *xi* (washed)	0.5 cup [9g]
Gan Jiang (Rhizoma Zingiberis)	9g
Huang Qin (Radix Scutellariae)	9g
Huang Lian (Rhizoma Coptidis)	3g
Ren Shen (Radix et Rhizoma Ginseng)	9g
Da Zao (Fructus Jujubae), *bo* (opened)	12 pieces [4 pieces]
Zhi Gan Cao (Radix et Rhizoma Glycyrrhizae Praeparata cum Melle)	9g [6g]

DOSAGE / PREPARATION / ADMINISTRATION

The source text advises to cook the ingredients in 10 cups [2,000 mL] of water until 6 cups [1,200 mL] of liquid remain. Discard the residue, and cook the strained decoction again until it is reduced to 3 cups [600 mL]. Take 1 cup [200 mL] of the warm decoction three times daily. Today, the decoction may be prepared using the doses suggested in brackets.

CHINESE THERAPEUTIC ACTIONS

1. Harmonizes the Stomach and corrects the reversed flow of qi
2. Disperses the interlocking of heat and cold and relieves epigastric distention

CLINICAL MANIFESTATIONS

Stomach qi disharmony: epigastric distention without pain, dry heaves, vomiting with or without vomitus, borborygmus, diarrhea, a thin, greasy tongue coating, and a wiry, rapid pulse.

VETERINARY CLINICAL APPLICATIONS

Chronic gastritis, chronic vomiting, reflux esophagitis, gastrointestinal ulcers, gastroenteritis, inflammatory bowel disease characterized by chronic vomiting, ulcerative colitis, diarrhea, nausea and vomiting due to motion sickness.

EXPLANATION

Ban Xia Xie Xin Tang (Pinellia Decoction to Drain the Epigastrium), first cited in *Shang Han Lun* (Discussion of Cold-Induced Disorders), is designed to correct the improper treatment of *shaoyang* syndrome with downward draining herbs, which results in injury to the yang qi of the middle *jiao* and the drawing of exterior pathogens into the interior. By this stage of the improper treatment, heat usually forms in the interior, resulting in the interlocking of heat and cold factors. The interlocking of heat and cold affects the normal ascending functioning of the Spleen and the descending functioning of the Stomach, causing borborygmus, diarrhea, and vomiting. It also creates a feeling of epigastric distention that is not painful and is soft on palpation.

Bàn Xià Xiè Xīn Tāng (Pinellia Decoction to Drain the Epigastrium)

Ban Xia Xie Xin Tang (Pinellia Decoction to Drain the Epigastrium)

Diagnosis	Clinical Signs	Treatment	Herbs
Stomach qi disharmony	• Epigastric distention and pain, borborygmus, diarrhea and vomiting: disharmony of the Stomach and Intestines with interlocking of heat and cold • Greasy tongue coating: damp accumulation • Wiry pulse: qi stagnation • Rapid pulse: interior heat	• Harmonizes the Stomach and corrects the reversed flow of qi • Disperses the interlocking of heat and cold and relieves epigastric distention	• *Ban Xia* (Rhizoma Pinelliae) disperses stagnation, relieves distention, directs reversed Stomach qi downward. • *Gan Jiang* (Rhizoma Zingiberis) warms the middle *jiao* and disperses cold accumulation. • *Huang Qin* (Radix Scutellariae) and *Huang Lian* (Rhizoma Coptidis) sedate heat and relieve distention. • *Ren Shen* (Radix et Rhizoma Ginseng), *Da Zao* (Fructus Jujubae) and *Zhi Gan Cao* (Radix et Rhizoma Glycyrrhizae Praeparata cum Melle) tonify the middle *jiao* and strengthen the Spleen.

A thin, white to yellow tongue coating may be present and suggests heat formation inside the body, and the greasy nature of the coating is the result of qi stagnation and damp accumulation. A wiry pulse is the result of epigastric distention and qi stagnation, and a rapid pulse indicates interior heat. This condition involves simultaneous excess and deficiency, heat and cold.

The chief herb, *Ban Xia* (Rhizoma Pinelliae), disperses stagnation, relieves distention, and directs reversed Stomach qi downward to relieve nausea and vomiting. The assistant herb, *Gan Jiang* (Rhizoma Zingiberis), warms the middle *jiao* and disperses cold accumulation. *Huang Qin* (Radix Scutellariae) and *Huang Lian* (Rhizoma Coptidis) sedate heat and relieve distention. *Ren Shen* (Radix et Rhizoma Ginseng), *Da Zao* (Fructus Jujubae), and *Zhi Gan Cao* (Radix et Rhizoma Glycyrrhizae Praeparata cum Melle) tonify the middle *jiao* and strengthen the Spleen. *Zhi Gan Cao* also harmonizes the warm and cold properties of the other herbs in this formula. This formula simultaneously disperses and directs downward, tonifies and sedates, clears heat, and warms the interior to restore the proper functioning of the Spleen and Stomach.

VETERINARY MODIFICATIONS

- For diarrhea and abdominal pain, add *Mu Xiang* (Radix Aucklandiae) and *Bai Shao* (Radix Paeoniae Alba).
- With vomiting and belching, add *Chen Pi* (Pericarpium Citri Reticulatae) and *Fu Ling* (Poria).
- With vomiting and phlegm accumulation, combine with *Er Chen Tang* (Two-Cured Decoction).
- With vomiting of food particles, combine with *Ping Wei San* (Calm the Stomach Powder).
- When there is food stagnation, add charred *Shan Zha* (Fructus Crataegi) and *Shen Qu* (Massa Fermentata).
- If there is a thick tongue coating, add *Hou Po* (Cortex Magnoliae Officinalis) and *Cang Zhu* (Rhizoma Atractylodis).
- If there is more deficiency, increase the dose of *Ren Shen* (Radix et Rhizoma Ginseng).

CAUTIONS / CONTRAINDICATIONS

- *Ban Xia Xie Xin Tang* is not suitable for epigastric distention and pain caused by accumulation of phlegm and heat, food stagnation, or qi stagnation.
- This formula should not be used in patients with nausea and vomiting caused by yin deficiency.[1]

PHARMACOLOGICAL EFFECTS

1. **Gastrointestinal**: *Ban Xia Xie Xin Tang* has been used to treat various types of gastrointestinal disorders. It has effects to normalize the upper and lower gastrointestinal system by raising the plasma levels of some hormones (somatostatin, motilin, and gastrin).[2]
2. **Antiulcer**: Administration of the formula was associated with protective effects in rats with gastric or duodenal ulcer, especially against ethanol-induced gastric injury. The mechanism of the protective effect was attributed to the strengthening and regeneration of the gastric membrane and the increase in gastric mucin content.[3,4,5] In addition, the alcohol extract of the formula inhibits intestinal peristalsis in mice.[6]
3. **Analgesic**: Administration of an alcohol extract of this formula at 10 g/kg was associated with analgesic effects in mice.[7]

HUMAN CLINICAL STUDIES AND RESEARCH

1. **Gastritis**: Modified *Ban Xia Xie Xin Tang* demonstrated 92.3% effectiveness in treating gastritis caused by bile acid regurgitation. The herbal treatment used *Ban Xia*

Bàn Xià Xiè Xīn Tāng (Pinellia Decoction to Drain the Epigastrium)

Xie Xin Tang as the base formula, with elimination of *Da Zao* (Fructus Jujubae), substitution of *Tai Zi Shen* (Radix Pseudostellariae) for *Ren Shen* (Radix et Rhizoma Ginseng), and the addition of *Bai Shao* (Radix Paeoniae Alba) and *Zhi Qiao* (Fructus Aurantii). Furthermore, *Bai Zhu* (Rhizoma Atractylodis Macrocephalae) and *Fu Ling* (Poria) were added for poor appetite; *Shen Qu* (Massa Fermentata) and *Zhe Shi* (Haematitum) for frequent belching; *Qing Pi* (Pericarpium Citri Reticulatae Viride) for pain with needling sensations; substitution of *Pao Jiang* (Rhizoma Zingiberis Praeparatum) for *Gan Jiang* (Rhizoma Zingiberis) for loose stools; *Bai He* (Bulbus Lilii) for fatigue and shortness of breath; and addition of *Fu Zi* (Radix Aconiti Lateralis Praeparata) and removal of *Ban Xia* (Rhizoma Pinelliae), *Tai Zi Shen* (Radix Pseudostellariae), and *Gan Jiang* (Rhizoma Zingiberis) for pain, perspiration and chills. Of 52 patients, the study reported complete recovery in 16 patients, marked improvement in 18 patients, moderate improvement in 14 patients, and no improvement in 4 patients.[8]

2. **Superficial gastritis**: Thirty patients with superficial gastritis were treated with modified *Ban Xia Xie Xin Tang* with 90% effectiveness. The formula included *Ban Xia* (Rhizoma Pinelliae) 9g, *Huang Lian* (Rhizoma Coptidis) 9g, *Huang Qin* (Radix Scutellariae) 9g, *Wu Ling Zhi* (Faeces Trogopteri) 4.5g, *Pu Huang* (Pollen Typhae) 4.5g, *Gan Jiang* (Rhizoma Zingiberis) 6g, *Hou Po* (Cortex Magnoliae Officinalis) 6g, *Shi Chang Pu* (Rhizoma Acori Tatarinowii) 6g, *Dang Shen* (Radix Codonopsis) 15g, *Long Kui* (Herba Solanum Nigrum) 15g, *Dan Shen* (Radix et Rhizoma Salviae Miltiorrhizae) 15g, *Da Zao* (Fructus Jujubae) 5 pieces, and *Gan Cao* (Radix et Rhizoma Glycyrrhizae) 3g.[9] Another study reported 95% effectiveness in treating superficial gastritis in 60 patients using *Ban Xia Xie Xin Tang* plus *Yan Hu Suo* (Rhizoma Corydalis), *Mu Xiang* (Radix Aucklandiae), *Chai Hu* (Radix Bupleuri), *Wu Zhu Yu* (Fructus Evodiae), *Pei Lan* (Herba Eupatorii), charred *Shan Zha* (Fructus Crataegi), charred *Shen Qu* (Massa Fermentata), and charred *Mai Ya* (Fructus Hordei Germinatus).[10]
3. **Chronic gastritis**: Use of modified *Ban Xia Xie Xin Tang* was associated with 92.31% effectiveness in treating 52 patients with chronic gastritis. In addition to the formula, modifications included the addition of *Zhi Shi* (Fructus Aurantii Immaturus) and *Hou Po* (Cortex Magnoliae Officinalis) for gastric fullness and distention; *Zhu Ru* (Caulis Bambusae in Taenia) and *Chen Pi* (Pericarpium Citri Reticulatae) for nausea and vomiting; *Bai Zhu* (Rhizoma Atractylodis Macrocephalae) and *Fu Ling* (Poria) for loose stools; *Di Huang* (Radix Rehmanniae) and *Hei Zhi Ma* (Semen Sesami Nigrum) for dry stools; *Yan Hu Suo* (Rhizoma Corydalis) for epigastric pain; *Hai Piao Xiao* (Endoconcha Sepiae) and calcined *Wa Leng Zi* (Concha Arcae) for acid reflux; *Long Dan* (Radix et Rhizoma Gentianae) for bitter taste in the mouth; *Ji Nei Jin* (Endothelium Corneum Gigeriae Galli) and *Shen Qu* (Massa Fermentata) for poor appetite; and *Huang Qi* (Radix Astragali) for fatigue. Of 52 patients, 18 had complete recovery, 30 had marked improvement, and 4 had no improvement.[11]
4. **Peptic ulcer disease**: One study reported marked success using modified *Ban Xia Xie Xin Tang* to treat peptic ulcer disease in 32 patients (18 with gastric and 14 with duodenal ulcers). In addition to the base formula, modifications included the addition of *Pao Jiang* (Rhizoma Zingiberis Praeparatum) to replace *Gan Jiang* (Rhizoma Zingiberis) in patients of bleeding; *Pao Jiang* (Rhizoma Zingiberis Praeparatum) and *Xiao Ji* (Herba Cirsii) for hematemesis; *Pao Jiang* (Rhizoma Zingiberis Praeparatum), *Xiao Ji* (Herba Cirsii), and *E Jiao* (Colla Corii Asini) for hematochezia; *Pao Jiang* (Rhizoma Zingiberis Praeparatum), *Xiao Ji* (Herba Cirsii), *E Jiao* (Colla Corii Asini) and *Bai Ji* (Rhizoma Bletillae) for hematochezia and hematemesis; and *Yan Hu Suo* (Rhizoma Corydalis) for abdominal pain. Of 32 patients, bleeding stopped in 21 patients after 4 packs of herbs, in 7 patients after 6 packs of herbs, and in 4 patients after 10 packs of herbs.[12]
5. **Reflux esophagitis**: An herbal formula that contained *Ban Xia Xie Xin Tang* plus *Zhu Ru* (Caulis Bambusae in Taenia), *Chen Xiang* (Lignum Aquilariae Resinatum) and *Zi Su Geng* (Caulis Perillae) was found to have good effect in treating 46 patients with reflux esophagitis. In addition to the base formula above, minor modifications were made by adding *Bai Shao* (Radix Paeoniae Alba) and *Wei Ling Xian* (Radix et Rhizoma Clematidis) for severe pain with difficulty swallowing; *Hai Piao Xiao* (Endoconcha Sepiae) and calcined *Wa Leng Zi* (Concha Arcae) for hyperacidity or duodenal ulcer; *Pu Gong Ying* (Herba Taraxaci) and *Zhi Zi* (Fructus Gardeniae) for burning in the stomach; *Chai Hu* (Radix Bupleuri) and *Jin Qian Cao* (Herba Lysimachiae) for cholecystitis or hypochondriac pain; and *Da Huang* (Radix et Rhizoma Rhei) and *Zhi Shi* (Fructus Aurantii Immaturus) for constipation. Of 46 patients, 8 had complete recovery, 34 had marked improvement, and 4 had no effect. The overall effectiveness was 91.3%.[13]
6. **Upper gastrointestinal bleeding**: According to one study, 39 patients with upper gastrointestinal bleeding were successfully treated with modified *Ban Xia Xie Xin Tang*. The average time needed to completely stop bleeding was 4.3 days, with a range of 3-6 days. The herbal treatment included the original formula with the addition of *Hua Rui Shi* (Ophicalcitum) 12g, *Ou Jie* (Nodus Nelumbinis Rhizomatis) 15g, and *Bai Ji* (Rhizoma Bletillae) 15g. Furthermore, *Mu Dan Pi* (Cortex Moutan), *Huang Qi* (Radix

Astragali), *Dang Gui* (Radix Angelicae Sinensis), *Sha Shen* (Radix Glehniae seu Adenophorae), *Yu Zhu* (Rhizoma Polygonati Odorati), and others were added as needed.[14]

7. **Gastroenteritis**: One study reported good results using modified *Ban Xia Xie Xin Tang* to treat acute gastroenteritis. In addition to the base formula, modifications were made as follows: double the dose of *Huang Lian* (Rhizoma Coptidis) if there are more than five bowel movements (diarrhea) per day; *Ge Gen* (Radix Puerariae Lobatae) for presence of excessive heat; *Sheng Jiang* (Rhizoma Zingiberis Recens) for nausea, vomiting, or feeling of coldness in the abdomen; and *Mu Xiang* (Radix Aucklandiae) for abdominal fullness. Of 100 patients, 78 had complete recovery, 14 had improvement, and 8 had no effect. The overall rate of effectiveness was 92%.[15]
8. **Stomach pain**: One study reported 94% effectiveness using this formula to treat 100 geriatric patients (ages 60 and over) with stomach pain caused by gastritis, stomach ulcer and duodenal ulcer.[16] In another study, 294 of 300 patients with stomach pain (caused by gastritis, or gastric or duodenal ulcers) had complete recovery using modified *Ban Xia Xie Xin Tang*.[17]
9. **Abdominal pain**: Use of *Ban Xia Xie Xin Tang* plus *Yan Hu Suo* (Rhizoma Corydalis), *Zhi Qiao* (Fructus Aurantii), and others to treat 36 children with abdominal pain was associated with complete recovery in 34 patients and improvement in 2 patients. The overall rate of effectiveness was 94.4%.[18]
10. **Irritable bowel syndrome (IBS)**: Administration of *Ban Xia Xie Xin Tang* plus *Chai Hu* (Radix Bupleuri), *Mu Xiang* (Radix Aucklandiae), *Bai Shao* (Radix Paeoniae Alba), and *Yan Hu Suo* (Rhizoma Corydalis) daily for 4 weeks in 37 patients with IBS was associated with complete recovery in 25 patients, improvement in 8 patients, and no effect in 4 patients. The overall effectiveness was 89.19%.[19] According to another study, 56 patients with IBS were treated with complete recovery in 35 patients (62.5%), improvement in 17 patients (30.36%), and no effect in 4 patients (7.14%). The herbal formula contained *Ban Xia Xie Xin Tang* plus *Bai Zhu* (Rhizoma Atractylodis Macrocephalae), *Mu Xiang* (Radix Aucklandiae) and *Bai Shao* (Radix Paeoniae Alba) as the base formula. Additional modifications included *Che Qian Zi* (Semen Plantaginis), *Bian Dou Yi* (Pericarpium Lablab Album), *Zhu Ling* (Polyporus) and *Ze Xie* (Rhizoma Alismatis) for loose stools; *Bai Tou Weng* (Radix Pulsatillae) and *Huang Bo* (Cortex Phellodendri Chinensis) for sticky stools with mucus; *Da Huang* (Radix et Rhizoma Rhei) for constipation; *Yi Yi Ren* (Semen Coicis) and *Huo Xiang* (Herba Agastaches) for dampness; *Bu Gu Zhi* (Fructus Psoraleae) for yang deficiency; *Sheng Jiang* (Rhizoma Zingiberis Recens) and *Zhu Ru* (Caulis Bambusae in Taenia) for nausea and vomiting; and the addition of *Hou Po* (Cortex Magnoliae Officinalis) and *Zhi Shi* (Fructus Aurantii Immaturus), and elimination of *Dang Shen* (Radix Codonopsis), *Bai Zhu* (Rhizoma Atractylodis Macrocephalae), and *Da Zao* (Fructus Jujubae) for abdominal distention, borborygmus, and pain that intensifies with pressure.[20]
11. **Ulcerative colitis**: Use of modified *Ban Xia Xie Xin Tang* was associated with 96.9% effectiveness in treating 33 patients with chronic ulcerative colitis. The base herbal formula contained this formula without *Da Zao* (Fructus Jujubae), and with the addition of *Da Huang* (Radix et Rhizoma Rhei). Furthermore, modifications based on individual conditions were made by adding *Mu Xiang* (Radix Aucklandiae), *Bai Shao* (Radix Paeoniae Alba), and *Dang Gui* (Radix Angelicae Sinensis) for abdominal pain; charred *Mu Dan Pi* (Cortex Moutan), charred *Di Huang* (Radix Rehmanniae), and charred *Huai Hua* (Flos Sophorae) for hematochezia; *Yi Yi Ren* (Semen Coicis) and *Ma Chi Xian* (Herba Portulacae) for severe diarrhea; *Sheng Ma* (Rhizoma Cimicifugae) for rectal tenesmus; *Chai Hu* (Radix Bupleuri) and *Zhi Qiao* (Fructus Aurantii) for hypochondriac fullness and pain; and the removal of *Huang Lian* (Rhizoma Coptidis) and the addition of *Bu Gu Zhi* (Fructus Psoraleae) and *Rou Gui* (Cortex Cinnamomi) for chronic diarrhea with soreness and coldness of the lower back and knees. Of 33 patients, 17 had complete recovery, 8 had marked improvement, 7 had moderate improvement, and 1 had no improvement.[21]
12. **Diarrhea**: Administration of 1 pack of *Ban Xia Xie Xin Tang* was effective in treating 20 of 25 patients with acute onset of diarrhea characterized by the presence of severe diarrhea, feeling of distention and oppression, and vomiting.[22]

HERB-DRUG INTERACTION

- **Cisplatin- and irinotecan-induced diarrhea**: Diarrhea induced by cisplatin (Platinol) and irinotecan (Camptosar) was effectively controlled with *Ban Xia Xie Xin Tang* (7.5 g/day) in patients with advanced non-small-cell lung cancer. In comparison with the control group, patients who received *Ban Xia Xie Xin Tang* showed a significant improvement in diarrhea grades (P=0.044), as well as a reduced frequency of diarrhea grades 3 and 4 (one patient versus ten patients; P=0.018).[23] The mechanisms of this action was attributed to accelerated healing of the intestinal tract, improved colonic water absorption, and decreased levels of colonic prostaglandin E2 (PGE2).[24] In another study, use of *Ban Xia Xie Xin Tang* was also found to be effective in preventing and controlling diarrhea induced by cisplatin and irinotecan (CPT-11) in patients with non-small-cell lung cancer. In comparison with the 23 patients in the control group that did not

Bàn Xià Xiè Xīn Tāng (Pinellia Decoction to Drain the Epigastrium)

receive any herbs, 18 patients in the herb group showed a significant improvement in diarrhea grades and reduced frequency of diarrhea grades. The therapeutic benefit of preventing and controlling diarrhea was attributed in part to baicalin, a beta-glucuronidase inhibitor.[25]

- **Irinotecan-induced diarrhea**: Numerous studies have shown that diarrhea induced by irinotecan (Camptosar) can be effectively controlled and treated with administration of *Ban Xia Xie Xin Tang*.[26,27,28]

TOXICOLOGY

Administration of *Ban Xia Xie Xin Tang* was associated with one case of pneumonitis in a 72-year-old woman. Upon admission to the hospital and discontinuation of the formula, the clinical signs were relieved, and the X-ray findings improved markedly. This is believed to be the first case of pulmonary hypersensitivity induced by *Ban Xia Xie Xin Tang* in Japan.[29]

SUGGESTED ACUPUNCTURE TREATMENT

1. Points: *Zhongwan* (CV 12), *Neiguan* (PC 6), *Tianshu* (ST 25), *Qihai* (CV 6), and *Housanli* (ST 36).
2. Technique: both tonification and sedation.

Sedate *Zhongwan* (CV 12) and *Neiguan* (PC 6) to remove heat in the Stomach and correct the reversed qi flow. Tonify *Tianshu* (ST 25), *Qihai* (CV 6), and *Housanli* (ST 36) to dispel cold and harmonize the Stomach and Intestines.

AUTHORS' COMMENTS

The original use of *Ban Xia Xie Xin Tang* aimed at treating Stomach qi disharmony caused by maltreatment of *shaoyang* syndrome with downward draining herbs. Today, the contemporary applications of this formula have been vastly expanded to include various gastrointestinal disorders characterized by the presence of hot and cold, exterior and interior factors, and disharmony of the Stomach and Intestines. These factors promote stagnation with heat in the Stomach and middle *jiao*, which interferes with the normal ascent of Spleen qi and descent of Stomach qi. The resulting clinical signs are a red tongue and, in severe cases, a thin white to yellow coating, a wiry pulse, and cold signs of borborygmus and diarrhea. The key to using this formula is the recognition of both heat and cold signs that are present at the same time. Cats that are exclusively fed a dry food diet loaded with grains such as corn, wheat and soybean often develop chronic vomiting and gastritis, and these animals do well when given this formula. These cats are diagnosed as having inflammatory bowel disease on stomach and intestinal biopsy. In chronic cases, it is often necessary to add herbs that further tonify the Spleen, such as *Fu Ling* (Poria) and *Bai Zhu* (Rhizoma Atractylodis Macrocephalae).

The herbs in this formula tonify the Spleen and Stomach, relieve bloating and nausea, and clear heat from the Stomach. This makes *Ban Xia Xie Xin Tang* ideal to treat animals that are stressed, taking multiple pharmaceutical drugs at the same time, and fed a suboptimal diet. Horses that colic at competitions are prime examples of this kind of patient. This situation is also common in hospitalized cancer patients and chronically-ill geriatric animals with multi-systemic diseases such cardiac, renal and inflammatory bowel conditions. It is effective in treating gastric bleeding and hematemesis secondary to aspirin, steroidal and non-steroidal anti-inflammatory drug administration; 7-10 days of treatment is typically sufficient. If sucralfate is also being given to treat gastrointestinal tract ulceration, it is best to give the herbal formula one hour prior to administration of this drug. In these cases, the addition of the herb *Fo Shou* (Fructus Citri Sarcodactylis) and *San Qi* (Radix et Rhizoma Notoginseng) can help resolve gastric and upper digestive tract ulceration.

Ban Xia Xie Xin Tang is based on *Xiao Chai Hu Tang* (Minor Bupleurum Decoction) without *Chai Hu* (Radix Bupleuri) and *Sheng Jiang* (Rhizoma Zingiberis Recens), and with the addition of *Huang Lian* (Rhizoma Coptidis) and *Gan Jiang* (Rhizoma Zingiberis). This is the best formula to treat epigastric pain caused by various kinds of digestive dysfunctions.

A question is often raised as to why *Ban Xia Xie Xin Tang*, a formula that treats epigastric bloating and pain, would contain *Ren Shen* (Radix et Rhizoma Ginseng), *Gan Cao* (Radix et Rhizoma Glycyrrhizae), and *Da Zao* (Fructus Jujubae), three tonic herbs that could create more stagnation. The answer is that in *Ban Xia Xie Xin Tang*, epigastric distention and pain are not caused by damp accumulation or stagnation, conditions that could be worsened with the use of tonic herbs. Instead, epigastric distention and pain occur as a result of the misuse of herbs that injure the middle *jiao*, thus creating disruption of Stomach functioning in addition to heat and cold stagnation in the middle *jiao*. In this case, *Ren Shen* (Radix et Rhizoma Ginseng), *Gan Cao* (Radix et Rhizoma Glycyrrhizae), and *Da Zao* (Fructus Jujubae) serve to protect the Spleen, restore normal digestive functioning, and restore *zheng* (upright) *qi* which was damaged by the use of downward draining herbs.

Bàn Xià Xiè Xīn Tāng (Pinellia Decoction to Drain the Epigastrium)

There are three "*Xie Xin Tang* (Drain the Epigastrium)" formulas that treat epigastric fullness and distention. Even though the main clinical signs are the same, the causes are different. Different causes in turn require different treatments. With minute changes in the composition and dosage of the formulas, their properties change as well.

- *Ban Xia Xie Xin Tang* treats epigastric distention (bloating) caused by interlocking of heat and cold.
- *Sheng Jiang Xie Xin Tang* (Fresh Ginger Decoction to Drain the Epigastrium) treats epigastric distention caused by interlocking of heat and water.
- *Gan Cao Xie Xin Tang* (Licorice Decoction to Drain the Epigastrium) treats epigastric distention caused by Stomach deficiency.

References

1. *Zhong Yao Ming Fang Yao Li Yu Ying Yong* (Pharmacology and Applications of Famous Herbal Formulas), 1989; 121-123.
2. Naito T, Itoh H, Yasunaga F, Takeyama M. Hange-shashin-to raises levels of somatostatin, motilin, and gastrin in the plasma of healthy subjects. Biol Pharm Bull. 2002 Mar; 25(3):327-31.
3. *Shan Xi Zhong Yi Xue Yuan Xue Bao* (Journal of Shanxi University School of Chinese Medicine), 1987; 10(3):11.
4. Li J, Takeda H, Inazu M, Hayashi M, Tsuji M, Ikoshi H, Takada K, Matsumiya T. Protective effects of Hange-shashin-to on water-immersion restraint stress-induced gastric ulcers. Methods Find Exp Clin Pharmacol. 1998 Jan-Feb; 20(1):31-7.
5. Kase Y, Yuzurihara M, Iizuka S, Ishige A, Komatsu Y. The effects of hange-shashin-to on gastric function in comparison with sho-saiko-to. Biol Pharm Bull. 1997 Nov; 20(11):1155-9.
6. *Hu Nan Zhong Yi Za Zhi* (Hunan Journal of Chinese Medicine), 1986; 5:21.
7. *Hu Nan Zhong Yi Za Zhi* (Hunan Journal of Chinese Medicine), 1986; 5:21.
8. *Zhe Jiang Zhong Yi Xue Yuan Xue Bao* (Journal of Zhejiang University of Chinese Medicine), 1997; 4:33.
9. *Fu Jian Zhong Yi Yao* (Fujian Chinese Medicine and Herbology), 1983; 1:27.
10. *Shan Xi Zhong Yi* (Shanxi Chinese Medicine), 1991; 12(3):128.
11. *Tian Jin Zhong Yi* (Tianjin Chinese Medicine), 1997; 1:15.
12. *Hei Long Jiang Zhong Yi Yao* (Heilongjiang Chinese Medicine and Herbology), 1996; 5:27.
13. *Hei Long Jiang Zhong Yi Yao* (Heilongjiang Chinese Medicine and Herbology), 1998; 3:30.
14. *Hu Bei Zhong Yi Za Zhi* (Hubei Journal of Chinese Medicine), 1987; 3:22.
15. *Zhe Jiang Zhong Yi Za Zhi* (Zhejiang Journal of Chinese Medicine), 1985; 4:155.
16. *Shang Hai Zhong Yi Yao Za Zhi* (Shanghai Journal of Chinese Medicine and Herbology), 1989; 10:31.
17. *Shan Xi Zhong Yi* (Shanxi Chinese Medicine), 1997; 7:299.
18. *Nei Meng Gu Zhong Yi Yao* (Traditional Chinese Medicine and Medicinals of Inner Mongolia), 1998; 4:14.
19. *Zhe Jiang Zhong Yi Xue Yuan Xue Bao* (Journal of Zhejiang University of Chinese Medicine), 1997; 3:29.
20. *Zhong Yi Ming Fang Lin Chuang Xin Yong* (Contemporary Clinical Applications of Classic Chinese Formulas), 2001; 303.
21. *Xin Zhong Yi* (New Chinese Medicine), 1997; 6:14.
22. *Si Chuan Zhong Yi* (Sichuan Chinese Medicine), 1989; 5:35.
23. Mori K, Kondo T, Kamiyama Y, Kano Y, Tominaga K. Preventive effect of Kampo medicine (Hangeshashin-to) against irinotecan-induced diarrhea in advanced non-small-cell lung cancer. Cancer Chemother Pharmacol. 2003 May;51(5):403-6. Epub 2003 Apr 09.
24. Kase Y, Hayakawa T, Aburada M, Komatsu Y, Kamataki T. Preventive effects of Hange-shashin-to on irinotecan hydrochloride-caused diarrhea and its relevance to the colonic prostaglandin E2 and water absorption in the rat. Jpn J Pharmacol. 1997 Dec; 75(4):407-13.
25. Mori K, Kondo T, Kamiyama Y, Kano Y, Tominaga K. Preventive effect of Kampo medicine (Hangeshashin-to) against irinotecan-induced diarrhea in advanced non-small-cell lung cancer. Cancer Chemotherapy & Pharmacology. 2003 May; 51(5):403-6.
26. Takasuna K, Kasai Y, Kitano Y, Mori K, Kobayashi R, Hagiwara T, Kakihata K, Hirohashi M, Nomura M, Nagai E, et al. Protective effects of kampo medicines and baicalin against intestinal toxicity of a new anticancer camptothecin derivative, irinotecan hydrochloride (CPT-11), in rats. Jpn J Cancer Res. 1995 Oct; 86(10):978-84.
27. Sakata Y, Suzuki H, Kamataki T. Preventive effect of TJ-14, a kampo (Chinese herb) medicine, on diarrhea induced by irinotecan hydrochloride (CPT-11). Gan To Kagaku Ryoho. 1994 Jul ;21(8):1241-4.
28. Mori K, Hirose T, Machida S, Tominaga K. Kampo medicines for the prevention of irinotecan-induced diarrhea in advanced non-small cell lung cancer. Gan To Kagaku Ryoho. 1998 Jul; 25(8):1159-63.
29. Oketani N, Saito H, Ebe T. Pneumonitis due to Hangeshashin-to. Nihon Kyobu Shikkan Gakkai Zasshi. 1996 Sep; 34(9):983-8.

Shēng Jiāng Xiè Xīn Tang
(Fresh Ginger Decoction to Drain the Epigastrium)
生薑瀉心湯
生姜泻心汤

Pinyin Name: *Sheng Jiang Xie Xin Tang*
Literal Name: Fresh Ginger Decoction to Drain the Epigastrium
Alternate Name: Pinellia and Ginger Combination
Original Source: *Shang Han Lun* (Discussion of Cold-Induced Disorders) by Zhang Zhong-Jing in the Eastern Han Dynasty

COMPOSITION

Ban Xia (Rhizoma Pinelliae), *xi* (washed)	0.5 cup [9g]
Sheng Jiang (Rhizoma Zingiberis Recens), *qie* (sliced)	12g [12g]
Gan Jiang (Rhizoma Zingiberis)	3g [3g]
Huang Qin (Radix Scutellariae)	9g [6g]
Huang Lian (Rhizoma Coptidis)	3g [3g]
Ren Shen (Radix et Rhizoma Ginseng)	9g [6g]
Da Zao (Fructus Jujubae), *bo* (opened)	12 pieces [4 pieces]
Zhi Gan Cao (Radix et Rhizoma Glycyrrhizae Praeparata cum Melle)	9g [6g]

DOSAGE / PREPARATION / ADMINISTRATION

The source text states to cook the ingredients in 10 cups [2,000 mL] of water until 6 cups [1,200 mL] of liquid remain. Discard the residue and cook the strained decoction again until it is reduced to 3 cups [600 mL]. Take 1 cup [200 mL] of the warm decoction three times daily. Today, the decoction may be prepared using the doses suggested in brackets.

CHINESE THERAPEUTIC ACTIONS

1. Harmonizes the Stomach and corrects the reversed flow of qi
2. Disperses the interlocking of heat and water and relieves epigastric distention

CLINICAL MANIFESTATIONS

Spleen and Stomach deficiencies with interlocking of heat and water in the interior: epigastric bloating and hardness, belching, foul breath, borborygmus, and diarrhea.

VETERINARY CLINICAL APPLICATIONS

Acute gastroenteritis, gastric ulcers, diarrhea, and dysentery.

EXPLANATION

Sheng Jiang Xie Xin Tang (Fresh Ginger Decoction to Drain the Epigastrium) was originally formulated for the following condition: individuals with exterior cold condition, who, after inappropriate treatment with diaphoretic methods to release exterior cold, now suffers

***Sheng Jiang Xie Xin Tang* (Fresh Ginger Decoction to Drain the Epigastrium)**

Diagnosis	Clinical Signs	Treatment	Herbs
Spleen and Stomach deficiencies with the interlocking of heat and water in the interior	Epigastric bloating and hardness, belching, foul breath, borborygmus and diarrhea	• Harmonizes the Stomach and corrects the reversed flow of qi • Disperses the interlocking of heat and water and relieves epigastric distention	• *Ban Xia* (Rhizoma Pinelliae) disperses stagnation, relieves distention, and directs reversed Stomach qi downward. • *Sheng Jiang* (Rhizoma Zingiberis Recens) warms the Stomach, stops nausea, and disperses water accumulation. • *Gan Jiang* (Rhizoma Zingiberis) warms the Stomach. • *Huang Qin* (Radix Scutellariae) and *Huang Lian* (Rhizoma Coptidis) sedate heat and relieve distention. • *Ren Shen* (Radix et Rhizoma Ginseng), *Da Zao* (Fructus Jujubae) and *Zhi Gan Cao* (Radix et Rhizoma Glycyrrhizae Praeparata cum Melle) tonify the middle *jiao* and strengthen the Spleen.

Shēng Jiāng Xiè Xīn Tāng
(Fresh Ginger Decoction to Drain the Epigastrium)

from damage to the middle *jiao*, deficiencies of the Spleen and Stomach, and interlocking of heat and water.

Sheng Jiang Xie Xin Tang aims at treating animals with Spleen and Stomach deficiencies, with the interlocking of heat and water in the interior. This formula is a modification of *Ban Xia Xie Xin Tang* (Pinellia Decoction to Drain the Epigastrium), with the addition of *Sheng Jiang* (Rhizoma Zingiberis Recens) and a reduction in the dose of *Gan Jiang* (Rhizoma Zingiberis). Because water and heat are interlocked, *Sheng Jiang* (Rhizoma Zingiberis Recens) warms the Stomach, stops nausea, and disperses water accumulation. *Gan Jiang* (Rhizoma Zingiberis) warms the Stomach, but the dose is reduced to avoid creating too much heat. Clinically, animals may show abdominal bloating and hardness, belching, foul breath, borborygmus, and diarrhea.

VETERINARY MODIFICATIONS

- With nausea and vomiting of clear fluids, add *Zhi Shi* (Fructus Aurantii Immaturus) and *Hou Po* (Cortex Magnoliae Officinalis).
- With diarrhea and abdominal pain, add *Bai Shao* (Radix Paeoniae Alba) and *Chen Pi* (Pericarpium Citri Reticulatae).
- If there is indigestion, add *Ping Wei San* (Calm the Stomach Powder).
- With belching and water retention in the middle *jiao*, add *Wu Ling San* (Five-Ingredient Powder with Poria).

HUMAN CLINICAL STUDIES AND RESEARCH

Epigastric distention: Use of modified *Sheng Jiang Xie Xin Tang* was effective in treating epigastric distention. Modifications included the elimination of *Sheng Jiang* (Rhizoma Zingiberis Recens) and *Ban Xia* (Rhizoma Pinelliae) for excess heat; and the elimination of *Huang Qin* (Radix Scutellariae) and *Huang Lian* (Rhizoma Coptidis) for excess cold. Of 245 cases, the study reported complete recovery in 187 cases, improvement in 45 cases, and no effect in 13 cases.

SUGGESTED ACUPUNCTURE TREATMENT

1. Points: *Zhongwan* (CV 12), *Neiguan* (PC 6), *Tianshu* (ST 25), *Qihai* (CV 6), *Housanli* (ST 36), *Sanyinjiao* (SP 6), and *Pangguangshu* (BL 28)
2. Technique: both tonification and sedation.

Sedate *Zhongwan* (CV 12) and *Neiguan* (PC 6) to remove heat in the Stomach and direct reversed flow of qi downward. Tonify *Tianshu* (ST 25), *Qihai* (CV 6), and *Housanli* (ST 36) to dispel cold and harmonize the Stomach and Intestines. *Sanyinjiao* (SP 6) and *Pangguangshu* (BL 28) help remove water accumulation.

Reference

1. *Zhe Jiang Zhong Yi Za Zhi* (Zhejiang Journal of Chinese Medicine), 1988; 2:75.

Gān Cǎo Xiè Xīn Tāng (Licorice Decoction to Drain the Epigastrium)

甘草瀉心湯
甘草泻心汤

Pinyin Name: *Gan Cao Xie Xin Tang*
Literal Name: Licorice Decoction to Drain the Epigastrium
Alternate Name: Pinellia and Licorice Combination
Original Source: *Shang Han Lun* (Discussion of Cold-Induced Disorders) by Zhang Zhong-Jing in the Eastern Han Dynasty

COMPOSITION

Ban Xia (Rhizoma Pinelliae), *xi* (washed)	0.5 cup [9g]
Gan Jiang (Rhizoma Zingiberis)	9g [6g]
Huang Qin (Radix Scutellariae)	9g [6g]
Huang Lian (Rhizoma Coptidis)	3g
Ren Shen (Radix et Rhizoma Ginseng)	9g [6g]
Da Zao (Fructus Jujubae), *bo* (opened)	12 pieces [4 pieces]
Zhi Gan Cao (Radix et Rhizoma Glycyrrhizae Praeparata cum Melle)	12g

Note: According to *Shang Han Lun* (Discussion of Cold-Induced Disorders), the source text, this formula does not contain *Ren Shen* (Radix et Rhizoma Ginseng). However, *Ren Shen* (Radix et Rhizoma Ginseng) is listed as an ingredient in many subsequent texts, such as *Jin Gui Yao Lue* (Essentials from the Golden Cabinet) by Zhang Zhong-Jing in the Eastern Han Dynasty, *Qian Jin Yao Fang* (Thousand Ducat Prescriptions) by Sun Si-Miao in 581-685 A.D., and *Wai Tai Mi Yao* (Arcane Essentials from the Imperial Library) by Wang Tao in 752 A.D. Based on historical data and formulary analysis, most texts now include *Ren Shen* (Radix et Rhizoma Ginseng) as an ingredient.

DOSAGE / PREPARATION / ADMINISTRATION

The source text instructs to cook the ingredients in 10 cups [2,000 mL] of water until 6 cups [1,200 mL] of liquid remain. Discard the residue and cook the strained decoction again until it is reduced to 3 cups [600 mL]. Take 1 cup [200 mL] of the warm decoction three times daily. Today, the decoction may be prepared using the doses suggested in brackets.

CHINESE THERAPEUTIC ACTIONS

1. Benefits qi and harmonizes the Stomach
2. Relieves epigastric distention and stops diarrhea

CLINICAL MANIFESTATIONS

Epigastric distention caused by Stomach deficiency and interlocking of heat and cold in the interior: epigastric distention and hardness, dry heaves, vomiting, irritability, borborygmus, and diarrhea with undigested food in the stool.

VETERINARY CLINICAL APPLICATIONS

Gastroenteritis, chronic gastritis, gastric or duodenal ulcers, chronic hepatitis, liver cirrhosis and motion sickness with nausea and vomiting.

EXPLANATION

Gan Cao Xie Xin Tang (Licorice Decoction to Drain the Epigastrium) was originally formulated for the following condition: patients with exterior cold condition, who after inappropriate treatment with downward draining herbs, now suffer from damage to the middle *jiao* and severe deficiencies of the Spleen and Stomach.

Gan Cao Xie Xin Tang is composed of *Ban Xia Xie Xin Tang* (Pinellia Decoction to Drain the Epigastrium), plus an extra 3g of *Zhi Gan Cao* (Radix et Rhizoma Glycyrrhizae Praeparata cum Melle), which is used in this formula to tonify the Stomach and treat diarrhea with undigested food in the stools. Please refer to *Ban Xia Xie Xin Tang* (Pinellia Decoction to Drain the Epigastrium) for an explanation of the etiology of this syndrome and the functions of the herbs in this formula.

Gān Cǎo Xiè Xīn Tāng (Licorice Decoction to Drain the Epigastrium)

***Gan Cao Xie Xin Tang* (Licorice Decoction to Drain the Epigastrium)**

Diagnosis	Clinical Signs	Treatment	Herbs
Epigastric distention caused by Stomach deficiency	Epigastric distention and hardness, dry heaves, vomiting, irritability, borborygmus, and diarrhea with undigested food in the stools	• Benefits qi and harmonizes the Stomach • Relieves epigastric distention and stops diarrhea	• *Ban Xia* (Rhizoma Pinelliae) disperses stagnation, relieves distention, and directs reversed Stomach qi downward to relieve nausea and vomiting. • *Gan Jiang* (Rhizoma Zingiberis) warms the middle *jiao* and disperses cold accumulation. • *Huang Qin* (Radix Scutellariae) and *Huang Lian* (Rhizoma Coptidis) sedate heat and relieve distention. • *Ren Shen* (Radix et Rhizoma Ginseng) and *Da Zao* (Fructus Jujubae) tonify the middle *jiao* and strengthen the Spleen. • A larger dose of *Zhi Gan Cao* (Radix et Rhizoma Glycyrrhizae Praeparata cum Melle) greatly tonifies the Stomach and treats diarrhea with undigested food in the stools.

VETERINARY MODIFICATIONS

- For diarrhea with abdominal pain, add *Mu Xiang* (Radix Aucklandiae) and *Bai Shao* (Radix Paeoniae Alba).
- With vomiting and belching, add *Chen Pi* (Pericarpium Citri Reticulatae) and *Fu Ling* (Poria).
- With vomiting and epigastric pain, combine with *San Huang Xie Xin Tang* (Three-Yellow Decoction to Sedate the Epigastrium).
- With vomiting with phlegm accumulation, combine with *Er Chen Tang* (Two-Cured Decoction).
- With vomiting of food particles, combine with *Ping Wei San* (Calm the Stomach Powder).

SUGGESTED ACUPUNCTURE TREATMENT

1. Points: *Zhongwan* (CV 12), *Neiguan* (PC 6), *Tianshu* (ST 25), *Qihai* (CV 6), and *Housanli* (ST 36).
2. Technique: tonification, moxibustion, and sedation.

Sedate *Zhongwan* (CV 12) and *Neiguan* (PC 6) to remove heat in the Stomach and direct reversed flow of qi downward. Tonify *Tianshu* (ST 25), *Qihai* (CV 6), and *Housanli* (ST 36) to dispel cold and harmonize the Stomach and Intestines. Apply moxibustion to *Qihai* (CV 6) to tonify the Stomach and ease pain.

Chapter 3 — Summary — Harmonizing Formulas

SECTION 1: *SHAOYANG* HARMONIZING FORMULAS

Name	Similarities	Differences
Xiao Chai Hu Tang (Minor Bupleurum Decoction)	Harmonize the exterior and interior to treat *shaoyang* syndrome	Standard formula to treat *shaoyang* syndrome: tonifies qi and strengthens the body
Chai Hu Gui Zhi Tang (Bupleurum and Cinnamon Twig Decoction)		Treats *taiyang* and *shaoyang* syndromes: dispels pathogenic factors from both stages
Chai Ling Tang (Bupleurum and Poria Decoction)		Treats *shaoyang* syndrome with water accumulation: dispels water stagnation, eliminates phlegm accumulation
Hao Qin Qing Dan Tang (Artemisia Annua and Scutellaria Decoction to Clear the Gallbladder)		Treats damp-heat in the Gallbladder: dispels dampness, dissolves phlegm

Xiao Chai Hu Tang is the standard formula to harmonize *shaoyang* syndrome, a condition characterized by the presence of pathogenic factors located between the exterior and interior. In addition, this formula also tonifies qi and strengthens the body.

Chai Hu Gui Zhi Tang (Bupleurum and Cinnamon Twig Decoction) treats both *taiyang* and *shaoyang* syndromes. It is formulated by combining two formulas together: *Xiao Chai Hu Tang* to treat *shaoyang* syndrome, and *Gui Zhi Tang* (Cinnamon Twig Decoction) to treat *taiyang* syndrome.

Chai Ling Tang (Bupleurum and Poria Decoction) treats *shaoyang* syndrome with accumulation of water, dampness, and phlegm. It is formulated by combining two formulas together: *Xiao Chai Hu Tang* to treat the *shaoyang* syndrome, and *Wu Ling San* (Five-Ingredient Powder with Poria) to treat water accumulation.

Hao Qin Qing Dan Tang (Artemisia Annua and Scutellaria Decoction to Clear the Gallbladder) cleanses the Gallbladder, harmonizes the Stomach, eliminates dampness, and dissolves phlegm. It is used to treat summer-heat invading the *shaoyang* with stagnation of dampness and phlegm. Hence, this formula is especially effective in treating *shaoyang* syndrome with severe interior heat accompanied by some dampness and phlegm.

Chapter 3 — Summary

SECTION 2: LIVER AND SPLEEN HARMONIZING FORMULAS

Name	Similarities	Differences
Si Ni San (Frigid Extremities Powder)	Regulate Liver qi circulation, relieve Liver qi stagnation	Circulates yang qi to relieve *shaoyin* syndrome with frigid extremities
Chai Hu Shu Gan Tang (Bupleurum Decoction to Spread the Liver)		Strongly activates qi circulation
Shu Gan Tang (Spread the Liver Decoction)		Strongly invigorates blood circulation
Chai Hu Qing Gan Tang (Bupleurum Decoction to Clear the Liver)		Clears heat from the Liver, Gallbladder, and *San Jiao* channels
Yi Gan San (Restrain the Liver Powder)		Clears Liver heat, nourishes Liver blood
Xiao Yao San (Rambling Powder)	Soothe the Liver and relieve qi stagnation, strengthen the Spleen, nourish the blood	Treats Liver qi stagnation
Jia Wei Xiao Yao San (Augmented Rambling Powder)		Treats Liver qi stagnation with heat and fire
Tong Xie Yao Fang (Important Formula for Painful Diarrhea)	Sedates the Liver, tonifies the Spleen	Dispels dampness and stops diarrhea

Si Ni San (Frigid Extremities Powder) ventilates the pathogens outward, relieves constraint, spreads Liver qi, and harmonizes the Liver and Spleen. It treats *shaoyin* syndrome characterized by frigid extremities, or disharmony of the Liver and Spleen. Clinical manifestations include cold extremities, epigastric and abdominal pain, and diarrhea.

Chai Hu Shu Gan Tang (Bupleurum Decoction to Spread the Liver) and ***Shu Gan Tang*** (Spread the Liver Decoction) both treat Liver qi stagnation with blood stasis characterized by hypochondriac pain.

- *Chai Hu Shu Gan San* has stronger effect to activate qi circulation.
- *Shu Gan Tang* is more effective to invigorate blood circulation and eliminate blood stasis.

Chai Hu Qing Gan Tang (Bupleurum Decoction to Clear the Liver) is a potent formula that clears heat in the Liver, Gallbladder, and *San Jiao* channels. Clinical manifestations may include fever, epistaxis, loss of hearing, and swelling of the lymph nodes.

Yi Gan San (Restrain the Liver Powder) treats a complex condition of both excess (Liver heat) and deficiency (Liver blood). Clinical signs include fever, easily frightened and scared, muscle spasms and contraction, clenching of the teeth, nervousness, irritability, restlessness, insomnia and seizures.

Xiao Yao San (Rambling Powder) nourishes the blood, smoothes the Liver, and strengthens the Spleen. It treats Liver qi stagnation (often due to blood deficiency) and deficiency of the Spleen. Clinical manifestations include hypochondriac pain, irritability, dry eyes, dandruff, poor hair coat and nail/hoof quality, poor digestion, poor appetite and lethargy.

Jia Wei Xiao Yao San (Augmented Rambling Powder) is formulated by adding *Mu Dan Pi* (Cortex Moutan) and *Zhi Zi* (Fructus Gardeniae) to *Xiao Yao San* (Rambling Powder). In comparison to the base formula, *Jia Wei Xiao Yao San* (Augmented Rambling Powder) has an enhanced effect to clear heat and sedate fire, and is more suitable for cases in which Liver qi stagnation is turning into Liver heat and fire.

Tong Xie Yao Fang (Important Formula for Painful Diarrhea) mainly treats abdominal pain and diarrhea caused by Liver overacting on the Spleen. The abdominal pain in this case usually persists after defecation.

Chapter 3 — Summary

SECTION 3: INTESTINE AND STOMACH HARMONIZING FORMULAS

Name	Similarities	Differences
Ban Xia Xie Xin Tang (Pinellia Decoction to Drain the Epigastrium)	"Drain the epigastrium" to relieve the feeling of epigastric distention	Eliminates the interlocking of heat and cold
Sheng Jiang Xie Xin Tang (Fresh Ginger Decoction to Drain the Epigastrium)		Eliminates the interlocking of water and heat
Gan Cao Xie Xin Tang (Licorice Decoction to Drain the Epigastrium)		Tonifies Stomach deficiency

Ban Xia Xie Xin Tang (Pinellia Decoction to Drain the Epigastrium), ***Sheng Jiang Xie Xin Tang*** (Fresh Ginger Decoction to Drain the Epigastrium), and ***Gan Cao Xie Xin Tang*** (Licorice Decoction to Drain the Epigastrium) are three formulas with similar names and functions: "*xie xin*" means "to drain the epigastrium."

- *Ban Xia Xie Xin Tang* treats epigastric distention caused by the interlocking of heat and cold. It activates qi stagnation, lowers the reversed flow of qi, and relieves epigastric distention and pain.
- *Sheng Jiang Xie Xin Tang* treats epigastric distention caused by the interlocking of water and heat. It eliminates water accumulation, disperses nodules, harmonizes the Stomach, and relieves epigastric distention and hardness.
- *Gan Cao Xie Xin Tang* treats epigastric distention caused by Stomach deficiency. It tonifies qi, stops diarrhea, harmonizes the Stomach, and relieves epigastric distention, pain and hardness.

Chapter 4

— Exterior- and Interior-Releasing Formulas

表里双解剂

刘完素 Lǐu Yuǎn-Sù

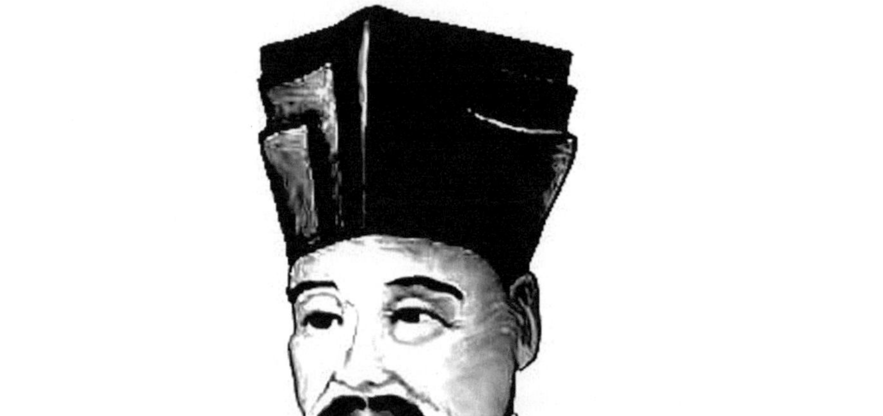

刘完素 Lǐu Yuǎn-Sù, 1120 – 1200.

刘完素 Lĭu Yuăn-Sù

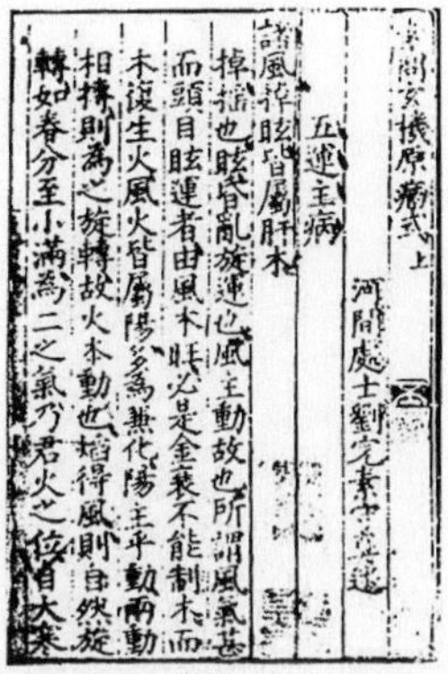
素問玄機原病式 上
河間處士劉完素守真述
五運主病
諸風掉眩皆屬肝木
掉搖也眩昏亂旋運也風主動故也所謂風氣甚
而頭目眩運者由風木旺必是金衰不能制木而
木復生火風火皆屬陽多為兼化陽主乎動兩動
相搏則為之旋轉故火本動也焰得風則自然旋
轉如春分至小滿為二之氣乃君火之位自大寒

黄帝素问宣明论方 *Huang Di Su Wen Xuan Ming Lun Fang* (Formulas from the Discussion Illuminating the Yellow Emperor's Basic Questions) in 1172.

One of the most famous physicians of the Song and Jin dynasties, Liu Yuan-Su was born in the dry environment of northern China. People in the region primarily ate meat and cheese, foods that are warm and create dampness. Liu practiced medicine largely in times of war, thus his clinical practice was mainly concerned with injuries, subsequent infections, and death. Because of those geographic and historical influences, Liu developed 火热论 *huo re lun* (discussion of fire and heat), and proposed the use of cool and cold substances to treat heat and fire disorders. Liu believed that among *liu yin* (the six exogenous factors of wind, cold, summer-heat, dampness, dryness, and fire), heat (including summer-heat) and fire are the dominant factors in causing disorders. Liu's works are important because they introduced a concept significantly different from the classic theories of *shang han* (cold damage) by Zhang Zhong-Jing, which had been the main school of thought up to that time.

Liu Yuan-Su wrote many books in his lifetime, among the most famous are:

- 黄帝素问宣明论方 *Huang Di Su Wen Xuan Ming Lun Fang* (Formulas from the Discussion Illuminating the Yellow Emperor's Basic Questions)
- 宣明论方 *Xuan Ming Lun Fang* (Discussion of Dispersing and Brightening Formulas)
- 伤寒直格方论 *Shang Han Zhi Ge Fang Lun* (Direct Investigations of Formulas for Cold-Induced Disorders)

Some sample herbal formulas found in the wealth of clinical information in these texts are:

- *Fang Feng Tong Sheng San* (Saposhnikovia Powder that Sagely Unblocks)
- *Liu Yi San* (Six-to-One Powder)
- *Gui Ling Gan Lu Yin* (Cinnamon and Poria Sweet Dew Decoction)
- *Di Huang Yin Zi* (Rehmannia Decoction)

Dynasties & Kingdoms	Year
Xia Dynasty 夏	2100-1600 BCE
Shang Dynasty 商	1600-1100 BCE
Zhou Dynasty 周	1100-221 BCE
Qin Dynasty 秦	221-207 BCE
Han Dynasty 漢	206 BCE-220
Three Kingdoms 三國	220-280
Western Jin Dynasty 西晉	265-316
Eastern Jin Dynasty 東晉	317-420
Northern and Southern Dynasties 北南朝	420-581
Sui Dynasty 隋	581-618
Tang Dynasty 唐	618-907
Five Dynasties 五代	907-960
Song Dynasty 宋	960-1279
Liao Dynasty 遼	916-1125
Jin Dynasty 金	**1115-1234**
Yuan Dynasty 元	1271-1368
Ming Dynasty 明	1368-1644
Qing Dynasty 清	1644-1911
Republic of China 中華民國	1912-Present Day
People's Republic of China 中華人民共和國	1949-Present Day

Table of Contents

Chapter 4 — Overview

表里双解剂

— Exterior- and Interior-Releasing Formulas

Definition: Exterior- and interior-releasing formulas simultaneously treat exterior and interior syndromes. They incorporate strategies such as *han fa* (sweating), *xia fa* (draining downward), *qing fa* (clearing), and *wen fa* (warming). These methods first appeared as parts of *ba fa* (eight treatment methods), as described in the *Huang Di Nei Jing* (Yellow Emperor's Inner Classic) in the first or second century, A.D.

Exterior- and interior-releasing formulas treat the concurrent presence of exterior and interior conditions. Exterior conditions are usually characterized by wind-cold or wind-heat, and treated with exterior-releasing herbs. Interior conditions are generally characterized by excess or deficiency, and heat or cold, and are treated with downward-draining, heat-clearing or interior-warming herbs. With this pattern, treating only the exterior syndrome will not relieve the interior syndrome, and treating only the interior syndrome will not release the exterior syndrome. Therefore, it is necessary to address and treat both at the same time. Careful pattern differentiation must be undertaken in order to choose correctly the right herbal formula. The type of pathogenic factor and its level of development and location (exterior or interior) within the body must be identified before the correct formula can be chosen. From biomedical perspectives, these formulas are commonly used to treat acute conditions such as pancreatitis, cholangiohepatitis and diarrhea that require immediate attention. Note: The condition of an (excess) exterior syndrome accompanied by interior deficiency is also addressed in Chapter 1: Exterior-Releasing Formulas.

SUBCATEGORIES OF ACTION

Exterior- and interior-releasing formulas are divided into three subcategories to reflect the nature of the disorders and characteristics of the formulas.

1. Exterior-Releasing and Interior-Attacking Formulas

These formulas are applicable when pathogenic factors present at both the exterior and in the interior. The exterior condition is usually characterized by wind-heat or wind-cold, while the interior condition is usually characterized by accumulation of heat or cold. Clinical signs include aversion to cold, fever, constipation, and a red tongue that, in severe cases, may have a white to yellow tongue coating.

Two types of herbs are commonly used to address this condition: exterior-releasing herbs such as *Ma Huang* (Herba Ephedrae), *Gui Zhi* (Ramulus Cinnamomi), *Jing Jie* (Herba Schizonepetae), *Fang Feng* (Radix Saposhnikoviae), *Chai Hu* (Radix Bupleuri), and *Bo He* (Herba Menthae); and downward draining herbs such as *Da Huang* (Radix et Rhizoma Rhei) and *Mang Xiao* (Natrii Sulfas). Exemplar formulas include *Da Chai Hu Tang* (Major Bupleurum Decoction) and *Fang Feng Tong Sheng San* (Saposhnikovia Powder that Sagely Unblocks).

2. Exterior-Releasing and Interior-Clearing Formulas

These formulas treat wind-heat or wind-cold at the exterior with heat formation in the interior. Common signs and symptoms are aversion to cold, fever, irritability, restlessness, thirst, diarrhea, and dyspnea.

Two types of herbs commonly used to address this condition are: exterior-releasing herbs such as *Ma Huang* (Herba Ephedrae), *Dan Dou Chi* (Semen Sojae Praeparatum), and *Ge Gen* (Radix

Chapter 4 — Overview

Puerariae Lobatae); and heat-clearing herbs such as *Huang Qin* (Radix Scutellariae), *Huang Lian* (Rhizoma Coptidis), *Huang Bo* (Cortex Phellodendri Chinensis), and *Shi Gao* (Gypsum Fibrosum). Representative formulas include *Ge Gen Huang Qin Huang Lian Tang* (Kudzu, Coptis, and Scutellaria Decoction) and *Shi Gao Tang* (Gypsum Decoction).

3. **Exterior-Releasing and Interior-Warming Formulas**
   These formulas are applicable when there is cold both at the exterior and in the interior. Clinical manifestations include aversion to cold, fever, coldness and pain in the epigastrium and abdomen, possibly a white tongue coating, and a slower pulse.

   Two types of herbs are commonly used to address this condition: exterior-releasing herbs such as *Ma Huang* (Herba Ephedrae) and *Bai Zhi* (Radix Angelicae Dahuricae); and interior-warming herbs such as *Gan Jiang* (Rhizoma Zingiberis) and *Rou Gui* (Cortex Cinnamomi). An exemplar formula is *Wu Ji San* (Five-Accumulation Powder).

CAUTIONS / CONTRAINDICATIONS

- Exterior- and interior-releasing formulas should be used only when both exterior and interior syndromes are present.
- Carefully differentiate exterior and interior syndromes on the basis of heat or cold, as well as excess or deficiency, before applying any of these formulas.
- Carefully adjust the doses of herbs in a formula according to the level of severity of the exterior and interior symptoms.
- When using formulas that contain *Ma Huang* (Herba Ephedrae), excessive panting, excessive increase in heart and respiratory rate and hyperactivity are indications that the dose of the formula used is too high and should be lowered or discontinued. As a species, cats are particularly sensitive to *Ma Huang* (Herba Ephedrae) and herbal formulas containing this herb should be used with caution.
- When using multiple herbal formulas, begin with the lowest therapeutic dose of each, especially if combining herbal medications with pharmaceutical drugs.

PHARMACOLOGICAL EFFECTS & CLINICAL APPLICATIONS

Similar to harmonizing formulas that treat *shaoyang* syndrome, exterior- and interior-releasing formulas treat both exterior and interior syndromes simultaneously. From the biomedical perspective, these formulas commonly treat liver disorders (hepatitis and fatty liver),[1,2] gallbladder disorders (cholecystitis and cholelithiasis),[3] pancreatic disorder (pancreatitis),[4] and gastrointestinal disorders (peptic ulcer, gastritis, gastric prolapse, diarrhea, dysentery, enteritis).[5,6,7,8,9,10] Exemplar formulas include *Da Chai Hu Tang* (Major Bupleurum Decoction) and *Ge Gen Huang Qin Huang Lian Tang* (Kudzu, Coptis, and Scutellaria Decoction).

References

1. *Shan Xi Zhong Yi* (Shanxi Chinese Medicine), 1989; 5:223.
2. *Fu Jian Zhong Yi Yao* (Fujian Chinese Medicine and Herbology), 1995; 6:43.
3. *Shan Dong Zhong Yi Za Zhi* (Shandong Journal of Chinese Medicine), 1987; 3:18.
4. *Bei Jing Zhong Yi Xue Yuan Xue Bao* (Journal of Beijing University School of Medicine), 1991; 14(4):12.
5. *Zhong Yi Fang Ji Xian Dai Yan Jiu* (Modern Study of Medical Formulas in Traditional Chinese Medicine), 1997; 434.
6. *Guang Dong Yi Xue* (Guangdong Medicine), 1993; 6:336.
7. *Zhe Jiang Zhong Yi Za Zhi* (Zhejiang Journal of Chinese Medicine), 1997; 10:441.
8. *Jiang Xi Zhong Yi Yao* (Jiangxi Chinese Medicine and Herbology), 1959; 6:28.
9. *Hu Bei Zhong Yi Za Zhi* (Hubei Journal of Chinese Medicine), 1983; 2:24.
10. *He Nan Zhong Yi* (Henan Chinese Medicine), 1992; 1:42.

Section 1

解表攻里剂

— Exterior-Releasing and Interior-Attacking Formulas

Dà Chái Hú Tāng (Major Bupleurum Decoction)

大柴胡湯
大柴胡汤

Pinyin Name: *Da Chai Hu Tang*
Literal Name: Major Bupleurum Decoction
Alternate Names: *Ta Tsai Hu Tang*, Major Bupleurum Combination
Original Source: *Jin Gui Yao Lue* (Essentials from the Golden Cabinet) by Zhang Zhong-Jing in the Eastern Han Dynasty

COMPOSITION

Chai Hu (Radix Bupleuri)	24g [15g]
Huang Qin (Radix Scutellariae)	9g
Da Huang (Radix et Rhizoma Rhei)	6g
Zhi Shi (Fructus Aurantii Immaturus), *zhi* (fried with liquid)	4 pieces [9g]
Bai Shao (Radix Paeoniae Alba)	9g
Ban Xia (Rhizoma Pinelliae), *xi* (washed)	0.5 cup [9g]
Sheng Jiang (Rhizoma Zingiberis Recens)	15g
Da Zao (Fructus Jujubae)	12 pieces [4 pieces]

DOSAGE / PREPARATION / ADMINISTRATION

The source text states to cook the ingredients in 12 cups [2,400 mL] of water until 6 cups [1,200 mL] of the liquid remain. Discard the residue and cook the strained decoction again to reduce it further. Take 1 cup [200 mL] of the warm decoction three times daily. Today, the decoction may be prepared using the doses suggested in brackets.

CHINESE THERAPEUTIC ACTIONS

1. Harmonizes *shaoyang* syndrome
2. Purges interior heat in *yangming* syndrome

CLINICAL MANIFESTATIONS

Shaoyang and *yangming* syndromes: recurring fever, continuous vomiting or gastric reflux, depression with restlessness, distention and pain in the epigastrium, constipation or discharge of fluids rectally, a red tongue, which in severe cases may have a white to yellow coating, and a wiry, forceful pulse.

VETERINARY CLINICAL APPLICATIONS

Acute cholangiohepatitis, cholelithiasis, cholecystitis, hepatic lipidosis in the cat, jaundice, acute pancreatitis, acute viral and toxic hepatitis, acute gastroenteritis, hyperlipidemia and constipation.

EXPLANATION

Da Chai Hu Tang (Major Bupleurum Decoction) treats *shaoyang* and *yangming* syndromes simultaneously by harmonizing the *shaoyang* stage and purging heat accumulation in the *yangming* stage. The clinical signs of intermittent fever and trembling, and continuous vomiting are all typical signs of a *shaoyang* pattern. Depression with restlessness, and a white to yellow tongue coating indicate a more severe form of *shaoyang* syndrome. Clinical signs indicating a *yangming* condition with excess heat include distention and pain in the epigastrium and constipation. In severe cases, the stool may become dry, hard and immobile, leading to discharge of fluids rectally. The yellow tongue coating indicates *yangming* heat in the body, and the wiry, forceful pulse indicates stagnation and the excess nature of this syndrome.

Dà Chái Hú Tāng (Major Bupleurum Decoction)

Da Chai Hu Tang **(Major Bupleurum Decoction)**

Diagnosis	Clinical Signs	Treatment	Herbs
Shaoyang and *yangming* syndromes	• Intermittent fever, trembling and continuous vomiting: *shaoyang* pattern • Distention and pain in the epigastrium and constipation: *yangming* syndrome • A red tongue with possibly a yellow tongue coating: heat in the body • Wiry, forceful pulse: stagnation and excess conditions	• Harmonizes *shaoyang* syndrome • Purges interior heat in *yangming* syndrome	• *Chai Hu* (Radix Bupleuri) and *Huang Qin* (Radix Scutellariae) harmonize *shaoyang* by releasing the exterior and clearing the interior. • *Da Huang* (Radix et Rhizoma Rhei) and *Zhi Shi* (Fructus Aurantii Immaturus) purge *yangming* Stomach heat and activate qi circulation. • *Bai Shao* (Radix Paeoniae Alba) harmonizes qi and blood. • *Ban Xia* (Rhizoma Pinelliae) and *Sheng Jiang* (Rhizoma Zingiberis Recens) direct the Stomach qi downward to relieve vomiting. • *Da Zao* (Fructus Jujubae) and *Sheng Jiang* (Rhizoma Zingiberis Recens) harmonize the herbs.

Normally, downward draining methods are prohibited in *shaoyang* syndrome, but unlike its typical manifestations, this is a combination of *shaoyang* and *yangming* syndromes. To effectively treat this set of clinical signs, both harmonizing and downward draining methods must be used in order to treat the exterior and interior simultaneously.

Da Chai Hu Tang is designed following the principles of two formulas: *Xiao Chai Hu Tang* (Minor Bupleurum Decoction) to harmonize *shaoyang,* and *Da Cheng Qi Tang* (Major Order the Qi Decoction) to drain heat from *yangming. Chai Hu* (Radix Bupleuri), the chief herb, combines with *Huang Qin* (Radix Scutellariae) to harmonize the *shaoyang* and clear Gallbladder heat. *Da Huang* (Radix et Rhizoma Rhei) and *Zhi Shi* (Fructus Aurantii Immaturus) purge *yangming* Stomach heat and activate qi circulation to relieve fullness and dispel hardened stools. *Bai Shao* (Radix Paeoniae Alba) combines with *Da Huang* (Radix et Rhizoma Rhei) to relieve the abdominal pain from constipation; also, *Bai Shao* (Radix Paeoniae Alba) softens the Liver to relieve depression and restlessness, and harmonizes qi and blood to help *Zhi Shi* (Fructus Aurantii Immaturus) relieve epigastric fullness and pain. *Ban Xia* (Rhizoma Pinelliae) and *Sheng Jiang* (Rhizoma Zingiberis Recens) direct Stomach qi downward to relieve vomiting. Finally, *Da Zao* (Fructus Jujubae) and *Sheng Jiang* (Rhizoma Zingiberis Recens) harmonize the *ying* (nutritive) and *wei* (defensive) levels, as well as all of the herbs.

For further explanation of the clinical signs of *shaoyang* and *yangming* patterns, please refer to *Xiao Chai Hu Tang* (Minor Bupleurum Decoction) and *Da Cheng Qi Tang* (Major Order the Qi Decoction).

VETERINARY MODIFICATIONS

- With excess dryness and heat in the *yangming* stage, add *Shi Gao* (Gypsum Fibrosum) and *Zhi Mu* (Rhizoma Anemarrhenae).
- With excess heat and toxicity, add *Jin Yin Hua* (Flos Lonicerae Japonicae), *Lian Qiao* (Fructus Forsythiae), and *Pu Gong Ying* (Herba Taraxaci).
- With abdominal bloating, add *Hou Po* (Cortex Magnoliae Officinalis), *Mu Xiang* (Radix Aucklandiae), and *Qing Pi* (Pericarpium Citri Reticulatae Viride).
- When there is severe pain, add *Yan Hu Suo* (Rhizoma Corydalis) and *Chuan Lian Zi* (Fructus Toosendan).
- For gastroenteritis and fever, add *Zhu Ru* (Caulis Bambusae in Taenia), *Sha Ren* (Fructus Amomi), and *Chen Pi* (Pericarpium Citri Reticulatae).
- For damp heat and jaundice, add *Yin Chen* (Herba Artemisiae Scopariae), *Zhi Zi* (Fructus Gardeniae), *Jin Qian Cao* (Herba Lysimachiae) or *Yin Chen Hao Tang* (Artemisia Scoparia Decoction).
- For gallstones, add *Jin Qian Cao* (Herba Lysimachiae), *Hai Jin Sha* (Spora Lygodii), *Yu Jin* (Radix Curcumae), and *Ji Nei Jin* (Endothelium Corneum Gigeriae Galli).

CAUTIONS / CONTRAINDICATIONS

- *Da Chai Hu Tang* is contraindicated in patients with Spleen and Stomach deficiencies.
- *Da Huang* (Radix et Rhizoma Rhei) should be prescribed in moderation in this formula. Use of *Da Huang* (Radix et Rhizoma Rhei) in excessive amounts, or for a prolonged period of time, may cause unnecessary depletion of body fluids, and can lead the disease deeper into the interior.
- Potential side effects associated with this formula include poor appetite, abdominal distention, diarrhea, and edema.

Dà Chái Hú Tāng (Major Bupleurum Decoction)

- Avoid cold or raw, pungent or spicy, and oily or greasy foods while taking this formula.[1]

PHARMACOLOGICAL EFFECTS

1. **Gastrointestinal**: Administration of *Da Chai Hu Tang* had marked antispasmodic and antiulcer effects on the gastrointestinal tract. According to laboratory experiments, the formula inhibited spasms and cramps of the smooth muscles of the intestines.[2] In addition, the herbs inhibited the production of gastric acid.[3] Lastly, administration of this formula in extract form at 250 mg/kg in rats was associated with a protective effect against damage to the stomach membrane induced by aspirin.[4]
2. **Hepatoprotective**: One study reported that *Da Chai Hu Tang* lowered elevated liver enzymes (SGPT and SGOT) and protected the liver from drug-induced damages.[5] Another study reported that *Da Chai Hu Tang* prevented the progression of acute liver injury induced by carbon tetrachloride by inhibiting enhanced lipid peroxidation and by improving disrupted active oxygen metabolism in the injured liver.[6]
3. **Cardiovascular**: The use of *Da Chai Hu Tang* has little or no impact on the cardiovascular system. There were minimal changes in blood pressure (both systolic and diastolic) and heart rate and rhythm.[7] There was, however, a slight drop of cholesterol and triglyceride levels.[8]
4. **Immunologic**: Administration of *Da Chai Hu Tang* enhanced the immune system. In mice with artificially suppressed immune systems, administration of the formula was associated with increased number of T-cells. There were, however, no significant changes with IgM and IgG.[9]
5. **Antibiotic**: *Da Chai Hu Tang* had a strong inhibitory effect *in vitro* against *Staphylococcus aureus* and *E. coli*.[10]
6. **Anti-inflammatory**: In mice with artificially-induced swelling and inflammation of the joints, the administration of *Da Chai Hu Tang* was determined to have an anti-inflammatory effect similar to aspirin.[11]
7. **Antihyperglycemic**: Administration of *Da Chai Hu Tang* was associated with a decreased blood glucose level at 30, 60, and 120 minutes after glucose loading in a tolerance test, and an increased serum insulin level at 120 minutes after glucose loading.
8. **Effect on lipid biosynthesis**: Administration of *Da Chai Hu Tang* was associated with decreased hepatic triglyceride biosynthesis and subsequent reduction in plasma VLDL levels.[12] According to another study, administering *Da Chai Hu Tang* to subjects with diets high in cholesterol was associated with significantly lower plasma and hepatic cholesterol levels.[13] Another study showed *Da Chai Hu Tang* to beneficially affect lipid metabolism by significantly increasing high-density lipoprotein-cholesterol (HDL) with little antihypertensive effect.[14] Lastly, *Da Chai Hu Tang* significantly reduced plasma triglyceride levels.[15]
9. **Antihyperlipidemic**: Administration of *Xiao Chai Hu Tang* (Minor Bupleurum Decoction) and *Da Chai Hu Tang* was associated with beneficial effects in treating rats with cholesterol-induced hypercholesterolemia and aging-induced hyperlipidemia. Both formulas reduced total liver cholesterol and inhibited increases of serum and liver triglyceride.[16]

HUMAN CLINICAL STUDIES AND RESEARCH

1. **Gallbladder disorders**: There have been numerous reports on the effect of *Da Chai Hu Tang* to treat gallbladder disorders, such as cholecystitis and cholelithiasis. In one report, 84 patients with gallbladder disorders (18 with cholecystitis and 73 with cholelithiasis) treated with modified *Da Chai Hu Tang* had complete recovery in 44 patients and improvement in 31 patients. The overall effectiveness was 89.28%.[17] In another report, 120 patients with cholelithiasis were treated with excellent results. The effectiveness was 88.2% for patients with stones in the bile duct, 78.5% for stones in the gallbladder, and 76.2% for stones in both the duct and the gallbladder.[18]
2. **Cholelithiasis**: *Da Chai Hu Tang* was used with good success to treat patients with gallstones after surgical removal of the gallbladder. The stones were successfully passed in 18 of 26 patients (69.2%). The duration of treatment ranged from 87-250 days.[19]
3. **Biliary ascariasis**: *Da Chai Hu Tang* has been shown in one study to effectively treat biliary ascariasis. Administration of modified *Da Chai Hu Tang* in decoction for an average of 15 days was associated with a 90.63% effectiveness in 32 patients. The researchers noted the formula to have marked anti-inflammatory, analgesic, cholagogic and antiparasitic effects. The herbal formula contained *Chai Hu* (Radix Bupleuri), *Huang Qin* (Radix Scutellariae), *Zhi Qiao* (Fructus Aurantii), *Ban Xia* (Rhizoma Pinelliae), *Bai Shao* (Radix Paeoniae Alba), *Sheng Jiang* (Rhizoma Zingiberis Recens), *Da Zao* (Fructus Jujubae), and *Da Huang* (Radix et Rhizoma Rhei). Strategies for modifications are as follows: for gallstones, add *Jin Qian Cao* (Herba Lysimachiae); and for jaundice, add *Yin Chen* (Herba Artemisiae Scopariae), *Zhi Zi* (Fructus Gardeniae), and *Da Huang* (Radix et Rhizoma Rhei) (post-decocted), and remove *Bai Shao* (Radix Paeoniae Alba), *Sheng Jiang* (Rhizoma Zingiberis Recens), and *Da Zao* (Fructus Jujubae).[20]
4. **Acute pancreatitis**: One study reported a pronounced effect using modified *Da Chai Hu Tang* to treat acute pancreatitis. The herbal treatment contained *Da Chai Hu Tang* plus *Xuan Ming Fen* (Natrii Sulfas Exsiccatus) 10g and *Zi Su Geng* (Caulis Perillae) 9g as the base formula.

Dà Chái Hú Tāng (Major Bupleurum Decoction)

Modifications included addition of *Chuan Lian Zi* (Fructus Toosendan) 6g and *Da Fu Pi* (Pericarpium Arecae) 9g for qi stagnation; *Huang Lian* (Rhizoma Coptidis) 6g and *Da Fu Pi* (Pericarpium Arecae) 9g for damp-heat in the Liver and Gallbladder; addition of *Chuan Lian Zi* (Fructus Toosendan) 6g, *Huang Lian* (Rhizoma Coptidis) 6g, *Zhu Ru* (Caulis Bambusae in Taenia) 9g, and removal of *Zhi Shi* (Fructus Aurantii Immaturus) for excess heat in the Liver and Stomach; and addition of *Chi Shao* (Radix Paeoniae Rubra) 9g, *Tao Ren* (Semen Persicae) 9g, *Hong Hua* (Flos Carthami) 9g, and *Wu Ling Zhi* (Faeces Trogopteri) 9g, and removal of *Xuan Ming Fen* (Natrii Sulfas Exsiccatus) and *Ban Xia* (Rhizoma Pinelliae) in the case of qi and blood stagnation. The study showed 98.5% effectiveness among 216 patients.[21] In another report, 84 patients with acute pancreatitis were treated with modified *Da Chai Hu Tang* with good results. Most clinical signs, such as abdominal pain, nausea, fever, and constipation, were resolved within 2-5 days. Laboratory results also confirmed the effectiveness of the treatment with blood amylase, urine amylase, and white blood cells returning to normal range in 2.9, 3.5, and 2 to 5 days, respectively.[22]

5. **Hepatitis**: In one study, 196 patients with acute icteric hepatitis treated with modified *Da Chai Hu Tang* recovered in 179 patients (asymptomatic with normal liver functions) and improved in 15 patients. The average duration of treatment was 25 days.[23]
6. **Fatty liver**: Use of modified *Da Chai Hu Tang* in 18 patients with fatty liver (6 months to 3 years history of illness) was associated with complete recovery in 5 patients, marked effect in 8 patients, slight improvement in 4 patients, and no effect in 1 case (94.4% effectiveness). The treatment protocol was to cook the herbs and drink the decoction in two equally-divided doses daily, for 30 days per course of treatment, with 7-10 days of rest in between courses, for a total of 2 courses. The base formula included *Chai Hu* (Radix Bupleuri) 12g, *Huang Qin* (Radix Scutellariae) 6-9g, *Ban Xia* (Rhizoma Pinelliae) 9g, *Bai Shao* (Radix Paeoniae Alba) 15g, *Zhi Shi* (Fructus Aurantii Immaturus) 6-9g, *Da Huang* (Radix et Rhizoma Rhei) 6-12g, *Dan Shen* (Radix et Rhizoma Salviae Miltiorrhizae) 15g, *Jue Ming Zi* (Semen Cassiae) 20g, and *Shan Zha* (Fructus Crataegi) 15g. Modifications included the addition of *Yu Jin* (Radix Curcumae) 10g and *Dan Shen* (Radix et Rhizoma Salviae Miltiorrhizae) 15g for chest and hypochondriac fullness and distention; *Fu Ling* (Poria) 15g and *Chen Pi* (Pericarpium Citri Reticulatae) 6g for nausea and vomiting; *Huang Jing* (Rhizoma Polygonati) 15g and *Shan Yao* (Rhizoma Dioscoreae) 20g for decreased intake of food and fatigue; *Da Huang* (Radix et Rhizoma Rhei) 12g, and *Di Huang* (Radix Rehmanniae) 15g for constipation with dry mouth and bitter taste; *Chuan Lian Zi* (Fructus Toosendan) 10g, and *Yan Hu Suo* (Rhizoma Corydalis) 10g for hypochondriac pain; and *Pu Huang* (Pollen Typhae) 9g and *Yin Chen* (Herba Artemisiae Scopariae) 15g for abnormal liver functions.[24]
7. **Hyperlipidemia**: Sixty-five patients with hyperlipidemia (49 had concurrent hypertension, 41 had concurrent diabetes) were treated with *Da Chai Hu Tang* with good results. The treatment protocol was to administer the herbs in granular extracts at 2.5g per dose, three times per day, for 16 weeks. At the conclusion of the study, the researchers stated that 71% of the patients had a moderate to significant reduction of serum cholesterol levels. Side effects reported in about 5% of the patients included poor appetite, abdominal distention, diarrhea, and edema.[25]
8. **Duodenal ulcer**: Thirty-four patients with duodenal ulcer were treated with *Da Chai Hu Tang* for 30 days with complete recovery in 23 patients, improvement in 9 patients, and no effect in 2 patients. The study reported an overall effectiveness rate of 94.1%.[26]
9. **Perforating ulcer**: In one study, 192 of 202 patients with acute perforating ulcer showed good response after treatment with *Da Chai Hu Tang*. Of 202 patients, only 20 still required surgery. The researchers were able to contact 75 of the patients for follow-up interviews 1-2 years later, and stated that there were no recurrences in 31 patients, significant improvement in 28 patients, and recurrence in 16 patients.[27]

HERB-DRUG INTERACTION

Aspirin- and ethanol-induced gastric lesions: Administration of *Da Chai Hu Tang* was associated with a notable effect to treat aspirin- and ethanol-induced gastric hemorrhagic lesions in rats. The gastroprotective effect of *Da Chai Hu Tang* was comparable to sucralfate (Carafate), cimetidine (Tagamet), and 16,16-dimethyl-prostaglandin E2 (DMPGE2).[28]

TOXICOLOGY

According to one case report in Japan, administration of *Dai-saiko-to* [*Da Chai Hu Tang*] was associated with one incidence of autoimmune hepatitis in one patient.[29] Note: Additional information on the medical history of this patient was unavailable at the time of publication.

SUGGESTED ACUPUNCTURE TREATMENT

1. Points: *Zuqiaoyin* (GB 44), *Zhiyang* (GV 9), *Qiuxu* (GB 40), *Housanli* (ST 36), *Pishu* (BL 20), *Weishu* (BL 21), *Dachangshu* (BL 25), *Zhangmen* (LR 13), *Shangjuxu* (ST 37), *Shangen* and *Tongguan*.
2. Technique: sedation or prick to bleed, or aquapuncture with vitamin B-12.

Dà Chái Hú Tāng (Major Bupleurum Decoction)

Zuqiaoyin (GB 44), the *jing* (well) point of the Gallbladder channel, sedates stagnation in the Liver and Gallbladder, clears heat, and nourishes yin. *Zhiyang* (GV 9) smoothes the qi flow in the chest and diaphragm. Both *Zuqiaoyin* (GB 44) and *Zhiyang* (GV 9) can be bled to sedate heat and remove stagnation. *Qiuxu* (GB 40) clears Liver and Gallbladder heat. *Housanli* (ST 36), *Pishu* (BL 20), and *Weishu* (BL 21) can be helpful in stimulating appetite. *Dachangshu* (BL 25), *Zhangmen* (LR 13), and *Shangjuxu* (ST 37) smooth the qi flow in the Stomach and Intestines to relieve constipation and abdominal distention. *Shangen* is a classical point used to stimulate appetite in the dog and cat, while *Tongguan* is used in a similar fashion for the horse.

AUTHORS' COMMENTS

Da Chai Hu Tang is used most often to treat acute cholangiohepatitis and hepatic lipidosis with jaundice in the cat and acute pancreatitis in the dog and cat. This formula contains *Da Huang* (Radix et Rhizoma Rhei) and should not be used for more than 3-5 days without re-evaluation and/or until loose stools are seen. For the treatment of cholangiohepatitis and hepatic lipidosis in the cat, it is often combined with *Yin Chen Wu Ling San* (Artemisia Scoparia and Five-Ingredient Powder with Poria). This formula can be combined with fluid therapy and antibiotics; however, herbs or formulas to harmonize the middle *jiao* are recommended when using combination therapy. *Da Chai Hu Tang* is usually followed with a formula such as *Jia Wei Xiao Yao San* (Augmented Rambling Powder) or *Xiao Yao San* (Rambling Powder), depending on the case.

In horses, practitioners will find *Da Chai Hu Tang* most useful in miniature horses and donkeys with acute cases of equine hyperlipemia, though it may be used in other cases of acute hepatitis, such as those that occur with plant toxicity. In both situations, severe anorexia is common, and the formula will likely have to be administered via nasogastric tube. It may also be advisable to combine the formula with 20-30% of *Liu Jun Zi Tang* (Six-Gentlemen Decoction) to prevent gastrointestinal upset. Intravenous fluid therapy, laxatives, and aquapuncture with vitamin B-12 injections are also helpful. This formula can also be useful in acute stages of gastritis brought on by an overdose of phenylbutazone and idiopathic duodenitis.

It should be noted that "pancreatitis" is a disease description of Western medicine, and the etiology of the disease is not well understood. In Chinese medicine, there are multiple patterns of disharmony which correspond to a diagnosis of pancreatitis: stagnation of Liver qi (acute and chronic pancreatitis), excess heat in the Spleen and Stomach (acute pancreatitis), damp-heat in the Liver and Gallbladder (acute pancreatitis), and weakness or deficiency of the Spleen (chronic pancreatitis and recovery stage of acute pancreatitis). Each of these patterns will require a different treatment approach.

- Liver qi stagnation: *Da Chai Hu Tang.*
- Damp-heat in the Liver and Gallbladder: *Da Chai Hu Tang* and *Long Dan Xie Gan Tang* (Gentiana Decoction to Drain the Liver).
- Excess heat in the Stomach and Intestines: *Da Cheng Qi Tang* (Major Order the Qi Decoction).
- Spleen deficiency: *Shen Ling Bai Zhu San* (Ginseng, Poria, and Atractylodes Macrocephala Powder).
- The first three formulas used to treat acute pancreatitis include the herb *Da Huang* (Radix et Rhizoma Rhei). Research has shown that this herb is key in the treatment of acute pancreatitis. *Da Huang* (Radix et Rhizoma Rhei) has been shown to have anti-inflammatory, antibacterial and cholagogic properties and can inhibit pancreatic enzyme activity.

A question is often raised as to how *Da Chai Hu Tang* can be used to treat both constipation and diarrhea. From a traditional Chinese medical perspective, the cause of constipation and diarrhea in this case is the same: excess heat in the Intestines that dries the stool and turns it into a hard, immobile mass. Accordingly, *Da Huang* (Radix et Rhizoma Rhei) and *Zhi Shi* (Fructus Aurantii Immaturus) are used to regulate qi and purge heat in the bowels. Because these two herbs dispel stagnation and heat in the Intestines, they can treat either constipation or diarrhea. Clearing or purging heat will resolve the root cause of the diarrhea. This is the same principle underlying *Da Cheng Qi Tang* (Major Order the Qi Decoction), in which a downward draining formula is used to purge watery diarrhea because fecal matter is still stagnant in the Intestines and has to be directed out. Note: Diarrhea in this case refers only to the passage of fluids rectally, and not the stool. This occurs because the stool is dry, hard and immobile, so the water in the Intestines has nowhere to go but to be excreted rectally as watery fluids.[30]

Although *Da Cheng Qi Tang* (Major Order the Qi Decoction) and *Da Chai Hu Tang* share the same principle of using *Da Huang* to purge damp-heat in excess *yangming fu* (hollow organs) syndrome, there are contrasting differences:

- *Da Cheng Qi Tang* is used for severe *yangming fu* excess condition with constipation and the four clinical signs of *pi* (distention), *man* (fullness), *zao* (dryness), and *shi* (hardness), along with a dry, red tongue body with a

Dà Chái Hú Tāng (Major Bupleurum Decoction)

yellow coating and abdominal pain that is worse with pressure.

- *Da Chai Hu Tang* treats *yangming fu* and *shaoyang* syndromes. The heat and constipation in cases that call for *Da Chai Hu Tang* is not as severe as that seen in *Da Cheng Qi Tang*. Consequently, a smaller dose of *Da Huang* is used in *Da Chai Hu Tang* to purge excess heat and treat constipation. If *Da Cheng Qi Tang* is used, there is a hidden danger that *zheng* (upright) *qi* may be damaged, and the disease may progress from being in between *shaoyang* and *yangming* stages, to moving deeper in the body.[31]

Xiao Chai Hu Tang (Minor Bupleurum Decoction) and *Da Chai Hu Tang* are both formulated to treat *shaoyang* stage disorder with intermittent fever and trembling, a bitter taste in the mouth, and chest and hypochondriac distention. Both formulas contain *Chai Hu* (Radix Bupleuri), *Huang Qin* (Radix Scutellariae), *Ban Xia* (Rhizoma Pinelliae), *Sheng Jiang* (Rhizoma Zingiberis Recens), and *Da Zao* (Fructus Jujubae) and are used to treat many of the same diseases. Despite similarities, they have contrasting differences:

- *Xiao Chai Hu Tang* contains *Chai Hu* (Radix Bupleuri) and *Huang Qin* (Radix Scutellariae) as chief herbs to harmonize the *shaoyang* stage. *Ren Shen* (Radix et Rhizoma Ginseng) is added to support the underlying constitutional deficiency and to prevent the pathogenic factor from moving further inward. It does not contain *Da Huang* (Radix et Rhizoma Rhei), allowing this formula to be used for a greater number of disorders and for a longer period of time than *Da Chai Hu Tang*.
- *Da Chai Hu Tang* is mainly used for *yangming fu* syndrome with excess heat and stool accumulation in the body. *Da Huang* (Radix et Rhizoma Rhei) and *Zhi Shi* (Fructus Aurantii Immaturus) serve to sedate heat in the *yangming* channel. The key differential diagnosis is continuous vomiting and constipation with abdominal pain.[32]

References

1. *Zhong Yao Ming Fang Yao Li Yu Ying Yong* (Pharmacology and Applications of Famous Herbal Formulas), 1989; 92-96.
2. *Yao Xue Za Zhi* (Journal of Medicinals), 1982; 102(4):371.
3. *Guo Wai Yi Xue* (Foreign Medicine), 1989; 11(3):55.
4. *Guo Wai Yi Xue* (Foreign Medicine), 1988; 10(5):36.
5. *Guo Wai Yi Xue Zhong Yi Zhong Yao Fen Ce* (Monograph of Chinese Herbology from Foreign Medicine), 1984, 6(2):58.
6. Ohta Y, Sasaki E, Nishida K, Kobayashi T, Nagata M, Ishiguro I. Preventive effect of dai-saiko-to (da-chai-hu-tang) extract on disrupted hepatic active oxygen metabolism in rats with carbon tetrachloride-induced liver injury. Am J Chin Med. 1995; 23(1):53-64.
7. *Guo Wai Yi Xue Zhong Yi Zhong Yao Fen Ce* (Monograph of Chinese Herbology from Foreign Medicine), 1995; 17(2):52.
8. *Zhong Yao Yao Li Yu Lin Chuang* (Pharmacology and Clinical Applications of Chinese Herbs), 1991; 7:1.
9. *Zhong Yi Fang Ji Xian Dai Yan Jiu* (Modern Study of Medical Formulas in Traditional Chinese Medicine), 1997; 432.
10. *Zhong Yi Za Zhi* (Journal of Chinese Medicine), 1955; 10:36.
11. *Yao Xue Za Zhi* (Journal of Medicinals), 1983; 103(4):466.
12. Yamamoto K, Ogawa Y, Yanagita T, Morito F, Fukushima N, Ozaki I, Mizuta T, Setoguchi Y, Sakai T. Pharmacological effects of dai-saiko-to on lipid biosynthesis in cultured human hepatocyte HepG2 cells. J Ethnopharmacol. 1995 Apr; 46(1):49-54.
13. Teramoto T, Matsushima T, Horie Y, Watanabe T. Production of apolipoprotein E-rich LDL by the liver. The effect of dietary cholesterol and some lipid lowering agents. Ann N Y Acad Sci. 1990; 598:301-7.
14. Saku K, Hirata K, Zhang B, Liu R, Ying H, Okura Y, Yoshinaga K, Arakawa K. Effects of Chinese herbal drugs on serum lipids, lipoproteins and apolipoproteins in mild to moderate essential hypertensive patients. J Hum Hypertens. 1992 Oct; 6(5):393-5.
15. Ying H, Saku K, Ando K, Okura Y, Yoshinaga K, Harada R, Hidaka K, Arakawa K. Effects of Chinese herbal drug, dai-saiko-to on plasma lipids, lipoproteins and liver lipid contents in guinea pig. Artery. 1991; 18(4):184-96.
16. Umeda M, Amagaya S, Ogihara Y. Effect of shosaikoto, daisaikoto and sannoshashinto (traditional Japanese and Chinese medicines) on experimental hyperlipidemia in rats. J Ethnopharmacol. 1989 Oct; 26(3):255-69.
17. *Yun Nan Zhong Yi Za Zhi* (Yunan Journal of Chinese Medicine), 1990; 11(4):18.
18. *Shan Dong Zhong Yi Za Zhi* (Shandong Journal of Chinese Medicine), 1987; 3:18.
19. *Zhong Yi Za Zhi* (Journal of Chinese Medicine), 1984; 5:46.
20. *Zhong Yi Ming Fang Lin Chuang Xin Yong* (Contemporary Clinical Applications of Classic Chinese Formulas), 2001; 61.
21. *Zhe Jiang Zhong Yi Za Zhi* (Zhejiang Journal of Chinese Medicine), 1988; 6:252.
22. *Bei Jing Zhong Yi Xue Yuan Xue Bao* (Journal of Beijing University School of Medicine), 1991; 14(4):12.
23. *Shan Xi Zhong Yi* (Shanxi Chinese Medicine), 1989; 5:223.
24. *Fu Jian Zhong Yi Yao* (Fujian Chinese Medicine and Herbology), 1995; 6:43.
25. *Xin Yao Yu Lin Chuang* (New Medicine and the Clinical Application), 1989; 38(4):61.
26. *Zhong Yi Fang Ji Xian Dai Yan Jiu* (Modern Study of Medical Formulas in Traditional Chinese Medicine), 1997; 434.
27. *Xin Yi Xue* (New Medicine), 1977; 10-11:482.
28. Takase H, Imanishi K, Miura O, Yumioka E, Watanabe H. Pharmacological studies on the effects of some traditional Chinese medicines on gastric functions. (3) The effects of oren-gedoku-to (OGT), san'o-syasin-to (SST), antyu-san (AS) and dai-saiko-to (DST) on ethanol- and aspirin-induced gastric lesions in rats. Nippon Yakurigaku Zasshi. 1988 May; 91(5):319-24.
29. Kamiyama T, Nouchi T, Kojima S, Murata N, Ikeda T, Sato C. Autoimmune hepatitis triggered by administration of an herbal medicine. American Journal of Gastroenterology. 1997 Apr; 92(4):703-4.
30. Wang MZ, et al. *Zhong Yi Xue Wen Da Ti Ku* (Questions and Answers on Traditional Chinese Medicine: Herbal Formulas).
31. Wang MZ, et al. *Zhong Yi Xue Wen Da Ti Ku* (Questions and Answers on Traditional Chinese Medicine: Herbal Formulas).
32. Wang MZ, et al. *Zhong Yi Xue Wen Da Ti Ku* (Questions and Answers on Traditional Chinese Medicine: Herbal Formulas).

Fáng Fēng Tōng Shèng Săn

(Saposhnikovia Powder that Sagely Unblocks)

防風通聖散
防风通圣散

Pinyin Name: *Fang Feng Tong Sheng San*
Literal Name: Saposhnikovia Powder that Sagely Unblocks
Alternate Names: *Fang Feng Tung Sheng San*, Siler Sage-Inspired Formula, Siler and Platycodon Formula
Original Source: *Huang Di Su Wen Xuan Ming Lun Fang* (Formulas from the Discussion Illuminating the Yellow Emperor's Basic Questions) by Liu Yuan-Su in 1172

COMPOSITION

Fang Feng (Radix Saposhnikoviae)	15g [6g]
Jing Jie (Herba Schizonepetae)	7.5-15g [3-6g]
Ma Huang (Herba Ephedrae)	15g [6g]
Bo He (Herba Menthae)	15g [6g]
Da Huang (Radix et Rhizoma Rhei), *zheng* (steamed) with liquor	15g [6g]
Mang Xiao (Natrii Sulfas), post-decocted	15g [6g]
Shi Gao (Gypsum Fibrosum)	30g [12g]
Huang Qin (Radix Scutellariae)	30g [12g]
Lian Qiao (Fructus Forsythiae)	15g [6g]
Jie Geng (Radix Platycodonis)	30g [12g]
Zhi Zi (Fructus Gardeniae), *tan* (charred to ash)	7.5-15g [3-6g]
Hua Shi (Talcum)	90g [20g]
Dang Gui (Radix Angelicae Sinensis)	15g [6g]
Chuan Xiong (Rhizoma Chuanxiong)	15g [6g]
Bai Shao (Radix Paeoniae Alba), *chao* (dry-fried)	15g [6g]
Bai Zhu (Rhizoma Atractylodis Macrocephalae)	7.5-15g [3-6g]
Gan Cao (Radix et Rhizoma Glycyrrhizae)	60g [10g]

DOSAGE / PREPARATION / ADMINISTRATION

The source text instructs to grind the ingredients into powder, and cook 6g of the powder with 3 slices of *Sheng Jiang* (Rhizoma Zingiberis Recens) in 1 large bowl of water until the liquid is reduced to 60%. Take the strained decoction while warm. Today, this formula may also be prepared as pills. For pills, grind all the ingredients, except *Hua Shi* (Talcum), into a fine powder, and sift evenly. Mix the powder with water to form into pills. Coat the pills with finely-powdered *Hua Shi* (Talcum), and polish and dry the pills. Take 6g of pills twice daily. Alternatively, this formula may be prepared as a decoction using the doses suggested in brackets above. *Cong Bai* (Bulbus Allii Fistulosi) may be added to enhance the exterior-releasing effect of the formula.

Note: The exact doses of *Jing Jie* (Herba Schizonepetae), *Bai Zhu* (Rhizoma Atractylodis Macrocephalae) and *Zhi Zi* (Fructus Gardeniae) are unclear. One reference specifies 2.5 *qian* (7.5g), while another instructs 5 *qian* (15g). We list both for reference purposes.

CHINESE THERAPEUTIC ACTIONS

1. Expels wind and releases the exterior
2. Clears interior heat and promotes defecation

CLINICAL MANIFESTATIONS

Exterior wind-heat syndrome with accumulation of interior heat: aversion to cold, high fever, red and painful eyes, coughing, dyspnea, thick and sticky nasal discharge and saliva, constipation, dark yellow-colored urine or dysuria. It also treats abscesses, sores, carbuncle, *chang feng* (intestinal wind), rectal fissures, rectal polyps, dermatitis, a red, greasy tongue, and a forceful, rapid or slippery to wiry pulse.

VETERINARY CLINICAL APPLICATIONS

Hypertension, itching, dermatitis, allergic dermatitis, abscesses, urticaria, upper respiratory infection and lymphoma.

EXPLANATION

Fang Feng Tong Sheng San (Saposhnikovia Powder that Sagely Unblocks) has three main functions: it releases

Fáng Fēng Tōng Shèng Sǎn

(Saposhnikovia Powder that Sagely Unblocks)

Fang Feng Tong Sheng San **(Saposhnikovia Powder that Sagely Unblocks)**

Diagnosis	Clinical Signs	Treatment	Herbs
Exterior wind-heat syndrome with accumulation of interior heat	• Aversion to cold and fever: exterior wind-heat • Red and painful eyes and dry mouth: wind-heat attacking upper body • Thick and sticky nasal discharge and saliva: exterior wind-heat damaging the body fluids • Coughing and dyspnea: heat affecting the Lung • Constipation and dysuria: interior heat consuming body fluids	• Expels wind and releases the exterior • Clears interior heat and promotes defecation	• *Fang Feng* (Radix Saposhnikoviae), *Jing Jie* (Herba Schizonepetae), *Ma Huang* (Herba Ephedrae) and *Bo He* (Herba Menthae) clear the exterior wind-heat. • *Da Huang* (Radix et Rhizoma Rhei) and *Mang Xiao* (Natrii Sulfas) purge interior heat and promote defecation. • *Shi Gao* (Gypsum Fibrosum), *Huang Qin* (Radix Scutellariae), *Lian Qiao* (Fructus Forsythiae), *Jie Geng* (Radix Platycodonis) and *Zhi Zi* (Fructus Gardeniae) clear Lung and Stomach heat. • *Hua Shi* (Talcum) dispels heat through urination and relieves dysuria. • *Dang Gui* (Radix Angelicae Sinensis), *Chuan Xiong* (Rhizoma Chuanxiong) and *Bai Shao* (Radix Paeoniae Alba) nourish the blood and activate blood circulation. • *Bai Zhu* (Rhizoma Atractylodis Macrocephalae) and *Gan Cao* (Radix et Rhizoma Glycyrrhizae) strengthen Spleen qi.

exterior wind-heat, clears interior heat, and drains downward. It is indicated for excess conditions at both the exterior (wind-heat) and interior (heat accumulation). Wind-heat at the exterior may cause exterior clinical signs such as aversion to cold and fever. Because both wind and heat tend to ascend and attack the upper body, they may cause clinical signs such as red and painful eyes. And since the Lung is the organ that is most vulnerable to exterior pathogenic factors and heat, the wind-heat factor may also damage the Lung and cause signs such as coughing and dyspnea. Thick, sticky nasal discharge and saliva indicate wind-heat damaging the exterior and the body fluids. Constipation and dysuria indicate excess heat in the interior damaging body fluids.

This formula uses *Fang Feng* (Radix Saposhnikoviae), *Jing Jie* (Herba Schizonepetae), *Ma Huang* (Herba Ephedrae), and *Bo He* (Herba Menthae) to clear the exterior wind-heat. *Da Huang* (Radix et Rhizoma Rhei) and *Mang Xiao* (Natrii Sulfas) purge interior heat and promote defecation. *Shi Gao* (Gypsum Fibrosum), *Huang Qin* (Radix Scutellariae), *Lian Qiao* (Fructus Forsythiae), *Jie Geng* (Radix Platycodonis), and *Zhi Zi* (Fructus Gardeniae) clear heat in the Lung and Stomach. *Hua Shi* (Talcum) dispels heat through urination and relieves dysuria. *Dang Gui* (Radix Angelicae Sinensis), *Chuan Xiong* (Rhizoma Chuanxiong), and *Bai Shao* (Radix Paeoniae Alba) nourish the blood and activate blood circulation. *Bai Zhu* (Rhizoma Atractylodis Macrocephalae) and *Gan Cao* (Radix et Rhizoma Glycyrrhizae) strengthen Spleen qi. These tonic herbs also prevent the heat-clearing and purgative herbs in this formula from injuring the body.

VETERINARY MODIFICATIONS

- For common cold or influenza caused by wind-cold, add *Qiang Huo* (Rhizoma et Radix Notopterygii).
- For common cold or influenza caused by wind-heat, add *Jin Yin Hua* (Flos Lonicerae Japonicae) and *Lian Qiao* (Fructus Forsythiae).
- When there is excess heat, add *Huang Lian* (Rhizoma Coptidis) and *Huang Bo* (Cortex Phellodendri Chinensis).
- With cough with excess phlegm, add *Ban Xia* (Rhizoma Pinelliae).
- For dermatological disorders without abscess and ulceration, combine with *Sheng Ma Ge Gen Tang* (Cimicifuga and Kudzu Decoction).
- For rectal fissure or polyps, add *Yi Zi Tang* (Yi Word Decoction).
- For dermatological disorders with abscess and ulceration, combine with *Pai Nong San* (Drain the Pus Powder).
- If accompanied by qi deficiency, add *Ren Shen* (Radix et Rhizoma Ginseng).

Fáng Fēng Tōng Shèng Săn

(Saposhnikovia Powder that Sagely Unblocks)

- With phlegm accumulation, add *Ban Xia* (Rhizoma Pinelliae).

CAUTIONS / CONTRAINDICATIONS

- *Fang Feng Tong Sheng San* is contraindicated in patients with deficiency or during gestation.
- This formula should be used with caution in patients having a sensitive gastrointestinal system because it contains strong downward draining herbs.

PHARMACOLOGICAL EFFECTS

1. **Cardiovascular**: According to laboratory experiments, administration of *Fang Feng Tong Sheng San* was associated with an inhibitory effect on the heart, reducing the heart rate, its contractile force, and blood pressure. It also has an anti-arrhythmic effect, as demonstrated in mice with aconitine-induced arrhythmia.[1]
2. **Metabolic**: Administration of *Fang Feng Tong Sheng San* in obese rats at 0.45 g/day for 11 weeks was effective in reducing cholesterol and triglycerides.[2]
3. **Thermogenic and anti-obesity**: Administration of *Fang Feng Tong Sheng San* suppressed body weight gain and prevented the elevation of serum triglyceride levels and body fat accumulation in female rats on a high fructose diet. The proposed mechanisms of actions included inhibition of triglyceride synthesis in the liver, enhancement of lipolysis in adipocytes and of thermogenesis in brown adipose tissue, and inhibition on the phosphodiesterase activity.[3,4]

HUMAN CLINICAL STUDIES AND RESEARCH

1. **Acute mastitis**: In one report, modified *Fang Feng Tong Sheng San* was effective in treating 97 out of 113 patients with acute mastitis.[5]
2. **Obesity**: In one study, 147 patients who were overweight were treated with both ear acupuncture and *Fang Feng Tong Sheng San* for 2 months. The study reported significant results in 27 patients (6.57 kg average in weight reduction), improvement in 93 patients (3.03 kg average in weight reduction), and no improvement in 27 patients (1.06 kg average in weight reduction). The maximum weight reduction was 11.5 kg in one patient.[6]
3. **Hyperlipidemia**: One study reported 80.1% effectiveness using modified *Fang Feng Tong Sheng San* to treat hyperlipidemia in 121 patients (average age of 53.41, with range of 35-72 years old). Modifications to the original formula were made as follows: addition of *Ban Xia* (Rhizoma Pinelliae) for drooling of saliva; addition of *Shi Chang Pu* (Rhizoma Acori Tatarinowii) and elimination of *Mang Xiao* (Natrii Sulfas) for deafness; and elimination of *Ma Huang* (Herba Ephedrae) for spontaneous sweating. Each course of treatment was 30 days. Of 121 patients, the study reported complete recovery in 69 patients, improvement in 28 patients, and no effect in 24 patients.[7] In another study, use of this formula was associated with 30% effectiveness in weight reduction in 68 patients. The study noted that the formula was most effective in female patients between 20 and 30 years of age.[8]
4. **Itching**: Use of modified *Fang Feng Tong Sheng San* in 40 geriatric patients with itching due to wind-heat was associated with great results. Of 40 patients, the study reported complete relief in 35 patients and no benefit in 5 patients. The duration of treatment was 2 weeks per course of treatment, for 2 courses total.[9]
5. **Acute conjunctivitis**: One study reported complete recovery of acute conjunctivitis in all 200 patients (74 unilateral, 126 bilateral) when treated with modified *Fang Feng Tong Sheng San*. Most patients showed improvements within 2-3 days, with duration of treatment ranging from 1 to 5 days. The herbal treatment contained this formula as the base, with the addition of *Hong Hua* (Flos Carthami) for red eyes; *Ji Li* (Fructus Tribuli), *Chan Tui* (Periostracum Cicadae), and *Man Jing Zi* (Fructus Viticis) for severe itching; *Bai Zhi* (Radix Angelicae Dahuricae), *Qiang Huo*, (Rhizoma et Radix Notopterygii), and *Mo Yao* (Myrrha) for severe pain; *Che Qian Zi* (Semen Plantaginis), and *Ze Xie* (Rhizoma Alismatis) for profuse eye secretions; *Pu Gong Ying* (Herba Taraxaci), *Jin Yin Hua* (Flos Lonicerae Japonicae), and *Yu Xing Cao* (Herba Houttuyniae) for redness and swelling of the eyes; elimination of *Mang Xiao* (Natrii Sulfas) if there was no constipation; and elimination of *Ma Huang* (Herba Ephedrae) for spontaneous or night sweating.[10]

TOXICOLOGY

Use of *Fang Feng Tong Sheng San* was associated with one incidence of pneumonitis in a 65-year-old man who complained of cough, fever, and dyspnea about one month after treatment with this formula. Upon discontinuation of this product, the patient recovered.[11]

SUGGESTED ACUPUNCTURE TREATMENT

1. Points: *Fengmen* (BL 12), *Zhizheng* (SI 7), *Quchi* (LI 11), *Hegu* (LI 4), *Dazhui* (GV 14), *Neiting* (ST 44), *Dachangshu* (BL 25), *Shangjuxu* (ST 37), and *Tianshu* (ST 25).
2. Technique: sedation.

Fengmen (BL 12) and *Zhizheng* (SI 7) disperse wind and relieve the exterior. *Quchi* (LI 11), *Hegu* (LI 4), *Dazhui* (GV 14), and *Neiting* (ST 44) clear *yangming* interior heat. *Dachangshu* (BL 25), *Shangjuxu* (ST 37), and *Tianshu* (ST 25) regulate the Intestines and bowel movement.

Fáng Fēng Tōng Shèng Săn

(Saposhnikovia Powder that Sagely Unblocks)

AUTHORS' COMMENTS

Fang Feng Tong Sheng San is literally translated as "Saposhnikovia Powder that Sagely Unblocks" because this formula is known to induce sweating without damaging the exterior and sedate heat without injuring the interior. This formula is used when exterior pathogens remain at the exterior but affect the interior at the same time; therefore, it must treat both conditions simultaneously.

Fang Feng Tong Sheng San has a strong downward draining action and can be used to treat interior toxic heat with exterior signs and has application to treat canine lymphoma from exterior wind-heat and interior dryness. In this pattern of lymphoma, the principles of treatment are to disperse wind, clear toxic heat, moisten dryness and disperse accumulation. This formula should be combined with *Zeng Ye Tang* (Increase the Fluids Decoction), *Bai Hua She She Cao* (Herba Hedyotis), *Ji Xue Teng* (Caulis Spatholobi) and *Shan Ci Gu* (Pseudobulbus Cremastrae seu Pleiones) to accomplish this goal. Once the stools become loose (typically in 5-7 days), decrease the amount of, or remove, *Da Huang* (Radix et Rhizoma Rhei) from the formula. If there is fever, add *Han Shui Shi* (Mirabilite), *Niu Huang* (Calculus Bovis) or *Shui Niu Jiao* (Cornu Bubali).

This formula can be used in horses in a similar fashion as *Yin Qiao San* (Honeysuckle and Forsythia Powder). The main difference is that appropriate use of this formula requires that there be clinical signs of interior heat as opposed to purely exterior signs. Examples include acute cases of influenza or rhinopneumonitis that have associated high fever and constipation. *Fang Feng Tong Sheng San* may also be used in severe cases of conjunctivitis and acute exacerbations of periodic ophthalmia.

Allergic dermatitis and skin rash can be treated effectively with *Fang Feng Tong Sheng San* and *Jing Fang Bai Du San* (Schizonepeta and Saposhnikovia Powder to Overcome Pathogenic Influences). For milder cases it can be combined with *Xiao Feng San* (Eliminate Wind Powder). Single herbs, such as *Di Fu Zi* (Fructus Kochiae), *Bai Xian Pi* (Cortex Dictamni), and *Ku Shen* (Radix Sophorae Flavescentis), can be added to further control pruritus.

References

1. *Zhong Yao Yao Li Yu Lin Chuang* (Pharmacology and Clinical Applications of Chinese Herbs), 1989; 5(3):3.
2. *Guo Wai Yi Xue* (Foreign Medicine), 1993; 15(3):53.
3. Morimoto Y, Sakata M, Ohno A, Maegawa T, Tajima S. Effects of bofu-tsusho-san, a traditional Chinese medicine, on body fat accumulation in fructose-loaded rats. Nippon Yakurigaku Zasshi. 2001 Jan; 117(1):77-86.
4. Yoshida T, Sakane N, Wakabayashi Y, Umekawa T, Kondo M. Thermogenic, anti-obesity effects of bofu-tsusho-san in MSG-obese mice. Int J Obes Relat Metab Disord. 1995 Oct; 19(10):717-22.
5. *Nei Meng Gu Zhong Yi Yao* (Traditional Chinese Medicine and Medicinals of Inner Mongolia), 1987; 2:43.
6. *Si Chuan Zhong Yi* (Sichuan Chinese Medicine), 1988; 2:26.
7. *Si Chuan Zhong Yi* (Sichuan Chinese Medicine), 1998; 5:31.
8. *Zhong Cheng Yao Yan Jiu* (Research of Chinese Patent Medicine), 1984; 4:36.
9. *Hei Long Jiang Zhong Yi Yao* (Heilongjiang Chinese Medicine and Herbology), 1992; 1:33.
10. *Hu Bei Zhong Yi Za Zhi* (Hubei Journal of Chinese Medicine), 1988; 5:29.
11. Matsushima H, Takayanagi N, Ubukata M, Tokunaga D, Mori S, Sato N, Kurashima K, Yanagisawa T, Sugita Y, Kawabata Y, Kanazawa M. A case of pneumonitis induced by Bofu-tsusho-san. Nihon Kokyuki Gakkai Zasshi. 2002 Dec; 40(12):955-9.

Section 2

解表清里剂
— Exterior-Releasing and Interior-Clearing Formulas

Gě Gēn Huáng Qín Huáng Lián Tāng

(Kudzu, Coptis, and Scutellaria Decoction)

葛根黄芩黄連湯
葛根黄芩黄连汤

Pinyin Name: *Ge Gen Huang Qin Huang Lian Tang*
Literal Name: Kudzu, Coptis, and Scutellaria Decoction
Alternate Names: *Ge Gen Qin Lian Tang, Ke Ken Huang Chin Huang Lien Tang*, Pueraria, Scute, and Coptis Decoction; Pueraria, Scutellaria and Coptis Decoction; Pueraria Coptis and Scute Combination
Original Source: *Shang Han Lun* (Discussion of Cold-Induced Disorders) by Zhang Zhong-Jing in the Eastern Han Dynasty

COMPOSITION

Ge Gen (Radix Puerariae Lobatae)	24g [15g]
Huang Qin (Radix Scutellariae)	9g
Huang Lian (Rhizoma Coptidis)	9g
Zhi Gan Cao (Radix et Rhizoma Glycyrrhizae Praeparata cum Melle)	6g

DOSAGE / PREPARATION / ADMINISTRATION

The source text states to cook *Ge Gen* (Radix Puerariae Lobatae) first in 8 cups [1,600 mL] of water until the liquid is reduced to 6 cups [1,200 mL]. Add the other ingredients and cook until the liquid is reduced to 2 cups [400 mL]. Take the warm, strained decoction in two equally-divided doses daily. Today, the decoction can be prepared using the dose of *Ge Gen* (Radix Puerariae Lobatae) suggested in brackets.

CHINESE THERAPEUTIC ACTIONS

1. Releases the exterior
2. Clears interior heat

CLINICAL MANIFESTATIONS

Wind-cold at the exterior with heat invading the interior: fever, nausea, vomiting, foul-smelling diarrhea, irritability, thirst, dyspnea with sweating, a red tongue and a superficial, rapid pulse.

VETERINARY CLINICAL APPLICATIONS

Acute diarrhea from exterior pathogen (micro-organisms) invasion, salmonellosis, Potomac horse fever, acute gastroenteritis following dietary indiscretion, food poisoning or garbage eating.

EXPLANATION

Ge Gen Huang Qin Huang Lian Tang (Kudzu, Coptis, and Scutellaria Decoction) was originally presented in *Shang Han Lun* (Discussion of Cold-Induced Disorders) for treating unresolved exterior wind-cold with heat invading the interior. This condition develops when the exterior condition is incorrectly treated with downward draining herbs, leading to continued presence of exterior heat (minor condition) and its transformation into interior heat (major condition). The interior heat may affect the Intestines and cause foul-smelling heat diarrhea, nausea and vomiting. Interior heat may rise to attack the upper body and cause irritability, a dry mouth, and thirst. The heat may damage the Lung to cause dyspnea and force body fluids out to the exterior, resulting in sweating. A red tongue and a superficial, rapid pulse indicate a heat condition.

To properly treat this condition, exterior-releasing herbs must be used to treat the unresolved exterior condition,

Gě Gēn Huáng Qín Huáng Lián Tāng

(Kudzu, Coptis, and Scutellaria Decoction)

Ge Gen Huang Qin Huang Lian Tang **(Kudzu, Coptis, and Scutellaria Decoction)**

Diagnosis	Clinical Signs	Treatment	Herbs
Unresolved exterior wind-cold with heat invading the interior	• Dyspnea: heat damaging the Lung • Irritability, a dry mouth, and thirst: interior heat consuming body fluids • Foul-smelling diarrhea with burning sensations, nausea, vomiting: damp-heat in the Intestines • Red tongue and a superficial, rapid pulse: heat condition	• Releases the exterior • Clears interior heat	• *Ge Gen* (Radix Puerariae Lobatae) dispels the exterior factors and lifts Spleen qi to relieve diarrhea. • *Huang Qin* (Radix Scutellariae) and *Huang Lian* (Rhizoma Coptidis) clear heat and dry dampness to relieve diarrhea. • *Zhi Gan Cao* (Radix et Rhizoma Glycyrrhizae Praeparata cum Melle) harmonizes the herbs and calms the middle *jiao*.

while interior heat-clearing herbs are used to sedate the interior. This formula contains *Ge Gen* (Radix Puerariae Lobatae) as the chief herb to dispel exterior factors, promote the production of body fluids to relieve the dry mouth and thirst, and direct Spleen qi upward to relieve diarrhea. *Huang Qin* (Radix Scutellariae) and *Huang Lian* (Rhizoma Coptidis) clear heat and dry dampness to relieve diarrhea. *Zhi Gan Cao* (Radix et Rhizoma Glycyrrhizae Praeparata cum Melle) harmonizes the herbs and calms the middle *jiao* to help relieve acute discomforts, such as burning sensations of the anus.

VETERINARY MODIFICATIONS

- When there is excess heat, add *Jin Yin Hua* (Flos Lonicerae Japonicae).
- With food stagnation, add *Mai Ya* (Fructus Hordei Germinatus), *Lai Fu Zi* (Semen Raphani), and *Shan Zha* (Fructus Crataegi).
- With vomiting, add *Ban Xia* (Rhizoma Pinelliae) and *Zhu Ru* (Caulis Bambusae in Taenia).
- With abdominal pain, add *Mu Xiang* (Radix Aucklandiae) and *Bai Shao* (Radix Paeoniae Alba).
- With abdominal pain and diarrhea, add *Bai Shao* (Radix Paeoniae Alba) and *Zhi Shi* (Fructus Aurantii Immaturus).
- For acute bacterial dysentery, add *Bai Tou Weng* (Radix Pulsatillae), *Mu Xiang* (Radix Aucklandiae), and *Qing Pi* (Pericarpium Citri Reticulatae Viride).
- If there is severe tenesmus, add *Mu Xiang* (Radix Aucklandiae) and *Bing Lang* (Semen Arecae).

CAUTIONS / CONTRAINDICATIONS

Ge Gen Huang Qin Huang Lian Tang is contraindicated in diarrhea caused by cold and deficiency with a deep, slow or weak pulse.

PHARMACOLOGICAL EFFECTS

1. **Antibacterial**: It has been demonstrated that decoction of *Ge Gen Huang Qin Huang Lian Tang* has an inhibitory effect *in vitro* against various microorganisms, especially *Staphylococcus aureus*, *Diplococcus pneumoniae*, and *Bacillus dysenteriae*.[1]
2. **Antipyretic**: In rabbits with artificially-induced fever, administration of *Ge Gen Huang Qin Huang Lian Tang* was associated with a marked effect to reduce fever, especially between 2-4 hours after ingestion. The treatment protocol was to administer 5 g/kg of the herbal decoction. In addition, the study noted that the effect of the herbs was comparable to 0.28 g/kg of aspirin.[2]
3. **Antiarrhythmic**: Intravenous injection of a *Ge Gen Huang Qin Huang Lian Tang* preparation was found to be effective in treating mice, rats, and rabbits with artificially-induced arrhythmia by injection of adrenaline and aconitine.[3]
4. **Gastrointestinal**: Administration of *Ge Gen Huang Qin Huang Lian Tang* in laboratory experiments has been associated with relieving diarrhea, slowing the peristalsis of the Intestines, and relieving spasms of the intestinal smooth muscles.[4]

HUMAN CLINICAL STUDIES AND RESEARCH

1. **Diarrhea**: *Ge Gen Huang Qin Huang Lian Tang* has been shown via many studies to effectively treat diarrhea arising from various causes, such as acute or chronic enteritis, postpartum diarrhea, food poisoning, and infectious diarrhea.[5] In one study, 202 infants with acute diarrhea were treated with intravenous fluids and oral ingestion of *Ge Gen Huang Qin Huang Lian Tang* with an overall effectiveness of 88.6%. The average time needed to stop diarrhea was 3.5 days.[6] Another study reported satisfactory results using this formula to treat 513 infants and children with diarrhea in the summer.[7]

Gě Gēn Huáng Qín Huáng Lián Tāng
(Kudzu, Coptis, and Scutellaria Decoction)

2. **Diarrhea during gestation**: Use of modified *Ge Gen Huang Qin Huang Lian Tang* in 30 pregnant women with diarrhea was associated with complete recovery in 25 patients, significant improvement in 4 patients, and no effect in 1 case. The herbal treatment contained this formula plus *Tu Si Zi* (Semen Cuscutae), *Sang Ji Sheng* (Herba Taxilli), and *Ai Ye* (Folium Artemisiae Argyi). Additional modifications included use of *Bai Shao* (Radix Paeoniae Alba) for restless fetus and *Shen Qu* (Massa Fermentata) for poor appetite. The herbs were given in decoction, in three equally-divided doses daily.[8]
3. **Salmonella infection**: Nineteen patients with acute salmonella infection were treated with complete recovery in 16 patients within 4 days, and 3 patients within 5 days.[9]
4. **Bacterial dysentery**: Forty patients with acute bacterial dysentery were treated with *Ge Gen Huang Qin Huang Lian Tang* with great success. The average recovery time was 1.15 days for reduction of fever, 4.51 days for relief of abdominal pain, 3.47 days for recovery of tenesmus, and 2.8 days for resolution of pus and blood in the stool. Overall, most patients reported stabilization of their condition within an average of 3.4 days.[10] Another study reported 96% effectiveness for treatment of acute bacterial dysentery in children using modified *Ge Gen Huang Qin Huang Lian Tang* via rectal enema. The treatment protocol was to cook the herbs in water to obtain 200 mL of herbal solution. Normal saline (300-500 mL) was used first to cleanse the intestines, prior to instilling 100 mL of the herbal solution. This procedure was repeated two times daily, for 3 days. Of 50 patients, the study reported significant improvement in 38 patients, improvement in 10 patients, and no benefit in 2 patients.[11]
5. **Amoebic dysentery**: One study reported 98.28% effectiveness using herbal therapy to treat 116 patients with amoebic dysentery. The herbal treatment contained *Ge Gen Huang Qin Huang Lian Tang* and *Bai Tou Weng Tang* (Pulsatilla Decoction), with addition of *Hou Po* (Cortex Magnoliae Officinalis) and *Huo Xiang* (Herba Agastaches), and removal of *Qin Pi* (Cortex Fraxini), as the base formula. Additional modifications included *Jin Yin Hua* (Flos Lonicerae Japonicae) for high fever; *Di Yu* (Radix Sanguisorbae) for the presence of blood in the stools; *Ban Xia* (Rhizoma Pinelliae) for nausea and vomiting; and *Bai Shao* (Radix Paeoniae Alba) for abdominal pain. The herbs were given in decoction daily in two equally-divided doses. The study reported complete recovery in 114 of 116 patients.[12]
6. **Enteritis**: Use of this formula plus *Bai Tou Weng* (Radix Pulsatillae), *Chi Shao* (Radix Paeoniae Rubra) and *Lian Qiao* (Fructus Forsythiae) was effective in treating all 22 infants with enteritis. The herbs were given via rectal instillation, 40-50 mL rectally two times daily for 3-7 days.[13]
7. **Ulcerative colitis**: Thirty patients with chronic ulcerative colitis were treated with *Ge Gen Huang Qin Huang Lian Tang* with recovery in 10 patients, significant improvement in 12 patients, and slight improvement in 3 patients. The treatment protocol was to flood the colon with 250 of the decoction one time daily for 15 days per course of treatment, for a total of 1-3 courses of treatment.[14] Another study reported 87.5% effectiveness using modified *Ge Gen Huang Qin Huang Lian Tang* to treat 32 patients with chronic ulcerative colitis characterized by Large Intestine damp-heat and Spleen and Stomach weakness and deficiency .[15]
8. **Gastritis**: Sixty patients with chronic superficial gastritis were treated with good results using *Ge Gen Huang Qin Huang Lian Tang* plus *Xiang Fu* (Rhizoma Cyperi), *Bai Shao* (Radix Paeoniae Alba), and *Huo Xiang* (Herba Agastaches). Additional modifications included use of *Bai Hua She She Cao* (Herba Hedyotis) for constipation; *Mu Xiang* (Radix Aucklandiae) for loose stools; calcined *Wa Leng Zi* (Concha Arcae) for acid reflux; and *Zhu Ru* (Caulis Bambusae in Taenia) and *Ban Xia* (Rhizoma Pinelliae) for nausea and vomiting. Additionally, for abdominal distention, *Da Fu Pi* (Pericarpium Arecae) was added and *Bai Shao* (Radix Paeoniae Alba) was removed; and for food stagnation, dry-fried *Lai Fu Zi* (Semen Raphani), *Shan Zha* (Fructus Crataegi), and *Shen Qu* (Massa Fermentata) were added, and *Bai Shao* (Radix Paeoniae Alba) was removed. The study reported relief of gastric pain in all patients within 1-2 weeks of herbal treatment. Of 60 patients, 32 had significant improvement and 28 had moderate improvement.[16]
9. **Fever**: One study reported 97% effectiveness using modified *Ge Gen Huang Qin Huang Lian Tang* to treat 200 children with fever. Modifications to this formula included *Qing Hao* (Herba Artemisiae Annuae) for fever in spring, *Shi Gao* (Gypsum Fibrosum) in summer, *Jie Geng* (Radix Platycodonis) in fall, and *Ma Huang* (Herba Ephedrae) in winter. The study reported improvement in 197 of 200 patients.[17]

TOXICOLOGY

The LD_{50} for alcohol extract of the formula via intravenous injection was 13.5 g/kg in mice. The cause of fatality was attributed to cardiovascular effects, with a decrease in heart rate and contractile force of the heart.[18]

SUGGESTED ACUPUNCTURE TREATMENT

1. Points: *Fengchi* (GB 20), *Quchi* (LI 11), *Neiting* (ST 44), *Shangyang* (LI 1), *Shaoze* (SI 1), *Changqiang* (GV 1),

Gě Gēn Huáng Qín Huáng Lián Tāng

(Kudzu, Coptis, and Scutellaria Decoction)

Dachangshu (BL 25), *Tianshu* (ST 25), *Dazhui* (GV 14), *Shixuan* (extra point), and *Weijian*.

2. Technique: sedation and prick to bleed.

Fengchi (GB 20), *Quchi* (LI 11), and *Neiting* (ST 44) disperse exterior pathogenic factors. *Neiting* (ST 44), *Quchi* (LI 11), and *Shaoze* (SI 1) may be bled to clear interior heat. *Changqiang* (GV 1), *Dachangshu* (BL 25), and *Tianshu* (ST 25) may be used to stop diarrhea. If there is high fever, prick and bleed *Dazhui* (GV 14) and *Shixuan* (extra point). *Weijian* ,a classical point, may be dry-needled or bled to release heat.

AUTHORS' COMMENTS

Clinically, *Ge Gen Huang Qin Huang Lian Tang* is safe for use in any condition involving heat in the Intestines, regardless of whether exterior clinical signs are present or not. It is most important, however, ***not*** to use it in animals with deficiency and cold of the Spleen and Stomach.

Ge Gen Huang Qin Huang Lian Tang and *Huo Xiang Zheng Qi San* (Agastache Powder to Rectify the Qi) are two excellent formulas to treat food poisoning and gastrointestinal infection.

- For damp-heat diarrhea due to food poisoning and grain overload enteritis, *Ge Gen Huang Qin Huang Lian Tang* is the herbal formula of choice.
- For cold-damp diarrhea due to food poisoning, *Huo Xiang Zheng Qi San* is the best formula.

Ge Gen Huang Qin Huang Lian Tang, *Shao Yao Tang* (Peony Decoction), and *Bai Tou Weng Tang* (Pulsatilla Decoction) are three commonly used formulas for diarrhea, but each with a very different etiology and emphasis.

- *Ge Gen Huang Qin Huang Lian Tang* treats exterior pathogen attacking the interior. Clinical signs include foul-smelling diarrhea, sweating (in species that sweat), a red tongue and a superficial, rapid pulse.
- *Shao Yao Tang* treats accumulation of damp-heat and toxins in the Large Intestine, leading to dysfunction and qi stagnation causing severe abdominal pain with blood and mucus in the stool, a greasy, yellow tongue coating, and a rapid, slippery pulse. The key sign for the use of this formula is tenesmus.
- *Bai Tou Weng Tang* treats accumulation of damp-heat and toxins in the Intestines at the *xue* (blood) level. The heat is more prominent than the dampness and is deep in the *xue* level, so more blood will be present in the stool. Clinical signs include bloody, explosive, foul smelling diarrhea, abdominal pain, tenesmus, mucus in the stool, a red tongue with a greasy coating, and a wiry, rapid pulse. Clinically, *Bai Tou Weng Tang* is used to treat more serious conditions than *Shao Yao Tang* and *Ge Gen Huang Qin Huang Lian Tang* and may be combined with either formula to treat more severe disease.

References

1. *Zhong Yi Fang Ji Xian Dai Yan Jiu* (Modern Study of Medical Formulas in Traditional Chinese Medicine), 1997; 458.
2. *Zhong Yao Yao Li Yu Lin Chuang* (Pharmacology and Clinical Applications of Chinese Herbs), 1985; 20.
3. *Ji Lin Zhong Yi Yao* (Jilin Chinese Medicine and Herbology), 1986; 6:30.
4. *Zhong Yi Fang Ji Xian Dai Yan Jiu* (Modern Study of Medical Formulas in Traditional Chinese Medicine), 1997; 460.
5. *Zhong Yi Fang Ji Xian Dai Yan Jiu* (Modern Study of Medical Formulas in Traditional Chinese Medicine), 1997; 461.
6. *Zhong Cheng Yao* (Study of Chinese Patent Medicine), 1989; 11(11):23.
7. *Jiang Xi Zhong Yi Yao* (Jiangxi Chinese Medicine and Herbology), 1959; 6:28.
8. *Hu Bei Zhong Yi Za Zhi* (Hubei Journal of Chinese Medicine), 1995; 5:33.
9. *Shi Yong Nei Ke Za Zhi* (Practical Journal of Internal Medicine), 1989; 3(3):12.
10. *Hei Long Jiang Zhong Yi Yao* (Heilongjiang Chinese Medicine and Herbology), 1995; 2:25.
11. *Zhe Jiang Zhong Yi Xue Yuan Xue Bao* (Journal of Zhejiang University of Chinese Medicine), 1998; 4:16.
12. *Hu Bei Zhong Yi Za Zhi* (Hubei Journal of Chinese Medicine), 1983; 2:24.
13. *He Nan Zhong Yi* (Henan Chinese Medicine), 1992; 1:42.
14. *Zhe Jiang Zhong Yi Za Zhi* (Zhejiang Journal of Chinese Medicine), 1992; 6:279.
15. *Xin Zhong Yi* (New Chinese Medicine), 2000; 10:19.
16. *Guang Dong Yi Xue* (Guangdong Medicine), 1993; 6:336.
17. *Xin Zhong Yi* (New Chinese Medicine), 1997; 9:45.
18. *Zhong Cheng Yao* (Study of Chinese Patent Medicine), 1992; 14(4):38.

Shí Gāo Tāng (Gypsum Decoction)

石膏湯
石膏汤

Pinyin Name: *Shi Gao Tang*
Literal Name: Gypsum Decoction
Original Source: *Wai Tai Mi Yao* (Arcane Essentials from the Imperial Library) by Wang Tao in 752 A.D.

COMPOSITION

Shi Gao (Gypsum Fibrosum)	6g
Ma Huang (Herba Ephedrae)	9g
Dan Dou Chi (Semen Sojae Praeparatum)	1 cup [9g]
Huang Qin (Radix Scutellariae)	6g
Huang Lian (Rhizoma Coptidis)	6g
Huang Bo (Cortex Phellodendri Chinensis)	6g
Zhi Zi (Fructus Gardeniae), *bo* (opened)	10 pieces [9g]

DOSAGE / PREPARATION / ADMINISTRATION

The source text instructs to cut the ingredients, cook them in 10 cups of water, and reduce the liquid to 3 cups. Take 1 cup of the warm, strained decoction three times daily. The source text advises to avoid consuming pork and coming into contact with cold water while taking this formula.

CHINESE THERAPEUTIC ACTIONS

1. Clears heat and eliminates toxins
2. Releases the exterior and induces sweating

CLINICAL MANIFESTATIONS

Unresolved exterior syndrome with interior heat in all three *jiaos*: high fever, no sweating, stiffness of movement, dry nose, thirst, restlessness, irritability, insomnia, confusion, petechiae and ecchymosis, and a slippery, rapid pulse.

VETERINARY CLINICAL APPLICATIONS

Fever, purpura hemorrhagica, and strangles

EXPLANATION

Shi Gao Tang (Gypsum Decoction) treats unresolved exterior syndrome with interior excess heat in all three *jiaos*. This syndrome often originates from *taiyang* syndrome. If the excess exterior symptoms in a *taiyang* syndrome are not relieved within a certain period of time, heat and toxins are created in the three *jiaos*, or all over the body. High fever, no sweating, stiffness of the body and the extremities, dry nose, thirst, restlessness, irritability and insomnia indicate excess at the exterior and heat in the interior. The heat and toxins may also cause skin hemorrhages by forcing the blood out of the blood vessels.

To effectively treat this syndrome, both exterior-releasing and interior-clearing methods need to be used. This formula contains *Shi Gao* (Gypsum Fibrosum) as the chief herb to clear excess heat and relieve the irritability. *Ma Huang* (Herba Ephedrae) and *Dan Dou Chi* (Semen Sojae Praeparatum) relieve exterior symptoms by inducing sweating. *Huang Lian* (Rhizoma Coptidis), *Huang*

***Shi Gao Tang* (Gypsum Decoction)**

Diagnosis	Clinical Signs	Treatment	Herbs
Unresolved exterior syndrome with interior heat in all three *jiaos*	• High fever, no sweating, stiffness of movement: unreleased exterior condition • Dry nose and thirst: interior heat consuming body fluids • Restlessness, irritability, insomnia: interior heat disturbing *shen* (spirit) • Petechiae and ecchymosis: heat forcing blood outwards • Slippery, rapid pulse: interior heat	• Clears heat and eliminates toxins • Releases the exterior and induces sweating	• *Shi Gao* (Gypsum Fibrosum) clears excess heat and relieves irritability. • *Ma Huang* (Herba Ephedrae) and *Dan Dou Chi* (Semen Sojae Praeparatum) relieve exterior symptoms via diaphoresis. • *Huang Qin* (Radix Scutellariae), *Huang Lian* (Rhizoma Coptidis), *Huang Bo* (Cortex Phellodendri Chinensis) and *Zhi Zi* (Fructus Gardeniae) sedate the heat and dispel toxins from all three *jiaos*.

Shí Gāo Tāng (Gypsum Decoction)

Qin (Radix Scutellariae), *Huang Bo* (Cortex Phellodendri Chinensis), and *Zhi Zi* (Fructus Gardeniae), four herbs in *Huang Lian Jie Du Tang* (Coptis Decoction to Relieve Toxicity), sedate heat and dispel toxins from all three *jiaos*. These four herbs also counter the warm nature of *Ma Huang* (Herba Ephedrae) and prevent it from creating heat in the body.

SUGGESTED ACUPUNCTURE TREATMENT

1. Points: *Dazhui* (GV 14), *Fengchi* (GB 20), *Hegu* (LI 4), *Quchi* (LI 11), *Waiguan* (TH 5), *Neiting* (ST 44), *Shangyang* (LI 1), *Guanchong* (TH 1), *Taiyang*, *Weijian*, and *Erjian*.
2. Technique: sedation and prick to bleed.

Dazhui (GV 14), *Fengchi* (GB 20), *Hegu* (LI 4), *Quchi* (LI 11), and *Waiguan* (TH 5) induce sweating and relieve exterior heat. Prick and bleed *Neiting* (ST 44), *Shangyang* (LI 1), and *Guanchong* (TH 1) to clear interior heat and eliminate heat toxins. *Taiyang*, *Weijian*, and *Erjian* are classical points to relieve heat.

AUTHORS' COMMENTS

Shi Gao Tang (Gypsum Decoction) is used to clear toxic heat (excess) in both the exterior and interior; however, its focus is on clearing interior toxic heat. Heat-clearing formulas have the ability to "clear heat and epidemic toxins," or "clear heat and eliminate toxic heat," depending on the individual Chinese medicine text. From a biomedical perspective, epidemic toxins or *wen yi* (warm epidemics) correspond to acute, infectious and contagious pathogens (e.g. bacteria, viruses, fungi) that can be catastrophic in nature and cause severe harm or death in a relatively short period of time. The term toxic heat may also include post-surgical septicemia and endotoxemia, toxicity due to drugs, plants, snake or insect envenomization, and systemic fungal infections. *Shi Gao Tang* can be used for any condition with exterior and interior signs with high fever. It contains all of the herbs found in *Huang Lian Jie Du Tang* (Coptis Decoction to Relieve Toxicity) and so can be used to treat many of the same diseases such as acute infections with appropriate clinical signs. However, it contains *Ma Huang* (Herba Ephedrae) to release the exterior through diaphoresis, and *Shi Gao* (Gypsum Fibrosum), which is very cold, to sedate fire.

Section 3

解表温里剂
— Exterior-Releasing and Interior-Warming Formulas

Wǔ Jī Sǎn (Five-Accumulation Powder)
五積散
五积散

Pinyin Name: Wu Ji San
Literal Name: Five-Accumulation Powder
Alternate Names: *Wu Chi San*, Five Accumulations Powder, Tangkuei and Magnolia Five Formula
Original Source: *Xian Shou Li Shang Xu Duan Mi Fang* (Secret Recipes for Treating Wounds and Bone-Setting Taught by Celestials) by Taoist Lin in 846 A.D.

COMPOSITION

Ma Huang (Herba Ephedrae)	180g
Bai Zhi (Radix Angelicae Dahuricae)	90g
Gan Jiang (Rhizoma Zingiberis)	120g
Rou Gui (Cortex Cinnamomi)	90g
Cang Zhu (Rhizoma Atractylodis)	600g
Hou Po (Cortex Magnoliae Officinalis)	120g
Chen Pi (Pericarpium Citri Reticulatae)	180g
Ban Xia (Rhizoma Pinelliae)	90g
Fu Ling (Poria)	90g
Dang Gui (Radix Angelicae Sinensis)	90g
Chuan Xiong (Rhizoma Chuanxiong)	90g
Bai Shao (Radix Paeoniae Alba)	90g
Jie Geng (Radix Platycodonis)	600g
Zhi Qiao (Fructus Citri Aurantii)	180g
Zhi Gan Cao (Radix et Rhizoma Glycyrrhizae Praeparata cum Melle)	90g

DOSAGE / PREPARATION / ADMINISTRATION

Source text instructions: grind the ingredients, except *Rou Gui* (Cortex Cinnamomi) and *Zhi Qiao* (Fructus Aurantii), into a coarse powder, dry-fry using low intensity fire until the color changes, and then remove from heat. Spread the powder and let it cool. Add the ground powder of *Rou Gui* (Cortex Cinnamomi) and *Zhi Qiao* (Fructus Aurantii), and mix them thoroughly. Cook 9g of this mixed powder with 3 slices of *Sheng Jiang* (Rhizoma Zingiberis Recens) in 1.5 bowls of water until 0.5 bowl of liquid remains. Take the strained decoction while warm.

CHINESE THERAPEUTIC ACTIONS

1. Releases the exterior
2. Warms the interior
3. Smoothes qi circulation and dissolves phlegm
4. Activates blood circulation and resolves accumulation

CLINICAL MANIFESTATIONS

Wind-cold at the exterior with five accumulations in the interior: fever, trembling, pain of the body, neck stiffness, lack of appetite, nausea, borborygmus, vomiting, and colic.

Wŭ Jī Săn (Five-Accumulation Powder)

VETERINARY CLINICAL APPLICATIONS

Gastroenteritis from cold foods or antibiotic use, gastrointestinal pain, anorexia, post-surgical nausea and vomiting, acute or chronic enteritis and arthritis.

EXPLANATION

Wu Ji San (Five-Accumulation Powder) treats five types of accumulations: cold, dampness, qi, blood, and phlegm. This syndrome of multiple stagnations can be attributed to the presence of excess cold at both the exterior and interior. Excess cold constricting the exterior can cause fever, trembling, and other exterior clinical signs. Because cold is stagnant in nature, it may obstruct qi and blood flow to cause soreness of the body and neck stiffness. Excess cold in the interior is often the result of improper dietary intake of raw or cold food that can obstruct qi and blood flow to cause accumulation of dampness and phlegm. The phlegm may obstruct the Lung qi, causing chest fullness. The presence of dampness and phlegm in the middle *jiao* damages the yang qi of the Spleen and Stomach; hence, appetite is affected. Various stagnations in the Stomach can cause the Stomach qi to rise abnormally, leading to nausea and vomiting. The abdominal and chest pains are caused by stagnation of both qi and blood.

To effectively treat this syndrome, the exterior cold has to be expelled with exterior-releasing herbs, and the interior cold removed with interior-warming herbs. In addition, aromatic and drying herbs should be used to dispel dampness and phlegm, and blood-activating herbs should be used to regulate the blood circulation.

Strong acrid and warm exterior-releasing herbs such as *Ma Huang* (Herba Ephedrae) and *Bai Zhi* (Radix Angelicae Dahuricae) release the exterior and induce sweating. *Ma Huang* (Herba Ephedrae) also ventilates the Lung to relieve chest fullness. *Gan Jiang* (Rhizoma Zingiberis) and *Rou Gui* (Cortex Cinnamomi) warm the interior and relieve pain. Together, these four herbs can effectively treat exterior and interior cold. *Cang Zhu* (Rhizoma Atractylodis) and *Hou Po* (Cortex Magnoliae Officinalis), both aromatic in nature, dry dampness and strengthen the Spleen. *Chen Pi* (Pericarpium Citri Reticulatae), *Ban Xia* (Rhizoma Pinelliae), and *Fu Ling* (Poria) dissolve phlegm and regulate qi flow. *Dang Gui* (Radix Angelicae Sinensis), *Chuan Xiong* (Rhizoma Chuanxiong), and *Bai Shao* (Radix Paeoniae Alba) regulate blood circulation and help relieve pain. *Jie Geng* (Radix Platycodonis) and *Zhi Qiao* (Fructus Aurantii) regulate qi flow to help dissolve phlegm. *Zhi Gan Cao* (Radix et Rhizoma Glycyrrhizae Praeparata cum Melle) harmonizes the middle *jiao*, strengthens the Spleen, and harmonizes the formula.

***Wu Ji San* (Five-Accumulation Powder)**

Diagnosis	Clinical Signs	Treatment	Herbs
Wind-cold at the exterior with five accumulations in the interior	• Fever, trembling, pain of the body, and neck stiffness: qi and blood stagnation due to exterior-excess wind-cold • Lack of appetite, borborygmus: damp and phlegm stagnation • Nausea and vomiting: reversed flow of Stomach qi due to stagnations • Abdominal and chest pain: qi and blood stagnation	• Releases the exterior • Warms the interior • Smoothes qi circulation and dissolves phlegm • Activates blood circulation and resolves accumulation	• *Ma Huang* (Herba Ephedrae) and *Bai Zhi* (Radix Angelicae Dahuricae) release the exterior and induce sweating. • *Gan Jiang* (Rhizoma Zingiberis) and *Rou Gui* (Cortex Cinnamomi) warm the interior and relieve pain. • *Cang Zhu* (Rhizoma Atractylodis) and *Hou Po* (Cortex Magnoliae Officinalis) dry dampness and strengthen the Spleen. • *Chen Pi* (Pericarpium Citri Reticulatae), *Ban Xia* (Rhizoma Pinelliae) and *Fu Ling* (Poria) dissolve phlegm and regulate qi circulation. • *Dang Gui* (Radix Angelicae Sinensis), *Chuan Xiong* (Rhizoma Chuanxiong) and *Bai Shao* (Radix Paeoniae Alba) regulate blood circulation and relieve pain. • *Jie Geng* (Radix Platycodonis) and *Zhi Qiao* (Fructus Aurantii) regulate qi flow to dissolve phlegm. • *Zhi Gan Cao* (Radix et Rhizoma Glycyrrhizae Praeparata cum Melle) harmonizes the middle *jiao*, strengthens the Spleen, and harmonizes the herbs.

Wǔ Jī Sǎn (Five-Accumulation Powder)

Because this formula activates qi and blood flow, warms the interior, and relieves pain, it is also effective in treating colic and abdominal pain caused by cold stagnation.

VETERINARY MODIFICATIONS

- With abdominal pain and food stagnation, add *Shan Zha* (Fructus Crataegi) and *Mai Ya* (Fructus Hordei Germinatus).
- If accompanied by pain, add *Qiang Huo* (Rhizoma et Radix Notopterygii), *Du Huo* (Radix Angelicae Pubescentis), and *Fang Feng* (Radix Saposhnikoviae).
- When there is pain in the entire body, add *Ru Xiang* (Gummi Olibanum), *Mo Yao* (Myrrha), and *Xi Xin* (Radix et Rhizoma Asari).
- With cough, add *Sang Bai Pi* (Cortex Mori) and *Ku Xing Ren* (Semen Armeniacae Amarum).
- With low back pain, add *Niu Xi* (Radix Achyranthis Bidentatae), *Du Zhong* (Cortex Eucommiae), and *Xiao Hui Xiang* (Fructus Foeniculi).
- If there is more interior cold, add *Wu Zhu Yu* (Fructus Evodiae).
- With severe food stagnation, add *Shan Zha* (Fructus Crataegi) and *Shen Qu* (Massa Fermentata).
- With dry heaves from Stomach qi reversal, add *Wu Zhu Yu* (Fructus Evodiae), *Ren Shen* (Radix et Rhizoma Ginseng), *Bai Zhu* (Rhizoma Atractylodis Macrocephalae), *Xiang Fu* (Rhizoma Cyperi), and *Sha Ren* (Fructus Amomi).
- For *lin zheng* (dysuria syndrome), add *Mu Tong* (Caulis Akebiae) and *Che Qian Zi* (Semen Plantaginis).

SUGGESTED ACUPUNCTURE TREATMENT

1. Points: *Fengchi* (GB 20), *Dazhui* (GV 14), *Quchi* (LI 11), *Hegu* (LI 4), *Zhongwan* (CV 12), *Housanli* (ST 36), *Mingmen* (GV 4), *Yinlingquan* (SP 9), *Fenglong* (ST 40), *Erding* and *Jiangye*.
2. Technique: tonification, sedation, and moxibustion.

Fengchi (GB 20), *Dazhui* (GV 14), *Quchi* (LI 11), and *Hegu* (LI 4) induce sweating and relieve the exterior factors. Moxibustion on *Zhongwan* (CV 12) and *Housanli* (ST 36) warms the middle *jiao* and tonifies qi. Moxibustion on *Mingmen* (GV 4) will warm yang and dispel cold. *Yinlingquan* (SP 9) strengthens the Spleen and dries dampness. *Fenglong* (ST 40) dissolves phlegm. *Erding* and *Jiangye* are classical points which improve gastrointestinal motility and ameliorate abdominal pain in horses.

RELATED FORMULA

***Wǔ Jī Sǎn* (Five-Accumulation Powder)**
五積散
五积散

Pinyin Name: *Wu Ji San*
Literal Name: Five-Accumulation Powder
Alternate Names: *Wu Chi San*, Five Accumulations Powder
Original Source: *Tai Ping Hui Min He Ji Ju Fang* (Imperial Grace Formulary of the Tai Ping Era) by the Imperial Medical Department in 1078-85

Ma Huang (Herba Ephedrae)	180g
Bai Zhi (Radix Angelicae Dahuricae)	90g
Gan Jiang (Rhizoma Zingiberis)	120g
Rou Gui (Cortex Cinnamomi)	90g
Cang Zhu (Rhizoma Atractylodis), *jin* (soaked) in rice water	720g
Hou Po (Cortex Magnoliae Officinalis)	120g
Chen Pi (Pericarpium Citri Reticulatae)	180g
Ban Xia (Rhizoma Pinelliae), *xi* (washed) 7 times	90g
Fu Ling (Poria)	90g
Dang Gui (Radix Angelicae Sinensis)	90g
Chuan Xiong (Rhizoma Chuanxiong)	90g
Bai Shao (Radix Paeoniae Alba)	90g
Jie Geng (Radix Platycodonis)	360g
Zhi Gan Cao (Radix et Rhizoma Glycyrrhizae Praeparata cum Melle)	90g
Zhi Qiao (Fructus Citri Aurantii), *chao* (dry-fried)	180g

These two formulas are essentially the same. Though they are derived from two different original sources, they have identical names and composition, but they differ in the doses and preparation of the ingredients. Clinically, the functions of these two formulas are very similar and can be used interchangeably. According to the source texts, their differences are as follows:

- *Wu Ji San* from *Xian Shou Li Shang Xu Duan Mi Fang* (Secret Recipes for Treating Wounds and Bone-Setting Taught by Celestials) treats patients with damages caused by five debilitations and seven damages (五劳七伤 *Wu Lao Qi Shang*).
- *Wu Ji San* from *Tai Ping Hui Min He Ji Ju Fang* (Imperial Grace Formulary of the Tai Ping Era) addresses external wind-cold due to exposure, and internal cold due to damages (外感风寒，内伤生冷 *Wai Gan Feng Han, Nei Shang Sheng Leng*).

AUTHORS' COMMENTS

Wu Ji San is literally named "five-accumulation powder" because it treats five types of accumulations: cold, dampness, qi, blood, and phlegm. It has application in the treatment of food stagnation with poor appetite, nausea and vomiting following abdominal surgery or as a result of antibiotic therapy. Antibiotics are cold from an energetic standpoint and can easily injure the middle *jiao*, resulting in qi and food stagnation. This situation can also arise

Wǔ Jī Sǎn (Five-Accumulation Powder)

from animals that undergo surgery and antibiotic therapy, have concurrent interior cold, and are then exposed to exogenous wind-cold pathogens while hospitalized. *Wu Ji San* can be used to treat wind-cold-damp *bi zheng* (painful obstruction syndrome) in the dog with modification.

This is a very effective formula for treating horses with colic, as cold is often a major contributor to stagnation in the middle *jiao*. For more effective pain control, combine with *Shao Fu Zhu Yu Tang* (Drive Out Blood Stasis in the Lower Abdomen Decoction).

Chái Hú Guì Zhī Gān Jiāng Tāng

(Bupleurum, Cinnamon Twig, and Ginger Decoction)

柴胡桂枝乾薑湯
柴胡桂枝干姜汤

Pinyin Name: *Chai Hu Gui Zhi Gan Jiang Tang*
Literal Name: Bupleurum, Cinnamon Twig, and Ginger Decoction
Alternate Name: Bupleurum Cinnamon and Ginger Combination
Original Source: *Shang Han Lun* (Discussion of Cold-Induced Disorders) by Zhang Zhong-Jing in the Eastern Han Dynasty

COMPOSITION

Chai Hu (Radix Bupleuri)	24g [15g]
Huang Qin (Radix Scutellariae)	9g
Tian Hua Fen (Radix Trichosanthis)	12g
Gui Zhi (Ramulus Cinnamomi)	9g [12g]
Gan Jiang (Rhizoma Zingiberis)	6g
Mu Li (Concha Ostreae), *ao* (simmered)	6g [20g]
Zhi Gan Cao (Radix et Rhizoma Glycyrrhizae Praeparata cum Melle)	6g [3g]

DOSAGE / PREPARATION / ADMINISTRATION

The source text states to cook the ingredients in 12 cups [2,400 mL] of water until the liquid is reduced to 6 cups [1,200 mL]. Discard the residue, and cook the strained decoction again until it is reduced to 3 cups [600 mL]. Take 1 cup [200 mL] of the warm decoction three times daily. Patients may feel slightly irritated after taking the first dose, but sweating is usually induced after taking the second dose, a sign that the condition is resolved. Today, the decoction may be prepared using the doses suggested in brackets.

CHINESE THERAPEUTIC ACTIONS

1. Harmonizes *shaoyang*
2. Warms interior and dispels water accumulation

CLINICAL MANIFESTATIONS

Shaoyang disorder with water accumulation in the interior: discomfort in the chest and hypochondrium, dysuria, thirst, absence of vomiting, intermittent fever, and irritability.

VETERINARY CLINICAL APPLICATIONS

Upper respiratory infection, kennel cough, pneumonia, bronchitis, hepatitis and cholecystitis.

Chái Hú Guì Zhī Gān Jiāng Tāng

(Bupleurum, Cinnamon Twig, and Ginger Decoction)

EXPLANATION

According to the source text, *Chai Hu Gui Zhi Gan Jiang Tang* (Bupleurum, Cinnamon Twig, and Ginger Decoction) treats patients who have had exterior condition for five to six days, and who have been treated unsuccessfully with exterior-releasing and downward draining methods. At this moment, the exterior condition is still unresolved, and the disease has moved interior. This condition is referred to as *shaoyang* disorder with water accumulation in the interior. *Shaoyang* disorders are typically described as "half-exterior and half-interior," with characteristic clinical signs such as intermittent fever and trembling, discomfort in the chest and hypochondrium, and irritability. In addition to *shaoyang* syndrome, water has accumulated in the interior. As normal water distribution becomes impaired, clinical signs such as thirst and dysuria occur.

Chai Hu (Radix Bupleuri) addresses the *shaoyang* stage of the disorder, harmonizing the "half-exterior and half-interior" condition and relieving fever and trembling. *Huang Qin* (Radix Scutellariae) clears damp-heat. *Tian Hua Fen* (Radix Trichosanthis) promotes generation of body fluids and relieves thirst, dry mouth, and dysuria. *Gui Zhi* (Ramulus Cinnamomi) eliminates the pathogenic factors that linger at the exterior, while *Gan Jiang* (Rhizoma Zingiberis) warms the interior to dispel cold. These two herbs also warm yang to dispel cold and eliminate water accumulation. *Mu Li* (Concha Ostreae) resolves phlegm and disperses the clumps. Lastly, *Zhi Gan Cao* (Radix et Rhizoma Glycyrrhizae Praeparata cum Melle) harmonizes the formula.

VETERINARY MODIFICATIONS

If there is difficulty with urination, add *Fu Ling* (Poria) and *Che Qian Zi* (Semen Plantaginis).

TOXICOLOGY

One case of interstitial pneumonia was reported in a 57-year-old man who had taken *Saikokeishikankyou-tou* (*Chai Hu Gui Zhi Gan Jiang Tang*) for one month and *Lycium halimifolium Mil* for two weeks. The diagnosis was confirmed when a lymphocyte stimulation test, skin test, and challenge test were all positive to these herbs. This was the first report on pneumonitis caused by this formula to be diagnosed by lymphocyte stimulation test, skin test, and challenge test.[1]

SUGGESTED ACUPUNCTURE TREATMENT

1. Points: *Fengchi* (GB 20), *Zhongwan* (CV 12), *Housanli* (ST 36), *Fenglong* (ST 40), *Yemen* (TH 2), and *Neiguan* (PC 6).
2. Technique: tonification and moxibustion.

Fengchi (GB 20) induces sweating and releases exterior pathogens. Moxibustion on *Zhongwan* (CV 12) and *Housanli* (ST 36) warms the middle *jiao* and tonifies qi. *Fenglong* (ST 40) dissolves phlegm. *Yemen* (TH 2) and *Neiguan* (PC 6) harmonize the interior and warm yang.

Reference

1. Heki U, Fujimura M, Ogawa H, Matsuda T, Kitagawa M. Pneumonitis caused by saikokeisikankyou-tou, an herbal drug. Internal Medicine. 1997 Mar; 36(3):214-7.

***Chai Hu Gui Zhi Gan Jiang Tang* (Bupleurum, Cinnamon Twig, and Ginger Decoction)**

Diagnosis	Clinical Signs	Treatment	Herbs
Shaoyang disorder with water accumulation in the interior	• Intermittent fever, trembling, and irritability: *shaoyang* disorder • Dysuria and thirst: damage of body fluids • Cold extremities and loose stools or diarrhea: cold condition	• Harmonizes and disperses clumps • Warms interior and dispels cold	• *Chai Hu* (Radix Bupleuri) harmonizes *shaoyang* condition of "half-exterior and half-interior." • *Huang Qin* (Radix Scutellariae) clears damp-heat and relieves the feeling of fullness and clumping. • *Tian Hua Fen* (Radix Trichosanthis) promotes generation of body fluids and relieves thirst, dry mouth and dysuria. • *Gui Zhi* (Ramulus Cinnamomi) eliminates the pathogenic factors that linger at the exterior. • *Gan Jiang* (Rhizoma Zingiberis) warms the interior to dispel cold. • *Mu Li* (Concha Ostreae) resolves phlegm and disperses the clumps. • *Zhi Gan Cao* (Radix et Rhizoma Glycyrrhizae Praeparata cum Melle) harmonizes the herbs.

Chapter 4 — Summary

— Exterior- and Interior-Releasing Formulas

SECTION 1: EXTERIOR-RELEASING AND INTERIOR-ATTACKING FORMULAS

Name	Similarities	Differences
Da Chai Hu Tang (Major Bupleurum Decoction)	Release the exterior and interior	Treats *shaoyang* and *yangming* syndromes
Fang Feng Tong Sheng San (Saposhnikovia Powder that Sagely Unblocks)		Treats exterior wind-heat syndrome with interior heat accumulation

Da Chai Hu Tang (Major Bupleurum Decoction) is the main formula to harmonize *shaoyang* and *yangming* syndromes. Key clinical manifestations include intermittent fever, trembling, pain of the epigastrium, constipation or diarrhea, and a wiry, forceful pulse.

Fang Feng Tong Sheng San (Saposhnikovia Powder that Sagely Unblocks) treats concurrent exterior and interior excess heat syndrome. Clinical manifestations include intermittent fever, trembling, constipation, red and painful eyes, thick and sticky nasal discharge, sore throat, coughing, dyspnea, and a dry mouth.

SECTION 2: EXTERIOR-RELEASING AND INTERIOR-CLEARING FORMULAS

Name	Similarities	Differences
Ge Gen Huang Qin Huang Lian Tang (Kudzu, Coptis, and Scutellaria Decoction)	Release the exterior and clear the interior	Releases wind-cold from the exterior, clears heat from the interior
Shi Gao Tang (Gypsum Decoction)		Clears heat from the upper, middle, and lower *jiaos*

Ge Gen Huang Qin Huang Lian Tang (Kudzu, Coptis, and Scutellaria Decoction) releases wind-cold from the exterior and clears heat from the interior. This formula mainly treats foul-smelling diarrhea or dysentery characterized by the presence of interior heat with an unresolved exterior condition. There is burning pain of the anus after defecation. The tongue is red, and the pulse is rapid.

Shi Gao Tang (Gypsum Decoction) clears heat in all three *jiaos*, eliminates heat and toxins, and dispels exterior factors through sweating. Clinical manifestations include high fever, trembling, heaviness and stiffness of the body and the extremities, dry nose, thirst, restlessness, and irritability.

Chapter 4 — Summary

SECTION 3: EXTERIOR-RELEASING AND INTERIOR-WARMING FORMULAS

Name	Similarities	Differences
Wu Ji San (Five-Accumulation Powder)	Release the exterior and warm the interior	Releases wind-cold from the exterior and dispels accumulation of cold, dampness, qi, blood, and phlegm in the interior
Chai Hu Gui Zhi Gan Jiang Tang (Bupleurum, Cinnamon Twig, and Ginger Decoction)		Harmonizes *shaoyang*, dispels water accumulation

Wu Ji San (Five-Accumulation Powder) treats concurrent exterior and interior cold syndrome. Clinical manifestations include fever and trembling without sweating, soreness of the body, neck stiffness, nausea, vomiting, and abdominal pain.

Chai Hu Gui Zhi Gan Jiang Tang (Bupleurum, Cinnamon Twig, and Ginger Decoction) treats *shaoyang* disorder with pain in the chest and hypochondrium. Key clinical signs include intermittent fever, trembling, pain in the chest and hypochondrium, irritability, dysuria, thirst, cold extremities, and loose stools or diarrhea.

Chapter 5

— Heat-Clearing Formulas

清热剂

叶桂 Yè Guì

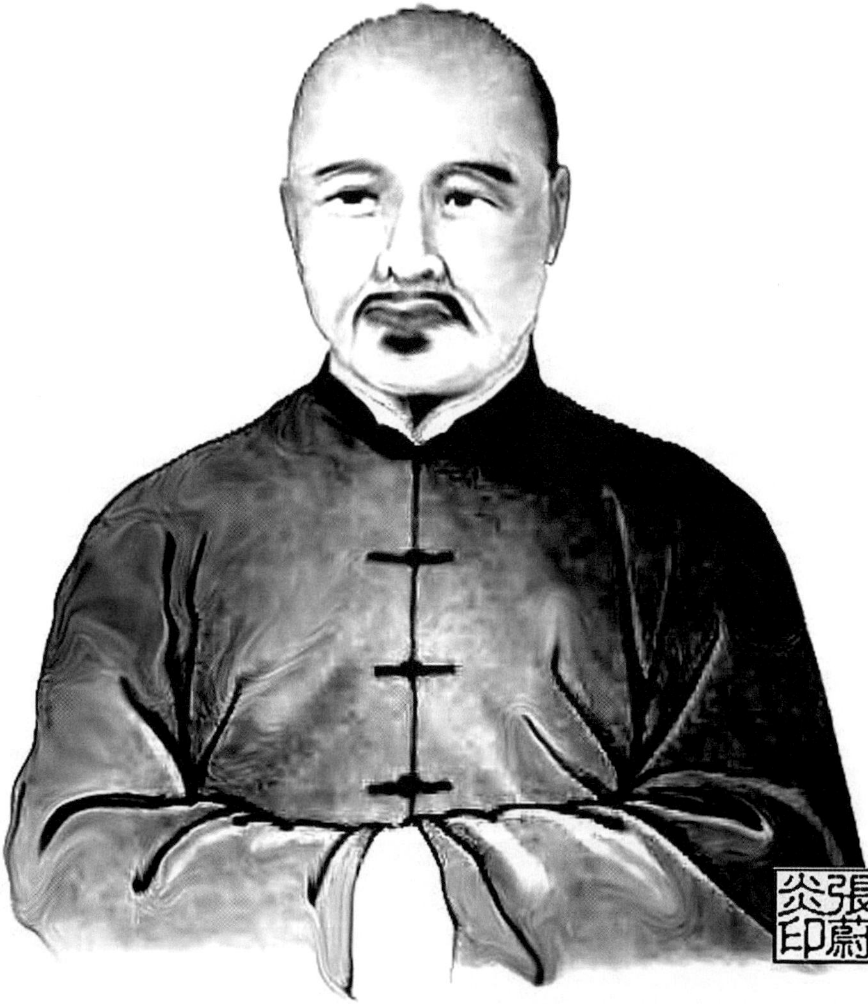

叶桂 Yè Guì, also known as 叶天士 Yè Tiān-Shì, 1666 – 1745.

叶桂 Yè Guì

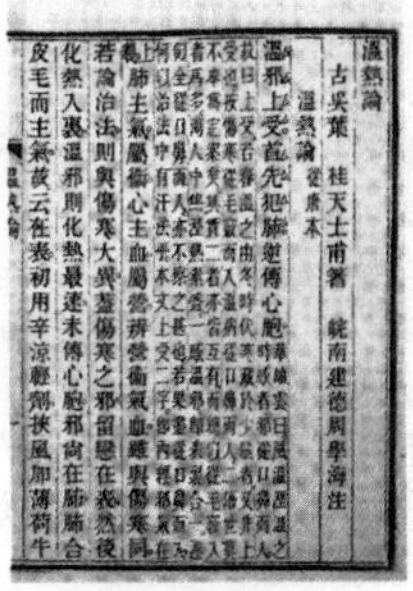

温热论 *Wen Re Lun* (Discussion of Warm and Hot Disorders).[1]

Ye Gui, also known as Ye Tian-Shi, was born into a long family lineage of physicians. His father and grandfather were famous pediatricians. Ye began to learn medicine from his father at the age of twelve. When his father passed away two years later, Ye apprenticed with other teachers. Being very intelligent and extremely diligent, Ye absorbed and integrated knowledge from his family and seventeen other masters over the next ten years, and became one of the best physicians in the country.

Ye lived in southern China and practiced medicine during a time when epidemics plagued the country. At the time, most doctors still followed the principles of 伤寒 *shang han* (cold damage), and had little success in treating epidemic illnesses. Observing this, Ye proposed the theories of 温病 *wen bing* (warm disease), and developed additional theories of *Wei Qi Ying Xue Bian Zheng* (Defensive, Qi, Nutritive, Blood Differentiation) and their corresponding treatment strategies.[2]

Ye dedicated his entire life to clinical practice, and did not have time to write about his work. His extraordinary knowledge was organized and published by his apprentices. The most famous works attributed to Ye Gui include 温热论 *Wen Re Lun* (Discussion of Warm and Hot Disorders) and 临证指南医案 *Lin Zheng Zhi Nan Yi An* (Case Histories from the Compass of Clinical Patterns). The first text focused on theories and treatment principles, and the second text detailed case studies. Credited as one of the most influential physicians in establishing the framework of *wen bing* (warm disease), Ye Gui significantly influenced the practice of traditional Chinese medicine today.

Dynasties & Kingdoms	Year
Xia Dynasty 夏	2100-1600 BCE
Shang Dynasty 商	1600-1100 BCE
Zhou Dynasty 周	1100-221 BCE
Qin Dynasty 秦	221-207 BCE
Han Dynasty 漢	206 BCE-220
Three Kingdoms 三國	220-280
Western Jin Dynasty 西晉	265-316
Eastern Jin Dynasty 東晉	317-420
Northern and Southern Dynasties 北南朝	420-581
Sui Dynasty 隋	581-618
Tang Dynasty 唐	618-907
Five Dynasties 五代	907-960
Song Dynasty 宋	960-1279
Liao Dynasty 遼	916-1125
Jin Dynasty 金	1115-1234
Yuan Dynasty 元	1271-1368
Ming Dynasty 明	1368-1644
Qing Dynasty 清	**1644-1911**
Republic of China 中華民國	1912-Present Day
People's Republic of China 中華人民共和國	1949-Present Day

1. Compiled and published between 1745 to 1766 by the apprentices of Ye Gui.
2. The diagnostic principles of *shang han* (cold damage) follow *Liu Jing Bian Zheng* (Six Stages Differentiation), from *taiyang*, through *yangming*, *shaoyang*, *taiyin*, and *shaoyin*, to *jueyin*. The diagnostic principles of *wen bing* (warm disease) follow *Wei Qi Ying Xue Bian Zheng* (Defensive, Qi, Nutritive, Blood Differentiation), from *wei* (defensive), *qi* (energy), and *ying* (nutritive) to *xue* (blood) levels. This latter set of diagnostic theories presented an alternative systematic perspective from which to evaluate the pathology of disease, and significantly expanded the practice of traditional Chinese medicine.

Table of Contents

Chapter 5 — Overview

清热剂 — Heat-Clearing Formulas

Definition: Heat-clearing formulas clear heat, purge fire, cool the blood, eliminate toxins, nourish yin, and clear deficiency heat. This method of treatment is known as *qing fa* (clearing), one of the *ba fa* (eight treatment methods) described in the *Huang Di Nei Jing* (Yellow Emperor's Inner Classic) in the first or second century A.D.

The terms heat and fire are frequently used interchangeably in many Chinese medicine texts; however, there are important distinctions. Heat-clearing formulas treat disorders characterized by warmth, heat and fire. These three factors are different manifestations of the same pathogenic factor: warmth represents a mild degree, heat a moderate degree, and fire an intense or extreme degree of heat. All three factors can be seen in exterior and interior heat syndromes, and can be treated by using cold herbs to clear heat. Fire or extreme heat more often consumes and impairs body fluids, leading to dryness, and is more likely to damage yin. The nature of fire is to rise and affect the head and upper parts of the body. Fire can cause bleeding disorders and blood stasis by damaging blood and scorching blood vessels, and is likely to affect the mind, causing *shen* (spirit) disturbance and behavioral disorders. Extreme fire can produce internal wind and cause seizure activity. Fire typically produces a higher fever as compared to warm or heat disorders. It should be noted that the term fire may also be used to describe conditions with gross visible clinical signs such as red eyes (Liver fire), stomatitis-gingivitis (Stomach fire), anxiety, insomnia, hyperactivity, and tongue ulcers (Heart fire), even when there are no obvious systemic signs of heat (fever) present.

The source of heat disorders may be externally contracted or internally generated. External sources primarily refer to the *liu yin* (six exogenous factors). Internal sources may include emotional stress, improper diet and/or overeating of damp and heat-engendering foods, and imbalance of the *zang fu* organs. Once generated, heat may reside in different levels of the body and affect various *zang fu* organs. The *zang fu* organs most frequently affected by heat include the Heart, Liver, Gallbladder, Lung, Stomach, and Intestines. The different levels include *qi* (energy), *ying* (nutritive), and *xue* (blood) levels.

Wei Qi Ying Xue Bian Zheng (Defensive, Qi, Nutritive, Blood Differentiation) is a pattern differentiation system for the diagnosis and treatment of exogenous diseases according to *Wen Bing* (Warm Disease) theories. During the Qing dynasty, Dr. Ye Gui introduced the theory that when warm diseases attack the body, they are transmitted through four different levels: the first level is the *wei* (defensive) level, which is associated with the surface of the body, then moving to the *qi* (energy) level, then to the *ying* (nutritive) level, and finally reaching the *xue* (blood) level, which is the deepest layer. In general, heat disorders become more severe and more difficult to treat the deeper they progress into the body. This pattern differentiation system is typically chosen for exogenous disorders that present with acute onset of fever, and provides a way to evaluate the depth, progression and severity of the disorder. It should be noted that in clinical practice, heat disorders do not always begin at the surface level and progress through each of the four levels in that order. The actual order and the initial level affected depends on the type of pathogen, the severity of the infection, the constitution and condition of the patients, and the therapy given.

Chapter 5 — Overview

Wei Qi Ying Xue Bian Zheng (Defensive, Qi, Nutritive, Blood Differentiation) system of diagnosis has been especially helpful in the evaluation and treatment of infectious diseases from a biomedical viewpoint. The clinical signs observed at the *wei* (defensive) level (prodromal stage of acute infectious diseases) relate to abnormalities in the body's defensive and compensatory capability, and there may be no detectable abnormalities on diagnostic tests. When the *qi* (energy) level is affected the signs seen are more severe and reflect disorders of metabolism and physiological dysfunction of internal organs and toxemia; diagnostic testing will frequently reveal abnormalities. In general, at the *wei* and *qi* levels the clinical signs are obvious and potentially reversible; the animal will usually recover if the infection is properly treated. However, once the disorder or infection progresses to involve the *ying* (nutritive) and *xue* (blood) levels, clinical signs may rapidly worsen with a decline in immune function and responsiveness, abnormalities in fluid, electrolyte and acid-base balance, abnormal central nervous system function, abnormal blood coagulation to include disseminated intravascular coagulation (DIC), systemic degeneration and necrosis of the tissues, and internal organ failure.

Heat-clearing formulas have the ability to "clear heat and epidemic toxins," or "clear heat and eliminate heat toxins," depending on the individual Chinese medicine text. From a biomedical perspective, epidemic toxins or *wen yi* (warm epidemics) correspond to acute, infectious and contagious pathogens (e.g. bacteria, viruses, fungi) which can be catastrophic in nature and cause severe harm or death in a relatively short period of time. These pathogenic factors are virulent and have a strong tendency to penetrate to the interior of the body to cause interior heat syndromes. In veterinary medicine, diseases such as leptospirosis, tick borne diseases, canine parvovirus, canine distemper, feline panleukopenia, Potomac horse fever, anthrax, viral encephalitis, pigeon fever, and strangles can be considered disorders characterized by epidemic toxins. In human medicine, examples of epidemic heat include plague, measles, encephalitis B, and sudden acute respiratory syndrome (SARS). In general, the term toxin or toxic heat implies infection, the presence of pus, sores, ulcerations, fistulas, necrosis, gangrene and development of abscesses either internally or externally. The term toxin or toxic heat may also include post-surgical septicemia and endotoxemia, toxicity due to drugs, plants, snake or insect envenomization and systemic fungal infections.

Heat-clearing herbal formulas may be categorized similarly to antimicrobial drugs in conventional medicine, as they are used to treat fever, infection and inflammation secondary to infectious and noninfectious pathogens. Heat-clearing herbs have been found to have potent antiviral, antibacterial, antifungal, antipyretic, antineoplastic and immune modulating effects clinically and *in vitro*. In addition, heat-clearing formulas do not select for microbial resistance, nor do they promote residual infection, damage intestinal microflora or negatively impact the immune system, as so many pharmaceutical drugs do.

Heat-clearing formulas can be combined with conventional antimicrobial therapy for synergistic effects to treat acute, chronic, and antibiotic resistant infections. Most heat-clearing herbal formulas contain herbs that are cold and bitter in nature, as are most antibiotics. Overdosing and/or the inappropriate, or prolonged use of heat-clearing herbal formulas will damage the Spleen and Stomach and consume qi and yin. When using heat-clearing formulas, many patients will require the use of herbs or formulas that support pre-existing Spleen and Stomach deficiencies caused by inappropriate diets and feeding practices, and this is especially true if they are used concurrently with antibiotics.

Heat-clearing formulas should be carefully prescribed, used only when necessary, and discontinued or modified as soon as the desired therapeutic results have been obtained. It is essential to correctly identify the pattern of illness in order to choose the correct category of herbal formula to correct the problem and avoid negative effects. It is recommended that the use of heat-clearing formulas not exceed two to six doses (2-3 days) without re-evaluation, especially if combined with

Chapter 5 — Overview

conventional antimicrobial therapy. Special care and caution additionally should be exercised when treating young, debilitated and geriatric animals. Heat-clearing formulas are contraindicated in yang deficient animals.

SUBCATEGORIES OF ACTION

Due to the complex nature of heat, six sub-categories of heat-clearing formulas have been created to delineate the specificity of the heat. Heat may be located in the *qi* (energy), *ying* (nutritive), and/or *xue* (blood) levels. It may affect different *zang* (solid) and *fu* (hollow) organs. Lastly, heat can have various intensities (warmth, heat, and fire) and characteristics (excess heat, deficiency heat, heat toxins, and epidemic toxins).

1. *Qi* (Energy) Level-Clearing Formulas

These formulas clear heat, reduce irritability, promote production of body fluids, and relieve thirst. They may be used to treat excess conditions (heat in the *qi* level), or complications of excess and deficiency conditions (heat in the *qi* level damaging qi, yin, and body fluids).

Heat attacking the *qi* level may produce signs and symptoms of high fever, irritability, thirst, profuse sweating in species which do, aversion to heat, a red tongue with white to yellow coating, and a forceful, rapid pulse. Herbs and formulas that commonly clear heat from the *qi* level include *Shi Gao* (Gypsum Fibrosum), *Zhi Mu* (Rhizoma Anemarrhenae), and *Bai Hu Tang* (White Tiger Decoction).

Heat in the *qi* level may damage qi, yin, and body fluids, causing signs and symptoms such as fever, profuse sweating, irritability, a dry mouth and tongue, a red tongue, and a rapid pulse. Herbs and formulas that commonly clear heat, tonify qi, and/or nourish yin include *Shi Gao* (Gypsum Fibrosum), *Ren Shen* (Radix et Rhizoma Ginseng), *Mai Dong* (Radix Ophiopogonis), and *Zhu Ye Shi Gao Tang* (Bamboo Leaves and Gypsum Decoction).

2. *Ying* (Nutritive) Level-Clearing and Blood-Cooling Formulas

These formulas clear heat in the *ying* (nutritive) level, cool heat in the *xue* (blood) level, disperse blood stasis, and eliminate toxins. Common clinical manifestations of heat in the *ying* level include: fever that worsens at night, with or without thirst, irritability, occasional dementia, hyperactivity, insomnia, red skin rash, a deep red tongue and rapid, thin pulse.

Shui Niu Jiao (Cornu Bubali) and *Di Huang* (Radix Rehmanniae) clear heat in the *ying* level. Moreover, because heat often attacks the *qi* (energy) level before it attacks the *ying* level, it is important to drive it outward using herbs that clear heat from the *qi* level, such as *Jin Yin Hua* (Flos Lonicerae Japonicae), *Lian Qiao* (Fructus Forsythiae), and *Zhu Ye* (Herba Phyllostachys). One exemplar formula is *Qing Ying Tang* (Clear the Nutritive Level Decoction), which focuses on clearing heat from the *ying* level via ventilating heat from the *qi* level.

Common clinical manifestations of heat in the *xue* (blood) level include: various types of bleeding, red skin rash, petechiae, ecchymosis, hematuria, hematochezia, hematemesis, epistaxis, hemoptysis, coma, insomnia, dementia, hyperactivity, a deep red to purple tongue, and a rapid pulse which can be wiry. In severe cases, extreme fire can lead to the development of internal wind and seizure activity. *Shui Niu Jiao* (Cornu Bubali) and *Di Huang* (Radix Rehmanniae) are frequently used to clear heat and cool the blood. Additionally, because heat in the *xue* level is often complicated by bleeding and blood stasis, it is important to cool the blood, stop bleeding, and disperse blood stasis using herbs such as *Mu Dan Pi* (Cortex Moutan) and *Chi Shao* (Radix Paeoniae Rubra). An exemplar formula is *Xi Jiao Di Huang Tang* (Rhinoceros Horn and Rehmannia Decoction).

3. *Qi* (Energy) and *Xue* (Blood) Levels-Clearing Formula

These formulas clear heat in the *qi* (energy) level, cool heat in the *xue* (blood) level, as well as purge fire and eliminate toxins. These formulas are suitable for treating excess heat and toxins, or epidemic toxins throughout the body affecting both the *qi* and *xue* levels. Common clinical manifestations

Chapter 5 — Overview

include high fever, irritability, strong thirst, various types of bleeding, red skin rash, petechiae, ecchymosis, hematuria, hematochezia, hematemesis, epistaxis, hemoptysis, coma, insomnia, dementia, hyperactivity, a deep red to purple tongue, and a pulse that may be any of the following: deep and rapid; deep, fine and rapid; or superficial, big and rapid. In these cases, herbs and formulas to clear heat from the *qi* and *xue* levels are used simultaneously.

Herbs that clear heat from the *qi* (energy) level include *Shi Gao* (Gypsum Fibrosum) and *Zhi Mu* (Rhizoma Anemarrhenae). Herbs that clear heat from the *xue* (blood) level include *Xi Jiao* (Cornu Rhinoceri) and *Di Huang* (Radix Rehmanniae). An exemplar formula is *Qing Wen Bai Du Yin* (Clear Epidemics and Overcome Pathogenic Influences Decoction).

4. **Heat-Clearing and Toxin-Eliminating Formulas**

These formulas clear heat, purge fire, and eliminate toxins. These formulas generally treat three main conditions: excess heat, fire, and toxins in all three *jiaos*; heat stagnation in the chest and diaphragm; and wind-heat and epidemic toxins invading the head and facial regions.

Excess heat, fire, and toxins in all three *jiaos* is characterized by fever, irritability, restlessness, insomnia, dry mouth and tongue, bleeding disorders, jaundice, skin rash, presence of pus, abscesses, cellulitis, a red tongue with a white to yellow coat and a rapid forceful pulse. *Huang Lian* (Rhizoma Coptidis), *Huang Qin* (Radix Scutellariae), *Zhi Zi* (Fructus Gardeniae), and *Lian Qiao* (Fructus Forsythiae) commonly clear heat, purge fire, and eliminate toxins. An excellent formula that clears excess heat in all three *jiaos* is *Huang Lian Jie Du Tang* (Coptis Decoction to Relieve Toxicity).

Stagnation of heat in the chest and diaphragm is characterized by fever, irritability, ulcerations of the mouth, gingiva and tongue, constipation, and dysuria. *Huang Lian* (Rhizoma Coptidis), *Huang Qin* (Radix Scutellariae), *Zhi Zi* (Fructus Gardeniae), and *Lian Qiao* (Fructus Forsythiae) clear heat, purge fire, and eliminate toxins. *Da Huang* (Radix et Rhizoma Rhei) and *Mang Xiao* (Natrii Sulfas) may be used to clear heat accumulated in the chest and diaphragm causing constipation and dysuria. An exemplar formula that guides and drains heat downward is *Liang Ge San* (Cool the Diaphragm Powder).

Wind-heat and epidemic toxins invading the head and facial regions are characterized by redness and painful swellings on the face, periorbital and temporal dermatitis, as well as a sore mouth and throat. *Niu Bang Zi* (Fructus Arctii), *Bo He* (Herba Menthae), and *Chan Tui* (Periostracum Cicadae) clear wind-heat and toxins affecting the upper parts of the body. *Pu Ji Xiao Du Yin* (Universal Benefit Decoction to Eliminate Toxin) is an excellent formula to dispel heat and toxins outward.

5. ***Zang Fu*-Clearing Formulas**

These formulas clear heat from the various *zang fu* organs and their associated channels and collaterals. Clinical signs vary, depending on the severity of the heat and the area affected.

- Heart heat is characterized by symptoms such as restlessness, irritability and *shen* (spirit) disturbance. Herbs and formulas that clear heat from the Heart channel include *Huang Lian* (Rhizoma Coptidis), *Zhi Zi* (Fructus Gardeniae), *Lian Zi Xin* (Plumula Nelumbinis), *Mu Tong* (Caulis Akebiae), and *Dao Chi San* (Guide Out the Red Powder).
- Liver and Gallbladder heat often presents with symptoms such as red, sore eyes, otitis, hypochondriac pain, and can produce aggressive behavior. Herbs and formulas that clear fire from the Liver and Gallbladder include *Long Dan* (Radix et Rhizoma Gentianae), *Xia Ku Cao* (Spica Prunellae), *Qing Dai* (Indigo Naturalis), and *Long Dan Xie Gan Tang* (Gentiana Decoction to Drain the Liver).
- Lung heat is characterized by symptoms such as coughing, tachypnea, epistaxis, and dyspnea. Herbs and formulas that clear heat from the Lung include *Huang Qin* (Radix Scutellariae), *Sang Bai Pi* (Cortex Mori), *Shi Gao* (Gypsum Fibrosum), *Zhi Mu* (Rhizoma Anemarrhenae), and *Xie Bai San* (Drain the White Powder).
- Stomach heat involves clinical manifestations of *cheilitis*, gingivitis-stomatitis and foul breath. Herbs and formulas that clear heat from the Spleen and Stomach include *Shi Gao* (Gypsum

Chapter 5 — Overview

Fibrosum), *Huang Lian* (Rhizoma Coptidis), *Xie Huang San* (Drain the Yellow Powder), and *Qing Wei San* (Clear the Stomach Powder).

- Heat in the Intestines may cause symptoms such as abdominal pain and tenesmus. Herbs and formulas that clear heat from the Intestines include *Bai Tou Weng* (Radix Pulsatillae), *Huang Lian* (Rhizoma Coptidis), *Huang Bo* (Cortex Phellodendri Chinensis), *Bai Tou Weng Tang* (Pulsatilla Decoction), and *Shao Yao Tang* (Peony Decoction).

6. **Deficiency-Heat Clearing Formulas**

These formulas nourish yin, clear deficiency heat, and relieve dryness. They mostly treat late stages of heat syndromes with damages of yin and body fluids. Common clinical manifestations include low-grade fever in the evenings, general weakness, irritability, dryness, insomnia, restlessness, panting excessively (especially at night), dry cough, constipation or dry feces, short urination, heat aversion, seeking cool surfaces/places, increased to ravenous appetite, increased thirst, trembling and jerking during sleep, poor hearing or deafness, hypersensitivity to acupuncture, a red tongue body with little to no coating, and a rapid, thready, thin pulse. Sometimes chronic deficiency heat patients may experience chronic, persistent low-grade fever.

Herbs that clear yin-deficient heat include *Bie Jia* (Carapax Trionycis), *Zhi Mu* (Rhizoma Anemarrhenae), *Di Huang* (Radix Rehmanniae), *Qing Hao* (Herba Artemisiae Annuae), and *Di Gu Pi* (Cortex Lycii). An exemplar formula is *Qing Hao Bie Jia Tang* (Artemisia Annua and Soft-Shelled Turtle Shell Decoction).

CAUTIONS / CONTRAINDICATIONS

Generally speaking, heat-clearing formulas should only be used when exterior symptoms have been resolved and heat has formed in the interior. If the heat is still located at the exterior, then the exterior-releasing method should be used. If the heat is located both at the exterior and in the interior, then use both exterior-releasing and heat-clearing methods. In addition, heat-clearing formulas should not be used on their own if stagnation or hardness has formed in the interior. In such cases, the downward-draining method should be used to eliminate the stagnation. Indeed, timing and correct differentiation of syndromes are very important factors in using heat-clearing formulas.

In addition, please pay attention to the following notes and precautions when prescribing heat-clearing formulas:

- Examine carefully whether the heat syndrome is of deficiency or excess type.
- Examine carefully which *zang fu* organ is most involved in the heat syndrome.
- Heat-clearing herbs may damage the Stomach and consume the yang, so it is often necessary to use Stomach-harmonizing herbs to prevent such side effects.
- Warm herbs are used as corrigent herbs in some heat-clearing formulas to neutralize the body's resistance to cold herbs; however, the dose of these warm herbs should be low.
- As soon as the desired therapeutic results have been obtained, the formula should be discontinued.

PHARMACOLOGICAL EFFECTS & CLINICAL APPLICATIONS

Heat-clearing formulas, as stated earlier, are divided into six subcategories based on their traditional therapeutic actions. Similarly, these six subcategories of formulas also have contrasting pharmacological effects and clinical applications.

1. ***Qi* (energy) level-clearing formulas** are used primarily to treat fever, with or without infection.
   - **Fever**: These formulas have marked antipyretic effects, and generally treat fever with or without infection.[1] *Bai Hu Tang* (White Tiger Decoction) is the representative formula, and it has been used to lower temperature associated with viral infection,[2] encephalitis B,[3] and epidemic hemorrhagic fever.[4]

Chapter 5 — Overview

- **Diabetes mellitus**: *Bai Hu Tang* (White Tiger Decoction) and *Bai Hu Jia Ren Shen Tang* (White Tiger plus Ginseng Decoction) both have marked hypoglycemic effects,[5,6] and have been used successfully to treat diabetes mellitus.[7,8]

2. ***Ying*** **(nutritive) level-clearing and blood-cooling formulas** are generally used to lower fever and stop bleeding.
   - **Fever**: *Qing Ying Tang* (Clear the Nutritive Level Decoction) and *Xi Jiao Di Huang Tang* (Rhinoceros Horn and Rehmannia Decoction) have shown marked antipyretic effects to lower body temperature in subjects with artificially-induced fever.[9,10] Clinically, they have been used as adjunct treatment to lower body temperature.
   - **Bleeding**: *Xi Jiao Di Huang Tang* (Rhinoceros Horn and Rehmannia Decoction) has an effect to stop bleeding and has been used successfully to treat thrombocytopenic purpura,[11,12] gastrointestinal bleeding,[13] epistaxis,[14] and other bleeding disorders.

3. **Formulas designed to clear heat from the *qi* (energy) and *xue* (blood)** levels can treat fever and infection. For example, *Qing Wen Bai Du Yin* (Clear Epidemics and Overcome Pathogenic Influences Decoction) may be used to treat epidemic hemorrhagic fever,[15] pyogenic infection,[16] and leptospirosis.[17]

4. **Heat-clearing and toxin-eliminating formulas** have remarkable antibiotic effects, and are commonly used to treat a wide variety of diseases associated with infection and inflammation.
   - **Infection**: Many of these formulas have excellent antibiotic effects, and have been used to treat various types of bacterial, viral, fungal, and other infections. These formulas have a wide range of clinical applications, including but not limited to common cold and influenza,[18] otitis media,[19] pneumonia,[20] bronchiectasis,[21] respiratory tract infection,[22] infectious parotitis,[23] tonsillitis,[24,25,26] pharyngitis,[27] encephalitis B,[28] cerebrospinal meningitis,[29] and epidemic hemorrhagic fever.[30] Representative formulas include *Huang Lian Jie Du Tang* (Coptis Decoction to Relieve Toxicity) and *Pu Ji Xiao Du Yin* (Universal Benefit Decoction to Eliminate Toxins).

5. ***Zang fu*****-clearing formulas** have excellent antibiotic and anti-inflammatory effects, and have been used to treat a wide variety of localized diseases characterized by infection and inflammation.
   - **Lung disorders**: These formulas have marked antibiotic effects, and have been used successfully to treat lung disorders such as cough,[31] whooping cough,[32] and pneumonia.[33,34] Exemplar formulas include *Xie Bai San* (Drain the White Powder) and *Bai Tou Weng Tang* (Pulsatilla Decoction).
   - **Stomach disorders**: These formulas have a marked influence to treat various types of stomach disorders, including but not limited to gastritis,[45,36] upper gastrointestinal bleeding,[37,38] erosive gastritis,[39] epigastric pain,[40] and gastroenteritis.[41] Exemplar formulas include *Long Dan Xie Gan Tang* (Gentiana Decoction to Drain the Liver), and *Yu Nu Jian* (Jade Woman Decoction).
   - **Liver disorders** (hepatitis) and **gallbladder disorders** (cholecystitis) may be treated with *Long Dan Xie Gan Tang* (Gentiana Decoction to Drain the Liver).[42,43]
   - **Intestinal disorders**: These formulas have been shown to treat various types of intestinal disorders characterized by infection and inflammation. Clinical applications include enteritis,[44] colitis,[45,46] ulcerative colitis,[47] dysentery,[48] bacterial dysentery,[49,50] and amoebic dysentery.[51] Two representative formulas are *Shao Yao Tang* (Peony Decoction) and *Bai Tou Weng Tang* (Pulsatilla Decoction).
   - **Kidney disorders**: *Qing Xin Lian Zi Yin* (Lotus Seed Decoction to Clear the Heart) has been used to successfully treat kidney disorders, such as glomerulonephritis,[52] pyelonephritis,[53] and nephrotic syndrome.[54]
   - **Eye disorders** (conjunctivitis) may be treated with *Bai Tou Weng Tang* (Pulsatilla Decoction).[55]
   - **Ear disorders** (otitis media) may be treated with *Long Dan Xie Gan Tang* (Gentiana Decoction to Drain the Liver).[56]
   - **Nose disorders** (epistaxis) may be treated with *Xie Bai San* (Drain the White Powder) and *Yu Nu Jian* (Jade Woman Decoction).[57,58]

Chapter 5 — Overview

- **Mouth and throat disorders**, such as stomatitis,[59,60] gingivitis,[61] periodontitis,[62] periodontal disease,[63] halitosis,[64] infectious parotitis,[65] pharyngitis,[66] and other oral cavity disorders,[67] may be treated with *Dao Chi San* (Guide Out the Red Powder), *Qing Wei San* (Clear the Stomach Powder), *Xie Huang San* (Drain the Yellow Powder), and *Yu Nu Jian* (Jade Woman Decoction).
- **Male disorders** (orchitis and prostatitis) may be treated with *Long Dan Xie Gan Tang* (Gentiana Decoction to Drain the Liver).[68,69]
- **Female disorders** (mastitis, cervicitis, polycystic ovary syndrome, and pelvic inflammatory disease) may be treated with *Long Dan Xie Gan Tang* (Gentiana Decoction to Drain the Liver) and *Bai Tou Weng Tang* (Pulsatilla Decoction).[70,71,72]
- **Urinary tract infection**: These formulas have a marked antibiotic activity, and have been used effectively to treat urinary tract infection. Three formulas that have been shown to effectively treat urinary tract infection are *Dao Chi San* (Guide Out the Red Powder),[73] *Long Dan Xie Gan Tang* (Gentiana Decoction to Drain the Liver),[74] and *Bai Tou Weng Tang* (Pulsatilla Decoction).[75]
- **Herpes**: *Dao Chi San* (Guide Out the Red Powder) and *Long Dan Xie Gan Tang* (Gentiana Decoction to Drain the Liver) have marked antiviral effects, and have been used to successfully treat herpes infections (oral herpes, genital herpes, and herpes zoster).[76,77,78]

6. **Deficiency-heat clearing formulas** are mainly used to treat yin deficiency, fever and infection.
   - **Fever**: These formulas are commonly used to treat fever of various causes, such as fever associated with cancer,[79,80] post-surgical fever,[81] and fever following bone fractures.[82] A representative formulas is *Qing Hao Bie Jia Tang* (Artemisia Annua and Soft-Shelled Turtle Shell Decoction).
   - **Infection**: Some formulas have antibiotic activity, and have been used to treat viral infections of the respiratory tract[83,84] and pulmonary tuberculosis.[85,86] An exemplar formula is *Qing Hao Bie Jia Tang* (Artemisia Annua and Soft-Shelled Turtle Shell Decoction).

References

1. *Yao Xue Tong Bao* (Report of Herbology), 1981; 3:61.
2. *Liao Ning Zhong Yi Za Zhi* (Liaoning Journal of Chinese Medicine), 1984; 4:54.
3. *Zhong Yi Za Zhi* (Journal of Chinese Medicine), 1958; 4:246.
4. *Liao Ning Yi Yao* (Liaoning Medicine and Herbology), 1975; 1:56.
5. Morimoto Y, Sakata M, Ohno A, Maegawa T, Tajima S. Effects of Byakko-ka-ninjin-to, Bofu-tsusho-san and Gorei-san on blood glucose level, water intake and urine volume in KKAy mice. Yakugaku Zasshi. 2002 Feb; 122(2):163-8.
6. Kimura I, Nakashima N, Sugihara Y, Fu-jun C, Kimura M. The antihyperglycaemic blend effect of traditional chinese medicine byakko-ka-ninjin-to on alloxan and diabetic KK-CA(y) mice. Phytother Res. 1999 Sep; 13(6):484-8.
7. *He Nan Zhong Yi Xue Yuan Xue Bao* (Journal of University of Henan School of Medicine), 1976; 3:34.
8. *He Nan Zhong Yi* (Henan Chinese Medicine), 1994; 5:266.
9. *Cheng Du Zhong Yi Xue Yuan Xue Bao* (Journal of Chengdu University of Traditional Chinese Medicine), 1995; 4:38.
10. *Zhong Yao Tong Bao* (Journal of Chinese Herbology), 1986; 11(1):51.
11. *Zhong Yi Za Zhi* (Journal of Chinese Medicine), 1958; 7:465.
12. *Zhong Yi Za Zhi* (Journal of Chinese Medicine), 1960; 7:22.
13. *Zhong Yi Za Zhi* (Journal of Chinese Medicine), 1980; 21(7):36.
14. *Shan Xi Zhong Yi* (Shanxi Chinese Medicine), 1989; 10(4):163.
15. *Yi Xue Yan Jiu Tong Xun* (Report of Medical Studies), 1986; (5):3.
16. *Shan Xi Yi Kan* (Shanxi Journal of Medicine), 1983; 4(4):13.
17. *Guang Xi Zhong Yi Yao* (Guangxi Chinese Medicine and Herbology), 1987; 3:6.
18. *Shan Dong Zhong Yi Za Zhi* (Shandong Journal of Chinese Medicine), 1991; (2):37.
19. *Zhong Yi Za Zhi* (Journal of Chinese Medicine), 1994; 35(10):608, 1988; 10:67.
20. *Fu Jian Zhong Yi Yao* (Fujian Chinese Medicine and Herbology), 1985; (2):43.
21. *Zhong Xi Yi Jie He Za Zhi* (Journal of Integrated Chinese and Western Medicine), 1985; 5:304.
22. *Guang Xi Zhong Yi Yao* (Guangxi Chinese Medicine and Herbology), 1989; (1):5.
23. *Zhong Yi Za Zhi* (Journal of Chinese Medicine), 1958; 7:463.
24. *Shan Dong Zhong Yi Za Zhi* (Shandong Journal of Chinese Medicine), 1984; 4:42.
25. *Jiang Su Zhong Yi* (Jiangsu Chinese Medicine), 1994; 4:166.
26. *Xin Zhong Yi* (New Chinese Medicine), 1990; (3):23.
27. *Zhe Jiang Zhong Yi Xue Yuan Xue Bao* (Journal of Zhejiang University of Chinese Medicine), 1996; 3:37.
28. *Fu Jian Zhong Yi Yao* (Fujian Chinese Medicine and Herbology), 1960; 6:7.
29. *Guang Dong Zhong Yi* (Guangdong Chinese Medicine), 1960; 6:296.
30. *Shan Xi Zhong Yi* (Shanxi Chinese Medicine), 1984; 3:16.

Chapter 5 — Overview

31. *Shi Yong Zhong Xi Yi Jie He Za Zhi* (Practical Journal of Integrated Chinese and Western Medicines), 1997; 3:239.
32. *Yi Fang Xin Jie* (New Explanation for Medical Formulas), 1980; 100.
33. *Shan Xi Zhong Yi* (Shanxi Chinese Medicine), 1995; 16(8):362.
34. *Zhe Jiang Zhong Yi Za Zhi* (Zhejiang Journal of Chinese Medicine), 1986; 12:551.
35. *Shang Hai Zhong Yi Za Zhi* (Shanghai Journal of Chinese Medicine), 1996; 6:38.
36. *Shan Xi Zhong Yi* (Shanxi Chinese Medicine), 1997; 4:14.
37. *Zhong Yi Fang Ji Xian Dai Yan Jiu* (Modern Study of Medical Formulas in Traditional Chinese Medicine), 1997; 322.
38. *Zhong Yi Ming Fang Lin Chuang Xin Yong* (Contemporary Clinical Applications of Classic Chinese Formulas), 2001; 186.
39. *Shi Yong Zhong Yi Za Zhi* (Journal of Practical Chinese Medicine), 1999; 2:10.
40. *Hu Bei Zhong Yi Za Zhi* (Hubei Journal of Chinese Medicine), 1998; 3:40.
41. *Hei Long Jiang Zhong Yi Yao* (Heilongjiang Chinese Medicine and Herbology), 1998; 5:54.
42. *Jiang Xi Yi Xue Yuan Xue Bao* (Medical Journal of Jiangxi University of Medicine), 1998; 3:123.
43. *Nei Meng Gu Zhong Yi Yao* (Traditional Chinese Medicine and Medicinals of Inner Mongolia), 1987; 6(2):42.
44. *Shang Hai Zhong Yi Yao Za Zhi* (Shanghai Journal of Chinese Medicine and Herbology), 1960; 6:254.
45. *Si Chuan Zhong Yi* (Sichuan Chinese Medicine), 1995; 7:28.
46. *Xin Zhong Yi* (New Chinese Medicine), 1996; 1:20.
47. *Si Chuan Zhong Yi* (Sichuan Chinese Medicine), 1995; 3:33.
48. *Hei Long Jiang Zhong Yi Yao* (Heilongjiang Chinese Medicine and Herbology), 1989; 6:29.
49. *Gan Su Zhong Yi* (Gansu Chinese Medicine), 1998; 2:13.
50. *Nan Jing Zhong Yi Yao Da Xue Xue Bao* (Journal of Nanjing University of Traditional Chinese Medicine and Medicinals), 1997; 5:311.
51. *Hu Bei Zhong Yi Za Zhi* (Hubei Journal of Chinese Medicine), 1983; 2:24.
52. *Shan Xi Zhong Yi* (Shanxi Chinese Medicine), 1998; 4:173.
53. *Shan Xi Zhong Yi* (Shanxi Chinese Medicine), 1998; 4:173.
54. *Shan Xi Zhong Yi* (Shanxi Chinese Medicine), 1998; 4:173.
55. *Zhong Yi Fang Ji Xian Dai Yan Jiu* (Modern Study of Medical Formulas in Traditional Chinese Medicine), 1997; 346-347.
56. *Zhong Cheng Yao Yan Jiu* (Research of Chinese Patent Medicine), 1985; 8:43.
57. *Hu Bei Zhong Yi Za Zhi* (Hubei Journal of Chinese Medicine), 1997; 4:35.
58. *Jiang Xi Zhong Yi Yao* (Jiangxi Chinese Medicine and Herbology), 1986; 5:18.
59. *Nei Meng Gu Zhong Yi Yao* (Traditional Chinese Medicine and Medicinals of Inner Mongolia), 1993; 12(3):27.
60. *He Bei Zhong Yi* (Hebei Chinese Medicine), 1989; 1:25.
61. *Shang Hai Zhong Yi Yao Za Zhi* (Shanghai Journal of Chinese Medicine and Herbology), 1994; 6:31.
62. *Hu Nan Zhong Yi Za Zhi* (Hunan Journal of Chinese Medicine), 1997; 5:36.
63. *Shan Dong Zhong Yi Za Zhi* (Shandong Journal of Chinese Medicine), 1996; 9:402.
64. *Shan Xi Zhong Yi* (Shanxi Chinese Medicine), 1996; 5:204.
65. *Shan Xi Zhong Yi* (Shanxi Chinese Medicine), 1991; (8):368.
66. *An Hui Zhong Yi Xue Yuan Xue Bao* (Journal of Anhui University School of Medicine), 1995; 2:21.
67. *Zhong Xi Yi Jie He Za Zhi* (Journal of Integrated Chinese and Western Medicine), 1989; 9(3):182.
68. *Zhong Yi Yao Yan Jiu* (Research of Chinese Medicine and Herbology), 1987; (4):39.
69. *Liao Ning Zhong Yi Za Zhi* (Liaoning Journal of Chinese Medicine), 1991; (6):32.
70. *Shi Yong Zhong Xi Yi Jie He Za Zhi* (Practical Journal of Integrated Chinese and Western Medicines), 1992; 4:245.
71. *Zhong Yi Yao Xin Xi* (Information on Chinese Medicine and Herbology), 1989; (6):38.
72. *Shang Hai Zhong Yi Za Zhi* (Shanghai Journal of Chinese Medicine), 1982; 12:17.
73. *Guang Xi Zhong Yi Yao* (Guangxi Chinese Medicine and Herbology), 1991; (3):104.
74. *Zhong Yi Fang Ji Xian Dai Yan Jiu* (Modern Study of Medical Formulas in Traditional Chinese Medicine), 1997; 321.
75. *Hei Long Jiang Zhong Yi Yao* (Heilongjiang Chinese Medicine and Herbology), 1986; 6:40.
76. *Nan Jing Zhong Yi Xue Yuan Xue Bao* (Journal of Nanjing University of Traditional Chinese Medicine), 1984; 4(2):90.
77. *Zhong Yi Za Zhi* (Journal of Chinese Medicine), 1987,; 6:34.
78. *Jiang Su Zhong Yi* (Jiangsu Chinese Medicine), 1993; (3):22.
79. *Fu Jian Zhong Yi Yao* (Fujian Chinese Medicine and Herbology), 1996; 1:21.
80. *Hu Nan Zhong Yi Za Zhi* (Hunan Journal of Chinese Medicine), 1997; 5:27.
81. *Zhong Yi Yao Xue Bao* (Report of Chinese Medicine and Herbology), 1995; 6:52.
82. *Zhe Jiang Zhong Yi Za Zhi* (Zhejiang Journal of Chinese Medicine), 1959; 9:34.
83. *Zhong Yi Fang Ji Xian Dai Yan Jiu* (Modern Study of Medical Formulas in Traditional Chinese Medicine), 1997; 351-352.
84. *Zhe Jiang Zhong Yi Za Zhi* (Zhejiang Journal of Chinese Medicine), 1992; 27(6):251.
85. *Zhe Jiang Zhong Yi Za Zhi* (Zhejiang Journal of Chinese Medicine), 1993; 28(5):206.
86. *Zhong Yi Fang Ji Xian Dai Yan Jiu* (Modern Study of Medical Formulas in Traditional Chinese Medicine), 1997; 350-351.

Section 1

清气分热剂
— Qi (Energy) Level-Clearing Formulas

Bái Hŭ Tang (White Tiger Decoction)
白虎湯
白虎汤

Pinyin Name: *Bai Hu Tang*
Literal Name: White Tiger Decoction
Alternate Names: *Pai Hu Tang*, Gypsum Decoction, Gypsum Combination
Original Source: *Shang Han Lun* (Discussion of Cold-Induced Disorders) by Zhang Zhong-Jing in the Eastern Han Dynasty

COMPOSITION

Shi Gao (Gypsum Fibrosum), *fen sui* (pulverized)	48g [30g]
Zhi Mu (Rhizoma Anemarrhenae)	18g [9g]
Zhi Gan Cao (Radix et Rhizoma Glycyrrhizae Praeparata cum Melle)	6g [3g]
Geng Mi (Semen Oryzae)	0.6 cup [9g]

DOSAGE / PREPARATION / ADMINISTRATION

The source text recommends to cook the ingredients in 10 cups [2,000 mL] of water until *Geng Mi* (Semen Oryzae) is fully cooked. Take 1 cup [200 mL] of the warm, strained decoction three times daily. Today, the decoction may be prepared using the doses suggested in brackets above.

CHINESE THERAPEUTIC ACTIONS

Clears heat and generates body fluids

CLINICAL MANIFESTATIONS

Yangming jing (channel) syndrome; excess heat in the *yangming qi* (energy) level: high fever, irritability, thirst with a strong desire to drink, profuse sweating, coughing, dyspnea, wheezing and aversion to heat, a red tongue and a rapid, bounding, forceful pulse.

VETERINARY CLINICAL APPLICATIONS

High fever, fever secondary to bacterial or viral infections, fever from infectious diseases, encephalitis, meningitis, pneumonia, lobar pneumonia, heat stroke, stomatitis, gingivitis, immune-mediated joint disease and diabetes mellitus.

EXPLANATION

Bai Hu Tang (White Tiger Decoction) treats generalized excess interior heat with damage to body fluids. Excess heat may form as a result of the migration of an exterior pathogen into the interior. A typical case is wind-cold traveling to the interior and transforming into heat. Because the disease location is in the interior and the factor is heat, there will be high fever without chills. Irritability is the result of heat attacking the *shen* (spirit). Heat in the interior may consume body fluids, causing thirst with a strong desire to drink. The interior heat may also force out body fluids, causing profuse sweating.

It is not appropriate to induce sweating to dispel the pathogenic factors because the heat is in the interior instead of the exterior. Neither is it suitable to approach this condition with purgative herbs because the heat has not yet attacked the *zang fu* and given rise to constipation. Heat-clearing herbs that are acrid and drying in nature should not be used because they may damage yin even further. The most appropriate treatment strategy is to clear heat and generate fluids with the use of sweet and cold herbs.

Bái Hǔ Tāng (White Tiger Decoction)

***Bai Hu Tang* (White Tiger Decoction)**

Diagnosis	Clinical Signs	Treatment	Herbs
Excess heat affecting *yangming jing* (channel) or *qi* (energy) level	• High fever with aversion to heat: excess heat in the interior • Thirst with a strong desire to drink: heat consuming body fluids • Profuse sweating: heat forcing body fluids outward • Red tongue and a bounding and forceful pulse: excess heat in the interior	• Clears heat • Generates body fluids	• *Shi Gao* (Gypsum Fibrosum) clears heat in *yangming jing* (channel) and *qi* (energy) level. • *Zhi Mu* (Rhizoma Anemarrhenae) clears interior excess heat, nourishes yin and moistens dryness. • *Zhi Gan Cao* (Radix et Rhizoma Glycyrrhizae Praeparata cum Melle) and *Geng Mi* (Semen Oryzae) tonify and protect the Stomach, and prevent the extreme coldness of *Shi Gao* (Gypsum Fibrosum) from injuring the middle *jiao*.

Shi Gao (Gypsum Fibrosum) is the chief herb because it is the most effective herb for clearing heat in *yangming jing* (channel) syndrome or *qi* (energy) level, which manifests as Lung and Stomach fire. *Shi Gao* (Gypsum Fibrosum) reduces fever and relieves irritability, while *Zhi Mu* (Rhizoma Anemarrhenae) helps to clear interior excess heat, as well as nourish yin and moisten dryness. Together, they relieve thirst and replenish fluids that are lost through sweating. *Shi Gao* (Gypsum Fibrosum) is stronger in clearing heat, while *Zhi Mu* (Rhizoma Anemarrhenae) is more effective in moistening dryness. *Zhi Gan Cao* (Radix et Rhizoma Glycyrrhizae Praeparata cum Melle) and *Geng Mi* (Semen Oryzae) tonify and protect the Stomach, and prevent the extreme coldness of *Shi Gao* (Gypsum Fibrosum) from injuring the middle *jiao*.

VETERINARY MODIFICATIONS

- When there is excess heat in the body consuming yin and body fluids, add *Mai Dong* (Radix Ophiopogonis).
- For gingivitis and toothache, add *Huang Lian* (Rhizoma Coptidis), *Huang Qin* (Radix Scutellariae) and *Bai Zhi* (Radix Angelicae Dahuricae).
- When accompanied by alternating fever and trembling, add *Chai Hu* (Radix Bupleuri) or *Xiao Chai Hu Tang* (Minor Bupleurum Decoction).
- For *wen bing* (warm diseases) with wind-heat invasion, add *Yin Qiao San* (Honeysuckle and Forsythia Powder).
- With high fever, thirst, irritability, dementia, and muscle twitching, add *Shui Niu Jiao* (Cornu Bubali) and *Gou Teng* (Ramulus Uncariae cum Uncis).
- With thirst, sweating, constipation, dark yellow urine, add *Da Huang* (Radix et Rhizoma Rhei) and *Mang Xiao* (Natrii Sulfas).
- With thirst due to *xiao ke* (wasting and thirsting) syndrome with Stomach heat, add *Tian Hua Fen* (Radix Trichosanthis), *Lu Gen* (Rhizoma Phragmitis), and *Mai Dong* (Radix Ophiopogonis).
- For skin lesions and burns, mix with sesame oil and apply topically.

CAUTIONS / CONTRAINDICATIONS

- *Bai Hu Tang* treats heat affecting *yangming jing* (channel), not *yangming fu* (hollow organs). *Yangming fu* (hollow organs) is treated with *Da Cheng Qi Tang* (Major Order the Qi Decoction).
- This formula is contraindicated in the following four situations: 1) fever and absence of sweating from an unresolved exterior condition; 2) a pulse that is fine or deep; 3) fever from blood deficiency evident by a bounding pulse that feels empty upon pressure; and 4) a "true-cold, false-heat" condition in which the interior yin rejects and repels yang to the exterior.

PHARMACOLOGICAL EFFECTS

1. **Antipyretic**: According to *in vitro* studies, *Bai Hu Tang* and its ingredients all have varying degrees of antipyretic effects in rabbits. Administration of the herbal treatment was associated with reduction of body temperature by 1.3°C with *Bai Hu Tang*, 1.2°C with both *Shi Gao* (Gypsum Fibrosum) and *Zhi Mu* (Rhizoma Anemarrhenae), 0.7°C with *Zhi Mu* (Rhizoma Anemarrhenae), and 0.3°C with *Shi Gao* (Gypsum Fibrosum). It was also noted that while *Shi Gao* (Gypsum Fibrosum) had a faster onset, *Zhi Mu* (Rhizoma Anemarrhenae) had a longer overall duration.[1]
2. **Immunostimulant**: Injection of *Bai Hu Tang* in mice was associated with an increased phagocytic effect for up to 6 hours.[2]

HUMAN CLINICAL STUDIES AND RESEARCH

1. **High fever**: *Bai Hu Tang* is commonly used as the first choice for treatment of febrile conditions. In one report, 50 patients with high fever who were treated with decoction of the formula experienced a reduction of temperature to normal within two days.[3] In another study, 69 patients

Bái Hǔ Tāng (White Tiger Decoction)

with fever caused by viral infection were treated with 87% effectiveness using modified *Bai Hu Tang*, with the removal of *Geng Mi* (Semen Oryzae) and *Gan Cao* (Radix et Rhizoma Glycyrrhizae), and the addition of *Ge Gen* (Radix Puerariae Lobatae) and *Chai Hu* (Radix Bupleuri).[4]

2. **Epidemic hemorrhagic fever**: Administration of modified *Bai Hu Tang* for 6-15 days was effective in reducing the duration of illness in all 40 patients with epidemic hemorrhagic fever.[5]
3. **Pneumonia**: Twenty patients with lobar pneumonia were treated with an injection of *Bai Hu Tang*; 13 patients had complete recovery, 4 patients had moderate improvement, and 3 patients experienced no change.[6]
4. **Encephalitis B**: One study of 78 patients with encephalitis B reported satisfactory results using *Bai Hu Tang* plus *Ban Lan Gen* (Radix Isatidis), *Lian Qiao* (Fructus Forsythiae), and *Ge Gen* (Radix Puerariae Lobatae). The patients were treated for 5 days per course of treatment. Of 78 patients, the study reported complete recovery in 69 patients, improvement in 4 patients, and fatality in 5 patients.[7] In another report, 31 patients with encephalitis B who were treated with a modification of the formula experienced a reduction of body temperature within the first day, resolution of most symptoms in the second day, and recovery in the third day.[8]
5. **Rheumatism**: Thirty-four patients with rheumatoid arthritis were treated with modified *Bai Hu Tang*. The rheumatism was characterized by redness, swelling, and pain, with duration of illness ranging from 2-36 days. Out of 34 patients, 8 had rheumatism in the upper extremities and 26 in the lower extremities. The treatment protocol was administration of the formula in decoction form one time daily. The study reported complete recovery in 23 patients, significant improvement in 7 patients, slight improvement in 2 patients, and no change in 2 patients.[9] Another study reported that administration of *Bai Hu Tang* plus *Zhi Chuan Wu* (Radix Aconiti Praeparata), *Ru Xiang* (Gummi Olibanum) and *Mo Yao* (Myrrha) was associated with complete relief in 22 of 28 patients with acute rheumatoid arthritis characterized by wind, dampness, and heat.[10]
6. **Diabetes mellitus**: Use of modified *Bai Hu Tang* in 268 patients was associated with recovery in 81 patients, significant effect in 58 patients, effectiveness in 110 patients, and no effect in 19 patients.[11] According to another study, 21 patients with diabetes mellitus were treated daily with an 800 to 1,000 mL decoction of *Bai Hu Tang* daily for approximately 6 months with 95% effectiveness. The dose of *Shi Gao* (Gypsum Fibrosum) may be increased to 120g if there is severe thirst.[12]

SUGGESTED ACUPUNCTURE TREATMENT

1. Points: *Neiting* (ST 44), *Hegu* (LI 4), *Quchi* (LI 11), *Shangyang* (LI 1), *Dazhui* (GV 14), *Taiyang*, *Weijian*, and *Erjian*.
2. Technique: sedation.

Neiting (ST 44), the *ying* (spring) point of the foot *yangming* channel, clears interior heat and harmonizes the Stomach. *Hegu* (LI 4), the *yuan* (source) point of the hand *yangming* channel, clears interior heat and leads the fire outward. *Quchi* (LI 11) and *Shangyang* (LI 1), the *he* (uniting) point and the *jing* (well) point of the hand *yangming* channel respectively, sedate accumulated heat in the *yangming* channel. *Dazhui* (GV 14) is very effective at clearing heat and reducing fever. *Taiyang*, *Weijian*, and *Erjian* are classical points to clear heat from the body.

RELATED FORMULA

Bái Hǔ Jiā Guì Zhī Tāng
(White Tiger plus Cinnamon Twig Decoction)
白虎加桂枝湯
白虎加桂枝汤

Pinyin Name: *Bai Hu Jia Gui Zhi Tang*
Literal Name: White Tiger plus Cinnamon Twig Decoction
Original Source: *Jin Gui Yao Lue* (Essentials from the Golden Cabinet) by Zhang Zhong-Jing in the Eastern Han Dynasty

Zhi Mu (Rhizoma Anemarrhenae)	18g [9g]
Zhi Gan Cao (Radix et Rhizoma Glycyrrhizae Praeparata cum Melle)	6g [3g]
Shi Gao (Gypsum Fibrosum)	48g [30g]
Geng Mi (Semen Oryzae)	0.2 cup [6g]
Gui Zhi (Ramulus Cinnamomi)	9g [5-9g]

The source text states to grind the ingredients into a coarse powder, and cook 15g of the powder in 1.5 large bowls of water until 80% of the liquid remains. Take the strained decoction while warm. Once sweating is induced, the condition will be resolved. Today, this formula may be prepared as a decoction using the doses suggested in brackets.

Bai Hu Jia Gui Zhi Tang (White Tiger plus Cinnamon Twig Decoction) is composed of *Bai Hu Tang* plus *Gui Zhi* (Ramulus Cinnamomi). With the addition of *Gui Zhi* (Ramulus Cinnamomi), this formula has the added functions to warm the channels and collaterals, and harmonize *ying* (nutritive) and *wei* (defensive) levels. It is often given

Bái Hŭ Tāng (White Tiger Decoction)

to patients with *bi zheng* (painful obstruction syndrome) caused by wind, dampness, and heat. Chief complaints are joint swelling, burning pain, and/or muscle pain. Secondary symptoms include fever, panting, irritability, thirst, a red tongue with white to yellow coating, and a wiry, rapid pulse. This formula can also be used for acute immune-mediated joint disease, such as *re bi* (heat painful obstruction) in the dog. If dampness is also a predominant factor, it can be combined with *Si Miao San* (Four-Marvel Powder). The formula should be changed or modified once the acute clinical signs have resolved, typically within four to six doses.

AUTHORS' COMMENTS

Bai Hu Tang treats heat in *yangming jing* (channel) syndrome according to *Shang Han Lun* (Discussion of Cold-Induced Disorders), and treats heat in *yangming qi* (energy) level according to *Wen Bing* (Warm Disease) theories. Although the names of the syndromes are different, they refer to the same condition: excess interior heat with damage to body fluids. *Bai Hu Tang* is the representative formula for treating excess heat in *yangming jing* (channel) syndrome and *yangming qi* (energy) level, two conditions characterized by the "four big's": "big fever" (high fever), "big sweating" (profuse sweating), "big thirst" (extreme thirst), and "big pulse" (surging, big, and forceful pulse). All of the "four big's" need not be present in order to prescribe this formula. Clinically, this formula can be applied if the animal has high fever, a forceful, big pulse and increased thirst. Horses may be treated on a dose-by-dose schedule to control fever in a similar matter as dipyrone, flunixin meglumine (Banamine), or phenylbutazone. In China, this formula has been used in injectable form to control high fevers which are unresponsive to other treatment.

Bai Hu Tang can be easily memorized by remembering that this formula is composed of four herbs and used to treat "four big's," the most important of which is big fever. It is not typically used alone and instead is combined with other herbs or formulas and has many diverse applications. It can be used to treat fever of unknown origin, and fevers due to exogenous pathogen invasion including infectious diseases. Topical applications of this formula can be used to promote healing of hot red skin rashes, necrotic tissue, non-healing wounds and burns, including those secondary to radiation treatment. It has a rapid onset of action, excellent antipyretic and anti-inflammatory properties, and has been shown to increase macrophage phagocytic activity *in vitro*. *Bai Hu Tang* can be used to treat diabetes mellitus with blazing Stomach heat, and later combined with *Xi Yang Shen* (Radix Panacis Quinquefolii) or *Yu Quan Wan* (Jade Spring Pill) at a lower dose once the intense Stomach fire has resolved. *Bai Hu Tang* is often combined with *Si Miao San* (Four-Marvel Powder) to treat acute *bi zheng* (painful obstruction syndrome) characterized by fever, hot, swollen joints, a red tongue with a white to yellow, greasy tongue coating, and a rapid, wiry to slippery pulse. This formula can be used for acute immune-mediated joint disease in the dog and should be changed or modified once the clinical signs have resolved, typically within four to six doses. Because it treats the channel, it is also useful for treating systemic lupus erythematosus, where heat in the Lung channel flares to create ulcerative lesions on the nose.

This formula is very cold and can easily cause gastrointestinal upset. It is recommended that herbal formulas such as *Liu Jun Zi Tang* (Six-Gentlemen Decoction) or *Xiang Sha Liu Jun Zi Tang* (Six-Gentlemen Decoction with Aucklandia and Amomum) be given concurrently to protect the middle *jiao*. *Bai Hu Tang* is for short term use only and fever can resolve in as little as two doses; it should be discontinued as soon as the clinical signs have resolved. *Zhu Ye Shi Gao Tang* (Bamboo Leaves and Gypsum Decoction) is often given following *Bai Hu Tang* once the heat has decreased substantially, when lingering or residual heat is present with damage to qi and yin. *Zhu Ye Shi Gao Tang* (Bamboo Leaves and Gypsum Decoction) is a formula that can clear heat and tonify qi and yin at the same time. *Bai Hu Tang* should not be used in cases in which there is little to no fever, a weak pulse, or yang deficiency.

References

1. *Yao Xue Tong Bao* (Report of Herbology), 1981; 3:61.
2. *Zhong Guo Zhong Yao Za Zhi* (People's Republic of China Journal of Chinese Herbology), 1989; 3:50.
3. *Jiang Su Zhong Yi Za Zhi* (Jiangsu Journal of Chinese Medicine), 1986; 1:9.
4. *Liao Ning Zhong Yi Za Zhi* (Liaoning Journal of Chinese Medicine), 1984; 4:54.
5. *Zhong Xi Yi Jie He Za Zhi* (Journal of Integrated Chinese and Western Medicine), 1987; 5:300.
6. *Liao Ning Yi Yao* (Liaoning Medicine and Herbology), 1975; 1:56.
7. *Tian Jin Yi Yao* (Tianjin Medicine and Herbology), 1980; 7:422.
8. *Zhong Yi Za Zhi* (Journal of Chinese Medicine), 1958; 4:246.
9. *Shang Hai Yi Yao Za Zhi* (Shanghai Journal of Medicine and Herbology), 1987; 3:24.
10. *He Bei Zhong Yi* (Hebei Chinese Medicine), 1989; 4:21.
11. *Shan Dong Zhong Yi Za Zhi* (Shandong Journal of Chinese Medicine), 1984; 5:23.
12. *He Nan Zhong Yi Xue Yuan Xue Bao* (Journal of University of Henan School of Medicine), 1976; 3:34.

Bái Hŭ Jiā Rén Shēn Tāng (White Tiger plus Ginseng Decoction)

白虎加人參湯
白虎加人参汤

Pinyin Name: *Bai Hu Jia Ren Shen Tang*
Literal Name: White Tiger plus Ginseng Decoction
Alternate Names: *Pai Hu Chia Jen Shen Tang*, Ginseng plus White Tiger Decoction, Ginseng and Gypsum Combination
Original Source: *Shang Han Lun* (Discussion of Cold-Induced Disorders) by Zhang Zhong-Jing in the Eastern Han Dynasty

COMPOSITION

Shi Gao (Gypsum Fibrosum), *fen sui* (pulverized)	48g [30g]
Zhi Mu (Rhizoma Anemarrhenae)	18g [9g]
Zhi Gan Cao (Radix et Rhizoma Glycyrrhizae Praeparata cum Melle)	6g [3g]
Geng Mi (Semen Oryzae)	0.6 cup [9g]
Ren Shen (Radix et Rhizoma Ginseng)	9g [10g]

DOSAGE / PREPARATION / ADMINISTRATION

The source text states to cook the ingredients in 10 cups [2,000 mL] of water until *Geng Mi* (Semen Oryzae) is fully cooked. Take 1 cup [200 mL] of the warm, strained decoction three times daily. Today, the decoction may be prepared using the doses suggested in brackets.

CHINESE THERAPEUTIC ACTIONS

1. Clears heat
2. Tonifies qi and generates body fluids

CLINICAL MANIFESTATIONS

Yangming jing (channel) syndrome or excess heat in the *yangming qi* (energy) level with qi and body fluid deficiencies: high fever, irritability, a dry mouth, thirst with a strong desire to drink, profuse sweating (horses), and a big, forceless pulse.

VETERINARY CLINICAL APPLICATIONS

High fever, bacterial or viral infections, encephalitis, meningitis, lobar pneumonia, and diabetes mellitus.

EXPLANATION

Bai Hu Jia Ren Shen Tang (White Tiger plus Ginseng Decoction) is composed of *Bai Hu Tang* (White Tiger Decoction) plus *Ren Shen* (Radix et Rhizoma Ginseng). It treats excess interior heat in *yangming jing* (channel) syndrome and *qi* (energy) level. Because heat may consume qi and dry up body fluids, corresponding symptoms such as thirst and profuse sweating will be present. Thus, in addition to using *Bai Hu Tang* (White Tiger Decoction) to clear heat and generate fluids, *Ren Shen* (Radix et Rhizoma Ginseng) is added to provide a stronger action to tonify qi and replenish body fluids.

VETERINARY MODIFICATIONS

- With restlessness, irritability, and thirst, add *Mai Dong* (Radix Ophiopogonis) and *Wu Wei Zi* (Fructus Schisandrae Chinensis).
- With more severe qi and yin deficiencies, replace *Ren Shen* (Radix et Rhizoma Ginseng) with *Xi Yang Shen* (Radix Panacis Quinquefolii).

PHARMACOLOGICAL EFFECTS

1. **Antidiabetic**: One study in mice confirmed that administration of *Bai Hu Jia Ren Shen Tang* was effective in treating polydipsia accompanied by diabetes mellitus. The herbs were given as food mixture for a total of 4 weeks.[1]
2. **Hypoglycemic**: Administration of *Bai Hu Jia Ren Shen Tang* was associated with marked effectiveness in reducing plasma glucose levels in both rabbits and mice.[2] Another study confirmed that both the individual ingredients and the formula had marked hypoglycemic effects in genetically obese diabetic mice.[3]
3. **Antipruritic**: Oral administration of *Bai Hu Jia Ren Shen Tang* (200 mg/kg) was associated with a marked effect to

***Bai Hu Jia Ren Shen Tang* (White Tiger plus Ginseng Decoction)**

Diagnosis	Signs and Symptoms	Treatment	Herbs
Yangming heat with qi and fluids deficiencies	• High fever, profuse sweating, and extreme thirst: *yangming* syndrome • Thirst and a forceless pulse: excess heat consuming qi and body fluids	• Clears heat • Tonifies qi and generates body fluids	• *Bai Hu Tang* (White Tiger Decoction) clears excess heat to treat *yangming* syndrome. • *Ren Shen* (Radix et Rhizoma Ginseng) tonifies qi and replenishes body fluids.

Bái Hŭ Jiā Rén Shēn Tāng (White Tiger plus Ginseng Decoction)

treat atopic dermatitis in mice. Therapeutic improvements included significantly reduced scratching frequency, and a decrease in skin temperature by 1.97°C. The study stated that this formula had an inhibitory effect on itching, and may be a useful antipruritic drug for atopic dermatitis.[4]

CLINICAL STUDIES AND RESEARCH

1. **Diabetes mellitus**: Use of *Bai Hu Jia Ren Shen Tang* lowered glucose levels in the blood and urine in patients with diabetes mellitus characterized by Stomach heat. This formula was effective in 56 of 64 patients (87.5% effectiveness).[5]
2. **Dry mouth and throat**: Administration of *Bai Hu Jia Ren Shen Tang* was effective in 12 of 15 patients in relieving dry mouth and throat.[6] Another study reported 80% effectiveness using *Bai Hu Jia Ren Shen Tang* to treat 30 patients with thirst caused by the use of antidepressant drugs.[7] *Bai Hu Jia Ren Shen Tang* facilitated salivary secretion to relieve dry mouth and throat by stimulating efferent activity of the autonomic nerve fibers innervating the sublingual glands in a dose-dependent manner.[8]

SUGGESTED ACUPUNCTURE TREATMENT

1. Points: *Neiting* (ST 44), *Hegu* (LI 4), *Dazhui* (GV 14), *Quchi* (LI 11), *Shangyang* (LI 1), *Housanli* (ST 36), *Sanyinjiao* (SP 6), *Taiyang*, *Weijian*, and *Erjian*.
2. Technique: sedation.

Neiting (ST 44), the *ying* (spring) point of the foot *yangming* channel, clears interior heat and harmonizes the Stomach. *Hegu* (LI 4), the *yuan* (source) point of the hand *yangming* channel, clears interior heat and leads fire outward. *Dazhui* (GV 14) clears heat from the body and is effective in reducing fever. *Quchi* (LI 11) and *Shangyang* (LI 1), the *he* (uniting) point and the *jing* (well) point of the hand *yangming* channel, respectively, sedate accumulated heat in the *yangming* channel. *Housanli* (ST 36) and *Sanyinjiao* (SP 6) tonify qi. *Taiyang*, *Weijian*, and *Erjian* are classical points effective in clearing heat from the body and reducing fever.

AUTHORS' COMMENTS

Bai Hu Jia Ren Shen Tang can be used to treat many of the same disorders as *Bai Hu Tang* (White Tiger Decoction); however it has the additional capability to treat qi deficiency in addition to clearing heat. It has been used to treat diabetes in the dog and cat characterized by Stomach heat with qi deficiency and excessive thirst. In the treatment of diabetes it can be modified as needed based on the clinical manifestations. However, *Bai Hu Jia Ren Shen Tang* is not for long term use and once therapeutic results have been obtained, it should be discontinued.

- For Stomach heat and yin deficiency, combine with *Yu Nu Jian* (Jade Woman Decoction).
- With Kidney yin deficiency, add *Liu Wei Di Huang Wan* (Six-Ingredient Pill with Rehmannia).
- For Kidney yin deficiency with heat, combine with *Zhi Bai Di Huang Wan* (Anemarrhena, Phellodendron, and Rehmannia Pill).
- With qi and yin deficiencies, add *Sheng Mai San* (Generate the Pulse Powder).
- With qi, yin and Kidney deficiencies and dryness, combine with *Yu Ye Tang* (Jade Fluid Decoction).
- With both yin and yang deficiencies, combined with *Jin Gui Shen Qi Wan* (Kidney *Qi* Pill from the Golden Cabinet).

Bai Hu Jia Gui Zhi Tang and *Gui Zhi Shao Yao Zhi Mu Tang* (Cinnamon Twig, Peony, and Anemarrhena Decoction) have been successfully used to treat *bi zheng* (painful obstruction syndrome) secondary to heat, and characterized by fever, severely painful, red, swollen joints, and difficult ambulation. This condition corresponds to the biomedical condition of immune-mediated polyarthritis. These formulas are not for long-term use and are typically combined with herbs or other formulas that clear toxic heat, cool and move the blood, nourish yin, and relieve pain.

References

1. Morimoto Y, Sakata M, Ohno A, Maegawa T, Tajima S. Effects of Byakko-ka-ninjin-to, Bofu-tsusho-san and Gorei-san on blood glucose level, water intake and urine volume in KKAy mice. Yakugaku Zasshi. 2002 Feb; 122(2):163-8.
2. *He Nan Zhong Yi* (Henan Chinese Medicine), 1994; 5:266.
3. Kimura I, Nakashima N, Sugihara Y, Fu-jun C, Kimura M. The antihyperglycaemic blend effect of traditional chinese medicine byakko-ka-ninjin-to on alloxan and diabetic KK-CA(y) mice. Phytother Res. 1999 Sep; 13(6):484-8.
4. Tohda C, Sugahara H, Kuraishi Y, Komatsu K. Inhibitory effect of Byakko-ka-ninjin-to on itch in a mouse model of atopic dermatitis. Phytother Res. 2000 May; 14(3):192-4.
5. *He Nan Zhong Yi* (Henan Chinese Medicine), 1994; 5:266.
6. *Guo Wai Yi Xue* (Foreign Medicine), 1992; 2:106.
7. *Zhong Yi Fang Ji Xian Dai Yan Jiu* (Modern Study of Medical Formulas in Traditional Chinese Medicine), 1997; 264.
8. Niijima A, Kubo M, Ichiki H, Komatsu Y, Maruno M, Okada M. Effect of byakko-ka-ninjin-to on the efferent activity of the autonomic nerve fibers innervating the sublingual gland of the rat. J Auton Nerv Syst. 1997 Mar 19; 63(1-2):46-50.

Zhú Yè Shí Gāo Tāng (Bamboo Leaves and Gypsum Decoction)

竹葉石膏湯
竹叶石膏汤

Pinyin Name: *Zhu Ye Shi Gao Tang*
Literal Name: Bamboo Leaves and Gypsum Decoction
Alternate Names: *Chu Yeh Shih Kao Tang*, Bamboo Leaves and Gypsum Combination
Original Source: *Shang Han Lun* (Discussion of Cold-Induced Disorders) by Zhang Zhong-Jing in the Eastern Han Dynasty

COMPOSITION

Zhu Ye (Herba Phyllostachys)	2 handfuls [15g]
Shi Gao (Gypsum Fibrosum)	48g [30g]
Ren Shen (Radix et Rhizoma Ginseng)	6g [5g]
Mai Dong (Radix Ophiopogonis)	1 cup [15g]
Ban Xia (Rhizoma Pinelliae), *xi* (washed)	0.5 cup [9g]
Zhi Gan Cao (Radix et Rhizoma Glycyrrhizae Praeparata cum Melle)	6g [3g]
Geng Mi (Semen Oryzae)	0.5 cup [15g]

Note: *Zhu Ye* (Herba Phyllostachys) and *Dan Zhu Ye* (Herba Lophatheri) have similar pinyin names and functions, and are sometimes used interchangeably. According to the source text, *Zhu Ye* (Herba Phyllostachys) is used in *Zhu Ye Shi Gao Tang* to clear heat and relieve irritability. Today, because *Zhu Ye* (Herba Phyllostachys) is not readily available, it is generally replaced with *Dan Zhu Ye* (Herba Lophatheri). In comparison, *Zhu Ye* (Herba Phyllostachys) is more effective in clearing Heart and Stomach heat, while *Dan Zhu Ye* (Herba Lophatheri) is better at clearing heat and promoting normal urination.

DOSAGE / PREPARATION / ADMINISTRATION

The source text states to cook all of the ingredients except *Geng Mi* (Semen Oryzae), in 10 cups [2,000 mL] of water until 6 cups [1,200 mL] of liquid remain. Discard the residue, add *Geng Mi* (Semen Oryzae) to the strained decoction and cook again until *Geng Mi* (Semen Oryzae) is fully cooked. Take 1 cup [200 mL] of the warm, strained decoction three times daily. Today, the decoction may be prepared using the doses suggested in brackets.

CHINESE THERAPEUTIC ACTIONS

1. Clears heat and generates body fluids
2. Tonifies qi and harmonizes the Stomach

CLINICAL MANIFESTATIONS

Lingering or residual heat resulting from *shang han* (cold damage), *wen bing* (warm diseases), or summer-heat with both qi and yin damage: fever, profuse sweating (horses), excessive panting, distention in the epigastrium, poor appetite, nausea, vomiting, dry mouth, gagging cough, increased thirst, irritability, insomnia, a red tongue with little to no coating, and a weak, rapid and thready pulse.

VETERINARY CLINICAL APPLICATIONS

Post-illness fever, bronchitis, pneumonia, gingivitis, stomatitis, nausea and vomiting secondary to chemotherapy, diabetes mellitus.

EXPLANATION

Zhu Ye Shi Gao Tang (Bamboo Leaves and Gypsum Decoction) is indicated in the late stage of *shang han* (cold damage), *wen bing* (warm diseases), or febrile diseases in which the heat has diminished substantially but there is still residual heat in the Lung and Stomach, and qi, yin and body fluids are damaged. Irritability, distention in the epigastrium, poor appetite, nausea, vomiting, profuse sweating and fever are indications that the heat has not been completely eliminated. Thirst, dry mouth and lips, a red tongue with little to no coating, and a weak, rapid, and thready pulse reflect consumption of yin and body fluids by heat.

This condition of lingering heat with underlying deficiencies must be treated carefully. Bitter and cold herbs that clear heat will not help generate body fluids and may further damage qi and yin. However, simply tonifying qi and yin will trap the residual heat inside. Therefore, the optimal treatment strategy is to sedate and tonify at the same time.

Zhu Ye (Herba Phyllostachys) and *Shi Gao* (Gypsum Fibrosum) clear interior heat to relieve fever and irritability. *Ren Shen* (Radix et Rhizoma Ginseng) and *Mai Dong* (Radix Ophiopogonis) tonify both qi and yin to promote generation of body fluids. *Ban Xia* (Rhizoma Pinelliae) corrects the reversed flow of Stomach qi to relieve nausea and vomiting. It also balances the tonic and cloying effects

Zhú Yè Shí Gāo Tāng (Bamboo Leaves and Gypsum Decoction)

Zhu Ye Shi Gao Tang (Bamboo Leaves and Gypsum Decoction)

Diagnosis	Clinical Signs	Treatment	Herbs
Lingering heat with qi and yin damage	• Irritability and insomnia: heat disturbing *shen* (spirit) • Fever and profuse sweating: lingering heat not yet cleared • Dry mouth and thirst: heat consuming body fluids • Epigastric distention, poor appetite, nausea, vomiting, dry heaves, dry cough: heat injuring Lung and Stomach qi • Red tongue with little to no coating: heat damaging qi and body fluids • Weak, rapid and thready pulse: deficiency condition	• Clears heat and generates body fluids • Tonifies qi and harmonizes the Stomach	• *Zhu Ye* (Herba Phyllostachys) and *Shi Gao* (Gypsum Fibrosum) clear interior heat. • *Ren Shen* (Radix et Rhizoma Ginseng) and *Mai Dong* (Radix Ophiopogonis) tonify qi and yin. • *Ban Xia* (Rhizoma Pinelliae) corrects the reversed flow of Stomach qi. • *Zhi Gan Cao* (Radix et Rhizoma Glycyrrhizae Praeparata cum Melle) and *Geng Mi* (Semen Oryzae) nourish the Stomach and harmonize the middle *jiao*.

of *Ren Shen* (Radix et Rhizoma Ginseng) and *Mai Dong* (Radix Ophiopogonis). *Zhi Gan Cao* (Radix et Rhizoma Glycyrrhizae Praeparata cum Melle) and *Geng Mi* (Semen Oryzae) nourish the Stomach and harmonize the middle *jiao*.

VETERINARY MODIFICATIONS

- With cough and dyspnea, add *Ku Xing Ren* (Semen Armeniacae Amarum).
- With cough and wheezing in pneumonia or bronchitis, add *Ma Huang* (Herba Ephedrae), *Ku Xing Ren* (Semen Armeniacae Amarum), *Huang Qin* (Radix Scutellariae), and *Yu Xing Cao* (Herba Houttuyniae).
- For deficiency condition with thirst, add *Huang Qi* (Radix Astragali) and *Wu Wei Zi* (Fructus Schisandrae Chinensis).

CAUTIONS / CONTRAINDICATIONS

Zhu Ye Shi Gao Tang is contraindicated in acute conditions of excess heat without underlying deficiencies. It is also contraindicated in animals with fever, dry heaves, and a greasy tongue coating caused by damp accumulation.

PHARMACOLOGICAL EFFECTS

Hypoglycemic: Administration of a water extract of *Zhu Ye Shi Gao Tang* at 500 mg/kg via intraperitoneal injection was associated with reduction of blood glucose level in mice. However, the hypoglycemic effect was significant only during the fasting state, and not during the normal state.[1]

HUMAN CLINICAL STUDIES AND RESEARCH

1. **Fever**: Forty-seven cases of fever (37.5-39.5°C / 99.5-103.1°F) with duration of illness from one week to three months and resistant to antibiotic therapy were treated with *Zhu Ye Shi Gao Tang*. The treatment protocol was daily administration of the formula as a decoction in three to five equally-divided doses for 1-5 days. Out of 47 cases, the study reported temperature of less than 37°C / 98.6°F in 40 cases.[2]
2. **Toothache**: In one report, 96 patients with toothache were divided into two groups and treated with modified *Zhu Ye Shi Gao Tang*. Group A of 60 patients received treatment within 3 days from the onset of illness, while Group B of 36 patients received treatment 4-6 days after the onset. The herbs were cooked twice to yield 2 batches of decoction, which were subsequently mixed together and taken before each meal. The study reported complete recovery in all 60 patients in group A, and only 30 out of 36 patients in group B. Complete recovery was defined as resolution of the symptoms, complete reduction of redness, swelling and pain, and normal chewing and eating without pain.[3]

SUGGESTED ACUPUNCTURE TREATMENT

1. Points: *Chize* (LU 5), *Neiguan* (PC 6), *Zhongwan* (CV 12), *Housanli* (ST 36), and *Sanyinjiao* (SP 6).
2. Technique: mainly tonification.

Chize (LU 5) and *Neiguan* (PC 6) clear interior heat, nourish fluids, and relieve irritability. *Zhongwan* (CV 12) harmonizes the middle *jiao* and corrects the reversed flow of Stomach qi. *Housanli* (ST 36) and *Sanyinjiao* (SP 6) nourish qi, yin, and body fluids.

AUTHORS' COMMENTS

Zhu Ye Shi Gao Tang may be used in combination with *Yu Nu Jian* (Jade Woman Decoction) for the treatment of diabetes mellitus in cats characterized by Stomach yin

Zhú Yè Shí Gāo Tāng (Bamboo Leaves and Gypsum Decoction)

deficiency and flaring of Stomach fire, with ulcerations in the mouth and a red tongue body. Gingivitis or stomatitis in the cat can be treated in combination with *Qing Wei San* (Clear the Stomach Powder) or *Yu Nu Jian* (Jade Woman Decoction). This formula can also treat bronchial pneumonia or bronchitis with low-grade fever, generalized dryness, cough, nausea, vomiting and poor appetite that has developed secondary to chronic infection, fever, and multiple courses of antibiotics. Similarly, *Zhu Ye Shi Gao Tang* may be used to treat gastric ulcers and gastritis in horses, which primarily derives from Stomach yin deficiency. Though *Yu Nu Jian* is the preferred formula for acute, active ulcerative conditions, *Zhu Ye Shi Gao Tang* is an acceptable substitute for mild gastritis or for upset stomach and anorexia that lingers after febrile disease or a course of medication. *Zhu Ye Shi Gao Tang* can be used to treat fever, nausea and vomiting from Stomach yin deficiency that develops secondary to poor diet, polypharmacy and chemotherapy in animals with cancer or chronic illness.

Zhu Ye Shi Gao Tang is derived from *Bai Hu Tang* (White Tiger Decoction), with the addition of *Ren Shen* (Radix et Rhizoma Ginseng) to tonify qi, *Mai Dong* (Radix Ophiopogonis) to nourish yin, *Ban Xia* (Rhizoma Pinelliae) to harmonize the Stomach, and the replacement of *Zhi Mu* (Rhizoma Anemarrhenae) with *Zhu Ye* (Herba Phyllostachys) to clear heat and relieve irritability.

Bai Hu Tang (White Tiger Decoction) and *Zhu Ye Shi Gao Tang* both clear heat and generate body fluids to treat heat in the *qi* (energy) level. Both formulas contain *Shi Gao* (Gypsum Fibrosum), *Geng Mi* (Semen Oryzae), and *Gan Cao* (Radix et Rhizoma Glycyrrhizae). The differences are as follows:

- *Bai Hu Tang* focuses on clearing heat, as it has *Zhi Mu* (Rhizoma Anemarrhenae) as the deputy herb to enhance the heat-clearing effect of *Shi Gao* (Gypsum Fibrosum). It is best for excess heat in the *qi* (energy) level manifesting in symptoms of high fever, irritability, thirst, profuse sweating, and a bounding and forceful pulse. It treats excess heat and generates body fluids at the same time.
- *Zhu Ye Shi Gao Tang* contains *Ren Shen* (Radix et Rhizoma Ginseng), *Mai Dong* (Radix Ophiopogonis), *Zhu Ye* (Herba Phyllostachys), and *Ban Xia* (Rhizoma Pinelliae) and is weaker in clearing heat but stronger in tonifying qi and nourishing yin. It is best for the post-febrile stage of lingering heat with qi and yin damage. Symptoms include heat sensation, sweating, increased thirst, shortness of breath, a red, dry tongue with little to no coating, and a deficient, rapid pulse.

Bai Hu Jia Ren Shen Tang (White Tiger plus Ginseng Decoction) and *Zhu Ye Shi Gao Tang* both treat patients with heat and deficiency. The differences are as follows:

- *Bai Hu Jia Ren Shen Tang* is for excess heat in the *yangming jing* (channel) syndrome or *yangming qi* (energy) level with qi and fluid deficiencies.
- *Zhu Ye Shi Gao Tang* is for lingering heat from *shang han* (cold damage), *wen bing* (warm diseases), or summer-heat, with injuries to both qi and yin.[4]

References

1. *Han Fang Yi Xue* (Kampo Medicine), 1981; 1:14.
2. *Yun Nan Zhong Yi Za Zhi* (Yunan Journal of Chinese Medicine), 1985; 4:20.
3. *Si Chuan Zhong Yi* (Sichuan Chinese Medicine), 1994; 10:52.
4. Wang MZ, et al. *Zhong Yi Xue Wen Da Ti Ku* (Questions and Answers on Traditional Chinese Medicine: Herbal Formulas).

Section 2

清营凉血剂
— Ying (Nutritive) Level-Clearing and Blood-Cooling Formulas

Qīng Yíng Tāng (Clear the Nutritive Level Decoction)
清營湯
清营汤

Pinyin Name: *Qing Ying Tang*
Literal Name: Clear the Nutritive Level Decoction
Original Source: *Wen Bing Tiao Bian* (Systematic Differentiation of Warm Disease) by Wu Ju-Tong in 1798

COMPOSITION

Xi Jiao (Cornu Rhinoceri), *chong fu* (taken drenched)	9g [2g]
Di Huang (Radix Rehmanniae)	15g [15-20g]
Mai Dong (Radix Ophiopogonis)	9g
Xuan Shen (Radix Scrophulariae)	9g
Jin Yin Hua (Flos Lonicerae Japonicae)	9g
Lian Qiao (Fructus Forsythiae)	6g
Huang Lian (Rhizoma Coptidis)	4.5g
Zhu Ye (Herba Phyllostachys)	3g [5g]
Dan Shen (Radix et Rhizoma Salviae Miltiorrhizae)	6g [9g]

Note: *Xi Jiao* (Cornu Rhinoceri) is derived from an endangered animal, and is rarely used as a medicinal substance today. Its discussion here is included primarily for academic purposes, to reflect the historical use of this substance in its original formulation. Most herbal products today have removed it completely, or replaced it with substitutes with similar functions.

Zhu Ye (Herba Phyllostachys) and *Dan Zhu Ye* (Herba Lophatheri) have similar pinyin names and functions, and are sometimes used interchangeably. According to the source text, *Zhu Ye* (Herba Phyllostachys) is used in *Qing Ying Tang* to clear Heart heat. Today, because *Zhu Ye* (Herba Phyllostachys) is not readily available, it is generally replaced with *Dan Zhu Ye* (Herba Lophatheri). In comparison, *Zhu Ye* (Herba Phyllostachys) is more effective in clearing Heart and Stomach heat, while *Dan Zhu Ye* (Herba Lophatheri) is better in clearing heat and promoting normal urination.

DOSAGE / PREPARATION / ADMINISTRATION

The source text states to cook the ingredients, except *Xi Jiao* (Cornu Rhinoceri), in 8 cups of water and reduce it down to 3 cups. Take 1 cup of the decoction three times daily with powdered *Xi Jiao* (Cornu Rhinoceri). Today, 2g of *Xi Jiao* (Cornu Rhinoceri) is generally replaced with 30g of *Shui Niu Jiao* (Cornu Bubali).

CHINESE THERAPEUTIC ACTIONS

1. Clears heat from the *ying* (nutritive) level
2. Nourishes yin and invigorates blood circulation

CLINICAL MANIFESTATIONS

Heat in the *ying* (nutritive) level: fever that worsens at night with or without thirst, irritability, occasional dementia, hyperactivity, insomnia, red skin rash, a dark red tongue, and a rapid, thin pulse.

VETERINARY CLINICAL APPLICATIONS

Septicemia, encephalitis, meningitis, uveitis, optic neuritis, dermatitis, infectious diseases with appropriate clinical signs.

Qīng Yíng Tāng (Clear the Nutritive Level Decoction)

EXPLANATION

Qing Ying Tang (Clear the Nutritive Level Decoction) is the representative formula for treating heat in the *ying* (nutritive) level, the third stage of the *Wei Qi Ying Xue Bian Zheng* (Defensive, Qi, Nutritive, Blood Differentiation). In the *ying* level, heat damages yin and causes *shen* (spirit) disturbance. Hence, *shen* disturbance is the key clinical manifestation of this syndrome. When yin is damaged, it gives rise to fever that worsens at night because yin cannot contain yang. Patients may have thirst or no thirst, depending on whether the heat has consumed body fluids or not. Signs of emerging red skin rash suggest that the heat is in the *ying* level but has not yet progressed to the *xue* (blood) level. If the heat were to progress to the *xue* level, it will congeal the blood and create blood stagnation, giving rise to large patches of petechiae and ecchymosis. A dark red and dry tongue and a rapid pulse suggest heat in the *ying* level damaging yin. To treat this syndrome, first clear heat from the *ying* level. Second, nourish the damaged yin. Finally, activate blood circulation to dispel heat stagnation and prevent the heat from progressing further into the *xue* level.

Xi Jiao (Cornu Rhinoceri), the chief herb, clears heat in the *ying* (nutritive) level and cools the blood in the *xue* (blood) level. *Di Huang* (Radix Rehmanniae), *Mai Dong* (Radix Ophiopogonis) and *Xuan Shen* (Radix Scrophulariae) clear deficiency heat and nourish yin and body fluids. *Jin Yin Hua* (Flos Lonicerae Japonicae), *Lian Qiao* (Fructus Forsythiae), and *Huang Lian* (Rhizoma Coptidis) clear heat and eliminate toxins. They assist the formula to bring heat and toxins from deeper aspects of the body (*ying* and *xue* levels) to the more superficial aspects (*qi* [energy] level) so that these toxins may be effectively cleared and eliminated. *Zhu Ye* (Herba Phyllostachys) clears the Heart and calms the *shen* (spirit) to relieve irritability. *Dan Shen* (Radix et Rhizoma Salviae Miltiorrhizae) invigorates blood circulation to remove blood stasis, and also assists the rest of the herbs in clearing heat.

VETERINARY MODIFICATIONS

With heat in both the *qi* (energy) and *ying* (nutritive) levels, add *Shi Gao* (Gypsum Fibrosum) and *Zhi Mu* (Rhizoma Anemarrhenae).

CAUTIONS / CONTRAINDICATIONS

Qing Ying Tang is contraindicated in cases of damp accumulation marked by a white, greasy tongue coating. Damp conditions cannot be treated with moistening and nourishing herbs.

PHARMACOLOGICAL EFFECTS

1. **Antipyretic**: In rabbits with artificially-induced fever, intraperitoneal injection of *Qing Ying Tang* at 5 mL/kg was associated with marked reduction of body temperature.[1]
2. **Antibiotic**: This formula exhibited an *in vitro* inhibitory effect against *Staphylococcus aureus, Staphylococcus albus, alpha-hemolytic streptococcus, beta-hemolytic streptococcus, Salmonella typhi, Bacillus paratyphosus,* and *Bacillus proteus.*[2]

HUMAN CLINICAL STUDIES AND RESEARCH

1. **Septicemia**: Ten patients with septicemia were treated with modified *Qing Ying Tang* with good results. The study reported complete reduction of temperature in all cases after an average of 12.6 days. All patients were followed

***Qing Ying Tang* (Clear the Nutritive Level Decoction)**

Diagnosis	Clinical Signs	Treatment	Herbs
Heat in the *ying* (nutritive) level	• Fever that worsens at night: interior heat damaging yin and *ying* (nutrition) • Irritability, dementia, insomnia and hyperactivity: heat attacking the *ying* level and disturbing *shen* (spirit) • Thirst: heat consuming body fluids • Red skin rash: heat in the *ying* level • A deep red and dry tongue: interior heat damaging yin • Rapid, thin pulse: heat condition	• Clears heat from the *ying* (nutrition) level • Nourishes yin	• *Xi Jiao* (Cornu Rhinoceri) clears heat in the *ying* (nutrition) level. • *Di Huang* (Radix Rehmanniae), *Mai Dong* (Radix Ophiopogonis) and *Xuan Shen* (Radix Scrophulariae) clear deficiency heat and nourish yin. • *Jin Yin Hua* (Flos Lonicerae Japonicae), *Lian Qiao* (Fructus Forsythiae), and *Huang Lian* (Rhizoma Coptidis) clear heat and eliminate toxins. • *Zhu Ye* (Herba Phyllostachys) clears the Heart and calms the *shen* (spirit) to relieve irritability. • *Dan Shen* (Radix et Rhizoma Salviae Miltiorrhizae) invigorates blood circulation.

Qīng Yíng Tāng (Clear the Nutritive Level Decoction)

up one year after the completion of the treatment with no recurrence.[3]

2. **Harada's syndrome**: Seven patients with Harada's syndrome of uveitis were treated with concurrent Western and herbal treatment. Herbal treatment included modification of *Qing Ying Tang*. Following 3 months of treatment, the study reported improvement in 6 out of 7 patients.[4]
3. **Psoriasis**: Eighty-seven patients with psoriasis were treated with both oral and topical application of herbs with marked improvement reported in 90.8% of the patients. The herbal formula used orally was modified *Qing Ying Tang*, and the topical herbal preparation contained *Bi Ma Zi* (Semen Ricini) 50g, *Ku Xing Ren* (Semen Armeniacae Amarum) 50g, *Qing Fen* (Calomelas) 50g, *Duan Shi Gao* (Gypsum Fibrosum Praeparatum) 50g, *Bai Fan* (Alumen) 50g, and *Bing Pian* (Borneolum Syntheticum) 20g. The herbs were ground into a fine powder and mixed with petroleum jelly to make a paste. Clinical improvements after oral and topical treatments included relief of itching, flaking, and restoration of normal skin color.[5] Another study of 5 psoriasis patients reported good results using the following formula in decoction form and administered daily: *Di Huang* (Radix Rehmanniae) 30g, *Huang Lian* (Rhizoma Coptidis) 20g, *Jin Yin Hua* (Flos Lonicerae Japonicae) 20g, *Lian Qiao* (Fructus Forsythiae) 20g, *Da Huang* (Radix et Rhizoma Rhei) 5g, *Zhu Ye* (Herba Phyllostachys) 15g, *Dan Shen* (Radix et Rhizoma Salviae Miltiorrhizae) 15g, *Xuan Shen* (Radix Scrophulariae) 15g, *Mu Tong* (Caulis Akebiae) 15g, *Shui Niu Jiao* (Cornu Bubali) 15g, and *Gan Cao* (Radix et Rhizoma Glycyrrhizae) 15g.[6]
4. **Optic neuritis**: One study reported good results using integrated treatments for 5 patients with acute optic neuritis. The herbal formula contained *Shui Niu Jiao* (Cornu Bubali), *Mu Dan Pi* (Cortex Moutan), *Dan Shen* (Radix et Rhizoma Salviae Miltiorrhizae), *Xuan Shen* (Radix Scrophulariae), *Huang Lian* (Rhizoma Coptidis), *Jin Yin Hua* (Flos Lonicerae Japonicae), *Lian Qiao* (Fructus Forsythiae), *Zhi Mu* (Rhizoma Anemarrhenae), *Bai Shao* (Radix Paeoniae Alba), *Jue Ming Zi* (Semen Cassiae), *Mai Dong* (Radix Ophiopogonis), *Dan Zhu Ye* (Herba Lophatheri), and others as needed. Dexamethasone 5mg was also given.[7]

SUGGESTED ACUPUNCTURE TREATMENT

1. Points: *Dazhui* (GV 14), *Taodao* (GV 13), *Quchi* (LI 11), *Hegu* (LI 4), *Shaoshang* (LU 11), *Rangu* (KI 2), *Yingu* (KI 10), *Xuehai* (SP 10), *Taiyang*, *Weijian*, and *Erjian*.
2. Technique: sedation.

Dazhui (GV 14) and *Taodao* (GV 13) clear heat from the *ying* (nutritive) level. *Quchi* (LI 11), *Hegu* (LI 4), and *Shaoshang* (LU 11) clear heat, eliminate heat toxins, and lead heat out of the body through the *qi* (energy) level. *Rangu* (KI 2) and *Yingu* (KI 10) nourish yin to help clear heat. *Xuehai* (SP 10) activates blood to help remove stagnant heat. *Taiyang*, *Weijian*, and *Erjian* are classical points used to clear heat. In more severe cases, it is often useful to bleed the points for greater effect.

AUTHORS' COMMENTS

From a clinical standpoint, disorders affecting the *qi* (energy) and *ying* (nutritive) levels have often already progressed to involve the *xue* (blood) level by the time of diagnosis. Many of these disorders are characterized by a high mortality despite conventional medical therapy and will result in the death of the animal without other effective treatment options. With this in mind, the following recommendations are made in an effort to provide practitioners, especially those in emergency medicine and critical care, with additional therapeutic options for patient care. Most animals in serious condition may be unable to take oral medications. In this situation, it is recommended to place an esophagostomy tube or pass a stomach tube to administer the herbal formula initially. These formulas are not readily available, but can be formulated in house or by any reputable Chinese herb company by request.

Qing Ying Tang, *Xi Jiao Di Huang Tang* (Rhinoceros Horn and Rehmannia Decoction), and *Qing Wen Bai Du Yin* (Clear Epidemics and Overcome Pathogenic Influences Decoction) are three herbal formulas which all contain *Di Huang* (Radix Rehmanniae) and *Xi Jiao* (Cornu Rhinoceri). All three clear heat (fever, infection and inflammation) and eliminate toxins.

- *Qing Ying Tang* clears heat and toxins from the *ying* (nutritive) level, and has the greatest ability to nourish yin, and has mild ability to invigorate the blood; it is classically used during the initial stages of heat attacking the *ying* level.
- *Xi Jiao Di Huang Tang* clears heat and toxins from the *xue* (blood) level, cools the blood, and disperses blood stagnation. It is used to treat more severe conditions with heat causing damage to the blood vessels and forcing blood out of the vessels, resulting in bleeding and coagulation disorders.
- *Qing Wen Bai Du Yin* clears heat and toxins in the *qi* (energy) and *xue* (blood) levels and purges fire. This formula has the greatest ability to clear heat and toxins, as it contains *Shi Gao* (Gypsum Fibrosum) and *Zhi Mu* (Rhizoma Anemarrhenae) in addition to other heat-clearing herbs, such as *Xuan Shen* (Radix Scrophulariae), *Jin Yin Hua* (Flos Lonicerae Japonicae), *Lian Qiao* (Fructus Forsythiae), *Huang Lian* (Rhizoma Coptidis) and *Zhu Ye* (Herba Phyllostachys).

Qīng Yíng Tāng (Clear the Nutritive Level Decoction)

These formulas contain many cold and bitter herbs and lack herbs to protect the middle *jiao*. It is recommended that single herbs or another formula be used concurrently to harmonize the middle *jiao* when using heat-clearing formulas. This recommendation is made primarily due to the nature of heat-clearing formulas, widespread Spleen-Stomach deficiencies in the small animal population from inappropriate diets and feeding practices, the sensitivity of the equine gastrointestinal tract, and the fact that most animals requiring these formulas are anorexic, weak and qi deficient. Formulas such as *Liu Jun Zi Tang* (Six-Gentlemen Decoction), *Xiang Sha Liu Jun Zi Tang* (Six-Gentlemen Decoction with Aucklandia and Amomum), *Bu Zhong Yi Qi Tang* (Tonify the Middle and Augment the Qi Decoction) and *Gui Pi Tang* (Restore the Spleen Decoction) may all be used, depending on the individual case.

- For a greasy tongue coating and a slippery pulse with signs of dampness, add *Ban Xia* (Rhizoma Pinelliae) and *Huo Xiang* (Herba Agastaches).
- To further increase the antimicrobial actions of these formula and promote cellular immunity, the following herbs may be added: *Ban Lan Gen* (Radix Isatidis) and/or *Da Qing Ye* (Folium Isatidis), *Pu Gong Ying* (Herba Taraxaci), *Bai Jiang Cao* (Herba cum Radice Patriniae), *Zi Hua Di Ding* (Herba Violae), *Bai Hua She She Cao* (Herba Hedyotis), *Yu Xing Cao* (Herba Houttuyniae) and *Chuan Xin Lian* (Herba Andrographis). Note: *Pu Gong Ying* (Herba Taraxaci) can interfere with the absorption of ciprofloxacin; thus the two should not be used concurrently.
- For heat and toxins in the skin from toxic heat and/or secondary to insect or snake bite, combine *Ban Bian Lian* (Herba Lobeliae Chinensis), *Bai Hua She She Cao* (Herba Hedyotis) and *Zi Hua Di Ding* (Herba Violae) and apply topically; all of these herbs may be administered orally.
- For bleeding disorders, add *Qing Dai* (Indigo Naturalis), *Bai Mao Gen* (Rhizoma Imperatae) and *San Qi* (Radix et Rhizoma Notoginseng).
- For qi deficiency with inability to control the blood in addition to reckless movement of hot blood, add *Ren Shen* (Radix et Rhizoma Ginseng) and *Huang Qi* (Radix Astragali).
- With severe yin deficiency and fluid depletion, add *Gou Qi Zi* (Fructus Lycii) and *Sha Shen* (Radix Glehniae seu Adenophorae).

References

1. *Cheng Du Zhong Yi Xue Yuan Xue Bao* (Journal of Chengdu University of Traditional Chinese Medicine), 1995; 4:38.
2. *Zhong Yi Za Zhi* (Journal of Chinese Medicine), 1981; 5:349.
3. *Zhong Yi Za Zhi* (Journal of Chinese Medicine), 1984; 2:42.
4. *Tian Jin Zhong Yi* (Tianjin Chinese Medicine), 1993; 3:38.
5. *Si Chuan Zhong Yi* (Sichuan Chinese Medicine), 1992; 3:36.
6. *Zhong Yi Yao Xue Bao* (Report of Chinese Medicine and Herbology), 1996; 6:42.
7. *Zhong Yi Ming Fang Lin Chuang Xin Yong* (Contemporary Clinical Applications of Classic Chinese Formulas), 2001; 661.

Xī Jiǎo Dì Huáng Tāng (Rhinoceros Horn and Rehmannia Decoction)

犀角地黃湯
犀角地黄汤

Pinyin Name: *Xi Jiao Di Huang Tang*
Literal Name: Rhinoceros Horn and Rehmannia Decoction
Original Source: *Bei Ji Qian Jin Yao Fang* (Thousands of Golden Prescriptions for Emergencies)

COMPOSITION

Xi Jiao (Cornu Rhinoceri)	3g [1.5-3g]
Di Huang (Radix Rehmanniae)	24g [30g]
Chi Shao (Radix Paeoniae Rubra)	9g [12g]
Mu Dan Pi (Cortex Moutan)	6g [9g]

Note: *Xi Jiao* (Cornu Rhinoceri) is derived from an endangered animal, and is rarely used as a medicinal substance today. Its discussion here is included primarily for academic purposes, to reflect the historical use of this substance in its original formulation. Most herbal products today have removed it completely, or replaced it with substitutes with similar functions.

The source text lists *Shao Yao* (Radix Paeoniae) as one of the ingredients, without specifying whether it is *Bai Shao* (Radix Paeoniae Alba) or *Chi Shao* (Radix Paeoniae Rubra). Today, most practitioners prefer to use *Chi Shao* (Radix Paeoniae Rubra) for its functions to clear heat and cool the blood.

DOSAGE / PREPARATION / ADMINISTRATION

The source text instructs to grind the ingredients coarsely. Cook the powdered herbs with 9 cups [1,800 mL] of water and reduce it to 3 cups [600 mL]. Take 1 cup [200 mL] of the decoction three times daily. Today, it is normally prepared as a decoction with the doses suggested in brackets. Moreover, the 1.5-3g of *Xi Jiao* (Cornu Rhinoceri) is generally replaced by 30g of *Shui Niu Jiao* (Cornu Bubali).

CHINESE THERAPEUTIC ACTIONS

1. Clears heat and eliminates toxins
2. Cools the blood and disperses blood stasis

CLINICAL MANIFESTATIONS

1. Heat in the *xue* (blood) level forcing blood out of the vessels: various types of bleeding disorders, red skin rash, petechiae, ecchymosis, hematuria, hematochezia, hematemesis, epistaxis and hemoptysis.
2. Blood stasis: a deep red to purple tongue and a rapid pulse which can be wiry.
3. Heat disturbing the Heart and *ying* (nutritive) level: coma, insomnia, dementia, and hyperactivity.

VETERINARY CLINICAL APPLICATIONS

Encephalitis, meningitis, disseminated intravascular coagulation (DIC), purpura hemorrhagica, septicemia, thrombocytopenia secondary to infectious disease, bacterial or viral infection causing heat and blood stasis in the *xue* (blood) level.

EXPLANATION

Xi Jiao Di Huang Tang (Rhinoceros Horn and Rehmannia Decoction) clears interior heat, cools the blood, and disperses blood stasis to treat heat in the *xue* (blood) level. Heat in the blood may force the blood to move recklessly, often out of the vessels. When the yang channels are injured, bleeding occurs outside of the vessels and manifests upward and outward as hematemesis, hemoptysis or epistaxis. When the yin channels are injured, blood moves downward, manifesting as hematuria and hematochezia. When the superficial channels are injured, there will be petechiae and ecchymosis present.

If blood stasis invades the Heart, then irritability and abnormal behavior may result. In addition, abdominal fullness and excretion of black, tarry stools may occur if blood stasis accumulates in the abdomen or the Intestines. If the tissues are severely attacked by heat, dark purplish petechiae and ecchymosis may appear on the skin.

Xi Jiao (Cornu Rhinoceri) enters directly into the *xue* (blood) level and clears heat in the Heart, cools the blood, and eliminates toxins. Combined, *Xi Jiao* (Cornu Rhinoceri) and *Di Huang* (Radix Rehmanniae) cool the blood and stop bleeding, as well as nourish yin and clear heat. *Chi Shao* (Radix Paeoniae Rubra) and *Mu Dan Pi* (Cortex Moutan) clear heat, cool the blood, and disperse blood stasis. This formula, therefore, cools the blood without causing blood stagnation.

Xī Jiǎo Dì Huáng Tāng (Rhinoceros Horn and Rehmannia Decoction)

Xi Jiao Di Huang Tang **(Rhinoceros Horn and Rehmannia Decoction)**

Diagnosis	Clinical Signs	Treatment	Herbs
Heat in the *xue* (blood) level	• Bleeding disorders: heat in the *xue* (blood) level forcing blood outward • Manic behavior and irritability: heat disturbing the Heart and *shen* (spirit) • Deep red to purple tongue and a rapid pulse which can be wiry: heat damaging yin and blood	• Clears heat and eliminates toxins • Cools the blood and disperses blood stasis	• *Xi Jiao* (Cornu Rhinoceri) clears heat, cools the blood, and eliminates toxins from the *ying* (nutritive) and *xue* (blood) levels. • *Di Huang* (Radix Rehmanniae) cools the blood, stops bleeding, nourishes yin, and clears heat. • *Chi Shao* (Radix Paeoniae Rubra) and *Mu Dan Pi* (Cortex Moutan) cool the blood and disperse blood stasis.

VETERINARY MODIFICATIONS

- With more epistaxis or vomiting of blood, add *Bai Mao Gen* (Rhizoma Imperatae) and *Ce Bai Ye* (Cacumen Platycladi).
- With more hematochezia, add *Huai Hua* (Flos Sophorae) and *Di Yu* (Radix Sanguisorbae).
- With more hematuria, add *Bai Mao Gen* (Rhizoma Imperatae) and *Xiao Ji* (Herba Cirsii).
- When there is aggressive behavior, add *Chai Hu* (Radix Bupleuri), *Huang Qin* (Radix Scutellariae), and *Zhi Zi* (Fructus Gardeniae).

CAUTIONS / CONTRAINDICATIONS

Xi Jiao Di Huang Tang should be used to treat only bleeding caused by heat in the *xue* (blood) level, leading to reckless movement of blood and bleeding from various parts of the body. It should not be used to treat bleeding caused by other reasons, such as constitutional deficiencies or external injuries.

PHARMACOLOGICAL EFFECTS

Antipyretic: In rabbits with artificially-induced fever, oral ingestion of *Xi Jiao Di Huang Tang* was effective in reducing the body temperature. The antipyretic effect has a slow onset of action (after 4 hours) but prolonged duration (up to 6 hours). The researchers characterized the antipyretic effect of *Xi Jiao Di Huang Tang* to be comparable to 0.2 mg/kg of aspirin.[1]

HUMAN CLINICAL STUDIES AND RESEARCH

1. **Upper gastrointestinal bleeding**: In one report, 39 patients with upper gastrointestinal bleeding diagnosed with Stomach heat were treated with either *Xie Xin Tang* (Drain the Epigastrium Decoction) or modified *Xi Jiao Di Huang Tang* with 100% effectiveness. The report stated that most patients stopped bleeding within 24 hours after taking the herbs.[2]
2. **Epistaxis**: Sixty-one patients with chronic epistaxis were treated with *Xi Jiao Di Huang Tang* with good results. The bleeding stopped in 28 patients after treatment, with no recurrence within 6 months of follow-up. The bleeding was reduced significantly in 25 patients, with much less recurrence and severity. Slight improvement was reported in 7 other cases, and no benefit in 1 case. The overall rate of effectiveness was 98.49%.[3]
3. **Thrombocytopenic purpura**: In one clinical study, 11 patients with primary thrombocytopenic purpura were treated with *Xi Jiao Di Huang Tang* with complete recovery in 6 patients, marked effect in 4 patients, and no effect (and eventual fatality) in 1 patient. The study reported that after administration of the herbal treatment, there was a significant reduction of bleeding time and gradual increase in platelets. The effect of the herbal formula was attributed to an initial change in permeability of the blood vessels, followed by stimulation and increased production of platelets.[4] Other studies also confirmed that *Xi Jiao Di Huang Tang* in the original or slightly modified form had marked effect for treatment of thrombocytopenic purpura.[5,6]
4. **Hepatitis**: In one report, 13 patients with hepatitis (characterized by Gallbladder stagnation) were treated with modified *Xi Jiao Di Huang Tang* for one month with improvement reported in 12 patients. Most patients showed a decrease in skin itching and reduction of jaundice.[7]

HERB-DRUG INTERACTION

Drug-induced allergic dermatitis: Administration of modified *Xi Jiao Di Huang Tang* was associated with good results in treating 38 patients with drug-induced allergic dermatitis. The treatment protocol was to administer the herbs in decoction form in two equally-divided doses daily in the morning and at night. The herbal formula used *Shui Niu Jiao* (Cornu Bubali) in place of *Xi Jiao* (Cornu Rhinoceri). Modifications were made by adding *Da Huang* (Radix et Rhizoma Rhei) for excess heat in the interior; and *Pu Gong Ying* (Herba Taraxaci), *Jin Yin Hua* (Flos Lonicerae Japonicae) and a larger dose of *Shui Niu Jiao* (Cornu Bubali) for toxins affecting the *ying* (nutritive) and *xue* (blood) levels. Of 38 cases, the study reported complete recovery in 33 cases and improvement in 5 cases.[8]

SUGGESTED ACUPUNCTURE TREATMENT

1. Points: *Dazhui* (GV 14), *Taodao* (GV 13), *Quchi* (LI 11), *Neiting* (ST 44), *Xuehai* (SP 10), *Geshu* (BL 17), *Rangu* (KI 2), *Yingu* (KI 10), *Duanxue* and *Tianping.*
2. Technique: sedation.

Dazhui (GV 14) and *Taodao* (GV 13) clear heat from the *ying* (nutritive) level. *Quchi* (LI 11) and *Neiting* (ST 44) sedate excess *yangming* heat. *Geshu* (BL 17) clears heat, cools the blood, and harmonizes the blood. *Xuehai* (SP 10) activates blood circulation and removes blood stasis. *Rangu* (KI 2) and *Yingu* (KI 10) nourish yin to help clear heat. *Duanxue* and *Tianping* are classical points for stopping hemorrhage.

AUTHORS' COMMENTS

Qing Ying Tang (Clear the Nutritive Level Decoction) and *Xi Jiao Di Huang Tang* both clear heat in the *ying* (nutritive) and *xue* (blood) levels and stop bleeding characterized by reckless movement of blood. Both formulas stop bleeding and contain blood-moving herbs to prevent the cold herbs from congealing the blood and creating further stagnation while clearing heat.

- *Qing Ying Tang* clears heat in the *ying* (nutritive) level and includes *Dan Shen* (Radix et Rhizoma Salviae Miltiorrhizae) to move blood and prevent the cold herbs from creating stagnation. It also helps to reduce petechiae and ecchymosis that may be present on the skin, marked by bleeding that is just beginning. The condition in this case is not as severe as that seen in *Xi Jiao Di Huang Tang.*
- *Xi Jiao Di Huang Tang* clears heat in the *xue* (blood) level. It contains *Chi Shao* (Radix Paeoniae Rubra) and *Mu Dan Pi* (Cortex Moutan) to move blood and to prevent the cold herbs from creating stagnation. They also assist the other heat-clearing herbs to cool the blood. Bleeding is more prominent and severe in this condition.

Qing Ying Tang (Clear the Nutritive Level Decoction) and *Xi Jiao Di Huang Tang* both contain *Xi Jiao* (Cornu Rhinoceri) and *Di Huang* (Radix Rehmanniae) as chief herbs. The differences between these two formulas are as follows:

- *Qing Ying Tang* focuses on bringing the heat out from the *ying* (nutritive) level and clearing it through the *qi* (energy) level. It is suitable for initial stages of heat attacking the *ying* level, and has herbs which tonify yin.
- *Xi Jiao Di Huang Tang* treats more severe conditions of heat attacking the *ying* and *xue* levels and forcing blood out of the vessels, manifesting in various types of bleeding and coagulation disorders.

Xi Jiao Di Huang Tang can be used alone but is more often modified and/or combined with other herbs or formula(s) that further treat heat and toxins, invigorate the blood, and tonify the middle *jiao*. For more information, see *Qing Ying Tang* (Clear the Nutritive Level Decoction).

References

1. *Zhong Yao Tong Bao* (Journal of Chinese Herbology), 1986; 11(1):51.
2. *Zhong Yi Za Zhi* (Journal of Chinese Medicine), 1980; 21(7):36.
3. *Shan Xi Zhong Yi* (Shanxi Chinese Medicine), 1989; 10(4):163.
4. *Zhong Yi Za Zhi* (Journal of Chinese Medicine), 1963; 11:12.
5. *Zhong Yi Za Zhi* (Journal of Chinese Medicine), 1958; 7:465.
6. *Zhong Yi Za Zhi* (Journal of Chinese Medicine), 1960; 7:22.
7. *Zhong Yi Za Zhi* (Journal of Chinese Medicine), 1983; 24(6):30.
8. *Hu Nan Zhong Yi Za Zhi* (Hunan Journal of Chinese Medicine), 1998; 1:39.

Section 3

气血两清剂

— Qi (Energy) and Xue (Blood) Levels-Clearing Formulas

Qīng Wēn Bài Dú Yǐn

(Clear Epidemics and Overcome Pathogenic Influences Decoction)

清瘟敗毒飲

清瘟败毒饮

Pinyin Name: *Qing Wen Bai Du Yin*

Literal Name: Clear Epidemics and Overcome Pathogenic Influences Decoction

Original Source: *Yi Zhen Yi De* (Achievements Regarding Epidemic Rashes) by Yu Shi-Yu in 1794

COMPOSITION

Shi Gao (Gypsum Fibrosum)	24-36g; 60-120g; 180-240g
Zhi Mu (Rhizoma Anemarrhenae)	
Huang Lian (Rhizoma Coptidis)	3-4.5g; 6-12g;12-18g
Huang Qin (Radix Scutellariae)	
Zhi Zi (Fructus Gardeniae)	
Xi Jiao (Cornu Rhinoceri)	6-12g; 9-15g; 18-24g
Di Huang (Radix Rehmanniae)	6-12g; 9-15g; 18-30g
Chi Shao (Radix Paeoniae Rubra)	
Mu Dan Pi (Cortex Moutan)	
Lian Qiao (Fructus Forsythiae)	
Xuan Shen (Radix Scrophulariae)	
Zhu Ye (Herba Phyllostachys), fresh	
Jie Geng (Radix Platycodonis)	
Gan Cao (Radix et Rhizoma Glycyrrhizae)	

Note: *Xi Jiao* (Cornu Rhinoceri) is derived from an endangered animal, and is rarely used as a medicinal substance today. Its discussion here is included primarily for academic purposes, to reflect the historical use of this substance in its original formulation. Most herbal products today have removed it completely, or replaced it with substitutes with similar functions.

DOSAGE / PREPARATION / ADMINISTRATION

The source text states to first cook *Shi Gao* (Gypsum Fibrosum), bring it to a boil multiple times (more than ten), and then add the remaining ingredients. Note: The three sets of doses correspond to small, medium and large doses for the four herbs listed. Doses for the other ten herbs are not available in the original source. Today, *Xi Jiao* (Cornu Rhinoceri) is generally replaced with *Shui Niu Jiao* (Cornu Bubali) with the following doses: 60-120g; 90-150g; and 180-240g.

CHINESE THERAPEUTIC ACTIONS

1. Clears heat and eliminates toxins
2. Purges fire and cools the blood

CLINICAL MANIFESTATIONS

Wen yi (warm epidemics) are characterized by excess heat and toxins in the *qi* (energy) and *xue* (blood) levels: high fever, irritability, strong thirst, various types of bleeding, red skin rash, petechiae, ecchymosis, hematuria, hematochezia, hematemesis, epistaxis, hemoptysis, coma, restlessness at night, dementia, hyperactivity, a dark red

Qīng Wēn Bài Dú Yǐn
(Clear Epidemics and Overcome Pathogenic Influences Decoction)

to purple tongue body with dry coating. The pulse may be any of the following: deep and rapid; deep, fine and rapid; or superficial, big and rapid.

VETERINARY CLINICAL APPLICATIONS

Epidemic pathogens, septicemia, encephalitis, meningitis, disseminated intravascular coagulation (DIC), thrombocytopenia, leptospirosis, septic arthritis, pneumonia, internal abscess, acute icteric jaundice, pyelonephritis, pyoderma, immune mediated skin disease, tick borne diseases (neorickettsia, babesia), toxoplasmosis, and insect or snake bite.

EXPLANATION

Wen yi (warm epidemics) are infectious or contagious diseases characterized by heat. In this case, excess heat and toxins affect the *qi* (energy) level and consume body fluids to cause high fever and extreme thirst. The heat and toxins may travel to the head and cause head pressing. If they travel to the Heart, abnormal behavior and dementia can occur. Eruptions of the skin, petechiae and ecchymosis, hematemesis, hematochezia, and epistaxis are all signs of heat in the *xue* (blood) level forcing the blood out of the vessels. In extreme cases, when too much blood is lost, extreme coldness or seizures may occur. A dark red to purple tongue body with dry coating is caused by the presence of excess heat and toxins inside the body damaging body fluids and blood stasis. The pulse may be superficial, big and rapid, or deep and rapid, depending on whether the *qi* or *xue* level is more adversely affected.

Qing Wen Bai Du Yin (Clear Epidemics and Overcome Pathogenic Influences Decoction) contains *Shi Gao* (Gypsum Fibrosum) and *Zhi Mu* (Rhizoma Anemarrhenae) to clear excess heat in the *qi* (energy) level and protect against further loss of body fluids. *Huang Lian* (Rhizoma Coptidis), *Huang Qin* (Radix Scutellariae), and *Zhi Zi* (Fructus Gardeniae) clear heat and eliminate toxins in all three *jiaos*. *Xi Jiao* (Cornu Rhinoceri), *Di Huang* (Radix Rehmanniae), *Chi Shao* (Radix Paeoniae Rubra), and *Mu Dan Pi* (Cortex Moutan) clear heat from the *xue* (blood) level and disperse blood stagnation, which may form after the blood is forced out of the vessels. *Lian Qiao* (Fructus Forsythiae) and *Xuan Shen* (Radix Scrophulariae) clear heat and eliminate toxins. *Zhu Ye* (Herba Phyllostachys) clears the Heart and calms the *shen* (spirit). *Jie Geng* (Radix Platycodonis) directs the formula to the upper *jiao* and disperses heat from the body. Finally, *Gan Cao* (Radix et Rhizoma Glycyrrhizae) clears heat and harmonizes the formula.

***Qing Wen Bai Du Yin* (Clear Epidemics and Overcome Pathogenic Influences Decoction)**

Diagnosis	Clinical Signs	Treatment	Herbs
Wen yi (warm epidemics) characterized by excess heat and toxins in the *qi* (energy) and *xue* (blood) levels	• High fever and extreme thirst: heat and toxins in the *qi* (energy) level consuming body fluids • Head pressing: heat and toxins traveling to the head • Abnormal behavior and dementia: heat and toxins traveling to the Heart • Bleeding disorders and eruptions of the skin: heat forcing the blood out of the vessels • A dark red to purple tongue body with dry coating: excess heat and toxins in the interior and blood stasis	• Clears heat and eliminates toxins • Purges fire and cools the blood	• *Shi Gao* (Gypsum Fibrosum) and *Zhi Mu* (Rhizoma Anemarrhenae) clear excess heat from the *qi* (energy) level. • *Huang Lian* (Rhizoma Coptidis), *Huang Qin* (Radix Scutellariae), and *Zhi Zi* (Fructus Gardeniae) clear heat and eliminate toxins in all three *jiaos*. • *Xi Jiao* (Cornu Rhinoceri), *Di Huang* (Radix Rehmanniae), *Chi Shao* (Radix Paeoniae Rubra), and *Mu Dan Pi* (Cortex Moutan) clear heat from the *xue* (blood) level and disperse blood stagnation. • *Lian Qiao* (Fructus Forsythiae) and *Xuan Shen* (Radix Scrophulariae) clear heat and eliminate toxins. • *Zhu Ye* (Herba Phyllostachys) clears the Heart and calms the *shen* (spirit). • *Jie Geng* (Radix Platycodonis) directs the formula to the upper *jiao* and disperses heat out of the body. • *Gan Cao* (Radix et Rhizoma Glycyrrhizae) clears heat and harmonizes the herbs.

Qīng Wēn Bài Dú Yǐn

(Clear Epidemics and Overcome Pathogenic Influences Decoction)

VETERINARY MODIFICATIONS

- If there is vomiting, add *Zhe Shi* (Haematitum) and *Zhu Ru* (Caulis Bambusae in Taenia).
- With constipation, add *Da Huang* (Radix et Rhizoma Rhei) and *Mang Xiao* (Natrii Sulfas).
- If accompanied by epistaxis, remove *Jie Geng* (Radix Platycodonis), and add *Bai Mao Gen* (Rhizoma Imperatae) and *Ce Bai Ye* (Cacumen Platycladi).
- When there are spasms, cramps and seizures, add *Gou Teng* (Ramulus Uncariae cum Uncis) and *Di Long* (Pheretima).

CAUTIONS / CONTRAINDICATIONS

- *Qing Wen Bai Du Yin* contains many bitter and cold herbs, and should not be used if the condition is not characterized by the presence of heat, fire and toxins.
- This formula should be used with caution in cases of yang deficiency, or in individuals with deficiency and cold of the Spleen and Stomach.

HUMAN CLINICAL STUDIES AND RESEARCH

1. **Epidemic hemorrhagic fever**: *Qing Wen Bai Du Yin* successfully treated 150 patients with epidemic hemorrhagic fever. The average time required to reduce fever to normal body temperature was 1.58 days. The mortality rate was less than 1%.[1]
2. **Pyogenic infection**: In one study, 113 patients with drug-resistent systemic pyogenic infection were treated with satisfactory results using modified *Qing Wen Bai Du Yin*. The study reported fatality in 20 of 113 patients.[2]
3. **Leptospirosis**: Use of modified *Qing Wen Bai Du Yin* was associated with 96% effectiveness in treating leptospirosis. The herbal formula contained *Shui Niu Jiao* (Cornu Bubali) 30g, *Shi Gao* (Gypsum Fibrosum) 30g, *Di Huang* (Radix Rehmanniae) 30g, *Tu Fu Ling* (Rhizoma Smilacis Glabrae) 30g, *Yi Yi Ren* (Semen Coicis) 30g, *Huang Lian* (Rhizoma Coptidis) 6g, *Zhi Mu* (Rhizoma Anemarrhenae) 10g, *Huang Qin* (Radix Scutellariae) 10g, *Zhi Zi* (Fructus Gardeniae) 10g, *Mu Dan Pi* (Cortex Moutan) 10g, and *Chi Shao* (Radix Paeoniae Rubra) 10g. One pack of herbs decocted in water was administered in two equally-divided doses. In severe cases, patients were given up to 2-3 packs of herbs per day. The study reported recovery in 65 of 68 patients using herbs, while the other three required additional drug treatment.[3]
4. **Coxarthritis**: One study reported effectiveness using modified *Qing Wen Bai Du Yin* to treat 13 patients with pyogenic coxarthritis. The patients were treated with up to 10 packs of herbs.[4]

SUGGESTED ACUPUNCTURE TREATMENT

1. Points: *Dazhui* (GV 14), *Zhiyang* (GV 9), *Quchi* (LI 11), *Housanli* (ST 36), *Neiting* (ST 44), *Quze* (PC 3), *Weizhong* (BL 40), *Taiyang, Weijian, Erjian, Xiongtang, Jingmai* and *jing* (well) points.
2. Technique: sedation. Two to three treatments per day.

Dazhui (GV 14) and *Zhiyang* (GV 9) sedate heat and control the yang of the body. *Quchi* (LI 11) and *Housanli* (ST 36) sedate excess heat. *Neiting* (ST 44) clears heat from both the organ and channel of the Stomach. *Quze* (PC 3) is the *he* (uniting) point of the Pericardium channel, and *Weizhong* (BL 40) is the *he* (uniting) point of the Urinary Bladder channel; they should be pricked to clear excess heat in the blood.

Taiyang, Weijian and *Erjian* are classical points that clear heat from the body. *Xiongtang* and *Jingmai* are classical equine points for clearing heat toxins. All of these points can be bled for greater effect. It is also common practice in horses to use hemoacupuncture at the *jing* (well) points for clearing heat.

AUTHORS' COMMENTS

Qing Wen Bai Du Yin has been used historically to treat *wen yi* (warm epidemics), conditions that correlate closely to biomedical disorders such as encephalitis, meningitis, septicemia, pyogenic infection, leptospirosis and other infectious diseases. Because these diseases vary drastically in severity, the ingredients of this formula differ in dose (up to 10 fold) dramatically. It is not readily available but can be formulated in house or by any reputable Chinese herbal company by request.

Qing Wen Bai Du Yin is a powerful antipyretic, anti-inflammatory and antimicrobial formula that follows the principles of three formulas used to clear heat and toxins, and to cool and invigorate the blood:

- *Bai Hu Tang* (White Tiger Decoction) to clear heat from the *qi* (energy) level.
- *Xi Jiao Di Huang Tang* (Rhinoceros Horn and Rehmannia Decoction) to clear heat from the *xue* (blood) level.
- *Huang Lian Jie Du Tang* (Coptis Decoction to Relieve Toxicity) to clear heat and eliminate toxins.

It should be noted that *Qing Wen Bai Du Yin* (Clear Epidemics and Overcome Pathogenic Influences Decoction) clears heat and toxins in the *qi* (energy) and *xue* (blood) levels and purges fire. It is a powerful formula to treat infectious disease and contains ***all*** of the herbs found in

Qīng Wēn Bài Dú Yǐn
(Clear Epidemics and Overcome Pathogenic Influences Decoction)

Xi Jiao Di Huang Tang (Rhinoceros Horn and Rehmannia Decoction) and can be used for cases with bleeding and coagulation disorders.

The following herbs have been shown to have inhibitory activity against leptospirosis, and can be added to this formula to improve treatment results for peracute management of the disease: *Ju Hua* (Flos Chrysanthemi), *Tu Fu Ling* (Rhizoma Smilacis Glabrae), *Chai Hu* (Radix Bupleuri), *Lian Qiao* (Fructus Forsythiae), *Ye Ju Hua* (Flos Chrysanthemi Indici), *Da Qing Ye* (Folium Isatidis), *Ban Lan Gen* (Radix Isatidis), *Yu Xing Cao* (Herba Houttuyniae), *Fu Ling* (Poria), *Hu Zhang* (Rhizoma et Radix Polygoni Cuspidati), *Huang Bo* (Cortex Phellodendri Chinensis), *Huang Qin* (Radix Scutellariae), *Huang Lian* (Rhizoma Coptidis) and *Zhi Zi* (Fructus Gardeniae). For more discussion on this formula, please refer to *Qing Ying Tang* (Clear the Nutritive Level Decoction).

References

1. *Yi Xue Yan Jiu Tong Xun* (Report of Medical Studies), 1986; (5):3.
2. *Shan Xi Yi Kan* (Shanxi Journal of Medicine), 1983; 4(4):13.
3. *Guang Xi Zhong Yi Yao* (Guangxi Chinese Medicine and Herbology), 1987; 3:6.
4. *Shan Xi Zhong Yi* (Shanxi Chinese Medicine), 1988; 4:152.

Section 4

清热解毒剂
— Heat-Clearing and Toxin-Eliminating Formulas

Huáng Lián Jiě Dú Tāng (Coptis Decoction to Relieve Toxicity)
黄連解毒湯
黄连解毒汤

Pinyin Name: *Huang Lian Jie Du Tang*
Literal Name: Coptis Decoction to Relieve Toxicity
Alternate Names: *Huang Lien Chieh Tu Tang*, Coptis and Scute Detoxifying Decoction, Coptis and Scute Combination
Original Source: *Wai Tai Mi Yao* (Arcane Essentials from the Imperial Library) by Wang Tao in 752 A.D.

COMPOSITION

Huang Qin (Radix Scutellariae)	6g
Huang Lian (Rhizoma Coptidis)	9g
Huang Bo (Cortex Phellodendri Chinensis)	6g
Zhi Zi (Fructus Gardeniae), *bo* (opened)	14 pieces [9g]

DOSAGE / PREPARATION / ADMINISTRATION

Coarsely cut the ingredients and cook the herbs in 6 cups [1,200 mL] of water until the liquid is reduced to 2 cups [400 mL]. Take the strained decoction in two equally-divided doses daily.

CHINESE THERAPEUTIC ACTIONS

Clears heat, purges fire and eliminates toxins

CLINICAL MANIFESTATIONS

Excess heat, fire and toxins in all three *jiaos*: fever, restlessness, irritability, a dry mouth and tongue, dementia, restlessness at night; febrile diseases causing bleeding with petechiae and ecchymosis, hematemesis, epistaxis, diarrhea, damp-heat jaundice; external abscesses, sores, cellulitis and boils with heat and toxins; a red tongue body with yellow tongue coating, and a rapid, forceful pulse.

VETERINARY CLINICAL APPLICATIONS

Fever, encephalitis, meningitis, hypertension, septicemia, peritonitis, pneumonia, otitis media, acute icteric jaundice, vaginitis, urinary tract infection, nephritis, acute bacterial diarrhea, post-surgical infection, bleeding disorders, anal gland abscess, acute laminitis, perianal fistula, pyoderma, bacterial and fungal rhinitis or sinusitis, systemic fungal infections, acute stomatitis or gingivitis and uveitis.

EXPLANATION

Huang Lian Jie Du Tang (Coptis Decoction to Relieve Toxicity) commonly treats excess heat, fire, and toxins in all three *jiaos*. Restlessness, irritability, and dementia are due to excess fire and toxins disturbing the *shen* (spirit). The presence of hematemesis and epistaxis are due to heat forcing the blood to travel upward and out of the body. Petechiae and ecchymosis are due to heat injuring the channels and collaterals forcing the blood to travel outwards to the skin. Jaundice results when the stagnant damp-heat inside the body vaporizes out to the skin. External abscesses, dermatitis and sores are due to the stagnant heat in the skin and muscles.

Although many clinical manifestations are indicated for this formula, the root cause for all of them is excess heat and fire in all three *jiaos*. In this formula, *Huang Qin* (Radix Scutellariae) clears Lung heat and sedates fire in the upper *jiao*, *Huang Lian* (Rhizoma Coptidis) sedates fire in the Heart and middle *jiao*, and *Huang Bo* (Cortex Phellodendri Chinensis) sedates fire in the lower *jiao*. *Zhi Zi* (Fructus Gardeniae) sedates fire in all three *jiaos* and guides the heat downward.

Huáng Lián Jiě Dú Tāng (Coptis Decoction to Relieve Toxicity)

Huang Lian Jie Du Tang (Coptis Decoction to Relieve Toxicity)

Diagnosis	Clinical Signs	Treatment	Herbs
Excess heat, fire and toxins in all three *jiaos*	• High fever: excess heat and fire • Restlessness, irritability and dementia: excess fire and toxins disturbing the *shen* (spirit) • Dry mouth and tongue: heat consuming body fluids • Hematemesis and epistaxis: heat forcing blood outward and upward • Petechiae and ecchymosis: heat injuring the channels and collaterals • Jaundice: stagnant damp-heat inside the body • External abscesses, dermatitis and sores: stagnant heat in the skin and muscles • Red tongue with a yellow tongue coating: heat and fire • Rapid, forceful pulse: excess condition of heat, fire and toxins	Clears heat, purges fire, and eliminates toxins	• *Huang Qin* (Radix Scutellariae) clears Lung heat and sedates fire in the upper *jiao*. • *Huang Lian* (Rhizoma Coptidis) sedates Heart fire and heat in the middle *jiao*. • *Huang Bo* (Cortex Phellodendri Chinensis) drains fire in the lower *jiao*. • *Zhi Zi* (Fructus Gardeniae) sedates fire in all three *jiaos* and guides heat downward.

VETERINARY MODIFICATIONS

- If there is constipation, add *Da Huang* (Radix et Rhizoma Rhei).
- With a dry mouth and throat, add *Mai Dong* (Radix Ophiopogonis) and *Wu Wei Zi* (Fructus Schisandrae Chinensis).
- With thirst and high fever, add *Shi Gao* (Gypsum Fibrosum) and *Zhi Mu* (Rhizoma Anemarrhenae).
- With jaundice and fever, add *Da Huang* (Radix et Rhizoma Rhei) and *Yin Chen* (Herba Artemisiae Scopariae).
- With tenesmus and hematochezia, add *Mu Xiang* (Radix Aucklandiae) and *Bing Lang* (Semen Arecae).
- With frequent urination or oliguria, add *Che Qian Zi* (Semen Plantaginis) and *Mu Tong* (Caulis Akebiae).
- With cough accompanied by pus and blood, add *Jie Geng* (Radix Platycodonis) or *Jie Geng Tang* (Platycodon Decoction).
- When there are abscesses and sores from accumulation of heat and toxins, add *Pu Gong Ying* (Herba Taraxaci), *Zi Hua Di Ding* (Herba Violae), or *Wu Wei Xiao Du Yin* (Five-Ingredient Decoction to Eliminate Toxins).
- With ulceration of the skin accompanied by swelling and pain, combine with *Pai Nong San* (Drain the Pus Powder).

CAUTIONS / CONTRAINDICATIONS

- *Huang Lian Jie Du Tang* is contraindicated in patients with yin deficiency manifesting in a cracked tongue or mirror tongue, and in patients in which excess fire is not present.
- Prolonged use of this formula may injure the Spleen and Stomach. It is not suitable for patients with weak constitutions. Furthermore, this formula should be stopped immediately if an animal begins to show signs of yin deficiency.

PHARMACOLOGICAL EFFECTS

1. **Antipyretic**: Administration of *Huang Lian Jie Du Tang* was associated with a reduction in body temperature in numerous *in vitro* and *in vivo* experiments. In one study in rabbits with artificially-induced fever, use of the formula was found to have a slow onset but prolonged duration of antipyretic effect. The effect started at approximately 2 hours after the administration, peaked after 4 hours, and continued for 6 hours.[1] In another report, the antipyretic effect of the formula was described as similar to aspirin, following a laboratory study that compared the antipyretic effect of the formula with aspirin and normal saline.[2]
2. **Gastrointestinal**: Administration of water extract of *Huang Lian Jie Du Tang* at room temperature was associated with a marked inhibitory effect on the peristalsis of the intestines in mice. Similarly, it was found to be effective in treating spasms and cramps of the intestines.[3] Lastly, one study reported *Huang Lian Jie Du Tang* as a beneficial therapy for inflammatory bowel disease such as colitis, as the use of this formula was associated with quicker healing of lesions, and a reduction of inflammatory cell infiltration in rats.[4]
3. **Antiulcer**: One study reported that administration of *Huang Lian Jie Du Tang* was associated with a dose-dependent effect to prevent the development of stress-induced and ethanol-induced gastric lesions.[5,6,7] The report proposed two mechanisms for this gastroprotective effect: increased

Huáng Lián Jiě Dú Tāng (Coptis Decoction to Relieve Toxicity)

ability of the gastric mucosa to synthesize prostaglandin,[8] and decreased secretion of gastric acid.[9,10]

4. **Antidiarrheal**: Administration of water extract of *Huang Lian Jie Du Tang* at room temperature was associated with marked effect in treating diarrhea in mice.[11]
5. **Hepatoprotective**: Use of *Huang Lian Jie Du Tang* was associated with a protective effect on the liver.[12] In rats intoxicated with carbon tetrachloride, administration of *Huang Lian Jie Du Tang* prevented the progression of the liver injury in a dose-dependent manner by inhibiting the serum and hepatic triglyceride accumulation, and scavenging free radicals formed in the liver.[13,14]
6. **Antioxidant**: *Huang Lian Jie Du Tang* had an antioxidant effect to protect red blood cell membranes from free radicals. This antioxidant effect was dose-dependent at concentrations of 5 to 500 mcg/mL. Clinical use of this formula (7.5 g/day via oral ingestion) was associated with a significant decrease in susceptibility of red blood cells to hemolysis in humans.[15]
7. **Analgesic and anti-inflammatory**: Administration of a water extract of *Huang Lian Jie Du Tang* reduced pain and inflammation in mice.[16] The anti-inflammatory effects were exerted mainly in the early stages of inflammation, where increased capillary permeability and migration of leucocytes occurred.[17]
8. **Antihypertensive**: Administration of *Huang Lian Jie Du Tang* was associated with effectiveness in lowering blood pressure, as documented in numerous reports.[18] Water extract of the formula administered via intravenous injection in rats was associated with reduction of blood pressure and increase of heart rate in a dose-dependant fashion.[19] In another study, *Huang Lian Jie Du Tang* ameliorated hypertension caused by sympathetic system dominance in anesthetized rats.[20]
9. **Antihyperlipidemic**: Administration of *Huang Lian Jie Du Tang* was associated with decreased serum total cholesterol and low-density lipoprotein cholesterol levels. The mechanism of this antihyperlipidemic activity was attributed to the inhibition of HMG-CoA reductase. Of all the herbs in *Huang Lian Jie Du Tang*, *Huang Lian* (Rhizoma Coptidis) was believed to be the most potent inhibitor.[21]
10. **Metabolic**: Daily administration of *Huang Lian Jie Du Tang* in mice was associated with effectiveness in reducing blood glucose and cholesterol levels.[22]
11. **Ocular**: One study reported that administration of *Xi Gan Ming Mu San* (Wash the Liver and Brighten the Eyes Powder) and *Huang Lian Jie Du Tang* was associated with significantly suppressing ($P < 0.001$) the elevation of aqueous flares induced by lipopolysaccharides in rabbits.[23]

HUMAN CLINICAL STUDIES AND RESEARCH

1. **Encephalitis B**: In one report, 56 patients with encephalitis B were treated with complete recovery in 51 patients and fatality in 4 patients. The average time for reduction of temperature was 4.9 days.[24]
2. **Cerebrospinal meningitis**: Twelve patients with infectious cerebrospinal meningitis were treated with complete recovery in 4 patients within 3 packs of herbs, in 2 patients after 4 packs, in 5 patients after 5 packs, and 1 patient after 6 packs. No long-term complications or sequelae were noted among all 12 patients.[25]
3. **Post-ischemic brain injury**: Administration of 3 herbal formulas minimized post-ischemic brain injury by inhibiting production of free radicals and lipid peroxidation. Three formulas that were found to be effective, both *in vitro* and *in vivo*, were *Huang Lian Jie Du Tang*, *Chai Hu Jia Long Gu Mu Li Tang* (Bupleurum plus Dragon Bone and Oyster Shell Decoction), and *Gui Zhi Fu Ling Wan* (Cinnamon Twig and Poria Pill).[26]
4. **Pneumonia**: In one report, 35 pediatric patients with viral pneumonia were effectively treated with modified *Huang Lian Jie Du Tang*. Most patients had significant reduction of body temperature, cough, and other symptoms within 10-18 days.[27]
5. **Otitis media**: In one clinical study, 50 patients with otitis media were treated topically with a modified *Huang Lian Jie Du Tang* preparation, 4-5 drops in the affected ear(s) three to four times daily. Out of 50 patients, the study reported complete recovery in 32 patients, improvement in 9 patients, no change in 7 patients, and discontinuation of treatment in 2 patients.[28]
6. **Vaginitis**: Topical application of a modified *Huang Lian Jie Du Tang* preparation one time daily for 5-7 days was successful in treating fungal or trichomonal vaginitis.[29]
7. **Bacterial dysentery**: In one report, 152 patients with bacterial dysentery characterized by the presence of mucus and blood in the stool were treated with rectal enema of a modified *Huang Lian Jie Du Tang* preparation which did not contain *Zhi Zi* (Fructus Gardeniae). Most patients exhibited marked reduction of temperature and other symptoms after just two procedures.[30]
8. **Prophylactic treatment against post-surgical infection**: *Huang Lian Jie Du Tang* has been used both before and after surgery with good success to prevent infection. Rectal instillation of the herbal solution prior to surgery on the colon effectively prevented infection and facilitated post-surgical recovery. The herbal formula contained *Huang Lian* (Rhizoma Coptidis) 30g, *Huang Qin* (Radix Scutellariae) 20g, *Huang Bo* (Cortex Phellodendri Chinensis) 20g, and *Zhi Zi* (Fructus Gardeniae) 30g. The treatment protocol was to cook the herbs in water twice, and the 2 resultant solutions mixed together (approximately 1,000 mL

Huáng Lián Jiě Dú Tāng (Coptis Decoction to Relieve Toxicity)

total), and instilled rectally while warm (35-40°C / 95-104°F).[31] In another study, administration of *Huang Lian Jie Du Tang* was associated with effectiveness in preventing infection in post-surgical patients. Of 50 patients who had various types of surgeries (primarily upper and lower extremities), use of herbs was successful in preventing infection in 48 patients, with use of antibiotic drugs needed in 2 patients.[32]

9. **Abscesses and sores**: One study reported good results using herbs topically to treat abscesses and sores in the lower extremities. The herbal treatment contained *Huang Lian* (Rhizoma Coptidis) 10g, *Huang Bo* (Cortex Phellodendri Chinensis) 10g, *Huang Qin* (Radix Scutellariae) 10g, *Bai Zhi* (Radix Angelicae Dahuricae) 15g, and *Tu Fu Ling* (Rhizoma Smilacis Glabrae) 20g. The herbs were cooked in water, and the solution was used as an herbal wash topically on the affected area for 20 minutes, three times daily.[33]
10. ***Lin zheng* (dysuria syndrome)**: One study reported 96.9% effectiveness using modified *Huang Lian Jie Du Tang* to treat 32 patients with various types of *lin zheng* (dysuria syndrome). The herbal treatment contained *Huang Lian* (Rhizoma Coptidis) 12g, *Huang Qin* (Radix Scutellariae) 10g, *Huang Bo* (Cortex Phellodendri Chinensis) 10g, *Che Qian Zi* (Semen Plantaginis) 10g, *Da Huang* (Radix et Rhizoma Rhei) 10g, *Zhi Zi* (Fructus Gardeniae) 9g, *Bai Jiang Cao* (Herba cum Radice Patriniae) 15g, and *Fen Bi Xie* (Rhizoma Dioscoreae Hypoglaucae) 12g. The treatment protocol was to cook the herbs in water, and administer the decoction in two equally-divided doses daily, for 7 days per course of treatment, for 1-2 courses total. During the herbal treatment, all patients were instructed to avoid foods that are pungent, hot, or sour. Of 32 patients, the study reported complete recovery in 22 patients, improvement in 9 patients, and no change in 1 patient.[34]
11. **Cataract surgery**: Use of *Huang Lian Jie Du Tang* and *Ge Gen Tang* (Kudzu Decoction) helped to reduce aqueous flare elevation after complicated cataract surgery. The treatment protocol was to administer *Huang Lian Jie Du Tang* (7.5 g/day) and *Ge Gen Tang* (Kudzu Decoction) (7.5 g/day) for 3 days before surgery, the day of surgery, and for 7 days after surgery. In comparison with the control group that did not receive herbs, oral administration of *Huang Lian Jie Du Tang* and *Ge Gen Tang* (Kudzu Decoction) decreases aqueous flare elevation after small-incision cataract surgery.[35]

HERB-DRUG INTERACTION

- **Drug-induced mucositis**: In 40 patients with acute leukemia treated with cytotoxic drugs, use of *Huang Lian Jie Du Tang* was associated with a marked effect to prevent iatrogenic mucositis, such as stomatitis and gastrointestinal mucosal injury. In the control group that did not receive herbs, the incidence was 71.6% for stomatitis, and 31.7% for diarrhea. In the herb group, the incidence was 27.9% for stomatitis, and 9.3% for diarrhea. The study concluded that *Huang Lian Jie Du Tang* had a significant preventive effect on mucositis caused by anticancer agents.[36]
- **Aspirin- and ethanol-induced gastric lesions**: Administration of *Huang Lian Jie Du Tang* was associated with success in treating aspirin- and ethanol-induced gastric hemorrhagic lesions in rats. The gastroprotective effect of *Huang Lian Jie Du Tang* was comparable to sucralfate (Carafate), cimetidine (Tagamet), and 16,16-dimethyl-prostaglandin E2 (DMPGE2).[37]

SUGGESTED ACUPUNCTURE TREATMENT

1. Points: All twelve *jing* (well) points, *Dazhui* (GV 14), *Shaochong* (HT 9), *Yuji* (LU 10), *Neiting* (ST 44), *Hegu* (LI 4), *Xingjian* (LR 2), *Yemen* (TH 2), *Geshu* (BL 17), *Weizhong* (BL 40), *Taiyang*, *Weijian* and *Erjian*.
2. Technique: sedation.

Pricking the twelve *jing* (well) points can quickly reduce excess heat; this is an especially effective method in the treatment of acute toxic laminitis. *Dazhui* (GV 14) clears heat from the entire body and is very effective for reducing fever. *Shaochong* (HT 9) sedates heat in the Heart. *Yuji* (LU 10) clears heat from the Lung. *Neiting* (ST 44) and *Hegu* (LI 4) clear heat from the *yangming* level. *Xingjian* (LR 2) sedates heat in the lower *jiao*. *Yemen* (TH 2) clears heat from three *jiaos*. *Geshu* (BL 17) and *Weizhong* (BL 40) clear heat, eliminate heat toxins, and reduce swelling and pain. The classical points *Taiyang*, *Weijian* and *Erjian* are effective at clearing heat and can be pricked to bleed in cases of extreme heat.

AUTHORS' COMMENTS

Huang Lian Jie Du Tang is one of the most commonly used formulas in veterinary medicine to treat infections due to bacteria, viruses or fungi. It can be thought of as having effects similar to a broad spectrum antibiotic from a biomedical perspective. The herbs, such as *Huang Lian* (Rhizoma Coptidis), *Huang Qin* (Radix Scutellariae) and *Huang Bo* (Cortex Phellodendri Chinensis), are the core herbs with antibiotic, anti-inflammatory, antipyretic effects in Chinese medicine as shown via modern pharmacological analysis. The translation of the word "*huang*" is yellow, and these three herbs are frequently referred to as the "yellow brothers" due to their color and because they are so often combined together to clear heat and fight infection. Clinical studies have shown synergistic antibiotic effects when these herbs are combined with the beta-lactam antibiotics, such as amoxicillin, ampicillin and cefotaxime.[38,39]

Huáng Lián Jiě Dú Tāng (Coptis Decoction to Relieve Toxicity)

According to Dr. Shen Yennan there are herbs that can be used preferentially to treat *zang fu* organs that have been damaged by fire to help improve clinical results:

- For Lung fire, use *Huang Qin* (Radix Scutellariae) and *Sang Bai Pi* (Cortex Mori).
- For Heart fire, use *Huang Lian* (Rhizoma Coptidis).
- For Stomach fire, use *Shi Gao* (Gypsum Fibrosum).
- For Liver fire, use *Zhi Zi* (Fructus Gardeniae).
- For Kidney fire, use *Zhi Mu* (Rhizoma Anemarrhenae).

Fungal infections can be a challenge to treat and are hard to dislodge once established in the body. The following herbs have shown antifungal effects and can be added to this or other formulas depending on the case to enhance treatment success against systemic fungal infections such as aspergillosis, cryptococcosis, blastomycosis, coccidioidomycosis and histoplasmosis: *Ren Dong Teng* (Caulis Lonicerae Japonicae), *Bai Tou Weng* (Radix Pulsatillae), *Huang Bo* (Cortex Phellodendri Chinensis), *Ku Shen* (Radix Sophorae Flavescentis), *Yu Xing Cao* (Herba Houttuyniae), *Mu Dan Pi* (Cortex Moutan), *Qing Hao* (Herba Artemisiae Annuae) and *Zi Cao* (Radix Arnebiae).

Huang Lian Jie Du Tang is a very cold and bitter formula and can easily injure the middle *jiao*. It is advisable to combine with a formula such as *Liu Jun Zi Tang* (Six-Gentlemen Decoction) or *Bu Zhong Yi Qi Tang* (Tonify the Middle and Augment the Qi Decoction) to prevent signs of abdominal discomfort, especially in horses and in patients on concurrent antibiotic drugs. Once the desired therapeutic results have been obtained the formula should be discontinued. A course of treatment should not exceed 5-7 days without re-evaluation or modification.

References

1. *Zhong Yao Tong Bao* (Journal of Chinese Herbology), 1986; 1:5.
2. *Zhong Cheng Yao* (Study of Chinese Patent Medicine), 1993; 8:29.
3. *Zhong Yi Fang Ji Xian Dai Yan Jiu* (Modern Study of Medical Formulas in Traditional Chinese Medicine), 1997; 280-283.
4. Zhou H, Mineshita S. The effect of Oren-gedoku-to on experimental colitis in rats. J Pharm Pharmacol. 1999 Sep; 51(9):1065-74.
5. Ohta Y, Kobayashi T, Nishida K, Sasaki E, Ishiguro I. Preventive effect of Oren-gedoku-to (Huanglian-Jie-Du-Tang) extract on the development of stress-induced acute gastric mucosal lesions in rats. J Ethnopharmacol. 1999 Nov 30; 67(3):377-84.
6. Ohta Y, Kobayashi T, Nishida K, Nagata M, Ishiguro I. Therapeutic effect of Oren-gedoku-to extract on stress-induced acute gastric mucosal lesions in rats. Phytother Res. 1999 Nov; 13(7):588-92.
7. Takase H, Inoue O, Saito Y, Yumioka E, Suzuki A. Roles of sulfhydryl compounds in the gastric mucosal protection of the herb drugs composing oren-gedoku-to (a traditional herbal medicine). Jpn J Pharmacol. 1991 Aug; 56(4):433-9.
8. Suenaga T, Shirakawa T, Harada N, Tao C, Yamasaki M, Komatsu H, Matsumoto N, Kida M, Kawamoto Y, Murakami Y, et al. Mechanism of protective effects of ouren-gedoku-to and san'ou-syashin-to on the gastric mucosa. Nippon Yakurigaku Zasshi. 1991 Oct; 98(4):319-25.
9. Takase H, Tatsumi Y, Miura O, Yumioka E, Suzuki A. The mechanism of the inhibitory effects of oren-gedoku-to (OGT) on gastric acid secretion in rats. Nippon Yakurigaku Zasshi. 1991 Feb; 97(2):97-103.
10. *Guo Wai Yi Xue* (Foreign Medicine), 1988; 5:36.
11. *Zhong Yi Fang Ji Xian Dai Yan Jiu* (Modern Study of Medical Formulas in Traditional Chinese Medicine), 1997; 280-283.
12. *Zhong Yi Yao Yan Jiu Can Kao* (Research and Discussion of Chinese Medicine and Herbology), 1975; 5:39.
13. Ohta Y, Sasaki E, Nishida K, Kongo M, Hayashi T, Nagata M, Ishiguro I. Inhibitory effect of Oren-gedoku-to (Huanglian-Jie-Du-Tang) extract on hepatic triglyceride accumulation with the progression of carbon tetrachloride-induced acute liver injury in rats. J Ethnopharmacol. 1998 May;61(1):75-80.
14. Ohta Y, Sasaki E, Nishida K, Hayashi T, Nagata M, Ishiguro I. Preventive effect of oren-gedoku-to (huanglian-jie-du-tang) extract on progression of carbon tetrachloride-induced acute liver injury in rats. Am J Chin Med. 1997;25(1):57-68.
15. Sekiya N, Shibahara N, Sakakibara I, Hattori N, Goto H, Terasawa K. Inhibitory effects of Oren-Gedoku-To (Huanglian-Jie-Du-Tang) on free radical-induced lysis of human red blood cells. Phytotherapy Research. 12003 Feb; 7(2):147-51.
16. *Zhong Yao Yao Li Yu Lin Chuang* (Pharmacology and Clinical Applications of Chinese Herbs), 1994; 6:9.
17. Wang LM, Yamamoto T, Wang XX, Yang L, Koike Y, Shiba K, Mineshita S. Effects of oren-gedoku-to and unsei-in, Chinese traditional medicines, on interleukin-8 and superoxide dismutase in rats. J Pharm Pharmacol. 1997 Jan;49(1):102-4.
18. *Zhong Yi Fang Ji Xian Dai Yan Jiu* (Modern Study of Medical Formulas in Traditional Chinese Medicine), 1997; 280-281.
19. *Guo Wai Yi Xue* (Foreign Medicine), 1982; 6:7.
20. Sanae F, Komatsu Y, Amagaya S, Chisaki K, Hayashi H. Effects of 9 Kampo medicines clinically used in hypertension on hemodynamic changes induced by theophylline in rats. Biol Pharm Bull. 2000 Jun; 23(6):762-5.
21. Kim YS, Jung EA, Shin JE, Chang JC, Yang HK, Kim NJ, Cho KH, Bae HS, Moon SK, Kim DH. Daio-Orengedokuto inhibits HMG-CoA reductase and pancreatic lipase. Biol Pharm Bull. 2002 Nov;25(11):1442-5.
22. *Guo Wai Yi Xue* (Foreign Medicine), 1987; 5:49.
23. Nagaki Y, Hayasaka S, Kadoi C, Matsumoto M, Nakamura N, Hayasaka Y. Effects of Orengedoku-to and Senkanmeimoku-to, traditional herbal medicines, on the experimental elevation of aqueous flare in pigmented rabbits. Am J Chin Med. 2001;29(1):141-7.
24. *Fu Jian Zhong Yi Yao* (Fujian Chinese Medicine and Herbology), 1960; 6:7.
25. *Guang Dong Zhong Yi* (Guangdong Chinese Medicine), 1960, 6:296.
26. Fushitani S, Minakuchi K, Tsuchiya K, Takasugi M, Murakami K. Studies on attenuation of post-ischemic brain injury by kampo medicines-inhibitory effects of free radical production. Yakugaku Zasshi. 1995 Aug;115(8):611-7.
27. *Jiang Su Zhong Yi* (Jiangsu Chinese Medicine), 1996; 2:3.
28. *Zhong Yi Za Zhi* (Journal of Chinese Medicine), 1994; 35(10):608.
29. *Xin Zhong Yi* (New Chinese Medicine), 1985, 4:23.
30. *Tian Jin Yi Yao* (Tianjin Medicine and Herbology), 1976; 6:294.
31. *Jiang Su Zhong Yi* (Jiangsu Chinese Medicine), 1998, 3:30.
32. *Hu Bei Zhong Yi Za Zhi* (Hubei Journal of Chinese Medicine), 1981, 4:30.
33. *Xin Zhong Yi* (New Chinese Medicine), 1998, 1:52.
34. *Shi Yong Zhong Yi Yao Za Zhi* (Journal of Practical Chinese Medicine and Medicinals), 1998, 12:19.
35. Ikeda N, Hayasaka S, Nagaki Y, Hayasaka Y, Kadoi C, Matsumoto M. Effects of traditional Sino-Japanese herbal medicines on aqueous

flare elevation after small-incision cataract surgery. J Ocul Pharmacol Ther. 2001 Feb;17(1):59-65.

36. Yuki F, Kawaguchi T, Hazemoto K, Asou N. Preventive effects of oren-gedoku-to (Huang-Lian-Jie-Du-Tang) on mucositis caused by anticancer agents in patients with acute leukemia. Gan To Kagaku Ryoho. 2003 Sep;30(9):1303-7.
37. Takase H, Imanishi K, Miura O, Yumioka E, Watanabe H. Pharmacological studies on the effects of some traditional Chinese medicines on gastric functions. (3) The effects of oren-gedoku-to (OGT), san'o-syasin-to (SST), antyu-san (AS) and dai-saiko-to (DST) on ethanol- and aspirin-induced gastric lesions in rats. Nippon Yakurigaku Zasshi. 1988 May;91(5):319-24.
38. *J Pharm Pharmacol* 2000 Mar;52(3):361-6.
39. Yang ZC, Wang BC, Yang XS, Wang Q, Ran L. The synergistic activity of antibiotics combined with eight traditional Chinese medicines against two different strains of Staphylococcus aureus. Colloids Surf B Biointerfaces. 2005 Mar 25;41(2-3):79-81. Epub 2004 Dec 18.

Huáng Lián Shàng Qīng Wán (Coptis Pill to Clear the Upper)

黃連上清丸

黄连上清丸

Pinyin Name: *Huang Lian Shang Qing Wan*
Literal Name: Coptis Pill to Clear the Upper
Alternate Names: *Huang Lien Shang Ching Wan*, Coptis Up-Clearing Pill, Coptis Phellodendron and Mint Formula
Original Source: *Si He Ting Ji Fang* (Collection of Formulas of Si He-Ting)

COMPOSITION

Huang Lian (Rhizoma Coptidis)	240g
Huang Qin (Radix Scutellariae)	240g
Huang Bo (Cortex Phellodendri Chinensis)	240g
Zhi Zi (Fructus Gardeniae)	240g
Da Huang (Radix et Rhizoma Rhei)	360g
Ju Hua (Flos Chrysanthemi)	120g
Jie Geng (Radix Platycodonis)	60g
Bo He (Herba Menthae)	120g
Jiang Huang (Rhizoma Curcumae Longae)	180g
Lian Qiao (Fructus Forsythiae)	180g
Xuan Shen (Radix Scrophulariae)	120g
Tian Hua Fen (Radix Trichosanthis)	60g
Ge Gen (Radix Puerariae Lobatae)	60g
Dang Gui (Radix Angelicae Sinensis)	120g
Chuan Xiong (Rhizoma Chuanxiong)	60g

DOSAGE / PREPARATION / ADMINISTRATION

Grind the ingredients into powder and mix with honey to form pills. Take 9g of pills with tea at bedtime.

CHINESE THERAPEUTIC ACTIONS

1. Clears heat and eliminates toxins
2. Purges fire and treats constipation

CLINICAL MANIFESTATIONS

Heat accumulation in all three *jiaos* with fire attacking the head: irritability, red eyes, a sore throat, ulcerations of the mouth and tongue, and painful urination.

VETERINARY CLINICAL APPLICATIONS

Fever, upper respiratory infection, stomatitis or gingivitis, glossitis, conjunctivitis, otitis media, yellow nasal

Huáng Lián Shàng Qīng Wán (Coptis Pill to Clear the Upper)

discharge, sinusitis, periodontal disease, toothache, red, hot skin rash, cellulitis of head and neck and front limbs, eosinophilic granuloma and urinary tract infection.

EXPLANATION

Huang Lian Shang Qing Wan (Coptis Pill to Clear the Upper) has a wide range of clinical applications, but is most effective in treating heat and fire in the upper *jiao* attacking the head. Heat and fire in the three *jiaos* are characterized by restlessness, irritability, and jaundice. As heat and fire move upward, they attack the head and the upper parts of the body, producing red eyes, a sore throat, and ulcerations of the mouth and tongue. As heat and fire travel downward, they affect both bowel movement and urination, leading to constipation and pain, as well as pain during urination.

Huang Lian (Rhizoma Coptidis), *Huang Qin* (Radix Scutellariae), *Huang Bo* (Cortex Phellodendri Chinensis), *Zhi Zi* (Fructus Gardeniae), and *Da Huang* (Radix et Rhizoma Rhei) are bitter and cold herbs that eliminate excess heat and fire in the upper, middle, and lower *jiaos. Huang Qin* (Radix Scutellariae) clears Lung heat and sedates fire in the upper *jiao*; *Huang Lian* (Rhizoma Coptidis) sedates fire in the Heart and middle *jiao*; *Huang Bo* (Cortex Phellodendri Chinensis) clears heat in the lower *jiao*; *Zhi Zi* (Fructus Gardeniae) sedates fire in all three *jiaos*; and *Da Huang* (Radix et Rhizoma Rhei) sedates fire and purges heat downward through defecation. *Ju Hua* (Flos Chrysanthemi), *Jie Geng* (Radix Platycodonis), *Bo He* (Herba Menthae), *Jiang Huang* (Rhizoma Curcumae Longae) and *Lian Qiao* (Fructus Forsythiae) dispel wind-heat and eliminate toxins from the exterior to relieve sore throat, red eyes, and ulcerations of the mouth and tongue. *Xuan Shen* (Radix Scrophulariae) and *Tian Hua Fen* (Radix Trichosanthis) clear heat and eliminate toxins. *Tian Hua Fen* (Radix Trichosanthis) and *Ge Gen* (Radix Puerariae Lobatae) promote generation of body fluids and prevent the cold and bitter herbs from damaging yin. *Dang Gui* (Radix Angelicae Sinensis) and *Chuan Xiong* (Rhizoma Chuanxiong) invigorate blood circulation, remove blood stasis, and relieve pain.

VETERINARY MODIFICATIONS

- With a dry mouth and throat, add *Mai Dong* (Radix Ophiopogonis) and *Wu Wei Zi* (Fructus Schisandrae Chinensis).
- With thirst and fever, add *Shi Gao* (Gypsum Fibrosum) and *Zhi Mu* (Rhizoma Anemarrhenae).
- With jaundice and fever, add *Yin Chen* (Herba Artemisiae Scopariae).
- With tenesmus and blood in the stool, add *Mu Xiang* (Radix Aucklandiae) and *Bing Lang* (Semen Arecae).
- With frequent urination and oliguria, add *Che Qian Zi* (Semen Plantaginis) and *Mu Tong* (Caulis Akebiae).

***Huang Lian Shang Qing Wan* (Coptis Pill to Clear the Upper)**

Diagnosis	Clinical Signs	Treatment	Herbs
Accumulation of heat in all three *jiaos* with fire attacking the head	• Red eyes, a sore throat and ulcerations of the mouth and tongue: heat and fire traveling to the head • Restlessness and irritability: heat and fire affecting the upper body • Constipation and dysuria: heat and fire affecting the lower body	• Clears heat and eliminates toxins • Purges fire and treats constipation	• *Huang Lian* (Rhizoma Coptidis), *Huang Qin* (Radix Scutellariae), *Huang Bo* (Cortex Phellodendri Chinensis) and *Zhi Zi* (Fructus Gardeniae) eliminate excess heat and fire in the upper, middle, and lower *jiaos*. • *Da Huang* (Radix et Rhizoma Rhei) sedates fire and purges heat downward through defecation. • *Ju Hua* (Flos Chrysanthemi), *Jie Geng* (Radix Platycodonis), *Bo He* (Herba Menthae), *Jiang Huang* (Rhizoma Curcumae Longae), and *Lian Qiao* (Fructus Forsythiae) dispel heat and eliminate toxins from the exterior. • *Xuan Shen* (Radix Scrophulariae) and *Tian Hua Fen* (Radix Trichosanthis) clear heat and eliminate toxins. • *Tian Hua Fen* (Radix Trichosanthis) and *Ge Gen* (Radix Puerariae Lobatae) promote generation of body fluids and prevent the cold and bitter herbs from damaging yin. • *Dang Gui* (Radix Angelicae Sinensis) and *Chuan Xiong* (Rhizoma Chuanxiong) invigorate blood circulation, remove blood stasis, and relieve pain.

Huáng Lián Shàng Qīng Wán (Coptis Pill to Clear the Upper)

SUGGESTED ACUPUNCTURE TREATMENT

1. Points: *Dazhui* (GV 14), *Quchi* (LI 11), *Neiting* (ST 44), *Xingjian* (LR 2), *Fengchi* (GB 20), *Hegu* (LI 4), *Yingxiang* (LI 20), *Waiguan* (TH 5), *Chize* (LU 5), and *Sanyinjiao* (SP 6).
2. Technique: sedation and bleeding

Sedate *Quchi* (LI 11), *Neiting* (ST 44), *Xingjian* (LR 2), and bleed *Dazhui* (GV 14) and ear apex [*Erjian*] to clear *San Jiao* heat. Sedate *Fengchi* (GB 20), *Hegu* (LI 4), *Yingxiang* (LI 20), and *Waiguan* (TH 5) to ventilate heat and toxins to the exterior. *Chize* (LU 5) nourishes yin and dissipates nodules; *Sanyinjiao* (SP 6) invigorates the blood. *Jingming* and *Jingshu* are used for conjunctivitis and uveitis.

AUTHORS' COMMENTS

Huang Lian Shang Qing Wan is most effective to treat toxic heat (bacterial infections) affecting the upper *jiao* (eyes, ears, nose, throat and skin of the face and head). It can be combined with antibiotics for a synergistic effect. It is for short-term use only and once therapeutic results have been obtained it should be discontinued. It is particularly useful in the treatment of acute flare up of periodontal disease, cat bite abscess involving the head and face, gingivitis or stomatitis and upper respiratory tract infection with yellow ocular or nasal discharge in the cat. It may also be used in horses for flares of periodic ophthalmia and conjunctivitis as well as dermatologic conditions such as scratches, rain rot, and summer itch.

Pǔ Jì Xiāo Dú Yǐn (Universal Benefit Decoction to Eliminate Toxin)

普濟消毒飲
普济消毒饮

Pinyin Name: *Pu Ji Xiao Du Yin*

Literal Name: Universal Benefit Decoction to Eliminate Toxin

Alternate Names: *Pu Chi Hsiao Tu Yin*, Universal Salvation Detoxifying Drink, Everyone's Detoxifying Decoction, Scute and Cimicifuga Combination

Original Source: *Dong Heng Shi Xiao Fang* (Tested and Effective Formulas by Dong Heng) by Dong Heng in 1266

COMPOSITION

Huang Qin (Radix Scutellariae), *chao* (dry-fried) with liquor	15g
Huang Lian (Rhizoma Coptidis), *chao* (dry-fried) with liquor	15g
Niu Bang Zi (Fructus Arctii)	3g
Lian Qiao (Fructus Forsythiae)	3g
Bo He (Herba Menthae)	3g
Jiang Can (Bombyx Batryticatus)	2.1g
Xuan Shen (Radix Scrophulariae)	6g
Ma Bo (Lasiosphaera seu Calvatia)	3g
Ban Lan Gen (Radix Isatidis)	3g
Jie Geng (Radix Platycodonis)	6g
Gan Cao (Radix et Rhizoma Glycyrrhizae)	6g
Chen Pi (Pericarpium Citri Reticulatae)	6g
Sheng Ma (Rhizoma Cimicifugae)	2.1g
Chai Hu (Radix Bupleuri)	6g
Ren Shen (Radix et Rhizoma Ginseng)	9g [3g]

Pǔ Jì Xiāo Dú Yǐn (Universal Benefit Decoction to Eliminate Toxin)

DOSAGE / PREPARATION / ADMINISTRATION

The source text states to grind the ingredients into powder, cook it in water, and take the warm decoction frequently in small amounts. It may also be formed into pills with honey, and dissolved under the tongue before swallowing. For patients with constipation, add *Da Huang* (Radix et Rhizoma Rhei). Today, this formula may be prepared as a decoction with the dose of *Ren Shen* (Radix et Rhizoma Ginseng) suggested in brackets. Note: One variation of this formula contains 6g of *Bo He* (Herba Menthae) and omits *Ren Shen* (Radix et Rhizoma Ginseng).

CHINESE THERAPEUTIC ACTIONS

1. Clears heat and eliminates toxins
2. Dispels wind and disperses pathogenic factors

CLINICAL MANIFESTATIONS

Wind, heat, and toxins in the upper *jiao* and head: redness, swelling and pain of the head and neck, red and swollen eyes, otitis media, purulent nasal discharge, fever, aversion to cold, a sore throat, thirst, a dry, red tongue, in severe cases a yellow tongue coating, and a rapid, forceful pulse.

VETERINARY CLINICAL APPLICATIONS

Feline and equine upper respiratory tract infection, puppy strangles, equine strangles, lymphadenitis, purulent naso-sinusitis, otitis media, purulent inflammation and abscess of the face and head, erysipelas, herpes, pyoderma of head and neck, and conjunctivitis.

EXPLANATION

Pu Ji Xiao Du Yin (Universal Benefit Decoction to Eliminate Toxins) treats conditions of wind, heat and toxins attacking the face and head. If the wind, heat, and toxins invade the head region, redness, swelling and pain of the face and head, swollen lymph nodes, sore throat, and thirst may result. Fever and aversion to cold suggest that the disease (wind-heat) is located at the exterior. The yellow tongue coating and rapid, forceful pulse suggest excess interior heat.

Huang Qin (Radix Scutellariae) and *Huang Lian* (Rhizoma Coptidis), the chief herbs of this formula, clear heat and eliminate toxins from the head. *Niu Bang Zi* (Fructus Arctii), *Lian Qiao* (Fructus Forsythiae), *Bo He* (Herba Menthae) and *Jiang Can* (Bombyx Batryticatus) disperse wind-heat accumulation in the head. *Xuan Shen* (Radix Scrophulariae), *Ma Bo* (Lasiosphaera seu Calvatia), and *Ban Lan Gen* (Radix Isatidis) clear heat and eliminate toxins. *Xuan Shen* (Radix Scrophulariae) also prevents the heat-clearing, damp-drying herbs from injuring yin. *Jie Geng* (Radix Platycodonis) and *Gan Cao* (Radix et Rhizoma Glycyrrhizae) synergistically relieve sore throat, thus helping the heat-clearing herbs. *Chen Pi*

***Pu Ji Xiao Du Yin* (Universal Benefit Decoction to Eliminate Toxin)**

Diagnosis	Clinical Signs	Treatment	Herbs
Wind, heat and toxins in the upper *jiao* and head	• Fever and aversion to cold: exterior wind-heat • Redness, swelling and pain of the face and head, red and swollen eyes, swollen lymph nodes and a sore throat: wind, heat and toxins invade the head region • Thirst: heat consuming body fluids • Dry, red tongue and yellow tongue coating: presence of heat and toxins • Rapid, forceful pulse: excess condition	• Clears heat and eliminates toxins • Dispels wind and disperses pathogenic factors	• *Huang Qin* (Radix Scutellariae) and *Huang Lian* (Rhizoma Coptidis) clear heat and eliminate toxins from the head. • *Niu Bang Zi* (Fructus Arctii), *Lian Qiao* (Fructus Forsythiae), *Bo He* (Herba Menthae), and *Jiang Can* (Bombyx Batryticatus) disperse wind-heat accumulation from the head. • *Xuan Shen* (Radix Scrophulariae), *Ma Bo* (Lasiosphaera seu Calvatia), and *Ban Lan Gen* (Radix Isatidis) clear heat and eliminate toxins. • *Jie Geng* (Radix Platycodonis) and *Gan Cao* (Radix et Rhizoma Glycyrrhizae) synergistically relieve sore throat. • *Chen Pi* (Pericarpium Citri Reticulatae) regulates qi circulation to reduce swelling and inflammation. • *Sheng Ma* (Rhizoma Cimicifugae) and *Chai Hu* (Radix Bupleuri) guide the other herbs upward to the head region. • *Ren Shen* (Radix et Rhizoma Ginseng) tonifies qi, and prevents the bitter and cold heat-clearing herbs from damaging the body.

Pǔ Jì Xiāo Dú Yǐn (Universal Benefit Decoction to Eliminate Toxin)

(Pericarpium Citri Reticulatae) regulates qi circulation to reduce swelling and inflammation. *Sheng Ma* (Rhizoma Cimicifugae) and *Chai Hu* (Radix Bupleuri), in addition to dispersing wind-heat, guide the other herbs upward to the head region where the condition is most critical. Finally, *Ren Shen* (Radix et Rhizoma Ginseng) tonifies qi, and prevents the bitter and cold heat-clearing herbs from damaging the body. Note: *Ren Shen* (Radix et Rhizoma Ginseng) may be removed from the formula when prescribed for individuals without underlying deficiencies.

VETERINARY MODIFICATIONS

- If the heat and toxins are severe, and for animals who are unresponsive to antibiotic drugs or have a stubborn infection, add one or more of the following: *Feng Wei Cao* (Herba Pteris), *Zi Hua Di Ding* (Herba Violae), *Hu Yao Huang* (Herba Leucas Mollissimae), *Da Ding Huang* (Caulis Euonymi), *Jin Yin Hua* (Flos Lonicerae Japonicae) and/or *Pu Gong Ying* (Herba Taraxaci).
- If there are more exterior symptoms, remove *Huang Qin* (Radix Scutellariae) and add *Jing Jie* (Herba Schizonepetae), *Fang Feng* (Radix Saposhnikoviae), *Chan Tui* (Periostracum Cicadae) and *Sang Ye* (Folium Mori).
- If the interior heat is severe, remove *Chai Hu* (Radix Bupleuri) and *Bo He* (Herba Menthae), and add *Jin Yin Hua* (Flos Lonicerae Japonicae) and *Qing Dai* (Indigo Naturalis), or *Shi Gao* (Gypsum Fibrosum) and *Huang Bo* (Cortex Phellodendri Chinensis).
- For nodules that are hard and difficult to reduce in size, add *Mu Dan Pi* (Cortex Moutan), *Bei Mu* (Bulbus Fritillariae), *Chi Shao* (Radix Paeoniae Rubra), *Si Gua Luo* (Retinervus Luffae Fructus) and *Xia Ku Cao* (Spica Prunellae).

CAUTIONS / CONTRAINDICATIONS

- *Pu Ji Xiao Du Yin* should be used with caution in patients with deficiencies of yin or body fluids, because this formula is bitter, cold, acrid and dispersing in nature.
- Avoid foods that are cold, raw or greasy while taking this formula.[1]

PHARMACOLOGICAL EFFECTS

Antibiotic: Numerous herbs in *Pu Ji Xiao Du Yin* have shown marked *in vitro* and *in vivo* antibacterial and antiviral effects.[2]

HUMAN CLINICAL STUDIES AND RESEARCH

1. **Epidemic hemorrhagic fever**: Administration of *Pu Ji Xiao Du Yin* was associated with improving the condition of 435 patients with epidemic hemorrhagic fever. The formula was described to be effective in reducing fever, preventing shock, relieving dysuria and anuria, and improving the overall treatment outcome.[3]
2. **Infectious parotitis**: Modified *Pu Ji Xiao Du Yin* was used successfully in treating 90 children with infectious parotitis (21 cases were diagnosed as wind-heat and 69 as accumulation of heat and toxins). According to the study, the average time was 2.8 days for the reduction of fever (ranging from 1-8 days) and 3.7 days for swelling of the parotid glands (ranging from 2-9 days).[4] Another study reported good results using modified *Pu Ji Xiao Du Yin* to treat all 100 patients (64 males and 36 females) with infectious parotitis. The study reported that more than 77% of patients had complete recovery within 4 days. The herbal treatment reduced the average duration of illness by 3-5 days.[5]
3. **Respiratory tract infection**: Modified *Pu Ji Xiao Du Yin* was used as an herbal decoction one time daily to treat 35 children with respiratory tract infections and high fever (>39°C / 102.2°F). Within 96 hours, 30 out of 35 patients experienced reduction of fever and other symptoms. The rate of effectiveness was 85.7%. The herbal formula contained *Huang Qin* (Radix Scutellariae), *Huang Lian* (Rhizoma Coptidis), *Ban Lan Gen* (Radix Isatidis), *Lian Qiao* (Fructus Forsythiae), *Sheng Ma* (Rhizoma Cimicifugae), *Ma Bo* (Lasiosphaera seu Calvatia), *Jie Geng* (Radix Platycodonis), *Xuan Shen* (Radix Scrophulariae), *Bo He* (Herba Menthae), *Niu Bang Zi* (Fructus Arctii), *Jiang Can* (Bombyx Batryticatus), *Chai Hu* (Radix Bupleuri), *Chen Pi* (Pericarpium Citri Reticulatae) and *Gan Cao* (Radix et Rhizoma Glycyrrhizae).[6]
4. **Myocarditis**: Modified *Pu Ji Xiao Du Yin* was used to treat 48 patients with acute viral myocarditis characterized by chest pain, tachypnea, feeling of oppression in the chest, palpitations, fever, headache, cough, sore throat, abdominal pain and diarrhea. The herbal decoction was administered one time daily for 15 days per course of treatment. The study reported that out of 48 patients, 16 had complete recovery, 28 showed marked improvement, and 4 showed no change.[7]
5. **Tonsillitis**: Use of modified *Pu Ji Xiao Du Yin* in decoction successfully treated acute suppurative tonsillitis. The herbal formula contained the following ingredients: *Jin Yin Hua* (Flos Lonicerae Japonicae) 15g, *Lian Qiao* (Fructus Forsythiae) 9g, *Ge Gen* (Radix Puerariae Lobatae) 9g, *Ban Lan Gen* (Radix Isatidis) 12g, *Shan Dou Gen* (Radix et Rhizoma Sophorae Tonkinensis) 9g, *Ma Bo* (Lasiosphaera seu Calvatia) 9g, *Jie Geng* (Radix Platycodonis) 9g, *Xuan Shen* (Radix Scrophulariae) 12g, *Shi Gao* (Gypsum Fibrosum) 30g, *Zhu Ye* (Herba Phyllostachys) 9g, and *Gan Cao* (Radix et Rhizoma Glycyrrhizae) 3g. The dosage was one pack of herbs daily for children 6 years of age or younger,

Pŭ Jì Xiāo Dú Yĭn (Universal Benefit Decoction to Eliminate Toxin)

and 3 packs of herbs in two days for children 7 years or older. The herbs were cooked in water to obtain 150 mL of decoction, and taken in two to three equally-divided doses. Of 57 patients with acute suppurative tonsillitis, 88% had normal body temperature within 3 days along with resolution of other signs and symptoms.[8]

6. **Conjunctivitis**: One study reported good results using *Pu Ji Xiao Du Yin* to treat acute conjunctivitis in 164 patients (306 affected eyes). The herbal formula contained *Huang Qin* (Radix Scutellariae), *Huang Lian* (Rhizoma Coptidis), *Chen Pi* (Pericarpium Citri Reticulatae), *Xuan Shen* (Radix Scrophulariae), *Chai Hu* (Radix Bupleuri), *Lian Qiao* (Fructus Forsythiae), *Ban Lan Gen* (Radix Isatidis), *Ma Bo* (Lasiosphaera seu Calvatia), *Niu Bang Zi* (Fructus Arctii), *Bo He* (Herba Menthae), *Jiang Can* (Bombyx Batryticatus), and *Sheng Ma* (Rhizoma Cimicifugae). *Chi Shao* (Radix Paeoniae Rubra) and *Chuan Xiong* (Rhizoma Chuanxiong) were added for early-stage conjunctivitis, and *Di Huang* (Radix Rehmanniae) and *Mu Dan Pi* (Cortex Moutan) were added for ocular bleeding. The herbs were given in decoction form daily. The study reported 98.7% effectiveness among 164 patients, with an average of 2.5 days to recovery.[9]
7. **Erysipelas**: One study reported 94.2% effectiveness in treating 52 patients with erysipelas with 2 weeks to 3 years of history of illness. The herbs were decocted, and their residue was applied topically to the affected area. Of 52 cases, the study reported complete recovery in 41 cases, improvement in 8 cases, and no effect in 3 cases.[10]

SUGGESTED ACUPUNCTURE TREATMENT

1. Points: *Waiguan* (TH 5), *Hegu* (LI 4), *Chize* (LU 5), *Yifeng* (TH 17), and *Jiache* (ST 6). For serious or acute conditions: add *Erheliao* (TH 22), *Guanchong* (TH 1), *Quchi* (LI 11), and *Shaoshang* (LU 11).
2. Technique: sedation.

Combine *Waiguan* (TH 5) and *Hegu* (LI 4) to dispel exterior heat and to clear interior heat. *Chize* (LU 5) clears excess Lung heat and will treat sore throat. *Yifeng* (TH 17) and *Jiache* (ST 6) sedate and disperse stagnant heat in the head. *Erheliao* (TH 22), *Waiguan* (TH 5), and *Guanchong* (TH 1) help clear heat, open the channels and collaterals, and reduce swelling. *Quchi* (LI 11), *Hegu* (LI 4), and *Shaoshang* (LU 11) clear heat and eliminate toxins.

Clinically, animals may show different clinical signs. For those who have high fever, add *Dazhui* (GV 14) and all twelve *jing* (well) points; for dementia and semi-unconsciousness, add *Renzhong* (GV 26); for headache, add *Xiaxi* (GB 43) and *Pishu* (BL 20); and for pain and swelling of the scrotum, add *Ququan* (LR 8) and *Taichong* (LR 3).

AUTHORS' COMMENTS

Pu Ji Xiao Du Yin is one of the best general herbal antibiotic formulas to treat infectious diseases (bacterial and viral infections). The name *Pu Ji Xiao Du Yin* literally means "Universal Benefit Decoction to Eliminate Toxins," which implies that this formula treats everyone [universal benefit] with infectious diseases [heat and toxins]. This formula is bitter, cold, acrid and dispersing in nature. It is contraindicated in yang-deficient patients, and should be used with herbs or formulas that harmonize the middle *jiao* in weak and debilitated animals with weak Spleen-Stomach function. This is the formula of choice to treat "puppy strangles," also known as juvenile cellulitis or juvenile pyoderma, which occurs from unknown causes in pups as young as one month of age to four months. This disease has several different presentations. It can present with an acute onset of small pimple-type lesions of the face, head and neck similar to classic pyoderma, whereas in other cases it develops as an abrupt, painful swelling of the eyelids, lips, ears, face, muzzle and ventral chin. In some cases, the swelling is so severe that the skin may crack and ooze serum. The lymph nodes of the head and neck typically become extremely swollen and painful, in particular the submandibular lymph nodes, which may drain to the skin surface. The eyelids may be swollen with yellow discharge, and the skin around the muzzle, under the chin and in the ears may ulcerate and develop draining sores. The disease is thought to be due to an immune system imbalance, as it is largely unresponsive to antibiotics, and is primarily treated with immunosuppressive doses of steroidal drugs. The clinical signs of puppy strangles correspond very well to the Chinese medicine pattern for which the formula *Pu Ji Xiao Du Yin* is well suited. Juvenile animals normally have immature Spleen function and will require the concurrent use of herbs or formulas which support the middle *jiao* during administration of this formula, or diarrhea will occur. The formula *Liu Jun Zi Tang* (Six-Gentlemen Decoction) or *Jian Pi Wan* (Strengthen the Spleen Pill) can be used, depending on the individual case. The average time for treatment is 10-14 days. The treatment of this disease with Chinese herbs is preferred over steroidal therapy, which, if administered at such a young age, can weaken or damage the immune system and the internal organs, and set the stage for future disharmony.

In horses, this formula is very useful to treat many different manifestations of upper respiratory disease. In treating a condition like *Streptococcus equi* (equine strangles), it is prudent to make sure abscesses are opened and draining before beginning treatment to prevent bastard strangles and interior abscesses from developing. Often, horses will

Pǔ Jì Xiāo Dú Yǐn (Universal Benefit Decoction to Eliminate Toxin)

continue to have submandibular lymph node swelling and pain, mucopurulent discharge from the nose, and cough even after treatment is completed. These cases will have toxins lodged in the throat, and are usually unresponsive to conventional medications. *Pu Ji Xiao Du Yin* is an excellent formula in both the acute and post-acute stage of disease and can lead to faster recovery from upper respiratory infection of both bacterial and viral origin.

References

1. *Zhong Yao Ming Fang Yao Li Yu Ying Yong* (Pharmacology and Applications of Famous Herbal Formulas), 1989; 143-145.
2. Chen J and Chen T. *Chinese Medical Herbology and Pharmacology*, Art of Medicine Press, 2004.
3. *Shan Xi Zhong Yi* (Shanxi Chinese Medicine), 1984; 3:16.
4. *Si Chuan Zhong Yi* (Sichuan Chinese Medicine), 1990; (5):25.
5. *Zhong Yi Za Zhi* (Journal of Chinese Medicine), 1958; 7:463.
6. *Guang Xi Zhong Yi Yao* (Guangxi Chinese Medicine and Herbology), 1989; (1):5.
7. *Zhong Guo Zhong Xi Yi Jie He Za Zhi* (Chinese Journal of Integrative Chinese and Western Medicine), 1993; 13(4):244.
8. *Shan Dong Zhong Yi Za Zhi* (Shandong Journal of Chinese Medicine), 1984; 4:42.
9. *Hei Long Jiang Zhong Yi Yao* (Heilongjiang Chinese Medicine and Herbology), 1995; 2:20.
10. *Hu Bei Zhong Yi Za Zhi* (Hubei Journal of Chinese Medicine), 1989; 5:11.

Sān Huáng Xiè Xīn Tāng

(Three-Yellow Decoction to Sedate the Epigastrium)

三黃瀉心湯

三黄泻心汤

Pinyin Name: *San Huang Xie Xin Tang*
Literal Name: Three-Yellow Decoction to Sedate the Epigastrium
Alternate Names: *Xie Xin Tang* (Drain the Epigastrium Decoction), *San Huang Hsieh Hsin Tang*, Three-Huang Heart-Draining Decoction, Coptis and Rhubarb Combination
Original Source: *Jin Gui Yao Lue* (Essentials from the Golden Cabinet) by Zhang Zhong-Jing in the Eastern Han Dynasty

COMPOSITION

Huang Qin (Radix Scutellariae)	3g [9g]
Huang Lian (Rhizoma Coptidis)	3g
Da Huang (Radix et Rhizoma Rhei)	6g

DOSAGE / PREPARATION / ADMINISTRATION

The source text states to cook the ingredients in 3 cups [600 mL] of water and reduce it to 1 cup [200 mL]. Take the warm, strained decoction immediately. Today, use the dose of *Huang Qin* (Radix Scutellariae) suggested in brackets.

CHINESE THERAPEUTIC ACTIONS

Purges fire and dries dampness

CLINICAL MANIFESTATIONS

Damp-heat in all three *jiao*s: hemoptysis, epistaxis, jaundice, irritability and restlessness, red eyes, swelling and pain of the eyes, tongue and mouth ulcerations, external abscesses and sores, and constipation.

VETERINARY CLINICAL APPLICATIONS

1. Bleeding disorders (hemoptysis, epistaxis, hemorrhoidal bleeding, intestinal bleeding, gastrointestinal bleeding, hematuria, uterine bleeding, subcutaneous bleeding).

Sān Huáng Xiè Xīn Tāng

(Three-Yellow Decoction to Sedate the Epigastrium)

2. Gastrointestinal disorders (gastroenteritis, stomatitis, habitual constipation, dysentery, hemorrhoids).
3. Dermatological diseases (furuncles, carbuncles, urticaria).
4. Liver and gallbladder disorders (hepatitis, jaundice).

EXPLANATION

San Huang Xie Xin Tang (Three-Yellow Decoction to Sedate the Epigastrium) is one of the strongest formulas for treating damp-heat accumulation throughout the body, including in the upper, middle, and/or lower *jiaos*. Heat in the blood will cause reckless movement of the blood, leading to bleeding from various parts of the body, as in hemoptysis and epistaxis. Damp-heat accumulation in the upper *jiao* causes irritability, restlessness, and a feeling of oppression in the chest. Damp-heat accumulation in the Liver causes jaundice, as well as redness, swelling, and pain of the eyes. Damp-heat accumulation in the Stomach causes a sore throat, and tongue and mouth ulcerations. Damp-heat accumulation in the lower *jiao* causes constipation. Damp-heat accumulation may also affect the skin, causing abscesses and sores. Clinically, damp-heat may affect many other parts of the body, manifesting in other signs and symptoms as well.

While damp-heat causes a wide variety of complications and disorders, the treatment strategy is rather simple. Only three herbs are required to manage and treat these conditions. *Huang Qin* (Radix Scutellariae), bitter and cold, enters the upper *jiao* to clear heat, purge fire, and dry dampness. *Huang Lian* (Rhizoma Coptidis), bitter and cold, enters the middle *jiao* to clear heat, purge fire, and dry dampness. *Da Huang* (Radix et Rhizoma Rhei), bitter and cold, enters the lower *jiao* to clear heat, purge fire, and eliminate toxins. All three herbs have a similar function of clearing damp-heat, yet they each focus on different parts of the body. The combination of these three herbs has a synergistic effect in relieving pain, stopping bleeding, reducing inflammation, and treating infection.

VETERINARY MODIFICATIONS

- With fever and thirst due to dryness and heat, add *Shi Gao* (Gypsum Fibrosum) and *Zhi Mu* (Rhizoma Anemarrhenae).
- For icteric jaundice, add *Yin Chen* (Herba Artemisiae Scopariae), *Zhi Zi* (Fructus Gardeniae), and *Che Qian Cao* (Herba Plantaginis).
- With bleeding gums, add *Mang Xiao* (Natrii Sulfas).
- For severe constipation, add *Mang Xiao* (Natrii Sulfas), *Zhi Shi* (Fructus Aurantii Immaturus), and *Hou Po* (Cortex Magnoliae Officinalis).
- With bleeding due to heat in the *xue* (blood) level, add *Mu Dan Pi* (Cortex Moutan) and *Di Huang* (Radix Rehmanniae).
- For severe abscesses and sores, add *Jin Yin Hua* (Flos Lonicerae Japonicae), *Lian Qiao* (Fructus Forsythiae), and *Zi Hua Di Ding* (Herba Violae).

CAUTIONS / CONTRAINDICATIONS

- *San Huang Xie Xin Tang* contains bitter and cold herbs that may damage the Spleen and Stomach. Thus, it should be discontinued when the desired effects are achieved. It should not be taken at large doses or for a prolonged period of time.
- This formula is contraindicated during pregnancy and nursing, and in animals with deficiency and cold of the Spleen and Stomach.[1]

PHARMACOLOGICAL EFFECTS

Gastroprotective: Use of *San Huang Xie Xin Tang* was found to have a protective effect on the gastrointestinal tract by inhibiting the gastric acid secretion via inhibition of H,K-ATPase activity. *San Huang Xie Xin Tang*, given

***San Huang Xie Xin Tang* (Three-Yellow Decoction to Sedate the Epigastrium)**

Diagnosis	Clinical Signs	Treatment	Herbs
Damp-heat in the three *jiaos*	• Irritability, restlessness: damp-heat in the upper *jiao* • Jaundice with redness, swelling and pain of the eyes: damp-heat in the Liver (middle *jiao*) • Sore throat and ulcerations of the tongue and mouth: damp-heat in the Stomach (middle *jiao*) • Constipation: damp-heat in the lower *jiao*	Purges fire and dries dampness	• *Huang Qin* (Radix Scutellariae) enters the upper *jiao* to clear heat, purge fire, and dry dampness. • *Huang Lian* (Rhizoma Coptidis) enters the middle *jiao* to clear heat, purge fire, and dry dampness. • *Da Huang* (Radix et Rhizoma Rhei) enters the lower *jiao* to clear heat, purge fire, and eliminate toxins.

Sān Huáng Xiè Xīn Tāng

(Three-Yellow Decoction to Sedate the Epigastrium)

30 minutes earlier, has a protective effect on the gastric mucosa against drugs such as aspirin, HCL-aspirin, and ethanol. However, it was found to be ineffective against gastric lesions induced by indomethacin.[2,3]

HUMAN CLINICAL STUDIES AND RESEARCH

1. **Gastrointestinal bleeding**: *San Huang Xie Xin Tang* was shown in many studies to effectively treat various types of gastrointestinal bleeding. In one study, administration of *San Huang Xie Xin Tang* in 60 patients (50 males and 10 females; between 14 and 70 years of age) was associated with treating gastrointestinal bleeding due to various causes (10 with gastritis, 35 with duodenal ulcer, 7 with gastric ulcer, and 8 with other causes). Of 60 cases, the study reported complete recovery in 50 cases, improvement in 9 cases, and voluntary discontinuation of treatment in 1 case (reason unknown).[4]
2. **Upper gastrointestinal bleeding**: Daily use of modified *San Huang Xie Xin Tang* in decoction was associated with complete recovery in 31 of 34 patients with acute and profuse bleeding from the upper gastrointestinal tract. The herbal formula contained *Da Huang* (Radix et Rhizoma Rhei) 10g, *Huang Lian* (Rhizoma Coptidis) 10g, *Huang Qin* (Radix Scutellariae) 12g, *Xian He Cao* (Herba Agrimoniae) 10g, *Ce Bai Ye* (Cacumen Platycladi) 15g, *Mu Dan Pi* (Cortex Moutan) 15g and *Xiao Ji* (Herba Cirsii) 15g. Individuals with severe loss of blood also received blood transfusions.[5]
3. **Lower gastrointestinal bleeding**: One study reported satisfactory results using modified *San Huang Xie Xin Tang* to treat 50 patients with hematochezia. The herbal formula contained *Da Huang* (Radix et Rhizoma Rhei) 15g, *Qian Cao* (Radix et Rhizoma Rubiae) 15g, *Zhi Zi* (Fructus Gardeniae) 10g, *Ou Jie* (Nodus Nelumbinis Rhizomatis) 10g, *Ce Bai Ye* (Cacumen Platycladi) 10g, *Huang Lian* (Rhizoma Coptidis) 10g, *Huang Qin* (Radix Scutellariae) 12g, and *Di Yu* (Radix Sanguisorbae) 12g. Furthermore, *Di Huang* (Radix Rehmanniae) and *Shi Hu* (Caulis Dendrobii) were added for individuals with a desire to drink water. Of 50 cases, the study reported complete recovery in 45 cases, improvement in 4 cases, and no change in 1 case.[6]
4. **Sleep apnea**: A 76-year-old male with obstructive sleep apnea syndrome was successfully treated with *San Huang Xie Xin Tang*. Polysomnography, performed before and after herbal treatment, showed a significant reduction in both the apnea index and the apnea plus hypopnea index. The mechanism for successful treatment of sleep apnea was attributed to alleviating upper airway resistance during sleep.[7]

SUGGESTED ACUPUNCTURE TREATMENT

1. Points: *Yuji* (LU 10), *Jianshi* (PC 5), *Quchi* (LI 11), *Neiting* (ST 44), *Tianshu* (ST 25), *Shangjuxu* (ST 37), *Weizhong* (BL 40), *Duanxue*, and *Tianping*.
2. Technique: sedation and bleeding.

Yuji (LU 10) and *Jianshi* (PC 5) clear heat in the upper *jiao*. *Quchi* (LI 11) and *Neiting* (ST 44) clear heat in the middle *jiao*. *Tianshu* (ST 25), *Shangjuxu* (ST 37), and bleeding on *Weizhong* (BL 40) clear heat in the lower *jiao*. *Duanxue* and *Tianping* are used to stop bleeding in horses and dogs, respectively.

AUTHORS' COMMENTS

San Huang Xie Xin Tang, when given in liquid form, can be used as a mouthwash for severe cases of gingivitis, stomatitis or glossitis in older animals when regular dental prophylaxis is contraindicated due to age and risk associated with anesthesia. In cats with chronic, painful stomatitis or gingivitis and anorexia, this formula, when used as a mouthwash, can bring relief in as little as two to three days. The mouthwash should be used at least twice daily for fastest relief. This formula is very bitter tasting and will need to be mixed with a small amount of honey in addition to water for successful administration.

San Huang Xie Xin Tang and *Huang Lian Jie Du Tang* (Coptis Decoction to Relieve Toxicity) both clear heat and eliminate toxins.

- *San Huang Xie Xin Tang*, with the addition of *Da Huang* (Radix et Rhizoma Rhei), has a purgative action in addition to its heat-clearing and detoxifying effects; therefore, it is more suitable for patients who have constipation caused by accumulation of heat and toxins.
- *Huang Lian Jie Du Tang* clears heat and eliminates toxins from all three *jiaos*.
- Both of these formulas can be used to treat severe bleeding disorders secondary to bacterial and viral disease by adding *Mu Dan Pi* (Cortex Moutan) and *Di Huang* (Radix Rehmanniae). If this combination therapy is required, the lowest dosage of each formula should be used initially and gradually increased only if no improvement is seen in two to six doses. It is highly recommended to use herbs and/or another formula to protect the middle *jiao* while using any of these formulas in combination.

Sān Huáng Xiè Xīn Tāng

(Three-Yellow Decoction to Sedate the Epigastrium)

References

1. *Zhong Yao Ming Fang Yao Li Yu Ying Yong* (Pharmacology and Applications of Famous Herbal Formulas), 1989; 139-141.
2. Lin WC, Tan TW. The role of gastric muscle relaxation in cytoprotection induced by San-Huang-Xie-Xin-Tang in rats. J Ethnopharmacol. 1994 Dec; 44(3):171-9.
3. Satoh K, Nagai F, Seto T, Yamauchi H. The effects of kampo-formulation and the constituting crude drugs, prescribed for the treatment of peptic ulcer on H,K-ATPase activity. Yakugaku Zasshi. 2001 Feb; 121(2):173-8.
4. *Guang Xi Zhong Yi Yao* (Guangxi Chinese Medicine and Herbology), 1985; 3(18).
5. *Yun Nan Zhong Yi Xue Yuan Xue Bao* (Journal of Yunnan University School of Medicine), 1996; 4:38.
6. *Xin Zhong Yi* (New Chinese Medicine), 1997; 6:46.
7. Hisanaga A, Saitoh O, Fukuda H, Kurokawa K, Okabe A, Tachibana H, Hagino H, Mita T, Yamashita I, Tsutsumi M, Kurachi M, Itoh T. Treatment of obstructive sleep apnea syndrome with a Kampo-formula, San'o-shashin-to: a case report. Psychiatry & Clinical Neurosciences. 1999 Apr; 53(2):303-5.

Section 5

清脏腑热剂
— Zang Fu-Clearing Formulas

Dǎo Chì Sǎn (Guide Out the Red Powder)

導赤散
导赤散

Pinyin Name: *Dao Chi San*
Literal Name: Guide Out the Red Powder
Alternate Names: *Tao Chih San*, Fire-Inducing Powder, Rehmannia and Akebia Formula
Original Source: *Xiao Er Yao Zheng Zhi Jue* (Craft of Medicinal Treatment for Childhood Disease Patterns) by Qian Yi in 1119

COMPOSITION

Mu Tong (Caulis Akebiae)	[6g]
Di Huang (Radix Rehmanniae)	[6g]
Gan Cao (Radix et Rhizoma Glycyrrhizae)	[6g]

DOSAGE / PREPARATION / ADMINISTRATION

The source text recommends to grind equal amounts of the ingredients into powder. Cook 9g of the powder with *Zhu Ye* (Herba Phyllostachys) in one large bowl of water until half of the liquid remains. Take the warm decoction after meals. Today, this formula may be prepared as a decoction with the doses suggested in brackets.

CHINESE THERAPEUTIC ACTIONS

1. Clears the Heart and nourishes yin
2. Promotes urination and relieves *lin zheng* (dysuria syndrome)

CLINICAL MANIFESTATIONS

Excess fire in the Heart channel: restlessness, irritability, thirst, desire to drink cold water, and mouth and tongue ulcerations. If the heat migrates from the Heart to the Small Intestine channel, dark-colored urine, hematuria or dysuria will occur.

VETERINARY CLINICAL APPLICATIONS

Idiopathic hematuria, dysuria, urethritis, cystitis, glomerulonephritis and gingivitis-stomatitis.

EXPLANATION

Dao Chi San (Guide Out the Red Powder) is a representative formula for treating excess fire in the Heart and Small Intestine channels. The Heart is the organ that houses the mind. If the Heart is attacked by heat, restlessness and irritability will develop. The desire to drink cold water results from an exuberance of heat traveling upwards. The tongue is the sensory organ of the Heart; therefore, excess fire in the Heart channel may cause mouth and tongue ulcerations. The Small Intestine has a yin/yang, exterior/interior relationship with the Heart; consequently, heat in the Heart may migrate to and affect the Small Intestine. As a result, urination disorders such as dysuria, dark-colored urine, or hematuria occur.

To effectively treat this heat syndrome, the Heart fire must be cleared and urination promoted to guide the heat downward and out of the body. The chief herb in this formula, *Mu Tong* (Caulis Akebiae) sedates Heart fire, promotes urination to lead heat out of the body, and relieves dysuria. *Di Huang* (Radix Rehmanniae) clears heat and nourishes yin. Together, they clear heat without damaging yin, and nourish yin without retaining heat. *Zhu Ye* (Herba Phyllostachys) clears Heart fire and relieves restlessness and irritability. *Gan Cao* (Radix et Rhizoma Glycyrrhizae) clears heat, eliminates toxins, and prevents

Dǎo Chì Sǎn (Guide Out the Red Powder)

***Dao Chi San* (Guide Out the Red Powder)**

Diagnosis	Clinical Signs	Treatment	Herbs
Excess fire in the Heart and/or Small Intestine channels	• Restlessness and irritability: heat attacking Heart and disturbing *shen* (spirit) • Thirst with a desire to drink cold water: heat consuming body fluids • Red mouth and tongue ulcerations: excess fire rising upward • Hematuria and dysuria with dark-colored urine: excess fire affecting the Heart and Small Intestine	• Clears the Heart and nourishes yin • Promotes urination and relieves *lin zheng* (dysuria syndrome)	• *Mu Tong* (Caulis Akebiae) sedates fire from the Heart and Small Intestine. • *Di Huang* (Radix Rehmanniae) clears heat and nourishes yin. • *Zhu Ye* (Herba Phyllostachys) clears Heart fire and relieves fidgeting and irritability. • *Gan Cao* (Radix et Rhizoma Glycyrrhizae) clears heat and eliminates toxins

the cold tendency of *Di Huang* (Radix Rehmanniae) and *Mu Tong* (Caulis Akebiae) from injuring the Stomach.

VETERINARY MODIFICATIONS

- With irritability and heat in the chest, add *Huang Lian* (Rhizoma Coptidis) and *Huang Qin* (Radix Scutellariae).
- For *xue lin* (bloody dysuria), add *Mo Han Lian* (Herba Ecliptae), *Xiao Ji* (Herba Cirsii), *Hou Po* (Cortex Magnoliae Officinalis), and *Qu Mai* (Herba Dianthi).
- For *re lin* (heat dysuria) characterized by frequent and painful urination, add *Feng Wei Cao* (Herba Pteris), *Bai Mao Gen* (Rhizoma Imperatae), *Shi Wei* (Folium Pyrrosiae), *Che Qian Zi* (Semen Plantaginis), and *Chi Fu Ling* (Poria Rubra).
- With fever and thirst, add *Hua Shi* (Talcum) and *Shi Gao* (Gypsum Fibrosum).
- With stomatitis and ulcerations in the mouth, add *Jin Yin Hua* (Flos Lonicerae Japonicae), *Lian Qiao* (Fructus Forsythiae), and *Huang Lian* (Rhizoma Coptidis).
- When there is cystitis, add *Huang Qin* (Radix Scutellariae), *Deng Xin Cao* (Medulla Junci), and *Zhi Zi* (Fructus Gardeniae).

CAUTIONS / CONTRAINDICATIONS

- *Dao Chi San* should be used with caution in patients with Stomach and Spleen deficiencies because most herbs in this formula are cold and may damage the digestive tract.
- This formula may not be appropriate for individuals with recurrent stomatitis.
- Avoid foods that are pungent, spicy, oily or greasy while taking this herbal formula.[1]

HUMAN CLINICAL STUDIES AND RESEARCH

1. **Urinary tract infection**: In one clinical trial, 95 out of 100 patients with urinary tract infection were treated successfully with *Dao Chi San*. Five women who did not respond were later determined to have mycotic infection.[2]
2. ***Lin zheng* (dysuria syndrome)**: Administration of modified *Dao Chi San* to 14 patients with *lin zheng* (dysuria syndrome) was associated with complete recovery in 10 cases, improvement in 2 cases, and no effect in 2 cases. The herbal treatment contained *Dao Chi San* plus *Jin Yin Hua* (Flos Lonicerae Japonicae), *Tu Fu Ling* (Rhizoma Smilacis Glabrae), *Dan Zhu Ye* (Herba Lophatheri), and *Zhi Zi* (Fructus Gardeniae) as the base formula, with the addition of *Qing Hao* (Herba Artemisiae Annuae) and *Chai Hu* (Radix Bupleuri) for fever; *Huo Xiang* (Herba Agastaches) and *Ban Xia* (Rhizoma Pinelliae) for nausea and vomiting; *Bai Mao Gen* (Rhizoma Imperatae) and a larger dose of *Zhi Zi* (Fructus Gardeniae) for hematuria; and *Che Qian Zi* (Semen Plantaginis) for edema.[3]
3. **Oral herpes**: Thirty patients with stomatitis due to oral herpes were treated with modified *Dao Chi San* with marked success. The herbal treatment used *Dao Chi San* as the base formula, with the addition of *Huang Lian* (Rhizoma Coptidis) and *Mai Dong* (Radix Ophiopogonis) for irritability, thirst and red tongue tip; and *Da Huang* (Radix et Rhizoma Rhei) and *Huang Qin* (Radix Scutellariae) for constipation. Out of 30 cases, the study reported marked improvement in 20 cases (within 2 days), moderate improvement in 8 cases (within 3 days), and no improvement in 2 cases.[4]
4. **Infectious parotitis**: Twenty-four patients with infectious parotitis (mumps) were treated with an herbal decoction with complete recovery in all cases. The herbal formula incorporated *Dao Chi San* with *Lian Qiao* (Fructus Forsythiae), *Huang Bo* (Cortex Phellodendri Chinensis), *Zhi Mu* (Rhizoma Anemarrhenae), *Hua Shi* (Talcum), *Ban Lan Gen* (Radix Isatidis), *Da Qing Ye* (Folium Isatidis), *Jin Yin Hua* (Flos Lonicerae Japonicae), *Dan Zhu Ye* (Herba Lophatheri), and *Zhi Zi* (Fructus Gardeniae). The duration of treatment ranged from 1 to 4 packs of herbs.[5]

Dăo Chì Săn (Guide Out the Red Powder)

SUGGESTED ACUPUNCTURE TREATMENT

1. Points: For excess heat in the Heart channel: *Zhongchong* (PC 9), *Waiguan* (TH 5), and *Hegu* (LI 4). For transmission of heat to the Small Intestine: *Pangguangshu* (BL 28), *Zhongji* (CV 3), *Yinlingquan* (SP 9), *Xingjian* (LR 2), and *Taixi* (KI 3).
2. Technique: sedation.

Zhongchong (PC 9) and *Waiguan* (TH 5) clear Heart fire. *Hegu* (LI 4) clears heat and eliminates toxins. *Pangguangshu* (BL 28) and *Zhongji* (CV 3) regulate urination and dispel heat according to the *shu* (transport) and *mu* (collecting) points principles. *Yinlingquan* (SP 9) helps regulate water circulation and urination. *Xingjian* (LR 2) sedates the Liver and relieves pain. *Taixi* (KI 3) nourishes yin and clears heat.

AUTHORS' COMMENTS

The key clinical signs that indicate the use of *Dao Chi San* include painful urination, hematuria, and ulcerations or sores in the mouth, especially on the tongue. These symptoms indicate that the heat in the Heart has transferred to the Small Intestine, thereby causing urinary dysfunction.

Dao Chi San is used to treat hematuria from Heart fire which empties into the Small Intestine and then into the Bladder resulting in hematuria. This condition can develop in cats with a fire constitution and that are under chronic stress. The most common causes of stress in cats are complete indoor confinement and living in a household with multiple cats. Chronic stress leads to Liver qi stagnation, which eventually turns to fire and then subsequently invades the Heart. The heat or fire flares upwards to cause ulceration of the tongue and mouth, and can also move downwards through the channels to the Small Intestine. The fire is transmitted to the Urinary Bladder, scorching the bladder walls and vasculature and causing bleeding with hematuria. This condition will not resolve unless the root cause is treated. These cats are often fractious and demonstrate significant anxiety; the tongue may be dark red to purple. The urine is often sterile and no crystals are seen. For the treatment of this condition, *Dao Chi San* is rarely used alone and is often combined with *Qing Xin Lian Zi Yin* (Lotus Seed Decoction to Clear the Heart).

Chronic Heart fire can lead to weakness of the Urinary Bladder and Kidney, and, over time, contribute to the development of urinary tract infection (UTI). This formula will require modification to improve its heat-clearing ability to treat UTI, and may be combined with *Ba Zheng San* (Eight-Herb Powder for Rectification) for this purpose. This condition is promoted and exacerbated by feeding a species inappropriate diet to cats, which are obligatory carnivores but often fed dry kibble diets high in processed grains and carbohydrates.

References

1. *Zhong Yao Ming Fang Yao Li Yu Ying Yong* (Pharmacology and Applications of Famous Herbal Formulas), 1989; 185-186.
2. *Guang Xi Zhong Yi Yao* (Guangxi Chinese Medicine and Herbology), 1991; (3):104.
3. *Cheng Du Zhong Yi Xue Yuan Xue Bao* (Journal of Chengdu University of Traditional Chinese Medicine), 1989; 2:29.
4. *Nan Jing Zhong Yi Xue Yuan Xue Bao* (Journal of Nanjing University of Traditional Chinese Medicine), 1984; 4(2):90.
5. *Shan Xi Zhong Yi* (Shanxi Chinese Medicine), 1991; (8):368.

Qīng Xīn Lián Zǐ Yǐn (Lotus Seed Decoction to Clear the Heart)

清心蓮子飲

清心莲子饮

Pinyin Name: *Qing Xin Lian Zi Yin*

Literal Name: Lotus Seed Decoction to Clear the Heart

Alternate Names: *Ching Hsin Lien Tzu Yin, Ching Xin Lian Zi Yin*, Lotus Seed Drink, Lotus Seed Combination

Original Source: *Tai Ping Hui Min He Ji Ju Fang* (Imperial Grace Formulary of the Tai Ping Era) by the Imperial Medical Department in 1078-85

COMPOSITION

Lian Zi (Semen Nelumbinis)	22.5g [15g]
Mai Dong (Radix Ophiopogonis)	15g [10g]
Huang Qin (Radix Scutellariae)	15g [10g]
Di Gu Pi (Cortex Lycii)	15g [10g]
Fu Ling (Poria)	22.5g [15g]
Che Qian Zi (Semen Plantaginis)	15g [10g]
Huang Qi (Radix Astragali), *mi zhi* (fried with honey)	22.5g [15g]
Ren Shen (Radix et Rhizoma Ginseng)	22.5g [15g]
Zhi Gan Cao (Radix et Rhizoma Glycyrrhizae Praeparata cum Melle)	15g [10g]

DOSAGE / PREPARATION / ADMINISTRATION

The source text states to grind the ingredients into powder. Cook 9g of the powder in 1.5 large bowl of water until 80% of the liquid remains. Cool the strained decoction and take it before meals on an empty stomach. Today, this formula may be prepared as a decoction with the doses suggested in brackets.

CHINESE THERAPEUTIC ACTIONS

1. Clears Heart fire
2. Tonifies qi and yin
3. Treats *lin zheng* (dysuria syndrome)

CLINICAL MANIFESTATIONS

Heart fire with qi and yin deficiencies and damp-heat in the lower *jiao*: irritability, restlessness, noise hypersensitivity, a dry mouth and tongue, fever, depression, dysuria, and chronic vaginal discharge.

VETERINARY CLINICAL APPLICATIONS

Behavioral disorder characterized by pacing at night, noise hypersensitivity, irritability and restlessness, nephrotic syndrome, chronic glomerulonephritis, chronic urinary tract infection, and urinary pain and difficulty from exhaustion and fatigue secondary to any of the following: overwork and/or over-breeding, cancer, surgery, chemotherapy, radiation, or as a result of chronic disease.

EXPLANATION

Qing Xin Lian Zi Yin (Lotus Seed Decoction to Clear the Heart) treats Heart fire with qi and yin deficiencies and damp-heat in the lower *jiao*. This complicated condition is often due to excessive stress, lack of exercise, and can follow any chronic long-term disorder where internal heat has been engendered. As a result of stress, physical overexertion, over breeding, or following chronic disease, there is excess heat and fire disturbing the Heart and a

***Qing Xin Lian Zi Yin* (Lotus Seed Decoction to Clear the Heart)**

Diagnosis	Clinical Signs	Treatment	Herbs
Heart fire with qi and yin deficiencies and damp-heat in the lower *jiao*	• Noise hypersensitivity, irritability, restlessness, and depression: Heart fire • Abnormal genitourinary functions: Kidney yin deficiency	• Clears Heart fire • Tonifies qi and yin • Treats *lin zheng* (dysuria syndrome)	• *Lian Zi* (Semen Nelumbinis) and *Mai Dong* (Radix Ophiopogonis) clear heat and fire from the Heart. • *Huang Qin* (Radix Scutellariae) and *Di Gu Pi* (Cortex Lycii) clear heat and relieve thirst. • *Fu Ling* (Poria) and *Che Qian Zi* (Semen Plantaginis) dispel damp-heat and promote normal urination. • *Huang Qi* (Radix Astragali), *Ren Shen* (Radix et Rhizoma Ginseng) and *Zhi Gan Cao* (Radix et Rhizoma Glycyrrhizae Praeparata cum Melle) tonify qi and facilitate recovery.

depletion of Kidney yin, leading to excess above and deficiency below with symptoms such as irritability, restlessness, depression, and abnormal genitourinary functions.

Lian Zi (Semen Nelumbinis) and *Mai Dong* (Radix Ophiopogonis) clear heat and fire from the Heart. *Huang Qin* (Radix Scutellariae) and *Di Gu Pi* (Cortex Lycii) clear heat and relieve thirst. *Fu Ling* (Poria) and *Che Qian Zi* (Semen Plantaginis) dispel damp-heat and promote normal urination. *Huang Qi* (Radix Astragali), *Ren Shen* (Radix et Rhizoma Ginseng), and *Zhi Gan Cao* (Radix et Rhizoma Glycyrrhizae Praeparata cum Melle) tonify qi and facilitate recovery.

VETERINARY MODIFICATIONS

- With prominent fire and severe deficiency, add *Zhi Mu* (Rhizoma Anemarrhenae) and *Huang Bo* (Cortex Phellodendri Chinensis).
- With fever, add *Chai Hu* (Radix Bupleuri) and *Bo He* (Herba Menthae).

CAUTIONS / CONTRAINDICATIONS

Qing Xin Lian Zi Yin is contraindicated in *lin zheng* (dysuria syndrome) or vaginitis caused by damp-heat in the Liver and Gallbladder.

PHARMACOLOGICAL EFFECTS

Hypoglycemic: According to a clinical study, administration of *Qing Xin Lian Zi Yin* was associated with a reduction of blood glucose level in patients with non-insulin dependant diabetes mellitus (NIDDM). Out of 20 patients who participated in the study, 84.2% showed a positive effect.[1]

HUMAN CLINICAL STUDIES AND RESEARCH

1. **Diabetes mellitus**: Administration of *Qing Xin Lian Zi Yin* was shown to be effective in the treatment of type II diabetes mellitus. The treatment protocol was to administer 10g of this formula in pills three times daily before meals, for 30 days per course of treatment. Of 50 cases, the study reported significant results in 21 cases, moderate results in 18 cases, and no effect in 11 cases.[2]
2. **Nephrotic syndrome**: One study reported good results using modified *Qing Xin Lian Zi Yin* to treat patients with nephrotic syndrome characterized by Kidney yin deficiency, Lung and Spleen qi deficiencies, and deficiency fire. The herbal formula contained *Di Gu Pi* (Cortex Lycii) 25g, *Huang Qin* (Radix Scutellariae) 15g, *Di Huang* (Radix Rehmanniae) 15g, *Tai Zi Shen* (Radix Pseudostellariae) 15g, *Huang Qi* (Radix Astragali) 15g, *Che Qian Zi* (Semen Plantaginis) 15g, *Mai Dong* (Radix Ophiopogonis) 12g, *Fu Ling* (Poria) 12g, *Chai Hu* (Radix Bupleuri) 10g, *Shan Zhu Yu* (Fructus Corni) 10g, *Bai Mao Gen* (Rhizoma Imperatae) 30g, *Shi Wei* (Folium Pyrrosiae) 30g, and *Gan Cao* (Radix et Rhizoma Glycyrrhizae) 6g. Additional modifications were made as needed based on the condition of the patients. The herbs were given for approximately six months to stabilize the condition.[3]
3. **Glomerulonephritis**: Administration of modified *Qing Xin Lian Zi Yin* was found to be effective in treating acute glomerulonephritis, characterized by Kidney qi and yin deficiencies accompanied by yin-deficient fire. The herbal formula contained *Di Gu Pi* (Cortex Lycii) 15g, *Huang Qin* (Radix Scutellariae) 10g, *Mai Dong* (Radix Ophiopogonis) 10g, *Lian Zi Xin* (Plumula Nelumbinis) 6g, *Gan Cao* (Radix et Rhizoma Glycyrrhizae) 6g, *Bai Mao Gen* (Rhizoma Imperatae) 30g, *Huang Qi* (Radix Astragali) 12g, *Che Qian Zi* (Semen Plantaginis) 12, *Shi Wei* (Folium Pyrrosiae) 20g, *Da Ji* (Herba Cirsii Japonici) 20g, and *Xiao Ji* (Herba Cirsii) 20g. The herbs were administered in decoction daily for approximately 5 months. Improvements were noted in most patients after about 15 packs of herbs. Clinical improvement included relief of night perspiration, improved appetite, improved sleeping pattern, and reduced number of cells in the urine. After the condition stabilized, the patients were then given *Liu Wei Di Huang Wan* (Six-Ingredient Pill with Rehmannia) for further consolidation.[4]
4. **Pyelonephritis**: One study reported success using modified *Qing Xin Lian Zi Yin* to treat pyelonephritis characterized by Heart and Kidney yin deficiencies with damp-heat affecting the Urinary Bladder. The herbal formula contained *Di Gu Pi* (Cortex Lycii) 15g, *Che Qian Zi* (Semen Plantaginis) 15g, *Bai He* (Bulbus Lilii) 15g, *Huang Qin* (Radix Scutellariae) 15g, *Mai Dong* (Radix Ophiopogonis) 12g, *Lian Zi* (Semen Nelumbinis) 12g, *Fu Ling* (Poria) 12g, *Bai Wei* (Radix et Rhizoma Cynanchi Atrati) 12g, *Pu Gong Ying* (Herba Taraxaci) 30g, *Huang Qi* (Radix Astragali) 20g, and *Yi Yuan San* (Benefit the Basal Powder) 18g. The above herbs were cooked in water and the decoction was taken daily, for 50 packs of herbs. The study reported normalization of all signs and symptoms, with no recurrence in follow-up exams.[5]

SUGGESTED ACUPUNCTURE TREATMENT

1. Points: *Tongli* (HT 5), *Daling* (PC 7), *Zhongji* (CV 3), *Ciliao* (BL 32), *Qihai* (CV 6), and *Housanli* (ST 36).
2. Technique: sedation and tonification.

Sedate *Tongli* (HT 5) and *Daling* (PC 7) to clear Heart fire and deficiency heat. Sedate *Zhongji* (CV 3) and *Ciliao* (BL 32) to dispel damp-heat and promote urination. Tonify *Qihai* (CV 6) and *Housanli* (ST 36) to tonify and regulate qi.

Qīng Xīn Lián Zǐ Yǐn (Lotus Seed Decoction to Clear the Heart)

AUTHORS' COMMENTS

Qing Xin Lian Zi Yin has a wide range of applications in veterinary medicine:

- For behavioral disorder in dogs with yin deficiency and heat, this formula can be combined with *Zhi Bai Di Huang Wan* (Anemarrhena, Phellodendron, and Rehmannia Pill).
- With deficiency of the Heart and Liver, it may be combined with *Suan Zao Ren Tang* (Sour Jujube Decoction).
- For aggression, combine with *Jia Wei Xiao Yao San* (Augmented Rambling Powder).
- For behavioral problems related to Heart fire in horses, combine with *Zhi Gan Cao Tang* (Honey-Fried Licorice Decoction) or *Tian Wang Bu Xin Dan* (Emperor of Heaven's Special Pill to Tonify the Heart).
- For hyperthyroidism and chronic renal disease in cats with extreme irritability and restlessness with a red tongue and no coating, it can be combined with *Zhi Bai Di Huang Wan* (Anemarrhena, Phellodendron, and Rehmannia Pill).
- For treatment of idiopathic hematuria in cats or dogs, it can be combined with *Dao Chi San* (Guide Out the Red Powder).

References

1. *Guo Wai Yi Xue* (Foreign Medicine), 1993; (4):36.
2. *Shi Yong Zhong Xi Yi Jie He Za Zhi* (Practical Journal of Integrated Chinese and Western Medicines), 1998; 6:523.
3. *Shan Xi Zhong Yi* (Shanxi Chinese Medicine), 1998; 4:173.
4. *Shan Xi Zhong Yi* (Shanxi Chinese Medicine), 1998; 4:173.
5. *Shan Xi Zhong Yi* (Shanxi Chinese Medicine), 1998; 4:173.

Lóng Dǎn Xiè Gān Tāng (Gentiana Decoction to Drain the Liver)

龍膽瀉肝湯
龙胆泻肝汤

Pinyin Name: *Long Dan Xie Gan Tang*
Literal Name: Gentiana Decoction to Drain the Liver
Alternate Names: *Lung Tan Hsieh Kan Tang*, Gentiana Liver-Draining Decoction (Pill), Gentiana Liver-Purging Decoction (Pill), Gentiana Combination
Original Source: *Yi Fang Ji Jie* (Analytical Collection of Medical Formulas) by Wang Ang in 1682

COMPOSITION

Long Dan (Radix et Rhizoma Gentianae), *chao* (dry-fried) with liquor	[6g]
Huang Qin (Radix Scutellariae), *chao* (dry-fried)	[9g]
Zhi Zi (Fructus Gardeniae), *chao* (dry-fried) with liquor	[9g]
Ze Xie (Rhizoma Alismatis)	[12g]
Mu Tong (Caulis Akebiae)	[9g]
Che Qian Zi (Semen Plantaginis)	[9g]
Di Huang (Radix Rehmanniae), *chao* (dry-fried) with liquor	[9g]
Dang Gui (Radix Angelicae Sinensis), *xi* (washed) with liquor	[3g]
Chai Hu (Radix Bupleuri)	[6g]
Gan Cao (Radix et Rhizoma Glycyrrhizae)	[6g]

Lóng Dǎn Xiè Gān Tāng (Gentiana Decoction to Drain the Liver)

DOSAGE / PREPARATION / ADMINISTRATION

The source text states to prepare the ingredients as a decoction. Note: Doses of herbs are unavailable from the source text. Suggested doses, however, are listed above in brackets.

CHINESE THERAPEUTIC ACTIONS

1. Purges excess fire in the Liver and Gallbladder
2. Clears damp-heat in the lower *jiao*

CLINICAL MANIFESTATIONS

1. Flaring of excess fire in the Liver and Gallbladder: miliary lesions of the face, head and neck; red, swollen eyes; hypochondriac pain; red, swollen, itchy, painful ears with sticky, thick discharge that may be foul smelling.
2. Damp-heat in the lower *jiao*: inflammation and dermatitis of the paws; hot, red, moist dermatitis and pruritis of the lateral body surface and/or perianal and inguinal region; swollen, painful and abscessed anal glands; dysuria, hematuria and yellow vaginal discharge.
3. Red tongue, which may have a white to yellow coating in severe cases, and a rapid, forceful wiry to slippery pulse.

VETERINARY CLINICAL APPLICATIONS

Aggression, acute cholangiohepatitis in cats, acute pancreatitis, hypertension, acute icteric hepatitis, acute urethritis, acute cystitis, acute pyelonephritis, acute orchitis, acute prostatitis, acute mastitis, acute conjunctivitis, acute uveitis, episcleritis, acute glaucoma, acute otitis media, allergic dermatitis, food allergy dermatitis, feline miliary dermatitis, dermatitis, pododermatitis, anal gland sacculitis, perianal fistula, hyperthyroidism and feline eosinophilic granuloma complex.

EXPLANATION

Long Dan Xie Gan Tang (Gentiana Decoction to Drain the Liver) treats excess fire in the Liver and Gallbladder. When excess fire in the Liver channel travels upward, it produces painful eyes and ears. When excess fire follows the channel to the hypochondriac region, pain can occur. When damp-heat is present it follows the Liver channel downward to the lower *jiao* to cause inflammation of the paws and hot, red, moist dermatitis and pruritis of the lateral body surface, ventral abdomen, perianal and inguinal region. Patients may also present with swollen, painful or abscessed anal glands, dysuria, hematuria, and yellow vaginal discharge.

Long Dan (Radix et Rhizoma Gentianae), an extremely bitter and cold herb, sedates fire in the Liver and Gallbladder and clears damp-heat in the lower *jiao. Huang Qin* (Radix Scutellariae) and *Zhi Zi* (Fructus Gardeniae) help *Long Dan* (Radix et Rhizoma Gentianae) sedate fire and damp-heat in all three *jiaos*. To minimize the bitter and cold herbs in this formula from damaging the stomach, *Huang Qin* (Radix Scutellariae) is dry-fried, and *Long Dan* (Radix et Rhizoma Gentianae) and *Zhi Zi* (Fructus Gardeniae) are dry-fried with liquor. *Ze Xie* (Rhizoma Alismatis), *Mu Tong* (Caulis Akebiae), and *Che Qian Zi* (Semen Plantaginis) dispel damp-heat through the urine. In this syndrome, blood and yin may be consumed as a result of both the excess fire and the bitter, cold herbs

***Long Dan Xie Gan Tang* (Gentiana Decoction to Drain the Liver)**

Diagnosis	Clinical Signs	Treatment	Herbs
Excess fire in the Liver and Gallbladder	• Painful eyes and ears with yellow to black discharge: excess fire traveling upward along the Liver channel • Hypochondriac pain: excess fire traveling along the Liver channel • Inflammation of the paws; hot, red, moist dermatitis and pruritis of the lateral body surface, ventral abdomen, perianal and inguinal region; swollen, painful or abscessed anal glands; dysuria, hematuria and yellow vaginal discharge: damp-heat traveling downward to the lower *jiao* • Red tongue, which may have a white to yellow coating in severe cases, and a rapid, forceful wiry to slippery pulse	• Purges excess fire in the Liver and Gallbladder • Clears damp-heat in the lower *jiao*	• *Long Dan* (Radix et Rhizoma Gentianae) sedates fire in the Liver and Gallbladder and clears damp-heat in the lower *jiao.* • *Huang Qin* (Radix Scutellariae) and *Zhi Zi* (Fructus Gardeniae) sedate fire and damp-heat in all three *jiaos*. • *Ze Xie* (Rhizoma Alismatis), *Mu Tong* (Caulis Akebiae) and *Che Qian Zi* (Semen Plantaginis) dispel damp-heat through the urine. • *Di Huang* (Radix Rehmanniae) and *Dang Gui* (Radix Angelicae Sinensis) nourish and protect yin and blood. • *Chai Hu* (Radix Bupleuri) regulates Liver qi and guides the herbs to the Liver. • *Gan Cao* (Radix et Rhizoma Glycyrrhizae) harmonizes the formula.

Lóng Dǎn Xiè Gān Tāng (Gentiana Decoction to Drain the Liver)

in this formula; therefore *Di Huang* (Radix Rehmanniae) and *Dang Gui* (Radix Angelicae Sinensis) are added to nourish and protect yin and blood. *Chai Hu* (Radix Bupleuri) regulates Liver qi and guides all of the herbs to the Liver. *Gan Cao* (Radix et Rhizoma Glycyrrhizae) harmonizes the formula.

VETERINARY MODIFICATIONS

- With constipation, add *Da Huang* (Radix et Rhizoma Rhei) and *Mang Xiao* (Natrii Sulfas).
- With dysuria, add *Yin Chen* (Herba Artemisiae Scopariae) and *Fu Ling* (Poria).
- If there is acute glaucoma, add *Xuan Shen* (Radix Scrophulariae) and *Qiang Huo* (Rhizoma et Radix Notopterygii).
- With redness, swelling and pain of the eyes, add *Chuan Xiong* (Rhizoma Chuanxiong) and *Ju Hua* (Flos Chrysanthemi).
- With urinary tract infection, add *Bian Xu* (Herba Polygoni Avicularis), *Qu Mai* (Herba Dianthi), *Bai Mao Gen* (Rhizoma Imperatae), and *Lian Qiao* (Fructus Forsythiae).
- When there is more visual disturbance, add *Ju Hua* (Flos Chrysanthemi) and *Jue Ming Zi* (Semen Cassiae), or *Xi Gan Ming Mu San* (Wash the Liver and Brighten the Eyes Powder).
- When there is more dampness, remove *Huang Qin* (Radix Scutellariae) and *Di Huang* (Radix Rehmanniae), and add *Hua Shi* (Talcum) and *Yi Yi Ren* (Semen Coicis), or *Ba Zheng San* (Eight-Herb Powder for Rectification).
- With vaginitis and itching in the inguinal regions, use *She Chuang Zi* (Fructus Cnidii) and *Ku Shen* (Radix Sophorae Flavescentis) topically as a wash on the affected area.

CAUTIONS / CONTRAINDICATIONS

- *Long Dan Xie Gan Tang* should be used with caution in animals with deficiency and cold in the Spleen and Stomach, since this formula is cold and may injure the Spleen and Stomach to cause vomiting or diarrhea.
- This formula is contraindicated in patients with yang, yin, and/or blood deficiencies.
- This formula is not recommended for prolonged use and should not be used unless there are clear signs of heat and dampness in the Liver and Gallbladder. It should not be used for longer than 7-14 days without re-evaluation or modification. Once the desired therapeutic effect is achieved, it should be discontinued.

PHARMACOLOGICAL EFFECTS

1. **Antibiotic**: Decoction of *Long Dan Xie Gan Tang* was associated with marked antibacterial effects, especially against beta-hemolytic streptococcus.[1]
2. **Anti-inflammatory**: Oral administration of *Long Dan Xie Gan Tang* in decoction was associated with marked anti-inflammatory effects in mice, with maximum effect observed 4 to 6 hours after ingestion. The mechanism of action is attributed to an inhibitive effect on blood vessel permeability.[2]
3. **Immunostimulant**: Oral administration of *Long Dan Xie Gan Tang* decoction at 50 g/kg was associated with increased phagocytic activity in mice within 3-6 hours.[3]
4. **Antiallergic**: Oral administration of *Long Dan Xie Gan Tang* decoction at 10 g/kg for 2 days was effective in minimizing shock and death caused by severe allergic reaction.[4]
5. **Cardiovascular**: *Long Dan Xie Gan Tang* was associated with marked hypotensive effects in anesthetized cats. The mechanisms of action were attributed to its effect of lowering heart rate, decreasing force of heart contraction, and dilation of blood vessels.[5]

HUMAN CLINICAL STUDIES AND RESEARCH

1. **Hypertension**: In one study, modified *Long Dan Xie Gan Tang* was used to treat patients with hypertension with 88.89% effectiveness.[6] In another report, it was mentioned that *Long Dan Xie Gan Tang* is most effective for hypertension with headache, irritability, insomnia, thirst, a bitter taste in the mouth, dysuria, and a wiry, rapid pulse.[7] Lastly, 100 hypertensive patients characterized by Liver fire rising had good results when treated with a herbal formula that contained *Long Dan Xie Gan Tang* plus *Xia Ku Cao* (Spica Prunellae), *Jue Ming Zi* (Semen Cassiae), *Gou Teng* (Ramulus Uncariae cum Uncis), and others.[8]
2. **Hepatitis**: *Long Dan Xie Gan Tang* was shown in many studies to be effective in treating hepatitis. In one study, 32 patients with non-icteric hepatitis were treated with *Long Dan Xie Gan Tang* with complete recovery in 27 patients, some improvement in 4 patients, and no change in one patient.[9] In another study, 30 patients with icteric hepatitis were treated with *Long Dan Xie Gan Tang* with good results. The study reported improvement in most patients within 3-9 days, with jaundice resolving after 21.5 days and liver enzymes returning to normal after 30.8 days.[10] Lastly, one study of 40 patients with icteric jaundice reported 87.5% effectiveness using modified *Long Dan Xie Gan Tang* in decoction for 14 days per course of treatment.[11]
3. **Cholecystitis**: In one report, 8 patients with acute cholecystitis were treated with complete recovery in all patients using *Long Dan Xie Gan Tang* with the addition of *Ku Lian Pi* (Cortex Meliae) and *Da Huang* (Radix et Rhizoma Rhei).[12] Another study reported similar success using *Long Dan Xie Gan Tang* with the addition of *Yin Chen* (Herba Artemisiae Scopariae) and *Da Huang* (Radix et Rhizoma Rhei).[13] Lastly, 81 patients with acute cholecystitis were

treated with 96.2% effectiveness using *Long Dan Xie Gan Tang* plus *Yin Chen* (Herba Artemisiae Scopariae), *Chuan Lian Zi* (Fructus Toosendan), and *Da Huang* (Radix et Rhizoma Rhei).[14]

4. **Gastritis**: Forty-seven patients with gastritis (characterized by damp-heat in the Spleen and Stomach, or Liver and Stomach heat) were treated with *Long Dan Xie Gan Tang* with significant improvement in 14 patients, moderate improvement in 31 patients, and no effect in 2 patients.[15]
5. **Erythromatosis (SLE)**: Thirty-five patients with erythromatosis were treated with good results using *Long Dan Xie Gan Tang* plus *Zhi Qiao* (Fructus Aurantii) and *Da Huang* (Radix et Rhizoma Rhei). Patients were given herbs three times daily, for 5 days (with 2 days of rest) per week, for 4 weeks per course of treatment, for 3 courses total. Of 35 patients, the study reported complete recovery in 24 patients, improvement in 8 patients and no benefit in 3 patients.[16]
6. **Urinary tract infection**: Eight patients with acute or chronic urinary tract infection were treated with *Long Dan Xie Gan Tang* with complete recovery in 6 patients and improvement in 2 patients.[17] In another report, 52 patients with acute or chronic pyelonephritis were treated with *Long Dan Xie Gan Tang* with complete recovery in 48 patients and improvement in 4 patients. The average time for recovery was 6.9 days.[18]
7. **Leukemia**: The effectiveness of *Long Dan Xie Gan Tang* was evaluated for treating acute leukemia characterized by damp-heat of the Liver and Gallbladder. Out of 26 patients with leukemia, 14 had significant improvement, 10 had moderate improvement, and 2 had no effect. The rate of effectiveness was 92.3% for the treatment. The herbal treatment included *Long Dan Xie Gan Tang* plus *Xia Ku Cao* (Spica Prunellae), *Ban Zhi Lian* (Herba Scutellariae Barbatae), and *Bai Hua She She Cao* (Herba Hedyotis) as the base formula. Modifications included addition of *Wu Wei Xiao Du Yin* (Five-Ingredient Decoction to Eliminate Toxins) and *Huang Lian Jie Du Tang* (Coptis Decoction to Relieve Toxicity) for excess heat; and *Xiang Sha Liu Jun Zi Tang* (Six-Gentlemen Decoction with Aucklandia and Amomum) for gastrointestinal disturbances.[19]
8. **Hyperthyroidism**: Eighteen hyperthyroid patients with elevated T3 and T4 were treated with *Long Dan Xie Gan Tang* with significant improvement in 6 patients, moderate improvement in 11 patients, and no change in 1 patient.[20]
9. **Diabetes mellitus**: According to one study, 36 patients with diabetes mellitus characterized by obesity and elevated cholesterol and triglyceride levels were treated with modified *Long Dan Xie Gan Tang* with significant improvement in 28 patients, moderate improvement in 5 patients, and slight improvement in 3 patients. The treatment protocol was to administer the decoction twice daily. The herbal treatment included *Huang Lian* (Rhizoma Coptidis), *Huang Qin* (Radix Scutellariae), *Long Dan* (Radix et Rhizoma Gentianae), *Zhi Zi* (Fructus Gardeniae), *Ze Xie* (Rhizoma Alismatis), *Mu Tong* (Caulis Akebiae), *Che Qian Zi* (Semen Plantaginis), *Di Huang* (Radix Rehmanniae), *Chai Hu* (Radix Bupleuri), *Fang Ji* (Radix Stephaniae Tetrandrae), *Can Sha* (Faeces Bombycis), and *Lian Zi Xin* (Plumula Nelumbinis).[21]
10. **Orchitis**: In one study using modified *Long Dan Xie Gan Tang*, 36 patients with acute orchitis were treated with significant improvement in all patients. Modifications were made based on the individual conditions. For swelling and pain of the testicles, *Yan Hu Suo* (Rhizoma Corydalis) and *Chuan Lian Zi* (Fructus Toosendan) were added. For swelling and hardening of the testicles, *Di Huang* (Radix Rehmanniae) was removed, and *Ju He* (Semen Citri Reticulatae), *Tao Ren* (Semen Persicae) and *Hong Hua* (Flos Carthami) were added. For hematuria, *Hu Zhang* (Rhizoma et Radix Polygoni Cuspidati) and *Bai Mao Gen* (Rhizoma Imperatae) were added. For frequent urination with burning sensation and pain, *Huang Bo* (Cortex Phellodendri Chinensis) and *Shi Wei* (Folium Pyrrosiae) were added. For orchitis with prostatitis, *Fen Bi Xie* (Rhizoma Dioscoreae Hypoglaucae) and *Li Zhi He* (Semen Litchi) were added. For those with concurrent *lin zheng* (dysuria syndrome) and urethritis, *Gan Cao* (Radix et Rhizoma Glycyrrhizae) was removed and *Tu Fu Ling* (Rhizoma Smilacis Glabrae) and *Bi Yu San* (Jasper Powder) were added.[22] In another report, 12 patients with orchitis were treated with complete recovery in all patients using *Long Dan Xie Gan Tang* with *Chuan Lian Zi* (Fructus Toosendan), *Yan Hu Suo* (Rhizoma Corydalis), and *Li Zhi He* (Semen Litchi).[23]
11. **Prostatitis**: Forty-four patients with prostatitis characterized by damp-heat were treated with modified *Long Dan Xie Gan Tang* with complete recovery in 16 patients, significant improvement in 12 patients, moderate improvement in 13 patients, and no effect in 3 patients. The overall rate of effectiveness was 93.2%. The herbal treatment contained *Long Dan Xie Gan Tang* as the base formula, with the addition of *Bai Jiang Cao* (Herba cum Radice Patriniae), *Pu Gong Ying* (Herba Taraxaci) and a large dose of *Long Dan* (Radix et Rhizoma Gentianae) for damp-heat with a bitter taste in the mouth; *Ze Lan* (Herba Lycopi), *Ru Xiang* (Gummi Olibanum), *Tao Ren* (Semen Persicae) and *Chi Shao* (Radix Paeoniae Rubra) for hardening of the prostate; and *Yin Yang Huo* (Herba Epimedii) and *Fen Bi Xie* (Rhizoma Dioscoreae Hypoglaucae) for sexual dysfunction.[24] In another report, 30 patients with chronic prostatitis were treated with modified *Long Dan Xie Gan Tang* with complete recovery in 18 patients, significant improvement in 8 patients, moderate improvement in 2

Lóng Dăn Xiè Gān Tāng (Gentiana Decoction to Drain the Liver)

patients, and no benefit in 2 patients. The overall rate of effectiveness was 93.3%.[25]

12. **Mastitis**: Use of *Long Dan Xie Gan Tang* produced complete recovery in 92 of 100 patients with mastitis characterized by redness, swelling and pain. The treatment protocol was to cook the herbs in water, and drink the decoction in three equally-divided doses (approximately 50 mL per dose) daily for 7 days.[26]
13. **Otitis media**: Eighty-five patients with chronic pyogenic otitis media were treated with an overall 89% success rate using *Long Dan Xie Gan Tang* with the addition of *Xin Yi Hua* (Flos Magnoliae) and *Cang Er Zi* (Fructus Xanthii).[27] In another report, 22 patients with acute pyogenic otitis media were treated with complete recovery in 14 patients, improvement in 6 patients, and no effect in 2 patients.[28] Lastly, one study of 20 patients with chronic otitis media due to damp-heat in the Liver and Gallbladder channels reported complete recovery in all patients using *Long Dan Xie Gan Tang*. The herbs were administered three times daily for 10 days per course of treatment, for 1-2 courses total.[29]

TOXICOLOGY

In acute toxicology studies, oral administration of the formula in mice at 26 g/kg showed no adverse reactions other than a short-term decrease in spontaneous physical activities (activities without a stimulus). No mortality was reported. With intravenous injection, the LD_{50} was determined to be 72g/kg.[30]

SUGGESTED ACUPUNCTURE TREATMENT

1. Points: *Fengchi* (GB 20), *Baihui* (GV 20), *Ganshu* (BL 18), *Danshu* (BL 19), *Yanglingquan* (GB 34), *Xingjian* (LR 2), *Zuqiaoyin* (GB 44), and *Yinlingquan* (SP 9).
2. Technique: sedation.

Combine *Fengchi* (GB 20) and *Baihui* (GV 20) to clear heat in the Liver and Gallbladder and to calm Liver wind. *Ganshu* (BL 18) and *Danshu* (BL 19) are the *shu* (transport) points on the back for the Liver and Gallbladder and will help to clear heat from these channels. *Yanglingquan* (GB 34) and *Xingjian* (LR 2) sedate excess fire in the Liver and Gallbladder. *Zuqiaoyin* (GB 44) clears heat from Liver and Gallbladder and nourishes Liver yin. *Yinlingquan* (SP 9) sedates damp-heat.

AUTHORS' COMMENTS

Long Dan Xie Gan Tang is one of the most commonly used formulas in veterinary medicine. It treats a large number of conditions caused by excess fire and damp-heat in the Liver and Gallbladder. Damp-heat conditions commonly develop in dogs and cats from insufficient exercise, chronic stress, and overeating of highly processed dry food diets containing corn, wheat, soybean, chemical additives and preservatives. Disease can develop anywhere along the Liver and Gallbladder channels from head to tail. A Spleen tonic is frequently used with *Long Dan Xie Gan Tang* as Spleen-Stomach deficiency is commonly seen with Liver fire and damp-heat conditions. *Liu Jun Zi Tang* (Six-Gentlemen Decoction), *Xiang Sha Liu Jun Zi Tang* (Six-Gentlemen Decoction with Aucklandia and Amomum), or *Shen Ling Bai Zhu San* (Ginseng, Poria, and Atractylodes Macrocephala Powder) can be selected, depending on the case.

Long Dan Xie Gan Tang can be safely used with steroidal anti-inflammatory drugs and antibiotics for an enhanced therapeutic effect. Antibiotics are considered cold from an energetic standpoint and thus can damage the Spleen and Stomach. Therefore, close monitoring of the animal's condition is recommended if both Chinese and allopathic therapies are administered, and if gastrointestinal problems develop, concurrent use of a Spleen/Stomach tonic is recommended.

Long Dan Xie Gan Tang is not for long-term use: a typical course of treatment is 7-14 days. If there is no improvement in that time then the animal should be re-evaluated and another formula administered. This formula can be used for up to 3 months for the treatment of chronic skin conditions provided the dose is low and other formulas to tonify the Spleen and Stomach, blood, and yin are given as needed.

Long Dan Xie Gan Tang can be combined with other formulas to treat the following conditions:

- For various kinds of lower *jiao* infections, such as bladder infection, urethritis, acute urinary tract infection, or infectious vaginitis, add *Ba Zheng San* (Eight-Herb Powder for Rectification).
- For acute glomerulonephritis, add *Ba Zheng San* (Eight-Herb Powder for Rectification), *Shui Ding Xiang* (Herba Ludwigiae Prostratae) and *Xian Feng Cao* (Herba Bidentis).
- For chronic nephritis, add *Ba Wei Di Huang Wan* (Eight-Ingredient Pill with Rehmannia).
- For acute hepatitis with fever, and jaundice with more heat than dampness, add *Yin Chen Hao Tang* (Capillaris Combination).
- For acute hepatitis without fever, but jaundice with more dampness than heat, add *Yin Chen Wu Ling San* (Capillaris and Hoelen Five).
- For acute pancreatitis, combine with *Li Jun Zi Tang* (Six Gentlemen Decoction).

5 HEAT-CLEARING FORMULAS

Lóng Dǎn Xiè Gān Tāng (Gentiana Decoction to Drain the Liver)

- For otitis externa/media, combine with *Si Miao San* (Four Marvel Pill).
- For feline miliary dermatitis, combine with *Li Jun Zi Tang* (Six Gentlemen Decoction).
- For allergic dermatitis with pruritis, combine with *Xiao Feng San* (eliminate Wind Powder).
- For canine food allergic dermatitis, combine with *Shen Ling Bai Zhu* San (Ginseng, Poria and Atractylodes Powder).
- For plasma cell pododermatitis in the cat, combine with *Shen Tong Zhu Yu Tang* (Drive Out Blood Stasis from a Painful Body Decoction); if qi and blood are deficient, combine with *Ren Shen Yang Ying Tang* (Ginseng Decoction to Nourish the Nutritive Qi).
- For damp-heat pododermatitis, with dark red or purple paw pads from blood stagnation combine with *Shen Tong Zhu Yu Tong* (Drive Out Blood Stasis from a Painful Body Decoction); with non-healing ulcers, combine with *Dang Gui Shao Yao San* (Tangkuei and Peony Powder); with more dampness, add *Si Miao San* (Four Marvel Pill); with Spleen qi and blood deficiency, add *Ba Zhen Tang* (Eight Treasure Decoction).
- For Liver yang rising and aggression, use with *Tian Ma Gou Teng Yin* (Gastrodia and Uncaria Decoction).
- For feline hyperthyroidism caused by flaring of Kidney fire, add *Zhi Bai Di Huang Wan* (Anemarrhena, Phellodendron, and Rehmannia Pill).
- With acute glaucoma, add *Ma Bian Cao* (Herba Verbenae), *Qian Li Guang* (Herba Senecionis Scandens), *Hu Zhang* (Rhizoma et Radix Polygoni Cuspidati), *Hu Yao Huang* (Herba Leucas Mollissimae), and *Ba Zheng San* (Eight-Herb Powder for Rectification).
- With acute equine periodic ophthalmia, combine with *Ming Mu Di Huang Wan* (Improve Vision Pill with Rehmannia).

Long Dan Xie Gan Tang, which drains damp-heat, contains blood-tonifying herbs such as *Di Huang* (Radix Rehmanniae) and *Dang Gui* (Radix Angelicae Sinensis) for three main reasons:

- First, this formula treats excess fire flaring upward in the Liver and Gallbladder channels, leading to red and painful eyes, hypochondriac pain, and swelling of the ears. It contains *Long Dan* (Radix et Rhizoma Gentianae), *Huang Qin* (Radix Scutellariae), and *Zhi Zi* (Fructus Gardeniae) to sedate excess fire. Damp-drying herbs such as these are likely to injure yin and cause more flaring of excess heat and Liver fire. Therefore, *Di Huang* (Radix Rehmanniae) and *Dang Gui* (Radix Angelicae Sinensis) are needed to prevent the heat-clearing, damp-drying herbs from damaging yin and blood.
- Second, this formula contains *Che Qian Zi* (Semen Plantaginis), *Mu Tong* (Caulis Akebiae), and *Ze Xie* (Rhizoma Alismatis) to drain damp-heat in the lower *jiao* to treat genital and perianal itching, turbid urine, and yellow leukorrhea (vaginal discharge). To prevent these herbs from excessively draining dampness and injuring yin and blood, *Di Huang* (Radix Rehmanniae) and *Dang Gui* (Radix Angelicae Sinensis) are added.
- Third, *Chai Hu* (Radix Bupleuri) is used in this formula as a channel-guiding and qi-regulating herb to spread Liver qi. To prevent any possible excessive drying caused by *Chai Hu* (Radix Bupleuri), *Di Huang* (Radix Rehmanniae) and *Dang Gui* (Radix Angelicae Sinensis) are added.[31]

References

1. *Zhong Yao Yao Li Du Li Yu Lin Chuang* (Pharmacology, Toxicology and Clinical Applications of Chinese Herbs); 1991; (1):5.
2. *Zhong Yi Fang Ji Xian Dai Yan Jiu* (Modern Study of Medical Formulas in Traditional Chinese Medicine), 1997; 318-319.
3. *Zhong Yi Fang Ji Xian Dai Yan Jiu* (Modern Study of Medical Formulas in Traditional Chinese Medicine), 1997; 318-319.
4. *Zhong Yao Yao Li Du Li Yu Lin Chuang* (Pharmacology, Toxicology and Clinical Applications of Chinese Herbs); 1991; (1):5.
5. *Zhong Yi Fang Ji Xian Dai Yan Jiu* (Modern Study of Medical Formulas in Traditional Chinese Medicine), 1997; 320.
6. *Ke Yan Tong Xun* (Journal of Science and Research); 1983; (2):1.
7. *Jiang Xi Zhong Yi Yao* (Jiangxi Chinese Medicine and Herbology); 1959; (10):18.
8. *Nan Jing Zhong Yi Xue Yuan Xue Bao* (Journal of Nanjing University of Traditional Chinese Medicine), 1986; 1:20.
9. *Xin Yi Yao Xue Za Zhi* (New Journal of Medicine and Herbology); 1978; 10:49.
10. *Ke Yan Tong Xun* (Journal of Science and Research); 1983; (2):13.
11. *Jiang Xi Yi Xue Yuan Xue Bao* (Medical Journal of Jiangxi University of Medicine), 1998; 3:123.
12. *Zhong Yi Fang Ji Xian Dai Yan Jiu* (Modern Study of Medical Formulas in Traditional Chinese Medicine), 1997; 321.
13. *Nei Meng Gu Zhong Yi Yao* (Traditional Chinese Medicine and Medicinals of Inner Mongolia), 1987; 6(2):42.
14. *Ji Lin Zhong Yi Yao* (Jilin Chinese Medicine and Herbology), 1997; 2:32.
15. *Shang Hai Zhong Yi Za Zhi* (Shanghai Journal of Chinese Medicine), 1996; 6:38.
16. *Zhong Yi Za Zhi* (Journal of Chinese Medicine), 1982; 4:269.
17. *Ke Yan Tong Xun* (Journal of Science and Research); 1983; (2):1.
18. *Zhong Yi Fang Ji Xian Dai Yan Jiu* (Modern Study of Medical Formulas in Traditional Chinese Medicine), 1997; 321.
19. *Zhong Yi Za Zhi* (Journal of Chinese Medicine), 1980; 21(4):276.
20. *Ke Yan Tong Xun* (Journal of Science and Research); 1983; (2):1.
21. *Zhong Yi Yao Xue Bao* (Report of Chinese Medicine and Herbology), 1995; (4):45.
22. *Hei Long Jiang Zhong Yi Yao* (Heilongjiang Chinese Medicine and Herbology), 1988; (6):44.
23. *Zhong Yi Yao Yan Jiu* (Research of Chinese Medicine and Herbology), 1987; (4):39.
24. *Fu Jian Zhong Yi Yao* (Fujian Chinese Medicine and Herbology), 1990; 21(1):9.
25. *Liao Ning Zhong Yi Za Zhi* (Liaoning Journal of Chinese Medicine), 1991; (6):32.
26. *Shi Yong Zhong Xi Yi Jie He Za Zhi* (Practical Journal of Integrated Chinese and Western Medicines), 1992; 4:245.
27. *Yi Xue Qing Kuang Jiao Liu* (Medical Information Exchange), 1975; (7):52.

Lóng Dǎn Xiè Gān Tāng (Gentiana Decoction to Drain the Liver)

28. *Shang Hai Yi Yao Za Zhi* (Shanghai Journal of Medicine and Herbology), 1985; (3):31.
29. *Zhong Cheng Yao Yan Jiu* (Research of Chinese Patent Medicine), 1985; 8:43.
30. *Zhong Yi Fang Ji Xian Dai Yan Jiu* (Modern Study of Medical Formulas in Traditional Chinese Medicine), 1997; 320.
31. Wang MZ, et al. *Zhong Yi Xue Wen Da Ti Ku* (Questions and Answers on Traditional Chinese Medicine: Herbal Formulas).

Xǐ Gān Míng Mù Sǎn (Wash the Liver and Brighten the Eyes Powder)

洗肝明目散

Pinyin Name: *Xi Gan Ming Mu San*
Literal Name: Wash the Liver and Brighten the Eyes Powder
Alternate Name: Gardenia and Vitex Combination
Original Source: *Wan Bing Hui Chun* (Restoration of Health from the Myriad Diseases) by Gong Ting-Xian in 1587

COMPOSITION

Dang Gui Wei (Extremitas Radix Angelicae Sinensis)
Chi Shao (Radix Paeoniae Rubra)
Chuan Xiong (Rhizoma Chuanxiong)
Di Huang (Radix Rehmanniae)
Huang Lian (Rhizoma Coptidis)
Huang Qin (Radix Scutellariae)
Zhi Zi (Fructus Gardeniae)
Shi Gao (Gypsum Fibrosum)
Qiang Huo (Rhizoma et Radix Notopterygii)
Fang Feng (Radix Saposhnikoviae)
Jie Geng (Radix Platycodonis)
Jing Jie (Herba Schizonepetae)
Bo He (Herba Menthae)
Jue Ming Zi (Semen Cassiae)
Lian Qiao (Fructus Forsythiae)
Man Jing Zi (Fructus Viticis)
Ji Li (Fructus Tribuli)
Ju Hua (Flos Chrysanthemi)
Gan Cao (Radix et Rhizoma Glycyrrhizae)

DOSAGE / PREPARATION / ADMINISTRATION

Grind equal amounts of the herbs into powder, cook in water, and take the warm, strained decoction after meals.

CHINESE THERAPEUTIC ACTIONS

1. Dispels wind-heat
2. Clears Liver heat and fire

CLINICAL MANIFESTATIONS

Wind-heat attacking the eyes: redness, swelling and pain of the eyes.

VETERINARY CLINICAL APPLICATIONS

Infectious keratitis, iritis, glaucoma, and acute conjunctivitis.

Xǐ Gān Míng Mù Sǎn (Wash the Liver and Brighten the Eyes Powder)

EXPLANATION

Xi Gan Ming Mu San (Wash the Liver and Brighten the Eyes Powder) treats various types of acute eye problems characterized by wind-heat. The presence of wind-heat encourages the rise of Liver heat and fire. Because wind and heat tend to travel upward, they cause symptoms such as redness, swelling, and pain of the eyes.

Dang Gui Wei (Extremitas Radix Angelicae Sinensis), *Chi Shao* (Radix Paeoniae Rubra), *Chuan Xiong* (Rhizoma Chuanxiong), and *Di Huang* (Radix Rehmanniae) tonify the blood, as well as activate and promote the circulation of blood. *Huang Lian* (Rhizoma Coptidis), *Huang Qin* (Radix Scutellariae), *Zhi Zi* (Fructus Gardeniae), and *Shi Gao* (Gypsum Fibrosum) clear heat from the body. *Qiang Huo* (Rhizoma et Radix Notopterygii), *Fang Feng* (Radix Saposhnikoviae), *Jie Geng* (Radix Platycodonis), *Jing Jie* (Herba Schizonepetae) and *Bo He* (Herba Menthae) are all lifting herbs that clear wind and lead the effects of the other herbs to the head. *Jue Ming Zi* (Semen Cassiae), *Lian Qiao* (Fructus Forsythiae), *Man Jing Zi* (Fructus Viticis), *Ji Li* (Fructus Tribuli), and *Ju Hua* (Flos Chrysanthemi) clear heat from the Liver channel, and are excellent herbs for addressing various types of eye disorders. Lastly, *Gan Cao* (Radix et Rhizoma Glycyrrhizae) harmonizes the formula.

VETERINARY MODIFICATIONS

- If there is more tearing as a result of wind-heat, add *Xia Ku Cao* (Spica Prunellae) and *Xiang Fu* (Rhizoma Cyperi).
- With Liver fire, add *Long Dan* (Radix et Rhizoma Gentianae) and *Chai Hu* (Radix Bupleuri), and remove *Bo He* (Herba Menthae).

PHARMACOLOGICAL EFFECTS

Ocular: One study reported that administration of *Xi Gan Ming Mu San* and *Huang Lian Jie Du Tang* (Coptis Decoction to Relieve Toxicity) was associated with significantly suppressed ($P < 0.001$) elevation of aqueous flare induced by lipopolysaccharides in rabbits.[1]

SUGGESTED ACUPUNCTURE TREATMENT

1. Points: *Sanyinjiao* (SP 6), *Xuehai* (SP 10), *Ganshu* (BL 18), *Quchi* (LI 11), *Taiyang* (extra point), *Longhui*, *Fengchi* (GB 20), *Waiguan* (TH 5), *Guangming* (GB 37), *Zhongdu* (LR 6), *Taichong* (LR 3), *Chengqi* (ST 1), *Jingming* (BL 1) and *Jingshu* (equine eye *shu* (transport) point).
2. Technique: even method and bleeding.

Sanyinjiao (SP 6), *Xuehai* (SP 10), and *Ganshu* (BL 18) nourish and invigorate the blood; sedation on *Quchi* (LI 11) and bleeding on *taiyang* (extra point) and the ear apex clear heat; *Longhui*, *Fengchi* (GB 20), and *Waiguan* (TH 5) dispel wind and lead qi up to the head; *Guangming* (GB 37), *Zhongdu* (LR 6), *Taichong* (LR 3), *Chengqi* (ST 1), *Jingming* (BL 1) and *Jingshu* clear Liver heat and benefit the eyes.

***Xi Gan Ming Mu San* (Wash the Liver and Brighten the Eyes Powder)**

Diagnosis	Clinical Signs	Treatment	Herbs
Wind-heat attacking the eyes	Redness, swelling and pain of the eyes: wind-heat attacking the eyes	• Dispels wind-heat • Clears Liver heat and fire	• *Dang Gui Wei* (Extremitas Radix Angelicae Sinensis), *Chi Shao* (Radix Paeoniae Rubra), *Chuan Xiong* (Rhizoma Chuanxiong) and *Di Huang* (Radix Rehmanniae) tonify the blood and promote blood circulation. • *Huang Lian* (Rhizoma Coptidis), *Huang Qin* (Radix Scutellariae), *Zhi Zi* (Fructus Gardeniae) and *Shi Gao* (Gypsum Fibrosum) clear heat from the body. • *Qiang Huo* (Rhizoma et Radix Notopterygii), *Fang Feng* (Radix Saposhnikoviae), *Jie Geng* (Radix Platycodonis), *Jing Jie* (Herba Schizonepetae) and *Bo He* (Herba Menthae) dispel wind. • *Jue Ming Zi* (Semen Cassiae), *Lian Qiao* (Fructus Forsythiae), *Man Jing Zi* (Fructus Viticis), *Ji Li* (Fructus Tribuli) and *Ju Hua* (Flos Chrysanthemi) clear heat from the Liver channel. • *Gan Cao* (Radix et Rhizoma Glycyrrhizae) harmonizes the formula.

Xǐ Gān Míng Mù Sǎn (Wash the Liver and Brighten the Eyes Powder)

AUTHORS' COMMENTS

Xi Gan Ming Mu San (Wash the Liver and Brighten the Eyes Powder) is typically prescribed for short-term use in veterinary medicine to treat acute eye disorders that are characterized by wind-heat (infection). The treatment of corneal damage from cat scratch in the dog is included here. It can be used with topical ophthalmic, anti-inflammatory (steroidal) and antibiotic medications. After the acute clinical signs have resolved, it is typical to follow this formula with a constitutional formula such as *Qi Ju Di Huang Wan* (Lycium Fruit, Chrysanthemum, and Rehmannia Pill) or *Ming Mu Di Huang Wan* (Improve Vision Pill with Rehmannia). *Xi Gan Ming Mu San* can be used to treat acute glaucoma secondary to uveitis in combination with conventional medications, depending on the case.

Xi Gan Ming Mu San and *Ming Mu Di Huang Wan* (Improve Vision Pill with Rehmannia) both improve and brighten vision.

- *Xi Gan Ming Mu San* is generally used for acute infection and inflammation of the eyes, characterized by wind-heat attacking the eyes.
- *Ming Mu Di Huang Wan* is more applicable for chronic deterioration of the eyes due to aging, characterized by Liver and Kidney yin deficiencies.

Reference

1. Nagaki Y, Hayasaka S, Kadoi C, Matsumoto M, Nakamura N, Hayasaka Y. Effects of Orengedoku-to and Senkanmeimoku-to, traditional herbal medicines, on the experimental elevation of aqueous flare in pigmented rabbits. Am J Chin Med. 2001; 29(1):141-7.

Xiè Bái Sǎn (Drain the White Powder)

瀉白散

泻白散

Pinyin Name: *Xie Bai San*

Literal Name: Drain the White Powder

Alternate Names: *Xie Fei San* (Drain the Lung Powder), White-Draining Formula, Morus and Lycium Formula

Original Source: *Xiao Er Yao Zheng Zhi Jue* (Craft of Medicinal Treatment for Childhood Disease Patterns) by Qian Yi in 1119

COMPOSITION

Sang Bai Pi (Cortex Mori), *chao* (dry-fried)	30g [15g]
Di Gu Pi (Cortex Lycii)	30g [15g]
Zhi Gan Cao (Radix et Rhizoma Glycyrrhizae Praeparata cum Melle)	3g [3g]

DOSAGE / PREPARATION / ADMINISTRATION

The source text states to grind the ingredients into powder. Cook the herbs with one pinch of *Geng Mi* (Semen Oryzae) in two small bowls of water until the liquid is reduced to 70%. Take the decoction before meals. Today, this formula may be prepared as a decoction with the doses suggested in brackets.

CHINESE THERAPEUTIC ACTIONS

1. Clears heat and sedates the Lung
2. Stops coughing and relieves dyspnea

CLINICAL MANIFESTATIONS

Lung heat: coughing, tachypnea, dyspnea, a red tongue body, and a fine, rapid pulse.

VETERINARY CLINICAL APPLICATIONS

Pneumonia, bacterial bronchitis, kennel cough, epistaxis, and asthma.

EXPLANATION

Xie Bai San (Drain the White Powder) treats Lung heat with reversed flow of Lung qi. As heat and fire accumulate

Xiè Bái Săn (Drain the White Powder)

***Xie Bai San* (Drain the White Powder)**

Diagnosis	Clinical Signs	Treatment	Herbs
Coughing caused by Lung heat	• Coughing, tachypnea and dyspnea: Lung heat causing reversed flow of Lung qi • Red tongue: heat in the body • Rapid, fine pulse: heat damaging yin	• Clears heat and sedates the Lung • Stops coughing and relieves dyspnea	• *Sang Bai Pi* (Cortex Mori) sedates Lung fire, clears stagnant heat, and corrects the reversed flow of Lung qi. • *Di Gu Pi* (Cortex Lycii) clears Lung heat. • *Geng Mi* (Semen Oryzae) and *Zhi Gan Cao* (Radix et Rhizoma Glycyrrhizae Praeparata cum Melle) nourish and strengthen Lung and Stomach qi.

in the Lung, they disturb the normal flow of Lung qi and cause it to rise abnormally, leading to coughing, tachypnea and dyspnea. A red tongue body with a yellow coating suggests accumulation of heat in the body, while a fine, rapid pulse suggests that the heat has damaged yin.

Sang Bai Pi (Cortex Mori) sedates Lung fire, clears Lung heat, and corrects the reversed flow of Lung qi. *Di Gu Pi* (Cortex Lycii) helps clear Lung heat. *Geng Mi* (Semen Oryzae) and *Zhi Gan Cao* (Radix et Rhizoma Glycyrrhizae Praeparata cum Melle) nourish and strengthen Lung and Stomach qi.

VETERINARY MODIFICATIONS

- For cough caused by dry heat, add *Bei Mu* (Bulbus Fritillariae), *Gua Lou Pi* (Pericarpium Trichosanthis), *Sha Shen* (Radix Glehniae seu Adenophorae), and *Ku Xing Ren* (Semen Armeniacae Amarum).
- With cough and wheezing, add *Ku Xing Ren* (Semen Armeniacae Amarum) and *Jie Geng* (Radix Platycodonis).
- With qi deficiency, add *Ren Shen* (Radix et Rhizoma Ginseng) and *Huang Qi* (Radix Astragali).
- With yin-deficient heat, add *Qing Hao* (Herba Artemisiae Annuae), *Bie Jia* (Carapax Trionycis), and *Yin Chai Hu* (Radix Stellariae).
- When there is Lung abscess, add *Bei Mu* (Bulbus Fritillariae), *Zi Wan* (Radix et Rhizoma Asteris), *Jie Geng* (Radix Platycodonis), *Dang Gui* (Radix Angelicae Sinensis), and *Gua Lou Zi* (Semen Trichosanthis).
- With more heat in the Lung, add *Huang Qin* (Radix Scutellariae) and *Zhi Mu* (Rhizoma Anemarrhenae).

CAUTIONS / CONTRAINDICATIONS

Xie Bai San is contraindicated in cases of cough caused by wind-cold or deficiency and cold.

HUMAN CLINICAL STUDIES AND RESEARCH

1. **Cough**: One study reported beneficial results using modified *Xie Bai San* to treat children with chronic cough. The herbal treatment used *Xie Bai San* as the base formula, and added *Zi Su Zi* (Fructus Perillae) and *Kuan Dong Hua* (Flos Farfarae) for individuals who have dyspnea; *Ban Xia* (Rhizoma Pinelliae) for profuse phlegm; *Shan Zha* (Fructus Crataegi) for poor appetite; and *Dong Gua Zi* (Semen Benincasae) for constipation.[1]
2. **Whooping cough**: Modified *Xie Bai San* was used to treat 63 patients with whooping cough with most reporting improved symptoms within 4-8 packs of herbs.[2]
3. **Pneumonia**: Fifty-eight children with pneumonia and cough were treated with modified *Xie Bai San* with 96.5% effectiveness. The study reported complete recovery in 48 cases, improvement in 8 cases, and no effect in 2 cases. The herbal treatment contained *Sang Bai Pi* (Cortex Mori) 6g, *Di Gu Pi* (Cortex Lycii) 6g, *Sha Shen* (Radix Glehniae seu Adenophorae) 6g, *Mai Dong* (Radix Ophiopogonis) 6g, *Huang Qin* (Radix Scutellariae) 3g, *Ku Xing Ren* (Semen Armeniacae Amarum) 3g, *Tao Ren* (Semen Persicae) 3g, *Bai Bu* (Radix Stemonae) 3g, *Chuan Bei Mu* (Bulbus Fritillariae Cirrhosae) 3g, *Bai Qian* (Rhizoma et Radix Cynanchi Stauntonii) 3g, *Ban Xia* (Rhizoma Pinelliae) 3g, *Gan Cao* (Radix et Rhizoma Glycyrrhizae) 1g, and *Shan Ci Gu* (Pseudobulbus Cremastrae seu Pleiones) 1-1.5g.[3]
4. **Epistaxis**: One study reported good results using modified *Xie Bai San* to treat 20 patients with nosebleeds. Modifications included the addition of *Sha Shen* (Radix Glehniae seu Adenophorae), *Yu Zhu* (Rhizoma Polygonati Odorati), *Mai Dong* (Radix Ophiopogonis), and *Sang Ye* (Folium Mori) for Lung dryness with yin deficiency; *Huang Qin* (Radix Scutellariae) and *Di Huang* (Radix Rehmanniae) for Lung heat; *Da Huang* (Radix et Rhizoma Rhei) and *Huang Lian* (Rhizoma Coptidis) for Stomach fire; and *Xi Yang Shen* (Radix Panacis Quinquefolii) and *Di Huang* (Radix Rehmanniae) for qi and yin deficiencies. Of 20 patients, 13 had complete recovery and 7 showed improvement.[4]

Xiè Bái Săn (Drain the White Powder)

SUGGESTED ACUPUNCTURE TREATMENT

1. Points: *Hegu* (LI 4), *Dazhui* (GV 14), *Zhongfu* (LU 1), *Kongzui* (LU 6), *Shanzhong* (CV 17), *Taixi* (KI 3), and *Xingjian* (LR 2).
2. Technique: sedation.

Hegu (LI 4) and *Dazhui* (GV 14) disperse heat in the Lung. *Zhongfu* (LU 1) and *Kongzui* (LU 6) smooth the qi flow of the Lung to relieve wheezing. *Shanzhong* (CV 17) corrects the reversed flow of Lung qi. *Taixi* (KI 3) and *Xingjian* (LR 2) clear deficiency heat. *Feishu* (BL 13) and *Yunmen* (LU 2) can be added for severe wheezing.

RELATED FORMULA

Tíng Lì Dà Zăo Xiè Fèi Tāng
(Descurainia and Jujube Decoction to Drain the Lung)
葶藶大棗瀉肺湯
葶苈大枣泻肺汤
Pinyin Name: *Ting Li Da Zao Xie Fei Tang*
Literal Name: Descurainia and Jujube Decoction to Drain the Lung
Original Source: *Jin Gui Yao Lue* (Essentials from the Golden Cabinet) by Zhang Zhong-Jing in the Eastern Han Dynasty

Ting Li Zi (Semen Descurainiae seu Lepidii), *ao* (simmered) until yellow and *dao* (pounded) into the size of a bullet	[6-9g]
Da Zao (Fructus Jujubae)	12 pieces [4 pieces]

The source text instructs to first cook 12 pieces of *Da Zao* (Fructus Jujubae) in 3 cups [600 mL] of water and reduce it to 2 cups [400 mL]. Discard *Da Zao* (Fructus Jujubae), add *Ting Li Zi* (Semen Descurainiae seu Lepidii), and cook again until it is reduced to 1 cup [200 mL]. Take the decoction immediately. Today, the decoction may be prepared using the doses suggested in brackets.

Ting Li Da Zao Xie Fei Tang (Descurainia and Jujube Decoction to Drain the Lung) primarily sedates the Lung, regulates water, corrects the reversed flow of Lung qi, and relieves dyspnea. Clinically, it is commonly used for coughing and dyspnea with chest fullness and profuse phlegm and saliva.

Xie Bai San and *Ting Li Da Zao Xie Fei Tang* (Descurainia and Jujube Decoction to Drain the Lung) both drain the Lung.

- *Xie Bai San* drains the Lung to relieve coughing caused by interior heat.
- *Ting Li Da Zao Xie Fei Tang* drains the Lung and relieves coughing caused by the accumulation of phlegm and water. This formula is used most often in the treatment of pulmonary edema and congestive heart failure in the dog and cat with Heart and Kidney deficiencies, in combination with *Zhen Wu Tang* (True Warrior Decoction).

AUTHORS' COMMENTS

Xie Bai San, literally meaning "Drain the White Powder," functions to drain heat from the Lung – the organ associated with the color white according to five elements theory.

Xie Bai San is a representative formula for treating cough caused by Lung heat. However, a question is sometimes raised that if *Xie Bai San* is formulated to sedate the Lung, why does the formula use *Sang Bai Pi* (Cortex Mori) and *Di Gu Pi* (Cortex Lycii), and not *Shi Gao* (Gypsum Fibrosum) and *Huang Qin* (Radix Scutellariae), to clear heat? Derived from the text *Xiao Er Yao Zheng Zhi Jue* (Craft of Medicinal Treatment for Childhood Disease Patterns), *Xie Bai San* was originally designed for children with Lung heat manifesting in both cough and dyspnea. *Huang Qin* (Radix Scutellariae) was not used because it can dry and damage yin in the process of clearing heat. *Shi Gao* (Gypsum Fibrosum) was also not selected because it is too strong for children's delicate internal organs. In contrast, *Sang Bai Pi* (Cortex Mori) and *Di Gu Pi* (Cortex Lycii) are more suitable, since they gently clear Lung heat and sedate Lung fire.[5]

Xie Bai San and *Ma Huang Xing Ren Gan Cao Shi Gao Tang* (Ephedra, Apricot Kernel, Licorice, and Gypsum Decoction) both clear Lung heat to relieve cough and wheezing, but have the following differences:

- *Xie Bai San* is designed for juvenile, geriatric and debilitated animals that have accumulation of heat and fire in the Lung, leading to qi reversal and gradual body fluid depletion. Aside from cough and wheezing, accompanying symptoms include yin-deficient heat and a fine, rapid pulse. Because the *zang fu* organs in young, old, and chronically ill animals are tender and/or deficient, they are much more susceptible to damage. For that reason, the draining herbs in this formula are milder in nature. *Sang Bai Pi* (Cortex Mori) and *Di Gu Pi* (Cortex Lycii) gently clear deficiency heat, while *Geng Mi* (Semen Oryzae) and *Gan Cao* (Radix et Rhizoma Glycyrrhizae) strengthen the Spleen and Stomach (earth element) to support the Lung (metal element). Together, the herbs clear heat without injuring yin and sedate the Lung without injuring *zheng* (upright) *qi*. In summary, *Xie Bai San* cools and nourishes the Lung and is more suitable for chronic cases of cough or wheezing with yin-deficient constitutions. It is often combined with other herbs or another formula to clear Lung heat as needed.

Xiè Bái Săn (Drain the White Powder)

- *Ma Huang Xing Ren Gan Cao Shi Gao Tang* is designed for wind-heat or wind-cold invasion leading to Lung heat accumulation, which then causes reversed flow of Lung qi. Besides the symptoms of cough and wheezing, it also treats fever, increased thirst and a rapid pulse. *Ma Huang* (Herba Ephedrae) is used to disperse external pathogenic factors, and is coupled with *Shi Gao* (Gypsum Fibrosum) to strongly sedate Lung and Stomach fire and also to generate body fluids. *Ku Xing Ren* (Semen Armeniacae Amarum) guides Lung qi downward, and further helps *Ma Huang* (Herba Ephedrae) regulate respiration. In summary, *Ma Huang Xing Ren Gan Cao Shi Gao Tang* sedates the Lung and ventilates qi, and is used mainly in cases of excess pathogenic factors (bacteria, viruses, etc) invading the Lung.[6]

References

1. *Shi Yong Zhong Xi Yi Jie He Za Zhi* (Practical Journal of Integrated Chinese and Western Medicines), 1997; 3:239.
2. *Yi Fang Xin Jie* (New Explanation for Medical Formulas), 1980; 100.
3. *Shan Xi Zhong Yi* (Shanxi Chinese Medicine), 1995; 16(8):362.
4. *Hu Bei Zhong Yi Za Zhi* (Hubei Journal of Chinese Medicine), 1997; 4:35.
5. Wang MZ, et al. *Zhong Yi Xue Wen Da Ti Ku* (Questions and Answers on Traditional Chinese Medicine: Herbal Formulas).
6. Wang MZ, et al. *Zhong Yi Xue Wen Da Ti Ku* (Questions and Answers on Traditional Chinese Medicine: Herbal Formulas).

Zuŏ Jīn Wán (Left Metal Pill)

左金丸

Pinyin Name: *Zuo Jin Wan*
Literal Name: Left Metal Pill
Alternate Name: *Yu Lian Wan* (Evodia and Coptis Pill)
Original Source: *Dan Xi Xin Fa* (Teachings of [Zhu] Dan-Xi) by Zhu Zhen-Heng in 1481

COMPOSITION

Huang Lian (Rhizoma Coptidis)	180g [9g]
Wu Zhu Yu (Fructus Evodiae)	15-30g [1.5g]

DOSAGE / PREPARATION / ADMINISTRATION

The source text states to grind the ingredients into powder and form into pills with water. Take 50 pills [6g] with warm, boiled water. Today, this formula may be prepared as a decoction with the doses suggested in brackets.

CHINESE THERAPEUTIC ACTIONS

1. Clears the Liver and purges fire
2. Corrects the reversed flow of Stomach qi and stops vomiting

CLINICAL MANIFESTATIONS

Liver fire overacting on the Stomach: hypochondriac pain, epigastric distention, acid regurgitation, nausea, vomiting, belching, a red tongue, and a wiry, rapid pulse.

VETERINARY CLINICAL APPLICATIONS

Acute and chronic gastritis, inflammatory bowel disease in the cat, peptic ulcer disease, *H. pylori* infection, acid regurgitation, erosive gastritis, epigastric pain, and hepatitis.

Zuǒ Jīn Wán (Left Metal Pill)

EXPLANATION

Zuo Jin Wan (Left Metal Pill) treats Liver fire overacting on the Stomach. Liver fire results from Liver qi stagnation. Fire in the Liver channel leads to hypochondriac pain. Because wood is the element that acts on earth, excess Liver fire overacts on the Stomach to cause Stomach heat and reversed flow of Stomach qi upward. As a result, patients may experience epigastric pain, acid regurgitation, and/or vomiting.

Huang Lian (Rhizoma Coptidis) purges Liver fire and clears Stomach heat to treat both the cause and the symptoms. *Wu Zhu Yu* (Fructus Evodiae) corrects the reversed flow of Stomach qi to stop vomiting. The dose ratio of *Huang Lian* (Rhizoma Coptidis) to *Wu Zhu Yu* (Fructus Evodiae) is to be kept at 6:1 for two important reasons. First, *Huang Lian* (Rhizoma Coptidis) is the chief herb and must be used at a large dose to effectively clear Liver fire and Stomach heat. However, *Huang Lian* (Rhizoma Coptidis) is bitter and cold, and may damage the body when used at large doses. Therefore, a small dose of warm *Wu Zhu Yu* (Fructus Evodiae) is used to balance the bitter and cold properties of *Huang Lian* (Rhizoma Coptidis).

The rationale for the composition of this formula can also be explained using the mother and son relationship from Five-Element Theory, which states that an excess condition of the mother element can be treated by sedating the son element. Thus, when the Liver (wood [mother] element) is in excess, the Heart (fire [son] element) can be sedated. So by using *Huang Lian* (Rhizoma Coptidis) to sedate Heart fire, one can indirectly treat Liver fire.

VETERINARY MODIFICATIONS

- With more severe acid regurgitation, add *Hai Piao Xiao* (Endoconcha Sepiae) and *Wa Leng Zi* (Concha Arcae).
- With more hypochondriac pain, add *Xiang Fu* (Rhizoma Cyperi), *Fo Shou* (Fructus Citri Sarcodactylis), or *Si Ni San* (Frigid Extremities Powder).
- With abdominal pain, add *Bai Shao* (Radix Paeoniae Alba).
- For dysentery with abdominal pain and spasms, add *Bai Shao* (Radix Paeoniae Alba) and *Gan Cao* (Radix et Rhizoma Glycyrrhizae).
- If there are stress ulcers, add *Xiao Yao San* (Rambling Powder) or *Jia Wei Xiao Yao San* (Augmented Rambling Powder).
- For *H. pylori* infection, add *Bai Hua She She Cao* (Herba Hedyotis).

CAUTIONS / CONTRAINDICATIONS

- *Zuo Jin Wan* is contraindicated in cases of deficiency cold.
- This formula should not be used to treat hypochondriac pain caused by Liver, Gallbladder, and blood deficiencies.
- This formula is contraindicated during pregnancy.[1]
- Avoid cold, raw and oily or greasy foods while taking this formula.[2]

PHARMACOLOGICAL EFFECTS

Gastrointestinal: Administration of a modified *Zuo Jin Wan* preparation was associated with protecting the stomach mucus membrane against sodium hydroxide, aspirin, and ethylamine hydrochloride in rats that have fasted for 24 hours. The dose of *Zuo Jin Wan* was 1 g/kg, and the formula was modified with the addition of one qi-regulating herb.[3]

HUMAN CLINICAL STUDIES AND RESEARCH

1. **Gastritis**: *Zuo Jin Wan* was evaluated for its effectiveness in treating gastric ulcer due to reflux of bile to the stomach. Out of 24 patients, there were 10 males and 14 females, with ages ranging from 24 to 68 years of age. The history of illness ranged from 6 months to 7 years. Clinical presentations included stomach and gastric pain, nausea, vomiting, abdominal distention, and poor appetite. The basic formula used to treat these patients included *Huang Lian* (Rhizoma Coptidis) 5g, *Wu Zhu Yu* (Fructus Evodiae) 3g, *Jiang Xiang* (Lignum Dalbergiae Odoriferae) 10g, *Zhi Qiao* (Fructus Aurantii) 10g, *Niu Xi* (Radix Achyranthis Bidentatae) 10g, and *Da Huang* (Radix et Rhizoma Rhei) 10g. Minor modifications were

***Zuo Jin Wan* (Left Metal Pill)**

Diagnosis	Clinical Signs	Treatment	Herbs
Liver fire overacting on the Stomach	• Hypochondriac pain: Liver fire • Epigastric distention, acid regurgitation, nausea, vomiting and belching: Liver fire overacting on the Stomach • Red tongue body: excess fire condition • Wiry, rapid pulse: Liver fire rising	• Clears the Liver and purges fire • Corrects the reversed flow of Stomach qi and stops vomiting	• *Huang Lian* (Rhizoma Coptidis) sedates Liver fire and clears Stomach heat. • *Wu Zhu Yu* (Fructus Evodiae) corrects the reversed flow of Stomach qi to stop vomiting.

Zuǒ Jīn Wán (Left Metal Pill)

made if necessary by adding *Chai Hu* (Radix Bupleuri), *Fo Shou* (Fructus Citri Sarcodactylis), *Zhi Zi* (Fructus Gardeniae), *Yu Jin* (Radix Curcumae), and *Gan Cao* (Radix et Rhizoma Glycyrrhizae) for Liver fire overacting on the Stomach; *Dang Gui* (Radix Angelicae Sinensis), *Xiang Fu* (Rhizoma Cyperi), and *Qing Pi* (Pericarpium Citri Reticulatae Viride) for irregular menstruation with breast distention; *Chi Shao* (Radix Paeoniae Rubra), *Bai Shao* (Radix Paeoniae Alba), *San Qi* (Radix et Rhizoma Notoginseng), and *Shi Xiao San* (Sudden Smile Powder) for blood stagnation; and the addition of *Dang Shen* (Radix Codonopsis), dry-fried *Bai Zhu* (Rhizoma Atractylodis Macrocephalae), *Zhi Gan Cao* (Radix et Rhizoma Glycyrrhizae Praeparata cum Melle), and *Da Zao* (Fructus Jujubae), and the elimination of *Da Huang* (Radix et Rhizoma Rhei), for Spleen and Stomach deficiencies. The duration of treatment ranged from 15 to 56 days. The study reported effectiveness in 20 patients (complete resolution of symptoms with normal endoscopy), moderate effect in 3 patients (resolution of symptoms with minimal ulceration based on endoscopy), and no benefit in 1 patient. The overall rate of effectiveness was 95.8%.[4] Another study reported that gastritis due to regurgitation of bile acid can be treated effectively using *Zuo Jin Wan* plus *Bai Hua She She Cao* (Herba Hedyotis), *Zhi Shi* (Fructus Aurantii Immaturus), and *Cang Zhu* (Rhizoma Atractylodis). The duration of treatment was 15 days per course of treatment, for a total of 2 courses. Of 39 patients, 20 had complete recovery, 16 had significant improvement, and 3 had no change.[5]

2. **Erosive gastritis**: Use of modified *Zuo Jin Wan* to treat 44 patients with erosive gastritis was associated with 95.8% effectiveness. The herbs were decocted in water, and taken in two equally-divided doses daily. The duration of treatment was 20 days per course, for 2 courses. Modifications to the herbal treatment were made by adding herbs as follows: *Zhi Qiao* (Fructus Aurantii) and *Hou Po* (Cortex Magnoliae Officinalis) for fullness and distention in the upper abdominal area; *Tian Hua Fen* (Radix Trichosanthis) and *Shi Hu* (Caulis Dendrobii) for dry mouth and tongue with hunger but no desire to eat; *Hai Piao Xiao* (Endoconcha Sepiae) and calcined *Wa Leng Zi* (Concha Arcae) for acid reflux; *Shen Qu* (Massa Fermentata), *Mai Ya* (Fructus Hordei Germinatus), and *Ji Nei Jin* (Endothelium Corneum Gigeriae Galli) for anorexia; *Huo Ma Ren* (Fructus Cannabis) and *Yu Li Ren* (Semen Pruni) for constipation; and *Dang Shen* (Radix Codonopsis) and *Bai Zhu* (Rhizoma Atractylodis Macrocephalae) for Spleen and Stomach deficiencies. Of 44 cases, the study reported complete recovery in 31 cases, improvement in 11 cases, and no effect in 2 cases.[6]
3. **Epigastric pain**: One study reported 96.4% effectiveness using *Zuo Jin Wan* plus *Ban Xia* (Rhizoma Pinelliae) and *Chen Pi* (Pericarpium Citri Reticulatae) to treat epigastric pain. Of 110 patients, 19 had complete recovery, 56 had significant improvement, 31 had moderate improvement, and 4 had no effect.[7]
4. ***H. pylori* infection**: Use of *Zuo Jin Wan* was associated with successful treatment in 86 of 133 patients (64.7%) with *H. pylori* infection. The treatment protocol was to administer one pill twice daily for 2 weeks per course of treatment, for 2 courses total.[8]

HERB-DRUG INTERACTION

Aspirin: Administration of *Zuo Jin Wan* in rats was found to have marked protective effect against aspirin-induced damages to the stomach mucus membrane.[9]

SUGGESTED ACUPUNCTURE TREATMENT

1. Points: *Yanglingquan* (GB 34), *Taichong* (LR 3), *Shangwan* (CV 13), *Liangqiu* (ST 34), and *Shenmen* (HT 7).
2. Technique: sedation.

Yanglingquan (GB 34) and *Taichong* (LR 3) sedate the Liver and Gallbladder. *Shangwan* (CV 13) and *Liangqiu* (ST 34) relieve chest congestion and harmonize the Stomach to relieve nausea and vomiting. *Shenmen* (HT 7) calms the mind.

AUTHORS' COMMENTS

Zuo Jin Wan is used to treat inflammatory bowel disease in the cat characterized by chronic, intermittent vomiting due to Liver fire invading the Stomach. The cats for which this formula is appropriate are typically exclusively fed dry cat food that contains grains that generate heat in the middle *jiao* and Liver. As the formula contains only two herbs, it can be readily made in-house, and some cats will eat the formula mixed into a small amount of food. *Zuo Jin Wan* can be used alone; however, it is more commonly combined with *Liu Jun Zi Tang* (Six-Gentlemen Decoction) or *Jia Wei Xiao Yao San* (Augmented Rambling Powder) to improve clinical efficacy depending on the case.

Zuo Jin Wan treats Liver fire overacting on the Stomach. There are two reasons why *Huang Lian* (Rhizoma Coptidis) is a more suitable herb than *Long Dan* (Radix et Rhizoma Gentianae) in this formula.

- *Huang Lian* (Rhizoma Coptidis) is better than *Long Dan* (Radix et Rhizoma Gentianae) at sedating Heart fire. Sedating the Heart will purge Liver fire according to the mother-son relationship in Five-Element Theory.
- The chief complaints are upper gastrointestinal symptoms. *Huang Lian* (Rhizoma Coptidis) is excellent at sedating

Zuǒ Jīn Wán (Left Metal Pill)

Stomach fire to treat acid regurgitation, burning pain, nausea, and vomiting. *Long Dan* (Radix et Rhizoma Gentianae) is an extremely bitter and cold herb, and although it can sedate Liver fire, it may damage the Stomach and cause more vomiting or nausea.[10]

References

1. *Zhong Yao Ming Fang Yao Li Yu Ying Yong* (Pharmacology and Applications of Famous Herbal Formulas), 1989; 189-191.
2. *Zhong Yao Ming Fang Yao Li Yu Ying Yong* (Pharmacology and Applications of Famous Herbal Formulas), 1989; 189-191.
3. *Zhong Yao Yao Li Yu Lin Chuang* (Pharmacology and Clinical Applications of Chinese Herbs), 1993; 9(4):9.
4. *Zhe Jiang Zhong Yi Za Zhi* (Zhejiang Journal of Chinese Medicine), 1993; 28(9):394.
5. *Shan Xi Zhong Yi* (Shanxi Chinese Medicine), 1997; 4:14.
6. *Shi Yong Zhong Yi Za Zhi* (Journal of Practical Chinese Medicine), 1999; 2:10.
7. *Hu Bei Zhong Yi Za Zhi* (Hubei Journal of Chinese Medicine), 1998; 3:40.
8. *Zhe Jiang Zhong Yi Za Zhi* (Zhejiang Journal of Chinese Medicine), 1997; 10:437.
9. *Zhong Yao Yao Li Yu Lin Chuang* (Pharmacology and Clinical Applications of Chinese Herbs), 1993; 9(4):9.
10. Wang MZ, et al. *Zhong Yi Xue Wen Da Ti Ku* (Questions and Answers on Traditional Chinese Medicine: Herbal Formulas).

Qīng Wèi Sǎn (Clear the Stomach Powder)

清胃散

Pinyin Name: *Qing Wei San*
Literal Name: Clear the Stomach Powder
Alternate Names: *Ching Wei San*, Stomach-Clearing Powder, Coptis and Rehmannia Formula
Original Source: *Lan Shi Mi Cang* (Secrets from the Orchid Chamber) by Li Gao in 1336

COMPOSITION

Huang Lian (Rhizoma Coptidis)	0.9-1.8g [3-6g]
Di Huang (Radix Rehmanniae)	0.9g [6-12g]
Mu Dan Pi (Cortex Moutan)	1.5g [9g]
Dang Gui (Radix Angelicae Sinensis)	0.9g [6g]
Sheng Ma (Rhizoma Cimicifugae)	3g [6-9g]

DOSAGE / PREPARATION / ADMINISTRATION

The source text states to grind the ingredients into powder. Cook the herbs in 1.5 bowls of water until 70% of the liquid remains. Take the strained decoction after it has cooled. The dose of *Huang Lian* (Rhizoma Coptidis) may be increased in the summer. Today, this formula may be prepared as a decoction with the doses suggested in brackets.

CHINESE THERAPEUTIC ACTIONS

1. Clears Stomach heat
2. Cools the blood

CLINICAL MANIFESTATIONS

Heat accumulation in the Stomach: toothache, with painful and swollen cheeks and oral cavity (lips and gum); swelling and ulcerations of the gum and/or bleeding gums; fever, foul breath, a dry mouth and tongue, a red tongue, and a slippery, big and rapid pulse.

VETERINARY CLINICAL APPLICATIONS

Stomatitis, ulcerative stomatitis, toothache, gingivitis, gingivitis-stomatitis complex in the cat, gastric ulcers in the horse, periodontal disease and halitosis.

Qīng Wèi Sǎn (Clear the Stomach Powder)

EXPLANATION

Qing Wei San (Clear the Stomach Powder) clears Stomach heat. Since the Stomach channel travels to the cheeks and gum region, Stomach heat results in toothache and painful cheeks. The *yangming* Stomach is the organ that has an abundance of qi and blood. Thus, heat in the Stomach affects the blood and causes blood to flow out of its vessels, leading to swelling, ulceration and/or bleeding of the gums. Foul breath and a dry mouth are the results of Stomach heat rising.

Qing Wei San (Clear the Stomach Powder) uses *Huang Lian* (Rhizoma Coptidis) as the chief herb to clear heat in the Stomach. *Di Huang* (Radix Rehmanniae) cools the blood and nourishes yin. *Mu Dan Pi* (Cortex Moutan) clears heat and cools the blood. *Di Huang* (Radix Rehmanniae) and *Mu Dan Pi* (Cortex Moutan) also assist *Dang Gui* (Radix Angelicae Sinensis) to nourish and harmonize the blood. *Sheng Ma* (Rhizoma Cimicifugae) has two functions in this formula: it assists *Huang Lian* (Rhizoma Coptidis) to disperse rising Stomach heat and eliminate toxins, and it guides the other herbs in this formula to the *yangming* channel.

VETERINARY MODIFICATIONS

- With constipation, add *Da Huang* (Radix et Rhizoma Rhei) and *Mang Xiao* (Natrii Sulfas), or *Da Cheng Qi Tang* (Major Order the *Qi* Decoction).
- When there is swelling and pain of the gums, add *Huang Qin* (Radix Scutellariae) and *Xuan Shen* (Radix Scrophulariae).
- With swelling, inflammation and pain, add *Zhi Mu* (Rhizoma Anemarrhenae) and *Gan Cao* (Radix et Rhizoma Glycyrrhizae).
- With stomatitis, add *Jin Yin Hua* (Flos Lonicerae Japonicae) and *Lian Qiao* (Fructus Forsythiae).
- If there is toothache, add *Bai Hu Tang* (White Tiger Decoction).
- With bleeding gums, add *Niu Xi* (Radix Achyranthis Bidentatae).

CAUTIONS / CONTRAINDICATIONS

Do not use *Qing Wei San* if the oral problems (toothache, swelling and pain of the gums, and gum bleeding) are caused by wind-cold, Kidney yin deficiency, or Kidney yin-deficient fire.

PHARMACOLOGICAL EFFECTS

1. **Anti-inflammatory**: In one laboratory study, injection of *Qing Wei San* was effective in reducing inflammation in rats. The injection given was a 5% solution with a dose of 10 mL/kg. Injection was given twice daily for 3 days.[1]
2. **Antibiotic**: Decoction of *Qing Wei San* was associated with mild inhibitory effects against *Staphylococcus aureus* and *Pseudomonas aeruginosa*, with a minimum inhibitory concentration (MIC) of 0.063 g/mL and 0.5 g/mL, respectively.[2]
3. **Immunostimulant**: In one experiment, oral ingestion of 0.5mL of a 0.5% solution of *Qing Wei San* for 3 days was associated with increased phagocytic activities by macrophages in mice.[3]

HUMAN CLINICAL STUDIES AND RESEARCH

1. **Stomatitis**: In one clinical study, 75 patients with recurrent ulcerations were treated with *Qing Wei San* with good results in all patients. The patients were instructed to gargle and swallow the decoction three to five times daily. The patients recovered within an average of 6 days, with a range of 3-9 days.[4]
2. **Gingivitis**: In one report, patients with gingivitis were treated with satisfactory results using a combination of *Qing Wei San* and *Yu Nu Jian* (Jade Woman Decoction).

***Qing Wei San* (Clear the Stomach Powder)**

Diagnosis	Clinical Signs	Treatment	Herbs
Stomach heat	• Toothache, foul breath, and painful and swollen cheeks and oral cavity: heat traveling up along the Stomach channel • Ulceration and/or bleeding of the gums: heat forcing the blood to flow out of its vessels • Dry mouth and tongue: Stomach heat consuming body fluids • Red tongue body: heat condition • Slippery, big and rapid pulse: heat condition	• Clears Stomach heat • Cools blood	• *Huang Lian* (Rhizoma Coptidis) sedates excess heat in the Stomach. • *Di Huang* (Radix Rehmanniae) cools the blood and nourishes yin. • *Mu Dan Pi* (Cortex Moutan) clears heat and cools the blood. • *Dang Gui* (Radix Angelicae Sinensis) nourishes the blood. • *Sheng Ma* (Rhizoma Cimicifugae) clears heat, eliminates toxins, and guides the formula to the *yangming* channel.

Qīng Wèi Săn (Clear the Stomach Powder)

Small modifications to the herbal formula were made as follows: *Da Huang* (Radix et Rhizoma Rhei) (post-decocted) for constipation; *Tian Hua Fen* (Radix Trichosanthis), *Lian Qiao* (Fructus Forsythiae), and *Zhu Ye* (Herba Phyllostachys) for severe gum swelling; and *Pu Huang* (Pollen Typhae), *Xian He Cao* (Herba Agrimoniae), *Bai Mao Gen* (Rhizoma Imperatae), and *Mo Han Lian* (Herba Ecliptae) for gum bleeding. Out of 103 cases, the study reported marked improvement in 94 cases (resolution of symptoms within 1 week) and moderate improvement in 9 cases (resolution of symptoms within 2 weeks).[5]

3. **Periodontitis**: Acute periodontitis in 56 patients was treated with marked success using *Qing Wei San* plus *Zhu Ye* (Herba Phyllostachys), *Lian Qiao* (Fructus Forsythiae), and *Tian Hua Fen* (Radix Trichosanthis). The herbs were given as decoction daily, and most patients experienced relief within 3-5 packs of herbs. Of 56 patients, the study reported complete relief in 32 cases, significant improvement in 19 cases, moderate improvement in 4 cases, and no effect in 1 case. The overall effectiveness was 98.2%.[6] Another study reported a marked effect using modified *Qing Wei San* to treat 52 patients with periodontitis. The herbal treatment contained *Qing Wei San* plus *Bai Hua She She Cao* (Herba Hedyotis) as the base formula, with addition of *Shi Gao* (Gypsum Fibrosum) and *Huang Lian* (Rhizoma Coptidis) for Stomach heat; *Bai Mao Gen* (Rhizoma Imperatae) and *Bai Ji* (Rhizoma Bletillae) for gum bleeding; *Sang Ji Sheng* (Herba Taxilli) and *Gou Ji* (Rhizoma Cibotii) for loose teeth; and *Da Huang* (Radix et Rhizoma Rhei) for constipation. After 7 days of herbal therapy, the study reported complete recovery in 41 cases, improvement in 8 cases, and no effect in 3 cases. The overall rate of effectiveness was 94%.[7]
4. **Periodontal disease**: Administration of *Qing Wei San* was associated with marked success in treating periodontal disease characterized by Stomach fire rising. The herbal treatment used *Qing Wei San* as the base formula, with the addition of *Da Huang* (Radix et Rhizoma Rhei) for constipation and *Yi Yi Ren* (Semen Coicis) and *Che Qian Zi* (Semen Plantaginis) for damp-heat. Of 58 cases, the study reported complete recovery in 38 cases, significant improvement in 15 cases, and slight improvement in 5 cases.[8]
5. **Halitosis**: One study reported good results using modified *Qing Wei San* to treat 32 patients with foul breath. In addition to the base formula, modifications were made as needed. For ulcerations of the mouth and tongue and redness, swelling, and pain of the gums, 30g of *Di Huang* (Radix Rehmanniae) was added, and the dose of *Huang Lian* (Rhizoma Coptidis) was increased to 15g. For abdominal distention and fullness, lack of appetite, belching and acid reflux, *Huang Qin* (Radix Scutellariae) and *Da Huang* (Radix et Rhizoma Rhei) were added, and *Dang Gui* (Radix Angelicae Sinensis) and *Sheng Ma* (Rhizoma Cimicifugae) were removed. For profuse, yellow sputum with chest and hypochondriac distention and pain, *Sheng Ma* (Rhizoma Cimicifugae) was removed, *Jin Yin Hua* (Flos Lonicerae Japonicae), *Di Gu Pi* (Cortex Lycii), and *Sang Bai Pi* (Cortex Mori) were added, and the dose of *Mu Dan Pi* (Cortex Moutan) was increased to 15g. The treatment protocol was to administer the herbs in decoction, for 6 packs of herbs per course of treatment, for 1-2 courses total. Of 32 cases, the study reported complete recovery in 31 cases and improvement in 1 case.[9]

TOXICOLOGY

In one acute toxicology study, no fatality was reported in mice following oral administration of a 100% solution of *Qing Wei San* at 0.4 mL per subject, a dose equivalent or greater than 150 times the normal adult dose in humans.[10]

SUGGESTED ACUPUNCTURE TREATMENT

1. Points: *Neiting* (ST 44), *Weishu* (BL 21), *Laogong* (PC 8), *Hegu* (LI 4), *Xiaguan* (ST 7), *Jiache* (ST 6) and *Xiaguan*.
2. Technique: sedation.

Neiting (ST 44) and *Weishu* (BL 21) sedate heat in the Stomach. *Laogong* (PC 8) clears Heart fire. *Hegu* (LI 4), *Xiaguan* (ST 7), and *Jiache* (ST 6) are combined to treat pain and swelling of the teeth, gums, lips, tongue, and cheeks. *Xiaguan* is a classical equine point used to help stomach ulceration.

AUTHORS' COMMENTS

Qing Wei San is commonly used for dental pain and acute gingivitis-stomatitis caused by Stomach heat, especially in the cat and horse. Stomach heat is a commonly seen problem in cats because they are often fed an exclusive diet of commercial dry cat food which contains high amounts of refined carbohydrates such as corn, wheat, and soybean. This type of diet is lacking in moisture and engenders development of damp-heat in the middle *jiao*. *Qing Wei San* is used to clear excess Stomach heat, and once it has been cleared, this formula is often followed with *Gan Lu Yin* (Sweet Dew Decoction) or *Yu Nu Jian* (Jade Woman Decoction).

In animals with chronic gingivitis-stomatitis with underlying Stomach and Kidney yin deficiencies, one of these two formulas may be given concurrently. Many horses are kept in stressful, confined environments, overfed concentrates, and overworked. This combination can result in Stomach yin deficiency and heat, resulting in a pattern

Qīng Wèi Săn (Clear the Stomach Powder)

most veterinarians will recognize as gastric ulcers. *Yu Nu Jian* is more commonly used in acute presentations, or after initial diagnosis for 30 to 60 days, whereas *Qing Wei San* is used for maintenance and prevention of recurrence. Either formula may be combined successfully with *Xiao Yao San* (Rambling Powder) to treat the Liver stagnation that is almost always present in these patients.

Qing Wei San, Yu Nu Jian (Jade Woman Decoction) and *Gan Lu Yin* (Sweet Dew Decoction) all clear heat and can be used to treat gingivitis and stomatitis, but these conditions have different underlying causes:

- *Qing Wei San* clears Stomach heat and cools the blood to treat toothache, gingivitis and stomatitis with bleeding gums and/or swollen cheeks.
- *Gan Lu Yin* clears damp-heat from the Spleen and Stomach and nourishes Stomach yin. It is used to treat gingivitis and stomatitis with red, swollen, pus-filled gums. It can treat conditions resulting from internal damage due to a poor diet or from exogenous pathogen invasion.
- *Yu Nu Jian* has the greatest ability to nourish Stomach yin; it also clears Stomach heat, treating both excess and deficiency. Symptoms include thirst, toothache, headache, pain at the withers, chronic colic, loose teeth and bleeding gums.

References

1. *Zhong Hua Kou Qiang Ke Za Zhi* (Chinese Journal of Stomatology), 1986; 1:44.
2. *Zhong Hua Kou Qiang Ke Za Zhi* (Chinese Journal of Stomatology), 1986; 1:44.
3. *Zhong Hua Kou Qiang Ke Za Zhi* (Chinese Journal of Stomatology), 1986; 1:44.
4. *He Bei Zhong Yi* (Hebei Chinese Medicine), 1989; 1:25.
5. *Shang Hai Zhong Yi Yao Za Zhi* (Shanghai Journal of Chinese Medicine and Herbology), 1994; 6:31.
6. *Zhong Yi Za Zhi* (Journal of Chinese Medicine), 1985; 7:65.
7. *Hu Nan Zhong Yi Za Zhi* (Hunan Journal of Chinese Medicine), 1997; 5:36.
8. *Shan Dong Zhong Yi Za Zhi* (Shandong Journal of Chinese Medicine), 1996; 9:402.
9. *Shan Xi Zhong Yi* (Shanxi Chinese Medicine), 1996; 5:204.
10. *Zhong Hua Kou Qiang Ke Za Zhi* (Chinese Journal of Stomatology), 1986; 1:44.

Yù Nǚ Jiān (Jade Woman Decoction)

玉女煎

Pinyin Name: Yu Nu Jian
Literal Name: Jade Woman Decoction
Alternate Names: *Yu Nu Chien*, Fairy Decoction, Rehmannia and Gypsum Decoction, Rehmannia and Gypsum Combination
Original Source: *Jing Yue Quan Shu* (Collected Treatises of [Zhang] Jing Yue) by Zhang Jie-Bin (Zhang Jing-Yue) in 1624

COMPOSITION

Shi Gao (Gypsum Fibrosum)	9-15g [15-30g]
Zhi Mu (Rhizoma Anemarrhenae)	4.5g
Shu Di Huang (Radix Rehmanniae Praeparata)	9-30g
Mai Dong (Radix Ophiopogonis)	6g
Chuan Niu Xi (Radix Cyathulae)	4.5g

DOSAGE / PREPARATION / ADMINISTRATION

Prepare the ingredients as a decoction with 1.5 bowls of water and cook until 70% of the liquid remains. The strained decoction may be taken warm or cool. The decoction may also be prepared using the dose of *Shi Gao* (Gypsum Fibrosum) suggested in brackets.

CHINESE THERAPEUTIC ACTIONS

1. Clears Stomach heat
2. Nourishes yin

CLINICAL MANIFESTATIONS

1. Stomach heat accompanied by yin deficiency: irritability, thirst, a dry mouth, toothache, gum bleeding, a red tongue

Yù Nǚ Jiān (Jade Woman Decoction)

body with a yellow, dry tongue coating, or little to no coating, and a rapid, thready pulse.

2. *Xiao ke* (wasting and thirsting) syndrome with excess hunger and thirst.

VETERINARY CLINICAL APPLICATIONS

Epistaxis, recurrent ulceration of the oral cavity, stomach ulcers, inflammatory bowel disease (IBD) with vomiting and nausea, gingivitis, stomatitis, halitosis, periodontal disease, pharyngitis and diabetes mellitus.

EXPLANATION

Yu Nu Jian (Jade Woman Decoction) treats excess in the *yangming* channel with deficiency in the *shaoyin* channel—in other words, excess Stomach heat with underlying yin deficiency. The Stomach channel travels to the head region, so Stomach heat may travel upward along the channel to cause toothache. If the heat forces blood out of the blood vessels, then gum bleeding may occur. Irritability, a dry mouth, and thirst are common clinical manifestations of excess heat injuring yin and body fluids. A red tongue body with a dry, yellow coating implies excess heat damaging yin.

Shi Gao (Gypsum Fibrosum), the chief herb, is excellent for clearing Stomach heat. Its sweet taste promotes the production of body fluids and its acrid nature disperses heat. *Shu Di Huang* (Radix Rehmanniae Praeparata), the deputy herb, is used to nourish yin. Combined, these two herbs clear excess heat and nourish deficient yin. *Zhi Mu* (Rhizoma Anemarrhenae) helps *Shi Gao* (Gypsum Fibrosum) to clear heat and moisten dryness. *Mai Dong* (Radix Ophiopogonis) helps *Shu Di Huang* (Radix Rehmanniae Praeparata) nourish yin. *Chuan Niu Xi* (Radix Cyathulae) leads Stomach heat downward to relieve the gum bleeding. This formula is also commonly used for excessive hunger caused by *xiao ke* (wasting and thirsting) syndrome.

VETERINARY MODIFICATIONS

- If the toothache is severe, add *Huang Lian* (Rhizoma Coptidis) and *Gan Cao* (Radix et Rhizoma Glycyrrhizae).
- With restlessness, irritability and thirst, add *Tian Dong* (Radix Asparagi) and *Di Huang* (Radix Rehmanniae).
- With vomiting of blood, add *Zhi Zi* (Fructus Gardeniae) and charred *Sheng Jiang* (Rhizoma Zingiberis Recens).
- If there is severe gum swelling and pain, add *Jin Yin Hua* (Flos Lonicerae Japonicae) and *Pu Gong Ying* (Herba Taraxaci); or add *Gan Lu Yin* (Sweet Dew Decoction).
- When bleeding gums are severe as a result of heat in the *xue* (blood) level, remove *Shu Di Huang* (Radix Rehmanniae Praeparata) and add *Di Huang* (Radix Rehmanniae), *Bai Mao Gen* (Rhizoma Imperatae), *Mo Han Lian* (Herba Ecliptae), and *Xuan Shen* (Radix Scrophulariae).
- With obvious infection of the gums, add *Ban Lan Gen* (Radix Isatidis) and *Da Qing Ye* (Folium Isatidis).
- With constipation, add *Da Huang* (Radix et Rhizoma Rhei) and *Mang Xiao* (Natrii Sulfas).
- With prominent yin deficiency, add *Bei Sha Shen* (Radix Glehniae) and *Shi Hu* (Caulis Dendrobii).
- With stomatitis and gingivitis, add *Qing Wei San* (Clear the Stomach Powder).

CAUTIONS / CONTRAINDICATIONS

Yu Nu Jian is contraindicated in cases of loose stools caused by deficiency and cold of the Spleen and Stomach.

PHARMACOLOGICAL EFFECTS

Hypoglycemic: In one experiment, oral administration of *Yu Nu Jian* at 5 mL/kg was associated with a gradual but sustained hypoglycemic effect in rabbits. The hypoglycemic effect was observed in these subjects between 3 to 9 hours after administration of the formula.[1]

Yu Nu Jian (Jade Woman Decoction)

Diagnosis	Clinical Signs	Treatment	Herbs
Stomach heat accompanied by yin deficiency	• Toothache: Stomach heat traveling upward along the Stomach channel • Gum bleeding: Stomach heat forcing blood out of the blood vessels • Irritability, a dry mouth, and thirst: excess heat injuring yin and body fluids • Red tongue body with a dry, yellow coating or little to no coating, and a thready, rapid pulse: heat damaging yin	• Clears Stomach heat • Nourishes yin	• *Shi Gao* (Gypsum Fibrosum) and *Zhi Mu* (Rhizoma Anemarrhenae) clear heat, generate body fluids, and moisten dryness. • *Shu Di Huang* (Radix Rehmanniae Praeparata) and *Mai Dong* (Radix Ophiopogonis) nourish Stomach yin. • *Chuan Niu Xi* (Radix Cyathulae) leads Stomach heat downward to relieve the gum bleeding.

Yù Nǔ Jiān (Jade Woman Decoction)

HUMAN CLINICAL STUDIES AND RESEARCH

1. **Gastrointestinal bleeding**: One study reported complete recovery in all 12 patients with upper gastrointestinal bleeding characterized by yin deficiency, with flushed face, dizziness, palpitations, poor sleeping patterns, warm sensations at the center of the palms and soles, hematemesis with profuse amount of bright red blood, a dry mouth with thirst, dark tarry stools, a red tongue body with little tongue coating, and a fine pulse. The herbal treatment contained *Yu Nu Jian* plus *Qian Cao* (Radix et Rhizoma Rubiae) as the base formula, with modifications as needed. For qi deficiency, *Dang Shen* (Radix Codonopsis) and *Tai Zi Shen* (Radix Pseudostellariae), or *Sheng Mai San* (Generate the Pulse Powder) were added. For severe bleeding, charred *Ce Bai Ye* (Cacumen Platycladi), *Mo Han Lian* (Herba Ecliptae), and *Zi Zhu* (Folium Callicarpae) were added.[2]
2. **Epistaxis**: Nosebleeds were successfully treated with an herbal formula containing *Yu Nu Jian* plus *Xian He Cao* (Herba Agrimoniae), *Ou Jie* (Nodus Nelumbinis Rhizomatis), *Di Huang* (Radix Rehmanniae), *Bai Mao Gen* (Rhizoma Imperatae) and *Qian Cao* (Radix et Rhizoma Rubiae). Of 55 patients with nosebleeds, 32 were diagnosed with Liver fire rising, 13 with Stomach fire, and 10 with yin-deficient heat. The herbs were given in decoction daily, for a total of 3-7 packs. The study reported complete recovery in 38 cases, marked effect in 14 cases, and no benefit in 3 cases.[3] In another study, 55 patients with nosebleeds were treated with complete recovery in 38 cases, improvement in 14 patients, and no effect in the rest. Most patients responded within 3-5 doses.[4]
3. **Recurrent ulceration of the oral cavity**: In one report, 32 patients with recurrent oral ulcerations were treated with modified *Yu Nu Jian* with satisfactory results. In addition to *Yu Nu Jian* as the base formula, modifications were made by adding: *Jin Yin Hua* (Flos Lonicerae Japonicae) and *Pu Gong Ying* (Herba Taraxaci) for gum swelling and pain; *Da Huang* (Radix et Rhizoma Rhei) and *Mang Xiao* (Natrii Sulfas) for constipation; *Zhi Zi* (Fructus Gardeniae) and *Huang Lian* (Rhizoma Coptidis) for Stomach fire; *Bei Sha Shen* (Radix Glehniae) and *Shi Hu* (Caulis Dendrobii) for yin deficiency; and *Suan Zao Ren* (Semen Ziziphi Spinosae) and *Shou Wu Teng* (Caulis Polygoni Multiflori) for poor sleeping patterns. Out of 32 patients, 15 showed complete recovery, 10 showed moderate improvement, and 7 showed no effect.[5]
4. **Oral cavity disorders**: Administration of *Yu Nu Jian* has been shown to effectively treat various types of oral cavity disorders. One report found *Yu Nu Jian* had a marked effect to treat swelling and pain of gums.[6] Modified *Yu Nu Jian* also showed marked success in treating 32 patients with recurrent stomatitis.[7] Lastly, use of this formula in 102 patients with toothache due to various causes was associated with complete relief in 68 cases and improvement in 34 cases.[8]
5. **Periodontal disease**: One study reported marked success using modified *Yu Nu Jian* to treat periodontal disease. Of 48 patients, the study reported complete recovery in 23 cases, marked effect in 20 cases, and slight improvement in 5 cases. The herbal treatment used *Yu Nu Jian* plus *Ku Shen* (Radix Sophorae Flavescentis) as the base formula, with addition of *Da Huang* (Radix et Rhizoma Rhei) for constipation and *Yi Yi Ren* (Semen Coicis) for damp-heat. The herbs were cooked in water, and the decoction was taken in two equally-divided doses.[9]
6. **Pharyngitis**: One study reported 93.44% effectiveness using modified *Yu Nu Jian* to treat 61 patients with chronic pharyngitis. In addition to using *Yu Nu Jian* as the base formula, modifications were made by adding *Huang Lian* (Rhizoma Coptidis) and *Zhi Zi* (Fructus Gardeniae) for irritability; *Bei Mu* (Bulbus Fritillariae) and *Tian Zhu Huang* (Concretio Silicea Bambusae) for cough with profuse phlegm; *Jin Yin Hua* (Flos Lonicerae Japonicae) and *Lian Qiao* (Fructus Forsythiae) for dry itchy throat with burning sensations; *Da Huang* (Radix et Rhizoma Rhei) for constipation; and *Chi Shao* (Radix Paeoniae Rubra) and *Mu Dan Pi* (Cortex Moutan) for swelling of the throat. The treatment protocol was to administer the herbs for 10 days per course of treatment, for 2-3 courses total. Of 61 cases, the study reported complete recovery in 9 cases, significant improvement in 23 cases, moderate improvement in 25 cases, and no effect in 4 cases.[10]
7. **Diabetes mellitus**: Use of modified *Yu Nu Jian* was associated with 86.5% effectiveness in treating 52 patients with adult-onset diabetes mellitus characterized by Stomach yin deficiency with dry heat. In addition to *Yu Nu Jian* as the base formula, *Zhi Bai Di Huang Wan* (Anemarrhena, Phellodendron, and Rehmannia Pill) was added for Kidney yin deficiency; *Sheng Mai San* (Generate the Pulse Powder) was added for qi and yin deficiencies; *Jin Gui Shen Qi Wan* (Kidney *Qi* Pill from the Golden Cabinet) was added for yin and yang deficiencies; *Ji Sheng Shen Qi Wan* (Kidney Qi Pill from Formulas that Aid the Living) was added for edema; and *Xiao Ke Fang* (Wasting and Thirsting Formula) for yin deficiency with dry heat.[11] Note: *Xiao Ke Fang* (Wasting and Thirsting Formula), as the name implies, is a formula that treats *xiao ke* (wasting and thirsting) syndrome. The exact composition of this formula was not available at the time of publication.

SUGGESTED ACUPUNCTURE TREATMENT

1. Points: *Weishu* (BL 21), *Neiting* (ST 44), *Pishu* (BL 20), *Sanyinjiao* (SP 6), *Hegu* (LI 4), *Xiaguan* (ST 7), *Jiache* (ST 6), and *Xiaguan*.

Yù Nǔ Jiān (Jade Woman Decoction)

2. Technique: Mainly sedation with some tonification.

Weishu (BL 21) and *Neiting* (ST 44) sedate heat in the Stomach. *Pishu* (BL 20) and *Sanyinjiao* (SP 6) strengthen the Spleen and facilitate water metabolism. *Hegu* (LI 4), *Xiaguan* (ST 7), and *Jiache* (ST 6) relieve pain and swelling of various parts of the head. *Xiaguan* is a classical equine point helpful in the treatment of stomach ulcers.

AUTHORS' COMMENTS

Yu Nu Jian clears excess Stomach heat and tonifies Stomach yin at the same time, and is most commonly used to treat gingivitis-stomatitis and diabetes mellitus. Because this formula both enriches yin and clears heat, it can be used to treat diabetes characterized by Stomach heat and accompanied by yin deficiency. Due to the large amount of *Shi Gao* (Gypsum Fibrosum) in the formula, it is not appropriate for long-term use without modification.

Perhaps the most common use of *Yu Nu Jian* in the horse is the treatment of stomach ulcers. This formula is used initially after a diagnosis has been made and there is either conformation or suspicion of unhealed ulcers in the stomach. As treatment progresses and usually after one or two months, the formula is changed to *Qing Wei San* (Clear the Stomach Powder) and *Xiao Yao San* (Rambling Powder) for maintenance. For the treatment of periodontal disease and gingivitis-stomatitis, *Yu Nu Jian* can be combined with *Qing Wei San* (Clear the Stomach Powder).

Yu Nu Jian and *Qing Wei San* (Clear the Stomach Powder) both treat Stomach fire flaring upward causing gingivitis, stomatitis, gum bleeding, thirst, a red tongue body and a yellow coating.

- *Yu Nu Jian* is indicated for Stomach fire with underlying Stomach and Kidney yin deficiencies. Consequently, the animal will feel more thirsty and dry, and the pulse will feel empty upon heavy pressure.
- *Qing Wei San* cools the blood and clears excess fire.
- Further discussion on equine stomach ulceration can be found in the discussion of *Qing Wei San* (Clear the Stomach Powder).

Yu Nu Jian is a versatile formula and can be combined with many different formulas in the treatment of diabetes mellitus in the dog and cat.

- With qi and yin deficiencies and dryness, it is often combined with *Yu Quan Wan* (Jade Spring Pill).
- With Stomach and/or Lung heat and Stomach yin deficiency, it can be combined with *Bai Hu Jia Ren Shen Tang* (White Tiger plus Ginseng Decoction).
- With yin deficiency, add *Liu Wei Di Huang Wan* (Six-Ingredient Pill with Rehmannia).
- If there is yin deficiency and deficiency fire, combine with *Zhi Bai Di Huang Wan* (Anemarrhena, Phellodendron, and Rehmannia Pill).
- With Kidney qi and yang deficiencies and signs of cold, it can be combined with *Jin Gui Shen Qi Wan* (Kidney Qi Pill from the Golden Cabinet).

References

1. *Zhong Yao Tong Bao* (Journal of Chinese Herbology), 1984; 6:33.
2. *Zhong Yi Ming Fang Lin Chuang Xin Yong* (Contemporary Clinical Applications of Classic Chinese Formulas), 2001; 186.
3. *Shang Hai Zhong Yi Yao Za Zhi* (Shanghai Journal of Chinese Medicine and Herbology), 1985; 19(6):39.
4. *Jiang Xi Zhong Yi Yao* (Jiangxi Chinese Medicine and Herbology), 1986; 5:18.
5. *Fu Jian Zhong Yi Yao* (Fujian Chinese Medicine and Herbology), 1983; 2:24.
6. *Zhong Yi Ming Fang Lin Chuang Xin Yong* (Contemporary Clinical Applications of Classic Chinese Formulas), 2001; 184.
7. *Fu Jian Zhong Yi Yao* (Fujian Chinese Medicine and Herbology), 1983; 14(2):24.
8. *Zhong Xi Yi Jie He Za Zhi* (Journal of Integrated Chinese and Western Medicine), 1989; 9(3):182.
9. *An Hui Zhong Yi Xue Yuan Xue Bao* (Journal of Anhui University School of Medicine), 1999; 6:37.
10. *An Hui Zhong Yi Xue Yuan Xue Bao* (Journal of Anhui University School of Medicine), 1995; 2:21.
11. *Hu Bei Zhong Yi Za Zhi* (Hubei Journal of Chinese Medicine), 1984; 6:33.

Gān Lù Yǐn (Sweet Dew Decoction)

甘露飲
甘露饮

Pinyin Name: *Gan Lu Yin*
Literal Name: Sweet Dew Decoction
Alternate Names: *Kan Lu Yin*, Sweet Combination Drink, Sweet Combination
Original Source: *Tai Ping Hui Min He Ji Ju Fang* (Imperial Grace Formulary of the Tai Ping Era) by the Imperial Medical Department in 1078-85

COMPOSITION

Di Huang (Radix Rehmanniae)
Shu Di Huang (Radix Rehmanniae Praeparata)
Mai Dong (Radix Ophiopogonis)
Tian Dong (Radix Asparagi)
Pi Pa Ye (Folium Eriobotryae)
Shi Hu (Caulis Dendrobii)
Zhi Qiao (Fructus Aurantii), *chao* (dry-fried)
Yin Chen (Herba Artemisiae Scopariae)
Huang Qin (Radix Scutellariae)
Zhi Gan Cao (Radix et Rhizoma Glycyrrhizae Praeparata cum Melle)

DOSAGE / PREPARATION / ADMINISTRATION

Grind equal amounts of the ingredients coarsely, and cook 6g of the powder in 1 bowl of water and reduce it to 80%. Take the warm, strained decoction after meals. For the treatment of loose teeth or swollen gums, swish the decoction in the mouth and then swallow it.

CHINESE THERAPEUTIC ACTIONS

1. Clears damp-heat
2. Nourishes yin

CLINICAL MANIFESTATIONS

Damp-heat in the Spleen and Stomach: swelling, inflammation and suppuration of the gums, stomatitis, ulcerations of the tongue, and toothache. Jaundice with edema, fever, constipation, and dysuria.

VETERINARY CLINICAL APPLICATIONS

Stomatitis, gingivitis, toothache, conjunctivitis, pancreatitis and jaundice.

EXPLANATION

Gan Lu Yin (Sweet Dew Decoction) treats damp-heat in the Spleen and Stomach. When damp-heat travels up the gastrointestinal tract, patients exhibit signs and symptoms in the oral cavity, such as swelling and suppuration of the gums, pain, stomatitis, and tongue ulcerations. If the damp-heat remains in the middle *jiao*, it may affect the adjacent organs, namely the Gallbladder, leading to jaundice, fever, and mild edema of the extremities. If the damp-heat travels downward, it affects urination and bowel movement, leading to dysuria and constipation.

Di Huang (Radix Rehmanniae), *Shu Di Huang* (Radix Rehmanniae Praeparata), *Mai Dong* (Radix Ophiopogonis) and *Tian Dong* (Radix Asparagi) nourish yin and clear heat simultaneously. The heat-clearing function of these herbs addresses the underlying cause of the disease, while the yin-nourishing function prevents the cold herbs from damaging the body. *Pi Pa Ye* (Folium Eriobotryae) harmonizes the Stomach and clears Stomach heat. *Zhi Qiao* (Fructus Aurantii) breaks up stagnant qi, and promotes normal bowel movement and urination. *Shi Hu* (Caulis Dendrobii) clears deficiency heat from the Stomach. The combination of *Zhi Qiao* (Fructus Aurantii) and *Shi Hu* (Caulis Dendrobii) regulates the Stomach and Intestines to promote normal function of the gastrointestinal tract and relieve constipation. *Yin Chen* (Herba Artemisiae Scopariae) clears damp-heat, and is one of the most effective herbs for treating jaundice. *Huang Qin* (Radix Scutellariae) clears excess fire and damp-heat to reduce inflammation and relieve ulceration. Lastly, *Zhi Gan Cao* (Radix et Rhizoma Glycyrrhizae Praeparata cum Melle) harmonizes the herbs.

Gān Lù Yǐn (Sweet Dew Decoction)

Gan Lu Yin (Sweet Dew Decoction)

Diagnosis	Clinical Signs	Treatment	Herbs
Damp-heat in the Spleen and Stomach	• Swelling, inflammation, suppuration and pain of the oral cavity: damp-heat in the Spleen and Stomach traveling upward • Jaundice: damp-heat affecting the Gallbladder in the middle *jiao* • Dysuria and constipation: damp-heat traveling downward	• Clears damp-heat • Nourishes yin	• *Di Huang* (Radix Rehmanniae), *Shu Di Huang* (Radix Rehmanniae Praeparata), *Mai Dong* (Radix Ophiopogonis), *Tian Dong* (Radix Asparagi), *Pi Pa Ye* (Folium Eriobotryae) and *Shi Hu* (Caulis Dendrobii) nourish yin and clear heat. • *Zhi Qiao* (Fructus Aurantii) breaks up stagnant qi, and promotes normal bowel movement and urination. • *Yin Chen* (Herba Artemisiae Scopariae) clears damp-heat. • *Huang Qin* (Radix Scutellariae) clears excess fire and damp-heat. • *Zhi Gan Cao* (Radix et Rhizoma Glycyrrhizae Praeparata cum Melle) harmonizes the herbs.

VETERINARY MODIFICATIONS

- With constipation, combine with *Da Cheng Qi Tang* (Major Order the Qi Decoction).
- With stomatitis and oral lesions, add *Huang Lian* (Rhizoma Coptidis), *Jin Yin Hua* (Flos Lonicerae Japonicae), and *Lian Qiao* (Fructus Forsythiae).

SUGGESTED ACUPUNCTURE TREATMENT

1. Points: *Jiexi* (ST 41), *Taixi* (KI 3), *Chize* (LU 5), *Housanli* (ST 36), *Gongsun* (SP 4), *Xingjian* (LR 2), and *Yinlingquan* (SP 9).
2. Technique: sedation.

Jiexi (ST 41), *Taixi* (KI 3), and *Chize* (LU 5) nourish yin and clear heat. *Housanli* (ST 36) and *Gongsun* (SP 4) regulate qi and remove stagnation. *Xingjian* (LR 2) and *Yinlingquan* (SP 9) purge heat and remove dampness.

AUTHORS' COMMENTS

Gan Lu Yin is commonly used for dental pain and acute gingivitis and stomatitis caused by Stomach damp-heat, especially in the cat. Stomach damp-heat is a commonly seen problem in this species because they are often fed an exclusive diet of commercial dry cat food which contains high amounts of refined carbohydrates such as corn, wheat, and soybean. This type of diet is lacking in moisture and engenders development of damp-heat in the middle *jiao*. *Qing Wei San* (Clear the Stomach Powder) can also be used to treat gingivitis and stomatitis in the cat; however, it does not have the yin nourishing capabilities of *Gan Lu Yin* to protect the Stomach. *Gan Lu Yin* can be used for a much longer period of time than *Qing Wei San* (Clear the Stomach Powder) for this reason. *Qing Wei San* (Clear the Stomach Powder) is better for acute cases with heat, while *Gan Lu Yin* is better for cases with yin deficiency, heat and dampness, or following treatment with *Qing Wei San* (Clear the Stomach Powder). For chronic gingivitis and stomatitis primarily caused by Stomach yin deficiency, *Yu Nu Jian* (Jade Woman Decoction) should be used.

Sháo Yào Tāng (Peony Decoction)

芍藥湯
芍药汤

Pinyin Name: *Shao Yao Tang*
Literal Name: Peony Decoction
Alternate Name: Peony Combination
Original Source: *Zheng Zhi Zhun Sheng* (Standards of Patterns and Treatments) by Wang Ken-Tang in 1602

COMPOSITION

Huang Lian (Rhizoma Coptidis)	15g [5-9g]
Huang Qin (Radix Scutellariae)	15g [9g]
Da Huang (Radix et Rhizoma Rhei)	9g [6g]
Dang Gui (Radix Angelicae Sinensis)	15g [9g]
Bai Shao (Radix Paeoniae Alba)	30g [15-20g]
Gan Cao (Radix et Rhizoma Glycyrrhizae), *chao* (dry-fried)	6g [5g]
Mu Xiang (Radix Aucklandiae)	6g [5g]
Bing Lang (Semen Arecae)	6g [5g]
Rou Gui (Cortex Cinnamomi)	7.5g [2-5g]

Note: The source text states to use *Shao Yao* (Radix Paeoniae) without specifying whether it should be *Bai Shao* (Radix Paeoniae Alba) or *Chi Shao* (Radix Paeoniae Rubra). *Bai Shao* (Radix Paeoniae Alba) is better at relieving pain and harmonizing the *ying* (nutritive) and *xue* (blood) levels, while *Chi Shao* (Radix Paeoniae Rubra) is more effective for clearing heat and cooling the blood. Thus, most scholars and clinicians agree that *Bai Shao* (Radix Paeoniae Alba) is a more suitable herb in *Shao Yao Tang*.

DOSAGE / PREPARATION / ADMINISTRATION

The source text states to grind the ingredients coarsely and cook 15g of the powder in two large bowls of water until one bowl of the liquid remains. Take the warm, strained decoction after meals. Today, this formula may be prepared as a decoction with the doses suggested in brackets.

CHINESE THERAPEUTIC ACTIONS

1. Harmonizes qi and blood
2. Clears heat and eliminates toxins

CLINICAL MANIFESTATIONS

Damp-heat diarrhea: abdominal pain, tenesmus, presence of mucus and blood in the stool, dark, scanty urine, a greasy, tongue coating, and a rapid, wiry to slippery pulse.

VETERINARY CLINICAL APPLICATIONS

Bacterial diarrhea, parvovirus diarrhea, acute gastroenteritis, and inflammatory bowel disease.

EXPLANATION

Shao Yao Tang (Peony Decoction) is the main formula used to treat diarrhea characterized by damp-heat in the Intestines. In this syndrome, dampness and heat stagnate in the Intestines, causing qi and blood stagnation. Qi and blood stagnation results in abdominal pain. Damp-heat injures the Intestines and causes the formation of mucus and blood in the stools, which, when defecated, appear white and red in color. Burning of the anus, tenesmus, and dark, scanty urine are due to damp-heat traveling downward.

The treatment plan for this syndrome is first to harmonize qi and blood, and then to dispel damp-heat and eliminate toxins. A heavy dose of *Bai Shao* (Radix Paeoniae Alba), along with *Dang Gui* (Radix Angelicae Sinensis), is used to harmonize the *ying* (nutritive) and *xue* (blood) levels. *Bai Shao* (Radix Paeoniae Alba) also works with *Gan Cao* (Radix et Rhizoma Glycyrrhizae), as seen in the formula *Shao Yao Gan Cao Tang* (Peony and Licorice Decoction), to relieve pain and other urgent symptoms.

Huang Lian (Rhizoma Coptidis) and *Huang Qin* (Radix Scutellariae), both bitter and cold, clear heat and dry dampness. *Mu Xiang* (Radix Aucklandiae) and *Bing Lang* (Semen Arecae) move qi to relieve stagnation. *Da Huang* (Radix et Rhizoma Rhei), as a supplement to *Huang Lian* (Rhizoma Coptidis) and *Huang Qin* (Radix Scutellariae), purges and drains heat downward. *Da Huang* (Radix et Rhizoma Rhei) also quickly removes harmful retention or stagnation in the body via defecation, thereby supplementing

Sháo Yào Tāng (Peony Decoction)

***Shao Yao Tang* (Peony Decoction)**

Diagnosis	Clinical Signs	Treatment	Herbs
Damp-heat dysentery	• Diarrhea, burning of the anus, tenesmus, and dark, scanty urine: damp-heat traveling downward • Abdominal pain: qi and blood stagnation • Stools with mucus and blood: damp-heat damaging the blood vessels • Greasy tongue coating and a rapid, wiry to slippery pulse: accumulation of damp-heat	• Harmonizes qi and blood • Clears heat and eliminates toxins	• *Huang Lian* (Rhizoma Coptidis) and *Huang Qin* (Radix Scutellariae) clear heat, eliminate toxins, and dry dampness. • *Da Huang* (Radix et Rhizoma Rhei) purges heat and drains heat downward. • *Dang Gui* (Radix Angelicae Sinensis) and *Bai Shao* (Radix Paeoniae Alba) regulate and harmonize *ying* (nutritive) and *xue* (blood) levels. • *Bai Shao* (Radix Paeoniae Alba) and *Gan Cao* (Radix et Rhizoma Glycyrrhizae) relieve spasms, cramps and pain. • *Mu Xiang* (Radix Aucklandiae) and *Bing Lang* (Semen Arecae) regulate and harmonize qi. • *Rou Gui* (Cortex Cinnamomi) restrains the bitter and cold herbs from injuring yin.

the qi-moving effect of *Mu Xiang* (Radix Aucklandiae) and *Bing Lang* (Semen Arecae). Although it is a purgative herb, *Da Huang* (Radix et Rhizoma Rhei) is necessary in this formula to drain stagnation to treat diarrhea and dysentery. *Rou Gui* (Cortex Cinnamomi) restrains the bitter and cold herbs from injuring yin and prevents them from constricting damp-heat inside the body. This formula focuses on treating the cause of the diarrhea and dysentery rather than just relieving the symptoms.

VETERINARY MODIFICATIONS

- With more blood than pus in the stool, change *Dang Gui* (Radix Angelicae Sinensis) to *Dang Gui Wei* (Extremitas Radix Angelicae Sinensis) and add *Mu Dan Pi* (Cortex Moutan).
- With food stagnation, remove *Gan Cao* (Radix et Rhizoma Glycyrrhizae), and add *Shan Zha* (Fructus Crataegi), *Mai Ya* (Fructus Hordei Germinatus), and *Shen Qu* (Massa Fermentata).
- With abdominal distention and pain, remove *Rou Gui* (Cortex Cinnamomi) and *Gan Cao* (Radix et Rhizoma Glycyrrhizae), and add *Zhi Shi* (Fructus Aurantii Immaturus), *Yan Hu Suo* (Rhizoma Corydalis), and *Wu Yao* (Radix Linderae).
- With increased bloody diarrhea, add *San Qi* (Radix et Rhizoma Notoginseng) and *Di Yu* (Radix Sanguisorbae).

CAUTIONS / CONTRAINDICATIONS

- *Shao Yao Tang* is not suitable for chronic diarrhea or diarrhea caused by deficiency and cold.
- Do not use this formula if the diarrhea is accompanied by exterior symptoms.

PHARMACOLOGICAL EFFECTS

1. **Gastrointestinal**: Administration of *Shao Yao Tang* was associated with stimulating the gastrointestinal tract and promoting expulsion of intestinal content. This effect was immediate and potent, with short duration. The potency of this action is directly proportional to the dose of the formula. It was noted that *Shao Yao Tang* did not have such an effect when *Bing Lang* (Semen Arecae) was removed from the formula.[1,2]
2. **Antibiotic**: Use of *Shao Yao Tang in vitro* was associated with an inhibiting effect on *Bacillus dysenteriae*, *E. coli*, *Pseudomonas aeruginosa*, *Bacillus proteus*, and *Staphylococcus aureus*. Interestingly, the formula has much less antibiotic effect without *Bing Lang* (Semen Arecae) even though when given individually, *Bing Lang* (Semen Arecae) does not have any antibiotic effect.[3]
3. **Anti-inflammatory**: Intraperitoneal injection of *Shao Yao Tang* in mice was associated with reducing swelling and inflammation.[4]

HUMAN CLINICAL STUDIES AND RESEARCH

1. **Dysentery**: There have been many reports on the efficacy of *Shao Yao Tang* for the treatment of dysentery. In one report, modified *Shao Yao Tang* was effective in treating all 25 infants with dysentery characterized by damp-heat. Most patients had complete recovery within 2-4 packs, with some needing up to 6 packs of herbs. The herbal treatment contained *Shao Yao Tang*, with the addition of *Bai Zhu* (Rhizoma Atractylodis Macrocephalae) and *Tai Zi Shen* (Radix Pseudostellariae) for chronic illness with qi deficiency; *Huo Xiang* (Herba Agastaches) and *Zhu Ru* (Caulis Bambusae in Taenia) for nausea and vomiting; and

Sháo Yào Tāng (Peony Decoction)

Bai Tou Weng (Radix Pulsatillae), *Pu Gong Ying* (Herba Taraxaci) and charred *Di Yu* (Radix Sanguisorbae) for severe bloody dysentery.[5]

2. **Bacterial dysentery**: *Shao Yao Tang* has been shown to be effective in treating bacterial dysentery in several studies. Modified *Shao Yao Tang* was effective in all 70 patients with bacterial dysentery.[6] According to another study, use of modified *Shao Yao Tang* was associated with 94% effectiveness in treating 50 patients with bacterial dysentery with high fever and bowel movements between 8-20 times per day.[7] Lastly, one study reported 98.9% effectiveness using modified *Shao Yao Tang* to treat 93 patients with bacterial dysentery. The herbal treatment contained *Shao Yao Tang* plus *Jin Yin Hua* (Flos Lonicerae Japonicae), *Di Yu* (Radix Sanguisorbae), *Bai Tou Weng* (Radix Pulsatillae), and *Yi Yi Ren* (Semen Coicis).[8]
3. **Colitis**: One study reported marked success using modified *Shao Yao Tang* to treat 48 patients with acute or chronic colitis. In addition to the base formula, the herbal treatment was modified by adding *Shan Zha* (Fructus Crataegi), *Gu Ya* (Fructus Setariae Germinatus), and *Mai Ya* (Fructus Hordei Germinatus) for undigested food in the stools; *Bai Zhu* (Rhizoma Atractylodis Macrocephalae), *Fu Ling* (Poria), *Shan Yao* (Rhizoma Dioscoreae), and *Bu Gu Zhi* (Fructus Psoraleae) for yang deficiency of the Spleen and Stomach; *Yi Yi Ren* (Semen Coicis) and *Bai Bian Dou* (Semen Lablab Album) for dampness; and eliminating *Rou Gui* (Cortex Cinnamomi) and adding *Zhi Shi* (Fructus Aurantii Immaturus) and *Hou Po* (Cortex Magnoliae Officinalis) for constipation with abdominal fullness. The duration of treatment was 5-10 packs of herbs for acute colitis, and 3-12 months for chronic colitis.[9]
4. **Ulcerative colitis**: Daily administration of modified *Shao Yao Tang* as rectal enema for one month was associated with resolution of all signs and symptoms in all 36 patients with ulcerative colitis. In addition to using *Shao Yao Tang* as the base formula, modifications included the addition of *Bai Tou Weng* (Radix Pulsatillae) and *Ma Chi Xian* (Herba Portulacae) for presence of pus and blood in the stools; *Huang Qi* (Radix Astragali), *Dang Shen* (Radix Codonopsis), and *E Jiao* (Colla Corii Asini) for qi and blood deficiencies; *Wu Mei* (Fructus Mume) and *Shi Liu Pi* (Pericarpium Granati) for chronic diarrhea; *Di Yu* (Radix Sanguisorbae) and *Bai Ji* (Rhizoma Bletillae) powder for severe hematochezia; a larger dose of *Bai Shao* (Radix Paeoniae Alba) for severe abdominal pain; and removal of *Mu Xiang* (Radix Aucklandiae) and *Bing Lang* (Semen Arecae) for absence of abdominal pain.[10]

TOXICOLOGY

In one experiment on the acute toxicology of *Shao Yao Tang*, oral administration of 100 g/kg of the formula caused fatality in 11 out of 12 mice within 72 hours. However, when *Bing Lang* (Semen Arecae) was removed from the formula, no fatality was reported at the same dose. The researchers concluded that the toxicity of the formula is due in part to *Bing Lang* (Semen Arecae).[11]

SUGGESTED ACUPUNCTURE TREATMENT

1. Points: *Changqiang* (GV 1), *Hegu* (LI 4), *Dachangshu* (BL 25), *Tianshu* (ST 25), *Shangjuxu* (ST 37), and *Yinlingquan* (SP 9).
2. Technique: sedation.

Changqiang (GV 1) is a local point to stop diarrhea. *Hegu* (LI 4) is the *yuan* (source) point of the Large Intestine channel. *Tianshu* (ST 25) is the *mu* (collecting) point of the Large Intestine, and *Dachangshu* (BL 25) is the *shu* (transport) point. *Shangjuxu* (ST 37) is the lower *he* (uniting) point of the Large Intestine. These four points clear heat and eliminate toxins in the Large Intestine. When combined with *Yinlingquan* (SP 9), which dissolves dampness, all four points harmonize qi and blood in the Large Intestine.

AUTHORS' COMMENTS

Shao Yao Tang is very effective for the treatment of acute onset and flare up of inflammatory bowel disease (IBD) in dogs and cats, characterized by blood and mucus in the stool. In horses, it can be used for diarrhea caused by clostridia and salmonella, as well as organisms like neorickettsia , and for diarrhea subsequent to grain overload. It can be safely used in combination with steroidal and antimicrobial medications.

Shao Yao Tang and *Bai Tou Weng Tang* (Pulsatilla Decoction) are both representative formulas for diarrhea. Both formulas treat similar signs and symptoms, but have distinctive differences:

- *Shao Yao Tang* treats diarrhea with mucus and blood (of equal amounts) in the stools caused by qi and blood stagnation with damp-heat accumulation. It harmonizes qi and blood while draining damp-heat accumulation. From a clinical perspective, this formula treats a less severe condition than *Bai Tou Weng Tang*.
- *Bai Tou Weng Tang* treats heat and toxins invading the *xue* (blood) level leading to foul-smelling, explosive diarrhea which is mostly bloody with little mucus. It has dual effects to bind the Intestines as well as to dispel toxins, and has a better ability to stop bleeding than *Shao Yao Tang*.[12]

Shao Yao Tang is often combined with *Ge Gen Huang Qin Huang Lian Tang* (Kudzu, Coptis, and Scutellaria Decoction) to treat acute inflammatory bowel disease or acute

Sháo Yào Tāng (Peony Decoction)

flare up of chronic disease with foul-smelling diarrhea with mucus and blood, continuous straining to defecate and increased urgency. The formulas are discontinued once the clinical signs have resolved, and a constitutional formula such as *Shen Ling Bai Zhu San* (Ginseng, Poria, and Atractylodes Macrocephala Powder) is often given.

Please refer to *Ge Gen Huang Qin Huang Lian Tang* (Kudzu, Coptis, and Scutellaria Decoction) for a comparative analysis with *Shao Yao Tang* and *Bai Tou Weng Tang* (Pulsatilla Decoction) in treating diarrhea.

References

1. *Jiang Su Zhong Yi* (Jiangsu Chinese Medicine), 1988; 9(6):34.
2. *Jiang Su Zhong Yi* (Jiangsu Chinese Medicine), 1959; 3:22.
3. *Jiang Su Zhong Yi* (Jiangsu Chinese Medicine), 1988; 9(6):34.
4. *Liao Ning Zhong Yi Za Zhi* (Liaoning Journal of Chinese Medicine), 1992; 19(9):43.
5. *Hei Long Jiang Zhong Yi Yao* (Heilongjiang Chinese Medicine and Herbology), 1989; 6:29.
6. *Liao Ning Yi Xue* (Liaoning Medicine), 1960; 95:23.
7. *Shi Yong Zhong Xi Yi Jie He Za Zhi* (Practical Journal of Integrated Chinese and Western Medicines), 1992; 12:764.
8. *Gan Su Zhong Yi* (Gansu Chinese Medicine), 1998; 2:13.
9. *Si Chuan Zhong Yi* (Sichuan Chinese Medicine), 1995; 7:28.
10. *Si Chuan Zhong Yi* (Sichuan Chinese Medicine), 1995; 3:33.
11. *Jiang Su Zhong Yi* (Jiangsu Chinese Medicine), 1988; 9(6):34.
12. Wang MZ, et al. *Zhong Yi Xue Wen Da Ti Ku* (Questions and Answers on Traditional Chinese Medicine: Herbal Formulas).

Bái Tóu Wēng Tāng (Pulsatilla Decoction)

白頭翁湯
白头翁汤

Pinyin Name: *Bai Tou Weng Tang*
Literal Name: Pulsatilla Decoction
Alternate Name: Anemone Combination
Original Source: *Shang Han Lun* (Discussion of Cold-Induced Disorders) by Zhang Zhong-Jing in the Eastern Han Dynasty

COMPOSITION

Bai Tou Weng (Radix Pulsatillae)	6g [15g]
Huang Lian (Rhizoma Coptidis)	9g [6g]
Huang Bo (Cortex Phellodendri Chinensis)	9g [12g]
Qin Pi (Cortex Fraxini)	9g [12g]

DOSAGE / PREPARATION / ADMINISTRATION

Cook the ingredients in 7 cups [1,400 mL] of water until 2 cups [400 mL] of the liquid remains. Take 1 cup [200 mL] of the warm, strained decoction. If the condition is not improved after the first dose, take another dose (1 cup or 200 mL). Today, the decoction may be prepared using the doses suggested in brackets.

CHINESE THERAPEUTIC ACTIONS

1. Clears heat and eliminates toxins
2. Cools the blood and stops diarrhea.

CLINICAL MANIFESTATIONS

Toxic-heat diarrhea: acute fever, abdominal pain, tenesmus, explosive bloody diarrhea with more blood than mucus and a foul odor, thirst with a strong desire to drink, dehydration, nausea, vomiting, a red tongue and a rapid, slippery pulse.

VETERINARY CLINICAL APPLICATIONS

Bacterial diarrhea, parvovirus diarrhea, acute gastroenteritis, Potomac horse fever, grain overload, hemorrhagic gastroenteritis (HGE) in the dog, intestinal abscess, and urinary tract infection.

Bái Tóu Wēng Tāng (Pulsatilla Decoction)

EXPLANATION

Bai Tou Weng Tang (Pulsatilla Decoction) treats toxic-heat diarrhea, with toxic heat affecting the *jueyin* channel. If the toxic heat injures the qi and blood of the Stomach and Intestines, there will be abdominal pain, nausea, vomiting, the presence of blood and pus in the stools, and tenesmus. Thirst with a strong desire to drink is caused by heat consuming body fluids, as well as by body fluid depletion from the diarrhea.

Bai Tou Weng (Radix Pulsatillae) clears heat and eliminates toxins in the *xue* (blood) level. *Huang Lian* (Rhizoma Coptidis) helps *Bai Tou Weng* (Radix Pulsatillae) clear heat and eliminate toxins. *Huang Bo* (Cortex Phellodendri Chinensis) sedates damp-heat in the lower *jiao*. Together, they clear damp-heat, eliminate toxins, and stop diarrhea and dysentery. *Qin Pi* (Cortex Fraxini), a cold, astringent herb, clears heat, dries dampness, and relieves diarrhea and dysentery.

VETERINARY MODIFICATIONS

- With urinary urgency and pain, add *Mu Tong* (Caulis Akebiae), *Bai Mao Gen* (Rhizoma Imperatae), and *Jin Qian Cao* (Herba Lysimachiae).
- With chills and fever, add *Ge Gen* (Radix Puerariae Lobatae), *Jing Jie* (Herba Schizonepetae), *Jin Yin Hua* (Flos Lonicerae Japonicae), and *Lian Qiao* (Fructus Forsythiae).
- With severe abdominal pain and tenesmus, add *Mu Xiang* (Radix Aucklandiae), *Bing Lang* (Semen Arecae), *Bai Shao* (Radix Paeoniae Alba), *Gan Cao* (Radix et Rhizoma Glycyrrhizae), and *Zhi Qiao* (Fructus Aurantii).
- For bacterial dysentery, add *Di Yu* (Radix Sanguisorbae), *Xian He Cao* (Herba Agrimoniae), and *Mu Xiang* (Radix Aucklandiae).
- For animals suffering from toxic-heat dysentery that cannot tolerate sedating and draining herbs alone because of blood and yin deficiencies, add *Gan Cao* (Radix et Rhizoma Glycyrrhizae) and *E Jiao* (Colla Corii Asini).
- To improve the heat clearing ability of the formula, it is recommended to add *Bai Jiang Cao* (Herba cum Radice Patriniae) and *Jin Yin Hua* (Flos Lonicerae Japonicae).
- For rectal prolapse from straining, add *Bu Zhong Yi Qi Tang* (Tonify the Middle and Augment the Qi Decoction).

CAUTIONS / CONTRAINDICATIONS

- *Bai Tou Weng Tang* treats heat-type dysentery, with toxic heat in the Intestines characterized by dark purplish blood. This formula is contraindicated in cases of chronic dysentery or diarrhea due to deficiency.
- This formula contains bitter and cold herbs which may injure the Spleen and Stomach. Therefore, it should not be taken at large doses or for a prolonged period of time.

PHARMACOLOGICAL EFFECTS

Antibiotic: Administration of *Bai Tou Weng Tang* in various doses was associated with an inhibitory effect *in vitro* against many different types of bacillus, staphylococcus, and other microorganisms.[1]

HUMAN CLINICAL STUDIES AND RESEARCH

1. **Bacterial dysentery**: In one clinical study, 249 patients with bacterial dysentery were effectively treated, with an average of 1-5 days for reduction of body temperature and normal bowel movement within 3 days.[2] In another report, modified *Bai Tou Weng Tang* was used to treat 100 patients with bacterial dysentery with a 97% effectiveness rate and no reports of significant side effects.[3] Lastly, one study reported success using modified *Bai Tou Weng Tang* as a rectal enema to treat 87 patients with chronic bacterial dysentery. The treatment protocol was to cook the herbs in 1,000 mL of water to yield 200 mL of an herbal solution. The herbal solution was instilled into the rectum at bedtime for 5 days, followed by 2 days of rest. This cycle was repeated 1-4 times as needed. The study reported complete recovery in 65 of 87 patients.[4]
2. **Amoebic dysentery**: In one report, 22 out of 25 patients with amoebic dysentery were treated with complete

***Bai Tou Weng Tang* (Pulsatilla Decoction)**

Diagnosis	Clinical Signs	Treatment	Herbs
Toxic-heat dysentery	• Explosive diarrhea, abdominal pain, tenesmus, and blood and pus in the stools with a foul odor: toxic heat in the Intestines • Thirst with a strong desire to drink: heat consuming body fluids • Red tongue: excess heat • Slippery, rapid pulse: excess heat	• Clears heat and eliminates toxins • Cools the blood and stops diarrhea	• *Bai Tou Weng* (Radix Pulsatillae) clears heat and eliminates toxins in the *xue* (blood) level. • *Huang Lian* (Rhizoma Coptidis) clears heat and eliminates toxins. • *Huang Bo* (Cortex Phellodendri Chinensis) clears damp-heat in the lower *jiao*. • *Qin Pi* (Cortex Fraxini) clears heat, dries dampness, and stops diarrhea and dysentery.

Bái Tóu Wēng Tāng (Pulsatilla Decoction)

recovery using modified *Bai Tou Weng Tang*. Out of 22 patients who had complete recovery, 5 responded within 11 doses, and 12 responded within 6-10 doses. The modifications included the addition of *Di Yu* (Radix Sanguisorbae) and *Ku Shen* (Radix Sophorae Flavescentis), and the removal of *Huang Lian* (Rhizoma Coptidis).[5] Another study reported complete recovery in 114 of 116 patients with amoebic dysentery using both *Bai Tou Weng Tang* and *Ge Gen Huang Qin Huang Lian Tang* (Kudzu, Coptis, and Scutellaria Decoction) with modifications. *Jin Yin Hua* (Flos Lonicerae Japonicae) was added for high fever with an aversion to cold. *Di Yu* (Radix Sanguisorbae) was added for blood in the stools. *Ban Xia* (Rhizoma Pinelliae) was added for nausea and vomiting. *Bai Shao* (Radix Paeoniae Alba) was added for abdominal pain.[6]

3. **Enteritis**: In one report, 144 patients with enteritis were treated with 95.8% effectiveness within 48 hours using *Bai Tou Weng Tang*.[7]
4. **Colitis**: One study reported 91.43% effectiveness using modified *Bai Tou Weng Tang* to treat 35 patients with colitis. In addition to using *Bai Tou Weng Tang* as the base formula, *Mu Dan Pi* (Cortex Moutan), *Dang Gui* (Radix Angelicae Sinensis) and charred *Jin Yin Hua* (Flos Lonicerae Japonicae) were added during acute episodes; and *Yan Hu Suo* (Rhizoma Corydalis), *Bai Zhu* (Rhizoma Atractylodis Macrocephalae), and *Tao Ren* (Semen Persicae) were added during remission. The treatment protocol was to administer the herbs twice daily, for 10 days per course of treatment, for 2 courses total. Of 35 cases, the study reported complete recovery in 14 cases, improvement in 18 cases, and no change in 3 cases.[8]
5. **Gastroenteritis**: One study reported complete recovery in 28 of 30 patients with gastroenteritis when treated with *Bai Tou Weng Tang*. The treatment protocol was to administer the herbs in capsule form three times daily, and relief was achieved in an average of 3 days.[9]
6. **Pneumonia**: In one report, 56 out of 67 patients with pneumonia were treated with complete recovery using modified *Bai Tou Weng Tang*. The 11 patients who did not respond, however, continued to deteriorate. In addition to *Bai Tou Weng Tang*, *Ku Xing Ren* (Semen Armeniacae Amarum), *Ma Huang* (Herba Ephedrae), *Yu Xing Cao* (Herba Houttuyniae), and *Da Qing Ye* (Folium Isatidis) were added for wind-heat attacking the Lung; *Di Huang* (Radix Rehmanniae), *Xuan Shen* (Radix Scrophulariae), *Di Gu Pi* (Cortex Lycii) and *Tian Hua Fen* (Radix Trichosanthis) for heat damaging the yin and body fluids; and *Di Huang* (Radix Rehmanniae), *Xuan Shen* (Radix Scrophulariae), *Sha Shen* (Radix Glehniae seu Adenophorae), *Dan Shen* (Radix et Rhizoma Salviae Miltiorrhizae), and *Bai Hua She She Cao* (Herba Hedyotis) for heat in the *qi* (energy) and *xue* (blood) levels.[10]
7. **Urinary tract infection**: Modified *Bai Tou Weng Tang* was used to treat 63 patients with various types of urinary tract infections. Of all patients, 19 had acute infection, 44 had chronic infection; 12 had urethra infections, 33 had bladder infections, and 18 had kidney infections. The study reported marked improvement in 29 cases, moderate improvement in 24 cases, and no effect in 10 cases.[11]
8. **Acute conjunctivitis**: Eighty-seven patients with acute conjunctivitis were treated with complete recovery within 1-3 doses. Out of 87 cases, 26 had complete recovery within 1 dose, 41 cases within 2 doses, and 20 cases within 3 doses. The herbal formula was modified by adding *Mu Zei* (Herba Equiseti Hiemalis).[12]

SUGGESTED ACUPUNCTURE TREATMENT

1. Points: *Tianshu* (ST 25), *Shangjuxu* (ST 37), *Hegu* (LI 4), *Dazhui* (GV 14), *Neiting* (ST 44), *Xuehai* (SP 10), *Taiyang*, *Weijian*, *Erjian*, *Duanxue*, and *Tianping*.
2. Technique: sedation.

Tianshu (ST 25), *Shangjuxu* (ST 37), and *Hegu* (LI 4) clear heat and stop dysentery. *Dazhui* (GV 14) sedates heat and eliminates heat and toxins. *Neiting* (ST 44) clears heat from the *yangming* organs. *Xuehai* (SP 10) clears heat from the blood. *Taiyang*, *Weijian*, and *Erjian* are classical points for clearing heat. *Duanxue* is a classical point for treating hemorrhage in horses. *Tianping* provides the same function in dogs.

AUTHORS' COMMENTS

Bai Tou Weng can be used to treat hemorrhagic gastroenteritis (HGE) in the dog. The cause of HGE is unknown, and the clinical signs of this disease closely match the Chinese medicine pattern of acute damp-heat diarrhea, for which this formula is effective. It may be safely combined with fluid therapy and/or antibiotics, and the use of this formula with conventional therapy will shorten recovery time and prevent recurrence of the disease. The same is true for the treatment of bloody diarrhea caused by parvovirus infection. This is an example of how one Chinese herbal formula can be used to treat two different diseases from a conventional medicine perspective because the *pattern* of the disease is the same in both cases. Likewise, severe hemorrhagic diarrhea in horses is most commonly seen in clostridial diarrhea, colitis (which may be caused by *Clostridium* in some cases), and Potomac horse fever. Although it can be caused by bacteria, neorickettsia, and/or pharmaceutical and environmental factors, all of these presentations may be treated with this formula. In severe cases in which there is a combination of both exterior and interior signs, *Bai Tou Weng Tang* may be combined with

Bái Tóu Wēng Tāng (Pulsatilla Decoction)

Ge Gen Huang Qin Huang Lian Tang (Kudzu, Coptis, and Scutellaria Decoction).

Shao Yao Tang (Peony Decoction) and *Bai Tou Weng Tang* both treat acute diarrhea.

- *Shao Yao Tang* treats damp-heat diarrhea resulting from qi and blood stagnation. It contains moving and purging herbs and does not contain any astringent, binding herbs to stop diarrhea. Its treatment strategy is to harmonize the qi and blood, as well as to clear damp-heat. It is used when there is more abdominal pain, straining and urgency from stagnation.
- *Bai Tou Weng Tang* is more suitable for treating explosive bloody diarrhea in which the toxic heat has extensively injured the blood. The treatment plan for heat dysentery is to clear heat, eliminate heat toxins, and cool the blood to relieve the dysentery. The formula includes herbs that bind the Intestines and stop diarrhea. It is used when there is primarily blood in the stool from damp-heat.

Please refer to *Ge Gen Huang Qin Huang Lian Tang* (Kudzu, Coptis, and Scutellaria Decoction) for a comparative analysis with *Shao Yao Tang* (Peony Decoction) and *Bai Tou Weng Tang* in treating diarrhea.

References

1. *Ha Er Bing Zhong Yi* (Haerbing Chinese Medicine), 1965; 8(3):34.
2. *Zhe Jiang Zhong Yi Za Zhi* (Zhejiang Journal of Chinese Medicine), 1957; 6:242.
3. *Zhe Jiang Zhong Yi Za Zhi* (Zhejiang Journal of Chinese Medicine), 1986; 4: 178.
4. *Nan Jing Zhong Yi Yao Da Xue Xue Bao* (Journal of Nanjing University of Traditional Chinese Medicine and Medicinals), 1997; 5:311.
5. *Zhong Yi Fang Ji Xian Dai Yan Jiu* (Modern Study of Medical Formulas in Traditional Chinese Medicine), 1997; 344-345.
6. *Hu Bei Zhong Yi Za Zhi* (Hubei Journal of Chinese Medicine), 1983; 2:24.
7. *Shang Hai Zhong Yi Yao Za Zhi* (Shanghai Journal of Chinese Medicine and Herbology), 1960; 6:254.
8. *Xin Zhong Yi* (New Chinese Medicine), 1996; 1:20.
9. *Hei Long Jiang Zhong Yi Yao* (Heilongjiang Chinese Medicine and Herbology), 1998; 5:54.
10. *Zhe Jiang Zhong Yi Za Zhi* (Zhejiang Journal of Chinese Medicine), 1986; 12:551.
11. *Hei Long Jiang Zhong Yi Yao* (Heilongjiang Chinese Medicine and Herbology), 1986; 6:40.
12. *Zhong Yi Fang Ji Xian Dai Yan Jiu* (Modern Study of Medical Formulas in Traditional Chinese Medicine), 1997; 346-347.

Section 6

清虚热剂 — Deficiency-Heat Clearing Formulas

Qīng Hāo Biē Jiǎ Tāng

(Artemisia Annua and Soft-Shelled Turtle Shell Decoction)

青蒿鱉甲湯
青蒿鳖甲汤

Pinyin Name: *Qing Hao Bie Jia Tang*
Literal Name: Artemisia Annua and Soft-Shelled Turtle Shell Decoction
Alternate Name: Artemisia Annua Decoction
Original Source: *Wen Bing Tiao Bian* (Systematic Differentiation of Warm Disease) by Wu Ju-Tong in 1798

COMPOSITION

Bie Jia (Carapax Trionycis)	15g
Qing Hao (Herba Artemisiae Annuae)	6g
Di Huang (Radix Rehmanniae)	12g
Zhi Mu (Rhizoma Anemarrhenae)	6g
Mu Dan Pi (Cortex Moutan)	9g

DOSAGE / PREPARATION / ADMINISTRATION

Cook the ingredients in 5 cups of water until it is reduced to 2 cups. Take 1 cup daily. Note: Cooking *Qing Hao* (Herba Artemisiae Annuae) at a high temperature for a prolonged period of time will destroy its active ingredients. Therefore, it should not be cooked with the rest of the herbs. Rather, for maximum effect, it should be steeped in hot water and served along with the decoction.

CHINESE THERAPEUTIC ACTIONS

Nourishes yin and vents interior deficiency heat

CLINICAL MANIFESTATIONS

Late-stage febrile diseases with extensive yin and body fluid deficiencies: low-grade fever in the evenings, general weakness, irritability, dryness, restlessness, panting excessively (especially at night), dry cough, constipation or dry feces, short urination, heat aversion, seeking cool surfaces/places, increased appetite (possibly to the point of being ravenous), increased thirst, trembling and jerking during sleep, hypersensitivity to acupuncture, a red tongue body with no coating, a rapid, thready, thin pulse, and a thin body condition.

VETERINARY CLINICAL APPLICATIONS

Fever of unknown origin, fever secondary to cancer, chemotherapy, or surgery, recovery from infectious disease, chronic pneumonia, chronic pyelonephritis and general yin deficiency.

EXPLANATION

Qing Hao Bie Jia Tang (Artemisia Annua and Soft-Shelled Turtle Shell Decoction) treats late-stage febrile diseases with extensive yin and body fluid deficiencies. Usually in late-stage febrile diseases, there is still some heat which has not been completely cleared, and now resides deep in the body. Moreover, yin and body fluids have been extensively injured and consumed by the heat pathogen, and produces a situation in which the insufficient yin fails to contain yang, resulting in low-grade fever at night. Since the body fluids are already depleted, there is an absence of sweating (in species which do sweat). A red tongue body with no coating and a rapid, thready, thin pulse suggest deficiency heat in the interior.

Because this is not a condition of excess heat in the *qi* (energy) level, strong heat-clearing herbs are not suitable.

Qīng Hāo Biē Jiǎ Tāng

(Artemisia Annua and Soft-Shelled Turtle Shell Decoction)

Qing Hao Bie Jia Tang **(Artemisia Annua and Soft-Shelled Turtle Shell Decoction)**

Diagnosis	Clinical Signs	Treatment	Herbs
Late-stage febrile diseases with extensive yin and body fluid deficiencies	• Low-grade fever in the evenings, general weakness, dryness, restlessness, panting excessively (especially at night), heat aversion, seeking cool surfaces/places, increased to ravenous appetite, and increased thirst: late stage of febrile diseases in which heat resides deep in the body with extreme yin and body fluid deficiencies • A red tongue body with little to no coating and a rapid, thready, thin pulse: deficiency heat in the interior	Nourishes yin and vents interior deficiency heat	• *Bie Jia* (Carapax Trionycis) nourishes yin and clears heat deep in the body. • *Qing Hao* (Herba Artemisiae Annuae) vents deficiency heat and leads it out of the body. • *Di Huang* (Radix Rehmanniae), *Zhi Mu* (Rhizoma Anemarrhenae) and *Mu Dan Pi* (Cortex Moutan) nourish yin and clear deficiency heat.

Neither are pure yin tonics called for since pure tonification will trap the remaining heat inside the body. The best treatment plan is to clear and vent the heat while nourishing yin. *Bie Jia* (Carapax Trionycis) nourishes yin to clear heat; it has the unique function of entering deeply into the *ying* (nutritive) and *xue* (blood) levels to search for and clear the remaining heat pathogen. *Qing Hao* (Herba Artemisiae Annuae), on the other hand, cannot enter into such a deep level. However, due to its aromatic property, it can vent the deficiency heat that *Bie Jia* (Carapax Trionycis) has cleared and guide it out of the body. *Di Huang* (Radix Rehmanniae) nourishes yin and clears heat. *Zhi Mu* (Rhizoma Anemarrhenae) moistens dryness and helps *Qing Hao* (Herba Artemisiae Annuae) and *Bie Jia* (Carapax Trionycis) clear deficiency heat. *Mu Dan Pi* (Cortex Moutan) is acrid and cold, and helps disperse and clear deficiency heat.

VETERINARY MODIFICATIONS

- With unremitting low-grade fever associated with chronic pyelonephritis, add *Bai Mao Gen* (Rhizoma Imperatae).
- With unremitting low-grade fever of unknown origin, add *Bai Wei* (Radix et Rhizoma Cynanchi Atrati), *Shi Hu* (Caulis Dendrobii) and *Di Gu Pi* (Cortex Lycii).
- For pneumonia and toxic heat lingering in the interior, add *Yin Chai Hu* (Radix Stellariae) and *Bai Wei* (Radix et Rhizoma Cynanchi Atrati).

CAUTIONS / CONTRAINDICATIONS

Qing Hao Bie Jia Tang is contraindicated in patients with yin deficiency and Liver wind rising.

HUMAN CLINICAL STUDIES AND RESEARCH

1. **Fever in cancer**: Administration of modified *Qing Hao Bie Jia Tang* has been shown in many studies to effectively reduce body temperature in cancer patients with fever. In one study, use of the modified formula in 25 cancer patients with fever (15-60 days with fever) was associated with significant effect in 10 patients, moderate effect in 10 patients, and no effect in 5 patients. The herbs were given in decoction daily for 10 packs of herbs per course of treatment. The herbal formula contained *Qing Hao* (Herba Artemisiae Annuae) 15g, *Bie Jia* (Carapax Trionycis) 20g, *Di Huang* (Radix Rehmanniae) 10g, *Zhi Mu* (Rhizoma Anemarrhenae) 10g, *Mu Dan Pi* (Cortex Moutan) 15g, *Chai Hu* (Radix Bupleuri) 10g, *Bai Shao* (Radix Paeoniae Alba) 10g, *Gan Cao* (Radix et Rhizoma Glycyrrhizae) 3g, and *Bai Hua She She Cao* (Herba Hedyotis) 30g. Modifications were made by adding *Tai Zi Shen* (Radix Pseudostellariae) 10g, *Di Gu Pi* (Cortex Lycii) 10g, and *Tian Hua Fen* (Radix Trichosanthis) 15g for *wu xin re* (five-center heat); *Fo Shou* (Fructus Citri Sarcodactylis) 10g, *Yu Zhi Zi* (Fructus Akebiae) 10g, *Chen Pi* (Pericarpium Citri Reticulatae) 6g, *Gu Ya* (Fructus Setariae Germinatus) 10g, *Mai Ya* (Fructus Hordei Germinatus) 10g, and *Ji Nei Jin* (Endothelium Corneum Gigeriae Galli) 6g for poor appetite; *Fu Xiao Mai* (Fructus Tritici Levis) 30g and *Mu Li* (Concha Ostreae) 30g for night perspiration; *Yan Hu Suo* (Rhizoma Corydalis) 10g, *Wu Yao* (Radix Linderae) 10g, and *Xu Chang Qing* (Radix et Rhizoma Cynanchi Paniculati) 10g for severe pain; *Chuan Bei Mu* (Bulbus Fritillariae Cirrhosae) 10g, *Kuan Dong Hua* (Flos Farfarae) 10g, *Yu Zhu* (Rhizoma Polygonati Odorati) 10g, *Mai Dong* (Radix Ophiopogonis) 10g, *Jie Geng* (Radix Platycodonis) 5g, and *Pi Pa Ye* (Folium Eriobotryae) 10g for cough with scanty sputum that is hard to expectorate; and *Gua Lou* (Fructus Trichosanthis) 30g, *Huo Ma Ren* (Fructus Cannabis) 10g, and processed *Da Huang* (Radix et Rhizoma Rhei) 10g for constipation.[1]
2. **Fever in lung cancer**: Twenty patients with fever associated with lung cancer were treated with modified *Qing Hao Bie Jia Tang* with 90% effectiveness in reducing body temperature. The duration of fever prior to treatment

Qīng Hāo Biē Jiǎ Tāng

(Artemisia Annua and Soft-Shelled Turtle Shell Decoction)

ranged from 10-50 days, with temperature ranging from 38-39°C / 100.4-102.2°F or above. In addition to fever, other clinical presentations included cough, sputum with blood, a dry mouth and throat, *wu xin re* (five-center heat), tidal fever, a red tongue body with a scanty tongue coating, and a fine, rapid pulse. The herbal treatment contained *Qing Hao* (Herba Artemisiae Annuae) 15g, *Bie Jia* (Carapax Trionycis) 20g (pre-decocted), *Di Huang* (Radix Rehmanniae) 20g, *Zhi Mu* (Rhizoma Anemarrhenae) 10g, *Mu Dan Pi* (Cortex Moutan) 10g, *Tian Hua Fen* (Radix Trichosanthis) 15g, *Bai He* (Bulbus Lilii) 15g, *Zao Xiu* (Rhizoma Paridis) 30g, and *Bai Hua She She Cao* (Herba Hedyotis) 30g. Modifications were made by adding *Bai Mao Gen* (Rhizoma Imperatae) 30g and *Xian He Cao* (Herba Agrimoniae) 30g for coughing of blood; *Gua Lou* (Fructus Trichosanthis) 15g and *Yu Jin* (Radix Curcumae) 15g for feeling of oppression and pain in the chest; *Fu Xiao Mai* (Fructus Tritici Levis) 30g and *Mu Li* (Concha Ostreae) 15g (pre-decocted) for night sweats; *Huo Ma Ren* (Fructus Cannabis) 30g for constipation; dry-fried *Shan Zha* (Fructus Crataegi) 10g and dry-fried *Mai Ya* (Fructus Hordei Germinatus) 15g for poor appetite; and *Shi Gao* (Gypsum Fibrosum) 30g and *Di Gu Pi* (Cortex Lycii) 15g for high fever. The herbs were given in decoction for 10 days per course of treatment. Of 20 patients, the study reported significant improvement in 12 patients, moderate improvement in 6 patients, and no change in 2 patients.[2]

3. **Fever after surgery**: In one study, 100 women with persistent post-surgical low-grade fever (37.3-38°C / 99.1-100.4°F) refractory to antibiotic therapy were treated with modified *Qing Hao Bie Jia Tang* with good results. The herbal formula contained *Di Huang* (Radix Rehmanniae) 15g, processed *Bie Jia* (Carapax Trionycis) 12g, *Qing Hao* (Herba Artemisiae Annuae) 10g, *Zhi Mu* (Rhizoma Anemarrhenae) 10g, *Mu Dan Pi* (Cortex Moutan) 10g, *Bai Wei* (Radix et Rhizoma Cynanchi Atrati) 10g, *Yin Chai Hu* (Radix Stellariae) 10g, *Bai Shao* (Radix Paeoniae Alba) 10g, and *Gan Cao* (Radix et Rhizoma Glycyrrhizae) 5g. The herbs were given in decoction one time daily, starting 5-10 days after surgery in 81 patients, and 11-15 days in 19 patients. Of 100 patients, 82 received only herbal therapy, and 18 received both herbal and antibiotic therapies. The study reported significant improvement in 70 patients, moderate improvement in 23 patients, and no effect in 7 patients.[3] In another study, 32 patients with post-surgical fever characterized by yin-deficient heat were treated with modified *Qing Hao Bie Jia Tang* with good results. Of 32 patients, the study reported normal body temperature in 8 patients after 1 day, 19 patients after 2 days, and 5 patients after 3 days.[4]
4. **Common cold**: Modified *Qing Hao Bie Jia Tang* was used with good results to treat common cold characterized by yin deficiency in 75 patients (48 males and 27 females, between 1 and 50 years of age, with 1-15 days of illness). The herbal formula contained *Qing Hao* (Herba Artemisiae Annuae) 10-15g, *Bie Jia* (Carapax Trionycis) 15-30g, *Sang Ye* (Folium Mori) 10-12g, *Tian Hua Fen* (Radix Trichosanthis) 10-12g, *Zhi Mu* (Rhizoma Anemarrhenae) 10-12g, and *Mu Dan Pi* (Cortex Moutan) 10-12g. Modifications were made as follows: *Tai Zi Shen* (Radix Pseudostellariae) for qi deficiency; *Bei Mu* (Bulbus Fritillariae) and *Bo He* (Herba Menthae) for cough, *Bai Wei* (Radix et Rhizoma Cynanchi Atrati) and *Mai Dong* (Radix Ophiopogonis) for severe yin deficiency; and *Ou Jie* (Nodus Nelumbinis Rhizomatis) and charred *Di Huang* (Radix Rehmanniae) for blood in the sputum. Out of 75 patients, 55 had complete recovery, 15 had significant improvement, and 5 had no benefit. The overall rate of effectiveness was 93.3%.[5]

SUGGESTED ACUPUNCTURE TREATMENT

1. Points: *Taixi* (KI 3), *Sanyinjiao* (SP 6), *Yinxi* (HT 6), *Shenmen* (HT 7), *Shenshu* (BL 23), *Dazhui* (GV 14), *Yongquan* (KI 1), *Ganshu* (BL 18), *Hegu* (LI 4), and *Neiting* (ST 44).
2. Technique: both tonification and sedation.

Taixi (KI 3) and *Sanyinjiao* (SP 6) nourish Kidney yin. *Yinxi* (HT 6) can help eliminate heat and excessive panting, while *Shenmen* (HT 7) can help to calm the *shen* (spirit) and restlessness. *Shenshu* (BL 23) and *Yongquan* (KI 1) control deficiency heat. *Ganshu* (BL 18) should be sedated to help clear deficiency heat. *Hegu* (LI 4) and *Neiting* (ST 44) sedate heat.

AUTHORS' COMMENTS

In addition to the clinical applications already mentioned, *Qing Hao Bie Jia Tang* can be combined with *Gan Mai Da Zao Tang* (Licorice, Wheat, and Jujube Decoction) to nourish yin, clear deficiency heat, nourish the Heart and calm the *shen* (spirit). Clinical applications of this combination include treatment of behavioral disorder characterized by touch and noise hypersensitivity, hiding, fearfulness, irritability, abrupt changes in behavior for no apparent reason, insomnia, anxiety, and pacing at night.

Qing Hao Bie Jia Tang and *Zhu Ye Shi Gao Tang* (Bamboo Leaves and Gypsum Decoction) are two formulas which can be used in combination in the treatment of severe yin deficiency and heat, with irritability, poor appetite, increased thirst, nausea, and dry heaves. Particularly this presentation and formula use would follow chemotherapy, radiation treatments, and recovery from febrile disorders

Qīng Hāo Biē Jiǎ Tāng
(Artemisia Annua and Soft-Shelled Turtle Shell Decoction)

(commonly pyelonephritis, pneumonia and chemotherapy) with persistent low-grade fever. Both formulas can also be used to treat advanced diabetes mellitus with severe yin and body fluid deficiencies and low-grade fever. From a biomedical perspective, residual low-grade fever due to deficiency heat is often diagnosed as bacterial infection and/or persistent infection, and these cases are typically treated with antibiotics, to which they are unresponsive. In these cases, one of these two formulas may be used to resolve the problem.

Qing Hao Bie Jia Tang and *Zhu Ye Shi Gao Tang* (Bamboo Leaves and Gypsum Decoction) both treat symptoms related to late-stage febrile disorders. Their differences are as follows:

- *Qing Hao Bie Jia Tang* more strongly nourishes yin and clears deficiency heat in the deeper parts of the body, and is more suitable for low-grade fever in the evenings. It nourishes yin and vents heat. Many of the animals for which this formula is appropriate have thin body condition despite a normal appetite and no signs of gastrointestinal upset.
- *Zhu Ye Shi Gao Tang* nourishes yin, benefits qi and harmonizes the Stomach. It is mainly used for late-stage febrile disorders with lingering fever that can occur any time during the day, accompanied by qi and yin deficiencies, and clinical signs of irritability, thirst, poor appetite, nausea, dry heaves vomiting, and sweating (in species which do sweat). *Zhu Ye Shi Gao Tang* nourishes both yin and qi and harmonizes the Stomach.[6]
- For more information, please see *Zhu Ye Shi Gao Tang* (Bamboo Leaves and Gypsum Decoction).

References

1. *Fu Jian Zhong Yi Yao* (Fujian Chinese Medicine and Herbology), 1996; 1:21.
2. *Hu Nan Zhong Yi Za Zhi* (Hunan Journal of Chinese Medicine), 1997; 5:27.
3. *Zhe Jiang Zhong Yi Za Zhi* (Zhejiang Journal of Chinese Medicine), 1981; 11:509.
4. *Zhong Yi Yao Xue Bao* (Report of Chinese Medicine and Herbology), 1995; 6:52.
5. *Zhong Yi Fang Ji Xian Dai Yan Jiu* (Modern Study of Medical Formulas in Traditional Chinese Medicine), 1997; 351-352.
6. Wang MZ, et al. *Zhong Yi Xue Wen Da Ti Ku* (Questions and Answers on Traditional Chinese Medicine: Herbal Formulas).

Zi Yin Jiàng Huǒ Tāng (Nourish Yin and Descend the Fire Decoction)

滋陰降火湯
滋阴降火汤

Pinyin Name: *Zi Yin Jiang Huo Tang*
Literal Name: Nourish Yin and Descend the Fire Decoction
Alternate Names: *Tzu Yin Chiang Huo Tang*, Phellodendron Decoction, Phellodendron Combination
Original Source: *Wan Bing Hui Chun* (Restoration of Health from the Myriad Diseases) by Gong Ting-Xian in 1587

COMPOSITION

Dang Gui (Radix Angelicae Sinensis), *xi* (washed) with liquor	3.6g
Bai Shao (Radix Paeoniae Alba), *xi* (washed) with liquor	6.9g
Shu Di Huang (Radix Rehmanniae Praeparata), *chao* (dry-fried) with ginger juice	3g
Tian Dong (Radix Asparagi)	3g
Mai Dong (Radix Ophiopogonis)	3g
Bai Zhu (Rhizoma Atractylodis Macrocephalae)	3g
Chen Pi (Pericarpium Citri Reticulatae)	2.1g
Zhi Gan Cao (Radix et Rhizoma Glycyrrhizae Praeparata cum Melle)	1.5g
Di Huang (Radix Rehmanniae)	2.4g
Zhi Mu (Rhizoma Anemarrhenae)	1.5g
Huang Bo (Cortex Phellodendri Chinensis), *chao* (dry-fried) with water and honey	1.5g

DOSAGE / PREPARATION / ADMINISTRATION

Cook the ingredients with 3 slices of *Sheng Jiang* (Rhizoma Zingiberis Recens) and 1 piece of *Da Zao* (Fructus Jujubae) in water to make a decoction. Add a small amount of *Zhu Li* (Succus Bambusae), *Tong Bian* (Infantis Urina) and the juice of *Sheng Jiang* (Rhizoma Zingiberis Recens) to the decoction prior to ingestion.

CHINESE THERAPEUTIC ACTIONS

1. Nourishes yin
2. Descends fire
3. Tonifies qi and blood

CLINICAL MANIFESTATIONS

Yin-deficient fire: low-grade fever in the evenings, general weakness, panting excessively (especially at night), dry cough, heat aversion, seeking cool surfaces/places, constipation, increased thirst, poor hearing or deafness, hypersensitivity to acupuncture, a dry mouth, a red tongue body with little to no coating, and a rapid, thready, thin pulse.

VETERINARY CLINICAL APPLICATIONS

Chronic bronchitis, cough in geriatric dogs, chronic glomerulonephritis, chronic renal insufficiency and diabetes mellitus.

EXPLANATION

Zi Yin Jiang Huo Tang (Nourish Yin and Descend the Fire Decoction) treats Kidney yin deficiency with Liver fire. Because of the underlying yin deficiency, the Kidney and Liver cannot be properly nourished and fire begins to rise upward. The fire usually disturbs the Stomach and Lung, leading to fever, cough, and a dry mouth and tongue.

This formula aims to nourish the underlying deficiency and control the excess. *Dang Gui* (Radix Angelicae Sinensis), *Bai Shao* (Radix Paeoniae Alba), and *Shu Di Huang* (Radix Rehmanniae Praeparata) tonify the blood. *Tian Dong* (Radix Asparagi) and *Mai Dong* (Radix Ophiopogonis) tonify yin. *Bai Zhu* (Rhizoma Atractylodis Macrocephalae), *Chen Pi* (Pericarpium Citri Reticulatae), *Zhi Gan Cao* (Radix et Rhizoma Glycyrrhizae Praeparata cum Melle), and *Da Zao* (Fructus Jujubae) tonify qi and activate qi circulation. *Di Huang* (Radix Rehmanniae), *Zhi Mu* (Rhizoma Anemarrhenae) and *Huang Bo* (Cortex Phellodendri Chinensis) are excellent herbs to guide the fire downward in cases involving underlying deficiency.

Zī Yīn Jiàng Huǒ Tāng (Nourish Yin and Descend the Fire Decoction)

Zi Yin Jiang Huo Tang (Nourish Yin and Descend the Fire Decoction)

Diagnosis	Clinical Signs	Treatment	Herbs
Yin-deficient fire	• Fever and cough: heat and fire rising upwards • Dry mouth and constipation: heat consuming body fluids • A red tongue body with little to no coating and a rapid, thready, thin pulse: deficiency and heat conditions	• Nourishes yin • Descends fire • Tonifies qi and blood	• *Dang Gui* (Radix Angelicae Sinensis), *Bai Shao* (Radix Paeoniae Alba) and *Shu Di Huang* (Radix Rehmanniae Praeparata) tonify the blood. • *Tian Dong* (Radix Asparagi) and *Mai Dong* (Radix Ophiopogonis) tonify yin. • *Bai Zhu* (Rhizoma Atractylodis Macrocephalae), *Chen Pi* (Pericarpium Citri Reticulatae), *Zhi Gan Cao* (Radix et Rhizoma Glycyrrhizae Praeparata cum Melle) and *Da Zao* (Fructus Jujubae) tonify qi and activate qi circulation. • *Di Huang* (Radix Rehmanniae), *Zhi Mu* (Rhizoma Anemarrhenae) and *Huang Bo* (Cortex Phellodendri Chinensis) clear deficiency fire.

VETERINARY MODIFICATIONS

- With wheezing and dyspnea with phlegm, add *Sang Bai Pi* (Cortex Mori), *Zi Wan* (Radix et Rhizoma Asteris), *Huang Qin* (Radix Scutellariae), and *Zhu Li* (Succus Bambusae).
- With cough and profuse sputum, add *Bei Mu* (Bulbus Fritillariae), *Kuan Dong Hua* (Flos Farfarae), and *Sang Bai Pi* (Cortex Mori).

SUGGESTED ACUPUNCTURE TREATMENT

1. Points: *Taiyuan (LU 9), Taixi* (KI 3), *Sanyinjiao* (SP 6), *Feishu* (BL 13), *Shenshu* (BL 23), *Tiantu* (CV 22), *Dingchuan*.
2. Technique: tonification

Taiyuan (LU 9) and *Feishu* (BL 13) tonify and disperse the Lung. *Taixi* (KI 3) and *Sanyinjiao* (SP 6) tonify yin. *Shenshu* (BL 23) is the *shu* (transport) point for the Kidney. *Tiantu* (CV 22) and the classical point *Dingchuan* stop cough.

AUTHORS' COMMENTS

Zi Yin Jiang Huo Tang is used to treat chronic coughing in the geriatric dog when no other cause for coughing can be found. Many older dogs have a dry, chronic cough, especially at night, and, despite a complete biomedical diagnostic evaluation, have no apparent reason for their coughing. In addition to coughing, from the owner's perspective many of these dogs also appear to have developed voice changes with a hoarse bark. This formula is similar to *Zhi Bai Di Huang Wan* (Anemarrhena, Phellodendron, and Rehmannia Pill) but focuses more on clearing deficiency heat, which is rising upward to scorch the Lung and throat. This formula is also effective in the treatment of concurrent chronic renal disease and bronchitis in the geriatric dog and cat. In horses, it is equally useful for treatment of younger patients and geriatrics. Horses, as fire animals and athletes, are predisposed to yin deficiency. Such patients will not only have a chronic cough and unresolved bronchitis but will be prone to fire attacking the Stomach creating signs of gastric ulceration.

Chapter 5 — Summary — Heat-Clearing Formulas

SECTION 1: *QI* (ENERGY) LEVEL-CLEARING FORMULAS

Name	Similarities	Differences
Bai Hu Tang (White Tiger Decoction)	Clear heat from the *qi* (energy) level	Generates body fluids
Bai Hu Jia Ren Shen Tang (White Tiger plus Ginseng Decoction)		Generates body fluids, tonifies qi
Zhu Ye Shi Gao Tang (Bamboo Leaves and Gypsum Decoction)		Generates body fluids, tonifies qi, harmonizes the Stomach

Bai Hu Tang (White Tiger Decoction) clears heat and promotes production of body fluids. It treats excessive heat from *yangming qi* (energy) level with high fever, profuse sweating (in horses), thirst, irritability, and a bounding and forceful pulse.

Bai Hu Jia Ren Shen Tang (White Tiger plus Ginseng Decoction) is formulated by adding *Ren Shen* (Radix et Rhizoma Ginseng) to *Bai Hu Tang* (White Tiger Decoction), which enables the formula to tonify qi.

Zhu Ye Shi Gao Tang (Bamboo Leaves and Gypsum Decoction) clears heat, nourishes yin, and tonifies qi to harmonize the Stomach. In comparison to *Bai Hu Tang* (White Tiger Decoction), this formula has a weaker heat-clearing effect, and therefore is used mostly to treat late-stage heat syndromes with damage to both qi and yin.

SECTION 2: *YING* (NUTRITIVE) LEVEL-CLEARING AND BLOOD-COOLING FORMULAS

Name	Similarities	Differences
Qing Ying Tang (Clear the Nutritive Level Decoction)	Clears heat from the *ying* (nutritive) level	Nourishes yin, invigorates blood circulation
Xi Jiao Di Huang Tang (Rhinoceros Horn and Rehmannia Decoction)	Clears heat and cools the blood in the *xue* (blood) level	Stops bleeding, disperses blood stasis

Qing Ying Tang (Clear the Nutritive Level Decoction) clears heat from the *ying* (nutritive) level, eliminates toxins, releases the heat, and nourishes yin. This formula is more appropriate for the initial stages of heat attacking the *ying* level, heat signs that worsen at night, and irritability.

Xi Jiao Di Huang Tang (Rhinoceros Horn and Rehmannia Decoction) clears heat, eliminates toxins, cools the blood, and disperses blood stagnation. This formula is suitable to treat more severe conditions of heat attacking the *xue* (blood) level, forcing blood out of the vessels and manifesting in various types of bleeding.

Chapter 5 — Summary

SECTION 3: *QI* (ENERGY) AND *XUE* (BLOOD) LEVELS-CLEARING FORMULA

Name	Actions
Qing Wen Bai Du Yin (Clear Epidemics and Overcome Pathogenic Influences Decoction)	Treats *wen yi* (warm epidemics) with heat and toxins in the *qi* (energy) and *xue* (blood) levels

Qing Wen Bai Du Yin (Clear Epidemics and Overcome Pathogenic Influences Decoction) clears heat, sedates fire, and eliminates toxins. It is a unique formula used to treat proliferation of heat toxins in both the *qi* (energy) and *xue* (blood) levels.

SECTION 4: HEAT-CLEARING AND TOXIN-ELIMINATING FORMULAS

Name	Similarities	Differences
Huang Lian Jie Du Tang (Coptis Decoction to Relieve Toxicity)	Clear heat, sedate fire, and eliminate toxins	Treats upper, middle, and lower *jiaos*
Huang Lian Shang Qing Wan (Coptis Pill to Clear the Upper)		Treats upper, middle, and lower *jiaos*, and the head
Pu Ji Xiao Du Yin (Universal Benefit Decoction to Eliminate Toxins)		Treats upper *jiao* and the head
San Huang Xie Xin Tang (Three-Yellow Decoction to Sedate the Epigastrium)		Clears heat and fire, drains damp-heat from the upper, middle, or lower *jiaos*

Huang Lian Jie Du Tang (Coptis Decoction to Relieve Toxicity) sedates fire and eliminates toxins. It is one of the most commonly used formulas to treat excess heat, fire, and toxins affecting all three *jiaos*.

Huang Lian Shang Qing Wan (Coptis Pill to Clear the Upper) clears heat, sedates fire, and eliminates toxins from the upper parts of the body and is most effective for heat and fire attacking the upper body and head, but it may also be used to treat heat affecting the upper, middle, and lower *jiaos*, and the head.

Pu Ji Xiao Du Yin (Universal Benefit Decoction to Eliminate Toxins) sedates fire and eliminates toxins in the upper *jiao* and head. It treats epidemic toxins in the head with a wind-heat diagnosis.

San Huang Xie Xin Tang (Three-Yellow Decoction to Sedate the Epigastrium) contains three "yellow" herbs to clear heat, purge fire, eliminate toxins and drain damp-heat from the upper, middle or lower *jiaos*. The three "yellow" herbs are *Huang Qin* (Radix Scutellariae), *Huang Lian* (Rhizoma Coptidis), and *Da Huang* (Radix et Rhizoma Rhei).

Chapter 5 — Summary

SECTION 5: *ZANG FU*-CLEARING FORMULAS

Name	Similarities	Differences
Dao Chi San (Guide Out the Red Powder)	Clear heat in the Heart and Small Intestine	Nourishes yin
Qing Xin Lian Zi Yin (Lotus Seed Decoction to Clear the Heart)		Tonifies qi and yin
Long Dan Xie Gan Tang (Gentiana Decoction to Drain the Liver)	Sedate excess fire in the Liver and Gallbladder	Clears damp-heat in the lower *jiao*
Xi Gan Ming Mu San (Wash the Liver and Brighten the Eyes Powder)	Clears Liver heat, dispels wind-heat	Treats eye disorders due to wind-heat and Liver heat
Xie Bai San (Drain the White Powder)	Clears Lung heat	Relieves coughing and dyspnea
Zuo Jin Wan (Left Metal Pill)	Clears Liver fire	Corrects the reversed flow of Stomach qi
Qing Wei San (Clear the Stomach Powder)	Clear Stomach heat and fire	Cools the blood
Yu Nu Jian (Jade Woman Decoction)		Nourishes yin
Gan Lu Yin (Sweet Dew Decoction)		Clears damp-heat in the Spleen and Stomach
Shao Yao Tang (Peony Decoction)	Clear damp-heat in the Intestines and stop dysentery	Harmonizes qi and blood
Bai Tou Weng Tang (Pulsatilla Decoction)		Cools the blood

Dao Chi San (Guide Out the Red Powder) and ***Qing Xin Lian Zi Yin*** (Lotus Seed Decoction to Clear the Heart) both clear heat from the Heart organ and channel. Heat in the Heart organ is characterized by symptoms such as restlessness and irritability. Heat in the Heart channel (and/or Small Intestines) is characterized by *lin zheng* (dysuria syndrome) with painful urination, cloudy urine, or blood-streaked urine.

- *Dao Chi San* calms Heart *shen* (spirit), cools the blood, promotes urination, and relieves dysuria. It treats heat in both the Heart and Small Intestine channels. It may be used for *lin zheng* (dysuria syndrome) with painful urination or blood-streaked urine.
- *Qing Xin Lian Zi Yin* clears heat in Heart (an excess condition in the upper *jiao*) and tonifies qi and Kidney yin (a deficient condition in the lower *jiao*). It may be used for *lin zheng* (dysuria syndrome) with turbid or cloudy urine.

Long Dan Xie Gan Tang (Gentiana Decoction to Drain the Liver) is a potent formula that purges excess fire in the Liver and Gallbladder channels. *Long Dan Xie Gan Tang* sedates Liver fire, drains damp-heat, and protects and nourishes Liver blood. It is mostly used for Liver fire flaring upward with damp-heat accumulation in the lower *jiao*.

Xi Gan Ming Mu San (Wash the Liver and Brighten the Eyes Powder) clears Liver heat and dispels wind-heat to treat various eye disorders.

Xie Bai San (Drain the White Powder) is a formula that clears Lung heat to relieve coughing, dyspnea, and coarse breathing.

Zuo Jin Wan* (Left Metal Pill), *Qing Wei San (Clear the Stomach Powder), ***Yu Nu Jian*** (Jade Woman Decoction), and ***Gan Lu Yin*** (Sweet Dew Decoction) all clear heat and treat stomach disorders.

- *Zuo Jin Wan* treats Liver fire overacting on the Stomach to address stomach disorders such as hypochondriac pain, epigastric bloating, acid regurgitation, nausea, and vomiting.
- *Qing Wei San* clears Stomach heat and cools the blood. It treats rising Stomach fire manifesting in toothache, gum bleeding, and swollen cheeks. It is used for acute conditions and should be discontinued once the clinical signs have resolved.

Chapter 5 — Summary

- *Yu Nu Jian* nourishes Stomach yin and clears Stomach heat to manage both excess and deficiency conditions, with symptoms such as increased thirst, gingivitis, stomatitis and periodontal disease.
- *Gan Lu Yin* clears damp-heat, cleanses the blood, and reduces inflammation. It treats damp-heat in the Spleen and Stomach with symptoms such as swelling, inflammation and suppuration of the gums and tongue, sore throat with inflammation and pain, stomatitis, tongue ulceration, and toothache.

Shao Yao Tang (Peony Decoction) and ***Bai Tou Weng Tang*** (Pulsatilla Decoction) both clear damp-heat in the Intestines to relieve diarrhea and dysentery.

- *Shao Yao Tang* (Peony Decoction) emphasizes harmonizing and activating qi and blood. It is more suitable for dysentery characterized by equal dampness and heat, with main signs and symptoms such as abdominal pain, tenesmus, and the presence of equal amounts of mucus and blood in the stools.
- *Bai Tou Weng Tang* (Pulsatilla Decoction) emphasizes cooling the blood to relieve dysentery. It is more suitable for treating bloody, explosive diarrhea characterized by more heat than dampness, with clinical signs of tenesmus, and the presence of more blood than mucus.

SECTION 6: DEFICIENCY-HEAT CLEARING FORMULAS

Name	Similarities	Differences
Qing Hao Bie Jia Tang (Artemisia Annua and Soft-Shelled Turtle Shell Decoction)	Clears deficiency heat, nourishes yin	Disperses deep, hidden deficiency heat
Zi Yin Jiang Huo Tang (Nourish Yin and Descend the Fire Decoction)	Clears deficiency heat, tonifies underlying deficiencies	Tonifies yin, qi and blood

Qing Hao Bie Jia Tang (Artemisia Annua and Soft-shelled Turtle Shell Decoction) nourishes yin and clears deficiency heat. It treats deficiency heat and deficiency fire syndromes, as well as late-stage heat syndromes (heat hidden in the yin).

Zi Yin Jiang Huo Tang (Nourish Yin and Descend the Fire Decoction) nourishes yin, tonifies qi and blood, and clears deficiency fire. It treats yin deficiency with fire from the Kidney and Liver.

Chapter 6

— Summer-Heat-Dispelling Formulas

祛暑剂

吴塘 Wú Táng

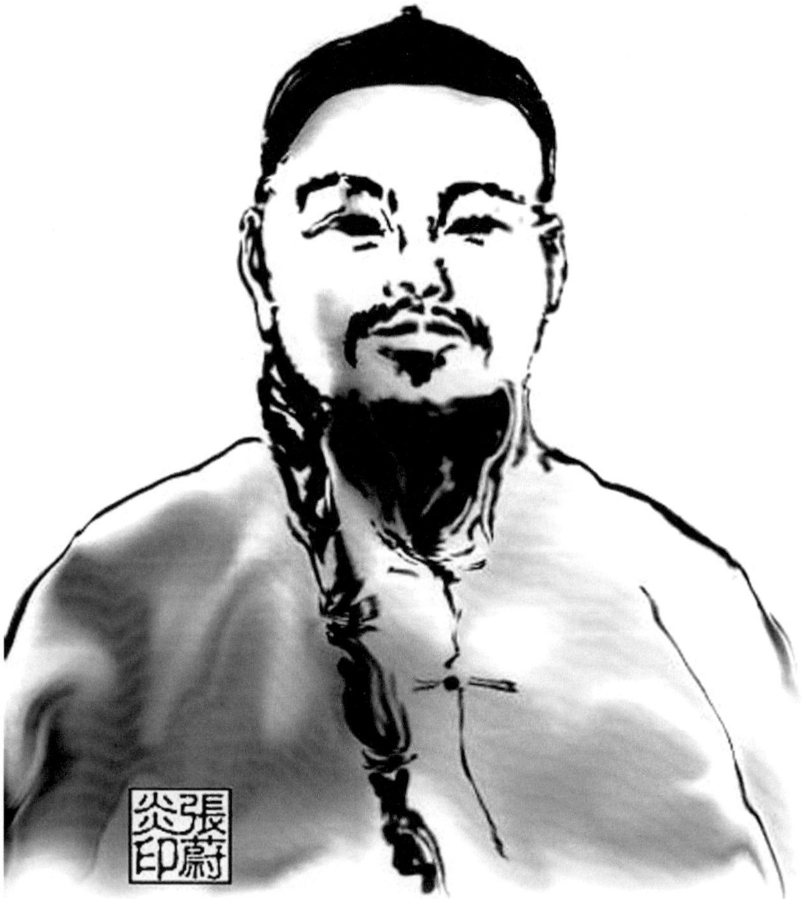

吴塘 Wú Táng, also known as 吴鞠通 Wú Jū-Tōng, 1758 – 1836.

吴塘 Wú Táng

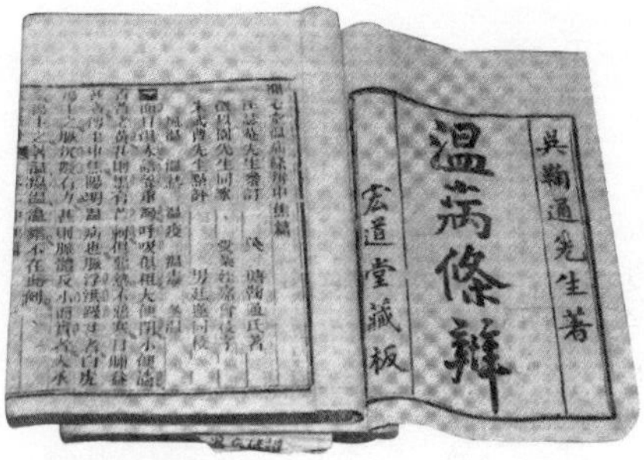

温病条辨 *Wen Bing Tiao Bian* (Systematic Differentiation of Warm Disease) in 1798.

Wu Tang was inspired to study medicine at nineteen years of age, when his father passed away from a warm disease epidemic. He was the most influenced in his pursuit of medicine by Wu You-Xing's *Wen Yi Lun* (Discussion of Epidemic Warm Diseases) and Ye Gui's *Wen Re Lun* (Discussion of Warm and Hot Disorders). Expanding beyond the theories of his predecessors, Wu proposed a new theory to treat *wen bing* (warm diseases): *San Jiao Bian Zheng* (Triple Burner Differentiation). He stated that *wen bing* (warm diseases) enters the body through the nose to affect the upper *jiao*, and the mouth to affect the middle *jiao*. If untreated, the disease will continue to deteriorate and affect the lower *jiao*.

Wu Tang was also the first to recommend specific herbal treatments based on *Wei Qi Ying Xue Bian Zheng* (Defensive, Qi, Nutritive, Blood Differentiation). He recommended *Yin Qiao San* (Honeysuckle and Forsythia Powder) for *wen bing* (warm diseases) affecting the *wei* (defensive) level, *Bai Hu Tang* (White Tiger Decoction) for *wen bing* (warm diseases) affecting the *qi* (energy) level, *Qing Ying Tang* (Clear the Nutritive Level Decoction) for disease that has progressed to the *ying* (nutritive) level, and *Xi Jiao Di Huang Tang* (Rhinoceros Horn and Rehmannia Decoction) for treatment at the *xue* (blood) level. Furthermore, he observed that the *wen bing* (warm diseases) strongly consume and damage yin and body fluids, and proposed using nourishing formulas to replenish the fluids and remedy the damage, such as *San Jia Fu Mai Tang* (Three-Shell Decoction to Restore the Pulse), *Da Ding Feng Zhu* (Major Arrest Wind Pearl) and *Xiao Ding Feng Zhu* (Minor Arrest Wind Pearl).

Wu Tang combined his academic and clinical experiences to publish *Wen Bing Tiao Bian* (Systematic Differentiation of Warm Diseases) in 1798. His greatest contribution to *wen bing* (warm diseases) is the integration of theories and treatment. While his predecessors (Wu You-Xing and Ye Gui) established the fundamental theories of *wen bing* (warm diseases), Wu Tang integrated the theories with clinically effective formulas, many of which are still in use today.

Examples of formulas written by Wu Tang include:

- *Sang Ju Yin* (Mulberry Leaf and Chrysanthemum Decoction)
- *Yin Qiao San* (Honeysuckle and Forsythia Powder)
- *Zeng Ye Cheng Qi Tang* (Increase the Fluids and Order the Qi Decoction)
- *Qing Ying Tang* (Clear the Nutritive Level Decoction)
- *Qing Hao Bie Jia Tang* (Artemisia Annua and Soft-Shelled Turtle Shell Decoction)
- *Qing Luo Yin* (Clear the Collaterals Decoction)
- *Xin Jia Xiang Ru Yin* (Newly-Augmented Mosla Decoction)
- *An Gong Niu Huang Wan* (Calm the Palace Pill with Cattle Gallstone)
- *Xing Su San* (Apricot Kernel and Perilla Leaf Powder)
- *Sang Xing Tang* (Mulberry Leaf and Apricot Kernel Decoction)
- *Sha Shen Mai Dong Tang* (Glehnia and Ophiopogonis Decoction)
- *Zeng Ye Tang* (Increase the Fluids Decoction)

Dynasties & Kingdoms	Year
Xia Dynasty 夏	2100-1600 BCE
Shang Dynasty 商	1600-1100 BCE
Zhou Dynasty 周	1100-221 BCE
Qin Dynasty 秦	221-207 BCE
Han Dynasty 漢	206 BCE-220
Three Kingdoms 三國	220-280
Western Jin Dynasty 西晉	265-316
Eastern Jin Dynasty 東晉	317-420
Northern and Southern Dynasties 北南朝	420-581
Sui Dynasty 隋	581-618
Tang Dynasty 唐	618-907
Five Dynasties 五代	907-960
Song Dynasty 宋	960-1279
Liao Dynasty 遼	916-1125
Jin Dynasty 金	1115-1234
Yuan Dynasty 元	1271-1368
Ming Dynasty 明	1368-1644
Qing Dynasty 清	**1644-1911**
Republic of China 中華民國	1912-Present Day
People's Republic of China 中華人民共和國	1949-Present Day

Table of Contents

Chapter 6 — Overview

祛暑剂 — Summer-Heat-Dispelling Formulas

Definition: Summer-heat-dispelling formulas, as the name implies, relieve summer-heat syndromes. Summer-heat, one of the *liu yin* (six exogenous factors), is the dominant exterior pathogenic factor during the hot and humid summer season. Summer-heat syndromes are characterized by the presence of heat and dampness, as well as by the consumption of, and damage to, qi and body fluids.

Summer-heat is a yang pathogen most prevalent in late summer and is characterized by the presence of heat and dampness, as well as the consumption of, and damage to, qi and body fluids. Those animals most susceptible to summer-heat syndrome include the very young (less than 4 months), geriatric, chronically ill, brachycephalic, obese, and performance animals that are expected to exert themselves during the hot summer months. Clinical manifestations of summer-heat syndromes include fever, thirst, restlessness, irritability, profuse sweating (in species that sweat), heavy panting, exercise intolerance, dysuria, yellow concentrated urine, a red tongue, and a forceful, rapid pulse. Summer-heat, in combination with dampness, is most common and these animals will present with hyperthermia, abdominal pain, vomiting, diarrhea, mental confusion or dullness, a lack of sweating where sweating is expected (in horses), a greasy, white tongue coating and a soft, rapid pulse, in addition to classic summer-heat signs. Summer-heat stroke is the most severe pattern of summer-heat, characterized by hyperthermia, loss of consciousness, and seizures. As a result of high fever and profuse sweating, qi and body fluids are often consumed and damaged. Therefore, optimal treatment of summer-heat syndromes requires the use of herbs that dispel summer-heat, tonify qi, and replenish body fluids.

From a biomedical perspective, the clinical signs of summer-heat syndrome correspond to heat stroke or hyperthermia. Animals that are confined or tied outdoors in the hot sun without shelter, left in vehicles that are parked in the sun with the windows rolled up, and animals that are over-worked in hot, humid climates without adequate rest and hydration often develop heat exhaustion or heat stroke. Bulldogs, pugs and other brachycephalic breeds are constitutionally predisposed to overheating, even with normal environmental temperatures, and are highly susceptible to heat stroke and summer-heat syndrome. These animals present with high body temperature (>105 °F), heavy panting or hyperventilation, thick saliva, vomiting, a red tongue, and a rapid pulse. As the condition worsens, animals often develop bloody diarrhea, may suddenly collapse, develop seizure, or go into a coma. During heat stroke, the animal becomes dehydrated and their blood viscosity increases to the point that the heart has difficulty pumping the abnormally "thick" blood through the blood vessels. The result is stagnation of blood, with clotting and death of tissues due to ischemic necrosis. In many cases, the body temperature has been dangerously high for so long that the brain and other body cells are irreparably damaged.

The use of summer-heat dispelling herbal formulas are not meant to replace emergency veterinary care but can be used in conjunction to help stabilize the animal, prevent the secondary effects of heat stroke, and promote recovery. The most common complications of heat stroke include cardiac arrhythmia, disseminated intravascular coagulation, cerebral edema and kidney failure. It is interesting to note that two common foods that are effective in treating summer-heat include watermelon (*Xi Gua* [Frucutus Citrulli]) and mung beans (*Lu Dou* [Semen Phaseoli Radiati]), which

Chapter 6 — Overview

are often consumed during the summer season. Some of the herbal formulas used to treat summer-heat contain *Xi Gua Cui Pi* (Exocarpium Citrulli), which is watermelon peel or rind.

Summer-heat formulas can also be used to treat acute exogenous pathogen invasion in the dog secondary to food poisoning from garbage eating, as well as to treat gastroenteritis from consumption of raw food, fast food, ice cream and ice cubes and from environmental pathogens acquired during a kennel stay. This condition is defined as damp-heat affecting the exterior and the digestive tract. Exogenous damp-heat causes fever and aversion to cold, and because damp-heat is also caused by ingestion of dirty, cold or raw food, the animal will show clinical signs of abdominal pain, nausea, vomiting and diarrhea.

SUBCATEGORIES OF ACTION

Summer-heat-dispelling formulas are divided into four subcategories to reflect the nature of the disorder and characteristics of the formulas. The four subcategories are as follows:

1. **Summer-Heat-Dispelling and Heat-Clearing Formulas**
   These formulas are designed to treat summer-heat syndromes with interior heat. Clinical manifestations include high fever, irritability, profuse sweating (in horses), excessive panting, and thirst. Herbs commonly used to dispel summer-heat include *Xi Gua Cui Pi* (Exocarpium Citrulli), *Jin Yin Hua* (Flos Lonicerae Japonicae), and *He Ye* (Folium Nelumbinis). An exemplar formula is *Qing Luo Yin* (Clear the Collaterals Decoction).

2. **Summer-Heat-Dispelling and Exterior-Releasing Formulas**
   These formulas are designed to relieve summer-heat in the interior and dispel any exterior factor (usually wind-cold) at the skin and muscle levels. Summer-heat and wind-cold occur together when animals try to cool down on hot summer days by drinking large volumes of cold water, and by standing or laying outside in the evening and at night. Bathing horses that have not sufficiently cooled down from exercise will also make them susceptible to this pattern. As a result, they contract both summer-heat and exterior wind-cold, and show clinical signs such as fever, aversion to cold, no sweating, no panting, irritability, and thirst. Commonly used herbs include *Huo Xiang* (Herba Agastaches), *Xiang Ru* (Herba Moslae) and *He Ye* (Folium Nelumbinis). An exemplar formula is *Xin Jia Xiang Ru Yin* (Newly-Augmented Mosla Decoction).

3. **Summer-Heat-Dispelling and Dampness-Draining Formulas**
   These formulas are designed to relieve summer-heat and dispel internal dampness simultaneously. Summer-heat and dampness often occur together in places subjected to both heat and humidity during the summer. Common clinical manifestations include fever, irritability, thirst, chest and hypochondriac discomfort, and dysuria. This condition is treated by the concurrent use of herbs that dispel summer-heat and drain dampness. Because internal dampness can be dispelled effectively through urination, herbs that regulate water and drain dampness are commonly used, such as *Hua Shi* (Talcum), *Fu Ling* (Poria), and *Ze Xie* (Rhizoma Alismatis). Representative formulas include *Liu Yi San* (Six-to-One Powder) and *Gui Ling Gan Lu Yin* (Cinnamon and Poria Sweet Dew Decoction).

4. **Summer-Heat-Dispelling and Qi-Benefiting Formulas**
   These formulas are used when summer-heat has damaged qi and body fluids extensively. Common clinical manifestations include fever, irritability, thirst, lethargy, weak breathing, profuse sweating, and a weak pulse. Herbs that benefit qi and nourish yin and body fluids are commonly used in these formulas, such as *Xi Yang Shen* (Radix Panacis Quinquefolii), *Ren Shen* (Radix et Rhizoma Ginseng), *Mai Dong* (Radix Ophiopogonis), *Shi Hu* (Caulis Dendrobii), and *Wu Wei Zi* (Fructus Schisandrae Chinensis). An exemplar formula is *Qing Shu Yi Qi Tang* (Clear Summer-Heat and Augment the Qi Decoction).

Chapter 6 — Overview

CAUTIONS / CONTRAINDICATIONS

As the name implies, summer-heat syndromes generally occur in the summer, and may be characterized by the presence of both heat and dampness. To properly treat this syndrome, herbs that clear heat and dispel dampness should be used simultaneously. However, use these herbs cautiously because inappropriate use of heat-clearing herbs may damage yin, while inappropriate use of damp-resolving herbs may dry up body fluids. Horses in particular should be monitored carefully for hydration status to avoid impaction.

PHARMACOLOGICAL EFFECTS & CLINICAL APPLICATIONS

Summer-heat dispelling formulas primarily treat disorders of the respiratory and gastrointestinal tracts.

- **Respiratory disorders**: These formulas have been used effectively to treat various lung disorders, such as common cold or influenza,[1] pneumonia,[2] whooping cough,[3] and wheezing and dyspnea.[4] Representative formulas include *Xin Jia Xiang Ru Yin* (Newly-Augmented Mosla Decoction), *Liu Yi San* (Six-to-One Powder), and *Qing Shu Yi Qi Tang* (Clear Summer-Heat and Augment the Qi Decoction).
- **Gastrointestinal disorders**: Diarrhea in infants, children and adults is frequently treated with good results using *Liu Yi San* (Six-to-One Powder) and *Gui Ling Gan Lu Yin* (Cinnamon and Poria Sweet Dew Decoction).[5,6]
- **Fever**: These formulas have been used effectively to treat fever in children and adults.[7,8,9] Exemplar formulas include *Xiang Ru San* (Mosla Powder) and *Xin Jia Xiang Ru Yin* (Newly-Augmented Mosla Decoction).

References

1. *Shang Hai Zhong Yi Yao Za Zhi* (Shanghai Journal of Chinese Medicine and Herbology), 1982; 8:35.
2. *Zhe Jiang Zhong Yi Za Zhi* (Zhejiang Journal of Chinese Medicine), 1984; 8:352.
3. *Shan Xi Zhong Yi* (Shanxi Chinese Medicine), 1986; 10: 441.
4. *Shan Xi Yi Kan* (Shanxi Journal of Medicine), 1992; 3:104.
5. *Ji Lin Zhong Yi Yao* (Jilin Chinese Medicine and Herbology), 1987; 6:24.
6. *Zhong Xi Yi Jie He Za Zhi* (Journal of Integrated Chinese and Western Medicine), 1985; 1:19.
7. *Fu Jian Zhong Yi Yao* (Fujian Chinese Medicine and Herbology), 1990; 2:14.
8. *Zhong Yi Ming Fang Lin Chuang Xin Yong* (Contemporary Clinical Applications of Classic Chinese Formulas), 2001; 708.
9. *Jiang Su Zhong Yi* (Jiangsu Chinese Medicine), 1999; 7:28.

Qīng Luò Yǐn (Clear the Collaterals Decoction)

清絡飲
清络饮

Pinyin Name: *Qing Luo Yin*
Literal Name: Clear the Collaterals Decoction
Original Source: *Wen Bing Tiao Bian* (Systematic Differentiation of Warm Diseases) by Wu Ju-Tong in 1798

COMPOSITION

Jin Yin Hua (Flos Lonicerae Japonicae), fresh	6g
Bian Dou Hua (Flos Lablab Album), fresh	6g
Xi Gua Cui Pi (Exocarpium Citrulli)	6g
He Ye (Folium Nelumbinis), fresh	6g
Si Gua Pi (Pericarpium Luffae)	6g
Zhu Ye (Herba Phyllostachys), fresh	6g

DOSAGE / PREPARATION / ADMINISTRATION

Cook the ingredients in 2 cups of water until 1 cup remains. Take the decoction twice daily.

CHINESE THERAPEUTIC ACTIONS

Clears heat and dispels summer-heat

CLINICAL MANIFESTATIONS

Summer-heat invading the Lung and *qi* (energy) level: mild fever, slight thirst, impaired vision, lethargy, a slightly red tongue.

VETERINARY CLINICAL APPLICATIONS

Upper respiratory infection in the summer, mild heat stroke, and prevention of heat stroke.

EXPLANATION

Qing Luo Yin (Clear the Collaterals Decoction) treats mild cases of summer-heat affecting the Lung and *qi* (energy) level. This condition occurs when mild summer-heat directly attacks the Lung, or it can be a residual condition of summer-heat that has not been dispelled after using exterior-releasing herbs. Summer-heat may affect the Lung and consume fluids, leading to thirst. Summer-heat may attack the *qi* (energy) level to cause mild fever. Summer-heat may travel to the head and cause mental dullness and confusion. A slightly red tongue suggests that this is a mild syndrome of heat.

Since the disorder is in the Lung and *qi* (energy) level, exterior-releasing herbs are not used. *Jin Yin Hua* (Flos Lonicerae Japonicae) and *Bian Dou Hua* (Flos Lablab Album), the chief herbs, are aromatic and can disperse and dispel summer-heat. *Xi Gua Cui Pi* (Exocarpium Citrulli) clears summer-heat. *Si Gua Pi* (Pericarpium Luffae) clears heat in the Lung and from its channel and collateral. *He Ye* (Folium Nelumbinis) disperses heat and dispels summer-heat. Because summer-heat can easily injure the Heart and disturb the *shen* (spirit), *Zhu Ye* (Herba Phyllostachys) is used to purge this heat through urination. Most of the herbs in this formula should be used in the fresh and aromatic form to enhance the summer-heat dispersing action. Because this formula is intended to treat mild cases of summer-heat syndrome, it can be taken regularly as an herbal tea during the summer to prevent summer-heat invasion.

***Qing Luo Yin* (Clear the Collaterals Decoction)**

Diagnosis	Clinical Signs	Treatment	Herbs
Summer-heat invading the Lung and *qi* (energy) level	• Mild fever: summer-heat invading the *qi* (energy) level • Increased thirst: summer-heat consuming body fluids • Impaired vision, lethargy: summer-heat blocking the sensory orifices • Slightly red tongue: early stage of heat condition	Clears heat and dispels summer-heat	• *Jin Yin Hua* (Flos Lonicerae Japonicae), *Bian Dou Hua* (Flos Lablab Album), *Xi Gua Cui Pi* (Exocarpium Citrulli), and *He Ye* (Folium Nelumbinis) clear summer-heat. • *Si Gua Pi* (Pericarpium Luffae) clears heat in the Lung and its channel and collateral. • *Zhu Ye* (Herba Phyllostachys) clears the Heart and purges heat through urination.

Qīng Luò Yǐn (Clear the Collaterals Decoction)

VETERINARY MODIFICATIONS

- With thirst, add *Tian Hua Fen* (Radix Trichosanthis), *Ge Gen* (Radix Puerariae Lobatae), and *Shi Hu* (Caulis Dendrobii).
- With fever, add *Shi Gao* (Gypsum Fibrosum) and *Zhi Mu* (Rhizoma Anemarrhenae).
- With summer-heat injuring the Lung manifesting in high-pitched cough with no sputum, add *Gan Cao* (Radix et Rhizoma Glycyrrhizae), *Jie Geng* (Radix Platycodonis), *Ku Xing Ren* (Semen Armeniacae Amarum) and *Mai Dong* (Radix Ophiopogonis).

CAUTIONS / CONTRAINDICATIONS

Qing Luo Yin treats only mild to moderate cases of summer-heat. It is insufficient for severe cases of summer-heat.

SUGGESTED ACUPUNCTURE TREATMENT

1. Points: *Xiangu* (ST 43), *Hegu* (LI 4), *Dazhui* (GV 14), *Waiguan* (TH 5), *Touwei* (ST 8), and *Taiyang* (extra point).
2. Technique: sedation.

Xiangu (ST 43), *Hegu* (LI 4), *Dazhui* (GV 14), and *Waiguan* (TH 5) disperse summer-heat. *Touwei* (ST 8) and *Taiyang* (extra point) dispel the exterior factors and relieve discomfort in the head. The tips of the ears and tail can also be treated with acupuncture to clear heat. Place an icepack behind the stifles over *Weizhong* (BL 40) for 10 minutes to reduce temperature.

AUTHORS' COMMENTS

Qing Luo Yin treats mild to moderate cases of summer-heat invading the Lung. This formula may be taken following prolonged exertion or exposure during the summer months, and for mild heatstroke. In more severe cases, it can be combined with *Sheng Mai San* (Generate the Pulse Powder) to tonify qi, promote the generation of body fluids, preserve yin, and stop sweating/panting. It may also be given in lower doses throughout the summer for prevention of heat strokes in brachycephalic dogs. *Qing Luo Yin* is not available ready made but can easily be formulated in-house; it contains watermelon rind as one of its ingredients.

Xiāng Rú Sǎn (Mosla Powder)

香薷散

Pinyin Name: *Xiang Ru San*
Literal Name: Mosla Powder
Alternate Names: *Hsiang Ju Yin, Xiang Ru Yin*, Elsholtzia Drink, Elsholtzia Decoction
Original Source: *Tai Ping Hui Min He Ji Ju Fang* (Imperial Grace Formulary of the Tai Ping Era) by the Imperial Medical Department in 1078-85

COMPOSITION

Xiang Ru (Herba Moslae)	480g [9g]
Hou Po (Cortex Magnoliae Officinalis), *zhi* (fried with ginger juice)	240g [6g]
Bai Bian Dou (Semen Lablab Album), *chao* (dry-fried)	240g [6g]

Note: Historically, "*Xiang Ru*" was derived from two sources: *Mosla chinensis* and *Elsholtzia splendens*. Both herbs have similar functions, and have been used interchangeably in the history of Chinese herbal medicine. In 2005, *Zhong Hua Ren Min Gong He Guo Yao Dian* (Pharmacopoeia of the People's Republic of China) identified *Mosla chinensis* as the official source of this herb. Therefore, *Xiang Ru* (Herba Moslae) is adopted as the standard nomenclature throughout this text.

DOSAGE / PREPARATION / ADMINISTRATION

The source text states to grind the ingredients into a coarse powder. Cook 9g of the powder with one large bowl of water and a small amount of grain-based liquor (approximately

Xiāng Rú Sǎn (Mosla Powder)

10% of the total volume) until 70% of the liquid remains. Discard the residue, and cool the strained decoction before ingestion. Today, this formula may be prepared as a decoction with the doses suggested in brackets, with or without the addition of grain-based liquor.

CHINESE THERAPEUTIC ACTIONS

1. Dispels summer-heat
2. Releases exterior cold
3. Resolves dampness and harmonizes the middle *jiao*

CLINICAL MANIFESTATIONS

Summer-heat syndrome with exterior cold and interior dampness: fever, aversion to cold, mental confusion and dullness, lethargy, anhidrosis, nausea, vomiting, diarrhea, abdominal pain, a white, greasy tongue coating, and a superficial pulse.

VETERINARY CLINICAL APPLICATIONS

Common cold, heat stroke, anhidrosis, gastroenteritis, bacterial dysentery secondary to garbage eating, and dietary indiscretion.

EXPLANATION

Xiang Ru San (Mosla Powder) treats summer-heat with exterior cold and interior dampness. More specifically, it treats exterior cold and interior dampness during the summer, a condition that often occurs when animals try to cool down on hot summer days by drinking excessive volumes of cold water and by sleeping outside in the evening and at night. As a result, they contract both dampness in the interior (from drinking cold liquids) and wind-cold at the exterior (by sleeping outside as the temperature cools down). Interior dampness blocks the qi flow to cause mental dullness, nausea, vomiting, diarrhea, lethargy, and abdominal pain. Fever and aversion to cold are common clinical signs caused by exterior wind-cold. A white, greasy tongue coating indicates damp accumulation in the interior, and a superficial pulse is a sign of an exterior condition.

Xiang Ru (Herba Moslae), aromatic and warm, dispels the exterior cold factor and resolves interior dampness. Frequently used in the summer to treat exterior wind-cold, *Xiang Ru* (Herba Moslae) has been called the "summer *Ma Huang* (Herba Ephedrae)." *Hou Po* (Cortex Magnoliae Officinalis) activates qi flow and dries interior dampness to relieve the feeling of heaviness and the stifling sensation in the chest. *Bai Bian Dou* (Semen Lablab Album) tonifies qi, strengthens the Spleen, and dries dampness.

VETERINARY MODIFICATIONS

- With nasal obstruction or discharge, add *Cong Chi Tang* (Scallion and Prepared Soybean Decoction).
- With cramps and spasms, add *Mu Gua* (Fructus Chaenomelis).
- With severe heat, add *Jin Yin Hua* (Flos Lonicerae Japonicae) and *Lian Qiao* (Fructus Forsythiae).
- When there is more dampness, add *Fu Ling* (Poria) and *Gan Cao* (Radix et Rhizoma Glycyrrhizae).
- If there is Spleen deficiency with *zhong* (central) *qi* deficiency, add *Ren Shen* (Radix et Rhizoma Ginseng), *Huang Qi* (Radix Astragali), *Bai Zhu* (Rhizoma Atractylodis Macrocephalae), and *Ju Hong* (Exocarpium Citri Rubrum).

CAUTIONS / CONTRAINDICATIONS

- *Xiang Ru San* is not suitable for animals that suffer from summer-heat with sweating or excessive panting, summer-heat with *wei* (defensive) *qi* deficiency with sweating or excessive panting, or summer-heat with irritability and thirst.
- This formula is not suitable for animals with exterior wind-heat conditions.[1]

PHARMACOLOGICAL EFFECTS

Effect on temperature regulation: Administration of *Xiang Ru San* was associated with a temporary reduction of body temperature in rats with artificially-induced fever. The effectiveness of the formula was increased when a small amount of alcohol was added to the water during

Xiang Ru San (Mosla Powder)

Diagnosis	Clinical Signs	Treatment	Herbs
Summer-heat syndrome with exterior cold and interior dampness	• Mental dullness, nausea, vomiting, diarrhea, lethargy, and abdominal pain: interior dampness • Fever and aversion to cold: exterior wind-cold • White, greasy tongue coating: damp accumulation • Superficial pulse: exterior condition	• Clears summer-heat • Releases exterior cold • Resolves dampness and harmonizes the middle *jiao*	• *Xiang Ru* (Herba Moslae) releases exterior cold. • *Hou Po* (Cortex Magnoliae Officinalis) activates qi flow and dries dampness. • *Bai Bian Dou* (Semen Lablab Album) tonifies qi, strengthens the Spleen, and dries dampness.

Xiāng Rú Sǎn (Mosla Powder)

the cooking process to enhance the extraction of essential oils.[2]

HUMAN CLINICAL STUDIES AND RESEARCH

1. **Fever**: Forty-five children with persistent fever (38-39°C / 100.4-102.2°F) longer than 10 days during the summer were treated with modified *Xiang Ru San* with success. Out of 45 cases, the study reported 14 cases with normal temperature after 1-3 days, 16 cases after 4-6 days, 12 cases after 7-9 days, and 3 cases with no effect after 10 days. *Xiang Ru San* was modified by adding *Ban Lan Gen* (Radix Isatidis), *Di Gu Pi* (Cortex Lycii), *Qing Hao* (Herba Artemisiae Annuae), and others as deemed necessary.[3]
2. **Hypokalemia**: Twenty-four patients with low potassium were treated with *Xiang Ru San* combined with *Liu Yi San* (Six-to-One Powder) and *Bo He* (Herba Menthae). After 2-4 doses, 19 returned to normal, 4 had some improvement, and 1 had no benefit.[4]

SUGGESTED ACUPUNCTURE TREATMENT

1. Points: *Fengchi* (GB 20), *Hegu* (LI 4), *Housanli* (ST 36), *Yinlingquan* (SP 9), *Erjian*, *Weijian*, and *Xiongtang*.
2. Technique: sedation.

Fengchi (GB 20) disperses exterior factors. *Hegu* (LI 4) relieves summer-heat. *Housanli* (ST 36) tonifies the middle *jiao* and resolves dampness. *Yinlingquan* (SP 9) strengthens the Spleen and eliminates dampness. Hemo-acupuncture at the classical points *Erjian*, *Weijian*, and *Xiongtang* clears excess heat.

RELATED FORMULAS

Sān Wù Xiāng Rú Yǐn **(Mosla Three Decoction)**
三物香薷飲
三物香薷饮
Pinyin Name: *San Wu Xiang Ru Yin*
Literal Name: Mosla Three Decoction
Original Source: *Zheng Zhi Zhun Sheng* (Standards of Patterns and Treatments) by Wang Ken-Tang in 1602

Xiang Ru (Herba Moslae)	[16g]
Hou Po (Cortex Magnoliae Officinalis)	[8g]
Bai Bian Dou (Semen Lablab Album)	[12g]

San Wu Xiang Ru Yin (Mosla Three Decoction) is taken as a decoction at room temperature because ingestion of warm decoction is sometimes associated with diarrhea. Note: Doses of herbs are unavailable from the source text. Suggested doses are listed above in brackets.

This formula primarily dispels summer-heat, eliminates toxins and stops diarrhea. It treats invasion of summer-heat with clinical signs such as fever, aversion to cold, irritability, abdominal pain, nausea and vomiting. Today, it may be used to treat enteritis, gastroenteritis, stomach flu, diarrhea, dysentery, and food poisoning.

This formula is used to treat sudden contraction of exterior condition during the summer. Because summer is characterized predominately by dampness and heat, the condition is defined as damp-heat affecting the exterior and the digestive tract. Damp-heat at the exterior causes fever and aversion to cold. Because damp-heat may be contracted via ingestion of cold or raw food, the animal may show abdominal pain, nausea, vomiting and diarrhea.

This is a rather simple formula containing only three herbs. *Xiang Ru* (Herba Moslae) is regarded as one of the best herbs to release the exterior during the summer. It releases the exterior via diaphoresis, and drains dampness via urination. In addition, *Hou Po* (Cortex Magnoliae Officinalis) strengthens the Spleen, and *Bai Bian Dou* (Semen Lablab Album) relieves diarrhea. Altogether, this formula dispels summer-heat from the exterior and interior, while strengthening the Spleen and Stomach simultaneously.

Shí Wèi Xiāng Rú Yǐn
(Ten-Ingredient Decoction with Mosla)
十味香薷飲
十味香薷饮
Pinyin Name: *Shi Wei Xiang Ru Yin*
Literal Name: Ten-Ingredient Decoction with Mosla
Original Source: *Zhou Hou Bei Ji Fang* (Emergency Formulas to Keep Up One's Sleeve) by Ge Hong in 341 A.D.

Xiang Ru (Herba Moslae)	30g
Ren Shen (Radix et Rhizoma Ginseng)	15g
Bai Zhu (Rhizoma Atractylodis Macrocephalae)	15g
Chen Pi (Pericarpium Citri Reticulatae)	15g
Fu Ling (Poria)	15g
Huang Qi (Radix Astragali)	15g
Hou Po (Cortex Magnoliae Officinalis)	15g
Mu Gua (Fructus Chaenomelis)	15g
Bai Bian Dou (Semen Lablab Album)	15g
Zhi Gan Cao (Radix et Rhizoma Glycyrrhizae Praeparata cum Melle)	15g

Shi Wei Xiang Ru Yin (Ten-Ingredient Decoction with Mosla) disperses summer-heat, harmonizes the Spleen and Stomach, and benefits qi. It treats summer-heat at the exterior with interior constitutional deficiency, manifesting in the following symptoms: exterior condition during the summer time, mental dullness or confusion, lethargy,

Xiāng Rú Sǎn (Mosla Powder)

fatigue, irritability, thirst, nausea, vomiting, and diarrhea. There may also be sweating and a weak pulse. The use of this formula is similar to *San Wu Xiang Ru Yin* (Mosla Three Decoction) to treat stomach flu, gastroenteritis, indigestion, and diarrhea as it contains all of the herbs in that formula in addition to herbs that tonify middle *jiao* deficiency. It can be used to consolidate treatment following *San Wu Xiang Ru Yin* (Mosla Three Decoction), once the acute clinical signs have resolved, and as the initial treatment for animals with obvious deficiency.

This formula uses herbs to clear summer-heat, harmonize the middle *jiao* and tonify qi. Aromatic and warm, *Xiang Ru* (Herba Moslae) disperses summer-heat from the exterior. *Hou Po* (Cortex Magnoliae Officinalis) resolves dampness and harmonizes the Stomach. *Bai Bian Dou* (Semen Lablab Album) resolves summer-heat and harmonizes the Spleen. *Ren Shen* (Radix et Rhizoma Ginseng) and *Huang Qi* (Radix Astragali) tonify qi and treat the underlying deficiency. *Huang Qi* (Radix Astragali) also strengthens *wei* (defensive) *qi* and stops sweating and panting. *Bai Zhu* (Rhizoma Atractylodis Macrocephalae), *Fu Ling* (Poria), and *Chen Pi* (Pericarpium Citri Reticulatae) strengthen the Spleen and Stomach, and relieve nausea, vomiting and diarrhea. *Mu Gua* (Fructus Chaenomelis) resolves dampness and promotes digestion. Lastly, *Gan Cao* (Radix et Rhizoma Glycyrrhizae) harmonizes the herbs.

AUTHORS' COMMENTS

These formulas can be used effectively to treat horses with anhidrosis, exercise-induced pulmonary hemorrhage (EIPH), and other forms of heat exhaustion in performance animals. In addition, all three formulas listed here can be used to treat acute gastroenteritis and bacterial dysentery from exogenous pathogen invasion characterized by wind, cold, and dampness during the summer months. *Xiang Ru San* and *San Wu Xiang Ru Yin* (Mosla Three Decoction) have the same ingredients, but are derived from different source texts. *Xiang Ru San* has specific doses and preparation methods for its ingredients, while the doses and preparation methods are unavailable for *San Wu Xiang Ru Yin* (Mosla Three Decoction). Because both formulas are used clinically, they are listed separately in this text. *San Wu Xiang Ru Yin* (Mosla Three Decoction) is available in prepared form and is the more common used formula in the dog and cat. Both *Xiang Ru San* and *San Wu Xiang Ru Yin* (Mosla Three Decoction) are used to treat the acute syndrome, and once the clinical signs resolve the formula should be discontinued. Treatment can be continued with *Shi Wei Xiang Ru Yin* (Ten-Ingredient Decoction with Mosla) that is readily available in prepared form to further consolidate the effects of treatment and strengthen the middle *jiao*.

References

1. *Zhong Yao Ming Fang Yao Li Yu Ying Yong* (Pharmacology and Applications of Famous Herbal Formulas), 1989; 50-51.
2. *Cheng Du Zhong Yi Xue Yuan Xue Bao* (Journal of Chengdu University of Traditional Chinese Medicine), 1992; 12(2):39.
3. *Fu Jian Zhong Yi Yao* (Fujian Chinese Medicine and Herbology), 1990; 2:14.
4. *Zhong Xi Yi Jie He Za Zhi* (Journal of Integrated Chinese and Western Medicine), 1988; 1:19.

Xīn Jiā Xiāng Rú Yǐn (Newly-Augmented Mosla Decoction)

新加香薷飲
新加香薷饮

Pinyin Name: *Xin Jia Xiang Ru Yin*
Literal Name: Newly-Augmented Mosla Decoction
Original Source: *Wen Bing Tiao Bian* (Systematic Differentiation of Warm Diseases) by Wu Ju-Tong in 1798

COMPOSITION

Xiang Ru (Herba Moslae)	6g
Bian Dou Hua (Flos Lablab Album), fresh	9g
Jin Yin Hua (Flos Lonicerae Japonicae)	9g
Lian Qiao (Fructus Forsythiae)	6g [9g]
Hou Po (Cortex Magnoliae Officinalis)	6g

Note: Historically, "*Xiang Ru*" was derived from two sources: *Mosla chinensis* and *Elsholtzia splendens*. Both herbs have similar functions, and have been used interchangeably in the history of Chinese herbal medicine. In 2005, *Zhong Hua Ren Min Gong He Guo Yao Dian* (Pharmacopoeia of the People's Republic of China) identified *Mosla chinensis* as the official source of this herb. Therefore, *Xiang Ru* (Herba Moslae) is adopted as the standard nomenclature throughout this text.

DOSAGE / PREPARATION / ADMINISTRATION

The source text states to cook the ingredients in 5 cups of water until 2 cups remain. Take 1 cup of the strained decoction. Once sweating has been induced, the formula should be discontinued. If sweating does not occur, take another cup of the decoction. If there is still no sweating, repeat the cooking steps above and administer another round of decoction. Today, the decoction may be prepared using the dose of *Lian Qiao* (Fructus Forsythiae) suggested in brackets.

CHINESE THERAPEUTIC ACTIONS

1. Dispels summer-heat
2. Releases exterior cold
3. Clears heat and resolves dampness

CLINICAL MANIFESTATIONS

Summer-heat disorders complicated by exterior cold and interior dampness: fever, aversion to cold, excessive panting, increased thirst, discomfort in the chest, a thick, white and greasy tongue coating, and a superficial, rapid pulse.

VETERINARY CLINICAL APPLICATIONS

Upper respiratory tract disease, fever of unknown origin in summer, anhidrosis, exercise-induced pulmonary hemorrhage (EIPH).

EXPLANATION

Xin Jia Xiang Ru Yin (Newly-Augmented Mosla Decoction), derived from *Xiang Ru San* (Mosla Powder), treats the type

***Xin Jia Xiang Ru Yin* (Newly-Augmented Mosla Decoction)**

Diagnosis	Clinical Signs	Treatment	Herbs
Summer-heat disorders complicated by exterior cold and interior dampness	• Fever, aversion to cold, and excessive panting: exterior cold • Increased thirst: summer-heat consuming yin and body fluids • Discomfort in the chest: dampness in the interior • White, greasy tongue coating: dampness in the interior • Superficial, rapid pulse: exterior cold and interior heat	• Dispels summer-heat • Releases the exterior • Clears heat and dampness	• *Xiang Ru* (Herba Moslae) releases the exterior cold factors and resolves interior dampness. • *Bian Dou Hua* (Flos Lablab Album), *Jin Yin Hua* (Flos Lonicerae Japonicae) and *Lian Qiao* (Fructus Forsythiae) clear summer-heat. • *Hou Po* (Cortex Magnoliae Officinalis) activates qi circulation and dries dampness.

Xīn Jiā Xiāng Rú Yǐn (Newly-Augmented Mosla Decoction)

of summer-heat disorder that is complicated by exterior cold and interior dampness factors. Animals that have this syndrome are usually first attacked by summer-heat. Before it is relieved, however, they are further invaded by exterior cold factor as a result of lack of shelter or other reasons. Because summer-heat is usually accompanied by dampness, interior dampness may arise as a result. Fever, aversion to cold, and lack of sweating or excessive panting are clinical manifestations associated with exterior cold. Increased thirst is the result of summer-heat damaging yin and body fluids. Discomfort in the chest, along with a white, greasy tongue coating, indicate dampness in the interior. A superficial, rapid pulse is caused by cold at the exterior and summer-heat in the interior.

To effectively treat this syndrome, one should release exterior cold, dispel interior summer-heat, and resolve interior dampness. *Xiang Ru* (Herba Moslae), aromatic and warm, dispels the exterior cold factor and dissolves interior dampness. Frequently used in the summer to treat exterior wind-cold, *Xiang Ru* has been called the "summer *Ma Huang* (Herba Ephedrae)." *Bian Dou Hua* (Flos Lablab Album), *Jin Yin Hua* (Flos Lonicerae Japonicae), and *Lian Qiao* (Fructus Forsythiae) penetrate to the interior to clear summer-heat, especially in the upper *jiao* or the *qi* (energy) level. *Hou Po* (Cortex Magnoliae Officinalis) activates qi circulation and dries dampness to clear the thick tongue coating and relieve the chest stuffiness and discomfort.

CAUTIONS / CONTRAINDICATIONS

Xin Jia Xiang Ru Yin is generally given as a warm decoction. However, the administration of this formula as a warm decoction has been occasionally associated with nausea and vomiting. In such circumstances, the decoction should be given at room temperature.[1]

HUMAN CLINICAL STUDIES AND RESEARCH

1. **Common cold or influenza in summer**: Modified *Xin Jia Xiang Ru Yin* was used to treat viral infection during the summer in 96 patients. The age of the patients ranged from 8-81 years of age, with average of 2.3 days of infection prior to receiving treatment. The study reported an average time of 1.77 days for reduction of fever, and 2.1 days for resolution of all other clinical signs.[2]
2. **Fever**: Concurrent use of *Xin Jia Xiang Ru Yin* and *Hao Qin Qing Dan Tang* (Artemisia Annua and Scutellaria Decoction to Clear the Gallbladder) was reported to have 94% effectiveness in treating fever. Of 50 cases, the study reported complete recovery in 24 cases, significant improvement in 17 cases, moderate improvement in 6 cases, and no effect in 3 cases.[3]
3. **Febrile disease in summer**: Use of modified *Xin Jia Xiang Ru Yin* to treat 31 patients with febrile diseases in the summer demonstrated 93.5% effectiveness. The study reported complete recovery in 21 cases, near-recovery in 8 cases, and moderate improvement in 2 cases.[4]

SUGGESTED ACUPUNCTURE TREATMENT

1. Points: *Fengchi* (GB 20), *Dazhui* (GV 14), *Xiangu* (ST 43), *Hegu* (LI 4), *Waiguan* (TH 5), *Housanli* (ST 36), *Erjian*, *Weijian*, and *Xiongtang*.
2. Technique: sedation.

Fengchi (GB 20) disperses exterior factors. *Dazhui* (GV 14), *Xiangu* (ST 43), and *Hegu* (LI 4) relieve summer-heat. *Waiguan* (TH 5) sedates heat in all three *jiaos*. *Housanli* (ST 36) tonifies the middle *jiao* and dissolves dampness. Hemoacupuncture at the classical points *Erjian*, *Weijian*, and *Xiongtang* clears excess heat.

AUTHORS' COMMENTS

Xiang Ru San (Mosla Powder) and *Xin Jia Xiang Ru Yin* both contain acrid and warm herbs, such as *Xiang Ru* (Herba Moslae) and *Hou Po* (Cortex Magnoliae Officinalis), to expel exterior pathogenic factors, disperse cold, and resolve dampness.

- *Xiang Ru San* is warmer in property, and is better for treating summer-heat disorders complicated by exterior cold and interior dampness.
- *Xin Jia Xiang Ru Yin* is slightly cooler in property, as it contains *Jin Yin Hua* (Flos Lonicerae Japonicae), *Bian Dou Hua* (Flos Lablab Album), and *Lian Qiao* (Fructus Forsythiae). It is better for summer-heat conditions with more heat signs (fever) and increased thirst.

References

1. *Hu Bei Zhong Yi Za Zhi* (Hubei Journal of Chinese Medicine), 1987; (5):44.
2. *Shang Hai Zhong Yi Yao Za Zhi* (Shanghai Journal of Chinese Medicine and Herbology), 1982; 8:35.
3. *Zhong Yi Ming Fang Lin Chuang Xin Yong* (Contemporary Clinical Applications of Classic Chinese Formulas), 2001; 708.
4. *Jiang Su Zhong Yi* (Jiangsu Chinese Medicine), 1999; 7:28.

Guì Líng Gān Lù Yǐn (Cinnamon and Poria Sweet Dew Decoction)

桂苓甘露飲
桂苓甘露饮

Pinyin Name: *Gui Ling Gan Lu Yin*
Literal Name: Cinnamon and Poria Sweet Dew Decoction
Original Source: *Huang Di Su Wen Xuan Ming Lun Fang* (Formulas from the Discussion Illuminating the Yellow Emperor's Basic Questions) by Liu Yuan-Su in 1172

COMPOSITION

Hua Shi (Talcum)	120g
Gan Cao (Radix et Rhizoma Glycyrrhizae)	60g
Fu Ling (Poria)	30g
Zhu Ling (Polyporus)	15g
Ze Xie (Rhizoma Alismatis)	30g
Rou Gui (Cortex Cinnamomi)	60g
Bai Zhu (Rhizoma Atractylodis Macrocephalae), *zhi* (fried with liquid)	15g
Shi Gao (Gypsum Fibrosum)	60g
Han Shui Shi (Mirabilite)	60g

DOSAGE / PREPARATION / ADMINISTRATION

Grind the ingredients into powder and take 9g with warm water, fresh spring water, or preferably with a decoction made from *Sheng Jiang* (Rhizoma Zingiberis Recens). For children, reduce the dose to 3g.

CHINESE THERAPEUTIC ACTIONS

1. Clears heat and dispels summer-heat
2. Regulates qi and dispels dampness

CLINICAL MANIFESTATIONS

Invasion of summer-heat and dampness: fever, irritability, thirst, dysuria, and sudden turmoil disorder with vomiting or diarrhea.

VETERINARY CLINICAL APPLICATIONS

Dysentery, diarrhea, vomiting, and allergy.

EXPLANATION

Gui Ling Gan Lu Yin (Cinnamon and Poria Sweet Dew Decoction) treats summer-heat syndrome accompanied by interior damp accumulation. Summer-heat rising upwards in the body causes fever. Summer-heat may also disturb the *shen* (spirit), causing irritability. If heat consumes body fluids, thirst occurs. Summer-heat may travel downwards to the lower *jiao*, causing dysuria. Vomiting and diarrhea occur if the dampness stagnates in the middle *jiao* and impairs the Spleen and Stomach's ability to separate the clear from the turbid.

In this formula, *Hua Shi* (Talcum) clears summer-heat and dampness through urination. *Gan Cao* (Radix et Rhizoma Glycyrrhizae) clears heat, harmonizes the Spleen and Stomach, and promotes the secretion of body fluids. *Rou Gui* (Cortex Cinnamomi) warms yang qi and helps the

***Gui Ling Gan Lu Yin* (Cinnamon and Poria Sweet Dew Decoction)**

Diagnosis	Clinical Signs	Treatment	Herbs
Summer-heat and dampness	• Fever: summer-heat rising upwards • Irritability and thirst: summer-heat consuming yin and disturbing the *shen* (spirit) • Dysuria: summer-heat travels downwards to the lower *jiao* • Vomiting and diarrhea: damp accumulation in the middle *jiao*	• Clears heat and dispels summer-heat • Regulates qi and dispels dampness	• *Hua Shi* (Talcum) and *Gan Cao* (Radix et Rhizoma Glycyrrhizae) dispel summer-heat and dampness. • *Fu Ling* (Poria), *Zhu Ling* (Polyporus), *Ze Xie* (Rhizoma Alismatis), *Rou Gui* (Cortex Cinnamomi) and *Bai Zhu* (Rhizoma Atractylodis Macrocephalae) regulate water circulation, dispel dampness, and disperse water accumulation. • *Shi Gao* (Gypsum Fibrosum) and *Han Shui Shi* (Mirabilite) clear heat and dispel summer-heat.

Guì Líng Gān Lù Yǐn (Cinnamon and Poria Sweet Dew Decoction)

urinary functioning of the lower *jiao*. *Fu Ling* (Poria), *Zhu Ling* (Polyporus) and *Ze Xie* (Rhizoma Alismatis) induce urination to dispel interior dampness and relieve dysuria. *Bai Zhu* (Rhizoma Atractylodis Macrocephalae) strengthens the Spleen, dries dampness, and regulates qi flow. Lastly, *Shi Gao* (Gypsum Fibrosum) and *Han Shui Shi* (Mirabilite), both extremely cold, clear heat and dispel summer-heat.

HUMAN CLINICAL STUDIES AND RESEARCH

Diarrhea: Administration of modified *Gui Ling Gan Lu Yin* along with adjustment in dietary habits showed 92.5% effectiveness in treating 80 children with diarrhea characterized by damp-heat. The herbal decoction contained *Fu Ling* (Poria), *Zhu Ling* (Polyporus), *Bai Zhu* (Rhizoma Atractylodis Macrocephalae), *Gan Cao* (Radix et Rhizoma Glycyrrhizae), *Gui Zhi* (Ramulus Cinnamomi), *Shi Gao* (Gypsum Fibrosum), *Han Shui Shi* (Mirabilite), and *Hua Shi* (Talcum) as the base formula. Modifications included the addition of *Ge Gen* (Radix Puerariae Lobatae) and *Jin Yin Hua* (Flos Lonicerae Japonicae) for the presence of an exterior syndrome. Of 80 cases, the study reported complete recovery in 49 cases, significant improvement in 22 cases, moderate improvement in 3 cases, and no change in 6 cases. The overall success rate was 92.5%.[1]

SUGGESTED ACUPUNCTURE TREATMENT

1. Points: *Dazhui* (GV 14), *Hegu* (LI 4), *Shaochong* (HT 9), *Weiyang* (BL 39), *Housanli* (ST 36), *Yinlingquan* (SP 9), and *Waiguan* (TH 5).
2. Technique: sedation.

Dazhui (GV 14) and *Hegu* (LI 4) sedate heat and eliminate toxins. *Shaochong* (HT 9) and *Weiyang* (BL 39) dispel summer-heat and dampness. *Housanli* (ST 36) and *Yinlingquan* (SP 9) activate qi circulation to dissolve dampness. *Waiguan* (TH 5) regulates the qi flow of the three *jiaos* and relieves interior heat.

AUTHORS' COMMENTS

Gui Ling Gan Lu Yin combines *Liu Yi San* (Six-to-One Powder) with *Wu Ling San* (Five-Ingredient Powder with Poria), *Shi Gao* (Gypsum Fibrosum), and *Han Shui Shi* (Mirabilite). It strongly clears heat and dispels dampness. It is mainly used for summer-heat with dampness in animals that have interior water retention manifesting in fever, thirst with a desire to drink, irritability, dysuria, vomiting, and/or diarrhea. It should be used cautiously in animals that are yin deficient, poorly hydrated, and living in dry environments.

References

1. *Zhong Xi Yi Jie He Za Zhi* (Journal of Integrated Chinese and Western Medicine), 1985; 1:19.

Qīng Shŭ Yi Qì Tāng

(Clear Summer-Heat and Augment the Qi Decoction)

清暑益氣湯
清暑益气汤

Pinyin Name: *Qing Shu Yi Qi Tang*
Literal Name: Clear Summer-Heat and Augment the Qi Decoction
Alternate Names: *Ching Shu I Chi Tang, Ching Shu Yi Chi Tang*, Summer-heat-clearing and Chi-tonifying Decoction, Astragalus and Atractylodes Combination
Original Source: *Wen Re Jing Wei* (Warp and Woof of Warm-Febrile Diseases) by Wang Meng-Ying in 1852

COMPOSITION

Xi Yang Shen (Radix Panacis Quinquefolii)	[5g]
Xi Gua Cui Pi (Exocarpium Citrulli)	[30g]
He Geng (Caulis Nelumbinis)	[15g]
Shi Hu (Caulis Dendrobii)	[15g]
Mai Dong (Radix Ophiopogonis)	[9g]
Zhi Mu (Rhizoma Anemarrhenae)	[6g]
Zhu Ye (Herba Phyllostachys)	[6g]
Huang Lian (Rhizoma Coptidis)	[3g]
Geng Mi (Semen Oryzae)	[15g]
Gan Cao (Radix et Rhizoma Glycyrrhizae)	[3g]

DOSAGE / PREPARATION / ADMINISTRATION

The herb doses are unavailable from the source text. Today, this formula may be prepared as a decoction with the doses suggested in brackets.

CHINESE THERAPEUTIC ACTIONS

1. Dispels summer-heat
2. Tonifies qi, nourishes yin, and generates body fluids

CLINICAL MANIFESTATIONS

Summer-heat damaging both qi and body fluids: fever, profuse sweating (horses), excessive panting, irritability, thirst, scanty, dark-colored urine, lethargy, shortness of breath, and a weak, rapid pulse.

VETERINARY CLINICAL APPLICATIONS

Upper respiratory tract infection in the summer, fever of unknown origin, adjunct treatment for heat stroke and post-heat stroke care.

EXPLANATION

Qing Shu Yi Qi Tang (Clear Summer-Heat and Augment the Qi Decoction) treats summer-heat syndromes with damage to both qi and body fluids. In this syndrome,

***Qing Shu Yi Qi Tang* (Clear Summer-Heat and Augment the Qi Decoction)**

Diagnosis	Clinical Signs	Treatment	Herbs
Summer-heat damaging both qi and body fluids	• Fever, excessive panting, and profuse sweating (horses): summer-heat forcing fluids out of the body • Irritability, thirst, and dark, scanty urine: summer-heat consuming body fluids • Lethargy and shortness of breath: summer-heat damaging qi • Weak, rapid pulse: presence of deficiency and excess	• Dispels summer-heat • Tonifies qi, nourishes yin, and generates body fluids	• *Xi Yang Shen* (Radix Panacis Quinquefolii) tonifies qi, yin, and body fluids. • *Xi Gua Cui Pi* (Exocarpium Citrulli) and *He Geng* (Caulis Nelumbinis) strongly clear summer-heat. • *Shi Hu* (Caulis Dendrobii) and *Mai Dong* (Radix Ophiopogonis) nourish yin and body fluids. • *Zhi Mu* (Rhizoma Anemarrhenae) and *Zhu Ye* (Herba Phyllostachys) clear heat to relieve irritability. • *Geng Mi* (Semen Oryzae) and *Gan Cao* (Radix et Rhizoma Glycyrrhizae) tonify qi.

Qīng Shǔ Yì Qì Tāng

(Clear Summer-Heat and Augment the Qi Decoction)

excess heat forces fluids out of the body, causing fever and profuse sweating. Profuse sweating may extensively consume and damage body fluids, leading to irritability, thirst, and dark, scanty urine. Qi travels with body fluids and may be lost and become deficient as a result of excess sweating. Lethargy and shortness of breath are both signs of qi deficiency. A weak, rapid pulse suggests qi deficiency and heat in the body.

Xi Yang Shen (Radix Panacis Quinquefolii), as a chief herb, clears heat and tonifies qi, yin and body fluids. *Xi Gua Cui Pi* (Exocarpium Citrulli), as the other chief herb of this formula, clears heat and resolves summer-heat. *He Geng* (Caulis Nelumbinis) helps *Xi Gua Cui Pi* (Exocarpium Citrulli) clear summer-heat. *Shi Hu* (Caulis Dendrobii) and *Mai Dong* (Radix Ophiopogonis) help *Xi Yang Shen* (Radix Panacis Quinquefolii) clear heat and nourish yin. *Zhi Mu* (Rhizoma Anemarrhenae) and *Zhu Ye* (Herba Phyllostachys) clear heat and relieve irritability. *Geng Mi* (Semen Oryzae) and *Gan Cao* (Radix et Rhizoma Glycyrrhizae) tonify qi and nourish the Stomach.

Although *Huang Lian* (Rhizoma Coptidis) is listed as an ingredient in this formula, use it cautiously as its bitter and cold nature may easily damage yin and body fluids. If the patient has only mild clinical signs of summer-heat but severe clinical signs of body fluids damage, omit *Huang Lian* (Rhizoma Coptidis) from the formula.

VETERINARY MODIFICATIONS

- When there is severe sweating in horses, add *Fu Xiao Mai* (Fructus Tritici Levis).
- With dysuria, add *Di Huang* (Radix Rehmanniae) and *Mu Tong* (Caulis Akebiae).
- With irritability, dryness and heat, add *Yin Chen* (Herba Artemisiae Scopariae) and *Zhi Zi* (Fructus Gardeniae).
- With deficiency of body fluids, add *Ge Gen* (Radix Puerariae Lobatae) and *Sha Shen* (Radix Glehniae seu Adenophorae).
- If there is qi deficiency, add *Ren Shen* (Radix et Rhizoma Ginseng) and *Huang Qi* (Radix Astragali).

CAUTIONS / CONTRAINDICATIONS

Qing Shu Yi Qi Tang is inappropriate in cases of summer-heat accompanied by dampness because it contains greasy yin-tonic herbs, such as *Mai Dong* (Radix Ophiopogonis) and *Zhi Mu* (Rhizoma Anemarrhenae).

HUMAN CLINICAL STUDIES AND RESEARCH

1. **Wheezing and dyspnea**: In one clinical study, 76 patients with wheezing and dyspnea during the summer were treated with modified *Qing Shu Yi Qi Tang*. The formula included *Xi Yang Shen* (Radix Panacis Quinquefolii) 20g, *Di Long* (Pheretima) 20g, *Shi Hu* (Caulis Dendrobii) 15g, *Mai Dong* (Radix Ophiopogonis) 15g, *Zhu Ye* (Herba Phyllostachys) 15g, *Zhi Mu* (Rhizoma Anemarrhenae) 15g, *Di Huang* (Radix Rehmanniae) 10g, *Gan Cao* (Radix et Rhizoma Glycyrrhizae) 10g, *Xi Gua Cui Pi* (Exocarpium Citrulli) 10g, and addition of others as deemed necessary per condition of the patient. The treatment protocol was to boil the herbs in water, and ingest the decoction in two equal portions. Out of 76 cases, the study reported stabilization in 22 cases (no wheezing or dyspnea for the entire year), significant improvement in 34 cases (no wheezing or dyspnea for the current season), moderate improvement in 15 cases (still requiring other treatment), and no effect in 5 cases. The overall rate of effectiveness was 93.4%.[1]
2. **Pneumonia**: Fourteen patients with pneumonia were treated with modified *Qing Shu Yi Qi Tang* with complete recovery in 12 patients and no benefit in 2 patients. The formula used included fresh *He Ye* (Folium Nelumbinis) 30g, fresh *Xi Gua Cui Pi* (Exocarpium Citrulli) 60g, *Zhu Ye* (Herba Phyllostachys) 12g, *Shi Hu* (Caulis Dendrobii) 12g, *Mai Dong* (Radix Ophiopogonis) 12g, *Zhi Mu* (Rhizoma Anemarrhenae) 12g, *Jin Yin Hua* (Flos Lonicerae Japonicae) 18g, *Lian Qiao* (Fructus Forsythiae) 18g, *Huang Qin* (Radix Scutellariae) 15g, *Lu Gen* (Rhizoma Phragmitis) 15g, *Pi Pa Ye* (Folium Eriobotryae) 24g, *Ren Shen* (Radix et Rhizoma Ginseng) 9-12g, *Gan Cao* (Radix et Rhizoma Glycyrrhizae) 6g, and the addition of others as deemed necessary per condition of the patient. Complete recovery was defined as reduction of body temperature to normal within 12-72 hours with normal count of white blood cells within 24-72 hours.[2]

SUGGESTED ACUPUNCTURE TREATMENT

1. Points: *Shaoshang* (LU 11), *Shaochong* (HT 9), *Taiyuan* (LU 9), *Waiguan* (TH 5), *Feishu* (BL 13), *Pishu* (BL 20), *Weishu* (BL 21), *Erjian*, *Weijian*, and *Xiongtang*.
2. Technique: both tonification and sedation.

Prick and bleed *Shaoshang* (LU 11), the *jing* (well) point of the Lung channel, to clear summer-heat. *Shaochong* (HT 9), the *jing* (well) point of the Heart channel, clears heat and revitalizes the *shen* (spirit). *Shaochong* (HT 9) is also combined with *Taiyuan* (LU 9) to nourish body fluids. *Waiguan* (TH 5), the *luo* (connecting) point of the *San Jiao* channel, clears heat in the three *jiaos*. *Feishu* (BL 13), *Pishu* (BL 20), and *Weishu* (BL 21) nourish qi and body fluids. To reduce fever, place a cold pack on the back of the stifle joint in the location of *Weizhong* (BL 40).

Qīng Shǔ Yì Qì Tāng

(Clear Summer-Heat and Augment the Qi Decoction)

Hemoacupuncture of the classical points *Erjian*, *Weijian*, and *Xiongtang* clears excess heat.

RELATED FORMULA

Qīng Shǔ Yì Qì Tāng

(Clear Summer-Heat and Augment the Qi Decoction)

清暑益氣湯
清暑益气汤

Pinyin Name: *Qing Shu Yi Qi Tang*

Literal Name: Clear Summer-Heat and Augment the Qi Decoction

Original Source: *Pi Wei Lun* (Discussion of the Spleen and Stomach) by Li Gao in 1249

Huang Qi (Radix Astragali)	3g [6g]
Cang Zhu (Rhizoma Atractylodis), *jin* (soaked)	3g [3g]
Sheng Ma (Rhizoma Cimicifugae)	3g [3g]
Ren Shen (Radix et Rhizoma Ginseng)	1.5g [1.5g]
Ze Xie (Rhizoma Alismatis)	1.5 [3g]
Shen Qu (Massa Fermentata), *chao* (dry-fried)	1.5g [3g]
Chen Pi (Pericarpium Citri Reticulatae)	1.5g [1.5g]
Bai Zhu (Rhizoma Atractylodis Macrocephalae)	1.5g [3g]
Mai Dong (Radix Ophiopogonis)	0.9g [3g]
Dang Gui (Radix Angelicae Sinensis)	0.9g [1g]
Zhi Gan Cao (Radix et Rhizoma Glycyrrhizae Praeparata cum Melle)	0.9g [1g]
Qing Pi (Pericarpium Citri Reticulatae Viride)	0.75g [1g]
Huang Bo (Cortex Phellodendri Chinensis), *xi* (washed) with liquor	0.6-0.9g [3g]
Ge Gen (Radix Puerariae Lobatae)	0.6g [6g]
Wu Wei Zi (Fructus Schisandrae Chinensis)	9 pieces [1.5g]

The source text states to grind the herbs into powder, and cook it in 2 large bowls of water until it is reduced to 1 bowl. Take the warm, strained decoction on an empty stomach. Today, this formula may be prepared as a decoction with the doses suggested in brackets.

This formula has the identical name as the previous formula, but they are derived from different sources and have slightly different compositions and applications. Therefore, it is very important that the two are not confused or used interchangeably. A comparative analysis of these two formulas is provided in the Authors' Comments section.

This formula clears summer-heat, dries dampness, benefits qi, and strengthens the Spleen. Clinically, it can be used for animals with exterior summer-heat and underlying chronic qi deficiency. Animals may show clinical signs such as thirst, panting, lethargy, lack of appetite, chest fullness, heaviness of the body, loose stools, dysuria, a greasy tongue coating, and a weak pulse.

AUTHORS' COMMENTS

These two formulas have identical names: the former is also known as Wang's *Qing Shu Yi Qi Tang*, and the latter is referred to as Li's *Qing Shu Yi Qi Tang*. Both formulas also have similar compositions and functions to clear summer-heat and augment the qi. Their differences are as follows:

- *Qing Shu Yi Qi Tang* from *Wen Re Jing Wei* (Warp and Woof of Warm-Febrile Diseases) by Wang Meng-Ying, treats summer-heat damaging both qi and body fluids. It should be used with caution in cases of summer-heat with dampness, as it contains rich, cloying herbs that can easily clog the qi mechanism in the middle *jiao*. It focuses more on nourishing yin and producing body fluid than on tonifying qi.
- *Qing Shu Yi Qi Tang* from *Pi Wei Lun* (Discussion of the Spleen and Stomach) by Li Gao, treats chronic qi deficiency complicated by exterior summer-heat. This formula focuses more on strengthening the Spleen and tonifying qi, than on nourishing yin and body fluids.
- Either can be used as an adjunct therapy for heat stroke to help improve survival rates. In cases of exercise-induced heat stroke in performance animals, environmental conditions should play an important factor in selecting a formula. In hot, dry climates like the desert southwest, *Qing Shu Yi Qi Tang* from either source may be the best choice, while in the humid southeast, a formula like *Xiang Ru San* (Mosla Powder) or one of its modifications may be more appropriate.

References

1. *Shan Xi Yi Kan* (Shanxi Journal of Medicine), 1992; 3:104.
2. *Zhe Jiang Zhong Yi Za Zhi* (Zhejiang Journal of Chinese Medicine), 1984; 8:352.

6 SUMMER-HEAT-DISPELLING FORMULAS

Chapter 6 — Summary

— Summer-Heat-Dispelling Formulas

Name	Similarities	Differences
Qing Luo Yin (Clear the Collaterals Decoction)	Dispels summer-heat, clears interior heat	Treats mild summer-heat syndromes
Xiang Ru San (Mosla Powder)	Dispel summer-heat, release the exterior	Treats summer-heat syndromes with cold and dampness
Xin Jia Xiang Ru Yin (Newly-Augmented Mosla Decoction)		Treats summer-heat syndromes with cold, dampness, and heat
Gui Ling Gan Lu Yin (Cinnamon and Poria Sweet Dew Decoction)	Dispels summer-heat, drains dampness	Moderate to strong in potency
Qing Shu Yi Qi Tang (Clear Summer-Heat and Augment the Qi Decoction)	Dispels summer-heat, tonifies qi, yin and body fluids	Treats summer-heat syndromes involving both excess and deficiency

Qing Luo Yin (Clear the Collaterals Decoction) relieves summer-heat and clears interior heat. The herbs in this formula are of light quality and thus can penetrate and clear interior heat. It is most suitable for treating mild summer-heat syndromes in which only the Lung is affected.

Xiang Ru San (Mosla Powder) and ***Xin Jia Xiang Ru Yin*** (Newly-Augmented Mosla Decoction) both relieve summer-heat and dispel exterior factors.
- *Xiang Ru San* is a warmer formula and is better for initial summer-heat syndromes with wind-cold and dampness.
- *Xin Jia Xiang Ru Yin* is a colder formula, and has a stronger effect to treat initial summer-heat syndromes with cold and dampness, but with indications of more heat.

Gui Ling Gan Lu Yin (Cinnamon and Poria Sweet Dew Decoction) relieves summer-heat and dispels dampness to treat summer-heat syndromes accompanied by dampness.

Qing Shu Yi Qi Tang (Clear Summer-Heat and Augment the Qi Decoction) treats summer-heat syndromes with extensive damage to qi and body fluids. It is the formula most often used to treat heat stroke and recovery from heat stroke in dogs.

Chapter 7

— Interior-Warming Formulas

温里剂

王叔和 Wāng Shū-Hē

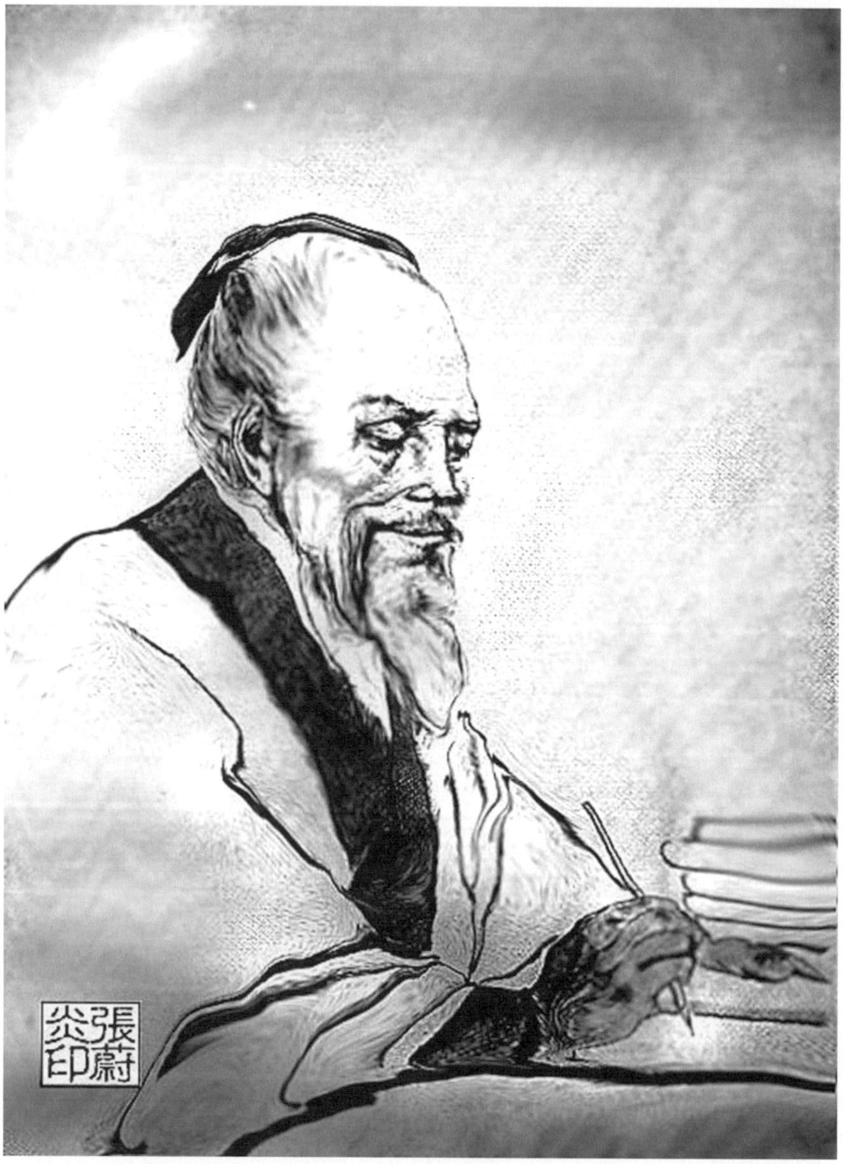

王叔和 Wāng Shū-Hē, third century.[1]

王叔和 Wāng Shū-Hē

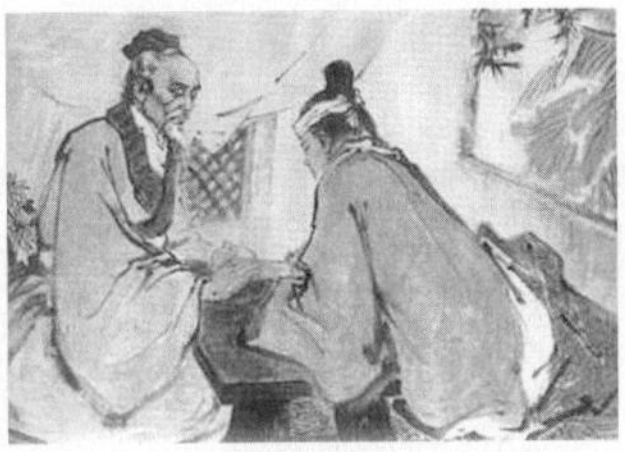
Wang Shu-He taking pulse of a patient.

Wang Shu-He is best known for preserving 伤寒杂病论 *Shang Han Za Bing Lun* (Discussion of Cold-Induced Disorders and Miscellaneous Diseases) by Zhang Zhong-Jing. Shortly after this text was published, it was lost during war time in the Eastern Han dynasty and the time of the Three Kingdoms. Realizing the tremendous importance of this text, Wang gathered bits and pieces of it wherever he could, re-organized it, and published it in two volumes:

- 伤寒论 *Shang Han Lun* (Discussion of Cold-Induced Disorders) emphasizes external disorders, classifying them according to *Liu Jing Bian Zheng* (Six Stages Differentiation).
- 金匮要略 *Jin Gui Yao Lue* (Essentials from the Golden Cabinet) focuses on internal and miscellaneous disease, classifying them according to *Ba Gang Bian Zheng* (Eight Principle Differentiation).

Without Wang's effort, Zhang Zhong-Jing's work would have been lost altogether, or, at best, incomplete.

Wang also wrote one of the most significant texts on pulse diagnosis, 脉经 *Mai Jing* (Pulse Classics). Though there were many references to pulse and their indications in historical texts before his time, most references were scattered and disorganized. After studying the *Nei Jing* (Inner Classic), the *Nan Jing* (Classic of Difficult Issues), *Shang Han Za Bing Lun* (Discussion of Cold-Induced Disorders and Miscellaneous Diseases) and references from Hua Tuo, Wang published *Mai Jing* (Pulse Classics), the first comprehensive text that systemically stated the proper definitions of pulse-related terminology and techniques for pulse diagnosis. It established the proper positions for pulse assessment and their relationship to the *zang fu* organs. It also clearly defined 24 different pulse qualities and their meanings. Lastly, it emphasized the importance of correlating the pulse to the age, sex, height, weight, and disease pattern of the patient.

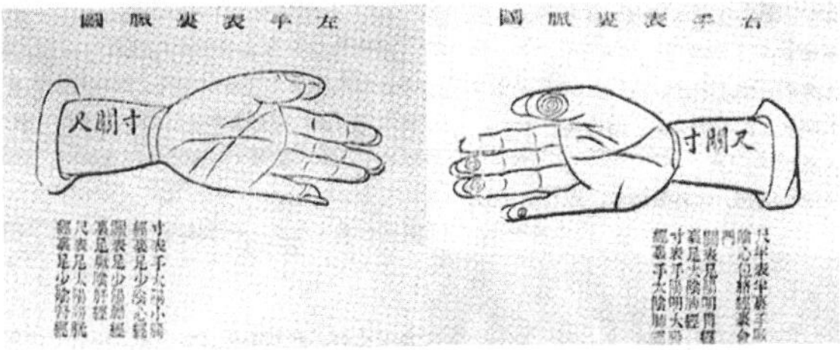
Pulse positions and definitions from 脉经 *Mai Jing* (Pulse Classics), third century.[2]

Dynasties & Kingdoms	Year
Xia Dynasty 夏	2100-1600 BCE
Shang Dynasty 商	1600-1100 BCE
Zhou Dynasty 周	1100-221 BCE
Qin Dynasty 秦	221-207 BCE
Han Dynasty 漢	206 BCE-220
Three Kingdoms 三國	**220-280**
Western Jin Dynasty 西晉	265-316
Eastern Jin Dynasty 東晉	317-420
Northern and Southern Dynasties 北南朝	420-581
Sui Dynasty 隋	581-618
Tang Dynasty 唐	618-907
Five Dynasties 五代	907-960
Song Dynasty 宋	960-1279
Liao Dynasty 潦	916-1125
Jin Dynasty 金	1115-1234
Yuan Dynasty 元	1271-1368
Ming Dynasty 明	1368-1644
Qing Dynasty 清	1644-1911
Republic of China 中華民國	1912-Present Day
People's Republic of China 中華人民共和國	1949-Present Day

1. Exact dates of birth and death are unknown.
2. Exact date of publication is unknown.

Table of Contents

Chapter 7 — Overview

溫里劑 — Interior-Warming Formulas

Definition: Interior-warming formulas warm the interior, raise yang, disperse cold, and dredge the channels and collaterals. This method of treatment is known as *wen fa* (warming), one of the *ba fa* (eight treatment methods) described in the *Huang Di Nei Jing* (Yellow Emperor's Inner Classic) in the first or second century, A.D.

Cold, one of the *liu yin* (six exogenous factors), is the primary environmental factor of winter, but can occur in other seasons as well. As a yin pathogenic factor it easily impairs the yang energies of the body, particularly the function of *wei* (defensive) *qi* and the transformational abilities of Kidney, Spleen and Heart yang. For this reason, interior cold is often associated with yang deficiency patterns. Cold causes sluggish flow of qi, blood and body fluids that result in accumulation and stagnation of these substances, causing pain and/or the development of masses.

Overall, cold impairs the maintenance of normal body temperature and metabolism of the whole body. Clinical signs of interior cold patterns vary, depending on the location and on what level of the body is affected. Cold can attack the superficial level of the body, invade the interior and affect the function of the middle *jiao*, and cause collapse of yang. These patterns are characterized by aversion to cold, warmth seeking, absence of thirst, cold extremities, loose stools and copious, clear urine. The tongue is often pale to purple in color, and the pulse may be deep, weak and slower in severe cases.

Interior cold can be externally contracted or internally generated, or both. Exogenous cold can attack the exterior or directly invade the interior of the body. Due to its constricting and stagnating nature, exogenous cold can lodge in the channels and collaterals of the body, impairing the flow of qi and blood, causing cramps, spasms and pain. If exogenous pathogenic cold is left untreated, or treated improperly (from excessive or prolonged use of cold herbs), it may penetrate to the interior. When exogenous cold penetrates directly to the interior, it preferentially invades the middle *jiao* where it disrupts the function of the middle *jiao* and the transformation and transportation of food and water. Many purebred animals have poor Kidney *jing* (essence) and constitutional yang deficiency, are fed a cold diet (raw or refrigerated), and commonly develop internally generated cold. Regardless of the etiological origin, interior cold must be treated with warm/hot herbs that warm the interior.

There are many causes of interior cold syndromes. In veterinary medicine, the most common causes of interior cold syndrome include: drug therapy (specifically antimicrobial drugs that are energetically cold and bitter), chronic illness (inflammatory bowel disease), chronic feeding of cold, refrigerated food (which consumes Spleen and Kidney yang), raw food diets in juvenile and geriatric animals, chronic overexposure to environmental cold from lack of adequate shelter, and qi deficiency in performance animals.

It is important to note that interior-warming herbs and herbs that tonify yang are not the same. Although these two categories of herbs share many similarities, they are different. Interior-warming herbs are hot, drying and acrid; their ability to disperse cold depends in part on their acrid nature, and most of these herbs enter the channels of the Spleen and Stomach. Yang-tonifying herbs are

Chapter 7 — Overview

mostly sweet, salty, and warm; they enter the Kidney channel to tonify Kidney yang and related deficiencies, and their sweet taste is indicative of their tonic nature. Interior-warming herbs largely function to warm Heart, Kidney and Spleen yang to drive out excess cold, while yang-tonifying herbs replenish Kidney yang, blood, and *jing* (essence), and strengthen tendons and bones.

Note: The presence of cold at the exterior (such as wind-cold) is treated with exterior-releasing herbs, which are discussed in Chapter 1: Exterior-Releasing Formulas. The presence of cold in the interior (interior cold) is treated with interior-warming formulas, which will be discussed in this chapter.

SUBCATEGORIES OF ACTION

Because interior cold syndromes manifest with different severities and in different locations, interior-warming formulas are differentiated into three sub-categories as follows:

1. **Middle-Warming and Cold-Dispelling Formulas**

These formulas are designed to treat deficiency cold syndromes affecting the middle *jiao*. The Spleen and Stomach reside in the middle *jiao* and belong to the Earth element. Together, they are responsible for the transformation and transportation of food, sending clear *gu* (food) *qi* to the upper *jiao* and turbid food particles to the lower *jiao*. If the yang qi of the middle *jiao* is weakened as a result of cold, the functioning of the Spleen and Stomach will be impaired. Main clinical manifestations include epigastric and abdominal pain, relief of pain with pressure and warmth, lethargy, fatigue, vomiting of saliva, coldness of the extremities, acid regurgitation, nausea, vomiting, diarrhea, loss of appetite, and lack of thirst. The tongue coating is usually white and slippery in more severe cases. The pulse may be deep and thin, or deep and slow.

Commonly used herbs in the middle-warming and cold-dispelling formulas are *Gan Jiang* (Rhizoma Zingiberis), *Wu Zhu Yu* (Fructus Evodiae), and *Hua Jiao* (Pericarpium Zanthoxyli). In addition, herbs that tonify qi and strengthen the Spleen are usually added to increase the effectiveness of the formulas, such as *Ren Shen* (Radix et Rhizoma Ginseng), *Bai Zhu* (Rhizoma Atractylodis Macrocephalae), and *Yi Tang* (Maltosum). Exemplar formulas include *Li Zhong Wan* (Regulate the Middle Pill), *Wu Zhu Yu Tang* (Evodia Decoction), *Xiao Jian Zhong Tang* (Minor Construct the Middle Decoction), and *Da Jian Zhong Tang* (Major Construct the Middle Decoction).

2. **Yang-Resuscitating Formulas**

These formulas recuperate depleted Heart and Kidney yang, and rescue animals from cardiovascular and respiratory collapse. They are used to treat exhausted yang qi, with cold affecting both the interior and the exterior. Because the preponderance of yin consumes yang, the following clinical signs appear: extremely cold limbs, aversion to cold, preference to curl up the body when lying down, vomiting, abdominal pain, diarrhea with undigested foods, extreme fatigue, and, in severe cases, profuse, cold sweating. The pulse will be either deep and thin, or deep and weak.

In order to rescue yang from depletion, large doses of hot and acrid herbs must be used. Frequently used herbs in this category include *Fu Zi* (Radix Aconiti Lateralis Praeparata), *Gan Jiang* (Rhizoma Zingiberis), and *Rou Gui* (Cortex Cinnamomi). Representative formulas that resuscitate yang include *Si Ni Tang* (Frigid Extremities Decoction) and *Hui Yang Jiu Ji Tang* (Restore and Revive the Yang Decoction).

In extreme cases, the depletion of yang and the abundance of cold in the interior will block the circulation of yang qi to the interior and redirect it to the exterior, giving rise to the condition of "true cold" (in the interior) and "false heat" (at the exterior). In addition to the clinical signs listed above, clinical manifestations of "false heat" may include dry heaves, irritability and restlessness. These animals may reject the warm decoction or interior-warming herbs by vomiting. In such cases, administer the decoction at room temperature, or add a small amount of cold herbs to the interior-warming formulas; these modifications usually help the animal to better tolerate the decoction.

Chapter 7 — Overview

3. **Channel-Warming and Cold-Dispersing Formulas**

These formulas treat exterior cold blocking and damaging the channels and collaterals in animals with underlying deficiencies of yang qi, yin and blood. Common clinical signs include extreme cold, numbness and pain of the extremities, reduced mobility of the joints, and formation of *yin* (deep-rooted) sores.

Using only acrid and hot herbs will not effectively treat such conditions. Instead, it is more appropriate to combine them with herbs that dispel cold, tonify the blood, and warm and unblock the channels and collaterals. Herbs commonly used include *Gui Zhi* (Ramulus Cinnamomi), *Xi Xin* (Radix et Rhizoma Asari), *Dang Gui* (Radix Angelicae Sinensis), *Bai Shao* (Radix Paeoniae Alba), *Huang Qi* (Radix Astragali), and *Shu Di Huang* (Radix Rehmanniae Praeparata). Exemplar formulas include *Dang Gui Si Ni Tang* (Tangkuei Decoction for Frigid Extremities), *Huang Qi Gui Zhi Wu Wu Tang* (Astragalus and Cinnamon Twig Five-Substance Decoction), and *Yang He Tang* (Yang-Heartening Decoction).

CAUTIONS / CONTRAINDICATIONS

- Interior-warming formulas are designed to disperse cold in the interior. If the cold is located at the exterior level, then exterior-releasing formulas should be used.
- It is extremely important to correctly diagnose the presence of cold in the body. Severe consequences can result if interior-warming formulas are used to treat excess heat syndromes.
- Interior-warming formulas can easily damage yin and blood and are contraindicated in animals with excess heat syndromes. Accurate pattern differentiation is essential for the safe and appropriate use of these formulas, and once clinical signs resolve, they should be stopped. Extra care and caution is advised in prescribing interior-warming formulas during the summer and in areas with hot climate.
- Because interior-warming formulas consist of acrid and warm herbs, they must be used carefully if the animal has yin deficiency or bleeding syndromes. Inappropriate use of interior warming herbs may easily create heat in the interior, further damaging yin and blood.
- Because a cold factor can easily damage yang and qi, it may be necessary to combine yang- and qi-tonifying herbs in interior-warming formulas.
- External factors should also be considered when prescribing interior-warming formulas. These formulas must be used with more caution during the summer, or in hot climates, and they must be discontinued immediately when the desired effects are achieved. On the other hand, they can be used at slightly larger doses, or for a longer period of time, during the winter or in cold climates.

PHARMACOLOGICAL EFFECTS & CLINICAL APPLICATIONS

Interior-warming formulas are divided into three subcategories, based on their traditional therapeutic actions. Similarly, these three subcategories of formulas also have contrasting pharmacological effects and clinical applications.

1. **Middle-warming and cold-dispelling formulas** treat deficiency and cold of the middle *jiao* (Spleen and Stomach). From the perspective of allopathic medicine, these formulas are most effective in treating disorders of the gastrointestinal tract.

- **Gastrointestinal disorders**: These formulas treat a wide variety of gastrointestinal disorders, including but not limited to nausea,[1] vomiting,[2] anorexia,[3] diarrhea,[4] dysentery,[5] constipation,[6] peptic ulcer,[7,8,9] gastritis (atrophic gastritis, superficial gastritis, gastritis with ulcer),[10] enteritis,[11] ulcerative colitis,[12,13] irritable bowel syndrome,[14] obstructive bowel diseases,[15] intestinal obstruction,[16] and post-operative ileus.[17] The mechanisms of action have been attributed in part to their antiulcer effects to inhibit the production of gastric acid,[18] their analgesic effects to relieve pain,[19] and their antiemetic effects to relieve nausea and vomiting.[20] Specific pharmacological effects vary depending on the formula and the disease. Representative formulas include *Li Zhong Wan* (Regulate the Middle Pill), *Fu Zi Li Zhong Wan* (Prepared Aconite Pill to Regulate the Middle), *Xiao Jian Zhong*

Chapter 7 — Overview

Tang (Minor Construct the Middle Decoction), and *Da Jian Zhong Tang* (Major Construct the Middle Decoction).

- **Others**: These formulas have also been used to treat other conditions that are associated with gastrointestinal disorders, such as stomatitis,[21] profuse salivation,[22] epigastric pain,[23] abdominal pain,[24,25] and a feeling of coldness in the abdomen.[26]

2. **Yang-resuscitating formulas** are used primarily to restore normal cardiovascular functions in animals that suffer acute cardiac collapse. They can also be used in animals that are having a hypoadrenal (Addisonian) crisis.
   - **Acute cardiac infarction**: *Si Ni Tang* (Frigid Extremities Decoction) has a marked effect on the cardiovascular system to increase the contractile force of the heart, increase blood pressure, and restore normal heart rhythm.[27] Clinically, it has been used to treat patients with acute cardiac infarction with good success.[28]

3. **Channel-warming and cold-dispersing formulas** treat exterior cold blocking and damaging the channels and collaterals. From the perspective of allopathic medicine, these formulas are most effective in treating pain.
   - **Pain**: These formulas are commonly used to treat many types and presentations of pain, such as cancer pain,[29] sciatica,[30] frostbite,[31,32] peripheral neuritis,[33,34] diabetic neuropathy,[35] periarthritis of shoulder,[36,37] frozen shoulder,[38] neck and shoulder stiffness and pain,[39] and general aches and pains.[40] Exemplar formulas include *Dang Gui Si Ni Tang* (Tangkuei Decoction for Frigid Extremities) and *Huang Qi Gui Zhi Wu Wu Tang* (Astragalus and Cinnamon Twig Five-Substance Decoction).

References

1. *Zhong Cheng Yao Yan Jiu* (Research of Chinese Patent Medicine), 1985; 1:46.
2. *Hu Nan Zhong Yi Za Zhi* (Hunan Journal of Chinese Medicine), 1998; 2:42.
3. *He Nan Zhong Yi* (Henan Chinese Medicine), 1998; 2:51.
4. *Gan Su Zhong Yi* (Gansu Chinese Medicine), 1993; 2:22.
5. *Shan Dong Zhong Yi Za Zhi* (*Shandong* Journal of Chinese Medicine), 1983; 2:21.
6. *Liao Ning Zhong Yi Za Zhi* (Liaoning Journal of Chinese Medicine), 1984; 4:29.
7. *An Hui Zhong Yi Xue Yuan Xue Bao* (Journal of Anhui University School of Medicine), 1988; 1:29.
8. *Zhe Jiang Zhong Yi Yao* (Zhejiang Chinese Medicine and Herbology), 1978; 2:9.
9. *Ji Lin Zhong Yi Yao* (Jilin Chinese Medicine and Herbology), 1996; 5:10.
10. *Jiang Xi Zhong Yi Yao* (Jiangxi Chinese Medicine and Herbology), 1981; 3:32.
11. *Shang Hai Zhong Yi Yao Za Zhi* (Shanghai Journal of Chinese Medicine and Herbology), 1984; 6:45.
12. *Zhong Yi Fang Ji Xian Dai Yan Jiu* (Modern Study of Medical Formulas in Traditional Chinese Medicine), 1997; 1:14.
13. *Bei Jing Zhong Yi* (Beijing Chinese Medicine), 1997; 1:19.
14. *Shi Yong Zhong Xi Yi Jie He Za Zhi* (Practical Journal of Integrated Chinese and Western Medicines), 1998; 6:560.
15. Ohya T, Usui Y, Arii S, Iwai T, Susumu T. Effect of dai-kenchu-to on obstructive bowel disease in children. Am J Chin Med. 2003; 31(1):129-35.
16. *Guo Wai Yi Xue* (Foreign Medicine), 1993; 15(5):39.
17. Hayakawa T, Kase Y, Saito K, Hashimoto K, Ishige A, Komatsu Y, Sasaki H. Effects of Dai-kenchu-to on intestinal obstruction following laparotomy. J Smooth Muscle Res. 1999 Apr; 35(2):47-54.
18. *Shan Dong Zhong Yi Za Zhi* (Shandong Journal of Chinese Medicine), 1984; 2:22.
19. *Zhong Cheng Yao* (Study of Chinese Patent Medicine), 1990; 5:25.
20. *Zhong Yi Fang Ji Xian Dai Yan Jiu* (Modern Study of Medical Formulas in Traditional Chinese Medicine), 1997; 378.
21. *Zhe Jiang Zhong Yi Za Zhi* (Zhejiang Journal of Chinese Medicine), 1992; 10:474.
22. *Guang Xi Zhong Yi Yao* (Guangxi Chinese Medicine and Herbology), 1992; 2:15.
23. *Shan Xi Zhong Yi* (Shanxi Chinese Medicine), 1984; 5(1):13.
24. *Shan Xi Zhong Yi* (Shanxi Chinese Medicine), 1992; 12:537.
25. *Ji Lin Zhong Yi Yao* (Jilin Chinese Medicine and Herbology), 1997; 2:19.
26. Nagano T, Itoh H, Takeyama M. Effects of Dai-kenchu-to on levels of 5-hydroxytryptamine (serotonin) and vasoactive intestinal peptides in human plasma. Biol Pharm Bull. 2000 Mar; 23(3):352-3.
27. *Zhong Yi Fang Ji Xian Dai Yan Jiu* (Modern Study of Medical Formulas in Traditional Chinese Medicine), 1997; 394-395.
28. *Tian Jin Yi Yao Tong Xun* (Publication of Tianjin Medicine and Herbology), 1972; 11:1.
29. *Zhong Yi Fang Ji Xian Dai Yan Jiu* (Modern Study of Medical Formulas in Traditional Chinese Medicine), 1997; 424.
30. *Hu Nan Zhong Yi Za Zhi* (Hunan Journal of Chinese Medicine), 1997; 2:48.
31. *Shan Dong Zhong Yi Za Zhi* (Shandong Journal of Chinese Medicine), 1984; 2:37.

Chapter 7 — Overview

32. *Shan Dong Zhong Yi Za Zhi* (Shandong Journal of Chinese Medicine), 1990; 3:49.
33. *Xin Zhong Yi* (New Chinese Medicine), 1996; 2:46.
34. *Zhong Yi Yao Xin Xi* (Information on Chinese Medicine and Herbology), 1998; 2:40.
35. *Hei Long Jiang Zhong Yi Yao* (Heilongjiang Chinese Medicine and Herbology), 1998; 4:17.
36. *Xin Zhong Yi* (New Chinese Medicine), 1987, 7:53.
37. *Si Chuan Zhong Yi* (Sichuan Chinese Medicine), 1993, 1:40.
38. *Si Chuan Zhong Yi* (Sichuan Chinese Medicine), 1989, 2:31.
39. *Shi Zhen Guo Yao Yan Jiu* (Research of Shizhen Herbs), 1999, 5:362.
40. *Hu Nan Zhong Yi Za Zhi* (Hunan Journal of Chinese Medicine), 1997, 6:29.

Section 1

温中祛寒剂

— Middle-Warming and Cold-Dispelling Formulas

Lǐ Zhōng Wán (Regulate the Middle Pill)

理中丸

Pinyin Name: *Li Zhong Wan*

Literal Name: Regulate the Middle Pill

Alternate Name: Ginseng and Ginger Combination

Original Source: *Shang Han Lun* (Discussion of Cold-Induced Disorders) by Zhang Zhong-Jing in the Eastern Han Dynasty

COMPOSITION

Gan Jiang (Rhizoma Zingiberis)	9g
Ren Shen (Radix et Rhizoma Ginseng)	9g
Bai Zhu (Rhizoma Atractylodis Macrocephalae)	9g
Zhi Gan Cao (Radix et Rhizoma Glycyrrhizae Praeparata cum Melle)	9g

DOSAGE / PREPARATION / ADMINISTRATION

The source text recommends to grind the ingredients into powder and form into pills with honey. The pills should resemble egg yolk in size. Take 1 pill with warm water three times during the day and twice at night. If ingestion of the pills does not create a feeling of warmth in the abdomen, then this formula may also be given as a decoction.

CHINESE THERAPEUTIC ACTIONS

1. Warms the middle *jiao* and dispels cold
2. Tonifies qi and strengthens the Spleen and Stomach

CLINICAL MANIFESTATIONS

1. Deficiency and cold of the middle *jiao*: absence of thirst, vomiting, diarrhea, abdominal pain, lack of appetite, and sudden turmoil disorder.
2. Bleeding due to yang deficiency: epistaxis, hematochezia, shortness of breath, lethargy, exercise intolerance, a pale pink to purple tongue, and a thin, weak pulse.

VETERINARY CLINICAL APPLICATIONS

Acute or chronic gastritis, gastric ulcers, chronic diarrhea, inflammatory bowel disease, gastroenteritis, nephropathy, male infertility, hypoadrenocorticism, and excessive salivation.

EXPLANATION

Li Zhong Wan (Regulate the Middle Pill) treats deficiency and cold of the middle *jiao*, where the Spleen and Stomach are located. The Spleen is responsible for transportation and transformation and raises the clear yang. The Stomach is responsible for accepting and digesting food and lowers the turbid yin. If the middle *jiao* is deficient as a result of coldness, the ascending and descending functions of the Spleen and Stomach may be impaired, causing diarrhea and vomiting. Abdominal pain is due to the presence of coldness. Lack of appetite is the result of deficiency of the middle *jiao* and impaired digestive functioning.

To treat this syndrome, use herbs to warm the middle *jiao*, dispel coldness, tonify Spleen qi, and invigorate the digestive function. *Gan Jiang* (Rhizoma Zingiberis), the chief herb, warms the middle *jiao* and dispels interior cold. *Ren Shen* (Radix et Rhizoma Ginseng) nourishes *yuan* (source) *qi*. *Bai Zhu* (Rhizoma Atractylodis Macrocephalae) strengthens the Spleen and dries dampness. *Zhi Gan Cao* (Radix et Rhizoma Glycyrrhizae Praeparata cum Melle) nourishes qi and harmonizes the middle *jiao*.

Li Zhong Wan can also be used to treat blood loss due to Spleen yang deficiency; a deficient Spleen fails to keep blood circulating within the vessels. Clinical manifestations include epistaxis, hematochezia, shortness of breath, lassitude, a pale face, and a fine pulse or a deficient, big

Lǐ Zhōng Wán (Regulate the Middle Pill)

***Li Zhong Wan* (Regulate the Middle Pill)**

Diagnosis	Clinical Signs	Treatment	Herbs
Deficiency and cold of the middle *jiao*	• Diarrhea and vomiting: deficiency and cold of the middle *jiao* impairing the normal ascending and descending functions of the Spleen and Stomach • Abdominal pain: cold in the middle *jiao*	• Warms the middle *jiao* and dispels cold • Tonifies qi and strengthens the Spleen	• *Gan Jiang* (Rhizoma Zingiberis) warms the middle *jiao* and dispels interior cold. • *Ren Shen* (Radix et Rhizoma Ginseng) nourishes *yuan* (source) *qi*. • *Bai Zhu* (Rhizoma Atractylodis Macrocephalae) strengthens the Spleen and dries dampness. • *Zhi Gan Cao* (Radix et Rhizoma Glycyrrhizae Praeparata cum Melle) nourishes qi and harmonizes the middle *jiao*.

pulse with little force. This syndrome of bleeding due to yang deficiency can be treated with *Li Zhong Wan*, with the addition of several other herbs such as *Huang Qi* (Radix Astragali), *Dang Gui* (Radix Angelicae Sinensis), and *E Jiao* (Colla Corii Asini); and the replacement of *Gan Jiang* (Rhizoma Zingiberis) with *Pao Jiang* (Rhizoma Zingiberis Praeparatum).

Li Zhong Wan may be used to treat clinical signs of yang deficiency of the middle *jiao* caused by excessive intake of cold food during the time of illness, or weakness after a major illness. Drooling of saliva or excessive production of foamy saliva following recovery from illness occurs when Spleen qi deficiency with cold fails to metabolize water. Body fluids thus flow upwards in the form of profuse saliva. *Li Zhong Wan* can be taken at a low dose for a prolonged period of time.

VETERINARY MODIFICATIONS

- With abdominal fullness and decreased intake of food, add *Shen Qu* (Massa Fermentata) and *Hou Po* (Cortex Magnoliae Officinalis).
- With abdominal pain, diarrhea, acid regurgitation, and a red tongue body with a white coating, add *Huang Lian* (Rhizoma Coptidis).
- With bloating of the abdomen, add *Wu Zhu Yu* (Fructus Evodiae), *Ding Xiang* (Flos Caryophylli), and *Gao Liang Jiang* (Rhizoma Alpiniae Officinarum).
- With nausea and vomiting due to cold in the Stomach, add *Ding Xiang* (Flos Caryophylli) and *Shi Di* (Calyx Kaki).
- With vomiting due to phlegm accumulation, add *Ban Xia* (Rhizoma Pinelliae) and *Fu Ling* (Poria).
- If there is severe vomiting, remove *Bai Zhu* (Rhizoma Atractylodis Macrocephalae); and add *Sheng Jiang* (Rhizoma Zingiberis Recens) and *Wu Zhu Yu* (Fructus Evodiae).
- With frequent diarrhea, add *Rou Dou Kou* (Semen Myristicae) and *He Zi* (Fructus Chebulae).
- With severe edema, add *Fu Ling* (Poria), *Ze Xie* (Rhizoma Alismatis), and *Dong Gua Pi* (Exocarpium Benincasae).
- If there is bleeding due to yang deficiency, add *E Jiao* (Colla Corii Asini), *San Qi* (Radix et Rhizoma Notoginseng), and charred *Ce Bai Ye* (Cacumen Platycladi).

CAUTIONS / CONTRAINDICATIONS

- *Li Zhong Wan* is contraindicated in animals with exterior wind invasion with fever.
- This formula contains many herbs that are warm and drying, and therefore is contraindicated in conditions characterized by interior heat with yin deficiency.
- This formula must be used with caution during pregnancy, as it contains many herbs that are warm and hot in nature.[1]

PHARMACOLOGICAL EFFECTS

1. **Antiulcer**: *Li Zhong Wan* has been shown to be beneficial in facilitating the healing of stomach ulcers. In one experiment, rats with artificially-induced ulcer were divided into herb and placebo groups. After 10 days of treatment, the herb group had only 3.57 mm^2 of ulceration, while the placebo group had 11.72 mm^2 of ulceration.[2]
2. **Adrenocortical**: The preliminary data showed that administration of *Li Zhong Wan* was associated with a regulating effect on the adrenal glands.[3]
3. **Effect on kidney function**: Administration of *Li Zhong Wan* was associated with a protective effect on kidney functions. In one study, continuous use of the formula for 1-3 months was effective in gradually reducing the amount of protein, cells, and blood urea nitrogen (BUN) in the urine.[4]

HUMAN CLINICAL STUDIES AND RESEARCH

1. **Epigastric pain**: Use of modified *Li Zhong Wan* was associated with marked results in treating 30 patients with epigastric pain characterized by deficiency and cold. The herbal treatment contained this formula plus *Huang Qi* (Radix Astragali), *Fu Ling* (Poria), *Chen Pi* (Pericarpium

Lǐ Zhōng Wán (Regulate the Middle Pill)

Citri Reticulatae), and *Cao Dou Kou* (Semen Alpiniae Katsumadai). Additional modifications were made as follows: double the dose of *Huang Qi* (Radix Astragali) for qi deficiency; *Rou Gui* (Cortex Cinnamomi) and *Fu Zi* (Radix Aconiti Lateralis Praeparata) for presence of cold; *Cang Zhu* (Rhizoma Atractylodis) and *Bai Bian Dou* (Semen Lablab Album) for dampness; *Dan Shen* (Radix et Rhizoma Salviae Miltiorrhizae), *Yan Hu Suo* (Rhizoma Corydalis), and *Chuan Lian Zi* (Fructus Toosendan) for stagnation; and *Bei Sha Shen* (Radix Glehniae), *Bai Shao* (Radix Paeoniae Alba), and *Shan Yao* (Rhizoma Dioscoreae) for yin deficiency. Of 30 patients, the study reported complete recovery in 5 patients within one month, and complete recovery in 20 patients and improvement in 5 patients within three months.[5]

2. **Gastritis**: Thirty patients with various types of gastritis (atrophic gastritis, superficial gastritis, gastritis with ulcer) were treated with *Li Zhong Wan*. The study reported complete relief of pain in 25 patients and partial relief of pain in 5 patients. Seventeen showed improvement based on endoscopy, and 13 showed no significant changes.[6]
3. **Bacterial dysentery**: Eighteen patients with chronic bacterial dysentery were treated with modification of *Li Zhong Wan* with complete recovery in 16 and improvement in 2 patients. The average duration of treatment was 12 days. The modification included addition of *Huang Lian* (Rhizoma Coptidis) and *Fu Ling* (Poria).[7]
4. **Enteritis**: Thirty patients with acute or chronic enteritis with diarrhea were treated with *Li Zhong Wan* for 3-10 days with significant improvement in 18 patients, moderate improvement in 8 patients, and no effect in 4 patients. The study reported an overall effectiveness rate of 86.6%.[8]
5. **Renal insufficiency**: Herbs were used to treat 15 patients (6 males and 9 females) with compromised kidney function, which included 12 patients of glomerulonephritis, polycystic kidney, kidney tuberculosis, and diabetic nephropathy. The herbal treatment included in extract 1.7 grams of *Li Zhong Wan* and 2.5 grams *Da Huang Gan Cao Tang* (Rhubarb and Licorice Decoction), given three times daily 30 minutes before meals for 3 months. The study reported an effectiveness rate of 66.7% after the first month, which was subsequently dropped to 40%. No significant side effects were reported.[9] (Note: *Da Huang Gan Cao Tang* (Rhubarb and Licorice Decoction) is not a commonly used formula, and is not discussed in detail in this text. The original source of this formula is *Shang Han Lun* (Discussion of Cold-Induced Disorders), with the following composition: *Da Huang* (Radix et Rhizoma Rhei) 12g and *Gan Cao* (Radix et Rhizoma Glycyrrhizae) 3g.)
6. **Male infertility**: In one study, *Li Zhong Wan* and *Ba Wei Di Huang Wan* (Eight-Ingredient Pill with Rehmannia) were combined together to treat 10 patients with male infertility. The study reported an increased production of seminal fluid (from 2.73 mL to 3.28 mL), in sperm count (from 1170/mL to 2185/mL), and in sperm motility (from 29.0% to 35.5%).[10]
7. **Excessive salivation**: Forty-two children (38 males and 4 females) with excessive salivation (20 days to 3 years history of illness) due to Spleen yang deficiency were treated with satisfactory results using modified *Li Zhong Wan*. The average age was 5.8 years (ranges from 3-9 years), and the average length of treatment was 4.6 packs of herbs in decoction. The herbs included *Dang Shen* (Radix Codonopsis) 10-18g, *Yi Zhi* (Fructus Alpiniae Oxyphyllae) 5-10g, *Gan Jiang* (Rhizoma Zingiberis) 5-8g, *Gan Cao* (Radix et Rhizoma Glycyrrhizae) 4-6g, and *Bai Zhu* (Rhizoma Atractylodis Macrocephalae) 8-10g. Modifications were made by adding *Sha Ren* (Fructus Amomi) 4-6g and *Ji Nei Jin* (Endothelium Corneum Gigeriae Galli) 5-8g for poor appetite and loose stools accompanied by long-term excessive salivation; and the addition of *Wu Mei* (Fructus Mume) 10-18g, *Shi Jun Zi* (Fructus Quisqualis) 7-10g, and *Hua Jiao* (Pericarpium Zanthoxyli) 4-6g, and removal of *Gan Cao* (Radix et Rhizoma Glycyrrhizae), for intestinal parasites with abdominal pain. After the treatment, 40 out of 42 patients showed complete recovery without any recurrence within 3 months.[11]
8. **Stomatitis**: One study reported effectiveness using modified *Li Zhong Wan* to treat recurrent stomatitis in 106 patients (47 males and 59 females, between 1-72 years of age, with 3 months to 24 years history of illness). In addition to this formula, modifications were made as follows: replacing *Ren Shen* (Radix et Rhizoma Ginseng) with *Dang Shen* (Radix Codonopsis) for severe Spleen deficiency; addition of *Rou Gui* (Cortex Cinnamomi) for cold; and addition of *Huang Lian* (Rhizoma Coptidis) for heat. The study reported complete recovery in all 106 patients after 2-17 days of treatment.[12]

SUGGESTED ACUPUNCTURE TREATMENT

1. Points: *Pishu* (BL 20), *Sanyinjiao* (SP 6), *Weishu* (BL 21), *Housanli* (ST 36), and *Zhongwan* (CV 12).
2. Technique: tonification and moxibustion.

Tonify *Pishu* (BL 20) and *Sanyinjiao* (SP 6) to nourish qi. Tonify and apply moxibustion on *Weishu* (BL 21) and *Housanli* (ST 36) to warm the middle *jiao*, disperse cold, and strengthen the middle *jiao*. Apply moxibustion on *Zhongwan* (CV 12) to activate the qi flow of the middle *jiao* and Stomach to relieve pain.

AUTHORS' COMMENTS

When discussing interior-warming formulas, it is important to remember that qi and yang are not two separate

Lǐ Zhōng Wán (Regulate the Middle Pill)

clinical entities; rather, they exist on a continuum. Yang deficiency is a more severe condition of cold than qi deficiency. Yang deficiency produces the same clinical signs as qi deficiency, but with additional signs of cold, such as cool extremities, ear tips and lumbar region; bloated and painful abdomen; and long, clear urination. Yang deficiency of the Spleen often includes Kidney yang deficiency. Accurate diagnosis is essential in deciding which formula to administer. Interior-warming formulas are hot and acrid and can further damage yin in patients with deficiency and heat. Unlike humans, dogs and cats may have significant yang deficiency without obvious signs of yang deficiency reflected in the tongue and pulse. It is rare for these species to show a classic wet, pale to purple tongue with a slow, deep pulse in most cases. Instead, it is recommended that practitioners comprehensively evaluate the history, clinical signs, and the tongue and pulse before diagnosing yang deficiency or discarding it as a possible diagnosis.

Li Zhong Wan is one of the most common formulas for treating deficiency and cold of the Spleen and Stomach in veterinary medicine. This formula was originally administered in pills, which usually have a slower onset of action. When necessary in acute or severe cases, this formula may first be given in decoction form, and then followed by pills when the condition stabilizes.

Deficiency cold of the Spleen and Stomach is commonly seen in animals that are fed exclusively refrigerated food, juvenile animals fed a cold, raw food diet, those on prolonged antibiotic therapy for chronic illness or following surgery (abdominal surgery in particular). It is also commonly seen in overworked performance animals, animals that live in cold environments without appropriate shelter, geriatric animals, valuable animals that are overbred, and constitutionally yang-deficient purebred animals.

It is normal for juvenile animals (less than 1 year of age) to have immature Spleen function. Because young animals cannot effectively process raw food, they need to have their food cooked and/or mixed with digestive enzymes to insure digestion of food until their Spleen matures. Feeding an exclusive raw food diet, or one that is cold and refrigerated on a regular basis, consumes Spleen qi and yang, leading to Spleen and/or Kidney yang deficiency over time. Kidney yang is the basis for all of the yang energies of the body. The same situation occurs in animals that are constantly exposed to environmental cold without shelter; in this case, exterior cold consumes the body's yang. Athletes are often not given adequate time for recuperation during a show season, which can lead to qi deficiency, among other things. Because qi is a yang substance and helps to warm the body, qi deficiency can lead to the accumulation of cold, especially if environmental conditions are concurrently cold. Overbreeding of animals frequently causes Kidney yang deficiency that eventually depletes Spleen yang as the Kidney "borrows" yang from the Spleen to maintain its normal functions. For this reason, it is often necessary to treat the Kidney at the same time as the Spleen to achieve good clinical results. This is especially true in older pets.

Antibiotics in general are classified as cold and bitter from an energetic perspective, according to Chinese medicine. Over time prolonged antimicrobial therapy can cool the middle *jiao* and consume Spleen yang, resulting in bleeding disorder, poor appetite, chronic vomiting and diarrhea. Animals on lifetime antimicrobial therapy for inflammatory bowel disease, chronic urinary tract or dermatological infections are often in this category. Animals that undergo abdominal surgery are further susceptible to cold from direct exposure of the gastrointestinal tract to environmental cold during the procedure.

Li Zhong Wan can be combined with *Jin Gui Shen Qi Wan* (Kidney Qi Pill from the Golden Cabinet) or *Ba Wei Di Huang Wan* (Eight-Ingredient Pill with Rehmannia) for the treatment of chronic renal failure, infertility, and hypoadrenocorticism. Some dogs with hypoadrenocorticism have signs of cold, chronic diarrhea and indigestion, despite adequate treatment with drugs that replace deficient mineralocorticoids. Of the two formulas, *Ba Wei Di Huang Wan* (Eight-Ingredient Pill with Rehmannia) is the warmest, as it contains *Rou Gui* (Cortex Cinnamomi), or cinnamon bark; while *Jin Gui Shen Qi Wan* (Kidney Qi Pill from the Golden Cabinet) contains *Gui Zhi* (Ramulus Cinnamomi), or cinnamon twig. If the animal shows signs of severe cold, the formula *Fu Zi Li Zhong Wan* (Prepared Aconite Pill to Regulate the Middle) should be given. This formula is *Li Zhong Wan* with the addition of *Fu Zi* (Radix Aconiti Lateralis Praeparata).

Li Zhong Wan and *Si Jun Zi Tang* (Four-Gentlemen Decoction) both treat Spleen qi deficiency with poor appetite, diarrhea, and other clinical signs. Both formulas contain qi-tonifying herbs such as *Ren Shen* (Radix et Rhizoma Ginseng), *Bai Zhu* (Rhizoma Atractylodis Macrocephalae), and *Zhi Gan Cao* (Radix et Rhizoma Glycyrrhizae Praeparata cum Melle). Despite these similarities, the differences are as follows:

- *Li Zhong Wan* is for deficiency with cold of the middle *jiao* (Spleen and Stomach), characterized by abdominal

Lǐ Zhōng Wán (Regulate the Middle Pill)

pain, vomiting, diarrhea, polyuria, cold limbs, intolerance to cold, and a deep, thin pulse. It is more warming overall than *Si Jun Zi Tang* (Four-Gentlemen Decoction).

- *Si Jun Zi Tang* is for Spleen qi deficiency, characterized by a sallow complexion, poor appetite, decreased dietary intake, fatigue, a pale tongue body, and a thin, moderate pulse.[13]

References

1. *Zhong Yao Ming Fang Yao Li Yu Ying Yong* (Pharmacology and Applications of Famous Herbal Formulas), 1989; 219-220.
2. *Shan Xi Yi Kan* (Shanxi Journal of Medicine), 1987; 7:333.
3. *Jiang Xi Zhong Yi Yao* (Jiangxi Chinese Medicine and Herbology), 1981; 3:32.
4. *Guo Wai Yi Xue* (Foreign Medicine), 1994; 6:30.
5. *Shan Xi Zhong Yi* (Shanxi Chinese Medicine), 1984; 5(1):13.
6. *Jiang Xi Zhong Yi Yao* (Jiangxi Chinese Medicine and Herbology), 1981; 3:32.
7. *Shan Dong Zhong Yi Za Zhi* (*Shandong* Journal of Chinese Medicine), 1983; 2:21.
8. *Shang Hai Zhong Yi Yao Za Zhi* (Shanghai Journal of Chinese Medicine and Herbology), 1984; 6:45.
9. *Guo Wai Yi Xue* (Foreign Medicine), 1994; 6:30.
10. *Zhong Yi Fang Ji Xian Dai Yan Jiu* (Modern Study of Medical Formulas in Traditional Chinese Medicine), 1997; 371.
11. *Guang Xi Zhong Yi Yao* (Guangxi Chinese Medicine and Herbology), 1992; 2:15.
12. *Zhe Jiang Zhong Yi Za Zhi* (Zhejiang Journal of Chinese Medicine), 1992; 10:474.
13. Wang MZ, et al. *Zhong Yi Xue Wen Da Ti Ku* (Questions and Answers on Traditional Chinese Medicine: Herbal Formulas).

Fù Zǐ Lǐ Zhōng Wán (Prepared Aconite Pill to Regulate the Middle)
附子理中丸

Pinyin Name: *Fu Zi Li Zhong Wan*
Literal Name: Prepared Aconite Pill to Regulate the Middle
Alternate Names: *Fu Tzu Li Chung Tang* (*Wan*), *Fu Zi Li Zhong Tang* (*Wan*), Aconite, Ginseng and Ginger Decoction (Pill); Aconite Middle-Regulating Decoction (Pill); Aconite Ginseng and Ginger Combination
Original Source: *Tai Ping Hui Min He Ji Ju Fang* (Imperial Grace Formulary of the Tai Ping Era) by the Imperial Medical Department in 1078-85

COMPOSITION

Fu Zi (Radix Aconiti Lateralis Praeparata), *pao* (blast-fried)	90g [9g]
Gan Jiang (Rhizoma Zingiberis), *pao* (blast-fried)	90g [9g]
Ren Shen (Radix et Rhizoma Ginseng)	90g [9g]
Bai Zhu (Rhizoma Atractylodis Macrocephalae), *cuo* (grated)	90g [9g]
Zhi Gan Cao (Radix et Rhizoma Glycyrrhizae Praeparata cum Melle)	90g [9g]

DOSAGE / PREPARATION / ADMINISTRATION

The source text states to grind the ingredients into a fine powder and form into pills with honey. Each pill should weigh 3 grams. Place and disintegrate 1 pill in one bowl of water, then cook it until 70% of the liquid remains. Take the warm decoction before meals on an empty stomach. For juveniles and neonates, divide the decoction into two to three separate doses. This formula may also be prepared as a decoction with the doses suggested in brackets.

CHINESE THERAPEUTIC ACTIONS

1. Warms yang and dispels cold
2. Tonifies qi and strengthens the Spleen

Fù Zǐ Lǐ Zhōng Wán (Prepared Aconite Pill to Regulate the Middle)

CLINICAL MANIFESTATIONS

Deficiency and cold of the Spleen and Stomach: warm seeking, extreme coldness of the body and the extremities, cool ear tips and lumbar region, weight loss, poor appetite, edema of the extremities, indigestion, borborygmus, severe epigastric and abdominal bloating and pain, nausea, vomiting, diarrhea, undigested food in the feces, a wet, pale to purple tongue, and a slow, weak, thin pulse.

VETERINARY CLINICAL APPLICATIONS

Inflammatory bowel disease, gastroenteritis, gastritis and peptic ulcer disease.

EXPLANATION

Fu Zi Li Zhong Wan (Prepared Aconite Pill to Regulate the Middle) combines *Fu Zi* (Radix Aconiti Lateralis Praeparata) and *Li Zhong Wan* (Regulate the Middle Pill). It warms the yang, dispels cold, benefits qi, and strengthens the Spleen. It is used for deficiency and cold secondary to yang deficiency of the Spleen and Stomach. Clinically, animals may show borborygmus, vomiting, diarrhea, muscle spasms, muscle stiffness in the extremities, and a white tongue coating.

In comparison to *Li Zhong Wan* (Regulate the Middle Pill), *Fu Zi Li Zhong Wan* more strongly warms yang and dispels cold. In this formula, *Fu Zi* (Radix Aconiti Lateralis Praeparata) dispels cold, tonifies yang, and warms the entire body. *Gan Jiang* (Rhizoma Zingiberis) warms the middle *jiao* and dispels interior cold. *Ren Shen* (Radix et Rhizoma Ginseng) nourishes *yuan* (source) *qi*. *Bai Zhu* (Rhizoma Atractylodis Macrocephalae) strengthens the Spleen and dries dampness. *Zhi Gan Cao* (Radix et Rhizoma Glycyrrhizae Praeparata cum Melle) nourishes qi and harmonizes the middle *jiao*.

VETERINARY MODIFICATIONS

- With severe deficiency and cold, add *Rou Gui* (Cortex Cinnamomi) and *Cang Zhu* (Rhizoma Atractylodis).
- With nausea and vomiting of phlegm and saliva, add *Ban Xia* (Rhizoma Pinelliae) and *Fu Ling* (Poria).
- With stagnation of phlegm and food, add *Wei Ling Tang* (Calm the Stomach and Poria Decoction).

CAUTIONS / CONTRAINDICATIONS

- *Fu Zi Li Zhong Wan* should be used with extreme caution in animals who have yin deficiency because the hot and dry herbs can further damage yin.
- This formula is contraindicated during pregnancy.[1]

PHARMACOLOGICAL EFFECTS

Analgesic: In one study, injection of *Fu Zi Li Zhong Wan* was associated with analgesic effects in mice.[2]

HUMAN CLINICAL STUDIES AND RESEARCH

1. **Peptic ulcer disease**: One study reported 91.5% effectiveness in the treatment of peptic ulcer characterized by deficiency and cold using *Fu Zi Li Zhong Wan*, *Huang Qi Jian Zhong Tang* (Astragalus Decoction to Construct the Middle), and others herbs as needed. Other herbs added included *Chai Hu* (Radix Bupleuri) and *Xiang Fu* (Rhizoma Cyperi) for a feeling of fullness and oppression in the chest and hypochondrium; *Yan Hu Suo* (Rhizoma Corydalis) and *Dan Shen* (Radix et Rhizoma Salviae Miltiorrhizae) for pain at a fixed location and purple tongue; *Chen Pi* (Pericarpium Citri Reticulatae) and *Fu Ling* (Poria) for fullness and distention of the epigastrium and a thick, greasy tongue coating; *Zhe Shi* (Haematitum) and *Xuan Fu Hua* (Flos Inulae) for nausea and vomiting; *Shen Qu* (Massa Fermentata), *Shan Zha* (Fructus Crataegi), *Gu Ya* (Fructus Setariae Germinatus) and *Mai Ya* (Fructus Hordei Germinatus) for poor appetite and indigestion. Of 59 patients, the study reported complete recovery in 37 patients, improvement in 17 patients, and no effect in 5 patients.[3]
2. **Ulcerative colitis**: Administration of modified *Fu Zi Li Zhong Wan* was effective in treating 78 patients with ulcerative colitis with a history of illness of 1-10 years.

Fu Zi Li Zhong Wan (Prepared Aconite Pill to Regulate the Middle)

Diagnosis	Clinical Signs	Treatment	Herbs
Deficiency and cold of the Spleen and Stomach	• Abdominal bloating and pain, borborygmus, diarrhea, undigested food in the feces, and vomiting: deficiency and cold of the Spleen and Stomach affecting the normal ascending and descending functions • Cold body and extremities, a pale, wet tongue, and a slow, weak pulse: cold in the middle *jiao* affecting the body and extremities	• Warms yang and dispels cold • Tonifies qi and strengthens the Spleen	• *Fu Zi* (Radix Aconiti Lateralis Praeparata) dispels cold, tonifies yang, and warms the entire body. • *Li Zhong Wan* (Regulate the Middle Pill) warms the middle *jiao*, tonifies qi and strengthens the Spleen and Stomach.

Fù Zǐ Lǐ Zhōng Wán (Prepared Aconite Pill to Regulate the Middle)

The herbal formula contained 12g each of *Fu Zi* (Radix Aconiti Lateralis Praeparata) (pre-decocted), *Gan Jiang* (Rhizoma Zingiberis), *Ren Shen* (Radix et Rhizoma Ginseng), *Zhi Gan Cao* (Radix et Rhizoma Glycyrrhizae Praeparata cum Melle), and *Bai Zhu* (Rhizoma Atractylodis Macrocephalae), and 8g each of *Chai Hu* (Radix Bupleuri) and *Sheng Ma* (Rhizoma Cimicifugae), and 20g of *He Zi* (Fructus Chebulae). For individuals with fever, abdominal pain, a yellow, greasy tongue coating and a slippery, rapid pulse, 30g of *Bai Tou Weng* (Radix Pulsatillae) and 10g of *Huang Bo* (Cortex Phellodendri Chinensis) was added, and *Gan Jiang* (Rhizoma Zingiberis) and *Fu Zi* (Radix Aconiti Lateralis Praeparata) were removed; for patients with poor appetite and abdominal distention, 20g each of charred *Shan Zha* (Fructus Crataegi), charred *Shen Qu* (Massa Fermentata), and charred *Mai Ya* (Fructus Hordei Germinatus) was added; and for severe early morning diarrhea, *Si Shen Wan* (Four-Miracle Pill) was added. The treatment protocol was to cook the herbs in decoction, and take the decoction in two equally-divided doses daily. The duration of treatment was between 7-40 packs of herbs. Of 78 patients, the study reported complete recovery in 34 patients, marked improvement in 35 patients, slight improvement in 7 patients, and no change in 2 patients.[4]

3. **Infantile diarrhea**: Thirty-six infants with ages ranging between under six months to three years with diarrhea refractory to drug treatment were treated with modified *Fu Zi Li Zhong Wan* with good results. The herbal formula included *Fu Zi* (Radix Aconiti Lateralis Praeparata) 3g, *Gan Jiang* (Rhizoma Zingiberis) 6g, *Dang Shen* (Radix Codonopsis) 10g, dry-fried *Bai Zhu* (Rhizoma Atractylodis Macrocephalae) 15g, *Fu Ling* (Poria) 15g, *Gui Zhi* (Ramulus Cinnamomi) 10g, *Zhu Ling* (Polyporus) 10g, *Ze Xie* (Rhizoma Alismatis) 6g, *Ying Su Ke* (Pericarpium Papaveris) 3g, *Cang Zhu* (Rhizoma Atractylodis) 6g, and *Chen Pi* (Pericarpium Citri Reticulatae) 6g. Modifications were made by adding 6g each of charred *Shan Zha* (Fructus Crataegi), charred *Shen Qu* (Massa Fermentata), and charred *Mai Ya* (Fructus Hordei Germinatus) for presence of undigested food in the stools; *Ge Gen* (Radix Puerariae Lobatae) 10g for fever; *Zhu Ru* (Caulis Bambusae in Taenia) 6g for nausea and vomiting; and *Mai Dong* (Radix Ophiopogonis) 6g and *Wu Wei Zi* (Fructus Schisandrae Chinensis) 6g for thirst. The treatment protocol was to cook the same herbs in water twice, mix the two batches of decoction together, and administer the decoction in four equally-divided doses. Of 36 patients, 25 had normal bowel movement within two packs of herbs, 9 within three packs, and 1 within four packs. However, one person required hospitalization because of continuous diarrhea and subsequent dehydration.[5]

SUGGESTED ACUPUNCTURE TREATMENT

1. Points: *Pishu* (BL 20), *Sanyinjiao* (SP 6), *Weishu* (BL 21), *Housanli* (ST 36), *Zhongwan* (CV 12), *Qihai* (CV 6), *Yaoyangguan* (GV 3), and *Mingmen* (GV 4).
2. Technique: tonification and moxibustion.

Tonify *Pishu* (BL 20) and *Sanyinjiao* (SP 6) to nourish qi. Tonify and apply moxibustion on *Weishu* (BL 21) and *Housanli* (ST 36) to warm the middle *jiao*, disperse cold, and strengthen the middle *jiao*. Apply moxibustion on *Zhongwan* (CV 12) to activate the qi flow of the middle *jiao* and Stomach to relieve pain. Apply moxibustion on *Qihai* (CV 6), *Yaoyangguan* (GV 3), and *Mingmen* (GV 4) to warm the Kidney and yang and enhance the interior-warming effect.

AUTHORS' COMMENTS

Fu Zi Li Zhong Wan is formulated by combining *Fu Zi* (Radix Aconiti Lateralis Praeparata) and *Li Zhong Wan* (Regulate the Middle Pill). The addition of *Fu Zi* (Radix Aconiti Lateralis Praeparata) makes it a stronger formula to tonify both Spleen and Kidney yang. Therefore, *Fu Zi Li Zhong Wan* is reserved for more severe coldness. In some animals, interior cold may be so severe that the addition of *Rou Gui* (Cortex Cinnamomi) is needed. As soon as severe cold signs resolve, formulas that are less warming should be used, such as *Li Zhong Tang* (Regulate the Middle Decoction), which can then be followed by *Xiang Sha Liu Jun Zi Tang* (Six-Gentlemen Decoction with Aucklandia and Amomum) or *Xiang Sha Liu Jun Zi Tang* (Six-Gentlemen Decoction with Cyperus and Amomum). Some of the most common applications for this formula include late-stage renal failure and diabetes in geriatric animals, late stages of *Cushing's* disease (hyperadrenocorticism) and hypoadrenocorticism.

Li Zhong Wan (Regulate the Middle Pill) and *Fu Zi Li Zhong Wan* have many similarities and differences:

- *Li Zhong Wan* is an interior-warming formula consisting of *Ren Shen* (Radix et Rhizoma Ginseng), *Gan Jiang* (Rhizoma Zingiberis), *Bai Zhu* (Rhizoma Atractylodis Macrocephalae), and *Zhi Gan Cao* (Radix et Rhizoma Glycyrrhizae Praeparata cum Melle). It warms the middle *jiao*, dispels cold, tonifies qi, and strengthens the Spleen. It is mainly used for digestive dysfunctions caused by deficiency and cold of the middle *jiao*, leading to clinical signs of diarrhea, vomiting, abdominal pain, poor appetite, and no desire to drink. Also, it is used for yang deficiency with loss of blood and preference for sleep. It can also treat excessive salivation with middle *jiao* deficiency and coldness.

Fù Zǐ Lǐ Zhōng Wán (Prepared Aconite Pill to Regulate the Middle)

- *Fu Zi Li Zhong Wan* is much more acrid and hot, as it contains *Fu Zi* (Radix Aconiti Lateralis Praeparata), one of the hottest herbs in the entire pharmacopeia. This formula warms and strengthens Spleen and Kidney yang. It is best for coldness and pain in the chest and abdomen, extreme coldness of the limbs and extremities, and muscle spasms and cramps. *Fu Zi Li Zhong Wan*, in comparison to *Li Zhong Wan*, is for more severe conditions of cold accumulation in the body.[6]

References

1. *Zhong Yao Ming Fang Yao Li Yu Ying Yong* (Pharmacology and Applications of Famous Herbal Formulas), 1989; 220-221.
2. *Zhong Cheng Yao* (Study of Chinese Patent Medicine), 1990; 5:25.
3. *An Hui Zhong Yi Xue Yuan Xue Bao* (Journal of Anhui University School of Medicine), 1988; 1:29.
4. *Zhong Yi Fang Ji Xian Dai Yan Jiu* (Modern Study of Medical Formulas in Traditional Chinese Medicine), 1997; 1:14.
5. *Gan Su Zhong Yi* (Gansu Chinese Medicine), 1993; 2:22.
6. Wang MZ, et al. *Zhong Yi Xue Wen Da Ti Ku* (Questions and Answers on Traditional Chinese Medicine: Herbal Formulas).

Wú Zhū Yú Tāng (Evodia Decoction)

吳茱萸湯
吴茱萸汤

Pinyin Name: *Wu Zhu Yu Tang*
Literal Name: Evodia Decoction
Alternate Names: *Wu Chu Yu Tang*, Evodia Fruit Decoction, Evodia Combination
Original Source: *Shang Han Lun* (Discussion of Cold-Induced Disorders) by Zhang Zhong-Jing in the Eastern Han Dynasty

COMPOSITION

Wu Zhu Yu (Fructus Evodiae), *xi* (washed) in liquid 7 times	1 cup [3-9g]
Sheng Jiang (Rhizoma Zingiberis Recens), *qie* (sliced)	18g [18g]
Ren Shen (Radix et Rhizoma Ginseng)	9g [6g]
Da Zao (Fructus Jujubae), *bo* (opened)	12 pieces [4 pieces]

DOSAGE / PREPARATION / ADMINISTRATION

The source text states to cook the ingredients in 7 cups [1,400 mL] of water until 2 cups [400 mL] of liquid remain. Take 0.7 cup [140 mL] of the warm, strained decoction three times daily. Today, the decoction may be prepared using the doses suggested in brackets. Note: Some patients may experience exacerbation of the clinical signs immediately after ingesting the herbs, which is a normal reaction and should abate in half an hour.

CHINESE THERAPEUTIC ACTIONS

1. Warms and tonifies the middle *jiao*
2. Corrects the reversed flow of qi and stops vomiting

CLINICAL MANIFESTATIONS

1. Vomiting as a result of deficiency and cold of the Stomach: nausea after eating, discomfort in the chest and diaphragm, epigastric pain, belching, and acid regurgitation. In horses, colic after eating or profuse, non-odorous reflux.
2. *Jueyin* dry heaves (vomiting of saliva only).
3. *Shaoyin* vomiting and diarrhea, with extremely cold extremities and severe restlessness and irritability.

VETERINARY CLINICAL APPLICATIONS

Acute and chronic vomiting secondary to cancer, post-operative vomiting, inflammatory bowel disease, and food poisoning.

Wú Zhū Yú Tāng (Evodia Decoction)

EXPLANATION

Wu Zhu Yu Tang (Evodia Decoction) treats vomiting due to deficiency and cold in the Stomach with rising of yin and cold upwards. This condition may be present in *yangming*, *shaoyin*, and *jueyin* disorders. In *yangming* disorder, deficiency and cold affect the Stomach and cause reversed flow of qi, leading to clinical signs such as vomiting, belching, and acid regurgitation. In *jueyin* disorder, yin and cold rise upwards to cause dry heaves and vomiting of saliva. In *shaoyin* disorder, yin and cold rise upwards to cause vomiting, while yang is deficient and cannot reach upwards or outwards, resulting in diarrhea with extremely cold distal extremities.

Wu Zhu Yu (Fructus Evodiae), acrid, bitter, and very warm, is the chief herb in this formula. It warms the Stomach, dispels cold, harmonizes the middle *jiao*, and corrects the reversed flow of qi. *Sheng Jiang* (Rhizoma Zingiberis Recens) warms the Stomach and relieves nausea and vomiting. *Ren Shen* (Radix et Rhizoma Ginseng) tonifies *yuan* (source) *qi* and strengthens the Stomach. *Da Zao* (Fructus Jujubae) tonifies qi and harmonizes the middle *jiao*. *Sheng Jiang* (Rhizoma Zingiberis Recens) and *Da Zao* (Fructus Jujubae) also harmonize and regulate the *ying* (nutritive) and *wei* (defensive) levels.

VETERINARY MODIFICATIONS

- If there is severe nausea and vomiting, add *Ban Xia* (Rhizoma Pinelliae), *Sha Ren* (Fructus Amomi), and *Fu Ling* (Poria).
- With abdominal pain, add *Bai Shao* (Radix Paeoniae Alba).
- With abdominal pain and extreme coldness, add *Si Ni Tang* (Frigid Extremities Decoction).
- With fullness and distention in the abdominal region, add *Sha Ren* (Fructus Amomi) and *Hou Po* (Cortex Magnoliae Officinalis).
- With involuntary salivation, nausea or dry heaves, add *Gan Jiang* (Rhizoma Zingiberis) and *Rou Gui* (Cortex Cinnamomi).
- If there is frequent acid regurgitation, add *Hai Piao Xiao* (Endoconcha Sepiae) and *Wa Leng Zi* (Concha Arcae).
- With irritability and extreme coldness, add *Fu Zi* (Radix Aconiti Lateralis Praeparata) and *Xi Xin* (Radix et Rhizoma Asari).

CAUTIONS / CONTRAINDICATIONS

- *Wu Zhu Yu Tang* is contraindicated in animals with vomiting and acid regurgitation caused by heat.
- This formula may be served at room temperature or administered via nasogastric tube, especially for animals who cannot keep the warm decoction down because of vomiting.
- According to one reference, use of this formula in decoction is occasionally associated with chest discomfort, and dizziness. These side effects, however, are self-limiting and generally resolve within 30 minutes without intervention.[1]

PHARMACOLOGICAL EFFECTS

1. **Antiemetic**: In one experiment, the administration of *Wu Zhu Yu Tang* was found to be effective in suppressing vomiting in pigeons with artificially-induced vomiting. The researchers noted that while *Wu Zhu Yu* (Fructus Evodiae) and *Sheng Jiang* (Rhizoma Zingiberis Recens) each have antiemetic effects, the potency is not as strong as *Wu Zhu Yu Tang*.[2]
2. **Gastrointestinal**: Administration of *Wu Zhu Yu Tang* was associated with a general inhibitory effect on the gastrointestinal system. In one experiment of two groups of mice who were given the same amount of food, the group that received herbs had significantly more food remaining in the stomach than the group that received placebo.[3] In another experiment, administration of *Wu Zhu Yu Tang* inhibited the production of gastric acid, and increased the pH in the stomach.[4]

HUMAN CLINICAL STUDIES AND RESEARCH

1. **Vomiting**: Use of *Wu Zhu Yu Tang* in 168 patients was associated with 91.7% effectiveness in relieving nausea

***Wu Zhu Yu Tang* (Evodia Decoction)**

Diagnosis	Clinical Signs	Treatment	Herbs
Deficiency and cold of the Stomach	• Vomiting, belching, and acid regurgitation: reversed flow of qi due to deficiency and cold of the Stomach • Discomfort in the chest and diaphragm, and epigastric pain: presence of cold in the middle *jiao*	• Warms and tonifies the middle *jiao* • Corrects the reversed flow of qi and stops vomiting	• *Wu Zhu Yu* (Fructus Evodiae) warms the Stomach, dispels cold, harmonizes the middle *jiao*, and corrects the reversed flow of qi. • *Sheng Jiang* (Rhizoma Zingiberis Recens) warms the Stomach and relieves nausea and vomiting. • *Ren Shen* (Radix et Rhizoma Ginseng) tonifies *yuan* (source) *qi* and strengthens the Stomach. • *Da Zao* (Fructus Jujubae) tonifies qi and harmonizes the middle *jiao*.

Wú Zhū Yú Tāng (Evodia Decoction)

and vomiting associated with cancer of the upper gastrointestinal tract. The treatment protocol was to administer the herbs in decoction daily, for 6 packs of herbs per course of treatment.[5] In another study, use of modified *Wu Zhu Yu Tang* was associated with 100% effectiveness in treating neurogenic vomiting in 68 patients who have 3 months to 3 years history of illness. Modifications to this formula included the addition of *Huo Xiang* (Herba Agastaches) and *Pei Lan* (Herba Eupatorii) for dampness with a white, greasy tongue coating; *Chen Xiang* (Lignum Aquilariae Resinatum) and *Qing Pi* (Pericarpium Citri Reticulatae Viride) for chest and hypochondriac fullness and pain; *Huang Lian* (Rhizoma Coptidis) and *Zhu Ru* (Caulis Bambusae in Taenia) for a red tongue body with irritability; and *Sha Ren* (Fructus Amomi) and *Mai Dong* (Radix Ophiopogonis) for chronic vomiting with Stomach yin deficiency. Of 68 patients, the study reported significant improvement in 53 patients and moderate improvement in 15 patients.[6]

2. **Nausea**: One study reported complete recovery in all 5 patients with nausea when treated with *Wu Zhu Yu Tang* plus *Shi Di* (Calyx Kaki), *Zhi Qiao* (Fructus Aurantii), and *Pi Pa Ye* (Folium Eriobotryae). The cause of nausea was determined to be weakness and deficiency of the Spleen and Stomach with accumulation of cold qi.[7]
3. **Ulcerative colitis**: Use of modified *Wu Zhu Yu Tang* was effective in treating chronic ulcerative colitis in 68 patients (between 20 and 58 years of age, with 1-12 years history of illness). In addition to the base formula, modifications were made as follows: *Chai Hu* (Radix Bupleuri) and *Ji Nei Jin* (Endothelium Corneum Gigeriae Galli) for Liver overacting on the Spleen; *Chuan Xiong* (Rhizoma Chuanxiong) and *Yan Hu Suo* (Rhizoma Corydalis) for a purple tongue with petechia spots and abdominal pain that worsens with pressure; *Bai Tou Weng* (Radix Pulsatillae) and *Qin Pi* (Cortex Fraxini) for damp-heat; *Xiao Hui Xiang* (Fructus Foeniculi) and *Fu Ling* (Poria) for damp-cold; *Shan Yao* (Rhizoma Dioscoreae) and dry-fried *Bai Bian Dou* (Semen Lablab Album) for Spleen and Stomach deficiencies; *Shen Qu* (Massa Fermentata) and dry-fried *Shan Zha* (Fructus Crataegi) for food stagnation; *Ba Ji Tian* (Radix Morindae Officinalis) and *Bu Gu Zhi* (Fructus Psoraleae) for Spleen and Kidney yang deficiencies; *Dan Shen* (Radix et Rhizoma Salviae Miltiorrhizae), *Rou Dou Kou* (Semen Myristicae), charred *Qian Cao* (Radix et Rhizoma Rubiae), and charred *Pu Huang* (Pollen Typhae) for blood stagnation due to chronic illness. The treatment protocol was to administer the herbs in decoction twice daily, for 30 days per course of treatment, for 1-2 courses total. Of 68 patients, the study reported complete recovery in 42 patients, improvement in 23 patients, and no effect in 3 patients.[8]
4. **Hypertension**: Forty-four patients (11 males and 33 females) ages between 40-67 with hypertension were treated with modified *Wu Zhu Yu Tang* with good success. Clinical presentation of these patients included hypertension with dizziness, and a feeling of swelling sensations and pain in the head. The treatment protocol was to administer the herbs in decoction twice daily. The formula included *Wu Zhu Yu* (Fructus Evodiae) 4g, *Ban Xia* (Rhizoma Pinelliae) 8g, *Dang Shen* (Radix Codonopsis) 10g, *Fu Ling* (Poria) 10g, *Fu Shen* (Poria Paradicis) 10g, *Bai Zhi* (Radix Angelicae Dahuricae) 10g, *Di Long* (Pheretima) 10g, *Jiang Can* (Bombyx Batryticatus) 10g, *Chai Hu* (Radix Bupleuri) 6g, *Qing Pi* (Pericarpium Citri Reticulatae Viride) 6g, *Chen Pi* (Pericarpium Citri Reticulatae) 6g, *Gou Teng* (Ramulus Uncariae cum Uncis) 30g, *Sheng Jiang* (Rhizoma Zingiberis Recens) 5-8 slices, *Da Zao* (Fructus Jujubae) 5-8 pieces, and *Zhi Gan Cao* (Radix et Rhizoma Glycyrrhizae Praeparata cum Melle) 4g. Other slight modifications were made as follows: addition of *Chuan Xiong* (Rhizoma Chuanxiong) 6g for a purple tongue; *Chan Tui* (Periostracum Cicadae) 5g for tinnitus; and removal of *Da Zao* (Fructus Jujubae) and addition of *Sha Ren* (Fructus Amomi) 3g and *Dou Kou* (Fructus Amomi Rotundus) 3g for a greasy tongue coating. Improvement was noted in most patients within 5 packs of herbs. Out of 44 patients, the study reported significant improvement in 34 patients, moderate improvement in 8 patients, and no effect in 2 patients. The overall rate of effectiveness was 95.45%.[9]

SUGGESTED ACUPUNCTURE TREATMENT

1. Points: *Pishu* (BL 20), *Weishu* (BL 21), *Housanli* (ST 36), *Zhongwan* (CV 12), *Guanyuan* (CV 4), and *Neiguan* (PC 6).
2. Technique: tonification and moxibustion.

Pishu (BL 20), *Weishu* (BL 21), *Housanli* (ST 36), and *Zhongwan* (CV 12) nourish the Spleen and Stomach and disperse cold. *Guanyuan* (CV 4) nourishes *yuan* (source) *qi* and *ying* (nutritive) *qi*. *Neiguan* (PC 6) regulates the qi flow of the Stomach and corrects the reversed flow of qi.

AUTHORS' COMMENTS

Wu Zhu Yu Tang has a wide range of therapeutic actions, and may be used to treat *yangming*, *shaoyin* and *jueyin* disorders. It has primary application to treat vomiting in veterinary medicine from both excess and deficiency cold. Provided a correct diagnosis has been made, vomiting should resolve in a few doses. It can be used for vomiting immediately after eating in dogs with cancer, and for vomiting post-operatively following gastrointestinal surgery or biopsy. Similarly, horses with reflux and small intestine ileus post surgery or those undergoing excessive

Wú Zhū Yú Tāng (Evodia Decoction)

antibiotic treatment may present with this pattern. The animals for which this formula is appropriate have a thick, white tongue coating and a pulse that is thin or slow, or thin and wiry.

Li Zhong Wan (Regulate the Middle Pill) and *Wu Zhu Yu Tang* both warm the middle *jiao* and dispel cold to treat abdominal pain, nausea, and diarrhea due to cold and deficiency of the middle *jiao*. Both formulas use *Ren Shen* (Radix et Rhizoma Ginseng) to tonify the Spleen and Stomach. Their differences are as follows:

- *Li Zhong Wan* warms the Stomach to dispel cold to treat vomiting, diarrhea, and excessive salivation. *Gan Jiang* (Rhizoma Zingiberis) and *Bai Zhu* (Rhizoma Atractylodis Macrocephalae) warm the Spleen and Stomach, and treat deficiency and cold of the middle *jiao*.
- *Wu Zhu Yu Tang* is specifically for deficiency and cold in the Liver and Stomach, with turbid yin rising and causing nausea and vomiting of white or yellow foam. The formula uses *Wu Zhu Yu* (Fructus Evodiae) to warm the Liver channel and redirect rebellious Stomach qi. It uses a heavy dose of *Sheng Jiang* (Rhizoma Zingiberis Recens) to complement the effects of *Wu Zhu Yu* (Fructus Evodiae).[10]

References

1. *Zhong Yao Ming Fang Yao Li Yu Ying Yong* (Pharmacology and Applications of Famous Herbal Formulas), 1989; 226-228.
2. *Zhong Yi Fang Ji Xian Dai Yan Jiu* (Modern Study of Medical Formulas in Traditional Chinese Medicine), 1997; 378.
3. *Zhong Yi Fang Ji Xian Dai Yan Jiu* (Modern Study of Medical Formulas in Traditional Chinese Medicine), 1997; 378.
4. *Zhong Yao Yao Li Yu Lin Chuang* (Pharmacology and Clinical Applications of Chinese Herbs), 1987; 3:49.
5. *Shan Xi Zhong Yi* (Shanxi Chinese Medicine), 1997; 1:9.
6. *Hu Nan Zhong Yi Za Zhi* (Hunan Journal of Chinese Medicine), 1998; 2:42.
7. *Zhong Cheng Yao Yan Jiu* (Research of Chinese Patent Medicine), 1985; 1:46.
8. *Bei Jing Zhong Yi* (Beijing Chinese Medicine), 1997; 1:19.
9. *Hei Long Jiang Zhong Yi Yao* (Heilongjiang Chinese Medicine and Herbology), 1995; 6:9.
10. Wang MZ, et al. *Zhong Yi Xue Wen Da Ti Ku* (Questions and Answers on Traditional Chinese Medicine: Herbal Formulas).

Xiǎo Jiàn Zhōng Tāng (Minor Construct the Middle Decoction)

小建中湯

小建中汤

Pinyin Name: *Xiao Jian Zhong Tang*
Literal Name: Minor Construct the Middle Decoction
Alternate Names: *Hsiao Chien Chung Tang, Xiao Jian Zhung Tang*, Minor Centre-Fortifying Decoction, Minor Middle-Strengthening Decoction, Minor Cinnamon and Peony Combination
Original Source: *Shang Han Lun* (Discussion of Cold-Induced Disorders) by Zhang Zhong-Jing in the Eastern Han Dynasty

COMPOSITION

Yi Tang (Maltosum)	1 cup [30g]
Gui Zhi (Ramulus Cinnamomi)	9g
Bai Shao (Radix Paeoniae Alba), *chao* (dry-fried) with liquor	18g
Zhi Gan Cao (Radix et Rhizoma Glycyrrhizae Praeparata cum Melle)	6g
Sheng Jiang (Rhizoma Zingiberis Recens), *qie* (sliced)	9g
Da Zao (Fructus Jujubae), *bo* (opened)	12 pieces [4 pieces]

Xiǎo Jiàn Zhōng Tāng (Minor Construct the Middle Decoction)

DOSAGE / PREPARATION / ADMINISTRATION

Cook the ingredients, except *Yi Tang* (Maltosum), in 7 cups [1,400 mL] of water until 3 cups [600 mL] of liquid remain. Filter and discard the herb residue, add *Yi Tang* (Maltosum) to the strained liquid, and allow it to dissolve using low heat. Take 1 cup [200 mL] of the warm, strained decoction three times daily. Today, the decoction is prepared by using the doses suggested in brackets, and by cooking the herbs twice. Filter and discard the herb residue, and dissolve *Yi Tang* (Maltosum) in the strained decoction. Take the warm decoction in two equally-divided doses.

CHINESE THERAPEUTIC ACTIONS

1. Tonifies and warms the middle *jiao*
2. Harmonizes the interior and relieves pain

CLINICAL MANIFESTATIONS

Deficiency and cold of the middle *jiao*: abdominal pain that decreases with warmth and pressure, a pale tongue and a fine, wiry and moderate pulse; restlessness, irritability, sore limbs, warm extremities, and a dry mouth and throat.

VETERINARY CLINICAL APPLICATIONS

Abdominal pain due to debility or overwork, chronic illness and gastritis, peptic ulcer disease, epigastric pain, habitual constipation and chronic active hepatitis.

EXPLANATION

Xiao Jian Zhong Tang (Minor Construct the Middle Decoction) treats deficiency and cold of the middle *jiao* with three clinical manifestations. Deficiency of the middle *jiao* may give rise to interior cold, which then produces abdominal pain. The pain usually improves with warmth and pressure. Deficiency and cold of the middle *jiao* also compromises the generation of qi and blood, which results in palpitations, fidgeting and irritability. Lastly, deficiency and cold of the middle *jiao* results in the inability of the Spleen to produce qi and blood. An insufficiency of qi and blood disrupts the harmony between the *ying* (nutritive) and *wei* (defensive) levels. Sore limbs occur as *ying* (nutritive) cannot properly nourish the muscles and warm extremities; and a dry mouth and throat occur when *wei* (defensive) *qi* leaks outwards. A pale tongue is a sign of deficiency, and a thin, wiry and moderate pulse suggests true deficiency and cold in the interior and pain.

Yi Tang (Maltosum), the chief herb, warms the middle *jiao*, tonifies Spleen qi, and nourishes Spleen yin. Furthermore, it softens the Liver to alleviate pain and moistens the Lung to relieve dryness. *Gui Zhi* (Ramulus Cinnamomi) warms yang and dispels cold. *Bai Shao* (Radix Paeoniae Alba) nourishes yin and blood, and relieves pain. *Zhi Gan Cao* (Radix et Rhizoma Glycyrrhizae Praeparata cum Melle) tonifies qi and helps *Yi Tang* (Maltosum) and *Gui Zhi* (Ramulus Cinnamomi) warm the middle and benefit qi. *Zhi Gan Cao* (Radix et Rhizoma Glycyrrhizae Praeparata cum Melle) also helps *Bai Shao* (Radix Paeoniae Alba) nourish the Liver and alleviate pain. *Sheng Jiang* (Rhizoma Zingiberis Recens) warms the Stomach and *Da Zao* (Fructus Jujubae) tonifies the Spleen. These two herbs also harmonize the *ying* (nutritive) and *wei* (defensive) levels. In summary, this formula warms and tonifies the middle *jiao*, which in turn alleviates the associated clinical signs characterized by deficiency and cold.

VETERINARY MODIFICATIONS

- With fatigue due to qi deficiency, add *Huang Qi* (Radix Astragali) and *Ren Shen* (Radix et Rhizoma Ginseng).

***Xiao Jian Zhong Tang* (Minor Construct the Middle Decoction)**

Diagnosis	Clinical Signs	Treatment	Herbs
Deficiency and cold of the middle *jiao*	• Abdominal pain that decreases with warmth and pressure: cold and deficiency of the middle *jiao* • Palpitations: qi and blood deficiencies • Sore limbs, warm extremities, and a dry mouth and throat: disharmony of *ying* (nutritive) and *wei* (defensive) levels • Pale tongue: deficiency • Thin, wiry and moderate pulse: deficiency and cold in the interior	• Tonifies and warms the middle *jiao* • Harmonizes the interior and relieves pain	• *Yi Tang* (Maltosum) warms the middle *jiao*, tonifies Spleen qi, and nourishes Spleen yin. • *Gui Zhi* (Ramulus Cinnamomi) warms yang and dispels cold. • *Bai Shao* (Radix Paeoniae Alba) nourishes yin and blood. • *Zhi Gan Cao* (Radix et Rhizoma Glycyrrhizae Praeparata cum Melle) tonifies qi, warms the middle *jiao*, and alleviates pain. • *Sheng Jiang* (Rhizoma Zingiberis Recens) and *Da Zao* (Fructus Jujubae) warm the Stomach and tonify the Spleen.

Xiăo Jiàn Zhōng Tāng (Minor Construct the Middle Decoction)

- With fatigue due to blood deficiency, add *Dang Gui* (Radix Angelicae Sinensis) and *Chuan Xiong* (Rhizoma Chuanxiong).
- If there is chronic weakness and blood deficiency add *Si Wu Tang* (Four-Substance Decoction); and with qi deficiency add *Si Jun Zi Tang* (Four-Gentlemen Decoction).

CAUTIONS / CONTRAINDICATIONS

- *Xiao Jian Zhong Tang* is contraindicated in cases of yin-deficient fire, and conditions characterized by middle *jiao* stagnation.
- This formula is not recommended for treating vomiting because the sweet herbs in this formula will create more stagnation and promote Stomach qi reversal.
- This formula is contraindicated in animals with intestinal parasites.

PHARMACOLOGICAL EFFECTS

1. **Antiulcer**: Administration of *Xiao Jian Zhong Tang* was associated with a protective effect on the stomach in rats. The beneficial effects are attributed to *Gui Zhi* (Ramulus Cinnamomi) for its effect to treat ulceration, *Bai Shao* (Radix Paeoniae Alba) for its effect to inhibit the production of gastric acid, and *Gan Cao* (Radix et Rhizoma Glycyrrhizae) and *Sheng Jiang* (Rhizoma Zingiberis Recens) for their effect to protect the mucous lining of the stomach.[1]
2. **Gastrointestinal**: Administration of *Xiao Jian Zhong Tang* was associated with a general inhibitory effect on the gastrointestinal system. According to a laboratory experiment, animals who received ingredients of *Xiao Jian Zhong Tang* responded with a decreased production of gastric acid and lowered rate of peristalsis.[2]

HUMAN CLINICAL STUDIES AND RESEARCH

1. **Gastrointestinal disorders**: In one report, 21 patients with various types of gastrointestinal disorders (11 with peptic ulcers, 8 with superficial gastritis, and 2 with atrophic gastritis) were treated with modified *Xiao Jian Zhong Tang* for 15 consecutive doses. The formula included *Bai Shao* (Radix Paeoniae Alba) 15g, *Gui Zhi* (Ramulus Cinnamomi) 10g, *Gan Jiang* (Rhizoma Zingiberis) 5g, *Da Zao* (Fructus Jujubae) 5 pieces, *Zhi Gan Cao* (Radix et Rhizoma Glycyrrhizae Praeparata cum Melle) 5g, *Dang Shen* (Radix Codonopsis) 10g, *Bai Zhu* (Rhizoma Atractylodis Macrocephalae) 10g, *Fo Shou* (Fructus Citri Sarcodactylis) 10g, and *Yi Tang* (Maltosum) 30g. The study reported significant improvement in pain reduction in 20 out of 21 patients.[3]
2. **Gastritis**: *Xiao Jian Zhong Tang* was reported in one study to have good effect to treat gastritis. Of 58 patients with chronic gastritis, 39 were diagnosed with atrophic gastritis and 19 with superficial gastritis. In addition to *Xiao Jian Zhong Tang*, modifications were made based on the individual conditions of the patients. For acid reflux, *Yi Tang* (Maltosum) was removed and *Wu Zhu Yu* (Fructus Evodiae), *Hai Piao Xiao* (Endoconcha Sepiae) and *Mu Li* (Concha Ostreae) were added. For pain at night, a purplish tongue with dark spots, *Yan Hu Suo* (Rhizoma Corydalis), *Chi Shao* (Radix Paeoniae Rubra), and *Dan Shen* (Radix et Rhizoma Salviae Miltiorrhizae) were added. For the presence of *H. pylori*, *Da Huang* (Radix et Rhizoma Rhei) and *Pu Huang* (Pollen Typhae) were added. For qi deficiency and generalized weakness, *Huang Qi* (Radix Astragali), *Fu Ling* (Poria), and *Bai Zhu* (Rhizoma Atractylodis Macrocephalae) were added. Out of 58 cases, the study reported complete recovery in 32 cases (55.5%), improvement in 18 cases (31.0%), and no benefit in 8 cases (13.8%). The overall rate of effectiveness was 86.2%.[4]
3. **Peptic ulcer disease**: Modified *Xiao Jian Zhong Tang* was used with good results in treating 31 of 35 patients with peptic ulcer and abdominal pain. No recurrence was noted amongst 31 patients in their one-year follow-up examination. The herbal treatment used *Xiao Jian Zhong Tang* plus *Gua Lou* (Fructus Trichosanthis), *Wu Zhu Yu* (Fructus Evodiae), and *Xie Bai* (Bulbus Allii Macrostemonis) as the base formula. For severe acid reflux, *Da Zao* (Fructus Jujubae) and *Yi Tang* (Maltosum) were removed and *Huang Lian* (Rhizoma Coptidis) and *Mu Li* (Concha Ostreae) were added. For nausea and vomiting, *Pao Jiang* (Rhizoma Zingiberis Praeparatum) was removed and *Ban Xia* (Rhizoma Pinelliae) and *Sheng Jiang* (Rhizoma Zingiberis Recens) were added. For frequent belching, *Xuan Fu Hua* (Flos Inulae), *Ban Xia* (Rhizoma Pinelliae), and *Zhe Shi* (Haematitum) were added. For feeling of chest and abdominal oppression and distention, *Da Zao* (Fructus Jujubae) was removed and *Hou Po* (Cortex Magnoliae Officinalis) and *Zhi Qiao* (Fructus Aurantii) were added. Lastly, *Fu Ling* (Poria) was added for palpitations and *Bai Zhu* (Rhizoma Atractylodis Macrocephalae) was added for loose stools.[5]
4. **Epigastric pain**: Numerous studies have shown that *Xiao Jian Zhong Tang* effectively treats epigastric pain due to various causes, including but not limited to chronic gastritis, gastric ulcer, duodenal ulcer, gastric prolapse, and others.[6,7]
5. **Abdominal pain**: *Xiao Jian Zhong Tang* was shown in two reports to effectively treat abdominal pain in infants and children between 3-10 years of age. Specific causes of abdominal pain were not stated in these reports.[8,9]
6. **Habitual constipation**: In one study, 11 patients with chronic habitual constipation were treated with modified *Xiao Jian Zhong Tang*. The formula included *Yi Tang* (Maltosum) 30g, *Bai Shao* (Radix Paeoniae Alba) 15g, *Gui Zhi* (Ramulus Cinnamomi) 6g, *Zhi Gan Cao* (Radix et

Xiǎo Jiàn Zhōng Tāng (Minor Construct the Middle Decoction)

Rhizoma Glycyrrhizae Praeparata cum Melle) 5g, and *Da Zao* (Fructus Jujubae) 5 pieces. The treatment protocol was to administer the herbs in decoction for seven days per course of treatment. The study reported success with all patients. Out of 11 patients, 4 responded within 1 course, 6 within 2 courses, and 1 after 5 courses. There were no recurrences in all patients in follow-up interviews 6 months after the termination of treatments.[10]

7. **Hepatitis B**: One study reported beneficial effect using modified *Xiao Jian Zhong Tang* to treat 68 patients with hepatitis B. The herbal treatment contained this formula plus *Sha Ren* (Fructus Amomi), *Ji Nei Jin* (Endothelium Corneum Gigeriae Galli), charred *Shan Zha* (Fructus Crataegi), charred *Shen Qu* (Massa Fermentata), and charred *Mai Ya* (Fructus Hordei Germinatus). Furthermore, modifications included addition of *Yin Chen* (Herba Artemisiae Scopariae), *Cang Zhu* (Rhizoma Atractylodis), *Pu Gong Ying* (Herba Taraxaci), and *Chui Pen Cao* (Herba Sedi) for damp-heat; *Dang Shen* (Radix Codonopsis), *Shan Yao* (Rhizoma Dioscoreae), *Bai Zhu* (Rhizoma Atractylodis Macrocephalae), and *Huang Qi* (Radix Astragali) for qi deficiency; *Bei Sha Shen* (Radix Glehniae), *Mai Dong* (Radix Ophiopogonis), *Gou Qi Zi* (Fructus Lycii), and *Yin Yang Huo* (Herba Epimedii) for yin deficiency; and other adjustments as needed. The duration of treatment was three months per course of treatment, for 1-2 courses. Of 68 cases, the study reported significant effect in 47 cases, moderate effect in 15 cases, and no effect in 6 cases. The overall rate of effectiveness was 91%.[11]

SUGGESTED ACUPUNCTURE TREATMENT

1. Points: *Pishu* (BL 20), *Zhangmen* (LR 13), *Tianshu* (ST 25), *Shangjuxu* (ST 37), *Xingjian* (LR 2), *Pishu* and *Qihaishu*.
2. Technique: tonification or moxibustion.

Pishu (BL 20) and *Zhangmen* (LR 13), the *shu* (transport) and *mu* (collecting) points of Spleen, nourish the Spleen, tonify qi, warm the middle *jiao*, and disperse cold. *Tianshu* (ST 25), the *mu* (collecting) point of the Large Intestine, is combined with *Shangjuxu* (ST 37), the lower *he* (uniting) point of the Large Intestine, to regulate qi and blood flow in the Large Intestine and relieve abdominal pain. *Xingjian* (LR 2) smoothes Liver qi flow to help relieve pain. *Pishu* and *Qihaishu* are classical points that strengthen the Spleen in horses.

RELATED FORMULA

Dāng Guī Jiàn Zhōng Tāng
(Tangkuei Decoction to Construct the Middle)
當歸建中湯
当归建中汤

Pinyin Name: *Dang Gui Jian Zhong Tang*
Literal Name: Tangkuei Decoction to Construct the Middle
Original Source: *Qian Jin Yi Fang* (Supplement to the Thousand Ducat Formulas) by Sun Si-Miao in 682 A.D.

Dang Gui (Radix Angelicae Sinensis)	12g
Gui Xin (Cortex Rasus Cinnamomi)	9g
Zhi Gan Cao (Radix et Rhizoma Glycyrrhizae Praeparata cum Melle)	6g
Bai Shao (Radix Paeoniae Alba), *chao* (dry-fried) with liquor	18g
Sheng Jiang (Rhizoma Zingiberis Recens), *qie* (sliced)	9g
Da Zao (Fructus Jujubae), *bo* (opened)	12 pieces [4 pieces]
Yi Tang (Maltosum)	18g

Cook the ingredients, except *Yi Tang* (Maltosum), in 10 cups [2,000 mL] of water until 3 cups [600 mL] of liquid remain. Filter and discard the herb residue, add *Yi Tang* (Maltosum) to the strained liquid, and allow it to dissolve over low intensity heat. Take 1 cup [200 mL] of the warm, strained decoction three times daily.

Dang Gui Jian Zhong Tang (Tangkuei Decoction to Construct the Middle) is composed of *Dang Gui* (Radix Angelicae Sinensis) and *Xiao Jian Zhong Tang*. It tonifies the blood, warms the middle *jiao*, and relieves pain. Clinically, patients may show abdominal pain, or lower abdominal pain that radiates to the lower back, in addition to all the clinical signs listed in *Xiao Jian Zhong Tang*. This formula may also be used in postpartum animals with generalized deficiency and weakness.

AUTHORS' COMMENTS

Abdominal pain may be caused by many different factors. Three potential causes and their diagnosis include: pain that worsens with pressure is considered acute and excess in nature; pain that lessens with pressure is regarded as deficient and chronic in nature; and pain that worsens with cold and lessens with warmth is cold in nature. *Xiao Jian Zhong Tang* is designed to treat abdominal pain due to yang deficiency of the middle *jiao*, with key clinical signs of abdominal pain that lessens with pressure and warmth, and a pale tongue. A common use for this formula and its variations is in performance animals. Both horses and dogs that are overworked may become qi deficient, which will lead to yang deficiency and the accumulation of cold. These animals may become lethargic, inappetent, and show mild signs of colic or bloating, which can be resolved with the correct administration of these formulas.

Xiǎo Jiàn Zhōng Tāng (Minor Construct the Middle Decoction)

There are four "*jian zhong tang* (construct the middle decoction)" formulas that have similar functions to warm and tonify the middle *jiao*.

- *Xiao Jian Zhong Tang* (Minor Construct the Middle Decoction) warms the yang of the middle *jiao*.
- *Huang Qi Jian Zhong Tang* (Astragalus Decoction to Construct the Middle) warms and tonifies qi of the middle *jiao*.
- *Dang Gui Jian Zhong Tang* (Tangkuei Decoction to Construct the Middle) harmonizes the blood and relieves pain.
- *Da Jian Zhong Tang* (Major Construct the Middle Decoction) redirects rising Stomach qi to treat nausea and vomiting.

Li Zhong Wan (Regulate the Middle Pill) and *Xiao Jian Zhong Tang* both warm the middle *jiao* and disperse cold to treat deficiency and cold of the middle *jiao*, manifesting in abdominal and epigastric coldness and pain. Their differences are as follows:

- *Li Zhong Wan* treats Spleen yang deficiency with excess cold accumulation. This formula has a greater qi-tonic effect than *Xiao Jian Zhong Tang*. Manifestations include diarrhea, vomiting, abdominal pain, and poor appetite. It is also suitable for yang deficiency with sudden blood loss, *xiong bi* (painful obstruction of the chest) syndrome, and excessive salivation in chronic diseases.
- *Xiao Jian Zhong Tang* warms the entire middle *jiao* and strengthens yang qi in the middle *jiao*. Animals usually also have yang deficiency of the middle *jiao* along with qi, blood, and yin deficiencies. The primary problem is pain. Other clinical signs include palpitations, irritability, and a dry mouth and throat. It can also treat qi, yin, and blood deficiencies with fatigue, palpitations, and shortness of breath usually seen in chronic, late-stage diseases.[12]

Gui Zhi Tang (Cinnamon Twig Decoction) and *Xiao Jian Zhong Tang* are both from *Shang Han Lun* (Discussion of Cold-Induced Disorders). They have essentially the same ingredients except for one herb, yet the difference in doses significantly changes the functions and indications of these formulas.

- *Gui Zhi Tang* contains 9g each of *Bai Shao* (Radix Paeoniae Alba) and *Gui Zhi* (Ramulus Cinnamomi). At equal doses, the emphasis of these two herbs is to dispel wind-cold and harmonize the *ying* (nutritive) and *wei* (defensive) levels to treat an exterior condition lingering in the *taiyang* channel.
- *Xiao Jian Zhong Tang* was originally derived from *Gui Zhi Tang* (Cinnamon Twig Decoction) with the addition of *Yi Tang* (Maltosum). The rest of the ingredients are exactly the same. *Xiao Jian Zhong Tang* contains 30g of *Yi Tang* (Maltosum) and 18g of *Bai Shao* (Radix Paeoniae Alba); whereas, there are only 9g in *Gui Zhi Tang* (Cinnamon Twig Decoction). With these two as the primary herbs used at higher doses, *Xiao Jian Zhong Tang* focuses on warming the middle *jiao*, tonifying deficiency, and relieving pain.[13]

References

1. *Guo Wai Yi Xue Zhong Yi Zhong Yao Fen Ce* (Monograph of Chinese Herbology from Foreign Medicine), 1983; 6:45.
2. *Shan Dong Zhong Yi Za Zhi* (Shandong Journal of Chinese Medicine), 1984; 2:22.
3. *Zhong Yi Za Zhi* (Journal of Chinese Medicine), 1981; 11:657.
4. *Shi Yong Zhong Xi Yi Jie He Za Zhi* (Practical Journal of Integrated Chinese and Western Medicines), 1998; 1:71.
5. *Zhe Jiang Zhong Yi Yao* (Zhejiang Chinese Medicine and Herbology), 1978; 2:9.
6. *Fu Jian Zhong Yi Yao* (Fujian Chinese Medicine and Herbology), 1990; 6:55.
7. *Zhong Yi Ming Fang Lin Chuang Xin Yong* (Contemporary Clinical Applications of Classic Chinese Formulas), 2001; 87-88.
8. *Shan Xi Zhong Yi* (Shanxi Chinese Medicine), 1992; 12:537.
9. *Ji Lin Zhong Yi Yao* (Jilin Chinese Medicine and Herbology), 1997; 2:19.
10. *Liao Ning Zhong Yi Za Zhi* (Liaoning Journal of Chinese Medicine), 1984; 4:29.
11. *Zhong Yi Fang Ji Xian Dai Yan Jiu* (Modern Study of Medical Formulas in Traditional Chinese Medicine), 1997; 385.
12. Wang MZ, et al. *Zhong Yi Xue Wen Da Ti Ku* (Questions and Answers on Traditional Chinese Medicine: Herbal Formulas).
13. Wang MZ, et al. *Zhong Yi Xue Wen Da Ti Ku* (Questions and Answers on Traditional Chinese Medicine: Herbal Formulas).

Huáng Qí Jiàn Zhōng Tāng

(Astragalus Decoction to Construct the Middle)

黃耆建中湯
黄芪建中汤

Pinyin Name: *Huang Qi Jian Zhong Tang*
Literal Name: Astragalus Decoction to Construct the Middle
Alternate Names: *Huang Chi Chien Chung Tang, Huang Qi Jian Zhung Tang*, Astragalus Centre-Fortifying Decoction, Astragalus Middle-Strengthening Decoction, Astragalus Combination
Original Source: *Jin Gui Yao Lue* (Essentials from the Golden Cabinet) by Zhang Zhong-Jing in the Eastern Han Dynasty

COMPOSITION

Yi Tang (Maltosum)	1 cup [30g]
Gui Zhi (Ramulus Cinnamomi)	9g
Bai Shao (Radix Paeoniae Alba), *chao* (dry-fried) with liquor	18g
Zhi Gan Cao (Radix et Rhizoma Glycyrrhizae Praeparata cum Melle)	6g
Sheng Jiang (Rhizoma Zingiberis Recens), *qie* (sliced)	9g
Da Zao (Fructus Jujubae), *bo* (opened)	12 pieces [4 pieces]
Huang Qi (Radix Astragali)	4.5g [12g]

DOSAGE / PREPARATION / ADMINISTRATION

Cook the ingredients, except *Yi Tang* (Maltosum), in 7 cups [1,400 mL] of water until 3 cups [600 mL] of liquid remain. Filter and discard the herb residue, add *Yi Tang* (Maltosum) to the strained liquid, and allow it to dissolve using low heat. Take 1 cup [200 mL] of the warm, strained decoction three times daily. Today, the decoction is prepared by using the doses suggested in brackets, and by cooking the herbs twice. Filter and discard the herb residue, and dissolve *Yi Tang* (Maltosum) in the strained decoction. Take the warm decoction in two equally-divided doses.

CHINESE THERAPEUTIC ACTIONS

1. Warms the middle *jiao* and tonifies qi
2. Harmonizes the interior and relieves pain

CLINICAL MANIFESTATIONS

Deficiency and cold of the middle *jiao* with severe qi deficiency: abdominal pain that decreases with warmth and pressure, and a pale tongue. There might be irritability, shortness of breath, lethargy, and dry mucous membranes.

VETERINARY CLINICAL APPLICATIONS

Peptic ulcer disease, gastritis, indigestion and anorexia following antibiotic therapy, gastric ulcer, anorexia, constipation, allergic rhinitis, leukopenia, delayed healing of wounds, and gangrene.

EXPLANATION

Huang Qi Jian Zhong Tang (Astragalus Decoction to Construct the Middle) is formulated by combining *Huang Qi* (Radix Astragali) and *Xiao Jian Zhong Tang* (Minor Construct the Middle Decoction). *Xiao Jian Zhong Tang* (Minor Construct the Middle Decoction) tonifies and warms the middle *jiao*, harmonizes the interior, and relieves pain. *Huang Qi* (Radix Astragali) tonifies qi to treat qi deficiency. Note: Please refer to *Xiao Jian Zhong Tang* (Minor Construct the Middle Decoction) for a complete explanation of this formula and its applications.

Huang Qi Jian Zhong Tang **(Astragalus Decoction to Construct the Middle)**

Diagnosis	Clinical Signs	Treatment	Herbs
Deficiency and cold of the middle *jiao* with severe qi deficiency	• Abdominal pain that decreases with warmth and pressure, a pale tongue and fine, wiry and moderate pulse: deficiency and cold of the middle *jiao* • Spontaneous sweating, shortness of breath and lethargy: qi deficiency	• Warms the middle *jiao* and tonifies qi • Harmonizes the interior and relieves pain	• *Xiao Jian Zhong Tang* (Minor Construct the Middle Decoction) tonifies and warms the middle *jiao*, harmonizes the interior, and relieves pain. • *Huang Qi* (Radix Astragali) tonifies qi.

Huáng Qí Jiàn Zhōng Tāng

(Astragalus Decoction to Construct the Middle)

VETERINARY MODIFICATIONS

- For generalized weakness following an illness, combine with *Si Jun Zi Tang* (Four-Gentlemen Decoction).
- For generalized weakness postpartum, combine with *Si Wu Tang* (Four-Substance Decoction).
- For generalized weakness following a wind-cold disorder, combine with *Yu Ping Feng San* (Jade Windscreen Powder).
- With abdominal fullness, add *Hou Po* (Cortex Magnoliae Officinalis), *Sha Ren* (Fructus Amomi), and *Mu Xiang* (Radix Aucklandiae).
- With vomitus of clear fluids, add *Wu Zhu Yu* (Fructus Evodiae), *Ban Xia* (Rhizoma Pinelliae), and *Gan Jiang* (Rhizoma Zingiberis).
- With edema, add *Bai Zhu* (Rhizoma Atractylodis Macrocephalae), *Fu Ling* (Poria), and *Ze Xie* (Rhizoma Alismatis).

PHARMACOLOGICAL EFFECTS

1. **Gastrointestinal**: Administration of *Huang Qi Jian Zhong Tang* was effective in suppressing the production of gastric acid, thereby promoting the recovery from gastric ulcers in rats.[1]
2. **Immunostimulant**: One study reported an increase in IgG from 12.4-24.5 mg/mL to 12.4-30 mg/mL (an average increase of 1.59 mg/mL; $p<0.05$) following ingestion of *Huang Qi Jian Zhong Tang* for 20 doses while treating gastrointestinal disorders.[2]

HUMAN CLINICAL STUDIES AND RESEARCH

1. **Peptic ulcer disease**: *Huang Qi Jian Zhong Tang* has been shown in many clinical studies to effectively treat gastric and duodenal ulcers. In one study, use of modified *Huang Qi Jian Zhong Tang* in 100 patients with peptic ulcer (gastric and duodenal ulcers) was associated with complete recovery in 85 patients, significant improvement in 13 patients, and no effect in 2 patients. The herbal treatment contained this formula plus *Hai Piao Xiao* (Endoconcha Sepiae) and *Bai Ji* (Rhizoma Bletillae). Additional modifications included *Yan Hu Suo* (Rhizoma Corydalis) for severe pain; *Zhi Qiao* (Fructus Aurantii) and *Chen Pi* (Pericarpium Citri Reticulatae) for fullness and distention in the chest and abdominal regions; *Wa Leng Zi* (Concha Arcae) and *Mai Ya* (Fructus Hordei Germinatus) for acid reflux; and *San Qi* (Radix et Rhizoma Notoginseng) for bleeding.[3] According to another study, 12 patients (4 with gastric ulcer, 4 with duodenal ulcer, and 4 with both gastric and duodenal ulcers) were treated with modified *Huang Qi Jian Zhong Tang* with marked success. In addition to this formula, *Huang Lian* (Rhizoma Coptidis) and *Wu Zhu Yu* (Fructus Evodiae) were added for acid reflux; *Fan Xie Ye* (Folium Sennae) for constipation; and charred *Shan Zha* (Fructus Crataegi), charred *Shen Qu* (Massa Fermentata), and charred *Mai Ya* (Fructus Hordei Germinatus) for food stagnation. Of 12 patients, the study reported complete recovery in 9 patients, improvement in 2 patients, and no benefit in 1 patient.[4]
2. **Antral gastritis**: One study reported 92.6% effectiveness in the treatment of chronic antral gastritis using *Huang Qi Jian Zhong Tang* plus *Dan Shen* (Radix et Rhizoma Salviae Miltiorrhizae), *Tao Ren* (Semen Persicae), *Yan Hu Suo* (Rhizoma Corydalis), and minus *Yi Tang* (Maltosum). Additional modifications were made as need. For Stomach yin deficiency, *Sha Shen* (Radix Glehniae seu Adenophorae) and *Mai Dong* (Radix Ophiopogonis) were added, and *Gan Jiang* (Rhizoma Zingiberis) and *Gui Zhi* (Ramulus Cinnamomi) were removed. For disharmony of the Liver and Stomach, *Chai Hu* (Radix Bupleuri) and *Xiang Fu* (Rhizoma Cyperi) were added. For accumulation of phlegm in the middle *jiao*, *Ban Xia* (Rhizoma Pinelliae) and *Chen Pi* (Pericarpium Citri Reticulatae) were added. For food stagnation, *Shen Qu* (Massa Fermentata) and *Shan Zha* (Fructus Crataegi) were added. Of 41 patients, the study reported complete recovery in 23 patients, significant improvement in 9 patients, slight improvement in 6 patients, and no change in 3 patients.[5]
3. **Atrophic gastritis**: Use of modified *Huang Qi Jian Zhong Tang* was associated with 96% effectiveness in treating 101 patients with 1-20 years history of atrophic gastritis. In addition to this formula, modifications were made to include *Dang Shen* (Radix Codonopsis) for deficiency and cold of the Spleen and Stomach; *Dan Shen* (Radix et Rhizoma Salviae Miltiorrhizae) and *Chuan Lian Zi* (Fructus Toosendan) for Liver qi stagnation; and *Bai He* (Bulbus Lilii) for Spleen and Stomach yin deficiencies. The duration of treatment was four weeks per course of treatment, for a total of three courses. Of 101 patients, the study reported complete recovery in 59 patients, significant improvement in 24 patients, moderate improvement in 14 patients, and no effect in 4 patients.[6]
4. **Anorexia**: One study reported complete recovery in 26 of 32 children with anorexia using *Huang Qi Jian Zhong Tang* plus dry-fried *Gu Ya* (Fructus Setariae Germinatus) and *Sha Ren* (Fructus Amomi) in decoction for one week per course of treatment.[7]
5. **Constipation**: Fifty patients with constipation characterized by deficiency were treated with good results using *Huang Qi Jian Zhong Tang* plus *Nu Zhen Zi* (Fructus Ligustri Lucidi) and *Dang Gui* (Radix Angelicae Sinensis). Additional modifications were made as follows: a larger dose of *Huang Qi* (Radix Astragali) for constipation with qi deficiency; a larger dose of *Dang Gui* (Radix Angelicae

Huáng Qí Jiàn Zhōng Tāng
(Astragalus Decoction to Construct the Middle)

Sinensis) for constipation with blood deficiency; *Fu Zi* (Radix Aconiti Lateralis Praeparata) and *Pao Jiang* (Rhizoma Zingiberis Praeparatum) for constipation with yang deficiency; *Rou Cong Rong* (Herba Cistanches), *Gou Qi Zi* (Fructus Lycii) and *Niu Xi* (Radix Achyranthis Bidentatae) for geriatric patients with soreness and weakness of the lower back and knees; and *Wu Wei Zi* (Fructus Schisandrae Chinensis) for presence of chloasma on the face. The treatment protocol was to administer the herbs in decoction form daily, for 10 days per course of treatment, for 1-2 courses total.[8]

6. **Irritable bowel syndrome (IBS)**: One study reported 92% effectiveness using modified *Huang Qi Jian Zhong Tang* to treat 50 patients with IBS. In addition to this formula, modifications were made by adding *Sha Ren* (Fructus Amomi) and *Lai Fu Zi* (Semen Raphani) for qi stagnation; *Huo Xiang* (Herba Agastaches), *Cang Zhu* (Rhizoma Atractylodis), and *Pei Lan* (Herba Eupatorii) for loose stools due to cold and dampness; *Sha Ren* (Fructus Amomi), *Gu Ya* (Fructus Setariae Germinatus) and *Ji Nei Jin* (Endothelium Corneum Gigeriae Galli) for food stagnation, poor appetite, and belching; *Chai Hu* (Radix Bupleuri) and *Fo Shou* (Fructus Citri Sarcodactylis) for Liver qi stagnation with hypochondriac pain; and *Fu Zi* (Radix Aconiti Lateralis Praeparata) and *Bu Gu Zhi* (Fructus Psoraleae) for soreness and weakness of the lower back and knees. The treatment protocol was to administer the herbs in decoction one time daily, for one month per course of treatment, for 1-4 courses total. Of 50 patients, the study reported complete recovery in 21 patients, significant improvement in 15 patients, moderate improvement in 10 patients, and no change in 4 patients.[9]
7. **Allergic rhinitis**: Sixty patients with allergic rhinitis were treated with significant improvement in 50 patients and moderate improvement in 10 patients. The herbal treatment contained *Huang Qi Jian Zhong Tang* plus *Ku Xing Ren* (Semen Armeniacae Amarum), *Gan Cao* (Radix et Rhizoma Glycyrrhizae), and *Ba Ji Tian* (Radix Morindae Officinalis). For individuals who showed presence of heat, *Huang Qin* (Radix Scutellariae) was added and *Ba Ji Tian* (Radix Morindae Officinalis) was removed. The herbs were given in decoction form one time daily, for between 7-20 days.[10]
8. **Otitis media**: One study reported good therapeutic effects using modified *Huang Qi Jian Zhong Tang* to treat chronic suppurative otitis media. In addition to this formula, modifications were made by adding *Long Dan* (Radix et Rhizoma Gentianae), *Che Qian Zi* (Semen Plantaginis), and *Jin Yin Hua* (Flos Lonicerae Japonicae) for profuse sticky ear discharge; *Huang Bo* (Cortex Phellodendri Chinensis), *Huang Lian* (Rhizoma Coptidis) and *Bai Jiang Cao* (Herba cum Radice Patriniae) for foul-smelling discharge; *Dang Gui* (Radix Angelicae Sinensis), *Yi Yi Ren* (Semen Coicis), *Bai Zhu* (Rhizoma Atractylodis Macrocephalae), and a large dose of *Jin Yin Hua* (Flos Lonicerae Japonicae) for profuse watery discharge; *Chuan Xiong* (Rhizoma Chuanxiong), *Man Jing Zi* (Fructus Viticis), *Bai Zhi* (Radix Angelicae Dahuricae) and *Pei Lan* (Herba Eupatorii); *Fang Feng* (Radix Saposhnikoviae), *Ji Li* (Fructus Tribuli), *Zhu Ru* (Caulis Bambusae in Taenia), and *Ban Xia* (Rhizoma Pinelliae) for nausea and dizziness. The treatment protocol was to cook the herbs in water and drink the decoction in two to three equally-divided doses. Of 30 patients, the study reported complete recovery in 10 patients, significant improvement in 14 patients, and no effect in 6 patients.[11]
9. **Leukopenia**: Twenty-six patients with decreased white blood cells count were effectively treated using *Huang Qi Jian Zhong Tang* plus *Huang Lian Jie Du Tang* (Coptis Decoction to Relieve Toxicity). In addition, *Bai Zhu* (Rhizoma Atractylodis Macrocephalae) and *Dang Gui* (Radix Angelicae Sinensis) were added for dizziness and fatigue; *Dang Shen* (Radix Codonopsis) and *Fu Ling* (Poria) for soreness and weakness of the extremities; *Shi Chang Pu* (Rhizoma Acori Tatarinowii) and *Yuan Zhi* (Radix Polygalae) for insomnia and palpitations; and *Huang Qi* (Radix Astragali) and *Huang Lian* (Rhizoma Coptidis) at large doses for frequent recurrences of infection. After 10-20 days of herbal therapy, the study reported complete recovery in 17 patients, improvement in 6 patients, and no benefit in 3 patients.[12]
10. **Athletic performance**: According to one study of 12 athletes randomly separated into a control group (treated with placebos) and the experimental group (treated with herbs), use of *Huang Qi Jian Zhong Tang* for 8 weeks was associated with effectively increasing time before exhaustion, positively influencing anaerobic threshold, and enhancing recovery from fatigue by increasing the uptake and the systemic utilization of oxygen.[13]
11. **Lead poisoning**: Use of this formula had a beneficial effect in treating 42 patients with chronic lead poisoning. Clinical improvements included relief of pain and reduced duration of treatment.[14]

TOXICOLOGY

According to one study on acute toxicology, the LD_{50} for subcutaneous injection of this formula in decoction form is 48 g/kg in mice.[15]

Huáng Qí Jiàn Zhōng Tāng
(Astragalus Decoction to Construct the Middle)

SUGGESTED ACUPUNCTURE TREATMENT

1. Points: *Pishu* (BL 20), *Zhangmen* (LR 13), *Tianshu* (ST 25), *Shangjuxu* (ST 37), *Xingjian* (LR 2), *Guanyuan* (CV 4), and *Housanli* (ST 36).
2. Technique: tonification or moxibustion.

Pishu (BL 20) and *Zhangmen* (LR 13), the *shu* (transport) and *mu* (collecting) points of Spleen, nourish the Spleen, tonify qi, warm the middle *jiao*, and disperse cold. *Tianshu* (ST 25), the *mu* (collecting) point of the Large Intestine, is combined with *Shangjuxu* (ST 37), the lower *he* (uniting) point of the Large Intestine, to regulate qi and blood flow in the Large Intestine and relieve abdominal pain. *Xingjian* (LR 2) smoothes Liver qi flow to help relieve pain. *Guanyuan* (CV 4) and *Housanli* (ST 36) tonify qi.

AUTHORS' COMMENTS

Huang Qi Jian Zhong Tang is called "Astragalus Decoction to Construct the Middle" because it builds the qi of the Spleen and Stomach, and is used when there is Spleen and Stomach qi deficiency present with cold signs. This formula can be used to treat animals that have signs of lethargy, fatigue, poor appetite, vomiting, loose stool, poor digestion from eating cold, refrigerated food, and/or following short- or long-term antibiotic therapy. It is helpful in restoring normal digestive function post-operatively, especially in geriatric, debilitated and chronically ill animals. It is commonly given to puppies and kittens that have weak digestion and poor immune function due to Kidney and Spleen deficiencies present from birth. A course of treatment in these cases is from ten days to several months in duration.

References

1. *Yao Xue Xue Bao* (Journal of Herbology), 1986; 7:440.
2. *Shang Hai Zhong Yi Yao Za Zhi* (Shanghai Journal of Chinese Medicine and Herbology), 1983; 2:28.
3. *Shan Xi Zhong Yi* (Shanxi Chinese Medicine), 1990; 8:345.
4. *Ji Lin Zhong Yi Yao* (Jilin Chinese Medicine and Herbology), 1996; 5:10.
5. *He Bei Zhong Yi* (Hebei Chinese Medicine), 1987; 1:28.
6. *Hu Bei Zhong Yi Za Zhi* (Hubei Journal of Chinese Medicine), 1991; 1:12.
7. *He Nan Zhong Yi* (Henan Chinese Medicine), 1998; 2:51.
8. *Xin Zhong Yi* (New Chinese Medicine), 1996; 3:30.
9. *Shi Yong Zhong Xi Yi Jie He Za Zhi* (Practical Journal of Integrated Chinese and Western Medicines), 1998; 6:560.
10. *Liao Ning Zhong Yi Za Zhi* (Liaoning Journal of Chinese Medicine), 1990; 5:39.
11. *Shan Xi Zhong Yi* (Shanxi Chinese Medicine), 1990; 6:20.
12. *Zhe Jiang Zhong Yi Za Zhi* (Zhejiang Journal of Chinese Medicine), 1995; 10:443.
13. Chen KT, Su CH, Hsin LH, Su YC, Su YP, Lin JG. Reducing fatigue of athletes following oral administration of huangqi jianzhong tang. Acta Pharmacologica Sinica. 23(8):757-61, 2002 Aug.
14. *Hu Nan Zhong Yi Za Zhi* (Hunan Journal of Chinese Medicine), 1989; 3:22.
15. *Yao Xue Xue Bao* (Journal of Herbology), 1986; 7:440.

Guī Qí Jiàn Zhōng Tāng

(Tangkuei and Astragalus Decoction to Construct the Middle)

歸耆建中湯
归芪建中汤

Pinyin Name: *Gui Qi Jian Zhong Tang*
Literal Name: Tangkuei and Astragalus Decoction to Construct the Middle
Alternate Name: Tangkuei and Astragalus Combination
Original Source: *Yi Fang Ji Jie* (Analytical Collection of Medical Formulas) by Wang Ang in 1682

COMPOSITION

Dang Gui (Radix Angelicae Sinensis)	12g
Huang Qi (Radix Astragali)	4.5g [12g]
Yi Tang (Maltosum)	1 cup [30g]
Bai Shao (Radix Paeoniae Alba), *chao* (dry-fried) with liquor	18g
Zhi Gan Cao (Radix et Rhizoma Glycyrrhizae Praeparata cum Melle)	6g
Gui Zhi (Ramulus Cinnamomi)	9g
Sheng Jiang (Rhizoma Zingiberis Recens), *qie* (sliced)	9g
Da Zao (Fructus Jujubae), *bo* (opened)	12 pieces [4 pieces]

DOSAGE / PREPARATION / ADMINISTRATION

Prepare the ingredients as a decoction. Today, the decoction may be prepared using the doses suggested in brackets.

CHINESE THERAPEUTIC ACTIONS

1. Tonifies qi and blood
2. Promotes generation of muscle tissues
3. Eases pain

CLINICAL MANIFESTATIONS

Abscesses and ulcerations with underlying qi and blood deficiencies: chronic abscesses and ulcerations characterized by mild inflammation, small amounts of pus, and pus discharge.

VETERINARY CLINICAL APPLICATIONS

Chronic abscess and ulceration of the skin, radiation burns, non-healing wounds, allergic rhinitis or sinusitis, postpartum weakness with abdominal coldness and pain.

EXPLANATION

Gui Qi Jian Zhong Tang (Tangkuei and Astragalus Decoction to Construct the Middle) treats chronic abscesses and ulcerations with underlying qi and blood deficiencies. Chronic abscesses or ulcerations are often complicated by inflammation and formation and discharge of pus in the local area. Inflammation causes irritation to the nerve endings and results in pain and muscle spasms. Due to the chronic nature of the illness, most of these animals also have underlying qi and blood deficiencies. This formula

***Gui Qi Jian Zhong Tang* (Tangkuei and Astragalus Decoction to Construct the Middle)**

Diagnosis	Clinical Signs	Treatment	Herbs
Abscesses and ulcerations with qi and blood deficiencies	Chronic abscesses and ulcerations that do not heal: qi and blood deficiencies	• Tonifies qi and blood • Promotes generation of muscle tissues • Eases pain	• *Dang Gui* (Radix Angelicae Sinensis) and *Huang Qi* (Radix Astragali) tonify blood and qi to treat the underlying deficiencies and facilitate recovery. • *Yi Tang* (Maltosum) tonifies deficiency and strengthens the middle *jiao*. • *Bai Shao* (Radix Paeoniae Alba) and *Zhi Gan Cao* (Radix et Rhizoma Glycyrrhizae Praeparata cum Melle) ease pain and relieve muscle spasms and cramps. • *Gui Zhi* (Ramulus Cinnamomi), *Sheng Jiang* (Rhizoma Zingiberis Recens) and *Da Zao* (Fructus Jujubae) warm the middle *jiao* and relieve pain.

Guī Qí Jiàn Zhōng Tāng

(Tangkuei and Astragalus Decoction to Construct the Middle)

tonifies the underlying qi and blood deficiencies, supplies nutrients to the affected area, and promotes generation of tissue to facilitate recovery.

Dang Gui (Radix Angelicae Sinensis) and *Huang Qi* (Radix Astragali) are the chief herbs; they tonify blood and qi to treat the underlying deficiencies and facilitate recovery. Moreover, *Dang Gui* (Radix Angelicae Sinensis) improves blood circulation to enhance healing and *Huang Qi* (Radix Astragali) promotes generation of flesh and new muscle tissues. Together, these two herbs effectively treat abscesses and ulcerations. *Yi Tang* (Maltosum) tonifies deficiency and strengthens the middle *jiao*. It supplies large amounts of essential nutrients to facilitate recovery from chronic illnesses. *Bai Shao* (Radix Paeoniae Alba) and *Zhi Gan Cao* (Radix et Rhizoma Glycyrrhizae Praeparata cum Melle), two herbs in *Shao Yao Gan Cao Tang* (Peony and Licorice Decoction), ease pain and relieve muscle spasms and cramps. Because patients with chronic qi and blood deficiencies may develop abdominal pain due to yang deficiency, warm herbs such as *Gui Zhi* (Ramulus Cinnamomi), *Sheng Jiang* (Rhizoma Zingiberis Recens), and *Da Zao* (Fructus Jujubae) are used to warm the middle *jiao* and relieve abdominal pain.

VETERINARY MODIFICATIONS

- If there are prominent signs of cold, add *Fu Zi* (Radix Aconiti Lateralis Praeparata) and *Xi Xin* (Radix et Rhizoma Asari).
- When there is infection of the abscesses and ulcerations, add *Wu Wei Xiao Du Yin* (Five-Ingredient Decoction to Eliminate Toxins).

SUGGESTED ACUPUNCTURE TREATMENT

1. Points: *Pishu* (BL 20), *Geshu* (BL 17), *Zhongwan* (CV 12), *Housanli* (ST 36), *Sanyinjiao* (SP 6), and *Guanyuan* (CV 4).
2. Technique: moxibustion and tonification.

Apply moxibustion on *Pishu* (BL 20) and *Geshu* (BL 17) to tonify qi and blood; on *Zhongwan* (CV 12) and *Guanyuan* (CV 4) to warm the middle *jiao*. Tonify *Housanli* (ST 36) and *Sanyinjiao* (SP 6) to nourish the blood.

AUTHORS' COMMENTS

Gui Qi Jian Zhong Tang is a variation of *Xiao Jian Zhong Tang* (Minor Construct the Middle Decoction), but it has additional ingredients and significantly different applications.

- *Xiao Jian Zhong Tang* also warms and tonifies the middle, but primarily treats yang deficiency of the middle *jiao* with abdominal pain.
- *Gui Qi Jian Zhong Tang*, as the name implies, contains *Dang Gui* (Radix Angelicae Sinensis) and *Huang Qi* (Radix Astragali) to "construct the middle" by tonifying the blood and qi, which, in turn, strengthen the body and enhance recovery from abscesses and ulcerations.

Dà Jiàn Zhōng Tāng (Major Construct the Middle Decoction)

大建中湯
大建中汤

Pinyin Name: *Da Jian Zhong Tang*
Literal Name: Major Construct the Middle Decoction
Alternate Names: *Ta Chien Chung Tang, Da Jian Zhung Tang*, Major Centre-Fortifying Decoction, Major Middle-Strengthening Decoction, Major Zanthoxylum Combintion
Original Source: *Jin Gui Yao Lue* (Essentials from the Golden Cabinet) by Zhang Zhong-Jing in the Eastern Han Dynasty

COMPOSITION

Hua Jiao (Pericarpium Zanthoxyli), *chao* (dry-fried)	0.2 cup [3g]
Gan Jiang (Rhizoma Zingiberis)	12g [4.5g]
Ren Shen (Radix et Rhizoma Ginseng)	6g

Dà Jiàn Zhōng Tāng (Major Construct the Middle Decoction)

DOSAGE / PREPARATION / ADMINISTRATION

Cook the ingredients in 4 cups [800 mL] of water until 2 cups [400 mL] of the liquid remain. Filter and discard the herb residue, add 1 cup [30g] of *Yi Tang* (Maltosum) to the strained liquid, and cook it over low heat until 1.5 cups [300 mL] of liquid remain. Take the warm, strained decoction in two equally-divided doses daily. The source text also recommends taking 2 cups [400 mL] of porridge between the two doses of herbs and throughout the day, and to cover the body with blankets. Today, the decoction is normally prepared by using the doses suggested in brackets and by cooking the herbs twice. Filter and discard the herb residue, and add 3g of *Yi Tang* (Maltosum) to the strained liquid. Take the warm decoction in two equally-divided doses.

CHINESE THERAPEUTIC ACTIONS

1. Tonifies and warms the middle *jiao*
2. Corrects the reversed flow of qi and relieves pain

CLINICAL MANIFESTATIONS

Yang deficiency of the middle *jiao* with proliferation of yin and cold: severe coldness and pain in the chest and paws/hooves, epigastric pain, vomiting with inability to eat, severe pain in the paws, a pale, wet tongue, and a thin, tight pulse. In severe cases, cold limbs, a hidden pulse, or the type of irregular peristalsis that sounds like water movement in the abdominal cavity may be present.

VETERINARY CLINICAL APPLICATIONS

Gastritis, gastric ulcer, duodenal ulcer, intestinal spasms, uncomplicated intestinal obstruction, obstructive bowel disease, post-operative ileus, and abdominal pain due to intestinal parasites.

EXPLANATION

Da Jian Zhong Tang (Major Construct the Middle Decoction) treats various pains/irregularities caused by yang deficiency and interior cold. Yang deficiency leads to yin excess, which then leads to proliferation of cold. Interior cold causes constriction and reversed flow of qi, resulting in severe coldness and pain in the chest and epigastrium, vomiting with inability to eat, and, in some cases, severe pain in the paws. The type of irregular peristalsis that sounds like water movement in the abdominal cavity is due to accumulation of water and cold in the abdomen. A pale, wet tongue suggests that the amount of water in the body is higher than normal as a result of deficiency of yang and cold accumulation.

This formula uses *Hua Jiao* (Pericarpium Zanthoxyli) as the chief herb. It is acrid and hot, and has functions to dispel cold and warm the Spleen and Stomach. *Gan Jiang* (Rhizoma Zingiberis) also warms the middle *jiao* and dispels cold. Together these two herbs raise the yang of the middle *jiao*, correct the reversed flow of qi, relieve pain, and stop vomiting. *Ren Shen* (Radix et Rhizoma Ginseng) and *Yi Tang* (Maltosum) both warm and tonify the Spleen and Stomach.

VETERINARY MODIFICATIONS

- With nausea and vomiting, add *Ban Xia* (Rhizoma Pinelliae) and *Sheng Jiang* (Rhizoma Zingiberis Recens).
- If there is severe coldness and pain in the chest and epigastric regions, add *Fu Zi* (Radix Aconiti Lateralis Praeparata) and *Xi Xin* (Radix et Rhizoma Asari).
- With coldness and pain in the abdominal region, combine with *Li Zhong Tang* (Regulate the Middle Decoction).
- With fullness and pain in the abdominal region, add *Hou Po* (Cortex Magnoliae Officinalis) and *Ku Xing Ren* (Semen Armeniacae Amarum).
- With nausea, vomiting, and severe abdominal pain, combine with *Ban Xia Xie Xin Tang* (Pinellia Decoction to Drain the Epigastrium).

***Da Jian Zhong Tang* (Major Construct the Middle Decoction)**

Diagnosis	Clinical Signs	Treatment	Herbs
Yang deficiency of the middle *jiao* with proliferation of yin and cold	• Severe coldness and pain in the chest, head and paws: proliferation of yin and cold causing constriction and stagnation • Vomiting with inability to eat: proliferation of yin and cold leading to reversed flow of qi upwards • Pale, wet tongue: water accumulation due to deficiency of yang and excess of cold • Thin, tight pulse: deficiency of yang and excess of cold	• Tonifies and warms the middle *jiao* • Corrects reversed flow of qi and relieves pain	• *Hua Jiao* (Pericarpium Zanthoxyli) and *Gan Jiang* (Rhizoma Zingiberis) warm the Spleen and Stomach and dispel cold. • *Ren Shen* (Radix et Rhizoma Ginseng) and *Yi Tang* (Maltosum) both warm and tonify the Spleen and Stomach.

Dà Jiàn Zhōng Tāng (Major Construct the Middle Decoction)

CAUTIONS / CONTRAINDICATIONS

- *Da Jian Zhong Tang* contains many warm herbs, and should not be used to treat abdominal pain characterized by excess heat, damp-heat, or yin-deficient heat.
- Due to the warm nature of this formula, overdose may lead to such side effects as non-productive cough, edema, nausea, and vomiting.

PHARMACOLOGICAL EFFECTS

1. **Gastrointestinal**: Administration of *Da Jian Zhong Tang* was associated with accelerated movement of the small intestine.[1] Increased intestinal motility occurred as a result of *Da Jian Zhong Tang* stimulating the cholinergic and 5-hydroxytryptamine-3 receptors.[2,3] The stimulating effect can be blocked by atropine, spantide, tetrodotoxin or capsazepine.[4] Another study reported that administration of *Da Jian Zhong Tang* has a dose-dependent effect to increase intestinal blood flow without affecting the mean arterial blood pressure. These studies suggested that *Da Jian Zhong Tang* may be useful in the treatment of uncomplicated post-operative adhesive intestinal obstruction and intestinal ischemia-related diseases.[5,6]
2. **Effect on gallbladder**: According to laboratory studies in rats, administration of *Da Jian Zhong Tang* was associated with a stimulating effect on the production of bile acid, starting after 30 minutes and ending 4 hours after the administration.[7]
3. **Uterine**: Administration of *Da Jian Zhong Tang* via intraduodenal or intravenous routes in anaesthetized rabbits was associated with intestinal motility but not the uterine motility. This suggests that *Da Jian Zhong Tang* has a selective stimulatory effect on the gastrointestinal tract, but not on the uterus. However, more studies are needed to determine whether *Da Jian Zhong Tang* could be administered during gestation.[8]

HUMAN CLINICAL STUDIES AND RESEARCH

1. **Intestinal obstruction**: In one report, 10 patients (6 males and 4 females, between 59 and 75 years of age, average age of 64.4 years) with intestinal obstruction due to adhesion were treated with herbs for prevention of recurrent attack. Out of 10 patients, 6 received *Da Jian Zhong Tang*, 4 received concurrent *Da Jian Zhong Tang* and *Xiao Jian Zhong Tang* (Minor Construct the Middle Decoction). The study reported that 9 out of 10 patients responded well with no recurrent attacks in 8, 12, and 15 months follow-up exams. The other patient continued to take the herbs, but experienced nausea and vomiting.[9]
2. **Obstructive bowel disease**: One study used *Da Jian Zhong Tang* to treat 46 pediatric patients with various obstructive bowel diseases accompanied with chronic constipation (post-operative ileus, large abdominal surgery, ano-rectal anomaly, Hirschsprung's disease, functional bowel obstructions, and SMA syndrome). The treatment protocol was to mix 0.1-0.15 g/kg of the formula with 5-10 mL of warm water, and administer orally two to three times a day. Of 46 cases, the study reported effective treatment in 39 cases (85%) and ineffective in 7 cases. No side effects were observed.[10]
3. **Post-operative ileus**: In one study, administration of *Da Jian Zhong Tang* was associated with marked effect to treat post-operative ileus, generally considered as an inevitable adverse consequence of abdominal surgical procedures. The treatment protocol was to administer 15g of *Da Jian Zhong Tang* orally daily for 14 days. Clinical improvements included reducing both the need for further surgery and the recurrence of post-operative ileus.[11] In another study, repeated administrations of *Da Jian Zhong Tang* (100 or 300 mg/kg) significantly inhibited the formation of intestinal obstruction, and prevented post-operative ileus following laparotomy. The mechanism of this effect was attributed to the gastroprokinetic and anti-inflammatory effects of the formula.[12]
4. **Post-surgical treatment**: In one study, *Da Jian Zhong Tang* was used to treat 23 patients with various types of complaints following an abdominal surgery. The study reported that the formula was effective in treating borborygmus, abdominal pain, and gastric distention associated with abdominal surgery.[13]
5. **Feelings of coldness in the abdomen**: *Da Jian Zhong Tang* has been used to treat yang deficiency and a feeling of coldness in the abdomen in traditional Chinese medicine. The pharmacological explanation of this application is attributed to the stimulatory effect of *Da Jian Zhong Tang* to increased 5-hydroxytryptamine (serotonin; 5-HT) levels and vasoactive intestinal peptide-immunoreactive substance secretion in the abdomen.[14]
6. **Ascariasis**: One report stated that administration of modified *Da Jian Zhong Tang* was effective in treating biliary ascariasis in 39 of 45 patients.[15] Another study reported successful treatment in all 8 patients with biliary ascariasis.[16]

HERB-DRUG INTERACTION

- **Antipsychotic drugs**: Eight patients with recurrent constipation and/or intestinal obstruction caused by use of antipsychotic drugs were treated with good success using *Da Jian Zhong Tang*. Of 8 cases, the study reported significant improvement in 4 cases, moderate improvement in 2 cases, and no change in 2 cases.[17]
- **Chlorpromazine-induced hypoperistalsis**: Chlorpromazine-induced hypoperistalsis can be treated effectively with *Da Jian Zhong Tang*, which has a dose-dependent effect to improve small intestinal peristalsis and distal colonic

Dà Jiàn Zhōng Tāng (Major Construct the Middle Decoction)

propulsion. *Hua Jiao* (Pericarpium Zanthoxyli) is believed to be the main ingredient that stimulates the cholinergic system, thereby enabling *Da Jian Zhong Tang* to improve chlorpromazine-induced hypoperistalsis.[18]

- **Morphine-induced constipation**: Administration of *Da Jian Zhong Tang* was found to be effective in alleviating severe constipation in cancer patients taking morphine to relieve pain. Use of *Da Jian Zhong Tang* did not alter the anti-nociceptive effect of morphine.[19]

SUGGESTED ACUPUNCTURE TREATMENT

1. Points: *Pishu* (BL 20), *Weishu* (BL 21), *Sanyinjiao* (SP 6), *Housanli* (ST 36), *Mingmen* (GV 4), *Zhongwan* (CV 12), and *Neiguan* (PC 6).
2. Technique: tonification and moxibustion.

Pishu (BL 20), *Weishu* (BL 21), *Sanyinjiao* (SP 6), and *Housanli* (ST 36) warm the middle *jiao* and tonify the Spleen. *Mingmen* (GV 4) tonifies *ming men* (life gate) fire to help dispel cold. *Zhongwan* (CV 12), combined with *Housanli* (ST 36), regulates the Stomach and relieves stagnation and pain. *Neiguan* (PC 6) relieves chest and abdominal pains and reverses the Stomach qi flow to relieve nausea and vomiting.

AUTHORS' COMMENTS

In theory, sweet herbs should not be administered to patients experiencing vomiting. *Da Jian Zhong Tang*, however, contains a large amount of *Yi Tang* (Maltosum) but does not create additional disharmony because the vomiting involved in this condition is not due to damp accumulation; rather, it is the result of cold accumulation disrupting the normal qi-lowering tendency of the Stomach. For this reason, *Yi Tang* (Maltosum) is used to harmonize the middle and relieve pain. Although it is sweet, it will not create more dampness and worsen the condition.

Xiao Jian Zhong Tang (Minor Construct the Middle Decoction) and *Da Jian Zhong Tang* both tonify and warm the middle to dispel cold and relieve pain. However, these two formulas have different compositions, functions, and indications.

- *Xiao Jian Zhong Tang* contains mainly sweet herbs to tonify, along with a large amount of the sour and slightly cold *Bai Shao* (Radix Paeoniae Alba) to relieve pain in the middle *jiao*. Its chief function is to tonify yang, qi, and blood, and warm the middle *jiao*.
- *Da Jian Zhong Tang* contains mainly acrid and sweet herbs to strengthen the middle *jiao*. It is weaker in harmonizing and tonifying but stronger in dispelling coldness. It is mainly used for middle *jiao* yang deficiency with excess cold accumulation.[20]

References

1. Satoh K, Kase Y, Hayakawa T, Murata P, Ishige A, Sasaki H. Dai-kenchu-to enhances accelerated small intestinal movement. Biol Pharm Bull. 2001 Oct; 24(10):1122-6.
2. Jin XL, Shibata C, Naito H, Ueno T, Funayama Y, Fukushima K, Matsuno S, Sasaki I. Intraduodenal and intrajejunal administration of the herbal medicine, dai-kenchu-tou, stimulates small intestinal motility via cholinergic receptors in conscious dogs. Dig Dis Sci. 2001 Jun; 46(6):1171-6.
3. Shibata C, Sasaki I, Naito H, Ueno T, Matsuno S. The herbal medicine Dai-Kenchu-Tou stimulates upper gut motility through cholinergic and 5-hydroxytryptamine 3 receptors in conscious dogs. Surgery. 1999 Nov; 126(5):918-24.
4. Satoh K, Hashimoto K, Hayakawa T, Ishige A, Kaneko M, Ogihara S, Kurosawa S, Yakabi K, Nakamura T. Mechanism of atropine-resistant contraction induced by Dai-kenchu-to in guinea pig ileum. Jpn J Pharmacol. 2001 May; 86(1):32-7.
5. Shibata C, Sasaki I, Naito H, Ueno T, Matsuno S. The herbal medicine Dai-Kenchu-Tou stimulates upper gut motility through cholinergic and 5-hydroxytryptamine 3 receptors in conscious dogs. Surgery. 1999 Nov; 126(5):918-24.
6. Murata P, Kase Y, Ishige A, Sasaki H, Kurosawa S, Nakamura T. The herbal medicine Dai-kenchu-to and one of its active components [6]-shogaol increase intestinal blood flow in rats. Life Sci. 2002 Mar 15; 70(17):2061-70.
7. *Zhong Xi Yi Jie He Za Zhi* (Journal of Integrated Chinese and Western Medicine), 1990; 10:638.
8. Murata P, Hayakawa T, Satoh K, Kase Y, Ishige A, Sasaki H. Effects of Dai-kenchu-to, a herbal medicine, on uterine and intestinal motility. Phytother Res. 2001 Jun; 15(4):302-6.
9. *Guo Wai Yi Xue* (Foreign Medicine), 1993; 15(5):39.
10. Ohya T, Usui Y, Arii S, Iwai T, Susumu T. Effect of dai-kenchu-to on obstructive bowel disease in children. Am J Chin Med. 2003; 31(1):129-35.
11. Itoh T, Yamakawa J, Mai M, Yamaguchi N, Kanda T. The effect of the herbal medicine dai-kenchu-to on post-operative ileus. J Int Med Res. 2002 Jul-Aug; 30(4):428-32.
12. Hayakawa T, Kase Y, Saito K, Hashimoto K, Ishige A, Komatsu Y, Sasaki H. Effects of Dai-kenchu-to on intestinal obstruction following laparotomy. J Smooth Muscle Res. 1999 Apr; 35(2):47-54.
13. *Guo Wai Yi Xue* (Foreign Medicine), 1993; 15(5):39.
14. Nagano T, Itoh H, Takeyama M. Effects of Dai-kenchu-to on levels of 5-hydroxytryptamine (serotonin) and vasoactive intestinal peptides in human plasma. Biol Pharm Bull. 2000 Mar; 23(3):352-3.
15. *Zhe Jiang Zhong Yi Za Zhi* (Zhejiang Journal of Chinese Medicine), 1964; 2:17.
16. *Zhong Xi Yi Jie He Za Zhi* (Journal of Integrated Chinese and Western Medicine), 1990; 10:638.
17. *Guo Wai Yi Xue* (Foreign Medicine), 1994; 16(2):28.
18. Satoh K, Kase Y, Yuzurihara M, Mizoguchi K, Kurauchi K, Ishige A. Effect of Dai-kenchu-to (Da-Jian-Zhong-Tang) on the delayed intestinal propulsion induced by chlorpromazine in mice. J Ethnopharmacol. 2003 May; 86(1):37-44.
19. Nakamura T, Sakai A, Isogami I, Noda K, Ueno K, Yano S.Abatement of morphine-induced slowing in gastrointestinal transit by Dai-kenchu-to, a traditional Japanese herbal medicine. Jpn J Pharmacol. 2002 Feb; 88(2):217-21.
20. Wang MZ, et al. *Zhong Yi Xue Wen Da Ti Ku* (Questions and Answers on Traditional Chinese Medicine: Herbal Formulas).

Section 2

回阳救逆剂
— Yang-Resuscitating Formulas

Sì Nì Tāng (Frigid Extremities Decoction)
四逆湯
四逆汤

Pinyin Name: *Si Ni Tang*
Literal Name: Frigid Extremities Decoction
Alternate Names: *Su Ni Tang*, Counterflow Cold Combination, Cold Limbs Decoction, Aconite Ginger and Licorice Combination
Original Source: *Shang Han Lun* (Discussion of Cold-Induced Disorders) by Zhang Zhong-Jing in the Eastern Han Dynasty

COMPOSITION

Sheng Fu Zi (Radix Aconiti Lateralis)	1 piece [6-9g]
Gan Jiang (Rhizoma Zingiberis)	4.5g [6-9g]
Zhi Gan Cao (Radix et Rhizoma Glycyrrhizae Praeparata cum Melle)	6g

Note: The original formula contains *Sheng Fu Zi* (Radix Aconiti Lateralis) to utilize its potent effects to dispel cold and restore yang. However, *Sheng Fu Zi* (Radix Aconiti Lateralis) is rather toxic, and is generally unavailable. Therefore, 20-30 grams of *Fu Zi* (Radix Aconiti Lateralis Praeparata) may be used to replace 5-10 grams of *Sheng Fu Zi* (Radix Aconiti Lateralis).

DOSAGE / PREPARATION / ADMINISTRATION

Cook the ingredients in 3 cups [600 mL] of water until 1.2 cups [240 mL] of the liquid remain. Take the warm, strained decoction in two equally-divided doses daily. For patients with a strong constitution, a large piece (15g) of *Sheng Fu Zi* (Radix Aconiti Lateralis) and 9g of *Gan Jiang* (Rhizoma Zingiberis) may be used. Today, the decoction may be prepared using the doses suggested in brackets. *Sheng Fu Zi* (Radix Aconiti Lateralis) should be cooked first for one hour before adding and cooking the other herbs. The decoction should be taken while warm.

CHINESE THERAPEUTIC ACTIONS

1. Restores depleted yang
2. Rescues from counterflow cold

CLINICAL MANIFESTATIONS

1. *Shaoyin* syndrome: severely cold extremities, aversion to cold, preference to curl up the body when lying down, lethargy, vomiting, absence of thirst, abdominal pain, diarrhea, a pale, wet tongue, and a weak, thin, deep and slow pulse.
2. Depletion of yang due to excessive sweating in *taiyang* syndrome.

VETERINARY CLINICAL APPLICATIONS

Cardiac failure, hypoadrenal shock (Addisonian crisis), equine Cushing's disease, and chronic severe vomiting and diarrhea secondary to gastroenteritis or dietary indiscretion.

EXPLANATION

Si Ni Tang (Frigid Extremities Decoction) is a standard formula used to treat *shaoyin* syndrome, in which coldness has progressed to the *shaoyin* stage and Kidney yang is diminished and depleted. This extreme imbalance of yin and yang causes disharmony at the exterior (icy cold extremities, aversion to cold, preference to curl up the body when lying down, lethargy) and in the interior (vomiting, absence of thirst, abdominal pain, and diarrhea with undigested food). A pale, wet tongue and an

Si Ni Tang (Frigid Extremities Decoction)

indistinct weak, deep, slow and thin pulse suggest depletion of yang and proliferation of yin and coldness.

Proper treatment of this condition requires high doses of acrid and hot interior-warming herbs to restore yang and rescue from counterflow cold. *Sheng Fu Zi* (Radix Aconiti Lateralis), the chief herb, is an essential herb for warming *ming men* (life gate) fire and raising Kidney yang. It warms all twelve channels immediately and strongly dispels interior cold. The fresh, unprocessed form is used here because interior cold must be dispelled at once. Due to the urgency of the situation, the fresh, unprocessed *Sheng Fu Zi* (Radix Aconiti Lateralis) is selected for its potent and drastic effect over the processed *Fu Zi* (Radix Aconiti Lateralis Praeparata). *Gan Jiang* (Rhizoma Zingiberis), the deputy herb, warms middle *jiao* yang and dispels interior cold. The warmth of *Sheng Fu Zi* (Radix Aconiti Lateralis) is further enhanced by the addition of *Gan Jiang* (Rhizoma Zingiberis). Lastly, *Zhi Gan Cao* (Radix et Rhizoma Glycyrrhizae Praeparata cum Melle) reduces the toxicity of *Sheng Fu Zi* (Radix Aconiti Lateralis), and moderates the harsh and warm properties of *Gan Jiang* (Rhizoma Zingiberis) and *Sheng Fu Zi* (Radix Aconiti Lateralis).

VETERINARY MODIFICATIONS

- When there is extreme coldness of the extremities, add *Xi Xin* (Radix et Rhizoma Asari) and *Gui Zhi* (Ramulus Cinnamomi).
- If there is abdominal pain due to cold, add *Gui Zhi* (Ramulus Cinnamomi) and *Bai Shao* (Radix Paeoniae Alba).
- With edema and palpitations, add *Ren Shen* (Radix et Rhizoma Ginseng) and *Fu Ling* (Poria).
- With edema or clear or white vaginal discharge from Spleen and Kidney yang deficiencies, add *Dang Shen* (Radix Codonopsis), *Fu Ling* (Poria), and *Ze Xie* (Rhizoma Alismatis).
- With diarrhea accompanied by undigested food, combine with *Li Zhong Tang* (Regulate the Middle Decoction).

CAUTIONS / CONTRAINDICATIONS

- *Si Ni Tang* is an extremely hot formula, and is contraindicated in cases of true-heat and false-cold conditions.
- This formula should be stopped immediately after the paws or hooves have warmed up.

PHARMACOLOGICAL EFFECTS

1. **Cardiovascular**: Administration of *Si Ni Tang* was associated with a marked influence on the cardiovascular system. In laboratory studies on rabbits, it increased the contractile force of the heart, increased blood pressure, and restored normal heart rhythm.[1]
2. **Immunostimulant**: Administration of *Si Ni Tang* was associated with an effect to enhance the immune system. In one experiment, the immune systems of rats were artificially suppressed with injection of hydrocortisone at 1.5 mg/100g/day for 7 days. The rats that also received the herbs in decoction were able to maintain their IgG count at a higher level in comparison to the rats that received only the hydrocortisone.[2]
3. **Analgesic and anti-inflammatory**: Intraperitoneal injection of *Si Ni Tang* was associated with marked analgesic and anti-inflammatory effects in rats.[3]
4. **Half-life**: According to pharmacokinetic studies using a two-compartment model, the half-life of *Si Ni Tang* is 5.8 hours.[4]

HUMAN CLINICAL STUDIES AND RESEARCH

1. **Acute cardiac infarction**: In one report, 105 patients with acute cardiac infarction characterized by collapse of yang were treated with *Si Ni Tang* or with slight modification without a single case of fatality. Of 105 patients, 10 received concurrent herbal and drug treatments. The therapeutic benefit was attributed to the effect of the formula to increase blood pressure and the contractile force of the heart.[5]
2. **Diarrhea**: Seventy children with diarrhea characterized by watery stools, cold extremities, a weak pulse, and a thin, white tongue coating were treated with a decoction

***Si Ni Tang* (Frigid Extremities Decoction)**

Diagnosis	Clinical Signs	Treatment	Herbs
Shaoyin syndrome	• Icy cold extremities, aversion to cold, preference to curl up the body when lying down, and lethargy: excess cold and yang deficiency at the exterior • Vomiting, absence of thirst, abdominal pain, and diarrhea with undigested food: excess cold and yang deficiency in the interior • Pale, wet tongue, and a slow pulse: depletion of yang and proliferation of yin and coldness	• Recuperates depleted yang • Rescues from counterflow cold	• *Sheng Fu Zi* (Radix Aconiti Lateralis) warms *ming men* (life gate) fire, raises Kidney yang, and warms all twelve channels and dispels interior coldness. • *Gan Jiang* (Rhizoma Zingiberis) warms middle *jiao* yang and dispels interior cold. • *Zhi Gan Cao* (Radix et Rhizoma Glycyrrhizae Praeparata cum Melle) harmonizes the formula.

Sì Nì Tāng (Frigid Extremities Decoction)

of *Si Ni Tang* with the addition of *Huang Lian* (Rhizoma Coptidis). Out of 70 cases, the study reported complete recovery in 58 cases (less than 3 bowel movements per day), slight improvement in 8 cases (less than 5 bowel movements per day), and no change in 4 cases. The average length of treatment was 4 days, and ranged from 1-7 days.[6]

TOXICOLOGY

In a toxicology study, *Si Ni Tang* was prepared using the herbs in the proportion of *Sheng Fu Zi* (Radix Aconiti Lateralis) : *Gan Jiang* (Rhizoma Zingiberis) : *Gan Cao* (Radix et Rhizoma Glycyrrhizae) as 4:3:3. The LD_{50} of *Si Ni Tang* in mice is 5.821 g/kg via intraperitoneal injection and 71.78 g/kg via oral ingestion. The LD_{50} for *Sheng Fu Zi* (Radix Aconiti Lateralis) is 17.42 g/kg via oral ingestion. The subject was able to tolerate a larger dose of *Sheng Fu Zi* (Radix Aconiti Lateralis) when given in a combination, indicating that *Gan Cao* (Radix et Rhizoma Glycyrrhizae) and *Gan Jiang* (Rhizoma Zingiberis) can effectively reduce the toxicity of *Sheng Fu Zi* (Radix Aconiti Lateralis). The reduced toxicity of the formula was not associated with changes in concentration of the alkaloids.[7]

SUGGESTED ACUPUNCTURE TREATMENT

1. Points: *Xinshu* (BL 15), *Pishu* (BL 20), *Guanyuanshu* (BL 26), *Shenshu* (BL 23), *Zhongwan* (CV 12), *Tianshu* (ST 25), and *Housanli* (ST 36).
2. Technique: tonification and moxibustion.

Xinshu (BL 15), *Pishu* (BL 20), and *Guanyuanshu* (BL 26) tonify the Spleen, Heart, qi, and blood. *Shenshu* (BL 23) warms Kidney yang and dispels cold. *Zhongwan* (CV 12), *Tianshu* (ST 25), and *Housanli* (ST 36) regulate the qi flow of the Stomach and Intestines to relieve vomiting and diarrhea.

RELATED FORMULAS

Sì Nì Jiā Rén Shēn Tāng
(Frigid Extremities Decoction plus Ginseng)
四逆加人參湯
四逆加人参汤
Pinyin Name: *Si Ni Jia Ren Shen Tang*
Literal Name: Frigid Extremities Decoction plus Ginseng
Original Source: *Shang Han Lun* (Discussion of Cold-Induced Disorders) by Zhang Zhong-Jing in the Eastern Han Dynasty

Ren Shen (Radix et Rhizoma Ginseng)	3g
Sheng Fu Zi (Radix Aconiti Lateralis)	1 piece [6-9g]
Gan Jiang (Rhizoma Zingiberis)	4.5g [6-9g]
Zhi Gan Cao (Radix et Rhizoma Glycyrrhizae Praeparata cum Melle)	6g [9g]

Cook the ingredients in 3 cups [600 mL] of water until 1.2 cups [240 mL] of the liquid remain. Take the warm, strained decoction in two equally-divided doses daily. Today, the decoction may be prepared using the doses suggested in brackets

Si Ni Jia Ren Shen Tang (Frigid Extremities Decoction plus Ginseng) combines *Si Ni Tang* with *Ren Shen* (Radix et Rhizoma Ginseng). *Ren Shen* (Radix et Rhizoma Ginseng) is added to tonify *yuan* (source) qi in patients with severe qi deficiency. This formula tonifies *yuan* (source) qi, recuperates depleted yang, and rescues the patient from collapse. Clinically, the patient may have shortness of breath and rapid breathing in addition to all the clinical signs listed in *Si Ni Tang*. It is appropriate for animals with cardiovascular and respiratory shock or compromise.

In comparison to *Si Ni Tang*, *Si Ni Jia Ren Shen Tang* (Frigid Extremities Decoction plus Ginseng) has a much stronger function to tonify *yuan* (source) qi. Therefore, it can be used on patients who have *shaoyin* cold syndrome complicated by shortness of breath and rapid breathing.

Shēn Fù Tāng
(Ginseng and Prepared Aconite Decoction)
參附湯
参附汤
Pinyin Name: *Shen Fu Tang*
Literal Name: Ginseng and Prepared Aconite Decoction
Original Source: *Zheng Ti Lei Yao* (Catalogued Essentials for Correcting the Body) by Bi Li-Zhai (Ji) in 1529

Ren Shen (Radix et Rhizoma Ginseng)	12g [9g]
Fu Zi (Radix Aconiti Lateralis Praeparata), *pao* (blast-fried)	9g [6g]

Prepare the ingredients as a decoction. Today, the decoction may be prepared using the doses suggested in brackets.

Shen Fu Tang (Ginseng and Prepared Aconite Decoction) is for the treatment of acute conditions only and treats collapse of yang qi with profuse sweating, cold lower extremities and paws, dizziness, shortness of breath, and even semi-unconsciousness. Collapse of yang qi occurs after severe illness with extreme deficiency, profuse bleeding in postpartum or *beng lou* (flooding and spotting) conditions, severe hemorrhage, and others.

This formula has only two ingredients. *Ren Shen* (Radix et Rhizoma Ginseng) tonifies *yuan* (source) qi and restore yang from collapse. *Fu Zi* (Radix Aconiti Lateralis Praeparata) warms yang qi and resuscitates the patient. This formula

Sì Nì Tāng (Frigid Extremities Decoction)

should be used only in emergency conditions. In severe instances, the doses listed above could be doubled. However, this formula only serves to quickly restore yang and should not be used once the patient has regained consciousness; otherwise, interior fire may be created. It can be used for animals with hypoadrenocorticism and hypoadrenal crisis, fulminant cardiac failure, and hypovolemic shock secondary to hemorrhage from vehicular trauma, post-partum hemorrhage or other causes of hypovolemia. It may be given via retention enema in animals unable to take oral medications.

AUTHORS' COMMENTS

The clinical signs associated with collapse of yang correspond to shock in conventional medicine, and include extreme weakness or collapse, semi-consciousness, cold extremities, vomiting, abdominal pain, tachycardia, cardiac arrhythmia and/or bradycardia. The tongue will be white and wet and the pulse weak and faint. *Si Ni Tang* is the representative formula for restoring depleted yang and rescuing animals from shock and cardiovascular collapse. This herbal formula can be given via retention enema in unconscious animals, and it is recommended that it be administered in liquid form to conscious animals.

Si Ni Tang (Frigid Extremities Decoction) and *Si Ni San* (Frigid Extremities Powder) are two formulas with similar names that must not be confused. These two formulas treat different syndromes (yang deficiency vs. qi stagnation) that share the same clinical signs (cold limbs/extremities).

- *Si Ni Tang* (Frigid Extremities Decoction): Yang deficiency with coldness will manifest not only in icy cold limbs/extremities, but cold everywhere in the body. Comparatively speaking, this type of cold is more severe and will not warm up when exposed to heat because there is an underlying deficiency of *ming men* (life gate) fire. Accompanying clinical signs include a withered *shen* (spirit), desire to sleep, intolerance to cold, preference to be in a fetal position, vomiting, abdominal pain, undigested food with diarrhea, and a deep, weak pulse. *Si Ni Tang* contains interior-warming herbs to warm Kidney yang and boost *ming men* (life gate) fire. in order to warm up the limbs/extremities.
- *Si Ni San* (Frigid Extremities Powder): Qi stagnation blocks and prevents yang qi from properly circulating to the extremities. Animals usually experience coldness below the stifles and elbows instead of the entire limbs. In general, these patients warm up faster when the extremities are exposed to heat and blood circulation is restored. Other accompanying signs include abdominal pain and discomfort, diarrhea, and a wiry pulse. In summary, the coldness is due to qi blockage instead of yang deficiency. *Si Ni San* is designed with qi-regulating herbs to harmonize and smooth Liver qi flow and open channel circulation to the extremities. This condition is often seen when pathogenic factors invade from the outside and get trapped in the *shaoyang* Liver/Gallbladder channels, coupled with qi stagnation. When yang qi is no longer blocked by qi stagnation, the symptom of cold limbs is relieved. [8]

References

1. *Zhong Yi Fang Ji Xian Dai Yan Jiu* (Modern Study of Medical Formulas in Traditional Chinese Medicine), 1997; 394-395.
2. *Zhong Yi Za Zhi* (Journal of Chinese Medicine), 1988; 10:59.
3. *Zhong Guo Zhong Yao Za Zhi* (People's Republic of China Journal of Chinese Herbology), 1992; 2:104.
4. *Zhong Guo Yi Yuan Yao Xue Za Zhi* (Chinese Hospital Journal of Herbology)logy, 1990; 11:487.
5. *Tian Jin Yi Yao Tong Xun* (Publication of Tianjin Medicine and Herbology), 1972; 11:1.
6. *Zhe Jiang Zhong Yi Za Zhi* (Zhejiang Journal of Chinese Medicine), 1981; 10:422.
7. *Zhe Jiang Zhong Yi Yao* (Zhejiang Chinese Medicine and Herbology), 1979; 7:246.
8. Wang MZ, et al. *Zhong Yi Xue Wen Da Ti Ku* (Questions and Answers on Traditional Chinese Medicine: Herbal Formulas).

Section 3

温经散寒剂
— Channel-Warming and Cold-Dispersing Formulas

Dāng Guī Sì Nì Tāng (Tangkuei Decoction for Frigid Extremities)
當歸四逆湯
当归四逆汤

Pinyin Name: *Dang Gui Si Ni Tang*
Literal Name: Tangkuei Decoction for Frigid Extremities
Alternate Names: *Tang Kuei Su Ni Tang, Tang Gui Si Ni Tang*, Tang-kuei and Counterflow Cold Decoction, Chinese Angelica Cold Limbs Decoction, Tangkuei and Jujube Combination
Original Source: *Shang Han Lun* (Discussion of Cold-Induced Disorders) by Zhang Zhong-Jing in the Eastern Han Dynasty

COMPOSITION

Dang Gui (Radix Angelicae Sinensis)	9g [12g]
Bai Shao (Radix Paeoniae Alba)	9g
Gui Zhi (Ramulus Cinnamomi)	9g
Xi Xin (Radix et Rhizoma Asari)	9g [1.5-3g]
Zhi Gan Cao (Radix et Rhizoma Glycyrrhizae Praeparata cum Melle)	6g
Da Zao (Fructus Jujubae), *bo* (opened)	25 pieces [8 pieces]
Mu Tong (Caulis Akebiae)	6g [3g]

Note: According to the source text, "*Tong Cao*" is stated as an ingredient in *Dang Gui Si Ni Tang*. The identity of this herb has been questioned, since "*Mu Tong*" and "*Tong Cao*" are two herbs with similar pinyin names and functions, and have been used interchangeably in the past. Both herbs have functions to promote urination and treat *lin zheng* (dysuria syndrome). However, *Mu Tong* (Caulis Akebiae) can open the channels and collaterals to treat pain, while *Tong Cao* (Medulla Tetrapanacis) can unblock and promote lactation. Therefore, based on the indications of the formula and the functions of these two herbs, most scholars and clinicians agree that *Mu Tong* (Caulis Akebiae) is a more suitable herb in *Dang Gui Si Ni Tang*.

DOSAGE / PREPARATION / ADMINISTRATION

Cook the ingredients in 8 cups [1,600 mL] of water until 3 cups [600 mL] of the liquid remain. Take 1 cup [200 mL] of the warm, strained decoction three times daily. Today, the decoction may be prepared using the doses suggested in brackets.

CHINESE THERAPEUTIC ACTIONS

1. Warms the channels and disperses cold
2. Nourishes the blood and opens the collaterals

CLINICAL MANIFESTATIONS

1. Invasion of cold with underlying deficiencies of yang qi and blood: icy cold paws/hooves, a pale tongue, and a deep, thin pulse, or a thin pulse that is barely palpable.
2. Cold factor attacking the channels and collaterals: pain at the flank, hips, hind limbs, and paws/hooves.

VETERINARY CLINICAL APPLICATIONS

Pain, rheumatoid arthritis, lumbar pain, navicular disease, chronic founder associated with equine Cushing's disease, cancer pain, frostbite, periarthritis of shoulder, peripheral neuritis, peptic ulcer disease, intestinal colic, and allergic rhinitis.

EXPLANATION

Dang Gui Si Ni Tang (Tangkuei Decoction for Frigid Extremities) treats invasion of cold with underlying deficiencies of yang qi and blood. The chief problem in

Dāng Guī Sì Nì Tāng (Tangkuei Decoction for Frigid Extremities)

this syndrome is icy cold lower extremities and feet, that may be caused by three factors. First, the yang qi is deficient, and therefore cannot warm the limbs and extremities. Second, blood is deficient and unable to nourish. Lastly, the properties of the pathogenic factor makes these areas colder. Invasion and accumulation of cold also obstructs the channels and collaterals, leading to pain at the flanks, hips, legs, and paws or hooves. A deep, thin pulse or a thin pulse that is barely palpable indicates invasion of cold with underlying deficiencies.

This formula uses *Dang Gui* (Radix Angelicae Sinensis) and *Bai Shao* (Radix Paeoniae Alba) to tonify and harmonize the blood. *Gui Zhi* (Ramulus Cinnamomi) and *Xi Xin* (Radix et Rhizoma Asari) warm the channels, dispel exterior and interior cold, and restore yang qi. *Zhi Gan Cao* (Radix et Rhizoma Glycyrrhizae Praeparata cum Melle) and *Da Zao* (Fructus Jujubae) strengthen the Spleen, tonify qi, and assist *Bai Shao* (Radix Paeoniae Alba) and *Dang Gui* (Radix Angelicae Sinensis) in producing blood. Finally, *Mu Tong* (Caulis Akebiae) opens the channels and collaterals to facilitate the circulation of qi and blood.

VETERINARY MODIFICATIONS

- With nausea and vomiting due to cold and deficiency of the Stomach, add *Wu Zhu Yu* (Fructus Evodiae) and *Sheng Jiang* (Rhizoma Zingiberis Recens).
- With painful extremities due to wind and dampness, add *Sang Ji Sheng* (Herba Taxilli) and *Wei Ling Xian* (Radix et Rhizoma Clematidis).
- With soreness and pain of the lower back, add *Niu Xi* (Radix Achyranthis Bidentatae) and *Du Zhong* (Cortex Eucommiae).
- With severe deficiency and cold, add *Fu Zi* (Radix Aconiti Lateralis Praeparata), *Gan Jiang* (Rhizoma Zingiberis) and *Huang Qi* (Radix Astragali).
- With pain in the hips, back, legs and feet caused by blood deficiency and cold accumulation, add *Xu Duan* (Radix Dipsaci), *Niu Xi* (Radix Achyranthis Bidentatae), *Ji Xue Teng* (Caulis Spatholobi) and *Mu Gua* (Fructus Chaenomelis).

CAUTIONS / CONTRAINDICATIONS

Dang Gui Si Ni Tang is contraindicated in animals with yin-deficient heat.

PHARMACOLOGICAL EFFECTS

Circulatory: Administration of *Dang Gui Si Ni Tang* in rabbits was associated with increased and improved blood perfusion to peripheral parts of the body with a relatively long duration of action.[1]

HUMAN CLINICAL STUDIES AND RESEARCH

1. **Pain**: Use of *Dang Gui Si Ni Tang* has been shown to effectively treat pain in many parts of the body due to various causes. One study reported success in the treatment of 52 postpartum women with general aches and pains using *Dang Gui Si Ni Tang* plus *Huang Qi* (Radix Astragali) and *Sang Zhi* (Ramulus Mori) for 20 days to 3 months.[2] Another study also reported success using modified *Dang Gui Si Ni Tang* for 2-6 weeks to treat 33 patients with pain in the lower back and legs.[3] Lastly, one study reported 93.1% effectiveness in 116 patients with *tong bi* (extremely painful obstruction) using *Dang Gui Si Ni Tang* plus *Huang Qi* (Radix Astragali), *Ji Xue Teng* (Caulis Spatholobi) and others as needed. The treatment protocol was to administer herbs in decoction form daily, for 10 days per course of treatment, for 2-8 courses total.[4]
2. **Cancer pain**: In one report, 50 patients with pain due to cancer were treated with modified *Dang Gui Si Ni Tang* with good results. The types of cancer included stomach (18 patients), esophageal (15 patients), lung (10 patients),

***Dang Gui Si Ni Tang* (Tangkuei Decoction for Frigid Extremities)**

Diagnosis	Clinical Signs	Treatment	Herbs
Invasion of cold with underlying deficiencies of yang qi and blood	• Icy cold lower extremities and paws: invasion of cold with underlying deficiencies of yang qi and blood • Pale tongue: presence of deficiency and cold • Deep, thin pulse or a thin pulse that is barely palpable: blood deficiency and invasion of cold	• Warms the channels and disperses cold • Nourishes the blood and opens the collaterals	• *Dang Gui* (Radix Angelicae Sinensis) and *Bai Shao* (Radix Paeoniae Alba) tonify and harmonize the blood. • *Gui Zhi* (Ramulus Cinnamomi) and *Xi Xin* (Radix et Rhizoma Asari) warm the channels, dispel exterior and interior cold, and restore yang qi. • *Zhi Gan Cao* (Radix et Rhizoma Glycyrrhizae Praeparata cum Melle) and *Da Zao* (Fructus Jujubae) strengthen the Spleen and tonify qi. • *Mu Tong* (Caulis Akebiae) opens the channels and collaterals to facilitate the circulation of qi and blood.

and liver (7 patients). The formula included *Dang Gui* (Radix Angelicae Sinensis) 30-50g, *Bai Shao* (Radix Paeoniae Alba) 50-100g, *Gui Zhi* (Ramulus Cinnamomi) 10-30g, *Xi Xin* (Radix et Rhizoma Asari) 6-15g, *Mu Tong* (Caulis Akebiae) 10-15g, *Gan Cao* (Radix et Rhizoma Glycyrrhizae) 10-12g, and *Da Zao* (Fructus Jujubae) 5-10 pieces. The herbs were cooked in water for 30 minutes to yield 600 mL of decoction. The treatment protocol was to ingest 150 mL of the decoction every 6 hours for 3 days. Out of 50 patients, the study reported marked improvement in 18 patients, moderate improvement in 24 patients, slight improvement in 3 patients, and no effect in 8 patients. The overall rate of effectiveness was 84%.[5]

3. **Sciatica**: In one study, 18 out of 20 patients with sciatica reported complete recovery using modified *Dang Gui Si Ni Tang* for 6-20 days. Those who had complete recovery did not have a recurrence for 1 year following the initial treatment. The formula included *Dang Gui* (Radix Angelicae Sinensis) 15g, *Niu Xi* (Radix Achyranthis Bidentatae) 15g, *Bai Shao* (Radix Paeoniae Alba) 30g, *Wei Ling Xian* (Radix et Rhizoma Clematidis) 30g, *Ji Xue Teng* (Caulis Spatholobi) 30g, *Gui Zhi* (Ramulus Cinnamomi) 10g, *Zhi Chuan Wu* (Radix Aconiti Praeparata) 10g, *Zhi Cao Wu* (Radix Aconiti Kusnezoffii Praeparata) 10g, *Ru Xiang* (Gummi Olibanum) 10g, *Mo Yao* (Myrrha) 10g, *Gan Cao* (Radix et Rhizoma Glycyrrhizae) 10g, and *Xi Xin* (Radix et Rhizoma Asari) 3g. Furthermore, 6g of *San Qi* (Radix et Rhizoma Notoginseng) was added for severe pain.[6] Another study reported 95.5% effectiveness in 31 patients with sciatica using herbs daily for 30 days per course of treatment. The herbal formula contained *Dang Gui Si Ni Tang* plus *Niu Xi* (Radix Achyranthis Bidentatae), *Mu Tong* (Caulis Akebiae), *Wu Shao She* (Zaocys), *Ru Xiang* (Gummi Olibanum) and *Mo Yao* (Myrrha).[7]
4. **Frostbite**: One hundred patients with I-II degree frostbite were treated with topical applications of *Dang Gui Si Ni Tang*. The herbal formula included *Dang Gui* (Radix Angelicae Sinensis) 20g, *Gui Zhi* (Ramulus Cinnamomi) 15g, *Bai Shao* (Radix Paeoniae Alba) 20g, *Xi Xin* (Radix et Rhizoma Asari) 5g, *Zhi Gan Cao* (Radix et Rhizoma Glycyrrhizae Praeparata cum Melle) 5g, *Mu Tong* (Caulis Akebiae) 10g, and *Sheng Jiang* (Rhizoma Zingiberis Recens) 10g. The treatment protocol was to cook the herbs in 500 mL of water. During the cooking process, the affected area was placed in the direction of the vapor for steam therapy. In addition, following the steam therapy, the affected area was soaked in the herbal solution for 15-20 minutes. One pack of herbs may be used up to four times for such topical treatment. The treatment was repeated twice daily, for a total of 6-8 treatments. The study reported improvement in all patients, with reduction of swelling and pain.[8]
5. **Peripheral neuritis**: In one report, 12 patients with peripheral neuritis were treated with good results using modified *Dang Gui Si Ni Tang*. Out of 12 patients, 6 had bilateral neuritis of upper extremities, 4 had bilateral neuritis of lower extremities, and 2 had neuritis in all four extremities. The formula included *Dang Gui* (Radix Angelicae Sinensis) 15g, *Bai Shao* (Radix Paeoniae Alba) 15g, *Da Zao* (Fructus Jujubae) 15g, *Mu Tong* (Caulis Akebiae) 15g, *Gui Zhi* (Ramulus Cinnamomi) 10g, *Xi Xin* (Radix et Rhizoma Asari) 10g, and *Zhi Gan Cao* (Radix et Rhizoma Glycyrrhizae Praeparata cum Melle) 5g. Modifications were made as follow: *Ji Xue Teng* (Caulis Spatholobi) 30g, *Zhi Chuan Wu* (Radix Aconiti Praeparata) 10g, and *Zhi Cao Wu* (Radix Aconiti Kusnezoffii Praeparata) 10g were added for severe pain; and *Wu Gong* (Scolopendra) 2 pieces, *Quan Xie* (Scorpio) 6g, and *Huang Qi* (Radix Astragali) 20g were added for numbness. The preparation procedure was to cook the herbs in 300 mL of water to yield 100 mL of decoction. The treatment protocol was to administer 50 mL of the decoction twice daily. Those with chronic illness were also treated with topical application of herbs in the form of an herbal wash made by cooking the herb residue from the decoction in water. Out of 12 patients, the study reported complete recovery in 9 patients and improvement in 3 patients. The average length of treatment was 11 days, ranging from 6 to 25 days.[9]
6. **Periarthritis of shoulder**: Administration of modified *Dang Gui Si Ni Tang* in 20 patients with periarthritis of shoulder was associated with complete recovery in 10 patients, improvement in 8 patients, and no effect in 2 patients. The treatment protocol was to cook the herbs in water, and drink the decoction in equally-divided doses twice daily for 15 days per course of treatment, for 1-2 courses total. The herbal treatment contained *Dang Gui Si Ni Tang* as the base formula, and added *Huang Qi* (Radix Astragali) for qi deficiency; *Hei Lao Hu* (Radix Kadsurae Coccineae) for blood stagnation; and *Wu Shao She* (Zaocys) for migratory pain.[10]
7. **Frozen shoulder**: One study reported complete recovery in 30 of 32 patients with frozen shoulder when treated with *Dang Gui Si Ni Tang* plus *Ji Xue Teng* (Caulis Spatholobi). The treatment protocol was to administer the herbs in decoction daily, for 12 days per course of treatment, for 1-3 courses total.[11]
8. **Allergic rhinitis**: Sixty-five patients with allergic rhinitis were treated with *Dang Gui Si Ni Tang* plus *Huang Qi* (Radix Astragali) and *Dang Shen* (Radix Codonopsis) with 90% effectiveness. Modifications were made as follow: *Xian Mao* (Rhizoma Curculiginis) was added for Kidney yang deficiency; *Bai Zhu* (Rhizoma Atractylodis Macrocephalae) and *Fu Ling* (Poria) for Spleen qi deficiency;

Dāng Guī Sì Nì Tāng (Tangkuei Decoction for Frigid Extremities)

and *Mai Dong* (Radix Ophiopogonis), *Wu Mei* (Fructus Mume) and *Tai Zi Shen* (Radix Pseudostellariae) for qi and yin deficiencies. The treatment protocol was to administer the decoction daily in the morning and at night, for 30 days per course of treatment, for 1-2 courses. Patients were advised to discontinue all other medications, and avoid all spicy and pungent foods. Of 65 patients, the study reported complete recovery in 38 patients, improvement in 21 patients, and no effect in 6 patients.[12]

9. **Post-surgical intestinal adhesion**: *Dang Gui Si Ni Tang* plus *Da Huang* (Radix et Rhizoma Rhei) was used to treat 108 patients with intestinal adhesion following such surgeries as removal of the appendix, gallbladder, and uterus. The herbs were cooked in 800 mL of water to yield 300 mL of decoction. The treatment protocol was to ingest 50 mL of decoction per dose, 5-6 times per day, for 5 days per course of treatment. Most patients were treated with 2-3 courses to control the pain and stabilize the condition. Out of 108 patients, the study reported complete recovery in 63 patients (asymptomatic for 3 months), significant improvement in 41 patients (mild pain only), and no change in 4 patients. The overall effectiveness rate was 96.3%.[13]

SUGGESTED ACUPUNCTURE TREATMENT

1. Points: *Guanyuan* (CV 4), *Taichong* (LR 3), *Zhongwan* (CV 12), and *Housanli* (ST 36).
2. Technique: tonification and moxibustion.

Guanyuan (CV 4), the intersecting point of the Liver, Spleen, Kidney, and *ren* (conception) channels, should be treated with needles and moxa to warm the blood and activate blood circulation. *Taichong* (LR 3) warms the channels and dispels cold from *jueyin*. *Zhongwan* (CV 12) and *Housanli* (ST 36) warm the middle *jiao*, raise yang qi, and dispel cold. For pain in specific areas, use local points.

AUTHORS' COMMENTS

Dang Gui Si Ni Tang can be used in diabetic animals with diabetic neuropathy, with blood deficiency and cold in the channels and collaterals. It is contraindicated in animals with yin deficiency and heat.

There are three "*si ni* (frigid extremities)" formulas that are commonly used. Although they share similar names, they have distinct functions.

- *Si Ni San* (Frigid Extremities Powder) is a harmonizing formula that treats cold extremities caused by the advancement of exterior pathogenic factor into the interior. Its main function is to harmonize the exterior and interior and remove stagnation.
- *Si Ni Tang* (Frigid Extremities Decoction) is an interior-warming formula that resuscitates yang. It is an extremely hot formula that treats very icy cold extremities caused by depletion of yang that is on the verge of collapse. The formula dispels cold, tonifies yang, and prevents collapse.
- *Dang Gui Si Ni Tang* (Tangkuei Decoction for Frigid Extremities) is an interior-warming formula that warms the channels and dispel cold. It treats cold extremities caused by cold, with underlying deficiencies of yang qi and blood. It dispels cold, warms the yang, nourishes the blood, and opens the channels and collaterals.

According to Dr. Chang Wei-Yen, *Dang Gui Si Ni Tang* can be used in a small amount to treat angina or cardiac infarction, since it has the effect to open the vessels. Furthermore, *Dang Gui Si Ni Tang* can be combined with *Xue Fu Zhu Yu Tang* (Drive Out Stasis in the Mansion of Blood Decoction) for maximum effect.

References

1. *Zhong Hua Yi Xue Za Zhi* (Chinese Journal of Medicine), 1981; 1:57.
2. *He Bei Zhong Yi* (Hebei Chinese Medicine), 1995; 4:15.
3. *Zhong Yi Ming Fang Lin Chuang Xin Yong* (Contemporary Clinical Applications of Classic Chinese Formulas), 2001; 336.
4. *Hu Nan Zhong Yi Za Zhi* (Hunan Journal of Chinese Medicine), 1997; 6:29.
5. *Zhong Yi Fang Ji Xian Dai Yan Jiu* (Modern Study of Medical Formulas in Traditional Chinese Medicine), 1997; 424.
6. *Hu Bei Zhong Yi Za Zhi* (Hubei Journal of Chinese Medicine), 1986; 2:39.
7. *Hu Nan Zhong Yi Za Zhi* (Hunan Journal of Chinese Medicine), 1997; 2:48.
8. *Shan Dong Zhong Yi Za Zhi* (Shandong Journal of Chinese Medicine), 1984; 2:37.
9. *Xin Zhong Yi* (New Chinese Medicine), 1996; 2:46.
10. *Xin Zhong Yi* (New Chinese Medicine), 1987; 7:53.
11. *Si Chuan Zhong Yi* (Sichuan Chinese Medicine), 1989; 2:31.
12. *Yun Nan Zhong Yi Zhong Yao Za Zhi* (Yunan Journal of Chinese Medicine and Medicinals), 1999; 4:29.
13. *Zhe Jiang Zhong Yi Za Zhi* (Zhejiang Journal of Chinese Medicine), 1995; 3:107.

Huáng Qí Guì Zhī Wǔ Wù Tāng

(Astragalus and Cinnamon Twig Five-Substance Decoction)

黄耆桂枝五物湯
黄芪桂枝五物汤

Pinyin Name: *Huang Qi Gui Zhi Wu Wu Tang*
Literal Name: Astragalus and Cinnamon Twig Five-Substance Decoction
Alternate Names: *Huang Chi Wu Wu Tang, Huang Qi Wu Wu Tang*, Astragalus Five-Component Decoction, Astragalus Five-Herbs Decoction, Astragalus Five Decoction, Astragalus and Cinnamon Five Herb Combination
Original Source: *Jin Gui Yao Lue* (Essentials from the Golden Cabinet) by Zhang Zhong-Jing in the Eastern Han Dynasty

COMPOSITION

Huang Qi (Radix Astragali)	9g [12g]
Gui Zhi (Ramulus Cinnamomi)	9g
Bai Shao (Radix Paeoniae Alba)	9g
Sheng Jiang (Rhizoma Zingiberis Recens)	18g [12g]
Da Zao (Fructus Jujubae)	12 pieces [4 pieces]

DOSAGE / PREPARATION / ADMINISTRATION

Cook the herbs in 6 cups [1,200 mL] of water until it is reduced to 2 cups [400 mL]. Take 0.7 cup [140 mL] of the warm, strained decoction in three equally-divided doses. Today, the decoction may be prepared using the doses suggested in brackets.

CHINESE THERAPEUTIC ACTIONS

1. Tonifies qi and warms the channels
2. Harmonizes the *ying* (nutritive) level and unblocks obstruction

CLINICAL MANIFESTATIONS

Xue bi (blood painful obstruction): stiffness of the extremities, and a wiry pulse.

VETERINARY CLINICAL APPLICATIONS

Periarthritis of the shoulders, neck and shoulder pain, peripheral neuritis, diabetic neuropathy, peripheral neuropathy, polyneuropathy, hemiplegia, muscle paralysis, facial paralysis, and frostbite.

EXPLANATION

Huang Qi Gui Zhi Wu Wu Tang (Astragalus and Cinnamon Twig Five-Substance Decoction) is designed to treat *xue bi* (blood painful obstruction). This condition begins in animals with underlying weakness and deficiency. When these patients are exposed to the wind, they experience obstruction of qi and blood circulation, which leads to localized stiffness of the limbs and extremities. In severe cases, there may be muscle aches and pains. The slightly wiry pulse is representative of blood stasis.

Huang Qi (Radix Astragali) tonifies *wei* (defensive) *qi* and consolidates the exterior. *Gui Zhi* (Ramulus Cinnamomi) disperses wind-cold and opens the channels. The combination of *Huang Qi* (Radix Astragali) and *Gui Zhi* (Ramulus Cinnamomi) tonifies qi, warms yang, harmonizes the blood, and opens the channels. *Bai Shao* (Radix Paeoniae Alba) nourishes the blood and harmonizes the *ying* (nutritive) level. The combination of *Gui Zhi* (Ramulus Cinnamomi) and *Bai Shao* (Radix Paeoniae Alba) also harmonizes the *ying* (nutritive) and *wei* (defensive) levels. *Sheng Jiang*

***Huang Qi Gui Zhi Wu Wu Tang* (Astragalus and Cinnamon Twig Five-Substance Decoction)**

Diagnosis	Clinical Signs	Treatment	Herbs
Xue bi (blood painful obstruction)	• Stiffness of the extremities: exterior wind blocking qi and blood circulation • Wiry pulse: blood stasis	• Tonifies qi and warms the channels • Harmonizes the channels and unblocks obstructions	• *Huang Qi* (Radix Astragali) tonifies *wei* (defensive) *qi* and consolidates the exterior. • *Gui Zhi* (Ramulus Cinnamomi) disperses wind-cold and opens the channels. • *Bai Shao* (Radix Paeoniae Alba) nourishes the blood and harmonizes the *ying* (nutritive) and *wei* (defensive) levels. • *Sheng Jiang* (Rhizoma Zingiberis Recens) dispels wind-cold. • *Da Zao* (Fructus Jujubae) tonifies qi and blood.

Huáng Qí Guì Zhī Wǔ Wù Tāng

(Astragalus and Cinnamon Twig Five-Substance Decoction)

(Rhizoma Zingiberis Recens) and *Gui Zhi* (Ramulus Cinnamomi) dispel wind-cold. *Da Zao* (Fructus Jujubae) tonifies qi and blood.

VETERINARY MODIFICATIONS

- With weak arms and hands, double the dose of *Gui Zhi* (Ramulus Cinnamomi).
- With weak knees and legs, add *Niu Xi* (Radix Achyranthis Bidentatae).
- For weak tendons, add *Mu Gua* (Fructus Chaenomelis).
- With deficiency of *yuan* (source) *qi*, add *Ren Shen* (Radix et Rhizoma Ginseng).
- With deficiency of yang, add *Fu Zi* (Radix Aconiti Lateralis Praeparata).
- With hemiparalysis affecting the left side, add *Dang Gui* (Radix Angelicae Sinensis).
- For hemiparalysis affecting the right side, double the dose of *Huang Qi* (Radix Astragali).
- For stiffness of the body, add *Dang Gui* (Radix Angelicae Sinensis) and *Fang Feng* (Radix Saposhnikoviae).
- With painful extremities, add *Bai Zhu* (Rhizoma Atractylodis Macrocephalae) and *Fang Ji* (Radix Stephaniae Tetrandrae).
- With stiffness and pain due to blood stagnation, combine with *Si Wu Tang* (Four-Substance Decoction).
- With stiffness and pain due to wind obstruction, combine with *Xu Ming Tang* (Prolong Life Decoction).
- If there is more wind, add *Fang Feng* (Radix Saposhnikoviae) and *Fang Ji* (Radix Stephaniae Tetrandrae).
- If there is more blood stasis, add *Tao Ren* (Semen Persicae) and *Hong Hua* (Flos Carthami).

HUMAN CLINICAL STUDIES AND RESEARCH

1. **Periarthritis of the shoulders**: Integrative treatment using herbs and *tui-na* was effective in treating 63 patients with periarthritis of the shoulders. The herbal formula contained *Huang Qi* (Radix Astragali) 15g, *Gui Zhi* (Ramulus Cinnamomi) 5g, *Chi Shao* (Radix Paeoniae Rubra) 5g, *Bai Shao* (Radix Paeoniae Alba) 5g, *Da Zao* (Fructus Jujubae) 5g, *Qiang Huo* (Rhizoma et Radix Notopterygii) 5g, *Du Huo* (Radix Angelicae Pubescentis) 5g, *Fang Feng* (Radix Saposhnikoviae) 5g, *Dang Gui* (Radix Angelicae Sinensis) 5g, *Chuan Xiong* (Rhizoma Chuanxiong) 5g, *Xi Xin* (Radix et Rhizoma Asari) 5g, and *Sheng Jiang* (Rhizoma Zingiberis Recens) 5g. Modifications were made as follow: *Zhi Chuan Wu* (Radix Aconiti Praeparata) 3-6g and *Zhi Cao Wu* (Radix Aconiti Kusnezoffii Praeparata) 3-6g were added for severe pain characterized by cold; *Xu Duan* (Radix Dipsaci) 9g and *Du Zhong* (Cortex Eucommiae) 9g were added for elderly patients with Liver and Kidney deficiencies; *Sang Zhi* (Ramulus Mori) 15g and *Shen Jin Cao* (Herba Lycopodii) 12g were added for stiff joints with limited range of motion; and *Di Long* (Pheretima) 9g and *Wu Shao She* (Zaocys) 30g were added for chronic arthritis. Of 63 patients, the study reported complete recovery in 26 patients, significant improvement in 31 patients, and moderate improvement in 6 patients. The duration of treatment varied from 14-48 days, with an average of 29 days.[1]
2. **Synovitis of the knees**: Thirty-eight patients with synovitis of the knees responded well to herbal treatment and physical therapy. Herbal treatment contained *Huang Qi Gui Zhi Wu Wu Tang* plus *Dang Gui* (Radix Angelicae Sinensis). The herbs were given in decoction daily, for three weeks per course of treatment. The duration of treatment varied from 14-42 days. Of 38 patients, 32 had complete recovery and 6 had moderate improvement.[2]
3. **Neck and shoulder pain**: One study reported marked effect using modified *Huang Qi Gui Zhi Wu Wu Tang* to treat 48 patients with neck and shoulder stiffness and pain. In addition to *Huang Qi Gui Zhi Wu Wu Tang* as the base formula, *Mu Gua* (Fructus Chaenomelis) was added for stiff muscles with limited mobility; *Dang Gui* (Radix Angelicae Sinensis) and *Chuan Xiong* (Rhizoma Chuanxiong) were added for stiffness; and *Ju Hua* (Flos Chrysanthemi) was added for dizziness. The herbs were given in decoction for 7 days per course of treatment. Of 48 patients, the study reported complete recovery in 20 patients, significant improvement in 18 patients and moderate improvement in 10 patients.[3]
4. ***Bi zheng* (painful obstruction syndrome)**: Use of *Huang Qi Gui Zhi Wu Wu Tang* was associated with good therapeutic effect to treat *bi zheng* (painful obstruction syndrome) characterized by yang deficiency and invasion cold and its subsequent obstruction of the channels and collaterals. The herbal treatment contained *Huang Qi Gui Zhi Wu Wu Tang* plus *Gu Sui Bu* (Rhizoma Drynariae), *Du Zhong* (Cortex Eucommiae), *Xu Duan* (Radix Dipsaci), and *Dang Gui* (Radix Angelicae Sinensis). Of 114 patients, the study reported significant improvement in 111 patients and no effect in 3 patients. The average duration of treatment was 5.4 packs of herbs, though the range was between 2 to 120 packs.[4]
5. **Peripheral neuritis**: *Huang Qi Gui Zhi Wu Wu Tang* was reported in several studies to effectively treat peripheral neuritis. According to one study, 51 patients with peripheral neuritis were effectively treated with *Huang Qi Gui Zhi Wu Wu Tang* plus *Sang Ji Sheng* (Herba Taxilli) and *Ji Xue Teng* (Caulis Spatholobi) as the base formula, with addition of *Mo Yao* (Myrrha) for severe pain; *Yi Yi Ren* (Semen Coicis) for swelling; *Tao Ren* (Semen Persicae)

Huáng Qí Guì Zhī Wǔ Wù Tāng

(Astragalus and Cinnamon Twig Five-Substance Decoction)

for dark purple skin appearance; *Jiang Huang* (Rhizoma Curcumae Longae) for neuritis in the upper limbs; and *Ren Shen Yang Ying Tang* (Ginseng Decoction to Nourish the Nutritive Qi) for neuritis in the lower limbs. Of 51 patients, the study reported complete recovery in 36 patients, improvement in 11 patients, and no effect in 4 patients.[5] According to another study, 198 patients with neuritis were treated with complete recovery in 195 patients, improvement in 2 patients, and no effect in 1 case. In addition to *Huang Qi Gui Zhi Wu Wu Tang*, *Sang Zhi* (Ramulus Mori), *Dang Gui* (Radix Angelicae Sinensis) and *Xi Xin* (Radix et Rhizoma Asari) were added for yang deficiency and cold obstruction; *Dang Gui* (Radix Angelicae Sinensis), *Ji Xue Teng* (Caulis Spatholobi) and *Sang Zhi* (Ramulus Mori) were added for blood deficiency; and *Ren Dong Teng* (Caulis Lonicerae Japonicae), *Tong Cao* (Medulla Tetrapanacis) and *Di Long* (Pheretima) were added, and *Gui Zhi* (Ramulus Cinnamomi) was removed for the presence of damp-heat.[6]

6. **Diabetic neuropathy**: One study reported 100% effectiveness using modified *Huang Qi Gui Zhi Wu Wu Tang* to treat diabetic neuropathy. The herbal treatment contained this formula plus *Jiang Can* (Bombyx Batryticatus), *Quan Xie* (Scorpio), *Wu Gong* (Scolopendra) and *Di Long* (Pheretima). Modifications included addition of *Sang Zhi* (Ramulus Mori) for burning sensations at the affected area; and *Fu Zi* (Radix Aconiti Lateralis Praeparata) for cold sensations. The herbs were given for 15 days per course of treatment. Of 30 patients, the study reported near-complete recovery in 13 patients, significant improvement in 10 patients, and moderate improvement in 7 patients.[7] Another study reported 85.71% effectiveness using modified *Huang Qi Gui Zhi Wu Wu Tang* to treat 42 patients with peripheral neuropathy. The herbal treatment contained *Huang Qi Gui Zhi Wu Wu Tang* plus *Dang Gui* (Radix Angelicae Sinensis), *Chi Shao* (Radix Paeoniae Rubra), *Ge Gen* (Radix Puerariae Lobatae), *Shan Yao* (Rhizoma Dioscoreae), *Shan Zhu Yu* (Fructus Corni), and *Ji Xue Teng* (Caulis Spatholobi) as the base formula. Additional modifications were made as needed to address complications of diabetes mellitus. The herbs were given for 10 days per course of treatment. Of 42 patients, the study reported significant improvement in 24 patients, moderate improvement in 12 patients, and no effect in 6 patients.[8]
7. **Frostbite**: Modified *Huang Qi Gui Zhi Wu Wu Tang* was reported in one study to effectively treat 566 patients with frostbite. The herbal treatment contained *Huang Qi Gui Zhi Wu Wu Tang* plus *Ji Xue Teng* (Caulis Spatholobi) and *Fu Zi* (Radix Aconiti Lateralis Praeparata) as the base formula. Modifications were made based on the area affected, and included addition of *Bai Zhi* (Radix Angelicae Dahuricae) and *Chuan Xiong* (Rhizoma Chuanxiong) for the face; *Jiang Huang* (Rhizoma Curcumae Longae) and *Gui Zhi* (Ramulus Cinnamomi) for upper limbs; *Niu Xi* (Radix Achyranthis Bidentatae) and *Du Huo* (Radix Angelicae Pubescentis) for lower limbs; *Tao Ren* (Semen Persicae), *Chuan Shan Jia* (Squama Manis) and *Dang Gui* (Radix Angelicae Sinensis) for bruises and swelling; *Fu Ling* (Poria), *Wu Shao She* (Zaocys), *Cang Zhu* (Rhizoma Atractylodis) and *Yi Yi Ren* (Semen Coicis) for blisters; *Xi Xin* (Radix et Rhizoma Asari), *Ru Xiang* (Gummi Olibanum) and *Cong Bai* (Bulbus Allii Fistulosi) for severe pain; *Di Long* (Pheretima), *Hai Feng Teng* (Caulis Piperis Kadsurae) and *Quan Xie* (Scorpio) for stiffness; and *Tu Fu Ling* (Rhizoma Smilacis Glabrae), *Da Xue Teng* (Caulis Sargentodoxae) and *Bai Jiang Cao* (Herba cum Radice Patriniae) for swelling, redness and pain. Of 566 patients, the study reported significant improvement in 453 patients and moderate improvement in 95 patients.[9]
8. **Restless leg syndrome**: Use of modified *Huang Qi Gui Zhi Wu Wu Tang* was associated with good results in treating 18 patients with restless leg syndrome. The herbal formula contained *Huang Qi* (Radix Astragali) 30g, *Gui Zhi* (Ramulus Cinnamomi) 12g, *Chuan Xiong* (Rhizoma Chuanxiong) 15g, *Dang Gui* (Radix Angelicae Sinensis) 12g, *Xi Xin* (Radix et Rhizoma Asari) 3g, *Di Long* (Pheretima) 12g, *Chuan Niu Xi* (Radix Cyathulae) 15g, *Bai Shao* (Radix Paeoniae Alba) 30g, and *Gan Cao* (Radix et Rhizoma Glycyrrhizae) 6g. Modifications were made by adding *Dan Shen* (Radix et Rhizoma Salviae Miltiorrhizae) 30g and *Ji Xue Teng* (Caulis Spatholobi) 30g for stiffness and weakness of the extremities with qi and blood deficiencies; *Tao Ren* (Semen Persicae) 9g, *Hong Hua* (Flos Carthami) 9g, and *Huang Qi* (Radix Astragali) 60g for stiffness and weakness of the extremities with qi deficiency and blood stagnation; and *Fu Zi* (Radix Aconiti Lateralis Praeparata) 12g and *Ma Huang* (Herba Ephedrae) 6g for cold extremities with yang deficiency. The herbs were given in decoction daily, with duration of treatment ranging from 6-25 packs of herbs. Of 18 patients, the study reported complete recovery in 12 patients, significant improvement in 3 patients, moderate improvement in 2 patients, and no change in 1 patient.[10]
9. **Pulmonary heart disease**: One study reported marked success using *Huang Qi Gui Zhi Wu Wu Tang* to treat 70 patients with pulmonary heart disease. Use of the formula was associated with elevated plasma levels of prealbumin, transferrin and fibronectin, and lowered levels of C-reactive protein, ceruloplasmin, haptoglobin, alpha 1-antitrypsin and alpha 1-acid glycoprotein. In comparison, in the control group, which did not receive any herbs,

Huáng Qí Guì Zhī Wǔ Wù Tāng

(Astragalus and Cinnamon Twig Five-Substance Decoction)

only the levels of ceruloplasmin and C-reactive protein decreased significantly. The study stated that *Huang Qi Gui Zhi Wu Wu Tang* may enhance the therapeutic effects for pulmonary heart disease, regulate the metabolism of plasma proteins, and improve the quality of life of such patients.[11]

SUGGESTED ACUPUNCTURE TREATMENT

1. Points: *Qihai* (CV 6), *Housanli* (ST 36), *Waiguan* (TH 5), *Shenmai* (BL 62), *Sanyinjiao* (SP 6), and *Hegu* (LI 4).
2. Technique: tonification.

Qihai (CV 6) and *Housanli* (ST 36) tonify qi; *Waiguan* (TH 5) and *Shenmai* (BL 62) open and warm the channels; *Sanyinjiao* (SP 6) nourishes yin; *Hegu* (LI 4) unblocks obstruction.

AUTHORS' COMMENTS

Dang Gui Si Ni Tang (Tangkuei Decoction for Frigid Extremities) and *Huang Qi Gui Zhi Wu Wu Tang* both warm the channels and dispel cold.

- *Dang Gui Si Ni Tang* is best at nourishing blood and opening the channels and collaterals.
- *Huang Qi Gui Zhi Wu Wu Tang* is mainly used for *bi zheng* (painful obstruction syndrome), since it is better at tonifying qi and warming the channels and collaterals.

References

1. *Si Chuan Zhong Yi* (Sichuan Chinese Medicine), 1993; 1:40.
2. *Gan Su Zhong Yi* (Gansu Chinese Medicine), 1993; 6:26.
3. *Shi Zhen Guo Yao Yan Jiu* (Research of Shizhen Herbs), 1999; 5:362.
4. *Hu Bei Zhong Yi Za Zhi* (Hubei Journal of Chinese Medicine), 1995; 6:11.
5. *Liao Ning Zhong Yi Za Zhi* (Liaoning Journal of Chinese Medicine), 1991; 1:36.
6. *Zhong Yi Yao Xin Xi* (Information on Chinese Medicine and Herbology), 1998; 2:40.
7. *He Bei Zhong Yi* (Hebei Chinese Medicine), 1998; 5:301.
8. *Hei Long Jiang Zhong Yi Yao* (Heilongjiang Chinese Medicine and Herbology), 1998; 4:17.
9. *Shan Dong Zhong Yi Za Zhi* (Shandong Journal of Chinese Medicine), 1990; 3:49.
10. *Shi Yong Zhong Yi Nei Ke Za Zhi* (Journal of Practical Chinese Internal Medicine), 1993; 3:43.
11. Che H, Luo K. Effects of huang qi wu wu decoction on plasma proteins in 70 patients of chronic pulmonary heart disease. Journal of Traditional Chinese Medicine. 2000 Dec; 20(4):254-7.

Chapter 7 — Summary

— Interior-Warming Formulas

SECTION 1: MIDDLE-WARMING AND COLD-DISPELLING FORMULAS

Name	Similarities	Differences
Li Zhong Wan (Regulate the Middle Pill)	Warm the middle *jiao*, dispel cold, tonify qi	Standard formula to treat deficiency and cold of the middle *jiao*
Fu Zi Li Zhong Wan (Prepared Aconite Pill to Regulate the Middle)		Stronger effect to tonify yang and dispel cold
Wu Zhu Yu Tang (Evodia Decoction)	Warms and tonifies the middle *jiao*, corrects the reversed flow of qi	Directs yin and cold downward
Xiao Jian Zhong Tang (Minor Construct the Middle Decoction)	Tonify and warm the middle *jiao*, dispel cold, relieve pain	Harmonizes the interior and relieves pain
Huang Qi Jian Zhong Tang (Astragalus Decoction to Construct the Middle)		Harmonizes the interior and relieves pain, tonifies qi
Gui Qi Jian Zhong Tang (Tangkuei and Astragalus Decoction to Construct the Middle)		Harmonizes the interior and relieves pain, tonifies qi and blood
Da Jian Zhong Tang (Major Construct the Middle Decoction)		Corrects the reversed flow of qi, strongly dispels cold and relieves pain

Li Zhong Wan (Regulate the Middle Pill) and ***Fu Zi Li Zhong Wan*** (Prepared Aconite Pill to Regulate the Middle) are formulas that warm the middle *jiao*, dispel cold, tonify qi, and strengthen the Spleen. They both treat deficiency and cold in the middle *jiao*.

- *Li Zhong Wan* is mainly used for digestive dysfunctions caused by deficiency and cold of the middle *jiao,* leading to clinical signs of diarrhea, vomiting, abdominal pain, poor appetite, and no desire to drink. Other applications include bleeding due to yang deficiency, and *xiong bi* (painful obstruction of the chest) due to deficiency and cold of the middle *jiao*.
- *Fu Zi Li Zhong Wan* contains *Fu Zi* (Radix Aconiti Lateralis Praeparata), and is a hotter and more acrid formula that warms and strengthens Spleen and Kidney yang. This formula is best for cold and pain in the chest and abdomen, extreme coldness of the limbs and extremities, and muscle spasms and cramps.

Wu Zhu Yu Tang (Evodia Decoction) warms and tonifies the middle *jiao*, corrects the reversed flow of qi, and stops vomiting. It mainly treats vomiting in the *yangming, shaoyin,* and *jueyin* levels. The focus is on deficiency and cold of the Stomach, accompanied by rising of yin and cold upward. Other clinical manifestations include fullness of the chest and gastralgia, acid regurgitation, diarrhea, cold limbs, and irritability.

Xiao Jian Zhong Tang (Minor Construct the Middle Decoction) harmonizes and warms the middle *jiao* to relieve pain. The emphasis of this formula is on tonifying middle *jiao* yang deficiency.

- ***Huang Qi Jian Zhong Tang*** (Astragalus Decoction to Construct the Middle) has the addition of *Huang Qi* (Radix Astragali), which tonifies qi. This formula is more suitable for yang deficiency of the middle *jiao,* complicated by qi deficiency.

Chapter 7 — Summary

- ***Gui Qi Jian Zhong Tang*** (Tangkuei and Astragalus Decoction to Construct the Middle) has the addition of both *Dang Gui* (Radix Angelicae Sinensis) and *Huang Qi* (Radix Astragali) to tonify the blood and qi. This is a good formula for treating chronic abscesses and ulcerations with underlying qi, blood, and yang deficiencies.

Da Jian Zhong Tang (Major Construct the Middle Decoction) relieves pain, corrects the reversed flow of qi, dispels cold, and warms the middle *jiao*. The emphasis of this formula is on reducing the proliferation of yin and cold and tonifying yang deficiency of the middle *jiao*.

Xiao Jian Zhong Tang (Minor Construct the Middle Decoction) and *Da Jian Zhong Tang* (Major Construct the Middle Decoction) both tonify and warm the middle *jiao* to dispel cold and relieve pain.

- *Xiao Jian Zhong Tang* emphasizes tonifying yang, qi, and blood, and warming the middle *jiao*.
- *Da Jian Zhong Tang* focuses mostly on dispelling cold and relieving pain.

SECTION 2: YANG-RESUSCITATING FORMULA

Name	Similarities	Differences
Si Ni Tang (Frigid Extremities Decoction)	Rescues yang from collapse	Restores depleted yang

Si Ni Tang (Frigid Extremities Decoction) restores depleted yang and rescue from counterflow cold. This is the main formula to rescue and restore yang in the *shaoyin* stage. This Kidney yang depletion manifests in cold extremities, preference to curl up when lying down, lethargic, vomiting, no thirst, abdominal pain, diarrhea, and a faint, fine pulse.

SECTION 3: CHANNEL-WARMING AND COLD-DISPERSING FORMULAS

Name	Similarities	Differences
Dang Gui Si Ni Tang (Tangkuei Decoction for Frigid Extremities)	Warm the channels and collaterals, disperse cold	Stronger effect to nourish the blood
Huang Qi Gui Zhi Wu Wu Tang (Astragalus and Cinnamon Twig Five-Substance Decoction)		Better function to tonify qi

Dang Gui Si Ni Tang (Tangkuei Decoction for Frigid Extremities) warms the channels and collaterals, disperses cold, and nourishes the blood. It is used for invasion of cold with deficiencies of blood and yang qi.

Huang Qi Gui Zhi Wu Wu Tang (Astragalus and Cinnamon Twig Five-Substance Decoction) tonifies qi and warms the channels and collaterals. It treats *xue bi* (blood painful obstruction) due to exterior wind invading and blocking qi and blood circulation.

Chapter 8

— Tonic Formulas

补益剂

钱乙 Qīan Yǐ

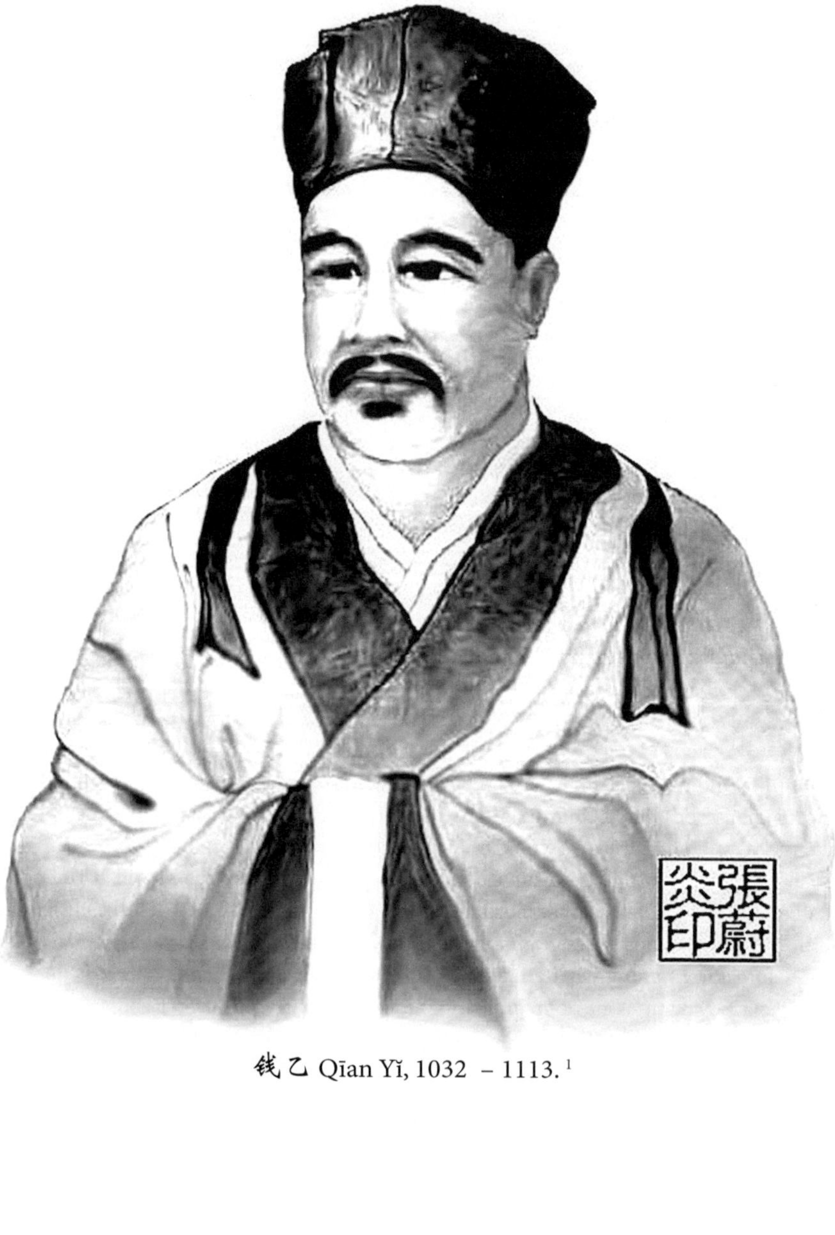

钱乙 Qīan Yǐ, 1032 – 1113.[1]

钱乙 Qīan Yǐ

Qian Yi became an orphan at the age of three: his father left home and his mother passed away. Qian was adopted by his aunt, and studied medicine with his uncle. Qian treated his aunt and uncle as his real parents, even after he was told his true family background.

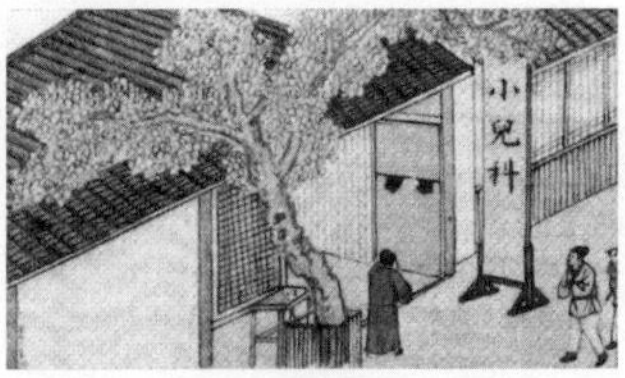

Painting of a pediatric clinic from the Song dynasty.

Qian studied and specialized in pediatrics for over 40 years. At one point, he successfully treated several children of the Imperial family, and was granted the position of 太医 the Supreme Physician. When he retired from the Imperial Palace and returned home, he began to compile his clinical experience. However, because he had *bi zheng* (painful obstruction syndrome) in his hands and could not write, his works were primarily organized by his apprentices. Finally in 1119, six years after his death, 小儿药症直决 *Xiao Er Yao Zheng Zhi Jue* (Craft of Medicinal Treatment for Childhood Disease Patterns) was published. This is considered to be the first and most authoritative text dedicated to pediatrics. In this text, Qian highlighted the importance of using "gentle and moistening" approaches to treat pediatric disorders, and opposed the use of potent herbs for drastic approaches such as attacking, purging, and even tonifying. Furthermore, he strongly emphasized the need to always balance the treatment with tonifying and sedating herbs simultaneously. This principle is reflected in one of his formulas that is among the most commonly used formulas today, *Liu Wei Di Huang Wan* (Six-Ingredient Pill with Rehmannia).[2]

Qian Yi is remembered as 儿科之圣 the Sage of Pediatrics.

Excellent formulas written by Qian Yi include:

- *Sheng Ma Ge Gen Tang* (Cimicifuga and Kudzu Decoction)
- *Xie Bai San* (Drain the White Powder)
- *Long Dan Xie Gan Tang* (Gentiana Decoction to Drain the Liver)
- *Dao Chi San* (Guide Out the Red Powder)
- *Xie Huang San* (Drain the Yellow Powder)
- *Liu Wei Di Huang Wan* (Six-Ingredient Pill with Rehmannia)
- *Bu Fei E Jiao Tang* (Tonify the Lung Decoction with Ass-Hide Gelatin)

Dynasties & Kingdoms	Year
Xia Dynasty 夏	2100-1600 BCE
Shang Dynasty 商	1600-1100 BCE
Zhou Dynasty 周	1100-221 BCE
Qin Dynasty 秦	221-207 BCE
Han Dynasty 漢	206 BCE-220
Three Kingdoms 三國	220-280
Western Jin Dynasty 西晉	265-316
Eastern Jin Dynasty 東晉	317-420
Northern and Southern Dynasties 北南朝	420-581
Sui Dynasty 隋	581-618
Tang Dynasty 唐	618-907
Five Dynasties 五代	907-960
Song Dynasty 宋	960-1279
Liao Dynasty 遼	**916-1125**
Jin Dynasty 金	1115-1234
Yuan Dynasty 元	1271-1368
Ming Dynasty 明	1368-1644
Qing Dynasty 清	1644-1911
Republic of China 中華民國	1912-Present Day
People's Republic of China 中華人民共和國	1949-Present Day

1. Approximate year of birth.
2. The most famous herbal formula by Qian Yi, *Liu Wei Di Huang Wan* (Six-Ingredient Pill with Rehmannia), is also the one that gave him most trouble. When he first prescribed *Liu Wei Di Huang Wan* (Six-Ingredient Pill with Rehmannia), he was ridiculed by his colleagues for deviating from the gold standards established by Zhang Zhong-Jing and his original formulation – *Jin Gui Shen Qi Wan* (Kidney Qi Pill from the Golden Cabinet). Finally when questioned, he explained that "*Jin Gui Shen Qi Wan* is for adults. Children have abundant yang qi, and if given hot herbs such as *Gui Zhi* (Ramulus Cinnamomi) and *Fu Zi* (Radix Aconiti Lateralis Praeparata), may suffer from heat and nosebleeds." This explanation silenced his critics, as it showed that not only did Qian Yi understand Zhang Zhong-Jing's teaching, he was knowledgeable and flexible enough to improve upon it. Today, *Liu Wei Di Huang Wan* (Six-Ingredient Pill with Rehmannia) is frequently used for both pediatric and geriatric patients.

Table of Contents

Table of Contents

Chapter 8 — Overview

补益剂 — Tonic Formulas

Definition: Tonic formulas supplement qi, blood, yin, yang, *jing* (essence), and body fluids to treat various patterns of deficiency syndromes and repair damage to *zang fu* organs. This method of treatment is known as *bu fa* (tonifying), one of the *ba fa* (eight treatment methods) described in the *Huang Di Nei Jing* (Yellow Emperor's Inner Classic) in the first or second century, A.D. Tonifying formulas are the most commonly prescribed category of Chinese herbal formula in veterinary medicine.

Deficiency syndromes refer primarily to insufficiencies of qi, blood, yin, yang, *jing* (essence), and body fluids. Although there are many causes of deficiency, the causes can all be categorized as either of prenatal (genetic) or postnatal (inappropriate diet, overwork, emotional stress, drug induced or chronic illness) origin. Aging and chronic illnesses are common causes of postnatal deficiency, and deficient patients are easily identified by their general appearance, characterized by poor body condition, weakness, and general lack of vitality. However, young animals may acquire deficiency conditions as well, although their presentation may be less obvious. Sporting animals may become deficient through overwork, and breeding stock (studs and multiparous females) will lose vital substances through overuse. Even house pets and pleasure horses can become deficient, if subjected to an improper diet and/or chronic drug therapy, which damages the Spleen and Stomach. Finally, both young and old will become deficient under chronic emotional stress.

It is essential that the diagnosis of deficiency is clear because formulas used to tonify deficiencies may exacerbate disorders caused by excess. A severe excess condition may exhibit clinical signs commonly associated with a deficiency condition (such as weakness, lethargy, weight loss, poor appetite). Not all deficient conditions are chronic, and not all chronic conditions are deficient. Hence, the root cause must be properly differentiated to determine whether excess should be treated simultaneously while tonifying identified deficiencies. Regardless of whether the origin is prenatal insufficiency or postnatal imbalance, these disorders are characterized by deficiencies of qi, blood, yin, yang, *jing* and body fluids in one or more of the five *zang* (solid organs).

In simple cases, herbs can be prescribed to directly treat the deficiency, such as qi-tonifying herbs to treat qi deficiency, and blood-tonifying herbs to treat blood deficiency. However, because qi, blood, yin and yang are mutually dependent, and the *zang* (solid) and *fu* (hollow) organs are closely connected to each other, deficiency syndromes usually do not occur independently. Rather, deficiency of one vital substance often affects others, leading to deficiency of multiple substances that affects more than one organ. Therefore, it is common to tonify qi and blood concurrently, or to supplement yin and yang simultaneously. Herbs that tonify qi, blood, and yang are generally sweet, and warm to hot in nature. Qi tonics primarily nourish the Lung and Spleen and enter the Lung and Spleen channels. Those that tonify blood mainly nourish Heart and Liver blood, and so enter the Liver and Heart channels, while those that tonify yang enter the Kidney channel. Herbs that tonify yin are mainly sweet, and cool or cold in temperature. They nourish and enter the Stomach, Lung, Kidney, and Liver channels; many of the herbs that enrich yin overlap these four organs.

Chapter 8 — Overview

Besides directly tonifying the deficiency, one could utilize other supplemental strategies to enhance the overall tonifying effect. Examples are as follows:

- The Spleen is considered to be the "mother of the five *zang* (solid organ) organs," responsible for the transformation and transportation of food and the source of all qi and blood after birth. In chronic deficiency syndromes, the Spleen and Stomach may become deficient and lead to a compromised ability to digest and absorb food and herbs. The rich, cloying nature of tonifying formulas can place further stress on the digestive system. To ensure that the herbal formulas are absorbed properly and to optimize the overall therapeutic effect, the Spleen and Stomach should be supported and fortified. When an animal exhibits signs of marked Spleen and Stomach deficiencies, it is often necessary to reduce the formula dosage for these reasons. Additionally, modern, commercial diets containing inappropriately high amounts of grains often already put the Spleen and Stomach at a disadvantage. Many dogs and cats have chronic Spleen deficiency from regular consumption of these high carbohydrate diets. Horses develop similar problems if fed diets with a high percentage of concentrates or grain mixtures with high molasses content. For these reasons, tonic formulas supporting the middle *jiao* are often required, and can be combined with a primary formula, to promote adequate digestion and the production of high quality food essence to nourish the *zang fu* organs and the whole body. Many equine practitioners may also add Spleen tonics prophylactically to prevent colic.
- Often a treatment strategy for deficiency is guided by the basic principle: "For deficiency, tonify the mother." The Five-Element theory treats deficiency syndromes by tonifying the "mother" organ to strengthen the "son" organ. For example, in the case of Liver deficiency, one can tonify the Kidney (water element, mother organ) to indirectly tonify the Liver (wood element, son organ). In the case of Lung deficiency, one can tonify the Spleen (earth element, mother organ) to indirectly tonify the Lung (metal element, son organ).
- Lastly, one theory posits the importance of tonifying the Kidney and Spleen to treat deficiency syndromes. The basis for this theory is that Kidney *jing* (essence) is the source of prenatal health, and Spleen qi is the source of postnatal health. The Kidney, "the root of prenatal life," and the Spleen, "the root of postnatal life," have a mutually engendering relationship. They protect, support and reinforce each other; because of this close relationship, if one is healthy, so will be the other. Likewise, if one organ is weak, the other will soon be compromised. Thus, tonification of these two organs will support the normal functions of all the other organs and promote the health of the entire body. This particular supplemental strategy for tonification of deficiency disorders in animals has proven to be very effective, especially in aging animals.

Although veterinarians may be asked to treat single- or multiple-substance deficiencies, such as prescribing a tonic for geriatric animals and athletes, it is more common to use tonic formulas in combination with a formula or formulas from other categories. As patients become deficient in vital substances, they will accumulate pathogens in the interior, or become susceptible to exterior pathogens. Examples include the accumulation of dampness as a result of Spleen qi deficiency, cold as a result of yang deficiency, and a predisposition to wind-heat and wind-cold invasions as a result of *wei* (defensive) *qi* deficiency. Pattern differentiation is essential in these types of cases, and, in particular, identification of combined excess and deficiency conditions is crucial, so as not to make the condition worse by incorrect treatment. In general, it is common practice to first drain or clear the excess, and then tonify the deficiency. Animals that are weak and debilitated may often require both tonification and drainage simultaneously. In aging and chronically ill animals, tonic herbal formulas are frequently combined with Chinese food therapy programs to consolidate treatment effects and prevent relapse of various deficiency conditions.

Chapter 8 — Overview

SUBCATEGORIES OF ACTION

Tonic formulas are divided into six subcategories based on function:

1. **Qi-Tonifying Formulas**

These formulas primarily treat Spleen and Lung qi deficiencies. Spleen qi deficiencies manifest symptoms that pertain to the Spleen's function of transforming qi from food. Lung qi deficiencies present as problems with respiration and the immune system. Common clinical manifestations of qi deficiency include lethargy, general weakness, fatigue, weak extremities, muscle wasting and the inability to maintain or gain weight, exercise intolerance, heaves and asthma, a weak vocalization loose stools, diarrhea, lack of appetite, predisposition to respiratory and skin disease, a pale tongue, and a weak and/or thin pulse. In severe cases, there may be prolapse of organs such as the uterus or rectum. Qi tonics are typically sweet and warm; they tend to promote dampness and heat and impair the function of the middle *jiao*. Thus, they are often combined with qi-regulating herbs to prevent these problems from occurring.

Qi-tonifying herbs, such as *Ren Shen* (Radix et Rhizoma Ginseng), *Dang Shen* (Radix Codonopsis), *Huang Qi* (Radix Astragali), *Bai Zhu* (Rhizoma Atractylodis Macrocephalae), and *Gan Cao* (Radix et Rhizoma Glycyrrhizae), are of primary importance in these formulas. Representative formulas include *Si Jun Zi Tang* (Four-Gentlemen Decoction), *Shen Ling Bai Zhu San* (Ginseng, Poria, and Atractylodes Macrocephala Powder), *Bu Zhong Yi Qi Tang* (Tonify the Middle and Augment the Qi Decoction), and *Sheng Mai San* (Generate the Pulse Powder).

2. **Blood-Tonifying Formulas**

These formulas contain blood-tonifying herbs to treat blood deficiency syndromes, which often affect the Heart and Liver. Common clinical manifestations of blood deficiency include pale gums, excessive dandruff, poor general hair coat, dry nails and hooves that have a tendency to split and crack, restlessness at night, arrhythmias, insomnia, dry stools, a dry, pale to pale pink tongue, and a rapid, weak, and thready pulse. Mares and bitches may experience abnormal estrus cycles, infertility, behavioral disorders, and discomfort surrounding estrus. Blood tonics, like yin tonics, can be cloying for the middle *jiao*; in cases in which there is Spleen qi deficiency, these herbs and/or formulas should be used with caution.

Herbs commonly used to tonify the blood include *Shu Di Huang* (Radix Rehmanniae Praeparata), *Dang Gui* (Radix Angelicae Sinensis), *Bai Shao* (Radix Paeoniae Alba), and *E Jiao* (Colla Corii Asini). Representative formulas include *Si Wu Tang* (Four-Substance Decoction), *Gui Pi Tang* (Restore the Spleen Decoction), and *Dang Gui Bu Xue Tang* (Tangkuei Decoction to Tonify the Blood).

3. **Qi- and Blood-Tonifying Formulas**

These formulas use qi- and blood-tonifying herbs to treat qi and blood deficiencies simultaneously. Clinical manifestations of qi and blood deficiencies include exercise intolerance, poor appetite, fatigue, weak extremities, muscle atrophy, a pale tongue that may be wet, and a rapid, weak, thin pulse.

Qi- and blood-tonifying formulas incorporate both qi-tonifying herbs such as *Ren Shen* (Radix et Rhizoma Ginseng), *Huang Qi* (Radix Astragali), and *Bai Zhu* (Rhizoma Atractylodis Macrocephalae), and blood-tonifying herbs such as *Shu Di Huang* (Radix Rehmanniae Praeparata), *Dang Gui* (Radix Angelicae Sinensis), and *Bai Shao* (Radix Paeoniae Alba). Representative formulas include *Ba Zhen Tang* (Eight-Treasure Decoction), *Shi Quan Da Bu Tang* (All-Inclusive Great Tonifying Decoction), and *Ren Shen Yang Ying Tang* (Ginseng Decoction to Nourish the Nutritive Qi). Because of the interdependency of qi and blood, these formulas are commonly prescribed in clinical practice.

4. **Yin-Tonifying Formulas**

These formulas treat yin deficiency syndromes with yin-tonifying herbs. Yin deficiency is often associated with the Liver and Kidney, and involves the following common clinical manifestations: low

Chapter 8 — Overview

body condition scores, emaciation, poor hearing, deafness, poor vision, painful and weak back and stifles, orthopedic and dental developmental abnormalities, lameness, dry feces, irritability, insomnia, restlessness, panting excessively (especially at night), short urination, cool seeking, dry eyes and mouth, increased appetite, increased thirst, trembling and jerking during sleep, hypersensitivity to acupuncture, a red tongue with little coating, and a rapid and thready pulse that is weaker on the left side. Yin-tonifying formulas are nourishing, and, as such, are rich and cloying in nature. Most of them contain herbs to promote the circulation of qi and body fluids, to prevent these formulas from impairing digestion and water metabolism. Even so, they should be used with caution, especially in animals with weakness of the middle *jiao*.

Herbs commonly used to treat yin deficiency include *Shu Di Huang* (Radix Rehmanniae Praeparata), *Mai Dong* (Radix Ophiopogonis), and *Tian Dong* (Radix Asparagi). Representative formulas include *Liu Wei Di Huang Wan* (Six-Ingredient Pill with Rehmannia), *Zuo Gui Wan* (Restore the Left [Kidney] Pill), and *Da Bu Yin Wan* (Great Tonify the Yin Pill).

5. **Yang-Tonifying Formulas**

These formulas use yang-tonifying herbs to treat Kidney yang deficiency. Common clinical manifestations of Kidney yang deficiency include soreness and pain of the back and stifles, weakness and pain of the extremities, weakness of the rear quarters, arthritis, degenerative joint disease, shivering, cardiac disease, chronic heaves or asthma, aversion to cold, coldness in the extremities, lumbar region and ears, laminitis without palpable heat, fecal and urinary incontinence, frequent urination, infertility, a pale pink to purple tongue that may be swollen and wet, and a deep, weak, thin pulse that is weaker on the right side. Yang tonic herbs can be very warm in nature, and thus should not be used in cases of yin deficiency with heat; they can easily consume and damage yin by further increasing internal heat.

Herbs that are commonly used to tonify yang include *Fu Zi* (Radix Aconiti Lateralis Praeparata), *Rou Gui* (Cortex Cinnamomi), *Du Zhong* (Cortex Eucommiae), *Ba Ji Tian* (Radix Morindae Officinalis), and *Bu Gu Zhi* (Fructus Psoraleae). Representative formulas include *Jin Gui Shen Qi Wan* (Kidney Qi Pill from the Golden Cabinet), and *You Gui Wan* (Restore the Right [Kidney] Pill).

6. **Yin- and Yang-Tonifying Formulas**

These formulas treat concurrent yin and yang deficiencies. The clinical signs are variable and include a combination of the clinical signs seen in both yin and yang deficiencies. Clinically, there will be a predominance of either yin or yang deficiency. The treatment strategy will depend on which deficiency is most predominant at the time, and the animal must be carefully monitored in order to make the appropriate changes or modifications to the herbal therapy over time.

Herbs that tonify yin include *Shu Di Huang* (Radix Rehmanniae Praeparata), *Mai Dong* (Radix Ophiopogonis), *Tian Dong* (Radix Asparagi), *Gui Ban* (Plastrum Testudinis), and *Zhi Mu* (Rhizoma Anemarrhenae). Herbs commonly used to tonify yang include *Fu Zi* (Radix Aconiti Lateralis Praeparata), *Rou Gui* (Cortex Cinnamomi), *Du Zhong* (Cortex Eucommiae), *Ba Ji Tian* (Radix Morindae Officinalis), and *Bu Gu Zhi* (Fructus Psoraleae). Representative formulas that tonify both yin and yang include *Di Huang Yin Zi* (Rehmannia Decoction) and *Gui Lu Er Xian Jiao* (Tortoise Shell and Deer Antler Syrup).

CAUTIONS / CONTRAINDICATIONS

- It is important to differentiate between deficient and excess conditions. While tonic herbs are prescribed to supplement deficiencies, clearing or draining herbs are used to eliminate excess conditions. Tonic herbs should not be used in excess conditions, as they will only worsen the condition. Clearing or draining herbs must not be used in cases of deficiency, as they will aggravate the condition by draining vital substances.
- Frequent or long-term use of tonic herbs may create stagnation. Animals with deficiencies of the middle *jiao* are often too weak to tolerate strong tonification and will often vomit and/or have diarrhea

Chapter 8 — Overview

when given tonic herbs. Therefore, tonic herbs should be combined with herbs that strengthen the Spleen, harmonize the Stomach, and move qi and blood to ensure minimal side effects.

- Tonic formulas are most effective when taken on an empty stomach or before meals for better absorption. However, many animals will not take herbs unless they are mixed into food, and are usually fed twice daily. In this case, it is best to give herbs mixed with the smallest amount of food possible, wait an hour, and then feed the remainder of the animal's food. In severe cases of deficiency, it is best to give tonic herbs three times daily, rather than twice.

PROCESSING

Most tonic herbs and formulas are cooked for a longer period of time at low temperature to ensure complete extraction of the active ingredients.

PHARMACOLOGICAL EFFECTS & CLINICAL APPLICATIONS

Tonic formulas are divided into six subcategories based on their traditional therapeutic actions. Moreover, these six subcategories have contrasting pharmacological effects and clinical applications.

1. **Qi-tonifying formulas** mainly treat Spleen and Lung qi deficiencies. Although they are certainly effective, there is little clinical research on general symptoms of qi deficiency, such as lethargy, general weakness, exercise intolerance, fatigue and weak extremities. Instead, most of the research focuses on treatment of specific biomedical disorders affecting the gastrointestinal system, such as gastritis, peptic ulcer, colitis, and irritable bowel syndrome.

   Many of these formulas are now used in cancer treatment, since they have demonstrated remarkable effects in alleviating the side effects associated with chemotherapy and radiation. Lastly, some formulas have antineoplastic effects based on performance during *in vitro* and *in vivo* studies.

- **Gastrointestinal disorders**: Qi-tonifying formulas treat a wide variety of gastrointestinal disorders. Pharmacologically, they have significant influence on the stomach and intestines, including but not limited to gastroprotective,[1] antiulcer effect,[2] a prokinetic action on gastric emptying,[3] and a regulatory effect on the intestines to either increase or decrease peristalsis.[4,5,6,7,8] Clinically, *Si Jun Zi Tang* (Four-Gentlemen Decoction) has been used to treat chronic gastritis,[9] peptic ulcer,[10,11] ulcerative colitis,[12] irritable bowel syndrome,[13] and epigastric or abdominal pain.[14] *Liu Jun Zi Tang* (Six-Gentlemen Decoction) has been used to treat abdominal pain,[15] gastritis,[16] duodenal ulcer,[17] indigestion,[18] and stomatitis.[19] *Shen Ling Bai Zhu San* (Ginseng, Poria, and Atractylodes Macrocephala Powder) has been used to address chronic colitis,[20] irritable bowel syndrome,[21] diarrhea,[22] and superficial gastritis.[23] Lastly, *Bu Zhong Yi Qi Tang* (Tonify the Middle and Augment the Qi Decoction) treats gastritis,[24] constipation,[25] and diarrhea.[26]
- **Morning sickness**: Three qi-tonifying formulas have been shown to treat nausea and vomiting. *Liu Jun Zi Tang* (Six-Gentlemen Decoction) is effective for morning sickness.[27] *Xiang Sha Liu Jun Zi Tang* (Six-Gentlemen Decoction with Aucklandia and Amomum) successfully treats morning sickness and anorexia.[28,29] *Bu Zhong Yi Qi Tang* (Tonify the Middle and Augment the Qi Decoction) relieves nausea and vomiting.[30]
- **Chronic fatigue syndrome**: *Bu Zhong Yi Qi Tang* (Tonify the Middle and Augment the Qi Decoction) has been used successfully to treat chronic fatigue syndrome.[31]
- **Supportive treatment for chemoprotective and radioprotective effect**: Many qi-tonifying formulas demonstrate beneficial effects to alleviate the side effects associated with chemotherapy and radiation. For example, *Si Jun Zi Tang* (Four-Gentlemen Decoction) has a hematopoietic effect to increase both white and red blood cell counts in subjects treated with radiation.[32,33] *Liu Jun Zi Tang* (Six-Gentlemen Decoction) has shown *in vitro* antineoplastic effect by inhibiting the growth of cancer cells in mice.[34] *Shen Ling Bai Zhu San* (Ginseng, Poria, and Atractylodes Macrocephala Powder) has been used successfully to relieve nausea and vomiting associated with chemotherapy and radiation.[35,36] Lastly, *Bu Zhong Yi Qi Tang* (Tonify the Middle and Augment the Qi Decoction) treats immunosuppression induced by mitomycin C, and leukopenia induced by cyclophosphamide.[37,38]

Chapter 8 — Overview

- **Cancer**: Most qi-tonifying formulas are used as supportive therapy during chemotherapy and radiation, as discussed above. However, some formulas also have direct antineoplastic effects. *Si Jun Zi Tang* (Four-Gentlemen Decoction) has been shown to inhibit the growth of tumor cells in mice with esophageal and lung cancer.[39] *Liu Jun Zi Tang* (Six-Gentlemen Decoction) has been shown to inhibit the growth of cancer cells in mice by increasing macrophages and natural killer cells.[40] Lastly, *Bu Zhong Yi Qi Tang* (Tonify the Middle and Augment the Qi Decoction) has antineoplastic effects by enhancing natural killer cell activity and suppressing the proliferation of certain cancer cells.[41,42]

2. **Blood-tonifying formulas** commonly treat a wide variety of disorders, including hematological, reproductive and dermatological disorders.
   - **Hematological disorders**: As the name implies, blood-tonifying formulas treat blood-related disorders, such as anemia,[43,44] leucopenia,[45,46] and thrombopenic purpura.[47,48] The mechanisms of these effects are attributed primarily to hematopoietic effects that increase blood cell production.[49,50] Formulas commonly used to treat hematological disorders include *Gui Pi Tang* (Restore the Spleen Decoction) and *Dang Gui Bu Xue Tang* (Tangkuei Decoction to Tonify the Blood).
   - **Obstetrics**: Several blood-tonifying formulas have been used to treat various pregnancy-related disorders and/or complications. For example, breeched presentation may be corrected with *Si Wu Tang* (Four-Substance Decoction) and *Dang Gui Shao Yao San* (Tangkuei and Peony Powder).[51,52] Habitual miscarriage may be prevented with a combination of *Dang Gui Shao Yao San* (Tangkuei and Peony Powder) and *Chai Ling Tang* (Bupleurum and Poria Decoction).[53,54]
   - **Infertility**: According to clinical studies, blood-tonifying formulas have been used successfully to treat infertility from various causes. Representative formulas include *Si Wu Tang* (Four-Substance Decoction),[55] *Tao Hong Si Wu Tang* (Four-Substance Decoction with Safflower and Peach Pit),[56] and *Dang Gui Shao Yao San* (Tangkuei and Peony Powder).[57]
   - **Dermatological disorders**: Many skin disorders have been treated successfully with blood-tonifying formulas. The clinical applications include itching,[58,59] psoriasis,[60,61,62] urticaria,[63,64] eczema, acne,[65] and chloasma.[66] Furthermore, some formulas have also been shown to effectively treat dermatitis induced by cosmetics and penicillin.[67,68] Representative formulas include *Si Wu Tang* (Four-Substance Decoction), *Tao Hong Si Wu Tang* (Four-Substance Decoction with Safflower and Peach Pit), and *Dang Gui Shao Yao San* (Tangkuei and Peony Powder), as they have antipruritic and anti-inflammatory effects to relieve itching and inflammation of the skin.[69,70]
   - **Others**: Blood-tonifying formulas may also be used for other conditions, such as cardiovascular (arrhythmia, angina pectoris, and hypotension),[71,72,73] ophthalmic (optic nerve atrophy, optic neuritis, and cataract),[74,75,76] hepatic disorders (hepatitis),[77] and many others.

3. **Qi- and blood-tonifying formulas** are composed of herbs that supplement qi and blood. The pharmacological effects of these formulas include those already mentioned above for qi-tonifying and blood-tonifying formulas, such as gastrointestinal disorders, hematological disorders, and reproductive disorders. Historically, these formulas have been used to treat pregnancy-related disorders, such as infertility,[78] habitual miscarriage,[79,80] morning sickness,[81] breeched presentation,[82] and postpartum care.[83]

   Today, several of these formulas have demonstrated marked chemoprotective and radioprotective effects, and are now commonly used as supportive treatments for patients with cancer.[84,85] These, however, are just some of the many clinical applications of qi- and blood-tonifying formulas. Representative formulas include *Ba Zhen Tang* (Eight-Treasure Decoction), *Shi Quan Da Bu Tang* (All-Inclusive Great Tonifying Decoction), and *Ren Shen Yang Ying Tang* (Ginseng Decoction to Nourish the Nutritive Qi).

4. **Yin-tonifying formulas** tonify yin and generate body fluids; they primarily treat disorders associated with Kidney, Liver, Lung, and Stomach yin deficiencies. These formulas treat an extremely wide

Chapter 8 — Overview

range and variety of disorders, and the summary below is only a brief attempt to identify the most common and significant applications.

- **Reproductive disorders**: Many yin-tonifying formulas have marked influences on the reproductive system, and have been used successfully to treat sexual and reproductive disorders, such as sexual dysfunction,[86,87] male infertility,[88,89] and female infertility.[90,91] The mechanisms of action vary, but have been attributed in part to the stimulation and regulation of both male and female sex hormones.[92,93] Exemplar formulas include *Liu Wei Di Huang Wan* (Six-Ingredient Pill with Rehmannia), *Zuo Gui Wan* (Restore the Left [Kidney] Pill), and *Er Xian Tang* (Two-Immortal Decoction).
- **Gynecological disorders**: Many yin-tonifying formulas have marked effects in treating gynecological disorders. For example, menopausal symptoms may be alleviated with *Liu Wei Di Huang Wan* (Six-Ingredient Pill with Rehmannia),[94] *Qi Ju Di Huang Wan* (Lycium Fruit, Chrysanthemum, and Rehmannia Pill),[95] and *Er Xian Tang* (Two-Immortal Decoction).[96] Premenstrual syndrome may be alleviated with *Yi Guan Jian* (Linking Decoction).[97] Uterine bleeding and amenorrhea may be treated with *Zuo Gui Wan* (Restore the Left [Kidney] Pill).[98,99]
- **Respiratory disorders**: Some yin-tonifying formulas have been used effectively to treat lung disorders. For example, *Liu Wei Di Huang Wan* (Six-Ingredient Pill with Rehmannia) has been used for bronchial asthma,[100] *Da Bu Yin Wan* (Great Tonify the Yin Pill) has been used for pulmonary tuberculosis,[101] and *Bu Fei E Jiao Tang* (Tonify the Lung Decoction with Ass-Hide Gelatin) has been used to treat cough due to various causes, such as asthma, bronchiectasis, bronchitis, pulmonary tuberculosis, and whooping cough.[102]
- **Gastrointestinal disorders**: Some yin-tonifying formulas have been used successfully to treat gastrointestinal disorders, such as atrophic gastritis,[103,104] peptic ulcer,[105] and chronic esophagitis.[106] The mechanisms of action has been attributed in part to the enhanced protection of the gastric mucosa.[107] Exemplar formulas include *Liu Wei Di Huang Wan* (Six-Ingredient Pill with Rehmannia) and *Yi Guan Jian* (Linking Decoction).
- **Diabetes mellitus**: Many yin-tonifying formulas successfully treat diabetes mellitus. Pharmacologically, these formulas effectively decrease plasma glucose levels.[108] Furthermore, some of these formulas continue to exert hypoglycemic effects in cases in which the pancreas has been surgically removed.[109] Clinically, formulas that have been used successfully in the treatment of diabetes mellitus include *Liu Wei Di Huang Wan* (Six-Ingredient Pill with Rehmannia),[110] *Zhi Bai Di Huang Wan* (Anemarrhena, Phellodendron, and Rehmannia Pill),[111] and *Mai Wei Di Huang Wan* (Ophiopogonis, Schisandra, and Rehmannia Pill).[112]
- **Hypertension**: Many yin-tonifying formulas have a marked influence on the cardiovascular system. Specifically, formulas that have been used to treat hypertension include *Liu Wei Di Huang Wan* (Six-Ingredient Pill with Rehmannia),[113] *Zhi Bai Di Huang Wan* (Anemarrhena, Phellodendron, and Rehmannia Pill),[114] *Qi Ju Di Huang Wan* (Lycium Fruit, Chrysanthemum, and Rehmannia Pill),[115,116] and *Yi Guan Jian* (Linking Decoction).[117]
- **Kidney disorders**: Some yin-tonifying formulas have shown nephroprotective effects, such as increasing blood perfusion to the kidneys, improving kidney function, and reducing the presence of protein and uric acid in the urine.[118] Clinically, *Liu Wei Di Huang Wan* (Six-Ingredient Pill with Rehmannia) has been used to treat chronic nephritis,[119] nephrotic syndrome,[120] chronic renal failure,[121] and periodic paralysis.[122] *Zhi Bai Di Huang Wan* (Anemarrhena, Phellodendron, and Rehmannia Pill) has been used to treat nephrotic syndrome.[123] Lastly, *Qi Ju Di Huang Wan* (Lycium Fruit, Chrysanthemum, and Rehmannia Pill) has been used to treat chronic nephritis.[124]
- **Liver disorders**: Some yin-tonifying formulas have hepatoprotective effects against damage induced by such substances as carbon tetrachloride, thioacetamide, and prednisolone.[125,126,127] Clinically, *Liu Wei Di Huang Wan* (Six-Ingredient Pill with Rehmannia) has been used to treat chronic hepatitis,[128] *Er Zhi Wan* (Two-Ultimate Pill) for hepatitis B,[129] and *Yi Guan Jian* (Linking Decoction) for liver diseases, such as hepatitis, liver cirrhosis, and liver cancer.[130,131]
- **Thyroid disorders**: *Liu Wei Di Huang Wan* (Six-Ingredient Pill with Rehmannia) has been used successfully to treat hyperthyroidism and thyroid adenoma.[132,133] *Yi Guan Jian* (Linking Decoction) has been used to treat hyperthyroidism.[134]

Chapter 8 — Overview

5. **Yang-tonifying formulas** mainly treat sexual, reproductive, prostate, and kidney disorders.
   - **Sexual and reproductive disorders**: Many yang-tonifying formulas have marked effects in treating sexual and reproductive disorders including sexual dysfunction,[135] male infertility,[136,137] and female infertility.[138,139] The pharmacological effects have been attributed in part to the stimulation and regulation of both male and female sex hormones.[140] Exemplar formulas include *Jin Gui Shen Qi Wan* (Kidney Qi Pill from the Golden Cabinet), *Ba Wei Di Huang Wan* (Eight-Ingredient Pill with Rehmannia), *Ji Sheng Shen Qi Wan* (Kidney Qi Pill from Formulas that Aid the Living), and *Zuo Gui Wan* (Restore the Left [Kidney] Pill).
   - **Prostate disorders**: Prostatic hypertrophy has been treated successfully with Kidney yang tonic formulas, such as *Jin Gui Shen Qi Wan* (Kidney Qi Pill from the Golden Cabinet) and *Ba Wei Di Huang Wan* (Eight-Ingredient Pill with Rehmannia).[141,142,143]
   - **Urinary disorders**: Yang-tonifying formulas are effective in treating urinary disorders (with or without enlarged prostate), such as dysuria, [144] frequent urination,[145] and urinary incontinence.[146] Representative formulas include *Jin Gui Shen Qi Wan* (Kidney Qi Pill from the Golden Cabinet) and *Ba Wei Di Huang Wan* (Eight-Ingredient Pill with Rehmannia).
   - **Kidney disorders**: Some yang-tonifying formulas treat kidney disorders. *Jin Gui Shen Qi Wan* (Kidney Qi Pill from the Golden Cabinet) has been used to treat chronic glomerulonephritis.[147] *You Gui Wan* (Restore the Right [Kidney] Pill) and *Ji Sheng Shen Qi Wan* (Kidney Qi Pill from Formulas that Aid the Living) have been used to treat nephrotic syndrome.[148,149]

6. **Yin- and yang-tonifying formulas**, as the name implies, treat concurrent yin and yang deficiencies. Two exemplar formulas, *Gui Lu Er Xian Jiao* (Tortoise Shell and Deer Antler Syrup) and *Qi Bao Mei Ran Wan* (Seven-Treasure Special Pill for Beautiful Whiskers), can treat a wide variety of disorders of yin and yang deficiencies, such as impotence,[150] male infertility,[151] and osteoporosis.[152,153]

References

1. Arakawa T, Higuchi K, Fujiwara Y, Watanabe T, Tominaga K, Hayakawa T, Kuroki T. Gastroprotection by Liu-Jun-Zi-Tang (TJ-43): possible mediation of nitric oxide but not prostaglandins or sulfhydryls. Drugs Under Experimental & Clinical Research. 1999; 25(5):207-10.
2. *Bei Jing Zhong Yi Yao Da Xue Xue Bao* (Journal of Beijing University of Medicine and Medicinals), 1994; 17(5):57.
3. Tatsuta M, Iishi H. Effect of treatment with liu-jun-zi-tang (TJ-43) on gastric emptying and gastrointestinal symptoms in dyspeptic patients. Aliment Pharmacol Ther. 1993 Aug; 7(4):459-62.
4. *Xin Zhong Yi* (New Chinese Medicine), 1978; 5:53.
5. *Nan Jing Zhong Yi Xue Yuan Xue Bao* (Journal of Nanjing University of Traditional Chinese Medicine), 1989; 1:36.
6. *Zhong Yi Fang Ji Xian Dai Yan Jiu* (Modern Study of Medical Formulas in Traditional Chinese Medicine), 1997; 499-500.
7. *Xin Yi Yao Xue Za Zhi* (New Journal of Medicine and Herbology), 1979; 3:129.
8. *Zhong Yao Yao Li Yu Lin Chuang* (Pharmacology and Clinical Applications of Chinese Herbs), 1987; 2:4.
9. *Zhong Yi Fang Ji Xian Dai Yan Jiu* (Modern Study of Medical Formulas in Traditional Chinese Medicine), 1997; 480-481.
10. *Xin Zhong Yi* (New Chinese Medicine), 1982; 11:12.
11. *Zhong Yi Za Zhi* (Journal of Chinese Medicine), 1980; 21(12):947.
12. *Zhong Yi Za Zhi* (Journal of Chinese Medicine), 1987; 10:28.
13. *Shang Hai Zhong Yi Za Zhi* (Shanghai Journal of Chinese Medicine), 1986; 1:12.
14. *He Nan Zhong Yi* (Henan Chinese Medicine), 1986; 3:1.
15. *Shan Xi Xin Zhong Yi* (New Shanxi Chinese Medicine), 1984; 1:23.
16. *Zhong Yi Ming Fang Lin Chuang Xin Yong* (Contemporary Clinical Applications of Classic Chinese Formulas), 2001; 160.
17. *Si Chuan Zhong Yi* (Sichuan Chinese Medicine), 1989; 2:21.
18. *Zhong Yi Ming Fang Lin Chuang Xin Yong* (Contemporary Clinical Applications of Classic Chinese Formulas), 2001; 161.
19. *Shi Yong Zhong Yi Za Zhi* (Journal of Practical Chinese Medicine), 1997; 2:11.
20. *Shan Dong Zhong Yi Za Zhi* (Shandong Journal of Chinese Medicine), 1991; 10(6):24.
21. *Shan Xi Zhong Yi* (Shanxi Chinese Medicine), 1998; 7:312.
22. *Xin Yi Yao Xue Za Zhi* (New Journal of Medicine and Herbology), 1979; 3:129.
23. *Zhong Yi Fang Ji Xian Dai Yan Jiu* (Modern Study of Medical Formulas in Traditional Chinese Medicine), 1997; 509.
24. *Jiang Su Zhong Yi Za Zhi* (Jiangsu Journal of Chinese Medicine), 1997; 11:514.
25. *Zhong Yi Fang Ji Xian Dai Yan Jiu* (Modern Study of Medical Formulas in Traditional Chinese Medicine), 1997; 529.
26. *Shi Yong Zhong Xi Yi Jie He Za Zhi* (Practical Journal of Integrated Chinese and Western Medicines), 1998; 3:262.
27. *Shang Hai Zhong Yi Yao Za Zhi* (Shanghai Journal of Chinese Medicine and Herbology), 1959; 7:48.
28. *Zhong Hua Fu Chan Ke Za Zhi* (Chinese Journal of Obstetrics and Gynecology), 1960; 8(1):33.
29. *Gan Su Zhong Yi Xue Yuan Xue Bao* (Journal of Gansu University of Chinese Medicine), 1995; 2:26.

Chapter 8 — Overview

30. *He Bei Zhong Yi* (Hebei Chinese Medicine), 1986; 6:13.
31. *Guo Wai Yi Xue Zhong Yi Zhong Yao Fen Ce* (Monograph of Chinese Herbology from Foreign Medicine), 1993; 15(6):27.
32. *Zhong Yi Fang Ji Xian Dai Yan Jiu* (Modern Study of Medical Formulas in Traditional Chinese Medicine), 1997; 477.
33. Hsu HY, Yang JJ, Lian SL, Ho YH, Lin CC. Recovery of the hematopoietic system by Si-Jun-Zi-Tang in whole body irradiated mice. J Ethnopharmacol. 1996 Nov; 54(2-3):69-75.
34. *Shi Yong Zhong Liu Xue Za Zhi* (Practical Journal of Cancer), 1987; 1(4):6.
35. *Zhong Yi Yao Xin Xi* (Information on Chinese Medicine and Herbology), 1995; 6:27.
36. *Gui Zhou Yi Yao* (Medicine and Medicinals from Guizhou), 1985; 3:7.
37. Kido T, Mori K, Daikuhara H, Tsuchiya H, Ishige A, Sasaki H. The protective effect of hochu-ekki-to (TJ-41), a Japanese herbal medicine, against HSV-1 infection in mitomycin C-treated mice. Anticancer Res. 2000 Nov-Dec; 20(6A):4109-13.
38. Kaneko M, Kawakita T, Kumazawa Y, Takimoto H, Nomoto K, Yoshikawa T. Accelerated recovery from cyclophosphamide-induced leukopenia in mice administered a Japanese ethical herbal drug, Hochu-ekki-to. Immunopharmacology. 1999 Nov; 44(3):223-31.
39. *Shang Hai Zhong Yi Yao Za Zhi* (Shanghai Journal of Chinese Medicine and Herbology), 1984; 1:2.
40. *Shi Yong Zhong Liu Xue Za Zhi* (Practical Journal of Cancer), 1987; 1(4):6.
41. Kao ST, Yeh CC, Hsieh CC, Yang MD, Lee MR, Liu HS, Lin JG. The Chinese medicine Bu-Zhong-Yi-Qi-Tang inhibited proliferation of hepatoma cell lines by inducing apoptosis via G0/G1 arrest. Life Sciences. 2001 Aug 17; 69(13):1485-96.
42. Cho JM, Sato N, Kikuchi K. Prophylactic anti-tumor effect of Hochu-ekki-to (TJ41) by enhancing natural killer cell activity. In Vivo. 1991 Jul-Aug; 5(4):389-91.
43. *Shan Xi Zhong Yi Xue Yuan Xue Bao* (Journal of Shanxi University School of Chinese Medicine), 1988; 1:29.
44. *Guo Wai Yi Yao Zhi Wu Yao Fen Ce* (Monograph of Foreign Botanical Medicine), 1993; 15(3):44.
45. *An Hui Zhong Yi Xue Yuan Xue Bao* (Journal of Anhui University School of Medicine), 1987; 6(3):43.
46. *Gan Su Zhong Yi* (Gansu Chinese Medicine), 1998; 5:28.
47. *Zhong Yi Za Zhi* (Journal of Chinese Medicine), 1984; 25(5):356.
48. *Bei Jing Zhong Yi Za Zhi* (Beijing Journal of Chinese Medicine), 1993; 3:227.
49. *Zhong Yao Yao Li Yu Lin Chuang* (Pharmacology and Clinical Applications of Chinese Herbs), 1992; 152.
50. *Hei Long Jiang Zhong Yi Yao* (Heilongjiang Chinese Medicine and Herbology), 1989; 4:41.
51. *Shan Xi Zhong Yi* (Shanxi Chinese Medicine), 1991; 7(3):22.
52. *Shan Xi Zhong Yi* (Shanxi Chinese Medicine), 1998; 12:534.
53. Fujii T, Kanai T, Kozuma S, Hamai Y, Hyodo H, Yamashita T, Miki A, Unno N, Taketani Y. Theoretical basis for herbal medicines, Tokishakuyaku-san and Sairei-to, in the treatment of autoimmunity-related recurrent abortion by correcting T helper-1/T helper-2 balance. American Journal of Reproductive Immunology. 2000 Dec; 44(6):342-6.
54. Fujii T. Herbal factors in the treatment of autoimmunity-related habitual abortion. Vitam Horm. 2002; 65:333-44.
55. *Zhong Yi Za Zhi* (Journal of Chinese Medicine), 1986; 10:35.
56. *He Bei Zhong Yi* (Hebei Chinese Medicine), 1998; 15(2):26.
57. *Zhong Cheng Yao Yan Jiu* (Research of Chinese Patent Medicine), 1984; (10):30.
58. *Zhong Yi Za Zhi* (Journal of Chinese Medicine), 1988; 8:608.
59. *Shi Yong Zhong Xi Yi Jie He Za Zhi* (Practical Journal of Integrated Chinese and Western Medicines), 1991; 4:41.
60. *Yun Nan Zhong Yi Za Zhi* (Yunan Journal of Chinese Medicine), 1985; 6:25.
61. *Shan Xi Zhong Yi* (Shanxi Chinese Medicine), 1990; 11(2):106.
62. *Zhong Yi Za Zhi* (Journal of Chinese Medicine), 1988; 29(5):366.
63. *Zhong Xi Yi Jie He Za Zhi* (Journal of Integrated Chinese and Western Medicine), 1991; 4:242.
64. *He Bei Zhong Yi* (Hebei Chinese Medicine), 1995; 17(4):47.
65. Higaki S, Toyomoto T, Morohashi M. Seijo-bofu-to, Jumi-haidoku-to and Toki-shakuyaku-san suppress rashes and incidental symptoms in acne patients. Drugs Exp Clin Res. 2002; 28(5):193-6.
66. *Bei Jing Zhong Yi Xue Yuan Xue Bao* (Journal of Beijing University School of Medicine), 1987; 5:36.
67. *Zhong Yi Yao Xin Xi* (Information on Chinese Medicine and Herbology), 1992; 9(5):36.
68. *Nei Meng Gu Zhong Yi Yao* (Traditional Chinese Medicine and Medicinals of Inner Mongolia), 1993; (3):1.
69. Dai Y, But PP, Chan YP, Matsuda H, Kubo M. Antipruritic and antiinflammatory effects of aqueous extract from Si-Wu-Tang. Biol Pharm Bull. 2002 Sep; 25(9):1175-8.
70. *Zhong Guo Zhong Yao Za Zhi* (People's Republic of China Journal of Chinese Herbology), 1994; 19(11):680.
71. *Shan Xi Yi Kan* (Shanxi Journal of Medicine), 1995; 15(9):399.
72. *Tian Jin Yi Yao* (Tianjin Medicine and Herbology), 1972; 26.
73. *Si Chuan Zhong Yi* (Sichuan Chinese Medicine), 1995; 9:20.
74. *Yan Ke Tong Xun* (Journal of Ophthalmology), 1987; 3:13.
75. *Zhong Yi Fang Ji Xian Dai Yan Jiu* (Modern Study of Medical Formulas in Traditional Chinese Medicine), 1997; 1103.
76. *Zhong Yi Fang Ji Xian Dai Yan Jiu* (Modern Study of Medical Formulas in Traditional Chinese Medicine), 1997; 1103.
77. *Zhong Yi Za Zhi* (Journal of Chinese Medicine), 1985; 5:32.
78. *Zhong Yi Fang Ji Xian Dai Yan Jiu* (Modern Study of Medical Formulas in Traditional Chinese Medicine), 1997; 639.
79. *Fu Jian Zhong Yi Yao* (Fujian Chinese Medicine and Herbology), 1960; 10:3.
80. *He Bei Zhong Yi* (Hebei Chinese Medicine), 1991; 13(3):24.
81. *Xin Jiang Zhong Yi Yao* (Xinjiang Chinese Medicine and Herbology), 1991; 1:32.
82. *Shan Dong Zhong Yi Za Zhi* (Shandong Journal of Chinese Medicine), 1996; 12:545.

Chapter 8 — Overview

83. Ushiroyama T, Sakuma K, Souen H, Nakai G, Morishima S, Yasuda K, Orino I, Ueki M. Therapeutic effects of Kyuki-chouketsu-in in restoring postpartum physical condition. American Journal of Chinese Medicine. 2003; 31(3):437-44.
84. Zee-Cheng RK. Shi-quan-da-bu-tang (ten significant tonic decoction), SQT. A potent Chinese biological response modifier in cancer immunotherapy, potentiation and detoxification of anticancer drugs. Methods Find Exp Clin Pharmacol. 1992 Nov; 14(9):725-36.
85. Miura S, Takimoto H, Yoshikai Y, Kumazawa Y, Yamada A, Nomoto K. Protective effect of Ren-Shen-Yang-Rong-Tang (Ninjin-youei-to) in mice with drug-induced leukopenia against Pseudomonas aeruginosa infection. Int J Immunopharmacol. 1992 Oct; 14(7):1249-57.
86. *Nan Jing Yi Xue Yuan Xue Bao* (Journal of Nanjing University of Medicine), 1988; 4:331.
87. *Si Chuan Zhong Yi* (Sichuan Chinese Medicine), 1995; 5:30.
88. *Hu Bei Zhong Yi Za Zhi* (Hubei Journal of Chinese Medicine), 1996; 2:24.
89. *Guang Xi Zhong Yi Yao* (Guangxi Chinese Medicine and Herbology), 1996; 2:43.
90. Chao SL, Huang LW, Yen HR. Pregnancy in premature ovarian failure after therapy using Chinese herbal medicine. Chang Gung Medical Journal. 2003 Jun; 26(6):449-52.
91. *Zhong Yi Fang Ji Xian Dai Yan Jiu* (Modern Study of Medical Formulas in Traditional Chinese Medicine), 1997; 766.
92. *Zhong Yi Fang Ji Xian Dai Yan Jiu* (Modern Study of Medical Formulas in Traditional Chinese Medicine), 1997; 709.
93. *Zhong Yi Ming Fang Lin Chuang Xin Yong* (Contemporary Clinical Applications of Classic Chinese Formulas), 2001; 205.
94. *Zhong Xi Yi Jie He Za Zhi* (Journal of Integrated Chinese and Western Medicine), 1986; 6:336.
95. *Shi Zhen Guo Yao Yan Jiu* (Research of Shizhen Herbs), 1998; 1:11.
96. *He Bei Zhong Yi* (Hebei Chinese Medicine), 1995; 17(4):14.
97. *Shan Xi Yi Kan* (Shanxi Journal of Medicine), 1992; 5:201.
98. *Hu Nan Zhong Yi Za Zhi* (Hunan Journal of Chinese Medicine), 1997; 3:57.
99. *Zhong Yi Za Zhi* (Journal of Chinese Medicine), 1984; 7:35.
100. *Shen De Yan Jiu* (Research of Kidney), 1981; 19.
101. *Xin Zhong Yi* (New Chinese Medicine), 1975; (4):40.
102. *Zhong Yi Fang Ji Xian Dai Yan Jiu* (Modern Study of Medical Formulas in Traditional Chinese Medicine), 1997; 6:25.
103. *Shan Xi Zhong Yi* (Shanxi Chinese Medicine), 1999; 4:161.
104. *Xin Jiang Zhong Yi Yao* (Xinjiang Chinese Medicine and Herbology), 1994; 4:13.
105. *Gui Zhou Yi Yao* (Medicine and Medicinals from Guizhou), 1991; 5:307.
106. *Zhong Yi Za Zhi* (Journal of Chinese Medicine), 1999; 4:243.
107. *Gui Yang Yi Xue Yuan Xue Bao* (Journal of Guiyang Medical University), 1986; 2:42.
108. *Guo Wai Yi Xue* (Foreign Medicine), 1986; 4:11.
109. *Zhong Yi Fang Ji Xian Dai Yan Jiu* (Modern Study of Medical Formulas in Traditional Chinese Medicine), 1997; 727.
110. *Hu Bei Zhong Yi Za Zhi* (Hubei Journal of Chinese Medicine), 1987; 3:14.
111. *Shang Hai Zhong Yi Yao Za Zhi* (Shanghai Journal of Chinese Medicine and Herbology), 1991; 10:23.
112. *Si Chuan Zhong Yi* (Sichuan Chinese Medicine), 1989; 3:25.
113. *Hei Long Jiang Zhong Yi Yao* (Heilongjiang Chinese Medicine and Herbology), 1987; 1:40.
114. *Zhong Cheng Yao* (Study of Chinese Patent Medicine), 1995; 4:51.
115. *Zhong Yao Yao Li Yu Lin Chuang* (Pharmacology and Clinical Applications of Chinese Herbs), 1992; 3:35.
116. *Xin Zhong Yi* (New Chinese Medicine), 1999; 3:12.
117. *Zhong Yi Za Zhi* (Journal of Chinese Medicine), 1983; 3:37.
118. *Zhong Yi Fang Ji Xian Dai Yan Jiu* (Modern Study of Medical Formulas in Traditional Chinese Medicine), 1997; 710.
119. *Jiang Xi Zhong Yi Yao* (Jiangxi Chinese Medicine and Herbology), 1998; 6:26.
120. *Zhe Jiang Zhong Yi Za Zhi* (Zhejiang Journal of Chinese Medicine), 1988; 6:244.
121. *Shi Yong Zhong Yi Nei Ke Za Zhi* (Journal of Practical Chinese Internal Medicine), 1993; 3:142.
122. *Zhong Yi Za Zhi* (Journal of Chinese Medicine), 1993; 1:61.
123. *Shi Yong Zhong Yi Za Zhi* (Journal of Practical Chinese Medicine), 1995; 6:10.
124. *Shi Yong Zhong Xi Yi Jie He Za Zhi* (Practical Journal of Integrated Chinese and Western Medicines), 1993; 1:41).
125. *Zhong Guo Yao Ke Da Xue Xue Bao* (Journal of University of Chinese Herbology), 1989; 6:951.
126. *Zhong Guo Zhong Yao Za Zhi* (People's Republic of China Journal of Chinese Herbology), 1992; (9):531.
127. *Zhong Yao Yao Li Yu Lin Chuang* (Pharmacology and Clinical Applications of Chinese Herbs), 1989; 6:14.
128. *Nei Meng Gu Zhong Yi Yao* (Traditional Chinese Medicine and Medicinals of Inner Mongolia), 1998; 1:4.
129. *Zhe Jiang Zhong Yi Xue Yuan Xue Bao* (Journal of Zhejiang University of Chinese Medicine), 1997; 3:35.
130. *Shan Xi Yi Kan* (Shanxi Journal of Medicine), 1989; 7:292.
131. *Fu Jian Zhong Yi Yao* (Fujian Chinese Medicine and Herbology; 1995; 4:33.
132. *Zhong Yi Fang Ji Xian Dai Yan Jiu* (Modern Study of Medical Formulas in Traditional Chinese Medicine), 1997; 712.
133. *Shan Xi Zhong Yi* (Shanxi Chinese Medicine), 1995; 16(11):485.
134. *Hu Bei Zhong Yi Za Zhi* (Hubei Journal of Chinese Medicine); 1999; 10:458.
135. *Guo Wai Yi Xue Zhong Yi Zhong Yao Fen Ce* (Monograph of Chinese Herbology from Foreign Medicine), 1991; 13(1):47.
136. *Guo Wai Yi Yao Zhi Wu Yao Fen Ce* (Monograph of Foreign Botanical Medicine), 1991; 1:45.
137. *Guo Wai Yi Xue Zhong Yi Zhong Yao Fen Ce* (Monograph of Chinese Herbology from Foreign Medicine), 1989; 5:26.
138. *Guo Wai Yi Yao Zhi Wu Yao Fen Ce* (Monograph of Foreign Botanical Medicine), 1991; 4:41.

Chapter 8 — Overview

139.Otani S, Usuki S, Iwasaki H, Inoue S, Yamashita K. Successful treatment of a infertile woman using hachimijiogan. Am J Chin Med. 1991; 19(2):145-54.

140.*Zhong Cheng Yao* (Study of Chinese Patent Medicine), 1993; 11:24.

141.*Han Fang Yi Xue* (Kampo Medicine), 1983; 5:14.

142.Sakamoto S, Kudo H, Kawasaki T, Kasahara N, Okamoto R. Effect of ba-wei-di-huang-wan (hachimi-jio-gan) on thymidine kinase and its isozyme activities in the prostate glands in rats. Am J Chin Med. 1988; 16(1-2):29-36.

143.Yoshimura K, Terai A, Arai Y. Two-week administration of low-dose Hachimi-jio-gan (Ba-Wei Di-Huang-Wan) for patients with benign prostatic hyperplasia. Hinyokika Kiyo. 2003 Sep; 49(9):509-14.

144.*Xin Zhong Yi* (New Chinese Medicine), 1997; 1:48.

145.*Zhong Yi Fang Ji Xian Dai Yan Jiu* (Modern Study of Medical Formulas in Traditional Chinese Medicine), 1997; 680.

146.*Xin Zhong Yi* (New Chinese Medicine), 1995; 27(1):50.

147.*Zhong Yi Za Zhi* (Journal of Chinese Medicine), 1956; 12:635.

148.*Shan Xi Zhong Yi* (Shanxi Chinese Medicine), 1997; 4:149.

149.*Shen De Yan Jiu* (Research of Kidney), 1981; 93.

150.*Fu Jian Zhong Yi Yao* (Fujian Chinese Medicine and Herbology), 1995; 26(3):59.

151.*Zhe Jiang Zhong Yi Za Zhi* (Zhejiang Journal of Chinese Medicine), 1995; 9:400.

152.Hsu H. Effectiveness of Gui Lu Er Xian Jiao (Tortoise Shell and Deer Antler Syrup) on treatment of osteoporosis. Clinic Medline of Taiwan

153.*Hu Nan Zhong Yi Za Zhi* (Hunan Journal of Chinese Medicine), 1999; 2:26.

Section 1

补气剂
— Qi-Tonifying Formulas

Sì Jūn Zǐ Tāng (Four-Gentlemen Decoction)

四君子湯
四君子汤

Pinyin Name: *Si Jun Zi Tang*
Literal Name: Four-Gentlemen Decoction
Alternate Names: *Szu Chun Tzu Tang, Si Jung Zi Tang,* Four Major Herb Decoction, Major Four Herb Combination
Original Source: *Tai Ping Hui Min He Ji Ju Fang* (Imperial Grace Formulary of the Tai Ping Era) by the Imperial Medical Department in 1078-85

COMPOSITION

Ren Shen (Radix et Rhizoma Ginseng)	[9g]
Bai Zhu (Rhizoma Atractylodis Macrocephalae)	[9g]
Fu Ling (Poria)	[9g]
Zhi Gan Cao (Radix et Rhizoma Glycyrrhizae Praeparata cum Melle)	[6g]

DOSAGE / PREPARATION / ADMINISTRATION

Grind equal amounts of the ingredients into a fine powder. Cook 6g of the powder in one large bowl of water until the liquid is reduced to 70%. The decoction may be taken any time during the day with an additional small pinch of salt. A small amount of *Sheng Jiang* (Rhizoma Zingiberis Recens) and *Da Zao* (Fructus Jujubae) may also be added to harmonize the formula.[1] Today, this formula may be prepared as a decoction with the doses suggested in brackets.

CHINESE THERAPEUTIC ACTIONS

1. Tonifies qi
2. Strengthens the Spleen

CLINICAL MANIFESTATIONS

Spleen and Stomach qi deficiencies: lethargy, weakness of the limbs, exercise intolerance, emaciation, weight loss, poor appetite, loose stools, a pale tongue, and a weak pulse.

VETERINARY CLINICAL APPLICATIONS

Gastrointestinal disorders such as gastric ulcers and exocrine pancreatic insufficiency, recovery from illness and surgery, supportive care for cancer, chronic illness, and post-partum recovery.

EXPLANATION

The Spleen and Stomach are the source of all qi and blood after birth (postnatal qi), as they are the most important organs for extracting nutrients and producing qi and blood. However, the Spleen and Stomach may be injured by an inappropriate diet, drugs, disease, or overwork. If these two organs become deficient and their digestive functions are affected, then the amount of qi produced will not be adequate. A lack of nourishment and qi deficiency result in weak vocalization, lethargy, and exercise intolerance. Poor appetite is the result of an impaired digestive system. Loose stools are the result of the Spleen's inability to direct the clear yang and water to the upper *jiao.* Since the Spleen is related to the muscles, Spleen deficiency can result in weakness of the limbs. A pale tongue and a weak pulse are common signs of qi deficiency.

Si Jun Zi Tang (Four-Gentlemen Decoction) uses *Ren Shen* (Radix et Rhizoma Ginseng) as the chief herb because it greatly tonifies *yuan* (source) *qi*, strengthens the Spleen, and nourishes the Stomach. *Bai Zhu* (Rhizoma Atractylodis Macrocephalae), the deputy herb, tonifies Spleen qi and dries dampness in the middle *jiao. Fu Ling* (Poria), the assistant, tonifies the middle *jiao* and dispels dampness. *Zhi Gan Cao* (Radix et Rhizoma Glycyrrhizae Praeparata

Sì Jūn Zǐ Tāng (Four-Gentlemen Decoction)

Si Jun Zi Tang **(Four-Gentlemen Decoction)**

Diagnosis	Clinical Signs	Treatment	Herbs
Spleen and Stomach qi deficiencies	• Weak vocalization, lethargy and exercise intolerance: Spleen and Stomach qi deficiencies and lack of nourishment • Loose stools: Spleen unable to guide the clear yang upward • Pale tongue and a weak pulse: qi deficiency	• Tonifies qi • Strengthens the Spleen	• *Ren Shen* (Radix et Rhizoma Ginseng) greatly tonifies *yuan* (source) *qi*, strengthens the Spleen, and nourishes the Stomach. • *Bai Zhu* (Rhizoma Atractylodis Macrocephalae) tonifies Spleen qi and dries dampness in the middle *jiao*. • *Fu Ling* (Poria) tonifies the middle *jiao* and dispels dampness. • *Zhi Gan Cao* (Radix et Rhizoma Glycyrrhizae Praeparata cum Melle) tonifies Spleen qi and harmonizes the herbs.

cum Melle), the envoy herb, tonifies Spleen qi and harmonizes the herbs.

Si Jun Zi Tang is a simple, yet extremely effective formula to tonify qi. It serves as the foundation for many qi-tonifying formulas that tonify the Spleen and nourish the Stomach to enable the production of qi and blood.

VETERINARY MODIFICATIONS

- For severe Spleen and Stomach qi deficiencies, add *Huang Qi* (Radix Astragali) and *Shan Yao* (Rhizoma Dioscoreae).
- With constipation due to qi deficiency, add *Dang Gui* (Radix Angelicae Sinensis) and *Huo Ma Ren* (Fructus Cannabis).
- With diarrhea due to deficiency and cold in the middle *jiao*, add *Li Zhong Tang* (Regulate the Middle Decoction).
- With postpartum diarrhea, add *Wu Mei* (Fructus Mume) and *Chen Pi* (Pericarpium Citri Reticulatae).
- With constant loose stools or diarrhea, add *He Zi* (Fructus Chebulae), *Huang Qi* (Radix Astragali) and *Bai Bian Dou* (Semen Lablab Album).
- With edema due to Spleen deficiency, add *Yi Yi Ren* (Semen Coicis), *Ze Xie* (Rhizoma Alismatis), and *Gui Zhi* (Ramulus Cinnamomi).
- With qi and blood deficiencies, combine with *Si Wu Tang* (Four-Substance Decoction).
- For malnutrition caused by yin deficiency, add *Gou Qi Zi* (Fructus Lycii) and *Nu Zhen Zi* (Fructus Ligustri Lucidi).
- For malnutrition caused by food stagnation, add *Mai Ya* (Fructus Hordei Germinatus).

CAUTIONS / CONTRAINDICATIONS

- *Si Jun Zi Tang*, while gentle, is slightly warm. Long-term use of this formula may cause a dry mouth, dry tongue, thirst, or irritability.
- This formula should be used with caution, or avoided in patients who have high fever, yin-deficient heat, excess heat, qi stagnation, body fluid deficiency, irritability, thirst, or constipation.

PHARMACOLOGICAL EFFECTS

1. **General**: Administration of *Si Jun Zi Tang* has been associated with a general effect to improve the health and well being of animal subjects. In mice with artificially-induced "Spleen deficiency" characterized by such symptoms as low body temperature, weight loss, decreased food intake, diarrhea, and inability to tolerate cold, ingestion of the formula reversed the symptoms and improved the overall health.[2]
2. **Gastrointestinal**: According to laboratory experiments in rabbits, administration of *Si Jun Zi Tang* was associated with a regulatory effect on the intestines. Depending on the condition of the subject, it either increased or decreased intestinal peristalsis.[3]
3. **Immunostimulant**: Administration of *Si Jun Zi Tang* was associated with an increase in T-lymphocytes, NK cells, and phagocytic activity of the macrophages.[4,5,6]
4. **Antineoplastic**: Administration of *Si Jun Zi Tang* was associated with an inhibitory effect on tumor cells in mice with esophageal and lung cancer.[7]
5. **Hematopoietic**: Administration of *Si Jun Zi Tang* in decoction for one week was associated with an increase in both white and red blood cells in rats.[8]
6. **Radioprotective**: One study reported recovery of the hematopoietic system in whole-body irradiated mice using *Si Jun Zi Tang*. Specific beneficial effects included an increase of leukocytes, erythrocytes, thrombocytes, and hematocrit. Moreover, the radioprotective function was more effective for leukocytes and thrombocytes than other hematocytes.[9]

HUMAN CLINICAL STUDIES AND RESEARCH

1. **Chronic gastritis**: In one clinical study, 32 patients with chronic superficial gastritis were treated with modified

Sì Jūn Zǐ Tāng (Four-Gentlemen Decoction)

Si Jun Zi Tang with good results. Out of 32 patients, 24 reported resolution of symptoms within 10 days, and 8 within 20 days. The formula used included the addition of *Zhi Qiao* (Fructus Aurantii), *Ji Nei Jin* (Endothelium Corneum Gigeriae Galli), *Huang Qi* (Radix Astragali), and others as deemed necessary.[10]

2. **Peptic ulcer disease**: One study of 126 peptic ulcer patients reported 97.6% effectiveness using *Si Jun Zi Tang* plus *Huang Qi* (Radix Astragali), *San Leng* (Rhizoma Sparganii), and *Hai Piao Xiao* (Endoconcha Sepiae) as the base formula, with the addition of *Chai Hu* (Radix Bupleuri), *Bai Shao* (Radix Paeoniae Alba), and *Zhi Zi* (Fructus Gardeniae) for Liver stagnation with Spleen deficiency; and *Si Ni San* (Frigid Extremities Powder) for Liver and Stomach disharmony. The treatment protocol was to give the herbs in decoction twice daily for 4-8 weeks per course of treatment.[11] In another report, 115 patients with peptic ulcer characterized by Spleen deficiency were treated with *Si Jun Zi Tang* with satisfactory results. *Fu Long Gan* (Terra Flava Usta) and *Bai Ji* (Rhizoma Bletillae) were added for individuals with bleeding ulcer. The overall effectiveness was 92.8%.[12]
3. **Ulcerative colitis**: Sixty patients with chronic ulcerative colitis were treated with herbs with complete recovery in 40 patients, significant improvement in 13 patients, moderate improvement in 5 patients, and no effect in 2 patients. The herbal treatment included *Si Jun Zi Tang* plus *Huang Qi* (Radix Astragali), *Dang Gui* (Radix Angelicae Sinensis), *Yan Hu Suo* (Rhizoma Corydalis), and others as deemed necessary. The herbs were made into pills, and were given three times daily.[13]
4. **Irritable bowel syndrome (IBS)**: One study reported 92.9% effectiveness using modified *Si Jun Zi Tang* to treat irritable bowel syndrome. Of 57 patients, the study reported significant improvement in 39 patients, moderate improvement in 14 patients, and no change in 4 patients. The base herbal formula included *Si Jun Zi Tang* plus *Pao Jiang* (Rhizoma Zingiberis Praeparatum), *Qin Pi* (Cortex Fraxini), and *Mu Xiang* (Radix Aucklandiae). Modifications were made by adding *Bai Shao* (Radix Paeoniae Alba) and *Yan Hu Suo* (Rhizoma Corydalis) for abdominal pain; *Chen Pi* (Pericarpium Citri Reticulatae) and dry-fried *Fang Feng* (Radix Saposhnikoviae) for abdominal pain causing urgent bowel movements; *Da Fu Pi* (Pericarpium Arecae) and *Zhi Qiao* (Fructus Aurantii) for feeling of incomplete evacuation after defecation; *Bai Tou Weng* (Radix Pulsatillae) and *Da Xue Teng* (Caulis Sargentodoxae) for mucus in the stools; *Cang Zhu* (Rhizoma Atractylodis) for profuse white mucus; *Di Yu* (Radix Sanguisorbae) and charred *Jin Yin Hua* (Flos Lonicerae Japonicae) for hematochezia; *Bu Gu Zhi* (Fructus Psoraleae) and *Rou Dou Kou* (Semen Myristicae) for 5 a.m. diarrhea; *Wu Bei Zi* (Galla Chinensis) and roasted *He Zi* (Fructus Chebulae) for frequent bowel movements with loose stools; *Rou Cong Rong* (Herba Cistanches) for constipation with yang deficiency; and *Shi Xiao San* (Sudden Smile Powder) for blood stagnation. The treatment protocol was to cook the herbs in water, and drink the decoction in three equally-divided doses daily.[14]
5. **Epigastric or abdominal pain**: Patients with epigastric or abdominal pain characterized by Spleen qi deficiency were treated with *Si Jun Zi Tang*. Out of 125 patients, the study reported recovery in 86 patients, significant improvement in 22 patients, and slight improvement in 17 patients.[15]
6. **Chronic hepatitis**: One hundred patients with chronic hepatitis were treated with complete recovery in 61 patients, improvement in 31 patients, and no benefit in 8 patients. The treatment protocol was to administer 40-60 packs of herbs in decoction. The herbal formulas included *Si Jun Zi Tang* plus *Dang Gui* (Radix Angelicae Sinensis), *Bai Shao* (Radix Paeoniae Alba), *Chai Hu* (Radix Bupleuri), and others as follows: *Huang Qi* (Radix Astragali) for qi deficiency; *Ji Nei Jin* (Endothelium Corneum Gigeriae Galli) and charred *Mai Ya* (Fructus Hordei Germinatus) for indigestion and poor appetite; *Lian Zi* (Semen Nelumbinis), *Shan Yao* (Rhizoma Dioscoreae), and *Ze Xie* (Rhizoma Alismatis) for loose stools; *Yan Hu Suo* (Rhizoma Corydalis) and *Yu Jin* (Radix Curcumae) for hypochondriac pain; *San Leng* (Rhizoma Sparganii), *E Zhu* (Rhizoma Curcumae), and *Bie Jia* (Carapax Trionycis) for splenomegaly and hepatomegaly; *Tao Ren* (Semen Persicae), *Hong Hua* (Flos Carthami), and *Yi Mu Cao* (Herba Leonuri) for blood stagnation; *Fo Shou* (Fructus Citri Sarcodactylis) and *Xiang Yuan* (Fructus Citri) for qi stagnation; *Yin Chen* (Herba Artemisiae Scopariae) for jaundice; and *Shi Hu* (Caulis Dendrobii), *Yu Zhu* (Rhizoma Polygonati Odorati), and *Xuan Shen* (Radix Scrophulariae) for yin deficiency.[16]

SUGGESTED ACUPUNCTURE TREATMENT

1. Points: *Pishu* (BL 20), *Weishu* (BL 21), *Housanli* (ST 36), *Tianshu* (ST 25), and *Qihai* (CV 6).
2. Technique: tonification.

Pishu (BL 20) nourishes Spleen yang. *Weishu* (BL 21) and *Housanli* (ST 36) tonify the middle *jiao* and harmonize the Stomach. *Tianshu* (ST 25) regulates the Stomach and Intestines. *Qihai* (CV 6) tonifies qi in general.

RELATED FORMULA

Bǎo Yuán Tāng (Preserve the Basal Decoction)
保元湯
保元汤
Pinyin Name: *Bao Yuan Tang*
Literal Name: Preserve the Basal Decoction

Sì Jūn Zǐ Tāng (Four-Gentlemen Decoction)

Original Source: *Bo Ai Xin Jian* (Manual of Universal Lover from the Heart) by Wei Zhi in 1525

Huang Qi (Radix Astragali)	6-9g
Ren Shen (Radix et Rhizoma Ginseng)	6-9g
Rou Gui (Cortex Cinnamomi)	1.5-2.1g
Zhi Gan Cao (Radix et Rhizoma Glycyrrhizae Praeparata cum Melle)	3g

Cook the herbs with 1 slice of *Sheng Jiang* (Rhizoma Zingiberis Recens) in water. Take the strained decoction while warm.

Bao Yuan Tang (Preserve the Basal Decoction) tonifies qi and warms yang. This formula is generally used for animals with Spleen and Stomach qi deficiencies, accompanied by the presence of cold and insufficiency of yang. Clinically, this formula also may be prescribed for juvenile animals with any condition characterized by yang and *yuan* (source) *qi* deficiencies, with clinical signs of lethargy, weakness, and intolerance to cold.

Bao Yuan Tang may be literally translated as "Preserve the Basal Decoction" or "Preserve the *yuan* (source) *qi* Decoction." *Ren Shen* (Radix et Rhizoma Ginseng), *Huang Qi* (Radix Astragali) and *Zhi Gan Cao* (Radix et Rhizoma Glycyrrhizae Praeparata cum Melle) are used to effectively tonify *zhong* (central) *qi* and *yuan* (source) *qi*. *Rou Gui* (Cortex Cinnamomi) is added to warm yang, dispel cold, and enhance the overall qi-tonifying effect.

Bao Yuan Tang has been used to tonify Heart qi-yang in cases of congestive heart failure and cardiomyopathy in the dog. With poor circulation and arrhythmia combine with *Xue Fu Zhu Yu Tang* (Drive Out Stasis in the Mansion of Blood Decoction) or substitute with *Zhi Gan Cao Tang* (Honey-Fried Licorice Decoction); with qi and yin deficiency combine with *Sheng Mai San* (Generate the Pulse Powder); and with Kidney yang deficiency and pulmonary edema combine with *Zhen Wu Tang* (True Warrior Decoction).

AUTHORS' COMMENTS

Tonic formulas that strengthen the Spleen and Stomach (middle *jiao*) are used more than any other group of tonification formulas in veterinary medicine. This is largely due to the practice of feeding dogs and cats commercially prepared diets that, while convenient and inexpensive, promote deficiency and/or dysfunction of the Spleen and Stomach and the other internal organs by extension. Similarly, most horses are managed in ways far different than their free-ranging ancestors and are fed diets high in concentrates that also negatively affect the Spleen and Stomach. The Spleen (pancreas) is considered to be the "mother of the five *zang* (solid organ) organs" and provides nutrition for the entire body after birth according to Chinese medicine. Commercial small-animal dry food diets that contain large amounts of damp- (corn, wheat, soybeans) and heat- (lamb, venison, buffalo) engendering foods easily overheat and damage the middle *jiao*, especially as these diets are often fed continuously for months and often times for years. Horses that are fed diets high in molasses and sugars, or that are given a high proportion of their diet as concentrate rather than forage, experience similar problems. Because of the importance of Spleen and Stomach tonics and their frequent use in animals, an in-depth review and comparison of their composition and actions is warranted.

The Spleen and Stomach are the root of postnatal qi, and the origin of qi and blood. It is only when these two organs are strong and the digestive functions are working properly that all the other organs and the rest of the body can be nourished, healthy, and be free of illnesses. *Si Jun Zi Tang* uses *Ren Shen* (Radix et Rhizoma Ginseng), a warm and sweet herb, to tonify Spleen and Stomach qi. *Bai Zhu* (Rhizoma Atractylodis Macrocephalae) and *Fu Ling* (Poria) tonify the Spleen and drain dampness, while *Zhi Gan Cao* (Radix et Rhizoma Glycyrrhizae Praeparata cum Melle), warm and sweet, functions to harmonize the middle *jiao* and tonify qi. These four herbs have gentle properties: they are not too hot, not too dry, gentle on the digestive system, and unlikely to create any side effects or adverse reactions—hence the name, Four Gentlemen. *Si Jun Zi Tang* can be modified according to different conditions of cold, heat, excess, or deficiency, to tonify Spleen and Stomach qi for the purpose of promoting overall bodily functions. Thus, *Si Jun Zi Tang* is the representative formula for tonifying qi. It treats Spleen and Stomach qi deficiencies caused by a variety of causes or with various complications, as long as it is modified accordingly.

Si Jun Zi Tang is often combined with other herbs or formulas in veterinary medicine to treat various gastrointestinal and/or lung disorders. The formulas listed below contain all of the herbs found in *Si Jun Zi Tang* and have similar functions. Knowledge of the modifications to this basic formula is important for a comprehensive understanding of each Spleen tonic formula, its specific actions, and how its use may be differentiated from the others.

- ***Liu Jun Zi Tang*** (Six-Gentlemen Decoction) strengthens the Spleen and Stomach, regulates qi, and stops vomiting. It has two additional herbs added to the base formula *Si Jun Zi Tang*: *Ban Xia* (Rhizoma Pinelliae) and *Chen*

Sì Jūn Zǐ Tāng (Four-Gentlemen Decoction)

Pi (Pericarpium Citri Reticulatae). These two additions strengthen its damp- and phlegm-dispelling properties. These two herbs are often included in formulas that treat damp-phlegm coughs. *Liu Jun Zi Tang* is frequently used to treat chronic bronchitis and coughing with clear phlegm. It has a better ability to strengthen the Spleen, dry dampness, and stop vomiting than *Xiang Sha Liu Jun Zi Tang* (Six-Gentlemen Decoction with Aucklandia and Amomum). It can be used for acute and chronic gastrointestinal disorders; prolonged use can cause generalized dryness, itching, and irritability.

- ***Xiang Sha Liu Jun Zi Tang*** (Six-Gentlemen Decoction with Aucklandia and Amomum) contains the same herbs as *Liu Jun Zi Tang* (Six-Gentlemen Decoction), but has two additional herbs added: *Mu Xiang* (Radix Aucklandiae) and *Sha Ren* (Fructus Amomi) to activate qi and treat deficiency of the middle *jiao* with cold and damp stagnation. These two herbs make the formula stronger at regulating qi, dispelling cold, and relieving abdominal pain, and make it warmer and more drying than *Liu Jun Zi Tang*. Animals should not be fed a raw food or cold diet while taking this formula. It is a stronger formula than *Xiang Sha Yang Wei Tang* (Nourish the Stomach Decoction with Aucklandia and Amomum) and is more effective to stop vomiting and diarrhea occurring postoperatively or secondary to antibiotic therapy, and for gastrointestinal problems from eating cold, damp or raw food.
- ***Xiang Sha Yang Wei Tang*** (Nourish the Stomach Decoction with Aucklandia and Amomum) primarily increases appetite in animals with middle *jiao* deficiency. It contains the herbs *Cang Zhu* (Rhizoma Atractylodis), *Sha Ren* (Fructus Amomi), and *Dou Kou* (Fructus Amomi Rotundus), which are aromatic herbs that dry dampness and help increase appetite. *Xiang Fu* (Rhizoma Cyperi), *Mu Xiang* (Radix Aucklandiae), and *Hou Po* (Cortex Magnoliae Officinalis) activate qi to dispel dampness. This formula has a stronger ability to stimulate appetite than *Xiang Sha Liu Jun Zi Tang*. It is especially useful in animals that act hungry, eat only a small amount, and then look and act uncomfortable. This formula can benefit animals that have bloating, borborygmus, belching, nausea and vomiting immediately after eating.
- ***Shen Ling Bai Zhu San*** (Ginseng, Poria, and Atractylodes Macrocephala Powder) tonifies qi and strengthens the Spleen, resolves dampness, and stops diarrhea. It contains herbs that strongly resolve dampness in cases of internally generated dampness from Spleen and Stomach qi deficiencies, causing impairment in the transportation and transformation functions. These herbs, *Shan Yao* (Rhizoma Dioscoreae) and *Lian Zi* (Semen Nelumbinis), treat diarrhea by assisting *Ren Shen* (Radix et Rhizoma Ginseng) in strengthening the Spleen and tonifying qi. *Bai Bian Dou* (Semen Lablab Album) and *Yi Yi Ren* (Semen Coicis) strengthen the Spleen and dispel dampness. *Sha Ren* (Fructus Amomi) awakens the Spleen and harmonizes the Stomach to regulate qi and resolve stagnation. *Jie Geng* (Radix Platycodonis) relieves chest fullness, and has an ascending function to help counteract diarrhea. *Shen Ling Bai Zhu San* (Ginseng, Poria, and Atractylodes Macrocephala Powder) is the herbal formula of choice in veterinary medicine to treat uncomplicated diarrhea due to Spleen qi deficiency and dampness, and to promote digestion when there is an inability to properly digest and absorb foods. It is also frequently used for chronic cough and/or chronic gagging with clear phlegm that arise as a result of damp accumulation.
- ***Qi Pi Wan*** (Guide the Spleen Pill) strengthens the Spleen and Stomach, promotes normal digestion, and treats food stagnation, diarrhea, and vomiting in animals with chronic Spleen and Stomach deficiencies. It contains *Shan Zha* (Fructus Crataegi) and *Chen Pi* (Pericarpium Citri Reticulatae) to regulate qi and promote normal appetite and digestion; *Lian Zi* (Semen Nelumbinis) to strengthen the Spleen and relieve diarrhea; *Ze Xie* (Rhizoma Alismatis) to drain dampness; and *Shan Yao* (Rhizoma Dioscoreae) to tonify the body and relieve thirst and diarrhea. It is especially effective for pancreatic diseases and maldigestion-malabsorption disorders with weight loss in constitutionally deficient young animals. It treats food accumulation and stagnation in deficient, debilitated and weak animals of all ages, and can be given long term with appropriate modifications.
- ***Bu Zhong Yi Qi Tang*** (Tonify the Middle and Augment the Qi Decoction) tonifies the middle *jiao* and benefits qi. It contains herbs that lift yang qi and treat prolapse of internal organs, strengthen *wei* (defensive) *qi*, and protect the exterior. It is used mainly for *chronic* problems. *Bu Zhong Yi Qi Tang* uses *Huang Qi* (Radix Astragali) as the chief herb because it tonifies *zhong* (central) *qi*. *Chai Hu* (Radix Bupleuri) and *Sheng Ma* (Rhizoma Cimicifugae) cause yang qi to ascend and lift prolapsed organs, while *Dang Gui* (Radix Angelicae Sinensis) nourishes and moves the blood. This formula is commonly chosen to treat rectal prolapse, chronic diarrhea, and fecal and urinary incontinence in the dog. The dosage of this formula is typically small, and the duration of treatment is prolonged. It can take up to 3 months or more to see clinically observable effects in chronic cases.
- ***Yi Qi Cong Ming Tang*** (Augment the Qi and Increase Acuity Decoction) tonifies qi and blood, raises yang qi, and benefits the eyes and ears. It tonifies the Spleen and Stomach, and raises yang qi like *Bu Zhong Yi Qi Tang* (Tonify the Middle and Augment the Qi Decoction). However, it has additional herbs that treat compromised

Sì Jūn Zǐ Tāng (Four-Gentlemen Decoction)

functioning and deterioration of the eyes and ears. It may be used to reverse deterioration, or preventively to maintain the acuity of both ears and eyes. *Huang Qi* (Radix Astragali), *Ge Gen* (Radix Puerariae Lobatae), *Sheng Ma* (Rhizoma Cimicifugae), and *Man Jing Zi* (Fructus Viticis) have an ascending function to lift yang qi and treat disorders of the upper parts of the body. When sufficient qi rises to the head, the normal functions of the eyes and ears will be restored. *Bai Shao* (Radix Paeoniae Alba) nourishes yin and harmonizes the blood. *Huang Bo* (Cortex Phellodendri) treats deficiency fire. It is used to treat diminished sight and hearing without inflammation in geriatric animals.

Si Jun Zi Tang and *Li Zhong Wan* (Regulate the Middle Pill) both treat Spleen qi deficiency with poor appetite, diarrhea, and other signs and symptoms. Both formulas contain qi-tonifying herbs such as *Ren Shen* (Radix et Rhizoma Ginseng), *Bai Zhu* (Rhizoma Atractylodis Macrocephalae), and *Zhi Gan Cao* (Radix et Rhizoma Glycyrrhizae Praeparata cum Melle). Although similar, their differences are as follows:

- *Si Jun Zi Tang* is indicated for Spleen qi deficiency, characterized by poor appetite, decreased food intake, fatigue, a pale tongue, and a weak pulse.
- *Li Zhong Wan* is for deficiency and cold of the middle *jiao* (Spleen and Stomach), characterized by abdominal pain, vomiting, diarrhea, polyuria, cold limbs, intolerance to cold, a pale pink to purple tongue, and a thin, weak pulse.[17]

References

1. *Yi Fang Ji Jie* (Analytical Collection of Medical Formulas), 1682.
2. *Shang Hai Di Er Yi Ke Da Xue Xue Bao* (Journal of Second Shanghai University College of Medicine), 1984; 3:7.
3. *Xin Zhong Yi* (New Chinese Medicine), 1978; 5:53.
4. *Zhong Cheng Yao Yan Jiu* (Research of Chinese Patent Medicine), 1981; 12:28.
5. *Zhong Yao Yao Li Yu Lin Chuang* (Pharmacology and Clinical Applications of Chinese Herbs), 1989; 5(5):24.
6. *Zhong Xi Yi Jie He Za Zhi* (Journal of Integrated Chinese and Western Medicine), 1984; 4(6):363.
7. *Shang Hai Zhong Yi Yao Za Zhi* (Shanghai Journal of Chinese Medicine and Herbology), 1984; 1:2.
8. *Zhong Yi Fang Ji Xian Dai Yan Jiu* (Modern Study of Medical Formulas in Traditional Chinese Medicine), 1997; 477.
9. Hsu HY, Yang JJ, Lian SL, Ho YH, Lin CC. Recovery of the hematopoietic system by Si-Jun-Zi-Tang in whole body irradiated mice. J Ethnopharmacol. 1996 Nov; 54(2-3):69-75.
10. *Zhong Yi Fang Ji Xian Dai Yan Jiu* (Modern Study of Medical Formulas in Traditional Chinese Medicine), 1997, 480-481.
11. *Xin Zhong Yi* (New Chinese Medicine), 1982; 11:12.
12. *Zhong Yi Za Zhi* (Journal of Chinese Medicine), 1980; 21(12):947.
13. *Zhong Yi Za Zhi* (Journal of Chinese Medicine), 1987; 10:28.
14. *Shang Hai Zhong Yi Za Zhi* (Shanghai Journal of Chinese Medicine), 1986; 1:12.
15. *He Nan Zhong Yi* (Henan Chinese Medicine), 1986; 3:1.
16. *He Bei Zhong Yi* (Hebei Chinese Medicine), 1987; 6:31.
17. Wang MZ, et al. *Zhong Yi Xue Wen Da Ti Ku* (Questions and Answers on Traditional Chinese Medicine: Herbal Formulas).

Liù Jūn Zǐ Tāng (Six-Gentlemen Decoction)

六君子湯
六君子汤

Pinyin Name: *Liu Jun Zi Tang*
Literal Name: Six-Gentlemen Decoction
Alternate Names: *Liu Chun Tzu Tang* (*Wan*), Six Major Herb Decoction (Pill), Six Gentlemen Decoction (Pill), Major Six Herb Combination
Original Source: *Fu Ren Liang Fang* (Fine Formulas for Women) by Chen Zi-Ming in 1237

COMPOSITION

Ren Shen (Radix et Rhizoma Ginseng)	6g [9g]
Bai Zhu (Rhizoma Atractylodis Macrocephalae)	6g [9g]
Fu Ling (Poria)	6g [9g]
Zhi Gan Cao (Radix et Rhizoma Glycyrrhizae Praeparata cum Melle)	3g [6g]
Chen Pi (Pericarpium Citri Reticulatae)	3g [9g]
Ban Xia (Rhizoma Pinelliae)	3g [12g]

DOSAGE / PREPARATION / ADMINISTRATION

The source text states to prepare the ingredients as a decoction with the addition of small amounts of *Sheng Jiang* (Rhizoma Zingiberis Recens) (3 slices) and *Da Zao* (Fructus Jujubae) (2 pieces). Today, the decoction may be prepared using the doses suggested in brackets.

CHINESE THERAPEUTIC ACTIONS

1. Strengthens the Spleen and Stomach
2. Regulates qi and stops vomiting

CLINICAL MANIFESTATIONS

Spleen and Stomach qi deficiencies accompanied by dampness and phlegm: lack of appetite, lethargy, exercise intolerance, fatigue, loose stools, nausea, vomiting, coughing of profuse, white, watery phlegm, a pale, wet tongue, and a deep, weak pulse.

VETERINARY CLINICAL APPLICATIONS

Treatment of gastrointestinal and pulmonary disorders: pancreatitis, cholangiohepatitis, cholangitis, diabetes mellitus, chronic gastritis, gastric ulcer, anorexia, poor digestion and weight loss in geriatric, weak and debilitated animals, chronic diarrhea, chronic vomiting, inflammatory bowel disease, chronic asthma, chronic bronchitis; also as supportive care for cancer, chronic disease, post-surgery, post-partum, and following chemotherapy or radiation therapy; and as a supplemental formula to aid in the digestion and absorption of other formulas.

EXPLANATION

Liu Jun Zi Tang (Six-Gentlemen Decoction) is derived from *Si Jun Zi Tang* (Four-Gentlemen Decoction), with the addition of *Ban Xia* (Rhizoma Pinelliae) and *Chen Pi* (Pericarpium Citri Reticulatae). It treats Spleen and Stomach deficiencies accompanied by damp and phlegm accumulation. Spleen and Stomach deficiencies cause poor digestion, fatigue, lethargy, exercise intolerance, lack of appetite, and loose stools. Damp accumulation blocks the normal descent of Stomach qi and causes qi reversal, manifested as nausea and vomiting. When the Spleen produces dampness, it is stored in the Lung. If dampness

***Liu Jun Zi Tang* (Six-Gentlemen Decoction)**

Diagnosis	Clinical Signs	Treatment	Herbs
Spleen and Stomach qi deficiencies accompanied by dampness and phlegm	• Poor appetite, lethargy, fatigue, exercise intolerance, loose stools, a pale, wet tongue, and a deep, weak pulse: Spleen and Stomach deficiencies • Nausea and vomiting: rebellious Stomach qi due to damp accumulation • Coughing: obstructed Lung qi circulation due to damp accumulation • Profuse, white, watery phlegm: damp and phlegm accumulation	• Strengthens the Spleen and Stomach • Regulates qi and stops vomiting	• *Si Jun Zi Tang* (Four-Gentlemen Decoction) tonifies qi and strengthens the Spleen and Stomach. • *Chen Pi* (Pericarpium Citri Reticulatae) dries dampness and regulates Lung qi to reduce profuse phlegm. • *Ban Xia* (Rhizoma Pinelliae) breaks up qi stagnation to relieve chest stuffiness, and redirects rebellious Stomach qi to relieve nausea and vomiting.

Liù Jūn Zǐ Tāng (Six-Gentlemen Decoction)

and phlegm accumulate and stagnate in the chest, they may interrupt the flow of Lung qi, resulting in coughing of profuse, white, watery phlegm.

Ren Shen (Radix et Rhizoma Ginseng), *Bai Zhu* (Rhizoma Atractylodis Macrocephalae), *Fu Ling* (Poria), and *Zhi Gan Cao* (Radix et Rhizoma Glycyrrhizae Praeparata cum Melle) tonify Spleen and Stomach qi, as explained in the section on *Si Jun Zi Tang* (Four-Gentlemen Decoction). *Chen Pi* (Pericarpium Citri Reticulatae) dries dampness and regulates Lung qi to reduce the profuse phlegm. *Ban Xia* (Rhizoma Pinelliae) breaks up qi stagnation to relieve chest stuffiness, and redirects rebellious Stomach qi to relieve nausea and vomiting.

VETERINARY MODIFICATIONS

- For deficiency and cold of the Spleen and Stomach, add *Wu Zhu Yu* (Fructus Evodiae), *Pao Jiang* (Rhizoma Zingiberis Praeparatum), and *Rou Gui* (Cortex Cinnamomi).
- For diarrhea due to Spleen deficiency, add *Shan Yao* (Rhizoma Dioscoreae) and *Qian Shi* (Semen Euryales).
- For diarrhea caused by deficiency and cold in the middle *jiao*, add *Li Zhong Tang* (Regulate the Middle Decoction).
- With mucus in the stools, add *Ge Gen* (Radix Puerariae Lobatae), *Bai Shao* (Radix Paeoniae Alba), and *Mu Xiang* (Radix Aucklandiae).
- With abdominal pain due to Spleen deficiency, add *Yan Hu Suo* (Rhizoma Corydalis), *Chai Hu* (Radix Bupleuri), *Bai Shao* (Radix Paeoniae Alba), and *Dang Gui* (Radix Angelicae Sinensis).
- If there is anorexia or poor appetite, add *Shan Zha* (Fructus Crataegi), *Shen Qu* (Massa Fermentata), and *Mai Ya* (Fructus Hordei Germinatus).
- If there are exterior signs and symptoms, add *Fang Feng* (Radix Saposhnikoviae) and *Zi Su Ye* (Folium Perillae).
- With generalized blood deficiency, add *Si Wu Tang* (Four-Substance Decoction).
- For poor appetite, add *Shen Qu* (Massa Fermentata).
- For *gan ji* (infantile malnutrition) caused by yin deficiency, add *Gou Qi Zi* (Fructus Lycii) and *Nu Zhen Zi* (Fructus Ligustri Lucidi).
- For *gan ji* (infantile malnutrition) caused by food stagnation, add *Mai Ya* (Fructus Hordei Germinatus).

CAUTIONS / CONTRAINDICATIONS

- *Liu Jun Zi Tang*, although gentle, is slightly warm. Long-term use of this formula may cause dry mouth, dry tongue, thirst, or irritability.
- This formula should be used with caution, or avoided, in animals with high fever, yin-deficient heat, excess heat, qi stagnation, body fluid deficiency, irritability, thirst, or constipation.
- Avoid feeding cold or raw, pungent or spicy, and oily or greasy foods.[1]

PHARMACOLOGICAL EFFECTS

1. **Gastrointestinal**: According to laboratory experiments in rabbits, administration of *Liu Jun Zi Tang* was associated with regulatory effects on the intestines. Depending on the condition of the subject, it will either increase or decrease intestinal peristalsis.[2] According to another study, *Liu Jun Zi Tang* promoted adaptive relaxation and provided symptom relief in patients with functional dyspepsia.[3] Lastly, one study reported *Liu Jun Zi Tang* to have a prokinetic action on gastric emptying to treat chronic dyspepsia.[4] In regards to plasma levels of gut-regulated peptide, administration of *Liu Jun Zi Tang* caused significant increases in plasma somatostatin and gastrin levels at 60 to 240 minutes compared with a placebo group.[5]
2. **Gastroprotective**: In one study in rats, use of *Liu Jun Zi Tang* had a dose-dependent effect and significantly inhibited gastric mucosal damage caused by absolute ethanol at doses over 500 mg/kg. The mechanism of this gastroprotective effect occurred partly through nitric oxide, not through prostaglandins or sulfhydryls.[6]
3. **Antineoplastic**: Subcutaneous injection of a modified *Liu Jun Zi Tang* preparation, followed by oral ingestion for 20 days was determined to have an inhibitory effect on the growth of cancer cells in mice. The mechanisms of action were attributed to an increase of macrophages and natural killer (NK) cells.[7]

HUMAN CLINICAL STUDIES AND RESEARCH

1. **Abdominal pain**: Patients with abdominal pain were treated with modified *Liu Jun Zi Tang* for 20 days. The causes of abdominal pain included chronic gastritis, gastric ulcer, and duodenal ulcer. The formula included the addition of *Yan Hu Suo* (Rhizoma Corydalis) and *Bai Shao* (Radix Paeoniae Alba). Out of 123 patients, the study reported significant improvement in 49 patients, moderate improvement in 65 patients, and no effect in 9 patients. The overall efficacy rate reported was 92.7%.[8]
2. **Gastritis**: According to one study, administration of *Liu Jun Zi Tang* to 207 patients with acute or chronic gastritis was associated with significant improvement in 62.9% and moderate improvement in 82.3% of patients. The treatment protocol was to administer 2.5g of the herbs in powder form, three times a day before meals.[9]
3. **Duodenal ulcer**: Administration of modified *Liu Jun Zi Tang* was effective in treating 31 patients with duodenal ulcer. The herbal treatment contained *Liu Jun Zi Tang* plus *Yan Hu Suo* (Rhizoma Corydalis), *Hai Piao Xiao* (Endoconcha Sepiae), and *Bai Zhi* (Radix Angelicae Dahuricae) as the base formula. Additional modifications were made

as follows: *Ru Xiang* (Gummi Olibanum) and *Mo Yao* (Myrrha) for severe pain; *Huang Lian* (Rhizoma Coptidis) for acid reflux and belching; *Zuo Jin Wan* (Left Metal Pill) for a bitter taste in the mouth, dry mouth, and acid reflux; *Si Ni San* (Frigid Extremities Powder) for hypochondriac pain; *Zhi Shi* (Fructus Aurantii Immaturus) for epigastric fullness and distention; and *Di Yu* (Radix Sanguisorbae) for hematochezia. The duration of treatment was 30 days per course of treatment. Of 31 patients, 9 had complete recovery, 11 had significant improvement, 8 had moderate improvement, and 3 had no improvement. The overall rate of effectiveness was 90.3%.[10]

4. **Indigestion**: One study reported 90.0% rate of effectiveness using modified *Liu Jun Zi Tang* to treat indigestion in 60 patients. In addition to the base formula, herbs were added as follows: *Wu Yao* (Radix Linderae), *Mu Xiang* (Radix Aucklandiae), and *Sha Ren* (Fructus Amomi) for qi stagnation; *Zhu Ru* (Caulis Bambusae in Taenia), *Huang Lian* (Rhizoma Coptidis), and *Pu Gong Ying* (Herba Taraxaci) for damp-heat; *Chi Shao* (Radix Paeoniae Rubra), *Dan Shen* (Radix et Rhizoma Salviae Miltiorrhizae), and *Dang Gui Wei* (Extremitas Radix Angelicae Sinensis) for chronic illness with blood stagnation, and processed *Huang Qi* (Radix Astragali) for qi deficiency. The duration of treatment was 30 days per course of treatment, for 2 courses total. Of 60 patients, the study reported complete recovery in 13 patients, significant improvement in 21 patients, moderate improvement in 14 patients, slight improvement in 6 patients, and no change in 6 patients.[11]
5. **Gastrointestinal disorder**: The use of *Liu Jun Zi Tang* has been associated with numerous benefits in treating gastrointestinal disorders, such as stomach prolapse, gastric pain, diarrhea, gastritis, and peptic ulcer.[12]
6. **Chronic bronchitis**: *Liu Jun Zi Tang* plus *Tu Si Zi* (Semen Cuscutae), *Wu Ling Zhi* (Faeces Trogopteri), and *Dan Shen* (Radix et Rhizoma Salviae Miltiorrhizae) effectively treated chronic bronchitis characterized by Spleen deficiency and phlegm obstruction in the Lung. The patients received 1 pack of herbs per day for a month, for a total of 30 packs. Of 30 patients, the study reported 93.3% rate of effectiveness.[13]
7. **Pain from liver cancer**: One study reported 87.7% effectiveness in relieving pain in 65 patients with liver cancer. The herbal formula contained *Liu Jun Zi Tang* plus *Hou Po* (Cortex Magnoliae Officinalis), *Dan Shen* (Radix et Rhizoma Salviae Miltiorrhizae), *Tu Bie Chong* (Eupolyphaga seu Steleophaga), *Shui Zhi* (Hirudo), *Wu Gong* (Scolopendra) and *Ma Qian Zi* (Semen Strychni).[14]

HERB-DRUG INTERACTION

- **Chemotherapy-induced side effects**: Administration of *Liu Jun Zi Tang* showed effectiveness in alleviating gastrointestinal side effects associated with chemotherapy. The base formula included *Liu Jun Zi Tang* plus *Shen Qu* (Massa Fermentata), *Hou Po* (Cortex Magnoliae Officinalis), and *Shan Yao* (Rhizoma Dioscoreae). Modifications include the addition of *Huang Lian* (Rhizoma Coptidis), *Zhu Ru* (Caulis Bambusae in Taenia), and *Sheng Jiang* (Rhizoma Zingiberis Recens) for continuous nausea and vomiting; *Cang Zhu* (Rhizoma Atractylodis), *Pei Lan* (Herba Eupatorii), and *Zhi Qiao* (Fructus Aurantii) for a thick, greasy tongue coating; and *Huang Qi* (Radix Astragali), *Ji Xue Teng* (Caulis Spatholobi), and *Yin Yang Huo* (Herba Epimedii) for qi deficiency, fatigue, and low white blood cell count. Patients were given herbs three times daily until the end of their chemotherapy treatment. Of 74 patients, the study reported complete relief in 49 patients, improvement in 24 patients, and no effect in 1 case. The rate of effectiveness was 98.6%.[15] In another study involving 110 patients on chemotherapy, use of *Liu Jun Zi Tang* plus *Huang Qi* (Radix Astragali) and *Yi Yi Ren* (Semen Coicis) was associated with relieving nausea and vomiting, and increased white blood cell count.[16]
- **Levofloxacin**: In a study of 8 healthy subjects, co-administrations of levofloxacin and *Liu Jun Zi Tang* did not cause any significant differences in any pharmacokinetic parameters, urinary recovery and renal clearance of levofloxacin. The study concluded that *Liu Jun Zi Tang* did not have a significant effect on the rate and extent of bioavailability, or renal excretion of levofloxacin.[17]
- **Ofloxacin**: A study of 7 volunteers in an open, random crossover fashion found no significant effect on the rate and extent of bioavailability of ofloxacin with co-administrations of *Liu Jun Zi Tang*, *Xiao Chai Hu Tang* (Minor Bupleurum Decoction), or *Chai Ling Tang* (Bupleurum and Poria Decoction).[18]

TOXICOLOGY

Use of *Liu Jun Zi Tang* has been associated with one case of pneumonitis in a 79-year-old woman who complained of dry cough and dyspnea on exertion after taking the herbs. At the time of publication, this is the only case of pulmonary hypersensitivity due to *Liu Jun Zi Tang* reported in the world.[19]

SUGGESTED ACUPUNCTURE TREATMENT

1. Points: *Pishu* (BL 20), *Weishu* (BL 21), *Housanli* (ST 36), *Tianshu* (ST 25), *Qihai* (CV 6), *Feishu* (BL 13), *Fenglong* (ST 40) and *Shangen* and *Mijiaogen*.
2. Technique: tonification.

Pishu (BL 20) nourishes Spleen yang. *Weishu* (BL 21) and *Housanli* (ST 36) tonify the middle *jiao* and harmonize the Stomach. *Tianshu* (ST 25) regulates the Stomach and

Liù Jūn Zǐ Tāng (Six-Gentlemen Decoction)

Intestines. *Qihai* (CV 6) tonifies qi in general. *Feishu* (BL 13) and *Fenglong* (ST 40) dispel dampness and phlegm. *Shangen* and *Mijiaogen* are classical points used to stimulate the appetite in dogs and horses, respectively.

AUTHORS' COMMENTS

Liu Jun Zi Tang is one of the most commonly used herbal formulas in veterinary medicine because of its large range of applications, and because of the prevalence of gastro-intestinal disease in domesticated animals due to poor and/or inappropriate diets and feeding practices. It follows the principle of cultivating the earth element (Spleen) to generate the metal element (Lung), according to Five-Element Theory.

- For supportive care and treatment of cholangiohepatitis or hepatic lipidosis in the cat with anorexia, combine with *Xiao Chai Hu Tang* (Minor Bupleurum Decoction).
- For dogs with Spleen qi deficiency and chronic cough with clear phlegm, combine with *Zi Wan* (Radix et Rhizoma Asteris), *Jie Geng* (Radix Platycodonis), and *Huang Qi* (Radix Astragali); and for animals with Kidney deficiency, combine with *Ren Shen Ge Jie San* (Ginseng and Gecko Powder).
- This formula can also be used to treat cats with Spleen deficiency and asthma characterized by cough with clear phlegm without heat signs. For chronic cases with qi deficiency, add *Bu Fei Tang* (Tonify the Lung Decoction); in cases with qi and yin deficiencies, combine with *Sheng Mai San* (Generate the Pulse Powder); and for animals with Kidney deficiency, combine with *Ren Shen Ge Jie San* (Ginseng and Gecko Powder).

Liu Jun Zi Tang and *Shen Ling Bai Zhu San* (Ginseng, Poria, and Atractylodes Macrocephala Powder) are both excellent Spleen tonics. The major differences between these two formulas are:

- *Liu Jun Zi Tang* contains *Chen Pi* (Pericarpium Citri Reticulatae) and *Ban Xia* (Rhizoma Pinelliae), which give the formula stronger effects in drying dampness and transforming phlegm. It can be used for both acute and chronic conditions.
- *Shen Ling Bai Zhu San* is better for chronic conditions with yin deficiency and loss of essence.
- These two formulas are frequently used to treat vomiting and diarrhea in animals undergoing chemotherapy or radiation therapy. *Liu Jun Zi Tang* is generally the first choice for treatment of vomiting, while *Shen Ling Bai Zhu San* is the first choice to treat diarrhea. For persistent vomiting, add *Sheng Jiang* (Rhizoma Zingiberis Recens), *Zhu Ru* (Caulis Bambusae in Taenia), and *Zi Su Geng* (Caulis Perillae). For chemotherapy patients with vomiting from Liver fire attacking the Stomach, combine *Liu Jun Zi Tang* with *Zuo Jin Wan* (Left Metal Pill).
- For a comparative discussion of Spleen tonic formulas, see *Si Jun Zi Tang* (Four-Gentlemen Decoction).

References

1. *Zhong Yao Ming Fang Yao Li Yu Ying Yong* (Pharmacology and Applications of Famous Herbal Formulas), 1989; 249-251.
2. *Nan Jing Zhong Yi Xue Yuan Xue Bao* (Journal of Nanjing University of Traditional Chinese Medicine), 1989; 1:36.
3. Hayakawa T, Arakawa T, Kase Y, Akiyama S, Ishige A, Takeda S, Sasaki H, Uno H, Fukuda T, Higuchi K, Kobayashi K. Liu-Jun-Zi-Tang, a kampo medicine, promotes adaptive relaxation in isolated guinea pig stomachs. Drugs Exp Clin Res. 1999; 25(5):211-8.
4. Tatsuta M, Iishi H. Effect of treatment with liu-jun-zi-tang (TJ-43) on gastric emptying and gastrointestinal symptoms in dyspeptic patients. Aliment Pharmacol Ther. 1993 Aug; 7(4):459-62.
5. Naito T, Itoh H, Yasunaga F, Takeyama M. Rikkunshi-to raises levels of somatostatin and gastrin in human plasma. Biol Pharm Bull. 2001 Jul; 24(7):841-3.
6. Arakawa T, Higuchi K, Fujiwara Y, Watanabe T, Tominaga K, Hayakawa T, Kuroki T. Gastroprotection by Liu-Jun-Zi-Tang (TJ-43): possible mediation of nitric oxide but not prostaglandins or sulfhydryls. Drugs Under Experimental & Clinical Research. 1999; 25(5):207-10.
7. *Shi Yong Zhong Liu Xue Za Zhi* (Practical Journal of Cancer), 1987; 1(4):6.
8. *Shan Xi Xin Zhong Yi* (New Shanxi Chinese Medicine), 1984; 1:23.
9. *Zhong Yi Ming Fang Lin Chuang Xin Yong* (Contemporary Clinical Applications of Classic Chinese Formulas), 2001; 160.
10. *Si Chuan Zhong Yi* (Sichuan Chinese Medicine), 1989; 2:21.
11. *Zhong Yi Ming Fang Lin Chuang Xin Yong* (Contemporary Clinical Applications of Classic Chinese Formulas), 2001; 161.
12. *Zhong Yi Fang Ji Xian Dai Yan Jiu* (Modern Study of Medical Formulas in Traditional Chinese Medicine), 1997; 493.
13. *Chong Qing Yi Yao* (Chongching Medicine and Herbology), 1994; 5:309.
14. *Jiang Su Zhong Yi* (Jiangsu Chinese Medicine), 1997; 6:23.
15. *Shi Yong Zhong Xi Yi Jie He Za Zhi* (Practical Journal of Integrated Chinese and Western Medicines), 1992; 9:528.
16. *Zhong Yi Yao Xin Xi* (Information on Chinese Medicine and Herbology), 1995; 6:27.
17. Hasegawa T, Yamaki K, Muraoka I, Nadai M, Takagi K, Nabeshima T. Effects of traditional Chinese medicines on pharmacokinetics of levofloxacin. Antimicrobial Agents & Chemotherapy. 1995 Sep; 39(9):2135-7.
18. Hasegawa T, Yamaki K, Nadai M, Muraoka I, Wang L, Takagi K, Nabeshima T. Lack of effect of Chinese medicines on bioavailability of ofloxacin in healthy volunteers. Int J Clin Pharmacol Ther. 1994 Feb; 32(2):57-61.
19. Maruyama Y, Maruyama M, Takada T, Haraguchi M, Uno K. A case of pneumonitis due to Rikkunshi-to. Nihon Kyobu Shikkan Gakkai Zasshi. 1994 Jan; 32(1):84-9.

Xiāng Shā Liù Jūn Zǐ Tāng

(Six-Gentlemen Decoction with Aucklandia and Amomum)

香砂六君子湯

香砂六君子汤

Pinyin Name: *Xiang Sha Liu Jun Zi Tang*

Literal Name: Six-Gentlemen Decoction with Aucklandia and Amomum

Alternate Names: *Hsiang Sha Liu Chun Tzu Tang*, Aucklandia and Amomum Gentlemen Decoction, Saussurea and Six-Major-Herb Decoction, Vladimiria and Cardamon Combination, Saussurea and Cardamon Combination

Original Source: *Gu Jin Ming Fang* (Famous Classic and Contemporary Formulas) by Luo Mei in 1675

COMPOSITION

Ren Shen (Radix et Rhizoma Ginseng)	3g
Bai Zhu (Rhizoma Atractylodis Macrocephalae)	6g
Fu Ling (Poria)	6g
Gan Cao (Radix et Rhizoma Glycyrrhizae)	2.1g
Ban Xia (Rhizoma Pinelliae)	3g
Chen Pi (Pericarpium Citri Reticulatae)	2.4g
Mu Xiang (Radix Aucklandiae)	2.1g
Sha Ren (Fructus Amomi)	2.4g

DOSAGE / PREPARATION / ADMINISTRATION

Prepare the ingredients as a decoction with 6g of *Sheng Jiang* (Rhizoma Zingiberis Recens).

CHINESE THERAPEUTIC ACTIONS

1. Tonifies qi, strengthens the Spleen, and harmonizes the Stomach
2. Regulates qi and warms the middle *jiao*

CLINICAL MANIFESTATIONS

Spleen and Stomach qi deficiencies accompanied by cold and damp stagnation in the middle *jiao*: lethargy, weakness of the limbs, exercise intolerance, lack of appetite, belching, bloating and pain of the abdomen and epigastrium after eating, vomiting, diarrhea, a pale tongue with possibly a greasy coating, and a weak, slippery pulse.

VETERINARY CLINICAL APPLICATIONS

Gastrointestinal and lung disorders: chronic gastritis, gastric ulcer, chronic gastroenteritis, post-surgical anorexia, vomiting and diarrhea, chronic bronchitis.

EXPLANATION

Xiang Sha Liu Jun Zi Tang (Six-Gentlemen Decoction with Aucklandia and Amomum) combines *Liu Jun Zi Tang* (Six-Gentlemen Decoction) with *Mu Xiang* (Radix Aucklandiae) and *Sha Ren* (Fructus Amomi) to treat deficiency of the middle *jiao* with cold and damp stagnation. Spleen and Stomach deficiencies weaken the digestive system, causing lethargy, weakness of the limbs, exercise intolerance, lack of appetite, belching, and general weakness. Accumulation of cold and dampness causes bloating and pain in the abdomen after eating. In addition, cold and dampness block Stomach qi from descending properly, causing vomiting. Moreover, as a result of Spleen deficiency, the normally ascending qi of the Spleen actually descends, resulting in loose stools or diarrhea.

Ren Shen (Radix et Rhizoma Ginseng), *Bai Zhu* (Rhizoma Atractylodis Macrocephalae), *Fu Ling* (Poria), and *Gan Cao* (Radix et Rhizoma Glycyrrhizae), four herbs from *Si Jun Zi Tang* (Four-Gentlemen Decoction), tonify Spleen and Stomach qi. *Ban Xia* (Rhizoma Pinelliae) and *Chen Pi* (Pericarpium Citri Reticulatae) break up qi and damp stagnation, and correct the reversed flow of Stomach qi. *Mu Xiang* (Radix Aucklandiae) and *Sha Ren* (Fructus Amomi) warm the middle *jiao* and activate qi circulation to dissolve damp accumulation and relieve fullness and pain.

VETERINARY MODIFICATIONS

- With lack of appetite, add *Mai Ya* (Fructus Hordei Germinatus) and *Shan Zha* (Fructus Crataegi).
- If there is abdominal bloating due to deficiency and cold, add *Fu Zi* (Radix Aconiti Lateralis Praeparata) and *Gan Jiang* (Rhizoma Zingiberis).
- For Spleen and Stomach qi deficiencies, add *Huang Qi* (Radix Astragali) and *Shan Yao* (Rhizoma Dioscoreae).
- With nausea, vomiting, and food retention, add *Huo Xiang* (Herba Agastaches) and *Zhu Ru* (Caulis Bambusae in Taenia).

Xiāng Shā Liù Jūn Zǐ Tāng

(Six-Gentlemen Decoction with Aucklandia and Amomum)

Xiang Sha Liu Jun Zi Tang **(Six-Gentlemen Decoction with Aucklandia and Amomum)**

Diagnosis	Clinical Signs	Treatment	Herbs
Spleen and Stomach qi deficiencies accompanied by cold and damp stagnation in the middle *jiao*	• Lethargy, weakness of the limbs, exercise intolerance, lack of appetite, bloating and abdominal pain after eating, belching, loose stools, a pale tongue with possibly a greasy coating, and weak, slippery pulse: Spleen and Stomach deficiencies • Nausea and vomiting: cold and damp stagnation in the Stomach	• Tonifies qi, strengthens the Spleen, and harmonizes the Stomach • Regulates qi and warms the middle *jiao*	• *Ren Shen* (Radix et Rhizoma Ginseng), *Bai Zhu* (Rhizoma Atractylodis Macrocephalae), *Fu Ling* (Poria), and *Gan Cao* (Radix et Rhizoma Glycyrrhizae) tonify Spleen and Stomach qi. • *Ban Xia* (Rhizoma Pinelliae) and *Chen Pi* (Pericarpium Citri Reticulatae) break up qi and damp stagnation and correct the reversed flow of qi. • *Mu Xiang* (Radix Aucklandiae) and *Sha Ren* (Fructus Amomi) warm the middle *jiao*, activate qi circulation, and relieve fullness and pain.

- With vomiting and diarrhea, combine with *Ping Wei San* (Calm the Stomach Powder).
- With vomiting and diarrhea due to deficiency and cold, combine with *Li Zhong Tang* (Regulate the Middle Decoction).

CAUTIONS / CONTRAINDICATIONS

Xiang Sha Liu Jun Zi Tang should not be given with raw and cold foods.[1]

PHARMACOLOGICAL EFFECTS

1. **Gastrointestinal**: According to laboratory experiments in rabbits, administration of *Xiang Sha Liu Jun Zi Tang* was associated with a regulatory effect on the intestines. Depending on the condition of the subject, it either increased or decreased intestinal peristalsis.[2]
2. **Antiulcer**: Administration of *Xiang Sha Liu Jun Zi Tang* was associated with a marked effect in preventing and treating stomach ulcer in rats. The mechanisms of action were attributed to promotion of normal stomach mucosa, and decreased production of gastric acid.[3]
3. **Immunostimulant**: Administration of *Xiang Sha Liu Jun Zi Tang* was associated with an increase of IgM, IgA, and T cells.[4,5]

HUMAN CLINICAL STUDIES AND RESEARCH

1. **Chronic atrophic gastritis**: *Xiang Sha Liu Jun Zi Tang* was used to treat patients with chronic atrophic gastritis characterized by deficiency and cold. Out of 25 cases, the study reported significant improvement with resolution of the symptoms in 18 cases, and moderate improvement with slight pain in 7 cases.[6] In another study, use of *Xiang Sha Liu Jun Zi Tang* plus *Shan Yao* (Rhizoma Dioscoreae) daily was associated with complete recovery in 12 of 14 patients with chronic atrophic gastritis characterized by Spleen qi deficiency.[7]
2. **Gastritis**: Use of *Xiang Sha Liu Jun Zi Tang* daily for 4 weeks per course of treatment was associated with marked effect to treat chronic gastritis in elderly patients. Of 23 patients, the study reported complete recovery in 9 cases, marked improvement in 12 cases, and no effect in 2 cases. The overall effectiveness was 91.3%.[8]
3. **Irritable bowel syndrome (IBS)**: In one study, 40 patients with irritable bowel syndrome were treated with marked improvement in 18 cases, moderate improvement in 16 cases, and no effect in 6 cases. The herbal treatment included this formula plus *Yan Hu Suo* (Rhizoma Corydalis), *Ru Xiang* (Gummi Olibanum), and *Mo Yao* (Myrrha). Furthermore, *Xiang Fu* (Rhizoma Cyperi) and *Yu Jin* (Radix Curcumae) were added for emotional distress; and *Pu Huang* (Pollen Typhae) and *Wu Ling Zhi* (Faeces Trogopteri) were added for menstrual pain. The treatment protocol was to administer the herbs for 2 weeks per course of treatment, for 1-3 courses total.[9]
4. **Stomatitis**: In one report, 30 patients with recurrent stomatitis were treated with modified *Xiang Sha Liu Jun Zi Tang* in decoction with complete recovery in all patients. The length of treatment varied from 4-20 packs of herbs. The herbal treatment contained *Xiang Sha Liu Jun Zi Tang*, with the addition of *Zhi Zi* (Fructus Gardeniae) for diarrhea with preference for warm drinks; *Huang Lian* (Rhizoma Coptidis), *Zhu Ye* (Herba Phyllostachys), and *Di Huang* (Radix Rehmanniae) for red tongue tip from Heart fire rising; and the addition of *Mu Dan Pi* (Cortex Moutan) and removal of *Ren Shen* (Radix et Rhizoma Ginseng) for dry throat with a bitter taste in the mouth.[10]
5. **Post-surgical diarrhea**: Administration of modified *Xiang Sha Liu Jun Zi Tang* was associated with 90.25% effectiveness in treating 113 patients with post-surgical

Xiāng Shā Liù Jūn Zǐ Tāng

(Six-Gentlemen Decoction with Aucklandia and Amomum)

diarrhea. The herbs were given in decoction daily for 2 weeks per course of treatment.[11]

6. **Anorexia**: Modified *Xiang Sha Liu Jun Zi Tang* was used to treat 33 children with anorexia with 94% effectiveness. The herbal treatment included this formula plus *Bing Lang* (Semen Arecae), *Lai Fu Zi* (Semen Raphani), charred *Ji Nei Jin* (Endothelium Corneum Gigeriae Galli), and charred *Shan Zha* (Fructus Crataegi). The treatment protocol was to administer the herbs daily, with 8 packs of herbs per course of treatment, followed by 3-5 days of rest, and then a second 8-pack course. Of 33 patients, the study reported marked effectiveness in 19 cases, moderate effectiveness in 12 cases, and no effect in 2 cases.[12]

TOXICOLOGY

In an acute toxicology study, oral ingestion of *Xiang Sha Liu Jun Zi Tang* in decoction at 0.4 mL/10g (equivalent to 80 g/kg of raw herbs) twice daily for 7 days did not cause any abnormal behavior in animal subjects. In fact, some subjects had an increase in body weight. The dose given to the subjects was equivalent to 434 times the normal adult dose in humans.[13]

SUGGESTED ACUPUNCTURE TREATMENT

1. Points: *Pishu* (BL 20), *Weishu* (BL 21), *Housanli* (ST 36), *Quchi* (LI 11), *Qihai* (CV 6), and *Zhongwan* (CV 12).
2. Technique: tonification.

Pishu (BL 20) nourishes Spleen yang. *Weishu* (BL 21) and *Housanli* (ST 36) tonify the middle *jiao* and harmonize the Stomach. *Tianshu* (ST 25) regulates the Stomach and Intestines. *Quchi* (LI 11) regulates qi and blood in *yangming* channels. *Qihai* (CV 6) tonifies qi in general. *Zhongwan* (CV 12) and *Qihai* (CV 6) enhance the qi flow of the abdomen and increase appetite.

RELATED FORMULA

Xiāng Shā Liù Jūn Zǐ Tāng
(Six-Gentlemen Decoction with Cyperus and Amomum)
香砂六君子湯
香砂六君子汤

Pinyin Name: *Xiang Sha Liu Jun Zi Tang*
Literal Name: Six-Gentlemen Decoction with Cyperus and Amomum
Original Source: *Yi Fang Ji Jie* (Analytical Collection of Medical Formulas) by Wang Ang in 1682

Ren Shen (Radix et Rhizoma Ginseng)	6g
Bai Zhu (Rhizoma Atractylodis Macrocephalae)	6g
Fu Ling (Poria)	6g
Zhi Gan Cao (Radix et Rhizoma Glycyrrhizae Praeparata cum Melle)	3g
Chen Pi (Pericarpium Citri Reticulatae)	3g
Ban Xia (Rhizoma Pinelliae)	3g
Xiang Fu (Rhizoma Cyperi)	6g
Sha Ren (Fructus Amomi)	6g

This formula is composed by adding *Xiang Fu* (Rhizoma Cyperi) and *Sha Ren* (Fructus Amomi) to *Liu Jun Zi Tang* (Six-Gentlemen Decoction). This formula strengthens the Spleen, harmonizes the Stomach, regulates qi circulation, and stops pain. It treats Spleen and Stomach qi deficiencies, accompanied by accumulation of cold and dampness in the middle *jiao*.

These two formulas have identical Chinese characters and pinyin names. They also have very similar ingredients, doses, and functions.

- In the primary formula, "*Xiang*" refers to *Mu Xiang* (Radix Aucklandiae), a qi-regulating herb that treats qi stagnation of the Spleen and Stomach. *Gan Cao* (Radix et Rhizoma Glycyrrhizae) is used to tonify qi and to harmonize the formula.
- In the related formula, "*Xiang*" refers to *Xiang Fu* (Rhizoma Cyperi), a qi-regulating herb that treats qi stagnation in the Liver and *San Jiao*. *Zhi Gan Cao* (Radix et Rhizoma Glycyrrhizae Praeparata cum Melle) is used to strongly tonify qi and harmonize the formula.

AUTHORS' COMMENTS

Xiang Sha Liu Jun Zi Tang treats gastrointestinal disorders characterized by cold and damp stagnation of the middle *jiao*, and by Spleen and Stomach deficiencies. The cold and damp stagnation present in these conditions may cause key clinical signs such as vomiting, belching, borborygmus, and abdominal pain. Cold and damp accumulation most often develops following surgery, secondary to feeding raw food diets in juvenile, weak, geriatric and debilitated animals with incompetent Spleen function, and following prolonged antibiotic use or chemotherapy. Cold accumulation is often an important factor in equine gastrointestinal disease due to common overuse of antibiotics and environmental exposure, and, as such, formulas like *Xiang Sha Liu Jun Zi Tang* and *Li Zhong Tang* (Regulate the Middle Decoction) are often preferred over *Liu Jun Zi Tang* (Six-Gentlemen Decoction). For a comparative discussion of Spleen tonic formulas, see *Si Jun Zi Tang* (Four-Gentlemen Decoction).

Xiāng Shā Liù Jūn Zǐ Tāng

(Six-Gentlemen Decoction with Aucklandia and Amomum)

References

1. *Zhong Yao Ming Fang Yao Li Yu Ying Yong* (Pharmacology and Applications of Famous Herbal Formulas), 1989; 405-406.
2. *Zhong Yi Fang Ji Xian Dai Yan Jiu* (Modern Study of Medical Formulas in Traditional Chinese Medicine), 1997; 499-500.
3. *Bei Jing Zhong Yi Yao Da Xue Xue Bao* (Journal of Beijing University of Medicine and Medicinals), 1994; 17(5):57.
4. *Liao Ning Zhong Yi Za Zhi* (Liaoning Journal of Chinese Medicine), 1982; 7:4.
5. *Shan Dong Zhong Yi Za Zhi* (Shandong Journal of Chinese Medicine), 1986; 27(11):53.
6. *Nan Jing Zhong Yi Xue Yuan Xue Bao* (Journal of Nanjing University of Traditional Chinese Medicine), 1987; 4:23.
7. *Liao Ning Zhong Yi Za Zhi* (Liaoning Journal of Chinese Medicine), 1982; 7:4.
8. *Shan Xi Zhong Yi Xue Yuan Xue Bao* (Journal of Shanxi University School of Chinese Medicine), 1999; 3:44.
9. *Hu Bei Zhong Yi Za Zhi* (Hubei Journal of Chinese Medicine), 1997; 3:15.
10. *Shan Dong Zhong Yi Za Zhi* (Shandong Journal of Chinese Medicine), 1991; 10(5):32.
11. *Fu Jian Zhong Yi Yao* (Fujian Chinese Medicine and Herbology), 1996; 3:34.
12. *Gan Su Zhong Yi Xue Yuan Xue Bao* (Journal of Gansu University of Chinese Medicine), 1995; 2:26.
13. *Zhong Yao Yao Li Yu Lin Chuang* (Pharmacology and Clinical Applications of Chinese Herbs), 1990; 6(2):5.

Xiāng Shā Yǎng Wèi Tāng

(Nourish the Stomach Decoction with Aucklandia and Amomum)

香砂養胃湯

香砂养胃汤

Pinyin Name: *Xiang Sha Yang Wei Tang*

Literal Name: Nourish the Stomach Decoction with Aucklandia and Amomum

Alternate Name: Cyperus and Cluster Combination

Original Source: *Wan Bing Hui Chun* (Restoration of Health from the Myriad Diseases) by Gong Ting-Xian in 1587

COMPOSITION

Ren Shen (Radix et Rhizoma Ginseng)	1.5g
Bai Zhu (Rhizoma Atractylodis Macrocephalae)	3g
Fu Ling (Poria)	2.4g
Zhi Gan Cao (Radix et Rhizoma Glycyrrhizae Praeparata cum Melle), a small amount	[0.6g]
Cang Zhu (Rhizoma Atractylodis), *zhi* (prepared) with rice water and *chao* (dry-fried)	2.4g
Sha Ren (Fructus Amomi)	2.4g
Dou Kou (Fructus Amomi Rotundus)	2.1g
Xiang Fu (Rhizoma Cyperi), *chao* (dry-fried)	2.4g
Mu Xiang (Radix Aucklandiae)	1.5g
Hou Po (Cortex Magnoliae Officinalis), *chao* (dry-fried) with ginger juice	2.4g
Chen Pi (Pericarpium Citri Reticulatae)	2.4g

DOSAGE / PREPARATION / ADMINISTRATION

Grind the herbs into powder, and cook the powder with *Sheng Jiang* (Rhizoma Zingiberis Recens) and *Da Zao* (Fructus Jujubae) to make a decoction.

CHINESE THERAPEUTIC ACTIONS

1. Strengthens the Spleen and dispels dampness
2. Improves appetite

Xiāng Shā Yǎng Wèi Tāng

(Nourish the Stomach Decoction with Aucklandia and Amomum)

Xiang Sha Yang Wei Tang **(Nourish the Stomach Decoction with Aucklandia and Amomum)**

Diagnosis	Clinical Signs	Treatment	Herbs
Low appetite caused by Spleen deficiency	• Lack of appetite: Spleen deficiency • Epigastric discomfort or distention: damp accumulation	• Strengthens the Spleen and dispels dampness • Improves appetite	• *Ren Shen* (Radix et Rhizoma Ginseng), *Bai Zhu* (Rhizoma Atractylodis Macrocephalae), *Fu Ling* (Poria), *Da Zao* (Fructus Jujubae), and *Zhi Gan Cao* (Radix et Rhizoma Glycyrrhizae Praeparata cum Melle) tonify Spleen qi. • *Cang Zhu* (Rhizoma Atractylodis), *Sha Ren* (Fructus Amomi), and *Dou Kou* (Fructus Amomi Rotundus) dry dampness and increase appetite. • *Xiang Fu* (Rhizoma Cyperi), *Mu Xiang* (Radix Aucklandiae), *Hou Po* (Cortex Magnoliae Officinalis), and *Chen Pi* (Pericarpium Citri Reticulatae) activate qi to dispel dampness. • *Sheng Jiang* (Rhizoma Zingiberis Recens) harmonizes the Stomach to increase appetite.

CLINICAL MANIFESTATIONS

Low appetite caused by Spleen deficiency: lack of appetite, abdominal bloating after eating, a pale tongue, and a weak, slippery pulse.

VETERINARY CLINICAL APPLICATIONS

Gastrointestinal disorders characterized by anorexia and poor appetite: cancer, feline hepatic lipidosis, chronic gastritis, gastroenteritis, gastric ulcer, idiopathic gastric hypomotility and bilious vomiting, and following chemotherapy or radiation therapy.

EXPLANATION

Spleen deficiency can lead to the formation of dampness, which causes loss of appetite because the transportation and transformation functions of the Spleen are impaired. *Xiang Sha Yang Wei Tang* (Nourish the Stomach Decoction with Aucklandia and Amomum) tonifies Spleen qi, dispels dampness, and activates qi circulation.

Ren Shen (Radix et Rhizoma Ginseng), *Bai Zhu* (Rhizoma Atractylodis Macrocephalae), *Fu Ling* (Poria), *Da Zao* (Fructus Jujubae), and *Zhi Gan Cao* (Radix et Rhizoma Glycyrrhizae Praeparata cum Melle) tonify Spleen qi. *Cang Zhu* (Rhizoma Atractylodis), *Sha Ren* (Fructus Amomi), and *Dou Kou* (Fructus Amomi Rotundus) are aromatic herbs that dry dampness and increase appetite. *Xiang Fu* (Rhizoma Cyperi), *Mu Xiang* (Radix Aucklandiae), *Hou Po* (Cortex Magnoliae Officinalis), and *Chen Pi* (Pericarpium Citri Reticulatae) activate qi to dispel dampness. *Sheng Jiang* (Rhizoma Zingiberis Recens) harmonizes the Stomach to improve appetite.

CAUTIONS / CONTRAINDICATIONS

Avoid raw and cold foods while taking *Xiang Sha Yang Wei Tang.*[1]

SUGGESTED ACUPUNCTURE TREATMENT

1. Points: *Pishu* (BL 20), *Weishu* (BL 21), *Zhongwan* (CV 12), *Housanli* (ST 36), *Sanyinjiao* (SP 6), *Qihai* (CV 6), *Zhangmen* (LR 13), *Gongsun* (SP 4) and *Shangen* and *Mijiaogan*.
2. Technique: tonification.

Since the main problem is Spleen deficiency, the selection of points centers around tonifying the Spleen. *Pishu* (BL 20) and *Weishu* (BL 21) tonify Spleen and Stomach yang to promote digestion. *Zhongwan* (CV 12), *Housanli* (ST 36), and *Sanyinjiao* (SP 6) restore the normal functions of the Spleen and Stomach, harmonize the middle *jiao*, and relieve fullness and distention. *Qihai* (CV 6) tonifies qi. Finally, *Zhangmen* (LR 13), the front *mu* (collecting) point of the Spleen, and *Gongsun* (SP 4) regulate Spleen qi. *Shangen* and *Mijiaogan* are classical points to stimulate appetite in the dog and horse, respectively.

AUTHORS' COMMENTS

Xiang Sha Yang Wei Tang is primarily used to promote appetite in animals with anorexia. It is a gentler formula than *Xiang Sha Liu Jun Zi Tang* (Six-Gentlemen Decoction with Aucklandia and Amomum), and has a weaker ability to stop vomiting but a stronger action to stimulate appetite. For a comparative discussion of Spleen tonic formulas, see *Si Jun Zi Tang* (Four-Gentlemen Decoction).

Reference

1. *Zhong Yao Ming Fang Yao Li Yu Ying Yong* (Pharmacology and Applications of Famous Herbal Formulas), 1989; 622-623.

Shēn Líng Bái Zhú Sǎn

(Ginseng, Poria, and Atractylodes Macrocephala Powder)

參苓白朮散
参苓白术散

Pinyin Name: *Shen Ling Bai Zhu San*
Literal Name: Ginseng, Poria, and Atractylodes Macrocephala Powder
Alternate Names: *Shen Ling Pai Chu San*, Ginseng, Poria and Bighead Atractylodes Powder; Ginseng and Atractylodes Formula
Original Source: *Tai Ping Hui Min He Ji Ju Fang* (Imperial Grace Formulary of the Tai Ping Era) by the Imperial Medical Department in 1078-85

COMPOSITION

Ren Shen (Radix et Rhizoma Ginseng)	960g [15g]
Bai Zhu (Rhizoma Atractylodis Macrocephalae)	960g [15g]
Fu Ling (Poria)	960g [15g]
Gan Cao (Radix et Rhizoma Glycyrrhizae), *chao* (dry-fried)	960g [9g]
Shan Yao (Rhizoma Dioscoreae)	960g [15g]
Lian Zi (Semen Nelumbinis)	480g [9g]
Bai Bian Dou (Semen Lablab Album), *jin* (soaked) in ginger juice and *chao* (dry-fried)	720g [12g]
Yi Yi Ren (Semen Coicis)	480g [9g]
Sha Ren (Fructus Amomi)	480g [6g]
Jie Geng (Radix Platycodonis), *chao* (dry-fried) to dark brown	480g [6g]

DOSAGE / PREPARATION / ADMINISTRATION

The source text states to grind the ingredients into a fine powder. Take 6g of the powder per dose with a decoction made from *Da Zao* (Fructus Jujubae). Adjust the dose accordingly for young animals. Today, this formula may be prepared as a decoction with the doses suggested in brackets.

CHINESE THERAPEUTIC ACTIONS

1. Tonifies qi and strengthens the Spleen
2. Resolves dampness and stops diarrhea

CLINICAL MANIFESTATIONS

Spleen and Stomach deficiencies with dampness: lethargy, fatigue, general weakness, diarrhea, vomiting, borborygmus, decreased appetite, weak extremities, weight loss, edema, chronic coughing with phlegm, a pale to pale pink tongue with possibly a white coating and scalloped edges, and a deep, weak pulse.

VETERINARY CLINICAL APPLICATIONS

Chronic gastrointestinal and lung disorders: chronic gastroenteritis, chronic diarrhea with undigested food in the stool, exocrine pancreatic insufficiency (EPI), diabetes mellitus, inflammatory bowel syndrome, nephritis, poor immune function, supportive therapy for chronic disease, cancer, nausea accompanying chemotherapy and radiation, debility after chronic illness, edema, damp-heat skin disorders, chronic cough with clear phlegm, white vaginal discharge, puppy vaginitis.

EXPLANATION

Shen Ling Bai Zhu San (Ginseng, Poria, and Atractylodes Macrocephala Powder) treats Spleen and Stomach deficiencies with damp accumulation. The Spleen and Stomach are in charge of transforming and transporting nutrients; deficiency in these two organs weakens the digestive function. As a result, food travels quickly through the body without being properly digested or absorbed, hence giving rise to loose stools or diarrhea. A weak digestive system may result in decreased appetite, weak extremities, and weight loss. Spleen deficiency usually causes damp accumulation, which, in turn, obstructs Lung qi, causing chronic coughing with phlegm and/or epigastric fullness and distention. Dampness can also obstruct Stomach qi, causing nausea and vomiting. The pale to pale pink tongue with possibly a white coating and scalloped edges and the deep, weak pulse indicate deficiency.

Ren Shen (Radix et Rhizoma Ginseng), *Bai Zhu* (Rhizoma Atractylodis Macrocephalae), *Fu Ling* (Poria), and *Gan Cao* (Radix et Rhizoma Glycyrrhizae) tonify qi and strengthen the Spleen and Stomach. *Shan Yao* (Rhizoma Dioscoreae) and *Lian Zi* (Semen Nelumbinis) treat diarrhea by assisting *Ren Shen* (Radix et Rhizoma Ginseng) in strengthening the Spleen and tonifying qi. *Bai Bian Dou*

Shēn Líng Bái Zhú Sǎn

(Ginseng, Poria, and Atractylodes Macrocephala Powder)

(Semen Lablab Album) and *Yi Yi Ren* (Semen Coicis) help *Bai Zhu* (Rhizoma Atractylodis Macrocephalae) and *Fu Ling* (Poria) strengthen the Spleen and dispel dampness. *Sha Ren* (Fructus Amomi) awakens the Spleen and harmonizes the Stomach to regulate qi and resolve stagnation. *Jie Geng* (Radix Platycodonis) relieves chest fullness, and has an ascending function to help counteract diarrhea. *Gan Cao* (Radix et Rhizoma Glycyrrhizae) harmonizes both the middle *jiao* and the formula.

VETERINARY MODIFICATIONS

- For frequent infections and weak immunity, combine with *Huang Qi* (Radix Astragali).
- With gagging of clear phlegm and chronic cough, add *Chen Pi* (Pericarpium Citri Reticulatae) and *Ban Xia* (Rhizoma Pinelliae).
- With edema, combine with *Wu Ling San* (Five-Ingredient Powder with Poria).
- For loose stools with abdominal pain due to cold, add *Gan Jiang* (Rhizoma Zingiberis) and *Rou Gui* (Cortex Cinnamomi).
- For loose stools with damp-heat, add *Huang Lian* (Rhizoma Coptidis), *Che Qian Zi* (Semen Plantaginis), and *Ze Xie* (Rhizoma Alismatis).
- With Spleen yang deficiency, add *Fu Zi Li Zhong Wan* (Prepared Aconite Pill to Regulate the Middle).
- For cough with phlegm accumulation, add *Ban Xia* (Rhizoma Pinelliae) and *Chen Pi* (Pericarpium Citri Reticulatae).
- For constant diarrhea, add *Qian Shi* (Semen Euryales) and *Mu Xiang* (Radix Aucklandiae).
- With frequent urination, add *Yi Zhi* (Fructus Alpiniae Oxyphyllae) and *Wu Yao* (Radix Linderae).
- For food retention, vomiting, and diarrhea, combine with *Ping Wei San* (Calm the Stomach Powder).
- For indigestion and weight loss, add dry-fried *Mai Ya* (Fructus Hordei Germinatus), *Shan Zha* (Fructus Crataegi), and *Shen Qu* (Massa Fermentata).

CAUTIONS / CONTRAINDICATIONS

- *Shen Ling Bai Zhu San* should be used with caution in the following conditions: yin-deficient fire and yin deficiency.
- Since this formula is slightly drying and warm in nature, it should be used with caution during pregnancy, and in animals with exterior or interior heat conditions.[1]

PHARMACOLOGICAL EFFECTS

Gastrointestinal: According to laboratory experiments in rabbits, administration of *Shen Ling Bai Zhu San* was associated with a regulatory effect on the intestines. Depending on the condition of the subject, it either increased or decreased the intestinal peristalsis.[2]

HUMAN CLINICAL STUDIES AND RESEARCH

1. **Superficial gastritis**: Use of modified *Shen Ling Bai Zhu San* in 32 patients with superficial gastritis was associated with 96.7% effectiveness. The herbal treatment contained *Ren Shen* (Radix et Rhizoma Ginseng), *Bai Zhu* (Rhizoma

***Shen Ling Bai Zhu San* (Ginseng, Poria, and Atractylodes Macrocephala Powder)**

Diagnosis	Clinical Signs	Treatment	Herbs
Spleen and Stomach deficiencies with dampness	• Diarrhea, borborygmus, decreased appetite, weak appearance: Spleen and Stomach qi deficiencies • Weak extremities and weight loss: Spleen and Stomach qi deficiencies unable to nourish the body and limbs • Epigastric distention and coughing with phlegm: damp accumulation blocking Lung qi circulation • Nausea and vomiting: damp accumulation obstructing Stomach qi circulation • A pale to pale pink tongue with possibly a white coating, and a deep, weak pulse: qi deficiency	• Tonifies qi and strengthens the Spleen • Resolves dampness and stops diarrhea	• *Ren Shen* (Radix et Rhizoma Ginseng), *Bai Zhu* (Rhizoma Atractylodis Macrocephalae), *Fu Ling* (Poria), and *Gan Cao* (Radix et Rhizoma Glycyrrhizae) tonify qi and strengthen the Spleen and Stomach. • *Shan Yao* (Rhizoma Dioscoreae) and *Lian Zi* (Semen Nelumbinis) strengthen the Spleen, tonify qi, and stop diarrhea. • *Bai Bian Dou* (Semen Lablab Album) and *Yi Yi Ren* (Semen Coicis) strengthen the Spleen and dispel dampness. • *Sha Ren* (Fructus Amomi) awakens the Spleen and harmonizes the Stomach to regulate qi and resolve stagnation. • *Jie Geng* (Radix Platycodonis) ventilates the Lung and relieves chest fullness. • *Gan Cao* (Radix et Rhizoma Glycyrrhizae) harmonizes the middle *jiao* and all of the herbs.

Shēn Líng Bái Zhú Sǎn

(Ginseng, Poria, and Atractylodes Macrocephala Powder)

Atractylodis Macrocephalae), *Fu Ling* (Poria), *Shan Yao* (Rhizoma Dioscoreae), *Gan Cao* (Radix et Rhizoma Glycyrrhizae), *Bai Bian Dou* (Semen Lablab Album), *Bai Shao* (Radix Paeoniae Alba), *Yan Hu Suo* (Rhizoma Corydalis), *Yi Yi Ren* (Semen Coicis), *Sha Ren* (Fructus Amomi), *Ying Su Ke* (Pericarpium Papaveris), and *Bai Ji* (Rhizoma Bletillae). Furthermore, modifications were made by adding *Wu Zhu Yu* (Fructus Evodiae) and *Gao Liang Jiang* (Rhizoma Alpiniae Officinarum) for cold; *Chai Hu* (Radix Bupleuri), *Huang Qin* (Radix Scutellariae), and *Huang Lian* (Rhizoma Coptidis) for Stomach heat; *Fu Zi* (Radix Aconiti Lateralis Praeparata) and *Rou Gui* (Cortex Cinnamomi) for deficiency and cold; *Shen Qu* (Massa Fermentata), *Shan Zha* (Fructus Crataegi) and *Mai Ya* (Fructus Hordei Germinatus) for food stagnation; *Chai Hu* (Radix Bupleuri), *Xiang Fu* (Rhizoma Cyperi) and *Dou Kou* (Fructus Amomi Rotundus) for qi stagnation; and *Dan Shen* (Radix et Rhizoma Salviae Miltiorrhizae), *Mo Yao* (Myrrha), and *E Zhu* (Rhizoma Curcumae) for blood stagnation. Of 32 cases, the study reported complete recovery in 15 cases, significant improvement in 9 cases, moderate improvement in 7 cases, and no effect in 1 case.[3]

2. **Diarrhea**: In one clinical study, 95 patients with diarrhea (negative for microorganism infection) were treated with modified *Shen Ling Bai Zhu San*. In addition to this formula, *Bu Zhong Yi Qi Tang* (Tonify the Middle and Augment the Qi Decoction) was given to patients with Spleen qi deficiency; *Fu Zi Li Zhong Wan* (Prepared Aconite Pill to Regulate the Middle) for Spleen yang deficiency; and *Si Shen Wan* (Four-Miracle Pill) for Spleen and Kidney yang deficiency. Out of 95 cases, the study reported significant improvement in 27 cases, moderate improvement in 41 cases, and no effect in 27 cases. The overall rate of effectiveness was 71.6%.[4]
3. **Chronic colitis**: Use of modified *Shen Ling Bai Zhu San* one time daily in decoction showed good results in treating chronic colitis characterized by Spleen deficiency and dampness. Modifications to the base formula included addition of *Mu Xiang* (Radix Aucklandiae), dry-fried *Zhi Qiao* (Fructus Aurantii), and dry-fried *Lai Fu Zi* (Semen Raphani) for qi stagnation; dry-fried *Gu Ya* (Fructus Setariae Germinatus), dry-fried *Mai Ya* (Fructus Hordei Germinatus), dry-fried *Shen Qu* (Massa Fermentata), and charred *Shan Zha* (Fructus Crataegi) for diarrhea; *Xiang Fu* (Rhizoma Cyperi), *Gao Liang Jiang* (Rhizoma Alpiniae Officinarum), and vinegar-fried *Yan Hu Suo* (Rhizoma Corydalis) for abdominal pain; *Bu Gu Zhi* (Fructus Psoraleae), roasted *Rou Dou Kou* (Semen Myristicae), and salt-fried *Wu Zhu Yu* (Fructus Evodiae) for deficiency and cold of the Spleen and Kidney; and *Huang Qi* (Radix Astragali), *Chai Hu* (Radix Bupleuri), and *Sheng Ma* (Rhizoma Cimicifugae) for diarrhea and rectal prolapse due to qi collapse. Out of 60 cases, the study reported complete recovery in 38 cases, significant improvement in 14 cases, slight improvement in 6 cases, and no effect in 2 cases. The overall rate of effectiveness was 97%.[5]
4. **Irritable bowel syndrome (IBS)**: Use of modified *Shen Ling Bai Zhu San* in 52 patients with irritable bowel syndrome was associated with 96.2% effectiveness. In addition to the base formula, modifications included addition of *Huang Qi* (Radix Astragali) and *He Zi* (Fructus Chebulae) for deficiency and weakness of the Spleen and Stomach; *Chai Hu* (Radix Bupleuri), *Yu Jin* (Radix Curcumae), and *Yan Hu Suo* (Rhizoma Corydalis) for Liver qi stagnation and Spleen deficiency; *Huang Lian* (Rhizoma Coptidis), *Pei Lan* (Herba Eupatorii), and *Bai Tou Weng* (Radix Pulsatillae) for Spleen deficiency with damp-heat; and *Bu Gu Zhi* (Fructus Psoraleae), *Rou Dou Kou* (Semen Myristicae), and *Wu Zhu Yu* (Fructus Evodiae) for Spleen and Kidney yang deficiency. The herbs were given in decoction daily, with duration of treatment ranging from 5-30 days (average of 18.1 days). Of 52 patients, the study reported complete recovery in 40 cases, improvement in 10 cases, and no effect in 2 cases.[6]
5. **Proctitis**: In one study, 12 patients with chronic proctitis were treated with *Shen Ling Bai Zhu San,* with complete recovery in 2 cases, remission in 4 cases, improvement in 5 cases, and no effect in 1 case. The overall rate of effectiveness was 91.67%. The herbal treatment contained *Shen Ling Bai Zhu San* plus *Sheng Ma* (Rhizoma Cimicifugae), *He Zi* (Fructus Chebulae), *Lian Zi* (Semen Nelumbinis), and *Wu Mei* (Fructus Mume). The treatment protocol was to cook the herbs and administer the decoction daily for 4 weeks.[7]
6. **Nephritis**: Administration of modified *Shen Ling Bai Zhu San* to 15 patients with nephritis was associated with significant improvement in 2 cases, moderate improvement in 4 cases, slight improvement in 2 cases, and no effect in 7 cases. Modifications to the original formula included the addition of *Di Huang* (Radix Rehmanniae), *Nu Zhen Zi* (Fructus Ligustri Lucidi), and *Gou Qi Zi* (Fructus Lycii) for nephritis characterized by Kidney yin deficiency; *Bai Mao Gen* (Rhizoma Imperatae), *Dan Shen* (Radix et Rhizoma Salviae Miltiorrhizae), *Chi Shao* (Radix Paeoniae Rubra), *Chuan Xiong* (Rhizoma Chuanxiong), and *Yi Mu Cao* (Herba Leonuri) for hematuria; and *Jin Yin Hua* (Flos Lonicerae Japonicae), *Huang Qin* (Radix Scutellariae), *Yu Xing Cao* (Herba Houttuyniae), *Pu Gong Ying* (Herba Taraxaci), and *Da Qing Ye* (Folium Isatidis) for upper respiratory tract infection characterized by damp-heat. The herbs were cooked in water, and the decoction taken in two equally-divided doses daily.[8]

Shēn Líng Bái Zhú Sǎn

(Ginseng, Poria, and Atractylodes Macrocephala Powder)

7. **Compromised immune system**: One study reported good results using modified *Shen Ling Bai Zhu San* to treat 48 patients with compromised immunity. In addition to the base formula, *Huang Qi* (Radix Astragali) was added for qi deficiency, *Chen Pi* (Pericarpium Citri Reticulatae) for qi stagnation, and *Yin Chen* (Herba Artemisiae Scopariae) for damp-heat. The treatment protocol was to administer the herbs in decoction one time daily, delivering 20 packs of herbs per course of treatment, for 1-3 courses total. The study reported gradual improvement over the courses of treatment, based on better tongue coating and normal pulse.[9] (Note: Specific details were unavailable on rate of effectiveness, and subjective and objective improvements.)
8. **Cognitive impairment**: Use of modified *Shen Ling Bai Zhu San* was associated with improvement in 33 of 47 children (32 males and 15 females, between 1-5 years of age) with slow mental development. The herbal treatment contained this formula plus *Bu Gu Zhi* (Fructus Psoraleae), *Yi Zhi* (Fructus Alpiniae Oxyphyllae), *He Shou Wu* (Radix Polygoni Multiflori), and *Rou Cong Rong* (Herba Cistanches). The treatment protocol was to cook the herbs in water and administer the decoction daily, for 4 packs of herbs per course of treatment, for 1-3 courses.[10]
9. **Rhinitis**: Administration of modified *Shen Ling Bai Zhu San* was associated with 92.7% effectiveness in treating 68 children with chronic rhinitis. The herbal treatment contained this formula plus *Huang Qi* (Radix Astragali), *Cang Er Zi* (Fructus Xanthii), and *Bai Zhi* (Radix Angelicae Dahuricae). Furthermore, modifications were made by adding *Huang Qi* (Radix Astragali) and *Jin Yin Hua* (Flos Lonicerae Japonicae) for profuse, yellow, and sticky nasal discharge; *Xin Yi Hua* (Flos Magnoliae) and *Shi Chang Pu* (Rhizoma Acori Tatarinowii) for severe nasal obstruction; *Tian Zhu Huang* (Concretio Silicea Bambusae), *Bai Jie Zi* (Semen Sinapis), and *Chen Pi* (Pericarpium Citri Reticulatae) for profuse sputum; *Fang Feng* (Radix Saposhnikoviae) for frequent infection; *Mai Ya* (Fructus Hordei Germinatus), *Gu Ya* (Fructus Setariae Germinatus), and *Shen Qu* (Massa Fermentata) for poor appetite and diarrhea; *Bai Mao Gen* (Rhizoma Imperatae), *Ce Bai Ye* (Cacumen Platycladi), and *Xian He Cao* (Herba Agrimoniae) for nosebleeds; and others as needed. Herbs were given in decoction daily for 10 days per course of treatment. Of 68 patients, the study reported complete recovery in 18 patients, marked improvement in 25 patients, moderate improvement in 20 patients, and no effect in 5 patients.[11]
10. ***Xiao ke* (wasting and thirsting) syndrome**: Administration of modified *Shen Ling Bai Zhu San* in 30 patients with *xiao ke* (wasting and thirsting) syndrome was associated with recovery in 11 patients, improvement in 17 patients, and no effect in 2 patients. In addition to the formula, modifications included the addition of *Shi Hu* (Caulis Dendrobii) for excessive thirst with a dry tongue and a white tongue coating; *Ze Xie* (Rhizoma Alismatis) and *Che Qian Zi* (Semen Plantaginis) for a white, greasy tongue coating and reduced frequency of urination; and *Shan Zhu Yu* (Fructus Corni) and *Wu Wei Zi* (Fructus Schisandrae Chinensis) for increased frequency of urination. The herbs were cooked in water, and the decoction was taken in two equally-divided doses daily for 1 month per course of treatment. All patients were instructed to control their diet. Those with a prescription for diabetes were instructed to continue using the drugs.[12]
11. **Edema**: Administration of *Shen Ling Bai Zhu San* was associated with complete recovery or significant improvement in 47 of 50 patients (10 males and 40 females, between 30-45 years of age) with edema. The treatment protocol was to cook the herbs in water, and administer the decoction in three equally-divided doses daily for 1 week per course of treatment, for 1-2 courses total.[13]

HERB-DRUG INTERACTION

Supportive therapy for chemotherapy and radiation: *Shen Ling Bai Zhu San* alleviated gastrointestinal side effects associated with chemotherapy and radiation treatments among 96 patients with mid-to-severe stages of cancer. Of 96 cases, the study reported significant effect in 33 cases, moderate effect in 46 cases, and no effect in 17 cases.[14]

SUGGESTED ACUPUNCTURE TREATMENT

1. Points: *Changqiang* (GV 1), *Pishu* (BL 20), *Weishu* (BL 21), *Housanli* (ST 36), *Sanyinjiao* (SP 6), *Yinlingquan* (SP 9), *Zhongwan* (CV 12), and *Tianshu* (ST 25).
2. Technique: tonification or moxibustion.

Changqiang (GV 1) regulates the middle *jiao* and stops diarrhea. *Pishu* (BL 20) and *Weishu* (BL 21) strengthen the Spleen and Stomach and regulate the Spleen qi flow. *Housanli* (ST 36) strengthens the Spleen and harmonizes the Stomach. *Sanyinjiao* (SP 6) and *Yinlingquan* (SP 9) nourish the Spleen and Stomach to relieve diarrhea. *Zhongwan* (CV 12), the *mu* (collecting) point of the Stomach, harmonizes the Stomach and dissolves damp accumulation. *Tianshu* (ST 25) regulates and strengthens the Spleen and Large Intestine.

AUTHORS' COMMENTS

Shen Ling Bai Zhu San is based on *Si Jun Zi Tang* (Four-Gentlemen Decoction), with the addition of *Shan Yao* (Rhizoma Dioscoreae), *Bai Bian Dou* (Semen Lablab

Shēn Líng Bái Zhú Sǎn

(Ginseng, Poria, and Atractylodes Macrocephala Powder)

Album), *Lian Zi* (Semen Nelumbinis), *Yi Yi Ren* (Semen Coicis), *Sha Ren* (Fructus Amomi), and *Jie Geng* (Radix Platycodonis). *Shen Ling Bai Zhu San* is a harmonious formula that is not too warm or too dry; it tonifies without creating stagnation, and drains dampness without injuring qi. It tonifies both the Lung and the Spleen, illustrating the concept of tonifying the metal element by strengthening the earth element.

Shen Ling Bai Zhu San has a wide range of applications, whether by itself or with slight modifications:

- It is a very effective formula for use in horses with chronic "cow-pie" diarrhea with undigested kernels of corn and/or oats in the manure. The stresses of showing and boarding, along with the damp accumulation that comes with modern feeding practices, very commonly lead to this type of deficiency. This is the perfect formula to address this condition.
- For puppies with vaginal discharge and Spleen qi deficiency, combine with *Cang Zhu* (Rhizoma Atractylodis), *Chen Pi* (Pericarpium Citri Reticulatae), *Ban Xia* (Rhizoma Pinelliae), *Sheng Ma* (Rhizoma Cimicifugae), *Chai Hu* (Radix Bupleuri), and *Sheng Jiang* (Rhizoma Zingiberis Recens).
- For the treatment of early Type II diabetes, combine with *Huang Qi* (Radix Astragali) and *Huang Jing* (Rhizoma Polygonati).
- For cats with asthma, and dogs with chronic bronchitis and Kidney deficiency, combine with *Su Zi Jiang Qi Tang* (Perilla Fruit Decoction for Directing Qi Downward).
- To treat skin rash and dermatitis caused by damp-heat in the Liver and Gallbladder channels, combine with *Long Dan Xie Gan Tang* (Gentiana Decoction to Drain the Liver).
- For dermatitis and pruritis caused by wind-heat, combine with *Xiao Feng San* (Eliminate Wind Powder).
- *Shen Ling Bai Zhu San* is often used in the support of chemotherapy and radiation therapy and can be combined with *Huang Qi* (Radix Astragali), *Wu Wei Zi* (Fructus Schisandrae Chinensis), *Mai Dong* (Radix Ophiopogonis), *Rou Gui* (Cortex Cinnamomi), *Dang Gui* (Radix Angelicae Sinensis), *Ji Xue Teng* (Caulis Spatholobi), *Shen Qu* (Massa Fermentata), *Shu Di Huang* (Radix Rehmanniae Praeparata), *Ci Wu Jia* (Radix et Rhizoma seu Caulis Acanthopanacis Senticosi), and *Zhi Qiao* (Fructus Aurantii) to improve clinical efficacy. It can also be combined with *Bu Zhong Yi Qi Tang* (Tonify the Middle and Augment the Qi Decoction). For animals that are difficult to medicate, or that are already taking numerous oral medications, this formula can be given and additional single herbs can be mixed into the food. The following herbs have adaptogenic, immune-strengthening and anticancer properties: *Dong Chong Xia Cao* (Cordyceps), *Ci Wu Jia* (Radix et Rhizoma seu Caulis Acanthopanacis Senticosi), *Ling Zhi* (Ganoderma), and *Yun Zhi* (Coriolus).
- For animals with poor appetite, add *Ji Nei Jin* (Endothelium Corneum Gigeriae Galli).
- For a comparative discussion of Spleen tonic formulas, see *Si Jun Zi Tang* (Four-Gentlemen Decoction).

Shen Ling Bai Zhu San, *Si Shen Wan* (Four-Miracle Pill), and *Tong Xie Yao Fang* (Important Formula for Painful Diarrhea) all bind the Intestines to treat diarrhea. The differences are as follows:

- *Shen Ling Bai Zhu San* is indicated for diarrhea characterized by Spleen qi deficiency with damp accumulation manifesting in fatigue, weakness of the limbs, and poor appetite. It can be seen in animals of any age: young animals with constitutional weakness of the middle *jiao*, animals with chronic illness, and those undergoing chemotherapy or radiation. It typically treats chronic problems
- *Si Shen Wan* treats diarrhea secondary to Spleen and Kidney yang deficiencies. It warms and tonifies Spleen and Kidney yang to stop chronic diarrhea. It is designed for animals with poor appetite, cold signs, and severe diarrhea that occurs in the early morning, is watery in consistency, and/or contains undigested food. It is most common in geriatric animals or those with chronic gastrointestinal disease.
- *Tong Xie Yao Fang* is used to treat stress-related diarrhea caused by Liver overacting on the Spleen; it tonifies the Spleen and spreads Liver qi. Animals often have poor appetite, flatulence, borborygmus, bloating, and straining with abdominal pain that is relieved with diarrhea. It is most often seen in animals that are high-strung or boarded frequently, in performance animals, and during the introduction of new pets into a household. Stress-related diarrhea can also develop in animals on prolonged drug therapy. It is primarily used for animals with acute signs; once the diarrhea resolves, it is advisable to administer a constitutional formula that is comprised of a formula to calm the *shen* (spirit).

References

1. *Zhong Yao Ming Fang Yao Li Yu Ying Yong* (Pharmacology and Applications of Famous Herbal Formulas), 1989; 251-252.
2. *Xin Yi Yao Xue Za Zhi* (New Journal of Medicine and Herbology), 1979; 3:129.
3. *Zhong Yi Fang Ji Xian Dai Yan Jiu* (Modern Study of Medical Formulas in Traditional Chinese Medicine), 1997; 509.
4. *Xin Yi Yao Xue Za Zhi* (New Journal of Medicine and Herbology), 1979; 3:129.
5. *Shan Dong Zhong Yi Za Zhi* (Shandong Journal of Chinese Medicine), 1991; 10(6):24.

Shēn Líng Bái Zhú Săn

(Ginseng, Poria, and Atractylodes Macrocephala Powder)

6. *Shan Xi Zhong Yi* (Shanxi Chinese Medicine), 1998; 7:312.
7. *Nan Jing Zhong Yi Yao Da Xue Xue Bao* (Journal of Nanjing University of Traditional Chinese Medicine and Medicinals), 1998; 5:318.
8. *Zhong Xi Yi Jie He Za Zhi* (Journal of Integrated Chinese and Western Medicine), 1987; 7:436.
9. *Ji Lin Zhong Yi Yao* (Jilin Chinese Medicine and Herbology), 1997; 4:14.
10. *Shan Xi Zhong Yi* (Shanxi Chinese Medicine), 1997; 8:348.
11. *Si Chuan Zhong Yi* (Sichuan Chinese Medicine), 1994; 11:55.
12. *Zhong Yi Yao Xue Bao* (Report of Chinese Medicine and Herbology), 1999; 4:23.
13. *Zhong Yi Yao Xue Bao* (Report of Chinese Medicine and Herbology), 1999; 4:23.
14. *Gui Zhou Yi Yao* (Medicine and Medicinals from Guizhou), 1985; 3:7.

Qǐ Pí Wán (Guide the Spleen Pill)

啟脾丸

启脾丸

Pinyin Name: *Qi Pi Wan*
Literal Name: Guide the Spleen Pill
Alternate Name: Lotus and Citrus Formula
Original Source: *Wan Bing Hui Chun* (Restoration of Health from the Myriad Diseases) by Gong Ting-Xian in 1587

COMPOSITION

Ren Shen (Radix et Rhizoma Ginseng)	30g
Fu Ling (Poria)	30g
Bai Zhu (Rhizoma Atractylodis Macrocephalae), *chao* (dry-fried)	30g
Zhi Gan Cao (Radix et Rhizoma Glycyrrhizae Praeparata cum Melle)	15g
Shan Zha (Fructus Crataegi)	15g
Chen Pi (Pericarpium Citri Reticulatae)	15g
Lian Zi (Semen Nelumbinis)	30g
Ze Xie (Rhizoma Alismatis)	15g
Shan Yao (Rhizoma Dioscoreae), *chao* (dry-fried)	30g

DOSAGE / PREPARATION / ADMINISTRATION

Grind the ingredients into powder, and mix with honey to form pills. The pills should resemble the size of *Wu Tong Zi* (Semen Firmianae), a small seed approximately 5 mm in diameter. Take 20-30 pills per dose with rice water on an empty stomach.

CHINESE THERAPEUTIC ACTIONS

1. Strengthens the Spleen and Stomach
2. Promotes normal digestion
3. Relieves diarrhea and vomiting

CLINICAL MANIFESTATIONS

Indigestion and food stagnation caused by Spleen and Stomach deficiencies: decreased appetite, diarrhea, foul breath, belching, abdominal pain, nausea, vomiting, a pale tongue and a weak, soft-to-slippery pulse.

VETERINARY CLINICAL APPLICATIONS

Chronic gastrointestinal disorders: indigestion, food stagnation and vomiting, diarrhea, poor appetite, weight loss, general weakness, exocrine pancreatic insufficiency (EPI), chronic gastroenteritis, chronic diarrhea, and infantile malnutrition.

EXPLANATION

Qi Pi Wan (Guide the Spleen Pill) treats patients with chronic Spleen and Stomach deficiencies, giving rise to various complaints of the digestive system, such as decreased appetite, belching, foul breath, nausea and

Qǐ Pí Wán (Guide the Spleen Pill)

Qi Pi Wan (Guide the Spleen Pill)

Diagnosis	Clinical Signs	Treatment	Herbs
Indigestion and food stagnation due to Spleen and Stomach deficiencies	• Nausea, vomiting, belching, foul breath, and abdominal pain: food stagnation and indigestion • Decreased appetite, diarrhea, a pale tongue, fatigue, lack of energy, and a weak, soft-to-slippery pulse: Spleen and Stomach deficiencies	• Strengthens the Spleen and Stomach • Promotes normal digestion and relieves diarrhea	• *Ren Shen* (Radix et Rhizoma Ginseng), *Fu Ling* (Poria), *Bai Zhu* (Rhizoma Atractylodis Macrocephalae), and *Zhi Gan Cao* (Radix et Rhizoma Glycyrrhizae Praeparata cum Melle) strengthen the Spleen and Stomach and restore normal digestive functions. • *Shan Zha* (Fructus Crataegi) and *Chen Pi* (Pericarpium Citri Reticulatae) regulate qi and promote normal appetite and digestion. • *Lian Zi* (Semen Nelumbinis) strengthens the Spleen and relieves diarrhea. • *Ze Xie* (Rhizoma Alismatis) resolves dampness. • *Shan Yao* (Rhizoma Dioscoreae) tonifies the body and relieves thirst and diarrhea.

vomiting, indigestion, abdominal pain, diarrhea, a pale tongue, and a weak, and soft to slippery pulse. In addition to digestive disorders, fatigue and lack of energy may be present as a result of poor absorption of nutrients.

Si Jun Zi Tang (Four-Gentlemen Decoction) is the foundation of this formula; its four constituents, *Ren Shen* (Radix et Rhizoma Ginseng), *Fu Ling* (Poria), *Bai Zhu* (Rhizoma Atractylodis Macrocephalae), and *Zhi Gan Cao* (Radix et Rhizoma Glycyrrhizae Praeparata cum Melle), strengthen the Spleen and Stomach and restore normal digestive functions. The addition of *Shan Zha* (Fructus Crataegi) and *Chen Pi* (Pericarpium Citri Reticulatae) regulates qi and promotes normal appetite and digestion. *Lian Zi* (Semen Nelumbinis) strengthens the Spleen and relieves diarrhea. *Ze Xie* (Rhizoma Alismatis) resolves dampness. *Shan Yao* (Rhizoma Dioscoreae) tonifies the body and relieves thirst and diarrhea.

VETERINARY MODIFICATIONS

- With more nausea, vomiting, and bloating, add *Zhi Shi* (Fructus Aurantii Immaturus) and *Ban Xia* (Rhizoma Pinelliae).
- With more abdominal pain and diarrhea, add *Mu Xiang* (Radix Aucklandiae) and *Sha Ren* (Fructus Amomi).
- For juvenile animals with poor Spleen function, add *Shi Jun Zi* (Fructus Quisqualis).

SUGGESTED ACUPUNCTURE TREATMENT

1. Points: *Housanli* (ST 36), *Pishu* (BL 20), *Zhongwan* (CV 12), *Taibai* (SP 3), *Tianshu* (ST 25), *Shenque* (CV 8), and *Yinlingquan* (SP 9).
2. Technique: moxibustion and tonification or aquapuncture with vitamin B12.

Apply moxibustion on *Housanli* (ST 36) and *Pishu* (BL 20) to tonify qi and strengthen the Spleen. *Zhongwan* (CV 12) regulates qi in the middle *jiao*. Tonify *Taibai* (SP 3) and *Tianshu* (ST 25), and apply moxibustion on *Shenque* (CV 8) to tonify the Spleen and Stomach and stop diarrhea. *Yinlingquan* (SP 9) dissolves dampness.

AUTHORS' COMMENTS

Qi Pi Wan is especially helpful in weak animals that cannot tolerate a strong formula to relieve food stagnation, such as *Bao He Wan* (Preserve Harmony Pill). This is a gentler formula, and can be given long term without further damaging the middle *jiao*. It was originally used to treat food stagnation and dampness in young animals with constitutional Spleen weakness; however, it can be used to treat deficient patients of any age.

- It can be combined with *Mai Ya* (Fructus Hordei Germinatus) and *Shen Qu* (Massa Fermentata) to improve clinical results to stimulate appetite in animals that have chronic disease, and/or are undergoing chemotherapy or radiation.
- It can be combined with *Xiao Chai Hu Tang* (Minor Bupleurum Decoction) to treat cats with cholangiohepatitis and dogs with liver failure or liver cancer with anorexia, in combination with acupuncture; *Yingxiang* (LI 20) and *Shangen* (the classical canine acupuncture point) are used with good results.
- For the treatment of exocrine pancreatic insufficiency, combine with *Sheng Ma* (Rhizoma Cimicifugae), *Chai Hu* (Radix Bupleuri), *Mai Ya* (Fructus Hordei Germinatus), and *Shen Qu* (Massa Fermentata), and mix with congee or rice porridge.
- For a comparative discussion of Spleen tonic formulas, see *Si Jun Zi Tang* (Four-Gentlemen Decoction).

Bŭ Zhōng Yì Qì Tāng

(Tonify the Middle and Augment the Qi Decoction)

補中益氣湯

补中益气汤

Pinyin Name: *Bu Zhong Yi Qi Tang*
Literal Name: Tonify the Middle and Augment the Qi Decoction
Alternate Names: *Pu Chung I Chi Tang (Wan), Bu Zhong Yi Chi Tang (Wan)*, Interior-Nourishing and Qi-Increasing Decoction (Pill), Middle-Reinforcing and Qi-Benefiting Decoction, Ginseng and Astragalus Combination
Original Source: *Pi Wei Lun* (Discussion of the Spleen and Stomach) by Li Gao in 1249

COMPOSITION

Huang Qi (Radix Astragali)	1.5-3g [15-30g]
Ren Shen (Radix et Rhizoma Ginseng)	0.9g [9g]
Bai Zhu (Rhizoma Atractylodis Macrocephalae)	0.9g [9g]
Zhi Gan Cao (Radix et Rhizoma Glycyrrhizae Praeparata cum Melle)	1.5g [15g]
Dang Gui (Radix Angelicae Sinensis), *bei* (stone-baked) with liquor	0.6g [6g]
Chen Pi (Pericarpium Citri Reticulatae)	0.6-0.9g [6-9g]
Chai Hu (Radix Bupleuri)	0.6-0.9g [6-9g]
Sheng Ma (Rhizoma Cimicifugae)	0.6-0.9g [6-9g]

DOSAGE / PREPARATION / ADMINISTRATION

Coarsely grind the ingredients into powder and cook the powder in 2 large bowls of water and reduce it to 1 large bowl. Take the warm, strained decoction between meals. Today, this formula may be prepared as a decoction with the doses suggested in brackets. It may also be administered as pills, by taking 10-15g of pills two to three times a day with warm, boiled water or ginger soup.

CHINESE THERAPEUTIC ACTIONS

1. Tonifies the middle *jiao* and benefits qi
2. Causes the yang qi to ascend and lifts prolapsed organs

CLINICAL MANIFESTATIONS

1. Spleen and Stomach qi deficiencies: poor appetite, spontaneous sweating in animals that sweat, thirst, exercise intolerance, lethargy, general weakness, fatigue, weakness of the extremities, loose stools, a pale tongue, and a deep, weak pulse.
2. Qi deficiency with prolapse of organs: prolapse of the rectum or uterus, chronic diarrhea or dysentery, and conditions characterized by the inability of yang qi to ascend.

VETERINARY CLINICAL APPLICATIONS

Chronic gastrointestinal, pulmonary, immune and other disorders: gastritis, inflammatory bowel disease, weight loss and cachexia, chronic diarrhea, vomiting, exocrine pancreatic insufficiency (EPI), chronic renal failure, chronic glomerulonephritis, endocrine disease, rectal prolapse, vaginal or uterine prolapse, fever of unknown origin, leukopenia, anemia, weak immunity, frequent infections, urinary dribbling and incontinence, fecal incontinence, megaesophagus, constipation, megacolon, myasthenia gravis, degenerative myelopathy, progressive retinal atrophy (PRA), corneal dystrophy, non-healing corneal ulcers, cataracts, immune-mediated hemolytic anemia (IHA), asthma, chronic bronchitis, supportive care for severe illness, post-partum weakness, and generalized deficiency in cancer patients receiving chemotherapy or radiation therapy.

EXPLANATION

The Spleen and Stomach, which are responsible for the transformation and transportation of food, are the source of qi and blood production. When these two organs become deficient and cannot carry out their normal functions, there will be poor appetite, exercise intolerance, lethargy, general weakness, fatigue, weakness of the extremities, and a pale tongue. Because of qi deficiency, the clear yang cannot ascend, leading to loose stools, diarrhea, and dysentery.

In severe cases of Spleen and Stomach deficiencies, the yang qi may be unable to hold the organs in their normal position, leading to prolapse of such internal organs as the stomach, uterus, and rectum. Furthermore, as yang qi, unable to ascend, sinks into yin, it causes spontaneous sweating, and a weak, deep pulse. Thirst is the result of qi deficiency, which is unable to transport fluids to the upper parts of the body.

Bǔ Zhōng Yì Qì Tāng

(Tonify the Middle and Augment the Qi Decoction)

Bu Zhong Yi Qi Tang (Tonify the Middle and Augment the Qi Decoction) uses *Huang Qi* (Radix Astragali) as the chief herb because it tonifies *zhong* (central) *qi* and causes the yang qi to ascend. It also strengthens *wei* (defensive) *qi* and protects the exterior. *Ren Shen* (Radix et Rhizoma Ginseng), *Bai Zhu* (Rhizoma Atractylodis Macrocephalae), and *Zhi Gan Cao* (Radix et Rhizoma Glycyrrhizae Praeparata cum Melle) strengthen the Spleen, benefit qi, and tonify the middle *jiao. Dang Gui* (Radix Angelicae Sinensis) tonifies the blood and enhances the production of qi. *Chen Pi* (Pericarpium Citri Reticulatae) regulates qi and harmonizes the Stomach. It also prevents the tonic herbs from creating stagnation in the middle *jiao*. *Chai Hu* (Radix Bupleuri) and *Sheng Ma* (Rhizoma Cimicifugae) cause yang qi to ascend and lift prolapsed organs.

VETERINARY MODIFICATIONS

- For chronic diarrhea, add *Shan Yao* (Rhizoma Dioscoreae), *Bai Bian Dou* (Semen Lablab Album), *Fu Ling* (Poria), and *Bu Gu Zhi* (Fructus Psoraleae).
- For chronic giardia infection, add *Qing Hao* (Herba Artemisiae Annuae) and *Da Suan* (Bulbus Alli Sativi).
- For diarrhea with cold and Spleen yang deficiency, add *Fu Zi* (Radix Aconiti Lateralis Praeparata) and *Pao Jiang* (Rhizoma Zingiberis Praeparatum); or *Li Zhong Wan* (Regulate the Middle Pill).
- For chronic prolapse of the rectum or uterus, add *Chi Shi Zhi* (Halloysitum Rubrum).
- With accompanying Liver qi stagnation, add *Xiao Yao San* (Rambling Powder).

CAUTIONS / CONTRAINDICATIONS

- *Bu Zhong Yi Qi Tang* is contraindicated in animals with significant yin deficiency or interior heat.
- As a general rule, the dose of this formula should be small. This formula consists of sweet and warm tonic herbs, which tend to be heavy and immobile in nature. Thus, a large dose of this formula may actually defeat the purpose of causing yang qi to ascend. For the individual ingredients, it is important keep the dose of *Huang Qi* (Radix Astragali) high to tonify qi, and the doses of *Chai Hu* (Radix Bupleuri) and *Sheng Ma* (Rhizoma Cimicifugae) should be just sufficient to raise yang qi.

PHARMACOLOGICAL EFFECTS

1. **Gastrointestinal**: According to laboratory experiments in rabbits, administration of *Bu Zhong Yi Qi Tang* was associated with a regulatory effect on the intestines. Depending on the condition of the subject, it will either increase or decrease intestinal peristalsis.[1]
2. **Influence on gastric acid secretion**: Administration of *Bu Zhong Yi Qi Tang* has a dose-dependent effect on the secretion of gastric acid. A small dose of the herb has little or no benefit on the secretion of gastric acid, while a large dose will significantly increase both gastric acid production and release.[2]
3. **Adaptogenic**: Administration of *Bu Zhong Yi Qi Tang* has been shown to increase the ability of animals to adapt to physical stress. In one experiment, administration of herbs for seven days increased the ability of mice to tread water longer when threatened with drowning. It was also noted that the subjects responded better to decoction than to pills.[3]

***Bu Zhong Yi Qi Tang* (Tonify the Middle and Augment the Qi Decoction)**

Diagnosis	Clinical Signs	Treatment	Herbs
Spleen and Stomach qi deficiencies with organ prolapse	• Poor appetite, fatigue, exercise intolerance, lethargy, general weakness, weakness of the extremities: Spleen and Stomach qi deficiencies • Loose stools, diarrhea, and dysentery: qi deficiency with failure of clear yang qi to ascend • Prolapse of internal organs, such as the stomach, uterus, and rectum: yang qi deficiency unable to lift internal organs • A pale tongue and a deep, weak pulse: Spleen and Stomach qi deficiencies	• Tonifies the middle *jiao* and benefits qi • Causes yang qi to ascend and lifts prolapsed organs	• *Huang Qi* (Radix Astragali) tonifies *zhong* (central) *qi*, causes yang qi to ascend, and strengthens *wei* (defensive) *qi*. • *Ren Shen* (Radix et Rhizoma Ginseng), *Bai Zhu* (Rhizoma Atractylodis Macrocephalae), and *Zhi Gan Cao* (Radix et Rhizoma Glycyrrhizae Praeparata cum Melle) strengthen the Spleen, benefit qi, and tonify the middle *jiao.* • *Dang Gui* (Radix Angelicae Sinensis) tonifies the blood. • *Chen Pi* (Pericarpium Citri Reticulatae) regulates qi and harmonizes the Stomach. • *Chai Hu* (Radix Bupleuri) and *Sheng Ma* (Rhizoma Cimicifugae) cause yang qi to ascend and lift prolapsed organs.

Bŭ Zhōng Yì Qì Tāng

(Tonify the Middle and Augment the Qi Decoction)

4. **Antiaging**: Administration of *Bu Zhong Yi Qi Tang* in mice was associated with a dose-dependent effect to improve endurance, learning, memory, neuromuscular coordination, and changes in the levels of monoamines (dopamine and noradrenaline) in the brain.[4]
5. **Immunostimulant**: Administration of *Bu Zhong Yi Qi Tang* has been associated with an immune-enhancing effect. According to one study, use of the formula was linked with increased T-lymphocyte count, elevated levels of IFN and IL-2, and increased NK cells and macrophage activity.[5] According to another study, *Bu Zhong Yi Qi Tang* enhances interleukin-18-induced cell-mediated immunity and may enhance host defense mechanisms against pathogens.[6]
6. **Antiallergic**: Administration of *Bu Zhong Yi Qi Tang* was associated with good results in treating allergies by suppressing IgE antibody production and inhibiting histamine release in type I allergic reactions in mice immunized with ovalbumin.[7] According to another study, the antiallergic effect was attributed mainly to inhibition of Th2 cell responses.[8]
7. **Anticancer**: In one study, use of *Bu Zhong Yi Qi Tang* was associated with a dose-dependent effect to inhibit the proliferation of human hepatoma cell lines (Hep3B, HepG2, and HA22T), but not normal human hepatocytes (Chang liver, CCL-13). The mechanism of this anticancer effect was attributed to the formula's ability to suppress the proliferation of hepatoma cells by inducing apoptosis via G0/G1 arrest.[9] Another study reported a marked prophylactic antitumor effect by enhancing the natural killer cell activity.[10]
8. **Radioprotective**: One study reported marked protective effects using *Bu Zhong Yi Qi Tang* in mice irradiated with high and low doses of gamma-rays. *Bu Zhong Yi Qi Tang* protected the jejunal crypts ($p < 0.0001$), increased the formation of the endogenous spleen colony ($p < 0.05$), and reduced the frequency of radiation-induced apoptosis ($p < 0.05$). The study also noted that while the individual ingredients also have radioprotective effects, the formula as a whole is much more effective. The study concluded that *Bu Zhong Yi Qi Tang* is a useful radioprotector, especially because it is a relatively non-toxic natural product.[11]
9. **Antibiotic**: Administration of *Bu Zhong Yi Qi Tang* was associated with marked effects to treat gastroduodenal diseases associated with *Helicobacter pylori* (*H. pylori*) infection. *Bu Zhong Yi Qi Tang* was found to be effective against *H. pylori* both *in vitro* and *in vivo*, and inhibited the growth of antibiotic-resistant strains of *H. pylori* as well as antibiotic-sensitive strains. In addition, concurrent use of *Bu Zhong Yi Qi Tang* and antibiotics completely eradicated the bacteria in mice. The antibiotic effect of *Bu Zhong Yi Qi Tang* was attributed partly to the induction of interferon.[12]
10. **Antiviral**: Administration of *Bu Zhong Yi Qi Tang* was associated with antiviral effects to treat mice infected with influenza virus. The mechanism of this antiviral effect was attributed to the enhancement of host immune responses, as the herbs do not have any inhibitory effect on the growth of influenza virus *in vitro*.[13]
11. **Effect on bone loss**: One study used *Bu Zhong Yi Qi Tang* and evaluated its effect on bone mass density in ovariectomized female rats at age 35 weeks. The subjects were given the formula by gastric tube for 8 weeks. The study reported that treatments using *Bu Zhong Yi Qi Tang* suppressed the ovariectomy-induced reduction of the bone mineral density in the whole and metaphysis of tibia. Furthermore, the study noted that there was a slight increase in serum levels of estradiol and progesterone maintaining bone mineral density values similar to that in the estradiol-treated ovariectomized rats, as well as the intact control rats. Based on this finding, the study suggested that *Bu Zhong Yi Qi Tang* prevented bone loss in ovariectomized rats because it elevated the serum levels of ovarian hormones slightly.[14]
12. **Antidepressive and antinociceptive**: Administration of *Bu Zhong Yi Qi Tang*, *Yi Gan San* (Restrain the Liver Powder), or *Chai Hu Jia Long Gu Mu Li Tang* (Bupleurum plus Dragon Bone and Oyster Shell Decoction) for 14 consecutive days showed both antidepressive and antinociceptive properties in mice.[15]

HUMAN CLINICAL STUDIES AND RESEARCH

1. **Stomach prolapse**: In one study, 40 patients with stomach prolapse characterized by Spleen and Stomach deficiencies were treated with modified *Bu Zhong Yi Qi Tang* with complete recovery in 21 patients, marked improvement in 16 patients, and no benefit in 3 patients. The herbal treatment contained *Bu Zhong Yi Qi Tang* with modifications as needed. With Liver and qi stagnation, *Dang Shen* (Radix Codonopsis) was removed and *Fo Shou* (Fructus Citri Sarcodactylis), *Xiang Fu* (Rhizoma Cyperi), and *Zi Su Geng* (Caulis Perillae) were added. With food stagnation, *Dang Gui* (Radix Angelicae Sinensis) was removed, and charred *Shan Zha* (Fructus Crataegi), charred *Shen Qu* (Massa Fermentata), charred *Mai Ya* (Fructus Hordei Germinatus), *Ji Nei Jin* (Endothelium Corneum Gigeriae Galli), and dry-fried *Lai Fu Zi* (Semen Raphani) were added. With Stomach heat, *Dang Shen* (Radix Codonopsis) was removed, and dry-fried *Huang Lian* (Rhizoma Coptidis), *Pu Gong Ying* (Herba Taraxaci), and *Da Huang* (Radix et Rhizoma Rhei) were added. For Stomach cold, *Dang Gui*

Bǔ Zhōng Yì Qì Tāng
(Tonify the Middle and Augment the Qi Decoction)

(Radix Angelicae Sinensis) was removed, and *Gan Jiang* (Rhizoma Zingiberis) and *Rou Gui* (Cortex Cinnamomi) were added. For Stomach yin deficiency, *Chai Hu* (Radix Bupleuri) and *Bai Zhu* (Rhizoma Atractylodis Macrocephalae) were removed, and *Sha Shen* (Radix Glehniae seu Adenophorae) and *Mai Dong* (Radix Ophiopogonis) were added. With blood stagnation, *Dang Shen* (Radix Codonopsis) and *Bai Zhu* (Rhizoma Atractylodis Macrocephalae) were removed, and *Tao Ren* (Semen Persicae), *Hong Hua* (Flos Carthami), and *Dan Shen* (Radix et Rhizoma Salviae Miltiorrhizae) were added.[16] In another study, modified *Bu Zhong Yi Qi Tang* was used to treat patients with stomach prolapse with good success. Out of 40 patients, the study reported complete recovery in 30 patients, improvement in 8 patients, and no benefit in 2 patients. The overall effectiveness rate was 95%.[17]

2. **Rectal prolapse**: Use of modified *Bu Zhong Yi Qi Tang* was successful in treating rectal prolapse in 68 patients with 3 months to 15 years history of illness. The herbal formula contained *Huang Qi* (Radix Astragali) 30g, *Ren Shen* (Radix et Rhizoma Ginseng) 20g, *Bai Zhu* (Rhizoma Atractylodis Macrocephalae) 5g, *Sheng Ma* (Rhizoma Cimicifugae) 5g, and *Chai Hu* (Radix Bupleuri) 5g. Modifications were made as follows: for frequent bowel movements with mucus and blood, add *Huang Lian* (Rhizoma Coptidis) 10g, *Chi Shi Zhi* (Halloysitum Rubrum) 10g, *Ying Su Ke* (Pericarpium Papaveris) 10g, and *Jin Ying Zi* (Fructus Rosae Laevigatae) 10g; for stubborn cough, add *Wu Wei Zi* (Fructus Schisandrae Chinensis) 15g, *Wu Bei Zi* (Galla Chinensis) 10g, and *Sang Bai Pi* (Cortex Mori) 10g; for constipation, add *Huo Ma Ren* (Fructus Cannabis) 15g and *Yu Li Ren* (Semen Pruni) 10g; for chronic illness with dry mouth and deficiency of body fluids, add *Shu Di Huang* (Radix Rehmanniae Praeparata) 15g, *Sha Shen* (Radix Glehniae seu Adenophorae) 15g, *Tian Dong* (Radix Asparagi) 15g, and *Yu Zhu* (Rhizoma Polygonati Odorati) 15g; and for profuse bleeding in the stools, add *Huai Hua* (Flos Sophorae) 10g, *Di Yu* (Radix Sanguisorbae) 15g, and *Ce Bai Ye* (Cacumen Platycladi) 15g.[18] Another study reported 94% effectiveness using modified *Bu Zhong Yi Qi Tang* to treat rectal prolapse. Modifications included the addition of *Wu Mei* (Fructus Mume), *Wu Bei Zi* (Galla Chinensis), and others as needed. Of 56 patients, the study reported significant improvement in 29 patients, moderate improvement in 24 patients, and no benefit in 3 patients.[19]
3. **Uterine prolapse**: One study reported good results using modified *Bu Zhong Yi Qi Tang* to treat 14 patients with prolapse of uterus. The herbal treatment contained *Bu Zhong Yi Qi Tang* as the base formula, with the addition of large doses of *Huang Qi* (Radix Astragali) and *Dang Shen* (Radix Codonopsis) for qi deficiency; *Xu Duan* (Radix Dipsaci) and *Du Zhong* (Cortex Eucommiae) for low back pain and frequent urination; and a large dose of *Zhi Qiao* (Fructus Aurantii) for those who did not respond well. After 9-18 packs of herbs, the study reported recovery in all 14 patients.[20]
4. **Gastritis**: Gastritis due to regurgitation of bile acid in 89 patients was treated with complete recovery in 19 patients, marked improvement in 32 patients, moderate improvement in 30 patients, and no benefit in 8 patients. The overall effectiveness was 90%. In addition to *Bu Zhong Yi Qi Tang* as the base formula, modifications included addition of *Zuo Jin Wan* (Left Metal Pill) for acid reflux; *Ban Xia* (Rhizoma Pinelliae) for belching; *Fu Ling* (Poria) and *Shan Yao* (Rhizoma Dioscoreae) for loose stools; *Da Huang* (Radix et Rhizoma Rhei) for constipation; and *Bai Shao* (Radix Paeoniae Alba) for stomach pain.[21]
5. **Nausea and vomiting**: In one report, 26 out of 30 patients with nausea and vomiting were treated with good results using modified *Bu Zhong Yi Qi Tang*.[22]
6. **Constipation**: Modified *Bu Zhong Yi Qi Tang* successfully treated constipation in geriatric patients with qi deficiency, postpartum women with qi and blood deficiency, and pregnant women.[23]
7. **Diarrhea**: One study reported good results using *Bu Zhong Yi Qi Tang* to treat geriatric patients with diarrhea characterized by Spleen deficiency. Out of the 33 patients, 16 were male and 17 were female, between 51-67 years of age, with 6 months to 15 years of illness. Patients were instructed to take herbs continuously for 1-1.5 months. The study reported complete recovery in 30 of 33 patients.[24]
8. **Fever**: Use of *Bu Zhong Yi Qi Tang* was effective in reducing fever secondary to chronic illness or postpartum weakness with qi and blood deficiencies. Of 20 patients treated, most reported a reduction of body temperature within 5 doses.[25] Another study on fever in 30 post-surgical patients reported 93.3% effectiveness using modified *Bu Zhong Yi Qi Tang* to reduce body temperature.[26]
9. **Leukopenia**: One study reported good results using modified *Bu Zhong Yi Qi Tang* in 80 patients (32 male, 48 female) with low white blood cell count due to various causes. In addition to the base formula, modifications included *Gu Ya* (Fructus Setariae Germinatus) and *Mai Ya* (Fructus Hordei Germinatus) for poor appetite; *Mai Dong* (Radix Ophiopogonis) and *Wu Wei Zi* (Fructus Schisandrae Chinensis) for palpitations; and *Cang Zhu* (Rhizoma Atractylodis) for damp. The herbs were cooked in water, and the decoction was taken in two equally-divided doses daily. Of 80 patients, the study reported a marked effect in 70 patients (> 2.0×10^9/L increase of WBC in 2 weeks); moderate improvement in 4 patients (1.0-1.9×10^9/L

Bŭ Zhōng Yì Qì Tāng

(Tonify the Middle and Augment the Qi Decoction)

increase of WBC in 2 weeks), and no benefit in 6 patients (<0.9 x 10^9/L increase of WBC in 2 weeks).[27]

10. **Compromised immunity in elderly persons**: Administration of *Bu Zhong Yi Qi Tang* was effective in improving immunological capacity in a group of elderly patients. Clinical improvements included significantly enhanced natural killer (NK) activity and serum IFN-gamma level. The treatment protocol was to administer 7.5g of the formula daily for at least 120 days.[28]
11. **Common cold**: In one report, 50 geriatric patients with constitutional deficiencies and common cold were treated successfully with modified *Bu Zhong Yi Qi Tang*. The modifications were as follows: *Jing Jie* (Herba Schizonepetae) was added for aversion to cold; *Fang Feng* (Radix Saposhnikoviae) and *Qiang Huo* (Rhizoma et Radix Notopterygii) for body ache; *Bai Zhi* (Radix Angelicae Dahuricae) was added for headache; *Bo He* (Herba Menthae) for dizziness; *Ju Hua* (Flos Chrysanthemi) for blurred vision; and *Yu Ping Feng San* (Jade Windscreen Powder) after the resolution of exterior symptoms. The average length of treatment was 37.5 days. Out of 50 patients, the study reported complete recovery in 48 patients (complete resolution of all symptoms without recurrence for 1 year).[29]
12. **Hypertension**: One study used *Bu Zhong Yi Qi Tang* to treat hypertension characterized by qi deficiency. The background of the 15 patients were as follows: 9 males and 6 females; between 45-49 years of age, with 3-10 years history of illness. After continuous herbal treatment for 1-3 months, the study reported stabilization of blood pressure and relief of symptoms in 13 patients, and no benefit in 2 patients.[30]
13. **Dysuria**: Modified *Bu Zhong Yi Qi Tang* was used with good results in treating 27 patients with postpartum dysuria. The modification included the addition of *Dong Kui Zi* (Semen Malvae), *Fu Ling* (Poria), and *Che Qian Zi* (Semen Plantaginis). The treatment duration was 1-3 days.[31]
14. **Frequent urination**: In one report, pregnant women with frequent urination were treated with great success using *Bu Zhong Yi Qi Tang* with the addition of *Xu Duan* (Radix Dipsaci), dry-fried *Bai Shao* (Radix Paeoniae Alba), *Di Huang* (Radix Rehmanniae), *Huang Qin* (Radix Scutellariae), and *Shan Yao* (Rhizoma Dioscoreae). Pregnancy continued smoothly with no complications or side effects.[32]
15. **Incontinence**: Modified *Bu Zhong Yi Qi Tang* was used with good results in treating 57 patients with incontinence due to postpartum or post-surgical procedures. Modifications included the addition of a large dose of *Huang Qi* (Radix Astragali), as well as the addition of *Yi Zhi* (Fructus Alpiniae Oxyphyllae), *Wu Wei Zi* (Fructus Schisandrae Chinensis), *Fu Pen Zi* (Fructus Rubi), *Sang Piao Xiao* (Ootheca Mantidis), and calcined *Long Gu* (Os Draconis). Out of 57 patients, the study reported recovery in 45 patients and improvement in 12 patients.[33]
16. **Seizures and epilepsy**: In one report, 54 patients with seizures were treated with good results using concurrent herb and drug therapy. The treatment protocol was to administer modified *Bu Zhong Yi Qi Tang* daily, for a duration ranging from 6 to 112 packs of herbal decoctions. The drugs were discontinued or reduced in dose only when the patients were stabilized. During the follow-up interviews, 35 patients had no recurrence within 1 year, 11 patients had no recurrence within 2 years, and 16 had reduced number of seizures. There was no benefit in 2 patients.[34]
17. **Myasthenia gravis**: One hundred patients with myasthenia gravis were treated with an 86% effective rate using *Bu Zhong Yi Qi Tang* combined with general Kidney tonics.[35]
18. **Male infertility**: Use of *Bu Zhong Yi Qi Tang* was 51.1% effective in improving sperm count and motility in a group of 45 men.[36] In another study involving 55 men, the formula was 67.3% effective in improving the sperm count, and 74.5% effective in improving the sperm motility.[37] Furthermore, use of this formula showed improved semen quality in 22 idiopathic infertile patients.[38] Lastly, one study reported favorable results (higher sperm motility) using *Bu Zhong Yi Qi Tang* to treat 14 patients with unexplained male infertility.[39]
19. **Allergic rhinitis**: *Bu Zhong Yi Qi Tang* can be combined with *Yu Ping Feng San* (Jade Windscreen Powder) or *Xin Yi San* (Magnolia Flower Powder) to effectively treat allergic rhinitis within 2 months.[40]
20. **Cataract**: Use of modified *Bu Zhong Yi Qi Tang* to treat 18 geriatric patients with cataracts was associated with 90.6% effectiveness. The base formula contained *Bu Zhong Yi Qi Tang* plus *Gou Qi Zi* (Fructus Lycii) and *Shu Di Huang* (Radix Rehmanniae Praeparata). The treatment protocol was to administer the herbs in decoction daily, for 6 days per course of treatment, followed by 1 day of rest, for 1 month.[41]
21. **Chronic hepatitis**: In a clinical study, modified *Bu Zhong Yi Qi Tang* was used to treat patients with chronic hepatitis characterized by Spleen qi deficiency or accumulation of dampness affecting the Spleen. The modification included the addition of *Yin Chen* (Herba Artemisiae Scopariae), *Cang Zhu* (Rhizoma Atractylodis), *Zhi Zi* (Fructus Gardeniae), *Zhu Ling* (Polyporus), *Fu Ling* (Poria), *Ze Xie* (Rhizoma Alismatis), *Huang Lian* (Rhizoma Coptidis), and *Hua Shi* (Talcum). The study reported significant results in 80 patients and moderate results in 2 patients.[42]
22. **Hepatoma**: Administration of *Bu Zhong Yi Qi Tang* had a dose-dependent effect to inhibit the proliferation of

Bǔ Zhōng Yì Qì Tāng

(Tonify the Middle and Augment the Qi Decoction)

human hepatoma cell lines (Hep3B, HepG2 and HA22T). The same formula, however, did not significantly inhibit the proliferation of normal human hepatocytes (Chang liver, CCL-13) at a concentration under 5,000 mcg/mL. The mechanism of this action was attributed to suppressed proliferation of hepatoma cells via G0/G1 cell cycle arrest and inhibition of DNA synthesis followed by apoptosis.[43]

23. **Hepatocellular carcinoma**: One study evaluated the cellular physiology of *Bu Zhong Yi Qi Tang* for the treatment of hepatocellular carcinoma. *In vitro* studies have shown that *Bu Zhong Yi Qi Tang* is capable of increasing granulocyte colony-stimulating-factor (G-CSF) and tumor necrosis factor-alpha (TNF-alpha) production by peripheral blood mononuclear cells. This effect was observed in both healthy volunteers and patients with hepatocellular carcinoma. Because of this unique effect to stimulate the production of TNF-alpha and G-CSF and activate the biological defensive mechanism, the researchers stated that *Bu Zhong Yi Qi Tang* may be beneficial for patients with hepatocellular carcinoma.[44]

HERB-DRUG INTERACTION

- **Mitomycin C-induced immunosuppression**: Administration of mitomycin C, a chemotherapy agent for cancer, is often associated with immunosuppression and infectious diseases. One study reported that *Bu Zhong Yi Qi Tang* had beneficial effects in mice, with improvements in spleen weight, number of colonies of granulocytes and macrophages forming in the bone-marrow cells, natural killer activity in splenocytes, and in susceptibility to lethal herpes simplex virus type-1 infection. The researchers concluded *Bu Zhong Yi Qi Tang* may be beneficial in immunocompromised patients receiving chemotherapeutic drugs.[45]
- **Cyclophosphamide-induced leukopenia**: Administration of *Bu Zhong Yi Qi Tang* (1000 mg/kg) in mice treated with cyclophosphamide significantly prevented leukopenia. *Bu Zhong Yi Qi Tang* enhanced the production of hematopoietic lymphokines, stimulated the proliferation of hematopoietic progenitor cells, and consequently accelerated recovery from leukopenia. *Bu Zhong Yi Qi Tang* also contributed a protective effect against bacterial infection by activating phagocyte cells.[46]
- **Radiation-induced hypotension**: According to one study, 30 patients between 25-50 years of age, who had worked in areas with high exposure to radiation, were treated for hypotension. The average blood pressure was 25 mmHg below normal. The patients were divided into three groups according to diagnosis of Spleen qi deficiency, qi and yang deficiencies, and qi and yin deficiencies. Patients in all three groups received *Bu Zhong Yi Qi Tang* as the base formula. *Fu Zi* (Radix Aconiti Lateralis Praeparata) and *Yin Yang Huo* (Herba Epimedii) were added for those who had qi and yang deficiencies. *Sheng Mai San* (Generate the Pulse Powder) was added for those who had qi and yin deficiencies. After 5 days of treatment, the study reported marked improvement in 47% of patients, moderate improvement in 40%, and no improvement in 13%. Marked improvement was defined as subjective improvement of symptoms according to the patients with an objective increase in blood pressure of 15-24 mmHg, and moderate improvement was defined as no significant changes in subjective symptoms, but an increase of 15 mmHg of blood pressure.[47]
- **Liver metabolism**: One study on the metabolic activity of different cytochrome P450 (CYP) isoforms reported *Bu Zhong Yi Qi Tang* to be a competitive inhibitor of CYP3A4 (Ki value of 0.65 mg/mL) and CYP2C9 (Ki value of 0.7-0.8 mg/mL), but not CYP2D6. The study concluded that because of this inhibitory effect on liver metabolism, care should be taken with concurrent use of *Bu Zhong Yi Qi Tang* and drugs.[48]

TOXICOLOGY

In an acute toxicology study, no fatality or abnormal reactions were noted in mice following oral ingestion of the formula at the dose of 166 g/kg twice daily for 3 days.[49]

SUGGESTED ACUPUNCTURE TREATMENT

1. Points: *Pishu* (BL 20), *Gaohuangshu* (BL 43), *Zhongwan* (CV 12), *Qihai* (CV 6), *Housanli* (ST 36), *Tianshu* (ST 25), *Guanyuan* (CV 4), and *Baihui* (GV 20).
2. Technique: Tonification. Moxibustion may also be used.

Pishu (BL 20), *Gaohuangshu* (BL 43), *Zhongwan* (CV 12), and *Qihai* (CV 6) tonify qi of the middle *jiao*. *Housanli* (ST 36) lifts qi of the middle *jiao* and relieves diarrhea, while *Tianshu* (ST 25) regulates the intestines and helps diarrhea. *Guanyuan* (CV 4) strengthens yang. *Baihui* (GV 20) causes yang qi to ascend and relieves qi depression or collapse.

AUTHORS' COMMENTS

Bu Zhong Yi Qi Tang is frequently used in veterinary medicine to treat a wide variety of body system disorders.

- For the treatment of myasthenia gravis with weakness in the dog, caused by the failure of the Spleen and Stomach to nourish the muscles, add *Gou Qi Zi* (Fructus Lycii), *Zhi Shi* (Fructus Aurantii Immaturus), *Jie Geng* (Radix Platycodonis), *Fu Ling* (Poria), *Huang Qin* (Radix Scutellariae), and *Dan Shen* (Radix et Rhizoma Salviae Miltiorrhizae).

Bŭ Zhōng Yì Qì Tāng

(Tonify the Middle and Augment the Qi Decoction)

- For the treatment of myasthenia gravis in young dogs with qi and yin deficiencies, combine with *Liu Wei Di Huang Wan* (Six-Ingredient Pill with Rehmannia) or *Zuo Gui Wan* (Restore the Left [Kidney] Pill). For dogs with Kidney qi and yang deficiencies, combine with *Jin Gui Shen Qi Wan* (Kidney Qi Pill from the Golden Cabinet). For dogs that have concurrent damp-heat, add *Si Miao San* (Four-Marvel Powder).
- To treat leukopenia secondary to chemotherapy with yin deficiency, add *Ji Xue Teng* (Caulis Spatholobi), *Nu Zhen Zi* (Fructus Ligustri Lucidi), *Qing Hao* (Herba Artemisiae Annuae), *Bie Jia* (Carapax Trionycis), and *Di Gu Pi* (Cortex Lycii).
- For poor appetite, bloating, and loose stools in horses with Cushing's disease, use *Bu Zhong Yi Qi Tang* to complement *You Gui Wan* (Restore the Right [Kidney] Pill).
- For the treatment of canine hypothyroidism with qi and yin deficiencies, combine with *Liu Wei Di Huang Wan* (Six-Ingredient Pill with Rehmannia).
- For degenerative myelopathy in the dog, combine with *Bu Yang Huan Wu Tang* (Tonify the Yang to Restore Five Decoction); for qi and yin deficiency, add *Sheng Mai San* (Generate the Pulse Powder).
- In the treatment of Addison's disease (hypoadrenocorticism) with hypotension, lethargy and inappetence, it can be combined with *Sheng Mai San* (Generate the Pulse Powder).
- For fibrocartilaginous emboli (FCE) in the dog, combine with either *Shen Tong Zhu Yu Tang* (Drive Out Blood Stasis from a Painful Body Decoction) or *Xue Fu Zhu Yu Tang* (Drive Out Stasis in the Mansion of Blood Decoction), depending on the case.
- For masticatory myositis in the dog, combine with *Shen Tong Zhu Yu Tang* (Drive Out Blood Stasis from a Painful Body Decoction) and add the following herbs to dispel toxic wind: *Quan Xie* (Scorpio), *Feng Fang* (Nidus Vespae), *Fang Feng* (Radix Saposhnikoviae), *Fang Ji* (Radix Stephaniae Tetrandrae), *Wei Ling Xian* (Radix et Rhizoma Clematidis), *Tian Nan Xing* (Rhizoma Arisaematis), and *Fu Zi* (Radix Aconiti Lateralis Praeparata). For dogs that have damp-heat, add *Si Miao San* (Four-Marvel Powder). This combination can be used until the clinical signs resolve, which can take up to 3 months; after resolution, it should be discontinued and a more constitutional formula chosen to consolidate the effects of treatment. For animals with significant atrophy, pneumoacupuncture is beneficial to restore normal muscle mass.
- For progressive retinal atrophy (PRA) due to qi and blood deficiency with stagnation, combine with *Xue Fu Zhu Yu Tang* (Drive Out Stasis in the Mansion of Blood Decoction) and *Si Wu Tang* (Four-Substance Decoction), or combine with *Tao Hong Si Wu Tang* (Four-Substance Decoction with Safflower and Peach Pit). With more yin deficiency, combine with *Qi Ju Di Huang Wan* (Lycium Fruit, Chrysanthemum, and Rehmannia Pill) and add *Dan Shen* (Radix et Rhizoma Salviae Miltiorrhizae).
- For the treatment of non-healing corneal ulcers or corneal dystrophy with blood deficiency and stagnation, combine with *Tong Qiao Huo Xue Tang* (Unblock the Orifices and Invigorate the Blood Decoction) and *Si Wu Tang* (Four-Substance Decoction); with Kidney and Liver yin deficiency, add *Qi Ju Di Huang Wan* (Lycium Fruit, Chrysanthemum, and Rehmannia Pill).
- For the treatment of cataracts in dogs with blood stasis and Spleen deficiency, combine with *Tao Hong Si Wu Tang* (Four-Substance Decoction with Safflower and Peach Pit) and add *Gou Qi Zi* (Fructus Lycii), *Shu Di Huang* (Radix Rehmanniae Praeparata), *Jue Ming Zi* (Semen Cassiae), *Gu Jing Cao* (Flos Eriocauli), *Shan Yao* (Rhizoma Dioscoreae), *Ju Hua* (Flos Chrysanthemi), *Xuan Shen* (Radix Scrophulariae), *Qing Xiang Zi* (Semen Celosiae), and *Shi Jue Ming* (Concha Haliotidis).
- For the treatment of chronic renal failure and glomerulonephritis with significant proteinuria, combine *Bu Zhong Yi Qi Tang* with *Dan Shen* (Radix et Rhizoma Salviae Miltiorrhizae), *Qian Shi* (Semen Euryales), *Yi Zhi* (Fructus Alpiniae Oxyphyllae), *Fu Pen Zi* (Fructus Rubi), and *Jin Ying Zi* (Fructus Rosae Laevigatae).
- For megaesophagus, combine with *Tao Hong Si Wu Tang* (Four-Substance Decoction with Safflower and Peach Pit) or *Xue Fu Zhu Yu Tang* (Drive Out Stasis in the Mansion of Blood Decoction), depending on the case.
- For megacolon in the cat due to qi and yin deficiencies, combine with *Zeng Ye Tang* (Increase the Fluids Decoction) to generate body fluids, moisten dryness, and unblock the bowels; and add the smallest therapeutic dose of *Da Huang* (Radix et Rhizoma Rhei) to help purge accumulation, in combination with subcutaneous or intravenous fluid therapy.
- For rectal prolapse that is chronic and severe, add astringent herbs such as *Wu Wei Zi* (Fructus Schisandrae Chinensis), *Jin Ying Zi* (Fructus Rosae Laevigatae), *Wu Bei Zi* (Galla Chinensis), or *Wu Mei* (Fructus Mume). If bleeding is a problem, add *Xian He Cao* (Herba Agrimoniae). If there is heat in the intestines, add *Huang Qin* (Radix Scutellariae), *Bai Shao* (Radix Paeoniae Alba) and *Huai Hua* (Flos Sophorae). With hard-to-pass sticky stools, add *Huo Ma Ren* (Fructus Cannabis) and *Feng Mi* (Mel).
- For urinary incontinence in the dog due to Spleen and Lung deficiencies, add *Mu Li* (Concha Ostreae), *Chen Pi* (Pericarpium Citri Reticulatae), *Yi Zhi* (Fructus Alpiniae Oxyphyllae), and *Wu Wei Zi* (Fructus Schisandrae Chinensis). Combine with *Suo Quan Wan* (Shut the Sluice

Bǔ Zhōng Yì Qì Tāng

(Tonify the Middle and Augment the Qi Decoction)

Pill) and *Fu Pen Zi* (Fructus Rubi) for Kidney qi deficiency; *You Gui Wan* (Restore the Right [Kidney] Pill) or *Jin Gui Shen Qi Wan* (Kidney Qi Pill from the Golden Cabinet) for Kidney yang deficiency; *Sang Piao Xiao San* (Mantis Egg-Case Powder) for Kidney and Heart qi deficiencies. Urinary incontinence can also be initially treated by combining *Bu Zhong Yi Qi Tang* with *Jin Suo Gu Jing Wan* (Metal Lock Pill to Stabilize the Essence), which is primarily an astringent formula. After the incontinence is under control, a constitutional or root formula to tonify underlying deficiencies is needed to consolidate the effects of treatment. For middle age and older dogs with yin deficiency, in which deficient yin causes weakness and deficiency heat forces urine out of the bladder with dribbling of urine, combine with *Zhi Bai Di Huang Wan* (Anemarrhena, Phellodendron, and Rehmannia Pill).

- For a comparative discussion of Spleen tonic formulas, see *Si Jun Zi Tang* (Four-Gentlemen Decoction).

It is often asked that if *Bu Zhong Yi Qi Tang* treats prolapsed organs, why are *Sheng Ma* (Rhizoma Cimicifugae) and *Chai Hu* (Radix Bupleuri) not used as chief herbs at larger doses to maximize the effects? There are two reasons why a large dose of these two herbs is inappropriate:

- First, the prolapse is caused by qi deficiency, so tonic herbs such as *Ren Shen* (Radix et Rhizoma Ginseng), *Bai Zhu* (Rhizoma Atractylodis Macrocephalae), and *Zhi Gan Cao* (Radix et Rhizoma Glycyrrhizae Praeparata cum Melle) must be used to treat the underlying deficiency, which is the root of the condition.
- Second, the primary function of *Chai Hu* (Radix Bupleuri) and *Sheng Ma* (Rhizoma Cimicifugae) is to release the exterior, and their secondary function is to lift prolapsed organs. If they are used at larger doses, their dispersing and exterior-releasing functions would override their lifting effect and injure the *zheng* (upright) *qi* of the body.[50]

Huang Qi (Radix Astragali) is the main ingredient in two important formulas, but with slightly different purposes:

- *Bu Zhong Yi Qi Tang* contains *Huang Qi* (Radix Astragali) to tonify qi and cause yang to ascend. It treats Spleen and Stomach qi deficiencies with prolapsed organs. Animals will exhibit fatigue, poor appetite, weight loss, chronic diarrhea, and spontaneous sweating.
- *Dang Gui Bu Xue Tang* (Tangkuei Decoction to Tonify the Blood) contains *Huang Qi* (Radix Astragali) at a dose five times higher than *Dang Gui* (Radix Angelicae Sinensis) to boost qi and generate blood. It is mainly used for blood deficiency with deficiency heat signs, spontaneous sweating, and a large, weak pulse.

References

1. *Zhong Yao Yao Li Yu Lin Chuang* (Pharmacology and Clinical Applications of Chinese Herbs), 1987; 2:4.
2. *Zhong Yao Yao Li Yu Lin Chuang* (Pharmacology and Clinical Applications of Chinese Herbs), 1988; 3:16.
3. *Zhong Yi Fang Ji Xian Dai Yan Jiu* (Modern Study of Medical Formulas in Traditional Chinese Medicine), 1997; 524.
4. Shih HC, Chang KH, Chen FL, Chen CM, Chen SC, Lin YT, Shibu ya A. Anti-aging effects of the traditional Chinese medicine bu-zhong-yi-qi-tang in mice. Am J Chin Med. 2000; 28(1):77-86.
5. *Zhong Yi Fang Ji Xian Dai Yan Jiu* (Modern Study of Medical Formulas in Traditional Chinese Medicine), 1997; 520-521.
6. Tamura R, Takahashi HK, Xue D, Kubo S, Saito S, Nishibori M, Iwagaki H, Tanaka N. Enhanced effects of combined bu-zhong-yi-qi-tang (TJ-41) and interleukin-18 on the production of tumour necrosis factor-alpha and interferon-gamma in human peripheral blood mononuclear cells. J Int Med Res. 2004 Jan-Feb; 32(1):25-32.
7. Suzuki T, Takano I, Nagai F, Fujitani T, Ushiyama K, Okubo T, Seto T, Ikeda S, Kano I. Suppressive effects of Hochu-ekki-to, a traditional Chinese medicine, on IgE production and histamine release in mice immunized with ovalbumin. Biol Pharm Bull. 1999 Nov; 22(11):1180-4.
8. Kaneko M, Kawakita T, Nomoto K. Inhibition of eosinophil infiltration into the mouse peritoneal cavity by a traditional Chinese medicine, Bu-zhong-yi-qi-tang (Japanese name: Hochu-ekki-to). Immunopharmacol Immunotoxicol. 1999 Feb; 21(1):125-40.
9. Kao ST, Yeh CC, Hsieh CC, Yang MD, Lee MR, Liu HS, Lin JG. The Chinese medicine Bu-Zhong-Yi-Qi-Tang inhibited proliferation of hepatoma cell lines by inducing apoptosis via G0/G1 arrest. Life Sciences. 2001 Aug 17; 69(13):1485-96.
10. Cho JM, Sato N, Kikuchi K. Prophylactic anti-tumor effect of Hochu-ekki-to (TJ41) by enhancing natural killer cell activity. In Vivo. 1991 Jul-Aug; 5(4):389-91.
11. Kim SH, Lee SE, Oh H, Kim SR, Yee ST, Yu YB, Byun MW, Jo SK. The radioprotective effects of bu-zhong-yi-qi-tang: a prescription of traditional Chinese medicine. Am J Chin Med. 2002; 30(1):127-37.
12. Xiaoqun Yan, Masakazu Kita, Masato Minami, Toshiro Yamamoto, Hiroko Kuriyama,Tomoyuki Ohno, Yoichiro Iwakura, and Jiro Imanishi. Antibacterial Effect of Kampo Herbal Formulation Hochu-Ekki-To (Bu-Zhong-Yi-Qi-Tang) on *Helicobacter pylori* Infection in Mice. Microbiol. Immunol. 2002; 46(7), 475-482.
13. Mori K, Kido T, Daikuhara H, Sakakibara I, Sakata T, Shimizu K, Amagaya S, Sasaki H, Komatsu Y. Effect of Hochu-ekki-to (TJ-41), a Japanese herbal medicine, on the survival of mice infected with influenza virus. Antiviral Res. 1999 Dec 15; 44(2):103-11.
14. Sassa S, Sakamoto S, Zhou YF, Mori T, Kikuchi T, Shinoda H. Preventive effects of a Chinese herbal medicine, hochu-ekki-to, on bone loss in ovariectomized rats. Medical Research Institute, Tokyo Medical and Dental University In Vivo. 2001 Jan-Feb; 15(1):25-8.
15. Koshikawa N, Imai T, Takahashi I, Yamauchi M, Sawada S, Kansaku A. Effects of Hochu-ekki-to, Yoku-kan-san and Saiko-ka-ryukotsu-borei-to on behavioral despair and acetic acid-induced writhing in mice. Methods Find Exp Clin Pharmacol. 1998 Jan-Feb; 20(1):47-51.
16. *Shi Yong Zhong Yi Za Zhi* (Journal of Practical Chinese Medicine), 1998; 8:20.
17. *Shang Hai Zhong Yi Yao Za Zhi* (Shanghai Journal of Chinese Medicine and Herbology), 1983; 12:20.
18. *Zhong Yi Yao Xue Bao* (Report of Chinese Medicine and Herbology), 1995; 3:42.
19. *Hu Nan Zhong Yi Za Zhi* (Hunan Journal of Chinese Medicine), 1997; 3:48.

Bŭ Zhōng Yì Qì Tāng

(Tonify the Middle and Augment the Qi Decoction)

20. *Shan Dong Yi Yao* (Shandong Medicine and Herbology), 1979; 4:43.
21. *Jiang Su Zhong Yi Za Zhi* (Jiangsu Journal of Chinese Medicine), 1997; 11:514.
22. *He Bei Zhong Yi* (Hebei Chinese Medicine), 1986; 6:13.
23. *Zhong Yi Fang Ji Xian Dai Yan Jiu* (Modern Study of Medical Formulas in Traditional Chinese Medicine), 1997; 529.
24. *Shi Yong Zhong Xi Yi Jie He Za Zhi* (Practical Journal of Integrated Chinese and Western Medicines), 1998; 3:262.
25. *Hunan Journal of Medicine and Herbology*, 1984; 6:35.
26. *Jiang Su Zhong Yi* (Jiangsu Chinese Medicine), 1995; 6:9.
27. *Shi Yong Zhong Yi Yao Za Zhi* (Journal of Practical Chinese Medicine and Medicinals), 1998; 6:13.
28. Kuroiwa A, Liou S, Yan H, Eshita A, Naitoh S, Nagayama A. Effect of a traditional Japanese herbal medicine, Hochu-ekki-to (Bu-Zhong-Yi-Qi Tang), on immunity in elderly persons. Int Immunopharmacol. 2004 Feb; 4(2):317-24.
29. *Zhe Jiang Zhong Yi Za Zhi* (Zhejiang Journal of Chinese Medicine), 1992; 10:444.
30. *Shi Yong Zhong Yi Yao Za Zhi* (Journal of Practical Chinese Medicine and Medicinals), 1998; 3:262.
31. *Shang Hai Zhong Yi Yao Za Zhi* (Shanghai Journal of Chinese Medicine and Herbology), 1983; 10:28.
32. *Xin Zhong Yi* (New Chinese Medicine), 1989; 4:47.
33. *Shan Xi Xin Zhong Yi* (New Shanxi Chinese Medicine), 1988; 6:258.
34. *Zhong Yi Fang Ji Xian Dai Yan Jiu* (Modern Study of Medical Formulas in Traditional Chinese Medicine), 1997; 532.
35. *Yi Xue Qing Kuang Jiao Liu* (Medical Information Exchange), 1975; 2:23.
36. *Zhong Xi Yi Jie He Za Zhi* (Journal of Integrated Chinese and Western Medicine), 1989; 4:242.
37. *Guo Wai Yi Xue Zhong Yi Zhong Yao Fen Ce* (Monograph of Chinese Herbology from Foreign Medicine), 1987; 4:16.
38. Furuya Y, Akashi T, Fuse H. Effect of Bu-zhong-yi-qi-tang on seminal plasma cytokine levels in patients with idiopathic male infertility. Arch Androl. 2004 Jan-Feb; 50(1):11-4.
39. Amano T, Hirata A, Namiki M. Effects of Chinese herbal medicine on sperm motility and fluorescence spectra parameters. Archives of Andrology. 1996 Nov-Dec; 37(3):219-24.
40. *He Bei Zhong Yi* (Hebei Chinese Medicine), 1989; 4:9.
41. Fu Jian Zhong Yi Yao (Fujian Chinese Medicine and Herbology), 1995; 2:12.
42. *He Bei Zhong Yi* (Hebei Chinese Medicine), 1984; 3:24.
43. Kao ST, Yeh CC, Hsieh CC, Yang MD, Lee MR, Liu HS, Lin JG. The Chinese medicine Bu-Zhong-Yi-Qi-Tang inhibited proliferation of hepatoma cell lines by inducing apoptosis via G0/G1 arrest. China Medical College Hospital, China Medical College, Taichung, Taiwan. Life Sciences. 2001 Aug 17; 69(13):1485-96.
44. Kao ST, Yang SL, Hsieh CC, Yang MD, Wang TF, Lin JG. Immunomodulation of Bu-Zhong-Yi-Qi-Tang on in vitro granulocyte colony-stimulating-factor and tumor necrosis factor-alpha production by peripheral blood mononuclear cells. Immunopharmacology & Immunotoxicology. 2000 Nov; 22(4):711-20.
45. Kido T, Mori K, Daikuhara H, Tsuchiya H, Ishige A, Sasaki H. The protective effect of hochu-ekki-to (TJ-41), a Japanese herbal medicine, against HSV-1 infection in mitomycin C-treated mice. Anticancer Res. 2000 Nov-Dec; 20(6A):4109-13.
46. Kaneko M, Kawakita T, Kumazawa Y, Takimoto H, Nomoto K, Yoshikawa T. Accelerated recovery from cyclophosphamide-induced leukopenia in mice administered a Japanese ethical herbal drug, Hochu-ekki-to. Immunopharmacology. 1999 Nov;44(3):223-31.
47. *Yun Nan Zhong Yi Za Zhi* (Yunan Journal of Chinese Medicine), 1983; (3):28.
48. Takahashi K, Uejima E, Morisaki T, Takahashi K, Kurokawa N, Azuma J. In vitro inhibitory effects of Kampo medicines on metabolic reactions catalyzed by human liver microsomes. Journal of Clinical Pharmacy & Therapeutics. 2003 Aug; 28(4):319-27.
49. *Xian Dai Shi Yong Yao Xue* (Practical Applications of Modern Herbal Medicine), 1989; 5:45.
50. Wang MZ, et al. *Zhong Yi Xue Wen Da Ti Ku* (Questions and Answers on Traditional Chinese Medicine: Herbal Formulas).

Yì Qì Cōng Míng Tāng (Augment the Qi and Increase Acuity Decoction)

益氣聰明湯
益气聪明汤

Pinyin Name: *Yi Qi Cong Ming Tang*
Literal Name: Augment the Qi and Increase Acuity Decoction
Alternate Names: *Yi Chi Cong Ming Tang, I Chi Chung Ming Tang*, Ginseng, Astragalus and Pueraria Decoction; Ginseng, Astragalus and Pueraria Combination
Original Source: *Dong Heng Shi Xiao Fang* (Tested and Effective Formulas by Dong Heng) by Dong Heng in 1266

COMPOSITION

Ren Shen (Radix et Rhizoma Ginseng)	15g
Huang Qi (Radix Astragali)	15g
Ge Gen (Radix Puerariae Lobatae)	9g
Sheng Ma (Rhizoma Cimicifugae)	9g
Man Jing Zi (Fructus Viticis)	4.5g
Bai Shao (Radix Paeoniae Alba)	3g
Huang Bo (Cortex Phellodendri Chinensis), *zhi* (fried with liquor) and *chao* (dry-fried) till yellow	3g
Zhi Gan Cao (Radix et Rhizoma Glycyrrhizae Praeparata cum Melle)	15g

DOSAGE / PREPARATION / ADMINISTRATION

Grind the herbs into a coarse powder, and cook 9g in two bowls of water until it is reduced to one bowl. Take the strained decoction while warm.

CHINESE THERAPEUTIC ACTIONS

1. Tonifies qi and blood
2. Lifts yang qi and benefits the eyes and ears

CLINICAL MANIFESTATIONS

Compromised visual and auditory functions: diminished acuity of the eyes and ears, impaired vision, decreased appetite, and chronic diarrhea.

VETERINARY CLINICAL APPLICATIONS

Cognitive dysfunction in the dog, deafness, diminished vision, cataract, and geriatric vestibular disease.

EXPLANATION

Yi Qi Cong Ming Tang (Augment the Qi and Increase Acuity Decoction) treats compromised functioning and deterioration of the eyes and ears. It may be used to reverse deterioration, or preventively to maintain the acuity of both ears and eyes.

Ren Shen (Radix et Rhizoma Ginseng) and *Huang Qi* (Radix Astragali) tonify qi and strengthen the Spleen and Stomach. *Ge Gen* (Radix Puerariae Lobatae), *Sheng Ma* (Rhizoma Cimicifugae), and *Man Jing Zi* (Fructus Viticis) have an ascending function to lift yang qi and treat disorders of the upper parts of the body. When sufficient qi rises to the head, the normal functions of the eyes and ears will be restored. *Bai Shao* (Radix Paeoniae Alba) nourishes yin and harmonizes the blood. *Huang Bo* (Cortex Phellodendri Chinensis) controls deficiency fire. Lastly, *Zhi*

***Yi Qi Cong Ming Tang* (Augment the Qi and Increase Acuity Decoction)**

Diagnosis	Clinical Signs	Treatment	Herbs
Deterioration of eye and ear functions	Diminished acuity of the eyes and ears, decreased appetite, and chronic diarrhea: qi and blood deficiencies	• Tonifies qi and blood • Lifts yang qi and benefits the eyes and ears	• *Ren Shen* (Radix et Rhizoma Ginseng) and *Huang Qi* (Radix Astragali) tonify qi and strengthen the Spleen and Stomach. • *Ge Gen* (Radix Puerariae Lobatae), *Sheng Ma* (Rhizoma Cimicifugae), and *Man Jing Zi* (Fructus Viticis) lift yang qi. • *Bai Shao* (Radix Paeoniae Alba) nourishes yin and harmonizes the blood. • *Huang Bo* (Cortex Phellodendri Chinensis) controls deficiency fire. • *Zhi Gan Cao* (Radix et Rhizoma Glycyrrhizae Praeparata cum Melle) harmonizes the herbs.

Yì Qì Cōng Míng Tāng (Augment the Qi and Increase Acuity Decoction)

Gan Cao (Radix et Rhizoma Glycyrrhizae Praeparata cum Melle) harmonizes the middle *jiao* and the other herbs in the formula.

VETERINARY MODIFICATIONS

- With impaired vision, add *Ju Hua* (Flos Chrysanthemi) and *Gou Qi Zi* (Fructus Lycii).
- With vestibular disease due to Kidney deficiency, add *Zhi Bai Di Huang Wan* (Anemarrhena, Phellodendron, and Rehmannia Pill), *Qi Ju Di Huang Wan* (Lycium Fruit, Chrysanthemum, and Rehmannia Pill) or *Yi Guan Jian* (Linking Decoction) depending on the case.

CAUTIONS / CONTRAINDICATIONS

- *Yi Qi Cong Ming Tang* is designed to treat compromised visual and auditory functions due to overall deterioration and deficiency. It should not be used if the eye and ear disorders are due to excess, such as Liver fire rising or damp-heat in the Liver and Gallbladder channels.[1]
- While taking this herbal formula, patients should avoid exposure to smoke and fire, and refrain from eating sour, cold, raw, oily or greasy foods.

HUMAN CLINICAL STUDIES AND RESEARCH

1. **Memory and Cognition**: *Yi Qi Cong Ming Tang* has been used with satisfactory effect in treating geriatric patients with gradual deterioration of cognitive functions. In another study, use of modified *Yi Qi Cong Ming Tang* was associated with both subjective and objective improvements in memory and cognitive performance in 30 geriatric patients with cerebral arteriosclerosis. The herbal treatment contained this formula plus *Tai Zi Shen* (Radix Pseudostellariae) and *Chi Shao* (Radix Paeoniae Rubra). The mechanism of action was attributed in part to the increased blood perfusion to the brain.[2]
2. **Vertigo**: Modified *Yi Qi Cong Ming Tang* was used to treat 52 geriatric patients with vertigo, with the history of illness ranging from 6 months to 3 years. The herbal treatment contained *Huang Qi* (Radix Astragali), *Dang Shen* (Radix Codonopsis), processed *Sheng Ma* (Rhizoma Cimicifugae), *Ge Gen* (Radix Puerariae Lobatae), *Man Jing Zi* (Fructus Viticis), *Huang Bo* (Cortex Phellodendri Chinensis), *Bai Shao* (Radix Paeoniae Alba), *Zhi Gan Cao* (Radix et Rhizoma Glycyrrhizae Praeparata cum Melle), *Tian Ma* (Rhizoma Gastrodiae), *Ban Xia* (Rhizoma Pinelliae), *Du Zhong* (Cortex Eucommiae), and *Niu Xi* (Radix Achyranthis Bidentatae). The treatment protocol was to cook the herbs in water, and administer the decoction in three equally-divided doses. Of 52 patients, the study reported complete recovery in 28 patients, improvement in 20 patients, and no benefit in 4 patients. The overall rate of effectiveness was 92.3%.[3]
3. **Otitis media**: One study reported good results for the treatment of suppurative otitis media using modified *Yi Qi Cong Ming Tang*. The herbal formula contained *Huang Qi* (Radix Astragali) 15g, *Ren Shen* (Radix et Rhizoma Ginseng) 15g, *Man Jing Zi* (Fructus Viticis) 9g, *Ge Gen* (Radix Puerariae Lobatae) 9g, *Bai Shao* (Radix Paeoniae Alba) 9g, *Huang Bo* (Cortex Phellodendri Chinensis) 6g, *Sheng Ma* (Rhizoma Cimicifugae) 6g, and *Zhi Gan Cao* (Radix et Rhizoma Glycyrrhizae Praeparata cum Melle) 6g. The herbs were given in decoction daily. Of 21 geriatric patients, the study reported complete recovery in 13 patients, moderate improvement in 6 patients, and no benefit in 2 patients.[4]

SUGGESTED ACUPUNCTURE TREATMENT

1. Points: *Housanli* (ST 36), *Qihai* (CV 6), *Ermen* (TH 21), *Jingming* (BL 1), *Sishencong* (extra point), *Guangming* (GB 37), *Sanyinjiao* (SP 6), and *Fuliu* (KI 7).
2. Technique: tonification.

Tonify *Housanli* (ST 36) and *Qihai* (CV 6) to supplement and invigorate qi. Tonify *Ermen* (TH 21), *Jingming* (BL 1), and *Sishencong* to lead qi to the upper body. *Guangming* (GB 37) benefits the eyes and harmonizes the Liver. Tonify *Sanyinjiao* (SP 6) and *Fuliu* (KI 7) to tonify yin and clear deficiency heat.

AUTHORS' COMMENTS

To treat cognitive dysfunction in the dog, combine *Yi Qi Cong Ming Tang* with *Dan Shen* (Radix et Rhizoma Salviae Miltiorrhizae), *Yin Xing Ye* (Folium Ginkgo), *San Qi* (Radix et Rhizoma Notoginseng), *Ci Wu Jia* (Radix et Rhizoma seu Caulis Acanthopanacis Senticosi), *Shu Di Huang* (Radix Rehmanniae Praeparata), *Gou Qi Zi* (Fructus Lycii), *He Shou Wu* (Radix Polygoni Multiflori), *Wu Wei Zi* (Fructus Schisandrae Chinensis), and *Chai Hu* (Radix Bupleuri). It can take up to 6 months before maximum clinical effects are observed. For a comparative discussion of Spleen tonic formulas, see *Si Jun Zi Tang* (Four-Gentlemen Decoction).

References

1. *Zhong Yao Ming Fang Yao Li Yu Ying Yong* (Pharmacology and Applications of Famous Herbal Formulas), 1989; 257-258.
2. *Shang Hai Zhong Yi Yao Za Zhi* (Shanghai Journal of Chinese Medicine and Herbology), 1991; 5:41.
3. *Yun Nan Zhong Yi Xue Yuan Xue Bao* (Journal of Yunnan University School of Medicine), 1993; 3:24.
4. *Shan Dong Yi Ke Da Xue Xue Bao* (Journal of Shandong University of Medicine), 1998; 3:197.

Shēng Mài Săn (Generate the Pulse Powder)

生脈散
生脉散

Pinyin Name: *Sheng Mai San*
Literal Name: Generate the Pulse Powder
Alternate Names: *Sheng Mai Yin* (Generate the Pulse Decoction), Ginseng and Ophiopogon Formula
Original Source: *Nei Wai Shang Bian Huo Lun* (Clarifying Doubts about Injury from Internal and External Causes) by Li Gao in 1247

COMPOSITION

Ren Shen (Radix et Rhizoma Ginseng)	1.5g [10g]
Mai Dong (Radix Ophiopogonis)	1.5g [10-15g]
Wu Wei Zi (Fructus Schisandrae Chinensis)	7 seeds [6g]

DOSAGE / PREPARATION / ADMINISTRATION

The source text states to prepare the ingredients as a decoction. It may be taken at any time of the day. Today, this formula is prepared by using larger doses of the ingredients, provided in brackets above, and cooking the herbs three times, and consuming the decoction within one day.

CHINESE THERAPEUTIC ACTIONS

1. Tonifies qi and promotes body fluid secretion
2. Astringes yin and stops sweating.

CLINICAL MANIFESTATIONS

1. Damaged qi and body fluids due to summer-heat and profuse sweating (in animals that sweat): a dry throat, thirst, irritability, lethargy, panting, and a fine, weak pulse.
2. Damaged qi and yin due to chronic coughing: coughing with scanty sputum, shortness of breath, a pale to red tongue and a thready, rapid or deep, weak pulse.

VETERINARY CLINICAL APPLICATIONS

Heatstroke, cardiomyopathy, congestive heart failure, arrhythmia, myocarditis, leukopenia, chronic cough, chronic bronchitis, hypoadrenocorticism and diabetes mellitus.

EXPLANATION

Sheng Mai San (Generate the Pulse Powder) treats deficiencies of qi and yin that may be caused by summer-heat inducing profuse sweating and damaging qi and body fluids. Damaged qi and yin in animals may also occur from chronic coughing, chronic disease, and chronic drug therapy. Qi deficiency is characterized by lethargy, exercise intolerance, fatigue, and shortness of breath. Yin deficiency is characterized by a dry mouth, thirst, irritability, cool-seeking behavior, coughing with scanty sputum, a pale to red tongue, and a thready, rapid or deep, weak pulse.

Ren Shen (Radix et Rhizoma Ginseng), the chief herb, tonifies *yuan* (source) *qi* and strengthens the Lung. *Mai Dong* (Radix Ophiopogonis) nourishes yin, replenishes body fluids lost through sweating, and relieves thirst and dry mouth. These two tonic herbs treat the root of the condition by replenishing what is lost and deficient. Lastly, *Wu Wei Zi* (Fructus Schisandrae Chinensis) astringes the Lung to stop sweating and arrest coughing.

VETERINARY MODIFICATIONS

- If there is more yin deficiency, use *Xi Yang Shen* (Radix Panacis Quinquefolii) instead of *Ren Shen* (Radix et Rhizoma Ginseng).

Sheng Mai San **(Generate the Pulse Powder)**

Diagnosis	Clinical Signs	Treatment	Herbs
Damages to qi, yin, and body fluids	• Dry mouth, cool-seeking behavior, thirst, and irritability: yin and body fluid deficiencies • Profuse sweating or spontaneous sweating, lethargy, exercise intolerance, fatigue, and shortness of breath: qi deficiency • A pale to red tongue with no coating: yin and body fluid deficiencies • A rapid, thready or deep, weak pulse: qi and yin deficiencies	• Tonifies qi and promotes body fluid secretion • Astringes yin and stops perspiration	• *Ren Shen* (Radix et Rhizoma Ginseng) tonifies *yuan* (source) *qi* and strengthens the Lung. • *Mai Dong* (Radix Ophiopogonis) nourishes yin and replenishes body fluids. • *Wu Wei Zi* (Fructus Schisandrae Chinensis) astringes the Lung to stop sweating and coughing.

Shēng Mài Sǎn (Generate the Pulse Powder)

- If there is a faint pulse and increased risk of shock, add a large dose of *Ren Shen* (Radix et Rhizoma Ginseng).
- For qi and yin deficiencies due to febrile disorder, add *Xuan Shen* (Radix Scrophulariae) and *Di Huang* (Radix Rehmanniae).
- For chronic respiratory disorder with coughing with phlegm secondary to qi and yin deficiencies, add *Ku Xing Ren* (Semen Armeniacae Amarum), *Chen Pi* (Pericarpium Citri Reticulatae), *Tao Ren* (Semen Persicae), *Zi Wan* (Radix et Rhizoma Asteris), *Huang Qi* (Radix Astragali), *Sang Bai Pi* (Cortex Mori) and *Shu Di Huang* (Radix Rehmanniae Praeparata).
- For chronic heart disorder with yin and yang deficiencies, add *Huang Qi* (Radix Astragali) and *Gan Cao* (Radix et Rhizoma Glycyrrhizae).

CAUTIONS / CONTRAINDICATIONS

- *Sheng Mai San* has an astringent action, and is contraindicated in animals with exterior syndromes or interior heat conditions.
- This formula is not recommended for chronic cough with Lung deficiency accompanied by an exterior syndrome.

PHARMACOLOGICAL EFFECTS

1. **Cardiovascular**: Administration of *Sheng Mai San* was associated with a marked effect on the cardiovascular system. In rabbits, it has a cardiotonic effect to increase the contractile force of heart tissues. It also prevents arrhythmia as demonstrated in laboratory experiments in rats. In addition, it increases blood perfusion to the coronary artery and the peripheral parts of the body.[1]
2. **Cardioprotective**: *Sheng Mai San* has a cardioprotective effect against post-ischemic myocardial dysfunction by opening the mitochondrial KATP channels.[2] It also reduces myocardial infarct size by activating protein kinase C and opening the mitochondrial KATP channel.[3] The lignan of *Wu Wei Zi* (Fructus Schisandrae Chinensis) is believed to be the major myocardial protective component in this formula.[4]
3. **Immunostimulant**: In mice, injection of *Sheng Mai San* at 0.4 mL per day for 5 days was associated with an increase in white blood cells and T-lymphocytes.[5]
4. **Central nervous system**: Administration of *Sheng Mai San* has a mild sedative effect on the central nervous system. It counters caffeine's stimulating effect.[6]
5. **Anti-inflammatory**: Administration of *Sheng Mai San* was associated with reduced swelling and inflammation in rats. The effect was attributed to the increased glucocorticoids production, because the formula had no benefit in subjects whose adrenal glands had been removed.[7]

HUMAN CLINICAL STUDIES AND RESEARCH

1. **Coronary artery disease**: In one report, 41 patients with coronary artery disease were treated with *Sheng Mai San* with subjective improvement noted in 78% of patients, and ECG improvement in 14.5% of patients.[8] Another study reported 66.7% effectiveness in 35 patients with coronary artery disease using 20 mL of *Sheng Mai San* in liquid form three times daily for 3 weeks per course of treatment.[9]
2. **Angina pectoris**: Patients with angina characterized by qi and yin deficiencies were treated with intravenous injection of *Sheng Mai San* for 14 days per course of treatment with good results. Of 53 patients, the study reported marked effect in 12 patients, improvement in 35 patients, and no benefit in 6 patients. The overall rate of effectiveness was 88.6%.[10]
3. **Myocardial infarction**: Twelve patients with acute myocardial infarction were treated with oral ingestion of *Sheng Mai San* plus *Dang Gui* (Radix Angelicae Sinensis), *Yan Hu Suo* (Rhizoma Corydalis), *Chi Shao* (Radix Paeoniae Rubra), *Huang Qi* (Radix Astragali), *Bai Zhu* (Rhizoma Atractylodis Macrocephalae), *Fu Ling* (Poria), *Tao Ren* (Semen Persicae), and *Hong Hua* (Flos Carthami). Out of 12 patients, the study reported complete recovery in 4 patients, improvement in 6 patients, and no benefit in 2 patients.[11]
4. **Coronary heart disease**: One study reported marked results using *Sheng Mai San* to treat patients with coronary heart disease (30 with angina pectoris and 68 with acute myocardial infarction). The administration of the herbs was found to increase the levels of superoxide dismutase (SOD) and decreased glutathione peroxidase (GSH-Px) and malondialdehyde (MDA) in blood. By acting as an effective free radical scavenger in minimizing the lipid peroxidation damage, *Sheng Mai San* was considered effective for prevention and treatment of coronary heart disease.[12]
5. **Arrhythmia**: In one study, 36 patients with arrhythmia characterized by qi and yin deficiencies were treated first by intravenous injection, followed by oral ingestion, of *Sheng Mai San*. The study reported an overall effectiveness rate of 83.4%.[13] In another study, *Sheng Mai San* was associated with 85.7% effectiveness in treating 21 patients with chronic bradyarrhythmia.[14]
6. **Viral myocarditis**: Sixty-three patients with viral myocarditis were treated with good results using *Sheng Mai San* plus *Chi Shao* (Radix Paeoniae Rubra), *Long Gu* (Os Draconis), and *Mu Li* (Concha Ostreae). The treatment protocol was to administer the herbs in decoction daily for 15 days per course of treatment, for 1-2 courses total. The overall rate of effectiveness was 90%.[15]

Shēng Mài Sǎn (Generate the Pulse Powder)

7. **Myocarditis**: Twenty patients with myocarditis (15 were refractory to drug treatment) were treated with both *Sheng Mai San* and *Gan Mai Da Zao Tang* (Licorice, Wheat, and Jujube Decoction). Out of 20 patients, the study reported marked improvement in 6 patients, moderate improvement in 10 patients, and no benefit in 4 patients.[16]
8. **Hypotension**: One study reported 97.32% effectiveness using *Sheng Mai San* plus *Dang Gui* (Radix Angelicae Sinensis), *Gui Zhi* (Ramulus Cinnamomi), and *E Jiao* (Colla Corii Asini) to treat hypotension. Of 112 patients, the study reported complete recovery in 78 patients, marked improvement in 23 patients, and slight improvement in 8 patients. The treatment protocol was to cook the herbs in water and drink the decoction in three equally-divided doses. The duration of treatment was 3 courses, with 10 days per course.[17] According to another study, 15 patients with primary hypotension were treated with *Sheng Mai San*. The study noted that the blood pressure began to increase after one week. After 4 weeks of treatment, the average increase in blood pressure was 14 mmHg for systolic and 6.7 mmHg for diastolic.[18]
9. **Shock**: In one report, 17 patients with shock due to infection were treated with an injection of *Sheng Mai San* with an overall 88.2% effectiveness.[19] In another report, 8 patients with shock due to excessive loss of blood were treated with *Sheng Mai San* with excellent effect in 5 patients, improvement in 2 patients, and no benefit in 1 patient.[20]
10. **Leukopenia**: Thirty-nine patients (21 males and 18 females, between 39-70 years of age) with leukopenia were treated with *Sheng Mai San* plus *Yu Zhu* (Rhizoma Polygonati Odorati), *Shi Hu* (Caulis Dendrobii), *Dang Gui* (Radix Angelicae Sinensis), and others as needed. The treatment protocol was to administer the herbs daily in decoction for 10 days per course of treatment, for 2-3 courses total. Of 39 patients, the study reported marked improvement in 14 patients, moderate improvement in 23 patients, and no benefit in 2 patients.[21]
11. **Infertility**: *Sheng Mai San* successfully treated infertility due to anovulation. The duration of treatment ranged from 1-6 months. Of 78 patients, the study reported pregnancy in 21 patients, normal ovulation in 17 patients, and no change in 40 patients.[22]
12. **Diabetes mellitus**: Twenty-one patients with diabetes were treated with 85.9% effectiveness using *Sheng Mai San* and *Liu Wei Di Huang Wan* (Six-Ingredient Pill with Rehmannia).[23]

TOXICOLOGY

In an acute toxicology study, no fatality or abnormal reactions were reported following intravenous injection at the dose of 0.4 g/20g. The LD_{50} was determined as 34.64 g/kg via injection.[24] In a chronic toxicology study, intravenous injection of the formula at 20 mL/kg/day for 15 days did not cause any abnormal reaction.[25]

SUGGESTED ACUPUNCTURE TREATMENT

1. Points: *Feishu* (BL 13), *Xinshu* (BL 15), *Shenshu* (BL 23), *Housanli* (ST 36), *Sanyinjiao* (SP 6), and *Yinxi* (HT 6).
2. Techniques: tonification and moxibustion.

Feishu (BL 13) nourishes Lung qi. *Xinshu* (BL 15) smoothes Heart qi flow and calms the *shen* (spirit). *Shenshu* (BL 23) nourishes Kidney and yin. *Housanli* (ST 36) and *Sanyinjiao* (SP 6) nourish qi and blood. *Yinxi* (HT 6) nourishes yin, calms the *shen*, and astringes the body to stop sweating.

AUTHORS' COMMENTS

Sheng Mai San consists of *Ren Shen* (Radix et Rhizoma Ginseng), *Mai Dong* (Radix Ophiopogonis), and *Wu Wei Zi* (Fructus Schisandrae Chinensis). It is a simple, yet powerful formula that can be combined with many other herbs or another formula to treat various disorders characterized by qi and yin deficiency. Its primary functions are to tonify qi, generate fluids, astringe yin, and generate the pulse. *Ren Shen* (Radix et Rhizoma Ginseng) is the essential ingredient in this formula because it is the most effective herb to warm the Heart, nourish *ying* (nutritive) level, and generate the pulse. *Ren Shen* (Radix et Rhizoma Ginseng) cannot be replaced with *Dang Shen* (Radix Codonopsis) as it can be in many other formulas, or this formula's clinical effectiveness will be significantly diminished.

In addition to the classic indication of qi and yin deficiencies, *Sheng Mai San* can be used to treat many other conditions:

- It can be used to tonify yin and qi following recovery from respiratory disease characterized by chronic coughing, such as pneumonia, frequent upper respiratory infections, chronic kennel cough, post-heartworm disease with cough due to pneumonitis, and can be combined with *Yu Ping Feng San* (Jade Windscreen Powder) to strengthen *wei* (defensive) *qi* to prevent recurrence of respiratory disease.
- *Sheng Mai San* may be used in horses with chronic cough from bronchitis or COPD. For bronchitis, it is often combined with *Bu Fei Tang* (Tonify the Lung Decoction), while COPD cases may benefit more from combination with *Ren Shen Ge Jie San* (Ginseng and Gecko Powder).
- This formula can be used to help dogs recover from hyperthermia or heat stroke. It is best given as a rectal suspension in obtunded dogs, and orally as a suspension in alert animals. It is important to give this formula as soon as possible for best results. Studies in rats indicate that this formula is best given every 3 hours to reduce the effects of heat stroke and prevent mortality.

Shēng Mài Săn (Generate the Pulse Powder)

- *Sheng Mai San* can be used in the treatment of cardiomyopathy and congestive heart failure in the dog and cat. It has been combined with conventional cardiac medications (diuretics, ACE-inhibitors, beta-blockers) without adverse effects. It can be combined with *Xue Fu Zhu Yu Tang* (Drive Out Stasis in the Mansion of Blood Decoction) to treat arrhythmia, promote normal circulation, and protect against the development of thromboembolism. Alternatively, it can be combined with *Dan Shen* (Radix et Rhizoma Salviae Miltiorrhizae).
- Research from China indicates that *Sheng Mai San* may have a protective effect on the myocardium from ischemic reperfusion injury. In dogs, gastric dilatation and volvulus (GDV) is an acute life threatening condition that is characterized by cardiogenic shock and hypoperfusion with consequent reperfusion injury Cardiac arrhythmias (typically ventricular) occur most frequently between 12 and 36 hours after the onset of GDV. Up to 50% of dogs with GDV develop these arrhythmias, with the highest mortality rate occurring during the first 7 days after surgery. Based on these findings, the use of *Sheng Mai San* to treat this condition should begin as soon as possible after diagnosis, and administration should be given every 6 hours thereafter for a minimum of one week.
- For dogs and horses with heart qi, yin and blood deficiencies, *Sheng Mai San* is frequently combined with *Zhi Gan Cao Tang* (Honey-Fried Licorice Decoction). The addition of *Huang Qi* (Radix Astragali) to these formulas helps tonify qi and prevent against infection, especially in older animals. It is interesting to note that *Sheng Mai San*, known as "Generate the Pulse Powder," and *Zhi Gan Cao Tang*, also known as *Fu Mai Tang* or "Pulse Reviving Decoction," have similar names and actions. *Zhi Gan Cao Tang*, however, contains herbs that strongly tonify the blood and fluids.
- For cancer patients undergoing chemotherapy with qi and yin deficiencies, *Sheng Mai San* can be combined with *Ba Zhen Tang* (Eight-Treasure Decoction). For animals that have non-healing wounds or poor wound healing after tumor removal, it can be combined with *Ren Shen Yang Ying Tang* (Ginseng Decoction to Nourish the Nutritive Qi).
- In China, this formula may also be given intravenously to treat cardio-pulmonary collapse and shock.

Sheng Mai San is also useful in treating many endocrine disorders:

- For diabetes mellitus in the dog or cat with qi and yin deficiencies, it can be combined with *Liu Wei Di Huang Wan* (Six-Ingredient Pill with Rehmannia) plus *Huang Qi* (Radix Astragali). For diabetic animals with excessive dryness, constipation and thirst, combine with *Zeng Ye Tang* (Increase the Fluids Decoction) and add additional herbs to tonify qi, enrich yin and engender fluids, such as *Huang Qi* (Radix Astragali), *Shu Di Huang* (Radix Rehmanniae Praeparata), *Tai Zi Shen* (Radix Pseudostellariae), *Huang Jing* (Rhizoma Polygonati), *Shan Yao* (Rhizoma Dioscoreae), and *Ge Gen* (Radix Puerariae Lobatae). In dogs with hyperadrenocorticism (Cushing's disease) and secondary heart failure, it can be given in combination with trilostane and/or lysodren without adverse effect.
- For dogs with hypoadrenocorticism (Addison's disease), combine with *Zhi Gan Cao Tang* (Honey-Fried Licorice Decoction). For cats with feline hyperthyroidism and secondary cardiomyopathy due to Heart and Kidney deficiencies, it can be combined with *Tian Wang Bu Xin Dan* (Emperor of Heaven's Special Pill to Tonify the Heart) to support and stabilize the animal prior to nuclear medicine therapy or surgery. These formulas can also be given to cats on oral antithyroid drugs (tapazole) without adverse effect.

References

1. *Zhong Yi Fang Ji Xian Dai Yan Jiu* (Modern Study of Medical Formulas in Traditional Chinese Medicine), 1997; 556-563.
2. Wang N, Minatoguchi S, Arai M, Uno Y, Nishida Y, Hashimoto K, Xue-Hai C, Fukuda K, Akao S, Takemura G, Fujiwara H. Sheng-Mai-San is protective against post-ischemic myocardial dysfunction in rats through its opening of the mitochondrial KATP channels. Circ J. 2002 Aug; 66(8):763-8.
3. Wang N, Minatoguchi S, Uno Y, Arai M, Hashimoto K, Hashimoto Y, Yamaguchi K, Fukuda K, Akao S, Fujiwara H. Treatment with sheng-mai-san reduces myocardial infarct size through activation of protein kinase C and opening of mitochondrial KATP channel. Am J Chin Med. 2001; 29(2):367-75.
4. Li PC, Poon KT, Ko KM. Schisandra chinensis-dependent myocardial protective action of sheng-mai-san in rats. Am J Chin Med. 1996; 24(3-4):255-62.
5. *Zhong Guo Bing Li Sheng Li Za Zhi* (Chinese Journal of Pathology and Biology), 1987; 3(1):38.
6. *Nei Meng Gu Zhong Yi Yao* (Traditional Chinese Medicine and Medicinals of Inner Mongolia), 1985; 4:35.
7. *Yao Xue Tong Bao* (Report of Herbology), 1984; 7:23.
8. *Zhe Jiang Zhong Yi Za Zhi* (Zhejiang Journal of Chinese Medicine), 1986; 21(9):400.
9. *Zhong Hua Xin Xue Guan Bing Za Zhi* (Chinese Journal of Cardiology), 1987; 3:144.
10. *Liao Ning Zhong Yi Za* Zhi (Liaoning Journal of Chinese Medicine), 1996; 10:451.
11. *Chang Chun Zhong Yi Xue Yuan Xue Bao* (Journal of Changchun University of Chinese Medicine), 1997; 2:13.
12. Lu BJ, Rong YZ, Zhao MH. Effect of sheng mai san on lipid peroxidation in acute myocardial infarction patients. Zhongguo Zhong Xi Yi Jie He Za Zhi. 1994 Dec; 14(12):712-4.
13. *Tian Jin Yi Xue Za Zhi* (Journal of Tianjin Medicine and Herbology), 1983; 1:43.
14. *Cheng Du Zhong Yi Xue Yuan Xue Bao* (Journal of Chengdu University of Traditional Chinese Medicine), 1981; 2:52.
15. *Shan Dong Zhong Yi Za Zhi* (Shandong Journal of Chinese Medicine), 1995; 5:207.
16. *Guang Zhou Zhong Yi Xue Yuan Xue Bao* (Journal of Guangzhou University of Chinese Medicine), 1984; 2:51.

Shēng Mài Sǎn (Generate the Pulse Powder)

17. *He Bei Zhong Yi* (Hebei Chinese Medicine), 1993; 2:11.
18. *Si Chuan Yi Xue* (Sichuan Medicine), 1981; 2:100.
19. *Nei Meng Gu Zhong Yi Yao* (Traditional Chinese Medicine and Medicinals of Inner Mongolia), 1985; 4:35.
20. *Zhong Hua Xin Xue Guan Bing Za Zhi* (Chinese Journal of Cardiology), 1980; 8(2):90.
21. *Tian Jin Zhong Yi* (Tianjin Chinese Medicine), 1996; 4:20.
22. *Zhong Yi Ming Fang Lin Chuang Xin Yong* (Contemporary Clinical Applications of Classic Chinese Formulas), 2001; 260-261.
23. *Si Chuan Yi Xue* (Sichuan Medicine), 1989; 7(12):20.
24. *Nei Meng Gu Zhong Yi Yao* (Traditional Chinese Medicine and Medicinals of Inner Mongolia), 1985; 4:35.
25. *Zhong Yao Yao Li Yu Lin Chuang* (Pharmacology and Clinical Applications of Chinese Herbs), 1987; 3(1):22.

Rén Shēn Gé Jiè Sǎn (Ginseng and Gecko Powder)

人參蛤蚧散

人参蛤蚧散

Pinyin Name: *Ren Shen Ge Jie San*
Literal Name: Ginseng and Gecko Powder
Alternate Name: Ginseng and Gecko Combination
Original Source: *Wei Sheng Bao Jian* (Precious Mirror of Health) by Luo Tian-Yi in the Yuan Dynasty

COMPOSITION

Ren Shen (Radix et Rhizoma Ginseng)	60g
Ge Jie (Gecko)	1 pair
Fu Ling (Poria)	60g
Sang Bai Pi (Cortex Mori)	60g
Ku Xing Ren (Semen Armeniacae Amarum), *chao* (dry-fried)	150g
Bei Mu (Bulbus Fritillariae)	60g
Zhi Mu (Rhizoma Anemarrhenae)	60g
Zhi Gan Cao (Radix et Rhizoma Glycyrrhizae Praeparata cum Melle)	150g

DOSAGE / PREPARATION / ADMINISTRATION

The source text instructs to grind the ingredients into a fine powder and store it in a porcelain container. Take the powdered formula with a small amount of water daily. Today, it is usually prepared as a powder. Take 6g with water on an empty stomach in the morning and evening.

Note: The source text specifies that *Ge Jie* (Gecko) should be processed first to remove its odor; this is done by soaking it in river water, and renewing the water daily, for five days. It is then fried until it turns yellow and crisp. Today, it is usually processed by washing and cleaning it with liquor. Then, bake it using mild heat until it turns dry and crisp, and then grind it into a fine powder.

CHINESE THERAPEUTIC ACTIONS

1. Tonifies qi and clears the Lung
2. Arrests cough and relieves wheezing

CLINICAL MANIFESTATIONS

Chronic consumptive Lung disease due to deficiency heat: chronic cough, wheezing, dyspnea, thick, yellow sputum with or without blood and pus, irritability, weight loss with or without facial edema, chronic lung atrophy, a red to purple tongue, and a superficial, weak, thin pulse.

VETERINARY CLINICAL APPLICATIONS

Chronic lung and respiratory disorders: chronic feline asthma, equine RAO, chronic bronchitis, emphysema, and chronic respiratory tract infection and chronic pneumonia.

Rén Shēn Gé Jiè Sǎn (Ginseng and Gecko Powder)

EXPLANATION

Ren Shen Ge Jie San (Ginseng and Gecko Powder) treats chronic consumptive Lung disease due to deficiency heat. This syndrome usually originates from chronic coughing, which may weaken the qi and lead to weight loss. The Lung controls the distribution of water throughout the body. When the Lung is deficient and cannot properly distribute water, water stagnates, and dampness and phlegm begin to accumulate. Damp and phlegm accumulation causes facial edema and coughing with sputum. Chronic coughing and heat may also damage the blood vessels, leading to bloody sputum. Damp and phlegm accumulation over time can create interior heat, which produces a red to purple tongue and gives rise to restlessness. A superficial, weak, thin pulse indicates severe Lung qi deficiency.

Ren Shen (Radix et Rhizoma Ginseng) tonifies *yuan* (source) *qi*, strengthens the Lung to improve respiration, and benefits the Spleen to eliminate dampness and phlegm. *Ge Jie* (Gecko), which enters the Lung and Kidney channels, tonifies the Lung to facilitate breathing, and aids the Kidney in grasping qi downward. Tonifying the Lung and Kidney is absolutely necessary in chronic coughing syndromes, which involve deficiency of both organs. *Fu Ling* (Poria) strengthens the Spleen, dispels dampness and phlegm, and relieves facial edema. *Sang Bai Pi* (Cortex Mori) and *Ku Xing Ren* (Semen Armeniacae Amarum) correct the reversed flow of Lung qi to stop coughing and wheezing. *Bei Mu* (Bulbus Fritillariae) clears Lung heat, dispels phlegm, and stops coughing. *Zhi Mu* (Rhizoma Anemarrhenae) clears Lung heat and nourishes the Kidney to assist in grasping the qi downward. *Zhi Gan Cao* (Radix et Rhizoma Glycyrrhizae Praeparata cum Melle) tonifies qi and harmonizes the herbs.

VETERINARY MODIFICATIONS

- With more phlegm accumulation, add *Lai Fu Zi* (Semen Raphani) and *Bai Jie Zi* (Semen Sinapis).
- With yin deficiency, add *Mai Dong* (Radix Ophiopogonis).
- With qi deficiency, add *Huang Qi* (Radix Astragali).
- With severe wheezing, coughing and dyspnea due to Lung and Kidney deficiencies, add *Dong Chong Xia Cao* (Cordyceps), *Wu Wei Zi* (Fructus Schisandrae Chinensis), *He Tao Ren* (Semen Juglandis), and *Bu Gu Zhi* (Fructus Psoraleae).
- With heat, add *Zhi Zi* (Fructus Gardeniae), *Lian Qiao* (Fructus Forsythiae), *Huang Qin* (Radix Scutellariae).
- With profuse bleeding with or without pus, add *Bai Mao Gen* (Rhizoma Imperatae), charred *Di Yu* (Radix Sanguisorbae) and charred *Ce Bai Ye* (Cacumen Platycladi).

CAUTIONS / CONTRAINDICATIONS

Ren Shen Ge Jie San is contraindicated in cases of cough and dyspnea caused by exterior conditions.

HUMAN CLINICAL STUDIES AND RESEARCH

Respiratory disorders: In one report, 30 geriatric patients with chronic respiratory disorders (asthma, chronic bronchitis, bronchial asthma) characterized by deficiency and cold were treated with modified *Ren Shen Ge Jie San* with good results. The modified formula contained *Ren Shen* (Radix et Rhizoma Ginseng) 20g, *San Qi* (Radix et Rhizoma Notoginseng) 20g, *Chuan Bei Mu* (Bulbus Fritillariae Cirrhosae) 30g, and *Ge Jie* (Gecko) 2 pieces. The formula was given as a fine powder, 1.5-2.0g per dose,

***Ren Shen Ge Jie San* (Ginseng and Gecko Powder)**

Diagnosis	Clinical Signs	Treatment	Herbs
Chronic consumptive Lung disease	• Chronic coughing with thick, yellow sputum: damp and phlegm accumulation affecting Lung qi circulation • Facial edema: Lung deficiency unable to distribute water evenly • Bloody sputum: chronic coughing and heat damaging the blood vessels • Superficial, weak, thin pulse: Lung qi deficiency	• Tonifies qi and clears the Lung • Arrests cough and relieves wheezing	• *Ren Shen* (Radix et Rhizoma Ginseng) strengthens the Lung and tonifies *yuan* (source) *qi*. • *Ge Jie* (Gecko) tonifies the Lung and Kidney to improve breathing. • *Fu Ling* (Poria) strengthens the Spleen. • *Sang Bai Pi* (Cortex Mori) and *Ku Xing Ren* (Semen Armeniacae Amarum) correct the reversed flow of Lung qi to stop coughing and wheezing. • *Bei Mu* (Bulbus Fritillariae) clears Lung heat, dispels phlegm, and stops coughing. • *Zhi Mu* (Rhizoma Anemarrhenae) clears Lung heat and nourishes the Kidney. • *Zhi Gan Cao* (Radix et Rhizoma Glycyrrhizae Praeparata cum Melle) tonifies qi and harmonizes the herbs.

8 TONIC FORMULAS

Rén Shēn Gé Jiè Sǎn (Ginseng and Gecko Powder)

two to three times daily. The study noted that the herbs effectively reduced or prevented asthma attacks in these patients.[1]

SUGGESTED ACUPUNCTURE TREATMENT

1. Points: *Feishu* (BL 13), *Pishu* (BL 20), *Housanli* (ST 36), *Taixi* (KI 3), *Taiyuan* (LU 9), *Fenglong* (ST 40), *Hegu* (LI 4), *Gaohuangshu* (BL 43), *Dingchuan*, *Qihaishu*, *Feimen*, and *Feipan*.
2. Technique: tonification.

Feishu (BL 13) tonifies Lung qi. *Pishu* (BL 20) and *Housanli* (ST 36) strengthen the Spleen, dissolve dampness, and harmonize the Stomach. *Taixi* (KI 3) is the source point for the Kidney and helps to anchor respiration. Combine *Taiyuan* (LU 9), the *yuan* (source) point of the Lung, with *Feishu* (BL 13) to tonify the Lung. *Fenglong* (ST 40) and *Hegu* (LI 4) dissolve dampness and phlegm, and harmonize the middle *jiao*. *Gaohuangshu* (BL 43) and *Dingchuan*, a classical point, are both essential points for treating chronic coughing and asthma. *Qihaishu*, *Feimen*, and *Feipan* are equine points that tonify the Lung and qi.

AUTHORS' COMMENTS

Ren Shen Ge Jie San is primarily used to treat *chronic* asthma or bronchitis caused by Lung and Kidney deficiencies, with phlegm-heat in the Lung. It is commonly used in horses, where heaves (RAO) cases seen by practitioners are often prolonged and stubborn in nature. This formula does not have a strong ability to clear heat; if heat is a prominent factor, other herbs or another formula should be added to address this problem.

For *acute* cases of asthma or relapse of chronic disease with heat, it is better to use *Ma Huang Xing Ren Gan Cao Shi Gao Tang* (Ephedra, Apricot Kernel, Licorice, and Gypsum Decoction). For acute asthma with cold, the formula *Xiao Qing Long Tang* (Minor Bluegreen Dragon Decoction) should be used. To treat chronic bronchial asthma due to Lung and Kidney deficiencies in cats, add *Dong Chong Xia Cao* (Cordyceps) to this formula. For chronic asthma with more Kidney qi and yang deficiencies, combine this formula with *Jin Gui Shen Qi Wan* (Kidney Qi Pill from the Golden Cabinet). Cats, as a species, are known to be difficult to medicate on a long-term basis. Unlike dogs, cats are also known to refuse food that has any type of medication mixed into it. This formula can be mixed in the cat's food for long-term control of asthma. Treatment should begin with a small dose and gradually increased over time. Even one time daily administration can produce beneficial effects in many of these cats. For animals with chronic bronchitis with qi and yin deficiencies and concurrent heart disease, it can be combined with *Sheng Mai San* (Generate the Pulse Powder). Many animals with chronic asthma and/or bronchitis have deficiencies of Lung, Kidney and Spleen. For animals with asthma and bronchitis with underlying Spleen deficiency and dampness, combine this formula with *Shen Ling Bai Zhu San* (Ginseng, Poria, and Atractylodes Macrocephala Powder) or *Er Chen Tang* (Two-Cured Decoction), depending on the case.

Ren Shen Ge Jie San and *Su Zi Jiang Qi Tang* (Perilla Fruit Decoction for Directing Qi Downward) have similar applications, and both are used to treat asthma and bronchitis caused by deficiency; both dispel phlegm to stop coughing.

- *Ren Shen Ge Jie San* is used for chronic asthma or bronchitis due to Lung and Kidney deficiencies and is used more in older animals and or those with persistent chronic disease.
- *Su Zi Jiang Qi Tang* is used to treat a mixed condition of excess and deficiency: excess above (phlegm in the Lung) and deficiency below (Kidney yang deficiency). It is commonly used as a transitional formula following an acute attack, and then tapered off and replaced with another formula that treats the root disorder. It can be used for a longer period time than other formulas to treat acute asthma, because it does not contain *Ma Huang* (Herba Ephedrae). It is used more often in younger animals.

References

1. *Jiang Su Zhong Yi* (Jiangsu Chinese Medicine), 1988; (3):25.

Bŭ Fèi Tāng (Tonify the Lung Decoction)

補肺湯
补肺汤

Pinyin Name: *Bu Fei Tang*
Literal Name: Tonify the Lung Decoction
Alternate Name: Ginseng and Aster Combination
Original Source: *Yong Lei Qian Fang* (Everlasting Categorization of Seal Formulas)

COMPOSITION

Huang Qi (Radix Astragali)	24g
Ren Shen (Radix et Rhizoma Ginseng)	9g
Sang Bai Pi (Cortex Mori)	12g
Zi Wan (Radix et Rhizoma Asteris)	9g
Wu Wei Zi (Fructus Schisandrae Chinensis)	6g
Shu Di Huang (Radix Rehmanniae Praeparata)	24g

DOSAGE / PREPARATION / ADMINISTRATION

Prepare this formula as a decoction.

CHINESE THERAPEUTIC ACTIONS

1. Tonifies Lung qi
2. Strengthens *wei* (defensive) *qi*

CLINICAL MANIFESTATIONS

Lung qi deficiency: cough, dyspnea, wheezing, exercise intolerance, fatigue, low energy, a weak voice, intolerance to cold, a pale tongue, and a deep, weak pulse.

VETERINARY CLINICAL APPLICATIONS

Chronic cough, asthma, and frequent respiratory infections.

EXPLANATION

Bu Fei Tang (Tonify the Lung Decoction) treats Lung qi deficiency characterized by wheezing, dyspnea, exercise intolerance, and fatigue. Animals with weak Lung qi are unable to control rhythmic respiration, and thus they have clinical signs such as wheezing, dyspnea, shortness of breath, and a weak voice. Wheezing and dyspnea may be due in part to Kidney deficiency, and its subsequent inability to grasp the qi. Deficient Lung qi is often accompanied by deficient *wei* (defensive) *qi*, which results in the body's inability to protect its exterior level. *Wei* (defensive) *qi* deficiency enables exterior cold factor to easily penetrate and constrict the Lung, causing cough, wheezing, dyspnea, and frequent infections. A pale tongue and a deep, weak pulse are indicative of qi deficiency.

Huang Qi (Radix Astragali) and *Ren Shen* (Radix et Rhizoma Ginseng) address the root of the illness by tonifying qi and strengthening *wei* (defensive) *qi*. *Sang Bai Pi* (Cortex Mori) guides Lung qi downward to relieve wheezing and dyspnea. *Zi Wan* (Radix et Rhizoma Asteris) moistens the Lung to relieve cough. *Wu Wei Zi* (Fructus Schisandrae Chinensis) astringes Lung qi and stops spontaneous

***Bu Fei Tang* (Tonify the Lung Decoction)**

Diagnosis	Clinical Signs	Treatment	Herbs
Lung qi deficiency	• Wheezing, dyspnea, fatigue, exercise intolerance, shortness of breath, and a weak voice: Lung qi deficiency • Intolerance to cold and frequent infections: *wei* (defensive) *qi* deficiency • Pale tongue and a weak, deep pulse: qi deficiency	• Tonifies Lung qi • Strengthens *wei* (defensive) *qi*	• *Huang Qi* (Radix Astragali) and *Ren Shen* (Radix et Rhizoma Ginseng) tonify qi and strengthen *wei* (defensive) *qi*. • *Sang Bai Pi* (Cortex Mori) guides Lung qi downward to relieve wheezing and dyspnea. • *Zi Wan* (Radix et Rhizoma Asteris) moistens the Lung to relieve cough. • *Wu Wei Zi* (Fructus Schisandrae Chinensis) constricts Lung qi and stops spontaneous perspiration. • *Shu Di Huang* (Radix Rehmanniae Praeparata) tonifies the Kidney and enhances its function to grasp the qi downward.

Bŭ Fèi Tāng (Tonify the Lung Decoction)

sweating. *Wu Wei Zi* (Fructus Schisandrae Chinensis) and *Shu Di Huang* (Radix Rehmanniae Praeparata) tonify the Kidney and enhance its function of grasping qi downward.

VETERINARY MODIFICATIONS

- With more phlegm, add *Jie Geng* (Radix Platycodonis).
- With more coughing, add *Zi Su Zi* (Fructus Perillae).
- With coughing and clear phlegm, combine with *Ning Sou Wan* (Quiet the Cough Pill).
- If there is severe qi deficiency, combine with *Si Jun Zi Tang* (Four-Gentlemen Decoction).
- With Kidney deficiency, combine with *Ren Shen Ge Jie San* (Ginseng and Gecko Powder).

CAUTIONS / CONTRAINDICATIONS

Avoid raw, uncooked, and cold types of foods while taking *Bu Fei Tang*.

SUGGESTED ACUPUNCTURE TREATMENT

1. Points: *Guanyuan* (CV 4), *Feishu* (BL 13), *Lieque* (LU 7), *Chize* (LU 5), *Taiyuan* (LU 9), *Shenshu* (BL 23), *Dingchuan*, *Qihaishu*, *Feimen*, and *Feipan*.
2. Technique: tonification and moxibustion.

Apply moxibustion on *Guanyuan* (CV 4) and *Feishu* (BL 13) to tonify qi and strengthen the *wei* (defensive) level. Tonify *Lieque* (LU 7), *Chize* (LU 5), and *Taiyuan* (LU 9) to tonify Lung qi and relieve wheezing. *Shenshu* (BL 23) strengthens the Kidney. *Dingchuan* is a classical point used to stop asthma and dyspnea. *Qihaishu*, *Feimen*, and *Feipan* are equine points that tonify the Lung and qi.

AUTHORS' COMMENTS

Bu Fei Tang, a modification of *Sheng Mai San* (Generate the Pulse Powder), is used to tonify the Lung in older animals, or in younger animals with chronic cough. These animals may often get frequent infections or recurrent respiratory disease, and their deficiency often is caused by overwork. The coughing in these cases is due to Lung deficiency and the inability of the Kidney to grasp and hold down the qi. The coughing may be dry in nature, or productive with clear phlegm. The phlegm is the result of the inability of the Lung to regulate water and send it down to the Kidney; on the other hand, a dry cough can arise because the Kidney is too weak to steam water upwards to moisten the Lung. It is common for animals that display this pattern to have underlying Spleen qi deficiency, which complicates the situation and contributes to the accumulation of phlegm in the Lung and inadequate production of food essence to nourish the Kidney. Other animals may have significant yin deficiency in addition to qi deficiency. In these cases, *Bu Fei Tang* can be combined with *Bai He Gu Jin Tang* (Lily Bulb Decoction to Preserve the Metal). After the clinical signs have resolved, *Bai He Gu Jin Tang* should be stopped or modified, or another formula given, to address the root cause of the condition. *Bu Fei Tang* may be used alone in mild cases of equine RAO, but is more often used as an adjunctive formula to *Ren Shen Ge Jie San* (Ginseng and Gecko Powder).

Section 2

补血剂
— Blood-Tonifying Formulas

Sì Wù Tāng (Four-Substance Decoction)
四物湯
四物汤

Pinyin Name: *Si Wu Tang*
Literal Name: Four-Substance Decoction
Alternate Names: *Szu Wu Tang*, Four Component Decoction, Four Herbs Decoction, Tangkuei Four Combination
Original Source: *Tai Ping Hui Min He Ji Ju Fang* (Imperial Grace Formulary of the Tai Ping Era) by the Imperial Medical Department in 1078-85

COMPOSITION

Shu Di Huang (Radix Rehmanniae Praeparata), *zheng* (steamed) with liquor	[12g]
Dang Gui (Radix Angelicae Sinensis), *jin* (soaked) and *chao* (dry-fried) with liquor	[9-12g]
Bai Shao (Radix Paeoniae Alba)	[9-12g]
Chuan Xiong (Rhizoma Chuanxiong)	[6-9g]

DOSAGE / PREPARATION / ADMINISTRATION

The source text states to coarsely grind equal amounts of the ingredients. Cook 9g of the powder in 1.5 large bowls of water and reduce it to 80%. Take the warm, strained decoction on an empty stomach. Today, it is usually prepared as a decoction with the doses suggested in brackets. Take the decoction in three equally divided doses three times daily (morning, noon and evening).

CHINESE THERAPEUTIC ACTIONS

1. Nourishes the blood
2. Regulates blood circulation

CLINICAL MANIFESTATIONS

1. General blood deficiency: pale mucous membranes, poor vision, red, dry eyes, chronic itching, dryness, dandruff and thin, dry, brittle hair coat, cracked hooves or paw pads, irritability, restlessness, insomnia, hyperactivity, inability to follow commands, a pale, dry tongue with a white tongue coating, and a thready, weak pulse.
2. Gestational and postpartum disorders: unstable fetus with bleeding, postpartum uterine bleeding with lower abdominal pain, chills and fever.

VETERINARY CLINICAL APPLICATIONS

Anemia, postpartum anemia, threatened abortion, infertility, insomnia, chronic nephritis, chronic itching and dermatitis, atopic dermatitis and urticaria.

EXPLANATION

Blood deficiency usually manifests in such signs as pale mucous membranes, a pale, dry tongue with a white tongue coating, and a thready, weak pulse. Other common clinical signs include pruritis, dryness, dandruff, thin, brittle hair coat, cracked hooves and paw pads; these signs are the result of the inability of the blood to nourish the skin and hair coat. The Liver stores blood; thus, insufficient blood in the Liver causes lack of nourishment in the upper body, leading to poor vision, red, dry eyes, and tinnitus. The Heart dominates the blood, and deficiency of blood leads to lack of nourishment to the *shen* (spirit), causing irritability, restlessness, hyperactivity, inability to follow commands, palpitations, and insomnia.

Si Wu Tang (Four-Substance Decoction) is indicated for deficiency or injury of the *chong* (thoroughfare) and *ren* (conception) channels with blood deficiency. The *chong* (thoroughfare) and *ren* (conception) channels are closely

Sì Wù Tāng (Four-Substance Decoction)

***Si Wu Tang* (Four-Substance Decoction)**

Diagnosis	Clinical Signs	Treatment	Herbs
Blood deficiency	• Pruritis, dryness, dandruff, thin, brittle hair coat, cracked hooves and paw pads, blurry vision, pale mucous membranes, a pale, dry tongue with a white tongue coating, and a thready, weak pulse: blood deficiency • Irritability, restlessness, hyperactivity, inability to follow commands, and insomnia: blood deficiency unable to nourish the Heart	• Nourishes the blood • Regulates blood circulation	• *Shu Di Huang* (Radix Rehmanniae Praeparata) tonifies yin and promotes blood production. • *Dang Gui* (Radix Angelicae Sinensis) tonifies the blood, activates blood circulation, and regulates the menses. • *Bai Shao* (Radix Paeoniae Alba) nourishes the blood, consolidates yin, and harmonizes the blood. • *Chuan Xiong* (Rhizoma Chuanxiong) activates and regulates blood circulation.

related to the blood and uterus, and deficiency of these two channels may result in lack of nourishment to the fetus, causing it to become unstable.

All of the herbs in this formula enter the *xue* (blood) level. *Shu Di Huang* (Radix Rehmanniae Praeparata), the chief herb, tonifies the blood. It also tonifies the Kidney, which generates the marrow necessary for increased blood production. When tonifying blood, it is essential to also move the blood to prevent stagnation. *Dang Gui* (Radix Angelicae Sinensis) tonifies the blood, activates blood circulation, and nourishes the Liver. *Bai Shao* (Radix Paeoniae Alba) nourishes the blood and consolidates yin. It harmonizes the blood in the *ying* (nutritive) level. *Chuan Xiong* (Rhizoma Chuanxiong) activates and regulates blood circulation, and prevents the tonic herbs from causing stagnation in the body.

VETERINARY MODIFICATIONS

- With qi deficiency, add *Ren Shen* (Radix et Rhizoma Ginseng) and *Huang Qi* (Radix Astragali).
- With severe qi deficiency, combine with *Si Jun Zi Tang* (Four-Gentlemen Decoction).
- With qi stagnation, add *Zhi Shi* (Fructus Aurantii Immaturus), *Hou Po* (Cortex Magnoliae Officinalis), *Xiang Fu* (Rhizoma Cyperi), and *Yu Jin* (Radix Curcumae).
- With fever from blood deficiency, add *Mu Dan Pi* (Cortex Moutan) and *Di Gu Pi* (Cortex Lycii).
- With wind and dry, pruritic, skin, add *Jing Jie* (Herba Schizonepetae), *Fang Feng* (Radix Saposhnikoviae) and *Dan Shen* (Radix et Rhizoma Salviae Miltiorrhizae).

CAUTIONS / CONTRAINDICATIONS

- *Si Wu Tang* should be used with caution in animals with deficiency of the Spleen and Stomach, because the rich, cloying, stagnating nature of *Shu Di Huang* (Radix Rehmanniae Praeparata) could affect digestion. Spleen tonics are often used concurrently when administering this formula; it should be avoided in animals with dampness or qi deficiency without modification.
- Although this formula treats blood deficiency, it is not suitable for animals that suffer from blood or qi collapse from hemorrhaging or acute blood loss. It should also be used with caution in cases of yin deficiency with heat, or those with middle *jiao* deficiency manifesting in diarrhea.
- This formula should be used with caution during pregnancy and at low doses in puppies and kittens and other juvenile animals.

PHARMACOLOGICAL EFFECTS

1. **Hematopoietic**: *Si Wu Tang*, *Si Jun Zi Tang* (Four-Gentlemen Decoction), and *Shi Quan Da Bu Tang* (All-Inclusive Great Tonifying Decoction), were given orally to mice to evaluate their effect for treatment of anemia. The study concluded that *Shi Quan Da Bu Tang* (All-Inclusive Great Tonifying Decoction) was most effective, followed by *Si Wu Tang*, and *Si Jun Zi Tang* (Four-Gentlemen Decoction).[1] The mechanism of action was attributed to increased activity of CSF.[2]
2. **Antiplatelet**: Administration of *Si Wu Tang* in mice was associated with a preventative effect on the formation of blood clots. The mechanism of action was attributed to its antiplatelet effect.[3,4]
3. **Radioprotective**: Administration of *Si Wu Tang* 5-120 minutes prior to exposure to X-ray was beneficial in minimizing the related side effects. Administration of the herbs afterwards, however, was not associated with any benefit. The protective effect of the herbs against radiation was attributed to its regulating effect on the immune system.[5] Another study reported significant protective effect against high and low dose of gamma-irradiation. Protective effects included reduced frequency of radiation-induced apoptosis ($p < 0.05$) and increased formation of endogenous spleen colonies ($p < 0.05$).[6]

Sì Wù Tāng (Four-Substance Decoction)

4. **Cognitive**: Administration of *Si Wu Tang* was associated with a dose dependant effect to improve memory and cognitive functions in rats. The dose given ranged from 0.5 to 1.0 g/kg of the dried herbs.[7]
5. **Antioxidant**: One study reports *Si Wu Tang* to have marked antioxidant and antiaging effects.[8]
6. **Cardiovascular**: According to one study on 7 healthy adult males (age, 22.3 +/- 1.8 years old), administration of *Si Wu Tang* induced an increase of diastolic blood pressure and mean blood pressure.[9]
7. **Antipruritic and anti-inflammatory**: One study reported *Si Wu Tang* to have marked antipruritic and anti-inflammatory effects for treatment of cutaneous pruritus, chronic inflammation, and other diseases. The mechanism of action was attributed to the inhibition of histamine release from mast cells in a concentration-dependent fashion.[10]
8. **Antitumor**: Administration of *Shi Quan Da Bu Tang* (All-Inclusive Great Tonifying Decoction) was associated with a preventive effect on endometrial carcinogenesis in mice. The antitumor effects of *Shi Quan Da Bu Tang* (All-Inclusive Great Tonifying Decoction) was attributed in part to the contents of *Si Wu Tang*, as the administration of these four herbs was found to have an inhibitory effect on estrogen-induced expression of c-fos, interleukin (IL)-1alpha and tumor necrosis factor (TNF)-alpha in uteri of ovariectomized mice.[11]

HUMAN CLINICAL STUDIES AND RESEARCH

1. **Infertility**: Use of modified *Si Wu Tang* was associated with good results to treat infertility. In addition to the base formula, *Zi Shi Ying* (Fluoritum), *Xian Mao* (Rhizoma Curculiginis), *Yin Yang Huo* (Herba Epimedii), *Tu Si Zi* (Semen Cuscutae), and *Fu Pen Zi* (Fructus Rubi) were added for Kidney yang deficiency; and *Nu Zhen Zi* (Fructus Ligustri Lucidi), *Mo Han Lian* (Herba Ecliptae), *Gou Qi Zi* (Fructus Lycii), *Wu Wei Zi* (Fructus Schisandrae Chinensis), *Xuan Shen* (Radix Scrophulariae), and *Mai Dong* (Radix Ophiopogonis) were added for Kidney yin deficiency. Each menstrual cycle was considered as one course of treatment (20 +/- 2 days). Herbs were not given during the period or if pregnancy was achieved. Successful pregnancy was reported once in 19 of 27 women. The average duration of treatment was 45 packs of herbs.[12]
2. **Insomnia**: Ten patients with insomnia were treated with herbs resulting in complete recovery in 6 patients (6-7 hours of sleep), moderate improvement in 3 patients (5-6 hours of sleep), and slight improvement in 1 patient. The herbal treatment combined *Si Wu Tang* with other herbs that invigorate blood circulation. The duration of treatment was one month or less.[13]
3. **Chronic nephritis**: It has been reported that patients with chronic nephritis characterized by proteinuria and hematuria responded well to the combination of *Si Wu Tang* and *Wu Ling San* (Five-Ingredient Powder with Poria). In a case report, two patients were successfully treated with herbs without recurrence for 5-7 years.[14]
4. **Headache due to trauma**: One study reported 96.2% effectiveness in treating 80 patients with headache due to trauma with an herbal formula that contained *Si Wu Tang*, *Huang Qi Gui Zhi Wu Wu Tang* (Astragalus and Cinnamon Twig Five-Substance Decoction), and others. Modifications included addition of *Xi Xin* (Radix et Rhizoma Asari) for severe pain; *Dang Shen* (Radix Codonopsis) for qi deficiency; *Bei Sha Shen* (Radix Glehniae) for yin deficiency; *Yin Yang Huo* (Herba Epimedii) for yang deficiency; and dry-fried *Shan Zha* (Fructus Crataegi) and *Ji Nei Jin* (Endothelium Corneum Gigeriae Galli) for poor appetite. Out of 80 patients, the study reported complete recovery in 48 patients, improvement in 29 patients, and no benefit in 3 patients.[15]
5. **Itching**: One study of 134 patients with skin itching reported 91.8% effectiveness when treated with *Si Wu Tang* plus *He Shou Wu* (Radix Polygoni Multiflori), *Wu Shao She* (Zaocys), and *Ji Li* (Fructus Tribuli).[16]
6. **Psoriasis**: One study consisting of 10 psoriasis patients reported successful results using as treatment *Si Wu Tang*, *Wu Shao She* (Zaocys), *Tu Bie Chong* (Eupolyphaga seu Steleophaga), *Qiang Huo* (Rhizoma et Radix Notopterygii), and others as needed.[17] According to another study, 13 patients with psoriasis were treated with complete recovery in 8 patients, improvement in 2 patients, and no benefit in 3 patients. The herbal formula included *Si Wu Tang* plus *Bai Xian Pi* (Cortex Dictamni), *Ku Shen* (Radix Sophorae Flavescentis), and *Da Zao* (Fructus Jujubae).[18]
7. **Urticaria**: Administration of a modified *Si Wu Tang* formula was found to be effective in treating both acute and chronic urticaria. The herbal formula contained *Si Wu Tang* plus *Chan Tui* (Periostracum Cicadae), *Gan Cao* (Radix et Rhizoma Glycyrrhizae), *Jiang Can* (Bombyx Batryticatus), and *Wu Shao She* (Zaocys). The treatment protocol was to administer the herbs in decoction, for 7-10 packs of herbs per course of treatment. Of 185 patients, the study reported complete recovery in 161 patients, improvement in 20 patients, and no benefit in 4 patients. Among 161 patients who had complete recovery, only 4 had recurrence within 1 year of follow-up.[19]
8. **Allergic rhinitis**: Forty-two patients with allergic rhinitis were treated with modified *Si Wu Tang* with good results. The herbs used included *Si Wu Tang* with additions such as *Cang Er Zi* (Fructus Xanthii), *Xin Yi Hua* (Flos Magnoliae), and *Xu Chang Qing* (Radix et Rhizoma Cynanchi Paniculati). *Ju Hua* (Flos Chrysanthemi) and *Bai Zhi* (Radix Angelicae Dahuricae) were added for headache; and *Yu Ping Feng San* (Jade Windscreen Powder) was

Sì Wù Tāng (Four-Substance Decoction)

added for *wei* (defensive) *qi* deficiency. The treatment protocol was to administer the herbs in decoction for 15 days per course of treatment, for a total of 2-4 courses. Out of 42 patients, the study reported complete recovery in 23 patients, marked improvement in 13 patients, and no benefit in 6 patients. The overall rate of effectiveness was 87.5%.[20]

HERB-DRUG INTERACTION

- **Penicillin-induced dermatitis**: Ten patients with dermatitis caused by penicillin were treated with herbs with complete recovery in 7 patients and improvement in 3 patients. The study also noted that the time required for recovery and improvement were shorter when treated with herbs in comparison with no treatment. The herbs used included *Si Wu Tang*, *Xie Bai San* (Drain the White Powder), and others as deemed necessary.[22]
- **Scopolamine-induced spatial cognitive deficits**: Administration of *Si Wu Tang* has a dose-dependent effect to reverse scopolamine-induced impairments in radial maze performance in mice.[23]

TOXICOLOGY

In acute toxicology studies in mice, oral administration of water or methyl alcohol extract of *Si Wu Tang* at 2 g/kg did not cause any fatality. No fatality was associated with intraperitoneal injection at 2 g/kg for the methyl alcohol extract, or 0.5 g/kg for the water extract. However, 60% fatality was reported with intraperitoneal injection at 1 g/kg for the water extract. The study concluded that the water extract of this formula is slightly more toxic than the alcohol extract.[24]

SUGGESTED ACUPUNCTURE TREATMENT

1. Points: *Pishu* (BL 20), *Weishu* (BL 21), *Housanli* (ST 36), *Xinshu* (BL 15), *Geshu* (BL 17), and *Sanyinjiao* (SP 6).
2. Technique: tonification.

Pishu (BL 20), *Weishu* (BL 21), and *Housanli* (ST 36) strengthen the Spleen and Stomach to increase blood production. *Xinshu* (BL 15) nourishes Heart blood. *Geshu* (BL 17) tonifies the blood. *Sanyinjiao* (SP 6) nourishes the Kidney, Spleen, and Liver.

AUTHORS' COMMENTS

The ancient tradition observes the four seasons as a natural cycle of genesis (spring), growth (summer), harvest (autumn) and storing (winter), respectively. Similarly, *Si Wu Tang* is formulated following the same principles. *Dang Gui* (Radix Angelicae Sinensis), sweet, warm and nourishing, represents genesis of blood like the spring sun. *Chuan Xiong* (Rhizoma Chuanxiong), acrid, warm and dispersing, corresponds to the growth and prospering energy of summer. *Bai Shao* (Radix Paeoniae Alba), sour and astringent, represents harvest in the autumn. Lastly, *Shu Di Huang* (Radix Rehmanniae Praeparata), rich and tonifying, implies storage of blood in winter. These four substances balance each other, similar to the way that the four seasons are balanced in nature.

Si Wu Tang is considered to be the representative formula for tonifying the blood. Although the source text states to use equal amounts of all four ingredients, the dose and use of each herb may be modified, depending on the condition of the individual patient. General guidelines for modifications are as follows:

- In patients with blood stagnation, *Bai Shao* (Radix Paeoniae Alba) should be replaced with *Chi Shao* (Radix Paeoniae Rubra).
- In patients with heat, *Shu Di Huang* (Radix Rehmanniae Praeparata) should be replaced with *Di Huang* (Radix Rehmanniae).
- In patients in whom *Shu Di Huang* (Radix Rehmanniae Praeparata) is not used because of its cloying nature, the dose of *Bai Shao* (Radix Paeoniae Alba) should be higher than that of *Dang Gui* (Radix Angelicae Sinensis). This is the general principle in balancing tonics: adjust the individual dose of the herbs to balance the herbal temperature so that the formula is not too warm or too cold.

Si Wu Tang is not typically used as a solitary formula in veterinary medicine; instead, it is combined with other herbs or formulas that use *Si Wu Tang* as a base from which to build a formula that is specific to the patient. It is commonly used to treat Liver blood deficiency, causing dry skin with dandruff, thin, brittle dry hair coat, and cracked and dry paw pads or hooves. Because of its relatively mild nature, it can be used in performance animals to promote a lustrous coat, and to aid in the re-growth of hair in bitches after they "blow coat" in estrus. It can also be used in the treatment of infertility caused by blood deficiency.

References

1. *Shan Xi Zhong Yi Xue Yuan Xue Bao* (Journal of Shanxi University School of Chinese Medicine), 1986; 2:40.
2. *Zhong Yao Yao Li Yu Lin Chuang* (Pharmacology and Clinical Applications of Chinese Herbs), 1992; 152.
3. *Zhong Cheng Yao* (Study of Chinese Patent Medicine), 1993; 15(1):44.
4. *Zhong Xi Yi Jie He Za Zhi* (Journal of Integrated Chinese and Western Medicine), 1981; 7(2):100.
5. *Zhong Yi Fang Ji Xian Dai Yan Jiu* (Modern Study of Medical Formulas in Traditional Chinese Medicine), 1997; 594.
6. Lee SE, Oh H, Yang JA, Jo SK, Byun MW, Yee ST, Kim SH. Radioprotective effects of two traditional Chinese medicine prescriptions: si-wu-tang and si-jun-zi-tang. Am J Chin Med. 1999; 27(3-4):387-96.

Sì Wù Tāng (Four-Substance Decoction)

7. *Guo Wai Yi Xue Zhong Yi Zhong Yao Fen Ce* (Monograph of Chinese Herbology from Foreign Medicine), 1992; 14(4):54.
8. *Liao Ning Zhong Yi Za Zhi* (Liaoning Journal of Chinese Medicine), 1992; 8:45.
9. Xu FH, Uebaba K. Effect of Kampo formulations (traditional Chinese medicine) on circulatory parameters. Acupuncture & Electro-Therapeutics Research. 1999; 24(1):11-28.
10. Dai Y, But PP, Chan YP, Matsuda H, Kubo M. Antipruritic and antiinflammatory effects of aqueous extract from Si-Wu-Tang. Biol Pharm Bull. 2002 Sep; 25(9):1175-8.
11. Tagami K, Niwa K, Lian Z, Gao J, Mori H, Tamaya T. Preventive effect of Juzen-taiho-to on endometrial carcinogenesis in mice is based on Shimotsu-to constituent. Biol Pharm Bull. 2004 Feb; 27(2):156-61.
12. *Zhong Yi Za Zhi* (Journal of Chinese Medicine), 1986; 10:35.
13. *Zhe Jiang Zhong Yi Za Zhi* (Zhejiang Journal of Chinese Medicine), 1988; 2:70.
14. *Hu Bei Zhong Yi Za Zhi* (Hubei Journal of Chinese Medicine), 1982; 4:32.
15. *Zhe Jiang Zhong Yi Xue Yuan Xue Bao* (Journal of Zhejiang University of Chinese Medicine), 1997; 3:41.
16. *Zhong Yi Za Zhi* (Journal of Chinese Medicine), 1988; 8:608.
17. *Zhe Jiang Zhong Yi Za Zhi* (Zhejiang Journal of Chinese Medicine), 1963; 2:29.
18. *Yun Nan Zhong Yi Za Zhi* (Yunan Journal of Chinese Medicine), 1985; 6:25.
19. *Zhong Xi Yi Jie He Za Zhi* (Journal of Integrated Chinese and Western Medicine), 1991; 4:242.
20. *Hei Long Jiang Zhong Yi Yao* (Heilongjiang Chinese Medicine and Herbology), 1991; 5:33.
21. *Nei Meng Gu Zhong Yi Yao* (Traditional Chinese Medicine and Medicinals of Inner Mongolia), 1993; (3):1.
22. Watanabe H, Ni JW, Ohta H, Ni XH, Matsumoto K. A kampo prescription, shimotsu-to, improves scopolamine-induced spatial cognitive deficits in rats. Yakubutsu Seishin Kodo. 1991 Jun; 11(3):215-22.
23. *Guo Wai Yi Xue Zhong Yi Zhong Yao Fen Ce* (Monograph of Chinese Herbology from Foreign Medicine), 1984; 5:305.

Táo Hóng Sì Wù Tāng

(Four-Substance Decoction with Safflower and Peach Pit)

桃紅四物湯
桃红四物汤

Pinyin Name: *Tao Hong Si Wu Tang*
Literal Name: Four-Substance Decoction with Safflower and Peach Pit
Alternate Names: *Tao Hung Szu Wu Tang*, Persica, Carthamus and Tang-kuei Decoction; Peach Kernel and Safflower plus Four Herbs; Tangkuei Four and Persica Carthamus Combination
Original Source: *Yi Zong Jin Jian* (Golden Mirror of the Medical Tradition) by Wu Qian in 1742

COMPOSITION

Shu Di Huang (Radix Rehmanniae Praeparata)	6g [15g]
Dang Gui (Radix Angelicae Sinensis)	6g [12g]
Bai Shao (Radix Paeoniae Alba), *chao* (dry-fried)	6g [10g]
Chuan Xiong (Rhizoma Chuanxiong)	3g [8g]
Tao Ren (Semen Persicae)	6g [6g]
Hong Hua (Flos Carthami)	3g [4g]

DOSAGE / PREPARATION / ADMINISTRATION

Prepare this formula as a decoction, and take three times a day, making sure to finish within one day. Today, the decoction may be prepared using the doses suggested in brackets.

CHINESE THERAPEUTIC ACTIONS

1. Nourishes the blood
2. Regulates blood circulation
3. Eliminates blood stasis

Táo Hóng Sì Wù Tāng

(Four-Substance Decoction with Safflower and Peach Pit)

CLINICAL MANIFESTATIONS

Blood deficiency with blood stagnation: irregular estrus cycle, back pain, a pale purple tongue, and a weak, wiry to choppy pulse.

VETERINARY CLINICAL APPLICATIONS

Infertility, irregular estrus cycles in breeding animals, lumbar pain occurring at estrus, diabetic neuropathy, non-healing bone fractures, progressive retinal atrophy, chronic superficial keratitis (CSK), non-healing corneal ulcer, optic neuritis, cataract, glaucoma, urticaria, itching, atopic dermatitis and seborrhea.

EXPLANATION

Tao Hong Si Wu Tang (Four-Substance Decoction with Safflower and Peach Pit) contains *Si Wu Tang* (Four-Substance Decoction) plus *Tao Ren* (Semen Persicae) and *Hong Hua* (Flos Carthami). The inclusion of these two herbs enables this formula to dispel blood stagnation in addition to tonifying the blood and regulating blood circulation. Historically, it has been used in human medicine for female patients who have early menstruation with excessive bleeding that is thick, sticky, and purplish in color, or bleeding with blood clots, and abdominal fullness and pain. Today, its clinical application has been extended to include many disorders characterized by both blood deficiency and blood stagnation.

VETERINARY MODIFICATIONS

- If there are more signs of stagnation and heat, add *Mu Dan Pi* (Cortex Moutan) and *Zhi Zi* (Fructus Gardeniae).
- With severe blood stasis, add *San Leng* (Rhizoma Sparganii) and *E Zhu* (Rhizoma Curcumae).
- For cerebrovascular accidents and complications, add *Huang Qi* (Radix Astragali), *Di Long* (Pheretima), *Niu Xi* (Radix Achyranthis Bidentatae), and *Gou Teng* (Ramulus Uncariae cum Uncis).
- For irregular estrous cycles, add *Yi Mu Cao* (Herba Leonuri), *Ze Lan* (Herba Lycopi), and *Zhi Gan Cao* (Radix et Rhizoma Glycyrrhizae Praeparata cum Melle).
- For atopic dermatitis, add *Huang Qi* (Radix Astragali), *Fang Feng* (Radix Saposhnikoviae), *Bai Xian Pi* (Cortex Dictamni), *Chan Tui* (Periostracum Cicadae), and *Ku Shen* (Radix Sophorae Flavescentis).
- For sore aching joints or injuries to tendons and ligaments, add *Ji Xue Teng* (Caulis Spatholobi) and *Niu Xi* (Radix Achyranthis Bidentatae).
- With abdominal pain from Liver cancer, add *Xiang Fu* (Rhizoma Cyperi) and *Yan Hu Suo* (Rhizoma Corydalis).

CAUTIONS / CONTRAINDICATIONS

- *Tao Hong Si Wu Tang* should be used with caution in animals with digestive weakness; it contains herbs that are rich and cloying. A Spleen tonic should be used as needed.
- This formula should also be used with caution in anemic animals with coldness, since this formula is cool by nature.
- Since this formula has strong actions to regulate blood circulation and eliminate blood stasis, it should be discontinued once the desired effects are achieved.
- This formula is contraindicated during pregnancy.
- This formula should be used with caution in animals with underlying qi and blood deficiencies.[1]
- *Tao Hong Si Wu Tang* is an ideal formula to tonify the blood, regulate blood circulation, and remove blood stagnation. It should be kept in mind, however, that because it moves the blood, it could cause excessive bleeding in some animals if used immediately prior to a surgical procedure. It is recommended to discontinue this formula at least 5 days prior to any surgical procedure.

PHARMACOLOGICAL EFFECTS

1. **Cardiovascular**: In an *in vitro* study, use of *Tao Hong Si Wu Tang* was shown to dilate the coronary artery and increase blood perfusion to cardiac muscles.[2]
2. **Antihyperlipidemic**: Administration of *Tao Hong Si Wu Tang* at 16 g/kg in rats was shown to decrease both total cholesterol and triglyceride levels.[3]
3. **Anti-inflammatory**: According to an *in vitro* study, oral administration of *Tao Hong Si Wu Tang* in rats at 8 g/kg and 16 g/kg was associated with marked anti-inflammatory effects similar to hydrocortisone 50 mg/kg. The study noted that the mechanisms of action of the herbs and the drug are very different. *Tao Hong Si Wu Tang* does not

***Tao Hong Si Wu Tang* (Four-Substance Decoction with Safflower and Peach Pit)**

Diagnosis	Clinical Signs	Treatment	Herbs
Blood deficiency with blood stagnation	Pale purple tongue with a weak, wiry or choppy pulse: blood deficiency with blood stagnation	• Nourishes the blood • Regulates blood circulation • Eliminates blood stasis	• *Si Wu Tang* (Four-Substance Decoction) tonifies the blood and regulates blood circulation. • *Tao Ren* (Semen Persicae) and *Hong Hua* (Flos Carthami) regulate blood circulation and eliminate blood stagnation.

Táo Hóng Sì Wù Tāng
(Four-Substance Decoction with Safflower and Peach Pit)

contribute to the negative feedback inhibition or the atrophy of the thymus or adrenal glands.[4]

HUMAN CLINICAL STUDIES AND RESEARCH

1. **Infertility**: Use of modified *Tao Hong Si Wu Tang* was effective in treating female infertility caused by blocked fallopian tubes. The herbal treatment consisted of *Tao Hong Si Wu Tang* plus *Xiang Fu* (Rhizoma Cyperi), *Shui Zhi* (Hirudo), *Lu Lu Tong* (Fructus Liquidambaris), *Dan Shen* (Radix et Rhizoma Salviae Miltiorrhizae), *San Qi* (Radix et Rhizoma Notoginseng) powder, and others. For Kidney deficiency, *Sang Shen* (Fructus Mori) and *Xu Duan* (Radix Dipsaci) are added. For dampness and phlegm, *Cang Zhu* (Rhizoma Atractylodis), *Chen Pi* (Pericarpium Citri Reticulatae), and *Ban Xia* (Rhizoma Pinelliae) were added, and *Shu Di Huang* (Radix Rehmanniae Praeparata) was removed. For damp-heat, *Huang Bo* (Cortex Phellodendri Chinensis), *Yi Yi Ren* (Semen Coicis), *Tu Fu Ling* (Rhizoma Smilacis Glabrae), and *Pu Gong Ying* (Herba Taraxaci) were added, and *Shu Di Huang* (Radix Rehmanniae Praeparata) was removed. Of 60 women, the study reported successful pregnancy in 31 patients, normal flow of egg in the fallopian tubes in 7 patients, and ectopic pregnancy in 1 patient. The overall rate of effectiveness was 80%.[5]
2. **Cerebral infarction**: Thirty-two patients with cerebral infarction were treated with complete recovery in 10 patients, significant improvement in 11 patients, moderate improvement in 9 patients, and no benefit in 2 patients. The herbal treatment contained *Tao Hong Si Wu Tang* plus *Ge Gen* (Radix Puerariae Lobatae), *Shui Zhi* (Hirudo) and *Huang Qi* (Radix Astragali).[6]
3. **Diabetic neuropathy**: Use of modified *Tao Hong Si Wu Tang* was associated with 96.4% effectiveness in treating peripheral neuropathy in 28 diabetic patients (22 with more than 5 years of illness, and 6 with less than 5 years of illness). The base formula contained *Tao Hong Si Wu Tang* plus *Huang Qi* (Radix Astragali), *Dang Shen* (Radix Codonopsis), *Huang Jing* (Rhizoma Polygonati) and *Gou Qi Zi* (Fructus Lycii). Additional modifications included *Xuan Shen* (Radix Scrophulariae) and *Huang Lian* (Rhizoma Coptidis) for irritability, thirst, polyphagia and polydypsia; and *Di Gu Pi* (Cortex Lycii) for *wu xin re* (five-center heat). Of 28 patients, the study reported complete recovery in 15 patients, moderate improvement in 9 patients, slight improvement in 3 patients, and no benefit in 1 patient.[7]
4. **Bone fractures**: Administration of an herbal formula was effective in reducing swelling and pain, and facilitating the recovery process. The herbal formula contained *Tao Hong Si Wu Tang* plus *Gu Sui Bu* (Rhizoma Drynariae), *Xu Duan* (Radix Dipsaci), *Zi Ran Tong* (Pyritum), *Tu Bie Chong* (Eupolyphaga seu Steleophaga), *Mu Xiang* (Radix Aucklandiae), and others as needed. Additional modifications included *Huang Bo* (Cortex Phellodendri Chinensis) for heat; unprocessed *Cao Wu* (Radix Aconiti Kusnezoffii) for cold; *Sang Zhi* (Ramulus Mori) for bone fractures in the upper extremities; and *Niu Xi* (Radix Achyranthis Bidentatae) for bone fractures in the lower extremities.[8]
5. **Allergic rhinitis**: Use of modified *Tao Hong Si Wu Tang* was shown to be effective in treating allergic rhinitis in 42 patients. The base formula contained *Tao Hong Si Wu Tang* plus *Cang Er Zi* (Fructus Xanthii), *Huang Qi* (Radix Astragali), *Fang Feng* (Radix Saposhnikoviae), and *Xin Yi Hua* (Flos Magnoliae). Modifications included addition of *Ma Huang* (Herba Ephedrae) and *Xi Xin* (Radix et Rhizoma Asari) for stuffy nose, frequent sneezing, and profuse watery nasal discharge; *Huang Qin* (Radix Scutellariae) and *Mu Dan Pi* (Cortex Moutan) for profuse yellow nasal discharge; *Fu Ling* (Poria), *Shan Yao* (Rhizoma Dioscoreae), and dry-fried *Bai Bian Dou* (Semen Lablab Album) for Spleen deficiency with poor appetite; *Nu Zhen Zi* (Fructus Ligustri Lucidi) and *Wu Wei Zi* (Fructus Schisandrae Chinensis) for Kidney deficiency; and *Jing Jie* (Herba Schizonepetae) and *Chan Tui* (Periostracum Cicadae) for itchy nose. The duration of treatment ranged between 6-20 days. Of 42 patients, the study reported complete recovery in 31 patients, improvement in 9 patients, and no benefit in 2 patients.[9]
6. **Optic nerve atrophy**: Twenty-eight patients (34 affected eyes) with glaucoma and atrophy of the optic nerve were treated with good results using the combination of herbs and vasodilators. The herbal treatment contained *Tao Hong Si Wu Tang* plus *Gou Qi Zi* (Fructus Lycii), *Dan Shen* (Radix et Rhizoma Salviae Miltiorrhizae), *Ren Shen* (Radix et Rhizoma Ginseng), *Bai Zhu* (Rhizoma Atractylodis Macrocephalae), and *Ju Hua* (Flos Chrysanthemi). The average duration of treatment was 69 packs of herbs.[10]
7. **Optic neuritis**: One study reported beneficial effect in 32 patients with optic neuritis using *Tao Hong Si Wu Tang* plus *Dan Shen* (Radix et Rhizoma Salviae Miltiorrhizae), *Zhi Qiao* (Fructus Aurantii), *Fu Ling* (Poria), *Tong Cao* (Medulla Tetrapanacis), and *Gan Cao* (Radix et Rhizoma Glycyrrhizae). The herbs were given in decoction daily.[11]
8. **Cataract**: One study reported 98.4% effectiveness using modified *Tao Hong Si Wu Tang* to treat 200 patients (381 affected eyes) with cataract. The herbal treatment contained this formula plus *Dan Shen* (Radix et Rhizoma Salviae Miltiorrhizae), *Gou Qi Zi* (Fructus Lycii), *Ju Hua* (Flos Chrysanthemi), *Ji Li* (Fructus Tribuli), *Chan Tui* (Periostracum Cicadae), *Ye Ming Sha* (Faeces Vespertilionis Murini), *Qing Xiang Zi* (Semen Celosiae), *Jue Ming Zi*

Táo Hóng Sì Wù Tāng
(Four-Substance Decoction with Safflower and Peach Pit)

(Semen Cassiae), *Ci Shi* (Magnetitum), *Shen Qu* (Massa Fermentata), *Sang Shen* (Fructus Mori), and *Chen Pi* (Pericarpium Citri Reticulatae). Effectiveness was defined as improvement of visual acuity.[12]

9. **Glaucoma**: Twelve patients (19 affected eyes) with glaucoma characterized by Liver stagnation were treated with recovery in 7 eyes, significant improvement in 4 eyes, moderate improvement in 5 eyes, and no benefit in 3 eyes. The herbal formula contained *Tao Hong Si Wu Tang* plus *Su Mu* (Lignum Sappan), *Qiang Huo* (Rhizoma et Radix Notopterygii), *Bu Gu Zhi* (Fructus Psoraleae), *Hua Shi* (Talcum), *Jie Geng* (Radix Platycodonis), *Zhi Qiao* (Fructus Aurantii), *Da Huang* (Radix et Rhizoma Rhei), and *Gan Cao* (Radix et Rhizoma Glycyrrhizae).[13]
10. **Urticaria**: One study reported 85.8% effectiveness using modified *Tao Hong Si Wu Tang* to treat chronic urticaria. The herbal treatment contained this formula plus *Jing Jie* (Herba Schizonepetae), *He Shou Wu* (Radix Polygoni Multiflori), *Zao Jiao Ci* (Spina Gleditsiae), *Chan Tui* (Periostracum Cicadae), and others as needed. Of 42 patients, the study reported recovery in 20 patients, significant improvement in 10 patients, moderate improvement in 6 patients, and no benefit in 6 patients.[14] In another study, use of modified *Tao Hong Si Wu Tang* to treat 24 patients with stubborn urticaria was associated with complete recovery in all 24 patients. The herbal treatment contained this formula plus *Jiang Can* (Bombyx Batryticatus) and *Chan Tui* (Periostracum Cicadae) as the base formula, with addition of others as needed. The duration of treatment ranged from 7 to 15 packs of herbs.[15]
11. **Itching**: One study reported 93.5% effectiveness using modified *Tao Hong Si Wu Tang* to treat itching. The herbal treatment contained this formula plus *He Shou Wu* (Radix Polygoni Multiflori), *Di Fu Zi* (Fructus Kochiae), *Bai Xian Pi* (Cortex Dictamni), and *Ji Li* (Fructus Tribuli). Of 92 patients, the study reported complete recovery in 53 patients, moderate improvement in 33 patients, and no benefit in 6 patients.[16]
12. **Eczema**: Administration of *Tao Hong Si Wu Tang* plus *Dan Shen* (Radix et Rhizoma Salviae Miltiorrhizae), *Chi Shao* (Radix Paeoniae Rubra), and *Mu Dan Pi* (Cortex Moutan) in 64 patients with eczema was associated with complete recovery in 53 patients, significant improvement in 5 patients, and slight improvement in 6 patients.[17]
13. **Psoriasis**: Administration of modified *Tao Hong Si Wu Tang* was associated with 93.7% effectiveness in treating 32 patients with psoriasis. In addition to this formula, modifications were made by adding *Jin Yin Hua* (Flos Lonicerae Japonicae), *Lian Qiao* (Fructus Forsythiae), *Pu Gong Ying* (Herba Taraxaci), *Zi Cao* (Radix Arnebiae), *Xuan Shen* (Radix Scrophulariae), and *Ban Lan Gen* (Radix Isatidis) for damaged skin with spots; *Fu Ling* (Poria), *Che Qian Zi* (Semen Plantaginis), *Bai Xian Pi* (Cortex Dictamni) and *Ku Shen* (Radix Sophorae Flavescentis) for damaged skin with geographic appearance; *Jin Yin Hua* (Flos Lonicerae Japonicae), *Lian Qiao* (Fructus Forsythiae), *Pu Gong Ying* (Herba Taraxaci), *Zi Cao* (Radix Arnebiae), *Fu Ling* (Poria), *Che Qian Zi* (Semen Plantaginis), *Bai Xian Pi* (Cortex Dictamni), and *Yi Yi Ren* (Semen Coicis) for psoriatic arthritis; *Jin Yin Hua* (Flos Lonicerae Japonicae), *Pu Gong Ying* (Herba Taraxaci), *Zi Cao* (Radix Arnebiae), and *Xuan Shen* (Radix Scrophulariae) for psoriasis with sores; and *Xuan Shen* (Radix Scrophulariae), *Sha Shen* (Radix Glehniae seu Adenophorae), *Mai Dong* (Radix Ophiopogonis), *Mu Dan Pi* (Cortex Moutan), *Bai Xian Pi* (Cortex Dictamni), *Ku Shen* (Radix Sophorae Flavescentis), *Fang Feng* (Radix Saposhnikoviae), *Chan Tui* (Periostracum Cicadae), *Wu Shao She* (Zaocys) and *Quan Xie* (Scorpio) during the remission period. Of 32 patients, the study reported complete recovery in 23 patients, improvement in 7 patients, and no benefit in 2 patients.[18]

HERB-DRUG INTERACTION

Cosmetics-induced dermatitis: One study reported good results in the treatment of dermatitis associated with the use of cosmetics using *Tao Hong Si Wu Tang* plus *Fang Feng* (Radix Saposhnikoviae), *Pu Gong Ying* (Herba Taraxaci), *Zi Hua Di Ding* (Herba Violae), and others. The herbs were given in decoction for 10 days per course of treatment. Most patients responded within 3-5 days, while some with severe conditions required up to 3 courses of treatment.[19]

SUGGESTED ACUPUNCTURE TREATMENT

1. Points: *Pishu* (BL 20), *Weishu* (BL 21), *Housanli* (ST 36), *Xinshu* (BL 15), *Geshu* (BL 17), *Sanyinjiao* (SP 6), and *Xuehai* (SP 10)
2. Technique: tonification.

Pishu (BL 20), *Weishu* (BL 21), and *Housanli* (ST 36) strengthen the Spleen and Stomach to tonify blood. *Xinshu* (BL 15) nourishes Heart blood. *Geshu* (BL 17) tonifies the blood. *Sanyinjiao* (SP 6) nourishes the Kidney, Spleen, and Liver. *Xuehai* (SP 10) activates blood circulation and removes blood stasis.

AUTHORS' COMMENTS

Tao Hong Si Wu Tang is designed to treat disorders characterized by blood deficiency with blood stagnation. The emphasis of the formula is to tonify the blood and eliminate blood stasis. To potentiate the effects of the formula, *Bai*

Táo Hóng Sì Wù Tāng
(Four-Substance Decoction with Safflower and Peach Pit)

Shao (Radix Paeoniae Alba) can be replaced with *Chi Shao* (Radix Paeoniae Rubra) to enhance the blood-activating effect, and *Shu Di Huang* (Radix Rehmanniae Praeparata) can be replaced with *Di Huang* (Radix Rehmanniae) to nourish the blood without creating more stagnation.

Tao Hong Si Wu Tang can be used to treat a variety of ophthalmologic disorders and pain conditions characterized by blood deficiency, and qi and blood stagnation.

- For progressive retinal atrophy with qi and blood stagnation, add *Mu Dan Pi* (Cortex Moutan), *Chong Wei Zi* (Fructus Leonuri), *Che Qian Zi* (Semen Plantaginis), *Yu Jin* (Radix Curcumae), *Dan Shen* (Radix et Rhizoma Salviae Miltiorrhizae), *Chai Hu* (Radix Bupleuri) and *Quan Xie* (Scorpio).
- For atrophy of the optic nerve, add *Dan Shen* (Radix et Rhizoma Salviae Miltiorrhizae), *Chong Wei Zi* (Fructus Leonuri), *Xia Ku Cao* (Spica Prunellae), and *Gan Cao* (Radix et Rhizoma Glycyrrhizae).
- For the treatment of chronic, superficial keratitis due to Liver fire, blood deficiency and stagnation, combine with *Shi Jue Ming* (Concha Haliotidis), *Jue Ming Zi* (Semen Cassiae), *Ju Hua* (Flos Chrysanthemi), *Che Qian Zi* (Semen Plantaginis), *Chi Shao* (Radix Paeoniae Rubra), *Zhi Qiao* (Fructus Aurantii), *Gou Qi Zi* (Fructus Lycii), *Zi Hua Di Ding* (Herba Violae), *Mi Meng Hua* (Flos Buddlejae), *Qing Xiang Zi* (Semen Celosiae), *Chai Hu* (Radix Bupleuri) and *Zhi Zi* (Fructus Gardeniae).
- For chronic, superficial keratitis due to Kidney yin deficiency with deficiency heat, combine with *Zhi Bai Di Huang Wan* (Anemarrhena, Phellodendron, and Rehmannia Pill) and add *Huang Jing* (Rhizoma Polygonati), *Gou Qi Zi* (Fructus Lycii), and *Che Qian Zi* (Semen Plantaginis).
- For non-healing corneal ulcers, combine with *Qi Ju Di Huang Wan* (Lycium Fruit, Chrysanthemum, and Rehmannia Pill) and add *Dan Shen* (Radix et Rhizoma Salviae Miltiorrhizae) and *Yu Jin* (Radix Curcumae).
- For the treatment of chronic glaucoma with Liver qi stagnation, combine with *Jia Wei Xiao Yao San* (Augmented Rambling Powder) and add *Yu Jin* (Radix Curcumae), *Xia Ku Cao* (Spica Prunellae) and *Dan Shen* (Radix et Rhizoma Salviae Miltiorrhizae).
- For chronic glaucoma with yin deficiency and fire, combine with *Zhi Bai Di Huang Wan* (Anemarrhena, Phellodendron, and Rehmannia Pill) and add *Shi Jue Ming* (Concha Haliotidis), *Chai Hu* (Radix Bupleuri), *Nu Zhen Zi* (Fructus Ligustri Lucidi), *Shi Hu* (Caulis Dendrobii) and *Dan Shen* (Radix et Rhizoma Salviae Miltiorrhizae).

Tao Hong Si Wu Tang is also a useful formula for pain associated with blood deficiency and blood stagnation.

- For lumbar pain associated with estrus in horses, use alone or in combination with *Shen Tong Zhu Yu Tang* (Drive Out Blood Stasis from a Painful Body Decoction). If behavioral signs are present (mania, irritability, excessive libido), combine with *Chai Hu Jia Long Gu Mu Li Tang* (Bupleurum plus Dragon Bone and Oyster Shell Decoction).
- For the treatment of diabetic neuropathy, add *Di Huang* (Radix Rehmanniae), *Dan Shen* (Radix et Rhizoma Salviae Miltiorrhizae), *Huang Qi* (Radix Astragali), *Yi Mu Cao* (Herba Leonuri) and *Ji Xue Teng* (Caulis Spatholobi).
- For the treatment of intervertebral disk disease in the dog with Kidney and Liver yin deficiencies and blood stasis, combine with *Si Wu Tang* (Four-Substance Decoction) and *Shen Tong Zhu Yu Tang* (Drive Out Blood Stasis from a Painful Body Decoction).

References

1. *Zhong Yao Ming Fang Yao Li Yu Ying Yong* (Pharmacology and Applications of Famous Herbal Formulas), 1989; 453-455.
2. *Jiang Su Zhong Yi Za Zhi* (Jiangsu Journal of Chinese Medicine), 1986; 12:541.
3. *Zhong Xi Yi Jie He Za Zhi* (Journal of Integrated Chinese and Western Medicine), 1988; 8(10):601.
4. *Zhong Guo Zhong Yao Za Zhi* (People's Republic of China Journal of Chinese Herbology), 1994; 19(11):680.
5. *He Bei Zhong Yi* (Hebei Chinese Medicine), 1995; 15(2):26.
6. *Zhong Yi Han Shou Tong Xun* (Reports of Chinese Medicine), 1992; 3:44.
7. *Shi Yong Zhong Yi Nei Ke Za Zhi* (Journal of Practical Chinese Internal Medicine), 1991; 5(2):73.
8. *Gui Yang Yi Xue Yuan Xue Bao* (Journal of Guiyang Medical University), 1983; 1:63.
9. *Zhong Yi Ming Fang Lin Chuang Xin Yong* (Contemporary Clinical Applications of Classic Chinese Formulas), 2001; 1:29.
10. *Yan Ke Tong Xun* (Journal of Ophthalmology), 1987; 3:13.
11. *Zhong Yi Fang Ji Xian Dai Yan Jiu* (Modern Study of Medical Formulas in Traditional Chinese Medicine), 1997; 1103.
12. *Zhong Yi Fang Ji Xian Dai Yan Jiu* (Modern Study of Medical Formulas in Traditional Chinese Medicine), 1997; 1103.
13. *Zhong Yi Za Zhi* (Journal of Chinese Medicine), 1983; 24(1):34.
14. *Bei Jing Zhong Yi* (Beijing Chinese Medicine), 1997; 5:31.
15. *He Bei Zhong Yi* (Hebei Chinese Medicine), 1995; 17(4):47.
16. *Shi Yong Zhong Xi Yi Jie He Za Zhi* (Practical Journal of Integrated Chinese and Western Medicines), 1991; 4:41.
17. *Zhong Yi Za Zhi* (Journal of Chinese Medicine), 1988; 29(5):366.
18. *Shan Xi Zhong Yi* (Shanxi Chinese Medicine), 1990; 11(2):106.
19. *Zhong Yi Yao Xin Xi* (Information on Chinese Medicine and Herbology), 1992; 9(5):36.

Dāng Guī Bǔ Xuè Tāng (Tangkuei Decoction to Tonify the Blood)

當歸補血湯
当归补血汤

Pinyin Name: *Dang Gui Bu Xue Tang*

Literal Name: Tangkuei Decoction to Tonify the Blood

Alternate Names: *Tang Kuei Pu Hsieh Tang*, Tang-kuei Blood-Nourishing Decoction, Chinese Angelica Blood-Tonifying Decoction, Tangkuei and Astragalus Combination

Original Source: *Nei Wai Shang Bian Huo Lun* (Clarifying Doubts about Injury from Internal and External Causes) by Li Gao in 1247

COMPOSITION

Huang Qi (Radix Astragali)	30g
Dang Gui (Radix Angelicae Sinensis), *xi* (washed) with liquor	6g

DOSAGE / PREPARATION / ADMINISTRATION

The source text states to coarsely grind the ingredients and cook the powder in water to make a decoction. Take the warm, strained decoction before meals on an empty stomach. Today, it is usually prepared as a decoction by cooking the herbs three times. The decoction is taken in three equally divided doses, three times daily in the morning, noon and evening.

CHINESE THERAPEUTIC ACTIONS

Tonifies qi and generates blood production

CLINICAL MANIFESTATIONS

Qi and blood deficiencies due to overexertion: excessive loss of blood after parturition or injury with fever, irritability and thirst with a desire to drink water, poor wound healing, a pale, dry tongue, and a large, weak pulse.

VETERINARY CLINICAL APPLICATIONS

Acute or chronic blood loss, anemia, leukopenia, purpura hemorrhagica, supportive therapy during chemotherapy or radiation treatment, insufficient lactation.

EXPLANATION

Dang Gui Bu Xue Tang (Tangkuei Decoction to Tonify the Blood) is designed to treat exertion-induced qi and blood deficiencies. Overexertion and overwork may damage qi and blood in the body, and lead to the floating of yang toward the exterior parts of the body. Clinical presentations include irritability and thirst with a desire to drink water. Since qi is deficient and the body is exhausted, wound healing is slow and the tongue is pale. A large, weak pulse indicates floating of yang and deficiency of qi and blood.

The productions of qi and blood are interdependent. Thus, both qi and blood tonics are used for optimal effect when treating deficiency. *Huang Qi* (Radix Astragali) and *Dang Gui* (Radix Angelicae Sinensis) tonify qi and blood. The dose of *Huang Qi* (Radix Astragali) is five times greater than *Dang Gui* (Radix Angelicae Sinensis) to greatly tonify *yuan* (source) *qi*, strengthen the Spleen, and ensure adequate production of blood. *Huang Qi* (Radix Astragali) also prevents the further leaking of yang and promotes the healing of wounds.

VETERINARY MODIFICATIONS

- For general blood deficiency, add *Shu Di Huang* (Radix Rehmanniae Praeparata), *He Shou Wu* (Radix Polygoni Multiflori), *Sang Ji Sheng* (Herba Taxilli), and *Bai Shao* (Radix Paeoniae Alba).
- For ulcerated sores that do not heal, add *Jin Yin Hua* (Flos Lonicerae Japonicae), *Lian Qiao* (Fructus Forsythiae), and *Tian Hua Fen* (Radix Trichosanthis).

CAUTIONS / CONTRAINDICATIONS

Dang Gui Bu Xue Tang is contraindicated in animals with excess heat or yin-deficient heat with tidal fever.

***Dang Gui Bu Xue Tang* (Tangkuei Decoction to Tonify the Blood)**

Diagnosis	Clinical Signs	Treatment	Herbs
Qi and blood deficiencies due to over-exertion	• Irritability and thirst with a desire to drink water: deficiencies of qi, blood and body fluids • Slow wound healing: qi and blood deficiencies • Pale, dry tongue and a large, weak pulse: qi and blood deficiencies with yang floating to the exterior	• Tonifies qi • Generates production of blood	• *Huang Qi* (Radix Astragali) tonifies qi. • *Dang Gui* (Radix Angelicae Sinensis) tonifies the blood.

Dāng Guī Bǔ Xuè Tāng (Tangkuei Decoction to Tonify the Blood)

PHARMACOLOGICAL EFFECTS

1. **Hematopoietic**: In experiments in mice, administration of *Dang Gui Bu Xue Tang* was associated with an increased red blood cell count.[1] It was noted that the formula was more effective than administering *Huang Qi* (Radix Astragali) or *Dang Gui* (Radix Angelicae Sinensis) individually with the same dose, implying that the formula has synergistic effect. Also, it was found that the herbs were more effective in increasing red blood cell count (but not white blood cells) when decocted for 90 minutes in comparison to 45 minutes.[2]
2. **Antiplatelet**: Use of *Dang Gui Bu Xue Tang* was found to be effective in blocking the aggregation of platelets and preventing the formation of blood clots.[3,4]
3. **Hepatoprotective**: Administration of *Dang Gui Bu Xue Tang* was associated with hepatoprotective effects against carbon tetrachloride in mice. The effects were attributed to increased blood circulation and increased regeneration of liver cells.[5]
4. **Immunostimulant**: In laboratory experiments in mice, the use of *Dang Gui Bu Xue Tang* was associated with an increase of phagocytic activities by macrophages. The effects of the herbs lasted up to 24 hours.[6]

HUMAN CLINICAL STUDIES AND RESEARCH

1. **Thrombopenic purpura**: Twenty-four patients with thrombopenic purpura were treated with modified *Dang Gui Bu Xue Tang* with recovery in 7 patients, marked improvement in 12 patients, and slight improvement in 5 patients. The average length of treatment was 64 days. The herbal treatment contained *Dang Gui Bu Xue Tang* plus *Xue Yu Tan* (Crinis Carbonisatus), *Gan Cao* (Radix et Rhizoma Glycyrrhizae), and *Xian He Cao* (Herba Agrimoniae) as the base formula. Additional modifications were made accordingly for qi deficiency, blood deficiency, yin deficiency, and yang deficiency.[7]
2. **Amenorrhea**: Thirty-seven women with amenorrhea due to abnormal development of the uterus were treated with the following herbal prescription with 91.89% effectiveness. The herbal treatment contained *Dang Gui Bu Xue Tang* plus *San Leng* (Rhizoma Sparganii), *E Zhu* (Rhizoma Curcumae), and *Dan Shen* (Radix et Rhizoma Salviae Miltiorrhizae) as the base formula. Additional modifications were made if necessary. The duration of treatment was 6 months. Of 37 patients, the study reported marked improvement in 23 patients, moderate improvement in 11 patients, and no benefit in 3 patients.[8]
3. **Leucopenia**: Twenty patients with leucopenia were treated with modified *Dang Gui Bu Xue Tang* with marked effect in 8 patients, moderate effect in 11 patients, and no effect in 1 patient. The formula contained *Dang Gui* (Radix Angelicae Sinensis), *Huang Qi* (Radix Astragali), *San Leng* (Rhizoma Sparganii), and *Gan Cao* (Radix et Rhizoma Glycyrrhizae). The treatment protocol was to administer the herbs one time daily for 3-4 weeks.[9]
4. **Insufficient lactation**: Use of modified *Dang Gui Bu Xue Tang* was successful in promoting lactation in 96 women within 3 months after delivery. The herbal treatment contained this formula plus *Ren Shen* (Radix et Rhizoma Ginseng). Furthermore, *Shi Gao* (Gypsum Fibrosum) was added in summer and *Gui Zhi* (Cortex Rasus Cinnamomi) was added in winter. The study reported 100% effectiveness, with most noticeable success when treatment began within one month of delivery.[10]
5. **Arthritis**: In one study, 51 patients with various presentations of arthritis were treated with modified *Dang Gui Bu Xue Tang* with good results. The base formula included *Dang Gui* (Radix Angelicae Sinensis), *Huang Qi* (Radix Astragali), *Gui Zhi* (Ramulus Cinnamomi), *Hai Feng Teng* (Caulis Piperis Kadsurae), *Qin Jiao* (Radix Gentianae Macrophyllae), and *Zhi Chuan Wu* (Radix Aconiti Praeparata). The modifications included the addition of *Fang Feng* (Radix Saposhnikoviae) and *Qiang Huo* (Rhizoma et Radix Notopterygii) for *xing bi* (mobile painful obstruction); *Fang Ji* (Radix Stephaniae Tetrandrae) and *Yi Yi Ren* (Semen Coicis) for *zhuo bi* (fixed painful obstruction); *Zhi Mu* (Rhizoma Anemarrhenae), *Shi Gao* (Gypsum Fibrosum), and *Ren Dong Teng* (Caulis Lonicerae Japonicae) for *re bi* (heat painful obstruction); and *Xi Xin* (Radix et Rhizoma Asari) for *tong bi* (extremely painful obstruction). The treatment protocol was to administer the herbs on a daily basis for 10 days per course of treatment, for a duration of 10-45 days. Out of 51 patients, the study reported recovery in 36 patients, improvement in 10 patients, and no benefit in 5 patients. The study noted that the formula was most effective for *tong bi* (extremely painful obstruction) and *zhuo bi* (fixed painful obstruction), and less effective for *re bi* (heat painful obstruction).[11]

HERB-DRUG INTERACTION

Chemotherapy- and radiation-induced leucopenia: One study reported 90.2% effectiveness using modified *Dang Gui Bu Xue Tang* to treat 102 patients with leucopenia due to chemotherapy and radiation. The herbal treatment contained this formula plus *Gou Qi Zi* (Fructus Lycii) and *Gu Sui Bu* (Rhizoma Drynariae). The average increase in white blood cell count was $1.665x10^9$/L, from $2.939x10^9$/L before herbal treatment to $4.600x10^9$/L after the treatment. Of 102 patients, the study reported significant improvement in 39 patients, moderate improvement in 53 patients, and no benefit in 10 patients.[12]

Dāng Guī Bǔ Xuè Tāng (Tangkuei Decoction to Tonify the Blood)

SUGGESTED ACUPUNCTURE TREATMENT

1. Points: *Qihai* (CV 6), *Guanyuan* (CV 4), *Gaohuangshu* (BL 43), *Pishu* (BL 20), *Housanli* (ST 36), *Shenshu* (BL 23), *Sanyinjiao* (SP 6), *Xinshu* (BL 15), and *Geshu* (BL 17).
2. Technique: tonification.

Qihai (CV 6), *Guanyuan* (CV 4), and *Gaohuangshu* (BL 43) tonify *yuan* (source) *qi*. *Pishu* (BL 20), *Housanli* (ST 36), *Shenshu* (BL 23), and *Sanyinjiao* (SP 6) tonify qi and nourish the blood. *Xinshu* (BL 15) and *Geshu* (BL 17) nourish and regulate the blood.

AUTHORS' COMMENTS

Dang Gui Bu Xue Tang (Tangkuei Decoction to Tonify the Blood) is generally used for the treatment of acute blood loss and anemia. It can also be combined with other herbs or formulas to provide supportive care for animals with cancer and other chronic diseases with blood deficiency and low red and white blood cell counts. It is often prescribed to replenish qi and blood following parturition.

It is often asked that if *Dang Gui Bu Xue Tang* is a blood-tonifying formula, why is the dose of *Huang Qi* (Radix Astragali), which is a qi tonic, five times greater than that of *Dang Gui* (Radix Angelicae Sinensis), which is a blood tonic? The answer is that the production of blood is directly dependent on an adequate supply of qi. In other words, to effectively tonify the blood, qi must be tonified first. That is why *Huang Qi* (Radix Astragali) is used at a dose five times greater than *Dang Gui* (Radix Angelicae Sinensis).[13]

Huang Qi (Radix Astragali) is the main ingredient in two important formulas with slightly different purposes:

- *Dang Gui Bu Xue Tang* contains *Huang Qi* (Radix Astragali) at a dose five times greater than that of *Dang Gui* (Radix Angelicae Sinensis) to boost qi and generate blood. It treats blood deficiency with deficiency heat signs, spontaneous sweating, and a large, weak pulse that is forceless upon pressure.
- *Bu Zhong Yi Qi Tang* (Tonify the Middle and Augment the Qi Decoction) uses *Huang Qi* (Radix Astragali) to tonify qi and lift yang. It treats Spleen and Stomach qi deficiencies with prolapsed organs. Animals will exhibit fatigue, exercise intolerance, poor appetite, chronic diarrhea, and spontaneous sweating.

References

1. *Hei Long Jiang Zhong Yi Yao* (Heilongjiang Chinese Medicine and Herbology), 1989; 4:41.
2. *Zhong Cheng Yao* (Study of Chinese Patent Medicine), 1991; 13(5):44.
3. *Zhong Yao Yao Li Yu Lin Chuang* (Pharmacology and Clinical Applications of Chinese Herbs), 1990; 6(5):40.
4. *Zhong Yao Yao Li Yu Lin Chuang* (Pharmacology and Clinical Applications of Chinese Herbs), 1993; 1.
5. *Zhong Yao Yao Li Yu Lin Chuang* (Pharmacology and Clinical Applications of Chinese Herbs), 1993; 9(4):4.
6. *Xin Yi Yao Xue Za Zhi* (New Journal of Medicine and Herbology), 1979; 3(5):27.
7. *Zhong Yi Za Zhi* (Journal of Chinese Medicine), 1984; 25(5):356.
8. *Shi Yong Zhong Xi Yi Jie He Za Zhi* (Practical Journal of Integrated Chinese and Western Medicines), 1991; 8:477.
9. *An Hui Zhong Yi Xue Yuan Xue Bao* (Journal of Anhui University School of Medicine), 1987; 6(3):43.
10. *Nei Meng Gu Zhong Yi Yao* (Traditional Chinese Medicine and Medicinals of Inner Mongolia), 1998; 4:12.
11. *He Bei Zhong Yi Za Zhi* (Hebei Journal of Chinese Medicine), 1986; 1:46.
12. *Gan Su Zhong Yi* (Gansu Chinese Medicine), 1998; 5:28.
13. Wang MZ, et al. *Zhong Yi Xue Wen Da Ti Ku* (Questions and Answers on Traditional Chinese Medicine: Herbal Formulas).

Guī Pí Tāng (Restore the Spleen Decoction)

歸脾湯
归脾汤

Pinyin Name: *Gui Pi Tang*
Literal Name: Restore the Spleen Decoction
Alternate Names: *Kuei Pi Tang*, Back to the Spleen Decoction, Ginseng and Longan Decoction, Ginseng and Longan Combination
Original Source: *Ji Sheng Fang* (Formulas to Aid the Living) by Yan Yong-He in 1253

COMPOSITION

Ren Shen (Radix et Rhizoma Ginseng)	15g [6g]
Huang Qi (Radix Astragali)	30g [12g]
Bai Zhu (Rhizoma Atractylodis Macrocephalae)	30g [9g]
Zhi Gan Cao (Radix et Rhizoma Glycyrrhizae Praeparata cum Melle)	7.5g [3g]
Dang Gui (Radix Angelicae Sinensis)	3g [9g]
Long Yan Rou (Arillus Longan)	30g [12g]
Fu Shen (Poria Pararadicis)	30g [9g]
Yuan Zhi (Radix Polygalae), *mi zhi* (fried with honey)	3g [6g]
Suan Zao Ren (Semen Ziziphi Spinosae), *chao* (dry-fried)	30g [12g]
Mu Xiang (Radix Aucklandiae), do not expose to heat	15g [6g]

Note: *Dang Gui* (Radix Angelicae Sinensis) and *Yuan Zhi* (Radix Polygalae) were not listed in the source text; they were added by Bi Li-Zhai in the 16th century in *Jiao Zhu Fu Ren Liang Fang* (Revised Fine Formulas for Women). *Dang Gui* (Radix Angelicae Sinensis) greatly enhances the effect to tonify blood, and *Yuan Zhi* (Radix Polygalae) strongly increases the efficacy of the formula to nourish the Heart and tranquilize the mind. Since the addition of these two herbs greatly enhances the overall effect, they are now accepted as standard ingredients in the formula.

DOSAGE / PREPARATION / ADMINISTRATION

The source text instructs to grind the ingredients coarsely. Cook 12g of the powder with 5 slices of *Sheng Jiang* (Rhizoma Zingiberis Recens) and 1 piece of *Da Zao* (Fructus Jujubae) in 1.5 large bowls of water until it is reduced to 70%. Take the warm, strained decoction at any time of the day. This formula may also be prepared as pills by mixing the powdered herbs with honey. Take 15g of pills per dose on an empty stomach three times daily with warm, boiled water. Today, this formula may be prepared as a decoction with the doses suggested in brackets.

CHINESE THERAPEUTIC ACTIONS

1. Tonifies qi and nourishes the blood
2. Strengthens the Spleen and nourishes the Heart

CLINICAL MANIFESTATIONS

1. Heart and Spleen deficiencies due to excessive worrying: arrhythmia, tachycardia, inability to concentrate and follow commands, restlessness at night, easily fatigued, poor appetite, lethargy, a pale, dry tongue, and a thready, weak pulse.
2. A deficient Spleen unable to keep the blood circulating within the vessels: petechiae and ecchymosis, hematochezia, hematuria, hematemesis, epistaxis and hemoptysis.

VETERINARY CLINICAL APPLICATIONS

Non-regenerative anemia, aplastic anemia, anemia secondary to cardiac disease, immune-mediated hemolytic anemia (IHA), immune-mediated thrombocytopenia (ITP), purpura hemorrhagica, post-operative weakness and recovery, behavioral disorder with restlessness, anxiety and fearfulness, fatigued and over-trained competitive animals, congestive heart failure, arrhythmia and tachycardia.

EXPLANATION

Gui Pi Tang (Restore the Spleen Decoction) is renowned for treating Heart (blood) and Spleen (qi) deficiencies. The common cause of this syndrome is excessive worrying and psychological stress that consume the blood and injure qi. Clinical signs of Heart (blood) deficiency include arrhythmia, tachycardia, inability to concentrate and follow commands, anxiety and insomnia. Clinical signs of Spleen (qi) deficiency include poor appetite, lethargy and bleeding disorders. A pale, dry tongue and a thready, weak pulse indicate qi and blood deficiencies.

This formula is also indicated for disorders in animals in which the Spleen fails to hold the blood within the vessels due to Spleen qi deficiency. Symptoms of bleeding, such

Guī Pí Tāng (Restore the Spleen Decoction)

as petechiae and ecchymosis, hematochezia, hematuria, hematemesis, epistaxis and hemoptysis, may occur.

Ren Shen (Radix et Rhizoma Ginseng), *Huang Qi* (Radix Astragali), *Bai Zhu* (Rhizoma Atractylodis Macrocephalae), and *Zhi Gan Cao* (Radix et Rhizoma Glycyrrhizae Praeparata cum Melle) warm and tonify Spleen qi. *Dang Gui* (Radix Angelicae Sinensis) and *Long Yan Rou* (Arillus Longan) nourish the Liver, tonify Heart blood, and regulate blood circulation. *Fu Shen* (Poria Paradicis), *Yuan Zhi* (Radix Polygalae) and *Suan Zao Ren* (Semen Ziziphi Spinosae) nourish the Heart and calm the *shen* (spirit). *Mu Xiang* (Radix Aucklandiae) moves qi and prevents the stagnating nature of the tonic herbs from impairing the Spleen and Stomach. *Sheng Jiang* (Rhizoma Zingiberis Recens) and *Da Zao* (Fructus Jujubae) harmonize the middle *jiao*. In short, this formula nourishes the Heart, strengthens the Spleen, and tonifies both qi and blood.

VETERINARY MODIFICATIONS

- With poor appetite, add *Chen Pi* (Pericarpium Citri Reticulatae) and *Ban Xia* (Rhizoma Pinelliae), *Sha Ren* (Fructus Amomi) and *Cang Zhu* (Rhizoma Atractylodis).
- If there is cough, add *Zi Wan* (Radix et Rhizoma Asteris) and *Jie Geng* (Radix Platycodonis).
- To tonify blood and stop bleeding, add *Shu Di Huang* (Radix Rehmanniae Praeparata) and *E Jiao* (Colla Corii Asini).

CAUTIONS / CONTRAINDICATIONS

- *Gui Pi Tang* is contraindicated in cases of interior heat or yin deficiency with a rapid pulse.
- This formula is relatively neutral in property and usually does not produce side effects even with long-term use.
- Avoid excessive physical exercise and feeding diets that are raw and cold in nature.

PHARMACOLOGICAL EFFECTS

1. **Antiulcer**: Use of *Gui Pi Tang* was effective in preventing stress-induced ulcer in mice. The mechanism of action was attributed to the regulatory effect of the herbs on the central nervous system to reduce the production and secretion of gastric acid.[1]
2. **Cognitive**: Use of *Gui Pi Tang* was effective in improving cognition in mice with impaired memory due to drugs, electric shock, or aging.[2]

HUMAN CLINICAL STUDIES AND RESEARCH

1. **Hepatitis**: In one report, 9 patients with hepatitis and thrombopenia were treated with modified *Gui Pi Tang* with recovery in 5 patients (asymptomatic with no recurrence within 2 years), improvement in 2 patients, and no benefit in 2 patients. Most patients began to notice improvement within 14-21 days of treatment.[3]
2. **Anemia**: In one study, 19 patients with anemia due to iron deficiency were treated with 79% effectiveness within one month.[4] In another study, 20 patients with anemia due to hemorrhage were treated for an average of 24 doses (ranges from 5-49 doses) of decoction with good results.[5] Lastly, its effectiveness is documented in patients with compromised kidney function with anemia and leucopenia.[6]
3. **Thrombopenic purpura**: In one study, 46 patients with primary thrombopenic purpura were treated with modified *Gui Pi Tang* with good results. The formula included *Huang Qi* (Radix Astragali) 15-30g, *Dang Gui* (Radix Angelicae Sinensis) 10-15g, *Di Huang* (Radix Rehmanniae) 10-30g, *Ce Bai Ye* (Cacumen Platycladi) 15-30g, *He Ye* (Folium Nelumbinis) 10-15g, dry-fried *Huai Hua* (Flos

***Gui Pi Tang* (Restore the Spleen Decoction)**

Diagnosis	Clinical Signs	Treatment	Herbs
Heart and Spleen deficiencies	• Tachycardia, arrhythmias, inability to concentrate and follow commands, anxiety, and insomnia: Heart blood deficiency • Poor appetite, lethargy and easily fatigued: Spleen qi deficiency • A pale, dry tongue: qi and blood deficiencies • Weak and thready pulse: qi and blood deficiencies	• Tonifies qi and nourishes the blood • Strengthens the Spleen and nourishes the Heart	• *Ren Shen* (Radix et Rhizoma Ginseng), *Huang Qi* (Radix Astragali), *Bai Zhu* (Rhizoma Atractylodis Macrocephalae), and *Zhi Gan Cao* (Radix et Rhizoma Glycyrrhizae Praeparata cum Melle) warm and tonify Spleen qi. • *Dang Gui* (Radix Angelicae Sinensis) and *Long Yan Rou* (Arillus Longan) nourish the Liver, tonify Heart blood, and regulate blood circulation. • *Fu Shen* (Poria Paradicis), *Yuan Zhi* (Radix Polygalae) and *Suan Zao Ren* (Semen Ziziphi Spinosae) nourish the Heart to calm the *shen* (spirit). • *Mu Xiang* (Radix Aucklandiae) moves qi and moderates the stagnating nature of the tonic herbs. • *Sheng Jiang* (Rhizoma Zingiberis Recens) and *Da Zao* (Fructus Jujubae) harmonize the middle *jiao*.

Guī Pí Tāng (Restore the Spleen Decoction)

Sophorae) 10-15g, *Shan Zhu Yu* (Fructus Corni) 10-30g, *San Qi* (Radix et Rhizoma Notoginseng) 2-6g given in powder separately, *Xian He Cao* (Herba Agrimoniae) 30g, *E Jiao* (Colla Corii Asini) 10-15g dissolved in decoction immediately before ingestion, and *Gan Cao* (Radix et Rhizoma Glycyrrhizae) 10g. The treatment protocol was to administer the herbs in decoction one time daily for one month per course of treatment. The average length of treatment was three courses. Out of 46 patients, the study reported marked effect in 11 patients (asymptomatic with normal platelet count for at least 3 months), improvement in 15 patients (asymptomatic with normal platelet count for at least 2 months), slight improvement in 11 patients (slight subjective and objective improvement) and no benefit in 9 patients. The overall rate of effectiveness was 80.4%.[7]

4. **Choroidopathy**: Use of modified *Gui Pi Tang* in 57 patients with choroidopathy was associated with complete recovery in 35 patients, improvement in 18 patients, and no benefit in 4 patients. The herbal treatment was based on *Gui Pi Tang*, with the removal of *Yuan Zhi* (Radix Polygalae) and *Long Yan Rou* (Arillus Longan), and the addition of *Gou Qi Zi* (Fructus Lycii), *Gu Jing Cao* (Flos Eriocauli), *Mi Meng Hua* (Flos Buddlejae), and others. Modifications were made as follows: for Liver and Kidney yin deficiencies, *Tai Zi Shen* (Radix Pseudostellariae), *Shan Zhu Yu* (Fructus Corni), *Di Huang* (Radix Rehmanniae), *Mu Dan Pi* (Cortex Moutan), and *Ju Hua* (Flos Chrysanthemi) were added, and *Dang Shen* (Radix Codonopsis) and *Mu Xiang* (Radix Aucklandiae) were removed; and for Liver qi stagnation, *Chai Hu* (Radix Bupleuri), *Yu Jin* (Radix Curcumae), *Bai Shao* (Radix Paeoniae Alba), and *Chuan Xiong* (Rhizoma Chuanxiong) were added, and *Dang Shen* (Radix Codonopsis) and *Huang Qi* (Radix Astragali) were removed.[8]

SUGGESTED ACUPUNCTURE TREATMENT

1. Points: *Xinshu* (BL 15), *Pishu* (BL 20), *Housanli* (ST 36), *Sanyinjiao* (SP 6), and *Shenmen* (HT 7).
2. Technique: tonification.

Xinshu (BL 15) and *Pishu* (BL 20) nourish and regulate blood circulation. *Housanli* (ST 36) tonifies Spleen qi and blood. *Sanyinjiao* (SP 6) nourishes yin and blood. *Shenmen* (HT 7) and *Xinshu* (BL 15) calm the *shen* (spirit) and nourish the blood.

AUTHORS' COMMENTS

Gui Pi Tang, literally "Restore the Spleen Decoction," has important functions to tonify qi, generate blood, and restore and normalize the transportation and transformation functions of the Spleen. It is vital to ensure that the Spleen functions properly, as it is the root of postnatal qi and the source of all qi and blood after birth.

Gui Pi Tang is commonly used to treat dogs with immune-mediated hemolytic anemia (IHA) and immune-mediated thrombocytopenia (ITP). Herbal formula treatment for this disease is highly effective and can help to decrease the high mortality rate seen; the mortality rates reported in dogs with IHA range from 20–75%. In dogs with ITP the mortality rate ranges from 10-30%, with a recurrence rate of 40%. *Gui Pi Tang* can be given with transfusions and/or in combination with steroidal, antimicrobial (doxycycline, enrofloxacin, cephalexin) and immunosuppressive drugs (azathioprine, cyclosporine, cytoxan), without adverse effects. Generally, the dose of steroids is gradually reduced over time, and the hematocrit and other blood parameters are closely monitored as the animal is weaned off steroids. Herbal formulas to treat hemolytic and platelet disorders typically require administration for a minimum of three months, with modifications made as needed. Therapy should be started as soon as possible for best results. *Gui Pi Tang* can be used alone, but may require modification, depending on the case. To stop bleeding, add *E Jiao* (Colla Corii Asini), *Pu Huang* (Pollen Typhae), *Xian He Cao* (Herba Agrimoniae), *Mo Han Lian* (Herba Ecliptae) and *Ou Jie (Nodus Nelumbinis Rhizomatis)*; with damp-heat, add *Dan Shen* (Radix et Rhizoma Salviae Miltiorrhizae), *Huang Lian* (Rhizoma Coptidis), *Zhi Zi* (Fructus Gardeniae), *Xuan Shen* (Radix Scrophulariae) and *Di Huang* (Radix Rehmanniae); with Spleen yang deficiency and cold, add *E Jiao* (Colla Corii Asini) and *Fu Zi* (Radix Aconiti Lateralis Praeparata).

Gui Pi Tang can be used to treat non-regenerative anemia seen in dogs with congestive heart failure with qi and blood deficiencies; it can be used long term without adverse effects. For the treatment of cardiac arrhythmia, *Long Gu* (Os Draconis) and *Dang Shen* (Radix Codonopsis) should be added.

Gui Pi Tang can address cases of chronic nasal bleeding in horses. Often these patients are not racehorses with exercise-induced pulmonary hemorrhage (EIPH), but instead are sport horses that have been overworked and are suffering from deficiencies of the Spleen, which compromise the Spleen's ability to hold blood in the vessels. These nosebleeds may or may not be associated with exertion and can result from both pulmonary and ethmoid hemorrhage.

Gui Pi Tang, *Si Wu Tang* (Four-Substance Decoction), and *Dang Gui Bu Xue Tang* (Tangkuei Decoction to Tonify the

Guī Pí Tāng (Restore the Spleen Decoction)

Blood) are three of the most commonly used formulas to tonify qi, and to nourish and generate blood. Their differences are as follows:

- *Gui Pi Tang* mainly strengthens the Spleen and tonifies qi to generate blood. It treats qi and blood deficiencies of the Spleen, as well as Heart deficiency patterns that manifest in clinical signs such as arrhythmia, tachycardia, inability to concentrate and follow commands, restlessness at night, easily fatigued, poor appetite, lethargy, a pale, dry tongue, and a thready, weak pulse. Because the Spleen is responsible for holding blood in the vessels, this formula is effective for bleeding disorders caused by Spleen deficiency. It is most often used for chronic problems in which Spleen qi deficiency has led to blood deficiency.
- *Si Wu Tang* focuses on the Liver and the *chong* (thoroughfare) and *ren* (conception) channels. It nourishes Liver blood and regulates the blood. It is the base formula for many other blood deficiency formulas and is not appropriate for acute blood loss. *Si Wu Tang* is composed of herbs that can be stagnating to the middle *jiao,* and thus it is often combined with herbs to promote digestion of this formula for best results.
- *Dang Gui Bu Xue Tang* tonifies qi and generates blood and is similar to *Gui Pi Tang* in that it tonifies the Spleen to generate blood. However, it is more appropriate for acute blood loss and is often combined with another formula to specifically treat the individual animal.

Gui Pi Tang and *Tian Wang Bu Xin Dan* (Emperor of Heaven's Special Pill to Tonify the Heart) both nourish the Heart and calm the *shen* (spirit) to treat palpitations, poor concentration, restlessness, and anxiety.

- *Gui Pi Tang* is designed for qi and blood deficiencies of the Spleen and Heart. Other than *shen* disturbance signs, animals will exhibit poor appetite, lethargy, exercise intolerance, fatigue, poor concentration, and other Spleen deficiency signs. In addition to tranquilizing herbs such as *Suan Zao Ren* (Semen Ziziphi Spinosae), *Fu Shen* (Poria Paradicis), *Long Yan Rou* (Arillus Longan), and *Yuan Zhi* (Radix Polygalae), this formula contains Spleen tonic herbs, such as *Ren Shen* (Radix et Rhizoma Ginseng), *Huang Qi* (Radix Astragali), *Bai Zhu* (Rhizoma Atractylodis Macrocephalae), and *Gan Cao* (Radix et Rhizoma Glycyrrhizae).
- *Tian Wang Bu Xin Dan* is indicated for disharmony of the Heart and Kidney, with Kidney yin and blood deficiencies unable to nourish the Heart, leading to Heart fire. Besides blood deficiency signs such as palpitations, forgetfulness and insomnia, there will be symptoms of Heart fire, such as irritability, ulcers on the tongue, and dry stools or constipation. This formula uses herbs that nourish yin and blood and have tranquilizing and calming effects, such as *Suan Zao Ren* (Semen Ziziphi Spinosae), *Bai Zi Ren* (Semen Platycladi), *Yuan Zhi* (Radix Polygalae), *Tian Dong* (Radix Asparagi), and *Mai Dong* (Radix Ophiopogonis).[9]

Gui Pi Tang, *Tian Wang Bu Xin Dan* (Emperor of Heaven's Special Pill to Tonify the Heart), and *Suan Zao Ren Tang* (Sour Jujube Decoction) all nourish and calm the *shen* (spirit) to treat palpitations, poor concentration, insomnia, anxiety, restlessness, and associated clinical signs.

- *Gui Pi Tang* tonifies qi, nourishes the blood, and strengthens the Spleen. The two organs involved are the Spleen and Heart. Symptoms include poor appetite, fatigue, lethargy, and possible bleeding disorders. The tongue is pale and dry, and the pulse is thready and weak. Affected animals can be of any age and include those with chronic disease, chronic Spleen qi deficiency from poor diet, anemia secondary to endoparasitism or flea infestation, etc.
- *Tian Wang Bu Xin Dan* nourishes yin and blood to tonify the Heart and calm the *shen*. Key organs involved are the Heart and Kidney. In addition to signs of *shen* disturbance, signs of yin and blood deficiencies include dry stools, a red tongue body with no coating, and a thready, rapid pulse. Most animals that suffer from Heart and Kidney deficiencies are usually older.
- *Suan Zao Ren Tang* nourishes the blood, calms the *shen*, clears heat, and relieves irritability. It treats Liver blood deficiency with flaring of deficiency fire causing *shen* disturbance. The key organ involved is the Liver, with signs of vertigo, irritability, and a thin, wiry pulse. Animals for which *Suan Zao Ren Tang* is appropriate are often under stress for prolonged periods of time and have depleted their Liver blood; this includes many breeding, show and performance animals.

Gui Pi Tang and *Bu Zhong Yi Qi Tang* (Tonify the Middle and Augment the Qi Decoction) both use *Ren Shen* (Radix et Rhizoma Ginseng), *Huang Qi* (Radix Astragali), *Bai Zhu* (Rhizoma Atractylodis Macrocephalae), and *Gan Cao* (Radix et Rhizoma Glycyrrhizae) to tonify qi and strengthen the Spleen. The difference is:

- The other herbs in *Gui Pi Tang* focus on nourishing the *shen* (spirit) and tonifying the blood. This formula targets the Heart and Spleen, and is used to treat bleeding disorders in addition to *shen* disturbance.
- The other herbs in *Bu Zhong Yi Qi Tang* lift yang and treat prolapse. This formula targets the Spleen and Stomach, and is mainly used for qi deficiency leading to organ prolapse.

References

1. *Tian Jin Zhong Yi* (Tianjin Chinese Medicine), 1995; 4:28.
2. *Zhong Yao Yao Li Yu Lin Chuang* (Pharmacology and Clinical Applications of Chinese Herbs), 1990; 6(5):2.
3. *Zhong Yi Za Zhi* (Journal of Chinese Medicine), 1985; 5:32.

Guī Pí Tāng (Restore the Spleen Decoction)

4. *Zhong Cheng Yao Yan Jiu* (Research of Chinese Patent Medicine), 1987; 5:20.
5. *Shan Xi Zhong Yi Xue Yuan Xue Bao* (Journal of Shanxi University School of Chinese Medicine), 1988; 1:29.
6. *Guo Wai Yi Yao Zhi Wu Yao Fen Ce* (Monograph of Foreign Botanical Medicine), 1993; 15(3):44.
7. *Bei Jing Zhong Yi Za Zhi* (Beijing Journal of Chinese Medicine), 1993; 3:227.
8. *Shi Yong Zhong Yi Za Zhi* (Journal of Practical Chinese Medicine), 1997; 6:5.
9. Wang MZ, et al. *Zhong Yi Xue Wen Da Ti Ku* (Questions and Answers on Traditional Chinese Medicine: Herbal Formulas).

Zhì Gān Cǎo Tāng (Honey-Fried Licorice Decoction)

炙甘草湯

炙甘草汤

Pinyin Name: *Zhi Gan Cao Tang*
Literal Name: Honey-Fried Licorice Decoction
Alternate Names: *Fu Mai Tang* (Restore the Pulse Decoction), *Chih Kan Tsao Tang*, Baked Licorice Decoction, Roasted Licorice Decoction, Licorice Combination
Original Source: *Shang Han Lun* (Discussion of Cold-Induced Disorders) by Zhang Zhong-Jing in the Eastern Han Dynasty

COMPOSITION

Zhi Gan Cao (Radix et Rhizoma Glycyrrhizae Praeparata cum Melle)	12g
Ren Shen (Radix et Rhizoma Ginseng)	6g
Da Zao (Fructus Jujubae), *bo* (opened)	30 pieces [5-10 pieces]
Di Huang (Radix Rehmanniae)	48g [30g]
Mai Dong (Radix Ophiopogonis)	0.5 cup [9g]
E Jiao (Colla Corii Asini)	6g
Huo Ma Ren (Fructus Cannabis)	0.5 cup [9g]
Sheng Jiang (Rhizoma Zingiberis Recens), *qie* (sliced)	9g
Gui Zhi (Ramulus Cinnamomi)	9g

DOSAGE / PREPARATION / ADMINISTRATION

Cook the ingredients, except *E Jiao* (Colla Corii Asini), in approximately 7 cups [1,400 mL] of grain-based liquor and 8 cups [1,600 mL] of water until it is reduced to 3 cups [600 mL]. Add *E Jiao* (Colla Corii Asini) to the warm, strained decoction and allow it to completely dissolve. Take 1 cup [200 mL] of the warm decoction three times a day. Today, this formula is usually prepared as decoction by cooking the ingredients in water to obtain a decoction. Use the doses suggested in brackets above. Add 10 mL of grain-based liquor to the warm, strained decoction. Separately dissolve *E Jiao* (Colla Corii Asini) in boiling water, and add it to the warm, strained decoction. Take the decoction in three equally divided doses and finish it within one day.

CHINESE THERAPEUTIC ACTIONS

1. Tonifies qi and nourishes yin
2. Tonifies the blood and restores the pulse

CLINICAL MANIFESTATIONS

1. Qi and blood deficiencies: a bound or intermittent pulse, arrhythmia, general weakness, irritability, anxiety, insomnia, exercise intolerance, and a dry, pale or red tongue.
2. Lung atrophy due to deficiency and consumption: dry coughing with little or no sputum, bloody streaks in the

Zhì Gān Cǎo Tāng (Honey-Fried Licorice Decoction)

sputum, shortness of breath, thin, poor body condition, constipation, and a dry tongue and mouth.

VETERINARY CLINICAL APPLICATIONS

Congestive heart failure, cardiomyopathy, arrhythmia, atrial fibrillation, hypotension and anemia.

EXPLANATION

Zhi Gan Cao Tang (Honey-Fried Licorice Decoction) treats a bound or intermittent pulse caused by qi and blood deficiencies. In this condition, qi is deficient and cannot flow freely, and blood is deficient and cannot nourish the Heart. Arrhythmia, general weakness, exercise intolerance, and a dry, pale or red tongue indicate qi deficiency. Insomnia, irritability, anxiety, a dry pale to red tongue and a thin, weak pulse, indicate yin and blood deficiencies. Dry coughing with little or no sputum, the presence of blood in the sputum, and a dry mouth and tongue suggest yin and body fluid deficiencies.

Zhi Gan Cao (Radix et Rhizoma Glycyrrhizae Praeparata cum Melle), *Ren Shen* (Radix et Rhizoma Ginseng), and *Da Zao* (Fructus Jujubae) tonify Heart and Spleen qi. *Di Huang* (Radix Rehmanniae), *Mai Dong* (Radix Ophiopogonis), *E Jiao* (Colla Corii Asini), and *Huo Ma Ren* (Fructus Cannabis) tonify Heart blood, nourish Lung yin, and replenish body fluids. *Sheng Jiang* (Rhizoma Zingiberis Recens), *Gui Zhi* (Ramulus Cinnamomi), and the grain-based alcohol activate yang and qi flow to restore the pulse.

This formula also can be used to treat Lung atrophy due to deficiency and consumption. This condition is characterized by Lung yin deficiency, with symptoms such as dry coughing with little or no sputum. However, if there are severe symptoms of yin deficiency, the doses of *Sheng Jiang* (Rhizoma Zingiberis Recens), *Gui Zhi* (Ramulus Cinnamomi) and grain-based alcohol should be decreased.

VETERINARY MODIFICATIONS

- If there is qi deficiency, add *Huang Qi* (Radix Astragali).
- With more severe fibrillation, add *Hu Po* (Succinum).
- With congestive heart failure, add *Sheng Mai San* (Generate the Pulse Powder).
- To enhance the overall functions of tonifying blood, yin, and body fluids, add *Bai Shao* (Radix Paeoniae Alba).
- If there is yang deficiency, add *Fu Zi* (Radix Aconiti Lateralis Praeparata).
- With restlessness, add *Suan Zao Ren* (Semen Ziziphi Spinosae) and *Bai Zi Ren* (Semen Platycladi).
- With generalized fatigue and deficiency, add *Tian Dong* (Radix Asparagi) and *Shu Di Huang* (Radix Rehmanniae Praeparata).
- With poor appetite and phlegm, add *Chen Pi* (Pericarpium Citri Reticulatae) and *Ban Xia* (Rhizoma Pinelliae).
- With cough due to Lung deficiency, add *Jie Geng* (Radix Platycodonis) and *Zhi Shi* (Fructus Aurantii Immaturus).
- With irritability and fearfulness, add *Huang Qi* (Radix Astragali) and *Wu Wei Zi* (Fructus Schisandrae Chinensis).
- For edema, add *Fu Ling* (Poria) and *Che Qian Zi* (Semen Plantaginis).

CAUTIONS / CONTRAINDICATIONS

Zhi Gan Cao Tang has a slight moistening and lubricating effect on the intestines. Therefore, it should be used with caution in animals with diarrhea and dysentery.[1]

***Zhi Gan Cao Tang* (Honey-Fried Licorice Decoction)**

Diagnosis	Clinical Signs	Treatment	Herbs
Bound or intermittent pulse with qi and blood deficiencies	• Bound or intermittent pulse with arrhythmia: qi deficiency unable to flow freely, and blood deficiency unable to nourish the Heart • General weakness, exercise intolerance, and thin, poor body condition: qi deficiency • Irritability, anxiety, insomnia, a dry, pale tongue, and a thin, weak pulse: yin and blood deficiencies • Dry coughing with little or no sputum, the presence of blood in the sputum, and a dry mouth and tongue: yin and body fluid deficiencies	• Tonifies qi and nourishes yin • Tonifies the blood and restores the pulse	• *Zhi Gan Cao* (Radix et Rhizoma Glycyrrhizae Praeparata cum Melle), *Ren Shen* (Radix et Rhizoma Ginseng) and *Da Zao* (Fructus Jujubae) tonify Heart and Spleen qi. • *Di Huang* (Radix Rehmanniae), *Mai Dong* (Radix Ophiopogonis), *E Jiao* (Colla Corii Asini), and *Huo Ma Ren* (Fructus Cannabis) tonify Heart blood, nourish Lung yin, and replenish body fluids. • *Sheng Jiang* (Rhizoma Zingiberis Recens), *Gui Zhi* (Ramulus Cinnamomi), and grain-based alcohol activate yang and qi flow to restore the pulse.

Zhì Gān Cǎo Tāng (Honey-Fried Licorice Decoction)

PHARMACOLOGICAL EFFECTS

1. **Cardiovascular**: Injection of a preparation of *Zhi Gan Cao Tang* was associated with an inhibitory effect on the cardiac tissues to lower the heart rate, reduce the contractile force of the heart, and decrease the blood perfusion to the coronary artery. Its inhibitory effect also counters the stimulating effect of adrenalin.[2] Additionally, administration of this formula was shown to have a protective effect against ischemia of the cardiac muscles.[3]
2. **Antiarrhythmic**: *Zhi Gan Cao Tang* has been shown in many studies to be beneficial in treating arrhythmia due to various causes. In one report, administration of the formula in many different animal subjects was effective in treating arrhythmia induced by drugs such as aconitine, $CaCl_2$, and adrenalin.[4]

HUMAN CLINICAL STUDIES AND RESEARCH

1. **Arrhythmia**: In a clinical study, patients with coronary heart disease and arrhythmia were divided into two groups. The first group of 23 patients received the normal dose of the herbs decocted in water and alcohol. The second group of 23 patients received only 25% the normal dose of the herbs decocted in water without alcohol. All patients were monitored for their signs (ECG) and symptoms (palpitations, shortness of breath, fatigue, and chest congestion). At the end of treatment, the study reported that out of 23 patients in the first group, 16 patients had complete recovery, 4 had marked improvement, and 3 showed no change. In comparison with the second group of 23 patients, 6 patients had complete recovery, 9 had marked improvement, and 8 showed no change. The overall rate of effectiveness was 87.1% in the first group, and 65.2% in the second group.[5]
2. **Angina pectoris**: One hundred and fifty patients with angina pectoris and coronary heart disease were treated with modified *Zhi Gan Cao Tang* with marked effect in 48 patients, improvement in 90 patients, and no change in 12 patients. The overall rate of effectiveness was 92%. Most patients began to notice improvement within 1-3 weeks. The herbal formula was based on *Zhi Gan Cao Tang*, with elimination of *Huo Ma Ren* (Fructus Cannabis) and *Sheng Jiang* (Rhizoma Zingiberis Recens), and the addition of *Gui Ban* (Plastrum Testudinis), *Wu Wei Zi* (Fructus Schisandrae Chinensis), and *Ji Xue Teng* (Caulis Spatholobi).[6]
3. **Viral myocarditis**: Use of *Zhi Gan Cao Tang* in 38 patients with viral myocarditis was associated with complete recovery in 30 patients, improvement in 4 patients, no change in 2 patients, and fatality in 2 patients.[7] Another report stated 87.5% effectiveness (21 of 24 patients) using this formula to treat viral myocarditis.[8]
4. **Hypotension**: Fifty patients with low blood pressure were treated with good results using modified *Zhi Gan Cao Tang*. Most patients responded within 1-2 weeks, while some needed up to 1 month of herbal therapy. The average length of treatment was 15.8 days.[9]

SUGGESTED ACUPUNCTURE TREATMENT

1. Points: *Taiyuan* (LU 9), *Feishu* (BL 13), *Gaohuangshu* (BL 43), *Pishu* (BL 20), *Housanli* (ST 36), *Sanyinjiao* (SP 6), *Taixi* (KI 3), *Geshu* (BL 17), and *Shentang* (BL 44).
2. Technique: tonification.

Taiyuan (LU 9) and *Feishu* (BL 13) nourish the Lung. *Gaohuangshu* (BL 43) is an essential point for all kinds of deficiency syndromes. *Pishu* (BL 20), *Sanyinjiao* (SP 6), and *Housanli* (ST 36) nourish the middle *jiao* to increase the production of blood. *Taixi* (KI 3) nourishes Kidney yin. *Geshu* (BL 17) and *Shentang* (BL 44) nourish the blood and Heart.

AUTHORS' COMMENTS

Historically, *Zhi Gan Cao Tang* is indicated for a bound pulse (结脉 *jie mai*, also translated as a knotted pulse, is a slow pulse with pulses at irregular intervals) and for an intermittent pulse (代脉 *dai mai*, which is a pulse interspersed with more relatively regular pauses). Because of its ability to restore normal rhythmic pulse, *Zhi Gan Cao Tang* is also known as 复脉汤 *Fu Mai Tang* (Restore the Pulse Decoction).

Zhi Gan Cao Tang and *Sheng Mai San* (Generate the Pulse Powder) both treat "pulse" disorders, but have the following similarities and differences:

- *Zhi Gan Cao Tang* treats a bound or intermittent pulse caused by qi and blood deficiencies and their subsequent inability to nourish Heart *shen* (spirit). Additional signs include arrhythmia, general weakness, irritability, anxiety, insomnia, exercise intolerance, a dry, pale or red tongue, and a thin, weak pulse. *Zhi Gan Cao Tang* nourishes Heart blood and tonifies Heart yang to "restore the pulse."
- *Sheng Mai San* treats a deficient, fine pulse caused by heat injuring qi and yin. Additional symptoms include profuse sweating, fatigue, exercise intolerance, a dry throat, and thirst. *Sheng Mai San* tonifies qi, promotes the production of body fluids, and astringes yin to "generate the pulse."[10]

Zhi Gan Cao Tang has excellent functions to tonify qi, replenish the blood, nourish yin, and warm yang. It can be used for the treatment of many cardiac conditions in the dog and horse that include atrial fibrillation and dilated cardiomyopathy (DCM) with qi and yin deficiencies.

Zhì Gān Căo Tāng (Honey-Fried Licorice Decoction)

- In equines with atrial fibrillation, it can be combined with *Gui Pi Tang* (Restore the Spleen Decoction). To improve clinical efficacy, add *Huang Qi* (Radix Astragali), *Dan Shen* (Radix et Rhizoma Salviae Miltiorrhizae), *Wu Wei Zi* (Fructus Schisandrae Chinensis), *Mu Li* (Concha Ostreae) and *Hong Jing Tian* (Radix et Rhizoma Rhodiolae Crenulatae).
- In dogs this formula has been found to be very effective in the treatment of congestive heart failure, with or without cardiac arrhythmias, due to qi and yin deficiencies. For this application, add *Huang Qi* (Radix Astragali) and *Dan Shen* (Radix et Rhizoma Salviae Miltiorrhizae). With these modifications, this formula can be used long term for periods of 6 months or more.
- This formula can be used for cancer patients undergoing chemotherapy with subsequent leukopenia, by adding *Suan Zao Ren* (Semen Ziziphi Spinosae), *Ji Xue Teng* (Caulis Spatholobi), *Huang Qi* (Radix Astragali) and *Gou Qi Zi* (Fructus Lycii). An increase in the red blood cell count can be seen as well when using this combination. It generally takes a minimum of 2 weeks to see measurable results.
- In animals with anemia and chronic cardiac disease, it can be given to restore normal red blood cell counts.

Zhi Gan Cao Tang and *Tian Wang Bu Xin Dan* (Emperor of Heaven's Special Pill to Tonify the Heart) both nourish yin and blood to treat palpitations, anxiety, insomnia, and dry stools.

- *Zhi Gan Cao Tang* addresses qi and blood deficiencies. Insufficiency of blood fails to nourish the Heart. When qi is deficient, the yang is weak and cannot generate the pulse, which leads to a bound or intermittent pulse. Thus, qi tonics must be used in conjunction with yin and blood tonics to generate the pulse. *Shu Di Huang* (Radix Rehmanniae Praeparata), *Sheng Jiang* (Rhizoma Zingiberis Recens), *E Jiao* (Colla Corii Asini), *Mai Dong* (Radix Ophiopogonis), and *Da Zao* (Fructus Jujubae) nourish yin and blood. *Ren Shen* (Radix et Rhizoma Ginseng) and *Zhi Gan Cao* (Radix et Rhizoma Glycyrrhizae Praeparata cum Melle) warm and tonify qi. *Gui Zhi* (Ramulus Cinnamomi) and *Sheng Jiang* (Rhizoma Zingiberis Recens) assist Heart yang to restore the pulse.
- *Tian Wang Bu Xin Dan* is suitable for Heart yin and blood deficiencies, with excess Heart yang flaring. Anxiety, decreased sleep, *shen* (spirit) disturbance with fearfulness and nervousness are the results of the *shen* not being nourished. Thus, nourishing herbs and *shen*-calming herbs are used together.[11]

References

1. *Zhong Yao Ming Fang Yao Li Yu Ying Yong* (Pharmacology and Applications of Famous Herbal Formulas), 1989; 299-300.
2. *Zhong Yao Yao Li Yu Lin Chuang* (Pharmacology and Clinical Applications of Chinese Herbs), 1994; 6:1.
3. *Zhong Yao Yao Li Yu Lin Chuang* (Pharmacology and Clinical Applications of Chinese Herbs), 1994; 4:5.
4. *Zhong Yi Fang Ji Xian Dai Yan Jiu* (Modern Study of Medical Formulas in Traditional Chinese Medicine), 1997; 622.
5. *Shan Xi Yi Kan* (Shanxi Journal of Medicine), 1995; 15(9):399.
6. *Tian Jin Yi Yao* (Tianjin Medicine and Herbology), 1972; 26.
7. *Jiang Su Zhong Yi Za Zhi* (Jiangsu Journal of Chinese Medicine), 1984; 5(1):25.
8. *Shang Hai Zhong Yi Yao Za Zhi* (Shanghai Journal of Chinese Medicine and Herbology), 1989; 5:36.
9. *Si Chuan Zhong Yi* (Sichuan Chinese Medicine), 1995; 9:20.
10. Wang MZ, et al. *Zhong Yi Xue Wen Da Ti Ku* (Questions and Answers on Traditional Chinese Medicine: Herbal Formulas).
11. Wang MZ, et al. *Zhong Yi Xue Wen Da Ti Ku* (Questions and Answers on Traditional Chinese Medicine: Herbal Formulas).

Dāng Guī Sháo Yào Sǎn (Tangkuei and Peony Powder)

當歸芍藥散
当归芍药散

Pinyin Name: *Dang Gui Shao Yao San*
Literal Name: Tangkuei and Peony Powder
Alternate Names: *Tang Kuei Shao Yao San*, Tang-kuei and Peony Formula, Tangkuei and Peony Formula
Original Source: *Jin Gui Yao Lue* (Essentials from the Golden Cabinet) by Zhang Zhong-Jing in the Eastern Han Dynasty

COMPOSITION

Dang Gui (Radix Angelicae Sinensis)	9g
Chuan Xiong (Rhizoma Chuanxiong)	24g [9g]
Bai Shao (Radix Paeoniae Alba)	48g
Bai Zhu (Rhizoma Atractylodis Macrocephalae)	12g
Fu Ling (Poria)	12g
Ze Xie (Rhizoma Alismatis)	24g

DOSAGE / PREPARATION / ADMINISTRATION

The source text states to grind the ingredients into a fine powder. Take 6g of powder per dose with a grain-based liquor three times daily. Today, this formula can also be given in decoction twice daily, with the dose of *Chuan Xiong* (Rhizoma Chuanxiong) suggested in brackets. Note: The source text states to use 24g of *Chuan Xiong* (Rhizoma Chuanxiong). Today, most practitioners and commercial products use only 9g.

CHINESE THERAPEUTIC ACTIONS

1. Nourishes the blood to soften the Liver
2. Strengthens the Spleen and resolves dampness

CLINICAL MANIFESTATIONS

Abdominal pain, with or without edema, due to disharmony of the Spleen and Liver and characterized by blood deficiency, Spleen deficiency, damp accumulation and qi stagnation: continuous cramping pain in the abdomen, anemia, diarrhea, vaginal discharge, fatigue, lack of energy, coldness of lower extremities, and edema.

VETERINARY CLINICAL APPLICATIONS

Abdominal pain secondary to the following: pregnancy, diarrhea, pancreatitis, cholangitis, urinary bladder and renal calculi, vaginal discharge, habitual abortion, infertility and anemia.

EXPLANATION

Dang Gui Shao Yao San (Tangkuei and Peony Powder) was originally formulated to treat abdominal pain and edema during pregnancy, characterized by blood deficiency and abnormal water circulation. Abdominal pain is generally considered to be the main indication for this formula. Due to the deficient nature of the illness, the abdominal pain is characterized as dull, cramping, and continuous but not severe. It is generally accompanied by coldness in the lower extremities. Since there is blood deficiency, patients could present with anemia, fatigue and lack of energy. If there is significant abnormal water circulation, animals may present with edema that develops most frequently in the hind legs.

***Dang Gui Shao Yao San* (Tangkuei and Peony Powder)**

Diagnosis	Clinical Signs	Treatment	Herbs
Abdominal pain with edema due to blood deficiency and abnormal water metabolism	• Anemia and coldness in the lower extremities: blood deficiency • Edema, vaginal discharge, and diarrhea: abnormal water metabolism with damp accumulation	• Nourishes the blood to soften the Liver • Strengthens the Spleen to regulate water metabolism	• *Dang Gui* (Radix Angelicae Sinensis) tonifies the blood and activates blood circulation. • *Chuan Xiong* (Rhizoma Chuanxiong) activates and regulates blood circulation. • *Bai Shao* (Radix Paeoniae Alba) nourishes the blood and consolidates yin. • *Bai Zhu* (Rhizoma Atractylodis Macrocephalae) and *Fu Ling* (Poria) strengthen the Spleen and resolve dampness. • *Fu Ling* (Poria) and *Ze Xie* (Rhizoma Alismatis) relieve edema.

Dāng Guī Sháo Yào Săn (Tangkuei and Peony Powder)

Dang Gui (Radix Angelicae Sinensis) tonifies the blood and activates blood circulation. It treats anemia and relieves abdominal pain. *Chuan Xiong* (Rhizoma Chuanxiong) activates and regulates blood circulation. *Bai Shao* (Radix Paeoniae Alba) nourishes the blood and consolidates yin. In addition, *Bai Shao* (Radix Paeoniae Alba) has an excellent effect to relieve spasms and cramps of both the skeletal and smooth muscles. It is commonly used in large quantities to relieve abdominal pain and cramps. *Bai Zhu* (Rhizoma Atractylodis Macrocephalae) and *Fu Ling* (Poria) strengthen the Spleen and resolve dampness. *Fu Ling* (Poria) and *Ze Xie* (Rhizoma Alismatis) have a diuretic action to relieve edema.

VETERINARY MODIFICATIONS

- If there is severe abdominal pain, add *Yan Hu Suo* (Rhizoma Corydalis), *Xiang Fu* (Rhizoma Cyperi) and *Ai Ye* (Folium Artemisiae Argyi).
- If there are more signs and symptoms of cold, add *Wu Zhu Yu* (Fructus Evodiae) and *Gui Zhi* (Ramulus Cinnamomi).

PHARMACOLOGICAL EFFECTS

1. **Endocrine**: Administration of *Dang Gui Shao Yao San* has a stimulating effect on the production and secretion of hormones.[1] One *in vitro* study reported that *Dang Gui Shao Yao San* stimulated preovulatory follicles before a luteinizing hormone (LH) surge to secrete progesterone, but it suppressed estradiol-17 beta secretion by growing preovulatory follicles before a LH surge.[2]
2. **Ovulatory**: Administration of *Dang Gui Shao Yao San* has marked effects on the endocrine system and the ovaries. In one experiment, the use of *Dang Gui Shao Yao San* at 0.5 g/kg successfully induced ovulation in 30% of the mice. In contrast, the use of gonadotropin-releasing hormone was associated with a 65% success rate in promoting ovulation. Lastly, the combination of herbs and drugs were 90% effective in inducing ovulation. The study suggested that the formula has either a direct or an indirect stimulating effect on the endocrine system.[3] Another study stated that *Dang Gui Shao Yao San* may treat ovulatory disorders by stimulating both steroidogenesis and the ovulatory process.[4]
3. **Effect on uterus**: Administration of *Dang Gui Shao Yao San* was associated with an increased uterine weight in rats. This effect is voided if the ovaries were surgically removed.[5] Other studies suggested that this formula is beneficial in fertility by promoting implantation and early growth.[6]
4. **Hemodynamic**: Administration of *Dang Gui Shao Yao San* was associated with a dual effect on the hemodynamics of the blood. In one study, continuous administration of the formula at 0.5 g/kg for 17 days was associated with decreased viscosity of the blood in pregnant rats. In another study, it was noted that the formula was effective at stopping bleeding in mice and reduces the amount of blood loss during an injury.[7]
5. **Immunostimulant**: Administration of *Dang Gui Shao Yao San* was associated with a significant increase in lymphocyte proliferation in aged rats. It also showed an antagonizing effect against the inhibition of isoprel on lymphocyte proliferation.[8]
6. **Radioprotective**: One study evaluated the protective effect of *Dang Gui Shao Yao San* in mice treated with single X-irradiation. The study found that this formula had a dose-dependent effect that protected mice and prevented hematopoietic injury from sublethal effects of radiation. *Dang Gui Shao Yao San* was given at doses of 10 and 20 mg/20g body weight, for 7 consecutive days before irradiation. Pretreatment of *Dang Gui Shao Yao San* increased the number of femoral spleen colony-forming units (CFU-S) that survived irradiation, and significantly ameliorated leukopenia, thrombocytopenia and the degression of hematocrits after irradiation.[9]
7. **Antioxidant**: In one study in rats, administration of *Dang Gui Shao Yao San* was associated with free radical scavenging activity, which contributed to its prophylactic effect against free radical-mediated neurological diseases associated with aging.[10]

HUMAN CLINICAL STUDIES AND RESEARCH

1. **Abdominal pain during pregnancy**: One study reported 96.5% effectiveness using *Dang Gui Shao Yao San* to treat 86 pregnant women with abdominal pain. The duration of treatment ranged from 3-14 days.[11]
2. **Infertility**: Twenty women with infertility were treated with *Dang Gui Shao Yao San* with a 100% success rate. All 20 women became pregnant and had normal pregnancy and delivery. According to other references, the success rate of the formula is approximately 55%.[12]
3. **Habitual miscarriage**: Two studies reported that use of *Dang Gui Shao Yao San* and *Chai Ling Tang* (Bupleurum and Poria Decoction) helped to prevent autoimmunity-related recurrent miscarriage by correcting T helper-1/ T helper-2 balance.[13,14]
4. **Luteal insufficiency**: Administration of *Dang Gui Shao Yao San* in women with luteal insufficiency was found to be effective in improving luteal insufficiency as determined by daily measurement of basal body temperature and plasma progesterone levels. In women with normal menstrual cycles, use of the formula did not cause any adverse effects on hormonal levels such as prolactin, gonadotropins, steroids, estrogens, pregnanediol and luteinizing hormone (LH). No side effects were reported. The researchers concluded that *Dang Gui Shao Yao San* improves luteal insufficiency in women but does not affect

Dāng Guī Sháo Yào Săn (Tangkuei and Peony Powder)

the hormonal levels of women with normal menstrual cycles.[15]

HERB-DRUG INTERACTION

- **Colchicine-induced learning impairment**: Concurrent administration of *Dang Gui Shao Yao San* and colchicine was associated with improvement in learning acquisition deficit induced by colchicine in rats. The action mechanism of *Dang Gui Shao Yao San* may be involved in the increase in the level of superoxide dismutase.[16]
- **Drug-induced menopause**: One study evaluated the therapeutic effects of certain herbal medicines on menopausal symptoms induced by gonadotropin-releasing hormone agonist therapy in Japanese women with endometriosis, adenomyosis, or leiomyoma. According to this study, menopausal symptoms induced by gonadotropin-releasing hormone agonist therapy in 13 patients were successfully treated with *Dang Gui Shao Yao San*, *Shao Yao Gan Cao Tang* (Peony and Licorice Decoction), *Gui Zhi Fu Ling Wan* (Cinnamon Twig and Poria Pill), *Jia Wei Xiao Yao San* (Augmented Rambling Powder), *Tao He Cheng Qi Tang* (Peach Pit Decoction to Order the Qi), or *Gui Zhi Tang* (Cinnamon Twig Decoction). Of 11 patients with hot flashes, *Dang Gui Shao Yao San* provided some relief in all 11 patients, and total relief in 4 patients. Most importantly, there were no significant changes in serum estradiol levels after treatment with these herbal medicines. The researchers concluded that these herbal medicines can be recommended for menopausal symptoms induced by gonadotropin-releasing hormone agonists without a negative effect on serum estradiol levels.[17]

TOXICOLOGY

This formula has little toxicity. No fatality was reported following oral ingestion of the formula at 8-10 g/kg in mice. Moreover, no abnormalities were observed in the fetus following oral administration of the formula at 8 g/kg/day for 7-17 days in pregnant rats.[18]

SUGGESTED ACUPUNCTURE TREATMENT

1. Points: *Sanyinjiao* (SP 6), *Guanyuan* (CV 4), *Zigong* (CV 19), *Housanli* (ST 36), *Yinlingquan* (SP 9), and *Gongsun* (SP 4).
2. Technique: moxibustion and tonification.

Apply moxibustion on *Sanyinjiao* (SP 6), *Guanyuan* (CV 4), and *Zigong* (CV 19) to tonify and invigorate the blood and relieve pain. *Housanli* (ST 36), *Yinlingquan* (SP 9), and *Gongsun* (SP 4) tonify the Spleen and resolve phlegm.

AUTHORS' COMMENTS

Dang Gui Shao Yao San was originally designed to treat abdominal pain with edema during pregnancy. Today, its clinical applications have been greatly expanded to include various reproductive and abdominal disorders caused by Liver and Spleen disharmony, and characterized by pain, blood deficiency and/or damp accumulation. It can be particularly useful in mares with a tendency to colic during the last few months of pregnancy. This formula is most often used in veterinary medicine to tonify the blood post-surgically, and in animals with chronic illness caused by Liver and Spleen disharmony. It is a well-balanced formula, has a mild nature, and can be used for prolonged periods of time to tonify Liver blood without further aggravating Spleen deficiency and stagnation from damp accumulation. For these reasons, it is also helpful in the treatment of chronic skin disease with damp-heat and blood deficiency in dogs.

References

1. *Chang Yong Zhong Yao Cheng Fen Yu Yao Li Shou Ce* (A Handbook of the Composition and Pharmacology of Common Chinese Drugs), 1997; vol. 1, 238.
2. Usuki S. Effects of hachimijiogan, tokishakuyakusan, keishibukuryogan, ninjinto and unkeito on estrogen and progesterone secretion in preovulatory follicles incubated in vitro. Am J Chin Med. 1991; 19(1):65-71.
3. *Guo Wai Yi Xue* (Foreign Medicine), 1988; 10(4):44.
4. Irahara M, Yasui T, Tezuka M, Ushigoe K, Yamano S, Kamada M, Aono T. Evidence that Toki-shakuyaku-san and its ingredients enhance the secretion of a cytokine-induced neutrophil chemoattractant (CINC/gro) in the ovulatory process. Methods Find Exp Clin Pharmacol. 2000 Dec; 22(10):725-30.
5. *Guo Wai Yi Xue* (Foreign Medicine), 1988; 10(5):8.
6. *Zhong Yi Fang Ji Xian Dai Yan Jiu* (Modern Study of Medical Formulas in Traditional Chinese Medicine), 1997; (1):238.
7. *Zhong Yi Fang Ji Xian Dai Yan Jiu* (Modern Study of Medical Formulas in Traditional Chinese Medicine), 1997; (1):238.
8. He HW, Wang CE, Xie Y. Effect of supplemented danggui shaoyao powder and its disassembled prescriptions on lymphocytes proliferation in aged rats. Zhongguo Zhong Xi Yi Jie He Za Zhi. 2003 Nov; 23(11):841-4.
9. Hsu HY, Lin CC. A preliminary study on the radioprotection of mouse hematopoiesis by dang-gui-shao-yao-san. J Ethnopharmacol. 1996 Dec; 55(1):43-8.
10. Ueda Y, Komatsu M, Hiramatsu M. Free radical scavenging activity of the Japanese herbal medicine toki-shakuyaku-san (TJ-23) and its effect on superoxide dismutase activity, lipid peroxides, glutamate, and monoamine metabolites in aged rat brain. Neurochem Res. 1996 Aug; 21(8):909-14.
11. *Zhong Yuan Yi Kan* (Resource Journal of Chinese Medicine), 1992; 5:36.
12. *Zhong Cheng Yao Yan Jiu* (Research of Chinese Patent Medicine), 1984; (10):30.
13. Fujii T, Kanai T, Kozuma S, Hamai Y, Hyodo H, Yamashita T, Miki A, Unno N, Taketani Y. Theoretical basis for herbal medicines, Tokishakuyaku-san and Sairei-to, in the treatment of autoimmunity-related recurrent abortion by correcting T helper-1/T helper-2 balance. American Journal of Reproductive Immunology. 2000 Dec; 44(6):342-6.

Dāng Guī Sháo Yào Săn (Tangkuei and Peony Powder)

14. Fujii T. Herbal factors in the treatment of autoimmunity-related habitual abortion. Vitam Horm. 2002; 65:333-44.
15. Usuki S, Higa TN, Soreya K. The improvement of luteal insufficiency in fecund women by tokishakuyakusan treatment. American Journal of Chinese Medicine. 2002; 30(2-3):327-38.
16. Lu MC. Danggui shaoyao san improve colchichine-induced learning acquisition impairment in rats. Acta Pharmacol Sin. 2001 Dec; 22(12): 1149-53.
17. Tanaka T. Effects of herbal medicines on menopausal symptoms induced by gonadotropin-releasing hormone agonist therapy. Clin Exp Obstet Gynecol. 2001; 28(1):20-3.
18. *Zhe Jiang Zhong Yi Za Zhi* (Zhejiang Journal of Chinese Medicine), 1987; 22(8):345.

Sháo Yào Gān Căo Tāng (Peony and Licorice Decoction)

芍藥甘草湯
芍药甘草汤

Pinyin Name: *Shao Yao Gan Cao Tang*
Literal Name: Peony and Licorice Decoction
Alternate Names: *Shao Yao Kan Tsao Tang*, Peony and Licorice Combination
Original Source: *Shang Han Lun* (Discussion of Cold-Induced Disorders) by Zhang Zhong-Jing in the Eastern Han Dynasty

COMPOSITION

Bai Shao (Radix Paeoniae Alba)	12g
Zhi Gan Cao (Radix et Rhizoma Glycyrrhizae Praeparata cum Melle)	12g

DOSAGE / PREPARATION / ADMINISTRATION

Cook both herbs in 3 cups [600 mL] of water and reduce it to 1.5 cups [300 mL]. Take the warm, strained decoction in two equally divided doses.

CHINESE THERAPEUTIC ACTIONS

1. Tonifies yin and blood
2. Replenishes body fluids

CLINICAL MANIFESTATIONS

Spasms and cramps due to yin, blood and body fluid deficiencies: smooth or skeletal muscle spasms and cramps in various parts of the body, and tightness of the tendons and ligaments.

VETERINARY CLINICAL APPLICATIONS

Spasms, cramps, shaking and trembling of the rear legs, stomach and intestinal cramps, acute back pain, gastric and abdominal pain, colitis, constipation, pain associated with cholelithiasis or urolithiasis.

EXPLANATION

Shao Yao Gan Cao Tang (Peony and Licorice Decoction) can relieve various pains, spasms, or cramps caused by deficiencies of yin, blood, and body fluids. These conditions may arise as a result of excessive sweating, high fever, excessive use of exterior-releasing herbs, overwork, and injury.

Bai Shao (Radix Paeoniae Alba) nourishes yin, tonifies the blood, and replenishes body fluids. *Zhi Gan Cao* (Radix et Rhizoma Glycyrrhizae Praeparata cum Melle) strengthens the Spleen and tonifies qi. Together, they relieve spasms and cramps due to deficiencies of yin, blood, and body fluids.

Sháo Yào Gān Cǎo Tāng (Peony and Licorice Decoction)

Shao Yao Gan Cao Tang (Peony and Licorice Decoction)

Diagnosis	Clinical Signs	Treatment	Herbs
Spasms and cramps	Spasms and/or cramps: deficiencies of yin, blood and body fluids	• Tonifies yin and blood • Replenishes body fluids	• *Bai Shao* (Radix Paeoniae Alba) nourishes yin, tonifies the blood, and replenishes body fluids. • *Zhi Gan Cao* (Radix et Rhizoma Glycyrrhizae Praeparata cum Melle) strengthens the Spleen and tonifies qi.

VETERINARY MODIFICATIONS

- For spasms and cramps of the extremities, add *Xi Xin* (Radix et Rhizoma Asari) and *Gan Jiang* (Rhizoma Zingiberis).
- If there is dysuria, add *Bai Zhu* (Rhizoma Atractylodis Macrocephalae) and *Fu Ling* (Poria).
- With back pain, add *Du Zhong* (Cortex Eucommiae), *Niu Xi* (Radix Achyranthis Bidentatae), and *Yan Hu Suo* (Rhizoma Corydalis).
- With neck and shoulder pain, add *Ge Gen* (Radix Puerariae Lobatae) or *Ge Gen Tang* (Kudzu Decoction).
- With severe pain, add *Yan Hu Suo* (Rhizoma Corydalis).
- For pain from bladder or kidney stones, add *Zhu Ling Tang* (Polyporus Decoction), *Hai Jin Sha* (Spora Lygodii), *Jin Qian Cao* (Herba Lysimachiae), and *Ji Nei Jin* (Endothelium Corneum Gigeriae Galli).

CAUTIONS / CONTRAINDICATIONS

- Use *Shao Yao Gan Cao Tang* with caution in animals with hypertension, since this formula contains a high dose of *Gan Cao* (Radix et Rhizoma Glycyrrhizae) and may cause water retention.
- Feeding cold or raw, pungent or spicy, and oily or greasy foods should be avoided.

PHARMACOLOGICAL EFFECTS

1. **Effect on the smooth muscles**: Administration of the formula had a marked inhibitory effect on the smooth muscles of the intestines in rabbits.[1]
2. **Effect on the skeletal muscles**: Administration of the formula had a marked effect to relax the skeletal muscles. Though the exact mechanism is not clear, part of the function is attributed to the lowered permeability of calcium and potassium across the cell membrane.[2]
3. **Analgesic**: In animal studies, *Shao Yao Gan Cao Tang* was very effective in relieving pain. In human studies, the formula was only slightly effective in relieving pain. The effectiveness increased significantly, however, when combined with acupuncture.[3]

HUMAN CLINICAL STUDIES AND RESEARCH

1. **Trigeminal neuralgia**: In one study, 42 patients with trigeminal neuralgia were treated with modified *Shao Yao Gan Cao Tang* for 7-25 packs of herbs with relief of pain in all patients. In a follow up one year later, 30 patients experienced no recurrences, while 12 patients experienced a relapse of neuralgia six months after the conclusion of herbal treatment that was less frequent and less severe. The formula was modified by adding *Suan Zao Ren* (Semen Ziziphi Spinosae) and *Mu Gua* (Fructus Chaenomelis).[4]
2. **Neuralgia**: One study reported relief of neuralgia in all 59 patients when they were treated with *Shao Yao Gan Cao Tang* using *Bai Shao* (Radix Paeoniae Alba) 50g and *Gan Cao* (Radix et Rhizoma Glycyrrhizae) 30g. The duration of treatment ranged from 3-24 packs of herbs. In follow-up exams one year later, 42 of 59 patients did not have any recurrences. However, recurrences reported in the other 17 patients were at lower frequency and severity of pain.[5]
3. **Restless leg syndrome**: In one study, 21 patients with restless leg syndrome were treated with modified *Shao Yao Gan Cao Tang* for 6-25 doses with complete recovery in all patients.[6] Another study reported 100% effectiveness among 54 patients (33 males and 21 females with 1 month to 11 years history of illness) with restless leg syndrome using *Shao Yao Gan Cao Tang* administered as tea three times daily for 2-9 packs of herbs. The herbal formula contained 15 grams each of *Bai Shao* (Radix Paeoniae Alba) and *Gan Cao* (Radix et Rhizoma Glycyrrhizae). The treatment protocol was to cook the herbs in 3 cups of water to yield 1 cup of decoction, which was then taken in two equally-divided doses.[7]
4. **Acute back pain**: In one study, 68 patients with acute back sprain were treated with *Shao Yao Gan Cao Tang* with complete recovery in 61 patients, moderate improvement in 6 patients, and no improvement in 1 patient. The herbal formula contained *Bai Shao* (Radix Paeoniae Alba) 20g, *Gan Cao* (Radix et Rhizoma Glycyrrhizae) 20g, and *San Qi* (Radix et Rhizoma Notoginseng) 6g. The herbs were given in decoction twice daily for 5 days.[8]
5. **Peptic ulcer disease**: In one study, 120 patients with peptic ulcer were treated with *Shao Yao Gan Cao Tang* with some success. The success rate was 63.5% for those diagnosed with deficiency and cold of the Spleen and Stomach, 74.4% for those diagnosed with Stomach yin deficiency, 84.6% for patients with qi and blood stagnation, and 66% for patients with Liver and Stomach disharmony.[9]
6. **Colitis**: One study reported 90.6% effectiveness in the treatment of chronic colitis using *Shao Yao Gan Cao Tang*

Sháo Yào Gān Cǎo Tāng (Peony and Licorice Decoction)

as a base formula, plus *Hua Jiao* (Pericarpium Zanthoxyli), *Da Xue Teng* (Caulis Sargentodoxae) and others. Modifications included addition of *Wu Zhu Yu* (Fructus Evodiae) and *Pao Jiang* (Rhizoma Zingiberis Praeparatum) for damp-cold; *Huang Lian* (Rhizoma Coptidis) and *Yi Yi Ren* (Semen Coicis) for damp-heat; *Da Huang* (Radix et Rhizoma Rhei) for constipation; *Wu Mei* (Fructus Mume) for diarrhea; and *Huai Hua* (Flos Sophorae) for hematochezia. Of 32 patients, 17 had significant improvement, 12 had moderate improvement, and 3 had no benefit.[10]

7. **Constipation**: Sixty patients with habitual constipation were treated with modified *Shao Yao Gan Cao Tang* with good results. *Bai Zhu* (Rhizoma Atractylodis Macrocephalae) was added for qi deficiency. *Fu Zi* (Radix Aconiti Lateralis Praeparata) was added for cold.[11]
8. **Gastric and abdominal pain**: In one study, 171 patients with gastric and abdominal pain due to various causes were treated with injection of the formula that contained a 4:1 ratio of *Bai Shao* (Radix Paeoniae Alba) and *Gan Cao* (Radix et Rhizoma Glycyrrhizae). The treatment was successful in 105 out of 120 patients with pain characterized by deficiency, and 26 out of 51 patients with pain characterized by excess.[12]
9. **Cholecystitis**: In one study, 36 patients with cholecystitis were treated with a large dose of *Shao Yao Gan Cao Tang* with good success. The formula contained 60-90g of *Bai Shao* (Radix Paeoniae Alba) and 15-30g of *Gan Cao* (Radix et Rhizoma Glycyrrhizae). *Chai Hu* (Radix Bupleuri), *Huang Qin* (Radix Scutellariae), and *Long Dan* (Radix et Rhizoma Gentianae) were added for alternation of fever and trembling. *Da Huang* (Radix et Rhizoma Rhei), *Di Huang* (Radix Rehmanniae) and *Xuan Shen* (Radix Scrophulariae) were added for constipation. *Chuan Lian Zi* (Fructus Toosendan), *Yu Jin* (Radix Curcumae), and *Yan Hu Suo* (Rhizoma Corydalis) were added for pain. *Tian Hua Fen* (Radix Trichosanthis) and *Mu Dan Pi* (Cortex Moutan) were added if there was a bitter taste in the mouth. *Mai Ya* (Fructus Hordei Germinatus) and *Shan Zha* (Fructus Crataegi) were added for poor appetite. *Huo Xiang* (Herba Agastaches), *Zhu Ru* (Caulis Bambusae in Taenia), and *Ban Xia* (Rhizoma Pinelliae) were added for nausea and vomiting. *Hou Po* (Cortex Magnoliae Officinalis) and *Zhi Qiao* (Fructus Aurantii) were added for abdominal fullness. *Wu Mei Wan* (Mume Pill) was added for the presence of parasites. *Yin Chen* (Herba Artemisiae Scopariae) and *Zhi Zi* (Fructus Gardeniae) were added for jaundice. The treatment protocol was to cook the herbs in decoction, and administer the decoction one time daily for 5 days per course of treatment. Out of 36 patients, the study reported complete recovery in 26 patients, moderate improvement in 8 patients, and no change in 2 patients.[13]
10. **Urolithiasis**: One study reported moderate success in the treatment of urinary stones using *Shao Yao Gan Cao Tang* plus *Dong Kui Zi* (Semen Malvae), *Hua Shi* (Talcum), *Che Qian Zi* (Semen Plantaginis), and others as the base formula. Of the 30 patients, 19 had kidney stones, 1 had bladder stones, and 19 had stones in the ureter. The study reported complete recovery in 19 patients, effectiveness in 10 patients, and no effect in 1 patient.[14]
11. **Diabetes mellitus**: In one clinical study, 36 patients with diabetes mellitus were treated with the formula with marked effect in 15 patients, moderate effect in 10 patients, and no effect in 11 patients. The study also noted that the effectiveness increased with prolonged duration of the treatment.[15]

HERB-DRUG INTERACTION

- **Neuroleptic-induced hyperprolactinemia**: According to a preliminary report, 11 schizophrenic patients with neuroleptic-induced hyperprolactinemia were treated with good success using *Shao Yao Gan Cao Tang*. After 4 weeks of herbal treatment, the mean plasma prolactin level decreased significantly from 28.9 +/- 14.5 ng/mL at baseline to 22.0 +/- 15.2 ng/mL. The potassium levels did not change significantly, and there were no adverse reactions or exacerbation of psychosis.[16]
- **Paclitaxel-induced myalgia/arthralgia**: Administration of both L-Glutamine and *Shao Yao Gan Cao Tang* showed effects to decrease paclitaxel-induced myalgia/arthralgia.[17]
- **Drug-induced menopause**: One study evaluated the therapeutic effects of certain herbal medicines on menopausal symptoms induced by gonadotropin-releasing hormone agonist therapy in Japanese women with endometriosis, adenomyosis, or leiomyoma. According to this study, menopausal symptoms induced by gonadotropin-releasing hormone agonist therapy in 13 patients were successfully treated using *Shao Yao Gan Cao Tang*, *Dang Gui Shao Yao San* (Tangkuei and Peony Powder), *Gui Zhi Fu Ling Wan* (Cinnamon Twig and Poria Pill), *Jia Wei Xiao Yao San* (Augmented Rambling Powder), *Tao He Cheng Qi Tang* (Peach Pit Decoction to Order the Qi) or *Gui Zhi Tang* (Cinnamon Twig Decoction). Most importantly, there were no significant changes in serum estradiol levels after treatment with these herbal medicines. The researchers concluded that these herbal medicines can be recommended for menopausal symptoms induced by gonadotropin-releasing hormone agonists without a negative effect on serum estradiol levels.[18]

TOXICOLOGY

According to toxicology studies in mice, the use of the formula created less side effects than the use of the herbs individually.[19]

Sháo Yào Gān Cǎo Tāng (Peony and Licorice Decoction)

SUGGESTED ACUPUNCTURE TREATMENT

1. Points: *Neiguan* (PC 6), *Zhongwan* (CV 12), *Tianshu* (ST 25), and *Shangjuxu* (ST 37).
2. Technique: sedation or even method.

Neiguan (PC 6) regulates qi and blood. *Zhongwan* (CV 12) is the *mu* (collecting) point of the Stomach, *Tianshu* (ST 25) is the *mu* (collecting) point of the Large Intestine, and *Shangjuxu* (ST 37) is the lower *he* (uniting) point of the Large Intestine. These points relieve abdominal cramps and spasms.

AUTHORS' COMMENTS

In the treatment of abdominal pain, *Shao Yao Gan Cao Tang* is not usually used alone but is combined with formulas that treat the root cause of the pain. It can be modified to treat persistent spasms, shaking and trembling of one or both rear legs in the dog, by adding *Niu Xi* (Radix Achyranthis Bidentatae), *Mu Gua* (Fructus Chaenomelis) and *Ji Xue Teng* (Caulis Spatholobi).

References

1. *Guo Wai Yi Xue* (Foreign Medicine), 1984; 6(1):58.
2. *He Nan Zhong Yi* (Henan Chinese Medicine), 1986; (6):15.
3. *Guo Wai Yi Xue* (Foreign Medicine), 1984; 6(1):58.
4. *Jiang Xi Yi Yao* (Jiangxi Medicine and Herbology), 1965; 5(7):909.
5. *Zhong Yi Ming Fang Lin Chuang Xin Yong* (Contemporary Clinical Applications of Classic Chinese Formulas), 2001; 313.
6. *Shan Dong Zhong Yi Za Zhi* (Shandong Journal of Chinese Medicine), 1986; (2):17.
7. *He Bei Zhong Yi* (Hebei Chinese Medicine), 1984; 3:29.
8. *Zhe Jiang Zhong Yi Za Zhi* (Zhejiang Journal of Chinese Medicine), 1995; (11):524.
9. *Chuan Dong Zhong Yi Za Zhi* (Chuandong Journal of Chinese Medicine), 1984; (2):22.
10. *Shang Hai Zhong Yi Yao Za Zhi* (Shanghai Journal of Chinese Medicine and Herbology), 1996; 10:18.
11. *Yun Nan Zhong Yi Za Zhi* (Yunan Journal of Chinese Medicine), 1983; (8):79.
12. *Fu Jian Zhong Yi Yao* (Fujian Chinese Medicine and Herbology), 1961; 9(4):44.
13. *Shi Yong Zhong Yi Za Zhi* (Journal of Practical Chinese Medicine), 1995; (4):10.
14. *Liao Ning Zhong Yi Za Zhi* (Liaoning Journal of Chinese Medicine), 1986; 3:29.
15. *Liao Ning Zhong Yi Za Zhi* (Liaoning Journal of Chinese Medicine), 1980; (9):36.
16. Yamada K, Kanba S, Murata T, Fukuzawa M, Terashi B, Yagi G, Asai M. Effectiveness of shakuyaku-kanzo-to in neuroleptic-induced hyperprolactinemia: a preliminary report. Psychiatry & Clinical Neurosciences. 1996 Dec; 50(6):341-2.
17. Hasegawa K, Mizutani Y, Kuramoto H, Nagao S, Masuyama H, Hongo A, Kodama J, Yoshinouchi M, Hiramatsu Y, Kudo T, Okuda H. The effect of L-Glutamine and Shakuyaku-Kanzo-to for paclitaxel-induced myalgia/arthralgia. Gan To Kagaku Ryoho. 2002 Apr; 29(4):569-74.
18. Tanaka T. Effects of herbal medicines on menopausal symptoms induced by gonadotropin-releasing hormone agonist therapy. Clin Exp Obstet Gynecol. 2001; 28(1):20-3.
19. *Zhong Yi Fang Ji De Yao Li Yu Ying Yong* (Pharmacology and Applications of Chinese Herbal Formulas), 1990; 296.

8 TONIC FORMULAS

Section 3

气血两补剂 — Qi- and Blood-Tonifying Formulas

Bā Zhēn Tāng (Eight-Treasure Decoction)
八珍湯
八珍汤

Pinyin Name: *Ba Zhen Tang*
Literal Name: Eight-Treasure Decoction
Alternate Names: *Pa Chen Tang (Wan), Ba Zhen Tang (Wan)*, Eight Jewel Decoction (Pill), Eight Treasures Decoction (Pill), Tangkuei and Ginseng Eight Combination
Original Source: *Zheng Ti Lei Yao* (Catalogued Essentials for Correcting the Body) by Bi Li-Zhai (Ji) in 1529

COMPOSITION

Ren Shen (Radix et Rhizoma Ginseng)	3g [3g]
Bai Zhu (Rhizoma Atractylodis Macrocephalae), *chao* (dry-fried)	3g [10g]
Fu Ling (Poria)	3g [8g]
Zhi Gan Cao (Radix et Rhizoma Glycyrrhizae Praeparata cum Melle), *chao* (dry-fried)	1.5g [5g]
Shu Di Huang (Radix Rehmanniae Praeparata), *ban* (blended) with liquor	3g [15g]
Dang Gui (Radix Angelicae Sinensis), *ban* (blended) with liquor	3g [10g]
Bai Shao (Radix Paeoniae Alba)	3g [8g]
Chuan Xiong (Rhizoma Chuanxiong)	3g [5g]

DOSAGE / PREPARATION / ADMINISTRATION

Cook the ingredients with 3 slices of *Sheng Jiang* (Rhizoma Zingiberis Recens) and 2 pieces of *Da Zao* (Fructus Jujubae) in 2 bowls of water until the liquid is reduced to 80%. Take the decoction before meals. Today, the decoction may be prepared using the doses suggested in brackets.

CHINESE THERAPEUTIC ACTIONS

Tonifies qi and blood

CLINICAL MANIFESTATIONS

Qi and blood deficiencies: general weakness, fatigue, poor appetite, dry skin, nails and hair coat, a pale tongue, and a thin, weak pulse.

VETERINARY CLINICAL APPLICATIONS

Anemia, dermatitis, itching, corneal ulcer, immune deficiency, recovery following: chronic illness, surgery, chemotherapy or radiation, and parturition.

EXPLANATION

Ba Zhen Tang (Eight-Treasure Decoction) was originally designed to treat qi and blood deficiencies caused by excessive bleeding. Today, however, this formula can be used in any condition involving qi and blood deficiencies, such as from chronic illnesses, or following the inappropriate use of clearing or draining herbs. Dry skin, nails and hair coat are signs of blood deficiency. General weakness, easily fatigued, and poor appetite are all due to qi deficiency. The tongue and pulse conditions described above indicate deficiencies of qi and blood.

Ba Zhen Tang (Eight-Treasure Decoction) combines *Si Jun Zi Tang* (Four-Gentlemen Decoction) and *Si Wu Tang* (Four-Substance Decoction). *Ren Shen* (Radix et Rhizoma Ginseng), *Bai Zhu* (Rhizoma Atractylodis Macrocephalae), *Fu Ling* (Poria), and *Zhi Gan Cao* (Radix et Rhizoma Glycyrrhizae Praeparata cum Melle) tonify qi. *Shu Di Huang* (Radix Rehmanniae Praeparata), *Dang Gui* (Radix Angelicae Sinensis), *Bai Shao* (Radix Paeoniae Alba), and *Chuan Xiong* (Rhizoma Chuanxiong) nourish the blood.

Bā Zhēn Tāng (Eight-Treasure Decoction)

***Ba Zhen Tang* (Eight-Treasure Decoction)**

Diagnosis	Clinical Signs	Treatment	Herbs
Qi and blood deficiencies	• General weakness, fatigue, and poor appetite: qi deficiency • Dry skin, nails and hair coat: blood deficiency • Pale tongue and a thin, weak pulse: deficiency condition	Tonifies qi and blood	• *Ren Shen* (Radix et Rhizoma Ginseng), *Bai Zhu* (Rhizoma Atractylodis Macrocephalae), *Fu Ling* (Poria) and *Zhi Gan Cao* (Radix et Rhizoma Glycyrrhizae Praeparata cum Melle) tonify qi. • *Shu Di Huang* (Radix Rehmanniae Praeparata), *Dang Gui* (Radix Angelicae Sinensis), *Bai Shao* (Radix Paeoniae Alba) and *Chuan Xiong* (Rhizoma Chuanxiong) nourish the blood. • *Sheng Jiang* (Rhizoma Zingiberis Recens) and *Da Zao* (Fructus Jujubae) harmonize the middle *jiao* to strengthen the Spleen and Stomach.

Sheng Jiang (Rhizoma Zingiberis Recens) and *Da Zao* (Fructus Jujubae) harmonize the middle *jiao* to strengthen the Spleen and Stomach and to counteract the potentially stagnating effect of the tonics.

Please refer to *Si Jun Zi Tang* (Four-Gentlemen Decoction) and *Si Wu Tang* (Four-Substance Decoction) for detailed explanations of these two formulas.

VETERINARY MODIFICATIONS

- With weakness and pain of the lower back, add *Niu Xi* (Radix Achyranthis Bidentatae) and *Du Zhong* (Cortex Eucommiae).
- For poor appetite, add *Shan Yao* (Rhizoma Dioscoreae), *Chen Pi* (Pericarpium Citri Reticulatae), and *Qian Shi* (Semen Euryales).
- For deficiencies of qi, blood and yang, add *Huang Qi* (Radix Astragali) and *Rou Gui* (Cortex Cinnamomi).
- For recurrent abortion or to prevent abortion, add *Sha Ren* (Fructus Amomi) and *Zi Su Ye* (Folium Perillae).

CAUTIONS / CONTRAINDICATIONS

- Avoid physical exhaustion and exposure to cold environments.
- *Ba Zhen Tang* is contraindicated in animals with heat or excess conditions.[1]

PHARMACOLOGICAL EFFECTS

1. **Hematopoietic**: In one experiment, it was determined that the administration of *Ba Zhen Tang* had a positive effect in treating mice with anemia due to profuse loss of blood. In comparison with the placebo group which did not receive any herbs, the mice that received the herbs for 10 days showed a significant increase of red blood cells. The study also noted that in normal subjects, use of *Ba Zhen Tang* caused only minor changes to the red blood cells and white blood cells.[2]
2. **Immunostimulant**: In one experiment, oral administration of *Ba Zhen Tang* daily for 7 days was associated with an increase in phagocytic activities by macrophages in mice.[3]
3. **Lymphatic**: In one laboratory experiment using mice, it was found that administration of *Ba Zhen Tang* was effective in countering the suppression of lymphocyte growth induced by hydrocortisone.[4]

HUMAN CLINICAL STUDIES AND RESEARCH

1. **Anemia**: In a clinical study, 102 patients with anemia characterized by qi and blood deficiencies were treated with *Ba Zhen Tang* with recovery in 8 patients, marked improvement in 45 patients, moderate improvement in 42 patients, and no change in 7 patients. The overall effectiveness was 93.1%. The evaluation of effectiveness was based on both subjective and objective findings.[5] According to another study, anemia due to bleeding ulcer was effectively treated using *Ba Zhen Tang* plus *Zi He Che* (Placenta Hominis), *E Jiao* (Colla Corii Asini), *Sha Ren* (Fructus Amomi), *Mu Xiang* (Radix Aucklandiae), and *Chen Pi* (Pericarpium Citri Reticulatae). Of 40 patients, the study reported complete recovery in 29 patients (72.5%), significant improvement in 10 patients (25%), and slight improvement in 1 patient (2.5%).[6]
2. **Thrombopenic purpura**: Modified *Ba Zhen Tang* was used to treat 42 patients (22 males and 20 females) with thrombopenic purpura. The causes of the illness included upper respiratory tract infection, enteritis, septicemia, and pyogenic otitis media. Out of 42 patients, the study reported recovery in 30 patients and improvement in 12 patients. Most patients responded within 5-6 days.[7]
3. **Post-surgical recovery**: In one study, 32 patients were divided into two groups for evaluation of post-surgical recovery. Group I received *Ba Zhen Tang*, and group II received standard antibiotic therapy. After treatment, the study reported the following findings: Patients in group I regained their appetite after approximately 24-28 hours,

Bā Zhēn Tāng (Eight-Treasure Decoction)

in comparison to the 48-52 hours for group II; and patients in group I felt normal 7-12 days after the surgery, in comparison to 8-25 days for patients in group II. In addition, all patients in group I had normal body temperature by day 5, but 3 patients in group II still had fever on the same date.[8]

4. **Prevention of miscarriage**: The effect of *Ba Zhen Tang* was evaluated for stabilization of pregnancy in 38 women (ages between 25-30 years) who had history of 2-5 miscarriages. The herbal formula included *Ba Zhen Tang* with addition of *Sha Ren* (Fructus Amomi) and *Zi Su Ye* (Folium Perillae). The study reported a 100% success rate in stabilizing the pregnancy to full term.[9]
5. **Itching**: Use of modified *Ba Zhen Tang* was effective in treating geriatric patients with constant skin itching. The formula contained *Ba Zhen Tang* with removal of *Ren Shen* (Radix et Rhizoma Ginseng), and addition of *Huang Qi* (Radix Astragali), *Chan Tui* (Periostracum Cicadae), *She Chuang Zi* (Fructus Cnidii), *Di Fu Zi* (Fructus Kochiae), *Bai Xian Pi* (Cortex Dictamni), and others as deemed necessary. Modifications included addition of *Nu Zhen Zi* (Fructus Ligustri Lucidi) for red tongue; *Dan Shen* (Radix et Rhizoma Salviae Miltiorrhizae) for chronic illness; and *Che Qian Zi* (Semen Plantaginis) for thick tongue coating. Of 36 patients, the study reported complete recovery in 20 patients (55.56%), improvement in 14 patients (38.89%) and no change in 2 patients (5.56%). The overall rate of effectiveness was 94.45%.[10]
6. **Corneal ulcer**: Thirty-six geriatric patients with corneal ulcer were treated with 88.9% effectiveness using modified *Ba Zhen Tang* plus antibiotic drugs. The herbal treatment used *Ba Zhen Tang* as the base, and added *Qian Shi* (Semen Euryales) and *Yi Yi Ren* (Semen Coicis) for Spleen qi deficiency; *He Shou Wu* (Radix Polygoni Multiflori), *Gou Qi Zi* (Fructus Lycii), *Shan Zhu Yu* (Fructus Corni), and *Shu Di Huang* (Radix Rehmanniae Praeparata) for Liver and Kidney deficiencies; and *Yi Zhi* (Fructus Alpiniae Oxyphyllae), *Ba Ji Tian* (Radix Morindae Officinalis), *Yin Yang Huo* (Herba Epimedii), and *Xian Mao* (Rhizoma Curculiginis) for Kidney qi deficiency. Antibiotic drugs were given locally and systemically. Of 36 patients, the study reported marked improvement in 12 patients, improvement in 20 patients, and no change in 4 patients.[11]
7. **Orbital optic neuritis**: *Ba Zhen Tang* effectively treated 14 patients with orbital optic neuritis. The average duration of treatment was 25.3 days.[12]
8. **Peripheral neuritis**: Thirteen patients with peripheral neuritis were treated with modified *Ba Zhen Tang*. The clinical presentation included numbness and pain of the upper and/or lower extremities. The modifications included addition of *Du Huo* (Radix Angelicae Pubescentis) and *Qiang Huo* (Rhizoma et Radix Notopterygii) for neuritis in the upper extremities; *Mu Gua* (Fructus Chaenomelis) and *Niu Xi* (Radix Achyranthis Bidentatae) for neuritis in the lower extremities; and elimination of *Shu Di Huang* (Radix Rehmanniae Praeparata) and *Gan Cao* (Radix et Rhizoma Glycyrrhizae) if there was fullness in the abdominal area with indigestion. Out of 13 patients, the study reported complete recovery in 11 patients and improvement in 2 patients. The average duration of treatment was 24 packs of the raw herbs in decoction (ranges from 12-36).[13]
9. **Organophosphorus-induced peripheral neuritis**: In one study, peripheral neuritis associated with acute organophosphorus poisoning was treated effectively using modified *Ba Zhen Tang*. The herbal treatment included *Ba Zhen Tang* plus *Gui Zhi* (Ramulus Cinnamomi) as the base formula. In addition, *Chi Shao* (Radix Paeoniae Rubra), *Dan Shen* (Radix et Rhizoma Salviae Miltiorrhizae), *Tao Ren* (Semen Persicae), and *Hong Hua* (Flos Carthami) were added for numbness of the extremities with dark blue/purple tongue; *Sang Zhi* (Ramulus Mori) for a feeling of heaviness in the upper extremities; *Niu Xi* (Radix Achyranthis Bidentatae) for a feeling of heaviness in the lower extremities; *Cang Zhu* (Rhizoma Atractylodis), *Fen Bi Xie* (Rhizoma Dioscoreae Hypoglaucae), *Huang Bo* (Cortex Phellodendri Chinensis), *Fang Ji* (Radix Stephaniae Tetrandrae), and *Mu Gua* (Fructus Chaenomelis) for a feeling of heaviness in the body and extremities; *Huang Bo* (Cortex Phellodendri Chinensis) and *Zhi Zi* (Fructus Gardeniae) for fever, a feeling of burning sensation and pain, irritability, and a red tongue; and *Gui Ban* (Plastrum Testudinis), *Mai Dong* (Radix Ophiopogonis), and *Zhi Mu* (Rhizoma Anemarrhenae) for tidal fever and night sweats. Out of 22 patients, 5 patients had complete recovery in 1 month, 5 patients had complete recovery in 2 months, 8 patients in 3 months, and 4 patients after 3 months.[14]

TOXICOLOGY

In an acute toxicology study, oral administration of the formula in decoction at 50 g/kg as a single dose did not cause any significant side effect in rats. In a chronic toxicology study, daily administration of the formula in decoction at 20 g/kg for 8 days did not cause any adverse reaction to the body weight, liver, adrenal glands, heart, uterus, or testicles. There was, however, a slight increase in the weight of the spleen.[15]

SUGGESTED ACUPUNCTURE TREATMENT

1. Points: *Xinshu* (BL 15), *Geshu* (BL 17), *Ganshu* (BL 18), *Qihai* (CV 6), *Pishu* (BL 20), *Weishu* (BL 21), *Housanli* (ST 36), and *Sanyinjiao* (SP 6).
2. Technique: tonification.

Bā Zhēn Tāng (Eight-Treasure Decoction)

Xinshu (BL 15), *Geshu* (BL 17), and *Ganshu* (BL 18) nourish the blood. *Qihai* (CV 6) nourishes qi. *Pishu* (BL 20), *Weishu* (BL 21), *Housanli* (ST 36), and *Sanyinjiao* (SP 6) nourish the middle *jiao* to increase qi and blood.

AUTHORS' COMMENTS

Ba Zhen Tang, *Shi Quan Da Bu Tang* (All-Inclusive Great Tonifying Decoction), and *Ren Shen Yang Ying Tang* (Ginseng Decoction to Nourish the Nutritive Qi) are three formulas that tonify qi and blood. These formulas are commonly used in veterinary medicine, and all three formulas tonify Spleen qi with *Ren Shen* (Radix et Rhizoma Ginseng), *Fu Ling* (Poria), *Bai Zhu* (Rhizoma Atractylodis Macrocephalae), and *Gan Cao* (Radix et Rhizoma Glycyrrhizae), and nourish the blood with *Dang Gui* (Radix Angelicae Sinensis), *Shu Di Huang* (Radix Rehmanniae Praeparata), and *Bai Shao* (Radix Paeoniae Alba). Their differences are as follows:

- *Ba Zhen Tang* combines *Si Jun Zi Tang* (Four-Gentlemen Decoction) and *Si Wu Tang* (Four-Substance Decoction) with *Sheng Jiang* (Rhizoma Zingiberis Recens) and *Da Zao* (Fructus Jujubae). It is a neutral-temperature tonic that tonifies qi and blood. Clinical signs include general weakness, poor appetite, fatigue, a pale tongue, and a thin, weak pulse. In animals, it can be used to treat acute and chronic anemia arising from the following situations: post-surgical, post-parturition, secondary to chronic renal insufficiency, blood loss from injury, infectious disease, toxic insult, drug induced, and non-regenerative anemia from chronic disease or illness. *Ba Zhen Tang* is the most commonly used qi and blood tonic in veterinary medicine for recovery from parturition, general illness and surgery. This is an excellent general-purpose tonic for performance animals, because it helps to replenish the deficiencies that occur with consistent athletic activity.
- *Shi Quan Da Bu Tang* combines *Ba Zhen Tang* with *Huang Qi* (Radix Astragali) and *Rou Gui* (Cortex Cinnamomi). The addition of these two single herbs changes the property of the formula from neutral to warm, making it more suitable for deficiency and cold conditions; it tonifies qi, blood and yang. Clinical signs include qi and blood deficiencies with poor appetite, back and stifle weakness, and slow healing wounds. This formula is often the choice to treat animals with cancer or chronic disease, with appropriate Chinese pattern differentiation. It can be used in many geriatric patients as a general tonic, purely for the sake of combating the effects of aging. *Shi Quan Da Bu Tang* has also been shown to have immunomodulatory, immunopotentiating, antineoplastic, antitumor and antimetastatic effects. Clinically, it has been found to have beneficial effects in dogs and cats by protecting against chemotherapy- and radiation-induced toxicities, stabilizing or improving white and red blood cell counts, and promoting wound healing in animals that have had mass removal or debulking surgeries with slow or poor healing. It is also beneficial for animals on chronic antimicrobial or steroidal therapy and animals with immune deficiency and secondary infections. Many animals with cancer undergoing chemotherapy or radiation therapy are often yin deficient, or become so after therapy with the development of significant deficiency fire. This formula is warming and should not be given indiscriminately to any animal with cancer. Chinese medicine pattern differentiation should be utilized to evaluate the appropriateness of this formula prior to its use or continued use over time.
- *Ren Shen Yang Ying Tang* is *Shi Quan Da Bu Tang* (All-Inclusive Great Tonifying Decoction) with the removal of *Chuan Xiong* (Rhizoma Chuanxiong), and the addition of *Chen Pi* (Pericarpium Citri Reticulatae), *Wu Wei Zi* (Fructus Schisandrae Chinensis), and *Yuan Zhi* (Radix Polygalae). *Wu Wei Zi* (Fructus Schisandrae Chinensis), *Ren Shen* (Radix et Rhizoma Ginseng), and *Huang Qi* (Radix Astragali) consolidate the exterior and prevent sweating. *Yuan Zhi* (Radix Polygalae) nourishes the Heart, calms the *shen* (spirit), and resolves phlegm to benefit the production of qi and blood. This formula is more suitable for animals with chronic qi and blood deficiencies with fatigue, general weakness, nausea, tendency to vomit with poor appetite, poor digestion, loose stools, weight loss, and *shen* disturbance that is characterized by clinical signs of an inability to calm down, nervousness, shaking, anxiety and fearfulness. These clinical manifestations often arise in animals that must undergo repetitive hospitalization for chemotherapy or radiation treatments. The emotional stress of treatment, in addition to drug-induced damage of qi, yin and blood by these treatments, strongly promotes the development of *shen* disturbance in many of these animals. *Ren Shen Yang Ying Tang* is also useful for animals recovering from chronic disease or illness. This formula can be used to treat chronic anemia, cancer, non-regenerative anemia seen with cardiac disease, and anemia and leukopenia secondary to radiation and chemotherapy. It is very effective in the treatment of non-healing wounds. This formula is neutral in nature and does not create heat or stagnation, when compared to other warm or heavy tonic formulas. These qualities make it ideal for long-term use in weak and debilitated animals.

References

1. *Zhong Yao Ming Fang Yao Li Yu Ying Yong* (Pharmacology and Applications of Famous Herbal Formulas), 1989; 296-297.
2. *Zhong Yi Fang Ji Xian Dai Yan Jiu* (Modern Study of Medical Formulas in Traditional Chinese Medicine), 1997; 629.
3. *Hu Nan Zhong Yi Za Zhi* (Hunan Journal of Chinese Medicine), 1994; 2:8.

8 TONIC FORMULAS

Bā Zhēn Tāng (Eight-Treasure Decoction)

4. *Zhong Guo Zhong Yao Za Zhi* (People's Republic of China Journal of Chinese Herbology), 1993; 18(4):495.
5. *Hu Nan Zhong Yi Za Zhi* (Hunan Journal of Chinese Medicine), 1994; 2:8.
6. *Jiang Xi Zhong Yi Yao* (Jiangxi Chinese Medicine and Herbology), 1997; 6:24.
7. *Zhong Guo Zhong Xi Yi Jie He Za Zhi* (Chinese Journal of Integrative Chinese and Western Medicine), 1994; 14(8):495.
8. *Zhong Xi Yi Jie He Za Zhi* (Journal of Integrated Chinese and Western Medicine), 1990; 10(5):319.
9. *Fu Jian Zhong Yi Yao* (Fujian Chinese Medicine and Herbology), 1960; 10:3.
10. *Shi Yong Zhong Yi Za Zhi* (Journal of Practical Chinese Medicine), 1999; 6:9.
11. *Fu Jian Zhong Yi Yao* (Fujian Chinese Medicine and Herbology), 1995; 4:57.
12. *Liao Ning Zhong Yi Za Zhi* (Liaoning Journal of Chinese Medicine), 1990; 12:26.
13. *Zhe Jiang Zhong Yi Za Zhi* (Zhejiang Journal of Chinese Medicine), 1992; 27(12):537.
14. *Zhong Yi Za Zhi* (Journal of Chinese Medicine), 1995; 12:725.
15. *Zhong Yi Fang Ji Xian Dai Yan Jiu* (Modern Study of Medical Formulas in Traditional Chinese Medicine), 1997; 630.

Shí Quán Dà Bŭ Tāng (All-Inclusive Great Tonifying Decoction)

十全大補湯

十全大补汤

Pinyin Name: *Shi Quan Da Bu Tang*
Literal Name: All-Inclusive Great Tonifying Decoction
Alternate Names: *Shih Chuan Ta Pu Tang (Wan)*, *Shi Quan Da Bu Tang (Wan)*, Complete Nourishment Decoction (Pill), Ten Strong Tonic Herbs Decoction (Pill), Ginseng and Tangkuei Ten Combination
Original Source: *Tai Ping Hui Min He Ji Ju Fang* (Imperial Grace Formulary of the Tai Ping Era) by the Imperial Medical Department in 1078-85

COMPOSITION

Ren Shen (Radix et Rhizoma Ginseng)	[8g]
Bai Zhu (Rhizoma Atractylodis Macrocephalae), *bei* (stone-baked)	[10g]
Fu Ling (Poria), *bei* (stone-baked)	[8g]
Zhi Gan Cao (Radix et Rhizoma Glycyrrhizae Praeparata cum Melle)	[5g]
Shu Di Huang (Radix Rehmanniae Praeparata), *xi* (washed) with liquor, *zheng* (steamed) and *bei* (stone-baked)	[8-15g]
Dang Gui (Radix Angelicae Sinensis), *xi* (washed)	[10g]
Bai Shao (Radix Paeoniae Alba)	[8g]
Chuan Xiong (Rhizoma Chuanxiong)	[5g]
Huang Qi (Radix Astragali)	[15g]
Rou Gui (Cortex Cinnamomi), do not expose to heat	[8g]

DOSAGE / PREPARATION / ADMINISTRATION

The source text states to grind equal amounts of the ingredients into a coarse powder. Cook 6g of the powder with 3 slices of *Sheng Jiang* (Rhizoma Zingiberis Recens) and 2 pieces of *Da Zao* (Fructus Jujubae) in 1 large bowl of water until the liquid is reduced to 70%. Take the warm decoction at any time during the day. Today, this formula may be prepared as a decoction with the doses suggested in brackets.

CHINESE THERAPEUTIC ACTIONS

Warms and tonifies qi and blood

Shí Quán Dà Bŭ Tāng (All-Inclusive Great Tonifying Decoction)

CLINICAL MANIFESTATIONS

1. Deficiencies of qi and blood accompanied by yang deficiency and cold manifestations: lethargy, poor appetite, intolerance to cold, a pale tongue and a thin, weak and deep pulse.
2. General deficiency of the body: deficient cough, poor appetite, weakness of the extremities and back, chronic ulcers, thin body condition.

VETERINARY CLINICAL APPLICATIONS

Regenerative and non-regenerative anemia, leukopenia, cancer, non-healing wounds, supportive care during chemotherapy/radiation therapy, recovery from chronic illness, supplemental formula for aging patients.

EXPLANATION

Shi Quan Da Bu Tang (All-Inclusive Great Tonifying Decoction) treats general deficiency and weakness of the body, conditions that may be caused by over-exertion, injuries, and chronic illnesses. The original text states that this formula has a wide range of effects and can be used to treat a variety of syndromes marked by qi and blood deficiencies with deficient qi progressing to cold signs and deficient yang.

This formula consists of *Si Jun Zi Tang* (Four-Gentlemen Decoction) and *Si Wu Tang* (Four-Substance Decoction), plus *Huang Qi* (Radix Astragali) and *Rou Gui* (Cortex Cinnamomi). *Ren Shen* (Radix et Rhizoma Ginseng), *Bai Zhu* (Rhizoma Atractylodis Macrocephalae), *Fu Ling* (Poria), and *Zhi Gan Cao* (Radix et Rhizoma Glycyrrhizae Praeparata cum Melle) tonify qi. *Shu Di Huang* (Radix Rehmanniae Praeparata), *Dang Gui* (Radix Angelicae Sinensis), *Bai Shao* (Radix Paeoniae Alba), and *Chuan Xiong* (Rhizoma Chuanxiong) nourish the blood. *Huang Qi* (Radix Astragali) tonifies qi and lifts yang qi to improve the general body condition. This herb also helps to speed the healing of wounds. *Rou Gui* (Cortex Cinnamomi) warms yang and dispels cold.

Please refer to *Si Jun Zi Tang* (Four-Gentlemen Decoction) and *Si Wu Tang* (Four-Substance Decoction) for detailed explanation of these two formulas.

VETERINARY MODIFICATIONS

- For animals with cold and weakness of the middle *jiao* with nausea and tendency to vomiting, add *Sheng Jiang* (Rhizoma Zingiberis Recens) and *Da Zao* (Fructus Jujubae).
- For malnutrition and emaciation with poor appetite: add *Shan Yao* (Rhizoma Dioscoreae) and *Qian Shi* (Semen Euryales).
- With sores and abscesses caused by qi and blood deficiencies, add *Zhi Qiao* (Fructus Aurantii), *Xiang Fu* (Rhizoma Cyperi), and *Lian Qiao* (Fructus Forsythiae).
- With fatigue due to Spleen deficiency, combine with *Gui Pi Tang* (Restore the Spleen Decoction).
- With palpitations, fear and fright, combine with *Yang Xin Tang* (Nourish the Heart Decoction).
- For *bi zheng* (painful obstruction syndrome), add *Niu Xi* (Radix Achyranthis Bidentatae) and *Xu Duan* (Radix Dipsaci).

CAUTIONS / CONTRAINDICATIONS

Because *Shi Quan Da Bu Tang* is a warm formula, it is contraindicated in animals with heat or excess conditions.

PHARMACOLOGICAL EFFECTS

1. **Immunostimulant**: Administration of *Shi Quan Da Bu Tang* was associated with immune-enhancing effects because it increases the number and/or the activities of the macrophages, B-lymphocytes, T-lymphocytes, and natural killer (NK) cells.[1]
2. **Hematopoietic**: In one study, the administration of *Shi Quan Da Bu Tang* for up to 10 days effectively treated mice with anemia caused by profuse blood loss. The use of this formula was associated with an increase in hemoglobin and red blood cells.[2] In another study, *Si Wu Tang* (Four-Substance Decoction), *Si Jun Zi Tang* (Four-Gentlemen Decoction) and *Shi Quan Da Bu Tang* were given orally to mice to evaluate their effect for treatment of anemia.

***Shi Quan Da Bu Tang* (All-Inclusive Great Tonifying Decoction)**

Diagnosis	Clinical Signs	Treatment	Herbs
Deficiencies of qi and blood accompanied by yang deficiency and cold manifestations	• Lethargy, poor appetite, intolerance to cold, a pale tongue and a thin, weak and deep pulse: qi and blood deficiency • Intolerance to cold: yang deficiency	Warms and tonifies qi and blood	• *Si Jun Zi Tang* (Four-Gentlemen Decoction) tonifies qi. • *Si Wu Tang* (Four-Substance Decoction) tonifies blood. • *Huang Qi* (Radix Astragali) tonifies qi and lifts yang. • *Rou Gui* (Cortex Cinnamomi) warms yang and dispels cold.

Shí Quán Dà Bǔ Tāng (All-Inclusive Great Tonifying Decoction)

The study concluded that *Shi Quan Da Bu Tang* was most effective, followed by *Si Wu Tang* and *Si Jun Zi Tang*.[3] The mechanism of action was attributed to increased activity of CSF.[4]

3. **Antineoplastic**: In one study in mice, the administration of *Shi Quan Da Bu Tang* was associated with an inhibitory effect on the growth of cancer cells. The mice that received the herbs survived longer in comparison with the control group. Also, it was noted that the use of herbs also minimized the side effects associated with chemotherapy treatments.[5]
4. **Antitumor and antimetastatic**: According to one *in vivo* study, use of *Shi Quan Da Bu Tang* was associated with marked antitumor and antimetastatic activities. Proposed mechanism of this action included enhancement of phagocytosis, cytokine induction, antibody production, and induction of the mitogenic activity of spleen cells. As a complement to western medical treatment, *Shi Quan Da Bu Tang* showed antitumor effects when combined with surgical excision, antitumor effects with or without other drugs, and protection against the deleterious effects of anticancer drugs as well as radiation-induced immunosuppression and bone marrow toxicity.[6] Specifically, in liver metastasis, one study reported that administration of *Shi Quan Da Bu Tang* had a dose-dependent inhibition of liver tumor colonies and significant enhancement of survival rate, without side effects, as compared with the untreated control.[7]
5. **Anticancer**: One study reported a promising preventative effect for endometrial cancers with use of *Shi Quan Da Bu Tang*. According to this study, this formula suppressed estradiol-17 beta (E2)-induced expression of c-fos/jun in uterine corpus and inhibited N-methyl-N-nitrosourea and E2-induced endometrial carcinogenesis in mice.[8] According to another study, *Shi Quan Da Bu Tang* suppressed primary melanocytic tumors through potentiation of T-cell-mediated antitumor cytotoxic immunity *in vivo*.[9]
6. **Antitumor**: Administration of *Shi Quan Da Bu Tang* was associated with a preventive effect on endometrial carcinogenesis in mice. The antitumor effect of *Shi Quan Da Bu Tang* was attributed in part to the contents of *Si Wu Tang*, as the administration of these four herbs was found to have an inhibitory effect on estrogen-induced expression of c-fos, interleukin (IL)-1alpha and tumor necrosis factor (TNF)-alpha in uteri of ovariectomized mice.[10]
7. **Antiaging**: One study found this formula to have marked anti-aging effects to prolong life expectancy in mice.[11]
8. **Effect on bone mass density**: Administration of *Shi Quan Da Bu Tang* for 19 weeks was effective in the prevention and treatment of osteoporosis in mice whose ovaries had been removed. In comparison with control groups (one receiving placebo and the other estradiol), *Shi Quan Da Bu Tang* was determined to be comparable in effect to estradiol, and significantly more effective than the placebo for prevention and treatment of osteoporosis.[12] This efficacy on prevention and treatment of osteoporosis was reproduced in another study that administered herbs for 49 days to rats with ovariectomy. In comparison with sham-operated rats, the bone mineral density (BMD) of tibia in ovariectomized rats decreased by 20%, but the BMD was unaffected in rats treated with *Shi Quan Da Bu Tang* or 17-beta-estradiol. The study concluded that *Shi Quan Da Bu Tang* is as effective as 17-beta-estradiol in preventing the development of bone loss induced by ovariectomy by preserving the fine particle surface of the bone.[13]
9. **Hepatoprotective**: Administration of *Shi Quan Da Bu Tang* was effective in treating N-nitrosomorpholine-induced hepatocarcinogenesis in male rats. The mechanism of action was attributed to the activation of the immune system.[14]

HUMAN CLINICAL STUDIES AND RESEARCH

1. **Post-surgical recovery**: Administration of *Shi Quan Da Bu Tang* has marked beneficial effects on gastric cancer patients during the post-operative recovery by improving interleukin 2 reactivity, natural killer activity, nutritional index, and bone mineral indices.[15]
2. **Cancer**: According to one report that screened and evaluated 116 herbal formulas for treatment of cancer, *Shi Quan Da Bu Tang* was determined to be the most effective as a potent biological response modifier. Clinical benefits of *Shi Quan Da Bu Tang* included extremely low toxicity, self-regulatory and synergistic actions of its components in immunomodulatory and immunopotentiating effects, enhanced therapeutic activity in chemotherapy and radiotherapy, inhibited recurrence of malignancies, prolonged survival, and reduced adverse toxicities of many anticancer drugs.[16]
3. **Anemia**: Administration of *Shi Quan Da Bu Tang* effectively increased hemoglobin, red blood cells, and platelets in 41 patients with post-surgical proteinemia.[17]
4. **Shwachman syndrome**: Use of *Shi Quan Da Bu Tang* was associated with beneficial effects in patients with Shwachman syndrome, a rare disease characterized by decreased ability to digest food because the cells of the pancreas do not work properly.[18]

HERB-DRUG INTERACTION

- **Chemotherapy- and radiation- induced toxicities**: *Shi Quan Da Bu Tang* was shown in one study to have a marked protective effect against chemotherapy and radiation in cancer patients, including but not limited to such drugs as mitomycin, cisplatin, carboplatin, cyclophosphamide,

Shí Quán Dà Bǔ Tāng (All-Inclusive Great Tonifying Decoction)

and 5-fluorouracil.[19] Moreover, many journals reported that *Shi Quan Da Bu Tang* demonstrated effectiveness as a supportive therapy for cancer patients treated with chemotherapy and/or radiation. In one study, 50 patients with cancer (stomach, large intestine and breast) who were treated with chemotherapeutic agents (FT-207, 5-FU, UFT, MMC, CDDP, and ADM) and this herbal formula for one month showed good tolerance for the treatments. In another report, 30 women with malignant cancer of the uterus and ovaries were treated with the herbal formula with marked improvement such as more energy, better appetite, and warmer extremities. Use of the formula has also shown effect to reverse bone marrow suppression induced by such drugs as MMC, Ara-C, and MTX. In one study with 26 patients, the use of the herbal formula inhibited the reduction of white blood cells and red blood cells associated with the drugs. It was noted in another study that the use of the herbal formula had a protective effect for white blood cells, red blood cells, and platelets against radiation treatment in 15 cancer patients. Lastly, administration of *Shi Quan Da Bu Tang* starting one week before chemotherapy was associated with 88% effectiveness in alleviating nausea and vomiting associated with EAP treatment (adriamycin, cisplatin and etoposide) for stomach and pancreatic cancer.[20]

- **Chemotherapy-induced toxicities**: One study reported significant benefits using *Shi Quan Da Bu Tang* in cancer patients treated with chemotherapeutic agents. *Shi Quan Da Bu Tang* potentiates the therapeutic effect of many anticancer drugs, such as mitomycin, cisplatin, cyclophosphamide and fluorouracil. It also counteracts adverse side effects of these anticancer drugs, such as gastrointestinal disturbances such as anorexia, nausea, vomiting, hepatotoxicity, immunosuppression, leukopenia, thrombocytopenia, anemia, and nephropathy.[21]
- **Chemotherapy- and radiation- induced neutropenia**: One study reported 84.32% effectiveness using *Shi Quan Da Bu Tang* to treat decreased white blood cell count induced by chemotherapy and/or radiation in 134 patients (39 with stomach cancer, 28 with lung cancer, 17 with breast cancer, 13 with rectal cancer, 12 with lymphatic cancer, 12 with liver cancer, 7 with bladder cancer, and others).[22]
- **Cyclophosphamide- or prednisolone-induced immunosuppression**: One study demonstrated that use of *Shi Quan Da Bu Tang* and *Ren Shen Yang Ying Tang* (Ginseng Decoction to Nourish the Nutritive Qi) effectively prolonged survival rate and life span in mice with candida infection associated with immunosuppression induced by cyclophosphamide or prednisolone.[23]
- **Carboplatin- or cisplatin-induced myelosuppression**: One study reported that administration of *Shi Quan Da Bu Tang* was effective in mice to prevent myelosuppression induced by nine-times intraperitoneal administration of 15 mg/kg carboplatin or 3.0 mg/kg cisplatin, without affecting the antitumor activities of these agents.[24]
- **Cisplatin-induced toxicities**: According to another study, daily administration of *Shi Quan Da Bu Tang* in mice was effective to protect against nephrotoxicity, immunosuppression, hepatic toxicity, and gastrointestinal toxicity caused by intraperitoneal administration of 3.0 mg/kg cisplatin nine times (on days 3, 4, 5, 6, 7, 8, 10, 11, and 12). Furthermore, the antitumor effect of cisplatin was not reduced.[25]
- **Cis-diamminedichloroplatinum-induced nephrotoxicity and bone marrow toxicity**: Administration of *Shi Quan Da Bu Tang* was effective in treating nephrotoxicity and bone marrow toxicity caused by intraperitoneal administration of cis-diamminedichloroplatinum (CDDP), a chemotherapeutic agent. Furthermore, use of the herbs did not affect the antitumor activity of CDDP. This beneficial effect is attributed in part to *Dang Gui* (Radix Angelicae Sinensis) and its constituent sodium L-malate.[26]
- **Interferon-induced toxicities**: One study reported a synergistic effect to potentiate the antitumor effect and decrease the toxicity using interferon-alpha and *Shi Quan Da Bu Tang* for treatment of lung metastasis of murine renal cell carcinoma. Interferon-alpha has been shown to significantly inhibit the metastasis of cancer cells, but is also associated with marked loss of body weight. This study demonstrated that the combination treatment of suboptimal doses of interferon-alpha and *Shi Quan Da Bu Tang* has marked effects to augment the antimetastatic effect without causing any loss of body weight, as compared to either treatment alone.[27]
- **Rifampin-induced neutropenia**: Administration of modified *Shi Quan Da Bu Tang* in 11 patients was effective in reversing neutropenia induced by rifampin within 7 days. The white blood cell count was below 3000 cells/mcl in 4 patients, and between 3000-4000 cells/mcl in 7 patients.[28]
- **Levofloxacin**: In a study of 8 healthy volunteers in an open, random crossover fashion, co-administrations of levofloxacin and *Shi Quan Da Bu Tang* did not cause any significant differences in any pharmacokinetic parameters, urinary recovery and renal clearance of levofloxacin. The study concluded that *Shi Quan Da Bu Tang* does not have a significant effect on the rate and extent of bioavailability or renal excretion of levofloxacin.[29]

TOXICOLOGY

In a toxicology study, the LD_{50} for the oral administration of the formula in herbal extract was 15 g/kg in mice. The herbal extract was prepared by cooking 1.5g of *Gan Cao* (Radix et Rhizoma Glycyrrhizae) and 3.0g of the other 9 herbs in 285 mL of water for 1 hour to yield 2.3g of

Shí Quán Dà Bǔ Tāng (All-Inclusive Great Tonifying Decoction)

herbal extract. The study concluded that the formula has very little toxicity.[30]

SUGGESTED ACUPUNCTURE TREATMENT

1. Points: *Xinshu* (BL 15), *Geshu* (BL 17), *Ganshu* (BL 18), *Qihai* (CV 6), *Pishu* (BL 20), *Weishu* (BL 21), *Housanli* (ST 36), *Sanyinjiao* (SP 6), *Feishu* (BL 13), *Shenshu* (BL 23), and *Guanyuan* (CV 4).
2. Techniques: tonification, with moxibustion on *Guanyuan* (CV 4).

Xinshu (BL 15), *Geshu* (BL 17), and *Ganshu* (BL 18) nourish blood. *Qihai* (CV 6) nourishes qi. *Pishu* (BL 20), *Weishu* (BL 21), *Housanli* (ST 36), and *Sanyinjiao* (SP 6) nourish the middle *jiao* to increase qi and blood. *Feishu* (BL 13), *Shenshu* (BL 23), and *Guanyuan* (CV 4) nourish qi and blood. Moxibustion on *Guanyuan* (CV 4) tonifies yang.

AUTHORS' COMMENTS

Shi Quan Da Bu Tang has been frequently used to protect against the adverse effects of chemotherapy and radiation therapy in dogs and cats with cancer. It has been found to be effective in stabilizing or improving white and red blood cell counts to resolve anemia and leukopenia. Many animals with cancer that undergo chemotherapy or radiation treatments are often yin deficient or become so during therapy with the development of significant deficiency fire. This formula is warming and should not be given indiscriminately to any animal with cancer. Chinese medicine pattern differentiation should be utilized to evaluate the appropriateness of this formula prior to its use or continued use over time. *Shi Quan Da Bu Tang* has been used to promote the quality of life and prolong survival time of dogs with hemangiosarcoma, lung adenocarcinoma, osteosarcoma and anal gland carcinoma and cats with intestinal adenocarcinoma. Depending on the case the anticancer effects of this formula can be enhanced by the addition of one or more of the following: *Qing Dai* (Indigo Naturalis), *Bai Hua She She Cao* (Herba Hedyotis), *Ban Zhi Lian* (Herba Scutellariae Barbatae), *Zao Xiu* (Rhizoma Paridis), *Dan Shen* (Radix et Rhizoma Salviae Miltiorrhizae), *San Leng* (Rhizoma Sparganii) and/or *E Zhu* (Rhizoma Curcumae) to detoxify, move the blood and resolve blood stasis to break up hardness.

- To improve the clinical results in the treatment of lung adenocarcinoma, add *Ban Zhi Lian* (Herba Scutellariae Barbatae), *Dong Chong Xia Cao* (Cordyceps) and *Dan Shen* (Radix et Rhizoma Salviae Miltiorrhizae). The addition of maitake mushroom (*Grifola frondosa*) is also recommended.
- This formula can be used for dogs and cats with alopecia that have lost their hair through chronic illness with qi and blood deficiencies by adding *He Shou Wu* (Radix Polygoni Multiflori), *Nu Zhen Zi* (Fructus Ligustri Lucidi), *Yuan Zhi* (Radix Polygalae), *Ji Xue Teng* (Caulis Spatholobi) and *Dan Shen* (Radix et Rhizoma Salviae Miltiorrhizae).
- For the recovery of dogs with fibrocartilaginous emboli (FCE) and paralysis, add *Gui Lu Er Xian Jiao* (Tortoise Shell and Deer Antler Syrup), *Lu Jiao* (Cornu Cervi), *Ci Wu Jia* (Radix et Rhizoma seu Caulis Acanthopanacis Senticosi), *Ji Xue Teng* (Caulis Spatholobi) and *Hong Hua* (Flos Carthami). Unless blood invigorating and stasis resolving herbs are added response to treatment will be marginal for this disease.
- *Shi Quan Da Bu Tang* can be used to promote wound healing in animals with poor immune function and healing following mass removal or debulking surgeries with slow or poor healing and in those on chronic antimicrobial or steroidal therapy with immune deficiency and secondary infection.

Function	Composition	Si Jun Zi Tang	Si Wu Tang	Ba Zhen Tang	Shi Quan Da Bu Tang
Tonifies qi	*Ren Shen* (Radix et Rhizoma Ginseng)	✓		✓	✓
	Bai Zhu (Rhizoma Atractylodis Macrocephalae)	✓		✓	✓
	Fu Ling (Poria)	✓		✓	✓
	Zhi Gan Cao (Radix et Rhizoma Glycyrrhizae Praeparata cum Melle)	✓		✓	✓
Tonifies blood	*Dang Gui* (Radix Angelicae Sinensis)		✓	✓	✓
	Chuan Xiong (Rhizoma Chuanxiong)		✓	✓	✓
	Bai Shao (Radix Paeoniae Alba)		✓	✓	✓
	Shu Di Huang (Radix Rehmanniae Praeparata)		✓	✓	✓
Warms and lifts yang	*Huang Qi* (Radix Astragali)				✓
	Rou Gui (Cortex Cinnamomi)				✓

Shí Quán Dà Bŭ Tāng (All-Inclusive Great Tonifying Decoction)

Si Jun Zi Tang (Four-Gentlemen Decoction), *Si Wu Tang* (Four-Substance Decoction), *Ba Zhen Tang* (Eight-Treasure Decoction), and *Shi Quan Da Bu Tang* (All-Inclusive Great Tonifying Decoction) illustrate the principles of combining formulas to treat various associated conditions.

References

1. *Zhong Yi Fang Ji Xian Dai Yan Jiu* (Modern Study of Medical Formulas in Traditional Chinese Medicine), 1997; 652-654.
2. *Zhong Xi Yi Jie He Za Zhi* (Journal of Integrated Chinese and Western Medicine), 1989; 9(10):622.
3. *Shan Xi Zhong Yi Xue Yuan Xue Bao* (Journal of Shanxi University School of Chinese Medicine), 1986; 2:40.
4. *Zhong Yao Yao Li Yu Lin Chuang* (Pharmacology and Clinical Applications of Chinese Herbs), 1992; 152.
5. *Zhong Yi Fang Ji Xian Dai Yan Jiu* (Modern Study of Medical Formulas in Traditional Chinese Medicine), 1997; 655.
6. Saiki I. A Kampo medicine "Juzen-taiho-to"--prevention of malignant progression and metastasis of tumor cells and the mechanism of action. Biological & Pharmaceutical Bulletin. 2000 Jun; 23(6):677-88.
7. Ohnishi Y, Fujii H, Hayakawa Y, Sakukawa R, Yamaura T, Sakamoto T, Tsukada K, Fujimaki M, Nunome S, Komatsu Y, Saiki I. Oral administration of a Kampo (Japanese herbal) medicine Juzen-taiho-to inhibits liver metastasis of colon 26-L5 carcinoma cells. Jpn J Cancer Res. 1998 Feb; 89(2):206-13.
8. Mori H, Niwa K, Zheng Q, Yamada Y, Sakata K, Yoshimi N. Cell proliferation in cancer prevention; effects of preventive agents on estrogen-related endometrial carcinogenesis model and on an in vitro model in human colorectal cells. Mutation Research. 2001 Sep 1; 480-481:201-7.
9. Dai Y, Kato M, Takeda K, Kawamoto Y, Akhand AA, Hossain K, Suzuki H, Nakashima I. T-cell-immunity-based inhibitory effects of orally administered herbal medicine juzen-taiho-to on the growth of primarily developed melanocytic tumors in RET-transgenic mice. J Invest Dermatol. 2001 Sep; 117(3):694-701.
10. Tagami K, Niwa K, Lian Z, Gao J, Mori H, Tamaya T. Preventive effect of Juzen-taiho-to on endometrial carcinogenesis in mice is based on Shimotsu-to constituent. Biol Pharm Bull. 2004 Feb; 27(2):156-61.
11. *Zhong Cheng Yao* (Study of Chinese Patent Medicine), 1991; 13(10):31.
12. *Guo Wai Yi Xue Zhong Yi Zhong Yao Fen Ce* (Monograph of Chinese Herbology from Foreign Medicine), 1991; 13(4):42.
13. Hidaka S, Okamoto Y, Nakajima K, Suekawa M, Liu SY. Preventive effects of traditional Chinese (Kampo) medicines on experimental osteoporosis induced by ovariectomy in rats. Calcif Tissue Int. 1997 Sep; 61(3):239-46.
14. Tatsuta M, Iishi H, Baba M, Nakaizumi A, Uehara H. Inhibition by shi-quan-da-bu-tang (TJ-48) of experimental hepatocarcinogenesis induced by N-nitrosomorpholine in Sprague-Dawley rats. Eur J Cancer. 1994; 30A(1):74-8.
15. Horie Y, Kato K, Kameoka S, Hamano K. Bu ji (hozai) for treatment of postoperative gastric cancer patients. Am J Chin Med. 1994; 22(3-4):309-19.
16. Zee-Cheng RK. Shi-quan-da-bu-tang (ten significant tonic decoction), SQT. A potent Chinese biological response modifier in cancer immunotherapy, potentiation and detoxification of anticancer drugs. Methods Find Exp Clin Pharmacol. 1992 Nov; 14(9):725-36.
17. *Zhong Xi Yi Jie He Za Zhi* (Journal of Integrated Chinese and Western Medicine), 1989; 10:622.
18. Hisha H, Kohdera U, Hirayama M, Yamada H, Iguchi-Uehira T, Fan TX, Cui YZ, Yang GX, Li Y, Sugiura K, Inaba M, Kobayashi Y, Ikehara S. Treatment of Shwachman syndrome by Japanese herbal medicine (Juzen-taiho-to): stimulatory effects of its fatty acids on hemopoiesis in patients. Stem Cells. 2002; 20(4):311-9.
19. Ikehara S, Kawamura H, Komatsu Y, Yamada H, Hisha H, Yasumizu R, Ohnishi-Inoue Y, Kiyohara H, Hirano M, Aburada M, et al. Effects of medicinal plants on hemopoietic cells. Adv Exp Med Biol. 1992; 319:319-30.
20. *Zhong Yi Fang Ji Xian Dai Yan Jiu* (Modern Study of Medical Formulas in Traditional Chinese Medicine), 1997, 658-659.
21. Zee-Cheng RK. Shi-quan-da-bu-tang (ten significant tonic decoction), SQT. A potent Chinese biological response modifier in cancer immunotherapy, potentiation and detoxification of anticancer drugs. Methods Find Exp Clin Pharmacol. 1992 Nov; 14(9):725-36.
22. *Shi Yong Zhong Xi Yi Jie He Za Zhi* (Practical Journal of Integrated Chinese and Western Medicines), 1995; 6:376.
23. Abe S, Ishibashi H, Tansho S, Hanazawa R, Komatsu Y, Yamaguchi H. Protective effect of oral administration of several traditional Kampo-medicines on lethal Candida infection in immunosuppressed mice. Nippon Ishinkin Gakkai Zasshi. 2000; 41(2):115-9.
24. Sugiyama K, Ueda H, Ichio Y. Protective effect of juzen-taiho-to against carboplatin-induced toxic side effects in mice. Biol Pharm Bull. 1995 Apr; 18(4):544-8.
25. Sugiyama K, Ueda H, Ichio Y, Yokota M. Improvement of cisplatin toxicity and lethality by juzen-taiho-to in mice. Biol Pharm Bull. 1995 Jan; 18(1):53-8.
26. Sugiyama K, Ueda H, Suhara Y, Kajima Y, Ichio Y, Yokota M. Protective effect of sodium L-malate, an active constituent isolated from Angelicae radix, on cis-diamminedichloroplatinum(II)-induced toxic side effect. Chem Pharm Bull (Tokyo). 1994 Dec; 42(12):2565-8.
27. Muraishi Y, Mitani N, Yamaura T, Fuse H, Saiki I. Effect of interferon-alpha A/D in combination with the Japanese and Chinese traditional herbal medicine juzen-taiho-to on lung metastasis of murine renal cell carcinoma. Anticancer Res. 2000 Sep-Oct; 20(5A):2931-7.
28. *Hu Bei Zhong Yi Za Zhi* (Hubei Journal of Chinese Medicine), 1981; 4:29.
29. Hasegawa T, Yamaki K, Muraoka I, Nadai M, Takagi K, Nabeshima T. Effects of traditional Chinese medicines on pharmacokinetics of levofloxacin. Antimicrobial Agents & Chemotherapy. 1995 Sep; 39(9):2135-7.
30. *He Han Yi Yao Xue Hui Zhi* (Hehan Journal of Medicine and Herbology), 1984; 1(1):68.

Rén Shēn Yǎng Yíng Tāng

(Ginseng Decoction to Nourish the Nutritive Qi)

人参養榮湯
人参养荣汤

Pinyin Name: *Ren Shen Yang Ying Tang*
Literal Name: Ginseng Decoction to Nourish the Nutritive Qi
Alternate Names: *Jen Shen Yang Yung Tang (Wan), Ren Shen Yang Rong Tang (Wan), Yang Ying Tang*, Ginseng Nutritive Decoction (Pill), Ginseng Nutrition Decoction (Pill), Nourish the Nutritive Qi Decoction, Ginseng and Rehmannia Combination
Original Source: *Tai Ping Hui Min He Ji Ju Fang* (Imperial Grace Formulary of the Tai Ping Era) by the Imperial Medical Department in 1078-85

COMPOSITION

Ren Shen (Radix et Rhizoma Ginseng)	30g [6g]
Huang Qi (Radix Astragali)	30g [12g]
Bai Zhu (Rhizoma Atractylodis Macrocephalae), *wei* (roasted)	30g [6g]
Shu Di Huang (Radix Rehmanniae Praeparata), *zhi* (prepared)	22.5g [9g]
Dang Gui (Radix Angelicae Sinensis)	30g [9g]
Bai Shao (Radix Paeoniae Alba)	90g [18g]
Wu Wei Zi (Fructus Schisandrae Chinensis)	22.5g [4g]
Fu Ling (Poria)	22.5g [4g]
Yuan Zhi (Radix Polygalae), *chao* (dry-fried)	15g [6g]
Chen Pi (Pericarpium Citri Reticulatae)	30g [6g]
Gui Xin (Cortex Rasus Cinnamomi)	30g [3g]
Zhi Gan Cao (Radix et Rhizoma Glycyrrhizae Praeparata cum Melle)	30g [3g]

DOSAGE / PREPARATION / ADMINISTRATION

Grind the ingredients into powder. Cook 12g of the powder with 3 slices of *Sheng Jiang* (Rhizoma Zingiberis Recens) and 2 pieces of *Da Zao* (Fructus Jujubae) in 1.5 bowls of water until the liquid is reduced to 70%. Take the strained decoction while warm. Today, the decoction may be prepared using the doses suggested in brackets.

CHINESE THERAPEUTIC ACTIONS

1. Tonifies both qi and blood
2. Nourishes the Heart and calms the *shen* (spirit)

CLINICAL MANIFESTATIONS

Exhaustion of the body due to consumptive diseases: lethargy, fatigue, general weakness, nausea, tendency to vomit with poor appetite, poor digestion and loose stools, weight loss, nervousness, anxiety, fearfulness, restlessness, insomnia, and dry mouth and skin.

VETERINARY CLINICAL APPLICATIONS

Anemia, emaciation, poor wound healing, weak immune system, cancer, canine hypoadrenocorticism, canine hypothyroidism, sudden acquired retinal degeneration (SARDS), progressive retinal atrophy (PRA) and lung carcinoma.

EXPLANATION

Ren Shen Yang Ying Tang (Ginseng Decoction to Nourish the Nutritive Qi) treats qi and blood deficiencies accompanied by Heart instability. This syndrome usually follows exhaustion of the body from chronic consumptive diseases, in which both the qi and the blood are depleted. Qi deficiency may lead to poor appetite, poor digestion, weight loss, lethargy, fatigue and general weakness. Blood deficiency leading to lack of nourishment to the Heart may cause nervousness, anxiety, fearfulness, restlessness, and insomnia. Depletion of blood may lead to yin or blood deficiency, causing the dry mouth and skin.

Ren Shen (Radix et Rhizoma Ginseng), *Huang Qi* (Radix Astragali), and *Bai Zhu* (Rhizoma Atractylodis Macrocephalae) tonify qi. *Shu Di Huang* (Radix Rehmanniae Praeparata), *Dang Gui* (Radix Angelicae Sinensis), and *Bai Shao* (Radix Paeoniae Alba) tonify the blood. *Wu Wei Zi* (Fructus Schisandrae Chinensis), *Fu Ling* (Poria), and *Yuan Zhi* (Radix Polygalae) nourish the Heart and calm the *shen* (spirit). *Chen Pi* (Pericarpium Citri Reticulatae) regulates qi flow and counteracts the stagnating properties of the tonic herbs. *Gui Xin* (Cortex Rasus Cinnamomi) tonifies yang and helps the regeneration of qi and blood. *Zhi Gan Cao* (Radix et Rhizoma Glycyrrhizae Praeparata

Rén Shēn Yǎng Yíng Tāng

(Ginseng Decoction to Nourish the Nutritive Qi)

***Ren Shen Yang Ying Tang* (Ginseng Decoction to Nourish the Nutritive Qi)**

Diagnosis	Clinical Signs	Treatment	Herbs
Exhaustion of the body due to consumptive diseases	• Lethargy, weakness, fatigue, and weight loss: qi deficiency • Nervousness, anxiety, fearfulness, insomnia, and restlessness: blood deficiency • Dry mouth and skin: yin and blood deficiencies	• Tonifies qi and blood • Nourishes the Heart and calms the *shen* (spirit)	• *Ren Shen* (Radix et Rhizoma Ginseng), *Huang Qi* (Radix Astragali), and *Bai Zhu* (Rhizoma Atractylodis Macrocephalae) tonify qi. • *Shu Di Huang* (Radix Rehmanniae Praeparata), *Dang Gui* (Radix Angelicae Sinensis), and *Bai Shao* (Radix Paeoniae Alba) tonify the blood. • *Wu Wei Zi* (Fructus Schisandrae Chinensis), *Fu Ling* (Poria), and *Yuan Zhi* (Radix Polygalae) nourish the Heart and calm the *shen*. • *Chen Pi* (Pericarpium Citri Reticulatae) regulates qi circulation. • *Gui Xin* (Cortex Rasus Cinnamomi) tonifies yang. • *Zhi Gan Cao* (Radix et Rhizoma Glycyrrhizae Praeparata cum Melle) harmonizes all of the herbs. • *Sheng Jiang* (Rhizoma Zingiberis Recens) and *Da Zao* (Fructus Jujubae) regulate the middle *jiao*.

cum Melle) tonifies qi and harmonizes the herbs. *Sheng Jiang* (Rhizoma Zingiberis Recens) and *Da Zao* (Fructus Jujubae) regulate the middle *jiao* and tonify qi and blood.

VETERINARY MODIFICATIONS

- With poor appetite, add *Cang Zhu* (Rhizoma Atractylodis) and *Hou Po* (Cortex Magnoliae Officinalis).
- With cough due to Lung deficiency and dryness, add *Chuan Bei Mu* (Bulbus Fritillariae Cirrhosae), *Ku Xing Ren* (Semen Armeniacae Amarum), and *Mai Dong* (Radix Ophiopogonis).
- With palpitations, fearfulness and anxiety, combine with *Yang Xin Tang* (Nourish the Heart Decoction).

PHARMACOLOGICAL EFFECTS

1. **Immunostimulant**: Administration of *Ren Shen Yang Ying Tang* in healthy male volunteers was associated with an increase in natural killer (NK) cells of up to 11% compared to the control group that did not receive any herbs.[1] In another study, administration of this formula at 15g/day for one week to healthy people was associated with an increase of NK cells activity. This study suggested that *Ren Shen Yang Ying Tang* may be useful in the prevention of carcinogenesis.[2] It also significantly (P less than 0.01) augmented the production of granulocyte-macrophage colony-stimulating factor (GM-CSF).[3]
2. **Antihyperlipidemic**: Administration of *Ren Shen Yang Ying Tang* was associated with a reduction of plasma triglyceride levels.[4]

HUMAN CLINICAL STUDIES AND RESEARCH

1. **Anemia**: In one study, 30 anemic patients (between age 30-55) were treated with iron supplements and *Ren Shen Yang Ying Tang* with satisfactory results.[5]
2. **Chronic fatigue syndrome**: *Ren Shen Yang Ying Tang* was used to treat 35 patients with chronic fatigue syndrome for over 6 months. The patients were treated for a total of 1-9 months. Out of 35 patients, the study reported improvement in 26 patients. No side effect or abnormal reactions were reported in the liver and kidneys.[6]
3. **Connective tissue diseases**: *Ren Shen Yang Ying Tang* was used to treat Raynaud's disease, scleroderma, mixed connective tissue disease (MCTD), and systemic lupus erythematosus (SLE). The treatment protocol was to administer 9g of the formula in extract daily for 4 weeks per course of treatment.[7]
4. **Nephritis**: One study reported 74% effectiveness (71 out of 94 patients) in using *Ren Shen Yang Ying Tang* to treat nephritis. Improvements included the gradual resolution of symptoms such as edema, thirst, fever, and dysuria.[8]
5. **Male infertility**: Concurrent use of *Ren Shen Yang Ying Tang* and *Gui Zhi Fu Ling Wan* (Cinnamon Twig and Poria Pill) for 3 months effectively treated male infertility in 19 patients by increasing sperm count, concentration, and motility.[9]
6. **Hepatitis C**: One study reported *Ren Shen Yang Ying Tang* to be very effective in treating chronic hepatitis C. The mechanism of this effect was attributed to an inhibitory effect on hepatitis C virus infection, and also from the

Rén Shēn Yǎng Yíng Tāng

(Ginseng Decoction to Nourish the Nutritive Qi)

protective effect on immunological hepatopathy. *Wu Wei Zi* (Fructus Schisandrae Chinensis) contains gomisin A, which is believed to be the most active herbal component of this formula for this indication.[10]

7. **Cancer**: In one study, 35 patients with cancer of the genitourinary tract were treated with integrative medicine. Following surgery and/or chemotherapy, all patients were given a liquid extract of *Ren Shen Yang Ying Tang* for 4-12 weeks. The study reported that the herbs enhanced recovery and minimized the side effects of standard surgery and/or chemotherapy treatments.[11]
8. **Lung carcinoma**: Administration of *Ren Shen Yang Ying Tang* had a positive effect on life expectancy for patients with lung carcinoma. It decreased tumor marker levels (CEA and CA19-9), relieved cough, and improved appetite. The treatment protocol was to administer 15g of extract per day for 7 weeks.[12]

HERB-DRUG INTERACTION

- **Cyclophosphamide- or 5-fluorouracil-induced leukopenia**: One study compared the effect of *Ren Shen Yang Ying Tang* and recombinant human granulocyte-colony stimulating factor (rhuG-CSF) on leukopenia induced by cyclophosphamide (CY) or 5-fluorouracil (5-FU). Leukopenia was induced by subcutaneous injection of 200 mg/kg of CY or 5-FU, and severe reduction of leukocyte numbers in the peripheral blood was observed. Treatment protocol was daily administration of *Ren Shen Yang Ying Tang* (1 g/kg/day) and rhuG-CSF (2 mcg/mouse/day). The study reported that administration of *Ren Shen Yang Ying Tang* and rhuG-CSF decreased the number of colony-forming units in the spleen (CFU-S) in drug-treated mice. *Ren Shen Yang Ying Tang* was more effective for improving host resistance against 5-FU, and rhuG-CSF was more effective against CY.[13]
- **Cyclophosphamide- or prednisolone-induced immunosuppression**: One study demonstrated that *Shi Quan Da Bu Tang* (All-Inclusive Great Tonifying Decoction) and *Ren Shen Yang Ying Tang* effectively prolonged survival rate and life span in mice with candida infection associated with immunosuppression induced by cyclophosphamide or prednisolone.[14]
- **Scopolamine**: One study reported that *Ren Shen Yang Ying Tang* was associated with improvement in scopolamine-induced impairment of passive avoidance response in mice by enhancing the cholinergic system.[15]

SUGGESTED ACUPUNCTURE TREATMENT

1. Points: *Xinshu* (BL 15), *Geshu* (BL 17), *Ganshu* (BL 18), *Qihai* (CV 6), *Pishu* (BL 20), *Weishu* (BL 21), *Housanli* (ST 36), *Sanyinjiao* (SP 6), and *Shenmen* (HT 7).
2. Technique: tonification.

Xinshu (BL 15), *Geshu* (BL 17), and *Ganshu* (BL 18) nourish the blood. *Qihai* (CV 6) nourishes qi. *Pishu* (BL 20), *Weishu* (BL 21), *Housanli* (ST 36), and *Sanyinjiao* (SP 6) nourish the middle *jiao* to tonify qi and blood. *Shenmen* (HT 7) calms the *shen* (spirit).

AUTHORS' COMMENTS

Ren Shen Yang Ying Tang is a commonly prescribed herbal formula because of its neutral thermal nature and broad-spectrum tonic effects.

- *Ren Shen Yang Ying Tang* can be used to treat atrial fibrillation with qi and blood deficiencies in dogs by the addition of *Dan Shen* (Radix et Rhizoma Salviae Miltiorrhizae), *Bai Zi Ren* (Semen Platycladi) and *E Jiao* (Colla Corii Asini). If Kidney and Heart qi and yang deficiencies are present, combine instead with *Shen Fu Tang* (Ginseng and Prepared Aconite Decoction) and *Dan Shen* (Radix et Rhizoma Salviae Miltiorrhizae).
- It has been used to prolong vision and slow the onset of blindness in progressive retinal atrophy (PRA) with qi and blood deficiencies in the dog; the addition of *Gou Qi Zi* (Fructus Lycii) and *Dan Shen* (Radix et Rhizoma Salviae Miltiorrhizae) will improve clinical results. For sudden-acquired retinal degeneration (SARDS) due to Liver qi stagnation and fire attacking the eyes, combine with *Jia Wei Xiao Yao San* (Augmented Rambling Powder) and add *Xia Ku Cao* (Spica Prunellae), *Ji Li* (Fructus Tribuli) and *Ju Hua* (Flos Chrysanthemi), *Chai Hu* (Radix Bupleuri), *Quan Xie* (Scorpio), *Yu Jin* (Radix Curcumae) and *Dan Shen* (Radix et Rhizoma Salviae Miltiorrhizae). This combination should be given as soon as possible after diagnosis and continued for one month. During this treatment interval the prognosis will become clear with the dog either recovering or becoming permanently blind.
- This formula has been used as an adjunct for the treatment of dogs with hypoadrenocorticism (Addison's disease) in combination with conventional mineralocorticoid supplementation (desoxycorticosterone, fludrocortisone) for prolonged periods of time without adverse effects. It has proven to be effective as a maintenance therapy for the treatment of Addison's disease; however, it must be given for several months before full clinical benefits can be appreciated. It may be given for years with appropriate modifications in these animals. For animals that are severely deficient, consider adding *Gui Lu Er Xian Jiao* (Tortoise Shell and Deer Antler Syrup). It is also useful for the treatment of early hypothyroidism in young animals; early intervention may reverse the disease to avoid permanent hypothyroidism and life-long replacement therapy.

Rén Shēn Yǎng Yíng Tāng

(Ginseng Decoction to Nourish the Nutritive Qi)

- *Ren Shen Yang Ying Tang* and *Yu Ping Feng San* (Jade Windscreen Powder) can be used together to enhance the immune system of animals with frequent infections. It is especially useful in the prevention of nosocomial (respiratory or gastrointestinal) infections in animals that are frequently hospitalized for cancer or other medical treatments, and in those that are immunosuppressed.
- For the treatment of non-healing or slow-healing wounds, it should be combined with *He Shou Wu* (Radix Polygoni Multiflori), *Dan Shen* (Radix et Rhizoma Salviae Miltiorrhizae) and *Ji Xue Teng* (Caulis Spatholobi) to more effectively and rapidly improve wound healing. *Ren Shen Yang Ying Tang* is one of the preferred tonic formulas for deficient patients, since its thermal nature is neutral and will not create heat or cold in animals, when taken over a long period of time. Also, it does not cause stagnation like many heavy tonics.

References

1. *Guo Wai Yi Xue Zhong Yi Zhong Yao Fen Ce* (Monograph of Chinese Herbology from Foreign Medicine), 1992; 14(2):52.
2. Kamei T, Kumano H, Beppu K, Iwata K, Masumura S. Response of healthy individuals to ninjin-yoei-to extract--enhancement of natural killer cell activity. American Journal of Chinese Medicine. 1998; 26(1):91-5.
3. Okamura S, Shimoda K, Yu LX, Omori F, Niho Y. A traditional Chinese herbal medicine, ren-shen-yang-rong-tang (Japanese name: ninjin-yoei-to) augments the production of granulocyte-macrophage colony-stimulating factor from human peripheral blood mononuclear cells in vitro. Int J Immunopharmacol. 1991; 13(5):595-8.
4. *He Han Yi Yao Xue Hui Zhi* (Hehan Journal of Medicine and Herbology), 1994; 44(5):207.
5. *Zhong Yi Fang Ji Xian Dai Yan Jiu* (Modern Study of Medical Formulas in Traditional Chinese Medicine), 1997; 4(1):73.
6. *He Han Yi Yao Xue Hui Zhi* (Hehan Journal of Medicine and Herbology), 1991; 8(3):414.
7. *Zhong Yi Fang Ji Xian Dai Yan Jiu* (Modern Study of Medical Formulas in Traditional Chinese Medicine), 1997; 639.
8. *Xin Zhong Yi Yao* (New Chinese Medicine and Medicinals), 1957; 1:24.
9. *Zhong Yi Fang Ji Xian Dai Yan Jiu* (Modern Study of Medical Formulas in Traditional Chinese Medicine), 1997; 639.
10. Cyong JC, Ki SM, Iijima K, Kobayashi T, Furuya M. Clinical and pharmacological studies on liver diseases treated with Kampo herbal medicine. American Journal of Chinese Medicine. 2000; 28(3-4):351-60.
11. *Xin Yao Yu Lin Chuang* (New Medicine and the Clinical Application), 1993; 42(4):91.
12. Kamei T, Kumano H, Iwata K, Nariai Y, Matsumoto T. The effect of a traditional Chinese prescription for a patient of lung carcinoma. Journal of Alternative & Complementary Medicine. 2000 Dec; 6(6):557-9.
13. Miura S, Takimoto H, Yoshikai Y, Kumazawa Y, Yamada A, Nomoto K. Protective effect of Ren-Shen-Yang-Rong-Tang (Ninjin-youei-to) in mice with drug-induced leukopenia against Pseudomonas aeruginosa infection. Int J Immunopharmacol. 1992 Oct; 14(7):1249-57.
14. Abe S, Ishibashi H, Tansho S, Hanazawa R, Komatsu Y, Yamaguchi H. Protective effect of oral administration of several traditional Kampo-medicines on lethal Candida infection in immunosuppressed mice. Nippon Ishinkin Gakkai Zasshi. 2000; 41(2):115-9.
15. Egashira N, Yuzurihara M, Hattori N, Sakakibara I, Ishige A. Ninjin-yoei-to (Ren-Shen-Yang-Rong-Tang) and Polygalae radix improves scopolamine-induced impairment of passive avoidance response in mice. Phytomedicine. 2003; 10(6-7):467-73.

Xiōng Guī Tiáo Xuè Yǐn

(Cnidium and Tangkuei Decoction to Regulate Blood)

芎歸調血飲
芎归调血饮

Pinyin Name: *Xiong Gui Tiao Xue Yin*
Literal Name: Cnidium and Tangkuei Decoction to Regulate Blood
Alternate Names: *Xiong Gui Bu Xue Tang* (Cnidium and Tangkuei Decoction to Tonify Blood), Cnidium and Rehmannia Combination
Original Source: *Wan Bing Hui Chun* (Restoration of Health from the Myriad Diseases) by Gong Ting-Xian in 1587

COMPOSITION

Dang Gui (Radix Angelicae Sinensis)
Chuan Xiong (Rhizoma Chuanxiong)
Shu Di Huang (Radix Rehmanniae Praeparata)
Bai Zhu (Rhizoma Atractylodis Macrocephalae)
Fu Ling (Poria)
Gan Cao (Radix et Rhizoma Glycyrrhizae)
Chen Pi (Pericarpium Citri Reticulatae)
Wu Yao (Radix Linderae)
Xiang Fu (Rhizoma Cyperi), *chao* (dry-fried) with *Tong Bian* (Infantis Urina)
Mu Dan Pi (Cortex Moutan)
Yi Mu Cao (Herba Leonuri)
Gan Jiang (Rhizoma Zingiberis), *chao* (dry-fried) to black

DOSAGE / PREPARATION / ADMINISTRATION

Cook the ingredients with 1 slice of *Sheng Jiang* (Rhizoma Zingiberis Recens) and 1 piece of *Da Zao* (Fructus Jujubae). Take the strained decoction while warm. For postpartum care, take this formula with a small amount of warm, grain-based liquor and *Tong Bian* (Infantis Urina). Note: The source text did not specify the doses of the herbs.

CHINESE THERAPEUTIC ACTIONS

1. Tonifies qi and blood
2. Harmonizes the Liver and Spleen

CLINICAL MANIFESTATIONS

Post-parturition complications: profuse bleeding, excessive loss of blood, irritability, aggression, fearfulness, distention of the hypochondrium, epigastric and abdominal pain, poor appetite, fever, and aversion to cold.

VETERINARY CLINICAL APPLICATIONS

Supportive treatment for various types of postpartum complications, such as anemia, retention of lochia, insufficient lactation, postpartum uterine bleeding, nausea and vomiting.

EXPLANATION

Xiong Gui Tiao Xue Yin (Cnidium and Tangkuei Decoction to Regulate Blood) treats various types of postpartum complications, including bleeding, qi and blood deficiencies, and disharmony of the Liver, Spleen, and Stomach. As a result of postpartum bleeding, patients are likely to have both qi and blood deficiencies. With Liver qi stagnation, animals experience behavioral disorders and fullness and distention of the hypochondrium. If Liver qi overacts on the Spleen and Stomach, epigastric and abdominal pain and poor appetite will occur. Lastly, because the condition is both excess and deficient in nature, patients also may experience both fever and aversion to cold.

Dang Gui (Radix Angelicae Sinensis), *Chuan Xiong* (Rhizoma Chuanxiong), and *Shu Di Huang* (Radix Rehmanniae Praeparata) tonify the blood and regulate blood circulation. *Bai Zhu* (Rhizoma Atractylodis Macrocephalae), *Fu Ling* (Poria), and *Gan Cao* (Radix et Rhizoma Glycyrrhizae) strengthen the Spleen and tonify qi. Together, they nourish underlying qi and blood deficiencies in postpartum women. *Chen Pi* (Pericarpium Citri Reticulatae), *Wu Yao* (Radix Linderae), and *Xiang Fu* (Rhizoma Cyperi) regulate qi circulation and unblock Liver qi stagnation. *Mu Dan Pi* (Cortex Moutan) and *Yi Mu Cao* (Herba Leonuri) cool the blood and stop bleeding. *Gan Jiang* (Rhizoma Zingiberis) warms the interior and dispels cold. *Da Zao* (Fructus Jujubae), *Gan Cao* (Radix et Rhizoma Glycyrrhizae), and *Sheng Jiang* (Rhizoma Zingiberis Recens) strengthen the middle *jiao* and harmonize the herbs. In short, this is an

Xiōng Guī Tiáo Xuè Yǐn

(Cnidium and Tangkuei Decoction to Regulate Blood)

***Xiong Gui Tiao Xue Yin* (Cnidium and Tangkuei Decoction to Regulate Blood)**

Diagnosis	Clinical Signs	Treatment	Herbs
Postpartum complications	• Postpartum bleeding: qi and blood deficiencies • Behavioral disorders, hypochondriac distention, easily frightened, irritability, and aggression: Liver qi stagnation • Epigastric and abdominal pain and poor appetite: Liver qi overacts on the Spleen and Stomach	• Tonifies qi and blood • Harmonizes the Liver and Spleen	• *Dang Gui* (Radix Angelicae Sinensis), *Chuan Xiong* (Rhizoma Chuanxiong) and *Shu Di Huang* (Radix Rehmanniae Praeparata) tonify the blood and regulate blood circulation. • *Bai Zhu* (Rhizoma Atractylodis Macrocephalae), *Fu Ling* (Poria) and *Gan Cao* (Radix et Rhizoma Glycyrrhizae) strengthen the Spleen and tonify qi. • *Chen Pi* (Pericarpium Citri Reticulatae), *Wu Yao* (Radix Linderae) and *Xiang Fu* (Rhizoma Cyperi) regulate qi circulation and unblock Liver qi stagnation. • *Mu Dan Pi* (Cortex Moutan) and *Yi Mu Cao* (Herba Leonuri) cool the blood and stop bleeding. • *Gan Jiang* (Rhizoma Zingiberis) warms the interior and dispels cold. • *Da Zao* (Fructus Jujubae), *Gan Cao* (Radix et Rhizoma Glycyrrhizae), and *Sheng Jiang* (Rhizoma Zingiberis Recens) strengthen the middle *jiao* and harmonize the herbs.

excellent formula for both treating and preventing various postpartum complications.

VETERINARY MODIFICATIONS

- With profuse and continuous bleeding, increase the dose of *Yi Mu Cao* (Herba Leonuri) and *Mu Dan Pi* (Cortex Moutan).
- With epigastric and abdominal bloating due to food stagnation, add *Zhi Shi* (Fructus Aurantii Immaturus), *Hou Po* (Cortex Magnoliae Officinalis), *Shan Zha* (Fructus Crataegi), and *Sha Ren* (Fructus Amomi).
- With pain in the lower abdomen, add *Yan Hu Suo* (Rhizoma Corydalis), *Tao Ren* (Semen Persicae), *Hong Hua* (Flos Carthami), and *Su Mu* (Lignum Sappan).
- With severe qi and blood deficiencies, add *Huang Qi* (Radix Astragali), or combine with *Dang Gui Bu Xue Tang* (Tangkuei Decoction to Tonify the Blood).
- With irritability, thirst and dryness, add *Di Huang* (Radix Rehmanniae) and *Huang Qin* (Radix Scutellariae).
- For *shen* (spirit) disturbance in which the animal becomes easily scared or frightened, add *Suan Zao Ren* (Semen Ziziphi Spinosae), *Yuan Zhi* (Radix Polygalae), and *Mai Dong* (Radix Ophiopogonis).

HUMAN CLINICAL STUDIES AND RESEARCH

Postpartum recovery: One study compared the effects of herbs and drugs on postpartum recovery and healing. The study enrolled 171 women who had normal deliveries, and randomly assigned them to the following two groups: 85 women who received *Xiong Gui Tiao Xue Yin* at a dose of 6.0 g/day, and 86 women who received ergometrine (methylergometrine maleate) at a dose of 0.375 mg/day. Overall, the study reported marked beneficial effects of this formula on physical recovery in the postpartum period, although its biopharmacological properties are not known.[1]

SUGGESTED ACUPUNCTURE TREATMENT

1. Points: *Sanyinjiao* (SP 6), *Housanli* (ST 36), *Qihai* (CV 6), *Taichong* (LR 3), *Ganshu* (BL 18), *Xuehai* (SP 10), and *Zhongwan* (CV 12).
2. Technique: tonification and moxibustion.

Sanyinjiao (SP 6) tonifies the blood and *Housanli* (ST 36) tonifies qi. *Qihai* (CV 6), *Taichong* (LR 3), and *Ganshu* (BL 18) regulate qi while *Xuehai* (SP 10) regulates the blood. Apply moxibustion on *Zhongwan* (CV 12) to strengthen the middle *jiao*.

Reference

1. Ushiroyama T, Sakuma K, Souen H, Nakai G, Morishima S, Yasuda K, Orino I, Ueki M. Therapeutic effects of Kyuki-chouketsu-in in restoring postpartum physical condition. American Journal of Chinese Medicine. 2003; 31(3):437-44.

Section 4

补阴剂
— Yin-Tonifying Formulas

Liù Wèi Dì Huáng Wán (Six-Ingredient Pill with Rehmannia)

六味地黄丸
六味地黄丸

Pinyin Name: *Liu Wei Di Huang Wan*
Literal Name: Six-Ingredient Pill with Rehmannia
Alternate Names: *Liu Wei Ti Huang Wan, Liu Wei Di Huang Wan, Di Huang Wan*, Six-Flavour Rehmannia Pill, Rehmannia Bolus with Six Herbs, Rehmannia Six Pills
Original Source: *Xiao Er Yao Zheng Zhi Jue* (Craft of Medicinal Treatment for Childhood Disease Patterns) by Qian Yi in 1119

COMPOSITION

Shu Di Huang (Radix Rehmanniae Praeparata)	240g [24g]
Shan Zhu Yu (Fructus Corni)	120g [12g]
Shan Yao (Rhizoma Dioscoreae)	120g [12g]
Ze Xie (Rhizoma Alismatis)	90g [9g]
Mu Dan Pi (Cortex Moutan)	90g [9g]
Fu Ling (Poria)	90g [9g]

DOSAGE / PREPARATION / ADMINISTRATION

Grind the ingredients into powder and form into small pills with honey. The pills should resemble the size of *Wu Tong Zi* (Semen Firmianae), a small seed approximately 5 mm in diameter. Take the pills on an empty stomach, three times daily with warm water. Today, it is usually prepared in pill form by mixing the powdered herbs with honey. Each pill should weigh approximately 15g. Take 1 pill three times daily on an empty stomach with warm, boiled water. This formula may also be prepared and administered in decoction form using the doses suggested in brackets.

CHINESE THERAPEUTIC ACTIONS

Nourishes Liver and Kidney yin

CLINICAL MANIFESTATIONS

1. Liver and Kidney yin deficiency: poor hearing, deafness, poor vision, painful and weak back and stifles, orthopedic and dental developmental abnormalities, lameness, dry feces, a red tongue with little coating, and a rapid and thready pulse that is weaker on the left.
2. Yin-deficient heat: irritability, restlessness, panting excessively (especially at night), short urination, seeking cool surfaces or places, dry eyes and mouth, increased appetite, increased thirst, trembling and jerking during sleep, and hypersensitivity to acupuncture.

VETERINARY CLINICAL APPLICATIONS

Chronic renal failure, chronic glomerulonephritis, chronic urinary tract infection, nephrotic syndrome, proteinuria, hypertension, chronic back pain, osteoarthritis, spondylosis, deafness, diabetes mellitus, hyperadrenocorticism, hypoadrenocorticism, hypothyroidism, cognitive dysfunction, neurological and musculoskeletal developmental abnormalities.

EXPLANATION

Kidney yin deficiency can be caused by fever, acute or chronic disease, bleeding, loss of body fluids, overuse of yang tonic herbs, overwork, stress, lack of rest, overbreeding, and deficiency of Kidney *jing* (essence). The Kidney governs the bones and produces marrow. The term marrow includes the bone marrow, spinal cord, and brain,

Liù Wèi Dì Huáng Wán (Six-Ingredient Pill with Rehmannia)

***Liu Wei Di Huang Wan* (Six-Ingredient Pill with Rehmannia)**

Diagnosis	Clinical Signs	Treatment	Herbs
Liver and Kidney yin deficiencies	• Poor hearing, deafness, dry eyes and mouth, poor vision, painful and weak back and stifles, neurological and orthopedic developmental abnormalities, lameness, and exercise intolerance: Liver and Kidney yin deficiencies • Irritability, restlessness, panting excessively (especially at night), dry feces, short urination, seeking cool surfaces/places, increased appetite, increased thirst, trembling and jerking during sleep, and hypersensitivity to acupuncture: yin-deficient heat	Nourishes Liver and Kidney yin	• *Shu Di Huang* (Radix Rehmanniae Praeparata) tonifies Kidney yin and *jing* (essence). • *Shan Zhu Yu* (Fructus Corni) nourishes the Liver and Kidney. • *Shan Yao* (Rhizoma Dioscoreae) tonifies the Spleen and Kidney. • *Ze Xie* (Rhizoma Alismatis) sedates the Kidney and causes turbidity to descend. • *Mu Dan Pi* (Cortex Moutan) sedates deficiency fire of the Liver. • *Fu Ling* (Poria) strengthens the Spleen and resolves dampness.

which is called "the sea of the marrow." Kidney deficiency can result in congenital and developmental diseases, such as hydrocephalus, canine hip dysplasia, elbow dysplasia, angular limb deformities, a delay or lack of closure of fontanels in young animals, and cervical spine abnormalities, which signifies prenatal *jing* deficiency and inadequate generation of marrow and bones. Weakness of the stifles and lower back and loose teeth are due to Kidney yin deficiency, since the lumbar area is the home of the Kidney, which controls the bones. The ear is the sensory organ that belongs to the Kidney; poor hearing and/or deafness may occur as a result of Kidney deficiency. Poor vision, dry eyes, conjunctivitis, and/or retinal atrophy are mainly caused by Liver yin and blood deficiencies, since the eyes are the sense organ of the Liver, and the Liver is said to open into the eyes. The Kidney stores *jing*, and when the Kidney becomes deficient, *jing* can leak out of the body in the urine or semen. Deficiency heat resulting from yin deficiency causes symptoms such as cool-seeking behavior, irritability, aggression, excessive panting, thirst, and dry eyes and mouth. A red tongue body with little or no coating and a rapid, thready pulse that is weaker on the left characterize yin deficiency.

Liu Wei Di Huang Wan (Six-Ingredient Pill with Rehmannia) consists of three tonic and three sedative herbs. *Shu Di Huang* (Radix Rehmanniae Praeparata), the chief herb, tonifies Kidney yin and *jing* (essence), and fills the marrow. *Shan Zhu Yu* (Fructus Corni) nourishes the Liver and Kidney and astringes *jing*. *Shan Yao* (Rhizoma Dioscoreae) tonifies the Spleen and Kidney and consolidates *jing*. Together, these three tonic herbs address deficiencies in the Kidney, Liver, and Spleen. *Ze Xie* (Rhizoma Alismatis) sedates the Kidney, causes turbidity to descend, and controls the stagnating effect of *Shu Di Huang* (Radix Rehmanniae Praeparata). *Mu Dan Pi* (Cortex Moutan) sedates deficiency fire of the Liver, as well as balances the astringent property of *Shan Zhu Yu* (Fructus Corni). *Fu Ling* (Poria) strengthens the Spleen, resolves dampness, and balances *Shan Yao* (Rhizoma Dioscoreae).

One significant characteristic of this formula is that it sedates and tonifies at the same time. The purpose of sedation is to eradicate the turbidity, and to prevent the stagnant properties of the tonic herbs from harming the body. The overall purpose of this formula, however, is to tonify, not to sedate. Therefore, the dose of the sedating herbs is lower than that of the tonic herbs.

VETERINARY MODIFICATIONS

- With urinary incontinence combine with *Jin Suo Gu Jing Wan* (Metal Lock Pill to Stabilize the Essence) or *Suo Quan Wan* (Shut the Sluice Pill).
- For bronchial asthma, combine with *Ren Shen Ge Jie San* (Ginseng and Gecko Powder).
- With yin-deficient fire, add *Zhi Mu* (Rhizoma Anemarrhenae) and *Huang Bo* (Cortex Phellodendri Chinensis).
- With Spleen qi deficiency with qi stagnation, add dry-fried *Bai Zhu* (Rhizoma Atractylodis Macrocephalae), *Sha Ren* (Fructus Amomi), and *Chen Pi* (Pericarpium Citri Reticulatae).
- For *xiao ke* (wasting and thirsting) syndrome, add *Tian Hua Fen* (Radix Trichosanthis).
- For hypertension, add *Sang Ye* (Folium Mori), *Di Long* (Pheretima), and *Niu Xi* (Radix Achyranthis Bidentatae).
- For chronic nephritis, add *Yi Mu Cao* (Herba Leonuri), *Tian Hua Fen* (Radix Trichosanthis), and *Dan Zhu Ye* (Herba Lophatheri).
- With restlessness, add *Suan Zao Ren* (Semen Ziziphi Spinosae) and *Bai Zi Ren* (Semen Platycladi).

Liù Wèi Dì Huáng Wán (Six-Ingredient Pill with Rehmannia)

- With weakness and pain of the lower back and knees, add *Niu Xi* (Radix Achyranthis Bidentatae) and *Du Zhong* (Cortex Eucommiae).

CAUTIONS / CONTRAINDICATIONS

- *Liu Wei Di Huang Wan* is rich and difficult to digest; use with caution in animals that have Spleen deficiency and damp-heat, as it may cause loose stools. If necessary, combine with a Spleen tonic formula.
- This formula is contraindicated in exterior conditions, high fever, or alternating chills and fever.

PHARMACOLOGICAL EFFECTS

1. **Reproductive**: In laboratory experiments, the use of *Liu Wei Di Huang Wan* was associated with an increase in the weight of the sex organs, such as the ovaries, uterus, and testicles. There was also an increase in sperm counts in the male subjects. In addition, after ingestion of the herbs for 10 days, there was an increase in sexual activity by up to 40%.[1]
2. **Metabolic**: In laboratory experiments, the use of *Liu Wei Di Huang Wan* for 6 weeks lowered plasma cholesterol and triglycerides significantly in rats with elevated levels. In addition, there was an increase of HDL. However, the formula had little effect on plasma cholesterol and triglyceride levels in healthy rats.[2] It was noted that the 3 herbs with "sedating effects", namely *Ze Xie* (Rhizoma Alismatis), *Mu Dan Pi* (Cortex Moutan), and *Fu Ling* (Poria), were effective in reducing the cholesterol levels. On the other hand, the 3 herbs with "tonic effect", namely *Shu Di Huang* (Radix Rehmanniae Praeparata), *Shan Zhu Yu* (Fructus Corni), and *Shan Yao* (Rhizoma Dioscoreae), were not effective in reducing the cholesterol levels.[3]
3. **Hypoglycemic**: In rats with diabetes, the use of *Liu Wei Di Huang Wan* lowered plasma glucose levels.[4] In follow-up studies, it was determined that the formula was effective in reducing plasma glucose levels even if the pancreas was surgically removed. Therefore, it was concluded that the hypoglycemic effect of *Liu Wei Di Huang Wan* was not dependant on pancreas function.[5]
4. **Immunostimulant**: According to one report, the use of *Liu Wei Di Huang Wan* was associated with an increase in white blood cell count and activity.[6] Furthermore, use of this formula reversed the immune suppression induced by dexamethasone.[7]
5. **Adaptogenic**: Administration of *Liu Wei Di Huang Wan* improved the physical performances of mice. After ingesting the herbs orally for 2 weeks, the mice were able to swim for 14.9 minutes, compared to 11.5 minutes for the placebo group that did not receive herbs.[8]
6. **Hepatoprotective and nephroprotective**: Administration of *Liu Wei Di Huang Wan* had protective effects on both the liver and kidneys. It has a hepatoprotective effect against damages induced by such substances as carbon tetrachloride, thioacetamide, and prednisolone.[9] It also increased blood perfusion to the kidneys, improved the kidney function, and reduced protein and uric acid in the urine.[10]
7. **Antiarrhythmic**: In laboratory experiments in rats, an extract of *Liu Wei Di Huang Wan* was found to be effective in treating arrhythmia induced by chloroform, aconitine, ouabain, and adrenalin.[11]
8. **Hypotensive**: In anesthetized rats, intraduodenal administration of *Liu Wei Di Huang Wan* in decoction was effective in reducing the blood pressure within 15 minutes. The mechanism of action was attributed to dilation of the blood vessels and reduction of peripheral resistance. The herbs did not affect the heart rate nor the contractile force of the heart.[12]

HUMAN CLINICAL STUDIES AND RESEARCH

1. **Diabetes mellitus**: *Liu Wei Di Huang Wan* is one of the most effective formulas for treating diabetes mellitus. One study reported 93.55% effectiveness using modified *Liu Wei Di Huang Wan* to treat 62 patients with non-insulin dependant diabetes. The herbal treatment was based on *Liu Wei Di Huang Wan* plus *Ge Gen* (Radix Puerariae Lobatae) and *Li Zhi He* (Semen Litchi) as the base formula. Modifications varied depending on the presentation of diabetes and its complications, and were made as follows: for hunger and increased food intake, add *Shi Gao* (Gypsum Fibrosum) and *Yu Zhu* (Rhizoma Polygonati Odorati); for thirst and increased water intake, add *Sha Shen* (Radix Glehniae seu Adenophorae) and *Tian Hua Fen* (Radix Trichosanthis); for shortness of breath and spontaneous sweating, add *Huang Qi* (Radix Astragali) and *Tai Zi Shen* (Radix Pseudostellariae); for clear urine with increased volume, add *Sang Piao Xiao* (Ootheca Mantidis), *Ba Ji Tian* (Radix Morindae Officinalis), and *Rou Gui* (Cortex Cinnamomi); cloudy urine and night sweats, add *Zhi Mu* (Rhizoma Anemarrhenae) and *Huang Bo* (Cortex Phellodendri Chinensis); for dizziness and swelling of the head, add *Gou Teng* (Ramulus Uncariae cum Uncis), *Bai Shao* (Radix Paeoniae Alba), and *Niu Xi* (Radix Achyranthis Bidentatae); for chest oppression and palpitations, add *Dan Shen* (Radix et Rhizoma Salviae Miltiorrhizae), *Yu Jin* (Radix Curcumae), and *Shi Chang Pu* (Rhizoma Acori Tatarinowii); for obesity, add *Pei Lan* (Herba Eupatorii) and *He Ye* (Folium Nelumbinis); for blurred vision, add *Gu Jing Cao* (Flos Eriocauli) and *Qing Xiang Zi* (Semen Celosiae); and for severe blood stagnation, add *Tao Ren* (Semen Persicae), *Hong Hua* (Flos Carthami), and *Shui Zhi* (Hirudo). The patients were given the herbs for 30 days per course of treatment. Of 62 patients, the study

Liù Wèi Dì Huáng Wán (Six-Ingredient Pill with Rehmannia)

reported complete recovery in 17 cases, improvement in 41 cases, and no effect in 4 cases.[13] In another study, 20 patients with adult-onset diabetes were treated with *Liu Wei Di Huang Wan* for 3-6 months with stabilization in 12 cases and improvement in 8 cases.[14] In another study, modified *Liu Wei Di Huang Wan* was used for 20 days to treat 53 patients with diabetes, with marked improvement in 46 cases, improvement in 5 cases, and no effect in 2 cases.[15] In addition, the use of herbs stabilized blood glucose in conjunction with insulin injection.[16] Lastly, one study reported that use of modified *Liu Wei Di Huang Wan* was associated with 89.2% effectiveness in 65 patients with non-insulin dependant diabetes mellitus.[17]

2. **Hypertension**: Administration of 5-10 packs of *Liu Wei Di Huang Wan* effectively reduced blood pressure in all 31 patients with primary hypertension. In follow-up visits one year later, 23 patients had normal blood pressure, and 8 still had hypertension.[18] In one case report, a patient with hypertension was treated with modified *Liu Wei Di Huang Wan* for 20 doses with good results. Blood pressure reduced from 160-180/110-120 mmHg to 140/90 mmHg. The patient continued to take the herbs for 6 months. The blood pressure did not elevate in any follow-up appointments up to 3 years later.[19]
3. **Hyperthyroidism**: Modified *Liu Wei Di Huang Wan* was used to treat patients with hyperthyroidism. Out of 31 patients, 28 had enlargement of the thyroid gland, 13 had protruding of the eyes, 29 had significant weight loss, and 28 had increased heart rate. After 15-20 doses of herbal treatment, the study reported symptomatic improvement in most patients.[20]
4. **Bronchial asthma**: In one report, 64 patients with bronchial asthma characterized by Kidney deficiency were treated with *Liu Wei Di Huang Wan* with good results.[21]
5. **Chronic nephritis**: Use of *Liu Wei Di Huang Wan* plus *Yu Mi Xu* (Stigma Maydis) was reported in one study to be effective in treating patients with chronic nephritis with hypertension and proteinuria.[22] The study found that administration of *Liu Wei Di Huang Wan* plus *Yu Mi Xu* (Stigma Maydis) in decoction daily for 3-24 months in 77 patients with chronic nephritis was associated with complete recovery in 22 cases, near-complete recovery in 36 cases, partial recovery in 13 cases, and no effect in 6 cases. The study noted that most patients with chronic nephritis had underlying Kidney yin deficiency and damp-heat.[23]
6. **Nephrotic syndrome**: Six patients with edema and proteinuria due to nephrotic syndrome were treated with modified *Liu Wei Di Huang Wan* for 50 days with good results. The study reported that edema and proteinuria were resolved in all patients.[24]
7. **Chronic renal failure**: In one study, 12 patients with chronic renal failure (8 with chronic nephritis, 2 with chronic glomerulonephritis, 1 with renal failure due to systemic lupus erythematosus, and 1 with renal failure due to atypical hemorrhagic fever) were treated with modified *Liu Wei Di Huang Wan* for 30-60 days with complete recovery in 8 cases, marked improvement in 3 cases, and slight improvement in 1 case. A modification to the original formula used a higher dose of *Shan Zhu Yu* (Fructus Corni).[25]
8. **Chronic hepatitis**: Use of modified *Liu Wei Di Huang Wan* in 65 patients with chronic hepatitis was associated with significant effect in 12 cases, improvement in 49 cases, and no effect in 4 cases. The treatment protocol was to use *Liu Wei Di Huang Wan* plus *Dang Gui* (Radix Angelicae Sinensis), *Bai Shao* (Radix Paeoniae Alba), and *Chuan Lian Zi* (Fructus Toosendan) as the base formula. For hypochondriac pain due to Liver qi stagnation, *Yan Hu Suo* (Rhizoma Corydalis), *Yu Jin* (Radix Curcumae), and *Chai Hu* (Radix Bupleuri) were added. For poor appetite, *Ji Nei Jin* (Endothelium Corneum Gigeriae Galli), *Shan Zha* (Fructus Crataegi), and *Shen Qu* (Massa Fermentata) were added. For a bitter taste in the mouth with a yellow tongue coating, *Zhi Zi* (Fructus Gardeniae) and *Huang Qin* (Radix Scutellariae) were added. For a red tongue body with a dry mouth, *Xuan Shen* (Radix Scrophulariae) and *Shi Hu* (Caulis Dendrobii) were added. For soreness and weakness of the lower back and knees, *Gou Qi Zi* (Fructus Lycii) and *Du Zhong* (Cortex Eucommiae) were added. For enlargement of the Liver and/or Spleen, *Tao Ren* (Semen Persicae), *Hong Hua* (Flos Carthami), and *Bie Jia* (Carapax Trionycis) were added. Lastly, for accumulation of water in the abdomen, *Shu Di Huang* (Radix Rehmanniae Praeparata) was removed, and *Bai Mao Gen* (Rhizoma Imperatae) and *Da Fu Pi* (Pericarpium Arecae) were added.[26]
9. **Infertility**: Modified *Liu Wei Di Huang Wan* was used to treat infertility in 42 patients (16 males and 26 females between the ages of 22 to 37). The duration of marriage of the patients ranged from 1-14 years. The treatment included the addition of *Rou Cong Rong* (Herba Cistanches), *Dan Shen* (Radix et Rhizoma Salviae Miltiorrhizae), *Tu Si Zi* (Semen Cuscutae), *Fen Bi Xie* (Rhizoma Dioscoreae Hypoglaucae), and others as deemed necessary. After 3-6 months of herbal treatment, the study reported marked results in 31 cases, moderate results in 9 cases, and no effect in 2 cases. [Note: criteria for evaluation were not given.][27]
10. **Frequent urination**: One study reported effectiveness in treating 46 of 47 children with frequent urination using modified *Liu Wei Di Huang Wan* as decoction one time daily. The duration of treatment ranged from 3-6 days.[28]

Líù Wèi Dì Huáng Wán (Six-Ingredient Pill with Rehmannia)

HERB-DRUG INTERACTION

Chemotherapy-induced toxicities: One study reported marked improvement using *Liu Wei Di Huang Wan* as an adjunct to chemotherapy. Clinical benefits included relief of nausea and vomiting, a decrease of hair loss and stomatitis, an improvement in appetite, and an increase in white blood cells, red blood cells, platelets, T-lymphocytes, and natural killer (NK) cells.[29]

TOXICOLOGY

According to one study, no abnormalities were noted in pregnant mice that received *Liu Wei Di Huang Wan* continuously throughout the third trimester.[30]

SUGGESTED ACUPUNCTURE TREATMENT

1. Points: *Ganshu* (BL 18), *Shenshu* (BL 23), *Pishu* (BL 20), *Taixi* (KI 3), *Zhaohai* (KI 6), *Yinlingquan* (SP 9), and *Xingjian* (LR 2).
2. Technique: tonification.

Ganshu (BL 18), *Shenshu* (BL 23), and *Pishu* (BL 20) tonify Liver, Kidney, and Spleen yin. *Taixi* (KI 3) and *Zhaohai* (KI 6) tonify Kidney yin. *Yinlingquan* (SP 9) strengthens the Spleen and eliminates dampness. *Xingjian* (LR 2) sedates Liver fire and other turbidity.

RELATED FORMULA

Ěr Lóng Zuǒ Cí Wán
(Pill for Deafness that Is Kind to the Left [Kidney])
耳聾左慈丸
耳聋左慈丸
Pinyin Name: *Er Long Zuo Ci Wan*
Literal Name: Pill for Deafness that Is Kind to the Left [Kidney]
Original Source: *Guang Wen Yi Lun* (Discussion of Widespread Warm Epidemics) by Dai Tian-Zhang in 1722

Shu Di Huang (Radix Rehmanniae Praeparata)	240g
Shan Zhu Yu (Fructus Corni)	120g
Shan Yao (Rhizoma Dioscoreae)	120g
Fu Ling (Poria)	90g
Mu Dan Pi (Cortex Moutan)	90g
Ze Xie (Rhizoma Alismatis)	90g
Ci Shi (Magnetitum), *duan* (calcined)	60g
Shi Chang Pu (Rhizoma Acori Tatarinowii)	45g
Wu Wei Zi (Fructus Schisandrae Chinensis)	15g

The source text states to grind the herbs into a fine powder, and mix with honey to make pills. Take 9g of pills with lightly salted water.

Er Long Zuo Ci Wan (Pill for Deafness that Is Kind to the Left [Kidney]) tonifies Liver and Kidney yin, and opens the sensory orifices (ear). It is based on *Liu Wei Di Huang Wan* with the addition of *Ci Shi* (Magnetitum), *Shi Chang Pu* (Rhizoma Acori Tatarinowii), and *Wu Wei Zi* (Fructus Schisandrae Chinensis). *Ci Shi* (Magnetitum) is commonly used to improve hearing. *Shi Chang Pu* (Rhizoma Acori Tatarinowii) opens the orifices and dispels phlegm that may be blocking the senses. *Wu Wei Zi* (Fructus Schisandrae Chinensis) prevents the leakage of *jing* (essence). Clinically, this formula treats impaired or diminished hearing, and deafness arising from Kidney deficiency. It also treats vertigo, red eyes, dry eyes and poor vision. If this formula is given early, as soon as hearing deficits are noticed, it can completely restore hearing. It can take up to 3 months for full clinical effects to be realized.

This formula can be used to restore hearing and prevent hearing loss with complete deafness in geriatric dogs, if administered as soon as the owner notices a problem with diminished hearing. This formula should be given continuously for a minimum of 90 days in order to achieve good therapeutic effect, and continued improvement can be seen for up to six months.

AUTHORS' COMMENTS

Kidney and Liver yin tonics are commonly prescribed every day by veterinarians that practice Chinese medicine. Kidney yin may be tonified using tonic formulas for a variety of deficiency syndromes and for damage to the *zang fu* organs. *Bu fa* (tonifying) is one of the *ba fa* (eight treatment methods) described in *Huang Di Nei Jing* (Yellow Emperor's Inner Classic); this text admonishes us to "tonify that which is deficient." It is essential that the diagnosis of deficiency is clear, because formulas used to tonify deficiencies may exacerbate disorders caused by excess. A severe excess condition may exhibit clinical signs commonly associated with a deficiency condition (such as lethargy, weight loss, lack of vitality). Not all deficient conditions are chronic, and not all chronic conditions are deficient. Hence, the root cause must be properly differentiated to determine whether excess should be treated simultaneously while tonifying identified deficiencies.

Deficiency syndromes usually do not occur independently and the weakness of one aspect of the body often affects another aspect, thus ultimately affecting more than one organ. Due to the integral relationship between yin and yang, tonifying one will fortify the other, but it may be more effective to nourish both concurrently. Therefore, many formulas that nourish yang will often contain ingredients to tonify yin as well. Often a treatment strategy for

Lìu Wèi Dì Huáng Wán (Six-Ingredient Pill with Rehmannia)

deficiency is guided by the basic principle: "for deficiency, tonify the mother." In other words, one should nourish the organ that precedes the deficient organ in the cycle of mutual generation. Thus, Kidney (the water element) is tonified to treat Liver (the wood element) deficiency. Yin-tonifying formulas are nourishing, and, as such, are rich and cloying in nature. Most of them contain herbs to promote the circulation of qi and body fluids to prevent the formulas from impairing digestion and water metabolism. Even so, they should be used with caution, especially in animals with weakness of the middle *jiao*. If an active pathogenic factor (bacterial or viral infection) is present, the use of tonifying formulas is contraindicated.

Chronic renal failure: *Liu Wei Di Huang Wan* has been shown to be clinically effective in the treatment of chronic renal failure in dogs and especially in cats. Efficacy of the formula is demonstrated by an improvement in renal parameters, which include BUN, creatinine and phosphorus. It has also shown positive effects in the treatment of proteinuria on repeat urinalysis and measurement of urine protein-creatinine ratio values. Beneficial effects can be seen within two weeks in attitude, energy and appetite; improvements in laboratory values are typically seen within three to four months, and continue up to 12 months. Phosphate binders, angiotensin-converting enzyme (ACE) inhibitors (enalapril, benazepril) and calcium channel antagonists (amlodipine, verapamil, diltiazem) have been given concurrently without adverse effects. For chronic renal failure with Spleen qi deficiency, combine with *Liu Jun Zi Tang* (Six-Gentlemen Decoction) or *Shen Ling Bai Zhu San* (Ginseng, Poria, and Atractylodes Macrocephala Powder); with anemia and qi and blood deficiency, combine with *Ba Zhen Tang* (Eight-Treasure Decoction); and with blood deficiency and stagnation, combine with *Tao Hong Si Wu Tang* (Four-Substance Decoction with Safflower and Peach Pit).

Nephrotic syndrome: *Liu Wei Di Huang Wan* and *Wu Ling San* (Five-Ingredient Powder with Poria) was used to treat a 10-year-old Golden Retriever with severe edema, hypoalbuminemia, and proteinuria. The dog was hospitalized and was given a plasma transfusion, and the herbal formula was administered immediately after hospitalization. After 8 days of treatment, the edema resolved and the dog was released. Treatment continued for another 14 months without relapse, and a good quality of life was maintained using *Liu Wei Di Huang Wan* plus *Du Zhong* (Cortex Eucommiae), *Shan Yao* (Rhizoma Dioscoreae), *Rou Cong Rong* (Herba Cistanches), *Ba Ji Tian* (Radix Morindae Officinalis), *Ren Shen* (Radix et Rhizoma Ginseng), *Dang Gui* (Radix Angelicae Sinensis), *Niu Xi* (Radix Achyranthis Bidentatae), *Wu Wei Zi* (Fructus Schisandrae Chinensis), and other herbs.

Diabetes Mellitus: *Liu Wei Di Huang Wan* can be used to treat both feline and canine diabetes. For diabetes with Stomach yin deficiency and heat, it can be combined with *Yu Nu Jian* (Jade Woman Decoction); with qi and yin deficiencies, it is often combined with *Sheng Mai San* (Generate the Pulse Powder). In animals with chronic Type I diabetes and peripheral neuropathy, it can be combined with *Bu Yang Huan Wu Tang* (Tonify the Yang to Restore Five Decoction).

Congenital portosystemic shunt: A combination of *Liu Wei Di Huang Wan* and *Xue Fu Zhu Yu Tang* (Drive Out Stasis in the Mansion of Blood Decoction) were used to treat congenital portosystemic shunt in a three-year old cat, as diagnosed by exploratory surgery and histopathology, with elevated bile acids (greater than 79 umol/L). Treatment for one year resulted in a return of bile acids to normal range and complete resolution of clinical signs.

Cerebellar disease: *Liu Wei Di Huang Wan* and *Shen Ling Bai Zhu San* (Ginseng, Poria, and Atractylodes Macrocephala Powder) were used to treat a cat that presented with an inability to stand, sit or walk, without falling over and that required hand feeding. The animal also had frequent vomiting episodes with weight loss. After 8 months of treatment, the animal was able to eat, sit, stand and ambulate on his own with moderate dysmetria.

Alopecia: For the treatment of alopecia that develops secondary to blood heat and hair loss, combine *Liu Wei Di Huang Wan* with *Si Wu Tang* (Four-Substance Decoction), *Er Zhi Wan* (Two-Ultimate Pill), *Xuan Shen* (Radix Scrophulariae), *Bai Fu Zi* (Rhizoma Typhonii), *Chi Shao* (Radix Paeoniae Rubra), and *Dan Shen* (Radix et Rhizoma Salviae Miltiorrhizae). If there is severe itching, add *Di Fu Zi* (Fructus Kochiae) and *Bai Xian Pi* (Cortex Dictamni).

Liu Wei Di Huang Wan is the representative formula to tonify Liver and Kidney yin, and is one of the most frequently prescribed formulas. Many herbal formulas that tonify Kidney yin are based on this formula. Below are the key similarities and differences among these tonic formulas:

- *Liu Wei Di Huang Wan* is the most basic Kidney and Liver yin tonic formula.
- *Mai Wei Di Huang Wan* (Ophiopogonis, Schisandra and Rehmannia Pill) is formulated with the addition of *Mai Dong* (Radix Ophiopogonis) and *Wu Wei Zi* (Fructus Schisandrae Chinensis). It nourishes yin, astringes the Lung, lowers reversed flow of Lung qi, and arrests wheezing.

Liù Wèi Dì Huáng Wán (Six-Ingredient Pill with Rehmannia)

- *Zhi Bai Di Huang Wan* (Anemarrhena, Phellodendron, and Rehmannia Pill) contains *Zhi Mu* (Rhizoma Anemarrhenae) and *Huang Bo* (Cortex Phellodendri Chinensis) to nourish yin and clear deficiency fire.
- *Qi Ju Di Huang Wan* (Lycium Fruit, Chrysanthemum, and Rehmannia Pill) has *Gou Qi Zi* (Fructus Lycii) and *Ju Hua* (Flos Chrysanthemi); it nourishes Kidney and Liver yin, and benefits the eyes to brighten vision.[31]

There are many herbal formulas that tonify Liver and Kidney yin. Their similarities and differences are as follows:

- *Liu Wei Di Huang Wan* is the most representative formula for tonifying yin. It nourishes and tonifies the Liver, Kidney, and Spleen.
- *Zuo Gui Wan* (Restore the Left [Kidney] Pill) replenishes Kidney *jing* (essence) and treats depleted *jing* and marrow. It is a pure yin-tonic formula without any sedating herbs to offset the heavy tonic effects. It has a stronger yin-tonifying effect than *Liu Wei Di Huang Wan*. However, because of its stagnating nature, it is usually not taken for a prolonged period of time.

Function	Composition	Liu Wei Di Huang Wan	Zhi Bai Di Huang Wan	Mai Wei Di Huang Wan	Qi Ju Di Huang Wan	Jin Gui Shen Qi Wan	Ba Wei Di Huang Wan
Tonifies Liver and Kidney yin	*Shu Di Huang* (Radix Rehmanniae Praeparata), *Shan Zhu Yu* (Fructus Corni) and *Shan Yao* (Rhizoma Dioscoreae)	✓	✓	✓	✓	✓*	✓
Lowers turbidity and resolves dampness	*Ze Xie* (Rhizoma Alismatis), *Mu Dan Pi* (Cortex Moutan) and *Fu Ling* (Poria)	✓	✓	✓	✓	✓	✓
Clears deficiency fire	*Zhi Mu* (Rhizoma Anemarrhenae) and *Huang Bo* (Cortex Phellodendri Chinensis)		✓				
Astringes the Lung and lowers reversed flow of qi	*Wu Wei Zi* (Fructus Schisandrae Chinensis) and *Mai Dong* (Radix Ophiopogonis)			✓			
Nourishes and benefits the eyes	*Gou Qi Zi* (Fructus Lycii) and *Ju Hua* (Flos Chrysanthemi)				✓		
Warms Kidney yang	*Gui Zhi* (Ramulus Cinnamomi) and *Fu Zi* (Radix Aconiti Lateralis Praeparata)					✓	
Strongly warms Kidney yang	*Rou Gui* (Cortex Cinnamomi) and *Fu Zi* (Radix Aconiti Lateralis Praeparata)						✓

* *Di Huang* (Radix Rehmanniae) is used in place of *Shu Di Huang* (Radix Rehmanniae Praeparata).

Liù Wèi Dì Huáng Wán (Six-Ingredient Pill with Rehmannia)

- *Da Bu Yin Wan* (Great Tonify the Yin Pill) nourishes yin, clears heat, anchors Liver yang, and is best for Kidney water depletion with deficiency heat flaming upwards that can manifest as hyperactivity, aggression, sleep disturbance, chronic, dry cough, and dry eyes, hair and skin. It is commonly combined with other herbal formulas to treat hypertension, diabetes, and hyperthyroidism.
- *Yi Guan Jian* (Linking Decoction) nourishes the middle *jiao* and smoothes Liver qi. It treats Liver and Kidney deficiency with Liver qi stagnation, causing acid regurgitation, and dry eyes, mouth and throat.
- *Shi Hu Ye Guang Wan* (Dendrobium Pill for Night Vision) causes Liver yang and wind to descend, nourishes yin, and brightens the eyes. It is best for visual disorders caused by Liver and Kidney yin deficiency with blood deficiency.
- *Qi Bao Mei Ran Wan* (Seven-Treasure Special Pill for Beautiful Whiskers) nourishes Kidney yin, tonifies Liver blood, and mainly treats hair disorders, such as hair loss, premature gray hair, and dry or brittle hair.
- *Gui Lu Er Xian Jiao* (Tortoise Shell and Deer Antler Syrup) tonifies Kidney yin and yang, *jing* (essence), and blood of the *du* (governing) and *ren* (conception) channels. This formula is useful for treating cats that are difficult to medicate with pills or capsules.
- *Er Zhi Wan* (Two-Ultimate Pill) is a balanced yin-tonic formula, not too warm or too cold, that mainly treats Kidney yin deficiency with dizziness and blurred vision.

References

1. *Zhong Yi Fang Ji Xian Dai Yan Jiu* (Modern Study of Medical Formulas in Traditional Chinese Medicine), 1997, 709
2. *Zhong Cheng Yao Yan Jiu* (Research of Chinese Patent Medicine), 1986, 12: 41
3. *Zhong Guo Yao Ke Da Xue Xue Bao* (Journal of University of Chinese Herbology), 1990, 4: 241
4. *Guo Wai Yi Xue* (Foreign Medicine), 1986, 4: 11
5. *Zhong Cheng Yao Yan Jiu* (Research of Chinese Patent Medicine), 1984, 11: 25
6. *Zhong Cheng Yao Yan Jiu* (Research of Chinese Patent Medicine), 1981, 12: 28
7. *Zhong Guo Mian Yi Xue Za Zhi* (Chinese Journal of Immunology), 1987, 5: 296
8. *Xin Yi Yao Xue Za Zhi* (New Journal of Medicine and Herbology), 1977, 7: 41
9. *Zhong Guo Yao Ke Da Xue Xue Bao* (Journal of University of Chinese Herbology), 1989, 6: 951
10. *Zhong Yi Fang Ji Xian Dai Yan Jiu* (Modern Study of Medical Formulas in Traditional Chinese Medicine), 1997, 710
11. *Zhong Yi Fang Ji Xian Dai Yan Jiu* (Modern Study of Medical Formulas in Traditional Chinese Medicine), 1997, 704
12. *Zhong Guo Yi Ke Da Xue Xue Bao* (Journal of University of Chinese Medicine), 1989, 6: 354
13. *He Bei Zhong Yi* (Hebei Chinese Medicine), 1999, 11: 35
14. *Yun Nan Yi Yao* (Yunan Medicine and Herbology), 1983, 3: 181
15. *Hu Bei Zhong Yi Za Zhi* (Hubei Journal of Chinese Medicine), 1987, 3: 14
16. *Zhong Hua Yi Xue Za Zhi* (Chinese Journal of Medicine), 1956, 6: 546
17. *Hu Bei Zhong Yi Za Zhi* (Hubei Journal of Chinese Medicine), 1992, 2: 20
18. *Hei Long Jiang Zhong Yi Yao* (Heilongjiang Chinese Medicine and Herbology), 1987, 1: 40
19. *Zhong Cheng Yao Yan Jiu* (Research of Chinese Patent Medicine), 1986, 10: 33
20. *Zhong Yi Fang Ji Xian Dai Yan Jiu* (Modern Study of Medical Formulas in Traditional Chinese Medicine), 1997, 712
21. *Shen De Yan Jiu* (Research of Kidney), 1981, 19
22. *Hu Nan Yi Yao Za Zhi* (Hunan Journal of Medicine and Herbology), 1978, 4: 26
23. *Jiang Xi Zhong Yi Yao* (Jiangxi Chinese Medicine and Herbology), 1998, 6: 26
24. *Zhe Jiang Zhong Yi Za Zhi* (Zhejiang Journal of Chinese Medicine), 1988, 6: 244
25. *Shi Yong Zhong Yi Nei Ke Za Zhi* (Journal of Practical Chinese Internal Medicine), 1993, 3: 142
26. *Nei Meng Gu Zhong Yi Yao* (Traditional Chinese Medicine and Medicinals of Inner Mongolia), 1998, 1: 4
27. *Cheng Du Zhong Yi Xue Yuan Xue Bao* (Journal of Chengdu University of Traditional Chinese Medicine), 1993, 1: 20
28. *Shang Hai Zhong Yi Yao Za Zhi* (Shanghai Journal of Chinese Medicine and Herbology), 1998, 6: 31
29. *Zhe Jiang Zhong Yi Xue Yuan Xue Bao* (Journal of Zhejiang University of Chinese Medicine), 1992, 1: 29
30. *Zhong Yi Fang Ji Xian Dai Yan Jiu* (Modern Study of Medical Formulas in Traditional Chinese Medicine), 1997, 710-711
31. Wang, MZ et al. *Zhong Yi Xue Wen Da Ti Ku* (Questions and Answers on Traditional Chinese Medicine: Herbal Formulas).

8 TONIC FORMULAS

Zhī Bǎi Dì Huáng Wán

(Anemarrhena, Phellodendron, and Rehmannia Pill)

知柏地黃丸
知柏地黄丸

Pinyin Name: *Zhi Bai Di Huang Wan*
Literal Name: Anemarrhena, Phellodendron, and Rehmannia Pill
Alternate Names: *Zhi Bo Di Huang Wan, Zi Bo Di Huang Wan, Zhi Bai Ba Wei Wan, Chih Po Ti Huang Wan,* Eight-Ingredient Pill with Anemarrhena and Phellodendron, Anemarrhena, Phellodendron and Rehmannia Formula
Original Source: *Yi Zong Jin Jian* (Golden Mirror of the Medical Tradition) by Wu Qian in 1742

COMPOSITION

Shu Di Huang (Radix Rehmanniae Praeparata)	240g [24g]
Shan Zhu Yu (Fructus Corni)	120g [12g]
Shan Yao (Rhizoma Dioscoreae)	120g [12g]
Ze Xie (Rhizoma Alismatis)	90g [9g]
Mu Dan Pi (Cortex Moutan)	90g [9g]
Fu Ling (Poria)	90g [9g]
Zhi Mu (Rhizoma Anemarrhenae)	60g [6g]
Huang Bo (Cortex Phellodendri Chinensis)	60g [6g]

DOSAGE / PREPARATION / ADMINISTRATION

Prepare and administer this formula as honey pills or in decoction form. The instructions for preparation and administration for this formula are the same as *Liu Wei Di Huang Wan* (Six-Ingredient Pill with Rehmannia). For decoction, use the doses suggested in brackets.

CHINESE THERAPEUTIC ACTIONS

1. Nourishes Liver and Kidney yin
2. Clears yin-deficient fire

CLINICAL MANIFESTATIONS

Yin-deficient fire of the Liver and Kidney: irritability, dryness, restlessness, panting excessively (especially at night), dry cough, dry feces, short urination, heat aversion, desire for cool surfaces/places, increased appetite, increased thirst, trembling and jerking during sleep, soreness of the back and stifles, poor hearing or deafness, hypersensitivity to acupuncture, a red tongue body with no coating, and a rapid, thready pulse that is weaker on the left side.

VETERINARY CLINICAL APPLICATIONS

Diabetes mellitus, nephrotic syndrome, hypertension, chronic renal failure, feline hyperthyroidism, and canine hyperadrenocorticism (Cushing's disease).

EXPLANATION

Zhi Bai Di Huang Wan (Anemarrhena, Phellodendron, and Rehmannia Pill) nourishes Liver and Kidney yin, and clears yin-deficient heat. This formula has similar actions as *Liu Wei Di Huang Wan* (Six-Ingredient Pill with Rehmannia) to tonify yin; however, it has a much stronger effect to clear yin-deficient fire of the Liver and Kidney, making

***Zhi Bai Di Huang Wan* (Anemarrhena, Phellodendron, and Rehmannia Pill)**

Diagnosis	Clinical Signs	Treatment	Herbs
Yin-deficient fire of the Liver and Kidney	• Dry cough, constipation or dry feces, short urination, heat aversion, seeking cool surfaces/places, increased thirst, trembling and jerking during sleep, soreness of the back and stifles, poor hearing or deafness, hypersensitivity to acupuncture, a red tongue body with no coating, and a rapid, thready pulse that is weaker on the left side: Liver and Kidney yin deficiency • Excessive panting, dryness, restlessness, increased appetite, increased thirst, and irritability: yin-deficient fire	• Nourishes Liver and Kidney yin • Clears yin-deficient fire	• *Liu Wei Di Huang Wan* (Six-Ingredient Pill with Rehmannia) nourishes Liver and Kidney yin. • *Zhi Mu* (Rhizoma Anemarrhenae) and *Huang Bo* (Cortex Phellodendri Chinensis) sedate yin-deficient fire of the Liver and Kidney.

Zhī Bǎi Dì Huáng Wán
(Anemarrhena, Phellodendron, and Rehmannia Pill)

it more effective for relieving heat signs such as excessive panting (especially at night), dryness, insomnia, restlessness, increased to ravenous appetite, increased thirst, and irritability.

This formula consists of the six herbs of *Liu Wei Di Huang Wan* (Six-Ingredient Pill with Rehmannia), which nourish Liver and Kidney yin, plus *Zhi Mu* (Rhizoma Anemarrhenae) and *Huang Bo* (Cortex Phellodendri Chinensis) to sedate yin-deficient fire of the Liver and Kidney. For a more detailed explanation of the clinical manifestations and the functions of each of the herbs in this formula, please refer to *Liu Wei Di Huang Wan* (Six-Ingredient Pill with Rehmannia).

VETERINARY MODIFICATIONS

- For thirst and irritability, add *Huang Qi* (Radix Astragali) and *Ren Shen* (Radix et Rhizoma Ginseng).
- If there is more soreness of the lower back, add *Niu Xi* (Radix Achyranthis Bidentatae) and *Du Zhong* (Cortex Eucommiae).
- With significant deficiency heat signs, add one or more of the following: *Bie Jia* (Carapax Trionycis), *Qing Hao* (Herba Artemisiae Annuae), *Di Huang* (Radix Rehmanniae) or *Di Gu Pi* (Cortex Lycii).
- With pacing and restlessness at night, combine with *Suan Zao Ren Tang* (Sour Jujube Decoction).

CAUTIONS / CONTRAINDICATIONS

Please refer to *Liu Wei Di Huang Wan* (Six-Ingredient Pill with Rehmannia).

HUMAN CLINICAL STUDIES AND RESEARCH

1. **Male infertility**: Use of modified *Zhi Bai Di Huang Wan* was associated with 92.2% effectiveness in treating 220 men with infertility. The herbal treatment contained this formula plus *Bai Hua She She Cao* (Herba Hedyotis), *Pu Gong Ying* (Herba Taraxaci), *Dan Shen* (Radix et Rhizoma Salviae Miltiorrhizae), *Fen Bi Xie* (Rhizoma Dioscoreae Hypoglaucae), *Mu Li* (Concha Ostreae), *Niu Xi* (Radix Achyranthis Bidentatae), and *Shi Chang Pu* (Rhizoma Acori Tatarinowii) as the base formula. Additional modifications were made as necessary according to the condition of the patients. For Kidney yin deficiency, *Di Huang* (Radix Rehmanniae) and *Mu Dan Pi* (Cortex Moutan) were removed, and *Ba Ji Tian* (Radix Morindae Officinalis), *Rou Cong Rong* (Herba Cistanches), *Yin Yang Huo* (Herba Epimedii), *Huang Qi* (Radix Astragali), and *Gou Qi Zi* (Fructus Lycii) were added. For more damp-heat, *Da Huang* (Radix et Rhizoma Rhei) and *Mu Tong* (Caulis Akebiae) were added. For stagnation, *Wang Bu Liu Xing* (Semen Vaccariae), *Chi Shao* (Radix Paeoniae Rubra), and processed *Chuan Shan Jia* (Squama Manis) were added. For Liver qi stagnation, *Chai Hu* (Radix Bupleuri) and *Yu Jin* (Radix Curcumae) were added. Of 220 cases, the study reported pregnancy in their partners in 171 cases, improvement in 32 cases, and no benefit in 17 cases.[1]
2. **Diabetes mellitus**: Administration of modified *Zhi Bai Di Huang Wan* in 80 patients with type II diabetes mellitus was associated with normalization in 15 cases, significant improvement in 45 cases, slight improvement in 15 cases, and no benefit in 5 cases. The herbal formula contained *Zhi Bai Di Huang Wan*, with the elimination of *Fu Ling* (Poria) and *Ze Xie* (Rhizoma Alismatis), and the addition of *Jiao Gu Lan* (Rhizoma seu Herba Gynostemmatis), *Sha Shen* (Radix Glehniae seu Adenophorae), *Gou Qi Zi* (Fructus Lycii), *Shi Hu* (Caulis Dendrobii), *Shi Gao* (Gypsum Fibrosum), and others as needed.[2] In another study, 22 patients with diabetes were treated with modified *Zhi Bai Di Huang Wan*. In addition to diabetes, 8 patients had other complications, such as urinary tract infections, hypertension, coronary heart disease, and conjunctivitis. The patients were instructed to make dietary changes and take herbs on a daily basis. Out of 22 cases, the study reported a marked effect in 15 cases, moderate improvement in 6 cases, and no benefit in 1 case.[3]
3. **Nephrotic syndrome**: In one study, 30 patients with nephrotic syndrome were treated with modified *Zhi Bai Di Huang Wan*. The age of the patients ranged from 15-61 years of age, with a history of kidney disorder from 3 days to 17 years. All patients received herbal treatment and dietary changes. Out of 30 cases, the study reported marked improvement in 18 cases, moderate improvement in 11 cases, and no benefit in 1 case. The herbal treatment contained this formula plus *Dan Shen* (Radix et Rhizoma Salviae Miltiorrhizae), *Yi Yi Ren* (Semen Coicis), *Xuan Shen* (Radix Scrophulariae), and *Yi Mu Cao* (Herba Leonuri). Additional modifications were made as needed. For Lung qi deficiency with frequent infection, *Yu Ping Feng San* (Jade Windscreen Powder) with a larger dose of *Huang Qi* (Radix Astragali) was added. For Spleen deficiency with dampness, *Dang Shen* (Radix Codonopsis), *Bai Zhu* (Rhizoma Atractylodis Macrocephalae), *Zhu Ling* (Polyporus), and *Che Qian Zi* (Semen Plantaginis) were added. For Liver yang rising, *Ju Hua* (Flos Chrysanthemi) and *Gou Teng* (Ramulus Uncariae cum Uncis) were added. For Liver and Kidney yin deficiencies, *Di Huang* (Radix Rehmanniae), *Gou Qi Zi* (Fructus Lycii), and *Mai Dong* (Radix Ophiopogonis) were added. For soreness and pain of the throat, *Shan Dou Gen* (Radix et Rhizoma Sophorae Tonkinensis) and *She Gan* (Rhizoma Belamcandae) were

Zhī Bǎi Dì Huáng Wán

(Anemarrhena, Phellodendron, and Rehmannia Pill)

added. For severe hematuria, *Pu Huang* (Pollen Typhae), charred *Huang Qin* (Radix Scutellariae), charred *Da Huang* (Radix et Rhizoma Rhei), and a large dose of *Bai Mao Gen* (Rhizoma Imperatae) were added. For seminal emissions, calcined *Long Gu* (Os Draconis), *Qian Shi* (Semen Euryales), and *Jin Ying Zi* (Fructus Rosae Laevigatae) were added. For dry stools and constipation, *He Shou Wu* (Radix Polygoni Multiflori), *Dang Gui* (Radix Angelicae Sinensis), *Rou Cong Rong* (Herba Cistanches), *Sang Shen* (Fructus Mori), and *Da Huang* (Radix et Rhizoma Rhei) were added. For edema, *Da Fu Pi* (Pericarpium Arecae) and *Che Qian Zi* (Semen Plantaginis) were added.[4]

4. **Hypertension**: In one study, 40 patients with hypertension were diagnosed and treated with *Zhi Bai Di Huang Wan*. Out of 40 patients, 30 were diagnosed with secondary hypertension and 10 with primary hypertension. All patients were evaluated for both objective and subjective improvement, including blood pressure, headache, dizziness, feeling increased pressure in the head, insomnia, a bitter taste in the mouth, irritability, and a feeling of warmth in the palms and soles. Out of 10 patients with primary hypertension, the study reported improvement in 6 cases and no benefit in 4 cases after 8-9 weeks of treatment. Out of 30 cases of secondary hypertension, the study reported improvement in 24 cases and no benefit in 6 cases after 4-5 weeks of treatment.[5]
5. **Epistaxis**: One study of 30 patients with stubborn nosebleeds reported good results using modified *Zhi Bai Di Huang Wan*. The herbal treatment contained the formula plus *Huang Qin* (Radix Scutellariae) and *Xiao Ji* (Herba Cirsii) as the base formula, with the addition of other herbs as needed. For wind-cold, *Fang Feng* (Radix Saposhnikoviae) and *Niu Xi* (Radix Achyranthis Bidentatae) were added. For wind-heat, *Sang Bai Pi* (Cortex Mori) and *Ju Hua* (Flos Chrysanthemi) were added. For Stomach fire rising, *Shi Hu* (Caulis Dendrobii) and *Mai Dong* (Radix Ophiopogonis) were added. For Liver fire rising, *Chai Hu* (Radix Bupleuri) and *Zi Wan* (Radix et Rhizoma Asteris) were added. For Liver and Kidney yin deficiencies with deficiency fire, *Gou Qi Zi* (Fructus Lycii) and *Di Gu Pi* (Cortex Lycii) were added. For Spleen deficiency and its inability to control blood circulation, *Huang Qi* (Radix Astragali) and *Tai Zi Shen* (Radix Pseudostellariae) were added. After 10 days of herbal treatment, the study reported complete recovery without recurrence for one year in 15 cases, improvement in 12 cases, and no benefit in 3 cases.[6]
6. **Dryness in geriatric patients**: Use of modified *Zhi Bai Di Huang Wan* showed good results in treating 24 geriatric patients with various complaints of dryness, such as a dry mouth, dry nose, constipation, etc.[7]

HERB-DRUG INTERACTION

Streptomycin-induced toxicities: Administration of *Zhi Bai Di Huang Wan* showed effectiveness in treating streptomycin-induced toxicities in 39 patients between 10-73 years of age. Within 3-8 days following streptomycin injection, toxicities appeared, such as dizziness, tinnitus, deafness, muscle spasms and cramps, loss of balance when walking, nausea, vomiting, thirst, a dry mouth and throat, irritability, quick to anger, fatigue, poor appetite, night sweats, and dry stools. The treatment protocol was to administer modified *Zhi Bai Di Huang Wan* daily. The duration of treatment ranged from 10 to 116 days, with an average of 63 days. Of 39 cases, the study reported complete recovery in 30 cases, marked improvement in 6 cases, and moderate improvement in 3 cases. The study also noted that patients who responded the most were ones who sought treatment immediately after experiencing streptomycin toxicities.[8]

TOXICOLOGY

In an acute toxicology study, it was determined that the LD_{50} for a preparation of *Zhi Bai Di Huang Wan* was 13.31 g/kg via intraperitoneal injection in mice. The study concluded that the formula had very little toxicity.[9]

SUGGESTED ACUPUNCTURE TREATMENT

1. Points: *Ganshu* (BL 18), *Pishu* (BL 20), *Shenshu* (BL 23), *Taixi* (KI 3), *Zhaohai* (KI 6), *Yinlingquan* (SP 9), *Xingjian* (LR 2), *Yinxi* (HT 6), and *Yingu* (KI 10).
2. Technique: tonification.

Ganshu (BL 18), *Pishu* (BL 20), and *Shenshu* (BL 23) tonify Liver, Spleen, and Kidney yin. *Taixi* (KI 3) and *Zhaohai* (KI 6) mainly tonify Kidney yin. *Yinlingquan* (SP 9) strengthens the Spleen and eliminates dampness. *Xingjian* (LR 2) sedates Liver fire and other turbidity. *Yinxi* (HT 6) and *Yingu* (KI 10) nourish yin and clear fire.

AUTHORS' COMMENTS

Animals with Kidney yin deficiency and deficiency heat often display general weakness and irritability. They may be restless, especially at night, vocalize, and pace about at night. Moreover, they often have dry mouth and tongue, dry flaky hair coat with patchy alopecia, increased thirst, and increased urination. Constipation, or dry, hard feces alternating with diarrhea, may occur, along with short duration of urination. Most of these animals are thin, have a ravenous appetite, and are hypersensitive to acupuncture. Other signs include weak and painful back, arthritis and spondylosis, poor eyesight, hearing impairment or deafness. The tongue is red with little or no coating, dry, and

Zhī Bǎi Dì Huáng Wán

(Anemarrhena, Phellodendron, and Rehmannia Pill)

often with cracks, and the pulse is rapid, thready and weak, especially on the left side.

As *Zhi Bai Di Huang Wan* is cooling in nature, and many of the animals that require this formula are older, it is important to recheck the animal on a regular basis, in order to prevent over administration of this formula and damage to the yang energies of the body.

- *Zhi Bai Di Huang Wan* is commonly used as a sole formula in cats with chronic renal failure characterized by yin deficiency and deficiency heat and hypertension. For dogs with hypertension, add *Gou Teng* (Ramulus Uncariae cum Uncis), *Niu Xi* (Radix Achyranthis Bidentatae), and *Xuan Shen* (Radix Scrophulariae).
- For animals with hematuria from deficiency heat and normal urinalysis (idiopathic hematuria), combine with *Nu Zhen Zi* (Fructus Ligustri Lucidi) and *Mo Han Lian* (Herba Ecliptae).
- For the treatment of chronic glaucoma, combine with *Dan Shen* (Radix et Rhizoma Salviae Miltiorrhizae), *Shi Jue Ming* (Concha Haliotidis), *Nu Zhen Zi* (Fructus Ligustri Lucidi), *Shi Hu* (Caulis Dendrobii), and *Ju Hua* (Flos Chrysanthemi).
- *Zhi Bai Di Huang Wan* is appropriate and effective for cats with hyperthyroidism caused by yin deficiency and deficiency heat. The cats for which this formula is appropriate show signs of heat that include pacing at night, loud vocalization, voracious appetite, and possibly constipation.

For the treatment of diabetes with Kidney and Stomach yin deficiencies and Stomach heat, combine with *Yu Nu Jian* (Jade Woman Decoction). The animals for which this combination is appropriate have clinical signs that include a predominance of polyphagia, constipation with dry stool, halitosis, stomatitis and gingivitis. The tongue will be red and dry with a yellow coating, and the pulse will be full and slippery. With more yin deficiency present, the pulse may be thinner, rapid and weak.

Liu Wei Di Huang Wan (Six-Ingredient Pill with Rehmannia), *Zhi Bai Di Huang Wan*, and *Da Bu Yin Wan* (Great Tonify the Yin Pill) all treat Liver and Kidney yin deficiencies with heat; however, their differences are as follows:

- *Liu Wei Di Huang Wan* is the basic formula, and has minimal ability to clear deficiency heat. It is a more balanced formula than *Da Bu Yin Wan* (Great Tonify the Yin Pill), and is more appropriate for weaker patients.
- *Zhi Bai Di Huang Wan* contains two additional herbs, *Zhi Mu* and *Huang Bo* to nourish yin and clear deficiency heat, and so has a greater ability to clear deficiency fire than *Liu Wei Di Huang Wan*.
- *Da Bu Yin Wan* has the strongest ability to treat deficiency fire rising upward, and it also has some ability to anchor Liver yang. Animals may have a rapid, forceful pulse since this formula is more appropriate for strong patients.

References

1. *Guang Xi Zhong Yi Yao* (Guangxi Chinese Medicine and Herbology), 1996; 2:43.
2. *Hu Nan Zhong Yi Za Zhi* (Hunan Journal of Chinese Medicine), 1997; 6:7.
3. *Shang Hai Zhong Yi Yao Za Zhi* (Shanghai Journal of Chinese Medicine and Herbology), 1991; 10:23.
4. *Shi Yong Zhong Yi Za Zhi* (Journal of Practical Chinese Medicine), 1995; 6:10.
5. *Zhong Cheng Yao* (Study of Chinese Patent Medicine), 1995; 4:51.
6. *He Bei Zhong Yi* (Hebei Chinese Medicine), 1995; 4:46.
7. *Ji Lin Zhong Yi Yao* (Jilin Chinese Medicine and Herbology), 1993; 3:24.
8. *He Nan Zhong Yi* (Henan Chinese Medicine), 1994; 6:366.
9. *Zhong Yao Yao Li Yu Lin Chuang* (Pharmacology and Clinical Applications of Chinese Herbs), 1992; 17:2.

Qǐ Jú Dì Huáng Wán

(Lycium Fruit, Chrysanthemum, and Rehmannia Pill)

杞菊地黄丸
杞菊地黃丸

Pinyin Name: *Qi Ju Di Huang Wan*
Literal Name: Lycium Fruit, Chrysanthemum, and Rehmannia Pill
Alternate Names: *Chi Chu Ti Huang Wan, Chi Ju Di Huang Wan*, Wolfberry, Chrysanthemum and Rehmannia Pill; Lycium, Chrysanthemum and Rehmannia Pill; Lycium, Chrysanthemum and Rehmannia Formula
Original Source: *Yi Ji* (Levels of Medicine)

COMPOSITION

Shu Di Huang (Radix Rehmanniae Praeparata)	240g [24g]
Shan Zhu Yu (Fructus Corni)	120g [12g]
Shan Yao (Rhizoma Dioscoreae)	120g [12g]
Ze Xie (Rhizoma Alismatis)	90g [9g]
Mu Dan Pi (Cortex Moutan)	90g [9g]
Fu Ling (Poria)	90g [9g]
Gou Qi Zi (Fructus Lycii)	90g [9g]
Ju Hua (Flos Chrysanthemi)	90g [9g]

DOSAGE / PREPARATION / ADMINISTRATION

Prepare and administer this formula as honey pills or in decoction form. The instructions for preparation and administration for this formula are the same as *Liu Wei Di Huang Wan* (Six-Ingredient Pill with Rehmannia). For decoction, use the doses suggested in brackets.

CHINESE THERAPEUTIC ACTIONS

Nourishes Liver and Kidney yin

CLINICAL MANIFESTATIONS

Liver and Kidney yin deficiencies with eye disorders: impaired vision, dry eyes, excessive tearing, chronic ocular discharge, and other signs of yin deficiencies stated in *Liu Wei Di Huang Wan* (Six-Ingredient Pill with Rehmannia).

VETERINARY CLINICAL APPLICATIONS

Progressive retinal atrophy (PRA), optic nerve atrophy, photosensitivity, redness, swelling and pain of eyes, impaired vision, excessive tearing, chronic mucoid ocular discharge, chronic glaucoma, hypertension and diabetes mellitus.

EXPLANATION

Qi Ju Di Huang Wan (Lycium Fruit, Chrysanthemum, and Rehmannia Pill), derived from *Liu Wei Di Huang Wan* (Six-Ingredient Pill with Rehmannia), tonifies Kidney and Liver yin, brightens the eyes, and improves vision. Formulas that treat the eye and improve vision generally tonify Kidney and Liver yin. Liver yin and blood keep the eyes moist and promote normal tear production, while Kidney yin is needed to nourish Liver yin based on Five-Element Theory. The eyes are often referred to as "the window of the Liver." Insufficiency of yin leads to dry eyes, impaired vision, retinal or optic nerve atrophy, and opacity and hardening of the lens of the eye. Many disorders or pathogenic factors that affect the Liver will often be transmitted to the eyes due to their close relationship. Excess Liver fire or Liver yang rising due to yin deficiency can lead to redness and burning of the eyes, and can result in hypertension that can cause bleeding and retinal detachment. In these cases, it is necessary to clear Liver heat, tonify Liver yin, or clear deficiency fire at the same time. Compared

***Qi Ju Di Huang Wan* (Lycium Fruit, Chrysanthemum, and Rehmannia Pill)**

Diagnosis	Clinical Signs	Treatment	Herbs
Liver and Kidney yin deficiencies with eye disorders	• Impaired vision, excessive tearing, and chronic ocular discharge: Liver and Kidney yin deficiency • Dry eyes: Liver and Kidney yin deficiencies unable to nourish the eyes	• Nourishes Liver and Kidney yin • Nourishes the eyes and improves visual functions	• *Liu Wei Di Huang Wan* (Six-Ingredient Pill with Rehmannia) nourishes Liver and Kidney yin. • *Gou Qi Zi* (Fructus Lycii) and *Ju Hua* (Flos Chrysanthemi) improve vision and treat various visual disorders.

Qǐ Jú Dì Huáng Wán

(Lycium Fruit, Chrysanthemum, and Rehmannia Pill)

to *Liu Wei Di Huang Wan*, this formula more strongly nourishes the Liver and benefits the eyes.

This formula consists of *Liu Wei Di Huang Wan* (Six-Ingredient Pill with Rehmannia) plus *Gou Qi Zi* (Fructus Lycii) and *Ju Hua* (Flos Chrysanthemi). *Liu Wei Di Huang Wan* (Six-Ingredient Pill with Rehmannia) tonifies Liver and Kidney yin. *Gou Qi Zi* (Fructus Lycii) and *Ju Hua* (Flos Chrysanthemi) improve vision and treat various eye disorders. For more information, please refer to *Liu Wei Di Huang Wan* (Six-Ingredient Pill with Rehmannia).

VETERINARY MODIFICATIONS

- For red eyes with swelling and pain, add *Zhi Mu* (Rhizoma Anemarrhenae) and *Huang Bo* (Cortex Phellodendri Chinensis).
- With diminished and dimmed vision, add *Dang Gui* (Radix Angelicae Sinensis) and *Huang Qi* (Radix Astragali).
- For the treatment of uveitis, add *Dan Shen* (Radix et Rhizoma Salviae Miltiorrhizae), *Chi Shao* (Radix Paeoniae Rubra), *Shi Jue Ming* (Concha Haliotidis) and *Ji Li* (Fructus Tribuli).

CAUTIONS / CONTRAINDICATIONS

Please refer to *Liu Wei Di Huang Wan* (Six-Ingredient Pill with Rehmannia).

PHARMACOLOGICAL EFFECTS

1. **Immunostimulant**: One study reported a mild immunostimulant effect associated with the use of *Qi Ju Di Huang Wan* in mice. It increased phagocytic activities of macrophages.[1]
2. **Hypoglycemic**: Administration of *Qi Ju Di Huang Wan* was associated with reduced plasma glucose levels and decreased daily intake of water. The treatment protocol was to administer 2.5 g/kg and 5.0 g/kg of the formula via oral ingestion one time daily for 4 months.[2]

HUMAN CLINICAL STUDIES AND RESEARCH

1. **Retinitis**: Use of *Qi Ju Di Huang Wan* in 140 patients with retinitis was associated with complete recovery in 22 patients, significant improvement in 21 patients, moderate improvement in 70 patients, and no benefit in 27 patients. The treatment protocol was to administer the herbs in decoction daily, for 3 weeks per course of treatment. The duration of treatment ranged from 30 to 118 days, with an average of 57 days.[3]
2. **Vitreous opacity**: One study reported success using modified *Qi Ju Di Huang Wan* to treat vitreous opacity in 34 patients (21 males and 13 females, between 38-76 years of age). The herbal formula contained *Gou Qi Zi* (Fructus Lycii) 15g, *Ju Hua* (Flos Chrysanthemi) 15g, *Shan Yao* (Rhizoma Dioscoreae) 15g, *Shan Zhu Yu* (Fructus Corni) 15g, *Shu Di Huang* (Radix Rehmanniae Praeparata) 20g, *Fu Ling* (Poria) 10g, *Ze Xie* (Rhizoma Alismatis) 10g, *Mu Dan Pi* (Cortex Moutan) 10g, *Tu Si Zi* (Semen Cuscutae) 10g, *Nu Zhen Zi* (Fructus Ligustri Lucidi) 10g, and *Jue Ming Zi* (Semen Cassiae) 10g. The treatment protocol was to cook the herbs in water, and administer the decoction in 2 equally-divided doses, two times daily for 30 days. Of 34 patients, the study reported significant improvement in 18 patients, moderate improvement in 11 patients, and no benefit in 5 patients. The overall rate of effectiveness was 85.29%.[4]
3. **Hypertension**: Two studies have shown that administration of *Qi Ju Di Huang Wan* was effective in treating primary hypertension characterized by Kidney yin deficiency. The duration of treatment was 8-12 weeks per course of treatment. Clinical results included reduction of blood pressure and resolution of subjective symptoms.[5,6]

SUGGESTED ACUPUNCTURE TREATMENT

1. Points: *Ganshu* (BL 18), *Shenshu* (BL 23), *Pishu* (BL 20), *Taixi* (KI 3), *Zhaohai* (KI 6), *Yinlingquan* (SP 9), *Xingjian* (LR 2), *Jingming* (BL 1), *Zanzhu* (BL 2), and *Yanglao* (SI 6).
2. Technique: tonification.

Ganshu (BL 18), *Shenshu* (BL 23), and *Pishu* (BL 20) tonify Liver, Kidney, and Spleen yin. *Taixi* (KI 3) and *Zhaohai* (KI 6) mainly tonify Kidney yin. *Yinlingquan* (SP 9) strengthens the Spleen and eliminates dampness. *Xingjian* (LR 2) sedates Liver fire and other turbidity. *Jingming* (BL 1), *Zanzhu* (BL 2), and *Yanglao* (SI 6) clarify vision.

AUTHORS' COMMENTS

Qi Ju Di Huang Wan is commonly used to treat ocular diseases in veterinary medicine.

- This formula was used to treat progressive retinal atrophy (PRA) in a four-year-old male neutered dachshund following diagnosis by a veterinary ophthalmologist. The formula was given routinely, with modifications as needed, and the animal still has day vision after three years of treatment.
- This formula is frequently used to treat keratoconjunctivitis sicca (KCS) in the dog. Continuous use for up to six months can improve or normalize tear production, as measured per Schirmer tear test (STT). The younger the animal when therapy is instituted, the more likely the tear production can be restored.
- For the treatment of glaucoma with hyperactive Liver yang, combine it with *Tian Ma Gou Teng Yin* (Gastrodia and Uncaria Decoction). Once ocular pressures are normal, discontinue *Tian Ma Gou Teng Yin* (Gastrodia and Uncaria

Qǐ Jú Dì Huáng Wán

(Lycium Fruit, Chrysanthemum, and Rehmannia Pill)

Decoction) and administer *Qi Ju Di Huang Wan* for maintenance.

- For non-healing corneal ulcers, including indolent ulcers, combine with *Tao Hong Si Wu Tang* (Four-Substance Decoction with Safflower and Peach Pit) and add *Dan Shen* (Radix et Rhizoma Salviae Miltiorrhizae) and *Yu Jin* (Radix Curcumae).
- This formula can be used to treat feline hyperthyroidism with qi and yin deficiencies, by combining it with *Sheng Mai San* (Generate the Pulse Powder). Some cats will tolerate this combination added to their food.
- This formula can be used to treat renal hypertension in cats; in some cases, therapy can be discontinued after three to four months of treatment if there is complete resolution of hypertension.
- For a comparative discussion of herbal formulas to treat ophthalmologic conditions, see *Zi Shen Ming Mu Tang* (Nourish the Kidney to Brighten the Eyes Decoction).

References

1. *Zhong Cheng Yao* (Study of Chinese Patent Medicine), 1990; 10:28.
2. *Zhong Yao Yao Li Yu Lin Chuang* (Pharmacology and Clinical Applications of Chinese Herbs), 1993; 9(4):2.
3. *An Hui Zhong Yi Xue Yuan Xue Bao* (Journal of Anhui University School of Medicine), 1989; 4:18.
4. *Zhong Yi Yao Xue Bao* (Report of Chinese Medicine and Herbology), 1995; 2:25.
5. *Zhong Yao Yao Li Yu Lin Chuang* (Pharmacology and Clinical Applications of Chinese Herbs), 1992; 3:35.
6. *Xin Zhong Yi* (New Chinese Medicine), 1999; 3:12.

Mài Wèi Dì Huáng Wán

(Ophiopogonis, Schisandra, and Rehmannia Pill)

麥味地黃丸
麦味地黄丸

Pinyin Name: *Mai Wei Di Huang Wan*
Literal Name: Ophiopogonis, Schisandra, and Rehmannia Pill
Alternate Names: *Ba Xian Chang Shou Wan* (Eight-Immortal Pill for Longevity), *Mai Wei Ti Huang Wan* (Ophiopogon-Flavoured Rehmannia Pill)
Original Source: *Yi Ji* (Levels of Medicine)

COMPOSITION

Shu Di Huang (Radix Rehmanniae Praeparata)	240g [24g]
Shan Zhu Yu (Fructus Corni)	120g [12g]
Shan Yao (Rhizoma Dioscoreae)	120g [12g]
Ze Xie (Rhizoma Alismatis)	90g [9g]
Mu Dan Pi (Cortex Moutan)	90g [9g]
Fu Ling (Poria)	90g [9g]
Mai Dong (Radix Ophiopogonis)	90g [9g]
Wu Wei Zi (Fructus Schisandrae Chinensis)	60g [6g]

Mài Wèi Dì Huáng Wán

(Ophiopogonis, Schisandra, and Rehmannia Pill)

DOSAGE / PREPARATION / ADMINISTRATION

Prepare and administer this formula as honey pills or in decoction form. The instructions for preparation and administration of this formula are the same as *Liu Wei Di Huang Wan* (Six-Ingredient Pill with Rehmannia). For decoction, use the doses suggested in brackets.

CHINESE THERAPEUTIC ACTIONS

1. Nourishes Liver and Kidney yin
2. Astringes Lung qi and nourishes Lung yin

CLINICAL MANIFESTATIONS

Kidney and Lung yin deficiencies: coughing, shortness of breath, constipation or dry feces, and the clinical manifestations of yin deficiency found in *Liu Wei Di Huang Wan* (Six-Ingredient Pill with Rehmannia).

VETERINARY CLINICAL APPLICATIONS

Diabetes mellitus, asthma, and chronic bronchitis.

EXPLANATION

Mai Wei Di Huang Wan (Ophiopogonis, Schisandra and Rehmannia Pill) is a variation of *Liu Wei Di Huang Wan* (Six-Ingredient Pill with Rehmannia), with the addition of *Mai Dong* (Radix Ophiopogonis) and *Wu Wei Zi* (Fructus Schisandrae Chinensis). *Liu Wei Di Huang Wan* (Six-Ingredient Pill with Rehmannia) tonifies Liver and Kidney yin. *Mai Dong* (Radix Ophiopogonis) and *Wu Wei Zi* (Fructus Schisandrae Chinensis) tonify Lung yin and stop coughing and shortness of breath.

PHARMACOLOGICAL EFFECTS

Hypoglycemic: In laboratory experiments, the use of *Mai Wei Di Huang Wan* had marked hypoglycemic effect if the plasma glucose level was between 180-350 mg/dl. However, it had little effect when the plasma glucose level was above 350 mg/dl.[1] While the exact mechanism of this hypoglycemic effect is not well understood, it has been determined that administration of this formula does not increase plasma insulin levels, and that it still had marked hypoglycemic effect in dogs whose pancreas had been surgically removed.[2]

HUMAN CLINICAL STUDIES AND RESEARCH

1. **Diabetes mellitus**: One study reported satisfactory results using *Mai Wei Di Huang Wan* to treat 20 patients with diabetes mellitus with elevated blood glucose levels (180-410 mg/dL), glucose in the urine (++ to +++), and ketone in the urine (in 8 of 20 patients).[3]
2. **Tidal fever and night perspiration**: In one study, 150 patients with tidal fever and night sweats associated with pulmonary tuberculosis were treated with good results. The herbal treatment contained *Mai Wei Di Huang Wan* plus *Sha Shen* (Radix Glehniae seu Adenophorae), *Bai He* (Bulbus Lilii), and *Yu Zhu* (Rhizoma Polygonati Odorati) as the base formula. *Huang Qi* (Radix Astragali) was added for qi deficiency; *Zi Wan* (Radix et Rhizoma Asteris) was added for dry cough, and *Shan Zhu Yu* (Fructus Corni) for severe night sweats. Of 150 patients, the study reported resolution of tidal fever and night sweats in 146 patients, and no effect in 4 patients.[4]

SUGGESTED ACUPUNCTURE TREATMENT

1. Points: *Ganshu* (BL 18), *Shenshu* (BL 23), *Pishu* (BL 20), *Taixi* (KI 3), *Zhaohai* (KI 6), *Yinlingquan* (SP 9), *Xingjian* (LR 2), *Feishu* (BL 13), and *Gaohuangshu* (BL 43).
2. Technique: tonification.

Ganshu (BL 18), *Shenshu* (BL 23), and *Pishu* (BL 20) tonify Liver, Kidney, and Spleen yin. *Taixi* (KI 3) and *Zhaohai* (KI 6) mainly tonify Kidney yin. *Yinlingquan* (SP 9) strengthens the Spleen and eliminates dampness.

***Mai Wei Di Huang Wan* (Ophiopogonis, Schisandra and Rehmannia Pill)**

Diagnosis	Clinical Signs	Treatment	Herbs
Kidney and Lung yin deficiencies accompanied by coughing	• General weakness, irritability, dryness, insomnia, restlessness, panting excessively (especially at night), heat aversion, seeking cool surfaces/places, increased to ravenous appetite, increased thirst, trembling and jerking during sleep, soreness of the back and stifles, poor hearing or deafness, a red tongue body with little or no coating, and a rapid, thready pulse that is weaker on the left: Liver and Kidney yin deficiencies • Coughing, shortness of breath, and constipation or dry feces: Lung yin deficiency	• Nourishes Liver and Kidney yin • Astringes and nourishes Lung yin to stop coughing	• *Liu Wei Di Huang Wan* (Six-Ingredient Pill with Rehmannia) nourishes Liver and Kidney yin. • *Mai Dong* (Radix Ophiopogonis) and *Wu Wei Zi* (Fructus Schisandrae Chinensis) tonify and astringe Lung yin.

Mài Wèi Dì Huáng Wán
(Ophiopogonis, Schisandra, and Rehmannia Pill)

Xingjian (LR 2) sedates Liver fire and other turbidity. *Feishu* (BL 13) and *Gaohuangshu* (BL 43) consolidate the Lung and Kidney.

AUTHORS' COMMENTS

Mai Wei Di Huang Wan can be used to treat chronic bronchitis in geriatric dogs, and in animals recovering from pneumonia with yin deficiency. Cats with chronic bronchial asthma with Lung and Kidney yin deficiencies can be given this formula, and it can be combined with *Ren Shen Ge Jie San* (Ginseng and Gecko Powder) to improve its ability to resolve cough and stabilize asthma. *Mai Wei Di Huang Wan* can be used in the treatment and management of canine hypoadrenocorticism with Kidney and Liver yin deficiencies, by adding *Huang Jing* (Rhizoma Polygonati), *Zhi Gan Cao* (Radix et Rhizoma Glycyrrhizae Praeparata cum Melle), *Gui Ban* (Plastrum Testudinis) and *Tu Si Zi* (Semen Cuscutae), and *Gou Qi Zi* (Fructus Lycii). This formula can be safely given in combination with conventional drugs that include injectable mineralocorticoids (Percorten) or oral drugs (Florinef).

Mai Wei Di Huang Wan is also used to treat various kidney diseases:

- For the treatment of chronic glomerulonephritis in dogs, combine with *Tai Zi Shen* (Radix Pseudostellariae), *Sang Ji Sheng* (Herba Taxilli), *Yi Mu Cao* (Herba Leonuri), *Qian Shi* (Semen Euryales), *Huo Xiang* (Herba Agastaches), and *Dan Shen* (Radix et Rhizoma Salviae Miltiorrhizae).
- With severe proteinuria, add *Huang Qi* (Radix Astragali), *Yi Zhi* (Fructus Alpiniae Oxyphyllae), and *Jin Ying Zi* (Fructus Rosae Laevigatae).
- Add *Xian Mao* (Rhizoma Curculiginis) and *Yin Yang Huo* (Herba Epimedii) for yin and yang deficiencies. This combination can be modified and given long term as needed.

References

1. *Zhong Yao Tong Bao* (Journal of Chinese Herbology), 1982; 6:32.
2. *Zhong Yi Fang Ji Xian Dai Yan Jiu* (Modern Study of Medical Formulas in Traditional Chinese Medicine), 1997; 727.
3. *Si Chuan Zhong Yi* (Sichuan Chinese Medicine), 1989; 3:25.
4. *Zhong Yi Yan Jiu* (Research of Chinese Medicine), 1992; 3:40.

Zuǒ Guī Wán (Restore the Left [Kidney] Pill)
左歸丸
左归丸

Pinyin Name: *Zuo Gui Wan*
Literal Name: Restore the Left [Kidney] Pill
Alternate Name: Cyathula and Rehmannia Formula
Original Source: *Jing Yue Quan Shu* (Collected Treatises of [Zhang] Jing Yue) by Zhang Jie-Bin (Zhang Jing-Yue) in 1624

COMPOSITION

Shu Di Huang (Radix Rehmanniae Praeparata)	240g [24g]
Gou Qi Zi (Fructus Lycii)	120g [12g]
Shan Zhu Yu (Fructus Corni)	120g [12g]
Gui Ban Jiao (Gelatinum Plastrum Testudinis), *chao* (dry-fried)	120g [12g]
Lu Jiao Jiao (Colla Cornus Cervi), *chao* (dry-fried)	120g [12g]
Tu Si Zi (Semen Cuscutae), *zhi* (prepared)	120g [12g]
Chuan Niu Xi (Radix Cyathulae), *xi* (washed) with liquor and *zheng* (steamed)	90g [9g]
Shan Yao (Rhizoma Dioscoreae), *chao* (dry-fried)	120g [12g]

Zuǒ Guī Wán (Restore the Left [Kidney] Pill)

DOSAGE / PREPARATION / ADMINISTRATION

The source text's instructions are to first steam *Shu Di Huang* (Radix Rehmanniae Praeparata) and smash it into a paste. Grind the other ingredients into powder, and mix it with the paste and honey to form small pills. Take one hundred or more pills with salted or boiled water before meals. Today, it is prepared by mixing the powdered herbs with honey to form pills, with each pill weighing about 15g. Take one pill on an empty stomach in the morning and at night with lightly salted water. This formula may also be prepared as a decoction using the doses suggested in brackets.

CHINESE THERAPEUTIC ACTIONS

1. Nourishes yin and replenishes marrow and *jing* (essence)
2. Tonifies the Kidney

CLINICAL MANIFESTATIONS

Kidney yin deficiency with depletion of marrow and *jing* (essence): mental dullness, confusion, disorientation, pacing at night, impaired hearing, soreness and weakness of the back and stifles, poor hair coat and weak constitution, developmental orthopedic and dental abnormalities, dribbling of urine, increased thirst, excessive panting, skin, hair coat, nails/claws, a red tongue with no coating, and a thready, rapid pulse.

VETERINARY CLINICAL APPLICATIONS

Infertility, idiopathic polyneuritis, canine hypothyroidism, canine hypoadrenocorticism, chronic renal failure, leukopenia, immune deficiency with chronic infections, developmental abnormalities, cognitive dysfunction and deafness.

EXPLANATION

Zuo Gui Wan (Restore the Left [Kidney] Pill) is designed to tonify Kidney yin and replenish marrow and *jing* (essence). Because the brain is the sea of marrow, marrow deficiency may result in confusion and disorientation; dogs may forget how to navigate stairs or find the doggie door. Kidney deficiency often causes deficiency of the lower body, leading to weak stifles and sore back. A dry mouth, skin, hair coat and claws/nails and thirst indicate general yin deficiency and insufficiency of body fluids. A red tongue with no coating indicates severe yin deficiency. A thready, rapid pulse is a typical sign of yin deficiency.

This formula uses *Shu Di Huang* (Radix Rehmanniae Praeparata) to tonify the Kidney, nourish yin, and replenish *jing* (essence). *Gou Qi Zi* (Fructus Lycii) nourishes the Liver, tonifies the Kidney, and improves vision. *Shan Zhu Yu* (Fructus Corni) has a sour taste, and astringes yin and body fluids to prevent further loss. *Gui Ban Jiao* (Colla Plastrum Testudinis) and *Lu Jiao Jiao* (Colla Cornus Cervi) are two animal substances that have a very strong effect in nourishing the Kidney and tonifying yin, yang and *jing* (essence). *Tu Si Zi* (Semen Cuscutae) combines with *Chuan Niu Xi* (Radix Cyathulae) to tonify the Kidney and strengthen the lower body to relieve sore low back and weak knees. *Shan Yao* (Rhizoma Dioscoreae) tonifies the Kidney and strengthens the Spleen.

VETERINARY MODIFICATIONS

- For dry cough with scanty sputum, add *Bai He* (Bulbus Lilii).
- With deficiency heat, add *Di Gu Pi* (Cortex Lycii), *Huang Bo* (Cortex Phellodendri Chinensis) and *Nu Zhen Zi* (Fructus Ligustri Lucidi).

***Zuo Gui Wan* (Restore the Left [Kidney] Pill)**

Diagnosis	Clinical Signs	Treatment	Herbs
Kidney yin deficiency with depletion of marrow and *jing* (essence)	• Mental dullness, confusion, disorientation, and pacing at night: marrow deficiency of the brain • Weak stifles, sore back, a dry mouth, skin, hair coat, nails/claws, and increased thirst: yin deficiency • Red tongue with no coating, and a thready, rapid pulse: severe yin deficiency	• Nourishes yin • Tonifies the Kidney	• *Shu Di Huang* (Radix Rehmanniae Praeparata) tonifies the Kidney, nourishes yin, and replenishes *jing*. • *Gou Qi Zi* (Fructus Lycii) nourishes the Liver, tonifies the Kidney, and improves vision. • *Shan Zhu Yu* (Fructus Corni) astringes yin and body fluids. • *Gui Ban Jiao* (Colla Plastrum Testudinis) and *Lu Jiao Jiao* (Colla Cornus Cervi) nourish the Kidney and tonify yin, yang and *jing* (essence). • *Tu Si Zi* (Semen Cuscutae) and *Chuan Niu Xi* (Radix Cyathulae) tonify the Kidney and strengthen the lower body to relieve sore back and weak knees. • *Shan Yao* (Rhizoma Dioscoreae) tonifies the Kidney and strengthens the Spleen.

Zuǒ Guī Wán (Restore the Left [Kidney] Pill)

- With blood deficiency, add *He Shou Wu* (Radix Polygoni Multiflori) and *Huang Jing* (Rhizoma Polygonati).
- With qi deficiency, add *Ren Shen* (Radix et Rhizoma Ginseng) and *Huang Qi* (Radix Astragali).

CAUTIONS / CONTRAINDICATIONS

- *Zuo Gui Wan* mostly consists of stagnating herbs that could produce dampness inside the body, causing symptoms such as indigestion, poor appetite and vomiting. For animals with weakness of the middle *jiao*, qi activating herbs such as *Sha Ren* (Fructus Amomi) and *Chen Pi* (Pericarpium Citri Reticulatae) should be added to prevent damp accumulation and gastrointestinal upset.
- This formula is not recommended for prolonged use, since most of the herbs are yin tonics that are stagnating in nature, and may impair Spleen and Stomach functions and cause vomiting, diarrhea or loose stools. *Liu Wei Di Huang Wan* (Six-Ingredient Pill with Rehmannia) is a more balanced and more suitable yin tonic for long-term use.

PHARMACOLOGICAL EFFECTS

Reproductive: Administration of *Zuo Gui Wan* in male mice had a dose-dependant effect to increase plasma testosterone levels and weight of the testicles.[1]

HUMAN CLINICAL STUDIES AND RESEARCH

1. **Infertility due to premature ovarian failure**: According to one case report, a woman with premature ovarian failure and secondary amenorrhea for 8 years was treated with good results. The patient began to ovulate 3 months after treatment with modified *Zuo Gui Wan*. The patient then switched to clomiphene citrate. During the eight-month treatment with clomiphene citrate, there was no ovulation or conception, and the concentrations of follicle stimulating hormone and luteinizing hormone were still in the postmenopausal range. The patient then switched back to modified *Zuo Gui Wan*, and pregnancy was reported in one month. Based on this finding, the researchers suggested that *Zuo Gui Wan* may restore ovarian function effectively and promptly, and offers another option for treating infertility in patients with premature ovarian failure. Note: Modified *Zuo Gui Wan* used in this report contained *Shu Di Huang* (Radix Rehmanniae Praeparata), *Shan Yao* (Rhizoma Dioscoreae), *Gou Qi Zi* (Fructus Lycii), *Shan Zhu Yu* (Fructus Corni), *Chuan Niu Xi* (Radix Cyathulae), *Tu Si Zi* (Semen Cuscutae), *Lu Jiao Jiao* (Colla Cornus Cervi), *Gui Ban Jiao* (Colla Plastrum Testudinis), *Yin Yang Huo* (Herba Epimedii), and *Ba Ji Tian* (Radix Morindae Officinalis).[2]
2. **Multiple neuritis**: In one study, 56 patients (between 15-58 years of age) with multiple neuritis were treated with modified *Zuo Gui Wan*. The history of illness ranged from 2 months to 1 year. The formula included *Shu Di Huang* (Radix Rehmanniae Praeparata) 20g, *Shan Yao* (Rhizoma Dioscoreae) 20g, *Sang Ji Sheng* (Herba Taxilli) 20g, *Shan Zhu Yu* (Fructus Corni) 15g, *Tu Si Zi* (Semen Cuscutae) 15g, *Gou Qi Zi* (Fructus Lycii) 15g, *Chuan Niu Xi* (Radix Cyathulae) 15g, *Du Zhong* (Cortex Eucommiae) 15g, *Wei Ling Xian* (Radix et Rhizoma Clematidis) 15g, *Qin Jiao* (Radix Gentianae Macrophyllae) 15g, *Dang Gui* (Radix Angelicae Sinensis) 15g, and *Chuan Xiong* (Rhizoma Chuanxiong) 10g. Other modifications were made if deemed necessary. The treatment protocol was to administer the herbs in decoction twice daily in the morning and at night. Out of 56 patients, the study reported recovery in 42 cases and improvement in 14 cases.[3]
3. **Polyneuritis**: Administration of modified *Zuo Gui Wan* in 56 patients with polyneuritis was associated with complete recovery in 42 cases and improvement in 14 cases. For Liver and Kidney deficiencies, *Dang Gui* (Radix Angelicae Sinensis) and *Chuan Xiong* (Rhizoma Chuanxiong) were removed, and *Zhi Mu* (Rhizoma Anemarrhenae) and *Gui Ban* (Plastrum Testudinis) were added. For Spleen and Stomach deficiencies, *Shu Di Huang* (Radix Rehmanniae Praeparata) and *Shan Zhu Yu* (Fructus Corni) were removed, and *Dang Shen* (Radix Codonopsis), *Huang Qi* (Radix Astragali), and *Fu Ling* (Poria) were added.[4]

SUGGESTED ACUPUNCTURE TREATMENT

1. Points: *Shenshu* (BL 23), *Taixi* (KI 3), *Guanyuan* (CV 4), *Sanyinjiao* (SP 6), *Qihai* (CV 6), and *Zhishi* (BL 52).
2. Technique: tonification.

Shenshu (BL 23) and *Taixi* (KI 3) tonify Kidney yin. *Guanyuan* (CV 4), the meeting point of the three foot yin channels and the *ren* (conception) channel, nourishes yin of the lower *jiao*. *Sanyinjiao* (SP 6) nourishes the Liver, Kidney, and Spleen. *Qihai* (CV 6) and *Zhishi* (BL 52) tonify qi and consolidate *jing* (essence).

RELATED FORMULA

Zuǒ Guī Yǐn (Restore the Left [Kidney] Decoction)
左歸飲
左归饮
Pinyin Name: *Zuo Gui Yin*
Literal Name: Restore the Left [Kidney] Decoction
Original Source: *Jing Yue Quan Shu* (Collected Treatises of [Zhang] Jing Yue) by Zhang Jie-Bing (Zhang Jing-Yue) in 1624

Shu Di Huang (Radix Rehmanniae Praeparata)	6-60g [9g]
Shan Yao (Rhizoma Dioscoreae)	6g
Gou Qi Zi (Fructus Lycii)	6g

Zuǒ Guī Wán (Restore the Left [Kidney] Pill)

Zhi Gan Cao (Radix et Rhizoma Glycyrrhizae Praeparata cum Melle)	3g
Fu Ling (Poria)	4.5g
Shan Zhu Yu (Fructus Corni)	3-6g [6g]

The source text states to cook the ingredients with two bowls of water until the liquid is reduced to 70%. Take the decoction between meals. Today, this formula may be prepared as a decoction with the doses suggested in brackets.

Zuo Gui Yin (Restore the Left [Kidney] Decoction) tonifies and benefits Kidney yin. Clinical manifestations include soreness of the back, a dry mouth and throat, thirst with desire to drink, a red tongue with no tongue coating, and a thready, rapid pulse.

Zuo Gui Wan (Restore the Left [Kidney] Pill) and *Zuo Gui Yin* (Restore the Left [Kidney] Decoction) have similar compositions and functions to treat Kidney yin deficiency.

- *Zuo Gui Wan* is a stronger formula, and is used for severe cases of Kidney yin deficiency.
- *Zuo Gui Yin* is less potent, and is used for mild to moderate cases of Kidney yin deficiency.

AUTHORS' COMMENTS

Zuo Gui Wan contains rich and cloying herbs. These properties should be considered when administering this formula to animals that have weak middle *jiao* function. In these animals, it is best to add some herbs to promote appropriate assimilation of the formula to avoid indigestion, vomiting and diarrhea. Once the clinical signs have resolved, a more balanced formula, such as *Liu Wei Di Huang Wan* (Six-Ingredient Pill with Rehmannia), can be given.

- *Zuo Gui Wan* can be used to treat cognitive dysfunction in the geriatric dog by combining with *Gui Pi Tang* (Restore the Spleen Decoction) and adding *Yin Xing Ye* (Folium Ginkgo) and *Dan Shen* (Radix et Rhizoma Salviae Miltiorrhizae).
- For the treatment and management of canine hypoadrenocorticism (Addison's disease) due to deficiency of *jing* (essence) and Kidney yin deficiency, add *Dang Gui* (Radix Angelicae Sinensis), *Ren Shen* (Radix et Rhizoma Ginseng), *Rou Cong Rong* (Herba Cistanches), *Du Zhong* (Cortex Eucommiae), *Rou Gui* (Cortex Cinnamomi), *Xian Mao* (Rhizoma Curculiginis), and *Bu Gu Zhi* (Fructus Psoraleae). This formula can be used for animals suspected of developing Addison's disease, or for those recovering from Addisonian crisis and also taking conventional mineralocorticoid and glucocorticoids. Once the animal is stable, it should be placed on maintenance formulas, such as *Mai Wei Di Huang Wan* (Ophiopogonis, Schisandra, and Rehmannia Pill), *Liu Wei Di Huang Wan* (Six-Ingredient Pill with Rehmannia), or *Ren Shen Yang Ying Tang* (Ginseng Decoction to Nourish the Nutritive Qi).
- For the treatment of deafness associated with aging, add *Shi Chang Pu* (Rhizoma Acori Tatarinowii), *Ci Shi* (Magnetitum), *Bu Gu Zhi* (Fructus Psoraleae), *Sang Shen* (Fructus Mori), and *Dan Shen* (Radix et Rhizoma Salviae Miltiorrhizae).
- For the treatment of female infertility in the dog with blood deficiency in the *chong* (thoroughfare) and *ren* (conception) channels, add *Bai Shao* (Radix Paeoniae Alba), *Dang Gui* (Radix Angelicae Sinensis), *Ji Xue Teng* (Caulis Spatholobi), *Xiang Fu* (Rhizoma Cyperi), and *Yi Mu Cao* (Herba Leonuri).
- For leukopenia due to deficiency of *jing* (essence) and blood, add *Ren Shen* (Radix et Rhizoma Ginseng), *Huang Qi* (Radix Astragali), *Da Zao* (Fructus Jujubae), *E Jiao* (Colla Corii Asini), and *Er Zhi Wan* (Two-Ultimate Pill).
- For weak, painful back in young animals due to poor *jing* (essence) and yin deficiency, add *Xu Duan* (Radix Dipsaci), *Gou Ji* (Rhizoma Cibotii), *Yin Yang Huo* (Herba Epimedii), *Yan Hu Suo* (Rhizoma Corydalis), and *Mo Yao* (Myrrha).

Liu Wei Di Huang Wan (Six-Ingredient Pill with Rehmannia) and *Zuo Gui Wan* are both designed to nourish yin, especially Kidney yin, with clinical manifestations of a red tongue with no tongue coating and a thready, rapid pulse. Both formulas contain *Shu Di Huang* (Radix Rehmanniae Praeparata), *Shan Yao* (Rhizoma Dioscoreae), and *Shan Zhu Yu* (Fructus Corni) to nourish the Liver and strengthen the Spleen. Their differences are as follows:

- *Liu Wei Di Huang Wan* is a moderate Kidney yin tonic. It contains three tonic herbs, listed above, and three sedating herbs: *Fu Ling* (Poria), *Ze Xie* (Rhizoma Alismatis), and *Mu Dan Pi* (Cortex Moutan), which clear turbid water from the Kidney, promote water excretion, and clear heat respectively. They prevent the tonic herbs from creating stagnating side effects. *Liu Wei Di Huang Wan* has a proper balance of tonifying and sedating herbs to prevent stagnation. This is a more harmonious and balanced formula that can be taken for a long period of time.
- *Zuo Gui Wan* is a very strong Kidney tonic, and is used for depletion of yin and *jing* (essence). It contains *Shu Di Huang* (Radix Rehmanniae Praeparata) at double the dose in *Liu Wei Di Huang Wan* (Six-Ingredient Pill with Rehmannia), making *Zuo Gui Wan* richer. Most of the herbs in this formula are Kidney yin and *jing* tonics, but there are no sedating herbs: *Tu Si Zi* (Semen Cuscutae), *Chuan Niu Xi* (Radix Cyathulae), *Gou Qi Zi* (Fructus Lycii), *Lu Jiao Jiao* (Colla Cornus Cervi), and *Gui Ban Jiao* (Colla Plastrum Testudinis). Therefore, it should be used to immediately

Zuǒ Guī Wán (Restore the Left [Kidney] Pill)

boost depleted yin and *jing*. However, this formula is not suitable for long-term use.[5]

Liu Wei Di Huang Wan (Six-Ingredient Pill with Rehmannia) differs from *Zuo Gui Wan* (Restore the Left [Kidney] Pill) in the same way *Ba Wei Di Huang Wan* (Eight-Ingredient Pill with Rehmannia) differs from *You Gui Wan* (Restore the Right [Kidney] Pill).

- *Zuo Gui Wan* and *You Gui Wan* both tonify the Kidney without sedation. Thus, they have a more potent and immediate tonifying effect, and are more suitable for treating acute and severe cases.
- *Liu Wei Di Huang Wan* and *Ba Wei Di Huang Wan* tonify and sedate the Kidney at the same time. They have a moderate tonifying effect, and are suitable for long-term use to treat chronic deficiency.

Zuo Gui Wan (Restore the Left [Kidney] Pill) and *You Gui Wan* (Restore the Right [Kidney] Pill) have similar names and functions. These formulas may be used singularly, or in combination.

- *Zuo Gui Wan* tonifies Kidney yin.
- *You Gui Wan* tonifies Kidney yang

Zuo Gui Wan and *You Gui Wan* are often used to treat endocrine disorders because of their ability to tonify Kidney *jing* (essence)—the root of all hormones in the body. Deficiency of *yuan* (source) *qi*, Kidney yang, or Kidney yin may all be involved in conditions characterized by deficient hormones from a Chinese medicine perspective. Which one (*yuan qi*, Kidney yang, or Kidney yin) is most deficient depends on the particular hormone involved, the age, sex, and constitution of the animal. [Note: Prenatal *jing* (essence) is the foundation of *yuan* (source) *qi*. *Yuan qi* is the active form of Kidney *jing* and is divided into primary yin and primary yang. It is distributed throughout the body by the *San Jiao* and is stored in the extraordinary vessels.]

References

1. *Zhong Yi Ming Fang Lin Chuang Xin Yong* (Contemporary Clinical Applications of Classic Chinese Formulas), 2001; 205.
2. Chao SL, Huang LW, Yen HR. Pregnancy in premature ovarian failure after therapy using Chinese herbal medicine. Chang Gung Medical Journal. 2003 Jun; 26(6):449-52.
3. *Zhong Hua Ren Min Gong He Guo Yao Dian* (Chinese Herbal Pharmacopoeia by People's Republic of China), 1995; 348.
4. *Zhong Yi Yao Xue Bao* (Report of Chinese Medicine and Herbology), 1993; 6:34.
5. Wang MZ, et al. *Zhong Yi Xue Wen Da Ti Ku* (Questions and Answers on Traditional Chinese Medicine: Herbal Formulas).

Dà Bǔ Yīn Wán (Great Tonify the Yin Pill)

大補陰丸

大补阴丸

Pinyin Name: *Da Bu Yin Wan*
Literal Name: Great Tonify the Yin Pill
Alternate Names: *Da Bu Wan* (Great Tonify Pill), *Ta Pu Yin Wan*, Major Yin-Nourishing Pill, Rehmannia Combination
Original Source: *Dan Xi Xin Fa* (Teachings of [Zhu] Dan-Xi) by Zhu Zhen-Heng in 1481

COMPOSITION

Shu Di Huang (Radix Rehmanniae Praeparata), *zheng* (steamed) with liquor	180g [18g]
Gui Ban (Plastrum Testudinis), *zhi* (fried with liquid) till crisp	180g [18g]
Huang Bo (Cortex Phellodendri Chinensis), *chao* (dry-fried) to brown	120g [12g]
Zhi Mu (Rhizoma Anemarrhenae), *jin* (soaked) in liquor and *chao* (dry-fried)	120g [12g]

Dà Bŭ Yīn Wán (Great Tonify the Yin Pill)

DOSAGE / PREPARATION / ADMINISTRATION

The source text instructs to grind the ingredients into powder, mix with honey and bone marrow from pigs' vertebrae, and form into pills. Take 70 pills with salted water on an empty stomach. Today, this formula is usually prepared by grinding all of the ingredients into a fine powder. Steam the bone marrow from the pigs' vertebrae until it is fully cooked, and then smash it into a paste. Mix the powdered herbs, marrow paste, and honey and form into pills. The pills should weigh 15g each. Take 1 pill in the morning and at night with lightly salted water. Today, this formula may be prepared as a decoction using the doses suggested in brackets.

CHINESE THERAPEUTIC ACTIONS

Nourishes yin and clears deficiency fire

CLINICAL MANIFESTATIONS

Liver and Kidney yin deficiencies with deficiency fire rising upward: irritability, aggression, dryness, restlessness, panting excessively (especially at night), dry cough, constipation or dry feces, short urination, heat aversion, seeking cool surfaces/places, increased to ravenous appetite, increased thirst, trembling and jerking during sleep, soreness of the back and stifles, atrophy and weakness of the extremities, poor hearing or deafness, hypersensitivity to acupuncture, a red tongue with no coating, and a rapid, thready pulse that is weaker on the left side.

VETERINARY CLINICAL APPLICATIONS

Diabetes mellitus, canine hyperadrenocorticism, feline hyperthyroidism, cognitive dysfunction, behavioral disorders, and renal failure.

EXPLANATION

Da Bu Yin Wan (Great Tonify the Yin Pill) is designed to treat Liver and Kidney yin deficiencies with deficiency fire rising upward. Yin deficiency may lead to deficiency fire rising, causing symptoms such as irritability, aggression, dryness, insomnia, restlessness, and panting excessively, especially at night. Atrophy and weakness of the stifles and legs are caused by Liver and Kidney yin deficiencies. If deficiency fire flares up to affect the Lung, coughing may occur; similarly, if the deficiency fire flares up to affect the Heart, it may cause irritability and sleep disturbance. A red tongue body with no coating is representative of yin deficiency. A rapid, thready and more forceful pulse may be present if the deficiency fire is severe and flares up, causing acute symptoms.

Shu Di Huang (Radix Rehmanniae Praeparata) tonifies yin and replenishes *jing* (essence). *Gui Ban* (Plastrum Testudinis) nourishes yin and anchors yang to control deficiency fire. Both greatly tonify the true yin of the body, and thus help control the rising of deficiency fire. *Huang Bo* (Cortex Phellodendri Chinensis) strongly sedates deficiency fire. *Zhi Mu* (Rhizoma Anemarrhenae) clears deficiency fire and moistens the Lung and Kidney. Indeed, this formula consists of strong tonics to nourish Liver and Kidney yin, and sedating herbs to control the rising of deficiency fire. Bone marrow and honey nourish yin, replenish *jing*, and generate body fluids.

VETERINARY MODIFICATIONS

- If there is more yin deficiency, add *Mai Dong* (Radix Ophiopogonis) and *Tian Dong* (Radix Asparagi).
- With cough with sputum that is difficult to expectorate, add *Bai Bu* (Radix Stemonae) and *Chuan Bei Mu* (Bulbus Fritillariae Cirrhosae).
- With cough or vomiting with blood, add *Xian He Cao* (Herba Agrimoniae), *Bai Mao Gen* (Rhizoma Imperatae), and *Ce Bai Ye* (Cacumen Platycladi).

Da Bu Yin Wan (Great Tonify the Yin Pill)

Diagnosis	Clinical Signs	Treatment	Herbs
Liver and Kidney yin deficiencies with deficiency fire rising upward	• Panting excessively (especially at night), dry cough, cool seeking: yin-deficient fire rising • Atrophy and weakness of the knees and legs: Liver and Kidney yin deficiencies unable to nourish the bones and tendons • Aggression, irritability, restlessness, and insomnia: yin-deficient fire disturbing the Heart • Red tongue with no coating and a rapid, thready pulse: yin-deficient fire rising	Nourishes yin and clears deficient fire	• *Shu Di Huang* (Radix Rehmanniae Praeparata) tonifies yin and replenishes *jing* (essence). • *Gui Ban* (Plastrum Testudinis) nourishes yin and anchors yang to control deficiency fire. • *Huang Bo* (Cortex Phellodendri Chinensis) strongly sedates deficiency fire. • *Zhi Mu* (Rhizoma Anemarrhenae) clears deficiency fire and moistens the Lung and Kidney.

Dà Bǔ Yīn Wán (Great Tonify the Yin Pill)

CAUTIONS / CONTRAINDICATIONS

- *Da Bu Yin Wan* is contraindicated in Spleen and/or Stomach deficiencies with loose stools and poor appetite.
- This formula is contraindicated in animals with excess heat and fire.
- Avoid feeding foods that are pungent and spicy.

HUMAN CLINICAL STUDIES AND RESEARCH

1. **Pulmonary tuberculosis**: In one study, modified *Da Bu Yin Wan* was used to treat 10 patients with coughing of blood due to pulmonary tuberculosis. The diagnosis according to traditional Chinese medicine was Lung and Kidney yin deficiencies leading to deficiency fire attacking the Lung. The herbal formula included *Di Huang* (Radix Rehmanniae) 12g, *Shu Di Huang* (Radix Rehmanniae Praeparata) 12g, charred *Zhi Zi* (Fructus Gardeniae) 6g, *Zhi Mu* (Rhizoma Anemarrhenae) 6g, *Gui Ban* (Plastrum Testudinis) 30g, *Mai Dong* (Radix Ophiopogonis) 15g, *Niu Xi* (Radix Achyranthis Bidentatae) 9g, *Pi Pa Ye* (Folium Eriobotryae) 9g, *Ce Bai Ye* (Cacumen Platycladi) 30g, and *Mo Han Lian* (Herba Ecliptae) 30g. Out of 10 patients, the study reported successful cessation of bleeding in 9 patients.[1]
2. **Urinary tract infection**: In one study, modified *Da Bu Yin Wan* effectively treated urinary tract infection. Modifications to the formula included the addition of *Qu Mai* (Herba Dianthi) and *Che Qian Zi* (Semen Plantaginis) for painful urination; *Zhi Qiao* (Fructus Aurantii) for lower abdominal distention and urinary urgency; *Fen Bi Xie* (Rhizoma Dioscoreae Hypoglaucae) and *Yi Yi Ren* (Semen Coicis) for hematuria; *Xuan Shen* (Radix Scrophulariae) and *Shi Hu* (Caulis Dendrobii) for a red tongue body and lack of fluids; and injection of *Chai Hu* (Radix Bupleuri) for high fever. The study reported a 77.7% success rate (70 out of 90 patients) in treating urinary tract infection.[2]

SUGGESTED ACUPUNCTURE TREATMENT

1. Points: *Ganshu* (BL 18), *Shenshu* (BL 23), *Taixi* (KI 3), *Zhaohai* (KI 6), *Feishu* (BL 13), *Yingu* (KI 10), and *Yinxi* (HT 6).
2. Technique: tonification.

Ganshu (BL 18), *Shenshu* (BL 23), *Taixi* (KI 3), and *Zhaohai* (KI 6) nourish yin to control fire. *Feishu* (BL 13) nourishes Lung yin. *Yingu* (KI 10) nourishes yin. *Yinxi* (HT 6) clears deficiency heat to relieve steaming bones sensations.

AUTHORS' COMMENTS

Da Bu Yin Wan nourishes yin, clears heat, anchors Liver yang, and is best for Kidney water depletion with deficiency heat flaming upward, which can manifest as hyperactivity, aggression, sleep disturbance, chronic dry cough, and dry eyes, hair and skin. It is commonly combined with other herbal formulas to treat yin deficiency and deficiency fire seen in hypertension, diabetes mellitus, and hyperthyroidism. The indications for its use are very similar to *Liu Wei Di Huang Wan* (Six-Ingredient Pill with Rehmannia). *Da Bu Yin Wan* is used for stronger patients that have more severe deficiency heat flaring upward. It is not for long-term use; once the deficiency fire has been controlled, the patient is usually given a more balanced long-term tonic, such as *Liu Wei Di Huang Wan* (Six-Ingredient Pill with Rehmannia).

Liu Wei Di Huang Wan (Six-Ingredient Pill with Rehmannia) and *Da Bu Yin Wan* both nourish yin.

- *Liu Wei Di Huang Wan* is a more balanced, neutral tonic to replenish Kidney yin.
- *Da Bu Yin Wan* strongly sedates deficiency fire with depletion of yin, and has a mild ability to anchor Liver yang.

Da Bu Yin Wan and *Sheng Mai San* (Generate the Pulse Powder) both treat cough caused by Lung deficiency. Their differences are as follows:

- *Da Bu Yin Wan* treats Lung and Kidney yin deficiencies with deficiency fire flaring. The clinical signs include irritability, aggression, restlessness, panting excessively (especially at night), dry cough, seeking cool surfaces/places, increased to ravenous appetite, increased thirst, a red tongue body with no coating, and a rapid, thready pulse that is weaker on the left.
- *Sheng Mai San* is best for Lung qi and yin deficiencies, as it benefits qi, generates body fluids, astringes yin, and stops sweating. It is best for animals with coughing with scanty sputum, shortness of breath, spontaneous sweating, a pale or red tongue, and a thready, rapid or deep, weak pulse.

References

1. *Xin Zhong Yi* (New Chinese Medicine), 1975; (4):40.
2. *Ji Lin Zhong Yi Yao* (Jilin Chinese Medicine and Herbology), 1998; 1:16.

Hŭ Qián Wán (Hidden Tiger Pill)

虎潛丸
虎潜丸

Pinyin Name: *Hu Qian Wan*
Literal Name: Hidden Tiger Pill
Alternate Name: Phellodendron Formula
Original Source: *Dan Xi Xin Fa* (Teachings of [Zhu] Dan-Xi) by Zhu Zhen-Heng in 1481

COMPOSITION

Huang Bo (Cortex Phellodendri Chinensis), *chao* (dry-fried) with liquor	240g
Zhi Mu (Rhizoma Anemarrhenae), *chao* (dry-fried) with liquor	60g
Gui Ban (Plastrum Testudinis), *zhi* (fried) with liquor	120g
Shu Di Huang (Radix Rehmanniae Praeparata)	60g
Bai Shao (Radix Paeoniae Alba)	60g
Hu Gu (Os Tigris), *zhi* (fried) with liquid	30g
Suo Yang (Herba Cynomorii)	45g
Chen Pi (Pericarpium Citri Reticulatae)	60g
Gan Jiang (Rhizoma Zingiberis)	15g

Note: *Hu Gu* (Os Tigris) is derived from an endangered animal, and is rarely used as a medicinal substance today. Its discussion here is included primarily for academic purposes, to reflect the historical use of this substance in its original formulation. Most herbal products today have removed it completely, or replaced it with *Zhu Gu* (Os Porcus), which has similar functions.

DOSAGE / PREPARATION / ADMINISTRATION

Grind the ingredients into powder and form into pills with grain-based alcohol. Today, this formula is usually prepared by mixing the powdered herbs with honey to form pills, which should weigh 10g each. Take 1 pill in the morning and at night with lightly salted water or warm water.

CHINESE THERAPEUTIC ACTIONS

1. Nourishes yin, and lowers and clears deficiency fire
2. Strengthens sinews and bones

CLINICAL MANIFESTATIONS

Weakness and atrophy of the bones and tendons associated with Liver and Kidney yin-deficient fire: weakness and soreness of the back, legs, and stifles; weakness of the sinews and bones; atrophy of the muscles, sinews, and bones in the extremities; a red tongue with little or no coating; and a thready, weak pulse.

VETERINARY CLINICAL APPLICATIONS

Hindquarter weakness, muscle atrophy of the extremities, degenerative myelopathy, peripheral neuropathy, back pain, intervertebral disk disease, muscle atrophy, chronic arthritis and spondylosis.

EXPLANATION

Hu Qian Wan (Hidden Tiger Pill) treats *wei zheng* (atrophy syndrome) with severe weakness and atrophy of the sinews and bones arising from Kidney yin deficiency, Liver blood deficiency, and yin-deficient fire. The Kidney controls the bones, and the Liver controls the sinews and tendons. If the Kidney and Liver are deficient, the bones and tendons may become weak and deficient as well. Deficiency fire dries yin and blood, causing malnourishment of the sinews. Prolonged lack of nourishment of the sinews leads to stiffness and spasms of the sinews, which can eventually progress to atrophy. Weak bones and tendons may lead to soreness of the back and stifles, as well as weak legs and weakening of the leg muscles. A red tongue with little or no coating indicates deficiency fire, and a thready, weak pulse suggests that the bones and tendons are becoming deficient.

Huang Bo (Cortex Phellodendri Chinensis) and *Zhi Mu* (Rhizoma Anemarrhenae) clear deficiency fire and strengthen yin of the lower *jiao*. *Gui Ban* (Plastrum Testudinis) nourishes Kidney yin, and replenishes *jing* (essence) and marrow. *Shu Di Huang* (Radix Rehmanniae Praeparata) and *Bai Shao* (Radix Paeoniae Alba) nourish yin and tonify the blood. *Hu Gu* (Os Tigris) strengthens the sinews and bones. *Suo Yang* (Herba Cynomorii) nourishes Kidney yang and *jing*. *Chen Pi* (Pericarpium Citri Reticulatae) and *Gan Jiang* (Rhizoma Zingiberis) strengthen the Spleen and harmonize

Hŭ Qián Wán (Hidden Tiger Pill)

***Hu Qian Wan* (Hidden Tiger Pill)**

Diagnosis	Clinical Signs	Treatment	Herbs
Wei (atrophy) syndrome with Liver and Kidney yin-deficient fire	• Weakness and soreness of the back, legs and stifles: Liver and Kidney yin deficiencies • Atrophy of the muscles, sinews and bones in the extremities: deficiency fire drying yin and blood, and causing malnourishment of the soft tissues • Red tongue with little or no coating and a thready, weak pulse: deficiency fire condition	• Nourishes yin and blood • Lowers and clears and deficiency fire • Strengthens sinews and bones	• *Huang Bo* (Cortex Phellodendri Chinensis) and *Zhi Mu* (Rhizoma Anemarrhenae) clear deficiency fire. • *Gui Ban* (Plastrum Testudinis) nourishes Kidney yin, tonifies the blood, and replenishes *jing* (essence) and marrow. • *Shu Di Huang* (Radix Rehmanniae Praeparata) and *Bai Shao* (Radix Paeoniae Alba) nourish yin and tonify the blood. • *Hu Gu* (Os Tigris) strengthens the sinews and bones. • *Suo Yang* (Herba Cynomorii) nourishes Kidney yang and *jing*. • *Chen Pi* (Pericarpium Citri Reticulatae) and *Gan Jiang* (Rhizoma Zingiberis) strengthen the Spleen and harmonize the middle *jiao*.

the middle *jiao* to prevent the cold and stagnating herbs from damaging the digestive system.

VETERINARY MODIFICATIONS

- If there is more deficiency heat, use *Di Huang* (Radix Rehmanniae) instead of *Shu Di Huang* (Radix Rehmanniae Praeparata) and add *Zhi Mu* (Rhizoma Anemarrhenae) and *Di Gu Pi* (Cortex Lycii).
- With atrophy and weakness of the muscles due to blood deficiency, add *Chuan Xiong* (Rhizoma Chuanxiong) and *Du Zhong* (Cortex Eucommiae).
- With atrophy and weakness of the muscles due to qi deficiency, add *Ren Shen* (Radix et Rhizoma Ginseng) and *Huang Qi* (Radix Astragali).
- With atrophy and weakness of the muscles due to *jing* (essence) deficiency, add *Lu Jiao Shuang* (Cornu Cervi Degelatinatum) and *Rou Cong Rong* (Herba Cistanches).

CAUTIONS / CONTRAINDICATIONS

Hu Qian Wan is contraindicated in patients with atrophy caused by damp-heat invasion.

HUMAN CLINICAL STUDIES AND RESEARCH

1. **Muscle atrophy and lateral spinal sclerosis**: It has been reported that *Hu Qian Wan* plus *Ren Shen* (Radix et Rhizoma Ginseng) and *Huang Qi* (Radix Astragali) is effective in treating muscle atrophy and lateral spinal sclerosis, especially if the conditions are characterized by yin and yang deficiencies.[a]
2. **Hypocalcemia**: Use of modified *Hu Qian Wan* was associated with good therapeutic effect in treating 15 patients with low plasma calcium levels following thyroidectomy. The formula contained *Huang Bo* (Cortex Phellodendri Chinensis) 12g, *Zhi Mu* (Rhizoma Anemarrhenae) 6g, *Suo Yang* (Herba Cynomorii) 6g, *Shu Di Huang* (Radix Rehmanniae Praeparata) 9g, *Bai Shao* (Radix Paeoniae Alba) 9g, *Gui Ban* (Plastrum Testudinis) 10g, *Chen Pi* (Pericarpium Citri Reticulatae) 10g, *Gan Jiang* (Rhizoma Zingiberis) 15g, *Long Gu* (Os Draconis) 18g, *Mu Li* (Concha Ostreae) 30g, *E Jiao* (Colla Corii Asini) 30g, and lamb 15g. Additional modifications were made if necessary. Of 15 cases, the study reported complete recovery in 8 cases, improvement in 4 cases, and no change in 3 cases.[2]

SUGGESTED ACUPUNCTURE TREATMENT

1. Points: *Ganshu* (BL 18), *Shenshu* (BL 23), *Xuanzhong* (GB 39), *Yangjiao* (GB 35), *Biguan* (ST 31), *Liangqiu* (ST 34), *Housanli* (ST 36), *Shenshu* (classical equine location), *Shenpeng* and *Shenjiao*.
2. Technique: tonification.

Ganshu (BL 18) and *Shenshu* (BL 23) tonify Liver and Kidney yin. *Xuanzhong* (GB 39), the *ba hui* (eight meeting) point that dominates the marrow, nourishes marrow and Kidney. *Yangjiao* (GB 35) nourishes the tendons. Because the *yangming* channel contains more qi and blood, it is the target channel for treating atrophy. Therefore, *Biguan* (ST 31), *Liangqiu* (ST 34), and *Housanli* (ST 36) are used to strengthen qi and blood. The classical equine points *Shenshu*, *Shenpeng*, and *Shenjiao* are commonly used for both pain and weakness of the hindquarters.

RELATED FORMULA

Hŭ Qián Wán (Hidden Tiger Pill)

虎濳丸
虎潜丸

Hŭ Qián Wán (Hidden Tiger Pill)

Pinyin Name: *Hu Qian Wan*
Literal Name: Hidden Tiger Pill
Original Source: *Yi Fang Ji Jie* (Analytical Collection of Medical Formulas) by Wang Ang in 1682

Huang Bo (Cortex Phellodendri Chinensis)	[240g]
Gui Ban (Plastrum Testudinis)	[120g]
Zhi Mu (Rhizoma Anemarrhenae)	[60g]
Shu Di Huang (Radix Rehmanniae Praeparata)	[60g]
Niu Xi (Radix Achyranthis Bidentatae)	[60g]
Bai Shao (Radix Paeoniae Alba)	[60g]
Suo Yang (Herba Cynomorii)	[45g]
Chen Pi (Pericarpium Citri Reticulatae)	[60g]
Hu Gu (Os Tigris)	[30g]
Gan Jiang (Rhizoma Zingiberis)	[15g]
Dang Gui (Radix Angelicae Sinensis)	[45g]

Note: *Hu Gu* (Os Tigris) is derived from an endangered animal, and is rarely used as a medicinal substance today. Its discussion here is included primarily for academic purposes, to reflect the historical use of this substance in its original formulation. Most herbal products today have removed it completely, or replaced it with *Zhu Gu* (Os Porcus), which has similar functions.

The source text states to grind the ingredients into powder and form into pills with lamb meat. Take the pills with lightly salted water. This formula nourishes yin, tonifies blood, and lowers and clears deficiency fire. It treats weakness and atrophy of the bones and tendons associated with Liver and Kidney yin-deficient fire.

Huang Bo (Cortex Phellodendri Chinensis) and *Zhi Mu* (Rhizoma Anemarrhenae) clear deficiency fire and strengthens yin of the lower *jiao*. *Gui Ban* (Plastrum Testudinis) nourishes yin and lamb strengthens yang. *Shu Di Huang* (Radix Rehmanniae Praeparata) and *Bai Shao* (Radix Paeoniae Alba) nourish yin, while *Dang Gui* (Radix Angelicae Sinensis) tonifies blood. *Hu Gu* (Os Tigris) strengthens the sinews and bones. *Suo Yang* (Herba Cynomorii) nourishes Kidney yang and *jing* (essence). *Chen Pi* (Pericarpium Citri Reticulatae) and *Gan Jiang* (Rhizoma Zingiberis) strengthen the Spleen and harmonize the middle *jiao* to prevent the cold and stagnating herbs from damaging the digestive system. Lastly, *Niu Xi* (Radix Achyranthis Bidentatae) strengthens the tendons and bones, and guides the formula downward to the affected areas.

These two formulas have the same names and similar ingredients.

- *Hu Qian Wan* from *Dan Xi Xin Fa* (Teachings of [Zhu] Dan-Xi) is considered to be the original formula, since it was formulated approximately 200 years earlier.
- *Hu Qian Wan* from *Yi Fang Ji Jie* (Analytical Collection of Medical Formulas) is more commonly used today, as it is a more balanced and more effective formula. It contains additional herbs, such as lamb to strengthen yang, *Dang Gui* (Radix Angelicae Sinensis) to tonify the blood, and *Niu Xi* (Radix Achyranthis Bidentatae) to guide the formula to the affected areas.

AUTHORS' COMMENTS

Hu Qian Wan has found applications in the treatment of degenerative myelopathy in dogs and in treating horses recovering from equine protozoal myeloencephalitis (EPM) infection. It should be given continuously for 3 months or more for full clinical effects. Degenerative myelopathy is often associated with blood stagnation secondary to qi deficiency, and in these cases, it should be combined with herbs to support the Spleen, as needed. With blood stagnation, combine with *Bu Yang Huan Wu Tang* (Tonify the Yang to Restore Five Decoction)

Hu Qian Wan, a formula designed to treat Liver and Kidney yin deficiencies with weakness of the bones and tendons, uses *Gan Jiang* (Rhizoma Zingiberis) for three important reasons:

- *Gan Jiang* (Rhizoma Zingiberis) counters the bitter and cold effects of *Huang Bo* (Cortex Phellodendri Chinensis).
- *Gan Jiang* (Rhizoma Zingiberis) assists *Chen Pi* (Pericarpium Citri Reticulatae) in warming the middle *jiao*, strengthening the Spleen, regulating qi, and harmonizing the Stomach. Together, these two herbs prevent the yin tonics from creating stagnation in the middle *jiao*.
- *Gan Jiang* (Rhizoma Zingiberis) facilitates the generation of blood. According to Master Zhu Dan-Xi, it enters the Lung to benefit Lung qi, and enters the Liver channel to assist blood tonics in generating blood.[c]

Hu Qian Wan and *Da Bu Yin Wan* (Great Tonify the Yin Pill) both tonify Kidney yin, sedate fire, and contain *Shu Di Huang* (Radix Rehmanniae Praeparata), *Gui Ban* (Plastrum Testudinis), *Huang Bo* (Cortex Phellodendri Chinensis), and *Zhi Mu* (Rhizoma Anemarrhenae). Their differences are:

- *Hu Qian Wan* nourishes yin, sedates fire, and strengthens tendons and bones to treat yin-deficient heat in the Liver and Kidney, with *jing* (essence) and blood deficiencies causing atrophy or degeneration of the bones, tendons, and connective tissues.
- *Da Bu Yin Wan* treats Liver and Kidney yin deficiencies with deficiency fire, and clinical signs of increased thirst,

Hŭ Qián Wán (Hidden Tiger Pill)

cool seeking, irritability, insomnia, excessive panting (especially at night), restlessness, possible aggressive behavior, a red tongue with little or no tongue coating, and a rapid, thin, forceful pulse.

References

1. *Shang Hai Zhong Yi Yao Za Zhi* (Shanghai Journal of Chinese Medicine and Herbology), 1985; 11:32.
2. *Zhe Jiang Zhong Yi Za Zhi* (Zhejiang Journal of Chinese Medicine), 1995; 30(11):495.
3. Wang MZ, et al. *Zhong Yi Xue Wen Da Ti Ku* (Questions and Answers on Traditional Chinese Medicine: Herbal Formulas).

Èr Zhì Wán (Two-Ultimate Pill)

二至丸

Pinyin Name: *Er Zhi Wan*
Literal Name: Two-Ultimate Pill
Alternate Name: Ligustrum and Eclipta Combination
Original Source: *Yi Fang Ji Jie* (Analytical Collection of Medical Formulas) by Wang Ang in 1682

COMPOSITION

Nu Zhen Zi (Fructus Ligustri Lucidi)	500g
Mo Han Lian (Herba Ecliptae)	500g

DOSAGE / PREPARATION / ADMINISTRATION

The source text specifies that *Nu Zhen Zi* (Fructus Ligustri Lucidi) should be picked at the winter solstice, and *Mo Han Lian* (Herba Ecliptae) at the summer solstice. Blend *Nu Zhen Zi* (Fructus Ligustri Lucidi) with honey and liquor and steam until it is fully cooked. Allow it to dry in a cool place without direct exposure to sunlight, then grind it into a fine powder, and filter it through a sieve. Cook *Mo Han Lian* (Herba Ecliptae) with *Sang Shen* (Fructus Mori) in water three times, discard the herb residue, and then cook the strained decoction further until it becomes a thick paste. Mix the powder and the paste with honey to form pills, which should weigh 15g each. Take 1 pill in the morning and 1 at night with warm, boiled water.

CHINESE THERAPEUTIC ACTIONS

1. Tonifies the Kidney and nourishes the Liver
2. Nourishes yin and blood

CLINICAL MANIFESTATIONS

Kidney and Liver yin deficiencies: impaired vision, soreness and weakness of the back and stifles, gradual atrophy of the lower limbs, jerking and trembling during sleep, restlessness, and premature graying of hair.

VETERINARY CLINICAL APPLICATIONS

Chronic glomerulonephritis, chronic renal failure and cognitive dysfunction with restlessness and pacing.

EXPLANATION

Er Zhi Wan (Two-Ultimate Pill) treats Kidney and Liver yin deficiencies. Because the Liver opens to the eyes, Liver yin deficiency may cause dizziness and blurred vision. The Kidney channel reaches to the throat and tongue area, which may become dry as a result of Kidney yin and blood deficiencies. Kidney yin deficiency could lead to instability of yang, which would then affect the *shen* (spirit) to cause insomnia and jerking and trembling during sleep. Since the Kidney is located in the lower back, Kidney deficiency may lead to weakness and soreness of the back and stifles. Atrophy of the lower limbs is due to Kidney *jing* (essence) deficiency and lack of nourishment.

Nu Zhen Zi (Fructus Ligustri Lucidi) tonifies both Liver and Kidney yin and brightens the eyes. *Mo Han Lian* (Herba Ecliptae) is sweet, sour, and cold. It nourishes yin and consolidates *jing* (essence). *Sang Shen* (Fructus Mori) nourishes yin and tonifies the blood, and strengthens the overall effect of the formula.

Èr Zhì Wán (Two-Ultimate Pill)

***Er Zhi Wan* (Two-Ultimate Pill)**

Diagnosis	Clinical Signs	Treatment	Herbs
Kidney and Liver yin deficiencies	• Impaired vision, premature gray hair, soreness and weakness of the back and stifles, and atrophy of the lower limbs: Kidney and Liver yin deficiencies • Restlessness and jerking and trembling during sleep: deficiency heat disturbing the *shen* (spirit).	• Tonifies the Kidney and nourishes the Liver • Nourishes yin and blood	• *Nu Zhen Zi* (Fructus Ligustri Lucidi) tonifies both Liver and Kidney yin. • *Mo Han Lian* (Herba Ecliptae) nourishes yin and consolidates *jing* (essence). • *Sang Shen* (Fructus Mori) nourishes yin and tonifies the blood.

CAUTIONS / CONTRAINDICATIONS

- *Er Zhi Wan* is contraindicated in patients with atrophy caused by damp-heat invasion.
- This formula should be used with caution in animals with diarrhea caused by deficiency and cold of the Spleen and Stomach.[1]

PHARMACOLOGICAL EFFECTS

1. **Immunostimulant**: Administration of *Er Zhi Wan* was associated with an immune-enhancing effect by increasing white blood cell and T-lymphocyte counts.[2] Use of the herbs was also effective in reversing immune-suppression induced by hydrocortisone.[3]
2. **Metabolic**: Administration of *Er Zhi Wan* at 20g per day for 60 days in rabbits was associated with a reduction in plasma cholesterol and triglyceride levels.[4]
3. **Antiplatelet and anticoagulant**: Administration of *Er Zhi Wan* in decoction was associated with both antiplatelet and anticoagulant effects in rabbits.[5]
4. **Hypoglycemic**: Administration of *Er Zhi Wan* was associated with a reduction in plasma glucose levels in mice. It significantly decreased the rise in plasma glucose levels associated with adrenalin.[6]
5. **Hepatoprotective**: Use of *Er Zhi Wan* was associated with marked hepatoprotective effects. In laboratory experiments in mice, it lowered liver enzyme levels and minimized liver damage induced by carbon tetrachloride.[7]

HUMAN CLINICAL STUDIES AND RESEARCH

1. **Chronic nephritis**: Sixteen patients with chronic nephritis characterized by Liver and Kidney yin deficiencies with heat in the *xue* (blood) level were successfully treated with modified *Er Zhi Wan* and *Qi Ju Di Huang Wan* (Lycium Fruit, Chrysanthemum, and Rehmannia Pill). Modifications were made as follows: *Gui Ban* (Plastrum Testudinis) and *Mai Dong* (Radix Ophiopogonis) for severe yin deficiency; *Long Dan* (Radix et Rhizoma Gentianae), *Xia Ku Cao* (Spica Prunellae), and *Huang Qin* (Radix Scutellariae) for Liver yang rising; and *Xian Mao* (Rhizoma Curculiginis) and *Yin Yang Huo* (Herba Epimedii) for yin and yang deficiencies. Out of 16 patients, the study reported recovery in 2 patients, improvement in 6 patients, slight improvement in 6 patients, and no improvement in 2 patients.[8]
2. **Aplastic anemia**: In one study, 74 patients with aplastic anemia were treated with modified *Er Zhi Wan* with a 71.7% rate of effectiveness. Treatments were modified as follows: *Ren Shen* (Radix et Rhizoma Ginseng), *E Jiao* (Colla Corii Asini), and *Huang Qi* (Radix Astragali) were added for qi and yin deficiencies; *Shu Di Huang* (Radix Rehmanniae Praeparata), *Tu Si Zi* (Semen Cuscutae), and *Dang Gui* (Radix Angelicae Sinensis) were added for Liver and Kidney yin deficiencies; and various herbs to tonify Spleen and Kidney yang were added if needed. In addition, pharmaceutical drugs were added for symptomatic treatment if necessary. Out of 74 patients, the study reported complete recovery in 11 patients, marked improvement in 27 patients, improvement in 15 patients, and no benefit in 21 patients.[9]
3. **Hepatitis B**: Modified *Er Zhi Wan* was used with good results to treat 80 patients with chronic hepatitis B characterized by Liver and Kidney yin deficiencies. The herbal treatments were modified as follows: *Yin Chen* (Herba Artemisiae Scopariae), *Chui Pen Cao* (Herba Sedi), and *Tu Fu Ling* (Rhizoma Smilacis Glabrae) were added for damp-heat; *Ban Lan Gen* (Radix Isatidis) and *Pu Gong Ying* (Herba Taraxaci) were added for heat; processed *Ji Nei Jin* (Endothelium Corneum Gigeriae Galli) and dry-fried *Gu Ya* (Fructus Setariae Germinatus) were added for poor appetite; and *Hu Zhang* (Rhizoma et Radix Polygoni Cuspidati) and processed *Da Huang* (Radix et Rhizoma Rhei) were added for constipation. At the conclusion of the study, 93.7% of patients had symptomatic improvement and 91.2% showed improvement in liver function.[10]

TOXICOLOGY

In a toxicology report, no fatality or poisoning was observed following oral administration of *Er Zhi Wan* at 80 g/kg in mice. Using intraperitoneal injection, the LD_{50} of the formula was 13.84 g/kg.[11]

Èr Zhì Wán (Two-Ultimate Pill)

SUGGESTED ACUPUNCTURE TREATMENT

1. Points: *Ganshu* (BL 18), *Shenshu* (BL 23), *Pishu* (BL 20), *Taixi* (KI 3), *Zhaohai* (KI 6), *Yinlingquan* (SP 9), and *Xingjian* (LR 2).
2. Technique: tonification.

Ganshu (BL 18), *Pishu* (BL 20), and *Shenshu* (BL 23) tonify Liver, Kidney, and Spleen yin. *Taixi* (KI 3) and *Zhaohai* (KI 6) mainly tonify Kidney yin. *Yinlingquan* (SP 9) strengthens the Spleen and eliminates dampness. *Xingjian* (LR 2) sedates Liver fire and other turbidity.

AUTHORS' COMMENTS

Most tonic formulas cannot be taken for long periods of time because of their stagnating nature and interference with middle *jiao* function. However, *Er Zhi Wan* is a mild and non-stagnating tonic formula, and can be taken for a long period of time if necessary. This formula is not typically used alone but, instead, is combined with another formula to strengthen or nourish Kidney and Liver yin and blood. The advantage to using this formula is that it can be easily added to another formula without causing stagnation, despite not being as strong a yin tonic as *Liu Wei Di Huang Wan* (Six-Ingredient Pill with Rehmannia) or *Da Bu Yin Wan* (Great Tonify the Yin Pill). It is easily added to formulas that treat conditions of chronic osteoarthritis, to nourish the Kidney and Liver. To improve cognitive dysfunction with insomnia, pacing at night, and restlessness, add *He Huan Hua* (Flos Albiziae), *Suan Zao Ren* (Semen Ziziphi Spinosae), *Bai Zi Ren* (Semen Platycladi), and *Shou Wu Teng* (Caulis Polygoni Multiflori).

References

1. *Zhong Yao Ming Fang Yao Li Yu Ying Yong* (Pharmacology and Applications of Famous Herbal Formulas), 1989; 315-316.
2. *Zhong Guo Zhong Yao Za Zhi* (People's Republic of China Journal of Chinese Herbology), 1992; (9):531.
3. *Zhong Yao Yao Li Yu Lin Chuang* (Pharmacology and Clinical Applications of Chinese Herbs), 1991; 6:1.
4. *Zhong Yao Tong Bao* (Journal of Chinese Herbology), 1983; 3:32.
5. *Xin Zhong Yi* (New Chinese Medicine), 1991; 6:51.
6. *Bei Jing Zhong Yi* (Beijing Chinese Medicine), 1993; 2:17.
7. *Zhong Guo Zhong Yao Za Zhi* (People's Republic of China Journal of Chinese Herbology), 1992; (9):531.
8. *Shi Yong Zhong Xi Yi Jie He Za Zhi* (Practical Journal of Integrated Chinese and Western Medicines), 1993; 1:41.
9. *Hu Nan Yi Yao Za Zhi* (Hunan Journal of Medicine and Herbology), 1983; 6:7.
10. *Zhe Jiang Zhong Yi Xue Yuan Xue Bao* (Journal of Zhejiang University of Chinese Medicine), 1997; 3:35.
11. *Xin Zhong Yi* (New Chinese Medicine), 1990; 11:51.

Yī Guàn Jiān (Linking Decoction)

一貫煎

一贯煎

Pinyin Name: *Yi Guan Jian*
Literal Name: Linking Decoction
Original Source: *Xu Ming Yi Lei An* (Continuation of Famous Physicians' Patients Organized by Categories) in *Liu Zhou Yi Hua* (Medical Dialogues from Liuzhou) by Wei Zhi-Xiu in the mid-16th century

COMPOSITION

Di Huang (Radix Rehmanniae)	18-45 [30g]
Bei Sha Shen (Radix Glehniae)	9g [10g]
Mai Dong (Radix Ophiopogonis)	9g [10g]
Dang Gui (Radix Angelicae Sinensis)	9g [10g]
Gou Qi Zi (Fructus Lycii)	9-18g [12g]
Chuan Lian Zi (Fructus Toosendan)	4.5g [5g]

Yī Guàn Jiān (Linking Decoction)

DOSAGE / PREPARATION / ADMINISTRATION

Prepare and administer this formula as a warm, strained decoction. Today, the decoction may be prepared using the doses suggested in brackets.

CHINESE THERAPEUTIC ACTIONS

1. Nourishes Kidney and Liver yin
2. Regulates Liver qi

CLINICAL MANIFESTATIONS

Liver and Kidney yin deficiencies accompanied by qi stagnation and blood dryness: pain in the chest, epigastric and hypochondriac regions, acid regurgitation, bilious vomiting, a dry, red tongue, and a rapid, weak, and thready or wiry pulse.

VETERINARY CLINICAL APPLICATIONS

Chronic elevation of liver enzymes, canine hyperadrenocorticism (Cushing's disease), gastric and duodenal ulcers, chronic hepatitis, liver cirrhosis, shaking and trembling of the rear legs, feline hyperthyroidism, and epilepsy.

EXPLANATION

Yi Guan Jian (Linking Decoction) treats Kidney and Liver yin deficiencies accompanied by Liver qi stagnation and blood dryness. The Liver smoothes the qi flow and disperses stagnation in the body. Chronic illness, overwork, over breeding, chronic drug therapy, and frequent or prolonged intake of aromatic herbs may all cause yin deficiency and blood dryness. If Liver yin is deficient and the Liver becomes malnourished, Liver qi may become stagnant and invasive. Liver qi stagnation can lead to pain in the chest, epigastric and hypochondriac regions. If Liver qi overacts on the Stomach, acid reflux or bilious vomiting may occur. A dry mouth and dry, red tongue body are the results of yin deficiency and its inability to reach and moisten the upper parts of the body. Occasionally, there could be a hernia as a result of qi stagnation in the Liver channel, which passes through the inguinal region. In severe cases of stagnation, masses may form. A rapid, weak, thready pulse suggests yin deficiency, and a rapid, weak, wiry pulse suggests yin deficiency and qi stagnation.

This formula uses *Di Huang* (Radix Rehmanniae) as the chief herb to tonify Liver and Kidney yin and nourish the blood. *Bei Sha Shen* (Radix Glehniae), *Mai Dong* (Radix Ophiopogonis), *Dang Gui* (Radix Angelicae Sinensis), and *Gou Qi Zi* (Fructus Lycii) are the deputy herbs that tonify yin, nourish the blood, generate body fluids, and soften the Liver. *Chuan Lian Zi* (Fructus Toosendan) serves as both assistant and envoy herb. It smoothes Liver qi circulation, and guides the rest of the herbs to the Liver channel. Since *Chuan Lian Zi* (Fructus Toosendan) is bitter and cold and may consume yin and blood, only a small amount is used.

VETERINARY MODIFICATIONS

- With insomnia, add *Bai Zi Ren* (Semen Platycladi), *Suan Zao Ren* (Semen Ziziphi Spinosae), and *Wu Wei Zi* (Fructus Schisandrae Chinensis).
- With abdominal pain, add *Bai Shao* (Radix Paeoniae Alba) and *Gan Cao* (Radix et Rhizoma Glycyrrhizae).
- With irritability and thirst, add *Zhi Mu* (Rhizoma Anemarrhenae) and *Shi Gao* (Gypsum Fibrosum).

CAUTIONS / CONTRAINDICATIONS

- *Yi Guan Jian* is contraindicated in animals with hypochondriac pain caused by Liver fire rising without underlying deficiency.
- This formula is inappropriate for animals with qi and blood stagnation or phlegm accumulation, since it contains many tonics that can create more stagnation or produce more dampness and phlegm.

***Yi Guan Jian* (Linking Decoction)**

Diagnosis	Clinical Signs	Treatment	Herbs
Liver and Kidney yin deficiencies accompanied by qi stagnation and blood dryness	• Chest and hypochondriac pain: Liver qi stagnation • Acid regurgitation and bilious vomiting: Liver qi overacting on the Stomach • Dry mouth and a dry, red tongue: yin deficiency unable to reach the upper parts of the body • Rapid, weak, thready pulse: yin deficiency • Rapid, weak, wiry pulse: yin deficiency with qi stagnation	• Nourishes Kidney and Liver yin • Regulates Liver qi	• *Di Huang* (Radix Rehmanniae) tonifies Liver and Kidney yin and nourishes the blood. • *Bei Sha Shen* (Radix Glehniae), *Mai Dong* (Radix Ophiopogonis), *Dang Gui* (Radix Angelicae Sinensis), and *Gou Qi Zi* (Fructus Lycii) tonify yin, nourish the blood, generate body fluids, and soften the Liver. • *Chuan Lian Zi* (Fructus Toosendan) smoothes Liver qi and relieves pain.

Yī Guàn Jiān (Linking Decoction)

PHARMACOLOGICAL EFFECTS

1. **Hepatoprotective**: In laboratory experiments in mice, the use of *Yi Guan Jian* was effective in reducing liver damage caused by carbon tetrachloride.[1]
2. **Antiulcer**: According to laboratory experiments in mice, administration of *Yi Guan Jian* was associated with a marked effect for treating gastric and duodenal ulcer. The mechanism of action is attributed to enhancing the protective effect of the gastric mucosa, as the formula did not inhibit or neutralize the stomach acid.[2]
3. **Adaptogenic**: In one experiment, daily administration of *Yi Guan Jian* for 7 days was effective at significantly increasing physical performance in mice.[3]

HUMAN CLINICAL STUDIES AND RESEARCH

1. **Gastric and duodenal ulcers**: In one study, 18 patients with gastrointestinal disorders (10 with gastric ulcer and 8 with duodenal ulcer) were treated with modified *Yi Guan Jian* for 90 days with complete recovery in 8 patients, improvement in 7 patients, and no benefit in 3 patients. The overall effectiveness rate was 83.2%.[4]
2. **Ovarian dysfunction**: Modified *Yi Guan Jian* was used to treat women with abnormal ovarian functions. The base formula included *Yi Guan Jian* plus *Chai Hu* (Radix Bupleuri), *Bai Shao* (Radix Paeoniae Alba), *Nu Zhen Zi* (Fructus Ligustri Lucidi), and *Mu Dan Pi* (Cortex Moutan). In addition, *Da Huang* (Radix et Rhizoma Rhei), *Shui Zhi* (Hirudo), and *Niu Xi* (Radix Achyranthis Bidentatae) were added for amenorrhea; processed *He Shou Wu* (Radix Polygoni Multiflori) and *E Jiao* (Colla Corii Asini) were added for decreased menstrual discharge with insomnia; *Yi Mu Cao* (Herba Leonuri) and *Wu Yao* (Radix Linderae) for abdominal pain with menstruation; *Du Zhong* (Cortex Eucommiae) and *Xu Duan* (Radix Dipsaci) were added for low back pain; and *Shan Zha* (Fructus Crataegi), *Bai Zhu* (Rhizoma Atractylodis Macrocephalae), and *Shan Yao* (Rhizoma Dioscoreae) were added for lack of appetite due to Spleen deficiency. Out of 38 patients, the study reported complete recovery of ovarian function in 26 patients, marked improvement in 8 patients, improvement in 3 patients, and no benefit in one patient.[5]
3. **Liver diseases**: Modifications of *Yi Guan Jian* have been used in numerous studies to treat liver diseases, such as hepatitis, liver cirrhosis, and liver cancer. In one study, 50 patients with chronic hepatitis were treated with good results using modified *Yi Guan Jian* with the addition of *Bai Shao* (Radix Paeoniae Alba) and *Yu Jin* (Radix Curcumae).[6] In another study, 85 patients with liver cirrhosis were treated with modified *Yi Guan Jian* with 81.1% effectiveness.[7]
4. **Liver cancer**: In one study, 41 patients with liver cancer characterized by Liver and Kidney yin deficiencies were treated with good results using *Yi Guan Jian* plus *Zhi Mu* (Rhizoma Anemarrhenae) and *Gui Ban* (Plastrum Testudinis) as the base formula. In addition, *Du Zhong* (Cortex Eucommiae), *Sang Ji Sheng* (Herba Taxilli), and *He Shou Wu* (Radix Polygoni Multiflori) were added for dizziness and tinnitus; *Zhi Zi* (Fructus Gardeniae) and *Yin Chen* (Herba Artemisiae Scopariae) were added for jaundice; *Ze Xie* (Rhizoma Alismatis), *Dan Shen* (Radix et Rhizoma Salviae Miltiorrhizae,) and *Yu Jin* (Radix Curcumae) were added for ascites; and *Gu Ya* (Fructus Setariae Germinatus), *Mai Ya* (Fructus Hordei Germinatus), and *Shan Zha* (Fructus Crataegi) were added for poor appetite. Out of 41 patients, the study reported marked improvement in 7 patients, moderate improvement in 30 patients, and no improvement in 4 patients.[8]
5. **Fever during late-stage liver cancer**: Modified *Yi Guan Jian* showed effectiveness in treating liver cancer with fever. The formula was modified as follows: *Chai Hu* (Radix Bupleuri), *Bai Shao* (Radix Paeoniae Alba), and *Dan Shen* (Radix et Rhizoma Salviae Miltiorrhizae) were added for marked hypochondriac pain; *Che Qian Zi* (Semen Plantaginis), *Fu Ling* (Poria), and *Ze Xie* (Rhizoma Alismatis) were added for edema, ascites, and decreased urination; *Huang Qi* (Radix Astragali) and *Bai Zhu* (Rhizoma Atractylodis Macrocephalae) were added for nausea, poor appetite, and fatigue; and *Yin Chen* (Herba Artemisiae Scopariae) and *Che Qian Zi* (Semen Plantaginis) were added for jaundice. Out of 28 patients, the study reported a marked effect in 15 patients, moderate effect in 9 patients, and no effect in 4 patients.[9]
6. **Hyperthyroidism**: In one study, 40 patients with hyperthyroidism were treated with modified *Yi Guan Jian* with good results. The herbal treatment was modified as follows: *Hai Zao* (Sargassum), *Kun Bu* (Thallus Eckloniae), and *Niu Xi* (Radix Achyranthis Bidentatae) were added for thyroid gland enlargement; *Zhi Mu* (Rhizoma Anemarrhenae) and *Shi Gao* (Gypsum Fibrosum) were added for restlessness, irritability and a dry mouth; *Xuan Shen* (Radix Scrophulariae), charred *Shan Zha* (Fructus Crataegi), charred *Shen Qu* (Massa Fermentata), and charred *Mai Ya* (Fructus Hordei Germinatus) for poor appetite and abdominal pain; *Huang Qi* (Radix Astragali) and *Zhi Gan Cao* (Radix et Rhizoma Glycyrrhizae Praeparata cum Melle) were added for shortness of breath and profuse perspiration; and *Che Qian Zi* (Semen Plantaginis), *Ze Xie* (Rhizoma Alismatis), *Da Fu Pi* (Pericarpium Arecae), and *Gui Zhi* (Ramulus Cinnamomi) were added for edema and hypertension. Out of 40 patients, the study reported recovery in 20 patients, marked improvement in 12 patients, and slight improvement in 8 patients.[10]
7. **Restless leg syndrome**: In one study, 20 patients with restless legs were treated with an herbal formula for 15 days per course of treatment with good results. The formula

Yī Guàn Jiān (Linking Decoction)

contained *Yi Guan Jian* with *Gou Teng* (Ramulus Uncariae cum Uncis) and fresh *Mu Li* (Concha Ostreae). Out of 20 patients, the study reported complete recovery in 13 patients, improvement in 5 patients, and no benefit in 2 patients.[11]

TOXICOLOGY

No abnormal reaction was observed following oral ingestion at 50 g/kg of *Yi Guan Jian* as a bolus dose in mice.[12]

SUGGESTED ACUPUNCTURE TREATMENT

1. Points: *Ganshu* (BL 18), *Shenshu* (BL 23), *Taixi* (KI 3), *Xuehai* (SP 10), *Sanyinjiao* (SP 6), and *Qimen* (LR 14).
2. Technique: tonification.

Ganshu (BL 18), *Shenshu* (BL 23), and *Taixi* (KI 3) tonify Liver and Kidney yin. *Xuehai* (SP 10) and *Sanyinjiao* (SP 6) nourish yin and blood to calm the Liver. Combine *Qimen* (LR 14), the *mu* (collecting) point of the Liver, with *Ganshu* (BL 18), the *shu* (transport) point of the Liver, to smooth and regulate Liver qi.

AUTHORS' COMMENTS

Yi Guan Jian is used to nourish Kidney and Liver yin, nourish blood and regulate Liver qi. It is used in animals with Liver and Kidney yin deficiencies, along with blood deficiency and dryness and accompanied by Liver qi stagnation. When Liver yin and blood become deficient, they are unable to nourish the Liver, resulting in qi stagnation that can cause pain in the stomach, chest and hypochondriac regions of the body, and which can attack the Spleen and Stomach, causing digestive problems. A lack of Liver yin and blood to nourish the tendons and ligaments can cause trembling and shaking of the rear legs. This clinical situation can develop from chronic drug administration and in chronic thirsting and wasting diseases (such as Cushing's disease in dogs), in feline hyperthyroidism, and can be a component of chronic degenerative suspensory desmitis in horses. For the treatment of trembling and shaking of the rear legs, combine with *Tian Ma Gou Teng Yin* (Gastrodia and Uncaria Decoction); in severe cases, these formulas may be further combined with *Gui Lu Er Xian Jiao* (Tortoise Shell and Deer Antler Syrup) and by adding *Ji Xue Teng* (Caulis Spatholobi).

The following question is sometimes raised: if *Yi Guan Jian* treats chest, epigastric, and hypochondriac pain characterized by Liver qi stagnation, why are yin and blood tonics used instead of qi-regulating herbs, such as *Zhi Shi* (Fructus Aurantii Immaturus) or *Chai Hu* (Radix Bupleuri)? The answer is that *Yi Guan Jian* is designed for patients that have both Liver qi stagnation and Kidney and Liver yin deficiencies. Because there is yin deficiency, it is not suitable to use *Zhi Shi* (Fructus Aurantii Immaturus) or *Chai Hu* (Radix Bupleuri), since they are both drying herbs that deplete yin and will further exacerbate the yin deficiency.[13]

Yi Guan Jian, a yin tonic formula, uses *Chuan Lian Zi* (Fructus Toosendan), a bitter and cold herb that may damage yin, for the following reasons:

- *Chuan Lian Zi* (Fructus Toosendan) regulates Liver qi, sedates Liver heat, and prevents the formation of fire. It prevents the yin and blood tonic herbs from causing stagnation in the middle *jiao*.
- While bitter and cold herbs, such as *Chuan Lian Zi* (Fructus Toosendan), can dry yin, this is not a concern because *Yi Guan Jian* contains many sweet and cold herbs, such as *Bei Sha Shen* (Radix Glehniae), *Mai Dong* (Radix Ophiopogonis), *Di Huang* (Radix Rehmanniae), *Gou Qi Zi* (Fructus Lycii), and *Dang Gui* (Radix Angelicae Sinensis). The sweet and cold herbs outnumber *Chuan Lian Zi* (Fructus Toosendan) and control its potentially adverse effects.[14]

Yi Guan Jian and *Xiao Yao San* (Rambling Powder) both treat hypochondriac distention and pain, but the etiologies contributing to this condition and the focus of the two formulas are quite different.

- *Yi Guan Jian* treats Liver and Kidney yin deficiencies with Liver qi stagnation. It nourishes yin and regulates Liver qi to treat dry mouth, acid regurgitation, mass development, and hernias.
- *Xiao Yao San* addresses Liver qi stagnation with blood and Spleen deficiencies. It is considered a harmonizing formula. Clinical signs include hypochondriac pain, alternating fever and trembling, anxiety, irritability, vertigo, a dry mouth and throat, lethargy, lack of appetite, pale pink tongue and a wiry, deficient pulse. *Xiao Yao San* regulates Liver qi, spreads stagnation, strengthens the Spleen, and nourishes the blood.[15]

Yi Guan Jian and *Si Ni San* (Frigid Extremities Powder) both treat hypochondriac pain.

- *Yi Guan Jian* treats hypochondriac pain caused by Kidney and Liver yin deficiencies.
- *Si Ni San* treats epigastric, abdominal, or hypochondriac pain caused by Liver qi stagnation, with yang qi pent up in the body.[16]

References

1. *Zhong Yao Yao Li Yu Lin Chuang* (Pharmacology and Clinical Applications of Chinese Herbs), 1989; 6:14.
2. *Gui Yang Yi Xue Yuan Xue Bao* (Journal of Guiyang Medical University), 1986; 2:42.

8 TONIC FORMULAS

3. *Zhong Yi Fang Ji Xian Dai Yan Jiu* (Modern Study of Medical Formulas in Traditional Chinese Medicine), 1997; 735.
4. *Gui Zhou Yi Yao* (Medicine and Medicinals from Guizhou), 1991; 5:307.
5. *Gui Yang Zhong Yi Xue Yuan Xue Bao* (Journal of Guiyang University of Traditional Chinese Medicine); 1998; 4:19.
6. *Hu Bei Zhong Yi Za Zhi* (Hubei Journal of Chinese Medicine), 1986; 5:51.
7. *Shan Xi Yi Kan* (Shanxi Journal of Medicine), 1989; 7:292.
8. *Fu Jian Zhong Yi Yao* (Fujian Chinese Medicine and Herbology; 1995; 4:33.
9. *Fu Jian Zhong Yi Yao* (Fujian Chinese Medicine and Herbology), 1999; 2:10.
10. *Hu Bei Zhong Yi Za Zhi* (Hubei Journal of Chinese Medicine); 1999; 10:458.
11. *Liao Ning Zhong Yi Za Zhi* (Liaoning Journal of Chinese Medicine), 1991; 4:40.
12. *Zhong Guo Zhong Yao Za Zhi* (People's Republic of China Journal of Chinese Herbology), 1989; 9:42.
13. Wang MZ, et al. *Zhong Yi Xue Wen Da Ti Ku* (Questions and Answers on Traditional Chinese Medicine: Herbal Formulas).
14. Wang MZ, et al. *Zhong Yi Xue Wen Da Ti Ku* (Questions and Answers on Traditional Chinese Medicine: Herbal Formulas).
15. Wang MZ, et al. *Zhong Yi Xue Wen Da Ti Ku* (Questions and Answers on Traditional Chinese Medicine: Herbal Formulas).
16. Wang MZ, et al. *Zhong Yi Xue Wen Da Ti Ku* (Questions and Answers on Traditional Chinese Medicine: Herbal Formulas).

Míng Mù Dì Huáng Wán (Improve Vision Pill with Rehmannia)

明目地黄丸

明目地黄丸

Pinyin Name: *Ming Mu Di Huang Wan*
Literal Name: Improve Vision Pill with Rehmannia
Original Source: *Shen Shi Yao Han* (Scrutiny of the Priceless Jade Case) by Fu Ren-Yu in 1644

COMPOSITION

Shu Di Huang (Radix Rehmanniae Praeparata)	120g
Di Huang (Radix Rehmanniae), *xi* (washed) with liquor	60g
Shan Yao (Rhizoma Dioscoreae)	60g
Ze Xie (Rhizoma Alismatis)	60g
Shan Zhu Yu (Fructus Corni), *xi* (washed) with liquor	60g
Mu Dan Pi (Cortex Moutan), *xi* (washed) with liquor	60g
Chai Hu (Radix Bupleuri)	60g
Fu Shen (Poria Paradicis), *zheng* (steamed) with milk	60g
Dang Gui (Radix Angelicae Sinensis), *xi* (washed) with liquor	60g
Wu Wei Zi (Fructus Schisandrae Chinensis)	60g

CHINESE THERAPEUTIC ACTIONS

1. Tonifies the Liver and Kidney
2. Brightens vision

CLINICAL MANIFESTATIONS

Diminished or blurred vision.

VETERINARY CLINICAL APPLICATIONS

Acute and chronic conjunctivitis, blepharitis, dry eyes (keratoconjunctivitis sicca, or KCS), uveitis, keratitis, early cataracts and epiphora in the dog, and periodic ophthalmia in the horse.

Míng Mù Dì Huáng Wán (Improve Vision Pill with Rehmannia)

***Ming Mu Di Huang Wan* (Improve Vision Pill with Rehmannia)**

Diagnosis	Clinical Signs	Treatment	Herbs
Diminished vision	Diminished or blurred vision: Liver and Kidney deficiencies	• Tonifies the Liver and Kidney • Brightens vision	• *Shu Di Huang* (Radix Rehmanniae Praeparata), *Shan Zhu Yu* (Fructus Corni) and *Shan Yao* (Rhizoma Dioscoreae) tonify Liver and Kidney yin. • *Ze Xie* (Rhizoma Alismatis), *Mu Dan Pi* (Cortex Moutan) and *Fu Ling* (Poria) resolve dampness and prevent stagnation. • *Di Huang* (Radix Rehmanniae) clears deficiency heat caused by yin deficiency. • *Chai Hu* (Radix Bupleuri) acts as a channel-guiding herb to the Liver, which opens to the eyes. • *Dang Gui* (Radix Angelicae Sinensis) nourishes the blood. • *Fu Shen* (Poria Paradicis) and *Wu Wei Zi* (Fructus Schisandrae Chinensis) calm the *shen* (spirit).

EXPLANATION

Ming Mu Di Huang Wan (Improve Vision Pill with Rehmannia) tonifies the Liver and Kidney and brightens vision. Clinically, it is used for diminished vision.

In this formula, *Shu Di Huang* (Radix Rehmanniae Praeparata) tonifies Kidney yin and *jing* (essence), and fills the marrow. *Shan Zhu Yu* (Fructus Corni) nourishes the Liver and Kidney and astringes *jing*. *Shan Yao* (Rhizoma Dioscoreae) tonifies the Spleen and Kidney and consolidates *jing*. *Ze Xie* (Rhizoma Alismatis) sedates the Kidney and causes turbidity to descend. *Mu Dan Pi* (Cortex Moutan) sedates deficiency fire of the Liver. *Fu Ling* (Poria) strengthens the Spleen and resolves dampness. *Di Huang* (Radix Rehmanniae) clears deficiency heat caused by yin deficiency. *Chai Hu* (Radix Bupleuri) acts as a channel-guiding herb to the Liver, which opens to the eyes. *Dang Gui* (Radix Angelicae Sinensis) nourishes Liver blood to treat visual disorders. *Fu Shen* (Poria Paradicis) and *Wu Wei Zi* (Fructus Schisandrae Chinensis) calm the *shen* (spirit).

VETERINARY MODIFICATIONS

- To clear deficiency fire, add *Huang Bo* (Cortex Phellodendri Chinensis).
- To clear Liver heat, add *Shi Jue Ming* (Concha Haliotidis), *Jue Ming Zi* (Semen Cassiae) and *Gu Jing Cao* (Flos Eriocauli).
- To soothe the Liver and brighten the eyes, add *Ji Li* (Fructus Tribuli).
- To cool and move blood add *Chi Shao* (Radix Paeoniae Rubra).
- To move blood, add *Dan Shen* (Radix et Rhizoma Salviae Miltiorrhizae) or *Mo Yao* (Myrrha).
- To clear heat and brighten the eyes, add *Ju Hua* (Flos Chrysanthemi).
- To clear damp-heat, add *Zhi Zi* (Fructus Gardeniae) and *Huang Qin* (Radix Scutellariae).

SUGGESTED ACUPUNCTURE TREATMENT

1. Points: *Fuliu* (KI 7), *Sanyinjiao* (SP 6), *Chize* (LU 5), and *Neiguan* (PC 6).
2. Technique: even method.

Fuliu (KI 7) nourishes the Kidney. *Sanyinjiao* (SP 6) tonifies the blood. *Chize* (LU 5) nourishes yin and clears deficiency heat. *Neiguan* (PC 6) calms the *shen* (spirit).

RELATED FORMULA

Míng Mù Dì Huáng Wán
(Improve Vision Pill with Rehmannia)
明目地黃丸
明目地黄丸
Pinyin Name: *Ming Mu Di Huang Wan*
Literal Name: Improve Vision Pill with Rehmannia
Alternate Name: Rehmannia Vision Formula
Original Source: *Zhong Hua Ren Min Gong He Guo Yao Dian* (Pharmacopoeia of the People's Republic of China) in 2005

Shu Di Huang (Radix Rehmanniae Praeparata)	160g
Mu Dan Pi (Cortex Moutan)	60g
Fu Ling (Poria)	60g
Gou Qi Zi (Fructus Lycii)	60g
Dang Gui (Radix Angelicae Sinensis)	60g
Ji Li (Fructus Tribuli)	60g
Shan Zhu Yu (Fructus Corni), *zhi* (fried with liquid)	80g
Shan Yao (Rhizoma Dioscoreae)	80g

Míng Mù Dì Huáng Wán (Improve Vision Pill with Rehmannia)

Ze Xie (Rhizoma Alismatis)	60g
Ju Hua (Flos Chrysanthemi)	60g
Bai Shao (Radix Paeoniae Alba)	60g
Shi Jue Ming (Concha Haliotidis), *duan* (calcined)	80g

Grind the herbs into a fine powder, and mix with 35-50g of honey per 100g of powdered herbs to make pills. This is the contemporary version of *Ming Mu Di Huang Wan* (Improve Vision Pill with Rehmannia). It has functions to tonify Liver and Kidney yin, clear Liver heat, and brighten the eyes. It is generally used to treat diminished or blurred vision with photophobia, and excessive tearing with exposure to wind.

These two formulas have identical names, but are derived from different sources and have slightly different functions:

- *Ming Mu Di Huang Wan,* from *Shen Shi Yao Han* (Scrutiny of the Priceless Jade Patient) by Fu Ren-Yu, improves vision by tonifying Liver and Kidney yin.
- *Ming Mu Di Huang Wan,* from *Zhong Hua Ren Min Gong He Guo Yao Dian* (Pharmacopoeia of the People's Republic of China), also improves vision by tonifying Liver and Kidney yin, but has the added function of clearing Liver heat.

AUTHORS' COMMENTS

Formulas that treat the eye and improve vision generally tonify Kidney and Liver yin. Liver yin and blood keep the eyes moist and promote normal tear production, and Kidney yin is needed to nourish Liver yin, according to the Five-Element Theory. Insufficient yin leads to poor tear production, impaired vision, and opacity and hardening of the lens of the eye. Many disorders or pathogenic factors that affect the Liver will often be transmitted to the eyes, due to their close relationship. Excess Liver fire or Liver yang rising caused by yin deficiency can lead to redness and burning of the eyes, and can result in hypertension that can cause bleeding and retinal detachment. In these cases, it is necessary to clear Liver heat, tonify Liver yin, or clear deficiency fire at the same time.

There are many tonic formulas that treat ophthalmologic disorders:

- *Ming Mu Di Huang Wan* (Improve Vision Pill with Rehmannia) treats ocular disorders caused by Kidney and Liver yin and blood deficiencies. It is one of the most commonly used ocular formulas in veterinary medicine. The emphasis of this formula is on nourishing yin; it has a mild ability to nourish the blood and minimal ability to tonify qi.
- *Qi Ju Di Huang Wan* (Lycium Fruit, Chrysanthemum, and Rehmannia Pill) treats chronic ocular disorders caused by Kidney and Liver yin deficiencies. It is essentially *Liu Wei Di Huang Wan* (Six-Ingredient Pill with Rehmannia) with *Gou Qi Zi* (Fructus Lycii) and *Ju Hua* (Flos Chrysanthemi) added to improve vision and treat various visual disorders. The emphasis of this formula is on nourishing Liver yin deficiency, which is the predominant imbalance.
- *Shi Hu Ye Guang Wan* (Dendrobium Pill for Night Vision) treats ocular disorders caused by Liver and Kidney yin deficiencies complicated by internal fire and wind. Liver and Kidney yin deficiencies are often accompanied by deficiency fire, which may cause photophobia and excessive tearing. Liver and Kidney yin deficiencies lead to an inability to nourish the eyes, resulting in impaired vision. The emphasis of this formula is on soothing the Liver, calming Liver wind, clearing heat, and nourishing yin.
- *Zi Yin Di Huang Wan* (Rehmannia Pill to Nourish Yin) treats ocular disorders caused by Liver fire rising, with underlying qi, blood and yin deficiencies. When Liver fire rises upward, it causes red, dry eyes and photophobia. This formula contains herbs that clear excess and deficiency heat, and dispel Liver qi stagnation. The emphasis of this formula is on nourishing yin, tonifying qi, clearing Liver fire, and relieving Liver qi stagnation.
- *Zi Shen Ming Mu Tang* (Nourish the Kidney to Brighten the Eyes Decoction) treats chronic ocular disorders caused by qi, blood and yin deficiencies. These deficiencies result in malnourishment of the eyes and deterioration of their functions. It contains herbs that clear wind and damp-heat, including *Zhi Zi* (Fructus Gardeniae), *Huang Lian* (Rhizoma Coptidis), *Man Jing Zi* (Fructus Viticis), and *Ju Hua* (Flos Chrysanthemi). This formula primarily nourishes yin and blood, as well as clears excess heat.
- *Yi Qi Cong Ming Tang* (Augment the Qi and Increase Acuity Decoction) treats chronic ocular disorders caused by qi and blood deficiencies, with gradual deterioration of the eyes and ears that are typically associated with the aging process. It should not be used if the eye and ear disorders are caused by excess factors, such as Liver fire rising or damp-heat in the Liver and Gallbladder channels. It is primarily a nourishing formula that treats deficient-types of eye disorders, and has no real ability to clear excess heat. This formula is used to reverse deterioration, or preventively to maintain the acuity of both ears and eyes. The emphasis of this formula is on tonifying qi and blood deficiencies to benefit the eyes and ears; it has minimal ability to nourish yin.

Shí Hú Yè Guāng Wán (Dendrobium Pill for Night Vision)

石斛夜光丸

Pinyin Name: *Shi Hu Ye Guang Wan*
Literal Name: Dendrobium Pill for Night Vision
Alternate Name: Night Vision Formula
Original Source: *Yuan Ji Qi Wei* (Explanation of the Subtitles of the Original Mechanism) by Ni Wei-De in 1370

COMPOSITION

Shi Hu (Caulis Dendrobii)	15g
Mai Dong (Radix Ophiopogonis)	30g
Tian Dong (Radix Asparagi), *bei* (stone-baked)	60g
Di Huang (Radix Rehmanniae)	30g
Shu Di Huang (Radix Rehmanniae Praeparata)	30g
Wu Wei Zi (Fructus Schisandrae Chinensis), *chao* (dry-fried)	15g
Tu Si Zi (Semen Cuscutae), *jin* (soaked) in liquor	21g
Gou Qi Zi (Fructus Lycii)	21g
Niu Xi (Radix Achyranthis Bidentatae), *jin* (soaked) in liquor	23g
Rou Cong Rong (Herba Cistanches)	15g
Ren Shen (Radix et Rhizoma Ginseng)	60g
Fu Ling (Poria)	60g
Zhi Gan Cao (Radix et Rhizoma Glycyrrhizae Praeparata cum Melle)	15g
Shan Yao (Rhizoma Dioscoreae)	21g
Zhi Qiao (Fructus Citri Aurantii), *chao* (dry-fried) with bran	15g
Chuan Xiong (Rhizoma Chuanxiong)	15g
Ju Hua (Flos Chrysanthemi)	21g
Ku Xing Ren (Semen Armeniacae Amarum)	23g
Fang Feng (Radix Saposhnikoviae)	15g
Jue Ming Zi (Semen Cassiae)	24g
Ji Li (Fructus Tribuli)	15g
Qing Xiang Zi (Semen Celosiae)	15g
Huang Lian (Rhizoma Coptidis)	15g
Xi Jiao (Cornu Rhinoceri), thin slices	15g
Ling Yang Jiao (Cornu Saigae Tataricae), thin slices	15g

Note: *Xi Jiao* (Cornu Rhinoceri) and *Ling Yang Jiao* (Cornu Saigae Tataricae) are derived from endangered animals, and are rarely used as medicinal substances today. The discussion here is included primarily for academic purposes, to reflect the historical use of these substances in their original formulations. Most herbal products today have removed them completely, or replaced them with substitutes that have similar functions.

DOSAGE / PREPARATION / ADMINISTRATION

Grind the ingredients into powder and filter it through a sieve. Mix the powdered herbs with honey to form pills. Take 30-50 pills with salted water or warm grain-based liquor. Today, this formula is prepared by mixing the powdered herbs with honey to form pills, each weighing 10g. Take 1 pill in the morning and at night with lightly salted water.

CHINESE THERAPEUTIC ACTIONS

1. Soothes the Liver and calms Liver wind
2. Nourishes yin and brightens vision

CLINICAL MANIFESTATIONS

Liver and Kidney yin deficiencies leading to rising of internal fire and wind: impaired vision, photophobia, red eyes, painful eyes, cloudy lens, and epiphora.

VETERINARY CLINICAL APPLICATIONS

Glaucoma, early cataracts, uveitis, hyphema, keratitis, conjunctivitis, and hypertension.

EXPLANATION

Shi Hu Ye Guang Wan (Dendrobium Pill for Night Vision) treats Liver and Kidney yin deficiencies complicated by internal fire and wind. Liver and Kidney yin deficiencies lead to an inability of these two organs to nourish the eyes,

Shí Hú Yè Guāng Wán (Dendrobium Pill for Night Vision)

resulting in impaired vision. Liver and Kidney yin deficiencies are often accompanied by deficiency fire, which may cause photophobia and excessive tearing. Clinically, this formula can be used to treat various eye disorders, such as glaucoma, cataract, and retinitis.

This formula consists of 25 herbs, which may be grouped into five different categories of functions: nourish the blood and body fluids; tonify Liver and Kidney yin; tonify the Lung and Spleen; calm internal wind and clear heat; and calm the Liver and purge the Heart. *Shi Hu* (Caulis Dendrobii), *Mai Dong* (Radix Ophiopogonis), *Tian Dong* (Radix Asparagi), *Di Huang* (Radix Rehmanniae), *Shu Di Huang* (Radix Rehmanniae Praeparata), and *Wu Wei Zi* (Fructus Schisandrae Chinensis) nourish the blood and generate body fluids. *Tu Si Zi* (Semen Cuscutae), *Gou Qi Zi* (Fructus Lycii), *Niu Xi* (Radix Achyranthis Bidentatae), and *Rou Cong Rong* (Herba Cistanches) nourish yin and tonify the Liver and Kidney. Because *gu* (food) *qi* constantly replenishes Kidney *jing* (essence), the Spleen and Lung should be tonified to ensure proper digestion and absorption. The four herbs that tonify the Spleen and Lung are *Ren Shen* (Radix et Rhizoma Ginseng), *Fu Ling* (Poria), *Zhi Gan Cao* (Radix et Rhizoma Glycyrrhizae Praeparata cum Melle), and *Shan Yao* (Rhizoma Dioscoreae). Liver and Kidney yin and blood deficiencies can give rise to internal wind and heat. To sedate heat and clear internal wind, this formula uses *Zhi Qiao* (Fructus Aurantii), *Chuan Xiong* (Rhizoma Chuanxiong), *Ju Hua* (Flos Chrysanthemi), *Ku Xing Ren* (Semen Armeniacae Amarum), *Fang Feng* (Radix Saposhnikoviae), *Jue Ming Zi* (Semen Cassiae), *Ji Li* (Fructus Tribuli), and *Qing Xiang Zi* (Semen Celosiae). Finally, *Huang Lian* (Rhizoma Coptidis), *Xi Jiao* (Cornu Rhinoceri), and *Ling Yang Jiao* (Cornu Saigae Tataricae) soothe the Liver, purge the Heart, and cool the blood.

CAUTIONS / CONTRAINDICATIONS

Avoid feeding pungent and spicy foods.[1]

SUGGESTED ACUPUNCTURE TREATMENT

1. Points: *Ganshu* (BL 18), *Shenshu* (BL 23), *Xuehai* (SP 10), *Sanyinjiao* (SP 6), *Fengchi* (GB 20), *Taichong* (LR 3), *Jingming* (BL 1), and *Zanzhu* (BL 2).
2. Technique: tonification.

Ganshu (BL 18) and *Shenshu* (BL 23) tonify the Liver and Kidney. *Xuehai* (SP 10) and *Sanyinjiao* (SP 6) tonify yin and blood to soften the Liver. *Fengchi* (GB 20) disperses wind, opens the collaterals, and increases blood flow to the head. *Taichong* (LR 3) regulates Liver qi. *Jingming* (BL 1) and *Zanzhu* (BL 2) are local points that brighten vision.

AUTHORS' COMMENTS

Shi Hu Ye Guang Wan is not readily available in granular form, but can be made in-house or formulated by any

***Shi Hu Ye Guang Wan* (Dendrobium Pill for Night Vision)**

Diagnosis	Clinical Signs	Treatment	Herbs
Liver and Kidney yin deficiencies leading to rising internal fire and wind	• Impaired vision and ocular disease: Liver and Kidney yin deficiencies unable to nourish the eyes • Photophobia and excessive tearing: Liver and Kidney yin deficiencies with rising of internal fire and wind	• Soothes the Liver and calms Liver wind • Nourishes yin and brightens vision	• *Shi Hu* (Caulis Dendrobii), *Mai Dong* (Radix Ophiopogonis), *Tian Dong* (Radix Asparagi), *Di Huang* (Radix Rehmanniae), *Shu Di Huang* (Radix Rehmanniae Praeparata) and *Wu Wei Zi* (Fructus Schisandrae Chinensis) nourish the blood and produce body fluids. • *Tu Si Zi* (Semen Cuscutae), *Gou Qi Zi* (Fructus Lycii), *Niu Xi* (Radix Achyranthis Bidentatae), and *Rou Cong Rong* (Herba Cistanches) nourish yin and tonify the Liver and Kidney. • *Ren Shen* (Radix et Rhizoma Ginseng), *Fu Ling* (Poria), *Zhi Gan Cao* (Radix et Rhizoma Glycyrrhizae Praeparata cum Melle) and *Shan Yao* (Rhizoma Dioscoreae) tonify the Spleen and Lung. • *Zhi Qiao* (Fructus Aurantii), *Chuan Xiong* (Rhizoma Chuanxiong), *Ju Hua* (Flos Chrysanthemi), *Ku Xing Ren* (Semen Armeniacae Amarum), *Fang Feng* (Radix Saposhnikoviae), *Jue Ming Zi* (Semen Cassiae), *Ji Li* (Fructus Tribuli) and *Qing Xiang Zi* (Semen Celosiae) clear heat and calm wind. • *Huang Lian* (Rhizoma Coptidis), *Xi Jiao* (Cornu Rhinoceri), and *Ling Yang Jiao* (Cornu Saigae Tataricae) soothe the Liver, purge the Heart, and cool the blood.

Shí Hú Yè Guāng Wán (Dendrobium Pill for Night Vision)

reputable herbal company. It can be purchased as a patent formula, but the ingredients may vary from the classical formula because some of the ingredients may not be available.

Reference

1. *Zhong Yao Ming Fang Yao Li Yu Ying Yong* (Pharmacology and Applications of Famous Herbal Formulas), 1989; 322-323.

Zī Yīn Dì Huáng Wán (Rehmannia Pill to Nourish Yin)

滋陰地黄丸
滋阴地黄丸

Pinyin Name: *Zi Yin Di Huang Wan*
Literal Name: Rehmannia Pill to Nourish Yin
Alternate Names: *Chih Yin Ti Huang Wan* (Yin-Nourishing Rehmannia Pill), *Shou Gan Di Huang Wan* (Cooked and Dried Rehmannia Pill); Rehmannia, Bupleurum and Scute Formula
Original Source: *Yi Fang Ji Jie* (Analytical Collection of Medical Formulas) by Wang Ang in 1682

COMPOSITION

Di Huang (Radix Rehmanniae)
Shu Di Huang (Radix Rehmanniae Praeparata)
Dang Gui (Radix Angelicae Sinensis)
Tian Dong (Radix Asparagi)
Ren Shen (Radix et Rhizoma Ginseng)
Gan Cao (Radix et Rhizoma Glycyrrhizae)
Huang Lian (Rhizoma Coptidis)
Huang Qin (Radix Scutellariae)
Di Gu Pi (Cortex Lycii)
Chai Hu (Radix Bupleuri)
Zhi Qiao (Fructus Aurantii)
Wu Wei Zi (Fructus Schisandrae Chinensis)

DOSAGE / PREPARATION / ADMINISTRATION

This formula is prepared and administered as pills.

CHINESE THERAPEUTIC ACTIONS

1. Nourishes yin
2. Tonifies qi and blood
3. Purges fire

Zī Yīn Dì Huáng Wán (Rehmannia Pill to Nourish Yin)

CLINICAL MANIFESTATIONS

Impaired vision: poor vision, red eyes, dry eyes, photophobia, chronic renal failure.

VETERINARY CLINICAL APPLICATIONS

Poor vision, blepharitis, acute and chronic conjunctivitis, keratoconjunctivitis sicca (KCS), and chronic renal failure.

EXPLANATION

Zi Yin Di Huang Wan (Rehmannia Pill to Nourish Yin) treats impaired vision caused by Liver fire rising with underlying qi, blood and yin deficiencies. When Liver fire rises upward, it causes red eyes, and increased sensitivity to light. Impaired vision and generalized weakness can be attributed to the underlying qi, blood and yin deficiencies.

Di Huang (Radix Rehmanniae) and *Shu Di Huang* (Radix Rehmanniae Praeparata) together nourish yin and tonify the blood. *Dang Gui* (Radix Angelicae Sinensis) tonifies the blood, *Tian Dong* (Radix Asparagi) nourishes yin, and *Ren Shen* (Radix et Rhizoma Ginseng) and *Gan Cao* (Radix et Rhizoma Glycyrrhizae) boost qi. *Huang Lian* (Rhizoma Coptidis) and *Huang Qin* (Radix Scutellariae) clear excess Liver fire, while *Di Gu Pi* (Cortex Lycii) controls deficiency heat. *Chai Hu* (Radix Bupleuri) and *Zhi Qiao* (Fructus Aurantii) dispel Liver qi stagnation. Lastly, *Wu Wei Zi* (Fructus Schisandrae Chinensis) tranquilizes the Heart and calms the *shen* (spirit).

CAUTIONS / CONTRAINDICATIONS

Avoid hot and spicy foods.

SUGGESTED ACUPUNCTURE TREATMENT

1. Points: *Sanyinjiao* (SP 6), *Xingjian* (LR 2), *Taichong* (LR 3), *Chize* (LU 5), *Housanli* (ST 36), and *Neiguan* (PC 6).
2. Technique: even method.

Sanyinjiao (SP 6) tonifies the blood. *Xingjian* (LR 2) sedates Liver fire. *Taichong* (LR 3) soothes the Liver. *Chize* (LU 5) nourishes yin and clears deficiency heat. *Housanli* (ST 36) tonifies qi. *Neiguan* (PC 6) tranquilizes the Heart and calms the *shen* (spirit).

AUTHORS' COMMENTS

Zi Yin Di Huang Wan can be used to treat dry eyes (keratoconjunctivitis sicca, or KCS) in the dog, and conjunctivitis with red, itchy eyes from Liver heat and Kidney deficiencies in the dog and cat. To improve clinical results with KCS, combine with *Tao Hong Si Wu Tang* (Four-Substance Decoction with Safflower and Peach Pit). To improve clinical results with conjunctivitis, add *Ju Hua* (Flos Chrysanthemi) and *Ji Li* (Fructus Tribuli).

***Zi Yin Di Huang Wan* (Rehmannia Pill to Nourish Yin)**

Diagnosis	Clinical Signs	Treatment	Herbs
Blurred and impaired vision	• Red eyes and increased sensitivity to light: Liver fire • Impaired vision and generalized weakness: qi, blood and yin deficiencies	• Nourishes yin • Tonifies qi and blood • Purges fire	• *Di Huang* (Radix Rehmanniae) and *Shu Di Huang* (Radix Rehmanniae Praeparata) nourish yin and tonify the blood. • *Dang Gui* (Radix Angelicae Sinensis) tonifies the blood. • *Tian Dong* (Radix Asparagi) nourishes yin. • *Ren Shen* (Radix et Rhizoma Ginseng) and *Gan Cao* (Radix et Rhizoma Glycyrrhizae) boost qi. • *Huang Lian* (Rhizoma Coptidis) and *Huang Qin* (Radix Scutellariae) clear excess Liver fire. • *Di Gu Pi* (Cortex Lycii) controls deficiency heat. • *Chai Hu* (Radix Bupleuri) and *Zhi Qiao* (Fructus Aurantii) dispel Liver qi stagnation. • *Wu Wei Zi* (Fructus Schisandrae Chinensis) tranquilizes the Heart and calms the *shen* (spirit).

Zī Shèn Míng Mù Tāng

(Nourish the Kidney to Brighten the Eyes Decoction)

滋腎明目湯
滋肾明目汤

Pinyin Name: *Zi Shen Ming Mu Tang*
Literal Name: Nourish the Kidney to Brighten the Eyes Decoction
Alternate Name: Chrysanthemum Combination
Original Source: *Wan Bing Hui Chun* (Restoration of Health from the Myriad Diseases) by Gong Ting-Xian in 1587

COMPOSITION

Di Huang (Radix Rehmanniae)	2 parts
Shu Di Huang (Radix Rehmanniae Praeparata)	2 parts
Dang Gui (Radix Angelicae Sinensis)	2 parts
Bai Shao (Radix Paeoniae Alba)	2 parts
Chuan Xiong (Rhizoma Chuanxiong)	2 parts
Ren Shen (Radix et Rhizoma Ginseng)	2 parts
Gan Cao (Radix et Rhizoma Glycyrrhizae)	1 part
Ju Hua (Flos Chrysanthemi)	2 parts
Man Jing Zi (Fructus Viticis)	2 parts
Huang Lian (Rhizoma Coptidis)	2 parts
Zhi Zi (Fructus Gardeniae)	2 parts
Bai Zhi (Radix Angelicae Dahuricae)	2 parts
Jie Geng (Radix Platycodonis)	2 parts

DOSAGE / PREPARATION / ADMINISTRATION

The source text states to cook the ingredients with a small amount of *Cha Ye* (Folium Camelliae) and *Deng Xin Cao* (Medulla Junci) in water, and take the strained decoction while warm. Note: The source text only provided the proportions of the herbs, not the exact doses.

CHINESE THERAPEUTIC ACTIONS

1. Nourishes yin
2. Tonifies qi and blood
3. Clears heat

CLINICAL MANIFESTATIONS

Impaired vision as a result of qi, blood and yin deficiencies: conjunctivitis, blepharitis, red eyes, itching and tearing of the eyes.

VETERINARY CLINICAL APPLICATIONS

Poor vision, blepharitis, acute and chronic conjunctivitis, glaucoma and early cataracts.

EXPLANATION

Chronic qi, blood and yin deficiencies often result in malnourishment of the eyes and deterioration of their functions, producing symptoms such as red, itchy eyes with ocular discharge and impaired vision.

Zi Shen Ming Mu Tang (Nourish the Kidney to Brighten the Eyes Decoction) tonifies qi and blood, nourishes yin, clears heat, and improves vision. *Di Huang* (Radix Rehmanniae) and *Shu Di Huang* (Radix Rehmanniae Praeparata) nourish yin. *Dang Gui* (Radix Angelicae Sinensis), *Bai Shao* (Radix Paeoniae Alba), and *Chuan Xiong* (Rhizoma Chuanxiong) tonify the blood and regulate blood circulation. *Ren Shen* (Radix et Rhizoma Ginseng) and *Gan Cao* (Radix et Rhizoma Glycyrrhizae) are added to tonify qi. Together, these six herbs address the underlying deficiencies. In addition, *Ju Hua* (Flos Chrysanthemi) and *Man Jing Zi* (Fructus Viticis) clear the Liver and improve vision. *Huang Lian* (Rhizoma Coptidis) and *Zhi Zi* (Fructus Gardeniae) clear damp-heat, which can give rise to red and painful eyes. *Bai Zhi* (Radix Angelicae Dahuricae) opens the orifices in the head. Moreover, *Bai Zhi* (Radix Angelicae Dahuricae) and *Jie Geng* (Radix Platycodonis) have ascending properties, and guide the therapeutic effects of the formula to the affected area. *Deng Xin Cao* (Medulla Junci) and *Cha Ye* (Folium Camelliae) eliminate excess water from the body.

Zī Shèn Míng Mù Tāng
(Nourish the Kidney to Brighten the Eyes Decoction)

***Zi Shen Ming Mu Tang* (Nourish the Kidney to Brighten the Eyes Decoction)**

Diagnosis	Clinical Signs	Treatment	Herbs
Impaired vision due to qi, blood and yin deficiencies	Impaired vision, itching and tearing of the eyes: qi, blood and yin deficiencies	• Nourishes yin • Tonifies qi and blood • Clears heat	• *Di Huang* (Radix Rehmanniae) and *Shu Di Huang* (Radix Rehmanniae Praeparata) nourish yin. • *Dang Gui* (Radix Angelicae Sinensis), *Bai Shao* (Radix Paeoniae Alba) and *Chuan Xiong* (Rhizoma Chuanxiong) tonify the blood and regulate blood circulation. • *Ren Shen* (Radix et Rhizoma Ginseng) and *Gan Cao* (Radix et Rhizoma Glycyrrhizae) tonify qi. • *Ju Hua* (Flos Chrysanthemi) and *Man Jing Zi* (Fructus Viticis) clear the Liver and improve vision. • *Huang Lian* (Rhizoma Coptidis) and *Zhi Zi* (Fructus Gardeniae) clear damp-heat and relieve redness and pain of the eyes. • *Bai Zhi* (Radix Angelicae Dahuricae) opens the orifices in the head. • *Jie Geng* (Radix Platycodonis) guides the formula upward to the affected area. • *Deng Xin Cao* (Medulla Junci) and *Cha Ye* (Folium Camelliae) promote the excretion of excess water from the body.

VETERINARY MODIFICATIONS

- With blood stasis, combine with *Tong Qiao Huo Xue Tang* (Unblock the Orifices and Invigorate the Blood Decoction).
- With acute conjunctivitis with more wind-heat, combine with *Yin Qiao San* (Honeysuckle and Forsythia Powder).
- With chronic infection and more deficiency, add *Huang Qi* (Radix Astragali) and *Gou Qi Zi* (Fructus Lycii).
- With excessive tearing, red eyes and pain caused by wind-heat, add *Fang Feng* (Radix Saposhnikoviae) and *Jing Jie* (Herba Schizonepetae).
- For impaired vision caused by Kidney yin deficiency, add *Liu Wei Di Huang Wan* (Six-Ingredient Pill with Rehmannia).
- For cataract and impaired vision with Kidney yang deficiency, add *Ba Wei Di Huang Wan* (Eight-Ingredient Pill with Rehmannia).
- For impaired vision due to deficiency of *jing* (essence), combine with *Gui Lu Er Xian Jiao* (Tortoise Shell and Deer Antler Syrup).

SUGGESTED ACUPUNCTURE TREATMENT

1. Points: *Sanyinjiao* (SP 6), *Fuliu* (KI 7), *Housanli* (ST 36), *Guangming* (GB 37), *Taichong* (LR 3), *Taiyang* (extra point), *Longhui* (extra point), *Yemen* (TH 2), and *Yinlingquan* (SP 9).
2. Technique: sedation and tonification.

Tonify *Sanyinjiao* (SP 6) and *Housanli* (ST 36) to tonify qi and blood. *Fuliu* (KI 7) nourishes the Kidney. Sedation on *Guangming* (GB 37) and *Taichong* (LR 3) clears Liver heat and improves vision. *Taiyang* and *Longhui* lead qi upward. Sedate *Yemen* (TH 2) and *Yinlingquan* (SP 9) to clear damp-heat.

Zī Shèn Tōng Ěr Tāng

(Nourish the Kidney to Unblock the Ears Decoction)

滋腎通耳湯

滋肾通耳汤

Pinyin Name: *Zi Shen Tong Er Tang*
Literal Name: Nourish the Kidney to Unblock the Ears Decoction
Alternate Name: Scute Combination
Original Source: *Wan Bing Hui Chun* (Restoration of Health from the Myriad Diseases) by Gong Ting-Xian in 1587

COMPOSITION

Di Huang (Radix Rehmanniae)
Dang Gui (Radix Angelicae Sinensis)
Chuan Xiong (Rhizoma Chuanxiong)
Bai Shao (Radix Paeoniae Alba)
Bai Zhi (Radix Angelicae Dahuricae)
Zhi Mu (Rhizoma Anemarrhenae), *chao* (dry-fried) with liquor
Huang Bo (Cortex Phellodendri Chinensis), *chao* (dry-fried) with liquor
Xiang Fu (Rhizoma Cyperi)
Chai Hu (Radix Bupleuri)
Huang Qin (Radix Scutellariae), *chao* (dry-fried) with liquor

DOSAGE / PREPARATION / ADMINISTRATION

Grate equal amounts of the herbs and cook them in water to make a decoction. Take the strained decoction while warm.

CHINESE THERAPEUTIC ACTIONS

1. Nourishes the Kidney
2. Tonifies the blood

CLINICAL MANIFESTATIONS

Impaired hearing: poor hearing.

VETERINARY CLINICAL APPLICATIONS

Deafness

EXPLANATION

Zi Shen Tong Er Tang (Nourish the Kidney to Unblock the Ears Decoction) treats hearing disorders caused by aging, infection, or accumulation of toxic substances. A common complaint is poor hearing. This formula is ideal for treating various types of hearing disorders, especially in geriatric animals.

Di Huang (Radix Rehmanniae), the chief herb, nourishes the Kidney and treats the underlying deficiency. *Dang Gui* (Radix Angelicae Sinensis), *Chuan Xiong* (Rhizoma Chuanxiong), and *Bai Shao* (Radix Paeoniae Alba) tonify the blood and regulate blood circulation. *Bai Zhi* (Radix Angelicae Dahuricae) has an ascending function, and

***Zi Shen Tong Er Tang* (Nourish the Kidney to Unblock the Ears Decoction)**

Diagnosis	Clinical Signs	Treatment	Herbs
Impaired hearing	Poor hearing: Kidney and blood deficiencies unable to nourish the ears	• Nourishes the Kidney • Tonifies the blood	• *Di Huang* (Radix Rehmanniae) nourishes the Kidney. • *Dang Gui* (Radix Angelicae Sinensis), *Chuan Xiong* (Rhizoma Chuanxiong) and *Bai Shao* (Radix Paeoniae Alba) tonify the blood and regulate blood circulation. • *Bai Zhi* (Radix Angelicae Dahuricae) guides the formula to the upper parts of the body. • *Zhi Mu* (Rhizoma Anemarrhenae) and *Huang Bo* (Cortex Phellodendri Chinensis) nourish yin and clear deficiency heat. • *Xiang Fu* (Rhizoma Cyperi) and *Chai Hu* (Radix Bupleuri) unblock Liver qi stagnation. • *Huang Qin* (Radix Scutellariae) clears heat and reduces inflammation.

Zī Shèn Tōng Ěr Tāng

(Nourish the Kidney to Unblock the Ears Decoction)

guides the formula to the upper parts of the body. *Zhi Mu* (Rhizoma Anemarrhenae) and *Huang Bo* (Cortex Phellodendri Chinensis) nourish yin and clear deficiency heat. *Xiang Fu* (Rhizoma Cyperi) and *Chai Hu* (Radix Bupleuri) unblock Liver qi stagnation. *Huang Qin* (Radix Scutellariae) clears heat and reduces inflammation.

VETERINARY MODIFICATIONS

- For hearing disorders caused by toxicity of drugs, add *Huang Qi* (Radix Astragali) and *Lu Xian Cao* (Herba Pyrolae).
- If there is discomfort in the chest and diaphragm, add *Qing Pi* (Pericarpium Citri Reticulatae Viride) and *Zhi Qiao* (Fructus Aurantii).

SUGGESTED ACUPUNCTURE TREATMENT

1. Points: *Sanyinjiao* (SP 6), *Touwei* (ST 8), *Shuaigu* (GB 8), *Tinggong* (SI 19), *Taichong* (LR 3), *Fuliu* (KI 7), and *Yemen* (TH 2).
2. Technique: tonification.

Sanyinjiao (SP 6) tonifies and invigorates the blood. Needle *Touwei* (ST 8) through to *Shuaigu* (GB 8) and *Tinggong* (SI 19) to lead qi upward to benefit the ears. *Taichong* (LR 3) regulates qi. *Fuliu* (KI 7) and *Yemen* (TH 2) nourish yin to clear deficiency heat.

AUTHORS' COMMENTS

Zi Shen Tong Er Tang and *Er Long Zuo Ci Wan* (Pill for Deafness that Is Kind to the Left [Kidney]) both can be used to restore hearing and prevent complete deafness in geriatric dogs, if administered as soon as the owner notices a problem with diminished hearing.

- *Zi Shen Tong Er Tang* treats hearing loss caused by aging, and impaired hearing that occurs secondary to infection or accumulation of toxic substances. It contains herbs to clear heat and nourish and invigorate the blood. It can be used to treat hearing loss from ototoxic drugs and hearing loss secondary to trauma.
- *Er Long Zuo Ci Wan* treats hearing loss secondary to Kidney deficiency that develops as a result of aging. It contains herbs to tonify the Kidney and to open the sensory orifices. This formula must be given for a prolonged period of time to achieve a good clinical response. A minimum of 3 months is needed to see a therapeutic effect, and continued improvement and restoration of hearing can be seen up to 6 months. This formula works best when given as soon as hearing loss is noticed by the owner. It will not restore hearing in dogs that are already completely deaf at initial consultation.

Section 5

补阳剂
— Yang-Tonifying Formulas

Jīn Guì Shèn Qì Wán (Kidney Qi Pill from the Golden Cabinet)

金匱腎氣丸
金匮肾气丸

Pinyin Name: *Jin Gui Shen Qi Wan*
Literal Name: Kidney Qi Pill from the Golden Cabinet
Alternate Names: *Shen Qi Wan* (Kidney Qi Pill), Kidney Qi Formula from the Golden Cabinet
Original Source: *Jin Gui Yao Lue* (Essentials from the Golden Cabinet) by Zhang Zhong-Jing in the Eastern Han Dynasty

COMPOSITION

Di Huang (Radix Rehmanniae)	24g
Shan Zhu Yu (Fructus Corni)	12g
Shan Yao (Rhizoma Dioscoreae)	12g
Fu Ling (Poria)	9g
Mu Dan Pi (Cortex Moutan)	9g
Ze Xie (Rhizoma Alismatis)	9g
Gui Zhi (Ramulus Cinnamomi)	3g
Fu Zi (Radix Aconiti Lateralis Praeparata), *pao* (blast-fried)	3g

DOSAGE / PREPARATION / ADMINISTRATION

Grind the ingredients into powder, mix the powder with honey and form into small pills resembling the size of *Wu Tong Zi* (Semen Firmianae), a small seed approximately 5 mm in diameter. Take 15-25 pills (6-10g) with a grain-based liquor twice daily.

CHINESE THERAPEUTIC ACTIONS

Warms and tonifies Kidney yang

CLINICAL MANIFESTATIONS

Kidney yang deficiency: weakness, warmth-seeking behavior, decreased energy level, back pain, weak legs, cold ear tips, lumbar region and rear quarters, polyuria, urinary incontinence, edema, loose stool, a pale, flabby tongue with a thin, white coating, or a pale pink to purple tongue, and a deep, weak, thin pulse, that is weaker on the right side.

VETERINARY CLINICAL APPLICATIONS

Endocrine disorders (diabetes mellitus and insipidus, hypoadrenocorticism, hypothyroidism); sexual and reproductive disorders (impotence, male and female infertility); genitourinary disorders (nephritis, amyloidosis, renal failure, chronic glomerulonephritis, proteinuria, urinary incontinence); cardiovascular disorders (congestive heart failure, cardiomyopathy); respiratory disorders (chronic bronchitis, asthma); and other conditions such as back pain and intervertebral disk disease.

EXPLANATION

Jin Gui Shen Qi Wan (Kidney Qi Pill from the Golden Cabinet) treats Kidney yang deficiency and/or deficiency of *ming men* (life gate) fire. Warmth-seeking behavior, back pain, cold ear tips and lumbar region, and weak limbs are caused by Kidney yang deficiency and its inability to warm the lower parts of the body. Kidney yang is also responsible for regulating water circulation and metabolism, and its deficiency may cause urinary incontinence and water retention, which can give rise to edema and *tan yin* (phlegm retention). Polyuria may occur if there is Kidney deficiency in patients with *xiao ke* (wasting and thirsting) syndrome. A pale pink to purple tongue that can be wet and swollen with teeth marks, and

Jīn Guì Shèn Qì Wán (Kidney Qi Pill from the Golden Cabinet)

***Jin Gui Shen Qi Wan* (Kidney Qi Pill from the Golden Cabinet)**

Diagnosis	Clinical Signs	Treatment	Herbs
Kidney yang deficiency	• Back pain, weak limbs, cold ear tips and lumbar region: Kidney yang deficiency unable to warm the lower parts of the body • Urinary incontinence, polyuria and peripheral edema: Kidney yang unable to regulate water circulation and metabolism • A pale pink to purple tongue that may be wet and swollen with teeth marks, and a deep, weak, thin pulse that is weaker on the right: Kidney yang deficiency	Warms and tonifies Kidney yang	• *Di Huang* (Radix Rehmanniae) tonifies Kidney yin and *jing* (essence). • *Shan Zhu Yu* (Fructus Corni) tonifies Kidney and Liver yin. • *Shan Yao* (Rhizoma Dioscoreae) tonifies the Kidney and Spleen. • *Fu Ling* (Poria), *Mu Dan Pi* (Cortex Moutan) and *Ze Xie* (Rhizoma Alismatis) sedate turbidity and prevent the greasiness of the tonic herbs from blocking the qi flow. • *Gui Zhi* (Ramulus Cinnamomi) and *Fu Zi* (Radix Aconiti Lateralis Praeparata) tonify Kidney yang.

a deep, weak, thin pulse that is weaker on the right indicate Kidney yang deficiency.

Jin Gui Shen Qi Wan is composed of *Liu Wei Di Huang Wan* (Six-Ingredient Pill with Rehmannia) with the addition of *Gui Zhi* (Ramulus Cinnamomi) and *Fu Zi* (Radix Aconiti Lateralis Praeparata). The strategy behind this formula is to tonify Kidney yin to raise Kidney yang, since yin and yang are mutually dependent. This formula uses *Di Huang* (Radix Rehmanniae) to tonify Kidney yin and *jing* (essence), *Shan Zhu Yu* (Fructus Corni) to tonify Kidney and Liver yin, and *Shan Yao* (Rhizoma Dioscoreae) to tonify the Kidney and Spleen. To tonify Kidney yang, this formula uses a small amount of *Gui Zhi* (Ramulus Cinnamomi) and *Fu Zi* (Radix Aconiti Lateralis Praeparata). Only a small amount of these two warming herbs are needed to ignite the *ming men* (life gate) fire and raise Kidney yang. *Ze Xie* (Rhizoma Alismatis), *Fu Ling* (Poria), and *Mu Dan Pi* (Cortex Moutan) sedate turbidity and prevent the greasiness of the tonic herbs from blocking the qi flow.

VETERINARY MODIFICATIONS

- With edema, add *Niu Xi* (Radix Achyranthis Bidentatae) and *Che Qian Zi* (Semen Plantaginis).
- With back pain and weak stifles, add *Niu Xi* (Radix Achyranthis Bidentatae) and *Du Zhong* (Cortex Eucommiae).
- For cataract and poor vision, add *Yi Qi Cong Ming Tang* (Augment the Qi and Increase Acuity Decoction).
- For yin deficiency and generalized atrophy, add *Huang Qi Jian Zhong Tang* (Astragalus Decoction to Construct the Middle).

CAUTIONS / CONTRAINDICATIONS

- *Jin Gui Shen Qi Wan* should be used with caution in animals that have poor appetite, loose stools, and chronic diarrhea caused by Spleen and Stomach deficiencies.
- This formula is contraindicated in animals with deficiency heat rising, with symptoms such as a dry mouth and throat, and a red tongue with a scanty tongue coating.
- Possible side effects of the formula that have been reported include stomach discomfort, constipation, itching, rash, palpitations, and an irregular heart beat.[1]
- Use of this formula is contraindicated during pregnancy.[2]

PHARMACOLOGICAL EFFECTS

1. **Antiaging**: In numerous laboratory experiments, administration of *Jin Gui Shen Qi Wan* was associated with general improvements in the health and well-being of the subjects. The effects of the herbs include increased tolerance to cold weather, decreased risk of cancer formation, lower incidence of muscle atrophy, and decreased plasma cholesterol and triglyceride levels.[3]
2. **Immunostimulant**: Administration of *Jin Gui Shen Qi Wan* in mice at 0.3g each was associated with enhanced immunity by increasing the number of lymphocytes.[4]
3. **Endocrine**: Administration of *Jin Gui Shen Qi Wan* in 21-day-old mice for 28 days was associated with a stimulating effect on the endocrine system as evident in the increased weight of the pituitary glands, hypothalamus, and other glands. The dosage given to mice was equivalent to 10 times the human dose, according to weight calculation.[5]
4. **Reproductive**: Administration of *Jin Gui Shen Qi Wan* in rats was associated with an increase in sperm count and sperm motility.[6]

Jīn Guì Shèn Qì Wán (Kidney Qi Pill from the Golden Cabinet)

HUMAN CLINICAL STUDIES AND RESEARCH

1. **Diabetes mellitus**: In one study, 38 patients with type II diabetes mellitus for 3 months to 20 years were treated with modified *Jin Gui Shen Qi Wan*. The base formula included *Fu Zi* (Radix Aconiti Lateralis Praeparata) 9g, *Rou Gui* (Cortex Cinnamomi) 5g, *Di Huang* (Radix Rehmanniae) 15g, *Shan Zhu Yu* (Fructus Corni) 15g, *Dan Shen* (Radix et Rhizoma Salviae Miltiorrhizae) 15g, *Shan Yao* (Rhizoma Dioscoreae) 30g, *Long Gu* (Os Draconis) 30g, *Mu Dan Pi* (Cortex Moutan) 10g, *Huang Qi* (Radix Astragali) 20g, *Fu Ling* (Poria) 12g, *Ze Xie* (Rhizoma Alismatis) 12g, and *Wu Bei Zi* (Galla Chinensis) 12g. Other modifications were made based on the patients' clinical presentation. The treatment protocol was to administer the herbs in decoction one time daily for 30 days per course of treatment. Out of 38 patients, the study reported marked improvement in 8 patients, moderate improvement in 16 patients, slight improvement in 12 patients, and no benefit in 2 patients. The overall rate of effectiveness was 94.7%.[7]
2. **Hypertension**: Use of modified *Jin Gui Shen Qi Wan* in 40 patients with primary hypertension characterized by Spleen and Kidney yang deficiencies was associated with reduction of blood pressure in 82.5% of patients.[8]
3. **Coronary artery disease**: In one study, 60 geriatric patients with coronary artery disease were divided into two groups: 40 received herbs and 20 received vitamin E capsules. After 1 month of treatment, the study reported that in the herb group, 16 had marked improvement, 14 had moderate improvement, 8 had slight improvement, and 2 had no benefit. In the vitamin E group, 3 had marked improvement, 8 had moderate improvement, 4 had slight improvement, and 5 had no benefit. Overall, the effectiveness rate was 95% for the herb group and 75% for the vitamin E group.[9]
4. **Asthma**: In one study, 19 patients with asthma were treated with *Jin Gui Shen Qi Wan* as a maintenance therapy. The study indicated that up to 89.5% of the patients noted improvement after using the herbs.[10] According to another study, use of *Jin Gui Shen Qi Wan* three times daily for 6 months or more was associated with 89.5% effectiveness to prevent asthma attacks among 19 patients with asthma.[11]
5. **Lumbago**: In one report, 27 patients (aged 35-80 years) with low back pain due to various causes were treated with *Jin Gui Shen Qi Wan* for 4 weeks, with marked improvement in 6 patients, moderate improvement in 11 patients, and slight improvement in 3 patients. The overall rate of effectiveness was 70%.[12]
6. **Male infertility**: Administration of *Jin Gui Shen Qi Wan* plus *Ren Shen* (Radix et Rhizoma Ginseng) at 7.5 g/day for 12 weeks showed effectiveness in treating 10 male infertility patients between 28-36 years of age. The study noted that 90 days of herbal treatment was required for significant changes in sperm count and motility.[13] In another study, 51 men with infertility due to low sperm count and motility were treated with 7.5 g/day of *Jin Gui Shen Qi Wan*. Out of 51 men, pregnancy was reported in over 80% of couples within 3 months.[14]
7. **Female infertility**: In one study, 27 women with infertility caused by elevated prolactin levels (above 30 ng/mL) were treated with 2.5-10g of *Jin Gui Shen Qi Wan*. After 3 months of herbal therapy, prolactin levels decreased in 18 out of 27 patients. In addition, the level was < 30 ng/mL in 15 patients. In follow up interviews 6 months later, 12 women had become pregnant. No abnormalities were noted with the mothers or with the fetuses.[15]
8. **Impotence**: One study reported 43.2% effectiveness using *Jin Gui Shen Qi Wan* to treat 37 patients with impotence. The treatment protocol was to administer *Jin Gui Shen Qi Wan* in pills, 5g twice daily for 4 weeks.[16]
9. **Urinary incontinence**: In one study, 13 patients with 3 months to 1 year of incontinence were treated with *Jin Gui Shen Qi Wan* with salted water one time daily in the morning, for 10 days per course of treatment. The study reported that 6 patients had complete recovery after taking the herbs for 10-20 days, 4 had marked improvement after 20-30 days, 2 had slight improvement after 30-40 days, and 1 had no benefit.[17]
10. **Chronic glomerulonephritis**: One study of 12 patients with chronic glomerulonephritis characterized by yang deficiency reported success (recovery in 10 patients and no benefit in 2 patients) using modified *Jin Gui Shen Qi Wan*. *Wu Jia Pi* (Cortex Acanthopanacis) was added for individuals with edema in the legs. The duration of treatment was 21-90 days.[18]
11. **Cataract**: Use of *Jin Gui Shen Qi Wan* demonstrated effectiveness in treating geriatric patients with cataract. The study reported an overall effectiveness rate of 80%, with improvement in visual acuity noted in 60% of patients and stabilization of glaucoma in 20% of patients. The treatment protocol was to administer 3g of herbs in pills per day in two equally-divided doses. The study also noted that better prognosis was noted in individuals who began herbal therapy early.[19]

HERB-DRUG INTERACTION

Prednisone-induced adverse reactions: According to one report, use of *Jin Gui Shen Qi Wan* was effective in treating side effects and adverse reactions associated with long-term use of prednisone, such as dizziness, weight gain, perspiration, and emotional disturbance.[20]

Jīn Guì Shèn Qì Wán (Kidney Qi Pill from the Golden Cabinet)

TOXICOLOGY

According to a toxicology study, *Jin Gui Shen Qi Wan* was determined to have little toxicity. In rats, *Jin Gui Shen Qi Wan* in powder extract form was given at dosages of 40 mg/kg and 200 mg/kg in decoction one time daily for 6 months, and no abnormalities were noted in general signs and symptoms, complete blood count, urine analysis, and functions of the internal and reproductive organs.[21]

SUGGESTED ACUPUNCTURE TREATMENT

1. Points: *Shenshu* (BL 23), *Taixi* (KI 3), *Mingmen* (GV 4), *Ganshu* (BL 18), *Pishu* (BL 20), *Yinlingquan* (SP 9), *Shenshu*, *Shenpeng*, and *Shenjiao*.
2. Techniques: tonification and moxibustion.

Shenshu (BL 23) and *Taixi* (KI 3) tonify the Kidney; moxibustion on these two points warms Kidney yang. *Mingmen* (GV 4) nourishes yang to produce Kidney qi. *Ganshu* (BL 18) and *Pishu* (BL 20) nourish the Liver and Spleen. *Yinlingquan* (SP 9) tonifies the Spleen and dispels dampness. *Shenshu*, *Shenpeng*, and *Shenjiao* are classical equine points that tonify Kidney qi.

AUTHORS' COMMENTS

Originally named "*Shen Qi Wan* (Kidney Qi Pill)" by Zhang Zhong-Jing in the Eastern Han Dynasty, this formula today is commonly referred to as *Jin Gui Shen Qi Wan* (Kidney Qi Pill from the Golden Cabinet). The reason for this change is to avoid confusion and errors, since there are at least 16 formulas with the identical name of "*Shen Qi Wan* (Kidney Qi Pill)," according to *Zhong Yi Fang Ji Da Ci Dian* (Grand Dictionary of Chinese Herbal Formulas).

Shen Qi Wan, literally Kidney Qi Pill, is so named because it uses only a small amount of *Gui Zhi* (Ramulus Cinnamomi) and *Fu Zi* (Radix Aconiti Lateralis Praeparata) to generate Kidney qi and ignite *ming men* (life gate) fire. Large doses of these two dry and hot herbs may not be appropriate because they may damage yin and consume fluids, leading to other adverse effects.

Jin Gui Shen Qi Wan is one of the most commonly used formulas for the treatment and management of endocrine disorders and many other conditions characterized by qi and yang deficiencies.

- For the treatment of late-stage Type I diabetes with qi and yang deficiencies and blood stasis, combine with *Bu Yang Huan Wu Tang* (Tonify the Yang to Restore Five Decoction) and add *Huang Jing* (Rhizoma Polygonati). If blood stagnation and blood deficiency are present, combine with *Tao Hong Si Wu Tang* (Four-Substance Decoction with Safflower and Peach Pit).
- For dogs with Addison's disease and qi and yang deficiencies, combine with *Si Jun Zi Tang* (Four-Gentlemen Decoction) for Spleen deficiency, or with *Liu Jun Zi Tang* (Six-Gentlemen Decoction) for qi deficiency and dampness.
- In horses, Cushing's disease presents mainly as a yang deficiency pattern more than anything else, with hirsutism, damp and cold accumulation, and polyuria/polydipsia predominating the pattern. Although the first choice in these cases is usually *You Gui Wan* (Restore the Right [Kidney] Pill), *Jin Gui Shen Qi Wan* could be chosen as well. Like dogs, equine patients are likely to have compromised Spleen function and will need support in the form of formulas such as *Liu Jun Zi Tang* or *Li Zhong Tang* (Regulate the Middle Decoction).
- For hypothyroidism in middle-age to older dogs with qi and yang deficiencies, it can be used alone in addition to conventional thyroid medications. It should be discontinued once the clinical signs resolve and thyroid levels are normal. To improve clinical results, it can be combined with *Dong Chong Xia Cao* (Cordyceps) and/or *Ci Wu Jia* (Radix et Rhizoma seu Caulis Acanthopanacis Senticosi).
- For the treatment of urinary incontinence and dribbling in geriatric dogs, combine with *Suo Quan Wan* (Shut the Sluice Pill) and add *Fu Pen Zi* (Fructus Rubi) and *Sang Piao Xiao* (Ootheca Mantidis).
- For the treatment of fecal incontinence, combine with *Bu Zhong Yi Qi Tang* (Tonify the Middle and Augment the Qi Decoction) and add *Chu Shi Zi* (Fructus Broussonetiae).
- This formula is one of the most commonly used and effective formulas for the treatment of feline chronic renal failure. It is used in moderate- to late-stage renal disease and improvement in the condition is evaluated by regular measurement of BUN and creatinine, in addition to quality of life. A decrease in renal values can be seen in 6-8 weeks on average, provided the cat is consistently medicated. It can be used for prolonged periods of time, and is often combined with Spleen tonics, such as *Liu Jun Zi Tang* (Six-Gentlemen Decoction), *Jian Pi Wan* (Strengthen the Spleen Pill), *Shen Ling Bai Zhu San* (Ginseng, Poria, and Atractylodes Macrocephala Powder), or *Bu Zhong Yi Qi Tang* (Tonify the Middle and Augment the Qi Decoction), depending on the case.
- For the treatment of nephrotic syndrome, combine with *Bu Zhong Yi Qi Tang* (Tonify the Middle and Augment the Qi Decoction); with anemia, add *Tao Hong Si Wu Tang* (Four-Substance Decoction with Safflower and Peach Pit), *San Leng* (Rhizoma Sparganii), *E Zhu* (Rhizoma Curcumae), *San Qi* (Radix et Rhizoma Notoginseng), *Yu Mi Xu* (Stigma Maydis), and *Yi Mu Cao* (Herba Leonuri). This combination can also be used to treat renal amyloidosis.

Jīn Guì Shèn Qì Wán (Kidney Qi Pill from the Golden Cabinet)

- For the treatment of chronic bronchial asthma with Lung and Kidney deficiencies, combine with *Ren Shen Ge Jie San* (Ginseng and Gecko Powder). To improve clinical results, add *Dong Chong Xia Cao* (Cordyceps).

References

1. *Zhong Yi Fang Ji Xian Dai Yan Jiu* (Modern Study of Medical Formulas in Traditional Chinese Medicine), 1997; 681-682.
2. *Zhong Yao Ming Fang Yao Li Yu Ying Yong* (Pharmacology and Applications of Famous Herbal Formulas), 1989; 325-329.
3. *Zhong Yi Fang Ji Xian Dai Yan Jiu* (Modern Study of Medical Formulas in Traditional Chinese Medicine), 1997; 669-670.
4. *Cheng Du Zhong Yi Xue Yuan Xue Bao* (Journal of Chengdu University of Traditional Chinese Medicine), 1985; 4:40.
5. *Zhong Yi Fang Ji Xian Dai Yan Jiu* (Modern Study of Medical Formulas in Traditional Chinese Medicine), 1997; 673.
6. *Zhong Cheng Yao* (Study of Chinese Patent Medicine), 1993; 11:24.
7. *Xin Zhong Yi* (New Chinese Medicine), 1995; 27(9):39.
8. *Yun Nan Zhong Yao Zhi* (Yunan Journal of Chinese Herbal Medicine), 1987; 6:9.
9. *Zhe Jiang Zhong Yi Za Zhi* (Zhejiang Journal of Chinese Medicine), 1993; 6:270.
10. *Yi Yao Wei Sheng* (Medicine, Medicinals, and Sanitation), 1977; 6:33.
11. *Zhong Cheng Yao Yan Jiu* (Research of Chinese Patent Medicine), 1988; 11:47.
12. *Han Fang Yi Xue* (Kampo Medicine), 1986; 12:32.
13. *Guo Wai Yi Xue* (Foreign Medicine), 1985; 1:46.
14. *Guo Wai Yi Yao Zhi Wu Yao Fen Ce* (Monograph of Foreign Botanical Medicine), 1991; 1:45.
15. *Guo Wai Yi Yao Zhi Wu Yao Fen Ce* (Monograph of Foreign Botanical Medicine), 1991; 4:41.
16. *Guo Wai Yi Xue Zhong Yi Zhong Yao Fen Ce* (Monograph of Chinese Herbology from Foreign Medicine), 1991; 13(1):47.
17. *Xin Zhong Yi* (New Chinese Medicine), 1995; 27(1):50.
18. *Zhong Yi Za Zhi* (Journal of Chinese Medicine), 1956; 12:635.
19. *Zhong Cheng Yao* (Study of Chinese Patent Medicine), 1990; 12:720.
20. *Zhong Yi Za Zhi* (Journal of Chinese Medicine), 1987; 28(1):45.
21. *Han Fang Yi Xue* (Kampo Medicine), 1985; 10:48.

Bā Wèi Dì Huáng Wán (Eight-Ingredient Pill with Rehmannia)

八味地黄丸

八味地黄丸

Pinyin Name: *Ba Wei Di Huang Wan*
Literal Name: Eight-Ingredient Pill with Rehmannia
Alternate Names: *Pa Wei Ti Huang Wan*, Eight-Flavour Rehmannia Pill, Rehmannia Bolus with Eight Herbs, Rehmannia Eight Formula
Original Source: *Yi Fang Ji Jie* (Analytical Collection of Medical Formulas) by Wang Ang in 1682

COMPOSITION

Shu Di Huang (Radix Rehmanniae Praeparata)	24g
Shan Zhu Yu (Fructus Corni)	12g
Shan Yao (Rhizoma Dioscoreae)	12g
Fu Ling (Poria)	9g
Mu Dan Pi (Cortex Moutan)	9g
Ze Xie (Rhizoma Alismatis)	9g
Rou Gui (Cortex Cinnamomi)	3g
Fu Zi (Radix Aconiti Lateralis Praeparata), *pao* (blast-fried)	3g

Bā Wèi Dì Huáng Wán (Eight-Ingredient Pill with Rehmannia)

DOSAGE / PREPARATION / ADMINISTRATION

Grind the ingredients into powder, and mix the powder with honey and form into small pills that resemble the size of *Wu Tong Zi* (Semen Firmianae), a small seed approximately 5 mm in diameter. Take 15-25 pills (6-10g) with a grain-based liquor twice daily.

CHINESE THERAPEUTIC ACTIONS

Warms and tonifies Kidney yang

CLINICAL MANIFESTATIONS

Kidney yang deficiency: weakness, warmth-seeking behavior, decreased energy level, back pain, weak legs, cold ear tips, lumbar region and rear quarters, polyuria, urinary incontinence, edema, loose stool, a pale to purple, wet, swollen tongue, and a deep, weak, thin pulse that is weaker on the right side.

VETERINARY CLINICAL APPLICATIONS

Endocrine disorders (diabetes mellitus and insipidus, hypoadrenocorticism, equine Cushing's disease, hypothyroidism); sexual and reproductive disorders (impotence, prostatic hypertrophy, male and female infertility); genitourinary disorders (nephritis, amyloidosis, renal failure, chronic glomerulonephritis, proteinuria, urinary incontinence); cardiovascular disorders (congestive heart failure, hypertension); respiratory disorders (chronic bronchitis, asthma); and other conditions such as back pain and intervertebral disk disease.

EXPLANATION

Ba Wei Di Huang Wan (Eight-Ingredient Pill with Rehmannia) is a modification of *Jin Gui Shen Qi Wan* (Kidney Qi Pill from the Golden Cabinet). *Di Huang* (Radix Rehmanniae) is replaced with *Shu Di Huang* (Radix Rehmanniae Praeparata) to enhance the yin-tonic effect. *Gui Zhi* (Ramulus Cinnamomi) is substituted with *Rou Gui* (Cortex Cinnamomi) to increase the yang-tonic function. This slightly revised formula, *Ba Wei Di Huang Wan*, is a warmer and slightly stronger yang tonic than *Jin Gui Shen Qi Wan*.

For additional information, please refer to *Jin Gui Shen Qi Wan* (Kidney Qi Pill from the Golden Cabinet) and *Liu Wei Di Huang Wan* (Six-Ingredient Pill with Rehmannia).

VETERINARY MODIFICATIONS

Same as for *Jin Gui Shen Qi Wan* (Kidney Qi Pill from the Golden Cabinet).

CAUTIONS / CONTRAINDICATIONS

Same as for *Jin Gui Shen Qi Wan* (Kidney Qi Pill from the Golden Cabinet).

PHARMACOLOGICAL EFFECTS

1. **Immunosuppressant**: In one study, use of *Ba Wei Di Huang Wan* for 9 days was associated with suppressed development of MRL/lpr autoimmune diseases in mice.[1,2]
2. **Effect on the prostate**: *Ba Wei Di Huang Wan* has been used to treat various prostate disorders with great success. One study analyzed the mechanism of *Ba Wei Di Huang Wan* and found that this formula acts as a weak androgen and enhances prostatic thymidine kinase activity, but also acts as an anti-androgen and reduces prostatic thymidine kinase activity in the presence of androgen in immature rats.[3]
3. **Effect on bone mass density**: In one study on the prevention and treatment of osteoporosis, *Ba Wei Di Huang Wan*, *Wen Jing Tang* (Warm the Channels Decoction), and *Shi Quan Da Bu Tang* (All-Inclusive Great Tonifying Decoction)

***Ba Wei Di Huang Wan* (Eight-Ingredient Pill with Rehmannia)**

Diagnosis	Clinical Signs	Treatment	Herbs
Severe Kidney yang deficiency	• Back pain, weak limbs, cold ear tips and lumbar region: Kidney yang deficiency unable to warm the lower parts of the body • Urinary incontinence, polyuria and peripheral edema: Kidney yang unable to regulate water circulation and metabolism • Pale to purple, wet, swollen tongue, and a deep, weak, thin pulse that is weaker on the right: Kidney yang deficiency	Strongly warms and tonifies Kidney yang	• *Shu Di Huang* (Radix Rehmanniae Praeparata) strongly tonifies Kidney yin and *jing* (essence). • *Shan Zhu Yu* (Fructus Corni) tonifies Kidney and Liver yin. • *Shan Yao* (Rhizoma Dioscoreae) tonifies the Kidney and Spleen. • *Fu Ling* (Poria), *Mu Dan Pi* (Cortex Moutan) and *Ze Xie* (Rhizoma Alismatis) sedate turbidity and prevent the greasiness of the tonic herbs from blocking the qi flow. • *Rou Gui* (Cortex Cinnamomi) and *Fu Zi* (Radix Aconiti Lateralis Praeparata) strongly tonify Kidney yang.

Bā Wèi Dì Huáng Wán (Eight-Ingredient Pill with Rehmannia)

were administered for 49 days to rats with ovariectomy. Compared to sham-operated rats, the bone mineral density (BMD) of tibia in ovariectomized rats decreased by 20%, but the BMD was unaffected in rats treated with herbs or 17-beta-estradiol. The study concluded that these three formulas were as effective as 17-beta-estradiol in preventing the development of bone loss induced by ovariectomy by preserving the fine particle surface of the bone.[4]

4. **Antihypertensive and nephroprotective**: Administration of *Ba Wei Di Huang Wan* for 5 weeks dose-dependently decreased systolic blood pressure in rats fed with a high-salt (2% NaCl) diet. This blood pressure reduction was associated with a decrease in cardiac mass and thickness of the aortic wall, increased urinary excretion of prostaglandin E2, improved glomerular filtration rate, and improved glomerulosclerosis and arterial injury in the kidney. The study stated that *Ba Wei Di Huang Wan* had both antihypertensive and nephroprotective effects.[5]
5. **Endocrine**: Administration of *Ba Wei Di Huang Wan* was shown both *in vitro* and *in vivo* to stimulate the testes and increase the production of testosterone.[6] Use of this formula also stimulated the corpus luteum and increased secretion of progesterone.[7]

HUMAN CLINICAL STUDIES AND RESEARCH

1. **Benign prostatic hyperplasia**: Use of *Ba Wei Di Huang Wan* for two weeks in 41 patients with benign prostatic hyperplasia was associated with significant improvements in emptying, weak stream, max flow rate, and total quality of life score, according to the International Prostate Symptom Score. Of 41 patients, 40% of patients responded well to *Ba Wei Di Huang Wan* therapy, although 2 did not finish administration as a result of epigastric discomfort.[8]
2. **Female infertility**: In one case report, use of bromocriptine was ineffective in treating one infertile hyperprolactinemic woman with a pituitary microadenoma. This woman was subsequently treated with *Ba Wei Di Huang Wan*, and succeeded in having a normal pregnancy and delivery.[9]
3. **Cataract and other eye diseases**: In one study, use of *Ba Wei Di Huang Wan* was associated with delaying cataract appearance by up to 13.9 years. The mechanism of this effect was attributed to inhibition of sodium-potassium ATPase activity and also the oxidation of lens protein.[10] According to another study in 12 healthy adults, administration of *Ba Wei Di Huang Wan* was associated with significant increase in the systolic flow velocity, diastolic flow velocity, and mean flow velocity in the central retinal artery. Because various eye diseases are associated with a decrease of blood flow in the central retinal artery, use of *Ba Wei Di Huang Wan* to increase blood flow provides positive effects for treatment of such eye diseases.[11]

SUGGESTED ACUPUNCTURE TREATMENT

1. Points: *Ganshu* (BL 18), *Shenshu* (BL 23), *Pishu* (BL 20), *Taixi* (KI 3), *Zhaohai* (KI 6), *Yinlingquan* (SP 9), *Xingjian* (LR 2), *Mingmen* (GV 4), *Shenshu*, *Shenpeng*, and *Shenjiao*.
2. Technique: tonification.

Ganshu (BL 18), *Shenshu* (BL 23), and *Pishu* (BL 20) tonify the yin of the Liver, Kidney, and Spleen. *Taixi* (KI 3) and *Zhaohai* (KI 6) mainly tonify Kidney yin. *Yinlingquan* (SP 9) strengthens the Spleen and eliminates dampness. *Xingjian* (LR 2) sedates Liver fire and other turbidity. *Mingmen* (GV 4) warms *ming men* (life gate) and tonifies Kidney yang. *Shenshu*, *Shenpeng*, and *Shenjiao* are classical equine points that tonify Kidney qi.

AUTHORS' COMMENTS

According to *Zhong Yi Fang Ji Da Ci Dian* (Grand Dictionary of Chinese Herbal Formulas), there are seven different formulas with the same name of *Ba Wei Di Huang Wan* (Eight-Ingredient Pill with Rehmannia). All were written by different authors in various texts and references. The formula listed here, which appeared in *Yi Fang Ji Jie* (Analytical Collection of Medical Formulas) by Wang Ang in 1682, is the most commonly used formulation today.

Jin Gui Shen Qi Wan (Kidney Qi Pill from the Golden Cabinet) and *Ba Wei Di Huang Wan* are essentially the same formula, except for a few minor differences.

- *Jin Gui Shen Qi Wan* uses *Di Huang* (Radix Rehmanniae) to moderately nourish Kidney yin, and *Gui Zhi* (Ramulus Cinnamomi) to mildly warm Kidney yang. Overall, it is a milder formula that gently tonifies both Kidney yin and yang.
- *Ba Wei Di Huang Wan* uses *Shu Di Huang* (Radix Rehmanniae Praeparata) to strongly tonify Kidney yin, and *Rou Gui* (Cortex Cinnamomi) to strongly warm and tonify Kidney yang. Overall, it potently tonifies both Kidney yin and yang.
- In veterinary medicine, the uses of this formula are the same as those for *Jin Gui Shen Qi Wan* (Kidney Qi Pill from the Golden Cabinet). For conditions in which cold signs are predominant, *Ba Wei Di Huang Wan* would be the formula of choice because it has a stronger action to tonify Kidney yin and yang.

References

1. Furuya Y, Kawakita T, Nomoto K. Suppressive effect of a traditional Japanese medicine, Hachimi-jio-gan (Ba-Wei-Di-Huang-Wan), on the hyperresponsiveness to IL-18 in autoimmune MRL/MPJ-lpr/lpr mice. Int Immunopharmacol. 2003 Mar; 3(3):365-73.
2. Furuya Y, Kawakita T, Nomoto K. Immunomodulating effect of a traditional Japanese medicine, hachimi-jio-gan (ba-wei-di-huang-wan), on Th1 predominance in autoimmune MRL/MP-lpr/lpr mice. Int Immunopharmacol. 2001 Mar; 1(3):551-9.

3. Sakamoto S, Kudo H, Kawasaki T, Kasahara N, Okamoto R. Effect of ba-wei-di-huang-wan (hachimi-jio-gan) on thymidine kinase and its isozyme activities in the prostate glands in rats. Am J Chin Med. 1988; 16(1-2):29-36.
4. Hidaka S, Okamoto Y, Nakajima K, Suekawa M, Liu SY. Preventive effects of traditional Chinese (Kampo) medicines on experimental osteoporosis induced by ovariectomy in rats. Calcif Tissue Int. 1997 Sep; 61(3):239-46.
5. Hirawa N, Uehara Y, Kawabata Y, Numabe A, Takada S, Nagoshi H, Gomi T, Ikeda T, Omata M. Hachimi-jio-gan extract protects the kidney from hypertensive injury in Dahl salt-sensitive rat. Am J Chin Med. 1996; 24(3-4):241-54.
6. Usuki S. Hachimijiogan produces testosterone in adult rat testes. Am J Chin Med. 1988; 16(3-4):93-105.
7. Usuki S. Effects of hachimijiogan, tokishakuyakusan and keishibukuryogan on progesterone secretions by corpus luteum. Am J Chin Med. 1987; 15(3-4):109-15.
8. Yoshimura K, Terai A, Arai Y. Two-week administration of low-dose Hachimi-jio-gan (Ba-Wei Di-Huang-Wan) for patients with benign prostatic hyperplasia. Hinyokika Kiyo. 2003 Sep; 49(9):509-14.
9. Otani S, Usuki S, Iwasaki H, Inoue S, Yamashita K. Successful treatment of a infertile woman using hachimijiogan. Am J Chin Med. 1991; 19(2):145-54.
10. Kamei A, Hisada T, Iwata S. The evaluation of therapeutic efficacy of hachimi-jio-gan (traditional Chinese medicine) to mouse hereditary cataract. J Ocul Pharmacol. 1988 Winter; 4(4):311-9.
11. Isobe H. Yamamoto K. Cyong JC. Effects of hachimi-jio-gan (ba-wei-di-huang-wan) on blood flow in the human central retinal artery. American Journal of Chinese Medicine. 2003; 31(3):425-35.

Jì Shēng Shèn Qì Wán

(Kidney Qi Pill from Formulas that Aid the Living)

濟生腎氣丸

济生肾气丸

Pinyin Name: *Ji Sheng Shen Qi Wan*
Literal Name: Kidney Qi Pill from Formulas that Aid the Living
Alternate Names: *Jia Wei Shen Qi Wan* (Augmented Kidney Qi Pill), *Chi Sheng Shen Qi Wan*, Life-Saving Renal Chi Pill, Life-Preserving Kidney-Qi Pill, Cyathula and Plantago Formula
Original Source: *Ji Sheng Fang* (Formulas to Aid the Living) by Yan Yong-He in 1253

COMPOSITION

Shu Di Huang (Radix Rehmanniae Praeparata)	15g [6g]
Shan Zhu Yu (Fructus Corni)	30g [6g]
Shan Yao (Rhizoma Dioscoreae), *chao* (dry-fried)	30g [6g]
Fu Ling (Poria)	30g [6g]
Mu Dan Pi (Cortex Moutan)	30g [6g]
Ze Xie (Rhizoma Alismatis)	30g [6g]
Fu Zi (Radix Aconiti Lateralis Praeparata), *pao* (blast-fried)	60g [9g]
Rou Gui (Cortex Cinnamomi), do not expose to heat	15g [3g]
Chuan Niu Xi (Radix Cyathulae), *jin* (soaked) with liquor	15g [6g]
Che Qian Zi (Semen Plantaginis), *zheng* (steamed) with liquor	30g [6g]

Jì Shēng Shèn Qì Wán

(Kidney Qi Pill from Formulas that Aid the Living)

DOSAGE / PREPARATION / ADMINISTRATION

Grind the ingredients into a fine powder, mix with honey and form into small pills. The pills should resemble *Wu Tong Zi* (Semen Firmianae), a small seed approximately 5 mm in diameter. Take 70 pills (9g) with rice soup on an empty stomach. Today, this formula may be prepared as a decoction using the doses suggested in brackets.

CHINESE THERAPEUTIC ACTIONS

1. Warms and tonifies Kidney yang
2. Regulates water and relieves edema

CLINICAL MANIFESTATIONS

Kidney yang deficiency with water accumulation: severe pitting peripheral edema, cold back, rear quarters and extremities, back pain, fatigue, weakness, and urinary difficulties.

VETERINARY CLINICAL APPLICATIONS

Peripheral edema, diabetes mellitus, nephrotic syndrome, chronic glomerulonephritis, dysuria, oliguria and infertility.

EXPLANATION

Ji Sheng Shen Qi Wan (Kidney Qi Pill from Formulas that Aid the Living) treats Kidney yang deficiency accompanied by water accumulation. Kidney yang deficiency is characterized by generalized decline in both physiological and physical functions, as a result of insufficiency of *ming men* (life gate) fire to warm the Kidney. Consequently, the animal will have compromises in endocrine, reproductive, renal, cardiovascular, and pulmonary functions. Moreover, Kidney yang deficiency may lead to abnormal water circulation and metabolism, resulting in peripheral edema and urinary difficulties. Affected animals will exhibit clinical signs such as coldness of the back, rear quarters and extremities, back pain, fatigue, weakness, and urinary incontinence

Ji Sheng Shen Qi Wan is comprised of *Liu Wei Di Huang Wan* (Six-Ingredient Pill with Rehmannia), plus *Rou Gui* (Cortex Cinnamomi), *Fu Zi* (Radix Aconiti Lateralis Praeparata), *Che Qian Zi* (Semen Plantaginis), and *Chuan Niu Xi* (Radix Cyathulae). *Liu Wei Di Huang Wan* (Six-Ingredient Pill with Rehmannia) tonifies the underlying Kidney yin deficiency. Hot in nature, *Fu Zi* (Radix Aconiti Lateralis Praeparata) and *Rou Gui* (Cortex Cinnamomi) tonify Kidney yang and warm the lower body. *Fu Zi* (Radix Aconiti Lateralis Praeparata) is an excellent herb to treat various chronic disorders with signs and symptoms of cold. *Rou Gui* (Cortex Cinnamomi) strengthens the Spleen and tonifies Kidney yang. It warms cold extremities, relieves abdominal cold and pain, and stops diarrhea. Lastly, *Chuan Niu Xi* (Radix Cyathulae) and *Che Qian Zi* (Semen Plantaginis) promote urination and relieve edema.

VETERINARY MODIFICATIONS

- With weakness and fatigue due to qi deficiency, add *Huang Qi* (Radix Astragali) and *Ren Shen* (Radix et Rhizoma Ginseng).
- For impotence and fertility disorders, add *Gui Ban* (Plastrum Testudinis) and *Lu Jiao Shuang* (Cornu Cervi Degelatinatum).
- With soreness and pain in the upper and lower back, add *Du Zhong* (Cortex Eucommiae) and *Gou Qi Zi* (Fructus Lycii).

CAUTIONS / CONTRAINDICATIONS

- *Ji Sheng Shen Qi Wan* is contraindicated in the following situations: yin-deficient fire, excess fire and damaged body fluids, and the presence of an exterior condition.[1]

***Ji Sheng Shen Qi Wan* (Kidney Qi Pill from Formulas that Aid the Living)**

Diagnosis	Clinical Signs	Treatment	Herbs
Kidney yang deficiency with water accumulation	• General decline in physiological and physical functions: Kidney yang deficiency with insufficiency of *ming men* (life gate) fire • Peripheral edema and urinary difficulties: Kidney yang deficiency unable to regulate water circulation and metabolism • Coldness of the back, rear quarters and extremities: Kidney yang deficiency unable to warm the body	• Warms and tonifies Kidney yang • Regulates water and relieves edema	• *Liu Wei Di Huang Wan* (Six-Ingredient Pill with Rehmannia) nourishes Liver and Kidney yin. • *Fu Zi* (Radix Aconiti Lateralis Praeparata) and *Rou Gui* (Cortex Cinnamomi) tonify Kidney yang and warm the lower body. • *Chuan Niu Xi* (Radix Cyathulae) and *Che Qian Zi* (Semen Plantaginis) promote urination and relieve edema.

Jì Shēng Shèn Qì Wán

(Kidney Qi Pill from Formulas that Aid the Living)

- Use of this formula is sometimes associated with gastrointestinal irritation. In one study, 5 out of 30 patients who took this formula reported gastrointestinal side effects. In another study, 4 out of 80 patients had similar reactions. In both studies, the gastrointestinal side effects were mild and self-limiting, and resolved spontaneously with discontinuation of the herbs.[2]

PHARMACOLOGICAL EFFECTS

Hypoglycemic: Administration of *Ji Sheng Shen Qi Wan* to 24 patients with diabetes mellitus with various complications was associated with a marked decrease in plasma glucose levels for two hours.[3]

HUMAN CLINICAL STUDIES AND RESEARCH

1. **Diabetic neuropathy**: Administration of *Ji Sheng Shen Qi Wan* in 44 patients with diabetic neuropathy was associated with marked symptomatic improvement, such as relief of pain, numbness, perspiration, and weakness in the lower back and legs. The treatment protocol was to administer the herbs in extract, at doses of 7.5g daily in three equally-divided doses, for 12 weeks or more.[4]
2. **Nephrotic syndrome**: One study reported 94% effectiveness using modified *Ji Sheng Shen Qi Wan* to treat 68 patients with nephrotic syndrome. Modifications included the addition of *Sang Bai Pi* (Cortex Mori) and *Bai Mao Gen* (Rhizoma Imperatae) for severe edema; *Yi Yi Ren* (Semen Coicis) and *Sha Ren* (Fructus Amomi) for abdominal fullness with poor appetite; *Zhi Mu* (Rhizoma Anemarrhenae) and *Huang Bo* (Cortex Phellodendri Chinensis) for Kidney yin-deficient fire; and *Wu Wei Xiao Du Yin* (Five-Ingredient Decoction to Eliminate Toxins) for red eyes and face with the presence of sores. Of 68 patients, the study reported complete recovery in 19 patients, improvement in 45 patients, and no change in 4 patients.[5]
3. **Infertility**: *Ji Sheng Shen Qi Wan* was reported in one study of 34 men to have a marked effect in treating male infertility by increasing sperm count and motility. The treatment protocol was to administer 7.5g per day of this formula for 3 months.[6] In another study, use of *Ji Sheng Shen Qi Wan* was associated with increased sperm count in 16 of 24 men with infertility.[7]
4. **Prostatic hypertrophy**: Administration of *Ji Sheng Shen Qi Wan* was beneficial in treating 23 patients with enlarged prostate who suffered from frequent and difficult urination. The treatment protocol was to administer 7.5 grams of the formula in extract form daily for 8 weeks. The study reported 84% effectiveness in treating frequent and difficult urination.[8]

SUGGESTED ACUPUNCTURE TREATMENT

1. Points: *Shenshu* (BL 23), *Pishu* (BL 20), *Taixi* (KI 3), *Zhaohai* (KI 6), *Yinlingquan* (SP 9), *Xingjian* (LR 2), *Mingmen* (GV 4), *Housanli* (ST 36), and *Qihai* (CV 6).
2. Technique: tonification.

Shenshu (BL 23) and *Pishu* (BL 20) tonify Liver, Kidney, and Spleen yin. *Taixi* (KI 3) and *Zhaohai* (KI 6) mainly tonify Kidney yin. *Yinlingquan* (SP 9) strengthens the Spleen and eliminates dampness. *Xingjian* (LR 2) sedates Liver fire and other turbidity. *Mingmen* (GV 4) warms *ming men* (life gate) fire and tonifies Kidney yang. *Housanli* (ST 36) and *Qihai* (CV 6) tonify qi and yang and remove water retention.

AUTHORS' COMMENTS

The veterinary uses of this formula are similar to *Jin Gui Shen Qi Wan* (Kidney Qi Pill from the Golden Cabinet). This formula, however, contains *Chuan Niu Xi* (Radix Cyathulae) and *Che Qian Zi* (Semen Plantaginis) to help regulate water circulation, thus making it more suited to resolve conditions with edema. *Ji Sheng Shen Qi Wan* can be used to treat renal failure and nephrotic syndrome with proteinuria, edema and general weakness, by combining it with *Bu Zhong Yi Qi Tang* (Tonify the Middle and Augment the Qi Decoction) and adding *Dong Chong Xia Cao* (Cordyceps) and *Dan Shen* (Radix et Rhizoma Salviae Miltiorrhizae). This formula is most useful in older horses with chronic limb edema caused by deficiencies in the Kidney.

Originally named "*Jia Wei Shen Qi Wan* (Augmented Kidney Qi Pill)" by Yan Yong-He in 1253, this formula today is commonly referred to as *Ji Sheng Shen Qi Wan* (Kidney Qi Pill from Formulas that Aid the Living). The reason for this change is to avoid confusion and errors, since there are many formulas with similar names according to *Zhong Yi Fang Ji Da Ci Dian* (Grand Dictionary of Chinese Herbal Formulas).

Jin Gui Shen Qi Wan (Kidney Qi Pill from the Golden Cabinet) and *Ji Sheng Shen Qi Wan* (Kidney Qi Pill from Formulas that Aid the Living) have similar names, but are derived from different sources and have slightly different functions:

- *Jin Gui Shen Qi Wan* has a balanced and stronger effect to tonify both Kidney yin and yang.
- *Ji Sheng Shen Qi Wan* has a stronger effect to tonify Kidney yang and promote urination.

Jì Shēng Shèn Qì Wán

(Kidney Qi Pill from Formulas that Aid the Living)

References

1. *Zhong Yao Ming Fang Yao Li Yu Ying Yong* (Pharmacology and Applications of Famous Herbal Formulas), 1989; 329-331.
2. *Zhong Yi Fang Ji Xian Dai Yan Jiu* (Modern Study of Medical Formulas in Traditional Chinese Medicine), 1997; 688.
3. *Zhong Yi Fang Ji Xian Dai Yan Jiu* (Modern Study of Medical Formulas in Traditional Chinese Medicine), 1997; 686-687.
4. *Guo Wai Yi Xue* (Foreign Medicine), 1992; 1:44.
5. *Shan Xi Zhong Yi* (Shanxi Chinese Medicine), 1997; 4:149.
6. *Guo Wai Yi Xue Zhong Yi Zhong Yao Fen Ce* (Monograph of Chinese Herbology from Foreign Medicine), 1995; 6:27.
7. *Guo Wai Yi Xue Zhong Yi Zhong Yao Fen Ce* (Monograph of Chinese Herbology from Foreign Medicine), 1989; 5:26.
8. *Han Fang Yi Xue* (Kampo Medicine), 1983; 5:14.

Yòu Guī Wán (Restore the Right [Kidney] Pill)

右歸丸

右归丸

Pinyin Name: *You Gui Wan*

Literal Name: Restore the Right [Kidney] Pill

Alternate Name: Eucommia and Rehmannia Formula

Original Source: *Jing Yue Quan Shu* (Collected Treatises of [Zhang] Jing Yue) by Zhang Jie-Bin (Zhang Jing-Yue) in 1624

COMPOSITION

Rou Gui (Cortex Cinnamomi)	60-120g [6-12g]
Fu Zi (Radix Aconiti Lateralis Praeparata), *zhi* (prepared)	60-180g [6-18g]
Shu Di Huang (Radix Rehmanniae Praeparata)	240g [24g]
Shan Zhu Yu (Fructus Corni), *chao* (dry-fried)	90g [9g]
Shan Yao (Rhizoma Dioscoreae), *chao* (dry-fried)	120g [12g]
Gou Qi Zi (Fructus Lycii), *chao* (dry-fried)	120g [12g]
Lu Jiao Jiao (Colla Cornus Cervi), *chao* (dry-fried)	120g [12g]
Tu Si Zi (Semen Cuscutae), *zhi* (prepared)	120g [12g]
Du Zhong (Cortex Eucommiae), *chao* (dry-fried) with ginger juice	120g [12g]
Dang Gui (Radix Angelicae Sinensis)	90g [9g]

DOSAGE / PREPARATION / ADMINISTRATION

Grind the ingredients into powder and mix it with honey to form small pills. Take 100 or more pills with boiled water. Today, it is prepared by mixing the powdered herbs with honey to form pills, with each pill weighing about 15g. Take 1 pill on an empty stomach in the morning and at night, with water. This formula may also be prepared as a decoction using the doses suggested in brackets.

CHINESE THERAPEUTIC ACTIONS

1. Warms and tonifies Kidney yang
2. Replenishes *jing* (essence) and tonifies the blood

CLINICAL MANIFESTATIONS

Kidney yang deficiency with diminished *ming men* (life gate) fire: low energy, decreased activity, lethargy, aversion to cold, cold extremities, impotence, low sperm count,

Yòu Guī Wán (Restore the Right [Kidney] Pill)

urinary incontinence, loose stools with undigested food, weakness of the back and stifles, and peripheral edema of the rear legs.

VETERINARY CLINICAL APPLICATIONS

Equine Cushing's disease, infertility, impotence, urinary incontinence, nephrotic syndrome, chronic nephritis, diabetes mellitus, bronchial asthma, back pain, canine hypothyroidism and hypoadrenocorticism (Addison's disease).

EXPLANATION

You Gui Wan (Restore the Right [Kidney] Pill) treats Kidney yang deficiency with diminished *ming men* (life gate) fire. Since *ming men* (life gate) fire is the source of yang, when it diminishes, the entire body will be affected. When Kidney yang is deficient, it is unable to warm the body, resulting in aversion to cold and cold extremities. In horses, this cold accumulation spurs the development of hirsutism and causes stagnation and laminitic pain so common in these patients. Kidney yang deficiency may lead to Spleen and Stomach yang deficiencies, resulting in low energy, decreased activity, lethargy, loose stools with undigested food, and the accumulation of dampness, most noticeable in equine patients; typically, equine patients will experience fat accumulation in the suborbital fossa, the crest of the neck, and ascites of the abdomen. In males, Kidney yang deficiency often leads to reproductive disorders, such as impotence and low sperm count. Kidney yang deficiency can affect urinary function and cause urinary disorders, such as urinary dribbling and incontinence. It can also impair the body's ability to regulate water metabolism, giving rise to edema of the lower legs and loose stools. Because the Kidney resides in the low back area, Kidney deficiency may cause weakness of the back and stifles. Chronic illness may consume the yang qi of the body, causing low energy and lethargy.

Rou Gui (Cortex Cinnamomi) and *Fu Zi* (Radix Aconiti Lateralis Praeparata) warm Kidney yang and raise *ming men* (life gate) fire. According to the yin-yang theory of mutual dependence, in order to effectively tonify Kidney yang, Kidney yin must also be nourished. Thus, this formula uses *Shu Di Huang* (Radix Rehmanniae Praeparata), *Shan Zhu Yu* (Fructus Corni), *Shan Yao* (Rhizoma Dioscoreae), and *Gou Qi Zi* (Fructus Lycii) to nourish Kidney yin and replenish *jing* (essence). *Lu Jiao Jiao* (Colla Cornus Cervi), *Tu Si Zi* (Semen Cuscutae), and *Du Zhong* (Cortex Eucommiae) warm Kidney yang, replenish *jing*, and tonify the Liver and Kidney to strengthen the bones and tendons. *Dang Gui* (Radix Angelicae Sinensis) tonifies the blood and nourishes the Liver.

VETERINARY MODIFICATIONS

- For severe indigestion, acid regurgitation, or decreased dietary intake, add *Gan Jiang* (Rhizoma Zingiberis).
- With abdominal pain, add *Wu Zhu Yu* (Fructus Evodiae).
- With soreness and pain of the lower back and knees, add *He Tao Ren* (Semen Juglandis).
- For impotence as a result of yang deficiency, add *Ba Ji Tian* (Radix Morindae Officinalis) and *Rou Cong Rong* (Herba Cistanches Deserticolae).
- For chronic diarrhea, add *Bu Gu Zhi* (Fructus Psoraleae), *Wu Wei Zi* (Fructus Schisandrae Chinensis), and *Rou Dou Kou* (Semen Myristicae).

CAUTIONS / CONTRAINDICATIONS

- Animals with weak middle *jiao* function should be supplemented with herbs or formula to support the Spleen and

***You Gui Wan* (Restore the Right [Kidney] Pill)**

Diagnosis	Clinical Signs	Treatment	Herbs
Kidney yang deficiency with diminished *ming men* (life gate) fire	• Low energy, decreased activity, lethargy, aversion to cold, and cold extremities: diminished *ming men* fire • Weakness of the back and knees, impotence, and low sperm count: Kidney yang deficiency • Urinary incontinence and edema of the legs: Kidney yang deficiency unable to regulate water circulation and metabolism	• Warms and tonifies Kidney yang • Replenishes *jing* (essence) and tonifies the blood	• *Rou Gui* (Cortex Cinnamomi) and *Fu Zi* (Radix Aconiti Lateralis Praeparata) warm Kidney yang and raise *ming men* fire. • *Shu Di Huang* (Radix Rehmanniae Praeparata), *Shan Zhu Yu* (Fructus Corni), *Shan Yao* (Rhizoma Dioscoreae), and *Gou Qi Zi* (Fructus Lycii) nourish Kidney yin and replenish *jing*. • *Lu Jiao Jiao* (Colla Cornus Cervi), *Tu Si Zi* (Semen Cuscutae), and *Du Zhong* (Cortex Eucommiae) warm Kidney yang, replenish *jing*, and tonify the Liver and Kidney. • *Dang Gui* (Radix Angelicae Sinensis) tonifies the blood and nourishes the Liver.

Yòu Guī Wán (Restore the Right [Kidney] Pill)

Stomach when taking this formula to avoid gastrointestinal upset.

- *You Gui Wan* is contraindicated in cases of Kidney deficiency and damp accumulation.
- Feeding cold and raw foods should be avoided.

PHARMACOLOGICAL EFFECTS

1. **Immunostimulant**: In one experiment, daily administration of the formula at 30 g/kg orally for 5 days was associated with increased phagocytic activity of the macrophages in mice.[1]
2. **Adaptogenic**: Use of *You Gui Wan* was associated with improved physical performance in various laboratory studies. In one study, oral administration of the formula at 20-30 g/kg for 5 days increased the duration of swimming in mice ($P<0.01$).[2]
3. **Cognitive**: One study reported improved cognition (improved memory and decreased repetition of errors) in mice that were administered *You Gui Wan* at 30 g/kg and 20 g/kg (dose based on dried herbs) for 5 days.[3]
4. **Antiplatelet**: In one study, oral administration of the formula at 20 g/kg for 5 days was associated with a mild antiplatelet effect.[4]
5. **Hepatoprotective**: In a laboratory experiment, oral administration of the formula at 20-30 g/kg for 5 days was effective in protecting against liver damage induced by injection of 0.1% carbon tetrachloride.[5]

HUMAN CLINICAL STUDIES AND RESEARCH

1. **Male infertility**: One study reported successful treatment in all 11 male patients with a history of infertility (the female partners became pregnant) using modified *You Gui Wan* in decoction.[6]
2. **Frequent urination**: Frequent urination in elderly patients was successfully treated using *You Gui Wan* plus *Suo Quan Wan* (Shut the Sluice Pill). In addition to these two formulas, others herbs were added as deemed necessary: *Dang Shen* (Radix Codonopsis) and *Huang Qi* (Radix Astragali) for Spleen and Lung qi deficiencies; *Chuan Xiong* (Rhizoma Chuanxiong) and *Dan Shen* (Radix et Rhizoma Salviae Miltiorrhizae) for blood stagnation; and *Gui Ban* (Plastrum Testudinis), *Niu Xi* (Radix Achyranthis Bidentatae), and *Zhi Mu* (Rhizoma Anemarrhenae) for yin deficiency. *Gui Lu Er Xian Jiao* (Tortoise Shell and Deer Antler Syrup) was given at the end to consolidate the treatment effect. The treatment protocol was to administer the herbs in decoction daily for 3 weeks per course of treatment. Of 64 patients, 17 had complete recovery, 21 showed significant improvement, 21 showed slight improvement, and 5 showed no change.[7]
3. **Nephrotic syndrome**: In one report, 6 patients with nephrotic syndrome who were unresponsive to drug treatment (steroids) were treated with herbs with satisfactory results. General progress included symptomatic improvement and a reduction of protein in the urine.[8]
4. **Bronchial asthma**: In a clinical study, long-term administration of *You Gui Wan* was successful in preventing asthma. The treatment protocol was to take the formula daily for 2 months prior to the seasonal changes starting in August. For patients who followed the protocol for 3 years, the success rate was between 83-95.5%. Moreover, 50% of the patients who were dependant on corticosteroids for prevention and treatment of asthma were able to discontinue the drugs.[9]
5. **Sciatica**: Use of modified *You Gui Wan* in 48 patients with sciatica was associated with complete recovery in 32 cases, significant improvement in 12 cases, and no benefit in 4 cases.[10]
6. **Hypertrophic myelitis**: Use of modified *You Gui Wan* successfully treated hypertrophic myelitis. The treatment protocol was to administer the herbs for 10-15 days per course of treatment, with duration ranging from 10-42 days. Of 48 patients, the study reported complete recovery in 31 cases and improvement in 17 cases. Most patients had relief of pain after 2-3 days, and resolution of all symptoms after 10 days.[11]

HERB-DRUG INTERACTION

Corticosteroid-induced immune suppression: One study found *You Gui Wan* to be effective in reversing corticosteroid-induced immune suppression in rats. The mechanism was attributed to the "yang-tonifying" effect of the formula, as subjects who use steroids for a long period of time often have "yang deficiency" signs and symptoms, such as edema, swelling, and immune-suppression.[12]

TOXICOLOGY

In an acute toxicology study, no fatality was reported in mice following oral ingestion of a bolus dose of 50 g/kg and 25 g/kg of raw herbs in decoction. No abnormalities were observed in follow-up observation for up to 7 days.[13]

SUGGESTED ACUPUNCTURE TREATMENT

1. Points: *Shenshu* (BL 23), *Taixi* (KI 3), *Ganshu* (BL 18), *Pishu* (BL 20), *Geshu* (BL 17), *Guanyuan* (CV 4), *Qihai* (CV 6), *Mingmen* (GV 4), *Shenshu*, *Shenpeng*, and *Shenjiao*.
2. Techniques: tonification and moxibustion.

Moxibustion on *Shenshu* (BL 23) and *Taixi* (KI 3) warms Kidney yang. *Ganshu* (BL 18) and *Pishu* (BL 20) nourish the Liver and strengthen the Spleen to help tonify the Kidney. *Geshu* (BL 17) nourishes the blood. *Qihai* (CV 6) tonifies qi and consolidates the Kidney. *Mingmen* (GV 4)

Yòu Guī Wán (Restore the Right [Kidney] Pill)

and *Guanyuan* (CV 4) nourish Kidney yang to tonify Kidney qi. *Shenshu*, *Shenpeng*, and *Shenjiao* are classical equine points that tonify Kidney qi.

RELATED FORMULA

Yòu Guī Yǐn (Restore the Right [Kidney] Decoction)
右歸飲
右归饮
Pinyin Name: *You Gui Yin*
Literal Name: Restore the Right [Kidney] Decoction
Original Source: *Jing Yue Quan Shu* (Collected Treatises of [Zhang] Jing Yue) by Zhang Jie-Bing (Zhang Jing-Yue) in 1624

Shu Di Huang (Radix Rehmanniae Praeparata)	6-60g [6-30g]
Shan Yao (Rhizoma Dioscoreae), *chao* (dry-fried)	6g
Shan Zhu Yu (Fructus Corni)	3g
Gou Qi Zi (Fructus Lycii)	6g
Zhi Gan Cao (Radix et Rhizoma Glycyrrhizae Praeparata cum Melle)	3-6g [6g]
Du Zhong (Cortex Eucommiae), *zhi* (prepared) with fresh ginger	6g
Rou Gui (Cortex Cinnamomi)	3-6g [6g]
Fu Zi (Radix Aconiti Lateralis Praeparata), *zhi* (prepared)	3-9g [9g]

Cook the ingredients in two large bowls of water until the liquid is reduced to 70%. Take the warm decoction between meals. Today, the decoction may be prepared using the doses suggested in brackets.

You Gui Yin (Restore the Right [Kidney] Decoction) warms Kidney yang and tonifies Kidney *jing* (essence). Clinically, patients may have low energy, lethargy, abdominal pain, lower back soreness, cold extremities, and a fine pulse.

AUTHORS' COMMENTS

You Gui Wan contains rich and cloying herbs that can produce dampness and indigestion in Spleen qi deficient animals. In these animals, it is best to add some herbs to promote appropriate assimilation of the formula to avoid gastrointestinal upset, vomiting and diarrhea. Once the clinical signs have resolved, a more balanced formula, such as *Jin Gui Shen Qi Wan* (Kidney Qi Pill from the Golden Cabinet) or *Liu Wei Di Huang Wan* (Six-Ingredient Pill with Rehmannia), can be given.

- *You Gui Wan* can be used in the treatment of hypoadrenocorticism (Addison's disease) with a predominance of yang deficiency; once the animal is stabilized, discontinue this formula and select a more balanced, long-term formula. For animals with Spleen deficiency, combine with *Bu Zhong Yi Qi Tang* (Tonify the Middle and Augment the Qi Decoction).
- For equine Cushing's disease with laminitis, combine with *Si Ni Tang* (Frigid Extremities Decoction) and *Shen Tong Zhu Yu Tang* (Drive Out Blood Stasis from a Painful Body Decoction). In milder cases with less foot pain, *Dang Gui Si Ni Tang* (Tangkuei Decoction for Frigid Extremities) may be used in place of *Si Ni Tang*. As symptoms improve, *You Gui Wan* may prove to be too warming, at which point, the dose can be decreased or the formula substituted with *Er Xian Tang* (Two-Immortal Decoction).
- For the treatment of urinary incontinence, combine with *Suo Quan Wan* (Shut the Sluice Pill) and add *Huang Qi* (Radix Astragali), *Fu Pen Zi* (Fructus Rubi), *Sang Piao Xiao* (Ootheca Mantidis), and *Jin Ying Zi* (Fructus Rosae Laevigatae).
- For the treatment of nephrotic syndrome with Kidney yang deficiency, combine with *Bu Zhong Yi Qi Tang* (Tonify the Middle and Augment the Qi Decoction) and add *Dong Chong Xia Cao* (Cordyceps), *San Qi* (Radix et Rhizoma Notoginseng), *Yu Mi Xu* (Stigma Maydis), and *Dan Shen* (Radix et Rhizoma Salviae Miltiorrhizae). With anemia, combine with *Tao Hong Si Wu Tang* (Four-Substance Decoction with Safflower and Peach Pit)

You Gui Wan differs from *Ba Wei Di Huang Wan* (Eight-Ingredient Pill with Rehmannia) in the same way that *Zuo Gui Wan* (Restore the Left [Kidney] Pill) differs from *Liu Wei Di Huang Wan* (Six-Ingredient Pill with Rehmannia).

- *You Gui Wan* and *Zuo Gui Wan* tonify the Kidney without sedation. They have a more potent and immediate tonifying effect, and are more suitable for treating acute and severe cases.
- *Ba Wei Di Huang Wan* and *Liu Wei Di Huang Wan* tonify and sedate the Kidney at the same time. They have a moderate tonifying effect, and are suitable for long-term use to treat chronic deficiencies.

You Gui Wan (Restore the Right [Kidney] Pill) and *Zuo Gui Wan* (Restore the Left [Kidney] Pill) have similar names and functions. These formulas may be used singularly, or in combination.

- *You Gui Wan* tonifies Kidney yang.
- *Zuo Gui Wan* tonifies Kidney yin.

You Gui Wan and *Zuo Gui Wan* can be used in combination to treat chronic renal failure in the dog and cat. Most of these animals are given herbal medication in the morning and evening, or every 12 hours. On this dosing schedule, *You Gui Wan* is administered in the morning and *Zuo Gui*

Yòu Guī Wán (Restore the Right [Kidney] Pill)

Wan in the evening, and these formulas can be combined with *Shen Ling Bai Zhu San* (Ginseng, Poria, and Atractylodes Macrocephala Powder) or *Liu Jun Zi Tang* (Six-Gentlemen Decoction). A Spleen tonic is often given in this treatment protocol for several reasons. The rich, cloying nature of these formulas can upset the middle *jiao* (many renal patients are already nauseous), and Spleen tonics are used to promote digestion of these formulas and protect the middle *jiao*. Spleen tonics are also used to nourish the Kidney and treat proteinuria. Proteinuria is associated with the inability of the Spleen to astringe *jing* (essence). Once the animal is stable, discontinue these formulas, and administer a maintenance formula combination, such as *Jin Gui Shen Qi Wan* (Kidney Qi Pill from the Golden Cabinet) and *Bu Zhong Yi Qi Tang* (Tonify the Middle and Augment the Qi Decoction).

References

1. *Zhong Yao Yao Li Yu Lin Chuang* (Pharmacology and Clinical Applications of Chinese Herbs), 1990; 6(4):6.
2. *Zhong Yao Yao Li Yu Lin Chuang* (Pharmacology and Clinical Applications of Chinese Herbs), 1990; 6(4):6.
3. *Zhong Yao Yao Li Yu Lin Chuang* (Pharmacology and Clinical Applications of Chinese Herbs), 1990; 6(4):6.
4. *Zhong Yao Yao Li Yu Lin Chuang* (Pharmacology and Clinical Applications of Chinese Herbs), 1990; 6(4):6.
5. *Zhong Yao Yao Li Yu Lin Chuang* (Pharmacology and Clinical Applications of Chinese Herbs), 1990; 6(4):6.
6. *He Bei Zhong Yi* (Hebei Chinese Medicine), 1988; 4:31.
7. *Xin Zhong Yi* (New Chinese Medicine), 1997; 1:48.
8. *Shen De Yan Jiu* (Research of Kidney), 1981; 93.
9. *Zhong Yi Za Zhi* (Journal of Chinese Medicine), 1981; (5):341.
10. *Si Chuan Zhong Yi* (Sichuan Chinese Medicine), 1985; 11:51.
11. *Hu Nan Zhong Yi Za Zhi* (Hunan Journal of Chinese Medicine), 1985; 3:27.
12. *Shan Xi Zhong Yi* (Shanxi Chinese Medicine), 1989; 6:277.
13. *Zhong Yao Yao Li Yu Lin Chuang* (Pharmacology and Clinical Applications of Chinese Herbs), 1990; 6(4):6.

Huán Shào Dān (Return to Youth Pill)

還少丹
还少丹

Pinyin Name: *Huan Shao Dan*
Literal Name: Return to Youth Pill
Alternate Names: *Huan Shao Tan*, Youth-Returning Formula, Lycium Formula
Original Source: *Yang Shi Mi Fang* (Secret Formulas of the Yang Family)

COMPOSITION

Rou Cong Rong (Herba Cistanches)	30g
Ba Ji Tian (Radix Morindae Officinalis)	30g
Xiao Hui Xiang (Fructus Foeniculi)	30g
Shu Di Huang (Radix Rehmanniae Praeparata)	15g
Shan Zhu Yu (Fructus Corni), *jin* (soaked) in liquor for 1 night and *bei* (stone-baked)	30g
Gou Qi Zi (Fructus Lycii)	15g
Du Zhong (Cortex Eucommiae), *zhi* (fried) with liquor and the juice of fresh ginger	30g
Chuan Niu Xi (Radix Cyathulae), *jin* (soaked) in liquor for 1 night and *bei* (stone-baked)	45g
Fu Ling (Poria)	30g
Shan Yao (Rhizoma Dioscoreae)	45g
Wu Wei Zi (Fructus Schisandrae Chinensis)	30g
Yuan Zhi (Radix Polygalae)	30g
Shi Chang Pu (Rhizoma Acori Tatarinowii)	30g
Da Zao (Fructus Jujubae)	15g
Chu Shi Zi (Fructus Broussonetiae)	30g

Huán Shào Dān (Return to Youth Pill)

DOSAGE / PREPARATION / ADMINISTRATION

Grind the ingredients into powder and mix with honey to form pills. The pills should resemble the size of *Wu Tong Zi* (Semen Firmianae), a small seed approximately 5 mm in diameter. Take 30 pills per dose three times daily on an empty stomach with a warm, grain-based liquor and/or warm, salted water. The source text states that improvement will be noted between 5 to 30 days of continuous use. It also states that this formula is safe for long-term use.

CHINESE THERAPEUTIC ACTIONS

1. Strengthens the Spleen, Stomach, Kidney and Heart
2. Tonifies qi, blood and *jing* (essence)
3. Warms yang

CLINICAL MANIFESTATIONS

Premature aging as a result of Spleen and Kidney deficiencies, with insufficiency of qi, blood, yang and *jing* (essence): decreased libido, generalized weakness and fatigue, anorexia, poor concentration, confusion, forgetfulness, and easily frightened.

VETERINARY CLINICAL APPLICATIONS

Diabetes mellitus, canine hypothyroidism, canine hypoadrenocorticism, poor constitution, recurrent infections, decreased libido, impotence, and premature aging.

EXPLANATION

Huan Shao Dan (Return to Youth Pill) treats premature aging in both males and females. Premature aging is commonly caused by excessive consumption of qi, blood, yang and *jing* (essence), with underlying deficiencies of the Spleen, Stomach, Heart and Kidney, which can be congenital in nature or brought about by poor diet, overbreeding, or overwork. Spleen and Stomach deficiencies result in an inadequate supply of qi, which manifests in symptoms such as generalized weakness, fatigue, and anorexia. Deficiencies of blood and Heart may lead to confusion, poor concentration, forgetfulness, and being easily frightened. Lastly, lack of *jing* is often accompanied by Kidney yang deficiency, which together manifest as decreased libido.

Rou Cong Rong (Herba Cistanches), *Ba Ji Tian* (Radix Morindae Officinalis), and *Xiao Hui Xiang* (Fructus Foeniculi) strengthen Spleen qi and Kidney yang. *Shu Di Huang* (Radix Rehmanniae Praeparata), *Shan Zhu Yu* (Fructus Corni) and *Gou Qi Zi* (Fructus Lycii) nourish the Kidney and benefit qi. *Du Zhong* (Cortex Eucommiae) and *Chuan Niu Xi* (Radix Cyathulae) tonify the Kidney and strengthen the knees and lower back. *Fu Ling* (Poria) and *Shan Yao* (Rhizoma Dioscoreae) strengthen the Spleen and dissolve dampness. *Wu Wei Zi* (Fructus Schisandrae Chinensis) reduces the loss of fluids from

***Huan Shao Dan* (Return to Youth Pill)**

Diagnosis	Clinical Signs	Treatment	Herbs
Premature aging as a result of Spleen and Kidney deficiencies, with insufficiency of qi, blood, yang and *jing* (essence)	• Generalized weakness, fatigue, and anorexia: deficiencies of qi, Spleen and Stomach • Poor concentration, confusion, forgetfulness, and being easily frightened: deficiencies of blood and Heart • Decreased libido: deficiencies of *jing* and Kidney	• Strengthens the Spleen, Stomach, Heart and Kidney • Tonifies qi, blood, and *jing* • Warms yang	• *Rou Cong Rong* (Herba Cistanches), *Ba Ji Tian* (Radix Morindae Officinalis), and *Xiao Hui Xiang* (Fructus Foeniculi) strengthen the Spleen and Kidney. • *Shu Di Huang* (Radix Rehmanniae Praeparata), *Shan Zhu Yu* (Fructus Corni), and *Gou Qi Zi* (Fructus Lycii) nourish the Kidney and benefit qi. • *Du Zhong* (Cortex Eucommiae) and *Chuan Niu Xi* (Radix Cyathulae) tonify the Kidney and strengthen the knees and lower back. • *Fu Ling* (Poria) and *Shan Yao* (Rhizoma Dioscoreae) strengthen the Spleen and dissolve dampness. • *Wu Wei Zi* (Fructus Schisandrae Chinensis) reduces the loss of fluids from the Kidney. • *Yuan Zhi* (Radix Polygalae) tonifies the Heart and calms the *shen* (spirit). • *Shi Chang Pu* (Rhizoma Acori Tatarinowii) opens the sensory orifices. • *Da Zao* (Fructus Jujubae) tonifies qi and blood. • *Chu Shi Zi* (Fructus Broussonetiae) warms and tonifies yang to strengthen the muscles and bones.

Huán Shào Dān (Return to Youth Pill)

the Kidney, namely seminal emissions. *Yuan Zhi* (Radix Polygalae) tonifies the Heart and calms the *shen* (spirit). *Shi Chang Pu* (Rhizoma Acori Tatarinowii) opens the sensory orifices and improves mental functions. *Da Zao* (Fructus Jujubae) tonifies qi and blood, and strengthens the Lung and Spleen. *Chu Shi Zi* (Fructus Broussonetiae) warms and tonifies yang to strengthen the muscles and bones. Taking the formula with salted water allows the salt to function as a channel-guiding substance to the Kidney, to enhance the Kidney-tonifying effect of this formula.

VETERINARY MODIFICATIONS

- If there is lack of appetite, add *Lian Zi* (Semen Nelumbinis) and *Qian Shi* (Semen Euryales), or combine with *Xiang Sha Liu Jun Zi Tang* (Six-Gentlemen Decoction with Aucklandia and Amomum) or *Xiang Sha Liu Jun Zi Tang* (Six-Gentlemen Decoction with Cyperus and Amomum).
- With more qi and yin deficiencies, add *Mai Dong* (Radix Ophiopogonis), *Ren Shen* (Radix et Rhizoma Ginseng), *Huang Qi* (Radix Astragali), and *Dang Gui* (Radix Angelicae Sinensis).

CAUTIONS / CONTRAINDICATIONS

- According to one report, use of *Huan Shao Dan* continuously for one month was associated with occasional side effects such as a dry mouth, constipation, and a feeling of warmth in the body. These reactions are self-limiting, and will resolve within 2 to 3 weeks. [1]
- Use of this formula is contraindicated during pregnancy. [2]

SUGGESTED ACUPUNCTURE TREATMENT

1. Points: *Pishu* (BL 20), *Shenshu* (BL 23), *Guanyuan* (CV 4), *Taixi* (KI 3), *Housanli* (ST 36), *Yinlingquan* (SP 9), *Zhishi* (BL 52), and *Tongli* (HT 5).
2. Technique: moxibustion and tonification.

Apply moxibustion on *Pishu* (BL 20), *Shenshu* (BL 23), and *Guanyuan* (CV 4) to strengthen the Spleen and Kidney. *Taixi* (KI 3), *Shenshu* (BL 23), and *Housanli* (ST 36) tonify the Kidney and strengthen the bones. *Yinlingquan* (SP 9) tonifies the Spleen and dissolves dampness. *Zhishi* (BL 52) and *Tongli* (HT 5) tonify the Heart and calm the *shen* (spirit).

AUTHORS' COMMENTS

Huan Shao Dan has application as a long-term maintenance and support formula used in an integrative approach to chronic diseases. It is a milder yang tonic than the others in this category, and does not contain hot herbs such as *Fu Zi* (Radix Aconiti Lateralis Praeparata) or *Rou Gui* (Cortex Cinnamomi). For this reason, it can be given longer term than formulas that do contain these herbs, without fear of injuring yin and blood. Disorders that can be treated include: endocrine disorders, chronic renal, cardiac or hepatic disease, chronic inflammatory bowel disease, young animals with premature aging, and poor constitution, breeding animals with low libido, and older animals that contract frequent infections. Many of these animals are taking chronic multiple medications. This formula is valuable because it can be given as a sole formula to animals whose owners are unwilling to give multiple herbal formulas. It is necessary to use a large dose of this formula for the maintenance and support of these conditions; using too small a dose will not produce the desired clinical effects. The combination of this formula with a blood-invigorating formula, such as *Xue Fu Zhu Yu Tang* (Drive Out Stasis in the Mansion of Blood Decoction) or *Dan Shen Yin* (Salvia Decoction), will greatly improve clinical results, especially in older animals.

References

1. *Zhong Guo Zhong Xi Yi Jie He Za Zhi* (Chinese Journal of Integrative Chinese and Western Medicine), 1992; 12(1):20.
2. *Zhong Yao Ming Fang Yao Li Yu Ying Yong* (Pharmacology and Applications of Famous Herbal Formulas), 1989; 345-346.

8 TONIC FORMULAS

Èr Xiān Tāng (Two-Immortal Decoction)

二仙湯
二仙汤

Pinyin Name: *Er Xian Tang*
Literal Name: Two-Immortal Decoction
Alternate Name: Curculigo and Epimedium Combination
Original Source: *Zhong Yi Fang Ji Lin Chuan Shou Ce* (Clinical Handbook of Chinese Herbal Formulae)

COMPOSITION

Xian Mao (Rhizoma Curculiginis)	9-15g
Yin Yang Huo (Herba Epimedii)	9-15g
Ba Ji Tian (Radix Morindae Officinalis)	9g
Huang Bo (Cortex Phellodendri Chinensis)	4.5-9g
Zhi Mu (Rhizoma Anemarrhenae)	4.5-9g
Dang Gui (Radix Angelicae Sinensis)	9g

DOSAGE / PREPARATION / ADMINISTRATION

Prepare this formula as a decoction and take it in two equally divided doses.

CHINESE THERAPEUTIC ACTIONS

1. Warms Kidney yang
2. Tonifies Kidney *jing* (essence)
3. Drains deficiency fire from the Kidney

CLINICAL MANIFESTATIONS

1. Kidney yang deficiency: weakness, warmth seeking, decreased energy level, back pain, weak legs, coldness in the ear tips, lumbar region and rear quarters, polyuria, urinary incontinence, edema, loose stools, a pale, flabby tongue with a thin, white coating, or a pale pink to purple tongue, and a deep, weak, thin pulse that is weaker on the right side.
2. Liver and Kidney yin deficiencies: poor hearing, deafness, poor vision, painful and weak back and stifles, orthopedic and dental developmental abnormalities, lameness, dry feces, a red tongue with little coating, and a rapid and thready pulse that is weaker on the left side.
3. Kidney yin and yang deficiencies with fire rising: lethargy, fatigue, increased urinary frequency, nervousness, irritability, aggression, excessive panting, especially at night.

VETERINARY CLINICAL APPLICATIONS

Infertility, feline hyperthyroidism, essential hypertension, chronic glomerulonephritis, chronic renal failure, chronic pyelonephritis, nephrotic syndrome, amyloidosis and polycystic kidneys.

EXPLANATION

Er Xian Tang (Two-Immortal Decoction) treats chronic and complicated disorders characterized by underlying Kidney yin and yang deficiencies, accompanied by deficiency fire rising. The clinical signs are variable, depending on the predominance of yin or yang deficiency present. As a result of the chronic nature of the illness, Kidney yin and yang become ever more deficient, and deficiency fire begins to rise to disturb the Heart, producing symptoms such as nervousness, irritability, aggression, restlessness, and excessive panting, especially at night.

***Er Xian Tang* (Two-Immortal Decoction)**

Diagnosis	Clinical Signs	Treatment	Herbs
Kidney yin and yang deficiencies with fire rising	• Dryness, cool seeking, increased thirst: Kidney yin deficiency • Fatigue, lethargy and urinary frequency: Kidney yang deficiency • Nervousness, irritability, aggression, and restlessness: deficiency fire rising to disturb the Heart	• Warms Kidney yang • Tonifies Kidney *jing* (essence) • Drains deficiency fire from the Kidney	• *Xian Mao* (Rhizoma Curculiginis), *Yin Yang Huo* (Herba Epimedii) and *Ba Ji Tian* (Radix Morindae Officinalis) warm Kidney yang and tonify Kidney *jing*. • *Huang Bo* (Cortex Phellodendri Chinensis) and *Zhi Mu* (Rhizoma Anemarrhenae) nourish Kidney yin and clear deficiency fire. • *Dang Gui* (Radix Angelicae Sinensis) nourishes the blood.

Èr Xiān Tāng (Two-Immortal Decoction)

The treatment strategy is to warm Kidney yang, tonify Kidney *jing* (essence), and drain deficiency fire. However, the selection of herbs and their doses is absolutely critical, because herbs that tonify yang may contribute to more heat and fire, and herbs that clear fire may further damage yin. *Xian Mao* (Rhizoma Curculiginis), *Yin Yang Huo* (Herba Epimedii), and *Ba Ji Tian* (Radix Morindae Officinalis) warm Kidney yang and tonify Kidney *jing*. *Yin Yang Huo* (Herba Epimedii) tonifies both Kidney yin and yang. *Huang Bo* (Cortex Phellodendri Chinensis) and *Zhi Mu* (Rhizoma Anemarrhenae) nourish Kidney yin and clear deficiency fire. *Dang Gui* (Radix Angelicae Sinensis) nourishes the blood and regulates the *chong* (thoroughfare) and *ren* (conception) channels to treat reproductive problems.

VETERINARY MODIFICATIONS

For insomnia, restlessness or pacing at night, add *Yuan Zhi* (Radix Polygalae) and *Suan Zao Ren* (Semen Ziziphi Spinosae).

PHARMACOLOGICAL EFFECTS

1. **Endocrine**: One study evaluated the effect of *Er Xian Tang* and its components on sex hormones in rats. The rats were divided into four groups: group one was the control, group two received *Er Xian Tang*, group three received Kidney and blood-tonifying herbs [*Xian Mao* (Rhizoma Curculiginis), *Yin Yang Huo* (Herba Epimedii), *Dang Gui* (Radix Angelicae Sinensis), and *Ba Ji Tian* (Radix Morindae Officinalis)] and group four received herbs that clear yin-deficient fire [*Huang Bo* (Cortex Phellodendri Chinensis) and *Zhi Mu* (Rhizoma Anemarrhenae)]. The treatment protocol was to administer 10 times the normal dose daily for 10 days, followed by 3 days of rest, and repeat again for a total of 6 months of treatment. At the end of the treatment period, the study reported that in comparison with the control group, rats that received herbs had a statistically significant increase in testosterone in male rats and estradiol in female rats, and a decrease in luteinizing-releasing hormone in both sexes.[1] (Note: Information on comparisons among the three herb groups was unavailable at the time of publication.)
2. **Antihypertensive**: Administration of *Er Xian Tang* was associated with a marked reduction in blood pressure in various laboratory studies. In one study, administration of the formula at 10 g/kg for 2 weeks was associated with a 9-15% reduction in blood pressure in rats. In another study, administration of the formula to anesthetized cats at 6 g/kg was associated with a 30% reduction in blood pressure 2 hours after the treatment. The researchers noted that *Huang Bo* (Cortex Phellodendri Chinensis) and *Yin Yang Huo* (Herba Epimedii) were the main ingredients responsible for the antihypertensive effects of the formula.[2]
3. **Antioxidant**: Administration of *Er Xian Tang* was associated with an anti-aging effect, an antioxidant effect, and reduction of free radicals.[3]

HUMAN CLINICAL STUDIES AND RESEARCH

1. **Infertility**: Administration of modified *Er Xian Tang* was successful in treating women with infertility due to irregular menstruation. Of the 26 women, 9 were between 25-27 years of age, 12 between 28-30 years of age, and 5 above 30 years of age. The treatment period ranged from 37 days to 1 year, with an average of 4-7 months. The study reported a success rate of 69.23% (18 pregnancies in 26 patients).[4]
2. **Nephropathy**: In one study, 60 children with a history of nephropathy from 3 days to 3 years were treated successfully with herbs. The children were divided into two groups: group one received prednisone, and group two received the prednisone with herbs. The herbal formula contained 10g of dry-fried *Bai Zhu* (Rhizoma Atractylodis Macrocephalae), and 6g each of *Xian Mao* (Rhizoma Curculiginis), *Yin Yang Huo* (Herba Epimedii), *Bu Gu Zhi* (Fructus Psoraleae), *Huang Qi* (Radix Astragali), *Rou Cong Rong* (Herba Cistanches), *Dan Shen* (Radix et Rhizoma Salviae Miltiorrhizae), and *Fang Feng* (Radix Saposhnikoviae). The herbs were given as decoction daily. After one year of treatment, the study reported that individuals in group two (drug and herb group) responded much better than group one (drug group), with alleviation of signs and symptoms. Upon follow-up 3-6 months after the discontinuation of treatment, group two had only 6.6% recurrence, while group one had 36.6% recurrence.[5]
3. **Aplastic anemia**: In one study of 84 patients, use of *Er Xian Tang* to warm and tonify the Spleen and Kidney was associated with good results in treating aplastic anemia. Of 84 patients, the total effective rate was 84.5%, and the remission rate was 47.6%. The mechanism of action was attributed to the nourishing effect of the formula and stimulation of hemopoiesis stem cell. The experiment showed that use of *Er Xian Tang* was associated with an increase in CFU-S and GM-CFU in the bone marrow.[6]

SUGGESTED ACUPUNCTURE TREATMENT

1. Points: *Taixi* (KI 3), *Zhaohai* (KI 6), *Sanyinjiao* (SP 6), *Mingmen* (GV 4), and *Shenshu* (BL 23).
2. Technique: tonification and moxibustion.

Taixi (KI 3) and *Zhaohai* (KI 6) nourish Kidney yin and clear deficiency fire. Apply moxibustion on *Mingmen* (GV 4) and *Shenshu* (BL 23) to tonify the Kidney. Moxibustion and needling on *Sanyinjiao* (SP 6) tonify and invigorate

Èr Xiān Tāng (Two-Immortal Decoction)

the blood, and harmonize both the *chong* (thoroughfare) and *ren* (conception) channels.

AUTHORS' COMMENTS

Er Xian Tang, literally "Two-Immortal Decoction," is aptly named for two reasons. First, the two chief herbs, *Xian Mao* (Rhizoma Curculiginis) and *Yin Yang Huo* (Herba Epimedii), effectively tonify the Kidney to prolong life. Second, it is called *Er Xian Tang* because the two chief herbs both contain "*Xian*" in their names: *Xian Mao* (Rhizoma Curculiginis) and *Xian Ling Pi* (Herba Epimedii). Note: "*Xian Ling Pi*" is an alternate pinyin name for *Yin Yang Huo* (Herba Epimedii).

Er Xian Tang is a formula that contains herbs to tonify Kidney yin, yang and *jing* (essence), as well as herbs to drain heat, which flares upward from deficiency. It treats chronic and complex disorders, and has clinically been found to halt and reverse early hyperthyroidism (mild elevation of T4) in the cat. For this application, the formula is modified by adding *Huang Qi* (Radix Astragali), *He Shou Wu* (Radix Polygoni Multiflori), *Mu Dan Pi* (Cortex Moutan), *Rou Cong Rong* (Herba Cistanches), *Tu Si Zi* (Semen Cuscutae), *Fu Ling* (Poria), and *Dan Shen* (Radix et Rhizoma Salviae Miltiorrhizae). This modified formula should be given for a minimum of 90 days to normalize T4 values. (On average, it can take 3-6 months to normalize values). In most cases, the dosage of the formula is decreased over time, and must be administered for one year or more before it can be discontinued.

Er Xian Tang can also be used for established cases of feline hyperthyroidism and it is reported to have antihypertensive effects; thus, it can be used to treat concurrent hypertension from yin deficiency with hyperactive Liver yang. For animals with significant hypertension and *shen* (spirit) disturbance, combine with *Jian Ling Tang* (Construct Roof Tiles Decoction). It can be combined with formulas to invigorate the blood, such as *Xue Fu Zhu Yu Tang* (Drive Out Stasis in the Mansion of Blood Decoction), to achieve more rapid clinical results.

In addition to *Er Xian Tang*, other formulas that treat hyperthyroidism are:

- For cats with early hyperthyroidism, chronic renal insufficiency and yin deficiency without signs of deficiency heat or hyperactive Liver yang, the formula *Qi Ju Di Huang Wan* (Lycium Fruit, Chrysanthemum, and Rehmannia Pill) can be used to reverse hyperthyroidism and protect against the development of hypertension and exacerbation of chronic to acute renal insufficiency.
- For cases with yin deficiency and deficiency heat, the formula *Zhi Bai Di Huang Wan* (Anemarrhena, Phellodendron, and Rehmannia Pill) can be used. If there are signs of significant heat, irritability, aggression and excessive vocalization, *Da Bu Yin Wan* (Great Tonify the Yin Pill) may be used. These formulas may also be used without adverse effects to support the kidneys in cats with chronic renal insufficiency while receiving conventional therapies, such as oral tapazole and nuclear medicine. All formulas that substantially tonify yin contain herbs that are rich and cloying and can easily upset the middle *jiao*. Herbs or herbal formulas that support the Spleen and Stomach should be given as needed in cats with deficiencies.

Er Xian Tang can also be used to treat many different chronic renal disorders as defined by conventional medicine, such as renal amyloidosis, polycystic kidneys, chronic glomerulonephritis, chronic renal failure, nephrotic syndrome and chronic pyelonephritis. This formula exemplifies the Chinese herbal principle that "many diseases may be treated with one formula," provided the pattern is the same in all of them. Any renal disorder characterized by deficiency of yin, yang and *jing* (essence) with deficiency fire can be treated with this formula as a base, with modifications made depending on the individual animal. The addition of another herbal formula, whether one that further tonifies yin and yang, such as *Gui Lu Er Xian Jiao* (Tortoise Shell and Deer Antler Syrup), or one that invigorates the blood, such as *Xue Fu Zhu Yu Tang* (Drive Out Stasis in the Mansion of Blood Decoction), can improve clinical results.

References

1. *Zhong Guo Yi Yao Xue Bao* (Chinese Journal of Medicine and Herbology), 1992; 7(5):24.
2. *Yi Xue Xue Bao* (Report of Medicine), 1962; 9(5):287.
3. *Zhong Guo Zhong Xi Yi Jie He Za Zhi* (Chinese Journal of Integrative Chinese and Western Medicine), 1995; 15(1):672.
4. *Zhong Yi Fang Ji Xian Dai Yan Jiu* (Modern Study of Medical Formulas in Traditional Chinese Medicine), 1997; 766.
5. *Zhe Jiang Zhong Yi Za Zhi* (Zhejiang Journal of Chinese Medicine), 1994; 29(8):379.
6. Lin L, Wu S, Tang J. Clinical observation and experimental study of the treatment of aplastic anemia by warming and tonifying the spleen and kidney. Zhong Xi Yi Jie He Za Zhi. 1990 May; 10(5):272-4, 259.

Section 6

阴阳两补剂

— Yin- and Yang-Tonifying Formulas

Guī Lù Èr Xiān Jiāo (Tortoise Shell and Deer Antler Syrup)

龜鹿二仙膠
龟鹿二仙胶

Pinyin Name: *Gui Lu Er Xian Jiao*
Literal Name: Tortoise Shell and Deer Antler Syrup
Alternate Names: *Gui Lu Er Xian Gao* (Tortoise Shell and Deer Antler Paste), Two Immortals Formula
Original Source: *Yi Bian* (Ordinary Medicine) by Wang San-Cai in 1587

COMPOSITION

Gui Ban (Plastrum Testudinis)	2,400g
Lu Jiao (Cornu Cervi)	4,800g
Ren Shen (Radix et Rhizoma Ginseng)	450g [750g]
Gou Qi Zi (Fructus Lycii)	900g [1,500g]

DOSAGE / PREPARATION / ADMINISTRATION

The source text specifically states to use fresh *Lu Jiao* (Cornu Cervi) from Pere David's deer (*Elaphurus davidianus*), and not from elk or red deer (*Cervus elaphus*). Cut *Lu Jiao* (Cornu Cervi) and crush *Gui Ban* (Plastrum Testudinis) into small pieces, and soak them in running water for 3 days. Simmer these two substances for 7 days to obtain a condensed extract. Separately simmer *Ren Shen* (Radix et Rhizoma Ginseng) and *Gou Qi Zi* (Fructus Lycii) to obtain a condensed extract. Mix these two batches of condensed extracts together, and simmer it over low intensity fire to make a condensed syrup. The preparation is finished when drops of the syrup crystallize. Take 4.5-9g of the syrup on an empty stomach every morning with a grain-based alcohol or lightly salted water. Today, this syrup may be prepared using the doses suggested in brackets.

CHINESE THERAPEUTIC ACTIONS

1. Replenishes yin and tonifies *jing* (essence)
2. Benefits qi and strengthens Kidney yang

CLINICAL MANIFESTATIONS

Kidney yin and yang deficiencies accompanied by blood and *jing* (essence) deficiencies of the *du* (governing) and *ren* (conception) channels: weight loss, cachexia, diarrhea, impotence, impaired vision, impaired hearing, soreness and weakness of the back and stifles, and a weak, thin pulse.

VETERINARY CLINICAL APPLICATIONS

Osteoarthritis, canine hypothyroidism, infertility, recovery from chronic illness, recovery from chemotherapy and radiation therapy, back pain, cervical pain, intervertebral disk disease, degenerative myelopathy and Addison's disease.

EXPLANATION

Gui Lu Er Xian Jiao (Tortoise Shell and Deer Antler Syrup) treats Kidney yin and yang deficiencies, as well as deficiencies of *jing* (essence) and blood of the *du* (governing) and *ren* (conception) channels. Because of its wide range of functions, this formula can treat a variety of disorders.

Lu Jiao (Cornu Cervi) enters the *du* (governing) channel and tonifies yang. *Gui Ban* (Plastrum Testudinis) enters the *ren* (conception) channel and tonifies yin. Together, these two animal substances have a synergistic effect to strongly tonify yin and yang, and to promote the generation of blood, *jing* (essence), and marrow. In addition, *Ren Shen* (Radix et Rhizoma Ginseng) tonifies *yuan* (source) *qi*, and *Gou Qi Zi* (Fructus Lycii) nourishes yin. Overall,

Guī Lù Èr Xiān Jiāo (Tortoise Shell and Deer Antler Syrup)

Gui Lu Er Xian Jiao (Tortoise Shell and Deer Antler Syrup)

Diagnosis	Clinical Signs	Treatment	Herbs
Kidney yin and yang deficiencies accompanied by insufficiencies of qi, blood and *jing* (essence)	• Weight loss, cachexia, diarrhea, poor vision and hearing: qi and blood deficiencies • Soreness and weakness of the back and stifles: Kidney yin and yang deficiencies	• Replenishes yin and tonifies *jing* • Benefits qi and strengthens Kidney yang	• *Gui Ban* (Plastrum Testudinis) and *Lu Jiao* (Cornu Cervi) tonify Kidney yin, yang, *jing*, and marrow. • *Ren Shen* (Radix et Rhizoma Ginseng) tonifies *yuan* (source) *qi*. • *Gou Qi Zi* (Fructus Lycii) nourishes yin and blood.

this is an excellent and comprehensive formula that tonifies yin, yang, qi, blood, *jing*, and marrow.

VETERINARY MODIFICATIONS

- For frequent infections as a result of generalized weakness and deficiency, add *Huang Qi Jian Zhong Tang* (Astragalus Decoction to Construct the Middle) or *Bu Zhong Yi Qi Tang* (Tonify the Middle and Augment the Qi Decoction).
- For recovery from chemotherapy or radiation therapy with anemia, add *Si Wu Tang* (Four-Substance Decoction) or *Ba Zhen Tang* (Eight-Treasure Decoction).
- For rear quarter atrophy and weakness, add *Ba Wei Di Huang Wan* (Eight-Ingredient Pill with Rehmannia) or *You Gui Wan* (Restore the Right [Kidney] Pill).
- For chronic intervertebral disk disease, add *Du Huo Ji Sheng Tang* (Angelica Pubescens and Taxillus Decoction) or with yang deficiency, add *You Gui Wan* (Restore the Right [Kidney] Pill).
- For delayed healing of wounds, sores and abscesses, add *Ren Shen Yang Ying Tang* (Ginseng Decoction to Nourish the Nutritive Qi) or *Shi Quan Da Bu Tang* (All-Inclusive Great Tonifying Decoction).
- For infertility caused by low sperm count or abnormal ovulation, add *Dong Chong Xia Cao* (Cordyceps) and *Rou Gui* (Cortex Cinnamomi).
- For impotence, add *Yin Yang Huo* (Herba Epimedii) and *Du Zhong* (Cortex Eucommiae).
- For osteoporosis, add *Xu Duan* (Radix Dipsaci) and *Gu Sui Bu* (Rhizoma Drynariae).

CAUTIONS / CONTRAINDICATIONS

- *Gui Lu Er Xian Jiao* should be used with caution in cases of Spleen and/or Stomach deficiencies.
- This formula is contraindicated in patients with interior heat or yang rising.

PHARMACOLOGICAL EFFECTS

It has been reported that modified *Gui Lu Er Xian Jiao* has numerous valuable therapeutic effects, including but not limited to adaptogenic, antihyperlipidemic, and immunologic.[1]

HUMAN CLINICAL STUDIES AND RESEARCH

1. **Osteoporosis**: In one clinical study, 28 women were given *Gui Lu Er Xian Jiao* to determine the effects of these herbs in treatment of osteoporosis. The women's age ranged from 36 to 67, with an average age of 48.8 years. Osteoporosis was diagnosed and confirmed using bone mass density (BMD). The treatment protocol was to administer 5 grams of powdered extract of the herbal formula twice daily for one year. BMD was measured before and at the end of the trial. After one year of herbal therapy, there was an average increase of 3.4% BMD among the 28 women. The researchers concluded the herbs to be effective in the treatment of osteoporosis.[2]
2. **Impotence**: In one clinical study, modified *Gui Lu Er Xian Jiao* was used to treat 826 patients with impotence. The age of the patients ranged from 17-55, and the duration of the condition ranged from 6 months to 8 years. Out of 826 patients, 608 were married and 218 were single. The formula included *Gui Ban Jiao* (Colla Plastrum Testudinis) 20g, *Lu Jiao Jiao* (Colla Cornus Cervi) 20g, *Yin Yang Huo* (Herba Epimedii) 30g, *Du Zhong* (Cortex Eucommiae) 10g, *Gou Qi Zi* (Fructus Lycii) 10g, *Shou Wu Teng* (Caulis Polygoni Multiflori) 30g, and others. Modifications included the addition of *Rou Gui* (Cortex Cinnamomi) and *Fu Zi* (Radix Aconiti Lateralis Praeparata) for feeling of coldness in the testicles, lower back, and legs; *Sha Ren* (Fructus Amomi), *Shan Yao* (Rhizoma Dioscoreae), and *Bai Zhu* (Rhizoma Atractylodis Macrocephalae) for poor appetite; *Suan Zao Ren* (Semen Ziziphi Spinosae), *Mai Dong* (Radix Ophiopogonis), and *Fu Shen* (Poria Paradicis) for excessive dreams at night; *Sang Shen* (Fructus Mori) and *Fu Pen Zi* (Fructus Rubi) for clear and profuse urination; and a larger dose of *Du Zhong* (Cortex Eucommiae) for incomplete erection. The formula was given orally as a decoction, and externally as steam therapy (by directing the steam to the penis). In addition, patients also received twice daily 30-50 mL of herbal wine made of *Ren Shen* (Radix et Rhizoma Ginseng) 20g and *Lu Rong* (Cornu Cervi Pantotrichum) 5g. Out of 826 cases, the study reported marked effects in 723 cases, improvement

Guī Lù Èr Xiān Jiāo (Tortoise Shell and Deer Antler Syrup)

in 82 cases, and no effect in 21 cases. The overall effectiveness rate was 97.48%. The duration of treatment was between 3-16 packs of raw herbs as decoction.[3]

3. **Hypotension**: One study reported good results using modified *Gui Lu Er Xian Jiao* to raise blood pressure. The herbal formula contained *Gui Lu Er Xian Jiao* plus *Dang Gui* (Radix Angelicae Sinensis), *Tu Si Zi* (Semen Cuscutae), *Shu Di Huang* (Radix Rehmanniae Praeparata) and others. The herbs were given in decoction daily, for 20 days per course of treatment, with 2 courses for most patients. Of 62 cases, the study reported complete recovery in 35 cases, moderate improvement in 19 cases, slight improvement in 6 cases, and no benefit in 2 cases.[4]

SUGGESTED ACUPUNCTURE TREATMENT

1. Points: *Shenshu* (BL 23), *Taixi* (KI 3), *Mingmen* (GV 4), *Guanyuan* (CV 4), *Qihai* (CV 6), *Sanyinjiao* (SP 6), *Pishu* (BL 20), and *Housanli* (ST 36).
2. Technique: tonification.

Shenshu (BL 23) and *Taixi* (KI 3) nourish Kidney yin and consolidate Kidney qi. *Mingmen* (GV 4) and *Guanyuan* (CV 4) strengthen yang, and with *Qihai* (CV 6), these three points tonify qi of the lower *jiao*. *Sanyinjiao* (SP 6) nourishes Liver, Spleen, and Kidney yin. *Pishu* (BL 20) and *Housanli* (ST 36) tonify the middle *jiao* and increase the volume of qi and blood.

AUTHORS' COMMENTS

Gui Lu Er Xian Jiao is not typically used alone in veterinary medicine, but instead is combined with many other formulas to tonify Kidney yin and yang, *jing* (essence), and to boost qi. It can be given for prolonged periods of time; however, because it contains herbs that are cloying or sticky, herbs or formulas that tonify and regulate the middle *jiao* should be given, as needed. *Lu Jiao Jiao* (Colla Cornus Cervi) and *Gui Ban* (Plastrum Testudinis) are derived from animals and, as such, have stronger tonifying effects on *jing* (essence) than herbs of plant origin. These herbs are thought to enter the eight extraordinary vessels, and thus are more effective in tonifying *jing* than plants, which are physiologically different from animals. This formula is most appropriate for conditions of deficiency, with little to no signs of excess.

- It can be used in the maintenance of dogs with Addison's disease on conventional medications, in combination with *Ren Shen Yang Ying Tang* (Ginseng Decoction to Nourish the Nutritive Qi) or *Jin Gui Shen Qi Wan* (Kidney Qi Pill from the Golden Cabinet).
- For the treatment of chronic renal failure in the dog, it can be combined with *Er Xian Tang* (Two-Immortal Decoction), *Dan Shen Yin* (Salvia Decoction) and *Dong Chong Xia Cao* (Cordyceps).
- For the treatment of degenerative myelopathy in the dog, combine with *Bu Zhong Yi Qi Tang* (Tonify the Middle and Augment the Qi Decoction), *Er Xian Tang* (Two-Immortal Decoction), *Lu Jiao* (Cornu Cervi), *Hong Hua* (Flos Carthami), and *Ji Xue Teng* (Caulis Spatholobi).
- For recurrent cervical pain, or cervical intervertebral disk disease with poor *jing*, combine with *Juan Bi Tang* (Remove Painful Obstruction Decoction) and *Shen Tong Zhu Yu Tang* (Drive Out Blood Stasis from a Painful Body Decoction).

References

1. *Fang Ji Xue* (Chinese Herbal Formulas), 1995; 284-286.
2. Hsu H. Effectiveness of Gui Lu Er Xian Jiao (Tortoise Shell and Deer Antler Syrup) on treatment of osteoporosis. Clinic Medline of Taiwan.
3. *Fu Jian Zhong Yi Yao* (Fujian Chinese Medicine and Herbology), 1995; 26(3):59.
4. *Guang Xi Zhong Yi Yao* (Guangxi Chinese Medicine and Herbology), 1996; 4:33.

Qī Bǎo Měi Rán Dān

(Seven-Treasure Special Pill for Beautiful Whiskers)

七寶美髯丹
七宝美髯丹

Pinyin Name: *Qi Bao Mei Ran Dan*
Literal Name: Seven-Treasure Special Pill for Beautiful Whiskers
Alternate Names: *Chi Pao Mei Jan Tan, Qi Bao Mei Ran Wan*, Seven-Treasury Beard-Blackening Formula, Seven-Treasure Pill for Beautiful Whiskers, Seven Treasures Formula
Original Source: *Yi Fang Ji Jie* (Analytical Collection of Medical Formulas) by Wang Ang in 1682

COMPOSITION

He Shou Wu (Radix Polygoni Multiflori), *zheng* (steamed) with *Hei Dou* (Semen Sojae) and sun-dried	480g [18g]
Gou Qi Zi (Fructus Lycii), *jin* (soaked) in liquor	240g [9g]
Tu Si Zi (Semen Cuscutae), *jin* (soaked) and *zheng* (steamed) in liquor	240g [9g]
Niu Xi (Radix Achyranthis Bidentatae), *jin* (soaked) in liquor	240g [9g]
Dang Gui (Radix Angelicae Sinensis), *xi* (washed) with liquor	240g [9g]
Bu Gu Zhi (Fructus Psoraleae), *ban* (blended) and *chao* (dry-fried) with *Hei Zhi Ma* (Semen Sesami Nigrum)	120g [6g]
Fu Ling (Poria), *ban* (blended) with milk	240g [18g]

DOSAGE / PREPARATION / ADMINISTRATION

The source text advises to prepare each herb as specified above. *He Shou Wu* (Radix Polygoni Multiflori) should be steamed and sun-dried nine times. Add *Fu Ling* (Poria) and *Niu Xi* (Radix Achyranthis Bidentatae) to *He Shou Wu* (Radix Polygoni Multiflori) on the seventh to ninth repetition of steaming and drying. Grind all seven herbs into powder and form into pills with honey. Take 1 pill (10g) in the morning and at night with a grain-based liquor or lightly salted water. Today, this formula may be prepared as a decoction with the doses suggested in brackets.

CHINESE THERAPEUTIC ACTIONS

1. Nourishes Kidney *jing* (essence)
2. Nourishes Liver blood

CLINICAL MANIFESTATIONS

Liver and Kidney deficiencies: premature aging, alopecia, loose teeth, pain and weakness of the back and stifles, and weak tendons and ligaments.

VETERINARY CLINICAL APPLICATIONS

Alopecia, premature aging, male infertility, impotence, low sperm count, decreased sperm motility, weakness of back and stifles, back and stifle pain, and weak tendons and ligaments.

EXPLANATION

Qi Bao Mei Ran Wan (Seven-Treasure Special Pill for Beautiful Whiskers) commonly treats premature aging that is caused by Kidney *jing* (essence) and Liver blood deficiencies. The Liver stores blood, and Liver blood

***Qi Bao Mei Ran Dan* (Seven-Treasure Special Pill for Beautiful Whiskers)**

Diagnosis	Clinical Signs	Treatment	Herbs
Liver blood and Kidney *jing* (essence) deficiencies	• Premature aging and gray hair, alopecia, and weak tendons and ligaments: Kidney *jing* and Liver blood deficiencies • Loose teeth, weak bones and joints: marrow deficiency secondary to Kidney deficiency • Soreness and weakness of the back and stifles: Kidney deficiency	• Nourishes Kidney *jing* • Nourishes Liver blood	• *He Shou Wu* (Radix Polygoni Multiflori) tonifies the Kidney and Liver and replenishes blood and *jing*. • *Gou Qi Zi* (Fructus Lycii), *Tu Si Zi* (Semen Cuscutae), and *Hei Zhi Ma* (Semen Sesami Nigrum) nourish the Liver and Kidney. • *Niu Xi* (Radix Achyranthis Bidentatae) tonifies the Kidney and Liver. • *Dang Gui* (Radix Angelicae Sinensis) tonifies the blood. • *Bu Gu Zhi* (Fructus Psoraleae) warms the yang. • *Fu Ling* (Poria) prevents the tonics herbs from creating stagnation.

Qī Bǎo Měi Rán Dān

(Seven-Treasure Special Pill for Beautiful Whiskers)

deficiency causes weak tendons and ligaments, as well as malnourishment of the hair, leading to premature graying of the hair and hair loss. The Kidney produces marrow, which nourishes the bones and teeth. Thus, if the Kidney is deficient, it fails to produce sufficient marrow, which may lead to weak bones and loose teeth. Soreness and weakness of the back and stifles are common clinical manifestations of Kidney deficiency.

He Shou Wu (Radix Polygoni Multiflori) is used heavily in this formula to tonify Kidney *jing* (essence). *Gou Qi Zi* (Fructus Lycii), *Tu Si Zi* (Semen Cuscutae), and *Hei Zhi Ma* (Semen Sesami Nigrum) nourish the Liver and Kidney to replenish Kidney *jing*. *Niu Xi* (Radix Achyranthis Bidentatae) tonifies the Kidney and Liver and strengthens the tendons and bones to relieve soreness and weakness of the back and stifles. *Dang Gui* (Radix Angelicae Sinensis) tonifies the blood. Since yin and yang are mutually interdependent, *Bu Gu Zhi* (Fructus Psoraleae) is used to warm the yang and balance yin and yang. By adding a yang-tonifying herb to this formula, the yin-tonifying herbs may become more active, thus promoting harmony between yin and yang inside the body. *Fu Ling* (Poria) promotes urination, helps the Spleen absorb the tonic herbs, and counters the greasy, stagnating properties of the tonic herbs.

VETERINARY MODIFICATIONS

- For alopecia, add *Huang Qi* (Radix Astragali) and *Shu Di Huang* (Radix Rehmanniae Praeparata).
- With back pain, combine with *Du Zhong* (Cortex Eucommiae) and *Sang Ji Sheng* (Herba Taxilli).
- With poor appetite and indigestion, add *Shan Yao* (Rhizoma Dioscoreae), *Bai Zhu* (Rhizoma Atractylodis Macrocephalae), *Shan Zha* (Fructus Crataegi), and *Mai Ya* (Fructus Hordei Germinatus).
- For more yin deficiency and deficiency heat, add *Zhi Mu* (Rhizoma Anemarrhenae), *Huang Bo* (Cortex Phellodendri Chinensis), *Mai Dong* (Radix Ophiopogonis), *Di Gu Pi* (Cortex Lycii), *Nu Zhen Zi* (Fructus Ligustri Lucidi), and *Wu Wei Zi* (Fructus Schisandrae Chinensis).

CAUTIONS / CONTRAINDICATIONS

- *Qi Bao Mei Ran Dan* contains many tonic herbs, and should be used with caution in cases of Spleen and Stomach deficiencies or damp and phlegm accumulation. Animals will commonly vomit on this formula unless herbs to regulate and tonify the middle *jiao* are added, such as *Zhi Qiao* (Fructus Aurantii), *Shan Yao* (Rhizoma Dioscoreae), *Bai Zhu* (Rhizoma Atractylodis Macrocephalae), *Shan Zha* (Fructus Crataegi), and *Mai Ya* (Fructus Hordei Germinatus). It should be avoided in animals with obvious damp conditions.
- The processed form of *He Shou Wu* (Radix Polygoni Multiflori) should be used to maximize the tonic effect, and to minimize its downward-draining effect. If the fresh, unprocessed form is used, animals may suffer from frequent episodes of loose stools and diarrhea.

PHARMACOLOGICAL EFFECTS

Cardiovascular: In one laboratory experiment, oral administration *Qi Bao Mei Ran Dan* in rabbits at 6 g/kg was associated with an antiplatelet effect two hours after the oral ingestion.[1]

HUMAN CLINICAL STUDIES AND RESEARCH

1. **Alopecia**: In one study, 24 patients with alopecia were treated with oral and topical applications of herbs with good results. All patients received *Qi Bao Mei Ran Dan* as the base formula, with modifications as needed. For individuals with mixed white and yellow hair that appear malnourished, *Huang Qi* (Radix Astragali) and *Shu Di Huang* (Radix Rehmanniae Praeparata) were added to *Qi Bao Mei Ran Dan* for oral ingestion. In addition, they were treated with an herbal solution topically made of *Ce Bai Ye* (Cacumen Platycladi) 500g, *Sang Shen* (Fructus Mori) 500g, and *Mu Gua* (Fructus Chaenomelis) 250g. For individuals with yellow hair that is short and thin, *Zhi Mu* (Rhizoma Anemarrhenae), *Huang Bo* (Cortex Phellodendri Chinensis), *Mai Dong* (Radix Ophiopogonis), and *Wu Wei Zi* (Fructus Schisandrae Chinensis) were added to *Qi Bao Mei Ran Dan* for oral ingestion. They were also instructed to wash their hair with an herbal solution made from *Sang Ye* (Folium Mori) 60g and *Ma Ye* (Folium Cannabis) 60g. Lastly, for white hair that falls out easily, *Nu Zhen Zi* (Fructus Ligustri Lucidi) and *Mo Han Lian* (Herba Ecliptae) were added for oral ingestion. In addition, they were instructed to wash their hair with an herbal solution made from *He Zi* (Fructus Chebulae) 2 pieces, *He Tao Ren* (Semen Juglandis) 2 pieces, and fresh *Ce Bai Ye* (Cacumen Platycladi) 30g.[2]
2. **Male infertility**: In one study, 36 male patients with infertility were treated with modified *Qi Bao Mei Ran Dan* with good results. The ages of the patients ranged from 23-41 years, with the duration of marriage between 1-10 years. The formula included *Chuan Niu Xi* (Radix Cyathulae) 9g, *Dang Gui* (Radix Angelicae Sinensis) 9g, *Bu Gu Zhi* (Fructus Psoraleae) 6g, *Fu Ling* (Poria) 6g, *He Shou Wu* (Radix Polygoni Multiflori) 12g, *Tu Si Zi* (Semen Cuscutae) 12g, *Gou Qi Zi* (Fructus Lycii) 12g, *Shu Di Huang* (Radix Rehmanniae Praeparata) 12g, and *Rou Gui* (Cortex Cinnamomi) 3g. In addition, *Du Zhong* (Cortex

Qī Bǎo Měi Rán Dān

(Seven-Treasure Special Pill for Beautiful Whiskers)

Eucommiae) 12g and *Sang Ji Sheng* (Herba Taxilli) 6g were added for soreness of the lower back and knees; *Zhi Mu* (Rhizoma Anemarrhenae) 6g and *Huang Bo* (Cortex Phellodendri Chinensis) 12g were added for irritability with a dry mouth. After continuous treatment for 20-30 days, pregnancy was reported within one year in 22 of 36 cases.[3]

3. **Aplastic anemia**: Use of modified *Qi Bao Mei Ran Dan* was effective in treating aplastic anemia. Of 38 patients, 15 were treated with herbs only and 23 were treated with herbs and drugs. Herbal treatment was based on *Qi Bao Mei Ran Dan*, and modifications varied depending on the differential diagnosis. For yin deficiency (20 cases), *Xuan Shen* (Radix Scrophulariae) 15g, *Mai Dong* (Radix Ophiopogonis) 15g, *Sang Shen* (Fructus Mori) 15g, *Can Sha* (Faeces Bombycis) 10g, *Shan Zhu Yu* (Fructus Corni) 10g, charred *Wu Mei* (Fructus Mume) 10g, charred *Zhi Zi* (Fructus Gardeniae) 10g, charred *Du Zhong* (Cortex Eucommiae) 10g, and charred *Zong Lu* (Petiolus Trachycarpi) were added. For yang deficiency (10 cases), *Xian Mao* (Rhizoma Curculiginis) 15g, *Rou Cong Rong* (Herba Cistanches) 15g, *Ba Ji Tian* (Radix Morindae Officinalis) 10g, *Yin Yang Huo* (Herba Epimedii) 10g, *Fu Zi* (Radix Aconiti Lateralis Praeparata) 6g, and *Lu Rong* (Cornu Cervi Pantotrichum) 6g were added. For yin and yang deficiency (8 cases), *Xiao Hui Xiang* (Fructus Foeniculi) 10g, *Xu Duan* (Radix Dipsaci) 10g, *Huang Jing* (Rhizoma Polygonati) 15g, and *Shan Yao* (Rhizoma Dioscoreae) 15g were added. The herbs were given in decoction daily, for 30 days per course of treatment, for a total of 3 courses. The study reported marked improvement in 20 of 38 patients.[4]
4. **Chronic infectious hepatitis**: In one study, 22 patients with chronic infectious hepatitis confirmed by Western medicine were treated successfully using modified *Qi Bao Mei Ran Dan*. The treatment protocol used this formula as the base, and added *Sha Ren* (Fructus Amomi) and *Hou Po* (Cortex Magnoliae Officinalis) for abdominal distention; *Huang Qi* (Radix Astragali) and *Dang Shen* (Radix Codonopsis) for fatigue; *Yan Hu Suo* (Rhizoma Corydalis) and *Chuan Lian Zi* (Fructus Toosendan) for hypochondriac pain; and *Bie Jia* (Carapax Trionycis) and *Mu Li* (Concha Ostreae) for hepatomegaly. The herbs were given daily for 2-3 months. Of 22 patients, the study reported complete recovery in 14 cases, improvement in 3 cases, and no effect in 5 cases. Complete recovery was defined as resolution of all symptoms with normal liver functions. Improvement included resolution of all symptoms with near normal liver functions.[5]

SUGGESTED ACUPUNCTURE TREATMENT

1. Points: *Ganshu* (BL 18), *Shenshu* (BL 23), *Taixi* (KI 3), *Geshu* (BL 17), *Pishu* (BL 20), and *Housanli* (ST 36).
2. Technique: tonification.

Ganshu (BL 18), *Shenshu* (BL 23), and *Taixi* (KI 3) strengthen the Liver and Kidney. *Shenshu* (BL 23) and *Geshu* (BL 17) nourish the blood and *jing* (essence). *Pishu* (BL 20) and *Housanli* (ST 36) nourish the middle *jiao* to provide more qi and blood.

AUTHORS' COMMENTS

Gui Lu Er Xian Jiao (Tortoise Shell and Deer Antler Syrup) and *Qi Bao Mei Ran Wan* both tonify Liver and Kidney deficiencies and are considered to be anti-aging formulas.

- *Gui Lu Er Xian Jiao* treats deficiencies of yin, yang, qi, and blood of the *ren* (conception) and *du* (governing) channels. *Lu Jiao* (Cornu Cervi) tonifies yang; *Gui Ban* (Plastrum Testudinis) tonifies yin; *Ren Shen* (Radix et Rhizoma Ginseng) boosts qi; and *Gou Qi Zi* (Fructus Lycii) nourishes the blood. All four herbs tonify, and this formula does not have any sedating or draining effect. It is particularly effective and useful to promote the healing of bone fractures and can be easily modified to accomplish this goal. It is also an excellent formula to help in recovery from chronic illness.
- *Qi Bao Mei Ran Wan* tonifies Liver and Kidney blood and *jing* (essence) with tonic herbs such as *He Shou Wu* (Radix Polygoni Multiflori), *Gou Qi Zi* (Fructus Lycii), *Niu Xi* (Radix Achyranthis Bidentatae), *Tu Si Zi* (Semen Cuscutae), and *Dang Gui* (Radix Angelicae Sinensis). *Fu Ling* (Poria), a mild draining herb, helps to balance the stagnating side effects of the tonic herbs. One of the main applications of *Qi Bao Mei Ran Wan* is for the treatment of alopecia; it also strengthens the organs and promote longevity.

References

1. *Zhong Yao Yao Li Yu Lin Chuang* (Pharmacology and Clinical Applications of Chinese Herbs), 1988; 4(4):8.
2. *Fu Jian Zhong Yi Yao* (Fujian Chinese Medicine and Herbology), 1983; 5:19.
3. *Zhe Jiang Zhong Yi Za Zhi* (Zhejiang Journal of Chinese Medicine), 1995; 9:400.
4. *Zhong Xi Yi Jie He Za Zhi* (Journal of Integrated Chinese and Western Medicine), 1990; 1:49.
5. *Zhe Jiang Zhong Yi Za Zhi* (Zhejiang Journal of Chinese Medicine), 1993; 4:150.

Dì Huáng Yǐn Zǐ (Rehmannia Decoction)

地黃飲子
地黄饮子

Pinyin Name: *Di Huang Yin Zi*
Literal Name: Rehmannia Decoction
Original Source: *Huang Di Su Wen Xuan Ming Lun Fang* (Formulas from the Discussion Illuminating the Yellow Emperor's Basic Questions) by Liu Yuan-Su in 1172

COMPOSITION

Shu Di Huang (Radix Rehmanniae Praeparata)	[12g]
Shan Zhu Yu (Fructus Corni)	[9g]
Rou Cong Rong (Herba Cistanches), *jin* (soaked) in liquor and *bei* (stone-baked)	[9g]
Ba Ji Tian (Radix Morindae Officinalis)	[9g]
Fu Zi (Radix Aconiti Lateralis Praeparata), *pao* (blast-fried)	[6g]
Rou Gui (Cortex Cinnamomi)	[6g]
Mai Dong (Radix Ophiopogonis)	[6g]
Shi Hu (Caulis Dendrobii)	[9g]
Wu Wei Zi (Fructus Schisandrae Chinensis)	[6g]
Shi Chang Pu (Rhizoma Acori Tatarinowii)	[6g]
Yuan Zhi (Radix Polygalae)	[6g]
Fu Ling (Poria)	[6g]

DOSAGE / PREPARATION / ADMINISTRATION

Grind equal amounts of the ingredients into powder. Cook 9g of the powder with 5 slices of *Sheng Jiang* (Rhizoma Zingiberis Recens), 1 piece of *Da Zao* (Fructus Jujubae), and 5-7 leaves of *Bo He* (Herba Menthae) in 1.5 bowls of water until the liquid is reduced to 80%. Take the decoction any time during the day. Today, this formula may be prepared as a decoction using the doses suggested in brackets.

CHINESE THERAPEUTIC ACTIONS

1. Tonifies Kidney yin and yang
2. Resolves phlegm and opens the orifices

CLINICAL MANIFESTATIONS

Paralysis, muscle atrophy of the extremities, hindquarter weakness, dry mouth without desire to drink, dry skin, pruritis, mental confusion, a pale tongue, and a deep, thin, weak pulse.

VETERINARY CLINICAL APPLICATIONS

Fibrocartilagenous emboli (FCE), post IVD herniation, paralysis and cognitive dysfunction.

EXPLANATION

Di Huang Yin Zi (Rehmannia Decoction) treats clinical signs of Kidney deficiency and deficiency yang rising. Kidney yin deficiency can lead to weakness of the bones and tendons, eventually resulting in leg paralysis. Kidney yin deficiency may also lead to rising of Liver yang, which can carry internal dampness and phlegm to the head, causing a dry mouth without desire to drink. Patients will have no desire to drink because there is no actual lack of body fluids. The tongue and pulse both indicate deficiency and dampness inside the body.

Shu Di Huang (Radix Rehmanniae Praeparata) and *Shan Zhu Yu* (Fructus Corni) nourish Kidney yin. *Rou Cong Rong* (Herba Cistanches) and *Ba Ji Tian* (Radix Morindae Officinalis) tonify and stabilize Kidney yang. *Fu Zi* (Radix Aconiti Lateralis Praeparata) and *Rou Gui* (Cortex Cinnamomi) warm the Kidney to cause floating yang to descend. *Mai Dong* (Radix Ophiopogonis), *Shi Hu* (Caulis Dendrobii), and *Wu Wei Zi* (Fructus Schisandrae Chinensis) nourish yin and body fluids. *Shi Chang Pu* (Rhizoma Acori Tatarinowii), *Yuan Zhi* (Radix Polygalae), and *Fu Ling* (Poria) connect and harmonize the Heart and Kidney, as well as dispel dampness and open the head orifices. *Bo He* (Herba Menthae) clears the head and opens the orifices. *Sheng Jiang* (Rhizoma Zingiberis Recens) and *Da Zao* (Fructus Jujubae) harmonize the herbs and enhance their tonic actions.

Dì Huáng Yǐn Zǐ (Rehmannia Decoction)

***Di Huang Yin Zi* (Rehmannia Decoction)**

Diagnosis	Clinical Signs	Treatment	Herbs
Paralysis and muscle atrophy with Kidney deficiency and deficient yang rising	• Paralysis and muscle atrophy: Kidney yin deficiency unable to nourish the bones and tendons • Mental confusion: damp and phlegm accumulation in the head • Pale tongue and a deep, thready, weak pulse: deficiency and dampness	• Tonifies Kidney yin and yang • Resolves phlegm and opens the orifices	• *Shu Di Huang* (Radix Rehmanniae Praeparata) and *Shan Zhu Yu* (Fructus Corni) nourish Kidney yin. • *Rou Cong Rong* (Herba Cistanches) and *Ba Ji Tian* (Radix Morindae Officinalis) tonify and stabilize Kidney yang. • *Fu Zi* (Radix Aconiti Lateralis Praeparata) and *Rou Gui* (Cortex Cinnamomi) warm the Kidney. • *Mai Dong* (Radix Ophiopogonis), *Shi Hu* (Caulis Dendrobii), and *Wu Wei Zi* (Fructus Schisandrae Chinensis) nourish yin and body fluids. • *Shi Chang Pu* (Rhizoma Acori Tatarinowii), *Yuan Zhi* (Radix Polygalae), and *Fu Ling* (Poria) connect and harmonize the Heart and Kidney, dispel dampness, and open the head orifices. • *Bo He* (Herba Menthae) clears the head and opens the orifices. • *Sheng Jiang* (Rhizoma Zingiberis Recens) and *Da Zao* (Fructus Jujubae) harmonize the herbs.

VETERINARY MODIFICATIONS

- For Kidney yang deficiency with coldness and pain in the back and stifles, add *Yin Yang Huo* (Herba Epimedii) and *Xian Mao* (Rhizoma Curculiginis).
- With qi deficiency, add *Huang Qi* (Radix Astragali) and *Ren Shen* (Radix et Rhizoma Ginseng).

CAUTIONS / CONTRAINDICATIONS

Di Huang Yin Zi is not recommended for animals with Liver yang rising, since the formula is warm and tonifying, and may worsen the Liver yang condition. Do not use in animals with pruritis and signs of excess.

HUMAN CLINICAL STUDIES AND RESEARCH

1. **Cerebrovascular diseases**: It has been shown in many studies that the use of *Di Huang Yin Zi* is an effective supportive treatment for patients with various types of cerebrovascular diseases. One study reported beneficial effect using this formula to treat 240 patients with cerebral embolism.[1] Another study reported good results using this formula to treat 67 patients with cerebrovascular accident.[2]
2. **Post-stroke sequelae**: Modified *Di Huang Yin Zi* was successful in treating 24 patients with various types of post-stroke sequelae.[3]
3. **Dementia**: Use of *Di Huang Yin Zi* in 50 patients with dementia was associated with significant improvement in 24 patients, moderate improvement in 21 patients, and no effect in 5 patients.[4]
4. **Diabetes mellitus**: One study reported 80% effectiveness using modified *Di Huang Yin Zi* to treat 20 patients with diabetes mellitus characterized by qi and yin deficiencies.[5]
5. **Itching**: Use of *Di Huang Yin Zi* was associated with 80.5% effectiveness in 180 patients to treat itching caused by Liver and Kidney deficiencies. Of 180 patients, the study reported complete recovery in 103 patients, significant improvement in 42 patients, and no benefit in 35 patients.[6]
6. **Myelanalosis**: According to several studies, use of modified *Di Huang Yin Zi* was associated with beneficial effects in patients with pain in the spinal cord caused by neurosyphilis. One formula that reported good success contained *Di Huang Yin Zi* plus *Lu Jiao Shuang* (Cornu Cervi Degelatinatum), *Gui Ban Jiao* (Colla Plastrum Testudinis), *Gou Qi Zi* (Fructus Lycii), *Suo Yang* (Herba Cynomorii), *Tian Ma* (Rhizoma Gastrodiae), and others.[7]

SUGGESTED ACUPUNCTURE TREATMENT

1. Points: *Shenshu* (BL 23), *Taixi* (KI 3), *Mingmen* (GV 4), *Qihaishu* (BL 24), *Xinshu* (BL 15), *Sanyinjiao* (SP 6), *Fenglong* (ST 40), *Yanglingquan* (GB 34), and *Huantiao* (GB 30).
2. Technique: tonification and moxibustion.

Shenshu (BL 23) and *Taixi* (KI 3) tonify Kidney yin, while moxibustion on *Mingmen* (GV 4) and *Qihaishu* (BL 24) strengthens Kidney yang. The combination of *Xinshu* (BL 15) and *Shenshu* (BL 23) connects and harmonizes the

Dì Huáng Yǐn Zǐ (Rehmannia Decoction)

Heart and Kidney channels. *Sanyinjiao* (SP 6) strengthens the Spleen and generates body fluids, while *Fenglong* (ST 40) dispels phlegm. *Yanglingquan* (GB 34) and *Huantiao* (GB 30) strengthen the tendons to relieve leg paralysis.

AUTHORS' COMMENTS

Di Huang Yin Zi is used to treat older animals with musculoskeletal disorders and clinical signs of Kidney deficiency and cognitive dysfunction. Kidney yin deficiency can lead to weakness of the bones and tendons, eventually resulting in leg paralysis. Patients for which this formula is indicated have a pale tongue with a white, slippery, tongue coating, and a deep, thin, weak pulse. It is a warming formula and should not be used in animals with Liver yang excess condition. To treat hindquarter weakness, combine with *Bu Yang Huan Wu Tang* (Tonify the Yang to Restore Five Decoction) or *Bu Zhong Yi Qi Tang* (Tonify the Middle and Augment the Qi Decoction).

References

1. *He Bei Zhong Yi* (Hebei Chinese Medicine), 1986; 1:12.
2. *Zhe Jiang Zhong Yi Xue Yuan Xue Bao* (Journal of Zhejiang University of Chinese Medicine), 1995; 4:8.
3. *Hei Long Jiang Zhong Yi Yao* (Heilongjiang Chinese Medicine and Herbology), 1995; 2:14.
4. *Bei Jing Zhong Yi* (Beijing Chinese Medicine), 1998; 1:13.
5. *Shang Hai Zhong Yi Za Zhi* (Shanghai Journal of Chinese Medicine), 1995; 8:28.
6. *Zhong Yi Za Zhi* (Journal of Chinese Medicine), 1983; 5:27.
7. *Zhong Yi Fang Ji Xian Dai Yan Jiu* (Modern Study of Medical Formulas in Traditional Chinese Medicine), 1997; 1265.

Chapter 8 — Summary — Tonic Formulas

SECTION 1: QI-TONIFYING FORMULAS

Name	Similarities	Differences
Si Jun Zi Tang (Four-Gentlemen Decoction)	Tonify qi, strengthen the Spleen and Stomach	Base formula to tonify qi and strengthen the middle *jiao*
Liu Jun Zi Tang (Six-Gentlemen Decoction)		Eliminates dampness and phlegm
Xiang Sha Liu Jun Zi Tang (Six-Gentlemen Decoction with Aucklandia and Amomum)		Eliminates dampness and phlegm, regulates qi circulation, relieves pain.
Xiang Sha Yang Wei Tang (Nourish the Stomach Decoction with Aucklandia and Amomum)		Regulates qi and dries dampness to increase appetite
Shen Ling Bai Zhu San (Ginseng, Poria, and Atractylodes Macrocephala Powder)	Tonify qi, strengthen the Spleen and Stomach, stop diarrhea	Resolves dampness
Qi Pi Wan (Guide the Spleen Pill)		Promotes digestion
Bu Zhong Yi Qi Tang (Tonify the Middle and Augment the Qi Decoction)	Tonify and raise qi, strengthen the Spleen and Stomach	Lifts yang qi and prolapsed organs
Yi Qi Cong Ming Tang (Augment the Qi and Increase Acuity Decoction)		Lifts yang qi and benefits the eyes and ears
Sheng Mai San (Generate the Pulse Powder)	Tonify Lung qi	Nourishes yin and body fluids
Ren Shen Ge Jie San (Ginseng and Gecko Powder)		Tonifies Lung and Kidney
Bu Fei Tang (Tonify the Lung Decoction)		Strengthens *wei* (defensive) *qi*

Si Jun Zi Tang (Four-Gentlemen Decoction) is the most commonly used and the most effective formula to tonify qi and strengthen the Spleen and Stomach. It treats Spleen and Stomach qi deficiencies arising from various causes or with various complications, and is often used as the base formula for many related conditions.

- ***Liu Jun Zi Tang*** (Six-Gentlemen Decoction) has the basic actions of *Si Jun Zi Tang* (Four-Gentlemen Decoction), but is stronger in dispelling dampness and phlegm.
- ***Xiang Sha Liu Jun Zi Tang*** (Six-Gentlemen Decoction with Aucklandia and Amomum) has the basic actions of *Liu Jun Zi Tang* (Six-Gentlemen Decoction) but is stronger in regulating qi, dispelling cold, and relieving pain.
- ***Xiang Sha Yang Wei Tang*** (Nourish the Stomach Decoction with Aucklandia and Amomum) primarily increases appetite in individuals with middle *jiao* deficiency.

Shen Ling Bai Zhu San (Ginseng, Poria, and Atractylodes Macrocephala Powder) and ***Qi Pi Wan*** (Guide the Spleen Pill) tonify qi, strengthen the Spleen and Stomach, and stop diarrhea.

- *Shen Ling Bai Zhu San* strongly resolves dampness in cases of Spleen and Stomach qi deficiencies causing impairment in the transportation and transformation functions.
- *Qi Pi Wan* promotes digestion in cases of Spleen and Stomach qi deficiencies, in which there is an inability to properly digest and absorb foods.

Bu Zhong Yi Qi Tang (Tonify the Middle and Augment the Qi Decoction) and ***Yi Qi Cong Ming Tang*** (Augment the Qi and Increase Acuity Decoction) strengthen the Spleen and Stomach, and tonify and raise yang qi.

- *Bu Zhong Yi Qi Tang* not only treats the usual symptoms of Spleen qi deficiency, it also lifts yang qi and treats prolapse of internal organs.

Chapter 8 — Summary

- *Yi Qi Cong Ming Tang* tonifies qi and blood, raises yang qi, and nourishes the Kidney and Liver. It tonifies underlying deficiencies and treats compromised visual and auditory functions.

Sheng Mai San (Generate the Pulse Powder), ***Ren Shen Ge Jie San*** (Ginseng and Gecko Powder), and ***Bu Fei Tang*** (Tonify the Lung Decoction) tonify Lung qi and treat lung disorders.

- *Sheng Mai San* tonifies qi, generates body fluids, astringes yin, and stops sweating. It treats excess heat or chronic cough damaging qi and yin.
- *Ren Shen Ge Jie San* tonifies qi, clears Lung heat, stops cough, and relieves wheezing. Lung qi deficiency is the cause of cough and the excess phlegm is due to the impairment of the transformation function of the Spleen. This formula can also be used for cough and dyspnea caused by the Kidney not being able to grasp the qi downward.
- *Bu Fei Tang* tonifies Lung qi to treat wheezing and dyspnea caused by Lung qi deficiency. It also strengthens *wei* (defensive) *qi* to relieve intolerance to cold.

SECTION 2: BLOOD-TONIFYING FORMULAS

Name	Similarities	Differences
Si Wu Tang (Four-Substance Decoction)	Tonify the blood, regulate blood circulation	Base formula to tonify the blood
Tao Hong Si Wu Tang (Four-Substance Decoction with Safflower and Peach Pit)		Eliminates blood stasis
Dang Gui Bu Xue Tang (Tangkuei Decoction to Tonify the Blood)		Tonifies qi and promotes the generation of blood
Gui Pi Tang (Restore the Spleen Decoction)	Tonify qi and blood	Strengthens the Spleen, nourishes the Heart
Zhi Gan Cao Tang (Honey-Fried Licorice Decoction)		Nourishes yin, restores the pulse
Dang Gui Shao Yao San (Tangkuei and Peony Powder)	Tonifies the blood	Softens the Liver, strengthens the Spleen to regulate water metabolism
Shao Yao Gan Cao Tang (Peony and Licorice Decoction)	Replenishes body fluids	Harmonizes the *ying* (nutritive) and *wei* (defensive) levels

Si Wu Tang (Four-Substance Decoction) is the basic formula for tonifying and regulating the blood. It treats general Liver blood deficiency with impairment of the *chong* (thoroughfare) and *ren* (conception) channels.

Tao Hong Si Wu Tang (Four-Substance Decoction with Safflower and Peach Pit) is formulated by adding *Tao Ren* (Semen Persicae) and *Hong Hua* (Flos Carthami) to *Si Wu Tang* (Four-Substance Decoction). The addition of these two herbs greatly enhances the effect of regulating blood circulation and eliminating blood stasis.

Dang Gui Bu Xue Tang (Tangkuei Decoction to Tonify the Blood) tonifies qi and blood in cases of acute or chronic blood loss. Clinical signs include irritability, thirst with a strong desire to drink, and slow healing of wounds.

Gui Pi Tang (Restore the Spleen Decoction) tonifies qi, nourishes the blood, strengthens the Spleen, and nourishes the Heart. It treats Heart and Spleen deficiencies. This formula can also be used for any type of bleeding disorder caused by the inability of the Spleen to hold the blood within the vessels, such as immune mediated thrombocytopenia (ITP) and immune-mediated hemolytic anemia (IHA).

Zhi Gan Cao Tang (Honey-Fried Licorice Decoction) treats a bound or intermittent pulse caused by qi and blood deficiencies. It is commonly used to treat cardiac conditions in veterinary medicine and can also be used to treat chronic Lung disorders with deficiency.

Chapter 8 — Summary

Dang Gui Shao Yao San (Tangkuei and Peony Powder) nourishes the blood, softens the Liver, strengthens the Spleen, and regulates water metabolism. It treats abdominal pain with edema caused by blood deficiency and abnormal water metabolism.

Shao Yao Gan Cao Tang (Peony and Licorice Decoction) harmonizes the *ying* (nutritive) and *wei* (defensive) levels and replenishes body fluids. It is most effective for spasms, shaking, and trembling of the extremities, caused by overwork with excessive sweating or deficiency of blood and body fluids.

SECTION 3: QI- AND BLOOD-TONIFYING FORMULAS

Name	Similarities	Differences
Ba Zhen Tang (Eight-Treasure Decoction)	Tonify qi and blood	Base formula to tonify qi and blood
Shi Quan Da Bu Tang (All-Inclusive Great Tonifying Decoction)		Tonifies qi, warms yang, dispels cold
Ren Shen Yang Ying Tang (Ginseng Decoction to Nourish the Nutritive Qi)		Nourishes the Heart and calms the *shen* (spirit)
Xiong Gui Tiao Xue Yin (Cnidium and Tangkuei Decoction to Regulate Blood)		Treats post-parturition complications

There are four formulas that effectively tonify qi and nourish blood:

- ***Ba Zhen Tang*** (Eight-Treasure Decoction) is formulated by combining *Si Jun Zi Tang* (Four-Gentlemen Decoction) and *Si Wu Tang* (Four-Substance Decoction) to tonify qi and blood. It is neutral in thermal property, and will not warm or cool the body.
- ***Shi Quan Da Bu Tang*** (All-Inclusive Great Tonifying Decoction) is formulated by adding *Huang Qi* (Radix Astragali) and *Rou Gui* (Cortex Cinnamomi) to *Ba Zhen Tang* (Eight-Treasure Decoction). The addition of these two herbs increases the overall warmth of the formula, and enhances the effects of benefiting qi, tonifying yang, and dispelling cold. This formula is suitable for qi and blood deficiencies, accompanied by the presence of interior cold.
- ***Ren Shen Yang Ying Tang*** (Ginseng Decoction to Nourish the Nutritive Qi) treats qi and blood deficiencies arising from chronic consumptive diseases. Chronic qi and blood deficiencies may lead to malnourishment and instability of the Heart. Thus, this formula contains herbs to nourish the Heart and calm the *shen* (spirit).
- ***Xiong Gui Tiao Xue Yin*** (Cnidium and Tangkuei Decoction to Regulate Blood) tonifies qi and blood, and treats postpartum complications such as uterine bleeding, anemia, retained lochia, and insufficient lactation.

Chapter 8 — Summary

SECTION 4: YIN-TONIFYING FORMULAS

Name	Similarities	Differences
Liu Wei Di Huang Wan (Six-Ingredient Pill with Rehmannia)	Tonify Liver and Kidney yin	Base formula to tonify Liver and Kidney yin
Zhi Bai Di Huang Wan (Anemarrhena, Phellodendron, and Rehmannia Pill)		Clears deficiency fire
Qi Ju Di Huang Wan (Lycium Fruit, Chrysanthemum, and Rehmannia Pill)		Brightens the eyes, treats eye disorders
Mai Wei Di Huang Wan (Ophiopogonis, Schisandra and Rehmannia Pill)		Astringes the Lung, redirects Lung qi downward
Zuo Gui Wan (Restore the Left [Kidney] Pill)	Tonifies Kidney yin	Replenishes bone marrow and Kidney *jing* (essence)
Da Bu Yin Wan (Great Tonify the Yin Pill)	Tonify Liver and Kidney yin, clear deficiency fire	Clears deficiency fire
Hu Qian Wan (Hidden Tiger Pill)		Strengthens the sinews and bones
Er Zhi Wan (Two-Ultimate Pill)	Tonify Liver and Kidney yin	Nourishes the blood
Yi Guan Jian (Linking Decoction)		Regulates the Liver qi
Ming Mu Di Huang Wan (Improve Vision Pill with Rehmannia)	Tonify Liver and Kidney yin, improve sensory functions	Tonifies Liver and Kidney yin to improve vision
Shi Hu Ye Guang Wan (Dendrobium Pill for Night Vision)		Calms Liver wind, treats eye disorders
Zi Yin Di Huang Wan (Rehmannia Pill to Nourish Yin)		Clears Liver fire, treats eye disorders
Zi Shen Ming Mu Tang (Nourish the Kidney to Brighten the Eyes Decoction)		Tonifies qi and blood, treats eye disorders
Zi Shen Tong Er Tang (Nourish the Kidney to Unblock the Ears Decoction)		Tonifies the blood, treats ear disorders

Liu Wei Di Huang Wan (Six-Ingredient Pill with Rehmannia) is the representative formula in the yin-tonics category. It tonifies Liver and Kidney yin, and strengthens the water element while controlling the wood element. Kidney yin deficiency and deficiency fire may manifest in signs such as poor hearing, deafness, poor vision, painful and weak back and stifles, orthopedic and dental developmental abnormalities, lameness, dry feces, irritability, restlessness, excessive panting (especially at night), short urination, preference for cool surfaces or places, dry eyes and mouth, increased appetite, increased thirst, trembling and jerking during sleep, hypersensitivity to acupuncture, a red tongue with little coating, and a rapid and thready pulse that is weaker on the left. Related formulas and their differential functions are as follows:

- ***Zhi Bai Di Huang Wan*** (Anemarrhena, Phellodendron, and Rehmannia Pill) is formulated by adding *Zhi Mu* (Rhizoma Anemarrhenae) and *Huang Bo* (Cortex Phellodendri Chinensis) to *Liu Wei Di Huang Wan* (Six-Ingredient Pill with Rehmannia). This formula nourishes yin and clears deficiency fire.
- ***Qi Ju Di Huang Wan*** (Lycium Fruit, Chrysanthemum, and Rehmannia Pill) is formulated by adding *Gou Qi Zi* (Fructus Lycii) and *Ju Hua* (Flos Chrysanthemi) to *Liu Wei Di Huang Wan* (Six-Ingredient Pill with Rehmannia). It nourishes Kidney and Liver yin and benefits the eyes to brighten vision.
- ***Mai Wei Di Huang Wan*** (Ophiopogonis, Schisandra and Rehmannia Pill) is formulated with the addition of *Mai Dong* (Radix Ophiopogonis) and *Wu Wei Zi* (Fructus Schisandrae Chinensis) to *Liu Wei Di Huang Wan* (Six-Ingredient Pill with Rehmannia). It nourishes yin, astringes the Lung, redirects Lung qi downward, and arrests wheezing.

Chapter 8 — Summary

Zuo Gui Wan (Restore the Left [Kidney] Pill) is a potent formula that tonifies Kidney yin, fills the bone marrow, and replenishes *jing* (essence). It contains primarily tonic herbs, which are not balanced by any sedating herbs. This is a strong tonic formula, and it is heavier and more stagnant in nature than *Liu Wei Di Huang Wan* (Six-Ingredient Pill with Rehmannia).

Da Bu Yin Wan (Great Tonify the Yin Pill) and ***Hu Qian Wan*** (Hidden Tiger Pill from the Analytic Collection) both tonify Liver and Kidney yin and clear deficiency fire.

- *Da Bu Yin Wan* treats yin deficiency of the Liver and Kidney, with flaring up of deficiency fire. Clinical manifestations include irritability, aggression, dryness, restlessness, panting excessively (especially at night), dry cough, constipation or dry feces, short urination, heat aversion, seeking cool surfaces/places, increased to ravenous appetite, increased thirst, trembling and jerking during sleep, soreness of the back and stifles, atrophy and weakness of the extremities, poor hearing or deafness, hypersensitivity to acupuncture, a red tongue with no coating, and a rapid, thready pulse that is weaker on the left.
- *Hu Qian Wan* nourishes yin, clears deficiency fire, and strengthens the bones and tendons. Weakness of bones and tendons are due to the lack of nourishment from Kidney yin. The clinical applications include soreness of lower back and knees, weakness of bones and tendons, and *wei zheng* (atrophy syndrome).

Er Zhi Wan (Two-Ultimate Pill) and ***Yi Guan Jian*** (Linking Decoction) tonify Liver and Kidney yin, nourish the blood, and moisten dryness.

- *Er Zhi Wan* tonifies Kidney and Liver yin deficiency and nourishes the blood. Key manifestations for this formula include impaired vision, soreness and weakness of the back and stifles, gradual atrophy of the lower limbs, and premature graying of hair.
- *Yi Guan Jian* tonifies Liver and Kidney yin, regulates Liver qi, nourishes the blood, and moistens dryness. Clinical manifestations include chest and hypochondriac pain, acid regurgitation, and a dry mouth.

There are many formulas that tonify Liver and Kidney yin, improve sensory (visual and auditory) functions, and treat eye and ear disorders.

- ***Ming Mu Di Huang Wan*** (Improve Vision Pill with Rehmannia) greatly tonifies Liver and Kidney yin to treat eye disorders.
- ***Shi Hu Ye Guang Wan*** (Dendrobium Pill for Night Vision) soothes the Liver, calms Liver wind, and nourishes yin to treat eye disorders.
- ***Zi Yin Di Huang Wan*** (Rehmannia Pill to Nourish Yin) tonifies Liver and Kidney yin and clears Liver fire to treat eye disorders.
- ***Zi Shen Ming Mu Tang*** (Nourish the Kidney to Brighten the Eyes Decoction) tonifies Liver and Kidney yin, nourishes qi and blood, and clears heat to treat eye disorders.
- ***Zi Shen Tong Er Tang*** (Nourish the Kidney to Unblock the Ears Decoction) tonifies Liver and Kidney yin to treat ear disorders.

Chapter 8 — Summary

SECTION 5: YANG-TONIFYING FORMULAS

Name	Similarities	Differences
Jin Gui Shen Qi Wan (Kidney Qi Pill from the Golden Cabinet)	Tonify Kidney yang, warm *ming men* (life gate) fire	Base formula to tonify Kidney yang
Ba Wei Di Huang Wan (Eight-Ingredient Pill with Rehmannia)		Slightly stronger function to tonify Kidney yang
Ji Sheng Shen Qi Wan (Kidney Qi Pill from Formulas that Aid the Living)		Regulates water and relieves edema
You Gui Wan (Restore the Right [Kidney] Pill)	Tonify Kidney yang and *jing* (essence)	Tonifies the blood
Huan Shao Dan (Return to Youth Pill)		Tonifies qi and blood, strengthens the Spleen, Stomach, Kidney, and Heart
Er Xian Tang (Two-Immortal Decoction)		Clears deficiency fire

Jin Gui Shen Qi Wan (Kidney Qi Pill from the Golden Cabinet) tonifies Kidney yang and warms *ming men* (life gate) fire. Clinical applications of this formula includes endocrine disorders (diabetes mellitus and insipidus, hypoadrenocorticism, hypothyroidism); reproductive disorders (impotence, male and female infertility); genitourinary disorders (nephritis, amyloidosis, renal failure, chronic glomerulonephritis, proteinuria, urinary incontinence); cardiovascular disorders (congestive heart failure, cardiomyopathy); respiratory disorders (chronic bronchitis, asthma); and other conditions such as back pain and intervertebral disk disease.

Ba Wei Di Huang Wan (Eight-Ingredient Pill with Rehmannia) is a modified formula that is slightly stronger than the original *Jin Gui Shen Qi Wan* (Kidney Qi Pill from the Golden Cabinet) in tonifying Kidney yang and warming *ming men* (life gate) fire. The clinical applications are the same as for *Jin Gui Shen Qi Wan.*

Ji Sheng Shen Qi Wan (Kidney Qi Pill from Formulas that Aid the Living) is very similar in composition to *Jin Gui Shen Qi Wan* (Kidney Qi Pill from the Golden Cabinet). It tonifies Kidney yang, but focuses more on regulating water circulation. It treats water accumulation caused by Kidney yang deficiency, with signs and symptoms such as severe pitting peripheral edema, cold rear quarters, dysuria or excessive urination.

You Gui Wan (Restore the Right [Kidney] Pill) tonifies Kidney yang, and nourishes *jing* (essence) and blood. This formula is indicated for chronic illness resulting in deficiency of Kidney yang and *ming men* (life gate) fire. This formula does not contain the "three sedative herbs;" hence, the tonifying action is stronger than that of *Jin Gui Shen Qi Wan* (Kidney Qi Pill from the Golden Cabinet).

Huan Shao Dan (Return to Youth Pill) is a comprehensive formula that tonifies qi, blood, Kidney yang and *jing* (essence). In addition, it strengthens the Spleen, Stomach, Kidney, and Heart. This formula is most effective for treating deterioration associated with normal or premature aging, with generalized weakness and deficiencies. It is also an appropriate formula for maintenance or recovery from chronic illness.

Er Xian Tang (Two-Immortal Decoction) tonifies Kidney yin and yang, replenishes Kidney *jing* (essence), and drains deficiency fire. This formula treats Kidney deficiency with deficiency fire rising, causing nervousness, irritability, fatigue, and a variety of Kidney deficiency clinical signs, depending on which type of deficiency is most predominant.

Chapter 8 — Summary

SECTION 6: YIN- AND YANG-TONIFYING FORMULAS

Name	Similarities	Differences
Gui Lu Er Xian Jiao (Tortoise Shell and Deer Antler Syrup)	Tonify Kidney yin and yang	Tonifies qi and blood, replenishes *jing* (essence)
Qi Bao Mei Ran Wan (Seven-Treasure Special Pill for Beautiful Whiskers)		Tonifies Liver blood, replenishes *jing* (essence)
Di Huang Yin Zi (Rehmannia Decoction)		Dissolves phlegm, opens the orifices

Gui Lu Er Xian Jiao (Tortoise Shell and Deer Antler Syrup) tonifies qi and blood, supplements Kidney yin and yang, and replenishes *jing* (essence). Clinical applications of this formula include osteoarthritis, hypothyroidism, infertility, recovery from chronic illness, recovery from chemotherapy and radiation therapy, back pain, cervical pain, intervertebral disk disease, degenerative myelopathy, and endocrine diseases.

Qi Bao Mei Ran Dan (Seven-Treasure Special Pill for Beautiful Whiskers) nourishes both Kidney *jing* (essence) and Liver blood to treat alopecia, premature aging, male infertility, impotence, low sperm count, decreased sperm motility, back and stifle weakness and pain, and tendon and ligament weakness.

Di Huang Yin Zi (Rehmannia Decoction) tonifies Kidney yin and yang, dissolves phlegm, and opens the orifices. Clinical manifestations include aphasia caused by a stiff tongue, leg paralysis, rear quarter weakness, cognitive dysfunction, a dry mouth without desire to drink, a pale tongue, and a deep, thin and weak pulse.

Chapter 9

— Shen-Calming Formulas

安神剂

扁鹊 Biǎn Què

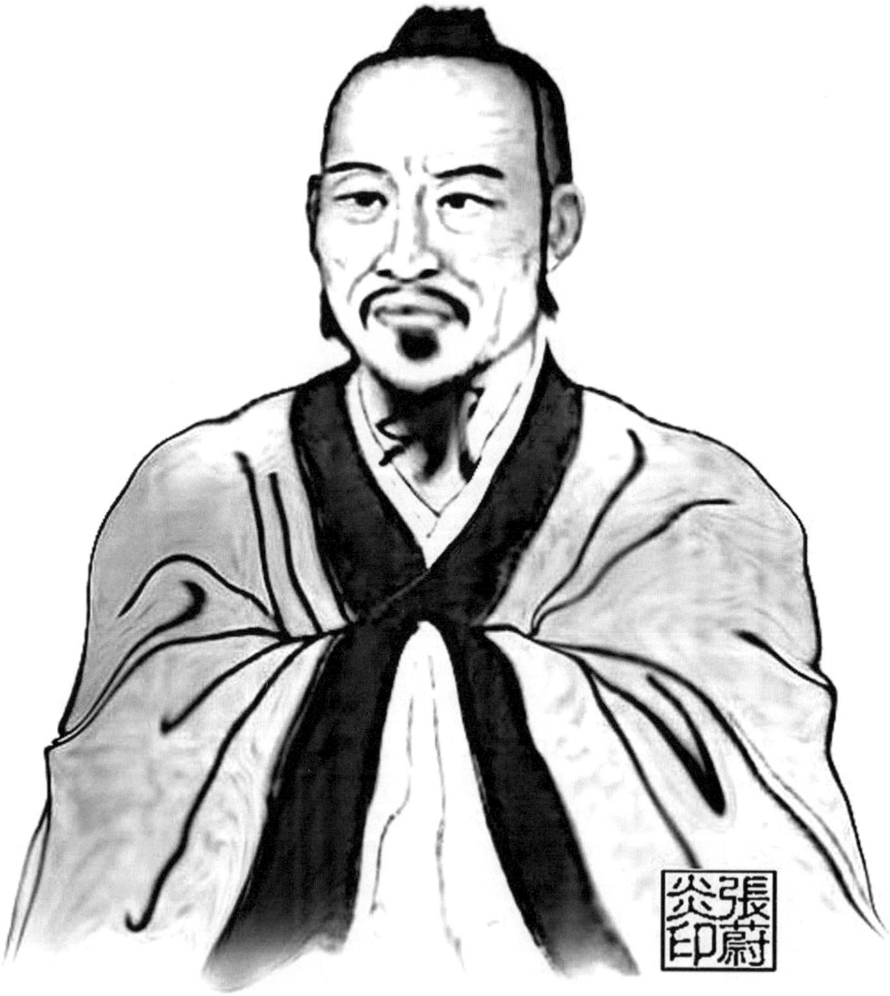

扁鹊 Biǎn Què, also known as 秦越人 Qìn Yuè-Rēn, 407 – 310 BCE. [1]

扁鹊 Biǎn Què

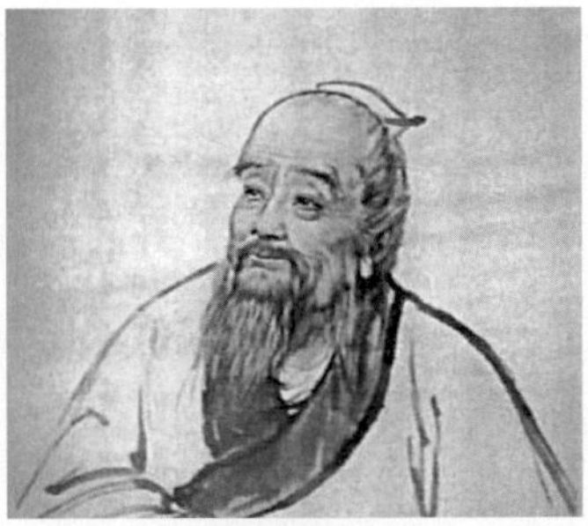

Bian Que

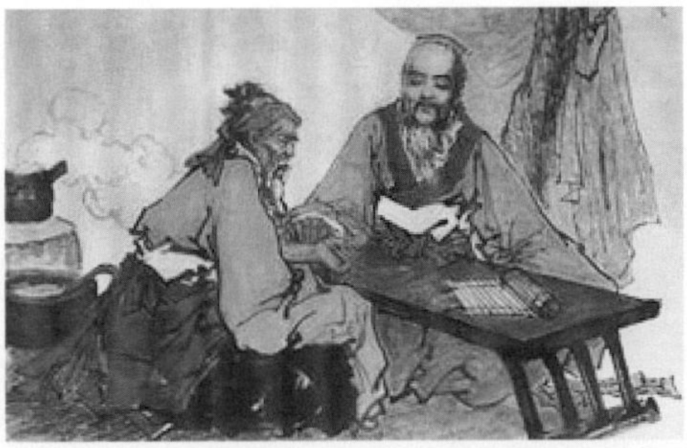

Bian Que taking pulse of a patient.

So far as can be determined from recorded history, Bian Que is the founder of traditional Chinese medicine. The first physician spoken of in Chinese historical texts, Bian Que lived in the fifth century BCE. Bian Que understood all aspects of medicine, including herbs, acupuncture, internal and external medicine, gynecology, pediatrics, geriatrics, and disorders of the five senses. He was particularly skilled in the four diagnostic skills, including *wang* (inspection), *wen* (listening), *wen* (inquiry) and *qie* (palpation).

Bian Que authored two major texts during his life: 扁鹊内经 *Bian Que Nei Jing* (Internal Medicine according to Bian Que) and 扁鹊外经 *Bian Que Wai Jing* (External Medicine according to Bian Que). Physicians during the Han dynasty claimed to have studied the works of Bian Que. Unfortunately, both texts have been lost to history, and we are left with folklore and legends of his life and accomplishments.

There is one story that offers particular insight into the medical philosophy of Bian Que. King of Wei asked Bian Que one day, "You and your two brothers are all experts in medicine, which of you is the best?" Bian Que replied, "My eldest brother is the best, followed by my second brother, and I am the last." The king then asked, "Then why is it that you are the most famous?" Bian Que answered, "My eldest brother cures a disease before it shows any symptoms. Since people do not see the disease, they do not recognize his ability. My second brother terminates a disease in its early stages. People assume he is only capable of treating minor illnesses, so he is merely known within this locality and its neighborhood. As for me, I treat a disease when it is already very severe and serious. When I perform blood-letting by injecting needles into vessels, or apply medical ointment on the skin, people think I am well versed in medicine. Therefore, I have become well known all over the country." The king was quite satisfied with his answer and said, "You've spoken wisely."

Dynasties & Kingdoms	Year
Xia Dynasty 夏	2100-1600 BCE
Shang Dynasty 商	1600-1100 BCE
Zhou Dynasty 周	**1100-221 BCE**
Qin Dynasty 秦	221-207 BCE
Han Dynasty 漢	206 BCE-220
Three Kingdoms 三國	220-280
Western Jin Dynasty 西晉	265-316
Eastern Jin Dynasty 東晉	317-420
Northern and Southern Dynasties 北南朝	420-581
Sui Dynasty 隋	581-618
Tang Dynasty 唐	618-907
Five Dynasties 五代	907-960
Song Dynasty 宋	960-1279
Liao Dynasty 遼	916-1125
Jin Dynasty 金	1115-1234
Yuan Dynasty 元	1271-1368
Ming Dynasty 明	1368-1644
Qing Dynasty 清	1644-1911
Republic of China 中華民國	1912-Present Day
People's Republic of China 中華人民共和國	1949-Present Day

1. Approximate years of birth and death.

Table of Contents

Chapter 9 — Overview

安神剂

— Shen-Calming Formulas

Definition: *Shen*-calming formulas act to calm the *shen* (spirit) and tranquilize the mind.

When animals have normal *shen* (spirit), they are bright and alert, the eyes are sparkling, and the mind is calm and peaceful. They are focused and purposeful in their actions, exhibit clarity of mental processes, and their sleep is normal. Healthy *shen* is necessary for normal behavior and reaction to environmental stimuli. *Shen* disturbance or disorder is a commonly diagnosed condition in veterinary medicine, and can occur in many different types of animals, including domestic and zoo animals and avian species. *Shen* disturbance can be excess or deficient in nature; it is common for elements of both to be present. The biomedically defined conditions of behavioral disorder and cognitive dysfunction are included in the definition of *shen* disturbance in Chinese medicine. The most common etiological factors in the development of *shen* disorders in animals are poor diet and feeding practices (lack of ancestral diet), inappropriate environment or habitat, and restrictions placed on the animal's behavior that prevent the animal from expressing normal innate behaviors. This can include a lack of socialization, abnormal confinement, isolation, over crowding, inadequate exercise, and suppression of other behaviors unique to the species. The presence and observation of *shen* disorders is nowhere more obvious than in zoo animals.

Shen-calming formulas can be used to treat behavioral disorders with clinical signs of irritability, aggression (growling, biting, clawing, attacking), anxiety, nervousness, hiding, fear-biting, touch hypersensitivity, noise sensitivity, repetitive compulsive behaviors (constant pacing, flank sucking, tail chasing), restlessness and pacing at night, insomnia, sleep disturbance (whining, jerking and vocalizing during sleep), hyperactivity, hyperexcitability, poor memory and concentration, inability to perform commands from the trainer or handler, general fearfulness, abnormal or excessive vocalization (whining, barking, howling, yowling), destructive (to the environment) and self-destructive behaviors (self-mutilation, over grooming, excessive chewing and licking, hair pulling, feather picking), mental dullness, disorientation, and depression.

Shen disorders can develop from dysfunction of the three *zang* (internal organs): the Heart, which governs the blood and stores *shen*; the Liver, which regulates qi and stores *hun* (ethereal soul); and the Kidney, which stores *zhi* (will-power) and provides water to balance the fire of the Heart. Imbalance of these organs contributes to the development of *shen* disturbance. In clinical practice, the organ affected depends on the constitution of the animal, environmental factors, diet and other disease factors. The majority of the herbal formulas that treat *shen* disorders contain herbs that enter the Heart and Liver channels. Acute emotional events or trauma easily affect the Heart, while the Liver is more involved in chronic stress situations.

The Heart is considered to be the most important *zang* organ in Chinese medicine because it regulates blood circulation and houses the mind. For *shen* to be strong and healthy, the Heart requires an adequate amount of blood and yin to nourish normal emotions and mental processes. In practice, many TCM practitioners do not differentiate between a lack of Heart yin and blood; yin and blood are from the same source, and often, when a lack of Heart blood in discussed, a lack of Heart yin is also implied. Animals with *shen* disturbance associated with deficiency of Heart yin

Chapter 9 — Overview

and blood may show clinical signs of sleep disturbance, insomnia, anxiety, poor memory, and be easily distracted, fearful, or hypersensitive to noise. These patients have a dry, pale to red tongue with cracks and little to no coating, and a rapid, thready, and weak pulse. Most herbal formulas that treat *shen* disturbance due to deficiency of Heart blood also include herbs to tonify Heart yin. According to the Five-Element Theory, a lack of Heart blood and yin can develop as a result of a lack of nourishment from the wood element (Liver), the mother of the Heart, and/or deficiency and lack of production of blood by its child, the earth element (Spleen). The Heart is a fire organ and dislikes heat; the *shen* of the Heart is easily disturbed by excess heat and fire in the body, and it is not uncommon for cancer patients undergoing weekly radiation and chemotherapy treatment to develop Heart blood and yin deficiencies. Chronic stress (boarding, grooming, competition, isolation, confinement), in combination with lack of exercise and being fed a high carbohydrate diet that engenders damp-heat, is a common cause of *shen* disturbance and behavioral disorders. These factors lead to Liver qi stagnation, Liver fire, and the development of Heart fire. This is especially true of animals with a fire or wood constitution. Chronic fire damages body fluids and leads to the development of phlegm. Phlegm fire obstructs the sensory orifices, causing severe *shen* disturbance and manic behavior. Animals affected by phlegm fire show a deep red tongue with white to yellow coating, and a forceful, rapid, and slippery to wiry pulse. In addition, they also exhibit behaviors such as self-mutilation, excessive vocalization, destructive behavior, restlessness, anxiety, hyperactivity, and repetitive compulsive disorders.

The Liver regulates the flow of qi throughout the entire body, stores the blood, and regulates digestion. Part of the Liver's regulatory function is the control and moderation of the emotions; the smooth flow of Liver qi is associated with normal emotional balance and well-being. If Liver qi flow is not smooth or becomes blocked, the animal can become irritable and aggressive, and respond inappropriately to its environment, people and other animals. Liver qi stagnation often develops from frustration due to isolation, over-confinement, boredom, over-training, chronic drug administration, lack of regular exercise, and inappropriate diet and feeding practices. Liver qi stagnation generates heat and leads to the development of Liver fire, which then attacks the Heart, causing emotional instability. Chronic Liver fire from stagnation can eventually consume Liver yin and blood, leading to Liver yin and blood deficiency. When yin becomes insufficient and cannot restrain and anchor Liver yang, it becomes hyperactive or mobile and ascends or rises. Ascendant hyperactive Liver yang, or "Liver yang rising," is a term used to describe a relative heat excess that develops from a deficiency of yin. This fire flares upward and results in the clinical signs of red eyes, outbursts of aggression, a dark red to purple tongue, and a rapid, wiry, and thin pulse.

Kidney yin is the source of yin for all of the *zang* (solid organ) of the body, and bestows cooling, resting and nourishing properties to the body. Kidney *jing* (essence) deficiency (poor genetics, chronic disease, chronic medications, aging), in combination with an inappropriate diet (dry, processed, heat- and dampness-engendering), often leads to an imbalance between the Heart and Kidney, with the subsequent development of Kidney yin deficiency and the generation of deficiency fire, which disturbs the *shen*. Animals with constitutional Kidney weakness are especially prone to this mechanism of *shen* disturbance. The clinical signs are the same as those seen in Heart yin and blood deficiency, but there will be additional signs of heat, such as an increased sensitivity to acupuncture, being easily frightened, excessive panting (especially at night), increased thirst, and sleep disturbance. The tongue is red with no coating, and it may have cracks, while the pulse is thready and rapid.

While there are many causes of *shen* (spirit) disturbance, the disturbance can nevertheless be categorized as either excess or deficient in nature.

- **Excess**-type *shen* disturbance may be caused externally by a sudden, terrifying experience or trauma, excessive environmental heat, an inappropriate diet, chronic drug therapy, or internally by Liver qi stagnation producing Liver fire. These conditions create an extreme upward blazing of

Chapter 9 — Overview

Heart fire and yang that cannot be cooled by Kidney water. In either case, these pathological factors disturb the *shen*, leading to clinical signs such as anxiety, irritability, restlessness, pacing, abnormal vocalization, destructive or self-destructive behavior, diminished hearing and/or sight, constipation, difficulty with urination, insomnia or disturbed sleep patterns, abnormal levels of fear and aggression, a red to purple tongue, and a thin, thready, rapid pulse. Because of the excess nature of the *shen* disturbance in these conditions, treatment usually involves herbs that clear heat and sedate the *shen*.

- **Deficient**-type *shen* disturbance may be caused by the following factors: diets that bring about qi and blood deficiencies; yin deficiency, secondary to chronic drug therapy; chemotherapy and radiation therapy; chronic disease; and normal aging. Such conditions lead to Heart, Kidney and Liver blood deficiencies, Heart blood and yin deficiency with malnourishment of the *shen,* and rising of deficiency fire in the interior. Clinical signs include palpitations, poor memory, deficiency-induced irritability and restlessness, insomnia, and an abnormal level of fear. Because of the deficient nature of the *shen* disturbance, the treatment methods should focus on nourishing the Heart and calming the *shen.* Canine cognitive disorder is typically categorized as a deficient type of *shen* disturbance, which commonly occurs in geriatric dogs with clinical signs of pacing, mental dullness, depression, inability to find the dog door, staring into space or at the wall, becoming trapped in small places with disorientation and inability to find a way out, and decreased or inappropriate response to environmental stimuli. The clinical signs will vary depending on the Chinese medicine pattern identified.

Although *shen* disturbance is categorized as either excess or deficient, both may occur separately or together, with or without complications. If both excess and deficiency clinical signs are observed, then both sedating and nourishing methods may be employed simultaneously. If complications are noted, select additional herbs accordingly. In most cases, treating *shen* disturbance will involve treating both the clinical signs and cause(s) concurrently. *Shen* disturbance may also be complicated by interior heat, phlegm accumulation, and blood stasis. These conditions are discussed in Chapter 5: Heat-Clearing Formulas, Chapter 18: Phlegm-Dispelling Formulas, and Chapter 13: Blood-Regulating Formulas, respectively.

Behavioral disorders in animals are often treated with sedative drugs to control or extinguish their undesirable behaviors. The difficulty with this is approach is that sedated animals are unable to express normal behaviors as well as the undesirable behaviors, or perform normally when called upon to do so. The type of drugs selected to control behavioral disorders in animals is a much debated topic among veterinary behaviorists, and, in fact, many of the behavioral disorders diagnosed in veterinary medicine are treated with the same drugs used to treat similar conditions in humans. One of the problems in deciding which drug to use is that for many of these drugs, it is still not fully known how they operate and exert their psychological effects. The problem with using drugs to treat behavioral and cognitive disorders is that unless the animal is chronically medicated, the behaviors can persist or recur. Also, the drugs may not produce therapeutic effects, or, if they do, the results are not long lasting. The use of Chinese herbs in recent years has been shown to safely and effectively treat behavioral disorders in domesticated and non-domesticated animals.

The use of any medication, whether conventional or herbal, is not considered to be a substitute for appropriate diet, regular exercise, environmental enrichment, and behavioral modification. The use of behavioral modification is especially critical in the management of behavioral disorders; an integrative approach produces superior clinical results than either modality used alone. A Chinese medicine approach is often chosen when pharmaceutical drugs are ineffective or produce unwanted or long-term side effects. Chinese medicine is also useful when polypharmacy is a concern, when conventional medication is contraindicated due to aging or weak organ systems, or prohibited in competition, and when the caretaker or owner wishes to use a more natural approach. In general, the use of Chinese herbal medicine to treat behavioral disorders should be considered as

Chapter 9 — Overview

an alternative to chronic medication, and for the prevention of unnecessary euthanasia of animals with behavioral disorders.

SUBCATEGORIES OF ACTION

Shen-calming formulas fall into two subcategories: **sedative** formulas that treat excess-type *shen* disturbance, and **nourishing** formulas that treat deficient-type *shen* disturbance.

1. **Sedative Formulas that Calm the *Shen* (Spirit)**

These formulas treat *shen* disorder caused by hyperactivity of Heart yang and flaring upward of Heart fire. Common clinical manifestations include irritability, restlessness, insomnia, palpitations, epilepsy, and abnormal levels of fear, fright and anger.

The following substances are used to treat excess-type *shen* disturbance: *Ci Shi* (Magnetitum), *Long Chi* (Dens Draconis), and *Zhen Zhu Mu* (Concha Margaritiferae) sedate and calm the *shen*; *Di Huang* (Radix Rehmanniae), *Shu Di Huang* (Radix Rehmanniae Praeparata), and *Dang Gui* (Radix Angelicae Sinensis) nourish yin and blood that may have been consumed by excess yang; and *Huang Lian* (Rhizoma Coptidis) clears excess heat and fire. An exemplar formula that sedates and calms the *shen* is *Zhen Zhu Mu Wan* (Mother of Pearl Pill).

2. **Nourishing Formulas that Calm the *Shen* (Spirit)**

These formulas treat *shen* disturbance with deficiency fire rising upward, caused by yin and blood deficiencies. Common clinical manifestations include deficiency type of irritability and restlessness, insomnia, dream-disturbed sleep, abnormal levels of fear, pacing at night, a red tongue with no tongue coating, and a rapid, thready pulse.

Treatment simultaneously calms the *shen* and nourishes yin and blood. Herbs that calm the *shen* include *Suan Zao Ren* (Semen Ziziphi Spinosae), *Bai Zi Ren* (Semen Platycladi), *Wu Wei Zi* (Fructus Schisandrae Chinensis), and *Xiao Mai* (Fructus Tritici). Herbs that nourish yin and blood include *Di Huang* (Radix Rehmanniae), *Zhi Mu* (Rhizoma Anemarrhenae), *Mai Dong* (Radix Ophiopogonis), and *Dang Gui* (Radix Angelicae Sinensis). Representative formulas include *Suan Zao Ren Tang* (Sour Jujube Decoction), *Tian Wang Bu Xin Dan* (Emperor of Heaven's Special Pill to Tonify the Heart), and *Gan Mai Da Zao Tang* (Licorice, Wheat, and Jujube Decoction).

CAUTIONS / CONTRAINDICATIONS

- Some sedative formulas that calm the *shen* (spirit) contain minerals or heavy metal substances. These formulas should not be taken for a long period of time, as they may injure the Spleen and Stomach. Furthermore, for animals that have constitutional Spleen and Stomach deficiencies, Spleen-tonifying and Stomach-harmonizing herbs should be added to prevent unwanted side effects.
- *Zhu Sha* (Cinnabaris), an ingredient traditionally used in some sedative formulas, is rarely utilized as a medicinal substance today. Its discussion here is included primarily for academic purposes, to reflect the historical use of this substance.

Chapter 9 — Overview

PHARMACOLOGICAL EFFECTS & CLINICAL APPLICATIONS

***Shen*-calming formulas** calm the *shen* (spirit) and tranquilize the mind. From allopathic medicine perspectives, these formulas primarily treat a wide variety of mental disorders. Note: The term "mental disorders" is used here loosely to describe a general and broad range of abnormal emotional, behavioral, and psychological conditions.

- **Mental disorders**: *Shen*-calming herbs and formulas primarily treat a wide range of mental disorders. General pharmacological effects include sedative and hypnotic effects on the central nervous system to suppress both mental and physical activities.[1,2,3] One formula also demonstrated marked effectiveness in reducing elevated levels of serum corticosterone caused by emotional stress (psychological stress and conditioned-fear stress).[4] Clinically, *shen*-calming formulas have been used successfully to treat a wide variety of emotional, behavioral, and psychological disorders, including, but not limited to, insomnia,[5,6,7,8] neurasthenia,[9,10] neurosis,[11] schizophrenia,[12,13] depression,[14] and hysteria.[15] Formulas frequently used to calm the *shen* and treat mental disorders include *Suan Zao Ren Tang* (Sour Jujube Decoction), *Tian Wang Bu Xin Dan* (Emperor of Heaven's Special Pill to Tonify the Heart), *Yang Xin Tang* (Nourish the Heart Decoction), and *Gan Mai Da Zao Tang* (Licorice, Wheat, and Jujube Decoction).
- **Others**: *Shen*-calming formulas have also been used to treat seizures and epilepsy,[16] impotence,[17] nocturnal emissions,[18] enuresis,[19] and menopause.[20]

References

1. *Guo Wai Yi Xue* (Foreign Medicine), 1992; 14(5):47.
2. *Zhong Yi Fang Ji Xian Dai Yan Jiu* (Modern Study of Medical Formulas in Traditional Chinese Medicine), 1997; 849-850.
3. Journal of Ethnopharmacology, 1986; 15:289.
4. Sasaki K, Suzuki K, Yoshizaki F, Ando T. Effect of saiko-ka-ryukotsu-borei-to on the stress-induced increase of serum corticosterone in mice. Biol Pharm Bull. 1995 Apr; 18(4):563-5.
5. *Tian Jin Zhong Yi* (Tianjin Chinese Medicine), 1999; 2:25.
6. *Shan Dong Yi Kan* (Shandong Medical Journal), 1965; 27.
7. *He Nan Zhong Yi* (Henan Chinese Medicine), 1992; 2:83.
8. *Zhe Jiang Zhong Yi Za Zhi* (Zhejiang Journal of Chinese Medicine), 1982; 9:412.
9. *Zhong Xi Yi Jie He Yan Jiu Zi Liao* (Research Information on Integration of Chinese and Western Medicine), 1976; 6:7.
10. *Jiang Su Yi Yao* (Jiangsu Journal of Medicine and Herbology), 1976; 1:47.
11. *Han Fang Yi Xue* (Kampo Medicine), 1986; 10(9):26.
12. *Shi Yong Zhong Xi Yi Jie He Za Zhi* (Practical Journal of Integrated Chinese and Western Medicines), 1998; 2:170.
13. *Shang Hai Yi Yao Za Zhi* (Shanghai Journal of Medicine and Herbology), 1982; 6:273.
14. *Liao Ning Zhong Yi Za Zhi* (Liaoning Journal of Chinese Medicine), 1984; 12:34.
15. *Zhong Yi Za Zhi* (Journal of Chinese Medicine), 1960; 2:32.
16. Hung-Ming W, Liu CS, Tsai JJ, Ko LY, Wei YH. Antioxidant and anticonvulsant effect of a modified formula of chaihu-longu-muli-tang. American Journal of Chinese Medicine. 30(2-3):339-46, 2002.
17. *Shan Xi Zhong Yi* (Shanxi Chinese Medicine), 1990; 11(5):224.
18. *Shi Yong Zhong Xi Yi Jie He Za Zhi* (Practical Journal of Integrated Chinese and Western Medicines), 1991; 12:729.
19. *Hu Bei Zhong Yi Za Zhi* (Hubei Journal of Chinese Medicine), 1986; 1:19.
20. *Fu Jian Zhong Yi Yao* (Fujian Chinese Medicine and Herbology), 1960; 10:17.

Section 1

重镇安神剂
— Sedative Formulas that Calm the Shen (Spirit)

Zhēn Zhū Mŭ Wán (Mother of Pearl Pill)
珍珠母丸

Pinyin Name: *Zhen Zhu Mu Wan*
Literal Name: Mother of Pearl Pill
Alternate Name: *Zhen Zhu Wan* (True Pearl Pill)
Original Source: *Pu Ji Ben Shi Fang* (Formulas of Universal Benefit from My Practice) by Xu Shu-Wei in 1132

COMPOSITION

Zhen Zhu Mu (Concha Margaritiferae), *yan* (ground) to powder	22.5g
Long Chi (Dens Draconis)	15g
Ren Shen (Radix et Rhizoma Ginseng)	30g
Dang Gui (Radix Angelicae Sinensis), *bei* (stone-baked)	45g
Shu Di Huang (Radix Rehmanniae Praeparata), *zheng* (steamed) with liquor	45g
Suan Zao Ren (Semen Ziziphi Spinosae), *chao* (dry-fried) and *yan* (ground) to small particles	30g
Bai Zi Ren (Semen Platycladi), *yan* (ground) to small particles	30g
Fu Shen (Poria Pararadicis)	15g
Xi Jiao (Cornu Rhinoceri), *bang* (scraped) into fine powder	15g
Chen Xiang (Lignum Aquilariae Resinatum)	15g

DOSAGE / PREPARATION / ADMINISTRATION

The source text states to grind the ingredients into powder, form into very small pills with honey, and coat the pills with *Zhu Sha* (Cinnabaris). The pills should resemble the size of *Wu Tong Zi* (Semen Firmianae), a small seed approximately 5 mm in diameter. Separately prepare a decoction of *Jin Bo* (gold foil), *Yin Bo* (silver foil), and *Bo He* (Herba Menthae). Take 40-50 pills with the strained decoction during the day and at bedtime.

Note: *Xi Jiao* (Cornu Rhinoceri) is derived from an endangered animal, and *Zhu Sha* (Cinnabaris) is a potentially toxic heavy metal. Both are rarely used as medicinal substances today. They are discussed here primarily for academic purposes, to reflect the historical use of these substances in its original formulation. Most herbal products today have removed them completely, or replaced them with substitutes with similar functions. For additional information on the toxicity, please refer to *Chinese Medical Herbology and Pharmacology* by John Chen and Tina Chen.

CHINESE THERAPEUTIC ACTIONS

1. Tranquilizes the Heart and calms the *shen* (spirit)
2. Nourishes yin and blood

CLINICAL MANIFESTATIONS

Hyperactivity of Liver yang with yin and blood deficiencies: behavioral disorders characterized by irritability, aggression, insomnia, and a fine, wiry pulse.

VETERINARY CLINICAL APPLICATIONS

Hypertension, behavioral disorder, epilepsy, seizure, and irritability associated with estrus.

EXPLANATION

Zhen Zhu Mu Wan (Mother of Pearl Pill) treats hyperactivity of Liver and Heart yang that is accompanied by underlying yin and blood deficiencies. The Heart is the organ that houses the mind. If yin and blood are deficient, then the *shen* (spirit) may become unstable, leading to night restlessness and palpitations. Deficiency of yin with hyperactivity of yang may affect the brain, causing seizure disorder.

Zhēn Zhū Mǔ Wán (Mother of Pearl Pill)

***Zhen Zhu Mu Wan* (Mother of Pearl Pill)**

Diagnosis	Clinical Signs	Treatment	Herbs
Hyperactivity of Liver yang with yin and blood deficiencies	• Emotional instability, night restlessness, and palpitations: insufficiency of yin and blood to nourish the *shen* (spirit) • Irritability, aggression, insomnia: hyperactivity of yang due to deficiency of yin	• Nourishes yin and blood • Tranquilizes the Heart and calms the *shen*	• *Zhen Zhu Mu* (Concha Margaritiferae) and *Long Chi* (Dens Draconis) subdue hyperactivity of Liver yang and calm Heart *shen*. • *Ren Shen* (Radix et Rhizoma Ginseng), *Dang Gui* (Radix Angelicae Sinensis) and *Shu Di Huang* (Radix Rehmanniae Praeparata) nourish qi, yin and blood. • *Suan Zao Ren* (Semen Ziziphi Spinosae), *Bai Zi Ren* (Semen Platycladi), and *Fu Shen* (Poria Paradicis) calm the *shen* and anchor *zhi* (will-power). • *Xi Jiao* (Cornu Rhinoceri) enters the *xue* (blood) level and cools the blood. • *Chen Xiang* (Lignum Aquilariae Resinatum) lowers hyperactive yang to help calm the *shen*.

Zhen Zhu Mu (Concha Margaritiferae) and *Long Chi* (Dens Draconis) subdue hyperactivity of Liver yang and calm Heart *shen* (spirit). *Zhen Zhu Mu* (Concha Margaritiferae) also enters the Heart and Liver channels, and guides the formula to these organs. *Ren Shen* (Radix et Rhizoma Ginseng), *Dang Gui* (Radix Angelicae Sinensis), and *Shu Di Huang* (Radix Rehmanniae Praeparata) nourish qi, yin, and blood. *Suan Zao Ren* (Semen Ziziphi Spinosae), *Bai Zi Ren* (Semen Platycladi), and *Fu Shen* (Poria Paradicis) calm the *shen* and anchor *zhi* (will-power). They also help to promote restful sleep. *Xi Jiao* (Cornu Rhinoceri) enters the *xue* (blood) level to cool the blood and relieves fright and palpitations. *Chen Xiang* (Lignum Aquilariae Resinatum) lowers hyperactive yang to help calm the *shen*. *Zhu Sha* (Cinnabaris) calms the *shen* and guides the formula to the Heart. *Jin Bo* (gold foil) and *Yin Bo* (silver foil) calm the *shen*. *Bo He* (Herba Menthae) soothes Liver qi and clears Liver fire.

CAUTIONS / CONTRAINDICATIONS

Zhen Zhu Mu Wan contains rich tonics, such as *Shu Di Huang* (Radix Rehmanniae Praeparata) and *Suan Zao Ren* (Semen Ziziphi Spinosae), and is not suitable for treating night restlessness and *shen* (spirit) disturbance caused by phlegm and heat.

SUGGESTED ACUPUNCTURE TREATMENT

1. Points: *Shenshu* (BL 23), *Taixi* (KI 3), *Sanyinjiao* (SP 6), *Shenmen* (HT 7), *Neiguan* (PC 6), *Jueyinshu* (BL 14), *Xinshu* (BL 15), *Geshu* (BL 17), *Taichong* (LR 3), *Anshen*, and *Dafengmen*.
2. Technique: even method.

Shenshu (BL 23) and *Taixi* (KI 3) nourish the Kidney and clear deficiency fire. *Sanyinjiao* (SP 6) nourishes qi and blood of the Spleen and Liver. *Shenmen* (HT 7) is the *yuan* (source) point of the Heart channel. *Jueyinshu* (BL 14) and *Xinshu* (BL 15) are the *shu* (transport) points on the back for the Pericardium and Heart and can help to calm *shen* (spirit). *Geshu* (BL 17) is the *shu* (transport) point for blood. *Neiguan* (PC 6) is the *luo* (connecting) point of the Pericardium channel. The combination of *Shenmen* (HT 7) and *Neiguan* (PC 6) effectively tranquilizes the mind. *Taichong* (LR 3) sedates the Liver to help calm the *shen*. *Anshen* and *Dafengmen* are classical points to calm the *shen*.

AUTHORS' COMMENTS

Zhen Zhu Mu Wan can be used to treat seizure disorder that develops secondary to hyperactivity of Liver and Heart yang, and that is accompanied by underlying yin and blood deficiencies. This formula is not commercially available and contains many substances that are not readily available and will need to be made in the clinic; thus, it is not commonly used for these reasons.

Chái Hú Jiā Lóng Gŭ Mŭ Lì Tāng

(Bupleurum plus Dragon Bone and Oyster Shell Decoction)

柴胡加龍骨牡蠣湯
柴胡加龙骨牡蛎汤

Pinyin Name: *Chai Hu Jia Long Gu Mu Li Tang*
Literal Name: Bupleurum plus Dragon Bone and Oyster Shell Decoction
Alternate Names: *Chai Hu Jia Long Mu Tang, Tsai Hu Chia Lung Ku Mu Li Tang,* Bupleurum and Dragon Bone Combination
Original Source: *Shang Han Lun* (Discussion of Cold-Induced Disorders) by Zhang Zhong-Jing in the Eastern Han Dynasty

COMPOSITION

Chai Hu (Radix Bupleuri)	12g
Huang Qin (Radix Scutellariae)	4.5g
Long Gu (Os Draconis)	4.5g
Mu Li (Concha Ostreae), *ao* (simmered)	4.5g
Qian Dan (Minium)	4.5g
Gui Zhi (Ramulus Cinnamomi)	4.5g
Da Huang (Radix et Rhizoma Rhei)	6g
Ban Xia (Rhizoma Pinelliae), *xi* (washed)	6-9g
Fu Ling (Poria)	4.5g
Ren Shen (Radix et Rhizoma Ginseng)	4.5g
Sheng Jiang (Rhizoma Zingiberis Recens), *qie* (sliced)	4.5g
Da Zao (Fructus Jujubae), *bo* (opened)	6 pieces

Note: *Qian Dan* (Minium), commonly known as lead oxide red, is a potentially toxic heavy metal and is rarely used as a medicinal substance today. Its discussion here is included primarily for academic purposes, to reflect the historical use of this substance in its original formulation. Most herbal products today have removed it completely, or replaced it with substitutes with similar functions, such as *Zhe Shi* (Haematitum), which also has a calming action.[1] For additional information on *Qian Dan* (Minium) and *Zhe Shi* (Haematitum), please refer to *Chinese Medical Herbology and Pharmacology* by John Chen and Tina Chen.

DOSAGE / PREPARATION / ADMINISTRATION

Cook all of the ingredients, except *Da Huang* (Radix et Rhizoma Rhei), in 8 cups [1,600 mL] of water until the decoction is reduced to 4 cups [800 mL]. Add *Da Huang* (Radix et Rhizoma Rhei), and bring the decoction to a quick boil. Take 1 cup [200 mL] of the warm, strained decoction.

CHINESE THERAPEUTIC ACTIONS

1. Harmonizes the *shaoyang*
2. Unblocks the three yang stages
3. Calms the *shen* (spirit)

CLINICAL MANIFESTATIONS

1. Disorder in the three yang stages (*taiyang, yangming,* and *shaoyang*): night restlessness, anxiety, palpitations, irritability, aggression, dysuria, stiffness in the entire body with inability to rotate the trunk, a red tongue body, and a rapid, wiry pulse.
2. *Shaoyang* syndrome: irritability, aggression, restlessness, dysuria, stiffness of the whole body, and difficulty in moving the body.

VETERINARY CLINICAL APPLICATIONS

Anxiety, aggression, repetitive and compulsive behaviors (constant pacing, flank sucking, tail chasing), restlessness, hyperexcitability and barking, inability to focus and perform or listen to the trainer, night restlessness, depression, abnormal vocalization (whining, barking, howling, yowling), destructive (to the local environment or other animals) and self-destructive behaviors (self-mutilation, over grooming, excessive chewing licking, hair pulling, feather picking), hypertension, hyperthyroidism, seizure disorder and epilepsy.

EXPLANATION

Chai Hu Jia Long Gu Mu Li Tang (Bupleurum plus Dragon Bone and Oyster Shell Decoction), first presented in *Shang Han Lun* (Discussion of Cold-Induced Disorders), was originally indicated for patients who received improper downward-draining treatment when their disorder is still

Chái Hú Jiā Lóng Gǔ Mǔ Lì Tāng

(Bupleurum plus Dragon Bone and Oyster Shell Decoction)

***Chai Hu Jia Long Gu Mu Li Tang* (Bupleurum plus Dragon Bone and Oyster Shell Decoction)**

Diagnosis	Clinical Signs	Treatment	Herbs
Disorder in the three yang stages	• Night restlessness, aggression, hyperexcitability, anxiety, and repetitive compulsive disorders: heat attacking the Heart and *shen* (spirit) • A feeling of stiffness in the entire body with an inability to rotate the trunk: heat in the *shaoyang* stage • Constipation and urinary difficulties: heat damaging body fluids • A red tongue body and rapid, wiry pulse: interior heat	• Harmonizes the *shaoyang* • Unblocks the three yang stages • Calms the *shen* (spirit)	• *Chai Hu* (Radix Bupleuri) and *Huang Qin* (Radix Scutellariae) clear heat from the *shaoyang* stage and harmonize the exterior and interior. • *Long Gu* (Os Draconis), *Mu Li* (Concha Ostreae) and *Qian Dan* (Minium) calm the *shen* to relieve anxiety, palpitations, and delirious speech. • *Gui Zhi* (Ramulus Cinnamomi) dispels exterior pathogenic factors. • *Da Huang* (Radix et Rhizoma Rhei) drains internal heat. • *Ban Xia* (Rhizoma Pinelliae) causes qi to descend. • *Fu Ling* (Poria) promotes smooth urination. • *Ren Shen* (Radix et Rhizoma Ginseng) strengthens the Spleen and calms the *shen.* • *Sheng Jiang* (Rhizoma Zingiberis Recens) and *Da Zao* (Fructus Jujubae) harmonize all of the herbs.

at the exterior and has not yet entered the *yangming* stage. As the result of improper downward-draining treatment, the pathogenic factor travels inward to penetrate the *taiyang, yangming,* and *shaoyang* levels.

These patients usually exhibit a wide array of complex heat signs and other clinical signs. The presence of heat in the chest produces a feeling of fullness and distention; heat attacking the Heart causes night restlessness, anxiety, and palpitations; heat in the *yangming* stage causes delirium; and heat in the *shaoyang* stage leads to a feeling of heaviness in the entire body with an inability to rotate the trunk. The improper use of downward-draining herbs may damage body fluids, thus causing constipation and urinary difficulties. A red tongue body and rapid, wiry pulse are also indicative of heat. While clinical presentations may vary between patients, the diagnostic feature is the *shen* (spirit) floating upward, as evident from clinical signs such as anxiety, irritability and aggression. The *shaoyang* syndrome discussed here is caused by the inappropriate use of downward-draining methods instead of exterior-releasing methods for illnesses at the *taiyang* stage. The inappropriate use of downward-draining methods may result in penetration of the pathogenic factors into the interior of the body, causing a syndrome that is both exterior and interior, deficient and excess. Chest fullness, irritability, and excitability are caused by fire in the *shaoyang* channel. *Shaoyang* syndrome may affect the water passages, causing dysuria. Delirium is the result of Stomach heat and *shaoyang* fire disturbing the Heart. Heaviness of the body is the result of the disrupted flow of yang qi.

Chai Hu Jia Long Gu Mu Li Tang is based on *Xiao Chai Hu Tang* (Minor Bupleurum Decoction), which is the representative formula for harmonizing *shaoyang* syndrome. (Please refer to the section on *Xiao Chai Hu Tang* for complete details.) *Chai Hu* (Radix Bupleuri) and *Huang Qin* (Radix Scutellariae) clear heat from the *shaoyang* stage and harmonize the exterior and interior. *Long Gu* (Os Draconis), *Mu Li* (Concha Ostreae) and *Qian Dan* (Minium) calm the *shen* (spirit) to relieve anxiety, aggression and hyperexcitability. *Gui Zhi* (Ramulus Cinnamomi) dispels exterior pathogenic factors, while *Da Huang* (Radix et Rhizoma Rhei) drains internal heat. *Ban Xia* (Rhizoma Pinelliae) guides the qi downward, while *Fu Ling* (Poria) promotes normal urination. Furthermore, *Fu Ling* (Poria) and *Ren Shen* (Radix et Rhizoma Ginseng) strengthen the Spleen and calm the *shen. Sheng Jiang* (Rhizoma Zingiberis Recens) and *Da Zao* (Fructus Jujubae) harmonize the formula.

VETERINARY MODIFICATIONS

- With hypertension, add *Gou Teng* (Ramulus Uncariae cum Uncis), *Ge Gen* (Radix Puerariae Lobatae), *Niu Xi* (Radix Achyranthis Bidentatae) and *Xia Ku Cao* (Spica Prunellae).
- With irritability add *Huang Lian* (Rhizoma Coptidis) and *Tian Hua Fen* (Radix Trichosanthis).

Chái Hú Jiā Lóng Gǔ Mǔ Lì Tāng

(Bupleurum plus Dragon Bone and Oyster Shell Decoction)

- With seizure disorder and epilepsy, add *Ling Zhi* (Ganoderma), *Tian Ma* (Rhizoma Gastrodiae), *Gou Teng* (Ramulus Uncariae cum Uncis) and *Xie Cao* (Radix et Rhizoma Valerianae).

CAUTIONS / CONTRAINDICATIONS

- For animals with a sensitive gastrointestinal system, remove *Da Huang* (Radix et Rhizoma Rhei), as this herb may cause loose stools.
- For animals with manic behavior and severe *shen* (spirit) disturbance, *Da Huang* (Radix et Rhizoma Rhei) should be given and the dose increased if possible.
- This formula should be used cautiously in those with Spleen and Stomach deficiencies, and may cause vomiting as *Long Gu* (Os Draconis) and *Mu Li* (Concha Ostreae) are hard to digest. Combine with Spleen tonic herbs or formula as needed to protect the middle *jiao*. It is best to begin with a low dose and work up to a higher dose.

PHARMACOLOGICAL EFFECTS

1. **Central nervous system**: Continuous administration of this formula for seven days was associated with increased sleeping time, decreased body temperature, and decreased spontaneous activity in rats.[2]
2. **Antidepressant**: Administration of *Chai Hu Jia Long Gu Mu Li Tang* in mice successfully treated depression induced by chronic stress, by restoring the normal functioning of the hypothalamo-pituitary-adrenal system and the prefrontal cortex. Furthermore, studies have demonstrated that *Chai Hu Jia Long Gu Mu Li Tang* significantly prevented chronic stress-induced decreases in extracellular concentrations of dopamine and serotonin in the prefrontal cortex.[3,4] Lastly, administration of *Chai Hu Jia Long Gu Mu Li Tang*, *Yi Gan San* (Restrain the Liver Powder) and *Bu Zhong Yi Qi Tang* (Tonify the Middle and Augment the Qi Decoction) for 14 consecutive days showed both antidepressive and antinociceptive properties in mice.[5]
3. **Endocrine**: A study evaluated the relationship between *Chai Hu Jia Long Gu Mu Li Tang* and serum corticosterone in mice. The study found *Chai Hu Jia Long Gu Mu Li Tang* to be effective in reducing elevated corticosterone caused by emotional stress (psychological stress and conditioned-fear stress), but not physical stress (immobilized stress, forced-swim stress, and electric-shock stress). The researchers concluded that *Chai Hu Jia Long Gu Mu Li Tang* is more effective for stress associated with psychological changes, and less effective for stress caused by physical changes.[6]
4. **Sedative and hypnotic**: Administration of *Chai Hu Jia Long Gu Mu Li Tang* was associated with marked reduction in locomotor activity, and dose-dependent prolongation in the duration of drug-induced sleep time. The study suggested *Chai Hu Jia Long Gu Mu Li Tang* as a useful therapy against sleep disorder caused by excitation.[7]
5. **Antihypertensive**: *Chai Hu Jia Long Gu Mu Li Tang* has been used clinically in the treatment of hypertension. The mechanism of this antihypertensive effect was attributed to the antipressor effect (inhibition of vasoconstriction induced by nor-adrenaline).[8,9]
6. **Metabolic**: Administration of the extract of the formula to mice at 0.4 g/kg for 12 months was associated with reduction of total cholesterol and triglyceride levels in both the liver and blood vessels.[10]
7. **Effects on hypercholesterolemia and atherosclerosis**: Use of *Chai Hu Jia Long Gu Mu Li Tang* in rabbits was associated with prevention of hypercholesterolemia and protection against atheromatous lesions by affecting apoE and LDL receptor mRNA gene expression in the liver.[11] According to another study, *Chai Hu Jia Long Gu Mu Li Tang* prevented arteriosclerosis by inhibiting the proliferation of vascular smooth muscle cells.[12]

HUMAN CLINICAL STUDIES AND RESEARCH

1. **Neurosis**: Thirty-two patients with neurosis were treated with this formula for two weeks, with significant improvement in 6 cases, moderate improvement in 6 cases, and slight improvement in 14 cases. The overall rate of effectiveness was 81.3%.[13]
2. **Depression**: Thirty-five patients (between 19-60 years of age) with depression were treated with *Chai Hu Jia Long Gu Mu Li Tang* plus *Sheng Tie Luo* (Frusta Ferri) with complete recovery in 15 cases, significant improvement in 10 cases, moderate improvement in 9 cases, and no improvement in 1 case. The formula was given in decoction daily for 30 days per course of treatment, and the duration of the treatment was between 14-90 days. The overall effectiveness rate was 97.1%.[14] According to another study, use of *Chai Hu Jia Long Gu Mu Li Tang* in 63 patients (15 males and 48 females) with depression was associated with recovery in 32 cases, improvement in 19 cases, and no effect in 12 cases.[15]
3. **Schizophrenia**: In one study, 67 patients with schizophrenia were divided into three groups. Group A contained 15 schizophrenic patients characterized by *shaoyang* disorder and treated with *Chai Hu Jia Long Gu Mu Li Tang*. Diazepam or chlordiazepoxide was given only if necessary to treat night restlessness. Group B had 31 schizophrenic patients characterized by *shaoyang* disorder who were treated with *Chai Hu Jia Long Gu Mu Li Tang* as the primary treatment, with the addition of chlorpromazine or chlorprothixene at low doses (200mg per day or less).

Chái Hú Jiā Lóng Gŭ Mŭ Lì Tāng
(Bupleurum plus Dragon Bone and Oyster Shell Decoction)

Group C had 21 schizophrenic patients characterized by *shaoyang* disorder with qi and blood stagnation; they were treated with modified *Chai Hu Jia Long Gu Mu Li Tang* as the primary treatment, with the addition of chlorpromazine or chlorprothixene at low doses (200mg per day or less). The modified formula used in Group C contained *Chai Hu* (Radix Bupleuri) 9g, *Huang Qin* (Radix Scutellariae) 9g, *Dang Gui* (Radix Angelicae Sinensis) 9g, *Chi Shao* (Radix Paeoniae Rubra) 9g, *Tao Ren* (Semen Persicae) 9g, *Hong Hua* (Flos Carthami) 9g, *Da Huang* (Radix et Rhizoma Rhei) 6-9g, *Chuan Xiong* (Rhizoma Chuanxiong) 6g, *Mu Li* (Concha Ostreae) 15g, *Sheng Jiang* (Rhizoma Zingiberis Recens) 6g, and *Da Zao* (Fructus Jujubae) 15g. The treatment protocol for herbs in all three groups was to cook the herbs in water, and administer the decoction daily for 30 days per course of treatment. Those who did not respond after the first course received a second course of treatment. Of 67 patients, the study reported complete recovery in 1 case, significant recovery in 35 cases, and improvement in 14 cases. The overall effectiveness was 76.1%.[16] Note: Comparative analysis of results among the three groups of patients was unavailable at the time of publication.

In another study, use of modified *Chai Hu Jia Long Gu Mu Li Tang* was associated with 86.67% effectiveness in treating 45 patients with schizophrenia. The herbal formula contained *Chai Hu* (Radix Bupleuri) 12g, *Long Gu* (Os Draconis) 20g, *Mu Li* (Concha Ostreae) 20g, *Dang Shen* (Radix Codonopsis) 15g, *Ban Xia* (Rhizoma Pinelliae) 12g, *Da Huang* (Radix et Rhizoma Rhei) 10g, *Fu Ling* (Poria) 12g, *Huang Qin* (Radix Scutellariae) 12g, *Gui Zhi* (Ramulus Cinnamomi) 6g, *Dan Shen* (Radix et Rhizoma Salviae Miltiorrhizae) 15g, *Sheng Jiang* (Rhizoma Zingiberis Recens) 3 slices, and *Da Zao* (Fructus Jujubae) 6 pieces. Most patients showed improvement after an average of 15 packs of herbs. Of 45 patients, the study reported significant improvement in 31 cases, moderate improvement in 8 cases, and no effect in 6 cases.[17]

4. **Hyperlipoproteinemia**: Modified *Chai Hu Jia Long Gu Mu Li Tang* showed marked effectiveness in treating hyperlipoproteinemia in 58 patients. The study divided all patients into three categories based on traditional Chinese medical diagnoses. Hyperlipoproteinemia characterized by dampness and phlegm was treated with this formula plus *Fu Ling* (Poria), *Bai Zhu* (Rhizoma Atractylodis Macrocephalae), *Ban Xia* (Rhizoma Pinelliae), and others. Hyperlipoproteinemia characterized by Liver qi stagnation was treated with this formula plus *Zhi Qiao* (Fructus Aurantii), *Bai Shao* (Radix Paeoniae Alba), *Yu Jin* (Radix Curcumae) and others. Hyperlipoproteinemia characterized by Liver qi stagnation and Spleen deficiency was treated by this formula plus *Zhi Qiao* (Fructus Aurantii), *Yan Hu Suo* (Rhizoma Corydalis), *Fo Shou* (Fructus Citri Sarcodactylis), and others. The duration of treatment was 3 months per course of treatment. The study reported an overall rate of effectiveness of 87.9%.[18] In addition, another study stated that *Chai Hu Jia Long Gu Mu Li Tang* may prevent the development of vascular complications in hyperlipidemia patients, as use of the herbs was associated with reduction of triglycerides, total cholesterol, CD62P, PMPs, sE-selectin, and anti-oxidized LDL antibody.[19]
5. **Seizures and epilepsy**: A study reported 88% effectiveness using modified *Chai Hu Jia Long Gu Mu Li Tang* to treat 50 patients with epilepsy. The herbal treatment was based on *Chai Hu Jia Long Gu Mu Li Tang* without *Qian Dan* (Minium). Modifications included addition of *Shi Chang Pu* (Rhizoma Acori Tatarinowii), *Yuan Zhi* (Radix Polygalae) and *Dan Nan Xing* (Arisaema cum Bile) for the presence of excessive amounts of phlegm; *Suan Zao Ren* (Semen Ziziphi Spinosae), *Shou Wu Teng* (Caulis Polygoni Multiflori) and *He Huan Pi* (Cortex Albiziae) for night restlessness due to deficiency and restlessness; *Shi Jue Ming* (Concha Haliotidis), *Gou Teng* (Ramulus Uncariae cum Uncis), *Sheng Tie Luo* (Frusta Ferri) and *Huang Lian* (Rhizoma Coptidis) for wind and yang rising; *Sha Shen* (Radix Glehniae seu Adenophorae), *Mai Dong* (Radix Ophiopogonis) and *Xuan Shen* (Radix Scrophulariae) for yin deficiency. Additional adjustments were also made, depending on the severity of the condition and age of the patients. Of 50 patients, the study reported near-recovery in 25 cases, improvement in 19 cases, and no effect in 6 cases.[20] Another study reported marked success using modified *Chai Hu Jia Long Gu Mu Li Tang* to treat 20 patients with seizures and epilepsy, reducing the seizure frequency from an average of 13.4 +/- 3.4 to 10.7 +/- 2.5 per month.[21]
6. **Night restlessness**: Thirty-six patients with night restlessness were treated with 88.9% effectiveness using modified *Chai Hu Jia Long Gu Mu Li Tang*. The herbal formula contained *Chai Hu* (Radix Bupleuri) 12-20g, *Long Gu* (Os Draconis) 20-30g, *Mu Li* (Concha Ostreae) 20-30g, *Huang Qin* (Radix Scutellariae) 10-15g, *Fu Ling* (Poria) 10-15g, *Ban Xia* (Rhizoma Pinelliae) 10-15g, *Da Huang* (Radix et Rhizoma Rhei) 6-10g, *He Huan Hua* (Flos Albiziae) 20g, *Da Zao* (Fructus Jujubae) 3-5 pieces, and *Sheng Jiang* (Rhizoma Zingiberis Recens) 3-5 slices. *Long Dan* (Radix et Rhizoma Gentianae) and *Zhi Zi* (Fructus Gardeniae) were added for Liver fire rising; *Shen Qu* (Massa Fermentata) and *Lai Fu Zi* (Semen Raphani) for Stomach disharmony; *Huang Lian* (Rhizoma Coptidis) and *E Jiao* (Colla Corii Asini) for yin-deficient fire; and *Dang Shen*

Chái Hú Jiā Lóng Gŭ Mŭ Lì Tāng

(Bupleurum plus Dragon Bone and Oyster Shell Decoction)

(Radix Codonopsis) and *Dang Gui* (Radix Angelicae Sinensis) for Heart and Spleen deficiencies. Of 36 patients, the study reported significant improvement in 19 cases, moderate improvement in 13 cases, and no effect in 4 cases. The overall rate of effectiveness was 88.9%.[22]

7. **Postischemic brain injury**: Administration of three herbal formulas minimized postischemic brain injury by inhibiting production of free radicals and generation of lipid peroxidation. The three formulas found to be effective, both *in vitro* and *in vivo*, were *Chai Hu Jia Long Gu Mu Li Tang*, *Huang Lian Jie Du Tang* (Coptis Decoction to Relieve Toxicity), and *Gui Zhi Fu Ling Wan* (Cinnamon Twig and Poria Pill).[23]

HERB-DRUG INTERACTION

- **Carbamazepine**: Researchers evaluated the possibility of pharmacokinetic interactions between *Chai Hu Jia Long Gu Mu Li Tang* and carbamazepine. After extensive examination in rats, the researchers found no significant differences in the serum protein binding of carbamazepine and carbamazepine-10,11-epoxide, its active metabolite. Furthermore, one-week pretreatment with *Chai Hu Jia Long Gu Mu Li Tang* (1 g/kg/day) did not affect the plasma concentration-time profile or any pharmacokinetic parameter of carbamazepine or its metabolite. The researchers concluded that oral co-administration of *Chai Hu Jia Long Gu Mu Li Tang* with carbamazepine appears to be pharmacokinetically safe.[24]
- **Theophylline**: Administration of theophylline is often accompanied by side effects such as tachycardia and central nervous system stimulation. According to one study in rats and mice, administration of *Chai Hu Jia Long Gu Mu Li Tang* concurrent with theophylline successfully suppressed the cardiovascular and central nervous systems to alleviate theophylline-induced tachycardia, locomotion, and convulsions.[25]

TOXICOLOGY

Qian Dan (Minium), lead oxide red (Pb_3O_4), is a potentially toxic substance. Acute poisoning may occur following a bolus dose of 15 grams; chronic poisoning has been reported following daily ingestion of 2 mg of this mineral.[26] Two cases of anemia have been reported with the use of *Chai Hu Jia Long Gu Mu Li Tang* that contained *Qian Dan* (Minium). The cause of this toxicity was attributed to *Qian Dan* (Minium), as anemia is a potential consequence of lead poisoning.[27] Note: For additional information on the toxicity of *Qian Dan* (Minium), please refer to *Chinese Medical Herbology and Pharmacology* by John Chen and Tina Chen.

SUGGESTED ACUPUNCTURE TREATMENT

1. Points: *Yangchi* (TH 4), *Neiguan* (PC 6), *Qiuxu* (GB 40), *Ligou* (LR 5), *Shenmen* (HT 7), and *Tianshu* (ST 25).
2. Technique: even method.

Yangchi (TH 4), the *yuan* (source) point of the *San Jiao* channel, regulates qi circulation in all three *jiaos* and harmonizes the *shaoyang*. *Neiguan* (PC 6), the *luo* (connecting) point of the Pericardium channel, regulates qi circulation, removes stagnation, and redirects the reversed flow of Stomach qi. *Qiuxu* (GB 40), the *yuan* (source) point of the Gallbladder channel, sedates heat in the *shaoyang* and leads the fire downward. *Ligou* (LR 5), the *luo* (connecting) point of the Liver channel, regulates the qi flow of the Liver and relieves stagnation. *Qiuxu* (GB 40) and *Ligou* (LR 5) are therefore combined to relieve heat and stagnation associated with the Gallbladder and Liver. Finally, *Shenmen* (HT 7) and *Tianshu* (ST 25) help relieve *shaoyang* syndrome by tranquilizing the mind and harmonizing the interior and exterior.

AUTHORS' COMMENTS

Many behavioral disorders are rooted in Liver qi stagnation or Liver fire, which can be treated with *Chai Hu Jia Long Gu Mu Li Tang*. This formula is extremely adept at treating show anxiety in performance animals. Because of the stress of travel, and the confinement that often accompanies both equine and canine athletes, Liver stagnation and imbalance in the *shaoyang* are common occurrences. *Chai Hu Jia Long Gu Mu Li Tang* does not excessively sedate *shen*, so most animals will have no decrease in performance while on this formula. However, it is also not strong enough alone to treat patients with severe behavioral disorders or with accompanying deficiencies. In these cases, the following combinations may be employed:

- In the treatment of irritability, anxiety, restlessness, and night restlessness with more Heart and Liver yin and blood deficiencies, this formula can be combined with *Suan Zao Ren Tang* (Sour Jujube Decoction).
- For animals with more anxiety, restlessness, nervousness, fearfulness and noise hypersensitivity, and more Heart and Kidney yin deficiencies and Heart blood deficiency, combine with *Tian Wang Bu Xin Dan* (Emperor of Heaven's Special Pill to Tonify the Heart).
- For animals with Liver heat, red eyes, irritability, aggression and unpredictable behavior, combine with *Jia Wei Xiao Yao San* (Augmented Rambling Powder).
- For animals that are destructive at home with a tendency to work themselves into hysterical behavior, and that are nervous, anxious and hyperexcitable with more Heart qi

Chái Hú Jiā Lóng Gŭ Mŭ Lì Tāng

(Bupleurum plus Dragon Bone and Oyster Shell Decoction)

and yin deficiencies and Liver qi stagnation, combine with *Gan Mai Da Zao Tang* (Licorice, Wheat, and Jujube Decoction)

- In the treatment of hyperthyroidism and hypertension in cats with Kidney yin deficiency, combine with *Tian Wang Bu Xin Dan* (Emperor of Heaven's Special Pill to Tonify the Heart); and with deficiency heat, combine with *Zhi Bai Di Huang Wan* (Anemarrhena, Phellodendron, and Rehmannia Pill).

References

1. *Zhong Yao Ming Fang Yao Li Yu Ying Yong* (Pharmacology and Applications of Famous Herbal Formulas), 1989; 372-373.
2. *Guo Wai Yi Xue* (Foreign Medicine), 1992; 14(5):47.
3. Mizoguchi K, Yuzurihara M, Ishige A, Aburada M, Tabira T. Saiko-ka-ryukotsu-borei-to, a herbal medicine, ameliorates chronic stress-induced depressive state in rotarod performance. Pharmacol Biochem Behav. 2003 May; 75(2):419-25.
4. Mizoguchi K, Yuzurihara M, Ishige A, Sasaki H, Tabira T. Saiko-ka-ryukotsu-borei-to, an herbal medicine, prevents chronic stress-induced disruption of glucocorticoid negative feedback in rats. Life Sci. 2002 Nov 22; 72(1):67-77.
5. Koshikawa N, Imai T, Takahashi I, Yamauchi M, Sawada S, Kansaku A. Effects of Hochu-ekki-to, Yoku-kan-san and Saiko-ka-ryukotsu-borei-to on behavioral despair and acetic acid-induced writhing in mice. Methods Find Exp Clin Pharmacol. 1998 Jan-Feb;20(1):47-51.
6. Sasaki K, Suzuki K, Yoshizaki F, Ando T. Effect of saiko-ka-ryukotsu-borei-to on the stress-induced increase of serum corticosterone in mice. Biol Pharm Bull. 1995 Apr; 18(4):563-5.
7. Iizuka S, Ishige A, Komatsu Y, Matsumiya T, Tsuji M, Takeda H. Effects of Saiko-ka-ryukotsu-borei-to on irritable characteristics in El mice. Methods Find Exp Clin Pharmacol. 1998 Jan-Feb; 20(1):19-26.
8. Okano H, Ohkubo C. Anti-pressor effect of a Chinese-Japanese herbal medicine, saiko-ka-ryukotsu-borei-to on hemodynamics in rabbits. In Vivo. 1999 Jul-Aug; 13(4):333-7.
9. Wei MJ, Shintani F, Kanba S, Yagi G, Asai M, Kato R, Nakaki T. Endothelium-dependent and -independent vasoactive actions of a Japanese kampo medicine, Saiko-ka-ryukotsu-borei-to. Biomed Pharmacother. 1997; 51(1):38-43.
10. *Zhong Yi Fang Ji Xian Dai Yan Jiu* (Modern Study of Medical Formulas in Traditional Chinese Medicine), 1997; (1): 203.
11. Yoshie F, Iizuka A, Kubo M, Komatsu Y, Matsumoto A, Itakura H, Takeda H, Matsumiya T, Kondo K. Protective effects of Saiko-ka-ryukotsu-borei-to (Chai-Hu-Jia-Long-Gu-Mu-Li-Tang) against atherosclerosis in Kurosawa and Kusanagi-hypercholesterolemic (KHC) rabbits. Pharmacol Res. 2001 May; 43(5):481-8.
12. Chung HJ, Kim DW, Maruyama I, Tani T. Effects of traditional Chinese formulations on rat carotid artery injured by balloon endothelial denudation. Am J Chin Med. 2003; 31(2):201-12.
13. *Han Fang Yi Xue* (Kampo Medicine), 1986; 10(9):26.
14. *Shan Dong Zhong Yi Za Zhi* (Shandong Journal of Chinese Medicine), 1984; (3):24.
15. *Liao Ning Zhong Yi Za Zhi* (Liaoning Journal of Chinese Medicine), 1984; 12:34.
16. *Zhong Xi Yi Jie He Za Zhi* (Journal of Integrated Chinese and Western Medicine), 1986; 12:753.
17. *Shi Yong Zhong Xi Yi Jie He Za Zhi* (Practical Journal of Integrated Chinese and Western Medicines), 1998; 2:170.
18. *Fu Jian Zhong Yi Yao* (Fujian Chinese Medicine and Herbology), 1997; 4:12.
19. Nomura S, Hattori N, Sakakibara I, Fukuhara S. Effects of Saiko-ka-ryukotsu-borei-to in patients with hyperlipidemia. Phytomedicine. 2001 May; 8(3):165-73.
20. *Si Chuan Zhong Yi* (Sichuan Chinese Medicine), 1998, 7:36.
21. Hung-Ming W, Liu CS, Tsai JJ, Ko LY, Wei YH. Antioxidant and anticonvulsant effect of a modified formula of chaihu-longu-muli-tang. American Journal of Chinese Medicine. 2002; 30(2-3):339-46.
22. *Tian Jin Zhong Yi* (Tianjin Chinese Medicine), 1999; 2:25.
23. Fushitani S, Minakuchi K, Tsuchiya K, Takasugi M, Murakami K. Studies on attenuation of post-ischemic brain injury by kampo medicines-inhibitory effects of free radical production. Yakugaku Zasshi. 1995 Aug; 115(8):611-7.
24. Ohnishi N, Nakasako S, Okada K, Umehara S, Takara K, Nagasawa K, Yoshioka M, Kuroda K, Yokoyama T. Studies on interactions between traditional herbal and Western medicines. IV: lack of pharmacokinetic interactions between Saiko-ka-ryukotsu-borei-to and carbamazepine in rats. Eur J Drug Metab Pharmacokinet. 2001 Jan-Jun; 26(1-2):129-35.
25. Sanae F, Hayashi H, Chisaki K, Komatsu Y. Effects of Saiko-ka-ryukotsu-borei-to, a Japanese Kampo medicine, on tachycardia and central nervous system stimulation induced by theophylline in rats and mice. Jpn J Pharmacol. 1999 Mar; 79(3):283-8.
26. *Xian Dai Zhong Yao Yao Li Xue* (Contemporary Pharmacology of Chinese Herbs), 1997; 1425.
27. *Si Chuan Zhong Yi* (Sichuan Chinese Medicine), 1987; 5(12):30.

Section 2

滋养安神剂

— Nourishing Formulas that Calm the Shen (Spirit)

Suān Zǎo Rén Tāng (Sour Jujube Decoction)

酸棗仁湯

酸枣仁汤

Pinyin Name: *Suan Zao Ren Tang*
Literal Name: Sour Jujube Decoction
Alternate Names: *Suan Zao Tang*, Zizyphus Combination
Original Source: *Jin Gui Yao Lue* (Essentials from the Golden Cabinet) by Zhang Zhong-Jing in the Eastern Han Dynasty

COMPOSITION

Suan Zao Ren (Semen Ziziphi Spinosae), *chao* (dry-fried)	2 cups [15-18g]
Chuan Xiong (Rhizoma Chuanxiong)	6g [3-5g]
Fu Ling (Poria)	6g [10g]
Zhi Mu (Rhizoma Anemarrhenae)	6g [8-10g]
Gan Cao (Radix et Rhizoma Glycyrrhizae)	3g

DOSAGE / PREPARATION / ADMINISTRATION

The source text states to first dry-fry *Suan Zao Ren* (Semen Ziziphi Spinosae), crack the seeds open, and then cook them with 8 cups [1,600 mL] of water until only 6 cups [1,200 mL] of the liquid remain. Add the other ingredients and cook until the liquid is further reduced to 3 cups [600 mL]. Take the warm, strained decoction in three equally divided doses.

Note: Proper processing of *Suan Zao Ren* (Semen Ziziphi Spinosae) is extremely important, as it will determine the overall effectiveness of this formula. According to the source text, *Suan Zao Ren* (Semen Ziziphi Spinosae) must be dry-fried first, and then the seeds should be crushed open, before placing them in water for cooking. Dry-frying the seeds enhances the effects of tonifying Liver blood and treating night restlessness; crushing them maximizes extraction of the active ingredients.[1]

CHINESE THERAPEUTIC ACTIONS

1. Nourishes the blood and calms the *shen* (spirit)
2. Clears heat and relieves irritability

CLINICAL MANIFESTATIONS

Liver blood deficiency with deficiency heat rising: irritability, night restlessness, dizziness, dry mouth and throat, cracked hooves, claws and nails, dandruff, dry skin and hair coat, a red, dry tongue and a thin, wiry pulse.

VETERINARY CLINICAL APPLICATIONS

Night restlessness, aggression, hyperactivity, obsessive-compulsive behaviors, irritability, geriatric vestibular disease and noise sensitivity.

EXPLANATION

Suan Zao Ren Tang (Sour Jujube Decoction) treats night restlessness characterized by Liver blood deficiency with deficiency heat rising, caused by over-exertion or chronic consumption. Cracked hooves, claws and nails, dandruff, dry skin and hair coat, and a dry mouth and throat are caused by blood deficiency and lack of adequate nourishment to the Heart. Animals with this syndrome may have yin deficiency and deficiency heat, which can cause irritability, palpitations, and night restlessness. Liver blood deficiency may contribute to hyperactivity of Liver yang, leading to dizziness.

Suān Zǎo Rén Tāng (Sour Jujube Decoction)

Suan Zao Ren Tang **(Sour Jujube Decoction)**

Diagnosis	Clinical Signs	Treatment	Herbs
Liver blood deficiency with deficiency heat rising	• Night restlessness and irritability: interior heat disturbing *shen* (spirit) and consuming yin • Cracked hooves, claws and nails, dandruff, dry skin and hair coat, and a dry mouth and throat: blood deficiency unable to nourish the Heart • Aggression, irritability, and dizziness: Liver blood deficiency with hyperactivity of Liver yang	• Nourishes the blood and calms the *shen* • Clears heat and relieves irritability	• *Suan Zao Ren* (Semen Ziziphi Spinosae) nourishes Liver blood and calms Heart *shen*. • *Chuan Xiong* (Rhizoma Chuanxiong) regulates Liver blood. • *Fu Ling* (Poria) tranquilizes the mind and calms the *shen*. • *Zhi Mu* (Rhizoma Anemarrhenae) nourishes yin and clears deficiency heat. • *Gan Cao* (Radix et Rhizoma Glycyrrhizae) clears heat and harmonizes all of the herbs.

Suan Zao Ren (Semen Ziziphi Spinosae), the chief herb of this formula, nourishes Liver blood and calms Heart *shen* (spirit). *Chuan Xiong* (Rhizoma Chuanxiong) regulates Liver blood. *Fu Ling* (Poria) tranquilizes the mind and calms the *shen*. *Zhi Mu* (Rhizoma Anemarrhenae) nourishes yin and clears deficiency heat. *Gan Cao* (Radix et Rhizoma Glycyrrhizae) clears heat and harmonizes all of the herbs in this formula.

VETERINARY MODIFICATIONS

- If there is qi deficiency, add *Ren Shen* (Radix et Rhizoma Ginseng) and *Huang Qi* (Radix Astragali Membranacei).
- With more yin deficiency and qi stagnation, combine with *Yi Guan Jian* (Linking Decoction).
- With severe night sweats, add *Mu Li* (Concha Ostreae) and *Fu Xiao Mai* (Fructus Tritici Levis).
- With irritability, thirst, and night restlessness, add *Mai Dong* (Tuber Ophiopogonis Japonici) and *Wu Wei Zi* (Fructus Schisandrae Chinensis).
- For night restlessness due to blood deficiency, add *Dang Gui* (Radix Angelicae Sinensis), *Shu Di Huang* (Radix Rehmanniae Glutinosae Conquitae), and *He Shou Wu* (Radix Polygoni Multiflori).
- With fright and palpitations, add *Yuan Zhi* (Radix Polygalae Tenuifoliae) and *Shi Chang Pu* (Rhizoma Acori Graminei).
- With palpitations and excessive vocalization and twitching while sleeping, or waking up at night due to Heart and Gallbladder deficiencies, add *Dang Shen* (Radix Codonopsis) and *Long Chi* (Dens Draconis).
- With deficiency fire flaring, remove *Chuan Xiong* (Rhizoma Chuanxiong) and add *Bai Shao* (Radix Paeoniae Alba), *Di Huang* (Radix Rehmanniae), and *Huang Lian* (Rhizoma Coptidis).

PHARMACOLOGICAL EFFECTS

Central nervous system: Administration of *Suan Zao Ren Tang* was associated with marked sedative and hypnotic effects. According to various experiments in mice, rats, guinea pigs, rabbits, dogs, and humans, administration of the formula decreased spontaneous physical activities, inhibited caffeine-induced stimulation, and potentiated the effects of sedative and hypnotic drugs.[2]

HUMAN CLINICAL STUDIES AND RESEARCH

Insomnia: Use of modified *Suan Zao Ren Tang* was associated with 91.7% effectiveness in treating insomnia. Modifications were made by adding *Long Dan* (Radix et Rhizoma Gentianae) and *Chai Hu* (Radix Bupleuri) for restlessness, irritability, anger, red eyes, a bitter taste in the mouth, red tongue, yellow tongue coating, and a wiry, rapid pulse; *Tao Ren* (Semen Persicae), *Hong Hua* (Flos Carthami), and *Shou Wu Teng* (Caulis Polygoni Multiflori) for blood stagnation; *E Jiao* (Colla Corii Asini), *Huang Bo* (Cortex Phellodendri Chinensis), and *Bie Jia* (Carapax Trionycis) for yin-deficient heat; *Dang Shen* (Radix Codonopsis), *Huang Qi* (Radix Astragali), and *He Huan Pi* (Cortex Albiziae) for qi and blood deficiencies; *Huang Qi* (Radix Astragali) and *Yuan Zhi* (Radix Polygalae) for Heart qi deficiency; and *Dan Nan Xing* (Arisaema cum Bile) and *Zhu Li* (Succus Bambusae) for profuse sputum. The herbs were given 30 minutes before bedtime. Of 72 patients, the study reported recovery in 47 cases, significant improvement in 12 cases, moderate improvement in 7 cases, and no effect in 6 cases.[3] In another study, 20 out of 31 patients (64.5%) reported improvement following ingestion of 2.5g of an extract preparation of *Suan Zao Ren Tang*. Improvement was defined as shorter time needed to fall asleep, better quality of sleep, and better energy during the following day.[4]

SUGGESTED ACUPUNCTURE TREATMENT

1. Points: *Ganshu* (BL 18), *Housanli* (ST 36), *Taixi* (KI 3), *Sanyinjiao* (SP 6), *Neiguan* (PC 6), *Shenmen* (HT 7), *Xingjian* (LR 2), *Anshen* and *Dafengmen*.

Suān Zǎo Rén Tāng (Sour Jujube Decoction)

2. Technique: tonification.

Ganshu (BL 18) and *Housanli* (ST 36) nourish both qi and blood. *Taixi* (KI 3) and *Sanyinjiao* (SP 6) nourish yin and blood of the Liver and Kidney. *Neiguan* (PC 6) and *Shenmen* (HT 7) together calm the *shen* (spirit). *Xingjian* (LR 2) clears Liver fire to calm the *shen*. *Anshen* and *Dafengmen* are classical veterinary acupuncture points to calm the *shen*.

AUTHORS' COMMENTS

Suan Zao Ren Tang is one of the most commonly used formulas for treating night restlessness caused by deficiency, irritability, and consumption. Key clinical signs include palpitations, dry mouth and throat, and a thin, wiry pulse. For dog owners with animals that keep them awake by repeatedly pacing the house or jumping on and off the bed, this formula can be very helpful for restoring harmony to the home. It is most effective if given an hour or two before the humans are expected to retire. For horses, this formula can be used for such daytime vices as weaving, stall walking, and repetitive wall kicking. It is also useful in performance horses that have developed irritability from overwork that depletes yin.

Suan Zao Ren and *Tian Wang Bu Xin Dan* (Emperor of Heaven's Special Pill to Tonify the Heart) are often used in combination to treat yin and blood deficiencies of *both* the Heart and Liver that result in behavioral disorder and/or night restlessness, especially in geriatric animals. It can be combined in a 1:1 ratio and re-evaluated in 2-4 weeks.

Suan Zao Ren Tang, *Tian Wang Bu Xin Dan* (Emperor of Heaven's Special Pill to Tonify the Heart), and *Gan Mai Da Zao Tang* (Licorice, Wheat, and Jujube Decoction) all treat sleep disorders, night restlessness, and anxiety caused by lack of nourishment to the Heart and leading to *shen* (spirit) disturbance.

- *Suan Zao Ren Tang* is best for nourishing Liver blood and clearing deficiency heat. Chief manifestations include aggression, irritability, night restlessness, and a dry mouth and throat.
- *Tian Wang Bu Xin Dan* is better for nourishing yin and blood caused by Kidney and Heart deficiencies. Chief manifestations include anxiety, being easily frightened, noise sensitivity, decreased sleep, palpitations, and poor concentration and focus.
- *Gan Mai Da Zao Tang* harmonizes the middle *jiao*, relieves pain, and treats yin deficiency of the *zang* organs with Liver qi stagnation and Heart deficiency. Chief manifestations include hyperexcitability, an inability to calm down, restlessness, and behavioral disorders of a repetitive (compulsive) nature.

Please refer to *Gui Pi Tang* (Restore the Spleen Decoction) for a comparison of the uses, similarities, and differences between *Tian Wang Bu Xin Dan* (Emperor of Heaven's Special Pill to Tonify the Heart) and *Suan Zao Ren Tang*.

References

1. *Zhe Jiang Zhong Yi Za Zhi* (Zhejiang Journal of Chinese Medicine), 1966; (1).
2. *Zhong Yi Fang Ji Xian Dai Yan Jiu* (Modern Study of Medical Formulas in Traditional Chinese Medicine), 1997; 849-850.
3. *He Nan Zhong Yi* (Henan Chinese Medicine), 1999; 6:9.
4. *Shan Dong Yi Kan* (Shandong Medical Journal), 1965, 27.

Tiān Wáng Bŭ Xīn Dān

(Emperor of Heaven's Special Pill to Tonify the Heart)

天王補心丹
天王补心丹

Pinyin Name: *Tian Wang Bu Xin Dan*
Literal Name: Emperor of Heaven's Special Pill to Tonify the Heart
Alternate Name: Ginseng and Zizyphus Formula
Original Source: *Jiao Zhu Fu Ren Liang Fang* (Revised Fine Formulas for Women) by Bi Li-Zhai in the 16th century

COMPOSITION

Di Huang (Radix Rehmanniae), *xi* (washed) with liquor	120g [12g]
Xuan Shen (Radix Scrophulariae)	15g [5g]
Tian Dong (Radix Asparagi)	30g [9g]
Mai Dong (Radix Ophiopogonis)	30g [9g]
Dan Shen (Radix et Rhizoma Salviae Miltiorrhizae)	15g [5g]
Dang Gui (Radix Angelicae Sinensis), *jin* (soaked) with liquor	30g [9g]
Ren Shen (Radix et Rhizoma Ginseng)	15g [5g]
Fu Ling (Poria)	15g [5g]
Suan Zao Ren (Semen Ziziphi Spinosae), *chao* (dry-fried)	30g [9g]
Wu Wei Zi (Fructus Schisandrae Chinensis)	30g [9g]
Bai Zi Ren (Semen Platycladi)	30g [9g]
Yuan Zhi (Radix Polygalae)	15g [5g]
Jie Geng (Radix Platycodonis)	15g [5g]

DOSAGE / PREPARATION / ADMINISTRATION

Grind the ingredients into powder and form into small pills with honey. The pills should resemble the size of *Wu Tong Zi* (Semen Firmianae), a small seed approximately 5 mm in diameter. Coat the pills with 9-15g of powdered *Zhu Sha* (Cinnabaris). Take 20-30 pills [9g] per dose on an empty stomach with either warm/hot boiled water or with a decoction of *Zhu Ye* (Herba Phyllostachys). Today, this formula may be prepared and administered as pills or decoction. For pills, take 9g per dose with warm/hot boiled water. For decoction, use the suggested doses in brackets above.

Note: *Zhu Sha* (Cinnabaris) is a potentially toxic heavy metal, and is rarely used as a medicinal substance today. Its discussion here is included primarily for academic purposes, to reflect the historical use of this substance in its original formulation. Most herbal products today have removed it completely, or replaced it with substitutes with similar functions. For additional information on the toxicity, please refer to *Chinese Medical Herbology and Pharmacology* by John Chen and Tina Chen.

CHINESE THERAPEUTIC ACTIONS

1. Nourishes yin and tonifies the blood
2. Tonifies the Heart and Kidney
3. Calms the *shen* (spirit)

CLINICAL MANIFESTATIONS

Heart and Kidney deficiencies with yin and blood insufficiencies: lethargy, generalized weakness and deficiency, irritability, night restlessness, palpitations, anxiety, nervousness, dry stools, mouth and tongue ulceration, a red dry tongue with little coating, and a thready, rapid pulse.

VETERINARY CLINICAL APPLICATIONS

Behavioral disorder, feline hyperthyroidism, night restlessness, mouth and tongue ulceration.

EXPLANATION

Tian Wang Bu Xin Dan (Emperor of Heaven's Special Pill to Tonify the Heart) is designed to treat Heart and Kidney deficiencies with yin and blood insufficiencies. Heart blood deficiency may lead to hyperactivity of yang, resulting in lack of concentration, irritability, night restlessness, and palpitations. Deficiency of blood may cause malnourishment of the body, leading to lethargy. Dry stools indicate yin deficiency with insufficient nourishment to the bowels. Since the tongue is the sensory organ that belongs to the Heart, Heart yin deficiency may lead to tongue ulcerations. A red tongue with little coating, and a thready, rapid pulse, both suggest yin deficiency.

Tiān Wáng Bǔ Xīn Dān

(Emperor of Heaven's Special Pill to Tonify the Heart)

Tian Wang Bu Xin Dan **(Emperor of Heaven's Special Pill to Tonify the Heart)**

Diagnosis	Clinical Signs	Treatment	Herbs
Heart and Kidney deficiencies with yin and blood insufficiencies	• Lack of focus, nervousness, and anxiety: Heart blood deficiency • Irritability and night restlessness: hyperactivity of yang due to Heart blood deficiency • Lethargy: malnourishment of the body due to blood deficiency • Dry stools: yin-deficient fire consuming body fluids • Tongue ulcerations: yin-deficient fire rising upward • Red tongue with little coating and a thready, rapid pulse: yin-deficient fire	• Nourishes yin and tonifies the blood • Tonifies the Heart and Kidney • Calms the *shen* (spirit)	• *Di Huang* (Radix Rehmanniae) tonifies yin and blood, moistens dryness and helps to control hyperactivity of yang. • *Xuan Shen* (Radix Scrophulariae), *Tian Dong* (Radix Asparagi), and *Mai Dong* (Radix Ophiopogonis) tonify yin to clear deficiency fire. • *Dan Shen* (Radix et Rhizoma Salviae Miltiorrhizae) and *Dang Gui* (Radix Angelicae Sinensis) tonify blood and activate blood circulation. • *Ren Shen* (Radix et Rhizoma Ginseng) and *Fu Ling* (Poria) tonify qi and calm the *shen*. • *Suan Zao Ren* (Semen Ziziphi Spinosae) and *Wu Wei Zi* (Fructus Schisandrae Chinensis) astringe the Heart qi to calm the *shen*. • *Bai Zi Ren* (Semen Platycladi), *Yuan Zhi* (Radix Polygalae) and *Zhu Sha* (Cinnabaris) nourish the Heart to calm the *shen*. • *Jie Geng* (Radix Platycodonis) leads all of the herbs to the upper *jiao*. • *Zhu Sha* (Cinnabaris) and *Zhu Ye* (Herba Phyllostachys) calm the *shen* and guide the formula to the Heart.

Di Huang (Radix Rehmanniae) is the chief herb in this formula. It tonifies yin and blood, helps to control hyperactivity of yang, and moistens dryness. It also nourishes Kidney water, and helps to control Heart fire. *Xuan Shen* (Radix Scrophulariae), *Tian Dong* (Radix Asparagi), and *Mai Dong* (Radix Ophiopogonis) tonify yin to clear deficiency fire. *Dan Shen* (Radix et Rhizoma Salviae Miltiorrhizae) and *Dang Gui* (Radix Angelicae Sinensis) tonify blood and activate blood circulation. *Ren Shen* (Radix et Rhizoma Ginseng) and *Fu Ling* (Poria) tonify qi and calm the *shen* (spirit). *Suan Zao Ren* (Semen Ziziphi Spinosae) and *Wu Wei Zi* (Fructus Schisandrae Chinensis) astringe Heart qi to calm the *shen*. *Bai Zi Ren* (Semen Platycladi), *Yuan Zhi* (Radix Polygalae), and *Zhu Sha* (Cinnabaris) nourish the Heart to calm the *shen*. *Jie Geng* (Radix Platycodonis) is a channel-guiding herb that leads all of the herbs to the upper *jiao*. *Zhu Sha* (Cinnabaris) and *Zhu Ye* (Herba Phyllostachys) calm the *shen* and guide the formula to the Heart.

VETERINARY MODIFICATIONS

- With ulcerations of the mouth and tongue, add *Huang Lian* (Rhizoma Coptidis) and *Mu Dan Pi* (Cortex Moutan Radicis); or combine with *Qing Wei San* (Clear the Stomach Powder).
- If there is constipation, add *Zhi Shi* (Fructus Immaturus Citri Aurantii) and *Hou Po* (Cortex Magnoliae Officinalis); or combine with *Ma Zi Ren Wan* (Hemp Seed Pill).
- With severe palpitations, night restlessness, add *Long Yan Rou* (Arillus Longanae Euphoriae) and *Shou Wu Teng* (Caulis Polygoni Multiflori).
- With inability to concentrate, or to enhance memory, add *Yuan Zhi* (Radix Polygalae), *Shi Chang Pu* (Rhizoma Acori Tatarinowii), and *Yin Xing Ye* (Folium Ginkgo).
- For severe night restlessness, add *Long Gu* (Os Draconis) and *Ci Shi* (Magnetitum).
- With dizziness, add *Chuan Xiong* (Rhizoma Chuanxiong) and *Bai Zhi* (Radix Angelicae Dahuricae).
- For irritability, aggression, night restlessness or restless sleep, add *Suan Zao Ren Tang* (Sour Jujube Decoction).

CAUTIONS / CONTRAINDICATIONS

- While taking *Tian Wang Bu Xin Dan*, avoid the following: cilantro, garlic, radishes, seafood, and liquor.
- This formula contains many rich tonics, which make it unsuitable for long-term use by animals that have Spleen

Tiān Wáng Bŭ Xīn Dān

(Emperor of Heaven's Special Pill to Tonify the Heart)

and Stomach deficiencies, or those with damp or phlegm accumulation.

- According to one report, use of this formula may cause occasional side effects such as indigestion, epigastric fullness and distention, mild diarrhea, skin rashes, and itching.[1]

PHARMACOLOGICAL EFFECTS

1. **Central nervous system**: Many herbs in *Tian Wang Bu Xin Dan* have marked sedative and hypnotic effects, including *Dang Gui* (Radix Angelicae Sinensis), *Fu Ling* (Sclerotium Poriae Cocos), *Yuan Zhi* (Radix Polygalae Tenuifoliae), *Bai Zi Ren* (Semen Biotae Orientalis), and *Suan Zao Ren* (Semen Ziziphi Spinosae). Furthermore, some of the herbs also improve cognitive functions, such as *Ren Shen* (Radix et Rhizoma Ginseng) and *Wu Wei Zi* (Fructus Schisandrae Chinensis).[2]
2. **Cardiovascular**: Laboratory experiments in mice showed administration of the formula to be beneficial in cases of shock, angina, arrhythmia, and hypoxia. The mechanisms of action are attributed to increased blood perfusion to the heart and increased resistance to hypoxia.[3]

HUMAN CLINICAL STUDIES AND RESEARCH

1. **Neurasthenia**: In one study, 218 patients with neurasthenia were treated with *Tian Wang Bu Xin Dan* with an overall 66.5% rate of effectiveness. The treatment protocol was to administer the herbs in pills, 10-15 pills (1 g/pill) three times daily before meals and at bedtime. The duration of treatment was 30 days per course.[4]
2. **Coronary heart disease**: *Tian Wang Bu Xin Dan* has beneficial effects in treating coronary heart disease, angina, hypotension, palpitations and insomnia. It was noted that the dose of *Ren Shen* (Radix et Rhizoma Ginseng) should be 15g or above to have significant impact.[5]
3. **Angina**: Use of modified *Tian Wang Bu Xin Dan* in 35 patients with angina was associated with complete recovery in 10 cases, improvement in 20 cases, and no effect in 5 cases. In addition to *Tian Wang Bu Xin Dan* as the base formula, modifications were made as needed. For a feeling of severe oppression in the chest, *Fo Shou* (Fructus Citri Sarcodactylis), *Zhi Shi* (Fructus Aurantii Immaturus), and *Tan Xiang* (Lignum Santali Albi) were added. For severe angina pain, a preparation containing *Su He Xiang* (Styrax) and *Bing Pian* (Borneolum Syntheticum) was added. For Heart yin deficiency, *Dang Shen* (Radix Codonopsis) was added. For insomnia, *Shou Wu Teng* (Caulis Polygoni Multiflori) and *He Huan Pi* (Cortex Albiziae) were added. For a thick, greasy tongue coating, *Gua Lou* (Fructus Trichosanthis) was added. And, for irregular heartbeat, *Zhi Gan Cao* (Radix et Rhizoma Glycyrrhizae Praeparata cum Melle) was added.[6]
4. **Viral myocarditis**: In one study of 23 patients with viral myocarditis, use of modified *Tian Wang Bu Xin Dan* daily for 1-3 courses of treatment (10 days per course) was associated with 95.6% effectiveness. In addition to *Tian Wang Bu Xin Dan*, intravenous infusion of *Dan Shen* (Radix et Rhizoma Salviae Miltiorrhizae) was given for cases of severe blood stagnation. Of 23 cases, the study reported complete recovery in 16 cases, moderate improvement in 6 cases, and no effect in 1 case.[7]
5. **Insomnia**: Administration of *Tian Wang Bu Xin Dan* showed marked effectiveness in the treatment of insomnia. Depending on the dose and dosage form, the rate of success ranged from 87-96%.[8]
6. **Impotence**: Administration of modified *Tian Wang Bu Xin Dan* effectively treated 30 of 37 patients with impotence. The herbal treatment was based on *Tian Wang Bu Xin Dan*, with the addition of *Zhu Ye* (Herba Phyllostachys), *Mu Tong* (Caulis Akebiae), and *Zhu Sha* (Cinnabaris) for ulcerations of the mouth and tongue as well as burning sensations and pain in the penis; *Jin Ying Zi* (Fructus Rosae Laevigatae) and *Qian Shi* (Semen Euryales) for premature ejaculation and seminal emission; and *Gan Mai Da Zao Tang* (Licorice, Wheat, and Jujube Decoction) for palpitations with fear and fright. In addition to herbs, patients were advised to control their emotions, avoid spicy and pungent foods, and not to engage in excessive sexual activity.[9]

TOXICOLOGY

Use of *Tian Wang Bu Xin Dan* has been associated with side effects such as a general feeling of warmth, thirst, rash and eczema of the entire body.[10] Note: These reactions are due to older formulations of the product containing *Zhu Sha* (Cinnabaris), a potentially toxic substance, in the coating of the pellets. Most products today do ***not*** contain *Zhu Sha* (Cinnabaris), and should not cause these side effects.

SUGGESTED ACUPUNCTURE TREATMENT

1. Points: *Shenshu* (BL 23), *Taixi* (KI 3), *Geshu* (BL 17), *Housanli* (ST 36), *Baihui* (GV 20), *Neiguan* (PC 6), *Shenmen* (HT 7), *Xinshu* (BL 15), *Anshen* and *Dafengmen*.
2. Technique: tonification.

Shenshu (BL 23) and *Taixi* (KI 3) nourish Kidney yin to clear deficiency heat. *Geshu* (BL 17) and *Housanli* (ST 36) nourish qi and blood. *Baihui* (GV 20), *Neiguan* (PC 6) and *Shenmen* (HT 7) are combined to calm the *shen* (spirit).

Tiān Wáng Bǔ Xīn Dān

(Emperor of Heaven's Special Pill to Tonify the Heart)

Xinshu (BL 15) nourishes the Heart to calm the *shen*. *Anshen* and *Dafengmen* are classical veterinary points to calm the *shen*.

RELATED FORMULAS

Tiān Wáng Bǔ Xīn Dān
(Emperor of Heaven's Special Pill to Tonify the Heart)
天王補心丹
天王补心丹
Pinyin Name: *Tian Wang Bu Xin Dan*
Literal Name: Emperor of Heaven's Special Pill to Tonify the Heart
Original Source: *She Sheng Mi Pou* (Secrets Investigations into Obtaining Health) by Hong Ji in 1638

Di Huang (Radix Rehmanniae), *xi* (washed) with liquor	120g
Ren Shen (Radix et Rhizoma Ginseng)	15g
Dan Shen (Radix et Rhizoma Salviae Miltiorrhizae), *chao* (dry-fried) lightly	15g
Xuan Shen (Radix Scrophulariae), *chao* (dry-fried) lightly	15g
Fu Ling (Poria)	15g
Wu Wei Zi (Fructus Schisandrae Chinensis), *hong* (baked)	30g
Yuan Zhi (Radix Polygalae), *chao* (dry-fried)	15g
Jie Geng (Radix Platycodonis)	15g
Dang Gui (Radix Angelicae Sinensis), *xi* (washed) with liquor	30g
Tian Dong (Radix Asparagi)	30g
Mai Dong (Radix Ophiopogonis)	30g
Bai Zi Ren (Semen Platycladi), *chao* (dry-fried)	30g
Suan Zao Ren (Semen Ziziphi Spinosae)	30g

This formula has functions to moisten yin, nourish the blood, tonify the Heart, and calm the *shen* (spirit). It is used to treat dry mouth and throat, ulcerations of the mouth and tongue, dry stools, a red tongue with a thin tongue coating, and thready, rapid pulse.

These two formulas have the same name, as well as similar functions and clinical applications.

- *Tian Wang Bu Xin Dan* from *Jiao Zhu Fu Ren Liang Fang* (Revised Fine Formulas for Women) is generally considered to be the representative formula, since this composition is the one most commonly used today.
- *Tian Wang Bu Xin Dan* from *She Sheng Mi Pou* (Secrets Investigations into Obtaining Health) is usually considered to be a related formula, but it was published approximately 200 years later. It has the same composition, but differs slightly in doses.

Bǎi Zǐ Yǎng Xīn Wán
(Biota Seed Pill to Nourish the Heart)
柏子養心丸
柏子养心丸
Pinyin Name: *Bai Zi Yang Xin Wan*
Literal Name: Biota Seed Pill to Nourish the Heart
Original Source: *Ti Ren Hui Bian* (Compilation of Materials of Benevolence for the Body) by Peng Yong-Guang in 1549

Bai Zi Ren (Semen Platycladi)	120g [12g]
Gou Qi Zi (Fructus Lycii)	90g [9g]
Mai Dong (Radix Ophiopogonis)	30g [5g]
Dang Gui (Radix Angelicae Sinensis)	30g [5g]
Shi Chang Pu (Rhizoma Acori Tatarinowii)	30g [5g]
Fu Shen (Poria Paradicis)	30g [5g]
Xuan Shen (Radix Scrophulariae)	60g [6g]
Shu Di Huang (Radix Rehmanniae Praeparata)	60g [6g]
Gan Cao (Radix et Rhizoma Glycyrrhizae)	15g [5g]

The source text states to grind the ingredients into powder and form into small pills with honey. The pills should resemble the size of *Wu Tong Zi* (Semen Firmianae), a small seed approximately 5 mm in diameter. Take 40-50 pills [6g] per dose. Today, this formula may be prepared as a decoction using the suggested doses in brackets.

The main actions of this formula are to nourish the Heart, calm the *shen* (spirit), tonify the Kidney, and nourish yin. *Bai Zi Yang Xin Wan* (Biota Seed Pill to Nourish the Heart) treats disharmony of the Heart and Kidney with deficiency of *ying* (nutrition) and blood, manifesting in clinical signs such as severe palpitations, excessive dreams, restlessness and dream-disturbed sleep, and lack of concentration. This formula focuses more on treating the root disorder (lack of harmony between the Heart-Fire and Kidney-Water) than does *Tian Wang Bu Xin Dan*.

AUTHORS' COMMENTS

In addition to treating night restlessness and behavioral disorder in the dog and cat, *Tian Wang Bu Xin Dan* is useful in treating feline hyperthyroidism with secondary hypertrophic cardiomyopathy. This formula can be used to strengthen the cat before undergoing radioiodine therapy, and can also be given following the treatment. The average duration of treatment is one to three months. It can be combined with *Chai Hu Shu Gan San* (Bupleurum Powder to Spread the Liver) to treat the Liver qi stagnation that often accompanies this condition. This formula contains many rich and cloying herbs, and can cause nausea and vomiting in cats which are Spleen deficient.

Tiān Wáng Bǔ Xīn Dān

(Emperor of Heaven's Special Pill to Tonify the Heart)

This is often the case in that many hyperthyroid cats are fed an exclusive commercial dry food diet and so have developed damp and phlegm accumulation in the middle *jiao*. In these cases, it can be combined with *Liu Jun Zi Tang* (Six-Gentlemen Decoction), and dietary therapy should be instituted.

In the authors' experience, *Tian Wang Bu Xin Dan* should be considered the formula of choice in treating behavioral disorders resulting from what might be called post-traumatic stress. This can occur in rescue animals coming from abusive situations, animals that have survived a severe physical trauma like a car accident or fire, or even an emotional trauma like losing a longtime companion. In such instances, the harmony between the Heart and Kidney is severely and acutely damaged and in need of repair. Clients should be counseled that such repair takes time and that treatment may take months of herbal therapy and may need concurrent behavioral training as well.

Tian Wang Bu Xin Dan and *Bai Zi Yang Xin Wan* (Biota Seed Pill to Nourish the Heart) both treat night restlessness. Their differences are as follows:

- *Tian Wang Bu Xin Dan* treats both the cause and the clinical signs of night restlessness by nourishing yin, tonifying the blood, benefiting qi, and calming the Heart. It is one of the most commonly used formulas for treating behavioral disorders characterized by anxiety, nervousness, noise sensitivity, and night restlessness arising from yin and blood deficiencies. It can be combined with *Suan Zao Ren* (Semen Ziziphi Spinosae), *Chai Hu Jia Long Gu Mu Li Tang* (Bupleurum plus Dragon Bone and Oyster Shell Decoction), or *Jia Wei Xiao Yao San* (Augmented Rambling Powder) for the treatment of behavioral disorder characterized by aggression.
- *Bai Zi Yang Xin Wan* is primarily a tonic formula that treats night restlessness by focusing more on treating the root disorder (lack of harmony between the Heart-Fire and Kidney-Water) than does *Tian Wang Bu Xin Dan.*

Tian Wang Bu Xin Dan and *Gui Pi Tang* (Restore the Spleen Decoction) both nourish the Heart and calm the *shen* (spirit) to treat palpitations, poor concentration, and night restlessness.

- *Tian Wang Bu Xin Dan* is indicated for patients with disharmony of the Heart and Kidney, in which a deficient Kidney yin is unable to nourish the Heart, and thus creates Heart fire. Besides blood deficiency signs of palpitations, lack of concentration, and night restlessness, clinical signs of Heart fire will also manifest, such as irritability, ulcers on the tongue, and dry stools or constipation. This formula uses herbs that not only nourish yin and blood, but also have tranquilizing and calming effects, such *Suan Zao Ren* (Semen Ziziphi Spinosae), *Bai Zi Ren* (Semen Platycladi), *Yuan Zhi* (Radix Polygalae), *Tian Dong* (Radix Asparagi), and *Mai Dong* (Radix Ophiopogonis).
- *Gui Pi Tang* is designed for patients that worry excessively, resulting in qi and blood deficiencies of the Spleen and Heart. Other than *shen* (spirit) disturbance signs, they will exhibit poor appetite, lethargy, exercise intolerance, spontaneous sweating, and other Spleen deficiency signs. Therefore, besides tranquilizing herbs such as *Suan Zao Ren* (Semen Ziziphi Spinosae), *Fu Shen* (Poria Paradicis), *Long Yan Rou* (Arillus Longan), and *Yuan Zhi* (Radix Polygalae), this formula contains Spleen tonic herbs, such as *Ren Shen* (Radix et Rhizoma Ginseng), *Huang Qi* (Radix Astragali), *Bai Zhu* (Rhizoma Atractylodis Macrocephalae), and *Gan Cao* (Radix et Rhizoma Glycyrrhizae). *Mu Xiang* (Radix Aucklandiae) is added to regulate qi and awaken the Spleen. This formula can also be used for bleeding or bruising due to a deficient Spleen not being able to retain the blood inside the vessels.[11]

Tian Wang Bu Xin Dan and *Zhi Gan Cao Tang* (Honey-Fried Licorice Decoction) both nourish yin and blood, and thus address the palpitations, anxiety, night restlessness, and dry stools.

- *Tian Wang Bu Xin Dan* is better for Heart yin and blood deficiencies with excess Heart yang flaring. Anxiety, decreased sleep, palpitations, withered *shen* (spirit), nocturnal emissions, and nervousness are the result of the *shen* not being nourished. Therefore, nourishing herbs as well as *shen*-calming herbs are used in this formula.
- *Zhi Gan Cao Tang* is mainly used for qi and blood deficiencies. Blood deficiency results in an inability to nourish the Heart. With the qi being deficient, the yang is weak and cannot generate the pulse, leading to a bounding or intermittent pulse. Qi tonics, along with yin and blood tonics, are used to generate the pulse. *Shu Di Huang* (Radix Rehmanniae Praeparata), *Sheng Jiang* (Rhizoma Zingiberis Recens), *E Jiao* (Colla Corii Asini), *Mai Dong* (Radix Ophiopogonis), and *Da Zao* (Fructus Jujubae) nourish yin and blood. *Ren Shen* (Radix et Rhizoma Ginseng) and *Zhi Gan Cao* (Radix et Rhizoma Glycyrrhizae Praeparata cum Melle) warm and tonify qi. *Gui Zhi* (Ramulus Cinnamomi) and *Sheng Jiang* (Rhizoma Zingiberis Recens) assist Heart yang to generate the pulse. This formula can also be used for Lung qi and yin deficiencies, manifesting in emaciation, shortness of breath, anxiety, poor sleep, and spontaneous sweating.[12]

Tiān Wáng Bǔ Xīn Dān
(Emperor of Heaven's Special Pill to Tonify the Heart)

References

1. *Zhong Yao Ming Fang Yao Li Yu Ying Yong* (Pharmacology and Applications of Famous Herbal Formulas), 1989; 318-319.
2. *Zhong Yi Fang Ji Xian Dai Yan Jiu* (Modern Study of Medical Formulas in Traditional Chinese Medicine), 1997; 853-854.
3. *Zhong Xi Yi Jie He Yan Jiu Zi Liao* (Research Information on Integration of Chinese and Western Medicine), 1976; 6:7.
4. *Zhong Xi Yi Jie He Yan Jiu Zi Liao* (Research Information on Integration of Chinese and Western Medicine), 1976; 6:7.
5. *Si Chuan Zhong Yi* (Sichuan Chinese Medicine), 1986; 1:48.
6. *Zhe Jiang Zhong Yi Za Zhi* (Zhejiang Journal of Chinese Medicine), 1998; 11:513.
7. *Zhong Guo Yi Yao Xue Bao* (Chinese Journal of Medicine and Herbology), 1998; 6:38.
8. *He Nan Zhong Yi* (Henan Chinese Medicine), 1992; 2:83.
9. *Shan Xi Zhong Yi* (Shanxi Chinese Medicine), 1990; 11(5):224.
10. *Zhong Yao Bu Liang Fan Ying Yu Zhi Liao* (Adverse Reactions and Treatment of Chinese Herbal Medicine), 1996; 60.
11. Wang MZ, et al. *Zhong Yi Xue Wen Da Ti Ku* (Questions and Answers on Traditional Chinese Medicine: Herbal Formulas).
12. Wang MZ, et al. *Zhong Yi Xue Wen Da Ti Ku* (Questions and Answers on Traditional Chinese Medicine: Herbal Formulas).

Gān Mài Dà Zǎo Tāng (Licorice, Wheat, and Jujube Decoction)
甘麥大棗湯
甘麦大枣汤

Pinyin Name: *Gan Mai Da Zao Tang*
Literal Name: Licorice, Wheat, and Jujube Decoction
Alternate Names: *Gan Cao Xiao Mai Da Zao Tang; Kan Mai Ta Tsao Tang; Kan Tsao Hsiao Mai Ta Tsao Tang; Gan Mai Da Zao Tang; Gan Zao Xiao Mai Da Zao Tang*; Licorice, Wheat, and Date Decoction; Licorice and Jujube Combination
Original Source: *Jin Gui Yao Lue* (Essentials from the Golden Cabinet) by Zhang Zhong-Jing in the Eastern Han Dynasty

COMPOSITION

Gan Cao (Radix et Rhizoma Glycyrrhizae)	9g
Xiao Mai (Fructus Tritici)	1 cup [9-15g]
Da Zao (Fructus Jujubae)	10 pieces [5-7 pieces]

DOSAGE / PREPARATION / ADMINISTRATION

The source text states to prepare the ingredients as a decoction using 6 cups [1,200 mL] of water and reduce the liquid to 3 cups [600 mL]. Take the warm, strained decoction in three equally divided doses daily. Today, the decoction may be prepared using the doses suggested in brackets.

CHINESE THERAPEUTIC ACTIONS

1. Nourishes the Heart and calms the *shen* (spirit)
2. Harmonizes the middle *jiao* and relieves acute conditions
3. Tonifies Spleen qi

CLINICAL MANIFESTATIONS

Anxiety, nervousness, irritability, hiding, aggression, hypersensitivity to noise and/or touch, disorientation, sleep disturbance (whining, jerking and vocalizing during sleep), hyperactivity, hyperexcitability, poor memory and concentration, inability to perform commands from the trainer or handler, a red, dry tongue with little coating, and a thready, rapid pulse

VETERINARY CLINICAL APPLICATIONS

Behavioral disorders and night restlessness.

Gān Mài Dà Zăo Tāng (Licorice, Wheat, and Jujube Decoction)

EXPLANATION

Gan Mai Da Zao Tang (Licorice, Wheat, and Jujube Decoction) specifically treats a Chinese medical condition called *zang zao* (restless organ) disorder. This condition is characterized by Heart blood deficiency and Liver qi stagnation. With Heart blood deficiency, the *shen* (spirit) becomes unstable and patients will show such clinical signs as sleep disturbance (whining, jerking and vocalizing during sleep), poor memory and concentration, and an inability to respond to commands from the trainer or handler. Because of Liver qi stagnation, the emotions of the patients become unstable. In mild cases, they may experience mood swings, irritability, and disorientation. In severe cases, they may exhibit aggression, hyperactivity and hyperexcitability. Clinically, this formula can be used to treat behavioral or emotional disorders characterized by deficiency.

Gan Cao (Radix et Rhizoma Glycyrrhizae) harmonizes the middle *jiao* and nourishes the Heart to relieve the acute condition. *Xiao Mai* (Fructus Tritici) nourishes the Heart and calms the *shen* (spirit). *Da Zao* (Fructus Jujubae) tonifies Spleen qi, relieves Liver qi stagnation, and nourishes the Heart. Combined, these three herbs tonify the Heart, relieve the acute condition, soften the Liver, relieve Liver qi stagnation, tranquilize the Heart, and calm the *shen*.

VETERINARY MODIFICATIONS

- When irritability and thirst are present, add *Mai Dong* (Radix Ophiopogonis) and *Wu Wei Zi* (Fructus Schisandrae Chinensis).
- With yin deficiency signs, add *Di Huang* (Radix Rehmanniae), *Bai Zi Ren* (Semen Platycladi), and *Bai He* (Bulbus Lilii).
- For night restlessness or pacing at night, add *He Huan Pi* (Cortex Albiziae), *Shou Wu Teng* (Caulis Polygoni Multiflori) and *Suan Zao Ren* (Semen Ziziphi Spinosae).
- With fear and fright, add *Bai Zi Ren* (Semen Platycladi) and *Fu Shen* (Poria Paradicis).
- For urinary incontinence during sleep, add *Sang Piao Xiao* (Ootheca Mantidis), *Yi Zhi* (Fructus Alpinia Oxyphyllae), and *Tu Si Zi* (Semen Cuscutae Chinensis).
- With dry stools, add *Hei Zhi Ma* (Semen Sesami Nigrum) and *He Shou Wu* (Radix Polygoni Multiflori).

PHARMACOLOGICAL EFFECTS

1. **Central nervous system**: In one study, daily administration of the formula at 2-4 g/kg per day for 7 days was associated with increased sleeping time. The formula was also effective in treating and preventing artificially-induced seizures in mice.[1]
2. **Musculoskeletal**: In one experiment, administration of the formula effectively inhibited the contraction of the smooth muscles, such as the intestines and the uterus, in mice.[2]

HUMAN CLINICAL STUDIES AND RESEARCH

1. ***Zang zao* (restless organ) disorder**: In one study of 38 patients (12 males and 26 females) with *zang zao* (restless organ) disorder, use of modified *Gan Mai Da Zao Tang* was associated with complete recovery in 28 cases, marked improvement in 7 cases, and no effect in 3 cases. The overall effectiveness was 92.1%. Modifications included the addition of *Bai He* (Bulbus Lilii) and *Di Huang* (Radix Rehmanniae) for restlessness, irritability, insomnia, dry mouth, and a red tongue body with little tongue coating; *Suan Zao Ren* (Semen Ziziphi Spinosae) and *Zhi Mu* (Rhizoma Anemarrhenae) for insomnia with excessive dreams, emotional instability, fidgeting, feeling of insecurity, and a wiry, rapid pulse; and *Huo Ma Ren* (Fructus Cannabis) and *Fu Ling* (Poria) for poor appetite and dry stools.[3]
2. **Insomnia**: In a clinical study, 110 patients with insomnia were treated with *Gan Mai Da Zao Tang* with the addition

***Gan Mai Da Zao Tang* (Licorice, Wheat, and Jujube Decoction)**

Diagnosis	Clinical Signs	Treatment	Herbs
Zang zao (restless organ) disorder	• Sleep disturbance (whining, jerking and vocalizing during sleep), poor memory and concentration, and an inability to respond to commands from the trainer or handler: Heart blood deficiency unable to nourish the *shen* (spirit) • Mood swings, irritability, and disorientation: Liver qi stagnation • Aggression, hyperactivity and hyperexcitability: severe Liver qi stagnation • Red, dry tongue with little coating and a rapid, thready pulse: dryness consuming yin	• Nourishes the Heart and calms the *shen* • Harmonizes the middle *jiao* and relieves acute conditions • Tonifies Spleen qi	• *Gan Cao* (Radix et Rhizoma Glycyrrhizae) harmonizes the middle *jiao* and nourishes the Heart. • *Xiao Mai* (Fructus Tritici) nourishes the Heart and calms the *shen*. • *Da Zao* (Fructus Jujubae) tonifies Spleen qi, relieves Liver stagnation, and nourishes the Heart.

Gān Mài Dà Zǎo Tāng (Licorice, Wheat, and Jujube Decoction)

of *Bai He* (Bulbus Lilii), *Di Huang* (Radix Rehmanniae Glutinosae) and *Shou Wu Teng* (Caulis Polygoni Multiflori) with good success. The overall effectiveness reported was 74.2%.[4]

3. **Hysteria**: One study reported marked success using herbs and acupuncture to treat hysteria. The herbal formula was given in decoction, and contained *Gan Cao* (Radix et Rhizoma Glycyrrhizae) 20g, *Da Zao* (Fructus Jujubae) 30 pieces, *Xiao Mai* (Fructus Tritici) 60g and *Wu Wei Zi* (Fructus Schisandrae Chinensis) 12g. Acupuncture points selected included *Hegu* (LI 4), *Renzhong* (GV 26), *Neiguan* (PC 6), and others to regulate qi and emotions. Of 60 patients, the study reported stabilization and resolution of all clinical signs , with no recurrence in follow-up visits 6 months after the conclusion of treatments.[5] According to another study, 27 patients with hysteria were treated with heavy doses of *Gan Mai Da Zao Tang* with recovery in 24 cases, marked improvement in 2 cases, slight improvement in 1 case, and no effect in 2 cases. The doses of the herbs used were *Gan Cao* (Radix et Rhizoma Glycyrrhizae) 24-45g, *Fu Xiao Mai* (Fructus Tritici Levis) 60g, and *Da Zao* (Fructus Zizyphi Jujubae) 10 pieces.[6] Lastly, 25 patients with hysteria were treated with *Gan Mai Da Zao Tang* plus electro-acupuncture (5 cases) with complete recovery in 22 cases, marked improvement in 2 cases, and slight improvement in 1 case.[7]
4. **Schizophrenia**: One report described *Gan Mai Da Zao Tang* with addition of *Long Gu* (Os Draconis) and *Mu Li* (Concha Ostreae) to be effective in treating 79 cases of schizophrenia. The duration of treatment was between 7-70 days. During the treatment period, 62 out of 79 patients were treated concurrently with a low dose of chlorpromazine (< 200mg per day). Out of 79 cases, the study reported recovery in 5 cases, marked effectiveness in 23 cases, moderate effects in 34 cases, and no effect in 17 cases.[8] According to another study, 146 schizophrenic patients were treated for 7-98 days with recovery in 11 cases, significant improvement in 44 cases, improvement in 64 cases, and no effect in 27 cases. The herbal treatment included *Gan Mai Da Zao Tang* plus wild-crafted *Bai He* (Bulbus Lilii) and *Di Huang* (Radix Rehmanniae). In addition, a small amount of chlorpromazine was given in 17 patients.[9]
5. **Enuresis**: A study of 28 children with bed-wetting characterized by deficiency and cold of the lower *jiao* treated with *Gan Mai Da Zao Tang* with addition of *Sang Piao Xiao* (Ootheca Mantidis), roasted *Yi Zhi* (Fructus Alpinia Oxyphyllae) and *Tu Si Zi* (Semen Cuscutae Chinensis) showed good results. After 10 days of herbal therapy, enuresis stopped in 13 cases. After 20 days of herbal therapy, enuresis stopped in all patients. In follow-up interviews 8-12 months later, only 2 out of 28 children had had any recurrence.[10]
6. **Chorea**: Fourteen children with chorea were treated with good success using *Gan Mai Da Zao Tang* plus *Gui Zhi Jia Long Gu Mu Li Tang* (Cinnamon Twig Decoction plus Dragon Bone and Oyster Shell) with modifications. The herbal formula contained the following ingredients: *Gan Cao* (Radix et Rhizoma Glycyrrhizae) 15g, *Fu Xiao Mai* (Fructus Tritici Levis) 30g, *Da Zao* (Fructus Jujubae) 10 pieces, *Gui Zhi* (Ramulus Cinnamomi) 12g, *Bai Shao* (Radix Paeoniae Alba) 15g, *Sheng Jiang* (Rhizoma Zingiberis Recens) 6g, *Long Gu* (Os Draconis) 30g, *Mu Li* (Concha Ostreae) 30g, *Yu Jin* (Radix Curcumae) 15g, *Gou Teng* (Ramulus Uncariae cum Uncis) 15g, *Qin Jiao* (Radix Gentianae Macrophyllae) 12g, and *Tian Ma* (Rhizoma Gastrodiae) 9g. The study reported recovery in 11 of 14 cases. The remaining three patients were also treated with drugs prior to recovery.[11]

SUGGESTED ACUPUNCTURE TREATMENT

1. Points: *Housanli* (ST 36), *Sanyinjiao* (SP 6), *Shenmen* (HT 7), *Renzhong* (GV 26), *Taichong* (LR 3), *Anshen* and *Dafengmen*.
2. Technique: both tonification and sedation.

Tonifying *Housanli* (ST 36), *Sanyinjiao* (SP 6), and *Shenmen* (HT 7) nourishes yin and moistens dryness to calm hysteria. Sedating *Renzhong* (GV 26) quickly tranquilizes the mind. *Taichong* (LR 3) regulates Liver qi and removes stagnation. *Anshen* and *Dafengmen* are classical points that calm *shen*.

AUTHORS' COMMENTS

Gan Mai Da Zao Tang can be used to treat animals that have sustained blood loss from toxicity, trauma or surgery, and then develop abnormal behavior. These animals are typically normal before the bleeding or hemorrhaging incident, but then have sudden bouts of fearfulness, inappropriate or exaggerated response to noise or changes in environment, and intermittent bouts of irritability and/or aggression. In cases of aggression, it can be combined with *Suan Zao Ren Tang* (Sour Jujube Decoction) or *Chai Hu Jia Long Gu Mu Li Tang* (Bupleurum plus Dragon Bone and Oyster Shell Decoction). This is a mild formula and can be used long term, especially in performance animals that are anxious and under chronic stress to perform on a regular basis, in dogs and cats that are poor travelers, or when introducing new dogs or pets into the household. Another good use for the formula is to mitigate excessive exuberance in dogs when greeting owners or other guests coming into the home. This can be especially helpful in

Gān Mài Dà Zǎo Tāng (Licorice, Wheat, and Jujube Decoction)

older dogs with laryngeal paralysis that may work themselves into a frenzy and have difficulty breathing. Because of the availability and nature of these herbs, it is not difficult to incorporate this formula as part of a home-cooked diet.

Xiao Mai (Fructus Tritici) and *Fu Xiao Mai* (Fructus Tritici Levis) are derived from the same plant, and have similar characteristics and functions. When both herbs are placed in water, *Xiao Mai* (Fructus Tritici) sinks and *Fu Xiao Mai* floats. *Xiao Mai* (Fructus Tritici) can nourish the Heart and calm the *shen*, while *Fu Xiao Mai* has astringent functions to stop sweating. The source text uses *Xiao Mai* (Fructus Tritici) to nourish the Heart to alleviate *shen* disturbance. Some contemporary texts recommend the use of *Fu Xiao Mai* (Fructus Tritici Levis) to treat yin-deficient heat and relieve spontaneous sweating and night sweats.

References

1. Journal of Ethnopharmacology, 1986, 15:289.
2. *Guo Wai Yi Xue Zhong Yi Zhong Yao Fen Ce* (Monograph of Chinese Herbology from Foreign Medicine), 1983; 3:53.
3. *Nan Jing Zhong Yi Yao Da Xue Xue Bao* (Journal of Nanjing University of Traditional Chinese Medicine and Medicinals), 1996; 6:22.
4. *Zhe Jiang Zhong Yi Za Zhi* (Zhejiang Journal of Chinese Medicine), 1982; 9:412.
5. *Shan Dong Zhong Yi Za Zhi* (Shandong Journal of Chinese Medicine), 1994; 5:237.
6. *Jiang Su Yi Yao* (Jiangsu Journal of Medicine and Herbology), 1978; 1:3.
7. *Zhong Yi Za Zhi* (Journal of Chinese Medicine), 1960; 2:32.
8. *Zhe Jiang Zhong Yi Za Zhi* (Zhejiang Journal of Chinese Medicine), 1982; 6:273.
9. *Shang Hai Yi Yao Za Zhi* (Shanghai Journal of Medicine and Herbology), 1982; 6:273.
10. *Hu Bei Zhong Yi Za Zhi* (Hubei Journal of Chinese Medicine), 1986; 1:19.
11. *Zhong Yi Za Zhi* (Journal of Chinese Medicine), 1986; 5:26.

Yǎng Xīn Tāng (Nourish the Heart Decoction)

養心湯

养心汤

Pinyin Name: *Yang Xin Tang*
Literal Name: Nourish the Heart Decoction
Alternate Names: *Yang Hsin Tang*, Heart-Nourishing Decoction, Astragalus and Zizyphus Combination
Original Source: *Ren Zhai Zhi Zhi* (Straight Directions of Benevolent Aid) by Yang Tu-Ying in 1264

COMPOSITION

Ren Shen (Radix et Rhizoma Ginseng)	0.3g
Huang Qi (Radix Astragali), *zhi* (fried with liquid)	15g
Bai Fu Ling (Poria Alba)	15g
Zhi Gan Cao (Radix et Rhizoma Glycyrrhizae Praeparata cum Melle)	12g
Dang Gui (Radix Angelicae Sinensis)	15g
Chuan Xiong (Rhizoma Chuanxiong)	15g
Fu Shen (Poria Paradicis)	15g
Yuan Zhi (Radix Polygalae), *yan* (drowned) in ginger juice and *bei* (stone-baked)	0.3g
Bai Zi Ren (Semen Platycladi)	0.3g
Wu Wei Zi (Fructus Schisandrae Chinensis)	0.3g
Suan Zao Ren (Semen Ziziphi Spinosae), *jin* (soaked) and *chao* (dry-fried) till aromatic	0.3g
Ban Xia Qu (Rhizoma Pinelliae Massa Fermentata)	15g
Rou Gui (Cortex Cinnamomi)	0.3g

Yǎng Xīn Tāng (Nourish the Heart Decoction)

DOSAGE / PREPARATION / ADMINISTRATION

The source text states to grind the ingredients into a coarse powder. Cook 9g of the powder with 5 slices of *Sheng Jiang* (Rhizoma Zingiberis Recens) and 2 pieces of *Da Zao* (Fructus Jujubae) in water, and take the warm, strained decoction before meals.

CHINESE THERAPEUTIC ACTIONS

1. Nourishes the Heart
2. Tonifies the blood and qi

CLINICAL MANIFESTATIONS

Heart blood deficiency: lethargy, exercise intolerance, palpitations, spontaneous sweating, night restlessness, easily frightened, hypersensitive to noise, poor memory and concentration, easily distracted, unable to obey trainer or handlers commands, restlessness, a pale pink tongue with thin, white coating, and a weak, thin pulse that may be irregular.

VETERINARY CLINICAL APPLICATIONS

Cardiomyopathy, congestive heart failure, mitral valve disease, cardiac arrhythmia, weak irregular pulse, fearfulness, poor athletic performance and concentration.

EXPLANATION

Yang Xin Tang (Nourish the Heart Decoction) treats blood and qi deficiencies and the subsequent inability to nourish the Heart. Because it is malnourished, the Heart cannot carry out its normal functions. Thus, there are clinical signs of Heart blood deficiency, such as lethargy, exercise intolerance, palpitations, spontaneous sweating and night restlessness. Furthermore, Heart blood deficiency may contribute to *shen* (spirit) disturbance, manifesting in clinical signs such as being easily scared or frightened, restlessness, hypersensitivity to noise, poor memory and concentration, being easily distracted, and an inability to obey the trainer's or handler's commands.

This formula contains many tonic herbs and focuses mainly on nourishing the Heart and replenishing the blood. Since production of blood requires an adequate amount of qi, this formula uses herbs to tonify qi and nourish the blood concurrently. *Ren Shen* (Radix et Rhizoma Ginseng), *Huang Qi* (Radix Astragali), *Bai Fu Ling* (Poria Alba), and *Zhi Gan Cao* (Radix et Rhizoma Glycyrrhizae Praeparata cum Melle) tonify qi. *Dang Gui* (Radix Angelicae Sinensis) and *Chuan Xiong* (Rhizoma Chuanxiong) replenish and move the blood. *Fu Shen* (Poria Paradicis), *Yuan Zhi* (Radix Polygalae), *Bai Zi Ren* (Semen Platycladi), *Wu Wei Zi* (Fructus Schisandrae Chinensis), and *Suan Zao Ren* (Semen Ziziphi Spinosae) calm the *shen* (spirit). *Ban Xia Qu* (Rhizoma Pinelliae Massa Fermentata) dries dampness and eliminates phlegm, which may form from the use of tonic herbs. *Rou Gui* (Cortex Cinnamomi) acts as a guiding herb to direct the therapeutic effects of the herbs to the Heart channel. *Sheng Jiang* (Rhizoma Zingiberis Recens) and *Da Zao* (Fructus Jujubae) harmonize the herbs in the formula.

VETERINARY MODIFICATIONS

- With fever and thirst, add *Mai Dong* (Radix Ophiopogonis) and *Zhu Ru* (Caulis Bambusae in Taenia).
- With yin-deficient heat, irritability and night restlessness, add *Zhi Mu* (Rhizoma Anemarrhenae) and *Huang Bo* (Cortex Phellodendri Chinensis).

***Yang Xin Tang* (Nourish the Heart Decoction)**

Diagnosis	Clinical Signs	Treatment	Herbs
Heart blood deficiency	• Poor memory and concentration, easily distracted, night restlessness, and spontaneous sweating: Heart blood deficiency • Fear, fright and restlessness: *shen* (spirit) disturbance	• Nourishes the Heart • Tonifies the blood	• *Ren Shen* (Radix et Rhizoma Ginseng), *Huang Qi* (Radix Astragali), *Bai Fu Ling* (Poria Alba) and *Zhi Gan Cao* (Radix et Rhizoma Glycyrrhizae Praeparata cum Melle) tonify qi. • *Dang Gui* (Radix Angelicae Sinensis) and *Chuan Xiong* (Rhizoma Chuanxiong) replenish and move the blood. • *Fu Shen* (Poria Paradicis), *Yuan Zhi* (Radix Polygalae), *Bai Zi Ren* (Semen Platycladi), *Wu Wei Zi* (Fructus Schisandrae Chinensis) and *Suan Zao Ren* (Semen Ziziphi Spinosae) calm the *shen* (spirit). • *Ban Xia Qu* (Rhizoma Pinelliae Massa Fermentata) dries dampness and eliminates phlegm. • *Rou Gui* (Cortex Cinnamomi) guides the herbs to the Heart channel. • *Sheng Jiang* (Rhizoma Zingiberis Recens) and *Da Zao* (Fructus Jujubae) harmonize all of the herbs.

Yǎng Xīn Tāng (Nourish the Heart Decoction)

- With poor memory and concentration and being easily frightened, add *Shi Chang Pu* (Rhizoma Acori Tatarinowii) and *Bai Shao* (Radix Paeoniae Alba).
- To prevent thromboembolic disease, combine with *Dan Shen* (Radix et Rhizoma Salviae Miltiorrhizae).

SUGGESTED ACUPUNCTURE TREATMENT

1. Points: *Housanli* (ST 36), *Xinshu* (BL 15), *Jueyinshu* (BL 14), *Sanyinjiao* (SP 6), *Neiguan* (PC 6), *Gongsun* (SP 4), *Shenmen* (HT 7), *Shanzhong* (CV 17), and *Fenglong* (ST 40).
2. Technique: tonification.

Tonify *Housanli* (ST 36), *Xinshu* (BL 15), and *Jueyinshu* (BL 14) to supplement qi. *Sanyinjiao* (SP 6) nourishes and invigorates the blood. *Neiguan* (PC 6), *Gongsun* (SP 4), *Shenmen* (HT 7), and *Shanzhong* (CV 17) tonify the Heart and calm the *shen* (spirit). *Fenglong* (ST 40) dissolves phlegm.

AUTHORS' COMMENTS

In addition to the treatment of *shen* (spirit) disorders, *Yang Xin Tang* is commonly used to nourish and support the Heart in dogs and cats that have weak, irregular pulse and cardiac arrhythmia secondary to valvular disease and cardiomyopathy. It is a well-balanced formula and can be used long term. To improve clinical results and for the prevention of thromboembolic disease, combine with *Xue Fu Zhu Yu Tang* (Drive Out Stasis in the Mansion of Blood Decoction) or *Zhi Gan Cao Tang* (Honey-Fried Licorice Decoction). These combinations can be given long term with excellent results and minor modifications over time. In contrast to *Tian Wang Bu Xin Dan* (Emperor of Heaven's Special Pill to Tonify the Heart), *Yang Xin Tang* is used more for the treatment of qi and blood deficiencies, rather than yin deficiency.

Yang Xin Tang, literally "Nourish the Heart Decoction," is a common generic name for a variety of formulas. There are at least 13 formulas with the exact same name documented in the history of Chinese herbal medicine, all with slightly different ingredients, doses, and indications. Some formulations contain more herbs to tonify qi, while others contain more herbs to tonify the blood; it is important to review all of the herbs in the formula before using.

Chapter 9 — Summary — Shen-Calming Formulas

SECTION 1: SEDATIVE FORMULAS THAT CALM THE *SHEN* (SPIRIT)

Name	Similarities	Differences
Zhen Zhu Mu Wan (Mother of Pearl Pill)	Tranquilize the mind and calm the *shen* (spirit)	Calms the Heart and Liver yang
Chai Hu Jia Long Gu Mu Li Tang (Bupleurum plus Dragon Bone and Oyster Shell Decoction)		Harmonizes the *shaoyang* and anchors the *shen*

Zhen Zhu Mu Wan (Mother of Pearl Pill), and ***Chai Hu Jia Long Gu Mu Li Tang*** (Bupleurum plus Dragon Bone and Oyster Shell Decoction) tranquilize the mind and calm the *shen* (spirit). The common symptoms are irritability, night restlessness, and palpitations.

- *Zhen Zhu Mu Wan* controls hyperactivity of Liver and Heart yang in animals with yin and blood deficiencies.
- *Chai Hu Jia Long Gu Mu Li Tang* harmonizes the *shaoyang*, calms and tranquilizes the body with heavy substances, dredges the yang, and purges heat. It is used for *shaoyang* stage in which the emotions are unstable, for high blood pressure, and for seizure disorder.

SECTION 2: NOURISHING FORMULAS THAT CALM THE *SHEN* (SPIRIT)

Name	Similarities	Differences
Suan Zao Ren Tang (Sour Jujube Decoction)	Nourish the blood and yin, tonify the Heart, calm the *shen* (spirit)	Tonifies Liver blood and restrains Liver yang
Tian Wang Bu Xin Dan (Emperor of Heaven's Special Pill to Tonify the Heart)		Nourishes Heart and Kidney yin, calms the *shen*
Gan Mai Da Zao Tang (Licorice, Wheat, and Jujube Decoction)		Treats *zang zao* (restless organ) disorder, calms the *shen*
Yang Xin Tang (Nourish the Heart Decoction)		Tonifies Heart blood

Suan Zao Ren Tang (Sour Jujube Decoction), ***Tian Wang Bu Xin Dan*** (Emperor of Heaven's Special Pill to Tonify the Heart), ***Gan Mai Da Zao Tang*** (Licorice, Wheat, and Jujube Decoction), and ***Yang Xin Tang*** (Nourish the Heart Decoction) all have the common functions of nourishing blood and yin, tonifying the Heart, and calming the *shen* (spirit).

- *Suan Zao Ren Tang* tonifies Liver blood to restrain hyperactive Liver yang, which can produce deficiency heat that disturbs the Heart and creates symptoms of irritability, aggression, night restlessness, palpitations, and a dry mouth and throat. The pulse is usually thin and wiry.
- *Tian Wang Bu Xin Dan* tonifies the blood, nourishes yin, and calms the *shen*. The two deficient organs addressed by this formula are the Heart and Kidney. Key clinical manifestations include fear of loud noises, irritability, and poor memory and concentration.
- *Gan Mai Da Zao Tang* is used for *zang zao* (restless organ) disorder and *shen* disturbance caused Liver qi stagnation and Heart blood deficiency. Usually, this formula is used to harmonize and relieve acute conditions of emotional instability, hyperexcitability and hysteria.
- *Yang Xin Tang* nourishes Heart blood and qi deficiency to treat cardiac disease, arrhythmia, night restlessness, fearfulness, poor memory and concentration, being easily distracted, and an inability to obey the trainer's or handler's commands.

Chapter 10

— Orifice-Opening Formulas

开窍剂

华佗 Huă Tuŏ

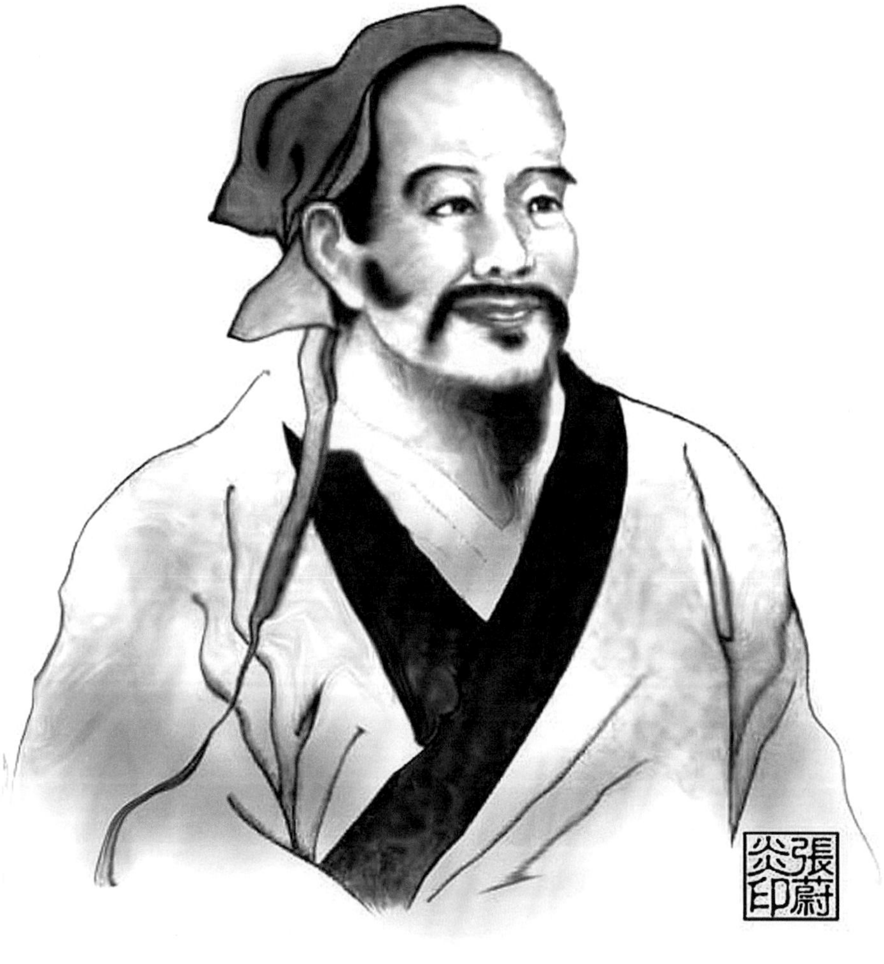

华佗 Huă Tuŏ, 110 – 207 CE.

华佗 Huă Tuŏ

Hua Tuo was born into a poor family. When Hua Tuo was seven years old, his father passed away, taking with him the only source of family income. Faced with financial hardship and poverty, Hua Tuo began to work in a local herbal pharmacy. While working there, Hua Tuo carefully observed the practice of medicine and pharmacy, and thus began the career of one of the best physicians in our profession.

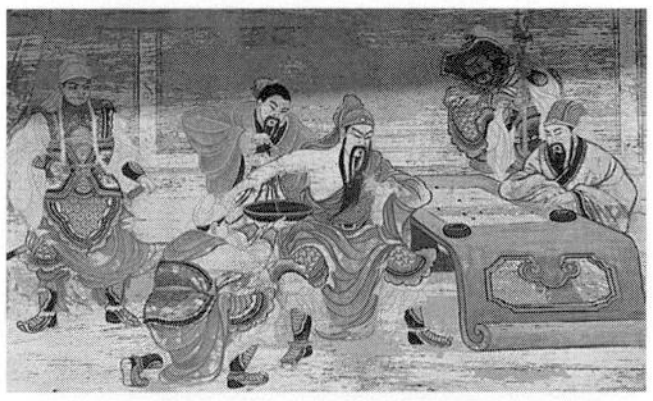

Hua Tuo performing arm surgery on 关羽 Guan Yu, one of the most famous generals in Chinese history.

Hua Tuo lived and practiced medicine during the end of the Eastern Han and beginning of the Three Kingdoms, a period of time characterized by political instability, with constant battles and turmoil. He sympathized with the common people whose lives were suppressed by the government, and dedicated his entire life to helping them. Therefore, Hua Tuo was also known as 'the physician of the people.' He preferred to treat the common folks of the world, and repeatedly refused to accept offers of the position of 太医 the Supreme Physician in the Imperial Palace.

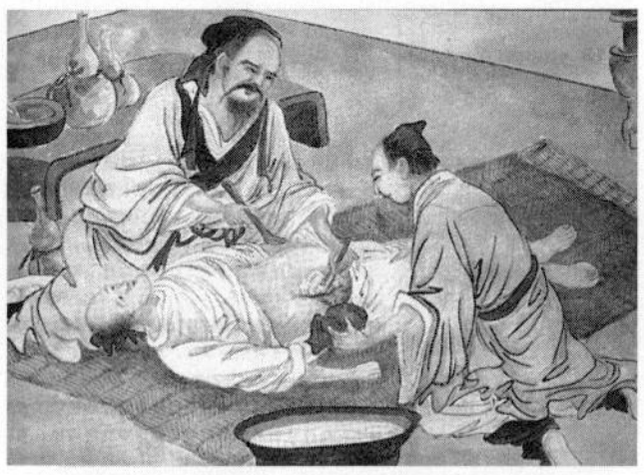

Hua Tuo performing abdominal surgery.

Hua Tuo is respected for being the first surgeon and the inventor of anesthesia in Traditional Chinese Medicine. He believed that for diseases that could not be treated with acupuncture and herbs, the only solution was surgery to remove the cause. It is well-documented that Hua Tuo frequently performed surgery on various parts of the body by using an herbal formula called 麻沸散 *Ma Fei San* (Numbing and Boiling Powder) for systemic anesthesia.[1]

Despite his outstanding achievements, there were always more patients than Hua Tuo could possibly care for in his practice. Thus, he began to wonder why people were always sick, and what would make them healthier. He concluded that chronic illnesses were due, in part, to lack of physical activity, and proposed regular exercise as a remedy. As part of Hua Tuo's strong emphasis on the importance of physical activity, he developed 五禽戏 *Wu Qin Xi* (Five Animal Frolics), an exercise that imitates the physical movement of tigers, deers, monkeys, bears and birds.

In his later years, Hua Tuo was called by the emperor of the Wei Kingdom, 曹操 Cāo Cáo,[2] to treat his "head wind" [presumably migraine headache] that had not responded to any of the treatments by many other physicians. By the insertion of just one needle, the chronic headache was alleviated. Cao was so impressed that he insisted on having Hua Tuo as his personal physician. Hua Tuo tactfully refused, claiming that he needed to return home to attend to his sick wife. Shortly after returning home, he was called again, and subsequently forced by Cao to return to the Imperial Palace. Cao had another severe headache wanted Hua Tuo to cure him, and would not let him leave the Imperial Palace. Hua Tuo stated that the headache was so severe that it could not be treated simply with herbs or acupuncture. The only cure would be to induce anesthesia, and surgically open the head to remove the cause of the headache. Cao thought Hua Tuo was making an attempt to assassinate him, and sentenced Hua Tuo to death. While in prison, Hua Tuo compiled all of his clinical experience in writing, and tried to give it to a prison guard for safe keeping. However, out of fear of Cao, the guard refused to do any favors or accept anything from Hua Tuo. In extreme anger and frustration, Hua Tuo burned his manuscripts, turning all his clinical knowledge to ashes. After Hua Tuo died, he was buried next to a flowing river of clear water – symbolizing that he was cleared from all wrong-doing.

Dynasties & Kingdoms	Year
Xia Dynasty 夏	2100-1600 BCE
Shang Dynasty 商	1600-1100 BCE
Zhou Dynasty 周	1100-221 BCE
Qin Dynasty 秦	221-207 BCE
Han Dynasty 漢	**206 BCE-220**
Three Kingdoms 三國	220-280
Western Jin Dynasty 西晉	265-316
Eastern Jin Dynasty 東晉	317-420
Northern and Southern Dynasties 北南朝	420-581
Sui Dynasty 隋	581-618
Tang Dynasty 唐	618-907
Five Dynasties 五代	907-960
Song Dynasty 宋	960-1279
Liao Dynasty 遼	916-1125
Jin Dynasty 金	1115-1234
Yuan Dynasty 元	1271-1368
Ming Dynasty 明	1368-1644
Qing Dynasty 清	1644-1911
Republic of China 中華民國	1912-Present Day
People's Republic of China 中華人民共和國	1949-Present Day

1. The exact composition of *Ma Fei San* (Numbing and Boiling Powder), similar to all of Hua Tuo's clinical knowledge, was lost when his manuscripts were burned to ashes. Many physicians have attempted to re-create the same formulation based on historical records, but none achieved the same clinical efficacy as Hua Tuo's. This formula is believed to have contained *Yang Jin Hua* (Flos Daturae), *Cao Wu* (Radix Aconiti Kusnezoffii), *Bai Zhi* (Radix Angelicae Dahuricae), *Dang Gui* (Radix Angelicae Sinensis), and *Chuan Xiong* (Rhizoma Chuanxiong), among others.
2. 曹操 Cāo Cáo was the emperor of the Wei Kingdom during the period of Three Kingdoms. Because these three kingdoms were at war constantly for approximately 60 years, Cao had many enemies and was consistently under the threat of assassination. So when Hua Tuo offered to cure Cao's headache by "cutting his head open" to perform brain surgery, Cao naturally assumed he was using medicine as an excuse to kill him, and subsequently sentenced Huo Tuo to death. This story, however, is considered to be folklore, as there is no confirmed historical record of exact motive and circumstances associated with Hua Tuo's death.

Table of Contents

Chapter 10 — Overview

开窍剂 — Orifice-Opening Formulas

Definition: Orifice-opening formulas are composed of aromatic herbs that open the sensory orifices, awaken the *shen* (spirit), and restore consciousness. Although "open the orifices" is not a specific treatment method listed in the *ba fa* (eight treatment methods) described in the *Huang Di Nei Jing* (Yellow Emperor's Inner Classic), cold orifice-opening formulas employ the *wen fa* (warming) method, and warm orifice-opening formulas utilize the *qing fa* (clearing) method to treat corresponding disorders.

Orifice-opening formulas are generally reserved for emergency, life-threatening conditions that include: acute encephalitis, acute meningitis, septicemia, seizure disorder, epilepsy, heat stroke, infectious diseases, uremia, acute hepatitis, and acute necrotizing pancreatitis. Many of these formulas contain herbs that are derived from endangered animals, such as *She Xiang* (Moschus) and *Xi Jiao* (Cornu Rhinoceri), and/or are potentially toxic heavy metals, such as *Zhu Sha* (Cinnabaris) and *Xiong Huang* (Realgar). These herbs are rarely used as medicinal substances today. Most herbal products today have removed them completely, or have replaced them with herbs with similar functions. Orifice-opening formulas are not typically available in ready-made form, and must be made in-house or formulated by a reputable Chinese herbal company, with appropriate substitutions for herbs that are no longer available or recommended. The discussion of these formulas is included here primarily for academic purposes; they are not commonly prescribed or used in veterinary medicine. Animals that present with conditions for which orifice-opening formulas are appropriate, generally require emergency care and close monitoring from a biomedical perspective.

Unconsciousness with closed sensory orifices is a condition that is divided, for purposes of assessment and treatment, into two main diagnostic categories: excess and deficiency. It is very important to distinguish between excess and deficiency when treating unconsciousness with closed sensory orifices. Excess disorders, such as *bi zheng* (closed disorder), may be treated with orifice-opening formulas to open the sensory orifices, awaken the *shen* (spirit), and restore consciousness. Deficiency disorders, such as *tuo zheng* (abandoned syndrome), must be treated with herbs that tonify qi and restore yang.

- *Bi zheng* (closed disorder) is an excess disorder characterized by the following manifestations: unconsciousness, muscle convulsions, stiff limbs, and a forceful pulse. Furthermore, the nature of *bi zheng* (closed disorder) can be either hot or cold. Hot *bi zheng* (closed disorder) is caused by heat toxins attacking the Pericardium, and is treated with cold orifice-opening formulas. Cold *bi zheng* (closed disorder) is caused by cold-phlegm or qi stagnation, which results in turbidity misting around the Heart. In this case, warm orifice-opening formulas should be administered.
- *Tuo zheng* (abandoned syndrome) is a deficiency disorder with manifestations such as cold limbs, sweating, extreme fatigue, open mouth, closed eyes, and enuresis. *Tuo zheng* (abandoned syndrome) should ***not*** be treated with herbs that open the orifices, as this will further accentuate the weakness and deficiency the animal is already experiencing. This deficient condition **must** be treated with herbs that tonify qi and restore yang.

Chapter 10 — Overview

Disorder	Primary Diagnosis	Secondary Diagnosis	Clinical Signs
Unconsciousness with closed sensory orifices	• *Bi zheng* (closed disorder)	• Hot *bi zheng* (closed disorder)	• High fever, unconsciousness, seizures and a forceful pulse
		• Cold *bi zheng* (closed disorder)	• Sudden unconsciousness, pale, bluish tongue, lips and mucous membranes, cold extremities, and a slow pulse
	• *Tuo zheng* (abandoned syndrome)		• Cold limbs, sweating, extreme fatigue, open mouth, closed eyes, and enuresis

Note: The pinyin names are exactly the same for 闭证 *bi zheng* (closed disorder) and 痹证 *bi zheng* (painful obstruction syndrome), although the Chinese characters are different. These two disorders have very different symptomology, diagnoses, and treatments, and should be correctly identified to ensure safe and effective treatment. Therefore, to avoid confusion, the term *bi zheng* (closed disorder) will be displayed with its English translation throughout the entire text, without abbreviation.

SUBCATEGORIES OF ACTION

Orifice-opening formulas are divided into two subcategories to reflect the differential diagnosis and treatment of hot and cold types of *bi zheng* (closed disorder).

1. **Cold Orifice-Opening Formulas**

These formulas treat hot *bi zheng* (closed disorder) caused by pathogenic heat toxins attacking the Pericardium and blocking the sensory orifices. The clinical signs include high fever, unconsciousness, and seizures. These formulas can also treat sudden unconsciousness due to *zhong feng* (wind stroke), or phlegm accumulation with heat signs and other clinical signs. In biomedical terminology, hot *bi zheng* (closed disorder) is often related to infectious diseases, meningitis, severe pneumonia, septicemia, heat stroke, liver diseases, or toxic uremia.

Herbs commonly used to open the sensory orifices include *Bing Pian* (Borneolum Syntheticum), *Shi Chang Pu* (Rhizoma Acori Tatarinowii), and *Yu Jin* (Radix Curcumae). To enhance the opening of the sensory orifices, herbs are added to clear heat, purge fire, cool the blood, and eliminate toxins, such as *Niu Huang* (Calculus Bovis), *Huang Lian* (Rhizoma Coptidis), and *Shi Gao* (Gypsum Fibrosum). Representative formulas include *An Gong Niu Huang Wan* (Calm the Palace Pill with Cattle Gallstone), *Zi Xue* (Purple Snow), and *Zhi Bao Dan* (Greatest Treasure Special Pill).

2. **Warm Orifice-Opening Formulas**

These formulas are used to treat cold *bi zheng* (closed disorder) in which unconsciousness is due to *zhong feng* (wind stroke), cold stroke, and phlegm accumulation. The main clinical manifestations include sudden unconsciousness, cold extremities, pale, bluish tongue, lips and mucous membranes, and a slow pulse. In allopathic terminology, cold *bi zheng* (closed disorder) is caused usually by cerebrovascular accidents and poisoning.

Commonly used herbs include *Su He Xiang* (Styrax) and *Bing Pian* (Borneolum Syntheticum). They are usually used together with acrid, warm, qi-regulating herbs to enhance their effects, such as *Xiang Fu* (Rhizoma Cyperi), *Ding Xiang* (Flos Caryophylli), and *Bi Bo* (Fructus Piperis Longi). Exemplar formulas include *Su He Xiang Wan* (Liquid Styrax Pill) and *Zi Jin Ding* (Purple Gold Special Pill).

CAUTIONS / CONTRAINDICATIONS

- *Tuo zheng* (abandoned syndrome), a deficiency disorder manifesting in cold limbs, sweating, extreme fatigue, open mouth, closed eyes, and enuresis, should be treated with herbs that tonify qi and restore yang. This condition must ***not*** be treated with orifice-opening formulas, which will only accentuate the underlying weakness and deficiency.

Chapter 10 — Overview

- Orifice-opening formulas are composed of acrid and aromatic herbs; therefore, prolonged use of these formulas will damage the *yuan* (source) *qi*. These formulas are generally reserved only for emergency use. Their use should be discontinued once the desired effects are achieved.
- These formulas are contraindicated during pregnancy.
- *Yangming fu* (hollow organ) excess syndrome with altered consciousness should be treated with cold formulas that drain downward, rather than with orifice-opening formulas.
- *Yangming fu* (hollow organ) excess syndrome with pathogenic heat attacking the Pericardium should be treated with orifice-opening formulas first, followed by cold formulas that drain downward, or both methods of treatment together, depending on the urgency of the condition.

PROCESSING

Orifice-opening formulas are usually prepared in pill form, powders, or injectables for two reasons. First, these herbs are aromatic in nature, and their effectiveness will be destroyed when processed with heat (such as in decoction). Second, they must be available immediately during an emergency. Having these formulas in pills, powders, or injections ensures immediate access to them. Decoction is inappropriate because it requires too much time to prepare. Moreover, decoctions cannot be prepared in advance because of their short shelf life and the difficulty of storing them for any useful period of time.

PHARMACOLOGICAL EFFECTS & CLINICAL APPLICATIONS

Orifice-opening herbs and formulas are generally reserved for acute, emergent cases of sudden unconsciousness, which may have a wide variety of causes. The pharmacological effects observed vary: some have a stimulant effect on the central nervous system, such as *Zhang Nao* (Camphora), which awakens patients from unconsciousness;[1] others have a sedative effect on the central nervous system, such as *Shi Chang Pu* (Rhizoma Acori Tatarinowii), which suppresses seizures and epileptic activities.[2] Other pharmacological effects include antipyretic effects to reduce body temperature,[3] and hypotensive effects to lower blood pressure.[4] Clinical applications of orifice-opening formulas include unconsciousness from encephalitis B, meningitis, toxic uremia, hepatitis, acute icteric hepatitis, acute pancreatitis, cerebrovascular accident, seizures, and convulsions.[5]

However, because of the acute and urgent nature of these illnesses, there are very few controlled clinical studies and research available for discussion. Exemplar formulas that open the sensory orifices include *An Gong Niu Huang Wan* (Calm the Palace Pill with Cattle Gallstone) and *Su He Xiang Wan* (Liquid Styrax Pill).

References

1. *Zhong Yao Xue* (Chinese Herbology), 1998; 989-991.
2. *Zhong Yi Fang Ji Xian Dai Yan Jiu* (Modern Study of Medical Formulas in Traditional Chinese Medicine), 1997; 870.
3. *Zhong Cheng Yao Yan Jiu* (Research of Chinese Patent Medicine), 1982; 5:23.
4. *Zhong Yi Fang Ji Xian Dai Yan Jiu* (Modern Study of Medical Formulas in Traditional Chinese Medicine), 1997; 871.
5. *Zhong Yi Fang Ji Xian Dai Yan Jiu* (Modern Study of Medical Formulas in Traditional Chinese Medicine), 1997; 871-874.

Section 1

凉开剂
— Cold Orifice-Opening Formulas

Ān Gōng Niú Huáng Wán (Calm the Palace Pill with Cattle Gallstone)
安宮牛黃丸
安宫牛黄丸

Pinyin Name: *An Gong Niu Huang Wan*
Literal Name: Calm the Palace Pill with Cattle Gallstone
Alternate Name: *Niu Huang Wan* (Cattle Gallstone Pill)
Original Source: *Wen Bing Tiao Bian* (Systematic Differentiation of Warm Diseases) by Wu Ju-Tong in 1798

COMPOSITION

Niu Huang (Calculus Bovis)	30g
She Xiang (Moschus)	7.5g
Xi Jiao (Cornu Rhinoceri)	30g
Huang Qin (Radix Scutellariae)	30g
Huang Lian (Rhizoma Coptidis)	30g
Zhi Zi (Fructus Gardeniae)	30g
Bing Pian (Borneolum Syntheticum)	7.5g
Yu Jin (Radix Curcumae)	30g
Zhu Sha (Cinnabaris)	30g
Zhen Zhu (Margarita)	15g
Xiong Huang (Realgar)	30g
Jin Bo (gold foil)	

Note: *Zhu Sha* (Cinnabaris) and *Xiong Huang* (Realgar) are potentially toxic heavy metals, and *Xi Jiao* (Cornu Rhinoceri) and *She Xiang* (Moschus) are derived from endangered animals. They are rarely used as medicinal substances today. The discussion of these substances here is included primarily for academic purposes, to reflect the historical use of these substances in its original formulation. Most herbal products today have removed them completely, or replaced them with substitutes with similar functions. For additional information on the toxicity of *Zhu Sha* (Cinnabaris) and *Xiong Huang* (Realgar), please refer to *Chinese Medical Herbology and Pharmacology* by John Chen and Tina Chen.

DOSAGE / PREPARATION / ADMINISTRATION

The source text states to grind the ingredients into a very fine powder and form into pills with honey. The pills should be 3g in weight, and are traditionally coated with *Jin Bo* (gold foil) and sealed with wax. For strong, otherwise healthy animals in severe condition, administer 1 pill, two to three times daily. For juvenile animals, give one-half pill, one time daily. If there is no response, a second dose may be given.

Today, this formula is prepared in four steps. First, process *Zhu Sha* (Cinnabaris), *Zhen Zhu* (Margarita), and *Xiong Huang* (Realgar) separately with the *shui fei* (refining with water) technique to obtain extremely fine powder. Second, grind *Niu Huang* (Calculus Bovis), *Xi Jiao* (Cornu Rhinoceri), *She Xiang* (Moschus), and *Bing Pian* (Borneolum Syntheticum) into a fine powder. Third, grind the remaining ingredients into powder. Finally, blend all of the herbal powders together and mix with *Feng Mi* (Mel) and water to form large pills. Dry the pills in a cool place without direct exposure to sunlight.

Ān Gōng Niú Huáng Wán (Calm the Palace Pill with Cattle Gallstone)

CHINESE THERAPEUTIC ACTIONS

1. Clears heat and opens the orifices
2. Dispels phlegm and eliminates toxins

CLINICAL MANIFESTATIONS

Febrile disorders with heat attacking the Pericardium and hot phlegm obstructing the orifices: high fever, irritability, coma, unconsciousness due to stroke, and convulsions.

VETERINARY CLINICAL APPLICATIONS

Fever, encephalitis, meningitis, dysentery, toxic uremia, hepatitis, acute icteric hepatitis, acute pancreatitis and seizures.

EXPLANATION

An Gong Niu Huang Wan (Calm the Palace Pill with Cattle Gallstone) is a representative formula for treating febrile disorders with heat attacking the Pericardium and hot phlegm obstructing the sensory orifices. The Heart, covered by the Pericardium, is the organ that houses the mind and controls the *shen* (spirit). If heat attacks the Pericardium, the patient may show *shen* disturbance, high fever, and irritability. If hot phlegm obstructs the sensory orifices and seizes the *shen*, the animal may lose consciousness, or go into a coma. Clinically, this formula is used to treat hot *bi zheng* (closed disorder) syndrome, as seen in stroke, coma, seizures, and epilepsy.

This formula uses *Niu Huang* (Calculus Bovis) to clear Heart heat, eliminate toxins, dispel phlegm, and open the orifices. *She Xiang* (Moschus) has a resuscitating function to open the sensory orifices and awaken the *shen* (spirit). Though *She Xiang* (Moschus) is a warm substance, it will not generate heat, as the formula contains many cold herbs at large doses. *Xi Jiao* (Cornu Rhinoceri) clears heat, cools the blood, and eliminates toxins. *Huang Qin* (Radix Scutellariae), *Huang Lian* (Rhizoma Coptidis), and *Zhi Zi* (Fructus Gardeniae) clear heat, purge fire, and eliminate toxins. *Bing Pian* (Borneolum Syntheticum) and *Yu Jin* (Radix Curcumae) enhance the resuscitating function of *She Xiang* (Moschus) to open the orifices and awaken the *shen*. *Zhu Sha* (Cinnabaris) and *Zhen Zhu* (Margarita) calm the *shen* and relieve fidgeting and irritability. *Xiong Huang* (Realgar) helps *Niu Huang* (Calculus Bovis) dispel phlegm and eliminate toxins. *Jin Bo* (gold foil) helps *Zhu Sha* (Cinnabaris) calm the *shen*. *Feng Mi* (Mel), as the envoy herb, regulates the middle *jiao* and strengthens the Stomach.

This formula can also be used to treat unconsciousness due to coma and convulsions, if the patient has the above clinical manifestations.

VETERINARY MODIFICATIONS

With heat entering the Pericardium and excess heat in the *fu* (hollow organs) manifesting in delirium, constipation, and thirst that cannot be relieved by the intake of water, administer 2 pills of *An Gong Niu Huang Wan* plus 9g of powdered *Da Huang* (Radix et Rhizoma Rhei) in warm water.

An Gong Niu Huang Wan (Calm the Palace Pill with Cattle Gallstone)

Diagnosis	Clinical Signs	Treatment	Herbs
Febrile disorder with heat attacking the Pericardium and hot phlegm obstructing the orifices	• *Shen* (spirit) disturbance, high fever, and irritability: heat attacking the Pericardium • Coma and unconsciousness: hot phlegm obstructing the sensory orifices	• Clears heat and opens the orifices • Dispels phlegm and eliminates toxins	• *Niu Huang* (Calculus Bovis) clears Heart heat, eliminates toxins, dispels phlegm, and opens the orifices. • *She Xiang* (Moschus) opens sensory orifices and awakens the *shen*. • *Xi Jiao* (Cornu Rhinoceri) clears heat, cools the blood, and eliminates toxins. • *Huang Qin* (Radix Scutellariae), *Huang Lian* (Rhizoma Coptidis) and *Zhi Zi* (Fructus Gardeniae) clear heat, purge fire, and eliminate toxins. • *Bing Pian* (Borneolum Syntheticum) and *Yu Jin* (Radix Curcumae) open the orifices and awaken the *shen*. • *Zhu Sha* (Cinnabaris), *Zhen Zhu* (Margarita), and *Jin Bo* (gold foil) calm the *shen* and relieve fidgeting and irritability. • *Xiong Huang* (Realgar) dispels phlegm and eliminates toxins. • *Feng Mi* (Mel) regulates the middle *jiao* and strengthens the Stomach.

Ān Gōng Niú Huáng Wán (Calm the Palace Pill with Cattle Gallstone)

CAUTIONS / CONTRAINDICATIONS

- *An Gong Niu Huang Wan* is contraindicated in cases of *zhong feng* (wind stroke) characterized by *tuo zheng* (abandoned syndrome).[1]
- Use of this formula is contraindicated during pregnancy.[2]

PHARMACOLOGICAL EFFECTS

1. **Central nervous system**: Laboratory experiments showed that administration of *An Gong Niu Huang Wan* had a sedative effect on the central nervous system by decreasing spontaneous physical activities and suppressing seizures.[3]
2. **Antipyretic**: Administration of the formula was effective in treating rabbits with artificially-induced fever. The antipyretic effect was observed one hour following ingestion, and lasted for 5-6 hours.[4]
3. **Anti-inflammatory**: In one study, the use of the formula was associated with marked effect to reduce swelling and inflammation. The effect was observed from 1 to 4.5 hours after administration.[5]
4. **Hypotensive**: In one experiment, intravenous injection of the formula was associated with an immediate drop of blood pressure of approximately 10-40 mmHg. The effect to lower blood pressure lasted for 3-5 minutes, with blood pressure returning to the previous level after 10 minutes.[6]

HUMAN CLINICAL STUDIES AND RESEARCH

1. **Fever**: One report described 8 cancer patients with high fevers of 39.1-41.5°C (102.4-106.7°F) for an average of 5.6 days. They were treated with *An Gong Niu Huang Wan*, and all patients stopped using analgesic and anti-inflammatory drugs during the herbal therapy. The treatment protocol was to administer one pill of the formula twice daily for 3-5 days. The study reported that the temperature was reduced to below 38°C (100.4°F) within 4-72 hours (average of 27.2 hours). The study concluded the formula to be effective in treating fever in cancer patients.[7]
2. **Others**: *An Gong Niu Huang Wan* has been used to treat encephalitis B, meningitis, dysentery, toxic uremia, hepatitis, acute icteric hepatitis, acute pancreatitis, cerebrovascular accident, seizures, and convulsions.[8]

TOXICOLOGY

In humans, the use of *An Gong Niu Huang Wan* has been associated with side effects such as palpitations, dull pain in the upper abdominal area, fear, fright, restlessness, irritability, facial edema, rashes, and dark purple appearance that starts at the lips and then spreads to the rest of the body. Long-term use or gross overdose (over 60 pills per dose) has been associated with nephritis, with clinical signs such as low back pain, decreased urination, red-colored urine, and the presence of protein and white blood cells in the urine.[9] Note: These reactions are usually attributed to *Zhu Sha* (Cinnabaris) and *Xiong Huang* (Realgar), two substances that are considered toxic.

SUGGESTED ACUPUNCTURE TREATMENT

1. Points: *Renzhong* (GV 26), *Zhongchong* (PC 9), *Shaochong* (HT 9), *Quze* (PC 3), *Weizhong* (BL 40), and *Fenglong* (ST 40).
2. Technique: sedation and prick to bleed.

The acupuncture treatment aims to quickly sedate excess heat and resuscitate the patient. *Renzhong* (GV 26) dispels wind and clears heat to open the orifices. *Zhongchong* (PC 9) is the *jing* (well) point of the Pericardium channel. *Shaochong* (HT 9) is the *jing* (well) point of the Heart channel. Both *Zhongchong* (PC 9) and *Shaochong* (HT 9) can be pricked and bled to sedate excess heat. *Quze* (PC 3) is the *he* (uniting) point of the Pericardium channel. *Weizhong* (BL 40) is the *he* (uniting) point of the Urinary Bladder channel. Both of them can be pricked and bled to sedate heat in the blood level. *Fenglong* (ST 40) disperses phlegm.

RELATED FORMULA

Niú Huáng Qīng Xīn Wán
(Cattle Gallstone Pill to Clear the Heart)
牛黃清心丸
牛黄清心丸
Pinyin Name: *Niu Huang Qing Xin Wan*
Literal Name: Cattle Gallstone Pill to Clear the Heart
Original Source: *Dou Zhen Shi Yi Xin Fa* (Teachings of Generations of Physicians about Pox) by Wan Quan in 1568

Niu Huang (Calculus Bovis)	0.75g
Zhu Sha (Cinnabaris)	4.5g
Huang Lian (Rhizoma Coptidis)	15g
Huang Qin (Radix Scutellariae)	9g
Zhi Zi (Fructus Gardeniae)	9g
Yu Jin (Radix Curcumae)	6g

Note: *Zhu Sha* (Cinnabaris) is a potentially toxic heavy metal, and is rarely used as a medicinal substance today. Its discussion here is included primarily for academic purposes, to reflect the historical use of this substance in its original formulation. Most herbal products today have removed it completely, or replaced it with substitutes with similar functions. For additional information on the toxicity, please refer to *Chinese Medical Herbology and Pharmacology* by John Chen and Tina Chen.

Ān Gōng Niú Huáng Wán (Calm the Palace Pill with Cattle Gallstone)

Grind the ingredients into a fine powder, and form into pills with flour and water. The pills should resemble corn kernels in size. Take 7-8 pills with a decoction of *Deng Xin Cao* (Medulla Junci). Today, this formula is normally prepared by mixing the powdered herbs with honey to form pills. The pills should weigh 1.5g each. Take 2 pills per dose two to three times daily. Adjust the doses for animals according to age and body weight.

Niu Huang Qing Xin Wan (Cattle Gallstone Pill to Clear the Heart) clears heat, eliminates toxins, opens the sensory orifices, and calms the *shen* (spirit). Clinically, this formula may be used for heat invading the Pericardium, leading to such clinical signs as delirium, semi-unconsciousness, feverish sensations, restlessness and irritability. This formula may also be used for infantile convulsions in which there is constant muscle contraction, and for *zhong feng* (wind stroke) with closed sensory orifices.

An Gong Niu Huang Wan and *Niu Huang Qing Xin Wan* (Cattle Gallstone Pill to Clear the Heart) have similar compositions, actions, and indications.

- *An Gong Niu Huang Wan* has a stronger action to tranquilize the *shen* (spirit) and open the sensory orifices; hence, it is more suitable for cases with such clinical signs as high fever, semiconsciousness, and delirium.
- *Niu Huang Qing Xin Wan* functions more strongly to clear heat and eliminate toxins, and is more suitable for cases with clinical signs such as feverish sensations and irritability.

AUTHORS' COMMENTS

An Gong Niu Huang Wan, *Zhi Bao Dan* (Greatest Treasure Special Pill), and *Zi Xue Dan* (Purple Snow Pill) are commonly referred to as "*San Bao* (Three Treasures)," as these are three of the most commonly used formulas to treat hot *bi zheng* (closed disorder).

- *An Gong Niu Huang Wan* is the coldest of the three formulas. It is most potent in clearing heat and eliminating toxins.
- *Zhi Bao Dan* is aromatic, and is the best for opening the sensory orifices to treat unconsciousness due to obstruction of phlegm and heat.
- *Zi Xue Dan* is most effective in calming Liver wind to treat seizures, epilepsy, and convulsions.

References

1. *Zhong Yao Ming Fang Yao Li Yu Ying Yong* (Pharmacology and Applications of Famous Herbal Formulas), 1989; 379-381.
2. *Zhong Yao Ming Fang Yao Li Yu Ying Yong* (Pharmacology and Applications of Famous Herbal Formulas), 1989; 379-381.
3. *Zhong Yi Fang Ji Xian Dai Yan Jiu* (Modern Study of Medical Formulas in Traditional Chinese Medicine), 1997; 870.
4. *Zhong Cheng Yao Yan Jiu* (Research of Chinese Patent Medicine), 1982; 5:23.
5. *Zhong Yi Fang Ji Xian Dai Yan Jiu* (Modern Study of Medical Formulas in Traditional Chinese Medicine), 1997; 871.
6. *Zhong Yi Fang Ji Xian Dai Yan Jiu* (Modern Study of Medical Formulas in Traditional Chinese Medicine), 1997; 871.
7. *Shi Yong Zhong Xi Yi Jie He Za Zhi* (Practical Journal of Integrated Chinese and Western Medicines), 1994; 7(9):545.
8. *Zhong Yi Fang Ji Xian Dai Yan Jiu* (Modern Study of Medical Formulas in Traditional Chinese Medicine), 1997; 871-874.
9. *Zhong Yao Bu Liang Fan Ying Yu Zhi Liao* (Adverse Reactions and Treatment of Chinese Herbal Medicine), 1996; 74.

Zhì Bǎo Dān (Greatest Treasure Special Pill)

至寶丹
至宝丹

Pinyin Name: *Zhi Bao Dan*
Literal Name: Greatest Treasure Special Pill
Original Sources: *Tai Ping Hui Min He Ji Ju Fang* (Imperial Grace Formulary of the Tai Ping Era) by the Imperial Medical Department in 1078-85

COMPOSITION

She Xiang (Moschus), *yan* (ground) to small particles	0.3g [7.5g]
Bing Pian (Borneolum Syntheticum), *yan* (ground) to small particles	0.3g [7.5g]
An Xi Xiang (Benzoinum), *ao* (simmered) into paste	45g
Xi Jiao (Cornu Rhinoceri), *yan* (ground) to small particles	30g
Niu Huang (Calculus Bovis), *yan* (ground) to small particles	0.3g [7.5g]
Dai Mao (Carapax Eretmochelydis Imbricatae), *yan* (ground) to small particles	30g
Jin Bo (gold foil)	50 leaves
Yin Bo (silver foil), *yan* (ground) to small particles	50 leaves
Zhu Sha (Cinnabaris), *yan* (ground) and *shui fei* (refined with water)	30g
Hu Po (Succinum), *yan* (ground) to small particles	30g
Xiong Huang (Realgar), *yan* (ground) and *shui fei* (refined with water)	30g

Note: *Zhu Sha* (Cinnabaris) and *Xiong Huang* (Realgar) are potentially toxic heavy metals, and *Xi Jiao* (Cornu Rhinoceri) and *She Xiang* (Moschus) are derived from endangered animals. They are rarely used as medicinal substances today. The discussion of these substances here is included primarily for academic purposes, to reflect the historical use of these substances in its original formulation. Most herbal products today have removed them completely, or replaced them with substitutes with similar functions. For additional information on the toxicity of *Zhu Sha* (Cinnabaris) and *Xiong Huang* (Realgar), please refer to *Chinese Medical Herbology and Pharmacology* by John Chen and Tina Chen.

DOSAGE / PREPARATION / ADMINISTRATION

Crush separately into fine powder *Xi Jiao* (Cornu Rhinoceri), *Dai Mao* (Carapax Eretmochelydis Imbricatae), *An Xi Xiang* (Benzoinum), and *Hu Po* (Succinum). *Zhu Sha* (Cinnabaris) and *Xiong Huang* (Realgar) are separately processed via the *shui fei* (refining with water) technique to obtain extremely fine powders. *Niu Huang* (Calculus Bovis), *She Xiang* (Moschus), and *Bing Pian* (Borneolum Syntheticum) are ground into powder. *Jin Bo* (gold foil) [25 leaves] and *Yin Bo* (silver foil) [50 leaves] are also ground into powder. Blend all of the powders together, place them through a sieve, and mix with honey to form pills. Coat the pills with the remaining 25 leaves of *Jin Bo* (gold foil). The pills should weigh 3g each. Give 1 pill, one time daily. Reduce the dose for young animals.

Note: The formulation today no longer uses *Jin Bo* (gold foil) or *Yin Bo* (silver foil), and has replaced *Xi Jiao* (Cornu Rhinoceri) with *Shui Niu Jiao* (Cornu Bubali).

CHINESE THERAPEUTIC ACTIONS

1. Clears heat and opens the sensory orifices
2. Dissolves turbidity and eliminates toxins

CLINICAL MANIFESTATIONS

1. Heat stroke, *zhong feng* (wind stroke), *wen bing* (warm diseases), and *bi zheng* (closed disorder) with obstruction of phlegm and heat: altered consciousness, irritability, restlessness, hoarse vocalization with profuse sputum, a red tongue with a greasy tongue coating, and a slippery, rapid pulse.
2. Seizures and epilepsy caused by obstruction of phlegm and heat.

VETERINARY CLINICAL APPLICATIONS

Stroke, heat stroke, coma, seizures and epilepsy, and encephalitis.

EXPLANATION

Zhi Bao Dan (Greatest Treasure Special Pill) treats various disorders characterized by obstruction of phlegm and heat in the interior. The phlegm and heat cover the Pericardium and block the sensory orifices. Due to the heat, there will be clinical signs of feverish sensations, irritability, and restlessness. Phlegm, which covers the Pericardium and

Zhì Bǎo Dān (Greatest Treasure Special Pill)

Zhi Bao Dan **(Greatest Treasure Special Pill)**

Diagnosis	Clinical Signs	Treatment	Herbs
Heat stroke, *zhong feng* (wind stroke), *wen bing* (warm diseases), and *bi zheng* (closed disorder) with obstruction by phlegm and heat	• Altered consciousness, irritability, and restlessness: heat and phlegm covering the Pericardium and blocking the sensory orifices • Hoarse vocalization with profuse sputum: phlegm and heat in the interior • Red tongue with a greasy tongue coating: phlegm and heat in the interior • Slippery, rapid pulse: phlegm and heat in the interior	• Clears heat and opens the sensory orifices • Dissolves turbidity and eliminates toxins	• *She Xiang* (Moschus), *Bing Pian* (Borneolum Syntheticum), and *An Xi Xiang* (Benzoinum) open the sensory orifices and dissolve turbidity. • *Xi Jiao* (Cornu Rhinoceri), *Niu Huang* (Calculus Bovis), and *Dai Mao* (Carapax Eretmochelydis Imbricatae) clear heat and eliminate toxins. • *Jin Bo* (gold foil), *Yin Bo* (silver foil), *Zhu Sha* (Cinnabaris), and *Hu Po* (Succinum) sedate the Heart and calm the *shen* (spirit). • *Xiong Huang* (Realgar) dispels phlegm and eliminates toxins.

blocks the sensory orifices, causes clinical signs such as altered consciousness and delirium.

This formula uses aromatic substances such as *She Xiang* (Moschus), *Bing Pian* (Borneolum Syntheticum), and *An Xi Xiang* (Benzoinum) to open the sensory orifices and dissolve turbidity. *Xi Jiao* (Cornu Rhinoceri), *Niu Huang* (Calculus Bovis), and *Dai Mao* (Carapax Eretmochelydis Imbricatae) clear heat and eliminate toxins. *Niu Huang* (Calculus Bovis) also treats seizures and epilepsy. *Jin Bo* (gold foil), *Yin Bo* (silver foil), *Zhu Sha* (Cinnabaris), and *Hu Po* (Succinum) sedate the Heart and calm the *shen* (spirit). *Xiong Huang* (Realgar) dispels phlegm and eliminates toxins.

VETERINARY MODIFICATIONS

For deficiency of *zheng* (upright) *qi*, administer *Zhi Bao San* with a decoction of *Ren Shen* (Radix et Rhizoma Ginseng).

CAUTIONS / CONTRAINDICATIONS

- *Zhi Bao Dan* is contraindicated in cases of yang excess and yin deficiency, as this formula has many acrid and drying herbs that may consume yin and body fluids.
- During pregnancy, this formula should only be used when absolutely necessary, and then, only with extreme caution.

SUGGESTED ACUPUNCTURE TREATMENT

1. Points: *Renzhong* (GV 26), *Baihui* (GV 20), *Dazhui* (GV 14), all twelve *jing* (well) points, *Laogong* (PC 8), *Shenmen* (HT 7), and *Fenglong* (ST 40).
2. Technique: sedation and bleeding.

Renzhong (GV 26) and *Baihui* (GV 20) open the orifices. Bleed *Dazhui* (GV 14) and the twelve *jing* (well) points to clear heat and open the orifices. Sedate *Laogong* (PC 8) and *Shenmen* (HT 7) to calm the *shen* (spirit). *Fenglong* (ST 40) dispels phlegm.

AUTHORS' COMMENTS

Zhi Bao Dan is a formula that traditionally has been used in humans. However, its use today in veterinary medicine is limited because most animals with such condition are treated in emergency rooms.

Zǐ Xuě (Purple Snow)

紫雪

紫雪

Pinyin Name: *Zi Xue*
Literal Name: Purple Snow
Alternate Name: *Zi Xue Dan* (Purple Snow Pill)
Original Source: *Wai Tai Mi Yao* (Arcane Essentials from the Imperial Library) by Wang Tao in 752 A.D.

COMPOSITION

Xi Jiao (Cornu Rhinoceri)	150g
Shi Gao (Gypsum Fibrosum)	1,500g
Han Shui Shi (Mirabilite)	1,500g
Hua Shi (Talcum)	1,500g
Xuan Shen (Radix Scrophulariae)	500g
Sheng Ma (Rhizoma Cimicifugae)	500g
She Xiang (Moschus), *yan* (ground) to small particles	1.5g
Mu Xiang (Radix Aucklandiae)	150g
Ding Xiang (Flos Caryophylli)	30g
Chen Xiang (Lignum Aquilariae Resinatum)	150g
Ling Yang Jiao (Cornu Saigae Tataricae)	150g
Zhu Sha (Cinnabaris), *shui fei* (refined with water) and *yan* (ground) to small particles	90g
Ci Shi (Magnetitum)	1,500g
Po Xiao (Sal Glauberis), *zhi* (prepared)	5,000g
Xiao Shi (Niter), *zhi* (prepared)	96g
Huang Jin (Gold)	3,000g
Zhi Gan Cao (Radix et Rhizoma Glycyrrhizae Praeparata cum Melle)	240g

Note: *Zhu Sha* (Cinnabaris) is a potentially toxic heavy metal, and *Ling Yang Jiao* (Cornu Saigae Tataricae), *She Xiang* (Moschus) and *Xi Jiao* (Cornu Rhinoceri) are derived from endangered animals. They are rarely used as a medicinal substance today. The discussion here is included primarily for academic purposes, to reflect the historical use of these substances in its original formulation. Most herbal products today have removed them completely, or replaced them with substitutes with similar functions. For additional information on the toxicity of *Zhu Sha* (Cinnabaris), please refer to *Chinese Medical Herbology and Pharmacology* by John Chen and Tina Chen.

Note: The source text states to use "*Qing Mu Xiang*" as one of the ingredients in this formula. However, it is believed that "*Qing Mu Xiang*" actually refers to *Mu Xiang* (Radix Aucklandiae) during that period. Therefore, most textbooks and clinicians now use *Mu Xiang* (Radix Aucklandiae) as the ingredient in this formula. Also, *Po Xiao* (Sal Glauberis) is usually replaced with *Mang Xiao* (Natrii Sulfas), which is more readily available. *Huang Jin* (Gold) is replaced with *Jin Bo* (gold foil), or removed from the formula.

DOSAGE / PREPARATION / ADMINISTRATION

Crush the mineral ingredients - *Shi Gao* (Gypsum Fibrosum), *Huang Jin* (Gold), *Han Shui Shi* (Mirabilite), *Hua Shi* (Talcum) and *Ci Shi* (Magnetitum) - into small particles and cook in water three times. Then, add the herbal ingredients - *Xuan Shen* (Radix Scrophulariae), *Mu Xiang* (Radix Aucklandiae), *Chen Xiang* (Lignum Aquilariae Resinatum), *Sheng Ma* (Rhizoma Cimicifugae), *Zhi Gan Cao* (Radix et Rhizoma Glycyrrhizae Praeparata cum Melle) and *Ding Xiang* (Flos Caryophylli) - and cook in water three times. Filter and discard the residues, and cook the strained decoction and reduce it to a condensed paste.

Mix into this paste powdered *Xiao Shi* (Niter) and *Po Xiao* (Sal Glauberis), and blend thoroughly. Allow it to dry and then grind it into a fine powder. Grate and grind the horns, *Xi Jiao* (Cornu Rhinoceri) and *Ling Yang Jiao* (Cornu Saigae Tataricae), into a fine powder. Process *Zhu Sha* (Cinnabaris) via the *shui fei* (refining with water) technique to obtain an extremely fine powder. Grind *She Xiang* (Moschus) into powder. Mix these powders together, and place them through a sieve to obtain the final powdered formula. Take 1.5-3g of the powder per

Zǐ Xuě (Purple Snow)

dose, two times daily. Reduce the dose for young animals. As the literal name of the formula implies, the finished product resembles "purple snow."

CHINESE THERAPEUTIC ACTIONS

1. Clears heat and opens the sensory orifices
2. Stops convulsions and calms the *shen* (spirit)

CLINICAL MANIFESTATIONS

Febrile disorders with heat attacking the Pericardium and the rising of Liver wind: high fever, irritability, restlessness, altered consciousness, thirst, dysuria, constipation, and epilepsy.

VETERINARY CLINICAL APPLICATIONS

Seizure disorders and epilepsy.

EXPLANATION

Zi Xue (Purple Snow) treats febrile disorders in which heat attacks the Pericardium and causes the rising of Liver wind. When heat attacks the Pericardium and disturbs the *shen* (spirit), there will be altered consciousness, delirium, irritability, and restlessness. The presence of heat in febrile disorders may also cause high fever, dysuria, and constipation. Heat may also stir Liver wind and cause it to rise upward, leading to seizures and epilepsy. Lastly, heat may dry up body fluids, causing thirst and dry lips.

Xi Jiao (Cornu Rhinoceri) clears heat from the Heart and eliminates toxins. Sweet and cold, *Shi Gao* (Gypsum Fibrosum), *Han Shui Shi* (Mirabilite), and *Hua Shi* (Talcum) clear heat, purge fire, and preserve yin. *Xuan Shen* (Radix Scrophulariae) and *Sheng Ma* (Rhizoma Cimicifugae) clear heat and eliminate toxins. *She Xiang* (Moschus), *Mu Xiang* (Radix Aucklandiae), *Ding Xiang* (Flos Caryophylli), and *Chen Xiang* (Lignum Aquilariae Resinatum) activate qi circulation and open the sensory orifices. *Ling Yang Jiao* (Cornu Saigae Tataricae) clears the Liver, calms Liver wind, and relieves convulsions. *Zhu Sha* (Cinnabaris) and *Ci Shi* (Magnetitum) are heavy substances that anchor the *shen* (spirit) and relieve irritability and restlessness. *Huang Jin* (Gold) sedates the Heart, calms the *shen*, and eliminates toxins. *Po Xiao* (Sal Glauberis) and *Xiao Shi* (Niter) clear heat and drain it downward. Lastly, *Zhi Gan Cao* (Radix et Rhizoma Glycyrrhizae Praeparata cum Melle) harmonizes the formula.

CAUTIONS / CONTRAINDICATIONS

- *Zi Xue* should be discontinued as soon as the desired effects are achieved. Prolonged use of this formula, or use

***Zi Xue* (Purple Snow)**

Diagnosis	Clinical Signs	Treatment	Herbs
Febrile disorders with heat attacking the Pericardium and the rising of Liver wind	• High fever, altered consciousness, delirium, irritability, and restlessness: heat attacking the Pericardium and disturbing the *shen* (spirit) • Seizures and epilepsy: heat stirring Liver wind upwards • Thirst and dry lips: heat consuming body fluids in the upper body • Dysuria and constipation: heat damaging body fluids in the lower body	• Clears heat and opens the sensory orifices • Stops convulsions and calms the *shen*	• *Xi Jiao* (Cornu Rhinoceri) clears heat from the Heart and eliminates toxins. • *Shi Gao* (Gypsum Fibrosum), *Han Shui Shi* (Mirabilite), and *Hua Shi* (Talcum) clear heat, purge fire, and preserve yin. • *Xuan Shen* (Radix Scrophulariae) and *Sheng Ma* (Rhizoma Cimicifugae) clear heat and eliminate toxins. • *She Xiang* (Moschus), *Mu Xiang* (Radix Aucklandiae), *Ding Xiang* (Flos Caryophylli) and *Chen Xiang* (Lignum Aquilariae Resinatum) activate qi circulation and open the orifices. • *Ling Yang Jiao* (Cornu Saigae Tataricae) clears the Liver, calms Liver wind, and relieves convulsions. • *Zhu Sha* (Cinnabaris) and *Ci Shi* (Magnetitum) are heavy substances that anchor the *shen* and relieve irritability and restlessness. • *Po Xiao* (Sal Glauberis) and *Xiao Shi* (Niter) clear heat and drain it downward. • *Huang Jin* (Gold) sedates the Heart, calms the *shen*, and eliminates toxins. • *Zhi Gan Cao* (Radix et Rhizoma Glycyrrhizae Praeparata cum Melle) harmonizes the formula.

Zǐ Xuě (Purple Snow)

at large doses, could cause such side effects as profuse sweating, nausea, vomiting, icy cold extremities, hurried respiration, palpitations, and dizziness.

- The use of this formula is contraindicated during pregnancy.[1]
- Avoid spicy, pungent, oily, and greasy foods while taking this formula.[2]

SUGGESTED ACUPUNCTURE TREATMENT

1. Points: *Shixuan* (extra point), *Dazhui* (GV 14), *Renzhong* (GV 26), *Shanzhong* (CV 17), *Taichong* (LR 3), *Shenmen* (HT 7), and *Weizhong* (BL 40).
2. Technique: bleeding and sedation.

Bleed *Shixuan* (extra point) and *Weizhong* (BL 40) and sedate *Dazhui* (GV 14) to purge heat. *Renzhong* (GV 26) and *Shanzhong* (CV 17) regulate qi and open the orifices. *Taichong* (LR 3) soothes the Liver. *Shenmen* (HT 7) calms the Heart.

AUTHORS' COMMENTS

Febrile disorders are often complicated by heat drying up body fluids. Therefore, it is important to note that this formula uses sweet and cold herbs, such as *Shi Gao* (Gypsum Fibrosum) and *Hua Shi* (Talcum), to clear heat and preserve body fluids, instead of bitter and cold herbs, such as *Huang Qin* (Radix Scutellariae) and *Huang Lian* (Rhizoma Coptidis), which clear heat but will damage yin and body fluids.

References

1. *Zhong Yao Ming Fang Yao Li Yu Ying Yong* (Pharmacology and Applications of Famous Herbal Formulas), 1989; 385-386.
2. *Zhong Yao Ming Fang Yao Li Yu Ying Yong* (Pharmacology and Applications of Famous Herbal Formulas), 1989; 385-386.

Section 2

温开剂
— Warm Orifice-Opening Formulas

Sū Hé Xiāng Wán (Liquid Styrax Pill)
蘇合香丸
苏合香丸

Pinyin Name: *Su He Xiang Wan*
Literal Name: Liquid Styrax Pill
Original Source: *Tai Ping Hui Min He Ji Ju Fang* (Imperial Grace Formulary of the Tai Ping Era) by the Imperial Medical Department in 1078-85

COMPOSITION

Su He Xiang (Styrax), *dun* (stewed)	30g
She Xiang (Moschus), *yan* (ground) to small particles	60g
Bing Pian (Borneolum Syntheticum), *yan* (ground) to small particles	30g
An Xi Xiang (Benzoinum), *ao* (simmered) the powder into paste	60g
Mu Xiang (Radix Aucklandiae)	60g
Tan Xiang (Lignum Santali Albi)	60g
Chen Xiang (Lignum Aquilariae Resinatum)	60g
Ru Xiang (Gummi Olibanum), *yan* (ground) to small particles	30g
Ding Xiang (Flos Caryophylli)	60g
Xiang Fu (Rhizoma Cyperi), *chao* (dry-fried)	60g
Bi Bo (Fructus Piperis Longi)	60g
Xi Jiao (Cornu Rhinoceri)	60g
Zhu Sha (Cinnabaris), *yan* (ground) and *shui fei* (refined with water)	60g
Bai Zhu (Rhizoma Atractylodis Macrocephalae)	60g
He Zi (Fructus Chebulae), *wei* (roasted)	60g

Note: *Zhu Sha* (Cinnabaris) is a potentially toxic heavy metal, and *Xi Jiao* (Cornu Rhinoceri) and *She Xiang* (Moschus) are derived from endangered animals. They are rarely used as medicinal substances today. The discussion here is included primarily for academic purposes, to reflect the historical use of these substances in its original formulation. Most herbal products today have removed them completely, or replaced them with substitutes with similar functions. For additional information on the toxicity of *Zhu Sha* (Cinnabaris), please refer to *Chinese Medical Herbology and Pharmacology* by John Chen and Tina Chen.

The source text states to use "*Qing Mu Xiang*" as one of the ingredients in this formula. However, it is believed that "*Qing Mu Xiang*" actually refers to *Mu Xiang* (Radix Aucklandiae) during that period. Therefore, most textbooks and clinicians now use *Mu Xiang* (Radix Aucklandiae) as one of the ingredients in this formula.

DOSAGE / PREPARATION / ADMINISTRATION

Grind separately *She Xiang* (Moschus), *Bing Pian* (Borneolum Syntheticum) and *Xi Jiao* (Cornu Rhinoceri) into fine powder and sift all of these powders together. Process *Zhu Sha* (Cinnabaris) separately via the *shui fei* (refining with water) method to obtain an extremely fine powder. Grind and blend all of the ingredients into powder. Separately simmer *An Xi Xiang* (Benzoinum) from powder into paste, and stew *Su He Xiang* (Styrax) from solid into liquid form, and then blend the paste and

Sū Hé Xiāng Wán (Liquid Styrax Pill)

the liquid together. Mix all of the ingredients (both powder and liquid) with honey to form large pills. Dry the pills in a cool place without direct exposure to sunlight. Give 1 pill, one to two times daily.

CHINESE THERAPEUTIC ACTIONS

1. Opens the sensory orifices with aromatic herbs
2. Activates qi circulation and stops pain

CLINICAL MANIFESTATIONS

Cold-type *bi zheng* (closed disorder) syndrome caused by stagnation of cold, qi and phlegm: sudden unconsciousness, extreme pain in the chest and abdomen, tetany, pale, bluish mucous membranes, tongue and lips, a white tongue coating, and a slow pulse.

VETERINARY CLINICAL APPLICATIONS

Acute congestive heart failure, cardiomyopathy, and cerebrovascular accident.

EXPLANATION

Su He Xiang Wan (Liquid Styrax Pill) is the representative formula for treating cold *bi zheng* (closed disorder) syndrome caused by stagnation of cold, qi and phlegm. Interior cold or phlegm obstruction may suddenly block the qi flow and "seize" Heart *shen* (spirit). As a result, acute and serious clinical signs such as sudden unconsciousness, lockjaw, and abdominal and chest pain occur. To effectively treat this syndrome, all three methods of cold-dispersing, qi-regulating, and phlegm-dissolving must be employed. This formula uses aromatic substances, such as *Su He Xiang* (Styrax), *She Xiang* (Moschus), *Bing Pian* (Borneolum Syntheticum), and *An Xi Xiang* (Benzoinum), to quickly open the sensory orifices. *Mu Xiang* (Radix Aucklandiae), *Tan Xiang* (Lignum Santali Albi), *Chen Xiang* (Lignum Aquilariae Resinatum), *Ru Xiang* (Gummi Olibanum), *Ding Xiang* (Flos Caryophylli), and *Xiang Fu* (Rhizoma Cyperi) activate qi circulation, dispel cold, and dissolve phlegm. *Bi Bo* (Fructus Piperis Longi) warms the interior and dispels cold. *Xi Jiao* (Cornu Rhinoceri) clears heat and eliminates toxins. *Zhu Sha* (Cinnabaris) quickly calms the *shen* (spirit) and stabilizes the mind. *Bai Zhu* (Rhizoma Atractylodis Macrocephalae) strengthens the Spleen and dispels dampness. *He Zi* (Fructus Chebulae) has a constricting effect to prevent the acrid and dispersing herbs of this formula from consuming too much *zheng* (upright) *qi*.

CAUTIONS / CONTRAINDICATIONS

- *Su He Xiang Wan* is contraindicated in cases of *tuo zheng* (abandoned syndrome) and hot *bi zheng* (closed disorder).
- Use of this formula is contraindicated during pregnancy.

SUGGESTED ACUPUNCTURE TREATMENT

1. Points: *Renzhong* (GV 26), *Neiguan* (PC 6), *Qihai* (CV 6), *Housanli* (ST 36), *Shanzhong* (CV 17), *Weiyang* (BL 39),

***Su He Xiang Wan* (Liquid Styrax Pill)**

Diagnosis	Clinical Signs	Treatment	Herbs
Cold-type *bi zheng* (closed disorder) syndrome due to stagnation of cold, qi and phlegm	• Sudden unconsciousness, lockjaw, and extreme pain in the chest and abdomen: cold *bi zheng* (closed disorder) • Pale, bluish mucous membranes, tongue and lips: cold • Pain in the chest and abdomen: qi and blood stagnation	• Opens the sensory orifices with aromatic herbs • Activates qi circulation and stops pain	• *Su He Xiang* (Styrax), *She Xiang* (Moschus), *Bing Pian* (Borneolum Syntheticum) and *An Xi Xiang* (Benzoinum) quickly open the sensory orifices. • *Mu Xiang* (Radix Aucklandiae), *Tan Xiang* (Lignum Santali Albi), *Chen Xiang* (Lignum Aquilariae Resinatum), *Ru Xiang* (Gummi Olibanum), *Ding Xiang* (Flos Caryophylli) and *Xiang Fu* (Rhizoma Cyperi) activate qi circulation, dispel cold, and dissolve phlegm. • *Bi Bo* (Fructus Piperis Longi) warms the interior and dispels cold. • *Xi Jiao* (Cornu Rhinoceri) clears heat and eliminates toxins. • *Zhu Sha* (Cinnabaris) quickly calms the *shen* (spirit) and stabilizes the mind. • *Bai Zhu* (Rhizoma Atractylodis Macrocephalae) strengthens the Spleen and dispels dampness. • *He Zi* (Fructus Chebulae) prevents the acrid and dispersing herbs of this formula from consuming too much *zheng* (upright) *qi*.

Sū Hé Xiāng Wán (Liquid Styrax Pill)

Taichong (LR 3), *Juque* (CV 14), *Fenglong* (ST 40), and *Shenque* (CV 8).

2. Technique: even method and moxibustion.

Renzhong (GV 26) enters the brain and opens the orifices to resuscitate the patient. *Neiguan* (PC 6), the *luo* (connecting) point of the Pericardium channel, regulates qi and blood flow to calm the mind. *Qihai* (CV 6) and *Housanli* (ST 36) strengthen Spleen qi, dry dampness, and activate qi circulation to relieve pain. *Shanzhong* (CV 17) regulates qi flow and relieves pain. *Weiyang* (BL 39) regulates the pathways of all three *jiaos*.

Depending on the patient's condition, the following points may be added: *Taichong* (LR 3) in cases of severe qi stagnation; *Juque* (CV 14) and *Fenglong* (ST 40) in cases of severe phlegm stagnation; and moxibustion on *Shenque* (CV 8) in cases of severe cold stagnation.

AUTHORS' COMMENTS

Su He Xiang Wan is a formula that traditionally has been used in humans. However, its use today in veterinary medicine is limited because most animals with such condition are treated in emergency rooms.

Zǐ Jīn Dìng (Purple Gold Special Pill)

紫金錠

紫金锭

Pinyin Name: *Zi Jin Ding*
Literal Name: Purple Gold Special Pill
Alternate Name: Calamus and Carthamus Formula
Original Source: *Pian Yu Xin Shu* (Text from Heart of Jade) by Wu Quan in the mid-16th century

COMPOSITION

She Xiang (Moschus)	9g
Shan Ci Gu (Pseudobulbus Cremastrae seu Pleiones)	90g
Xiong Huang (Realgar)	30g
Qian Jin Zi (Semen Euphorbiae), frost	30g
Hong Da Ji (Radix Knoxiae)	45g
Zhu Sha (Cinnabaris)	30g
Wu Bei Zi (Galla Chinensis)	90g

Note: *Zhu Sha* (Cinnabaris) and *Xiong Huang* (Realgar) are potentially toxic heavy metals, and *She Xiang* (Moschus) is derived from an endangered animal. They are rarely used as medicinal substances today. The discussion here is included primarily for academic purposes, to reflect the historical use of these substances in its original formulation. Most herbal products today have removed them completely, or replaced them with substitutes with similar functions. For additional information on the toxicity, please refer to *Chinese Medical Herbology and Pharmacology* by John Chen and Tina Chen.

Zǐ Jīn Dìng (Purple Gold Special Pill)

DOSAGE / PREPARATION / ADMINISTRATION

Grind the ingredients into powder and form into tablets with sticky rice paste. For topical application, crush the tablets and mix with water, and apply locally. Today, *Xiong Huang* (Realgar) and *Zhu Sha* (Cinnabaris) are processed with the *shui fei* (refining with water) technique to obtain extremely fine powder. *Shan Ci Gu* (Pseudobulbus Cremastrae seu Pleiones), *Wu Bei Zi* (Galla Chinensis), and *Hong Da Ji* (Radix Knoxiae) are crushed into powder. *She Xiang* (Moschus) is also crushed into powder. All of these powders are sifted together and mixed with the frost of *Qian Jin Zi* (Semen Euphorbiae). Mix the sticky rice powder with water and form into a dough. Steam the dough, and mix with the herbal powder, and form into tablets. Dry the tablets in a cool place without direct exposure to sunlight. For internal use, administer 0.6-1.5g of tablets, twice daily. For topical use, crush the tablets, mix with vinegar, and apply to the affected area.

CHINESE THERAPEUTIC ACTIONS

1. Dissolves phlegm and opens the sensory orifices
2. Dispels filth and fetidness and eliminates toxins
3. Reduces swelling and relieves pain

CLINICAL MANIFESTATIONS

Accumulation of filth, fetidness, phlegm and turbidity: epigastric and abdominal distention, pain, nausea, vomiting and diarrhea. This formula may be applied topically to treat abscesses and sores.

VETERINARY CLINICAL APPLICATIONS

Nausea and vomiting from gastrointestinal infections, sepsis following gastrointestinal surgery and dehiscence, ruptured bowel, intestinal abscess, and ruptured gallbladder.

EXPLANATION

Zi Jin Ding (Purple Gold Special Pill) has a wide range of applications, and was used in the past to treat disorders characterized by accumulation of filth, fetidness, phlegm and turbidity leading to stagnation of qi. Clinical presentations include feeling of epigastric and abdominal distention, oppression and pain, nausea, vomiting, and diarrhea, and abscesses and sores when applied topically.

In this formula, *She Xiang* (Moschus) opens the sensory orifices, activates qi circulation, and relieves pain. *Shan Ci Gu* (Pseudobulbus Cremastrae seu Pleiones) clears heat and reduces swellings. *Xiong Huang* (Realgar) dispels filth and fetidness and eliminates toxins. *Qian Jin Zi* (Semen Euphorbiae) and *Hong Da Ji* (Radix Knoxiae) eliminate phlegm and reduce swellings. *Zhu Sha* (Cinnabaris) calms the *shen* (spirit). *Wu Bei Zi* (Galla Chinensis) astringes the Intestines to relieve diarrhea. It also prevents the drastic and harsh herbs from damaging the body.

CAUTIONS / CONTRAINDICATIONS

Zi Jin Ding should be used with caution during gestation, since *She Xiang* (Moschus) has potent dispersing effect. It should be used with caution and with reduced dose in young, debilitated and geriatric animals, since some ingredients in this formula are potentially toxic.

AUTHORS' COMMENTS

Zi Jin Ding can also be applied topically on abscesses and sores to reduce swelling and disperse nodules.

***Zi Jin Ding* (Purple Gold Special Pill)**

Diagnosis	Clinical Signs	Treatment	Herbs
Accumulation of filth, fetidness, phlegm and turbidity	Epigastric and abdominal distention, oppression and pain, nausea, vomiting and diarrhea	• Dissolves phlegm and opens the sensory orifices • Dispels filth and fetidness and eliminates toxins • Reduces swellings and relieves pain	• *She Xiang* (Moschus) opens the sensory orifices, activates qi circulation, and relieves pain. • *Shan Ci Gu* (Pseudobulbus Cremastrae seu Pleiones) clears heat and reduces swellings. • *Xiong Huang* (Realgar) dispels filth and fetidness and eliminates toxins. • *Qian Jin Zi* (Semen Euphorbiae) and *Hong Da Ji* (Radix Knoxiae) eliminate phlegm and reduce swellings. • *Zhu Sha* (Cinnabaris) calms the *shen* (spirit). • *Wu Bei Zi* (Galla Chinensis) astringes the Intestines to relieve diarrhea.

Chapter 10 — Summary — Orifice-Opening Formulas

SECTION 1: COLD ORIFICE-OPENING FORMULAS

Name	Similarities	Differences
An Gong Niu Huang Wan (Calm the Palace Pill with Cattle Gallstone)	Open the sensory orifices, treat hot *bi zheng* (closed disorder)	Clears heat and eliminates toxins
Zhi Bao Dan (Greatest Treasure Special Pill)		Opens the sensory orifices, calms the *shen* (spirit)
Zi Xue (Purple Snow)		Calms Liver wind, relieves convulsions

An Gong Niu Huang Wan (Calm the Palace Pill with Cattle Gallstone), ***Zhi Bao Dan*** (Greatest Treasure Special Pill), and ***Zi Xue*** (Purple Snow) are generally considered to be the three representative formulas for treating heat-type *bi zheng* (closed disorder).

- *An Gong Niu Huang Wan* clears heat, eliminates toxins, opens the sensory orifices, and calms the *shen* (spirit). It mainly treats febrile disorders in which heat attacks the Pericardium and heat-phlegm obstructs the orifices.
- *Zhi Bao Dan* has potent functions to open the sensory orifices and calms the *shen* (spirit). It treats *bi zheng* (closed disorder) syndrome caused by heat-phlegm obstruction. It is also effective in treating infantile seizures, epilepsy, and convulsions caused by heat-phlegm obstruction.
- *Zi Xue* strongly calms Liver wind and stops convulsions, but has mild effects to clear heat, eliminate toxins, open the sensory orifices, and calm the *shen* (spirit). Thus, it is mostly used to treat febrile disorders in which heat attacks the Pericardium, giving rise to seizures, epilepsy, and convulsions.

SECTION 2: WARM ORIFICE-OPENING FORMULAS

Name	Similarities	Differences
Su He Xiang Wan (Liquid Styrax Pill)	Open the sensory orifices, treat cold *bi zheng* (closed disorder)	Activates qi circulation, dispels cold, stops pain
Zi Jin Ding (Purple Gold Special Pill)		Dissolves phlegm, dispels filth and fetidness, eliminates toxins

Su He Xiang Wan (Liquid Styrax Pill) and ***Zi Jin Ding*** (Purple Gold Special Pill) are two warm formulas with similar functions to open the sensory orifices and treat cold *bi zheng* (closed disorder).

- *Su He Xiang Wan* has additional functions to activate qi circulation, dispel cold, and stop pain. It treats cases of altered consciousness due to cold *bi zheng* (closed disorder), with stagnation of cold, qi and phlegm. Clinical manifestations include sudden unconsciousness, lockjaw, and extreme pain in the chest and abdomen.
- *Zi Jin Ding* has additional functions to dissolve phlegm, dispel filth and fetidness, and eliminate toxins. It treats gastrointestinal disorders characterized by accumulation of filth, fetidness, phlegm, and turbidity. Clinical manifestations include epigastric and abdominal distention, oppression and pain, nausea, vomiting, and diarrhea.

Chapter 11

— Astringent Formulas

固涩剂

傅山 Fù Shán

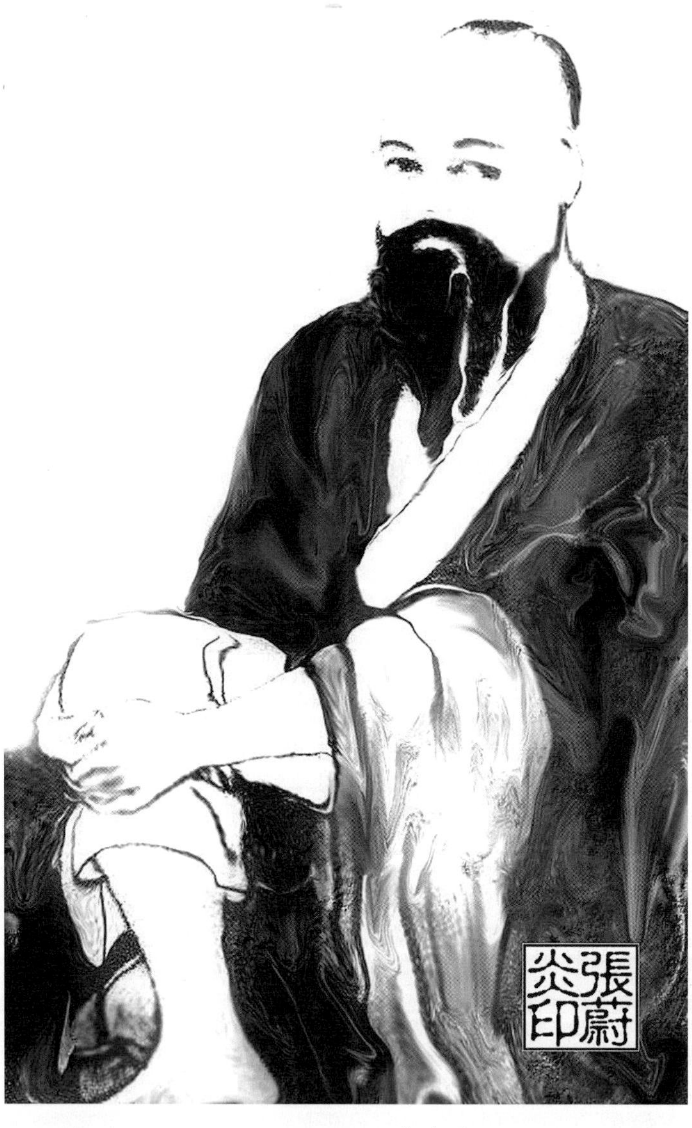

傅山 Fù Shán, also known as 傅青主 Fù Qíng-Zhǔ, 1607 - 1684.

傅山 Fù Shán

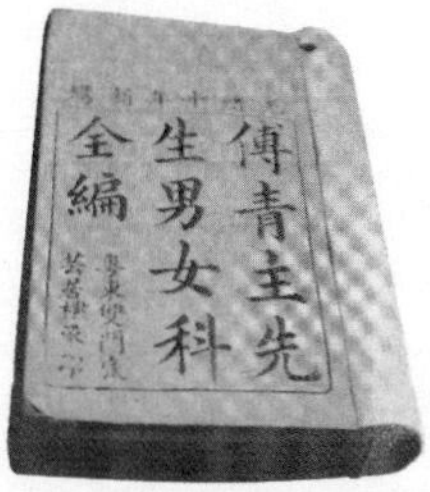

傅青主男科 *Fu Qing Zhu Nan Ke* (Men's Diseases According to Fu Qing-Zhu) and 傅青主女科 *Fu Qing Zhu Nu Ke* (Women's Diseases According to Fu Qing-Zhu), combined.

Fu Shan, also known as Fu Qing-Zhu,[1] is one of the most famous physicians from the Ming and Qing dynasties. He mastered the medical texts published before his time, and experimented with many *Yan Fang* (Time-Tested Formulas) from doctors during his own period of time. After many years of searching for and experimenting with regional remedies, Fu Shan discovered many unconventional, yet effective, herbal therapies. He concluded that it is extremely important to be completely open-minded when practicing medicine: "Do not be restricted to just one school of thought when making the diagnosis [whether *shang han* (cold damage) or *wen bing* (warm diseases)], and do not be confined to a fixed formula when prescribing medicine." By this, he set a strong example for practitioners to modify and customize each treatment as needed.

Fu Shan is known for having cared for his patients above and beyond his duty as a physician. He would frequently treat the poor and homeless for free, pay for their herbal medicines, and even give them money for food and shelter. When he died at the age of 78, thousands of people came from near and far to attend his funeral, to show their appreciation for his compassion and skills as a physician.

Fu Shan specialized in both men's and women's health, and significantly influenced the treatment of male and female disorders in Traditional Chinese Medicine. He wrote many books, and is best known for *Fu Qing Zhu Nan Ke* (Men's Diseases According to Fu Qing-Zhu) and *Fu Qing Zhu Nu Ke* (Women's Diseases According to Fu Qing-Zhu). Many of the formulas discussed in these texts are still in use today, such as *Wan Dai Tang* (End Discharge Decoction), *Bao Chan Wu You Fang* (Preserve Pregnancy and Care-Free Decoction), and *Sheng Hua Tang* (Generation and Transformation Decoction).

Dynasties & Kingdoms	Year
Xia Dynasty 夏	2100-1600 BCE
Shang Dynasty 商	1600-1100 BCE
Zhou Dynasty 周	1100-221 BCE
Qin Dynasty 秦	221-207 BCE
Han Dynasty 漢	206 BCE-220
Three Kingdoms 三國	220-280
Western Jin Dynasty 西晉	265-316
Eastern Jin Dynasty 東晉	317-420
Northern and Southern Dynasties 北南朝	420-581
Sui Dynasty 隋	581-618
Tang Dynasty 唐	618-907
Five Dynasties 五代	907-960
Song Dynasty 宋	960-1279
Liao Dynasty 遼	916-1125
Jin Dynasty 金	1115-1234
Yuan Dynasty 元	1271-1368
Ming Dynasty 明	**1368-1644**
Qing Dynasty 清	1644-1911
Republic of China 中華民國	1912-Present Day
People's Republic of China 中華人民共和國	1949-Present Day

1. Fu Shan was multi-talented. In addition to being an excellent physician, he was a expert in art, poetry, calligraphy, and martial arts. He was also a patriot in and soldier for the Ming dynasty, and led many revolts against the Qing dynasty. Eventually when the Ming dynasty collapsed, he retreated to the mountains to quietly practice medicine. To avoid being tracked down and prosecuted, he changed his name to Fu Qing-Zhu, which is why all his publications carry this pseudonym.

Table of Contents

Chapter 11 — Overview

固澀剂 — Astringent Formulas

Definition: Astringent formulas have actions to stabilize, bind (consolidate and astringe), and stop the loss of qi, blood, *jing* (essence) and body fluids, and treat syndromes of leakage and discharge. The term astringe, as it pertains to therapeutic action, refers to the property of these herbs to cause contraction of body tissues and prevent the loss of substances.

Qi, blood, *jing* (essence), and body fluids are fundamental substances of the body that support and maintain life. These four substances are responsible for the physiological activities of the *zang fu* organs; they nourish and support the entire body and are necessary for the maintenance of good health. Qi, blood, *jing* (essence), and body fluids are continuously consumed and replaced during the course of daily life, and require balance between consumption and replacement. If there is over-consumption, lack of production, or continuous loss of these vital substances then organ function is impaired and disease can develop. The loss of qi, blood, *jing* (essence), or body fluids results in a variety of clinical signs, depending on the cause and location of the disorder, and may include: spontaneous sweating (in species that sweat), chronic coughing, urinary incontinence, chronic diarrhea, and vaginal discharge.

Astringent formulas treat disorders characterized by underlying deficiency with the inability to produce qi, blood, *jing* (essence), or body fluids, and complicated by the continuous loss of these substances in the absence of exogenous pathogenic factors. The focus of astringent formulas is on treating the clinical signs, or branch, of disorders and not the root or underlying deficiencies. In most cases, both cause and clinical signs are treated concurrently by using tonic and astringent herbs. In cases of severe loss of qi, blood, *jing* (essence), or body fluids, astringent herbs are used first to stop the immediate loss, followed by the use of tonic herbs to regenerate and replace these substances. Finally, in the case of qi and yang depletion, high doses of qi and yang-tonifying herbs should be used to restore qi and yang [*see* Chapter 6: Interior-Warming Formulas].

These formulas should ***not*** be used in treating conditions in which exogenous pathogens are present, since failure to eliminate the pathogens first can cause them to be trapped internally and cause chronic or lingering disease. In severe cases, exogenous pathogens and syndromes of leakage and discharge can be treated simultaneously, if necessary.

SUBCATEGORIES OF ACTION

Astringent formulas are divided into five subcategories according to their different therapeutic actions and clinical applications.

1. **Exterior-Stabilizing Formula to Stop Sweating**
These formulas are designed to treat spontaneous sweating caused by *wei* (defensive) *qi* deficiency. Repeated bouts of infectious respiratory disease are often treated with formulas in this category. *Huang Qi* (Radix Astragali) and *Bai Zhu* (Rhizoma Atractylodis Macrocephalae) tonify *wei* (defensive) *qi* to stop spontaneous sweating. One exemplar formula that treats spontaneous sweating is *Yu Ping Feng San* (Jade Windscreen Powder).

Chapter 11 — Overview

2. **Lung-Restraining Formula to Relieve Cough**
   This formula is designed to treat chronic cough with Lung qi and yin deficiencies. The clinical signs of this condition include shortness of breath, spontaneous sweating, and a deficient, rapid pulse. In this case, astringent and tonic herbs are used together to treat the "symptoms" and the "cause." For example, *Wu Wei Zi* (Fructus Schisandrae Chinensis) and *Wu Mei* (Fructus Mume) restrain the Lung and relieve cough, while *Ren Shen* (Radix et Rhizoma Ginseng) and *E Jiao* (Colla Corii Asini) tonify qi and nourish yin. One representative formula is *Jiu Xian San* (Nine-Immortal Powder).

3. **Intestines-Binding Formula to Stop Leakage**
   These formulas treat diarrhea, dysentery, and, in severe cases, fecal incontinence, characterized by chronic deficiency and cold of the Spleen and Kidney. Astringent herbs that bind the Intestines to stop diarrhea and dysentery include *Chi Shi Zhi* (Halloysitum Rubrum), *Rou Dou Kou* (Semen Myristicae), *He Zi* (Fructus Chebulae), and *Wu Wei Zi* (Fructus Schisandrae Chinensis). Tonic herbs that address deficiency and cold of the Spleen and Kidney include *Bu Gu Zhi* (Fructus Psoraleae), *Rou Gui* (Cortex Cinnamomi), *Gan Jiang* (Rhizoma Zingiberis), *Ren Shen* (Radix et Rhizoma Ginseng), and *Bai Zhu* (Rhizoma Atractylodis Macrocephalae). An exemplar formula includes *Si Shen Wan* (Four-Miracle Pill).

4. ***Jing* (Essence)-Stabilizing Formulas to Stop Leakage**
   Formulas in this subcategory treat problems such as urinary incontinence, or enuresis due to Kidney deficiency. Kidney deficiency characterized by leakage of urine with signs such as urinary incontinence or enuresis, may be treated with herbs and formulas such as *Sang Piao Xiao* (Ootheca Mantidis), *Sang Piao Xiao San* (Mantis Egg-Case Powder), and *Suo Quan Wan* (Shut the Sluice Pill).

5. **Womb-Stabilizing Formulas to Stop Leakage**
   These formulas treat chronic vaginal discharge. These conditions are generally characterized by Spleen and Kidney deficiencies and treatment needs to be modified accordingly, as these conditions often occur with complications. Clinical manifestations include soreness and pain of the lower back, odorless, clear, and thin vaginal discharge that is white or straw-colored, a pale tongue and a weak, thin pulse. Commonly used herbs include *Cang Zhu* (Rhizoma Atractylodis), *Bai Zhu* (Rhizoma Atractylodis Macrocephalae), and *Jing Jie Sui Tan* (Spica Schizonepetae Carbonisata). Representative formulas include *Wan Dai Tang* (End Discharge Decoction) and *Ba Wei Dai Xia Fang* (Eight-Ingredient Formula for Leukorrhea).

CAUTIONS / CONTRAINDICATIONS

- Astringent formulas are not suitable if the loss of qi, blood, *jing* (essence), or body fluids is caused by excess syndromes with pathogenic factors residing in the interior. Examples include sweating due to heat, coughing due to phlegm retention, nocturnal emission due to fire, and diarrhea and dysentery due to damp-heat. These are some syndromes not suitable for treatment with astringent formulas, since the use of astringent herbs may trap the pathogenic factors inside the body, further aggravating the condition.
- Astringent formulas are primarily used to treat clinical signs to stop the loss of qi, blood, *jing* (essence), or body fluids temporarily. It is important to also use tonic herbs to address the underlying deficiency to resolve the disorder and prevent chronic problems.

PHARMACOLOGICAL EFFECTS & CLINICAL APPLICATIONS

Astringent formulas stop the loss of qi, blood, *jing* (essence), or body fluids from various parts of the body. From a biomedical perspective, these formulas treat respiratory, kidney, intestinal, genitourinary and reproductive disorders.

Chapter 11 — Overview

1. **Exterior-stabilizing formulas** that stop sweating are designed to treat spontaneous sweating. They also have effects to address respiratory and kidney disorders.
   - **Sweating**: *Yu Ping Feng San* (Jade Windscreen Powder) has been used effectively to treat both spontaneous and night sweating.[1,2]
   - **Prevention of respiratory tract infection**: *Yu Ping Feng San* (Jade Windscreen Powder) is also frequently used for the prevention of respiratory tract infection,[3] as it has marked immunostimulant and antiviral effects.[4,5]
   - **Nephritis**: *Yu Ping Feng San* (Jade Windscreen Powder) has been shown to have nephroprotective effects,[6] and has been used effectively to treat nephritis.[7]

2. **Lung-restraining formulas** are used mainly to treat cough.
   - **Cough**: *Jiu Xian San* (Nine-Immortal Powder) effectively suppresses cough, as many of its ingredients have antitussive and expectorant effects, such as *Ying Su Ke* (Pericarpium Papaveris),[8] *Kuan Dong Hua* (Flos Farfarae),[9] and *Jie Geng* (Radix Platycodonis).[10]

3. **Intestines-binding formulas** that stop leakage are used primarily to treat intestinal disorders marked by the loss of fluids, such as diarrhea and dysentery.
   - **Diarrhea and dysentery**: These formulas have been used with great success to treat diarrhea,[11,12,13] dysentery,[14,15] and colitis.[16,17] The mechanism of this antidiarrheal effect is attributed in part to the inhibition of intestinal peristalsis and increased reabsorption of water.[18] An exemplar formula is *Si Shen Wan* (Four-Miracle Pill).

4. ***Jing*** **(essence)-stabilizing formulas** that stop leakage are primarily used to treat urinary incontinence and enuresis.
   - **Urinary disorders**: These formulas are effective in the treatment of urinary disorders, such as enuresis,[19,20] frequent urination,[21,22] and urinary incontinence.[23] The mechanism of action is attributed in part to the antidiuretic effects of the formula.[24] Exemplar formulas include *Sang Piao Xiao San* (Mantis Egg-Case Powder) and *Suo Quan Wan* (Shut the Sluice Pill).

5. **Womb-stabilizing formulas** that stop leakage are mainly used to treat reproductive disorders.
   - **Gynecological disorders**: *Wan Dai Tang* (End Discharge Decoction) is used to address many gynecological disorders, such as leukorrhea,[25] chronic cervicitis,[26] and acute or chronic vaginitis.[27]

References

1. *Zhe Jiang Zhong Yi Za Zhi* (Zhejiang Journal of Chinese Medicine), 1992; 8:378.
2. *Fu Jian Zhong Yi Yao* (Fujian Chinese Medicine and Herbology), 1966; 3:37.
3. *Zhong Yi Za Zhi* (Journal of Chinese Medicine), 1982; 1:37.
4. *Zhong Yao Yao Li Yu Lin Chuang* (Pharmacology and Clinical Applications of Chinese Herbs), 1990; 6(3):7.
5. *Jiang Xi Zhong Yi Yao* (Jiangxi Chinese Medicine and Herbology), 1989; 6:40.
6. *Zhong Xi Yi Jie He Za Zhi* (Journal of Integrated Chinese and Western Medicine), 1986; 4:299.
7. *Zhong Yi Za Zhi* (Journal of Chinese Medicine), 1992; 33(5):24.
8. *Zhong Cao Yao Xue* (Study of Chinese Herbal Medicine), 1976; 355.
9. *Zhong Yao Yao Li Yu Ying Yong* (Pharmacology and Applications of Chinese Herbs), 1983; 1132.
10. *Zhong Yao Yao Li Yu Ying Yong* (Pharmacology and Applications of Chinese Herbs), 1983; 866.
11. *Zhong Yi Fang Ji Xian Dai Yan Jiu* (Modern Study of Medical Formulas in Traditional Chinese Medicine), 1997; 807-808.
12. *Zhe Jiang Zhong Yi Za Zhi* (Zhejiang Journal of Chinese Medicine), 1993; 9:395.
13. *Shan Xi Zhong Yi* (Shanxi Chinese Medicine), 1990; 1:30.
14. *Jiang Su Zhong Yi Za Zhi* (Jiangsu Journal of Chinese Medicine), 1987; 5:17.
15. *Hu Nan Zhong Yi Za Zhi* (Hunan Journal of Chinese Medicine), 1994; 4:38.
16. *Cheng Du Zhong Yi Xue Yuan Xue Bao* (Journal of Chengdu University of Traditional Chinese Medicine), 1989; 4:27.
17. *Nei Meng Gu Zhong Yi Yao* (Traditional Chinese Medicine and Medicinals of Inner Mongolia), 1987; 5:8.
18. *Zhong Cheng Yao Yan Jiu* (Research of Chinese Patent Medicine), 1981; 9:31.

Chapter 11 — Overview

19. *Shan Xi Zhong Yi* (Shanxi Chinese Medicine), 1997; 1:31.
20. *Jiang Su Zhong Yi* (Jiangsu Chinese Medicine), 1994; 4:14.
21. *Fu Jian Zhong Yi Yao* (Fujian Chinese Medicine and Herbology), 1998; 6:24.
22. *Hei Long Jiang Zhong Yi Yao* (Heilongjiang Chinese Medicine and Herbology), 1990; 1:33.
23. *Bei Jing Zhong Yi* (Beijing Chinese Medicine), 1997; 2:55.
24. *Zhong Yi Fang Ji Xian Dai Yan Jiu* (Modern Study of Medical Formulas in Traditional Chinese Medicine), 1997; 823.
25. *Shang Hai Zhong Yi Yao Za Zhi* (Shanghai Journal of Chinese Medicine and Herbology), 1991; 12:17.
26. *Jiang Su Zhong Yi* (Jiangsu Chinese Medicine), 1987; 4:17.
27. *Xin Zhong Yi* (New Chinese Medicine), 1997; 11:31.

Section 1

固表止汗剂
— Exterior-Stabilizing Formulas to Stop Sweating

Yù Píng Fēng Sǎn (Jade Windscreen Powder)
玉屏風散
玉屏风散

Pinyin Name: *Yu Ping Feng San*
Literal Name: Jade Windscreen Powder
Alternate Names: Jade Wind-Barrier Formula, Jade Screen Powder, Astragalus and Siler Formula
Original Source: *Dan Xi Xin Fa* (Teachings of [Zhu] Dan-Xi) by Zhu Zhen-Heng in 1481

COMPOSITION

Huang Qi (Radix Astragali)	30g [6g]
Bai Zhu (Rhizoma Atractylodis Macrocephalae)	60g [12g]
Fang Feng (Radix Saposhnikoviae)	30g [6g]

DOSAGE / PREPARATION / ADMINISTRATION

The source text states to grind the ingredients into powder. Cook 9g of the powdered herbs and 3 slices of *Sheng Jiang* (Rhizoma Zingiberis Recens) in 1.5 large bowls of water to make a decoction. Today, this formula may be prepared as a decoction with the doses suggested in brackets, with the addition of 3 slices of *Sheng Jiang* (Rhizoma Zingiberis Recens) and 1 piece of *Da Zao* (Fructus Jujubae).[1]

CHINESE THERAPEUTIC ACTIONS

1. Tonifies *wei* (defensive) *qi*
2. Consolidates the exterior
3. Stops spontaneous sweating

CLINICAL MANIFESTATIONS

Wei (defensive) *qi* deficiency: panting, aversion to wind and cold, increased susceptibility to invasion of exterior pathogens, a pale pink to red tongue, and a weak, superficial pulse.

VETERINARY CLINICAL APPLICATIONS

Prevention and/or treatment of the following diseases: infectious respiratory disease, seasonal epidemic diseases, recurrent herpes virus infection in cats, recurrent bronchopneumonia, allergic rhinitis, abnormal sweating, and glomerulonephritis.

EXPLANATION

Yu Ping Feng San (Jade Windscreen Powder) is commonly used to treat spontaneous sweating or increased susceptibility to invasion by exterior pathogens, as a result of deficiency of *wei* (defensive) *qi*. *Wei qi* resides at the exterior of the body, and regulates the skin pores and protects the body from invasion by exterior pathogenic factors. If *wei qi* becomes deficient, body fluids may leak out of the body through the open skin pores, resulting in spontaneous sweating. Deficiency of *wei qi* can compromise the defensive function of the skin, thus increasing the animal's susceptibility to invasion of exterior pathogens. A pale pink to red tongue and a weak, superficial pulse all indicate qi deficiency.

This formula uses a large dose of *Huang Qi* (Radix Astragali) to strengthen *wei* (defensive) *qi* at the exterior and increase the body's defense against foreign pathogenic factors. *Bai Zhu* (Rhizoma Atractylodis Macrocephalae) assists *Huang Qi* (Radix Astragali) in strengthening the exterior to stop spontaneous sweating. *Fang Feng* (Radix Saposhnikoviae) dispels any exterior pathogenic factors, especially wind. This formula has a unique check and balance: the use of an exterior-releasing herb, *Fang Feng* (Radix Saposhnikoviae), prevents retention of pathogenic

Yù Píng Fēng Sǎn (Jade Windscreen Powder)

Yu Ping Feng San (Jade Windscreen Powder)

Diagnosis	Clinical Signs	Treatment	Herbs
Wei (defensive) *qi* deficiency	• Spontaneous sweating (horses, others): leakage of body fluids due to deficiency of *wei* (defensive) *qi* • Aversion to wind and cold and increased susceptibility to exterior conditions: deficiency of *wei* (defensive) *qi* unable to protect the exterior • Pale pink to red tongue and a superficial pulse: qi deficiency	• Tonifies *wei* (defensive) *qi* • Protects the exterior • Stops spontaneous sweating	• *Huang Qi* (Radix Astragali) strengthens *wei* (defensive) *qi* at the exterior and increases the body's defense. • *Bai Zhu* (Rhizoma Atractylodis Macrocephalae) strengthens the exterior and stops spontaneous sweating. • *Fang Feng* (Radix Saposhnikoviae) dispels any exterior pathogenic factors.

factors trapped by a qi-tonifying herb, *Huang Qi* (Radix Astragali); and the use of a qi-tonifying herb prevents any damage to the body that may be induced by the use of an exterior-releasing herb. Thus, using an exterior-releasing herb, in conjunction with a tonic herb, prevents exterior pathogenic factors from being trapped in the interior and causing harm.

Yu Ping Feng San has functions to tonify *wei* (defensive) *qi*, protect the exterior, release exterior pathogenic factors, and stop sweating. It is commonly used to treat animals that frequently contract respiratory diseases, as well as for protection against contagious disease in performance animals under stress or traveling.

VETERINARY MODIFICATIONS

- For wind-cold, add *Cang Zhu* (Rhizoma Atractylodis) and *Qiang Huo* (Rhizoma et Radix Notopterygii).
- For common cold in constitutionally deficient animals, add *Jing Jie* (Herba Schizonepetae), *Zi Su Ye* (Folium Perillae), and *Dang Shen* (Radix Codonopsis).
- With skin eruptions, add *Dang Gui* (Radix Angelicae Sinensis) and *Bai Shao* (Radix Paeoniae Alba).
- With chronic or allergic sinusitis, add *Xin Yi Hua* (Flos Magnoliae) and *Cang Er Zi* (Fructus Xanthii); or combine with *Cang Er Zi San* (Xanthium Powder).
- With fatigue due to qi deficiency, add *Ren Shen* (Radix et Rhizoma Ginseng) and *Gan Cao* (Radix et Rhizoma Glycyrrhizae).

CAUTIONS / CONTRAINDICATIONS

- *Yu Ping Feng San* is contraindicated in animals with exterior syndrome. It should be used only for spontaneous sweating without exterior syndrome.
- Animals should be protected from exposure to wind and cold, and prevented from eating raw, cold and or greasy foods when given this formula.[2]
- According to one report, the use of this formula was associated with mild dry mouth in 8 out of 127 patients. Dry mouth appeared within the first 10 days of use, and was self-limiting and resolved between days 11 to 20. No other abnormalities were noted.[3]

PHARMACOLOGICAL EFFECTS

1. **Immunostimulant**: Administration of *Yu Ping Feng San* has been associated with increased immunity. According to one study, the use of this formula increased IgG and IgA in mice.[4] Another study reported that the use of this formula for 2 to 3 months increased NK cell count and activities.[5]
2. **Antiviral**: According to one *in vitro* study, *Yu Ping Feng San* has demonstrated inhibition on the replication of influenza A viruses.[6]
3. **Nephroprotective**: According to one study, administration of *Yu Ping Feng San* in rabbits was associated with marked reduction of creatinine in comparison with the control group which did not receive any herbs. *Yu Ping Feng San*, however, did not have any statistically-significant effect on proteinuria in the same subjects.[7]

HUMAN CLINICAL STUDIES AND RESEARCH

1. **Prevention of respiratory tract infection**: According to one study, *Yu Ping Feng San* was evaluated for its effect in preventing recurrent respiratory tract infection in 32 children who have had a history of frequent infections. The treatment protocol was to administer *Yu Ping Feng San* for 14 weeks prior to winter. The study reported an overall effectiveness of 96.9%. Furthermore, the study noted that there was an increase in IgA, but no significant changes to IgG or IgM.[8]
2. **Allergic rhinitis**: According to one study, the use of modified *Yu Ping Feng San* was associated with good results to treat 495 patients with allergic rhinitis characterized by deficiency of the exterior. Of 495 patients, the study reported significant improvement in 293 cases, improvement in 120 cases, and no effect in 79 cases. The rate of effectiveness was 84%. Information was unavailable on 3 individuals who did not complete the study.[9]

Yù Píng Fēng Săn (Jade Windscreen Powder)

3. **Sweating**: In one study, 88 children with profuse sweating were treated with satisfactory results using modified *Yu Ping Feng San*. Modifications were made based on traditional Chinese medical diagnosis. For qi deficiencies, *Da Zao* (Fructus Jujubae) 15g, *Nuo Mi Gen* (Radix Oryzae Glutinosae) 9g, calcined *Mu Li* (Concha Ostreae) 30g, and calcined *Long Gu* (Os Draconis) 30g were added. For qi and yin deficiencies, *Wu Wei Zi* (Fructus Schisandrae Chinensis) 4.5g and *Dang Gui* (Radix Angelicae Sinensis) 9g were added.[10]
4. **Nephritis**: According to one study, administration of modified *Yu Ping Feng San* was associated with beneficial effect in 29 of 33 patients. The treatment protocol was to administer the herbs in powder form, 9 grams three times daily for 3 consecutive days followed by 4 days of rest per week, for 6 months. The herbal formula contained *Huang Qi* (Radix Astragali) 20g, *Bai Zhu* (Rhizoma Atractylodis Macrocephalae) 15g, *Fang Feng* (Radix Saposhnikoviae) 12g, *Chen Pi* (Pericarpium Citri Reticulatae) 9g, *Lian Qiao* (Fructus Forsythiae) 40g, *Tu Fu Ling* (Rhizoma Smilacis Glabrae) 50g, and *Qiang Huo* (Rhizoma et Radix Notopterygii) 10g.[11]
5. **Facial paralysis**: According to one study, concurrent use of *Yu Ping Feng San* and *Bu Yang Huan Wu Tang* (Tonify the Yang to Restore Five Decoction) for treatment of facial paralysis in 49 patients was associated with complete recovery in 32 cases, significant improvement in 15 cases, and moderate improvement in 2 cases.[12]

TOXICOLOGY

Yu Ping Feng San has very little toxicity. According to one study on acute toxicology, administration of this formula at 100 g/kg in mice did not cause any abnormal reactions or fatalities.[13] According to another study on chronic toxicology in mice, oral administration of this formula at 15 g/kg/day for 14 days did not cause any abnormal reactions of the internal organs (heart, lung, liver, kidneys, and stomach). However, some mild side effects were observed, such as diarrhea.[14]

SUGGESTED ACUPUNCTURE TREATMENT

1. Points: *Qihai* (CV 6), *Housanli* (ST 36), *Yinxi* (HT 6), and *Houxi* (SI 3).
2. Technique: even method.

Qihai (CV 6) is an essential point to tonify the general qi of the body. *Housanli* (ST 36) tonifies both qi and blood. Combined together, these two points tonify qi and strengthen the exterior. Since sweat is the body fluid that belongs to the Heart, *Yinxi* (HT 6), the *xi* (cleft) point of the Heart channel, is used to stop sweating. *Houxi* (SI 3), the *shu* (stream) point of the Small Intestine channel, helps stop sweating. Also, since *Houxi* (SI 3) enters the *du* (governing) channel, which governs the yang of the body, *Houxi* (SI 3) warms and activates the yang to provide protection at the exterior.

AUTHORS' COMMENTS

Yu Ping Feng San is the key formula for tonifying and consolidating *wei* (defensive) *qi* and prevents the invasion of *liu yin* (six exogenous factors). Clinically, it treats animals with a compromised immune system and can be used prophylactically to prevent infectious diseases by boosting the immune system. *Yu Ping Feng San* can be used preventatively in kennels or catteries to prevent outbreaks of infectious respiratory disease. It is commonly used to prevent contraction of respiratory infection in horses that travel frequently and over long distances to compete. During acute outbreaks, it can be combined with *Yin Qiao San* (Honeysuckle and Forsythia Powder), and should initially be used in a 1:2 ratio.

Yu Ping Feng San can be combined with *Gui Zhi Tang* (Cinnamon Twig Decoction) for acute wind attack and treatment of seasonal allergic rhinitis. It can also be combined with *Cang Er Zi San* (Xanthium Powder) in a 1:1 ratio for the treatment of chronic nasal discharge commonly seen in young horses secondary to rhinopneumonitis and influenza infections.

Yu Ping Feng San is used to strengthen the body's overall defenses *before* an illness begins. It takes time to tonify qi and consolidate the body's defense system. Because this formula helps build the body's defenses in advance of an illness, it should be administered prior to the onset of illness or potential exposure to pathogens. It can require up to 3 months for full beneficial effects to be realized (e.g. decrease in frequency or severity of illness) and should be given for prolonged periods of time in between chronic infections to prevent their recurrence. Following 3 months of continuous use, it can be given for 2 weeks out of each month to prevent against infectious respiratory disease.

Yu Ping Feng San, *Sheng Mai San* (Generate the Pulse Powder), and *Ren Shen Yang Ying Tang* (Ginseng Decoction to Nourish the Nutritive Qi) can all be used to enhance the immune system of animals that frequently catch colds.

- *Yu Ping Feng San* tonifies *wei* (defensive) *qi.*
- *Sheng Mai San* (Generate the Pulse Powder) tonifies qi and generates body fluids.
- *Ren Shen Yang Ying Tang* tonifies qi and blood.

Yù Píng Fēng Sǎn (Jade Windscreen Powder)

Yu Ping Feng San and *Gui Zhi Tang* (Cinnamon Twig Decoction) both treat spontaneous sweating and aversion to wind, but have completely different clinical applications.

- *Yu Ping Feng San* is an astringent formula that treats spontaneous sweating and aversion to wind. However, these clinical signs are due to *wei* (defensive) *qi* deficiency with inability to consolidate the exterior. Besides leakage of body fluids, other clinical signs include frequent catching of infectious respiratory diseases, generalized weakness, and a deficient pulse. *Yu Ping Feng San* is designed for animals that have not yet contracted an exterior condition.
- *Gui Zhi Tang* is an exterior-releasing formula designed to treat wind-cold invasion with disharmony between the *ying* (nutritive) and *wei* (defensive) levels, causing clinical signs such as fever, aversion to cold, sweating, nasal congestion, and a superficial pulse. *Gui Zhi Tang* is formulated to treat animals that have already contracted an exterior wind-cold condition.[15]

References

1. *Shi Yi De Xiao Fang* (Effective Formulas from Generations of Physicians) by Wei Yi-Lin in 1345.
2. *Zhong Yao Ming Fang Yao Li Yu Ying Yong* (Pharmacology and Applications of Famous Herbal Formulas), 1989; 349-350.
3. *Zhong Yao Ming Fang Yao Li Yu Ying Yong* (Pharmacology and Applications of Famous Herbal Formulas), 1989; 349-350.
4. *Zhong Yao Yao Li Yu Lin Chuang* (Pharmacology and Clinical Applications of Chinese Herbs), 1990; 6(3):7.
5. *Zhong Xi Yi Jie He Za Zhi* (Journal of Integrated Chinese and Western Medicine), 1990; 12:22.
6. *Jiang Xi Zhong Yi Yao* (Jiangxi Chinese Medicine and Herbology), 1989; 6:40.
7. *Zhong Xi Yi Jie He Za Zhi* (Journal of Integrated Chinese and Western Medicine), 1986; 4:299.
8. *Zhong Yi Za Zhi* (Journal of Chinese Medicine), 1982; 1:37.
9. *Zhong Yi Za Zhi* (Journal of Chinese Medicine), 1989; 10:32.
10. *Zhe Jiang Zhong Yi Za Zhi* (Zhejiang Journal of Chinese Medicine), 1992; 8:378.
11. *Zhong Yi Za Zhi* (Journal of Chinese Medicine), 1992; 33(5):24.
12. *Shan Xi Zhong Yi* (Shanxi Chinese Medicine), 1989; 11:496.
13. *Zhong Yi Fang Ji Xian Dai Yan Jiu* (Modern Study of Medical Formulas in Traditional Chinese Medicine), 1997; 786.
14. *Zhong Yi Fang Ji Xian Dai Yan Jiu* (Modern Study of Medical Formulas in Traditional Chinese Medicine), 1997; 1:5.
15. Wang MZ, et al. *Zhong Yi Xue Wen Da Ti Ku* (Questions and Answers on Traditional Chinese Medicine: Herbal Formulas).

Section 2

斂肺止咳剂
— Lung-Restraining Formula to Relieve Cough

Jiŭ Xiān Săn (Nine-Immortal Powder)
九仙散

Pinyin Name: *Jiu Xian San*
Literal Name: Nine-Immortal Powder
Original Source: *Yi Xue Zheng Zhuan* (True Lineage of Medicine) by Yu Tian-Min in 1515

COMPOSITION

Ying Su Ke (Pericarpium Papaveris), *mi zhi* (fried with honey)	6g
Wu Wei Zi (Fructus Schisandrae Chinensis)	1.5g [3g]
Wu Mei (Fructus Mume)	1 piece [6g]
Ren Shen (Radix et Rhizoma Ginseng), *dun* (stewed) separately	1.5g [3g]
E Jiao (Colla Corii Asini)	1.5g [3g]
Kuan Dong Hua (Flos Farfarae)	1.5g [3g]
Bei Mu (Bulbus Fritillariae)	1.5g [3g]
Sang Bai Pi (Cortex Mori)	1.5g [3g]
Jie Geng (Radix Platycodonis)	1.5g [3g]

Note: *Ying Su Ke* (Pericarpium Papaveris), commonly known as opium poppy husks, is a highly regulated substance and is generally unavailable in most developed countries.

DOSAGE / PREPARATION / ADMINISTRATION

The source text states to grind all of the ingredients into powder. Cook the powdered herbs with 3 slices of *Sheng Jiang* (Rhizoma Zingiberis Recens) in two large bowls of water until it is reduced down to one bowl. Take the warm, strained decoction. Today, this formula may be prepared as a decoction with the doses suggested in brackets.

CHINESE THERAPEUTIC ACTIONS

1. Restrains the Lung and stops coughing
2. Benefits qi and nourishes yin

CLINICAL MANIFESTATIONS

Chronic coughing with Lung yin and qi deficiencies: chronic, persistent coughing, severe coughing leading to wheezing, dyspnea, a red tongue, and a weak, thready, rapid pulse.

VETERINARY CLINICAL APPLICATIONS

Pulmonary tuberculosis, chronic bronchitis, and chronic coughing.

EXPLANATION

Jiu Xian San (Nine-Immortal Powder) is designed to treat chronic coughing with Lung yin and qi deficiencies. Chronic coughing injures the Lung, causing wheezing, dyspnea and shortness of breath. Chronic coughing also consumes qi and prevents the skin pores from closing, leading to spontaneous sweating in species that sweat, such as horses. Chronic coughing may also deplete yin, leading to deficiency heat, and manifesting in the form of a red tongue and a weak, thready, rapid pulse.

Ying Su Ke (Pericarpium Papaveris) in this formula is used to restrain the Lung and stop coughing. *Wu Wei Zi* (Fructus Schisandrae Chinensis) and *Wu Mei* (Fructus Mume) help restrain the Lung to stop coughing. *Ren Shen* (Radix et Rhizoma Ginseng) tonifies Lung qi. *Wu Wei Zi* (Fructus Schisandrae Chinensis) also assists *Ren Shen* (Radix et Rhizoma Ginseng) to tonify qi. *E Jiao* (Colla Corii Asini) nourishes Lung yin. *Kuan Dong Hua* (Flos Farfarae) and

Jiŭ Xiān Săn (Nine-Immortal Powder)

***Jiu Xian San* (Nine-Immortal Powder)**

Diagnosis	Clinical Signs	Treatment	Herbs
Chronic coughing with damage of Lung yin and qi	• Chronic coughing, wheezing, and shortness of breath: Lung yin and qi deficiencies • Spontaneous sweating: Lung qi deficiency unable to close skin pores • A red tongue and a weak, thready and rapid pulse: deficiency heat	• Astringes the Lung and stops coughing • Benefits qi and nourishes yin	• *Ying Su Ke* (Pericarpium Papaveris) restrains the Lung and stops coughing. • *Wu Wei Zi* (Fructus Schisandrae Chinensis) and *Wu Mei* (Fructus Mume) restrain the Lung to stop coughing. • *Ren Shen* (Radix et Rhizoma Ginseng) tonifies Lung qi. • *E Jiao* (Colla Corii Asini) nourishes Lung yin. • *Kuan Dong Hua* (Flos Farfarae) and *Bei Mu* (Bulbus Fritillariae) cause Lung qi to descend, stop coughing and wheezing, and dissolve phlegm. • *Sang Bai Pi* (Cortex Mori) clears the Lung to stop coughing and wheezing. • *Jie Geng* (Radix Platycodonis) relieves coughing, dissolves phlegm, and guides the other herbs upward to the Lung.

Bei Mu (Bulbus Fritillariae) descend Lung qi, stop coughing and wheezing, and dissolve phlegm. *Sang Bai Pi* (Cortex Mori) clears the Lung to stop coughing and wheezing. *Jie Geng* (Radix Platycodonis), in addition to relieving cough and dissolving phlegm, guides all the other herbs upward to the Lung.

VETERINARY MODIFICATIONS

- With wheezing and dyspnea due to Lung and Kidney deficiencies, add *Shu Di Huang* (Radix Rehmanniae Praeparata), *Shan Zhu Yu* (Fructus Corni), *Shan Yao* (Rhizoma Dioscoreae), and *He Tao Ren* (Semen Juglandis).
- With loose stools and indigestion due to Spleen deficiency, add *Bai Zhu* (Rhizoma Atractylodis Macrocephalae), *Shan Yao* (Rhizoma Dioscoreae), and *Fu Ling* (Poria).
- If *Ying Su Ke* (Pericarpium Papaveris) is unavailable, substitute with *Gua Lou* (Fructus Trichosanthis) and *Chen Pi* (Pericarpium Citri Reticulatae) to treat profuse phlegm.

CAUTIONS / CONTRAINDICATIONS

- *Jiu Xian San* has a tonic effect, and, as such, it is not appropriate for coughing caused by exterior conditions with fever and aversion to cold. The use of tonic herbs may complicate the illness by drawing the pathogenic factors from the exterior to the interior.
- Since this formula has a strong astringent action, it is not indicated for cases of coughing with copious phlegm, as the astringent effect may trap the pathogenic factors inside.
- Overdose or long-term usage of *Ying Su Ke* (Pericarpium Papaveris) may result in numerous side effects and adverse reactions, as this herb is potentially toxic and addictive. For additional information, please refer to *Chinese Medical Herbology and Pharmacology* by John Chen and Tina Chen.

SUGGESTED ACUPUNCTURE TREATMENT

1. Points: *Feishu* (BL 13), *Gaohuangshu* (BL 43), *Taiyuan* (LU 9), and *Zhongfu* (LU 1)
2. Technique: tonification.

Feishu (BL 13) nourishes the Lung and regulates the qi flow of the Lung. *Gaohuangshu* (BL 43) nourishes yin and supplements the deficient Lung. *Taiyuan* (LU 9), the *yuan* (source) point of the Lung channel, nourishes and regulates Lung qi to relieve coughing. *Zhongfu* (LU 1), the *mu* (collecting) point of the Lung, regulates the qi flow of the Lung and relieves coughing and wheezing. *Feishu* (BL 13) and *Zhongfu* (LU 1) are combined according to the *shu* (transport) and *mu* (collecting) points principle to regulate Lung qi and correct the reversed flow of Lung qi.

AUTHORS' COMMENTS

Jiu Xian San is designed to treat chronic coughing with Lung yin and qi deficiencies following infectious tracheobronchitis, chronic bronchitis, and recurrent pneumonia secondary to megaesophagus and laryngeal paralysis. It is also useful for pneumonitis that may develop after treatment for heartworm.

Section 3

涩肠固脱剂

— Intestines-Binding Formula to Stop Leakage

Sì Shén Wán (Four-Miracle Pill)

四神丸

Pinyin Name: *Si Shen Wan*
Literal Name: Four-Miracle Pill
Original Source: *Zheng Zhi Zhun Sheng* (Standards of Patterns and Treatments) by Wang Ken-Tang in 1602

COMPOSITION

Bu Gu Zhi (Fructus Psoraleae)	120g [12g]
Rou Dou Kou (Semen Myristicae)	60g [6g]
Wu Zhu Yu (Fructus Evodiae), *jin* (soaked) and *chao* (dry-fried)	30g [3g]
Wu Wei Zi (Fructus Schisandrae Chinensis)	60g [6g]

DOSAGE / PREPARATION / ADMINISTRATION

The source text states to cook 100 pieces of *Da Zao* (Fructus Jujubae) with 240g of *Sheng Jiang* (Rhizoma Zingiberis Recens). Save only the fruit of *Da Zao* (Fructus Jujubae), and remove and discard the seeds, *Sheng Jiang* (Rhizoma Zingiberis Recens) and the decoction. Separately grind the rest of the ingredients into powder. Blend the fruit of *Da Zao* (Fructus Jujubae) and the powdered ingredients to form small pills. The source text recommends taking 50-70 pills with water before meal or on an empty stomach. Today, this formula is usually prepared and administered in pills. Take 6-9g of pills, once or twice daily. This formula may be prepared as a decoction with the doses suggested in brackets.

CHINESE THERAPEUTIC ACTIONS

1. Warms and tonifies the Spleen and Kidney
2. Binds the Intestines and stops diarrhea

CLINICAL MANIFESTATIONS

Deficiency and cold of the Spleen and Kidney: early morning diarrhea at around 5 a.m. (daybreak diarrhea), chronic watery diarrhea with undigested food, poor appetite, abdominal pain and coldness, pain and weakness of the lower back, cold limbs, lethargy, fatigue, a pale, wet tongue, and a deep, weak pulse.

VETERINARY CLINICAL APPLICATIONS

Chronic diarrhea with incontinence and leakage of stool, inflammatory bowel disease, and dysenteric disorders.

EXPLANATION

Si Shen Wan (Four-Miracle Pill) is particularly famous for treating early morning diarrhea at around 5 a.m. Early morning diarrhea is caused by the failure of the yang qi to ascend in the early morning. Pain and weakness of the lower back indicates Kidney yang deficiency. Fatigue, lethargy, and loss of appetite reflect Spleen yang deficiency. Abdominal pain, cold extremities, a pale, wet tongue and a deep, weak pulse are caused by accumulation of cold and the inability of yang to warm the body.

Bu Gu Zhi (Fructus Psoraleae), the chief herb of this formula, warms the Kidney and invigorates *ming men* (life gate) fire. *Rou Dou Kou* (Semen Myristicae) warms the Spleen and Kidney and binds the Intestines to stop diarrhea. *Wu Zhu Yu* (Fructus Evodiae) warms the Spleen and Stomach. It also disperses cold and relieves the abdominal pain. *Wu Wei Zi* (Fructus Schisandrae Chinensis) warms and binds the Intestines. *Sheng Jiang* (Rhizoma Zingiberis Recens) dispels cold and regulates water. *Da Zao* (Fructus Jujubae) nourishes the Spleen and Stomach.

Sì Shén Wán (Four-Miracle Pill)

Si Shen Wan (Four-Miracle Pill)

Diagnosis	Clinical Signs	Treatment	Herbs
Deficiency and cold of the Spleen and Kidney	• Early morning diarrhea: failure of the yang qi to ascend in the early morning • Pain and weakness of the lower back: Kidney yang deficiency • Lethargy, fatigue, loss of appetite, a pale, wet tongue, and a deep, weak pulse: Spleen yang deficiency • Abdominal pain and cold extremities: accumulation of cold	• Warms and tonifies the Spleen and Kidney • Binds the intestines and stops diarrhea	• *Bu Gu Zhi* (Fructus Psoraleae) warms the Kidney and invigorates *ming men* (life gate) fire. • *Rou Dou Kou* (Semen Myristicae) warms the Spleen and the Kidney and binds the Intestines to stop diarrhea. • *Wu Zhu Yu* (Fructus Evodiae) warms the Spleen and the Stomach to relieve pain. • *Wu Wei Zi* (Fructus Schisandrae Chinensis) warms and binds the Intestines to stop diarrhea. • *Sheng Jiang* (Rhizoma Zingiberis Recens) dispels cold and regulates water. • *Da Zao* (Fructus Jujubae) nourishes the Spleen and Stomach.

VETERINARY MODIFICATIONS

- For rectal prolapse, add *Huang Qi* (Radix Astragali) and *Sheng Ma* (Rhizoma Cimicifugae); or *Bu Zhong Yi Qi Tang* (Tonify the Middle and Augment the Qi Decoction).
- For pain of the back and coldness of the limbs, add *Rou Gui* (Cortex Cinnamomi) and *Fu Zi* (Radix Aconiti Lateralis Praeparata); or *You Gui Wan* (Restore the Right [Kidney] Pill).
- With lower abdominal pain, add *Xiao Hui Xiang* (Fructus Foeniculi) and *Mu Xiang* (Radix Aucklandiae).

CAUTIONS / CONTRAINDICATIONS

- *Si Shen Wan* contains tonic and astringent herbs to treat chronic diarrhea and dysentery due to deficiency. It is contraindicated in diarrhea caused by damp-heat accumulation or food stagnation.
- Avoid raw and cold foods while taking this formula.

PHARMACOLOGICAL EFFECTS

Antidiarrheal: *Si Shen Wan* has been shown to have marked antidiarrheal effect according to many studies and reports. The mechanism of this antidiarrheal effect has been attributed to its action to inhibit the intestinal peristalsis.[1]

HUMAN CLINICAL STUDIES AND RESEARCH

1. **Diarrhea**: Many studies have shown *Si Shen Wan* to effectively treat diarrhea due to various reasons. One study reported complete recovery in 24 of 28 patients with 5 a.m. diarrhea when treated with *Si Shen Wan* plus *Pao Jiang* (Rhizoma Zingiberis Praeparatum), *Bai Zhu* (Rhizoma Atractylodis Macrocephalae), *Huang Qi* (Radix Astragali), *Fu Zi* (Radix Aconiti Lateralis Praeparata), and *Rou Gui* (Cortex Cinnamomi). The duration of treatment ranged from 12 to 36 packs of herbs.[2]
2. **Dysentery**: One study reported good results using *Si Shen Wan* plus *Tong Xie Yao Fang* (Important Formula for Painful Diarrhea) to treat dysentery characterized by Liver stagnation and Spleen deficiency. Clinical presentations included abdominal pain, hematochezia, rectal tenesmus, absence of fever and thirst, fatigue, aversion to cold, poor appetite, sallow facial appearance, emaciated complexion, white tongue coating, and a deep, fine pulse. The herbal formula contained *Bu Gu Zhi* (Fructus Psoraleae), *Wu Zhu Yu* (Fructus Evodiae), roasted *Rou Dou Kou* (Semen Myristicae), *Chen Pi* (Pericarpium Citri Reticulatae), *Fang Feng* (Radix Saposhnikoviae), *Mu Xiang* (Radix Aucklandiae), *Bai Shao* (Radix Paeoniae Alba), *Bai Zhu* (Rhizoma Atractylodis Macrocephalae), *Huang Lian* (Rhizoma Coptidis), *Gan Cao* (Radix et Rhizoma Glycyrrhizae), and *Wu Wei Zi* (Fructus Schisandrae Chinensis). The study reported complete recovery in all 14 patients.[3]
3. **Irritable bowel syndrome**: One study reported a 93% success rate using *Si Shen Wan* and *Shen Ling Bai Zhu San* (Ginseng, Poria, and Atractylodes Macrocephala Powder) to treat alternation of diarrhea and constipation with abdominal pain in 30 patients with irritable bowel syndrome.[4]
4. **Colitis**: One study of colitis associated with diarrhea reported satisfactory results using modified *Si Shen Wan*. Patients were divided into early, middle and late stage of colitis with diarrhea. The formula for early stage contained *Wu Zhu Yu* (Fructus Evodiae) 10g, *Bu Gu Zhi* (Fructus Psoraleae) 20g, *Wu Wei Zi* (Fructus Schisandrae Chinensis) 10g, *Pao Jiang* (Rhizoma Zingiberis

Sì Shén Wán (Four-Miracle Pill)

Praeparatum) 5g, *Da Huang* (Radix et Rhizoma Rhei) 12g, *Hou Po* (Cortex Magnoliae Officinalis) 15g, and *Fu Zi* (Radix Aconiti Lateralis Praeparata) 10g. The formula for middle stage contained *Si Shen Wan* plus *Huang Bo* (Cortex Phellodendri Chinensis) 12g, *Cang Zhu* (Rhizoma Atractylodis) 15g, and *Huang Lian* (Rhizoma Coptidis) 15g. The formula for late stage contained *Si Shen Wan* plus *He Zi* (Fructus Chebulae) 12g and *Ying Su Ke* (Pericarpium Papaveris) 10g. The study reported 96.6% effectiveness among 100 patients.[5]

5. **Enuresis**: One study reported complete recovery in all 20 patients with enuresis when treated with *Si Shen Wan* plus *Yi Zhi* (Fructus Alpiniae Oxyphyllae). The duration of treatment ranged from 1 to 4 packs of herbs, with an average of 2 to 3 packs. No recurrence was reported in all 20 patients during follow up interview one year later.[6]
6. **Seminal emission**: One study reported marked improvement using modified *Si Shen Wan* to treat all 15 patients with seminal emission characterized by Spleen and Kidney yang deficiencies. Clinical presentations include pale face, fatigue, lack of energy, dizziness, tinnitus, soreness and weakness of the lower back and knees, frequent seminal emission, white and greasy tongue coating, and a deep, weak pulse. The herbal treatment contained *Rou Dou Kou* (Semen Myristicae) 12g, *Wu Wei Zi* (Fructus Schisandrae Chinensis) 12g, *Bu Gu Zhi* (Fructus Psoraleae) 30g, *Da Zao* (Fructus Jujubae) 30g, *Shan Zhu Yu* (Fructus Corni) 30g, *Wu Zhu Yu* (Fructus Evodiae) 6g, *Sheng Jiang* (Rhizoma Zingiberis Recens) 10g, and *Bai Shao* (Radix Paeoniae Alba) 24g. The duration of treatment was 15 packs of herbs.[7]
7. **Constipation**: One study reported marked effect using *Si Shen Wan* plus *Hua Jiao* (Pericarpium Zanthoxyli) and *Liu Huang* (Sulfur) to treat constipation characterized by deficiency and cold. Of 62 patients, the study reported complete recovery in 18 cases, marked improvement in 32 cases, and no effect in 12 cases.[8]

SUGGESTED ACUPUNCTURE TREATMENT

1. Points: *Pishu* (BL 20), *Shenshu* (BL 23), *Mingmen* (GV 4), *Guanyuan* (CV 4), *Dachangshu* (BL 25), *Tianshu* (ST 25), *Baihui* and *Hegu* (LI 4).
2. Technique: tonification and moxibustion.

Pishu (BL 20) warms Spleen yang and nourishes the yin and blood. *Shenshu* (BL 23) and *Mingmen* (GV 4) tonify Kidney yang to indirectly warm Spleen yang and regulate water metabolism in the body. *Guanyuan* (CV 4) nourishes the qi and blood and consolidates body fluids. *Dachangshu* (BL 25) and *Tianshu* (ST 25) are combined according to the *shu* (transport) and *mu* (collecting) points principle; this combination effectively regulates the qi flow of the Intestines and consolidates the Intestines to prevent further diarrhea. *Baihui* raises yang and astringes the intestines. *Hegu* (LI 4), the *yuan* (source) point of the Large Intestine channel, harmonizes the qi and blood in the Intestines to relieve diarrhea.

Note: *Baihui* is an acupuncture point in traditional Chinese veterinary medicine. Though the pinyin name is the same as *Baihui* (GV 20) in human, they are not the same points.

AUTHORS' COMMENTS

Si Shen Wan is literally known as "Four-Miracle Pill" because the four herbs in the formula readily and miraculously treat early morning diarrhea due to Spleen and Kidney yang deficiencies. For cases with nausea, vomiting, and severe abdominal pain from cold, it can be combined with *Li Zhong Wan* (Regulate the Middle Pill). For animals with renal failure and chronic diarrhea, it can be combined with *Jin Gui Shen Qi Wan* (Kidney Qi Pill from the Golden Cabinet) to further warm and tonify Kidney yang.

Si Shen Wan, *Shen Ling Bai Zhu San* (Ginseng, Poria, and Atractylodes Macrocephala Powder), and *Tong Xie Yao Fang* (Important Formula for Painful Diarrhea) all bind the Intestines and treat diarrhea.

- *Si Shen Wan* treats Spleen and Kidney yang deficiencies; it warms and tonifies yang to stop chronic diarrhea. It is designed for severe diarrhea that occurs in the early morning, characterized by watery stool that contains undigested food. This pattern of diarrhea occurs most often in geriatric animals. These animals tend to be depressed, minimally responsive, lay curled up, and want be left alone. There are often other disorders present concurrently in these animals.
- *Shen Ling Bai Zhu San* is for Spleen qi-deficiency diarrhea with damp accumulation, accompanied by fatigue, weakness of the limbs, and poor appetite. This pattern of diarrhea is common in animals of any age.
- *Tong Xie Yao Fang* treats abdominal pain and diarrhea caused by the Liver overacting on the Spleen. It tonifies the Spleen and spreads Liver qi. This formula stops stress-related diarrhea, which makes accurate history an important factor in choosing this formula. Animals will have signs of Liver qi stagnation with abdominal bloating, tenesmus, and abdominal pain that is relieved after the diarrhea.

Sì Shén Wán (Four-Miracle Pill)

References

1. *Zhong Cheng Yao Yan Jiu* (Research of Chinese Patent Medicine), 1981; 9:31.
2. *Shan Xi Zhong Yi* (Shanxi Chinese Medicine), 1990; 5:224.
3. *Hu Nan Zhong Yi Za Zhi* (Hunan Journal of Chinese Medicine), 1994; 4:38.
4. *Shan Xi Zhong Yi* (Shanxi Chinese Medicine), 1990; 1:30.
5. *Nei Meng Gu Zhong Yi Yao* (Traditional Chinese Medicine and Medicinals of Inner Mongolia), 1987; 5:8.
6. *Zhong Yi Za Zhi* (Journal of Chinese Medicine), 1982; 2:14.
7. *Cheng Du Zhong Yi Xue Yuan Xue Bao* (Journal of Chengdu University of Traditional Chinese Medicine), 1990; 1:33.
8. *Zhong Cheng Yao* (Study of Chinese Patent Medicine), 1989; 4:45.

Section 4

涩精止遗剂
— Jing (Essence)-Stabilizing Formulas to Stop Leakage

Jīn Suǒ Gù Jīng Wán (Metal Lock Pill to Stabilize the Essence)
金鎖固精丸
金锁固精丸

Pinyin Name: *Jin Suo Gu Jing Wan*
Literal Name: Metal Lock Pill to Stabilize the Essence
Alternate Names: *Chin Suo Ku Ching Wan*, Golden Lock Essence-Securing Pill, Golden Lock Pill for Consolidating the Essence, Lotus Stamen Formula
Original Source: *Yi Fang Ji Jie* (Analytical Collection of Medical Formulas) by Wang Ang in 1682

COMPOSITION

Sha Yuan Zi (Semen Astragali Complanati), *chao* (dry-fried)	60g [12g]
Qian Shi (Semen Euryales), *zheng* (steamed)	60g [12g]
Lian Xu (Stamen Nelumbinis)	60g [12g]
Long Gu (Os Draconis), *zhi* (fried with liquid) till crisp	30g [10g]
Mu Li (Concha Ostreae), *zhu* (boiled) in lightly salted water for 24 hours and *duan* (calcined) into powder	30g [10g]

DOSAGE / PREPARATION / ADMINISTRATION

The source text states to grind the ingredients into powder and form into pills with powdered *Lian Zi* (Semen Nelumbinis). Take the pills with salted water. Today this formula may be given in pills or decoction. For pills, take 9g per dose, once or twice daily with water or lightly salted water. For decoction, use the suggested doses in brackets.

CHINESE THERAPEUTIC ACTIONS

Tonifies the Kidney and stabilizes the *jing* (essence)

CLINICAL MANIFESTATIONS

Urinary incontinence and/or spermatorrhea caused by Kidney deficiency: seminal emission, frequent urination, lack of energy, weak and painful rear quarters and lumbar region, impaired hearing, a pale pink tongue, and a weak, thin pulse.

VETERINARY CLINICAL APPLICATIONS

Urinary incontinence, spermatorrhea, sexual dysfunction, enuresis, diarrhea, and prevention of pregnancy loss.

EXPLANATION

Jin Suo Gu Jing Wan (Metal Lock Pill to Stabilize the Essence) was originally formulated to treat spermatorrhea and/or nocturnal emissions caused by Kidney deficiency. Kidney is the organ that stores *jing* (essence). If the Kidney is deficient, then the *jing* may become unstable and leak out of the body, resulting in seminal emissions and/or spermatorrhea. In addition to Kidney *jing* deficiency, Kidney yin and yang may be deficient as well, leading to urinary incontinence, urine dripping, lethargy, weak, painful rear quarters and lumbar region, impaired hearing, a pale pink tongue, and a weak, thin pulse.

Sha Yuan Zi (Semen Astragali Complanati), the chief herb of this formula, is used to tonify the Kidney and stabilize *jing* (essence). *Lian Zi* (Semen Nelumbinis) and *Qian Shi* (Semen Euryales) help the chief herb tonify the Kidney and stabilize *jing*. *Lian Xu* (Stamen Nelumbinis), prepared *Long Gu* (Os Draconis), and calcined *Mu Li* (Concha Ostreae) are used mainly to stabilize the leaking *jing*.

Jīn Suǒ Gù Jīng Wán (Metal Lock Pill to Stabilize the Essence)

***Jin Suo Gu Jing Wan* (Metal Lock Pill to Stabilize the Essence)**

Diagnosis	Clinical Signs	Treatment	Herbs
Urinary incontinence, and/or spermatorrhea due to Kidney deficiency	• Urinary incontinence, and/or spermatorrhea: loss of *jing* (essence) due to Kidney deficiency • Weak and painful rear quarters and lumbar region and impaired hearing: Kidney yin and yang deficiencies	Tonifies the Kidney and stabilizes the *jing* (essence)	• *Sha Yuan Zi* (Semen Astragali Complanati) tonifies the Kidney and stabilizes the *jing* (essence). • *Lian Zi* (Semen Nelumbinis) and *Qian Shi* (Semen Euryales) tonify the Kidney and stabilize the *jing*. • *Lian Xu* (Stamen Nelumbinis), *Long Gu* (Os Draconis) and *Mu Li* (Concha Ostreae) stabilize and stop the leaking *jing*.

Since this formula concentrates on consolidating the *jing* (essence), it may be used to temporarily stop urinary incontinence and seminal emissions or spermatorrhea. However, it lacks strength in tonifying the Kidney; hence, once the urinary incontinence, spermatorrhea and/or seminal emissions are stopped, Kidney tonic herbs should be used.

VETERINARY MODIFICATIONS

- For severe urinary incontinence, add *Sang Piao Xiao* (Ootheca Mantidis), *Jin Ying Zi* (Fructus Rosae Laevigatae) and *Wu Wei Zi* (Fructus Schisandrae Chinensis).
- With Kidney yang deficiency, add *Jin Gui Shen Qi Wan* (Kidney Qi Pill from the Golden Cabinet).
- With Kidney yin deficiency, add *Liu Wei Di Huang Wan* (Six-Ingredient Pill with Rehmannia).
- With yin-deficient fire, add *Zhi Bai Di Huang Wan* (Anemarrhena, Phellodendron, and Rehmannia Pill).
- With irritability and insomnia, add *Suan Zao Ren* (Semen Ziziphi Spinosae) and *Bai Zi Ren* (Semen Platycladi).
- With irritability and thirst from yin deficiency, add *Mai Dong* (Radix Ophiopogonis) and *Ren Shen* (Radix et Rhizoma Ginseng).
- With cold signs, add *Rou Gui* (Cortex Cinnamomi) and *Fu Zi* (Radix Aconiti Lateralis Praeparata).
- With soreness and pain of the back, add *Du Huo Ji Sheng Tang* (Angelica Pubescens and Taxillus Decoction).
- With impotence, add *Yin Yang Huo* (Herba Epimedii) and *Suo Yang* (Herba Cynomorii); or *Huan Shao Dan* (Return to Youth Pill).
- With vaginal discharge add *Fu Ling* (Poria) and *Yi Yi Ren* (Semen Coicis).

CAUTIONS / CONTRAINDICATIONS

Jin Suo Gu Jing Wan contains many astringent herbs, and is therefore contraindicated in urinary incontinence caused by Heart fire, Liver fire, Kidney yin-deficient fire, or damp-heat in the lower *jiao*. It is used to treat urinary incontinence secondary to deficiency.

HUMAN CLINICAL STUDIES AND RESEARCH

1. **Reproductive**: According to one report, *Jin Suo Gu Jing Wan* was used with good results to treat one patient with a three-year history of severe spermatorrhea accompanied by night sweating, fatigue, sore lower back, low libido, impotence, premature ejaculation, and nocturnal emission. The treatment protocol was to administer 15 pills of *Jin Suo Gu Jing Wan* three times daily for one month.[1]
2. **Diarrhea**: One report stated that *Jin Suo Gu Jing Wan* can effectively treat diarrhea associated with chronic enteritis characterized by Spleen and Kidney deficiencies.[2]
3. **Myasthenia gravis**: One study reported marked success using *Jin Suo Gu Jing Wan* to treat one person with myasthenia gravis. Clinical manifestations included drooping eyelids, fatigue, lack of power in all four limbs, difficulty with chewing, shortness of breath, insomnia, spermatorrhea, low back pain, feeling of coldness in the legs, and red tongue with scanty tongue coating. The treatment protocol was to administer 12 grams of *Jin Suo Gu Jing Wan* three times daily with lightly salted water. Improvement was noted after two weeks of herbal therapy.[3]

SUGGESTED ACUPUNCTURE TREATMENT

1. Points: *Mingmen* (GV 4), *Shenshu* (BL 23), *Qihai* (CV 6), *Zhishi* (BL 52), *Sanyinjiao* (SP 6), and *Zhongji* (CV 3).
2. Technique: tonification and moxibustion.

Mingmen (GV 4) warms the Kidney and consolidates *jing* (essence) to stop its leakage. *Shenshu* (BL 23) nourishes Kidney yin and *jing*. *Qihai* (CV 6) tonifies the qi and warms the yang to ascend the qi and relieve the downward flow of body fluids. *Zhishi* (BL 52) nourishes *jing*; it is an experiential point for treating spermatorrhea and impotence. *Mingmen* (GV 4), *Shenshu* (BL 23), *Qihai* (CV 6), and *Zhishi* (BL 52) tonify and consolidate *jing*. *Sanyinjiao* (SP 6) nourishes yin to clear deficiency fire. *Zhongji* (CV 3) warms the lower *jiao* to relieve further leakage of *jing*.

Jīn Suǒ Gù Jīng Wán (Metal Lock Pill to Stabilize the Essence)

AUTHORS' COMMENTS

Jin Suo Gu Jing Wan is most commonly used in the treatment of urinary incontinence in dogs. It can also be used to help prevent pregnancy loss in dogs as a result of weakness and leakage of Kidney *jing* (essence). It is not typically effective as a sole formula to treat urinary incontinence and should be combined with qi or yang tonic herbs or formulas to treat this condition. For the treatment of urinary incontinence, it can be combined with *Suo Quan Wan* (Shut the Sluice Pill), *Sang Piao Xiao San* (Mantis Egg-Case Powder), *Jin Gui Shen Qi Wan* (Kidney Qi Pill from the Golden Cabinet), or *Bu Zhong Yi Qi Tang* (Tonify the Middle and Augment the Qi Decoction), depending on the animal.

References

1. *Hu Nan Zhong Yi Za Zhi* (Hunan Journal of Chinese Medicine), 1987; 3:46.
2. *Hu Bei Zhong Yi Za Zhi* (Hubei Journal of Chinese Medicine), 1985; 2:41.
3. *Xin Zhong Yi* (New Chinese Medicine), 1973; 5:30.

Sāng Piāo Xiāo Sǎn (Mantis Egg-Case Powder)

桑螵蛸散

Pinyin Name: *Sang Piao Xiao San*
Literal Name: Mantis Egg-Case Powder
Alternate Names: *Sang Piao Hsiao San*, Mantis Egg-Case Formula, Mantis Formula
Original Source: *Ben Cao Yan Yi* (Extension of the Materia Medica) by Kou Zong-Shi in 1116

COMPOSITION

Sang Piao Xiao (Ootheca Mantidis)	30g [9g]
Long Gu (Os Draconis)	30g [15g]
Gui Ban (Plastrum Testudinis), *chu zhi* (fried with vinegar)	30g [15g]
Ren Shen (Radix et Rhizoma Ginseng)	30g [9g]
Dang Gui (Radix Angelicae Sinensis)	30g [9g]
Yuan Zhi (Radix Polygalae)	30g [6g]
Shi Chang Pu (Rhizoma Acori Tatarinowii)	30g [6g]
Fu Shen (Poria Pararadicis)	30g [12g]

DOSAGE / PREPARATION / ADMINISTRATION

The source text states to grind the ingredients into powder and take 6g at bedtime, along with a decoction made from *Ren Shen* (Radix et Rhizoma Ginseng). Today, this formula is usually taken [6g at bedtime] with a decoction made from *Dang Shen* (Radix Codonopsis). This formula may also be prepared as a decoction with the doses suggested in brackets.

CHINESE THERAPEUTIC ACTIONS

1. Regulates and tonifies the Heart and Kidney
2. Stabilizes *jing* (essence) and stops seminal emissions

CLINICAL MANIFESTATIONS

Heart and Kidney deficiencies: urinary incontinence, frequent urination, seminal emissions, enuresis, confusion and disorientation, a pale tongue, and a weak, thin pulse.

Sāng Piāo Xiāo Săn (Mantis Egg-Case Powder)

VETERINARY CLINICAL APPLICATIONS

Chronic nephritis, cystitis, urinary incontinence, and seminal emissions.

EXPLANATION

Sang Piao Xiao San (Mantis Egg-Case Powder) is designed to treat the various clinical manifestations caused by Heart and Kidney deficiencies. According to Five-Element theory, the Kidney belongs to the water element and the Heart belongs to the fire element. If the Kidney (water) and the Heart (fire) cannot exist in harmony, then both organs may exhaust themselves. Kidney deficiency would lead to leaking of *jing* (essence), resulting in seminal emissions. Since the Kidney has an important function in regulating urination, deficiency of the Kidney would lead to urinary incontinence, enuresis and frequent urination. In addition, deficiency of the Heart may cause instability of the *shen* (spirit), leading to confusion and disorientation.

To effectively treat this syndrome, the Heart and Kidney should be tonified and their harmonious relationship should be restored. *Sang Piao Xiao* (Ootheca Mantidis), the chief substance of this formula, tonifies the Kidney, nourishes *jing* (essence), and stops seminal emissions. *Long Gu* (Os Draconis) calms the *shen* (spirit) and stabilizes *jing*. *Gui Ban* (Plastrum Testudinis) nourishes yin and tonifies the Heart and Kidney. *Ren Shen* (Radix et Rhizoma Ginseng) tonifies *yuan* (source) *qi*, and *Dang Gui* (Radix Angelicae Sinensis) nourishes blood. *Yuan Zhi* (Radix Polygalae) and *Shi Chang Pu* (Rhizoma Acori Tatarinowii) calm and anchor the *shen* to restore harmony between the Heart and Kidney. *Fu Shen* (Poria Paradicis) calms the *shen*.

VETERINARY MODIFICATIONS

- With generalized fatigue and deficiency, add *Huang Qi* (Radix Astragali).
- With Liver and Kidney yin deficiencies, add *Liu Wei Di Huang Wan* (Six-Ingredient Pill with Rehmannia).

CAUTIONS / CONTRAINDICATIONS

Sang Piao Xiao San contains many tonic and astringent herbs to treat loss of *jing* (essence) and body fluids due to Heart and Kidney deficiencies. This formula is not suitable for treating seminal emission and frequent urination due to damp-heat in the lower *jiao*.

HUMAN CLINICAL STUDIES AND RESEARCH

1. **Frequent urination**: According to one study, administration of *Sang Piao Xiao San* in decoction was associated with good results in treating frequent urination in 51 children (between 3 to 6 years of age, with 2 to 20 days history of illness). The clinical presentations included frequent urination with dripping, clear urine, no feelings of pain during urination, pale tongue with thin, white coating, and a fine, weak pulse. Of 51 patients, the study reported recovery in 2 cases after 2 days, 4 cases after 3 days, 14 cases after 4 days, 21 cases after 5 days, 6 cases after 6 days, and 2 cases after 7 days. Information was unavailable on individuals who did not complete the study.[1]
2. **Enuresis**: One study reported satisfactory results using modified *Sang Piao Xiao San* to treat bedwetting in 56 children (between 4 to 14 years of age, with 3 months to 10 years of history). The herbal formula contained processed *Huang Qi* (Radix Astragali) 10g, dry-fried *Dang Shen* (Radix Codonopsis) 10g, *Sang Piao Xiao* (Ootheca Mantidis) 15g, *Long Gu* (Os Draconis) 10g, dry-fried *Sheng Ma* (Rhizoma Cimicifugae) 10g, *Yi*

***Sang Piao Xiao San* (Mantis Egg-Case Powder)**

Diagnosis	Clinical Signs	Treatment	Herbs
Heart and Kidney deficiencies	• Urinary incontinence, enuresis and frequent urination: Kidney deficiency unable to control urination • Seminal emissions: leaking of *jing* (essence) due to Kidney deficiency • Confusion and disorientation: Heart deficiency unable to nourish *shen* (spirit)	• Regulates and tonifies the Heart and the Kidney • Stabilizes *jing* (essence) and stops seminal emissions	• *Sang Piao Xiao* (Ootheca Mantidis) tonifies the Kidney, nourishes the *jing* (essence) and stops seminal emissions. • *Long Gu* (Os Draconis) calms the *shen* (spirit) and stabilizes the *jing* (essence). • *Gui Ban* (Plastrum Testudinis) nourishes yin and tonifies the Heart and Kidney. • *Ren Shen* (Radix et Rhizoma Ginseng) and *Dang Gui* (Radix Angelicae Sinensis) tonify qi and blood. • *Yuan Zhi* (Radix Polygalae), *Shi Chang Pu* (Rhizoma Acori Tatarinowii), and *Fu Shen* (Poria Paradicis) calm the *shen* (spirit) to restore harmony to the Heart and Kidney.

Sāng Piāo Xiāo Sǎn (Mantis Egg-Case Powder)

Zhi (Fructus Alpiniae Oxyphyllae) 10g, and *Shan Yao* (Rhizoma Dioscoreae) 10g. The treatment protocol was to administer the herbs in decoction daily, for 10 days per course of treatment. The duration of treatment ranged from 7 to 23 days, with an average of 3 weeks. Of 56 children, the study reported complete recovery in 34 cases (no bedwetting for 3 months), significant improvement in 20 cases (reduced frequency of bedwetting within 3 months) and no effect in 2 cases. The overall effectiveness was 96.5%.[2]

3. **Constipation**: Use of *Sang Piao Xiao San* was associated with satisfactory results in treating constipation in 27 elderly patients (19 males and 8 females, between 56 to 86 years of age, with 10 months to 9 years history of illness). The clinical presentation included difficulty passing stools, with one bowel movement every 4 to 8 days. The herbal formula contained *Sang Piao Xiao* (Ootheca Mantidis) 12g, *Long Gu* (Os Draconis) 21g, *Qian Shi* (Semen Euryales) 15g, *Dang Shen* (Radix Codonopsis) 10g, *Gui Ban* (Plastrum Testudinis) 10g, *Dang Gui* (Radix Angelicae Sinensis) 10g, *Shi Chang Pu* (Rhizoma Acori Tatarinowii) 10g, and *Yuan Zhi* (Radix Polygalae) 10g. Furthermore, modifications were made by adding *Huang Qi* (Radix Astragali), *Bai Zhu* (Rhizoma Atractylodis Macrocephalae) and a larger dose of *Dang Shen* (Radix Codonopsis) for qi deficiency; *Bie Jia* (Carapax Trionycis) and a larger dose of *Gui Ban* (Plastrum Testudinis) for yin deficiency; *E Jiao* (Colla Corii Asini) and a larger dose of *Dang Gui* (Radix Angelicae Sinensis) for blood deficiency; *Huang Bo* (Cortex Phellodendri Chinensis) and *Zhi Mu* (Rhizoma Anemarrhenae) for frequent and painful urination with dark color urination; and *Yi Zhi* (Fructus Alpiniae Oxyphyllae), *Jin Ying Zi* (Fructus Rosae Laevigatae) and larger doses of *Sang Piao Xiao* (Ootheca Mantidis) and *Qian Shi* (Semen Euryales) for frequent urination with clear urine. The duration of treatment ranged from 7 to 25 days. Of 27 patients, the study reported complete recovery in 20 cases, improvement in 5 cases, and no effect in 2 cases.[3]

SUGGESTED ACUPUNCTURE TREATMENT

1. Points: *Shenshu* (BL 23), *Taixi* (KI 3), *Guanyuan* (CV 4), *Xinshu* (BL 15), *Shenmen* (HT 7), *Pishu* (BL 20), *Pangguangshu* (BL 28), and *Zhongji* (CV 3).
2. Technique: tonification.

Shenshu (BL 23), *Taixi* (KI 3), and *Guanyuan* (CV 4) tonify the Kidney. *Xinshu* (BL 15) and *Shenmen* (HT 7) nourish the Heart and calm the *shen* (spirit). Combined together, all of the above five points harmonize the Heart and Kidney. *Pishu* (BL 20) nourishes the qi of the middle *jiao*. *Pangguangshu* (BL 28) and *Zhongji* (CV 3) are combined according to the *shu* (transport) and *mu* (collecting) points principle to regulate the qi flow to stop the leakage of fluids.

AUTHORS' COMMENTS

Sang Piao Xiao San is the representative formula for treating loss of *jing* (essence) and body fluids caused by Heart and Kidney deficiencies. It can be used to treat urinary incontinence in dogs, and seems to be most effective in puppies having difficulties in house training or incontinence appearing shortly after a spay or neuter. It can be combined with *Suo Quan Wan* (Shut the Sluice Pill) to treat urinary incontinence in older dogs with qi and yang deficiencies, depending on the clinical signs. In cases of severe urinary incontinence, *Fu Pen Zi* (Fructus Rubi) and *Jin Ying Zi* (Fructus Rosae Laevigatae) can be added.

References

1. *Hei Long Jiang Zhong Yi Yao* (Heilongjiang Chinese Medicine and Herbology), 1990; 1:33.
2. *Jiang Su Zhong Yi* (Jiangsu Chinese Medicine), 1994; 4:14.
3. *Zhe Jiang Zhong Yi Xue Yuan Xue Bao* (Journal of Zhejiang University of Chinese Medicine), 1993; 2:27.

11

ASTRINGENT FORMULAS

Suō Quán Wán (Shut the Sluice Pill)

縮泉丸
缩泉丸

Pinyin Name: *Suo Quan Wan*
Literal Name: Shut the Sluice Pill
Alternate Name: Shut the Sluice Formula
Original Source: *Fu Ren Liang Fang* (Fine Formulas for Women) by Chen Zi-Ming in 1237

COMPOSITION

Yi Zhi (Fructus Alpiniae Oxyphyllae)	[9g]
Wu Yao (Radix Linderae)	[6g]

DOSAGE / PREPARATION / ADMINISTRATION

The source text states to grind equal amounts of *Yi Zhi* (Fructus Alpiniae Oxyphyllae) and *Wu Yao* (Radix Linderae) into powder. Separately cook powdered *Shan Yao* (Rhizoma Dioscoreae) [9-15g] with grain-based liquor until it becomes an herbal paste. Combine the powder and the paste to form pills. Take 70 pills per dose with salted, grain-based liquor or rice soup. Today, this formula is usually administered by giving 6g of pills per dose, once or twice a day with water. This formula may also be prepared as a decoction with the doses suggested in brackets.

CHINESE THERAPEUTIC ACTIONS

1. Warms the Kidney and dispels cold
2. Controls frequent urination and stops enuresis

CLINICAL MANIFESTATIONS

Frequent urination and enuresis caused by deficiency and cold of the lower *jiao*: frequent and prolonged urination, and dripping of urine after urination.

VETERINARY CLINICAL APPLICATIONS

Frequent urination, urinary dribbling, urinary incontinence, enuresis, and fecal incontinence.

EXPLANATION

Suo Quan Wan (Shut the Sluice Pill) is designed to treat urinary disorders caused by deficiency and cold of the lower *jiao*. The Kidney has the functions of regulating urination and dispelling turbid water out of the body. If Kidney qi is deficient and cold starts to accumulate in the Urinary Bladder, then urinary disorders such as frequent urination, urinary incontinence, and enuresis may occur.

In this formula, *Yi Zhi* (Fructus Alpiniae Oxyphyllae) warms the Kidney and Spleen to stop frequent urination and enuresis. *Wu Yao* (Radix Linderae) warms the lower *jiao* and disperses cold to restore the normal urinary functions of the Kidney and Urinary Bladder. *Shan Yao* (Rhizoma Dioscoreae) strengthens the Spleen and tonifies the Kidney to treat the underlying deficiency. It also stabilizes the *jing* (essence). These herbs are warm but not drying, and work to treat deficiency and cold and restore normal urination.

Even though *Suo Quan Wan* is effective, it is only mild to moderate in potency. In severe cases of urinary incontinence, frequent urination and enuresis, additional tonic and astringent herbs are called for to ensure adequate treatment.

***Suo Quan Wan* (Shut the Sluice Pill)**

Diagnosis	Clinical Signs	Treatment	Herbs
Frequent urination and enuresis	Urinary incontinence, dripping of urine after urination, and enuresis: deficiency and cold of the lower *jiao*	• Warms the Kidney and dispels cold • Controls frequent urination and stops enuresis	• *Yi Zhi* (Fructus Alpiniae Oxyphyllae) tonifies and warms the Kidney to stop frequent urination and enuresis. • *Wu Yao* (Radix Linderae) warms the lower *jiao* and disperses cold to restore the normal urinary function of the Kidney and Urinary Bladder. • *Shan Yao* (Rhizoma Dioscoreae) strengthens the Spleen and tonifies the Kidney to treat the underlying deficiencies.

Suō Quán Wán (Shut the Sluice Pill)

VETERINARY MODIFICATIONS

- In cases with more yang deficiency and cold, add *Gui Zhi* (Ramulus Cinnamomi).
- To improve the astringent action, add *Fu Pen Zi* (Fructus Rubi), *Jin Ying Zi* (Fructus Rosae Laevigatae), and/or *Sang Piao Xiao* (Ootheca Mantidis).

CAUTIONS / CONTRAINDICATIONS

Animals taking *Suo Quan Wan* should avoid pungent foods.[1]

PHARMACOLOGICAL EFFECTS

Antidiuretic: According to one study, use of *Suo Quan Wan* in healthy rats was associated with marked antidiuretic effect. Furthermore, there was a reduced concentration in the urine of sodium and chloride, but increased concentration of potassium.[2]

HUMAN CLINICAL STUDIES AND RESEARCH

1. **Frequent urination**: *Suo Quan Wan* has been shown in many studies to effectively treat frequent urination in children. According to one study, administration of this formula in powder form was associated with 93.75% effectiveness. Of 32 children, the study reported complete recovery in 27 cases, improvement in 3 cases, and no effect in 2 cases.[3] Another study also reported good results for treatment of frequent urination using *Suo Quan Wan* plus *Jin Ying Zi* (Fructus Rosae Laevigatae) and *Huang Qi* (Radix Astragali) as the base formula.[4]
2. **Urinary incontinence**: The use of modified *Suo Quan Wan* was shown in one study to have good effect to treat urinary and bowel incontinence in post-stroke patients. The herbal treatment contained this formula plus *Sang Piao Xiao* (Ootheca Mantidis), *Shan Zhu Yu* (Fructus Corni), *Bu Gu Zhi* (Fructus Psoraleae), *Tu Si Zi* (Semen Cuscutae) and *Huang Qi* (Radix Astragali) as the base formula. Furthermore, *Rou Dou Kou* (Semen Myristicae), *Wu Zhu Yu* (Fructus Evodiae) and *Wu Wei Zi* (Fructus Schisandrae Chinensis) were added for bowel incontinence; *Shi Chang Pu* (Rhizoma Acori Tatarinowii), *Yu Jin* (Radix Curcumae), *Yuan Zhi* (Radix Polygalae) and *Dan Nan Xing* (Arisaema cum Bile) were added for speech difficulties; *Tao Ren* (Semen Persicae), *Hong Hua* (Flos Carthami), *Di Long* (Pheretima), *Chi Shao* (Radix Paeoniae Rubra) and a larger dose of *Huang Qi* (Radix Astragali) for sallow facial appearance, fatigue, and weakness and paralysis of the extremities.[5]
3. **Enuresis**: According to one study, the use of *Suo Quan Wan* plus *Sang Piao Xiao* (Ootheca Mantidis), *Long Gu* (Os Draconis) and other herbs was associated with 95% effectiveness in treating 20 children with enuresis. Of 20 patients, 12 had complete recovery, 7 had improvement, and 1 had no effect.[6]

TOXICOLOGY

According to one toxicology study, administration of *Suo Quan Wan* at 10 g/kg, 15 g/kg and 20 g/kg daily (proportionally 50, 75 and 100 times the normal dose in human adults) for 2 days did not cause any abnormal reactions within 7 days of the observation period.[7]

SUGGESTED ACUPUNCTURE TREATMENT

1. Points: *Shenshu* (BL 23), *Mingmen* (GV 4), and *Pishu* (BL 20).
2. Technique: tonification and moxibustion.

Shenshu (BL 23) and *Mingmen* (GV 4) warm the Kidney and dispel cold. Moxibustion on these two points can increase the *ming men* (life gate) fire. *Pishu* (BL 20) warms the Spleen to increase the transformation and transportation of water and fluids.

AUTHORS' COMMENTS

Suo Quan Wan is effective in treating mild cases of urinary incontinence in dogs. In severe cases with more cold and deficiency of qi and yang, it can be combined with *Jin Gui Shen Qi Wan* (Kidney Qi Pill from the Golden Cabinet) or *You Gui Wan* (Restore the Right [Kidney] Pill).

Sang Piao Xiao San (Mantis Egg-Case Powder), *Jin Suo Gu Jing Wan* (Metal Lock Pill to Stabilize the Essence), and *Suo Quan Wan* can all be used to treat urinary incontinence and frequent urination.

- *Sang Piao Xiao San* tonifies, but is not warm in property. It tonifies the Heart and Kidney to treat urinary incontinence, frequent urination, and enuresis. It is not typically used alone to treat urinary incontinence in dogs; instead, combine it with additional herbs or another formula that tonifies and warms Kidney qi and yang.
- *Jin Suo Gu Jing Wan* tonifies the Kidney and stabilizes the *jing* (essence) to treat urinary incontinence. It can be combined with *Suo Quan Wan* for increased clinical efficacy.
- *Suo Quan Wan* warms the Kidney to treat urinary incontinence, frequent urination, dribbling urine, and enuresis caused by deficiency and cold. This formula is warm, but not drying, and has a mild effect. It can be used as a single formula in simple, uncomplicated cases of mild urinary incontinence. If the clinical signs are severe, other herbs or another formula will need to be added to achieve maximum clinical effect.

Suō Quán Wán (Shut the Sluice Pill)

References

1. *Zhong Yao Ming Fang Yao Li Yu Ying Yong* (Pharmacology and Applications of Famous Herbal Formulas), 1989; 352-353.
2. *Zhong Yi Fang Ji Xian Dai Yan Jiu* (Modern Study of Medical Formulas in Traditional Chinese Medicine), 1997; 823.
3. *Ji Lin Zhong Yi Yao* (Jilin Chinese Medicine and Herbology), 1998; 2:28.
4. *Fu Jian Zhong Yi Yao* (Fujian Chinese Medicine and Herbology), 1998; 6:24.
5. *Bei Jing Zhong Yi* (Beijing Chinese Medicine), 1997; 2:55.
6. *Shan Xi Zhong Yi* (Shanxi Chinese Medicine), 1997; 1:31.
7. *Xin Zhong Yi* (New Chinese Medicine), 1991; 12:49.

Section 5

固崩止带剂
— Womb-Stabilizing Formulas to Stop Leakage

Wán Dài Tāng (End Discharge Decoction)
完帶湯
完带汤

Pinyin Name: *Wan Dai Tang*
Literal Name: End Discharge Decoction
Alternate Names: *Wan Tai Tang*, Treating Morbid Leukorrhea Decoction, Atractylodes and Dioscorea Combination
Original Source: *Fu Qing Zhu Nu Ke* (Women's Diseases According to Fu Qing-Zhu) by Fu Shan in 1827

COMPOSITION

Bai Zhu (Rhizoma Atractylodis Macrocephalae), *chao* (dry-fried) with soil	30g
Shan Yao (Rhizoma Dioscoreae), *chao* (dry-fried)	30g
Ren Shen (Radix et Rhizoma Ginseng)	6g
Cang Zhu (Rhizoma Atractylodis), *zhi* (prepared)	9g
Chen Pi (Pericarpium Citri Reticulatae)	1.5g
Che Qian Zi (Semen Plantaginis), *chao* (dry-fried) with liquor	9g
Bai Shao (Radix Paeoniae Alba), *chao* (dry-fried) with liquor	15g
Chai Hu (Radix Bupleuri)	1.8g
Jing Jie Sui Tan (Spica Schizonepetae Carbonisata)	1.5g
Gan Cao (Radix et Rhizoma Glycyrrhizae)	3g

DOSAGE / PREPARATION / ADMINISTRATION

The source text states to prepare the ingredients as a decoction.

CHINESE THERAPEUTIC ACTIONS

1. Tonifies the middle *jiao* and strengthens the Spleen
2. Dissolves dampness and stops abnormal vaginal discharge

CLINICAL MANIFESTATIONS

Abnormal vaginal discharge caused by Spleen deficiency and Liver qi stagnation, accompanied by dampness and turbidity in the lower *jiao*: odorless, clear, and thin vaginal discharge that is white or light yellow in color, lethargy, loose stools, a pale tongue, and a soft, weak pulse.

VETERINARY CLINICAL APPLICATIONS

Puppy vaginitis and abnormal vaginal discharge.

EXPLANATION

Wan Dai Tang (End Discharge Decoction) is designed to treat abnormal vaginal discharge caused by Spleen qi deficiency and Liver qi stagnation. Vaginal discharge is associated with the *dai* (girdle) channel that encircles the lower trunk like a belt. The *dai* channel is intimately associated with the Liver and Spleen, and if there is obstruction of the *dai* (girdle) channel, vaginal discharge can occur. Stagnation of Liver qi may lead to the Liver overacting on the Spleen, causing Spleen deficiency. Deficiency of the Spleen may cause production and accumulation of dampness and turbidity, which usually travel to the lower *jiao* because of their heavy and descending character, and result in vaginal discharge. Since there is no heat or infection, the vaginal discharge will be clear, thin, odorless, and white or light yellow in color. Lethargy, loose stools, a pale tongue, and a soft, weak pulse indicate qi deficiency and dampness accumulation.

Wán Dài Tāng (End Discharge Decoction)

***Wan Dai Tang* (End Discharge Decoction)**

Diagnosis	Clinical Signs	Treatment	Herbs
Abnormal vaginal discharge caused by Spleen deficiency and Liver qi stagnation	• Abnormal vaginal discharge (clear, thin, odorless and white or light yellowish in color): Spleen deficiency with dampness and turbidity • Pale tongue, lethargy, and loose stools: Spleen deficiency • A soft, weak pulse: Spleen deficiency with dampness accumulation	• Tonifies middle *jiao* and strengthens the Spleen • Dissolves dampness and stops vaginal discharge	• *Bai Zhu* (Rhizoma Atractylodis Macrocephalae) and *Shan Yao* (Rhizoma Dioscoreae) strengthen the Spleen and dry dampness. • *Ren Shen* (Radix et Rhizoma Ginseng) tonifies qi. • *Cang Zhu* (Rhizoma Atractylodis) and *Chen Pi* (Pericarpium Citri Reticulatae) activate qi flow and dry dampness. • *Che Qian Zi* (Semen Plantaginis) resolves dampness through urination. • *Bai Shao* (Radix Paeoniae Alba) softens the Liver. • *Chai Hu* (Radix Bupleuri) ascends the yang and activates Liver qi flow. • *Jing Jie Sui Tan* (Spica Schizonepetae Carbonisata) stops vaginal discharge. • *Gan Cao* (Radix et Rhizoma Glycyrrhizae) harmonizes all of the herbs.

This formula uses dry-fried *Bai Zhu* (Rhizoma Atractylodis Macrocephalae) and *Shan Yao* (Rhizoma Dioscoreae) in heavy dosages to carry out two important functions. First, these two herbs strengthen the Spleen and tonify qi to facilitate the water metabolism function. Second, both herbs dry dampness and help reduce vaginal discharge. *Ren Shen* (Radix et Rhizoma Ginseng) tonifies qi. *Cang Zhu* (Rhizoma Atractylodis) and *Chen Pi* (Pericarpium Citri Reticulatae) activate the qi flow and dry dampness. These two herbs also prevent the tonifying herbs from creating additional dampness and stagnation. *Che Qian Zi* (Semen Plantaginis) resolves dampness through urination. *Bai Shao* (Radix Paeoniae Alba) softens the Liver. *Chai Hu* (Radix Bupleuri) ascends the yang and activates Liver qi flow. *Jing Jie Sui Tan* (Spica Schizonepetae Carbonisata) has the function to stop vaginal discharge. *Gan Cao* (Radix et Rhizoma Glycyrrhizae) harmonizes all of the herbs in this formula.

VETERINARY MODIFICATIONS

- For vaginal discharge characterized by cold, add *Li Zhong Tang* (Regulate the Middle Decoction).
- For vaginal discharge characterized by heat, add *Huang Lian Jie Du Tang* (Coptis Decoction to Relieve Toxicity).
- For vaginal discharge secondary to chronic illness and deficiency, add *Long Gu* (Os Draconis) and *Mu Li* (Concha Ostreae).
- For vaginal discharge that is yellow, add *Huang Bo* (Cortex Phellodendri Chinensis) and *Long Dan* (Radix et Rhizoma Gentianae).
- For chronic vaginal discharge that is white or clear, add *Lu Jiao Shuang* (Cornu Cervi Degelatinatum).
- With Spleen deficiency, add *Huang Qi* (Radix Astragali) and *Bai Bian Dou* (Semen Lablab Album).
- With blood deficiency, add *Shu Di Huang* (Radix Rehmanniae Praeparata) and *Dang Gui* (Radix Angelicae Sinensis).

CAUTIONS / CONTRAINDICATIONS

Wan Dai Tang is contraindicated in yellow or foul-smelling vaginal discharge caused by damp-heat, unless appropriately modified.

PHARMACOLOGICAL EFFECTS

Anti-inflammatory: One study reported marked effect in reducing inflammation using *Wan Dai Tang* in mice given via intraperitoneal injection.[1]

HUMAN CLINICAL STUDIES AND RESEARCH

1. **Vaginal discharge**: One study reported improvement to complete recovery using modified *Wan Dai Tang* to treat 50 women with vaginal discharge. The herbal formula contained *Tai Zi Shen* (Radix Pseudostellariae) 10g, charred *Bai Zhu* (Rhizoma Atractylodis Macrocephalae) 15g, processed *Cang Zhu* (Rhizoma Atractylodis) 6g, *Che Qian Zi* (Semen Plantaginis) 10g, *Zhi Gan Cao* (Radix et Rhizoma Glycyrrhizae Praeparata cum Melle) 3g, *Chen Pi* (Pericarpium Citri Reticulatae) 6g, *Chai Hu* (Radix Bupleuri) 3g, charred *Jing Jie* (Herba Schizonepetae) 2g, alcohol-fried *Bai Shao* (Radix Paeoniae Alba) 12g,

Wán Dài Tāng (End Discharge Decoction)

Shan Yao (Rhizoma Dioscoreae) 30g, *Qian Shi* (Semen Euryales) 12g, *Bai Guo* (Semen Ginkgo) 7 pieces, and others as deemed necessary. The duration of treatment ranged from 5 to 14 packs of herbs.[2]

2. **Cervicitis**: According to one study, administration of modified *Wan Dai Tang* in decoction daily for 15 to 46 packs of herbs was effective in treating chronic cervicitis. Of 47 women, the study reported complete recovery in 25 cases, improvement in 18 cases, and no effect in 4 cases.[3]
3. **Vaginitis**: According to one study, the use of modified *Wan Dai Tang* was associated with good effect to treat acute or chronic vaginitis caused by *Candida albicans*. Modifications to the original formula were made by adding *Di Fu Zi* (Fructus Kochiae) and *Bai Xian Pi* (Cortex Dictamni) for itching in the genital region; *Mu Tong* (Caulis Akebiae), *Zhi Zi* (Fructus Gardeniae) and *Zhi Mu* (Rhizoma Anemarrhenae) for burning sensations and pain; *Qu Mai* (Herba Dianthi) and *Hua Shi* (Talcum) for frequent urination with pain; *Yu Xing Cao* (Herba Houttuyniae) and *Huang Bo* (Cortex Phellodendri Chinensis) for yellow discharge; *Xu Duan* (Radix Dipsaci) and *Du Zhong* (Cortex Eucommiae) for low back pain; and *Bu Gu Zhi* (Fructus Psoraleae), *Wu Wei Zi* (Fructus Schisandrae Chinensis), *Rou Dou Kou* (Semen Myristicae) and *Wu Zhu Yu* (Fructus Evodiae) for chronic illness. Of 31 patients, the study reported complete recovery in 28 cases, significant improvement in 2 cases, and no effect in 1 case.[4]
4. **Irritable bowel syndrome (IBS)**: One study reported 92% effectiveness using modified *Wan Dai Tang* to treat 24 patients with IBS. In addition to the base formula, *Cang Zhu* (Rhizoma Atractylodis) and *Pu Gong Ying* (Herba Taraxaci) were added for more damp-heat; *Wu Zhu Yu* (Fructus Evodiae) and *Rou Dou Kou* (Semen Myristicae) for more deficiency and cold; *Mu Xiang* (Radix Aucklandiae) and *Gua Lou* (Fructus Trichosanthis) for abdominal distention; *Sheng Ma* (Rhizoma Cimicifugae) and *Bai Zhi* (Radix Angelicae Dahuricae) for frequent diarrhea; *Da Huang* (Radix et Rhizoma Rhei) for constipation; *Mu Xiang* (Radix Aucklandiae) and *Bing Lang* (Semen Arecae) for feeling of incomplete evacuation after defecation; and *Yi Zhi* (Fructus Alpiniae Oxyphyllae) and *Bu Gu Zhi* (Fructus Psoraleae) for chronic illness. Of 24 patients, the study reported complete recovery in 17 cases, improvement in 5 cases, and no effect in 2 cases.[5]

SUGGESTED ACUPUNCTURE TREATMENT

1. Points: *Housanli* (ST 36), *Sanyinjiao* (SP 6), *Daimai* (GB 26), *Qihai* (CV 6), *Baihuanshu* (BL 30), and *Ligou* (LR 5).
2. Technique: mainly tonification, supplemental sedation if needed.

Housanli (ST 36) and *Sanyinjiao* (SP 6) strengthen the Spleen to dissolve dampness. *Daimai* (GB 26) consolidates the *dai* (girdle) channel to stop vaginal discharge. *Qihai* (CV 6) tonifies qi, regulates the *ren* (conception) channel, and disperses dampness. *Baihuanshu* (BL 30) assists the function of the Urinary Bladder to eliminate dampness from the lower *jiao*. *Ligou* (LR 5) smoothes the Liver qi to disperse qi and blood stagnation within the body.

AUTHORS' COMMENTS

Wan Dai Tang can be used to treat puppy vaginitis. Puppies 6 weeks to 8 months of age are usually affected, and the condition is characterized by sticky, white or yellowish vaginal discharge that is mild to copious. The vaginal discharge can occur intermittently and can last for weeks to months. Some puppies may have vulvitis or develop perivulvar dermatitis. Cytology and culture of the discharge often show suppurative inflammation. However, no organisms are typically identified. The condition is considered to be benign from a biomedical perspective; the etiology is unknown, and no definitive treatment is available. The cause of the disease from a Chinese medicine perspective is Spleen qi deficiency and Liver qi stagnation, brought about by feeding a poor diet in combination with stress. This is the pattern of vaginitis for which this formula is ideally suited. *Wan Dai Tang* can also be used in adult dogs with similar clinical presentation. However, unless steps are taken to change the diet from dampness-engendering food (typical of high carbohydrate, kibbled food) to food that is more species appropriate, the condition will continue to be promulgated and resolution difficult to obtain, especially in older dogs.

Older mares may develop a similar pattern. There may not be visible discharge, but ultrasound will show pooling of fluid in the uterus. Organisms will not be present on culture of the fluid, though mares will often have difficulty becoming pregnant. Dietary issues are not the cause here, as it is in dogs, but aging or multiple pregnancies create deficiencies that lead to the discharge. The addition of a tonic formula, such as *Ba Zhen Tang* (Eight-Treasure Decoction), can be useful in restoring normal tone and function to the uterus and vagina.

Wan Dai Tang and *Long Dan Xie Gan Tang* (Gentiana Decoction to Drain the Liver) both treat vaginal discharge.

- *Wan Dai Tang* is reserved for vaginal discharge that is white and not foul-smelling, and that is caused by Spleen deficiency, Liver qi stagnation, and accumulation of dampness.

Wán Dài Tāng (End Discharge Decoction)

- *Long Dan Xie Gan Tang* is used only for yellow, thick, and foul-smelling vaginal discharge, caused by damp-heat attacking the Liver channel.[6]

References

1. *Liao Ning Zhong Yi Za Zhi* (Liaoning Journal of Chinese Medicine), 1992; 6:43.
2. *Shang Hai Zhong Yi Yao Za Zhi* (Shanghai Journal of Chinese Medicine and Herbology), 1991; 12:17.
3. *Jiang Su Zhong Yi* (Jiangsu Chinese Medicine), 1987; 4:17.
4. *Xin Zhong Yi* (New Chinese Medicine), 1997; 11:31.
5. *Zhe Jiang Zhong Yi Za Zhi* (Zhejiang Journal of Chinese Medicine), 1996; 10:445.
6. Wang MZ, et al. *Zhong Yi Xue Wen Da Ti Ku* (Questions and Answers on Traditional Chinese Medicine: Herbal Formulas).

Bā Wèi Dài Xià Fāng (Eight-Ingredient Formula for Leukorrhea)

八味带下方

八味带下方

Pinyin Name: *Ba Wei Dai Xia Fang*
Literal Name: Eight-Ingredient Formula for Leukorrhea
Alternate Names: *Pa Wei Tai Hsia Fang*, Eight-Taste Discharging Formula, Tangkuei Eight Herb Formula
Original Source: *Meika Hosen* (A Selection of Famous Physicians' Prescriptions) by Yoshine Hirai

COMPOSITION

Tu Fu Ling (Rhizoma Smilacis Glabrae)	4g
Jin Yin Hua (Flos Lonicerae Japonicae)	2g
Dang Gui (Radix Angelicae Sinensis)	5g
Chuan Xiong (Rhizoma Chuanxiong)	3g
Fu Ling (Poria)	3g
Mu Tong (Caulis Akebiae)	3g
Chen Pi (Pericarpium Citri Reticulatae)	2g
Da Huang (Radix et Rhizoma Rhei)	0.5-1g

DOSAGE / PREPARATION / ADMINISTRATION

Unavailable.

CHINESE THERAPEUTIC ACTIONS

1. Clears heat and eliminates toxins
2. Dries dampness

CLINICAL MANIFESTATIONS

Vaginal discharge characterized by damp-heat in the lower *jiao*: vaginal discharge with yellow, white, or bloody discharge, generalized itching, sores, dermatitis and discomfort in the perivulvar, perianal and urogenital region.

VETERINARY CLINICAL APPLICATIONS

Acute or chronic vaginal discharge that is yellow, white, or red in color, trichomonal vaginal discharge, and sores, dermatitis and generalized itching of the perivulvar, perianal and urogenital region.

EXPLANATION

Ba Wei Dai Xia Fang (Eight-Ingredient Formula for Leukorrhea) is designed to treat acute or chronic vaginal discharge caused by damp-heat and toxins in the lower *jiao*. Effective treatment must focus on clearing damp-heat and toxins from the affected area.

Bā Wèi Dài Xià Fāng (Eight-Ingredient Formula for Leukorrhea)

***Ba Wei Dai Xia Fang* (Eight-Ingredient Formula for Leukorrhea)**

Diagnosis	Clinical Signs	Treatment	Herbs
Vaginal discharge	Vaginal discharge that is yellow, white or red in color; dermatitis, and sores of the perivulvar, perianal and urogenital regions: damp-heat in the lower *jiao*	• Clears heat and eliminates toxins • Dries dampness	• *Tu Fu Ling* (Rhizoma Smilacis Glabrae) and *Jin Yin Hua* (Flos Lonicerae Japonicae) clear heat and remove toxins. • *Dang Gui* (Radix Angelicae Sinensis) and *Chuan Xiong* (Rhizoma Chuanxiong) nourish the blood and prevent the drying and draining herbs from consuming yin. • *Fu Ling* (Poria), *Mu Tong* (Caulis Akebiae) and *Chen Pi* (Pericarpium Citri Reticulatae) clear damp-heat. • *Da Huang* (Radix et Rhizoma Rhei) drains pathogenic heat from the body.

In this formula, *Tu Fu Ling* (Rhizoma Smilacis Glabrae) and *Jin Yin Hua* (Flos Lonicerae Japonicae) clear heat and remove toxins. *Dang Gui* (Radix Angelicae Sinensis) and *Chuan Xiong* (Rhizoma Chuanxiong) nourish the blood and prevent the drying and draining herbs from consuming yin. *Fu Ling* (Poria), *Mu Tong* (Caulis Akebiae), and *Chen Pi* (Pericarpium Citri Reticulatae) clear damp-heat. *Da Huang* (Radix et Rhizoma Rhei) drains pathogenic heat from the body.

VETERINARY MODIFICATIONS

- With itching and pain in the urogenital region due to damp-heat, add *Huang Lian Jie Du Tang* (Coptis Decoction to Relieve Toxicity).
- For severe bacterial vaginitis, combine with *Long Dan Xie Gan Tang* (Gentiana Decoction to Drain the Liver).
- With blood deficiency and generalized weakness, add *Si Wu Tang* (Four-Substance Decoction).

CAUTIONS / CONTRAINDICATIONS

Animals with a sensitive gastrointestinal tract may need to take *Ba Wei Dai Xia Fang* without *Da Huang* (Radix et Rhizoma Rhei), as this herb may cause diarrhea and stomach discomfort.

SUGGESTED ACUPUNCTURE TREATMENT

1. Points: *Ligou* (LR 5), *Xingjian* (LR 2), *Xuehai* (SP 10), *Sanyinjiao* (SP 6), *Ciliao* (BL 32), *Yinlingquan* (SP 9), and *Zhongji* (CV 3).
2. Technique: even method and sedation.

Sedation on *Ligou* (LR 5), *Xingjian* (LR 2), and *Xuehai* (SP 10) clear heat and eliminate toxins. Even method on *Sanyinjiao* (SP 6) and *Ciliao* (BL 32) nourish blood and prevent the drying and draining herbs from consuming yin. Even method on *Yinlingquan* (SP 9) and *Zhongji* (CV 3) removes dampness and reduces vaginal discharge.

AUTHORS' COMMENTS

There are four readily available formulas that are used to treat vaginal discharge in veterinary medicine. Their similarities and differences are as follows.

- *Si Miao San* (Four-Marvel Powder) treats acute or chronic vaginal discharge caused by Spleen deficiency and dampness. It is often the initial formula of choice to treat puppy vaginitis.
- *Wan Dai Tang* (End Discharge Decoction) is designed to treat chronic vaginal discharge caused by Spleen qi deficiency and Liver qi stagnation. It is often the initial formula chosen to treat older animals.
- *Ba Wei Dai Xia Fang* (Eight-Ingredient Formula for Leukorrhea) treats acute or chronic vaginal discharge caused by damp-heat and toxins in the lower *jiao*. It can be used for post-partum infections and bacterial infections.
- *Long Dan Xie Gan Tang* (Gentiana Decoction to Drain the Liver) treats acute vaginal discharge characterized by heat and dampness in the Liver and Gallbladder channels and the lower *jiao*. It can be used for post-partum infections and bacterial infections, but is not intended for long-term use. Once the clinical signs resolve, one of the other formulas should be given, depending on the case.

Chapter 11 — Summary

— Astringent Formulas

SECTION 1: EXTERIOR-STABILIZING FORMULA TO STOP SWEATING

Name	Similarities	Differences
Yu Ping Feng San (Jade Windscreen Powder)	Stabilizes the exterior, stops Sweating	Tonifies *wei* (defensive) *qi* to stop spontaneous sweating

Yu Ping Feng San (Jade Windscreen Powder) tonifies qi and strengthens the exterior *wei* (defensive) level. It is used for spontaneous sweating caused by *wei* (defensive) *qi* deficiency. It is also effective in strengthening *wei qi* and preventing frequent contraction of exterior wind-cold.

SECTION 2: LUNG-RESTRAINING FORMULA TO RELIEVE COUGH

Name	Similarities	Differences
Jiu Xian San (Nine-Immortal Powder)	Restrains the Lung	Tonifies Lung qi and yin

Jiu Xian San (Nine-Immortal Powder) restrains the Lung, tonifies qi and yin, and stops coughing. It is used for chronic cough and shortness of breath due to Lung qi and yin deficiencies.

SECTION 3: INTESTINES-BINDING FORMULA TO STOP LEAKAGE

Name	Similarities	Differences
Si Shen Wan (Four-Miracle Pill)	Binds the Intestines, stops diarrhea and dysentery	Warms and tonifies the Spleen and Kidney; stronger warming and tonifying effect

Si Shen Wan (Four-Miracle Pill) has the action to warm and tonify the Spleen and Kidney to stop diarrhea. This formula is especially effective for 5 a.m. diarrhea caused by Kidney yang deficiency. Clinical manifestations include early morning diarrhea, loss of appetite, soreness of the lower back, abdominal pain, cold extremities, lack of energy, a pale, wet tongue, and a weak, deep pulse.

Chapter 11 — Summary

SECTION 4: *JING* (ESSENCE)-STABILIZING FORMULAS TO STOP LEAKAGE

Name	Similarities	Differences
Jin Suo Gu Jing Wan (Metal Lock Pill to Stabilize the Essence)	Restrain and stop the leakage of *jing* (essence)	Tonifies the Kidney
Sang Piao Xiao San (Mantis Egg-Case Powder)		Tonifies the Heart and Kidney
Suo Quan Wan (Shut the Sluice Pill)		Warms the Kidney and astringes the Urinary Bladder

Jin Suo Gu Jing Wan (Metal Lock Pill to Stabilize the Essence) tonifies the Kidney and stabilizes the *jing* (essence). It treats urinary incontinence, and spermatorrhea and/or seminal emissions caused by Kidney deficiency, with clinical signs such as lethargy, weak and painful rear quarters and lumbar region, impaired hearing, a pale pink tongue, and a weak, thin pulse.

Sang Piao Xiao San (Mantis Egg-Case Powder) tonifies the Heart and Kidney. It is used to treat deficiency of both the Heart and Kidney, with clinical manifestations such as seminal emissions, urinary incontinence, enuresis, and frequent urination.

Suo Quan Wan (Shut the Sluice Pill) warms the Kidney and astringes the Urinary Bladder. It is used for Kidney qi deficiency with accumulation of cold in the Urinary Bladder, causing urinary incontinence, dripping urine, enuresis, and frequent, clear and prolonged urination.

SECTION 5: WOMB-STABILIZING FORMULAS TO STOP LEAKAGE

Name	Similarities	Differences
Wan Dai Tang (End Discharge Decoction)	Resolve dampness, stop vaginal discharge	Tonifies qi, strengthens the Spleen, regulates Liver qi
Ba Wei Dai Xia Fang (Eight-Ingredient Formula for Leukorrhea)		Clears damp-heat and toxins in the lower *jiao*

Wan Dai Tang (End Discharge Decoction) stops vaginal discharge due to Spleen deficiency and Liver qi stagnation. Clinical manifestations include odorless, clear, and thick vaginal discharge that is white or light yellow in color, pale face, and lethargy.

Ba Wei Dai Xia Fang (Eight-Ingredient Formula for Leukorrhea) treats vaginal discharge due to damp-heat and toxins in the lower *jiao*. Clinical manifestations include vaginal discharge with yellow, white, or red discharge, generalized itching sores, dermatitis and discomfort in the perivulvar, perianal and urogenital regions, abdominal pain, soreness of the lower back, and slight anemia.

Chapter 12

— Qi-Regulating Formulas

理气剂

李时珍 Lǐ Shí-Zhēn

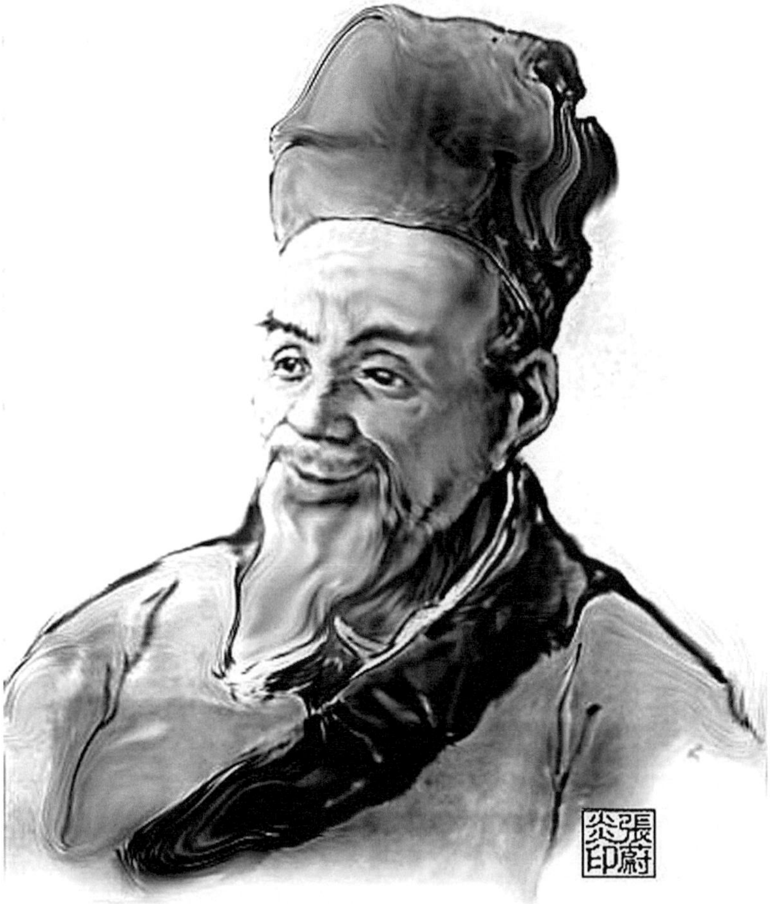

李时珍 Lǐ Shí-Zhēn, 1518 – 1593.

李时珍 Lǐ Shí-Zhēn

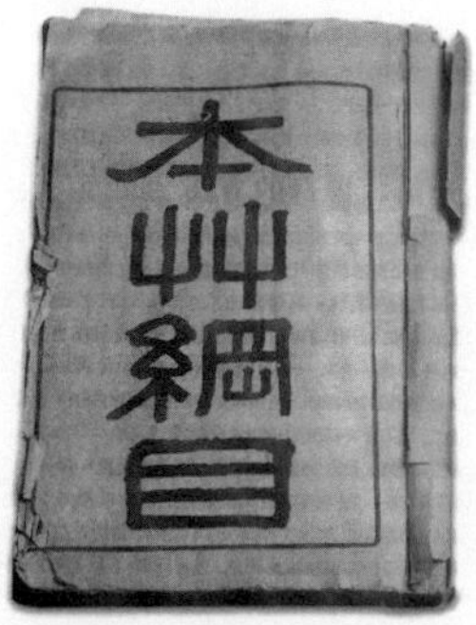

本草纲目 *Ben Cao Gang Mu* (Materia Medica) in 1596.

Li Shi-Zhen was born into a long family lineage of physicians. However, his father refused to allow him to study medicine in his youth because at that time, physicians were held in low social esteem and had poor economic status. Li remained interested in medicine, and after years of insistence, his father finally agreed, and began to teach Li medicine when he was 23 years old. Li made tremendous advances in the next fifteen years. When he was 38, he was called to the Imperial Palace to become 太医 the Supreme Physician. Three years later, he was promoted to Chief Supreme Physician. However, he disliked the politics of serving in the Imperial Palace, and resigned one year later to return home.

In Li's years of studying and practicing, he noticed many errors, omissions, and repetitions among herbal texts. Realizing that such errors create malpractice and jeopardize lives, he embarked on a life-long journey to research and rewrite the records of herbal medicine. During the research process, Li interviewed physicians and pharmacists, lived with hunters and farmers, and personally cultivated and tested many herbs, all to ensure accuracy in the information. In 1578, when Li Shi-Zhen was 60 years old, he finished the *Ben Cao Gang Mu* (Materia Medica) after 27 years of work. This was the most comprehensive of all herbal texts prior to the 17th century: it documented 1,892 medicinal substances (1,195 plants, 340 animals, and 357 mineral substances) classified into 6 sections, 52 scrolls, and 60 categories.

Ironically, Li spent his entire adult life in compiling the *Ben Cao Gang Mu* (Materia Medica), yet during his life time he found no one willing to invest the money to publish it. He eventually donated it to the Imperial Palace before he passed away, hoping that it would be preserved and passed on to future generations. Finally in 1596, three years after his death, it was published in Nanjing. Today, the *Ben Cao Gang Mu* (Materia Medica) is still considered one of the most important herbal texts, and has been translated into many languages, including English, Japanese, German, French and Russian.

Dynasties & Kingdoms	Year
Xia Dynasty 夏	2100-1600 BCE
Shang Dynasty 商	1600-1100 BCE
Zhou Dynasty 周	1100-221 BCE
Qin Dynasty 秦	221-207 BCE
Han Dynasty 漢	206 BCE-220
Three Kingdoms 三國	220-280
Western Jin Dynasty 西晉	265-316
Eastern Jin Dynasty 東晉	317-420
Northern and Southern Dynasties 北南朝	420-581
Sui Dynasty 隋	581-618
Tang Dynasty 唐	618-907
Five Dynasties 五代	907-960
Song Dynasty 宋	960-1279
Liao Dynasty 遼	916-1125
Jin Dynasty 金	1115-1234
Yuan Dynasty 元	1271-1368
Ming Dynasty 明	**1368-1644**
Qing Dynasty 清	1644-1911
Republic of China 中華民國	1912-Present Day
People's Republic of China 中華人民共和國	1949-Present Day

Table of Contents

Chapter 12 — Overview

理气剂

— Qi-Regulating Formulas

Definition: Qi-regulating formulas activate qi circulation to treat qi stagnation and restore the normal flow of qi. These formulas typically regulate qi in two general ways. First, they promote normal qi flow and unblock or eliminate qi stagnation; second, they direct rebellious or reversed qi flow to descend downward in the proper direction.

Normal qi flow is essential for good health. Qi circulates and provides warmth and protection, moves the blood, and ensures normal health and function of the *zang fu* organs and the four limbs. When disease develops in any region, channel or organ, the flow of qi is usually disrupted first. Qi flow disorders impair the movement of food, fluid and/or blood, depending on the location. Severe qi stagnation can lead to qi-flow reversal, that is, qi moving in the wrong direction. Qi stagnation does not typically occur in isolation and is usually accompanied by stagnation of blood (as the flow of one depends on the other), phlegm, food, or other substances. In addition, the presence of qi stagnation in one organ can impair the function of other organs. The *zang fu* organs most commonly affected by qi disorders are the Lung (cough, wheezing, dyspnea, exercise intolerance), the Liver (hypochondriac pain, irritability, aggression, red eyes, formation of cysts and nodules), and the Spleen and Stomach (nausea, acid regurgitation, belching, poor appetite, vomiting, abdominal bloating and irregular defecation). In veterinary medicine, qi disorders can develop from psychological stress, prevention of normal species behavior, lack of regular exercise, inappropriate diet, trauma, chronic drug therapy, exogenous pathogen invasion, qi deficiency, and blood stagnation. Qi disorders can also develop in animals that are constitutionally predisposed (Wood animal).

Qi disorders are generally characterized by deficiency (qi deficiency) or excess (qi stagnation and reversed qi flow). These conditions may occur independently or concurrently. Qi deficiency is treated with qi-tonifying formulas (*see* Chapter 8: Tonic Formulas). Qi stagnation is smoothed with qi-moving formulas. Reversed flow of qi is corrected with qi-descending formulas. If the qi disorder is characterized by both qi stagnation and reversed qi flow, then qi-moving and qi-descending formulas must be prescribed together. Similarly, in animals with underlying qi deficiency, the use of qi-regulating formulas should be accompanied by qi-tonifying herbs and/or formulas to prevent further loss of qi. Addressing only one of these aspects will aggravate the other, so treatment must take into account both conditions and balance tonification and movement of qi. Herbs that regulate qi are warming, bitter, and acrid; these qualities are what cause qi to disperse and move outwards, and most of these herbs enter the channels of the Spleen, Stomach, Liver, and Lung. Qi and yin are easily injured by the acrid, dry, and warm nature of these formulas, and they should be discontinued as soon as the clinical signs resolve.

SUBCATEGORIES OF ACTION

Qi-regulating formulas are divided into two subcategories: 1) qi-moving and 2) qi-descending formulas.

1. Qi-Moving Formulas

These formulas activate qi circulation and disperse qi stagnation. Qi stagnation usually does not occur as an isolated condition or disorder. Qi stagnation is usually accompanied by stagnation of

Chapter 12 — Overview

blood, phlegm, food, and other substances. Furthermore, qi stagnation in one organ may affect the normal functioning of another organ. Therefore, many qi-moving formulas are designed to treat qi stagnation with these complications. Qi stagnation is often seen in Spleen/Stomach and Liver syndromes.

Spleen and Stomach qi stagnation result in epigastric and abdominal clinical signs such as: distention and fullness, low appetite, nausea, vomiting, acid regurgitation, hiccups, belching, and constipation. Herbs commonly used to move Spleen and Stomach qi include *Chen Pi* (Pericarpium Citri Reticulatae), *Hou Po* (Cortex Magnoliae Officinalis), *Mu Xiang* (Radix Aucklandiae), *Zhi Shi* (Fructus Aurantii Immaturus), and *Sha Ren* (Fructus Amomi). Representative formulas for these purposes include *Yue Ju Wan* (Escape Restraint Pill) and *Hou Po Wen Zhong Tang* (Magnolia Bark Decoction for Warming the Middle).

Liver qi stagnation results in one or more disorders in the three *jiaos*: chest and hypochondriac distention, irritability, aggression, red eyes, and abdominal bloating. Herbs commonly used to soothe Liver qi and unblock stagnation include *Xiang Fu* (Rhizoma Cyperi), *Wu Yao* (Radix Linderae), *Chuan Lian Zi* (Fructus Toosendan), *Qing Pi* (Pericarpium Citri Reticulatae Viride), and *Yu Jin* (Radix Curcumae). Representative formulas that move Liver qi include *Ban Xia Hou Po Tang* (Pinellia and Magnolia Bark Decoction) and *Ju He Wan* (Tangerine Seed Pill).

2. **Qi-Descending Formulas**

These formulas are designed to direct reversed flow of qi downward, which often occurs as a result of stagnation or obstruction (such as qi stagnation or phlegm obstruction). The Lung and Stomach are most likely to be affected by reversed qi flow.

Reversed flow of Lung qi leads to coughing, wheezing, shortness of breath, and dyspnea. Herbs that help direct Lung qi downward include *Zi Su Zi* (Fructus Perillae), *Ku Xing Ren* (Semen Armeniacae Amarum), *Zi Wan* (Radix et Rhizoma Asteris), and *Hou Po* (Cortex Magnoliae Officinalis). Exemplar formulas include *Su Zi Jiang Qi Tang* (Perilla Fruit Decoction for Directing Qi Downward) and *Ding Chuan Tang* (Arrest Wheezing Decoction).

Reversed flow of Stomach qi may lead to acid regurgitation, nausea, vomiting, and hiccups. Herbs that redirect Stomach qi include *Xuan Fu Hua* (Flos Inulae), *Ban Xia* (Rhizoma Pinelliae), *Chen Pi* (Pericarpium Citri Reticulatae), *Ding Xiang* (Flos Caryophylli), *Zhe Shi* (Haematitum), *Shi Di* (Calyx Kaki), and *Zhu Ru* (Caulis Bambusae in Taenia). One exemplar formula is *Ju Pi Zhu Ru Tang* (Tangerine Peel and Bamboo Shaving Decoction).

CAUTIONS/CONTRAINDICATIONS

- Deficiency conditions, such as qi deficiency, must not be treated with qi-regulating herbs, which will further consume and injure the qi. These conditions must be treated with qi-tonifying herbs.
- Excess conditions, such as qi stagnation or reversed flow of qi, must not be treated with qi-tonifying formulas, which will only cause more stagnation. These conditions must be treated with qi-regulating herbs.
- Qi-regulating formulas often include acrid, drying, and aromatic herbs that consume qi and injure body fluids; thus, excessive or prolonged use is not recommended, especially in geriatric animals and those with yin-deficient fire or qi deficiency.

PHARMACOLOGICAL EFFECTS & CLINICAL APPLICATIONS

Qi-regulating formulas are divided into two subcategories based on differing traditional therapeutic actions: qi-moving and qi-descending. These subcategories of formulas appropriately have contrasting pharmacological effects and clinical applications.

1. From a traditional Chinese medicine perspective, **qi-moving formulas** activate qi circulation and disperse qi stagnation to treat Spleen/Stomach and Liver imbalances. From a biomedical perspective, these formulas treat gastrointestinal disorders, emotional disorders, and globus hystericus.

Chapter 12 — Overview

- **Gastrointestinal disorders**: Qi-moving formulas treat gastrointestinal disorders, such as peptic ulcer disease,[1,2] enteritis,[3] and swallowing disorders.[4,5] Exemplar formulas include *Yue Ju Wan* (Escape Restraint Pill), *Jin Ling Zi San* (Melia Toosendan Powder), and *Ban Xia Hou Po Tang* (Pinellia and Magnolia Bark Decoction).
- **Emotional disorders**: Qi-moving formulas have been used successfully in the treatment of various mental and psychiatric disorders, including but not limited to depression,[6] schizophrenia,[7]neurosis,[8] hysteria,[9] stress and depression,[10] panic disorder,[11] and *dian kuang* (mania and withdrawal).[12] Exemplar formulas include *Yue Ju Wan* (Escape Restraint Pill) and *Ban Xia Hou Po Tang* (Pinellia and Magnolia Bark Decoction).
- **Globus hystericus**: Known as *mei he qi* (plum-pit *qi*) in traditional Chinese medicine, this is a condition characterized by the feeling that there is a foreign substance obstructing the throat and which cannot be expectorated or swallowed. Globus hystericus, and related conditions such as pharyngeal paraesthesia and swallowing disorders, can be treated effectively with formulas such as *Yue Ju Wan* (Escape Restraint Pill) and *Ban Xia Hou Po Tang* (Pinellia and Magnolia Bark Decoction).[13,14,15]

2. **Qi-descending formulas** are designed to direct reversed flow of Lung or Stomach qi downward. From allopathic medical perspectives, these formulas treat respiratory and gastrointestinal disorders, and globus hystericus.
   - **Respiratory disorders**: Many of these formulas exert marked influence on the respiratory tract. Pharmacological effects include antitussive,[16,17] antiallergic,[18] and antiasthmatic.[19] Clinically, these formulas have been successfully used to treat cough and wheezing,[20] asthma,[21,22] bronchopneumonia,[23] and bronchial asthma.[24] Exemplar formulas include *Su Zi Jiang Qi Tang* (Perilla Fruit Decoction for Directing Qi Downward), *Ding Chuan Tang* (Arrest Wheezing Decoction), and *Si Mo Tang* (Four Milled-Herbs Decoction).
   - **Gastrointestinal disorders**: Clinical applications of qi-descending formulas include nausea and vomiting,[25,26,27] morning sickness,[28,29] peptic ulcer disease,[30] and gastritis.[31] Exemplar formulas include *Su Zi Jiang Qi Tang* (Perilla Fruit Decoction for Directing Qi Downward), *Xuan Fu Dai Zhe Shi Tang* (Inula and Hematite Decoction), and *Ding Xiang Shi Di Tang* (Clove and Persimmon Calyx Decoction).
   - **Globus hystericus**: Qi-descending formulas also treat globus hystericus. Specifically, *Su Zi Jiang Qi Tang* (Perilla Fruit Decoction for Directing Qi Downward) treats *mei he qi* (plum-pit *qi*),[32] and *Xuan Fu Dai Zhe Shi Tang* (Inula and Hematite Decoction) is used for pharyngeal neurosis.[33]

References

1. *Hu Nan Zhong Yi Za Zhi* (Hunan Journal of Chinese Medicine), 1989; 5(1):9.
2. *Shi Yong Zhong Yi Yao Za Zhi* (Journal of Practical Chinese Medicine and Medicinals), 1995; 6:15.
3. *Fu Jian Zhong Yi Yao* (Fujian Chinese Medicine and Herbology), 1984; 4:54.
4. Iwasaki K, Wang Q,. Nakagawa T, Suzuki T, Sasaki H. The traditional Chinese Medicine *Banxia Houpo Tang* improves swallowing reflex. Phytomedicine. 6(2):103-6, 1999 May.
5. Iwasaki K, Wang Q, Seki H, Satoh K, Takeda A, Arai H, Sasaki H. The effects of the traditional chinese medicine, "Banxia Houpo Tang (Hange-Koboku To)" on the swallowing reflex in Parkinson's disease. Department of Geriatric Medicine, Tohoku University School of Medicine, Sendai, Japan. Phytomedicine. 7(4):259-63, 2000 Jul.
6. *Zhong Yi Fang Ji Xian Dai Yan Jiu* (Modern Study of Medical Formulas in Traditional Chinese Medicine), 1997; 922-923.
7. *Jiang Su Zhong Yi* (Jiangsu Chinese Medicine), 1994; 2:35.
8. *Si Chuan Zhong Yi* (Sichuan Chinese Medicine), 1986; 4(5):18..
9. *Guo Wai Yi Xue Zhong Yi Zhong Yao Fen Ce* (Monograph of Chinese Herbology from Foreign Medicine), 1985; 4:41
10. Naito T, Itoh H, Takeyama M. Some gastrointestinal function regulatory Kampo medicines have modulatory effects on human plasma adrenocorticotropic hormone and cortisol levels with continual stress exposure. Biological & Pharmaceutical Bulletin. 26(1):101-4, 2003 Jan.
11. Mantani N, Hisanaga A, Kogure T, Kita T, Shimada Y, Terasawa K. Four cases of panic disorder successfully treated with Kampo (Japanese herbal) medicines: Kami-shoyo-san and Hange-koboku-to. Psychiatry & Clinical Neurosciences. 56(6):617-20, 2002 Dec.
12. *Jiang Xi Zhong Yi Yao* (Jiangxi Chinese Medicine and Herbology), 1989; 20(4):34.

Chapter 12 — Overview

13. *Zhong Guo Zhong Xi Yi Jie He Za Zhi* (Chinese Journal of Integrative Chinese and Western Medicine), 1993; 3:11.
14. *Yun Nan Zhong Yi Za Zhi* (Yunan Journal of Chinese Medicine), 1992; 13(5):16.
15. *Zhe Jiang Zhong Yi Za Zhi* (Zhejiang Journal of Chinese Medicine), 1983; 8:345.
16. *Zhong Yao Yao Li Yu Lin Chuang* (Pharmacology and Clinical Applications of Chinese Herbs), 1992; 8(5):13.
17. *Zhong Cheng Yao Yan Jiu* (Research of Chinese Patent Medicine), 1986; 11:27.
18. Kao ST, Chang CH, Chen YS, Chiang SY, Lin JG. Effects of Ding-Chuan-Tang on bronchoconstriction and airway leucocyte infiltration in sensitized guinea pigs. Immunopharmacol Immunotoxicol. 2004 Feb; 26(1):113-24.
19. *Zhe Jiang Zhong Yi Za Zhi* (Zhejiang Journal of Chinese Medicine), 1989; 24(3):123.
20. *Zhong Yi Za Zhi* (Journal of Chinese Medicine), 1964; 10:32.
21. *Hu Bei Zhong Yi Za Zhi* (Hubei Journal of Chinese Medicine), 1997; 19(2):17.
22. *Zhe Jiang Zhong Yi Za Zhi* (Zhejiang Journal of Chinese Medicine), 1987; 22(1):508.
23. *Jiang Xi Zhong Yi Yao* (Jiangxi Chinese Medicine and Herbology), 1992; 23(1):28.
24. *Xin Yi Xue* (New Medicine), 1972; 9:14.
25. *Zhong Yi Yao Yan Jiu* (Research of Chinese Medicine and Herbology), 1995; 2:31.
26. *Hei Long Jiang Zhong Yi Yao* (Heilongjiang Chinese Medicine and Herbology), 1991; 3:19.
27. *Xin Zhong Yi* (New Chinese Medicine), 1995; 7:48.
28. *Xin Jiang Zhong Yi Yao* (Xinjiang Chinese Medicine and Herbology), 1995; 4:20.
29. *Tian Jin Zhong Yi* (Tianjin Chinese Medicine), 1989; 3:5.
30. *Liao Ning Zhong Yi Za Zhi* (Liaoning Journal of Chinese Medicine), 1991; 18(1):20.
31. *Shi Yong Zhong Xi Yi Jie He Za Zhi* (Practical Journal of Integrated Chinese and Western Medicines), 1990; 3(31):152.
32. *Si Chuan Zhong Yi* (Sichuan Chinese Medicine), 1984; 2(1):46.
33. *Shang Hai Zhong Yi Yao Za Zhi* (Shanghai Journal of Chinese Medicine and Herbology), 1984; 4:18.

Section 1

行气剂
— Qi-Moving Formulas

Yuè Jú Wán (Escape Restraint Pill)
越鞠丸

Pinyin Name: *Yue Ju Wan*
Literal Name: Escape Restraint Pill
Alternate Names: *Yue Chu Wan* (Stagnation-Relieving Pill), *Xiong Zhu Wan* (Cyperus and Atractylodes Pill), Ligusticum Chuanxiong and Atractylodes Pill, Cyperus and Atractylodes Combination
Original Source: *Dan Xi Xin Fa* (Teachings of [Zhu] Dan-Xi) by Zhu Zhen-Heng in 1481

COMPOSITION

Xiang Fu (Rhizoma Cyperi)	[6g]
Chuan Xiong (Rhizoma Chuanxiong)	[6g]
Zhi Zi (Fructus Gardeniae)	[6g]
Cang Zhu (Rhizoma Atractylodis)	[6g]
Shen Qu (Massa Fermentata)	[6g]

DOSAGE / PREPARATION / ADMINISTRATION

The source text instructions are to grind equal amounts of the ingredients into powder and form into pills with water. The pills should resemble *Lu Dou* (Semen Phaseoli Radiati) in size. Take 6-9g of pills with warm water. Today, this formula may be prepared as a decoction with the doses suggested in brackets above.

CHINESE THERAPEUTIC ACTIONS

Regulates qi and relieves constraint

CLINICAL MANIFESTATIONS

Qi stagnation: distention and oppression in the chest and diaphragm, epigastric and abdominal bloating and pain, acid regurgitation, indigestion, nausea, vomiting, and belching with a fetid odor.

VETERINARY CLINICAL APPLICATIONS

Chronic vomiting, bilious vomiting, food stagnation, acid regurgitation, indigestion, gastric ulcer, infertility, infectious hepatitis, cholecystitis, and cholelithiasis.

EXPLANATION

Yue Ju Wan (Escape Restraint Pill) treats mild to moderate cases of constraint, in which qi stagnation has led to other complications, such as stagnation of blood, phlegm, heat, dampness, and food. If the qi is stagnant in the chest and abdomen, it will not be able to ascend or descend freely; consequently, chest distention and oppression, as well as abdominal bloating and pain, may occur. Qi stagnation of the Spleen and Stomach may lead to indigestion and reversed flow of Stomach qi, with clinical signs such as acid regurgitation, nausea, and vomiting.

Since the underlying cause of these clinical signs is qi stagnation, the primary focus of treatment is to relieve this stagnation. This formula uses *Xiang Fu* (Rhizoma Cyperi) to activate qi circulation and relieve qi stagnation. *Chuan Xiong* (Rhizoma Chuanxiong) activates blood circulation to dispel blood stagnation. *Zhi Zi* (Fructus Gardeniae) clears heat and sedates fire. *Cang Zhu* (Rhizoma Atractylodis) dries dampness to clear damp and phlegm stagnation. *Shen Qu* (Massa Fermentata) promotes digestion and clears food stagnation.

This formula emphasizes the relief of qi stagnation. Once the qi can circulate smoothly, other stagnations will be resolved. However, if there are any complications or changes in the condition, select additional herbs and adjust the doses accordingly.

Yuè Jú Wán (Escape Restraint Pill)

Yue Ju Wan (Escape Restraint Pill)

Diagnosis	Clinical Signs	Treatment	Herbs
Qi stagnation	• Chest distention and/or oppression and abdominal bloating and/or pain: qi stagnation in the chest and abdomen • Acid regurgitation, nausea and vomiting: reversed flow of Stomach qi due to qi stagnation	Regulates qi and relieves constraint	• *Xiang Fu* (Rhizoma Cyperi) activates qi circulation and relieves qi stagnation. • *Chuan Xiong* (Rhizoma Chuanxiong) activates blood circulation to dispel blood stagnation. • *Zhi Zi* (Fructus Gardeniae) clears heat and sedates fire. • *Cang Zhu* (Rhizoma Atractylodis) dries dampness to clear phlegm stagnation. • *Shen Qu* (Massa Fermentata) promotes digestion and clears food stagnation.

VETERINARY MODIFICATIONS

- For severe qi stagnation, bloating, distention, and sighing, add *Mu Xiang* (Radix Aucklandiae), *Zhi Qiao* (Fructus Aurantii), and *Hou Po* (Cortex Magnoliae Officinalis); or combine with *Xiao Yao San* (Rambling Powder).
- When there is severe blood stagnation, add *Tao Ren* (Semen Persicae), *Hong Hua* (Flos Carthami), and *Chi Shao* (Radix Paeoniae Rubra); or combine with *Xue Fu Zhu Yu Tang* (Drive Out Stasis in the Mansion of Blood Decoction).
- With more dampness, add *Fu Ling* (Poria) and *Ze Xie* (Rhizoma Alismatis).
- With more phlegm, add *Ban Xia* (Rhizoma Pinelliae) and *Gua Lou* (Fructus Trichosanthis).
- With more food stagnation, add *Mai Ya* (Fructus Hordei Germinatus) and *Shan Zha* (Fructus Crataegi); or combine with *Bao He Wan* (Preserve Harmony Pill).
- With more fire, add *Huang Qin* (Radix Scutellariae) and *Huang Lian* (Rhizoma Coptidis).

CAUTIONS / CONTRAINDICATIONS

Yue Ju Wan is contraindicated in cases of generalized weakness and qi deficiency with abdominal bloating, loose stools, and lack of appetite.

HUMAN CLINICAL STUDIES AND RESEARCH

1. **Psychiatric disorders**: According to various reports, *Yue Ju Wan* has been used successfully to treat various psychiatric disorders, such as depression, schizophrenia, and neurosis. According to one study, use of *Yue Ju Wan* was associated with 94.4% effectiveness in treating 72 patients with psychiatric disorders. The treatment protocol was to administer 6g of this formula in pills, twice daily. For those who did not respond to initial treatment, the herbs were given in decoction, and the formulation was modified as follows: with more dampness, *Fu Ling* (Poria) and *Bai Zhi* (Radix Angelicae Dahuricae) were added; for more fire, *Qing Dai* (Indigo Naturalis) was added; for more phlegm, *Ban Xia* (Rhizoma Pinelliae) and *Dan Nan Xing* (Arisaema cum Bile) were added; for more blood stagnation, *Tao Ren* (Semen Persicae) and *Hong Hua* (Flos Carthami) were added; for more qi stagnation, *Mu Xiang* (Radix Aucklandiae) and *Bing Lang* (Semen Arecae) were added; and for more food stagnation, *Shan Zha* (Fructus Crataegi) and *Sha Ren* (Fructus Amomi) were added. Of 72 patients, the study reported complete recovery in 51 cases, improvement in 17 cases, and no benefit in 4 cases.[1,2,3]
2. **Peptic ulcer disease**: Use of modified *Yue Ju Wan* achieved an 88% rate of effectiveness in treating gastric and duodenal ulcers. The herbal formula contained *Cang Zhu* (Rhizoma Atractylodis) 10g, *Xiang Fu* (Rhizoma Cyperi) 10g, *Chuan Xiong* (Rhizoma Chuanxiong) 10g, dry-fried *Zhi Zi* (Fructus Gardeniae) 10g, *Chai Hu* (Radix Bupleuri) 10g, *Shen Qu* (Massa Fermentata) 15g, *Bai Shao* (Radix Paeoniae Alba) 20g, *Ying Su Ke* (Pericarpium Papaveris) 6g, and others as needed. The treatment protocols include giving the herbs in decoction daily, for 20 days per course of treatment, for 3 courses total (with a resting period of 5 days between courses). Of 50 patients, the study reported complete recovery in 19 cases, improvement in 25 cases, and no effect in 6 cases.[4]

SUGGESTED ACUPUNCTURE TREATMENT

1. Points: *Neiguan* (PC 6), *Shanzhong* (CV 17), *Ligou* (LR 5), *Yinlingquan* (SP 9), *Yanglingquan* (GB 34), *Housanli* (ST 36), *Zulinqi* (GB 41), *Taichong* (LR 3), *Quchi* (LI 11), and *Xiawan* (CV 10)
2. Technique: even method.

Neiguan (PC 6) smoothes qi flow in the three *jiaos* and breaks down qi stagnation in the chest. *Shanzhong* (CV 17) regulates qi flow in the chest and relieves chest congestion. *Ligou* (LR 5), the *luo* (connecting) point of the Liver

Yuè Jú Wán (Escape Restraint Pill)

channel, regulates the Liver to smooth qi and blood flow. *Yinlingquan* (SP 9) dissolves dampness to strengthen the Spleen, *Yanglingquan* (GB 34) and *Housanli* (ST 36) regulate Stomach qi, and *Zulinqi* (GB 41) and *Taichong* (LR 3) regulate Liver qi and resolve Liver qi stagnation. *Quchi* (LI 11) sedates heat, and *Xiawan* (CV 10) dissolves food stagnation.

AUTHORS' COMMENTS

Yue Ju Wan is the representative formula for treating the six stagnations of qi, blood, phlegm, food, dampness and fire. In this syndrome, qi stagnation is the primary condition, while stagnations of blood, phlegm, food, dampness and fire are secondary. "越鞠 *Yue ju*," which figuratively means "to escape from restraint" or "to overcome an obstacle," refers to the ability of this formula to help the body overcome restrained qi. Once the qi flows smoothly, other stagnations will slowly be resolved.

Yue Ju Wan contains five herbs to treat six stagnations: *Xiang Fu* (Rhizoma Cyperi) activates qi circulation, *Chuan Xiong* (Rhizoma Chuanxiong) invigorates blood circulation; *Zhi Zi* (Fructus Gardeniae) clears fire; *Cang Zhu* (Rhizoma Atractylodis) dries dampness; and *Shen Qu* (Massa Fermentata) eliminates food stagnation. Since the phlegm is formed secondary to the stagnations of qi, blood, dampness and food, the phlegm will also be resolved when the other stagnations are eliminated. However, for more acute or severe conditions, herbs that transform phlegm may be added, such as *Ban Xia* (Rhizoma Pinelliae).

In veterinary medicine, this formula is used to treat conditions of the gastrointestinal tract characterized by poor appetite, belching, nausea, vomiting, food stagnation and indigestion. Animals for which the use of this formula is appropriate have a purple to red tongue with a greasy, white or yellow coating and a rapid, slippery to wiry pulse. Horses, which are commonly of Wood constitution, are very prone to qi stagnation and, as equine practitioners are all too familiar with, prone to gastrointestinal distress. *Yue Ju Wan* and *Xiao Yao San* (Rambling Powder) are both commonly used in equine practice. *Xiao Yao San* (Rambling Powder) is employed when Liver qi stagnation is at the forefront, causing patterns such as stomach ulcers, and *Yue Ju Wan* is used when the Liver may not be the primary culprit, and stagnation may be present in both yin and yang organs, or even the *San Jiao*. Clinical signs may include chronic bloating and colic, flank or girth pain, irritability, and other signs of stagnation.

In humans, *Yue Ju Wan* is commonly prescribed for depression with accompanying signs of indigestion. Animals that become withdrawn and uninterested in social play and/or work and have signs of indigestion, inappetence, or abdominal discomfort may also benefit from this formula.

References

1. *Zhong Yi Fang Ji Xian Dai Yan Jiu* (Modern Study of Medical Formulas in Traditional Chinese Medicine), 1997; 922-923.
2. *Jiang Su Zhong Yi* (Jiangsu Chinese Medicine), 1994; 2:35.
3. *Si Chuan Zhong Yi* (Sichuan Chinese Medicine), 1986; 4(5):18.
4. *Hu Nan Zhong Yi Za Zhi* (Hunan Journal of Chinese Medicine), 1989; 5(1):9.

Bàn Xià Hòu Pò Tāng (Pinellia and Magnolia Bark Decoction)

半夏厚樸湯
半夏厚朴汤

Pinyin Name: *Ban Xia Hou Po Tang*

Literal Name: Pinellia and Magnolia Bark Decoction

Alternate Names: *Pan Hsia Hou Pu Tang, Ban Xia Hou Pu Tang*, Pinellia and Magnolia Decoction, Pinellia and Magnolia Combination

Original Source: *Jin Gui Yao Lue* (Essentials from the Golden Cabinet) by Zhang Zhong-Jing in the Eastern Han Dynasty

COMPOSITION

Ban Xia (Rhizoma Pinelliae)	1 cup [12g]
Hou Po (Cortex Magnoliae Officinalis)	9g
Fu Ling (Poria)	12g
Sheng Jiang (Rhizoma Zingiberis Recens)	15g [9g]
Zi Su Ye (Folium Perillae)	6g

DOSAGE / PREPARATION / ADMINISTRATION

The source text states to cook the ingredients in 7 cups [1,400 mL] of water and reduce it to 4 cups [800 mL]. Take the warm, strained decoction in four equally divided doses, three times during the day and one time at night. Today, the decoction may be prepared using the doses suggested in brackets.

CHINESE THERAPEUTIC ACTIONS

1. Activates qi and disperses stagnation
2. Directs reversed flow of qi downward
3. Dissolves phlegm and resolves nodules

CLINICAL MANIFESTATIONS

Mei he qi (plum-pit *qi*): a sensation that a foreign object (such as a plum pit) is stuck in the throat and cannot be spit out or swallowed, difficulty in swallowing food, coughing, gagging, vomiting, a moist, greasy tongue, and a wiry or slippery pulse.

VETERINARY CLINICAL APPLICATIONS

Behavioral disorders characterized by anxiety, hyperactivity, nervousness and fearfulness; tracheitis, bronchitis, vomiting, and tracheal and laryngeal cancer.

EXPLANATION

Mei he qi (plum-pit *qi*) is a condition in which there is a feeling of having a foreign substance (such as a plum pit) obstructing the throat, and that this substance cannot be expectorated or swallowed. Since there is no physical obstruction, the feeling cannot be relieved by expectorating or swallowing. This condition usually begins with the formation of Liver qi stagnation caused by emotional disturbances. As Liver qi stagnates, it also interferes with the qi flow in the Lung and Stomach. As a result of qi stagnation, body fluids accumulate and eventually lead to phlegm obstruction. This condition of qi stagnation and phlegm obstruction affects various parts of the body, including the throat (in humans it causes a feeling that there

***Ban Xia Hou Po Tang* (Pinellia and Magnolia Bark Decoction)**

Diagnosis	Clinical Signs	Treatment	Herbs
Mei he qi (plum-pit *qi*)	• A feeling that there is a foreign substance obstructing the throat and causing hard swallowing or gagging: qi stagnation and phlegm obstruction • Coughing, and chest and hypochondriac fullness: phlegm accumulation in the Lung • Vomiting: phlegm accumulation in the Stomach	• Activates qi and disperses stagnation • Directs the reversed flow of qi downward • Dissolves phlegm	• *Ban Xia* (Rhizoma Pinelliae) dissolves and disperses phlegm and restores the descending function of the Stomach. • *Hou Po* (Cortex Magnoliae Officinalis) activates qi to clear phlegm obstruction, and reverses ascending Lung and Stomach qi. • *Fu Ling* (Poria) eliminates dampness and phlegm through diuresis. • *Sheng Jiang* (Rhizoma Zingiberis Recens) harmonizes the Stomach. • *Zi Su Ye* (Folium Perillae) regulates Lung qi flow and smoothes Liver qi circulation.

Bàn Xià Hòu Pò Tāng (Pinellia and Magnolia Bark Decoction)

is a foreign object stuck in the throat), Lung (coughing and fullness of the chest and hypochondrium), and Stomach (vomiting). In animals, the feeling of something lodged in the throat causes frequent, hard swallowing and gagging up of white phlegm.

Ban Xia Hou Po Tang (Pinellia and Magnolia Bark Decoction) contains *Ban Xia* (Rhizoma Pinelliae) as the chief herb to dissolve and disperse phlegm, and restore the descending function of the Stomach to relieve vomiting. *Hou Po* (Cortex Magnoliae Officinalis) activates qi to help *Ban Xia* (Rhizoma Pinelliae) clear the phlegm obstruction; it also directs the reversed flow of Lung and Stomach qi downward to relieve fullness, coughing and vomiting. *Fu Ling* (Poria) helps *Ban Xia* (Rhizoma Pinelliae) eliminate dampness and phlegm through diuresis. *Sheng Jiang* (Rhizoma Zingiberis Recens) disperses stagnation, harmonizes the Stomach, and relieves vomiting. Aromatic *Zi Su Ye* (Folium Perillae) regulates the Lung qi flow and smoothes Liver qi.

VETERINARY MODIFICATIONS

- With more phlegm and saliva with gagging up of white phlegm, add *Chen Pi* (Pericarpium Citri Reticulatae) and *Gan Cao* (Radix et Rhizoma Glycyrrhizae).
- When there is cough and dyspnea, add *Bei Mu* (Bulbus Fritillariae) and *Ku Xing Ren* (Semen Armeniacae Amarum).
- When the qi stagnation is severe, add *Xiang Fu* (Rhizoma Cyperi), *Yu Jin* (Radix Curcumae); or *Chai Hu Shu Gan Tang* (Bupleurum Decoction to Spread the Liver).
- With throat spasms and heavy swallowing, add *Zhi Shi* (Fructus Aurantii Immaturus) and *Jie Geng* (Radix Platycodonis).
- With deficiency and cold of the Stomach, add *Wu Zhu Yu* (Fructus Evodiae).
- With red eyes, anxiety and irritability due to Liver qi stagnation, add *Chai Hu* (Radix Bupleuri), *Yu Jin* (Radix Curcumae), *Xiang Fu* (Rhizoma Cyperi), and *Qing Pi* (Pericarpium Citri Reticulatae Viride).

CAUTIONS / CONTRAINDICATIONS

- *Ban Xia Hou Po Tang* is not suitable for yin-deficient patients with a red tongue and no tongue coating because many herbs in this formula are acrid, bitter, warm, and drying.
- Animals with internal heat due to qi stagnation should not be given this formula.

PHARMACOLOGICAL EFFECTS

1. **Sedative**: Administration of this formula in rats at 4 g/kg/day for 6 days was associated with a reduction of spontaneous physical activities. The effect was more obvious in a dark environment, and less in a bright one. The sedative effect lasted for approximately 2 days upon discontinuation of the herbal therapy. Another report states that the use of this formula at 2-4 g/kg prolonged sleeping time induced by phenobarbitals.[1]
2. **Antiallergic**: According to one report, use of *Ban Xia Hou Po Tang* was effective in treating contact dermatitis in mice.[2]
3. **Effect on the throat**: *Ban Xia Hou Po Tang* has been used with great success to treat various disorders of the throat, such as *mei he qi* (plum-pit *qi*), a hoarse voice, swallowing reflex, and others. The mechanism of this effect was attributed to stimulation of neuropeptidergic nerves locally.[3]
4. **Anxiolytic**: According to one study, administration of *Ban Xia Hou Po Tang* was associated with a marked anxiolytic effect in mice. The effect was attributed to the component honokiol from *Hou Po* (Cortex Magnoliae Officinalis), because administration of the formula without *Hou Po* did not have any anxiolytic effect.[4]

HUMAN CLINICAL STUDIES AND RESEARCH

1. ***Mei he qi*** (plum-pit *qi*): Administration of *Ban Xia Hou Po Tang* plus *Wu Zhu Yu* (Fructus Evodiae) and *Huang Lian* (Rhizoma Coptidis) in 74 patients with plum-pit *qi* was associated with complete recovery in 9 cases, improvement in 24 cases, and no effect in 41 cases.[5]
2. **Pharyngeal paraesthesia**: Use of modified *Ban Xia Hou Po Tang* was effective in treating pharyngeal paraesthesia. In addition to *Ban Xia Hou Po Tang* as the base formula, modifications were made by adding *Xiang Fu* (Rhizoma Cyperi), *Chen Pi* (Pericarpium Citri Reticulatae), and *Gua Lou* (Fructus Trichosanthis) for individuals with emotional stress and instability with a feeling of fullness and distention in the chest and hypochondrium; and *Huang Qi* (Radix Astragali), *Sha Shen* (Radix Glehniae seu Adenophorae), *Huang Lian* (Rhizoma Coptidis), *Huang Qin* (Radix Scutellariae), *Da Zao* (Fructus Jujubae), and *Mu Dan Pi* (Cortex Moutan) for individuals with qi and yin deficiencies due to chronic illness with fatigue, lack of energy, irritability, and insomnia. Of 34 patients, the study reported complete recovery in 8 cases, significant improvement in 20 cases, moderate improvement in 4 cases, and no effect in 2 cases. The overall effectiveness was 84.1%.[6]
3. **Swallowing disorder in aspiration pneumonia**: One study evaluated the therapeutic effect of *Ban Xia Hou Po Tang* for treatment of depressed swallowing reflex in patients with aspiration pneumonia. Of 32 geriatric patients (mean age 74.2 +/- 1.7 years), 24 were treated with herbs (7.5 g/day) and 12 with placebo. After 4 weeks

of treatment, the herb group responded much better than the placebo group, using various measurements of swallowing reflex. The researchers suggested that *Ban Xia Hou Po Tang* improves the impaired swallowing reflex and may help to prevent aspiration pneumonia in the elderly.[7]

4. **Enteritis**: One study reported good results using *Ban Xia Hou Po Tang* plus *Ping Wei San* (Calm the Stomach Powder) to treat acute enteritis. The herbal formula contained *Zi Su Geng* (Caulis Perillae) 6g, *Ban Xia* (Rhizoma Pinelliae) 6g, *Hou Po* (Cortex Magnoliae Officinalis) 4-6g, *Cang Zhu* (Rhizoma Atractylodis) 4-6g, *Fu Ling* (Poria) 9g, and *Gan Cao* (Radix et Rhizoma Glycyrrhizae) 3g. Of 129 patients, the study reported complete recovery in 81 cases, significant improvement in 42 cases, and improvement in 6 cases.[8]
5. ***Dian kuang* (mania and withdrawal)**: One study reported good results using modified *Ban Xia Hou Po Tang* to treat 21 patients with *dian kuang* (mania and withdrawal). The herbal formula contained *Ban Xia* (Rhizoma Pinelliae) 10g, *Hou Po* (Cortex Magnoliae Officinalis) 10g, *Fu Ling* (Poria) 10g, *Zi Su Geng* (Caulis Perillae) 7g, *Zhen Zhu Mu* (Concha Margaritiferae) 10g, *He Huan Pi* (Cortex Albiziae) 10g, *Jiu Jie Chang Pu* (Rhizoma Anemones Altaicae) 10g, *Dan Zhu Ye* (Herba Lophatheri) 5g, *Lian Zi Xin* (Plumula Nelumbinis) 10g, and others as needed. The duration of treatment ranged from 10 to 45 days. The study reported recovery in 19 of 21 cases, with 2 cases needing chlorpromazine as addition therapy.[9]
6. **Hysteria**: One study reported successful treatment in 103 of 104 patients with hysteria characterized by phlegm stagnation using modified *Ban Xia Hou Po Tang*. The duration of treatment ranged from 5-27 days. During follow-up visits 7 years later, the study reported stabilization in 91 of 94 who returned.[10]
7. **Stress and depression**: One study evaluated the clinical usefulness of herbal formulas for the treatment of stress and depression by examining the modulatory effects of the herbs on the hypothalamo-pituitary-adrenal axis and autonomic nervous function. Of several formulas tested, three were found to be effective in lowering plasma ACTH and cortisol levels under stress. The study stated that the modulatory effects of these formulas might be beneficial in treating stress-related diseases. Three formulas found to be effective were *Liu Jun Zi Tang* (Six-Gentlemen Decoction), *Ban Xia Xie Xin Tang* (Pinellia Decoction to Drain the Epigastrium), and *Ban Xia Hou Po Tang*.[11]
8. **Panic disorder**: Four patients diagnosed with panic disorder with agoraphobia in accordance with the Diagnostic and Statistical Manual of Mental Disorders (DSM) criteria were successfully treated with herbal medicine. Two patients were treated with *Ban Xia Hou Po Tang*, and two with *Jia Wei Xiao Yao San* (Augmented Rambling Powder). Both formulas successfully relieved panic attacks, anticipatory anxiety, and agoraphobia. The study concluded that these formulas may be useful as additional or alternative treatments for panic disorder.[12]

SUGGESTED ACUPUNCTURE TREATMENT

1. Points: *Taichong* (LR 3), *Shanzhong* (CV 17), *Fenglong* (ST 40), and *Shenmen* (HT 7).
2. Techniques: both tonification and sedation.

Taichong (LR 3), the *yuan* (source) point of the Liver channel, is combined with *Shanzhong* (CV 17) to smooth Liver qi and break up stagnation in the chest. *Fenglong* (ST 40) regulates qi flow to dissolve phlegm. *Shenmen* (HT 7) calms the *shen* (spirit) to tranquilize the mind.

AUTHORS' COMMENTS

Ban Xia Hou Po Tang can be used to treat behavioral disorders, acute vomiting with phlegm, and tracheal tumors (osteochondroma) and laryngeal tumors (lymphosarcoma). Treatment of these conditions require the addition of single herbs and/or formulas.

- For behavioral disorder with anxiety, restlessness and insomnia, combine with *Gan Mai Da Zao Tang* (Licorice, Wheat, and Jujube Decoction).
- For acute gastroenteritis and vomiting, combine with *Ping Wei San* (Calm the Stomach Powder).
- To help dissolve phlegm and reduce laryngeal and tracheal tumors, combine with *Xue Fu Zhu Yu Tang* (Drive Out Stasis in the Mansion of Blood Decoction).
- For throat pain secondary to cancer, add *Xuan Shen* (Radix Scrophulariae), *Jie Geng* (Radix Platycodonis), *Chuan Lian Zi* (Fructus Toosendan), and *Yan Hu Suo* (Rhizoma Corydalis).

References

1. *Zhong Yi Fang Ji Xian Dai Yan Jiu* (Modern Study of Medical Formulas in Traditional Chinese Medicine), 1997; 934.
2. *Guo Wai Yi Xue Zhong Yi Zhong Yao Fen Ce* (Monograph of Chinese Herbology from Foreign Medicine), 1982; 6:46.
3. Naito T, Itoh H, Takeyama M. Effects of Hange-koboku-to (Banxia-houpo-tang) on neuropeptide levels in human plasma and saliva. Biol Pharm Bull. 2003 Nov; 26(11):1609-13.
4. Kuribara H, Kishi E, Hattori N, Okada M, Maruyama Y. The anxiolytic effect of two oriental herbal drugs in Japan attributed to honokiol from magnolia bark. J Pharm Pharmacol. 2000 Nov; 52(11):1425-9.
5. *Zhe Jiang Zhong Yi Za Zhi* (Zhejiang Journal of Chinese Medicine), 1983; 8:345.
6. *Zhong Guo Zhong Xi Yi Jie He Za Zhi* (Chinese Journal of Integrative Chinese and Western Medicine), 1993; 3:11.
7. Iwasaki K, Wang Q, Nakagawa T, Suzuki T, Sasaki H. The traditional Chinese medicine banxia houpo tang improves swallowing reflex. Phytomedicine. 1999 May; 6(2):103-6.

8. *Fu Jian Zhong Yi Yao* (Fujian Chinese Medicine and Herbology), 1984; 4:54.
9. *Jiang Xi Zhong Yi Yao* (Jiangxi Chinese Medicine and Herbology), 1989; 20(4):34.
10. *Guo Wai Yi Xue Zhong Yi Zhong Yao Fen Ce* (Monograph of Chinese Herbology from Foreign Medicine), 1985; 4:41.
11. Naito T, Itoh H, Takeyama M. Some gastrointestinal function regulatory Kampo medicines have modulatory effects on human plasma adrenocorticotropic hormone and cortisol levels with continual stress exposure. Biological & Pharmaceutical Bulletin. 2003 Jan; 26(1):101-4.
12. Mantani N, Hisanaga A, Kogure T, Kita T, Shimada Y, Terasawa K. Four cases of panic disorder successfully treated with Kampo (Japanese herbal) medicines: Kami-shoyo-san and Hange-koboku-to. Psychiatry & Clinical Neurosciences. 2002 Dec; 56(6):617-20.

Hòu Pò Wēn Zhōng Tāng

(Magnolia Bark Decoction for Warming the Middle)

厚樸溫中湯

厚朴温中汤

Pinyin Name: *Hou Po Wen Zhong Tang*

Literal Name: Magnolia Bark Decoction for Warming the Middle

Alternate Name: Magnolia Combination

Original Source: *Nei Wai Shang Bian Huo Lun* (Clarifying Doubts about Injury from Internal and External Causes) by Li Gao in 1247

COMPOSITION

Hou Po (Cortex Magnoliae Officinalis), *zhi* (prepared) with ginger	30g
Chen Pi (Pericarpium Citri Reticulatae)	30g
Mu Xiang (Radix Aucklandiae)	15g
Cao Dou Kou (Semen Alpiniae Katsumadai)	15g
Gan Jiang (Rhizoma Zingiberis)	2.1g
Fu Ling (Poria)	15g
Zhi Gan Cao (Radix et Rhizoma Glycyrrhizae Praeparata cum Melle)	15g

DOSAGE / PREPARATION / ADMINISTRATION

The source text recommends grinding the ingredients into a coarse powder. Cook 15g of the powder and 3 slices of *Sheng Jiang* (Rhizoma Zingiberis Recens) in 2 large bowls of water until it is reduced to one bowl. Take the warm, strained decoction before meals.

CHINESE THERAPEUTIC ACTIONS

1. Warms the middle *jiao* and activates qi circulation
2. Dries dampness and relieves abdominal fullness

CLINICAL MANIFESTATIONS

Damp-cold affecting the Spleen and Stomach: epigastric and abdominal bloating and/or pain, low appetite, belching, acid regurgitation, weakness of the extremities, diarrhea, lethargy, a swollen, pale purple tongue with a sticky, white coating, and a deep, slippery pulse.

VETERINARY CLINICAL APPLICATIONS

Poor appetite, chronic gastritis, chronic vomiting, chronic colitis, inflammatory bowel syndrome, and vaginal discharge.

Hòu Pò Wēn Zhōng Tāng

(Magnolia Bark Decoction for Warming the Middle)

EXPLANATION

Hou Po Wen Zhong Tang (Magnolia Bark Decoction for Warming the Middle) treats various clinical signs caused by damp-cold in the Spleen and Stomach. Dampness has a greasy and sticky character, while cold is constricting and stagnating by nature. When combined, these two factors slow the circulation of qi and disrupt the ascending and descending functions of the Spleen and Stomach. As a result, abdominal fullness and pain, poor appetite, and lethargy manifest.

This formula contains *Hou Po* (Cortex Magnoliae Officinalis) to activate qi, dry dampness, and reduce distention and fullness. *Chen Pi* (Pericarpium Citri Reticulatae) and *Mu Xiang* (Radix Aucklandiae) activate qi and relieve pain. *Cao Dou Kou* (Semen Alpiniae Katsumadai) warms the middle *jiao*, dispels cold, dries dampness, and eliminates phlegm. *Gan Jiang* (Rhizoma Zingiberis) and *Sheng Jiang* (Rhizoma Zingiberis Recens) warm the Spleen and Stomach to dispel cold. *Fu Ling* (Poria) and *Zhi Gan Cao* (Radix et Rhizoma Glycyrrhizae Praeparata cum Melle) dispel dampness and strengthen the middle *jiao*.

Because the emphasis of this formula is on warming the middle *jiao*, it is also effective in treating nausea, vomiting, and epigastric pain resulting from cold invading the Stomach.

VETERINARY MODIFICATIONS

- With abdominal pain and diarrhea, add *Cang Zhu* (Rhizoma Atractylodis) and *Sha Ren* (Fructus Amomi).
- With nausea and vomiting of clear watery vomitus, add *Ban Xia* (Rhizoma Pinelliae) and *Bai Zhu* (Rhizoma Atractylodis Macrocephalae).
- For food stagnation, add *Shan Zha* (Fructus Crataegi) and *Shen Qu* (Massa Fermentata).
- When accompanied by a cold body and extremities due to deficiency and cold, add *Fu Zi* (Radix Aconiti Lateralis Praeparata) and *Rou Gui* (Cortex Cinnamomi).
- With edema and a feeling of heaviness in the body, add *Da Fu Pi* (Pericarpium Arecae).
- If there is severe pain, add *Rou Gui* (Cortex Cinnamomi) and *Gao Liang Jiang* (Rhizoma Alpiniae Officinarum).

CAUTIONS / CONTRAINDICATIONS

Avoid cold and raw foods while taking *Hou Po Wen Zhong Tang*.

SUGGESTED ACUPUNCTURE TREATMENT

1. Points: *Zhongwan* (CV 12), *Housanli* (ST 36), *Daheng* (SP 15), *Gongsun* (SP 4), and *Yinlingquan* (SP 9).
2. Techniques: sedation and moxibustion.

Zhongwan (CV 12) is the *mu* (collecting) point of the Stomach, while *Housanli* (ST 36) is the *he* (uniting) point of the Stomach. The combination of these two points smoothes Stomach qi and relieves chest and abdominal congestion. *Daheng* (SP 15) and *Gongsun* (SP 4) strengthen the Spleen to relieve stagnation. *Yinlingquan* (SP 9) strengthens the Spleen by drying dampness. Moxibustion on select points warms the body and dries dampness.

***Hou Po Wen Zhong Tang* (Magnolia Bark Decoction for Warming the Middle)**

Diagnosis	Clinical Signs	Treatment	Herbs
Damp-cold affecting the Spleen and Stomach	• Epigastric and abdominal bloating or pain, a swollen, pale purple tongue with a sticky, white coating, and a deep, slippery pulse: damp-cold in the Spleen and Stomach • Low appetite and lethargy: damp-cold accumulation affecting digestive functions	• Warms the middle *jiao* and activates qi circulation • Dries dampness and relieves abdominal fullness	• *Hou Po* (Cortex Magnoliae Officinalis) activates qi, dries dampness, and reduces distention and fullness. • *Chen Pi* (Pericarpium Citri Reticulatae) and *Mu Xiang* (Radix Aucklandiae) activate qi and relieve pain. • *Cao Dou Kou* (Semen Alpiniae Katsumadai) warms the middle *jiao*, dispels cold, dries dampness, and eliminates phlegm. • *Gan Jiang* (Rhizoma Zingiberis) and *Sheng Jiang* (Rhizoma Zingiberis Recens) warm the Spleen and Stomach to dispel cold. • *Fu Ling* (Poria) and *Zhi Gan Cao* (Radix et Rhizoma Glycyrrhizae Praeparata cum Melle) dispel dampness and strengthen the middle *jiao*.

Hòu Pò Wēn Zhōng Tāng

(Magnolia Bark Decoction for Warming the Middle)

AUTHORS' COMMENTS

Hou Po Wen Zhong Tang focuses on warming the middle *jiao*, dispelling cold, and drying dampness. This formula treats disruption of the qi mechanism of the Spleen and Stomach secondary to damp-cold invasion. Damp-cold impairs the ascending and descending functions of these organs, which results in abdominal bloating and clinical signs of lethargy, poor appetite, belching, weak limbs, vomiting of clear fluid, and loose stools. This condition can develop from feeding a cold, raw food diet to juvenile or geriatric animals, from antibiotic use, and following gastrointestinal surgery. Many cases of equine Cushing's disease exhibit signs that correlate to damp and cold accumulation in the middle *jiao* arising from Kidney yang deficiency. *Hou Po Wen Zhong Tang* can be used to supplement these patients specifically for the clinical signs of anorexia and bloating. It can also treat inflammatory bowel syndrome in geriatric animals with abdominal bloating and pain, a swollen, pale purple tongue with a white coating, and a deep, slippery pulse. The key clinical sign for the use of this formula is abdominal bloating accompanied by the presence of cold signs.

Section 2

降气剂 — Qi-Descending Formulas

Sū Zǐ Jiàng Qì Tāng

(Perilla Fruit Decoction for Directing Qi Downward)

蘇子降氣湯

苏子降气汤

Pinyin Name: *Su Zi Jiang Qi Tang*
Literal Name: Perilla Fruit Decoction for Directing Qi Downward
Alternate Names: *Su Tzu Chiang Chi Tang, Su Zi Jiang Chi Tang*, Perilla Seed Decoction, Perilla Seed Combination
Original Source: *Tai Ping Hui Min He Ji Ju Fang* (Imperial Grace Formulary of the Tai Ping Era) by the Imperial Medical Department in 1078-85

COMPOSITION

Zi Su Zi (Fructus Perillae)	75g [9g]
Ban Xia (Rhizoma Pinelliae), *xi* (washed) with liquid 7 times	75g [9g]
Hou Po (Cortex Magnoliae Officinalis), *chao* (dry-fried) with ginger juice	30g [6g]
Qian Hu (Radix Peucedani)	30g [6g]
Rou Gui (Cortex Cinnamomi)	45g [3g]
Dang Gui (Radix Angelicae Sinensis)	45g [6g]
Gan Cao (Radix et Rhizoma Glycyrrhizae)	60g [6g]

DOSAGE / PREPARATION / ADMINISTRATION

The source text recommends grinding the ingredients into a fine powder. Cook 6g of the powder with 2 slices of *Sheng Jiang* (Rhizoma Zingiberis Recens), 1 piece of *Da Zao* (Fructus Jujubae), and 5 leaves [2g] of *Zi Su Ye* (Folium Perillae) in 1.5 large bowls of water until the liquid is reduced to 80% (1.2 large bowls). Take the hot, strained liquid any time during the day. Today, this formula may be prepared as a decoction with the doses suggested in brackets.

CHINESE THERAPEUTIC ACTIONS

1. Directs Lung qi downward to relieve wheezing
2. Eliminates phlegm and stops coughing

CLINICAL MANIFESTATIONS

Upper excess with lower deficiency syndrome: abundant phlegm and watery sputum; wheezing, coughing, shortness of breath, dyspnea, abnormal respiration that is more pronounced on exhalation than inhalation, fullness of the chest and diaphragm; possibly a sore back and weak legs, and, in severe cases, edema of the limbs may be present; a pale tongue and a weak, slippery or wiry pulse.

VETERINARY CLINICAL APPLICATIONS

Feline bronchial asthma, chronic bronchitis, equine RAO (recurrent airway obstruction), bronchiectasis, and pulmonary emphysema.

EXPLANATION

Su Zi Jiang Qi Tang (Perilla Fruit Decoction for Directing Qi Downward) is indicated for respiratory problems characterized by upper excess and lower deficiency. Upper excess refers to phlegm accumulation in the Lung, affecting the flow of Lung qi and causing fullness and oppression in the chest and diaphragm. Lower deficiency refers to deficiency of Kidney yang. Under normal conditions, the Kidney assists Lung qi to descend. However, when Kidney yang is deficient, the Lung qi may no longer be able to descend properly, and wheezing or shortness

Sū Zǐ Jiàng Qì Tāng

(Perilla Fruit Decoction for Directing Qi Downward)

***Su Zi Jiang Qi Tang* (Perilla Fruit Decoction for Directing Qi Downward)**

Diagnosis	Clinical Signs	Treatment	Herbs
Upper-excess, lower-deficiency syndrome	• Phlegm and sputum, wheezing, coughing, shortness of breath, dyspnea, and chest and hypochondriac fullness and oppression: phlegm accumulation [excess] in the Lung [upper] • Back soreness, lassitude, and weakness and edema of the lower extremities: yang deficiency of the Kidney [lower]	• Directs Lung qi downward to relieve wheezing • Eliminates phlegm and stops coughing	• *Zi Su Zi* (Fructus Perillae) directs Lung qi downward, eliminates phlegm, and relieves coughing and wheezing. • *Ban Xia* (Rhizoma Pinelliae), *Hou Po* (Cortex Magnoliae Officinalis), and *Qian Hu* (Radix Peucedani) eliminate phlegm and relieve coughing and wheezing. • *Rou Gui* (Cortex Cinnamomi) warms Kidney yang to grasp qi downwards. • *Dang Gui* (Radix Angelicae Sinensis) nourishes the blood to balance the acrid and drying herbs. • *Sheng Jiang* (Rhizoma Zingiberis Recens) and *Zi Su Ye* (Folium Perillae) disperse cold and ventilate the Lung. • *Gan Cao* (Radix et Rhizoma Glycyrrhizae) and *Da Zao* (Fructus Jujubae) harmonize the herbs.

of breath may occur. Clinically, inhalation will be shorter than exhalation. Also, Kidney deficiency may result in back pain and leg weakness. Moreover, edema may occur because Kidney yang is no longer able to regulate the water metabolism, leaving the fluids to accumulate and form edema in the extremities, especially the lower limbs.

To treat upper excess, the reversed qi flow must be corrected, and phlegm must be eliminated. To treat lower deficiency, Kidney yang must be reinforced. The chief herb of this formula, *Zi Su Zi* (Fructus Perillae), directs Lung qi downward, eliminates phlegm, and relieves coughing and wheezing. *Ban Xia* (Rhizoma Pinelliae), *Hou Po* (Cortex Magnoliae Officinalis), and *Qian Hu* (Radix Peucedani) eliminate phlegm and relieve coughing and wheezing. Together, these four herbs treat the "upper excess." *Rou Gui* (Cortex Cinnamomi) warms Kidney yang to treat the "lower deficiency." By warming and tonifying the Kidney, *Rou Gui* (Cortex Cinnamomi) enables the Kidney to grasp qi, pull it downward and facilitate inhalation. *Dang Gui* (Radix Angelicae Sinensis) nourishes the blood to balance the acrid and drying herbs. *Sheng Jiang* (Rhizoma Zingiberis Recens) and *Zi Su Ye* (Folium Perillae) disperse cold and ventilate the Lung. *Gan Cao* (Radix et Rhizoma Glycyrrhizae) and *Da Zao* (Fructus Jujubae) harmonize the formula.

VETERINARY MODIFICATIONS

- For qi deficiency, add *Ren Shen* (Radix et Rhizoma Ginseng) and *Wu Wei Zi* (Fructus Schisandrae Chinensis).
- For deficiency and cold, add *Huang Qi* (Radix Astragali) and increase the dose of *Rou Gui* (Cortex Cinnamomi).
- With cough and dyspnea due to reversed flow of qi, add *Chen Xiang* (Lignum Aquilariae Resinatum).
- With cough and dyspnea due to wind-cold, add *Ding Chuan Tang* (Arrest Wheezing Decoction).
- When there is nausea, add *Zhe Shi* (Haematitum).
- With nausea, vomiting, and drooling of saliva, add *Fu Ling* (Poria) and *Jie Geng* (Radix Platycodonis).
- With chest and epigastric fullness and oppression, add *Huang Qin* (Radix Scutellariae) and *Chai Hu* (Radix Bupleuri).

CAUTIONS / CONTRAINDICATIONS

- *Su Zi Jiang Qi Tang* is warm and drying, and is mainly used to reverse the flow of Lung qi and eliminate dampness and phlegm. It is not suitable for coughing or wheezing due to Lung deficiency; likewise, it is not suitable for wheezing due to heat and phlegm accumulation in the Lung.
- This formula is contraindicated in animals with yin-deficient heat.
- Animals that take this formula should avoid exposure to cold and wind, and should not be fed raw, cold, oily and greasy foods.[1]

PHARMACOLOGICAL EFFECTS

Respiratory: According to one study, administration of *Su Zi Jiang Qi Tang* in mice was associated with marked antitussive, antiasthmatic, and anti-inflammatory effects.[2]

12 QI-REGULATING FORMULAS

Sū Zǐ Jiàng Qì Tāng

(Perilla Fruit Decoction for Directing Qi Downward)

HUMAN CLINICAL STUDIES AND RESEARCH

Cough and wheezing: One study reported marked success using *Su Zi Jiang Qi Tang* to treat various respiratory disorders, such as bronchial asthma, chronic bronchitis, pulmonary emphysema, and others.[3]

SUGGESTED ACUPUNCTURE TREATMENT

1. Points: *Pishu* (BL 20), *Feishu* (BL 13), *Chize* (LU 5), *Lieque* (LU 7), *Fenglong* (ST 40), *Shanzhong* (CV 17), *Dingchuan*, *Shenshu* (BL 23), and *Taixi* (KI 3).
2. Techniques: tonification and sedation.

Because the Spleen produces phlegm and the Lung stores phlegm, *Pishu* (BL 20) and *Feishu* (BL 13) are used to tonify the Spleen and Lung to stop the production and eliminate the storage of phlegm. *Chize* (LU 5) and *Lieque* (LU 7) sedate the Lung to correct the reversed flow of Lung qi. *Fenglong* (ST 40) dissolves phlegm. *Shanzhong* (CV 17) and *Dingchuan*, a classical point, regulate qi flow in the chest. *Shenshu* (BL 23) and *Taixi* (KI 3) tonify the Kidney to strengthen its qi-descending function.

AUTHORS' COMMENTS

Phlegm accumulation and bronchoconstriction with obstruction of Lung qi flow are primary features of feline bronchial asthma. Chronic asthma can lead to irreversible airway disease and the development of pulmonary emphysema. Phlegm accumulation in the Lung commonly results from feeding inappropriate diets to cats. Commercial cat foods, especially dry kibbled foods, contain high levels of carbohydrates in the form of grains, notably corn, wheat, and soybean that are inappropriate for this species. Cats are obligatory carnivores and have minimal ability to process diets high in carbohydrates. Many commercial feline diets also contain additives, dyes and preservatives that are detrimental to the Spleen and Stomach functions. Feline diets that contain high levels of carbohydrates, dyes and/or preservatives weaken Spleen function, resulting in heat and dampness that eventually turn into phlegm. This phlegm is then stored in the Lung. According to the *Huang Di Nei Jing* (Yellow Emperor's Inner Classic), the Kidney (the root of prenatal life) and the Spleen (the root of postnatal life) mutually support and protect each other; when one is weak, the other will soon be weakened also. Appropriate food therapy is essential for the successful treatment of asthma in cats in addition to herbal medications and acupuncture.

Cats that are born with poor Kidney *jing* (essence) [genetics] are predisposed to the development of Kidney qi and yang deficiencies early in life (1-2 years of age). This is particularly true of purebred cats. Kidney qi and yang are required for normal Lung function and water metabolism. A lack of Kidney qi and yang results in the inability of the Kidney to grasp or root the Lung qi (manifesting as cough and dyspnea) and to transform water (manifesting as edema). This combination of disease factors can lead to the condition for which this formula is intended: "upper excess and lower deficiency."

It is important to remember that the primary focus of *Su Zi Jiang Qi Tang* is to treat upper excess or phlegm (which is treated with four herbs), and the secondary focus is on treating lower deficiency or Kidney qi-yang (which is addressed with only one herb.) For cats or dogs with moderate to severe Kidney qi and yang deficiencies and an inability of the Kidney to grasp the qi and transform water, it is recommended that this formula be combined with other herbs or formulas to warm and tonify Kidney qi and yang. This formula should not be used in cats with yin-deficient heat because of its warm, acrid and drying nature.

Dong Chong Xia Cao (Cordyceps) is used to treat Lung and Kidney deficiencies and comes in granular extract form that can be mixed into cat food. It can be combined with *Su Zi Jiang Qi Tang* to improve clinical results. It can also be used for treating feline asthma in cats that refuse acupuncture and herbal therapy. The vast majority of cats will reject food with herbal medication added to it. However, *Dong Chong Xia Cao* (Cordyceps) has a pleasant odor and mild taste and is accepted when mixed in food by many finicky cats as the sole treatment for their asthma or allergic bronchitis. Herbal medication, acupuncture and Chinese veterinary food therapy can be successfully used to control and resolve asthma in young purebred animals (especially Persian and Siamese cats one to two years of age). The recommended dose is 3 grams daily, initially divided into morning and evening meals and adjusted over time, depending on the response.

In combination with feeding a species-appropriate diet, the successful treatment of feline asthma lies in the ability to differentiate excess (typically seen in acute attacks) from deficiency (typically chronic) disease, and determine whether heat or cold predominates. During periods of remission in which there are no acute signs, the focus of the treatment should be on addressing the root of the disorder by nourishing the Lung, Spleen and Kidney as needed. During acute attacks, the focus of the treatment should be on eliminating the branch (pathogenic factors of wind, cold, heat, phlegm. etc) and ventilating the Lung

Sū Zǐ Jiàng Qì Tāng

(Perilla Fruit Decoction for Directing Qi Downward)

to control respiratory distress. For animals that are weak, geriatric or chronically debilitated, treatment will need to address both the root and the branch simultaneously.

There are many formulas that can be used in the treatment of feline asthma. They make up two major categories: formulas that release the exterior (Chapter 1) and that regulate qi (Chapter 12). Below are some general guidelines that may be helpful in choosing the appropriate formula. These guidelines are used in conjunction with tongue and pulse evaluation:

- *Su Zi Jiang Qi Tang* is used to treat mixed excess and deficiency, manifesting as phlegm above and Kidney deficiency below. It is commonly used as a transitional formula following an acute attack and then switched to a formula that treats the root disorder. As this formula does not contain *Ma Huang* (Herba Ephedrae), it can be used for a longer period time than the other formulas.
- For acute asthma attack due to wind-heat, use *Ma Huang Xing Ren Gan Cao Shi Gao Tang* (Ephedra, Apricot Kernel, Licorice, and Gypsum Decoction). This formula treats excess heat from an exogenous pathogen that invades the Lung, causing stagnation of qi and the development of fever and phlegm.
- For acute asthma attack brought on by wind-cold, use *Xiao Qing Long Tang* (Minor Bluegreen Dragon Decoction). This formula treats the exterior and the interior at the same time. It simultaneously releases the exterior and clears phlegm caused by wind-cold invasion. It is contraindicated in heat conditions.
- For cats that have chronic asthma and suffer an acute attack from invasion of wind-cold with pre-existing phlegm-heat in the Lung, use *Ding Chuan Tang* (Arrest Wheezing Decoction). This formula is unique in that it can treat hot phlegm in the Lung in the face of wind-cold. The heat signs predominate in these cases, and the signs of wind-cold are typically mild (nasal congestion, sneezing and aversion to cold). *Ding Chuan Tang* is the best formula for treating animals that contract wind-cold with pre-existing hot phlegm in the Lung, which the exterior constriction abruptly makes worse.
- In general, cats are notoriously difficult to medicate. Furthermore, cats as a species are sensitive to *Ma Huang* (Herba Ephedrae), and the administration of formulas that contain this herb is even more challenging. In the authors' experience, the use of teapills has been very successful in both short- and long-term use, and the dosage can easily be adjusted. In addition, teapills are less potent than concentrated granular formulations, and are safe to begin therapy, especially in acute asthma cases when the use of *Ma Huang* (Herba Ephedrae) is essential for good clinical results.

References

1. *Zhong Yao Ming Fang Yao Li Yu Ying Yong* (Pharmacology and Applications of Famous Herbal Formulas), 1989; 406-407.
2. *Zhong Yao Yao Li Yu Lin Chuang* (Pharmacology and Clinical Applications of Chinese Herbs), 1992; 8(5):13.
3. *Zhong Yi Za Zhi* (Journal of Chinese Medicine), 1964; 10:32.

Dìng Chuǎn Tāng (Arrest Wheezing Decoction)

定喘湯
定喘汤

Pinyin Name: *Ding Chuan Tang*
Literal Name: Arrest Wheezing Decoction
Alternate Names: *Ting Chuen Tang, Din Chuan Tang*, Asthma-Stopping Decoction, Asthma-Relieving Decoction, Mahuang and Ginkgo Combination
Original Source: *She Sheng Zhong Miao Fang* (Marvelous Formulas for the Health of Multitudes) by Zhang Shi-Che in 1550

COMPOSITION

Ma Huang (Herba Ephedrae)	9g
Bai Guo (Semen Ginkgo), *zha* (crushed) and *chao* (dry-fried) till yellow	21 kernels [9g]
Zi Su Zi (Fructus Perillae)	6g
Ku Xing Ren (Semen Armeniacae Amarum)	4.5g [9g]
Ban Xia (Rhizoma Pinelliae)	9g
Kuan Dong Hua (Flos Farfarae)	9g
Sang Bai Pi (Cortex Mori)	9g
Huang Qin (Radix Scutellariae)	4.5g [6g]
Gan Cao (Radix et Rhizoma Glycyrrhizae)	3g

DOSAGE / PREPARATION / ADMINISTRATION

The source text recommends decocting the ingredients in three bowls of water until two bowls of liquid remain. Take one bowl of decoction per dose, twice daily at any time during the day. The source text prohibits the use of ginger in the decoction. Today, the decoction may be prepared with the doses suggested in brackets.

CHINESE THERAPEUTIC ACTIONS

1. Ventilates the Lung and directs Lung qi downward
2. Dispels phlegm and relieves wheezing

CLINICAL MANIFESTATIONS

Wind-cold constricting the exterior and phlegm-heat accumulation in the interior: thick, sticky, yellow sputum that is difficult to expectorate, abundant phlegm; tachypnea, coughing, wheezing, dyspnea; a red to purple, greasy tongue and a slippery, rapid pulse.

VETERINARY CLINICAL APPLICATIONS

Feline bronchial asthma, tracheitis, acute and chronic bronchitis, bronchopneumonia and acute exacerbation of chronic low-grade aspiration pneumonia secondary to megaesophagus, and laryngeal paralysis surgery in dogs.

EXPLANATION

Ding Chuan Tang (Arrest Wheezing Decoction) is one of the most commonly used formulas to treat wheezing and dyspnea caused by exterior wind-cold and interior phlegm-heat. Animals suffering from this syndrome

***Ding Chuan Tang* (Arrest Wheezing Decoction)**

Diagnosis	Clinical Signs	Treatment	Herbs
Wind-cold at the exterior and phlegm-heat in the interior	• Abundant phlegm, rapid breathing, and thick, sticky, yellow sputum: phlegm-heat accumulation in the interior • Coughing, wheezing and dyspnea: reversed flow of Lung qi • Red to purple, greasy tongue and a slippery, rapid pulse: phlegm-heat accumulation in the interior	• Ventilates the Lung and redirects Lung qi • Dispels phlegm and relieves wheezing	• *Ma Huang* (Herba Ephedrae) releases the exterior wind-cold factor and ventilates the Lung. • *Bai Guo* (Semen Ginkgo) eliminates phlegm and astringes Lung qi. • *Zi Su Zi* (Fructus Perillae), *Ku Xing Ren* (Semen Armeniacae Amarum), *Ban Xia* (Rhizoma Pinelliae), and *Kuan Dong Hua* (Flos Farfarae) eliminate phlegm and direct the reversed flow of qi downward. • *Sang Bai Pi* (Cortex Mori) and *Huang Qin* (Radix Scutellariae) clear Lung heat. • *Gan Cao* (Radix et Rhizoma Glycyrrhizae) harmonizes the herbs.

Dìng Chuǎn Tāng (Arrest Wheezing Decoction)

usually already have interior phlegm prior to wind-cold attack. When the wind-cold factor attacks the exterior and constricts the Lung, the dispersing and descending functions of the Lung may be further inhibited, causing phlegm stagnation and heat. The tongue coating and pulse both indicate heat and phlegm accumulation in the body.

In this formula, *Ma Huang* (Herba Ephedrae) releases the exterior wind-cold factor and dilates the Lung to relieve wheezing and dyspnea. *Bai Guo* (Semen Ginkgo) eliminates phlegm and astringes Lung qi to relieve wheezing. The astringent effect of *Bai Guo* (Semen Ginkgo) also prevents *Ma Huang* (Herba Ephedrae) from over-venting the Lung and leading to the loss of Lung qi. The dispersing effect of *Ma Huang* (Herba Ephedrae) prevents *Bai Guo* (Semen Ginkgo) from retaining the disease in the body. *Zi Su Zi* (Fructus Perillae), *Ku Xing Ren* (Semen Armeniacae Amarum), *Ban Xia* (Rhizoma Pinelliae), and *Kuan Dong Hua* (Flos Farfarae) eliminate phlegm and direct the reversed flow of qi downward to relieve wheezing and coughing. *Sang Bai Pi* (Cortex Mori) and *Huang Qin* (Radix Scutellariae) clear Lung heat and relieve wheezing and coughing. *Gan Cao* (Radix et Rhizoma Glycyrrhizae) harmonizes the formula.

VETERINARY MODIFICATIONS

- For sputum that is thick and difficult to expectorate, add *Gua Lou* (Fructus Trichosanthis), *Dan Nan Xing* (Arisaema cum Bile), and *Zhe Bei Mu* (Bulbus Fritillariae Thunbergii).
- For wheezing and dyspnea due to excessive phlegm, combine with *Chen Pi* (Pericarpium Citri Reticulata), *Ting Li Zi* (Semen Descurainiae seu Lepidii) and *Wu Wei Zi* (Fructus Schisandrae Chinensis).
- With irritability and thirst, add *Mai Dong* (Radix Ophiopogonis) and *Di Gu Pi* (Cortex Lycii).
- With profuse sputum, add *Fu Hai Shi* (Pumice), *Ju Hong* (Exocarpium Citri Rubrum), and *Gua Lou Pi* (Pericarpium Trichosanthis).
- When there is severe Lung heat with fever, add *Shi Gao* (Gypsum Fibrosum) and *Yu Xing Cao* (Herba Houttuyniae).

CAUTIONS / CONTRAINDICATIONS

- Without appropriate clinical findings, *Ding Chuan Tang* should be used with caution during the very first stage of a wind invasion that manifests in dyspnea without sweating or other signs of wind-cold.
- This formula is contraindicated in chronic wheezing or cough caused by Lung and Kidney yin deficiencies.

PHARMACOLOGICAL EFFECTS

1. **Antiasthmatic**: Intraperitoneal injection of *Ding Chuan Tang* was shown to be effective in relieving asthma. The formula had no antiasthmatic effect when *Bai Guo* (Semen Ginkgo) was removed; but did have a significantly stronger antiasthmatic effect when the dose of *Bai Guo* was doubled. The study concluded that *Bai Guo* is an essential ingredient for this function.[1] The mechanism of its antiasthmatic effect was attributed to the formula's ability to blend histamine and acetylcholine, decrease contraction of external trachea smooth muscle, and promote secretion of phenol red in the respiratory tract.[2] Another study stated that *Ding Chuan Tang* may be used as a prophylactic treatment against allergen-induced asthma and airway inflammation via its bronchodilating influence and its ability to inhibit eosinophils in the airway.[3]
2. **Expectorant**: Intraperitoneal injection of *Ding Chuan Tang* in mice was shown to have a marked expectorant effect.[4]
3. **Antitussive**: According to one study, use of *Ding Chuan Tang* was associated with suppressing cough in mice.[5]

HUMAN CLINICAL STUDIES AND RESEARCH

1. **Asthma**: Modified *Ding Chuan Tang* was effective in treating 36 patients with severe asthma. The herbal treatment contained *Ding Chuan Tang* plus *Dan Nan Xing* (Arisaema cum Bile), *Di Long* (Pheretima), *Yu Xing Cao* (Herba Houttuyniae), *Mian Hua Gen* (Radix Gossypii), *Fang Feng* (Radix Saposhnikoviae), and others. Antibiotic drugs were given in cases of severe infection. Of 36 patients, the study reported complete recovery in 24 cases, marked improvement in 10 cases, and no effect in 2 cases. The rate of effectiveness was 94.5%.[6]
2. **Asthma with bronchitis**: Use of modified *Ding Chuan Tang* showed good results in treating asthma associated with bronchitis in 63 infants (2 years of age or below, with more than 10 days of illness). The formula contained *Ma Huang* (Herba Ephedrae) 3g, *Huang Qin* (Radix Scutellariae) 4g, *Zi Su Zi* (Fructus Perillae) 4g, *Ku Xing Ren* (Semen Armeniacae Amarum) 4g, *Sang Bai Pi* (Cortex Mori) 4g, *Bai Guo* (Semen Ginkgo) 4g, *Ban Xia* (Rhizoma Pinelliae) 4g, *Kuan Dong Hua* (Flos Farfarae) 4g, *She Gan* (Rhizoma Belamcandae) 4g, *Jie Geng* (Radix Platycodonis) 4g, *Ban Lan Gen* (Radix Isatidis) 12g, and *Gan Cao* (Radix et Rhizoma Glycyrrhizae) 2g. [The dose listed is for a 2 year old. Adjust the dose accordingly for infants under 2 years of age.] The herbs were given in decoction twice daily, for 7 days per course of treatment. Of 63 infants, the study reported complete recovery in 59 cases, improvement in 3 cases, and no benefit in 1 case. The rate of effectiveness was 98.4%.[7]

Dìng Chuǎn Tāng (Arrest Wheezing Decoction)

3. **Bronchopneumonia**: Administration of daily decoction of modified *Ding Chuan Tang* was effective in treating 34 patients with bronchopneumonia. The study reported resolution of cough and wheezing after an average of 4.61 days (range of 2.02 to 7.20 days) and complete recovery after 7.88 days (range of 4.66 to 11.70 days).[8]
4. **Bronchial asthma**: One study reported 97% effectiveness using modified *Ding Chuan Tang* to treat 100 patients with chronic bronchial asthma. The herbal formula contained *Ding Chuan Tang* plus *Yu Xing Cao* (Herba Houttuyniae), *Pu Gong Ying* (Herba Taraxaci), and others as needed. The treatment protocol was to administer the herbs in decoction form for 10 days per course of treatment. Of 100 patients, the study reported significant improvement in 83 cases and moderate improvement in 14 cases. The study described *Ding Chuan Tang* to have marked antiasthmatic, antitussive, and expectorant effects.[9]

TOXICOLOGY

According to one acute toxicology study, administration of *Ding Chuan Tang* at 150 g/kg in a bolus dose did not cause any abnormal reaction in dietary habits or physical activities.[10]

SUGGESTED ACUPUNCTURE TREATMENT

1. Point: *Feishu* (BL 13), *Fengmen* (BL 12), *Chize* (LU 5), *Lieque* (LU 7), *Shanzhong* (CV 17), *Fenglong* (ST 40), and *Shaoshang* (LU 11).
2. Techniques: sedation and bleeding.

Feishu (BL 13), *Fengmen* (BL 12), *Chize* (LU 5), and *Lieque* (LU 7) dilate the Lung to relieve coughing and wheezing. *Shanzhong* (CV 17) regulates qi in the chest and reverses rising Lung qi. *Fenglong* (ST 40) dissolves phlegm. *Shaoshang* (LU 11) should be pricked and bled to reduce Lung heat.

AUTHORS' COMMENTS

Ding Chuan Tang can be used for cats that have chronic bronchial asthma with pre-existing phlegm-heat in the Lung and that suffer an acute attack from invasion of wind-cold (abrupt change of weather or acute upper respiratory infection). This formula also has veterinary application in the treatment of chronic bronchitis, and acute exacerbation of chronic aspiration pneumonia secondary to laryngeal paralysis surgery and megaesophagus in dogs. Many of these dogs have chronic low-grade bronchopneumonia with retained phlegm and heat in the Lung. They are exquisitely sensitive to abrupt changes in environmental temperatures and highly susceptible to exterior pathogen invasion. *Ding Chuan Tang* is unique in that it can treat hot phlegm in the Lung in the face of wind-cold signs; the signs of interior heat typically predominate. It is common to add herbs, such as *Yu Xing Cao* (Herba Houttuyniae) and *Pu Gong Ying* (Herba Taraxaci), to this formula to enhance its effects and prevent and treat infection.

The medical history of dogs is important in determining the appropriate use of *Ding Chuan Tang* in these cases. These animals will usually have a pre-existing chronic cough with hard-to-expectorate, thick, yellow mucus and a record of repeated courses of antibiotics and emergency room visits. The dog owner may describe the coughing as choking, gagging or rattling. This formula should be discontinued once the clinical signs resolve, which can generally take 7-10 days. If there are fever and Lung heat present, discontinue this formula and give *Ma Huang Xing Ren Gan Cao Shi Gao Tang* (Ephedra, Apricot Kernel, Licorice, and Gypsum Decoction) and *Yin Qiao San* (Honeysuckle and Forsythia Powder). In moderate to severe acute cases with persistent coughing, gagging and wheezing with copious, yellow phlegm, the inclusion of *Yin Qiao San* is essential for remission of clinical signs to prevent repeated hospitalization, which often results in a decision to euthanize the animal by the owner. During periods of remission, the formula *Yu Ping Feng San* (Jade Windscreen Powder), which tonifies the Lung and *wei qi*, is recommended to help prevent a recurrence.

References

1. *Zhe Jiang Zhong Yi Za Zhi* (Zhejiang Journal of Chinese Medicine), 1989; 24(3):123.
2. Li Z, Li T. Pharmacological study on asthma-relieving decoction (dingchuan tang) treating asthma. Zhong Yao Cai. 1999 Aug; 22(8):411-3.
3. Kao ST, Chang CH, Chen YS, Chiang SY, Lin JG. Effects of Ding-Chuan-Tang on bronchoconstriction and airway leucocyte infiltration in sensitized guinea pigs. Immunopharmacol Immunotoxicol. 2004 Feb; 26(1):113-24.
4. *Zhong Cheng Yao* (Study of Chinese Patent Medicine), 1986; 11:27.
5. *Zhong Cheng Yao Yan Jiu* (Research of Chinese Patent Medicine), 1986; 11:27.
6. *Hu Bei Zhong Yi Za Zhi* (Hubei Journal of Chinese Medicine), 1997; 19(2):17.
7. *Zhe Jiang Zhong Yi Za Zhi* (Zhejiang Journal of Chinese Medicine), 1992; 27(3):109.
8. *Jiang Xi Zhong Yi Yao* (Jiangxi Chinese Medicine and Herbology), 1992; 23(1):28.
9. *Xin Yi Xue* (New Medicine), 1972; 9:14.
10. *Zhe Jiang Zhong Yi Za Zhi* (Zhejiang Journal of Chinese Medicine), 1989; 24(3):123.

Jú Pí Zhú Rú Tāng (Tangerine Peel and Bamboo Shaving Decoction)

橘皮竹茹湯
橘皮竹茹汤

Pinyin Name: *Ju Pi Zhu Ru Tang*
Literal Name: Tangerine Peel and Bamboo Shaving Decoction
Alternate Names: *Chu Pi Tsu Ju Tang, Ju Pi Zu Ru Tang*, Citrus and Bamboo Shaving Decoction, Citrus and Bamboo Combination
Original Source: *Jin Gui Yao Lue* (Essentials from the Golden Cabinet) by Zhang Zhong-Jing in the Eastern Han Dynasty

COMPOSITION

Chen Pi (Pericarpium Citri Reticulatae)	2 cups [12g]
Zhu Ru (Caulis Bambusae in Taenia)	2 cups [12g]
Ren Shen (Radix et Rhizoma Ginseng)	3g [3g]
Sheng Jiang (Rhizoma Zingiberis Recens)	24g [9g]
Da Zao (Fructus Jujubae)	30 pieces [5 pieces]
Gan Cao (Radix et Rhizoma Glycyrrhizae)	15g [6g]

DOSAGE / PREPARATION / ADMINISTRATION

The source text suggests cooking all of the ingredients in 10 cups [2,000 mL] of water until it is reduced to 3 cups [600 mL]. Take 1 cup of the warm decoction three times daily. Today, the decoction may be prepared using the doses suggested in brackets above.

CHINESE THERAPEUTIC ACTIONS

1. Counters reversed flow of qi to relieve vomiting
2. Tonifies qi and harmonizes the middle

CLINICAL MANIFESTATIONS

Reversed flow of Stomach qi due to deficiency and heat: belching, dry heaves, gagging, retching and vomiting.

VETERINARY CLINICAL APPLICATIONS

Nausea and vomiting secondary to surgery, radiation and chemotherapy.

EXPLANATION

Ju Pi Zhu Ru Tang (Tangerine Peel and Bamboo Shaving Decoction) treats belching, dry heaves, retching and vomiting due to deficiency and heat of the Stomach. It contains herbs that tonify Stomach deficiency, clear heat, and correct the reversed flow of Stomach qi.

In this formula, *Chen Pi* (Pericarpium Citri Reticulatae) regulates qi, harmonizes the Stomach, and relieves belching, gagging, vomiting and retching. *Zhu Ru* (Caulis Bambusae in Taenia) clears Stomach heat. *Ren Shen* (Radix et Rhizoma Ginseng) nourishes qi and strengthens the Stomach. Together with *Chen Pi* (Pericarpium Citri Reticulatae), *Ren Shen* (Radix et Rhizoma Ginseng) can tonify qi without causing stagnation. *Sheng Jiang* (Rhizoma Zingiberis Recens) harmonizes the Stomach to stop nausea and vomiting. The warm nature of *Sheng Jiang* (Rhizoma Zingiberis Recens) also balances the cold influence of *Zhu Ru* (Caulis Bambusae in Taenia). *Da Zao* (Fructus Jujubae) and *Gan Cao* (Radix et Rhizoma Glycyrrhizae) help *Ren Shen* (Radix et Rhizoma Ginseng) to tonify qi

Ju Pi Zhu Ru Tang (Tangerine Peel and Bamboo Shaving Decoction)

Diagnosis	Clinical Signs	Treatment	Herbs
Reversed flow of Stomach qi due to deficiency and heat	Belching, nausea, and vomiting: Reversed flow of Stomach qi	• Corrects reversed flow of qi to relieve vomiting • Benefits qi and clears heat	• *Chen Pi* (Pericarpium Citri Reticulatae) regulates qi and harmonizes the Stomach. • *Zhu Ru* (Caulis Bambusae in Taenia) clears Stomach heat. • *Ren Shen* (Radix et Rhizoma Ginseng) nourishes qi and strengthens the Stomach. • *Sheng Jiang* (Rhizoma Zingiberis Recens) harmonizes the Stomach. • *Da Zao* (Fructus Jujubae) and *Gan Cao* (Radix et Rhizoma Glycyrrhizae) tonify qi and harmonize the middle *jiao*.

Jú Pí Zhú Rú Tāng (Tangerine Peel and Bamboo Shaving Decoction)

and harmonize the middle *jiao*. This formula was formulated carefully to benefit qi without creating stagnation and to clear deficiency heat without creating unnecessary cold in the body.

VETERINARY MODIFICATIONS

- For Stomach yin deficiency accompanied by thirst, add *Mai Men Dong Tang* (Ophiopogonis Decoction).
- For Stomach heat and Stomach qi and yin deficiencies, add *Mai Dong* (Radix Ophiopogonis), *Fu Ling* (Poria), *Ban Xia* (Rhizoma Pinelliae), and *Pi Pa Ye* (Folium Eriobotryae).
- When there is Stomach heat but no qi deficiency, add *Shi Di* (Calyx Kaki), and remove *Ren Shen* (Radix et Rhizoma Ginseng), *Gan Cao* (Radix et Rhizoma Glycyrrhizae), and *Da Zao* (Fructus Jujubae).
- For Stomach heat causing Stomach qi reversal, add *Huang Lian* (Rhizoma Coptidis).
- With phlegm, add *Ban Xia* (Rhizoma Pinelliae) and *Fu Ling* (Poria).

CAUTIONS / CONTRAINDICATIONS

Ju Pi Zhu Ru Tang is not suitable for gagging, retching or vomiting due to excess heat or deficiency cold.

CLINICAL STUDIES AND RESEARCH

Erosive esophagitis: One study report 88.2% effectiveness using *Ju Pi Zhu Ru Tang* to treat patients with erosive esophagitis.[1]

HERB-DRUG INTERACTION

Chemotherapy-induced nausea and vomiting: One study reported a beneficial effect using modified *Ju Pi Zhu Ru Tang* to treat nausea and vomiting induced by chemotherapy. The herbal formula contained *Ren Shen* (Radix et Rhizoma Ginseng) 10g, *Dan Zhu Ye* (Herba Lophatheri) 30g, *Chen Pi* (Pericarpium Citri Reticulatae) 10g, *Sheng Jiang* (Rhizoma Zingiberis Recens) 20g, and *Da Zao* (Fructus Jujubae) 30g. The treatment protocol was to cook one pack of herbs in water to obtain 250 mL of decoction, which was administered in six to eight equally divided doses daily. Five packs of herbs were given per course of treatment. Those with severe nausea and vomiting were also given 1g of charred salt to hold in the mouth to help to relieve nausea and vomiting.[2]

SUGGESTED ACUPUNCTURE TREATMENT

1. Points: *Weishu* (BL 21), *Zhongwan* (CV 12), *Shanzhong* (CV 17), *Housanli* (ST 36), *Xiangu* (ST 43), *Geshu* (BL 17), and *Neiguan* (PC 6).
2. Techniques: tonification and sedation.

Weishu (BL 21) and *Zhongwan* (CV 12) are combined according to the *shu* (transport) and *mu* (collecting) principle (combination of back and front points) to nourish Stomach qi. Adding *Shanzhong* (CV 17) helps to direct reversed flow of qi downward. *Housanli* (ST 36) strengthens the Stomach and regulates Stomach qi. Sedate *Xiangu* (ST 43) to clear Stomach heat. *Geshu* (BL 17) corrects the reversed flow of Stomach qi to relieve hiccups and retching, and *Neiguan* (PC 6) regulates the middle *jiao*.

RELATED FORMULA

Jú Pí Zhú Rú Tāng
(Tangerine Peel and Bamboo Shaving Decoction)
橘皮竹茹湯
橘皮竹茹汤
Pinyin Name: *Ju Pi Zhu Ru Tang*
Literal Name: Tangerine Peel and Bamboo Shaving Decoction
Original Source: *Ji Sheng Fang* (Formulas to Aid the Living) by Yan Yong-He in 1253

Chi Fu Ling (Poria Rubra)	30g
Chen Pi (Pericarpium Citri Reticulatae)	30g
Pi Pa Ye (Folium Eriobotryae)	30g
Mai Dong (Radix Ophiopogonis)	30g
Zhu Ru (Caulis Bambusae in Taenia)	30g
Ban Xia (Rhizoma Pinelliae), *xi* (washed) with liquid 7 times	30g
Ren Shen (Radix et Rhizoma Ginseng)	15g
Zhi Gan Cao (Radix et Rhizoma Glycyrrhizae Praeparata cum Melle)	15g

The source text states to grind the herbs into a coarse powder. Cook 12g of the powder and 5 slices of *Sheng Jiang* (Rhizoma Zingiberis Recens) with 1.5 large bowls of water until it is reduced to 80%. Take the warm, strained decoction at any time during the day.

The main actions of this formula are to correct the reversed flow of qi, harmonize the Stomach, and clear heat. The animal may have Stomach heat along with clinical signs such as gagging, vomiting, thirst, and a picky appetite.

This formula has the same name as the previous formula, but is derived from a different source and has a different composition and application. Therefore, it is important that the two are not confused or used interchangeably.

- *Ju Pi Zhu Ru Tang* from *Jin Gui Yao Lue* (Essentials from the Golden Cabinet) is indicated for vomiting due to Stomach heat and accompanied by Stomach qi deficiency.

Jú Pí Zhú Rú Tāng (Tangerine Peel and Bamboo Shaving Decoction)

- *Ju Pi Zhu Ru Tang* from *Ji Sheng Fang* (Formulas to Aid the Living) treats vomiting due to Stomach heat, but accompanied by qi and yin deficiencies.

AUTHORS' COMMENTS

Historically used to treat hiccups in humans, *Ju Pi Zhu Ru Tang* can be used for nausea and vomiting secondary to radiation and chemotherapy in veterinary medicine. It is a mild formula that can be used in older and deficient animals without further damaging qi and yin. It also can be used for nausea, belching and vomiting following abdominal surgery and can be given to horses via nasogastric tube to stimulate appetite and prevent small intestinal ileus.

Hou Po Wen Zhong Tang (Magnolia Bark Decoction for Warming the Middle) and *Ju Pi Zhu Ru Tang* treat gastrointestinal disorders with similar clinical presentations.

- *Hou Po Wen Zhong Tang* treats gastrointestinal disorders that occur as a result of damp-cold.
- *Ju Pi Zhu Ru Tang* treats disorders that are caused by Stomach heat and deficiency.

References

1. *Zhong Yi Yao Xin Xi* (Information on Chinese Medicine and Herbology), 1988; 5:19.
2. *Hei Long Jiang Zhong Yi Yao* (Heilongjiang Chinese Medicine and Herbology), 1991; 3:19.

Chapter 12 — Summary

— Qi-Regulating Formulas

SECTION 1: QI-MOVING FORMULAS

Name	Similarities	Differences
Yue Ju Wan (Escape Restraint Pill)	Regulates qi circulation to relieve constraint	Treats stagnation of qi, blood, phlegm, fire, dampness, and food
Ban Xia Hou Po Tang (Pinellia and Magnolia Bark Decoction)	Activates qi circulation, dissolves phlegm, directs the reversed flow of qi downward	Treats *mei he qi* (plum-pit *qi*) and phlegm stagnation
Hou Po Wen Zhong Tang (Magnolia Bark Decoction for Warming the Middle)	Activates qi circulation, warms the middle *jiao*	Dispels damp-cold in the Spleen and Stomach

Yue Ju Wan (Escape Restraint Pill) treats stagnation of qi, blood, phlegm, fire, dampness, and food. Because qi stagnation is the main cause of all the other stagnations, this formula is placed in the qi-regulating category. Clinical manifestations include abdominal fullness and pain, acid regurgitation, nausea, vomiting, and indigestion.

Ban Xia Hou Po Tang (Pinellia and Magnolia Bark Decoction) activates qi, disperses stagnation, reverses the flow of ascending qi, and dissolves phlegm. In humans, it is used to treat *mei he qi* (plum-pit *qi*). In veterinary medicine, it is used to treat behavioral disorders characterized by anxiety, hyperactivity, nervousness and fearfulness. Additional applications include tracheitis, bronchitis, vomiting, and tracheal and laryngeal cancer.

Hou Po Wen Zhong Tang (Magnolia Bark Decoction for Warming the Middle) mainly treats abdominal bloating and pain due to qi stagnation and damp-cold in the Spleen and Stomach.

Chapter 12 — Summary

SECTION 2: QI-DESCENDING FORMULAS

Name	Similarities	Differences
Su Zi Jiang Qi Tang (Perilla Fruit Decoction for Directing Qi Downward)	Direct the reversed flow of Lung qi downward, relieve cough, wheezing, and dyspnea	Eliminates phlegm, warms the Kidney
Ding Chuan Tang (Arrest Wheezing Decoction)		Releases exterior wind-cold, eliminates interior hot phlegm
Ju Pi Zhu Ru Tang (Tangerine Peel and Bamboo Shaving Decoction)	Directs the reversed flow of Stomach qi downward, relieves nausea and vomiting	Tonifies Stomach qi, clears Stomach heat

Su Zi Jiang Qi Tang (Perilla Fruit Decoction for Directing Qi Downward) is used mainly for upper-excess and lower-deficiency syndrome. In this syndrome, upper excess refers to phlegm accumulation in the Lung, and lower deficiency refers to Kidney yang deficiency. Clinical manifestations include excess phlegm and sputum, wheezing, coughing, shortness of breath, back pain, lethargy, a pale tongue, and a weak, slippery or wiry pulse.

Ding Chuan Tang (Arrest Wheezing Decoction) ventilates the Lung, corrects the reversed flow of qi, relieves wheezing, and clears heat and phlegm. It is used for wheezing caused by wind-cold constricting the exterior and phlegm-heat brewing in the interior. Clinical manifestations include rapid breathing, excess phlegm, thick, yellow sputum, coughing, wheezing, a red to purple, greasy tongue, and a slippery, rapid pulse.

Ju Pi Zhu Ru Tang (Tangerine Peel and Bamboo Shaving Decoction) nourishes qi, clears heat, and redirects Stomach qi to relieve gagging, retching and vomiting. This formula is used for dry heaves, and vomiting and retching due to deficiency and heat of the Stomach.

Chapter 13

— Blood-Regulating Formulas

理血剂

王清任 Wāng Qíng-Rèn

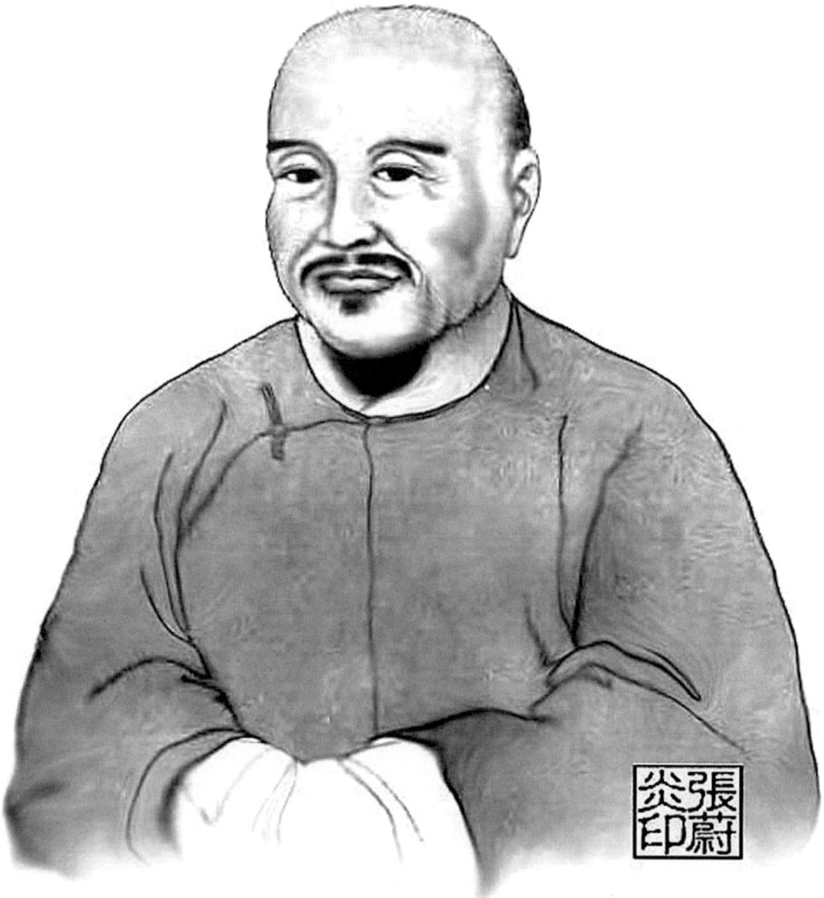

王清任 Wāng Qíng-Rèn, 1768 – 1831.

王清任 Wāng Qīng-Rèn

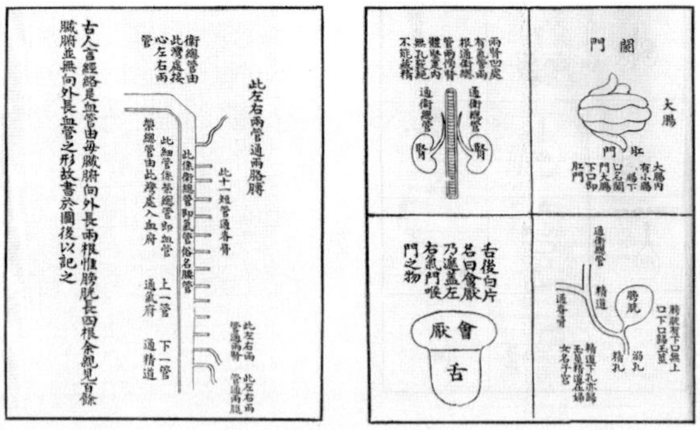

医林改错 *Yi Lin Gai Cuo* (Corrections of Errors Among Physicians) in 1830, with illustrations and explanations of internal organs.

Wang Qing-Ren was born during the Qing dynasty. He grew up studying martial arts, and later pursued the study of traditional Chinese medicine. Because of his martial arts background, he had a good understanding of human anatomy.

Wang suspected many errors in the ancient texts.[1] He was the first person of his era to question traditional wisdom. To confirm his opinions, he personally observed the internal organs of corpses of executed convicts, and the deserted bodies of children who had died from epidemics.[2] After years of observation, Wang published *Yi Lin Gai Cuo* (Corrections of Errors Among Physicians) in 1830. In this text, he drew 25 precise illustrations of human anatomy from different angles and depth. Furthermore, based on his findings, he accurately pointed out many errors among medical texts at the time, such as the presence of the pancreas and diaphragm; corrected the mistaken notion that the liver was in the left hypochondrium; and stated that it is the brain that thinks (not the heart). Wang also said that "treating diseases without knowing the internal organs is like a blind man walking in the dark." Wang was harshly criticized for his boldness, and his works were not recognized for a long time.

Wang parlayed his uncommon understanding of human anatomy to develop the use of blood-moving formulas to treat blood stasis disorders. His outstanding formulas for treatment of blood stasis affecting different parts of the body include:

- *Tong Qiao Huo Xue Tang* (Unblock the Orifices and Invigorate the Blood Decoction)
- *Xue Fu Zhu Yu Tang* (Drive Out Stasis in the Mansion of Blood Decoction)
- *Ge Xia Zhu Yu Tang* (Drive Out Blood Stasis Below the Diaphragm Decoction)
- *Shao Fu Zhu Yu Tang* (Drive Out Blood Stasis in the Lower Abdomen Decoction)
- *Shen Tong Zhu Yu Tang* (Drive Out Blood Stasis from a Painful Body Decoction)
- *Bu Yang Huan Wu Tang* (Tonify the Yang to Restore Five Decoction)

Dynasties & Kingdoms	Year
Xia Dynasty 夏	2100-1600 BCE
Shang Dynasty 商	1600-1100 BCE
Zhou Dynasty 周	1100-221 BCE
Qin Dynasty 秦	221-207 BCE
Han Dynasty 漢	206 BCE-220
Three Kingdoms 三國	220-280
Western Jin Dynasty 西晉	265-316
Eastern Jin Dynasty 東晉	317-420
Northern and Southern Dynasties 北南朝	420-581
Sui Dynasty 隋	581-618
Tang Dynasty 唐	618-907
Five Dynasties 五代	907-960
Song Dynasty 宋	960-1279
Liao Dynasty 遼	916-1125
Jin Dynasty 金	1115-1234
Yuan Dynasty 元	1271-1368
Ming Dynasty 明	1368-1644
Qing Dynasty 清	**1644-1911**
Republic of China 中華民國	1912-Present Day
People's Republic of China 中華人民共和國	1949-Present Day

1. In Chinese culture, it is extremely disrespectful to cut [dissect] the human body, which is considered a gift from heaven. Therefore, ancient Chinese physicians learned human anatomy from illustrations in the *Nei Jing* (Inner Classic), and accepted it as universal truth.
2. Wang claimed in his writing that he only observed, but did not cut or dissect, human bodies. The corpses were deserted bodies of executed convicts or dead children, whose bodies were torn open by wild animals. Therefore, he did not commit any act of disrespect to those dead individuals.

Table of Contents

Chapter 13 — Overview

理血剂 — Blood-Regulating Formulas

Definition: Blood-regulating formulas invigorate blood circulation, remove blood stasis, and/or stop bleeding. They are used to treat blood stagnation and to stop bleeding.

There are two major categories of blood-regulating formulas: 1) blood-invigorating and stasis-removing formulas and 2) stop-bleeding formulas. Blood-invigorating and stasis-removing formulas promote blood circulation to treat disorders arising from impaired flow (stagnation) or obstruction (stasis) of blood in the channels and internal organs; this includes extravasated blood that has accumulated within the body. Blood stagnation and blood stasis represent progressive stages of blood flow impairment. Stop-bleeding formulas treat hemorrhage or spillage of blood. This commonly develops from excess, such as when heat forces blood out of the vessels, as well as deficiencies, such as when qi is too weak to contain the blood or when the vessels are damaged by yin-deficient heat. Both patterns can be externally contracted or internally generated. Herbal formulas to stop bleeding from traumatic injury also have wide application in veterinary medicine.

Blood in Chinese medicine is defined as a fundamental substance that contains *ying* qi (nutritive qi), which continuously circulates in the vessels of the body. *Ying* qi nourishes and moistens the whole body and the *zang fu* organs and is a vital component in the generation of blood. To effectively treat and manage blood disorders, one must keep in mind the intimate relationship between qi and blood. There is an adage: "blood is the mother of qi, and qi is the commander of blood." Because of this close relationship, a disorder of one typically leads to a disorder of the other. Blood circulates throughout the body to provide nourishment (*gu* [food] *qi*) for the functional activities of all the different types of qi in the body. Because *gu qi* is the basic material for the generation of all the qi of the body, production of qi is inseparable from blood. Blood carries qi throughout the body, and is said to be the dwelling place or home of qi. From a clinical perspective, qi loss will follow acute blood loss (blood desertion), and signs of both qi and blood deficiency will be seen. Shock from acute hemorrhage corresponds to the clinical manifestation of acute loss of blood *and* qi in Chinese medicine. According to the *Huang Di Nei Jing* (Yellow Emperor's Inner Classic) in the first or second century A.D., "if blood and qi are not harmonious hundreds of diseases can form."

Qi generates blood, moves the blood, and holds the blood in the vessels. Qi is the motivating force for the generation of blood; all steps in the production of blood require the transforming functions of qi. If qi is deficient, the ability to generate the blood is weak, which is why qi tonic herbs are commonly included in blood tonic formulas. Qi transports blood to the entire body; without qi to propel the blood it is unable to circulate normally and stagnates. This is in accordance with the adage "when qi moves, blood follows, and if qi stagnates, blood congeals." Thus, in the treatment of blood stagnation or stasis, one usually must treat qi stagnation as well. Qi holds the blood within the vessels; without the holding function of qi, blood can escape or leak out. Qi contains the blood in the vessels so it can continuously circulate and provide oxygen and nutrition to the tissues and carry away the byproducts of metabolism. Bleeding disorders develop when qi becomes deficient and unable to hold the blood within the vessels. In cases of life threatening hemorrhage (blood desertion), the qi must be secured.

Chapter 13 — Overview

Blood stagnation and stasis can be caused by deficient or stagnant qi. Qi is said to lead the blood, and without sufficient qi, blood stagnates and congeals. Cold disorders cause constriction that slows and inhibits the free movement of blood, while heat disorders can damage the vessels and cause obstruction of blood flow, as well as force the blood out of the vessels. In addition, acute and chronic traumatic injury, surgery, parturition, cancer, chronic disease, immune-mediated diseases, and cardiovascular disease may also affect the free flow of blood. Specific diseases seen in veterinary medicine, in which blood stagnation and stasis are common, include: diabetes mellitus, intervertebral disk disease, fibrocartilaginous emboli, feline hypertrophic cardiomyopathy, aortic thrombo-embolism, degenerative myelopathy, retained placenta, and polycythemia vera. Phlegm, which is energetically "sticky," often complicates and exacerbates conditions of blood stagnation/stasis. Phlegm and blood stagnation/stasis or entanglement is a major pathology in the development of cancer. From a clinical perspective, blood stagnation and stasis are generally associated with the formation of masses and pain. Clinical signs vary, depending on the etiology and location, and include: unmoving, sharp, stabbing pain unrelieved by warmth and worse with pressure, tumors, cysts, a dark red to purple tongue, and a rapid and wiry or choppy pulse. Other signs may include acute middle or lower abdominal pain, loss of appetite and emaciation, hemiplegia, paralysis, atrophy of the limbs, and frequent urination or incontinence. Formulas that dispel blood stasis or stagnation are quite strong and should be used with caution in debilitated or geriatric animals, or those with patterns of deficiency. Prolonged use of blood-invigorating and stasis-removing herbs will consume qi and blood, especially at large dosages; qi- and blood-tonifying herbs are often added to these formulas for this reason.

Conditions characterized by excessive bleeding or hemorrhage arise from external and internal causes. Patterns are differentiated based on duration, location (upper, middle, lower *jiao*), temperature (hot or cold), deficiency or excess, and the *zang fu* organs affected. Bleeding as the primary clinical sign is usually caused by excess heat entering the blood, *zang fu* organs intimately associated with the blood (i.e., Liver, Spleen, Heart) and/or the nutritive levels of the body, or is caused by deficiency (yin and/or qi). Heat easily burns and damages the vessels, causing the blood to move recklessly and escape the vessels. Yin-deficient heat and dryness can cause bleeding with hemoptysis, and Spleen qi deficiency can lead to hemolytic anemia or thrombocytopenia with petechiae and ecchymosis. The clinical signs of bleeding vary, but, in general, bleeding that involves excess patterns present acutely with profuse amounts of bright red blood accompanied by a red tongue and a rapid pulse. Other common clinical manifestations include epistaxis, hemoptysis, hematemesis, hematochezia, hematuria, hematoma, petechiae and ecchymosis. Bleeding related to deficiency presents as chronic bleeding of small volume with a dull or darker red color and accompanied by a pale tongue and a weak, thin pulse. Common conditions in veterinary medicine characterized by bleeding or hemorrhage include: immune-mediated disease (hemolytic anemia, thrombocytopenia), infectious disease, toxin ingestion (zinc, copper, lead, onions, rodenticide), drugs (acetaminophen, cephalosporins, tapazole), neoplasia, clotting disorders (*von Willebrand disease* [*vWD*]), canine hemorrhagic gastroenteritis, exercise induced pulmonary hemorrhage (EIPH) in horses, traumatic injury, surgery and parturition.

In summary, there are a variety of etiologies that contribute to disorders of the blood (blood deficiency, blood stagnation or stasis, blood heat, and loss of blood or bleeding), and these conditions may occur independently or concurrently. Blood deficiency is treated with blood-tonifying formulas (*see* Chapter 8: Tonic Formulas); blood stagnation is treated with blood-invigorating and stasis-removing formulas; and bleeding is treated with stop-bleeding formulas. Differential diagnosis of blood disorders is extremely important for patient safety and treatment success. One must determine the severity of the blood disorder (acute or chronic), the cause of the disorder, the character of the condition (the presence of cold, heat, excess, or deficiency), and which internal organs are most affected. In emergency situations (e.g., acute and severe bleeding), it is more important to address the acute signs first (i.e., stop the bleeding) and stabilize the animal before addressing the underlying or

Chapter 13 — Overview

root cause. In non-emergent situations (e.g., chronic and mild blood disorders), one should focus on identification and treatment of the underlying cause of the condition, or address both the cause and the clinical signs concurrently. In general, it is recommended that herbs that invigorate the blood and dispel blood stasis be discontinued 3-5 days prior to any surgical procedure, and then administration can be resumed 3-5 days post-operatively.

SUBCATEGORIES OF ACTION

Blood-regulating formulas are divided into two subcategories: blood-invigorating and stasis-removing formulas, and stop-bleeding formulas.

1. **Blood-Invigorating and Stasis-Removing Formulas**

These formulas are suitable for treating blood stagnation, and are commonly used to treat acute and chronic traumatic injuries, surgery, parturition, chronic disease, immune-mediated diseases, cardiovascular disease, retained placenta, hemiplegia and cancer. Clinical manifestations of blood stagnation include sharp, stabbing pain at a fixed location, pain that intensifies with pressure, and stiffness and hardness at the affected area upon palpation. The tongue is usually dark red to purple, and may have prominent or pronounced petechia in severe cases, and the pulse may be wiry or choppy.

Because conditions involving blood stagnation are often complex, other herbs are usually added to enhance the overall effectiveness of the treatment. If the blood stasis is accompanied by qi stagnation, qi-regulating herbs are added to promote normal qi circulation. If the blood stasis is generating heat, both blood-invigorating and heat-clearing herbs should be used at the same time. If blood stasis is caused by cold, the addition of herbs that warm the channels and disperse cold enhances the treatment effect. Finally, chronic stagnation may contribute to qi and blood deficiencies, thus requiring the use of qi- and blood-tonifying herbs.

Herbs commonly used to invigorate blood circulation and remove blood stasis include *Chuan Xiong* (Rhizoma Chuanxiong), *Tao Ren* (Semen Persicae), *Hong Hua* (Flos Carthami), *Chi Shao* (Radix Paeoniae Rubra), and *Dan Shen* (Radix et Rhizoma Salviae Miltiorrhizae). Exemplar formulas include *Tao He Cheng Qi Tang* (Peach Pit Decoction to Order the Qi), *Xue Fu Zhu Yu Tang* (Drive Out Stasis in the Mansion of Blood Decoction), *Fu Yuan Huo Xue Tang* (Revive Health by Invigorating the Blood Decoction), *Wen Jing Tang* (Warm the Channels Decoction), *Sheng Hua Tang* (Generation and Transformation Decoction), and *Shi Xiao San* (Sudden Smile Powder).

2. **Stop-Bleeding Formulas**

In veterinary medicine, these formulas are used to treat various types of bleeding characterized by epistaxis, hemoptysis, hematemesis, hematochezia, hematuria, hematoma, petechiae and ecchymosis. These formulas also treat conditions such as immune-mediated disease (hemolytic anemia, thrombocytopenia), infectious disease, toxin ingestion (zinc, copper, lead, onions, rodenticide), drugs (acetaminophen, cephalosporins, tapazole), neoplasia, clotting disorders (*von Willebrand disease* [*vWD*]), canine hemorrhagic gastroenteritis, exercise induced pulmonary hemorrhage (EIPH) in horses, traumatic injury, surgery and parturition.

Proper management of bleeding is rather complicated, as there are many factors that must be considered, such as its characteristics (cold or hot, deficiency or excess), location (upper or lower body), and urgency (acute or chronic). For example, bleeding caused by heat in the *xue* (blood) level and leading to the reckless movement of blood needs to be treated with herbs that cool the blood and stop bleeding; bleeding due to deficiency and damage to the *chong* (thoroughfare) and *ren* (conception) channels is treated with herbs that tonify the blood and stop bleeding. In addition, bleeding in the upper parts of the body should be treated with an additional proportion of herbs that guide the blood downward; and bleeding in the lower parts of the body should be treated with herbs that lift upward. Furthermore, in acute and severe cases of bleeding, it is more important to treat the clinical signs first and stop the bleeding, than it is to initially address the underlying cause; while in chronic cases, it is more important to address the underlying cause. Lastly, profuse bleeding

Chapter 13 — Overview

may contribute to the collapse of qi, and this condition must be treated first by herbs that restore and rescue *yuan* (source) *qi* from collapse.

Herbs commonly used to stop bleeding caused by heat include *Ce Bai Ye* (Cacumen Platycladi), *Xiao Ji* (Herba Cirsii), *Bai Mao Gen* (Rhizoma Imperatae), and *Di Yu* (Radix Sanguisorbae). Herbs used to stop bleeding caused by cold include *Pao Jiang* (Rhizoma Zingiberis Praeparatum), *Ai Ye* (Folium Artemisiae Argyi), and *Fu Long Gan* (Terra Flava Usta). Herbs commonly used to stop bleeding accompanied by blood stasis include *San Qi* (Radix et Rhizoma Notoginseng) and *Pu Huang* (Pollen Typhae). Furthermore, bleeding in the upper parts of the body should be treated with a small amount of herbs that guide the blood downward, such as *Niu Xi* (Radix Achyranthis Bidentatae) and *Da Huang* (Radix et Rhizoma Rhei); bleeding in the lower parts of the body should be treated with herbs that lift upward, such as charred *Jing Jie* (Herba Schizonepetae), charred *Sheng Ma* (Rhizoma Cimicifugae), and *Huang Qi* (Radix Astragali).

Exemplar formulas that stop bleeding include *Shi Hui San* (Ten Partially-Charred Substances Powder), *Huai Hua San* (Sophora Japonica Flower Powder), *Huang Tu Tang* (Yellow Earth Decoction), and *Jiao Ai Tang* (Ass-Hide Gelatin and Mugwort Decoction).

CAUTIONS / CONTRAINDICATIONS

- Use of blood-invigorating herbs may consume and damage qi and blood, especially if used at large doses or for an extended period of time. Therefore, qi- and blood-tonifying herbs are often added to protect the body from such adverse effects.
- Blood-regulating formulas have moving and dispersing effects and should be used with extreme caution in pregnancy and in animals with known bleeding disorders (Dobermans).
- Blood-activating herbs must be used cautiously, as overdose or prolonged use may contribute to more bleeding. If bleeding is accompanied by blood stasis (such as in a trauma), then blood-activating herbs should be used to clear any residual blood stagnation in the body.
- Herbs that stop bleeding should not be given at large doses or for prolonged periods of time, as such uses may contribute to the development of blood stasis.
- Astringent herbs and formulas must be used with caution in cases of bleeding, as their binding and retaining effects may contribute to blood stasis.
- Bleeding in the upper parts of the body should not be treated with herbs that have ascending or lifting characteristics. Bleeding in the lower parts of the body should not be treated with herbs that have descending or sinking characteristics.

PHARMACOLOGICAL EFFECTS & CLINICAL APPLICATIONS

Blood-regulating formulas are divided into two subcategories: blood-invigorating and stasis-removing formulas, and stop-bleeding formulas. These two subcategories of formulas have distinct characteristics in Chinese herbal medicine; they also have contrasting differences in Western pharmacology and clinical applications.

1. **Blood-invigorating and stasis-removing formulas** have a wide variety of pharmacological effects and clinical applications. The main applications are as follows:

- **Clotting disorders**: Many blood-invigorating and stasis-removing herbs have been shown to have marked hematological effects. For example, *Dan Shen* (Radix et Rhizoma Salviae Miltiorrhizae) and *Chi Shao* (Radix Paeoniae Rubra) have anticoagulant effects; *Dan Shen* (Radix et Rhizoma Salviae Miltiorrhizae), *Chuan Xiong* (Rhizoma Chuanxiong) and *Hong Hua* (Flos Carthami) have antiplatelet effects; and *San Leng* (Rhizoma Sparganii) and *E Zhu* (Rhizoma Curcumae) have thrombolytic effects.[1] Similarly, blood-invigorating and stasis-removing formulas have marked anticoagulant, antiplatelet, and thrombolytic effects.[2,3,4,5,6,7] Clinical applications of these formulas include stroke,[8,9] ischemic stroke,[10] cerebral infarction,[11] post-stroke sequelae,[12] and deep vein thrombosis.[13] Exemplar formulas include *Xue Fu Zhu Yu Tang* (Drive Out Stasis in the Mansion of Blood Decoction) and *Bu Yang Huan Wu Tang* (Tonify the Yang to Restore Five Decoction).

Chapter 13 — Overview

- **Cardiovascular disorders**: Many blood-invigorating and stasis-removing herbs and formulas have been shown to exert profound influence on the cardiovascular system. They dilate blood vessels, decrease blood pressure, and increase blood perfusion to smaller blood vessels.[14,15] Clinical applications include cardiac angina,[16] ischemia,[17] bradyarrhythmia,[18] and coronary heart disease.[19] Exemplar formulas include *Xue Fu Zhu Yu Tang* (Drive Out Stasis in the Mansion of Blood Decoction) and *Bu Yang Huan Wu Tang* (Tonify the Yang to Restore Five Decoction).
- **Hyperlipidemia**: Many blood-invigorating and stasis-removing herbs and formulas have been shown to lower plasma cholesterol and triglyceride levels.[20,21,22] These formulas may be used to treat hyperlipidemia,[23] arteriosclerosis,[24] and atherosclerosis.[25,26] They also are used to treat associated clotting and cardiovascular disorders. Exemplar formulas include *Xue Fu Zhu Yu Tang* (Drive Out Stasis in the Mansion of Blood Decoction) and *Bu Yang Huan Wu Tang* (Tonify the Yang to Restore Five Decoction).
- **Gynecological and obstetric disorders:** One of the most common and effective uses of blood-invigorating and stasis-removing formulas is in the treatment of gynecological and obstetric disorders. Clinical applications include uterine bleeding,[27,28] premenstrual syndrome,[29] dysmenorrhea,[30,31] amenorrhea,[32,33] anovulation,[34] infertility (male and female),[35,36,37,38] ectopic pregnancy,[39,40] endometriosis,[41,42,43] hysteromyoma,[44,45] uterine myomas,[46] uterine leiomyomas,[47] adnexitis,[48] oophoritic cyst,[49] hyperplasia of mammary glands,[50] and retention of lochia.[51] Exemplar formulas include *Shao Fu Zhu Yu Tang* (Drive Out Blood Stasis in the Lower Abdomen Decoction), *Shi Xiao San* (Sudden Smile Powder), *Wen Jing Tang* (Warm the Channels Decoction), *Ai Fu Nuan Gong Wan* (Mugwort and Cyperus Pill for Warming the Womb), *Sheng Hua Tang* (Generation and Transformation Decoction), and *Gui Zhi Fu Ling Wan* (Cinnamon Twig and Poria Pill).
- **Pain**: Many blood-invigorating and stasis-removing herbs are well-documented for their analgesic and anti-inflammatory effects.[52,53,54,55,56] Clinical applications include sciatica,[57,58] arthritis,[59] rheumatoid arthritis,[60] lumbago,[61] and many others. Exemplar formulas include *Shen Tong Zhu Yu Tang* (Drive Out Blood Stasis from a Painful Body Decoction), *Fu Yuan Huo Xue Tang* (Revive Health by Invigorating the Blood Decoction), *Zheng Gu Zi Jin Dan* (Purple and Gold Pill for Righteous Bones), and *Huo Luo Xiao Ling Dan* (Fantastically Effective Pill to Invigorate the Collaterals).
- **Traumatic injuries**: These formulas also treat traumatic injuries, such as concussion,[62,63,64] bone fractures,[65,66] and various external and sports injuries.[67] Exemplar formulas that treat traumatic injuries include *Tong Qiao Huo Xue Tang* (Unblock the Orifices and Invigorate the Blood Decoction), *Fu Yuan Huo Xue Tang* (Revive Health by Invigorating the Blood Decoction), *Zheng Gu Zi Jin Dan* (Purple and Gold Pill for Righteous Bones), and *Qi Li San* (Seven-Thousandths of a Tael Powder).
- **Liver, gallbladder, and pancreatic disorders**: These formulas may be used for certain liver, gallbladder, and pancreatic disorders, such as hepatitis,[68,69,70] hepatic hemangioma,[71] liver abscess,[72] cholecystitis,[73] and pancreatitis.[74] Exemplar formulas include *Tao He Cheng Qi Tang* (Peach Pit Decoction to Order the Qi), *Ge Xia Zhu Yu Tang* (Drive Out Blood Stasis Below the Diaphragm Decoction), and *Fu Yuan Huo Xue Tang* (Revive Health by Invigorating the Blood Decoction).
- **Kidney disorders**: Some blood-invigorating and stasis-removing formulas have been used successfully to treat various kidney disorders, such as pyelonephritis,[75] renal insufficiency,[76] chronic nephritis,[77] and renal colic caused by stones.[78] Exemplar formulas include *Tao He Cheng Qi Tang* (Peach Pit Decoction to Order the Qi) and *Bu Yang Huan Wu Tang* (Tonify the Yang to Restore Five Decoction).

2. **Stop-bleeding formulas** are used primarily for their hemostatic effect to stop bleeding.
- **Bleeding**: These formulas may be used to treat all types of bleeding disorders, including but not limited to epistaxis and hemoptysis in the upper body, hematemesis in the middle body, and hematochezia, hematuria, abnormal uterine bleeding, and bleeding hemorrhoids in the lower body.[79,80,81,82] Furthermore, they treat acute bleeding from external injuries, such as trauma or

Chapter 13 — Overview

sports injuries, or chronic bleeding from internal illnesses such as bleeding ulcers.[83,84] These hemostatic herbs and formulas increase platelets and facilitate the clotting cascade.[85] Representative formulas that stop bleeding include *Shi Hui San* (Ten Partially-Charred Substances Powder), *Huai Hua San* (Sophora Japonica Flower Powder), *Huang Tu Tang* (Yellow Earth Decoction), and *Jiao Ai Tang* (Ass-Hide Gelatin and Mugwort Decoction).

References

1. Chen J, Chen T. Chinese Medical Herbology and Pharmacology. Art of Medicine Press. 2004.
2. *Zhe Jiang Zhong Yi Za Zhi* (Zhejiang Journal of Chinese Medicine), 1988; 23(7):319.
3. *Zhong Hua Nei Ke Xue Za Zhi* (Journal of Chinese Internal Medicine), 1977; 2(2):79.
4. *Zhong Yi Ming Fang Lin Chuang Xin Yong* (Contemporary Clinical Applications of Classic Chinese Formulas), 2001; 144.
5. *Zhong Cheng Yao Yan Jiu* (Research of Chinese Patent Medicine), 1983; 8:31.
6. *Hu Nan Zhong Yi Xue Yuan Xue Bao* (Journal of Hunan University of Traditional Chinese Medicine), 1989; 9:545.
7. *Yun Nan Zhong Yi Za Zhi* (Yunan Journal of Chinese Medicine), 1992; 13(1):23.
8. Lin CC, Yen FL, Hsu FF, Lin JM. Anti-hypercholesterolaemia, antioxidant activity and free radical scavenger effects of traditional Chinese medicine prescriptions used for stroke. Journal of Pharmacy & Pharmacology. 2000 Nov ; 52(11):1387-93.
9. *Liao Ning Zhong Yi Za Zhi* (Liaoning Journal of Chinese Medicine), 1984; 9:26.
10. *Zhong Yi Za Zhi* (Journal of Chinese Medicine), 1984; 9:45.
11. *Zhe Jiang Zhong Yi Za Zhi* (Zhejiang Journal of Chinese Medicine), 1997; 7:317.
12. *Guang Dong Yi Xue* (Guangdong Medicine), 1992; 13(1):39.
13. *Jiang Su Zhong Yi* (Jiangsu Chinese Medicine), 1998; 2:33.
14. *Zhong Yao Yao Li Yu Lin Chuang* (Pharmacology and Clinical Applications of Chinese Herbs), 1993; 9(1):8.
15. *Zhong Guo Yi Yao Xue Bao* (Chinese Journal of Medicine and Herbology), 1990; 5(4):33.
16. *Xin Yi Yao Xue Za Zhi* (New Journal of Medicine and Herbology), 1976; 5:41.
17. *Zhe Jiang Zhong Yi Za Zhi* (Zhejiang Journal of Chinese Medicine), 1997; 10:445.
18. *Zhe Jiang Zhong Yi Xue Yuan Xue Bao* (Journal of Zhejiang University of Chinese Medicine), 1992; 16(3):19.
19. *Tian Jin Zhong Yi* (Tianjin Chinese Medicine), 1993; 5:22.
20. *Zhe Jiang Zhong Yi Za Zhi* (Zhejiang Journal of Chinese Medicine), 1988; 23(7):319.
21. *Shan Xi Zhong Yi* (Shanxi Chinese Medicine), 1988; 9(3):126.
22. *Zhong Xi Yi Jie He Za Zhi* (Journal of Integrated Chinese and Western Medicine), 1988; 8(10):601.
23. *Zhong Xi Yi Jie He Za Zhi* (Journal of Integrated Chinese and Western Medicine), 1988; 8(10):601.
24. *Shan Dong Zhong Yi Za Zhi* (Shandong Journal of Chinese Medicine), 1991; 10(2):26.
25. *Hu Nan Zhong Yi Za Zhi* (Hunan Journal of Chinese Medicine), 1993; 9(1):41.
26. *Jiang Su Zhong Yi* (Jiangsu Chinese Medicine), 1992; 13(5):16.
27. *Shi Yong Zhong Xi Yi Jie He Za Zhi* (Practical Journal of Integrated Chinese and Western Medicines), 1993; 6(6):380.
28. *Hu Bei Zhong Yi Za Zhi* (Hubei Journal of Chinese Medicine), 1990; 4:17.
29. *Guo Wai Yi Xue* (Foreign Medicine), 1980; 2(4):185.
30. *Zhe Jiang Zhong Yi Za Zhi* (Zhejiang Journal of Chinese Medicine), 1964; 11:17.
31. *He Bei Zhong Yi* (Hebei Chinese Medicine), 1991; 3:16.
32. *Shan Xi Zhong Yi* (Shanxi Chinese Medicine), 1991; 12(5):200.
33. Ushiroyama T, Tsubokura S, Ikeda A, Ueki M. The effect of unkei-to on pituitary gonadotropin secretion and ovulation in anovulatory cycles of young women. Am J Chin Med. 1995; 23(3-4):223-30.
34. Ushiroyama T, Ikeda A, Sakai M, Hosotani T, Suzuki Y, Tsubokura S, Ueki M. Effects of unkei-to, an herbal medicine, on endocrine function and ovulation in women with high basal levels of luteinizing hormone secretion. Journal of Reproductive Medicine. 2001 May; 46(5):451-6.
35. *Hu Nan Yi Yao Za Zhi* (Hunan Journal of Medicine and Herbology), 1983; 3:52.
36. *He Nan Zhong Yi* (Henan Chinese Medicine), 1985; 3:29.
37. Yang CC, Chen JC, Chen GW, Chen YS, Chung JG. Effects of Shao-Fu-Zhu-Yu-Tang on motility of human sperm. American Journal of Chinese Medicine. 2003; 31(4):573-9.

Chapter 13 — Overview

38. *Shan Xi Zhong Yi* (Shanxi Chinese Medicine), 1995; 11(5):20.
39. *Hu Bei Zhong Yi Za Zhi* (Hubei Journal of Chinese Medicine), 1982; 16(5):48.
40. *Xin Zhong Yi* (New Chinese Medicine), 1984; 11:33.
41. *Shang Hai Zhong Yi Yao Za Zhi* (Shanghai Journal of Chinese Medicine and Herbology), 1993; 2:16.
42. *Zhong Xi Yi Jie He Za Zhi* (Journal of Integrated Chinese and Western Medicine), 1988; 10:639.
43. *Jiang Su Zhong Yi* (Jiangsu Chinese Medicine), 1990; 8:14.
44. *Bei Jing Zhong Yi* (Beijing Chinese Medicine), 1987; 5:34.
45. *Shan Xi Zhong Yi* (Shanxi Chinese Medicine), 1997; 11:508.
46. Sakamoto S, Yoshino H, Shirahata Y, Shimodairo K, Okamoto R. Pharmacotherapeutic effects of kuei-chih-fu-ling-wan (keishi-bukuryo-gan) on human uterine myomas. Am J Chin Med. 1992; 20(3-4):313-7.
47. Sakamoto S, Mitamura T, Iwasawa M, Kitsunai H, Shindou K, Yagishita Y, Zhou YF, Sassa S. Conservative management for perimenopausal women with uterine leiomyomas using Chinese herbal medicines and synthetic analogs of gonadotropin-releasing hormone. In Vivo. 1998 May-Jun; 12(3):333-7.
48. *Hu Bei Zhong Yi Za Zhi* (Hubei Journal of Chinese Medicine), 1987; 5:14.
49. *Xin Zhong Yi* (New Chinese Medicine), 1995; 8:40.
50. *Shan Xi Zhong Yi* (Shanxi Chinese Medicine), 1994; 2:52.
51. *He Nan Zhong Yi* (Henan Chinese Medicine), 1993; 4:35.
52. *Zhong Yao Yan Jiu* (Research of Chinese Herbology), 1993; 6(4):15.
53. *Zhong Yao Yao Li Yu Lin* Chuang (Pharmacology and Clinical Applications of Chinese Herbs), 1987; 37.
54. *Zhong Yao Yan Jiu* (Research of Chinese Herbology), 1993; 6(4):15.
55. *Zhong Cheng Yao Yan Jiu* (Research of Chinese Patent Medicine), 1987; 3:45.
56. *Shang Hai Zhong Yi Yao Za Zhi* (Shanghai Journal of Chinese Medicine and Herbology), 1985; 10:29.
57. *Si Chuan Zhong Yi* (Sichuan Chinese Medicine), 1985; 11:50.
58. *Zhong Yi Fang Ji Xian Dai Yan Jiu* (Modern Study of Medical Formulas in Traditional Chinese Medicine), 1997; 1012.
59. Yun *Nan Zhong Yao Zhi* (Yunan Journal of Chinese Herbal Medicine), 1989; 3:46.
60. *Bei Jing Zhong Yi Za Zhi* (Beijing Journal of Chinese Medicine), 1988; 6:35.
61. *Guang Xi Zhong Yi Yao* (Guangxi Chinese Medicine and Herbology), 1987; 2:47.
62. *Shan Xi Zhong Yi* (Shanxi Chinese Medicine), 1991; 12(11):511.
63. *Shan Xi Zhong Yi* (Shanxi Chinese Medicine), 1993; 14(5):222.
64. *Zhe Jiang Zhong Yi Za Zhi* (Zhejiang Journal of Chinese Medicine), 1996; 5:301.
65. *Zhong Yi Fang Ji Xian Dai Yan Jiu* (Modern Study of Medical Formulas in Traditional Chinese Medicine), 1997; 999.
66. *Zhong Hua Wai Ke Za Zhi* (Chinese Journal of External Medicine), 1962; 5:305.
67. *Jiang Su Zhong Yi* (Jiangsu Chinese Medicine), 1963; 5:13.
68. *Zhong Yi Ming Fang Lin Chuang Xin Yong* (Contemporary Clinical Applications of Classic Chinese Formulas), 2001; 561.
69. *Jiang Su Zhong Yi* (Jiangsu Chinese Medicine), 1995; 7:10.
70. *Xin Yi Yao Xue Za Zhi* (New Journal of Medicine and Herbology), 1978; 9:44.
71. *Jiang Su Zhong Yi* (Jiangsu Chinese Medicine), 1997; 8:21.
72. *Zhong Guo Zhong Xi Yi Jie He Za Zhi* (Chinese Journal of Integrative Chinese and Western Medicine), 1993; 8:491.
73. *Shan Dong Zhong Yi Za Zhi* (Shandong Journal of Chinese Medicine), 1993; 12(3):28.
74. *Shi Yong Zhong Yi Yao Za Zhi* (Journal of Practical Chinese Medicine and Medicinals), 1994; 10(4):27.
75. *Ji Lin Zhong Yi Yao* (Jilin Chinese Medicine and Herbology), 1986; 4:10.
76. *Gan Su Zhong Yi* (Gansu Chinese Medicine), 1993; 6(4):26.
77. *Shi Yong Zhong Yi Nei Ke Za Zhi* (Journal of Practical Chinese Internal Medicine), 1990; 4(3):123.
78. *Hu Nan Yi Yao Za Zhi* (Hunan Journal of Medicine and Herbology), 1984; 3:44.
79. *Fu Jian Zhong Yi Yao* (Fujian Chinese Medicine and Herbology), 1960; 4:27.
80. *Hei Long Jiang Zhong Yi Yao* (Heilongjiang Chinese Medicine and Herbology), 1985; 3:43.
81. *Zhong Hua Fu Chan Ke Za Zhi* (Chinese Journal of Obstetrics and Gynecology), 1959; 5:413.
82. *Fu Jian Zhong Yi Yao* (Fujian Chinese Medicine and Herbology), 1991; 22(3):12.
83. *Zhe Jiang Zhong Yi Za Zhi* (Zhejiang Journal of Chinese Medicine), 1958; 7:21.
84. *Zhe Jiang Zhong Yi Yao* (Zhejiang Chinese Medicine and Herbology), 1963; 7:4.
85. Chen J, Chen T. Chinese Medical Herbology and Pharmacology. Art of Medicine Press. 2004.

Section 1

活血祛瘀剂
— Blood-Invigorating and Stasis-Removing Formulas

Táo Hé Chéng Qì Tāng (Peach Pit Decoction to Order the Qi)
桃核承氣湯
桃核承气汤

Pinyin Name: *Tao He Cheng Qi Tang*
Literal Name: Peach Pit Decoction to Order the Qi
Alternate Names: *Tao He Cheng Chi Tang, Tao Ren Cheng Qi Tang, Tao Jen Cheng Chi Tang*, Persica Qi-Infusing Decoction, Peach Kernel Purgative Decoction, Persica and Rhubarb Combination
Original Source: *Shang Han Lun* (Discussion of Cold-Induced Disorders) by Zhang Zhong-Jing in the Eastern Han Dynasty

COMPOSITION

Tao Ren (Semen Persicae)	50 pieces [12g]
Da Huang (Radix et Rhizoma Rhei)	12g
Gui Zhi (Ramulus Cinnamomi)	6g
Mang Xiao (Natrii Sulfas)	6g
Zhi Gan Cao (Radix et Rhizoma Glycyrrhizae Praeparata cum Melle)	6g

DOSAGE / PREPARATION / ADMINISTRATION

The source text states to cook all of the ingredients, except *Mang Xiao* (Natrii Sulfas), in 7 cups [1,400 mL] of water until the liquid is reduced to 2.5 cups [500 mL]. Discard the residue, add *Mang Xiao* (Natrii Sulfas), and bring the decoction to a slight boil. Take 0.5 cup [100 mL] of the warm, strained decoction three times daily after meals. This formula may cause loose stools.

CHINESE THERAPEUTIC ACTIONS

Breaks up blood stasis and drains it downward

CLINICAL MANIFESTATIONS

Blood accumulation in the lower *jiao*: acute lower abdominal pain, irritability, thirst, fever at night, and mania in severe cases.

VETERINARY CLINICAL APPLICATIONS

Cholecystitis, pyelonephritis, diabetes mellitus, acute pelvic inflammation, and retained placenta.

EXPLANATION

According to the *Shang Han Lun* (Discussion of Cold-Induced Disorders), *Tao He Cheng Qi Tang* (Peach Pit Decoction to Order the Qi) was originally formulated to treat blood stagnation in the lower *jiao* from a *taiyang* disorder that was not relieved of exterior pathogens, with the pathogens traveling along the channel pathway to transform into heat in the interior. The heat then stagnates with the blood in the lower *jiao*, resulting in lower *jiao* blood stasis. Acute lower abdominal pain is due to the blood stasis in the lower *jiao*. Delirium, irritability, thirst, fever at night, and mania are due to heat in the *xue* (blood) level. Because the water passages are not affected, urination is still normal. Today, this formula has found multiple applications to treat blood stagnation/stasis in the lower *jiao* from a variety of causes unrelated to *taiyang* disorder.

Tao He Cheng Qi Tang consists of *Tiao Wei Cheng Qi Tang* (Regulate the Stomach and Order the Qi Decoction) plus *Tao Ren* (Semen Persicae) and *Gui Zhi* (Ramulus Cinnamomi). In this formula, *Tao Ren* (Semen Persicae) breaks up and dispels blood stagnation. *Da Huang* (Radix et Rhizoma Rhei) drains the heat and blood stagnation downward. These two herbs, which together dispel blood stasis and heat, are the chief herbs in this formula. *Gui Zhi* (Ramulus Cinnamomi) opens the channels and collaterals to

Táo Hé Chéng Qì Tāng (Peach Pit Decoction to Order the Qi)

***Tao He Cheng Qi Tang* (Peach Pit Decoction to Order the Qi)**

Diagnosis	Clinical Signs	Treatment	Herbs
Accumulation of blood in the lower *jiao*	• Acute lower abdominal pain: blood stasis in the lower *jiao* • Delirium, irritability, and mania: heat disturbing the *shen* (spirit) • Thirst and fever at night: heat consuming yin and body fluids	Breaks up blood stasis and drains it downward	• *Tao Ren* (Semen Persicae) breaks up and dispels blood stagnation. • *Da Huang* (Radix et Rhizoma Rhei) drains heat and stagnation downward. • *Gui Zhi* (Ramulus Cinnamomi) opens the channels and collaterals to dispel blood stasis. • *Mang Xiao* (Natrii Sulfas) drains heat. • *Zhi Gan Cao* (Radix et Rhizoma Glycyrrhizae Praeparata cum Melle) supplements qi, regulates the middle *jiao*, and lessens the harsh effects of the other herbs.

help *Tao Ren* (Semen Persicae) dispel blood stasis. *Mang Xiao* (Natrii Sulfas) drains heat and softens any hardness to help *Da Huang* (Radix et Rhizoma Rhei) drain downward. *Zhi Gan Cao* (Radix et Rhizoma Glycyrrhizae Praeparata cum Melle), besides supplementing qi and harmonizing the middle *jiao*, lessens the harsh effects of the other herbs to prevent injury to the qi.

VETERINARY MODIFICATIONS

- With blood deficiency, add *Dang Gui* (Radix Angelicae Sinensis) and *Bai Shao* (Radix Paeoniae Alba).
- With blood stagnation, add *San Qi* (Radix et Rhizoma Notoginseng) and *Chi Shao* (Radix Paeoniae Rubra).
- With qi stagnation, add *Xiang Fu* (Rhizoma Cyperi), *Wu Yao* (Radix Linderae), *Qing Pi* (Pericarpium Citri Reticulatae Viride), and *Mu Xiang* (Radix Aucklandiae).
- With constipation, add *Zhi Shi* (Fructus Aurantii Immaturus) and *Hou Po* (Cortex Magnoliae Officinalis).
- With restlessness and thirst, add *Huang Lian* (Rhizoma Coptidis) and *Huang Qin* (Radix Scutellariae).
- With oliguria, add *Che Qian Zi* (Semen Plantaginis), *Fu Ling* (Poria), and *Mu Tong* (Caulis Akebiae).
- With bleeding, add *Di Huang* (Radix Rehmanniae) and *Bai Mao Gen* (Rhizoma Imperatae).
- With distention and pain due to qi stagnation, add *Xiang Fu* (Rhizoma Cyperi) and *Zhi Qiao* (Fructus Aurantii).
- With trauma-related pain, add *Chi Shao* (Radix Paeoniae Rubra), *Dang Gui Wei* (Extremitas Radix Angelicae Sinensis), *Hong Hua* (Flos Carthami), and *Su Mu* (Lignum Sappan).
- With fire flaring upward manifesting in red eyes and vomiting of blood, add *Di Huang* (Radix Rehmanniae), *Mu Dan Pi* (Cortex Moutan), *Zhi Zi* (Fructus Gardeniae), and *Niu Xi* (Radix Achyranthis Bidentatae).
- With gallstones, add *Jin Qian Cao* (Herba Lysimachiae), *Hai Jin Sha* (Spora Lygodii), *Yu Jin* (Radix Curcumae), and *Ji Nei Jin* (Endothelium Corneum Gigeriae Galli).

CAUTIONS / CONTRAINDICATIONS

- *Tao He Cheng Qi Tang* should be used only when the wind-cold pathogen is no longer present at the exterior. Therefore, if exterior clinical signs are still present, exterior-releasing methods need to be employed before this formula can be given.
- Because this formula strongly breaks up blood stagnation and dispels heat, a careful diagnosis should be made before applying this strong formula.
- This formula is contraindicated during pregnancy.
- Use of this formula is occasionally associated with side effects that include nausea, vomiting, and diarrhea.[1]

PHARMACOLOGICAL EFFECTS

1. **Purgative**: One study reported marked success using *Tao He Cheng Qi Tang* to induce bowel movements in constipated mice. The first bowel movement was generally reported within 4 hours after the administration of the herbs.[2]
2. **Antiplatelet and anticoagulant**: According to various *in vitro* studies, administration of *Tao He Cheng Qi Tang* has been associated with inhibiting platelet aggregation, inhibiting coagulation, and decreasing blood viscosity.[3,4]
3. **Antihyperlipidemic**: Administration of *Tao He Cheng Qi Tang* in animal subjects was associated with reduced plasma lipoprotein and triglyceride levels.[5]
4. **Hypoglycemic**: According to one study, administration of *Tao He Cheng Qi Tang* on an empty stomach to diabetic rats was associated with decreased plasma levels of glucose and insulin.[6]
5. **Anti-inflammatory**: Administration of *Tao He Cheng Qi Tang* in animal subjects was associated with reduced

swelling and inflammation. The anti-inflammatory effect was attributed primarily to *Da Huang* (Radix et Rhizoma Rhei) and *Gan Cao* (Radix et Rhizoma Glycyrrhizae).[7,8]

HUMAN CLINICAL STUDIES AND RESEARCH

1. **Cholecystitis**: Use of modified *Tao He Cheng Qi Tang* was associated with 94% effectiveness in treating cholecystitis in 100 patients (47 males and 53 females, between 19-54 years of age, with 1 day to 13 months history of illness). The herbal treatment contained *Tao Ren* (Semen Persicae), *Da Huang* (Radix et Rhizoma Rhei), *Gui Zhi* (Ramulus Cinnamomi), *Gan Cao* (Radix et Rhizoma Glycyrrhizae), *Huang Lian* (Rhizoma Coptidis), *Huang Qin* (Radix Scutellariae), and *Zhi Shi* (Fructus Aurantii Immaturus). The treatment protocol was to administer the decoction every 6 hours in acute cases, and twice daily in chronic cases. The duration of treatment ranged from 5-27 days. Of 100 patients, the study reported complete recovery in 23 cases, remission in 64 cases, improvement in 7 cases, and no effect in 6 cases.[9]
2. **Hepatitis**: Administration of *Tao He Cheng Qi Tang* and *Chai Ling Tang* (Bupleurum and Poria Decoction) in 10 patients with chronic active hepatitis was associated with significant reduction of liver enzymes and symptomatic improvements.[10]
3. **Enteroparalysis**: One study reported marked effectiveness using modified *Tao He Cheng Qi Tang* to treat 20 patients with enteroparalysis associated with traumatic injuries to the thoracic or lumbar spine. For patients with a severe condition, the formula was modified by removing *Gui Zhi* (Ramulus Cinnamomi) and adding *Zhi Shi* (Fructus Aurantii Immaturus), *Hou Po* (Cortex Magnoliae Officinalis), *Fan Xie Ye* (Folium Sennae), and others as needed. For those who did not have a bowel movement after the initial herbal treatment, 30 grams each of *Da Huang* (Radix et Rhizoma Rhei) and *Xuan Ming Fen* (Natrii Sulfas Exsiccatus) were added. The herbs were cooked in water, and the herbal solution (approximately 600 mL) was given via rectal enema. The study reported marked effect in most patients to induce bowel movement.[11]
4. **Pyelonephritis**: Use of modified *Tao He Cheng Qi Tang* was effective in treating 46 patients with chronic pyelonephritis. The formula was modified based on the condition of each individual patient. For individuals with diarrhea, *Mang Xiao* (Natrii Sulfas) was removed. For frequent and urgent urination, *Hua Shi* (Talcum) was added. For lower abdominal pain, a large dose of *Gui Zhi* (Ramulus Cinnamomi) or *Tian Tai Wu Yao San* (Top-Quality Lindera Powder) was added. Of 46 patients, the study reported significant improvement in 24 cases and improvement in 15 cases.[12]
5. **Renal insufficiency**: Administration of modified *Tao He Cheng Qi Tang* in 18 patients with renal insufficiency was associated with marked improvements in BUN, SCr, and CO_2CP. The herbal formula was given one time daily, and contained the following ingredients: *Tao Ren* (Semen Persicae), *Da Huang* (Radix et Rhizoma Rhei), *Gui Zhi* (Ramulus Cinnamomi), *Zhi Gan Cao* (Radix et Rhizoma Glycyrrhizae Praeparata cum Melle), *Huang Qi* (Radix Astragali), *Fu Zi* (Radix Aconiti Lateralis Praeparata), *Ze Xie* (Rhizoma Alismatis), *Yi Mu Cao* (Herba Leonuri), and *Nu Zhen Zi* (Fructus Ligustri Lucidi).[13]
6. **Renal colic**: One study reported pain relief using *Tao He Cheng Qi Tang* to treat renal colic caused by stones. The treatment protocol was to administer the herbs in decoction (1 pack per day, with decoction given in three equally-divided doses). The study reported relief of pain in all 11 patients within 2-3 days.[14]
7. **Diabetes mellitus**: One study reported 79% effectiveness using *Tao He Cheng Qi Tang* to treat 106 patients with type II diabetes mellitus. The mechanism was attributed to the formula's ability to stimulate the beta-islet cells of the pancreas to produce more insulin.[15,16]
8. **Schizophrenia**: Use of *Tao He Cheng Qi Tang* was associated with beneficial effect in all 10 patients with schizophrenia that was characterized by blood stagnation in the lower *jiao*.[17]

HERB-DRUG INTERACTION

Drug-induced menopause: One study evaluated the therapeutic effects of certain herbal medicines on menopausal clinical signs induced by gonadotropin-releasing hormone agonist therapy in Japanese women with endometriosis, adenomyosis, or leiomyoma. According to this study, 13 menopausal patients were successfully treated with *Tao He Cheng Qi Tang*, *Dang Gui Shao Yao San* (Tangkuei and Peony Powder), *Shao Yao Gan Cao Tang* (Peony and Licorice Decoction), *Gui Zhi Fu Ling Wan* (Cinnamon Twig and Poria Pill), *Jia Wei Xiao Yao San* (Augmented Rambling Powder), or *Gui Zhi Tang* (Cinnamon Twig Decoction). Most importantly, there were no significant changes in serum estradiol levels after treatment with these herbal medicines. The researchers concluded that these herbal medicines could be recommended for menopausal clinical signs induced by gonadotropin-releasing hormone agonists without a negative effect on serum estradiol levels.[18]

SUGGESTED ACUPUNCTURE TREATMENT

1. Points: *Quchi* (LI 11), *Hegu* (LI 4), *Weizhong* (BL 40), *Xuehai* (SP 10), *Geshu* (BL 17), *Zhaohai* (KI 6), *Lieque* (LU 7), *Shangjuxu* (ST 37), and *Housanli* (ST 36).
2. Technique: sedation.

Táo Hé Chéng Qì Tāng (Peach Pit Decoction to Order the Qi)

Quchi (LI 11) and *Hegu* (LI 4) clear interior *yangming* heat. *Weizhong* (BL 40) sedates heat in the *xue* (blood) level. *Xuehai* (SP 10) and *Geshu* (BL 17) activate blood and break up blood stagnation. *Zhaohai* (KI 6) nourishes water to restrain fire in the body. *Lieque* (LU 7), the *luo* (connecting) point of the Lung channel, enters the Large Intestine and the lower *jiao* to sedate heat. *Shangjuxu* (ST 37), the lower *he* (uniting) point of the Large Intestine, smoothes Large Intestine qi. *Housanli* (ST 36) nourishes the qi of the middle *jiao* to prevent injuries to the Stomach as a result of activating blood.

AUTHORS' COMMENTS

Tao He Cheng Qi Tang strongly moves the blood and contains *Da Huang* (Radix et Rhizoma Rhei); thus, treatment should begin with a low dose and gradually increase. This formula should be regarded as a blood-moving purgative and is typically not given for longer than 3 days at one time. It should not be given on an empty stomach and should be discontinued as soon as the desired clinical effects have been achieved. Moreover, it should not be used in the presence of exterior syndromes.

Tao He Cheng Qi Tang was used originally to treat blood stasis in the lower *jiao*. Today, its clinical application in veterinary medicine has been expanded, as this formula has been proven effective in treating other conditions characterized by blood stasis, such as:

- Traumatic injuries (pelvic fractures, vehicular trauma, bite wounds, sacrococcygeal injuries) to the hind quarters with bruising and severe pain that limit physical movement, accompanied by difficult defecation or urination. It can be combined with *Yan Hu Suo* (Rhizoma Corydalis), *Hong Hua* (Flos Carthami) and *Chi Shao* (Radix Paeoniae Rubra) to help relieve pain and improve clinical efficacy.
- Blood stagnation secondary to chronic urinary tract infection (UTI), multiple urinary bladder surgeries for cystic calculi, and cancer of the urinary bladder with the presence of dark purple blood clots and straining to urinate.
- For retained placenta, it can take up to 48 hours to expel retained placenta and clinical results can be improved by adding *Hong Hua* (Flos Carthami).
- For the treatment of pancreatitis with blood stagnation and abdominal pain with fever, it can be combined with *Huang Lian Jie Du Tang* (Coptis Decoction to Relieve Toxicity). The lowest therapeutic dosage of each herbal formula is combined in a 1:1 ratio. For animals with concurrent Spleen qi deficiency, it should be combined with herbs or an additional formula to tonify and protect the middle *jiao*.
- For the treatment of acute cholangiohepatitis or cholangitis, combine with *Yin Chen* (Herba Artemisiae Scopariae) and *Zhi Zi* (Fructus Gardeniae). In cases in which there is more dampness and less heat, combine with *Yin Chen Wu Ling San* (Artemisia Scoparia and Five-Ingredient Powder with Poria).

References

1. *Zhong Yao Ming Fang Yao Li Yu Ying Yong* (Pharmacology and Applications of Famous Herbal Formulas), 1989; 451-453.
2. *Zhong Cheng Yao* (Study of Chinese Patent Medicine), 1990; 11:24.
3. *Zhe Jiang Zhong Yi Za Zhi* (Zhejiang Journal of Chinese Medicine), 1988; 23(7):319.
4. *Yao Xue Za Zhi* (Journal of Medicinals), 1983; 103(7):313.
5. *Zhe Jiang Zhong Yi Za Zhi* (Zhejiang Journal of Chinese Medicine), 1988; 23(7):319.
6. *Xin Zhong Yi* (New Chinese Medicine), 1988; 20(4):53.
7. *Han Fang Yi Xue* (Kampo Medicine), 1984; 1:11.
8. *Guo Wai Yi Xue* (Foreign Medicine), 1971; 9(2):48.
9. *Shan Dong Zhong Yi Za Zhi* (Shandong Journal of Chinese Medicine), 1993; 12(3):28.
10. *Zhong Yi Ming Fang Lin Chuang Xin Yong* (Contemporary Clinical Applications of Classic Chinese Formulas), 2001; 561.
11. *Xin Zhong Yi* (New Chinese Medicine), 1984; 2:34.
12. *Ji Lin Zhong Yi Yao* (Jilin Chinese Medicine and Herbology), 1986; 4:10.
13. *Gan Su Zhong Yi* (Gansu Chinese Medicine), 1993; 6(4):26.
14. *Hu Nan Yi Yao Za Zhi* (Hunan Journal of Medicine and Herbology), 1984; 3:44.
15. *Zhong Guo Zhong Xi Yi Jie He Za Zhi* (Chinese Journal of Integrative Chinese and Western Medicine), 1992; 12(2):74.
16. *Zhong Guo Zhong Yi Yao Xue Bao* (Chinese Journal of Chinese Medicine and Herbology), 1993; 8(5):50.
17. *Shan Xi Zhong Yi* (Shanxi Chinese Medicine), 1983; 3(3):14.
18. Tanaka T. Effects of herbal medicines on menopausal symptoms induced by gonadotropin-releasing hormone agonist therapy. Clin Exp Obstet Gynecol. 2001; 28(1):20-3.

Tōng Qiào Huó Xuè Tāng

(Unblock the Orifices and Invigorate the Blood Decoction)

通竅活血湯
通窍活血汤

Pinyin Name: *Tong Qiao Huo Xue Tang*
Literal Name: Unblock the Orifices and Invigorate the Blood Decoction
Original Source: *Yi Lin Gai Cuo* (Corrections of Errors Among Physicians) by Wang Qing-Ren in 1830

COMPOSITION

Chi Shao (Radix Paeoniae Rubra)	3g
Chuan Xiong (Rhizoma Chuanxiong)	3g
Tao Ren (Semen Persicae), *yan* (ground) till muddy	9g
Hong Hua (Flos Carthami)	9g
Lao Cong (Herba Allii Fistulosi), *qie* (sliced)	3 pieces [3-6g]
Sheng Jiang (Rhizoma Zingiberis Recens)	9g
She Xiang (Moschus)	0.15g
Da Zao (Fructus Jujubae)	7 pieces [5g]
Grain-based liquor	250g

Note: *She Xiang* (Moschus) is derived from an endangered animal and is rarely used as a medicinal substance today. Its discussion here is included primarily for academic purposes, to reflect the historical use of this substance in its original formulation. Most herbal products today have removed it completely, or replaced it with substitutes with similar functions.

DOSAGE / PREPARATION / ADMINISTRATION

The source text states to cook all of the ingredients, except *She Xiang* (Moschus), in a large bowl of water. Discard the residue, add *She Xiang* (Moschus) and grain-based liquor to the strained decoction, and bring it to a boil twice. Take the warm decoction before bedtime. Today, this formula may be prepared as a decoction with the doses suggested in brackets, with the addition of a small amount of grain-based liquor.

CHINESE THERAPEUTIC ACTIONS

Activates blood circulation and opens the sensory orifices

CLINICAL MANIFESTATIONS

Blood stagnation in the head and face: head and dental pain, dizziness, poor hearing, hair loss and dry eyes.

VETERINARY CLINICAL APPLICATIONS

Post-concussion, ototoxicity, chronic sinusitis, traumatic proptosis, hyphema, keratoconjunctivitis sicca (KCS), and cerebrovascular accident.

EXPLANATION

The main actions of *Tong Qiao Huo Xue Tang* (Unblock the Orifices and Invigorate the Blood Decoction) are to activate blood circulation and remove blood stagnation in the head and facial regions. It can be used for various

Tong Qiao Huo Xue Tang **(Unblock the Orifices and Invigorate the Blood Decoction)**

Diagnosis	Clinical Signs	Treatment	Herbs
Blood stagnation in the head and face	• Head pain: blood stagnation in the head • Poor hearing: blood stagnation blocking the sensory orifices	• Activates blood circulation • Opens the sensory orifices	• *Chi Shao* (Radix Paeoniae Rubra), *Chuan Xiong* (Rhizoma Chuanxiong), *Tao Ren* (Semen Persicae), and *Hong Hua* (Flos Carthami) activate blood circulation and eliminate blood stasis. • *Lao Cong* (Herba Allii Fistulosi) unblocks stagnation and promotes the circulation of yang qi. • *She Xiang* (Moschus) opens the sensory orifices and restores their normal functions. • *Sheng Jiang* (Rhizoma Zingiberis Recens) and *Da Zao* (Fructus Jujubae) harmonize the herbs.

Tōng Qiào Huó Xuè Tāng

(Unblock the Orifices and Invigorate the Blood Decoction)

conditions characterized by blood stagnation in the head and face.

In this formula, *Chi Shao* (Radix Paeoniae Rubra), *Chuan Xiong* (Rhizoma Chuanxiong), *Tao Ren* (Semen Persicae), and *Hong Hua* (Flos Carthami) all activate blood circulation and eliminate blood stasis. *Lao Cong* (Herba Allii Fistulosi) unblocks stagnation and promotes the circulation of yang qi. *She Xiang* (Moschus) opens the sensory orifices and restores their normal functions. *Sheng Jiang* (Rhizoma Zingiberis Recens) and *Da Zao* (Fructus Jujubae) harmonize the herbs.

HUMAN CLINICAL STUDIES AND RESEARCH

1. **Concussion**: One study reported a marked effect using modified *Tong Qiao Huo Xue Tang* to treat concussion. The herbal formula contained *Chuan Xiong* (Rhizoma Chuanxiong) 20g, *Niu Xi* (Radix Achyranthis Bidentatae) 20g, *Fu Ling* (Poria) 20g, *Huang Jing* (Rhizoma Polygonati) 20g, *Mu Dan Pi* (Cortex Moutan) 20g, *Tao Ren* (Semen Persicae) 10g, *Hong Hua* (Flos Carthami) 10g, *Tu Bie Chong* (Eupolyphaga seu Steleophaga) 10g, *Shi Chang Pu* (Rhizoma Acori Tatarinowii) 10g, *Bai Zhi* (Radix Angelicae Dahuricae) 6g, *Xi Xin* (Radix et Rhizoma Asari) 3g, and *Bo He* (Herba Menthae) 3g. Of 61 patients, the study reported complete recovery in 14 cases after 4-6 packs of herbs, and in 47 cases after 8-14 packs.[1]
2. **Carbon monoxide poisoning**: Use of modified *Tong Qiao Huo Xue Tang* was effective in treating 11 patients with carbon monoxide poisoning. The herbal formula contained *She Xiang* (Moschus) 6g, *Chi Shao* (Radix Paeoniae Rubra) 30g, *Chuan Xiong* (Rhizoma Chuanxiong) 30g, *Tao Ren* (Semen Persicae) 30g, *Hong Hua* (Flos Carthami) 30g, *Dan Shen* (Radix et Rhizoma Salviae Miltiorrhizae) 30g, *Yu Jin* (Radix Curcumae) 30g, *Huang Qi* (Radix Astragali) 50g, *Dang Gui* (Radix Angelicae Sinensis) 50g, *Shi Chang Pu* (Rhizoma Acori Tatarinowii) 20g, and others. The herbs were ground into a fine powder and placed into capsules. The treatment protocol was to administer 3g of herbs in capsules twice daily after meals with an herbal tea made by cooking 3 slices of *Sheng Jiang* (Rhizoma Zingiberis Recens), 3 pieces of *Cong Bai* (Bulbus Allii Fistulosi), and 7 pieces of *Da Zao* (Fructus Jujubae) in equal portions of water and grain-based liquor. The herbs were given for 1 month per course of treatment. Of 11 patients, the study reported significant improvement in 7 cases, moderate improvement in 3 cases, and no improvement in 1 case. No side effects were reported.[2]

SUGGESTED ACUPUNCTURE TREATMENT

Xinshu (BL 15), *Geshu* (BL 17), *Xuehai* (SP 10), *Shangxing* (GV 23), *Longhui*, and *Hegu* (LI 4) effectively remove blood stagnation in the head.

AUTHORS' COMMENTS

Tong Qiao Huo Xue Tang can be used to treat traumatic proptosis to resolve blood stagnation after the globe has been replaced and intraocular hemorrhage has stopped; it works to resolve post-traumatic blood stagnation and promote the restoration of vision. Treatment can generally be started 5 days after the initial injury and used continuously for the following 2-3 weeks. It also has application in restoring hearing loss caused by the use of ototoxic drugs administered orally or applied topically as ear wash. It can be combined with *Yin Qiao San* (Honeysuckle and Forsythia Powder) and/or *Cang Er Zi San* (Xanthium Powder) to treat stubborn cases of sinusitis. In young animals that present with KCS, it can be combined with *Qi Ju Di Huang Wan* (Lycium Fruit, Chrysanthemum, and Rehmannia Pill) to help promote normal tear production in these cases. It can take 3-4 months to see the full clinical effects with this combination. If there is heat present, it should be combined with *Ming Mu Di Huang Wan* (Improve Vision Pill with Rehmannia).

Tong Qiao Huo Xue Tang is closely related to the formula *Xue Fu Zhu Yu Tang* (Drive Out Stasis in the Mansion of Blood Decoction); it was designed to treat conditions characterized by blood stagnation affecting the head and face. It originally contained *She Xiang* (Moschus) to open the sensory orifices to help restore the functions of sight and hearing. As this substance is no longer available because of its CITES status, it has been replaced by other herbs in some formulations; however, these replacement herbs are not considered to be as effective as the original. It also contains *Cong Bai* (Bulbus Allii Fistulosi), or spring scallions, which are warming and should be used with caution in yin and blood deficient animals. For these reasons, *Tong Qiao Huo Xue Tang* is not used as frequently as *Xue Fu Zhu Yu Tang* (Drive Out Stasis in the Mansion of Blood Decoction), a formula that is commonly used to treat the condition of blood stagnation affecting the chest.

The uses of *Xue Fu Zu Yu Tang* (Drive Out Stasis in the Mansion of Blood Decoction) have been greatly expanded since it was first developed; it can be used to treat conditions of blood stagnation involving the head, face and general circulation, in addition to the treatment of

Tōng Qiào Huó Xuè Tāng

(Unblock the Orifices and Invigorate the Blood Decoction)

conditions involving blood stagnation in the chest. The uses for *Tong Qiao Huo Xue Tang* in veterinary medicine are also very similar to that of *Xue Fu Zhu Yu Tang* because the two formulas have in common four herbs that move the blood: *Tao Ren* (Semen Persicae), *Hong Hua* (Flos Carthami), *Chuan Xiong* (Rhizoma Chuanxiong), and *Chi Shao* (Radix Paeoniae Rubra). *Xue Fu Zu Yu Tang*, however, contains two herbs that protect yin and blood from being injured: *Dang Gui* (Radix Angelicae Sinensis) and *Di Huang* (Radix Rehmanniae). Moreover, it has *Chai Hu* (Radix Bupleuri), *Zhi Qiao* (Fructus Aurantii) and *Jie Geng* (Radix Platycodonis) to move and regulate qi and to relieve Liver qi stagnation. For most cases then, *Xue Fu Zhu Yu Tang* is the formula of choice for treating conditions of the head and face, not *Tong Qiao Huo Xue Tang*.

References

1. *Shan Xi Zhong Yi* (Shanxi Chinese Medicine), 1991; 12(11):511.
2. *Shan Xi Zhong Yi* (Shanxi Chinese Medicine), 1990; 6(5):25.

Xuè Fǔ Zhú Yū Tāng

(Drive Out Stasis in the Mansion of Blood Decoction)

血府逐瘀湯
血府逐瘀汤

Pinyin Name: *Xue Fu Zhu Yu Tang*
Literal Name: Drive Out Stasis in the Mansion of Blood Decoction
Alternate Names: *Hsieh Fu Chu Yu Tang*, Blood-House Blood Stasis-Dispelling Decoction, Persica and Carthamus Combination
Original Source: *Yi Lin Gai Cuo* (Corrections of Errors Among Physicians) by Wang Qing-Ren in 1830

COMPOSITION

Tao Ren (Semen Persicae)	12g
Hong Hua (Flos Carthami)	9g
Di Huang (Radix Rehmanniae)	9g
Dang Gui (Radix Angelicae Sinensis)	9g
Chi Shao (Radix Paeoniae Rubra)	6g
Chuan Xiong (Rhizoma Chuanxiong)	4.5g
Chai Hu (Radix Bupleuri)	3g
Zhi Qiao (Fructus Citri Aurantii)	6g
Jie Geng (Radix Platycodonis)	4.5g
Chuan Niu Xi (Radix Cyathulae)	9g
Gan Cao (Radix et Rhizoma Glycyrrhizae)	6g

DOSAGE / PREPARATION / ADMINISTRATION

Prepare as a decoction.

CHINESE THERAPEUTIC ACTIONS

1. Activates blood circulation and dispels blood stagnation
2. Activates qi circulation and relieves pain

Xuè Fŭ Zhú Yū Tāng

(Drive Out Stasis in the Mansion of Blood Decoction)

CLINICAL MANIFESTATIONS

Blood stagnation in the chest and obstructed blood circulation: chronic, stabbing pain at a fixed location in the chest and/or the head, hypochondriac pain, dry heaves or vomiting after intake of water, palpitations, restless sleep, irritability, a dark red to purple tongue that may have petechiae spots, and a rapid, choppy or wiry, thready pulse.

VETERINARY CLINICAL APPLICATIONS

Head trauma, concussion, post-concussion syndrome, pneumothorax, physical injury to the chest, heart base tumor, cardiovascular disease, congestive heart failure, cardiomyopathy, arrhythmia, cardiac ischemia, bradyarrhythmia, hypertension, thromboembolic disease, stroke, cerebrovascular accident, temporomandibular joint dysplasia, craniomandibular osteopathy, masticatory myositis, temporal muscle atrophy, vasculitis secondary to snake bite, polyneuritis, cancer of the brain, nose, and liver, chronic non-healing wounds, hyperlipidemia, cholangiohepatitis and pancreatitis.

EXPLANATION

Xue Fu Zhu Yu Tang (Drive Out Stasis in the Mansion of Blood Decoction) treats various clinical manifestations induced by blood stagnation in the chest [the mansion of blood]. Blood stagnation in the chest may cause stabbing pain at a fixed location in the chest and hypochondrium. Blood stagnation may cause pain in the body, which, in turn, may lead to restlessness and irritability. Chronic blood stagnation may contribute to Liver qi stagnation, which, when overacting on the Stomach, may cause dry heaves and vomiting. Furthermore, chronic blood stasis contributes to heat formation, causing palpitations, irritability and restless sleep. A dry, dark red to purple tongue that may have petechiae spots and a rapid, choppy or wiry, thready pulse both indicate blood stagnation.

The design of this formula uses the principles of two formulas: *Tao Hong Si Wu Tang* (Four-Substance Decoction with Safflower and Peach Pit) to nourish the blood, activate blood circulation, and eliminate blood stasis; and *Si Ni San* (Frigid Extremities Powder) to activate qi circulation, harmonize the blood, and soothe the Liver.

In this formula, *Tao Ren* (Semen Persicae) and *Hong Hua* (Flos Carthami) are used to break up blood stagnation and activate blood circulation. *Di Huang* (Radix Rehmanniae), *Dang Gui* (Radix Angelicae Sinensis), *Chi Shao* (Radix Paeoniae Rubra), and *Chuan Xiong* (Rhizoma Chuanxiong) nourish the blood, activate blood circulation, and clear heat. *Chai Hu* (Radix Bupleuri) smoothes Liver qi to relieve chest pain. *Zhi Qiao* (Fructus Aurantii) regulates qi in the chest and the upper *jiao*. *Jie Geng* (Radix Platycodonis) guides all of the herbs upward to the chest. *Chuan Niu Xi* (Radix Cyathulae) unblocks stagnation in the blood vessels and guides blood downward. *Gan Cao*

***Xue Fu Zhu Yu Tang* (Drive Out Stasis in the Mansion of Blood Decoction)**

Diagnosis	Clinical Signs	Treatment	Herbs
Blood stagnation in the chest and obstructed blood circulation	• Chronic, stabbing pain at a fixed location in the chest and head, and hypochondriac pain: blood stagnation in the chest • Dry heaves and vomiting: reversed flow of Stomach qi due to blood stagnation • Palpitations, restless sleep, and irritability: *shen* (spirit) disturbance caused by blood stagnation • A dark red to purple tongue that may have petechiae spots and a rapid, choppy or wiry, thready pulse: blood stagnation	• Activates blood circulation and dispels blood stagnation • Activates qi and relieves pain	• *Tao Ren* (Semen Persicae) and *Hong Hua* (Flos Carthami) break up blood stagnation and activate blood circulation. • *Di Huang* (Radix Rehmanniae), *Dang Gui* (Radix Angelicae Sinensis), *Chi Shao* (Radix Paeoniae Rubra), and *Chuan Xiong* (Rhizoma Chuanxiong) nourish the blood, activate blood circulation, and clear heat. • *Chai Hu* (Radix Bupleuri) smoothes Liver qi, and *Zhi Qiao* (Fructus Aurantii) regulates qi in the chest and the upper *jiao*. • *Jie Geng* (Radix Platycodonis) guides all of the herbs upward to the chest. • *Chuan Niu Xi* (Radix Cyathulae) unblocks stagnation in the blood vessels and guides blood downward. • *Gan Cao* (Radix et Rhizoma Glycyrrhizae) harmonizes the formula.

Xuè Fŭ Zhú Yū Tāng

(Drive Out Stasis in the Mansion of Blood Decoction)

(Radix et Rhizoma Glycyrrhizae) harmonizes the formula. Overall, this formula has the unique and valuable attributes of activating blood circulation and dispelling blood stasis without injuring the blood, while also soothing the Liver and relieving qi stagnation without consuming qi.

VETERINARY MODIFICATIONS

- To improve ability to resolve blood stagnation and/or stasis add one or more of the following: *Dan Shen* (Radix et Rhizoma Salviae Miltiorrhizae), *Shui Zhi* (Hirudo) or *Di Long* (Pheretima).
- To improve pain relief, add *Yan Hu Suo* (Rhizoma Corydalis).
- With post-head trauma complications, add *Quan Xie* (Scorpio) and *Gao Ben* (Rhizoma et Radix Ligustici).
- With sinusitis and pain due to heat and blood stagnation, add *Bai Zhi* (Radix Angelicae Dahuricae), *Ban Lan Gen* (Radix Isatidis) and *Shi Gao* (Gypsum Fibrosum).
- With vestibular disease, add *Ju Hua* (Flos Chrysanthemi), *Gou Teng* (Ramulus Uncariae cum Uncis), and *Xia Ku Cao* (Spica Prunellae).
- With blood stagnation and yin deficiency, add *Liu Wei Di Huang Wan* (Six-Ingredient Pill with Rehmannia).
- With blood stagnation and yin-deficient heat, add *Zhi Bai Di Huang Wan* (Anemarrhena, Phellodendron, and Rehmannia Pill).
- With blood stagnation and qi deficiency, add *Ren Shen* (Radix et Rhizoma Ginseng) and *Huang Qi* (Radix Astragali).
- With cardiac arrhythmia, add *Fu Shen* (Poria Paradicis) and *Bai Zi Ren* (Semen Platycladi).
- With more chest pain, add *Dan Shen* (Radix et Rhizoma Salviae Miltiorrhizae), *Yan Hu Suo* (Rhizoma Corydalis) and *Jiang Xiang* (Lignum Dalbergiae Odoriferae).
- With liver cancer, add *Yu Jin* (Radix Curcumae), *Dan Shen* (Radix et Rhizoma Salviae Miltiorrhizae), *Chuan Lian Zi* (Fructus Toosendan) and *Bai Hua She She Cao* (Herba Hedyotis).
- To dissolve blood clots in animals with thromboembolism, add *Shui Zhi* (Hirudo), *Meng Chong* (Tabanus), *Da Huang* (Radix et Rhizoma Rhei), and *Tu Bie Chong* (Eupolyphaga seu Steleophaga).
- With neck and shoulder stiffness and pain, add *Ge Gen* (Radix Puerariae Lobatae), *Yan Hu Suo* (Rhizoma Corydalis) and *Qiang Huo* (Rhizoma et Radix Notopterygii).

CAUTIONS / CONTRAINDICATIONS

- *Xue Fu Zhu Yu Tang* is contraindicated in pregnancy because this formula strongly activates blood circulation and removes blood stasis.
- If this formula is to be taken for a prolonged period of time, blood-tonic herbs should be added accordingly.

PHARMACOLOGICAL EFFECTS

1. **Antiplatelet and anticoagulant**: Administration of *Xue Fu Zhu Yu Tang* was associated with a marked antiplatelet effect in animal subjects.[1,2] It also inhibits the formation of blood clots.[3] Lastly, it improves blood circulation by decreasing blood viscosity.[4]
2. **Cardiovascular**: Administration of *Xue Fu Zhu Yu Tang* was associated with reduced blood pressure, a response attributed to its effect to inhibit the rhythm and contractility of the heart. Furthermore, it has a regulatory effect on the blood vessels, causing them to relax or constrict.[5,6]
3. **Antihyperlipidemic**: Administration of *Xue Fu Zhu Yu Tang* in male rats at 16g/kg was associated with a reduction of plasma cholesterol levels. However, it did not affect the plasma glucose or triglyceride levels.[7]

HUMAN CLINICAL STUDIES AND RESEARCH

1. **Cardiac ischemia**: One study reported 89.3% effectiveness using modified *Xue Fu Zhu Yu Tang* to treat elderly patients with cardiac ischemia. Of 84 patients, the study reported significant improvement in 29 cases, moderate improvement in 46 cases, and no effect in 9 cases. The duration ranged from 1-3 courses of treatment.[8]
2. **Bradyarrhythmia**: One study reported 92.8% effectiveness using modified *Xue Fu Zhu Yu Tang* in decoction daily to treat 28 patients with bradyarrhythmia. The herbal treatment contained *Tao Ren* (Semen Persicae) 10g, *Dang Gui* (Radix Angelicae Sinensis) 10g, *Chi Shao* (Radix Paeoniae Rubra) 10g, *Niu Xi* (Radix Achyranthis Bidentatae) 10g, *Fu Zi* (Radix Aconiti Lateralis Praeparata) 10g, *Gua Lou Pi* (Pericarpium Trichosanthis) 10g, *Hong Hua* (Flos Carthami) 5g, *Chuan Xiong* (Rhizoma Chuanxiong) 5g, *Jie Geng* (Radix Platycodonis) 5g, *Gan Cao* (Radix et Rhizoma Glycyrrhizae) 3g, and *Huang Qi* (Radix Astragali) 15g. Of 28 patients, the study reported complete recovery in 14 cases, improvement in 12 cases, and no effect in 2 cases.[9]
3. **Pneumothorax**: One study reported complete recovery in all 12 patients with pneumothorax after 2-4 weeks of treatment with *Xue Fu Zhu Yu Tang*.[10]
4. **Hepatitis**: Administration of modified *Xue Fu Zhu Yu Tang* in decoction in 81 patients with chronic hepatitis was associated with complete recovery in 67 cases, improvement in 8 cases, and no effect in 6 cases. The overall effectiveness was 92.6%. In addition to the base formula, modifications were made as follows: *Huang Qin* (Radix Scutellariae) and *Zhi Zi* (Fructus Gardeniae) were added for dry mouth with bitter taste, yellow urine, and

Xuè Fǔ Zhú Yū Tāng

(Drive Out Stasis in the Mansion of Blood Decoction)

yellow greasy tongue coating; *Fu Ling* (Poria) and *Bai Zhu* (Rhizoma Atractylodis Macrocephalae) were added for abdominal fullness, loose stools, and a pale tongue body with a white coating; and *Shu Di Huang* (Radix Rehmanniae Praeparata) and *Gou Qi Zi* (Fructus Lycii) for *wu xin re* (five-center heat), soreness and weakness of the lower back and knees, and a red tongue body with a thin coating.[11]

5. **Pancreatitis**: One study reported complete recovery in 128 patients using integrated treatments of herbs and drugs. The herbal treatment included modified *Xue Fu Zhu Yu Tang* in decoction daily for 7 days per course of treatment. Western treatment included drugs and intravenous fluids (specific details were unavailable). Instructions were also given to follow a low-fat, high-protein, and high carbohydrate diet. The study reported complete recovery in all 128 patients within 3 courses of treatment.[12]
6. **Insomnia**: Use of modified *Xue Fu Zhu Yu Tang* was associated with 93.5% effectiveness in treating 31 patients with stubborn insomnia. The base formula contained *Xue Fu Zhu Yu Tang*, with addition of *Shou Wu Teng* (Caulis Polygoni Multiflori) and *Hu Po* (Succinum), and elimination of *Chai Hu* (Radix Bupleuri) and *Chuan Xiong* (Rhizoma Chuanxiong). Modifications were made based on the condition of the patients. *Dang Shen* (Radix Codonopsis) and *Huang Qi* (Radix Astragali) were added for qi deficiency; *Shu Di Huang* (Radix Rehmanniae Praeparata) and *E Jiao* (Colla Corii Asini) were added for blood deficiency; *Gou Qi Zi* (Fructus Lycii) and *Shan Zhu Yu* (Fructus Corni) were added for yin deficiency; and *Chen Pi* (Pericarpium Citri Reticulatae) and *Ban Xia* (Rhizoma Pinelliae) were added to clear hot phlegm.[13]
7. **Phlebitis**: Administration of modified *Xue Fu Zhu Yu Tang* has been shown to effectively treat phlebitis. In addition to the base formula, *Mu Dan Pi* (Cortex Moutan) was added for redness and swelling associated with heat in the *xue* (blood) level; *San Qi* (Radix et Rhizoma Notoginseng) was added for blood vessel pain with swelling and inflammation; and *Huang Qi* (Radix Astragali) was added for a fine, weak pulse. Each course of treatment was 7 days. Of 38 patients, the study reported significant benefit in 8 cases, moderate improvement in 29 cases, and no effect in 1 case.[14] Another study reported marked effects using herbs orally and topically to treat phlebitis. The herbal formula for oral ingestion contained *Xue Fu Zhu Yu Tang* plus *Zhe Bei Mu* (Bulbus Fritillariae Thunbergii) and *Di Long* (Pheretima), and was given daily for 15 days per course of treatment. Herbs also were applied topically to the affected area twice daily to relieve pain. Of 12 patients, the study reported complete recovery in 9 cases, improvement in 2 cases, and no effect in 1 case. The overall effectiveness was 92%.[15]
8. **Mammary gland hyperplasia**: According to one study, 104 patients with mammary gland hyperplasia were treated with complete recovery in 68 cases and moderate improvement in 27 cases (91.4% effectiveness). The herbal treatment contained *Xue Fu Zhu Yu Tang* as the base formula, with the addition of *San Leng* (Rhizoma Sparganii) and *E Zhu* (Rhizoma Curcumae), and removal of *Di Huang* (Radix Rehmanniae) and *Jie Geng* (Radix Platycodonis). Other herbs were added if deemed necessary.[16]
9. **Pelvic inflammatory disease**: One study reported 92% effectiveness using modified *Xue Fu Zhu Yu Tang* to treat 60 patients with chronic pelvic inflammatory disease. Modifications included the addition of *Xiao Hui Xiang* (Fructus Foeniculi) and *Pao Jiang* (Rhizoma Zingiberis Praeparatum) for cold sensations in the lower abdomen; *Pu Gong Ying* (Herba Taraxaci) and *Zi Hua Di Ding* (Herba Violae) for toxic heat; and *Yi Yi Ren* (Semen Coicis) for dampness. Of 60 patients, the study reported complete recovery in 24 cases, improvement in 31 cases, and no response in 5 cases.[17]
10. **Concussion**: One study reported 92.3% effectiveness for 12 patients with concussion using modified *Xue Fu Zhu Yu Tang*. The herbal treatment contained this formula plus *Shi Chang Pu* (Rhizoma Acori Tatarinowii) 10g, *Yuan Zhi* (Radix Polygalae) 15g, *Dan Shen* (Radix et Rhizoma Salviae Miltiorrhizae) 25g, *Mai Dong* (Radix Ophiopogonis) 16g, and *Suan Zao Ren* (Semen Ziziphi Spinosae) 13g. The herbs were given in decoction daily.[18]
11. **Stroke**: Benefit in the prevention and treatment of stroke and ischemia has been associated with many Chinese herbal formulas, including *Xue Fu Zhu Yu Tang*, *Bu Yang Huan Wu Tang* (Tonify the Yang to Restore Five Decoction), *Xiao Xu Ming Tang* (Minor Prolong-Life Decoction), and *Chai Hu Jia Long Gu Mu Li Tang* (Bupleurum plus Dragon Bone and Oyster Shell Decoction). The mechanisms of these beneficial effects were attributed to anti-hypercholesterolemia, antioxidant activity, and free radical scavenger effects of these formulas.[19]
12. **Cerebral atherosclerosis**: Sixty-three patients were treated with excellent results using modified *Xue Fu Zhu Yu Tang* plus ear acupuncture. The herbal treatment contained *Dang Gui* (Radix Angelicae Sinensis) 15-20g, *Di Huang* (Radix Rehmanniae) 5g, *Tian Ma* (Rhizoma Gastrodiae) 5g, *Tao Ren* (Semen Persicae) 9g, *Zhi Qiao* (Fructus Aurantii) 9g, *Chuan Xiong* (Rhizoma Chuanxiong) 9g, *Hong Hua* (Flos Carthami) 6g, *Chai Hu* (Radix Bupleuri) 6g, *Gan Cao* (Radix et Rhizoma Glycyrrhizae) 6g, *Niu Xi* (Radix Achyranthis Bidentatae)

Xuè Fǔ Zhú Yū Tāng

(Drive Out Stasis in the Mansion of Blood Decoction)

10g, *Chi Shao* (Radix Paeoniae Rubra) 10g, and *Dan Shen* (Radix et Rhizoma Salviae Miltiorrhizae) 15-30g. The duration of treatment ranged from 1-6 months. Of 63 patients, the study reported complete recovery in 42 cases, improvement in 13 cases, and no effect in 8 cases.[20]

13. **Hyperlipidemia**: Use of *Xue Fu Zhu Yu Tang* was associated with 95% effectiveness in reducing cholesterol and triglyceride levels. Of 20 patients, the study reported significant improvement in 11 cases, moderate improvement in 8 cases, and no effect in 1 case.[21]
14. **Schizophrenia**: According to one study of 66 schizophrenic patients with 3 months to 23 years history of illness, use of modified *Xue Fu Zhu Yu Tang* was associated with marked beneficial effects. The herbal treatment contained *Chai Hu* (Radix Bupleuri) 15g, *Hong Hua* (Flos Carthami) 10g, *Chi Shao* (Radix Paeoniae Rubra) 30g, *Chuan Xiong* (Rhizoma Chuanxiong) 15g, *Dan Shen* (Radix et Rhizoma Salviae Miltiorrhizae) 30g, and *Jiang Xiang* (Lignum Dalbergiae Odoriferae) 15g. Modifications were made by adding *Xiang Fu* (Rhizoma Cyperi) to regulate qi, *Da Huang* (Radix et Rhizoma Rhei) to clear heat, *Fu Ling* (Poria) and *Bai Zhu* (Rhizoma Atractylodis Macrocephalae) to strengthen the Spleen, and *Dang Shen* (Radix Codonopsis) and *Huang Qi* (Radix Astragali) to tonify qi. The treatment protocol was to cook the herbs in water and administer the decoction in two equally-divided doses daily for 8 weeks per course of treatment. In addition to Chinese herbs, a small dose of antipsychotic medication (selection depended on the condition of the patient) was given daily.[22]
15. **Endometriosis**: Use of *Xue Fu Zhu Yu Tang* was associated with 94% effectiveness in the treatment of 83 patients with endometriosis, using herbs orally and rectally. The herbal formula for oral ingestion contained *Dang Gui* (Radix Angelicae Sinensis) 9g, *Di Huang* (Radix Rehmanniae) 9g, *Hong Hua* (Flos Carthami) 9g, *Chi Shao* (Radix Paeoniae Rubra) 9g, *Niu Xi* (Radix Achyranthis Bidentatae) 9g, *Zhi Qiao* (Fructus Aurantii) 6g, *Jie Geng* (Radix Platycodonis) 6g, *Chuan Xiong* (Rhizoma Chuanxiong) 6g, *Gan Cao* (Radix et Rhizoma Glycyrrhizae) 6g, *Chai Hu* (Radix Bupleuri) 3g, and *Tao Ren* (Semen Persicae) 12g. Modifications were made by adding *Xi Xin* (Radix et Rhizoma Asari) and *Fu Zi* (Radix Aconiti Lateralis Praeparata) for blood stagnation with cold; *Chuan Lian Zi* (Fructus Toosendan), *Pu Huang* (Pollen Typhae), and *Wu Ling Zhi* (Faeces Trogopteri) for qi and blood stagnation; *Da Xue Teng* (Caulis Sargentodoxae) and *Bai Jiang Cao* (Herba cum Radice Patriniae) for blood stagnation with heat; *Huang Qi* (Radix Astragali), *Dang Shen* (Radix Codonopsis), and *Mu Xiang* (Radix Aucklandiae) for blood stagnation with qi deficiency; *San Leng* (Rhizoma Sparganii) and *E Zhu* (Rhizoma Curcumae) for nodules and cysts; and *Yin Yang Huo* (Herba Epimedii), *Xian Mao* (Rhizoma Curculiginis) and *Tu Si Zi* (Semen Cuscutae) for infertility. The herbs were given as decoction in two equally-divided doses. Herbs also were given as rectal enema one time daily, with an herbal solution made from *San Leng* (Rhizoma Sparganii) 10g, *E Zhu* (Rhizoma Curcumae) 10g, *Da Xue Teng* (Caulis Sargentodoxae) 12g, *Zao Jiao Ci* (Spina Gleditsiae) 12g, *Feng Fang* (Nidus Vespae) 12g, *Chi Shao* (Radix Paeoniae Rubra) 12g, and *Tao Ren* (Semen Persicae) 6g. Of 83 patients, the study reported complete recovery in 41 cases, significant improvement in 27 cases, moderate improvement in 10 cases, and no improvement in 5 cases.[23]

SUGGESTED ACUPUNCTURE TREATMENT

1. Points: *Weishu* (BL 21), *Housanli* (ST 36), *Sanyinjiao* (SP 6), *Xinshu* (BL 15), *Geshu* (BL 17), *Xuehai* (SP 10), *Neiguan* (PC 6), *Gongsun* (SP 4), *Yangchi* (TH 4), and *Xingjian* (LR 2).
2. Techniques: tonification and sedation.

Weishu (BL 21), *Housanli* (ST 36), *Sanyinjiao* (SP 6), *Xinshu* (BL 15), *Geshu* (BL 17), and *Xuehai* (SP 10) activate qi, break up blood stagnation, and nourish both qi and blood. *Neiguan* (PC 6) and *Gongsun* (SP 4) relieve chest congestion. *Yangchi* (TH 4) regulates *shaoyang* qi. *Xingjian* (LR 2) regulates Liver qi. Combined, these points relieve blood stagnation and pain.

AUTHORS' COMMENTS

Xue Fu Zhu Yu Tang was used originally to treat blood stasis in the chest and upper *jiao*. Today, its clinical application has been expanded, and this formula has been proven effective in treating a wide variety of conditions in veterinary medicine characterized by blood stagnation and stasis affecting the head, including:

- adenocarcinoma and fibrosarcoma of the nasal cavity
- masticatory myositis
- chronic corneal ulcers and corneal degeneration
- pancreatitis
- chronic cholangiohepatitis, cholecystitis.
- pneumothorax, broken ribs and other physical injury to the chest
- head trauma and concussion secondary to vehicular or blunt trauma, or fighting
- cardiovascular disease: congestive heart failure (CHF), cardiomyopathy, and arrhythmia. It supports normal blood circulation in animals with cardiovascular disease and is an effective herbal supplement for cardiac health

Xuè Fǔ Zhú Yū Tāng

(Drive Out Stasis in the Mansion of Blood Decoction)

and as a preventative measure against development of thromboembolism in patients with cardiomyopathy.

Furthermore, with appropriate additions and/or modifications, *Xue Fu Zhu Yu Tang* is also effective in treating the following conditions:

- For chronic sinusitis, add *Yin Qiao San* (Honeysuckle and Forsythia Powder) or *Cang Er Zi San* (Xanthium Powder), depending on the condition. To improve the formula's ability to clear heat and toxins, add herbs such as *Yu Xing Ca* (Herba Houttuyniae), *Zi Hua Di Ding* (Herba Violae), *Ma Bian Cao* (Herba Verbenae), *Chuan Xin Lian* (Herba Andrographis), *Da Qing Ye* (Folium Isatidis), and *Ban Lan Gen* (Radix Isatidis).
- For brain tumors, add *Quan Xie* (Scorpio), *Wu Gong* (Scolopendra), *Jiang Can* (Bombyx Batryticatus), *Di Long* (Pheretima), *Ji Xue Teng* (Caulis Spatholobi), and *Bai Hua She She Cao* (Herba Hedyotis).
- For liver cancer, combine with *Ge Xia Zhu Yu Tang* (Drive Out Blood Stasis Below the Diaphragm Decoction) in equal amounts.
- For progressive retinal atrophy, combine with *Qi Ju Di Huang Wan* (Lycium Fruit, Chrysanthemum, and Rehmannia Pill).
- For thromboembolic disease, combine with *Dan Shen* (Radix et Rhizoma Salviae Miltiorrhizae) and *Shui Zhi* (Hirudo).

There are four "*zhu yu tang* (drive out stasis decoction)" formulas that are commonly used for similar conditions. All four formulas contain *Chuan Xiong* (Rhizoma Chuanxiong), *Dang Gui* (Radix Angelicae Sinensis), *Tao Ren* (Semen Persicae), and *Hong Hua* (Flos Carthami) as key ingredients to activate the blood, eliminate blood stasis, and relieve pain. Their main differences are as follows:

- *Xue Fu Zhu Yu Tang* (Drive Out Stasis in the Mansion of Blood Decoction) treats qi and blood stagnation in the upper *jiao* to alleviate pain in the chest and hypochondrium. It has actions to relieve Liver qi stagnation and regulate the qi mechanism. It has less ability to relieve pain than the other formulas in this class and will require modification as needed to address conditions with significant pain.
- *Ge Xia Zhu Yu Tang* (Drive Out Blood Stasis Below the Diaphragm Decoction) treats qi and blood stagnation in the middle *jiao* to alleviate pain below the diaphragm, including the Liver and upper abdominal area.
- *Shao Fu Zhu Yu Tang* (Drive Out Blood Stasis in the Lower Abdomen Decoction) treats pain and qi and blood stagnation with cold in the lower *jiao*; it is also used to address infertility and mass formation in the lower *jiao*. It contains *Rou Gui* (Cortex Cinnamomi), *Xiao Hui Xiang* (Fructus Foeniculi), and *Gan Jiang* (Rhizoma Zingiberis) and is very warming; thus, it should not be used without modification in animals with yin deficiency and heat.
- *Shen Tong Zhu Yu Tang* (Drive Out Blood Stasis from a Painful Body Decoction) treats qi and blood stagnation with painful obstruction of the channels, collaterals and the whole body. It is commonly used to treat acute and/or chronic pain in the whole body (generalized) arising from blood stagnation/stasis in the extremities and joints.

References

1. *Zhong Yao Yao Li Yu Lin Chuang* (Pharmacology and Clinical Applications of Chinese Herbs), 1993; 9(1):8.
2. *Zhong Hua Nei Ke Xue Za Zhi* (Journal of Chinese Internal Medicine), 1977; 2(2):79.
3. *Zhong Yao Yao Li Yu Lin Chuang* (Pharmacology and Clinical Applications of Chinese Herbs), 1993; 9(5):9.
4. *Zhong Guo Yi Yao Xue Bao* (Chinese Journal of Medicine and Herbology), 1990; 5(4):33.
5. *Zhong Yao Yao Li Yu Lin Chuang* (Pharmacology and Clinical Applications of Chinese Herbs), 1993; 9(1):8.
6. *Zhong Guo Yi Yao Xue Bao* (Chinese Journal of Medicine and Herbology), 1990; 5(4):33.
7. *Shan Xi Zhong Yi* (Shanxi Chinese Medicine), 1988; 9(3):126.
8. *Zhe Jiang Zhong Yi Za Zhi* (Zhejiang Journal of Chinese Medicine), 1997; 10:445.
9. *Zhe Jiang Zhong Yi Xue Yuan Xue Bao* (Journal of Zhejiang University of Chinese Medicine), 1992; 16(3):19.
10. *He Nan Zhong Yi* (Henan Chinese Medicine), 1990; 10(1):33.
11. *Jiang Su Zhong Yi* (Jiangsu Chinese Medicine), 1995; 7:10.
12. *Shi Yong Zhong Yi Yao Za Zhi* (Journal of Practical Chinese Medicine and Medicinals), 1994; 10(4):27.
13. *Xin Zhong Yi* (New Chinese Medicine), 1996; 8:32.
14. *Zhe Jiang Zhong Yi Za Zhi* (Zhejiang Journal of Chinese Medicine), 1997; 4:157.
15. *Shi Yong Zhong Yi Nei Ke Za Zhi* (Journal of Practical Chinese Internal Medicine), 1992; 6(3):21.
16. *Tian Jin Zhong Yi* (Tianjin Chinese Medicine), 1986; 5:18.
17. *Gan Su Zhong Yi* (Gansu Chinese Medicine), 1995; 4:34.
18. *Shan Xi Zhong Yi* (Shanxi Chinese Medicine), 1993; 14(5):222.
19. Lin CC, Yen FL, Hsu FF, Lin JM. Anti-hypercholesterolaemia, antioxidant activity and free radical scavenger effects of traditional Chinese medicine prescriptions used for stroke. Journal of Pharmacy & Pharmacology. 2000 Nov; 52(11):1387-93.
20. *Hu Nan Zhong Yi Za Zhi* (Hunan Journal of Chinese Medicine), 1993; 9(1):41.
21. *Zhong Xi Yi Jie He Za Zhi* (Journal of Integrated Chinese and Western Medicine), 1988; 8(10):601.
22. *Zhong Guo Zhong Xi Yi Jie He Za Zhi* (Chinese Journal of Integrative Chinese and Western Medicine), 1993; 13(7):397.
23. *Shang Hai Zhong Yi Yao Za Zhi* (Shanghai Journal of Chinese Medicine and Herbology), 1993; 2:16.

Gé Xià Zhú Yū Tāng

(Drive Out Blood Stasis Below the Diaphragm Decoction)

膈下逐瘀湯
膈下逐瘀汤

Pinyin Name: *Ge Xia Zhu Yu Tang*
Literal Name: Drive Out Blood Stasis Below the Diaphragm Decoction
Alternate Name: Tangkuei and Corydalis Combination
Original Source: *Yi Lin Gai Cuo* (Corrections of Errors Among Physicians) by Wang Qing-Ren in 1830

COMPOSITION

Tao Ren (Semen Persicae), *yan* (ground) until muddy	9g
Hong Hua (Flos Carthami)	9g
Dang Gui (Radix Angelicae Sinensis)	9g
Chuan Xiong (Rhizoma Chuanxiong)	6g
Mu Dan Pi (Cortex Moutan)	6g
Chi Shao (Radix Paeoniae Rubra)	6g
Zhi Qiao (Fructus Citri Aurantii)	4.5g
Wu Yao (Radix Linderae)	6g
Xiang Fu (Rhizoma Cyperi)	4.5g
Wu Ling Zhi (Faeces Trogopteri), *chao* (dry-fried)	9g
Yan Hu Suo (Rhizoma Corydalis)	3g
Gan Cao (Radix et Rhizoma Glycyrrhizae)	9g

DOSAGE / PREPARATION / ADMINISTRATION

Prepare as a decoction.

CHINESE THERAPEUTIC ACTIONS

1. Activates blood circulation and dispels blood stagnation
2. Activates qi circulation and relieves pain

CLINICAL MANIFESTATIONS

Blood stagnation below the diaphragm: palpable mass in the abdomen caused by blood stasis.

VETERINARY CLINICAL APPLICATIONS

Acute and chronic cholangiohepatitis, liver cirrhosis, cholecystitis, liver cancer, jaundice, splenomegaly, prostatic hypertrophy, heart base tumor (chemodectoma, aortic body tumor), cardiac hemangiosarcoma, and tumors of the intestines and urinary bladder.

EXPLANATION

Ge Xia Zhu Yu Tang (Drive Out Blood Stasis Below the Diaphragm Decoction) activates qi and blood circulation, removes blood stagnation, and relieves pain in the region below the diaphragm. Because blood stagnation below the diaphragm is the underlying cause of the illness, the animal may experience severe pain and swelling. Additionally, blood stagnation often presents as a mass or hardness in the abdominal region. The animal may show clinical signs such as fixed abdominal pain and a palpable mass in the abdomen.

Tao Ren (Semen Persicae) and *Hong Hua* (Flos Carthami) break up blood stagnation and activate blood circulation. These two herbs have synergistic effects and are often used together. *Dang Gui* (Radix Angelicae Sinensis) and *Chuan Xiong* (Rhizoma Chuanxiong) nourish the blood and activate blood circulation. The pairing of these herbs points to the fact that blood-tonifying herbs are commonly combined with blood-activating herbs to prevent tonification from turning into stagnation. *Mu Dan Pi* (Cortex Moutan) and *Chi Shao* (Radix Paeoniae Rubra) clear heat, cool the blood, and dispel blood stagnation. Because blood stagnation and qi stagnation often occur simultaneously, *Zhi Qiao* (Fructus Aurantii), *Wu Yao* (Radix Linderae), and *Xiang Fu* (Rhizoma Cyperi) are employed to activate and regulate qi circulation. *Zhi Qiao* (Fructus Aurantii) breaks up stagnation; *Wu Yao* (Radix Linderae) stimulates peristalsis of the intestines; and *Xiang Fu* (Rhizoma Cyperi) relieves pain. Because patients with blood stasis often experience severe pain, *Wu Ling Zhi* (Faeces Trogopteri) and *Yan Hu Suo* (Rhizoma Corydalis) are added to dispel blood stasis and relieve pain. Lastly, *Gan Cao* (Radix et Rhizoma Glycyrrhizae) tonifies qi and harmonizes the herbs in this formula.

Gé Xià Zhú Yū Tāng

(Drive Out Blood Stasis Below the Diaphragm Decoction)

Ge Xia Zhu Yu Tang **(Drive Out Blood Stasis Below the Diaphragm Decoction)**

Diagnosis	Clinical Signs	Treatment	Herbs
Blood stagnation below the diaphragm	Abdominal pain in a fixed location, and the presence of a mass or hardness in the abdomen: blood stagnation in the middle *jiao* area	• Activates blood circulation and dispels blood stagnation • Activates qi circulation and relieves pain	• *Tao Ren* (Semen Persicae) and *Hong Hua* (Flos Carthami) break up blood stagnation and activate blood circulation. • *Dang Gui* (Radix Angelicae Sinensis) and *Chuan Xiong* (Rhizoma Chuanxiong) nourish the blood and activate blood circulation. • *Mu Dan Pi* (Cortex Moutan) and *Chi Shao* (Radix Paeoniae Rubra) clear heat, cool the blood, and dispel blood stagnation. • *Zhi Qiao* (Fructus Aurantii), *Wu Yao* (Radix Linderae), and *Xiang Fu* (Rhizoma Cyperi) regulate qi circulation and relieve pain. • *Wu Ling Zhi* (Faeces Trogopteri) and *Yan Hu Suo* (Rhizoma Corydalis) dispel blood stasis and relieve pain. • *Gan Cao* (Radix et Rhizoma Glycyrrhizae) tonifies qi and harmonizes all of the herbs in this formula.

VETERINARY MODIFICATIONS

- With qi deficiency, add *Si Jun Zi Tang* (Four-Gentlemen Decoction).
- For chronic hepatitis, jaundice and liver cirrhosis, combine with *Yin Chen Wu Ling San* (Artemisia Scoparia and Five-Ingredient Powder with Poria), *Jia Wei Xiao Yao San* (Augmented Rambling Powder), or *Xiao Chai Hu Tang* (Minor Bupleurum Decoction). *San Qi* (Radix et Rhizoma Notoginseng), *E Zhu* (Rhizoma Curcumae), and *Bie Jia* (Carapax Trionycis) are also useful and can be added to these formulas.
- For liver cancer, add *Xiao Chai Hu Tang* (Minor Bupleurum Decoction), *Ban Zhi Lian* (Herba Scutellariae Barbatae), *San Leng* (Rhizoma Sparganii) and *Bai Hua She She Cao* (Herba Hedyotis).
- For cirrhosis of the liver and hepatitis, add *Chai Hu* (Radix Bupleuri), *Ban Lan Gen* (Radix Isatidis), *Huang Jing* (Rhizoma Polygonati), *Huang Qi* (Radix Astragali), *Gou Qi Zi* (Fructus Lycii), and *Ren Shen* (Radix et Rhizoma Ginseng).
- For nasal adenocarcinoma, combine with *San Zhong Kui Jian Tang* (Disperse the Swelling and Break the Hardness Decoction) and *Xia Ku Cao* (Spica Prunellae).
- For chronic cholecystitis, combine with *Yin Chen Wu Ling San* (Artemisia Scoparia and Five-Ingredient Powder with Poria), *Huang Lian Jie Du Tang* (Coptis Decoction to Relieve Toxicity), and *Jin Yin Hua* (Flos Lonicerae Japonicae).
- For bladder tumors, combine with *Bie Jia* (Carapax Trionycis), *E Zhu* (Rhizoma Curcumae), and *San Leng* (Rhizoma Sparganii).

CAUTIONS / CONTRAINDICATIONS

Use of this formula is contraindicated during pregnancy.[1]

HUMAN CLINICAL STUDIES AND RESEARCH

1. **Hematoporphyria**: Use of *Ge Xia Zhu Yu Tang* was associated with complete recovery in all 8 patients with hematoporphyria characterized by qi and blood stagnation, with clinical signs such as hypochondriac or upper abdominal pain that intensifies at night, and urine with red, yellow, or coffee-ground color.[2]
2. **Hepatitis**: Use of *Ge Xia Zhu Yu Tang* in 25 patients with chronic active hepatitis was associated with alleviating pain, improving appetite, resolving jaundice, and relieving ascites.[3]
3. **Hepatic hemangioma**: Use of *Ge Xia Zhu Yu Tang* plus *Meng Chong* (Tabanus) and *San Leng* (Rhizoma Sparganii) was associated with 86% effectiveness in treating hepatic hemangioma. Modifications to the base formula were made as follows: *Huang Qi* (Radix Astragali), *Shan Yao* (Rhizoma Dioscoreae), and *Dan Shen* (Radix et Rhizoma Salviae Miltiorrhizae) for chronic hepatitis; *Bie Jia* (Carapax Trionycis) and *Mu Li* (Concha Ostreae) for liver cirrhosis; *Chai Hu* (Radix Bupleuri), *Huang Qin* (Radix Scutellariae), and *Yu Jin* (Radix Curcumae) for chronic cholecystitis; and *Jiang Xiang* (Lignum Dalbergiae Odoriferae), *Mu Xiang* (Radix Aucklandiae), and *Shan Zha* (Fructus Crataegi) for epigastric pain. Of 32 patients, the study reported complete recovery in 12 cases, significant improvement in 5 cases, moderate improvement in 12 cases, and no benefit in 3 cases.[4]

Gé Xià Zhú Yū Tāng

(Drive Out Blood Stasis Below the Diaphragm Decoction)

4. **Prostatic hypertrophy**: One study reported 90% effectiveness using modified *Ge Xia Zhu Yu Tang* to treat 22 patients with prostatic hypertrophy. The herbal treatment was based on this formula, with the addition of *Hua Shi* (Talcum) and the removal of *Wu Ling Zhi* (Faeces Trogopteri) and *Yan Hu Suo* (Rhizoma Corydalis). Furthermore, *Nu Zhen Zi* (Fructus Ligustri Lucidi), *Shan Zhu Yu* (Fructus Corni) and *Wu Wei Zi* (Fructus Schisandrae Chinensis) were added for Kidney yin deficiency; *Gui Zhi* (Ramulus Cinnamomi) and *Mu Hu Die* (Semen Oroxyli) were added for Kidney qi deficiency; and *Dang Shen* (Radix Codonopsis) and *Huang Qi* (Radix Astragali) were added for qi deficiency. Of 22 patients, the study reported recovery in 17 cases, improvement in 3 cases, and no effect in 2 cases.[5]
5. **Chronic colitis**: Use of modified *Ge Xia Zhu Yu Tang* in 75 patients with chronic colitis was associated with complete recovery in 63 cases, significant improvement in 9 cases, and improvement in 3 cases. The duration of treatment ranged from 3-9 days in most cases, with some cases requiring up to 40 days to resolve. The herbal formula contained *Dang Gui* (Radix Angelicae Sinensis) 9-12g, *Chi Shao* (Radix Paeoniae Rubra) 6-9g, *Xiang Fu* (Rhizoma Cyperi) 6-9g, *Wu Yao* (Radix Linderae) 6-9g, *Wu Ling Zhi* (Faeces Trogopteri) 6-9g, *Zhi Qiao* (Fructus Aurantii) 6-9g, *Hong Hua* (Flos Carthami) 6g, and *Chuan Xiong* (Rhizoma Chuanxiong) 6g. Furthermore, modifications were made by adding *Dang Shen* (Radix Codonopsis) 9-12g and *Yi Yi Ren* (Semen Coicis) 12-15g for chronic illness; *Da Huang* (Radix et Rhizoma Rhei) 6-9g and *Huo Ma Ren* (Fructus Cannabis) 9-12g for difficulties with bowel movement; *Bai Jiang Cao* (Herba cum Radice Patriniae) 9-12g for deficiency heat; *Fu Zi* (Radix Aconiti Lateralis Praeparata) 3-5g for deficiency and cold; and *Da Huang* (Radix et Rhizoma Rhei), *Bai Tou Weng* (Radix Pulsatillae) and *Ma Chi Xian* (Herba Portulacae) for chronic ulcerative colitis with rectal tenesmus and mucous and blood in the stools.[6]
6. **Peptic ulcer disease**: One study reported that modified *Ge Xia Zhu Yu Tang* was effective in treating gastric or duodenal ulcer in 30 patients (24 males and 6 females, between 20-60 years of age, with 1-18 years history of illness). The herbal treatment contained *Dang Gui* (Radix Angelicae Sinensis) 10g, *Chi Shao* (Radix Paeoniae Rubra) 5g, *Wu Ling Zhi* (Faeces Trogopteri) 5g, *Chuan Xiong* (Rhizoma Chuanxiong) 4g, *Tao Ren* (Semen Persicae) 5g, *Mu Dan Pi* (Cortex Moutan) 5g, *Wu Yao* (Radix Linderae) 6g, *Yan Hu Suo* (Rhizoma Corydalis) 10g, *Gan Cao* (Radix et Rhizoma Glycyrrhizae) 8g, *Xiang Fu* (Rhizoma Cyperi) 10g, and *Zhi Qiao* (Fructus Aurantii) 5g. After 3 months of herbal treatment in 30 patients, the study reported significant improvement in 18 cases, moderate improvement in 9 cases, and no effect in 3 cases.[7]

SUGGESTED ACUPUNCTURE TREATMENT

1. Points: *Weishu* (BL 21), *Housanli* (ST 36), *Sanyinjiao* (SP 6), *Xinshu* (BL 15), *Geshu* (BL 17), *Xuehai* (SP 10), *Taichong* (LR 3), *Yanglingquan* (GB 34), and *Qimen* (LR 14).
2. Techniques: tonification and sedation

Tonify *Weishu* (BL 21), *Housanli* (ST 36), *Sanyinjiao* (SP 6), *Xinshu* (BL 15), *Geshu* (BL 17), and *Xuehai* (SP 10) to activate qi, break up blood stagnation, and nourish qi and blood. Sedate *Xinshu* (BL 15), *Geshu* (BL 17), *Xuehai* (SP 10), *Taichong* (LR 3), *Yanglingquan* (GB 34), and *Qimen* (LR 14) to remove blood stagnation below the diaphragm.

AUTHORS' COMMENTS

Ge Xia Zhu Yu Tang treats conditions of blood stasis located below the diaphragm, including conditions involving palpable, fixed abdominal masses. The clinical applications of this formula in veterinary medicine have been expanded to include: treatment of various tumors of the abdomen, relief of persistent abdominal pain post-surgery, and acute and chronic liver disease.

According to Dr. Chang Wei-Yen, *Ge Xia Zhu Yu Tang* can be combined with *Xue Fu Zhu Yu Tang* (Drive Out Stasis in the Mansion of Blood Decoction), *Zhe Chong Yin* (Break the Conflict Decoction), *Shui Zhi* (Hirudo), and *Yan Hu Suo* (Rhizoma Corydalis) to treat chronic blood stasis of the whole body manifesting in pain and other complex, difficult-to-treat conditions.

References

1. *Zhong Yao Ming Fang Yao Li Yu Ying Yong* (Pharmacology and Applications of Famous Herbal Formulas), 1989; 516-518.
2. *Xin Zhong Yi* (New Chinese Medicine), 1976; 4:35.
3. *Xin Yi Yao Xue Za Zhi* (New Journal of Medicine and Herbology), 1978; 9:44.
4. *Jiang Su Zhong Yi* (Jiangsu Chinese Medicine), 1997; 8:21.
5. *Si Chuan Zhong Yi* (Sichuan Chinese Medicine), 1998; 1:36.
6. *Shan Xi Zhong Yi* (Shanxi Chinese Medicine), 1991; 7(5):16.
7. *Xin Zhong Yi* (New Chinese Medicine), 1976; 4:35.

Shào Fù Zhú Yū Tāng

(Drive Out Blood Stasis in the Lower Abdomen Decoction)

少腹逐瘀湯
少腹逐瘀汤

Pinyin Name: *Shao Fu Zhu Yu Tang*
Literal Name: Drive Out Blood Stasis in the Lower Abdomen Decoction
Alternate Name: Fennel Seed and Corydalis Combination
Original Source: *Yi Lin Gai Cuo* (Corrections of Errors Among Physicians) by Wang Qing-Ren in 1830

COMPOSITION

Dang Gui (Radix Angelicae Sinensis)	9g
Chuan Xiong (Rhizoma Chuanxiong)	3g
Chi Shao (Radix Paeoniae Rubra)	6g
Wu Ling Zhi (Faeces Trogopteri), *chao* (dry-fried)	6g
Pu Huang (Pollen Typhae)	9g
Yan Hu Suo (Rhizoma Corydalis)	3g
Mo Yao (Myrrha)	6g
Gan Jiang (Rhizoma Zingiberis), *chao* (dry-fried)	0.6g [3g]
Xiao Hui Xiang (Fructus Foeniculi), *chao* (dry-fried)	7 pieces [1.5g]
Rou Gui (Cortex Cinnamomi)	3g

DOSAGE / PREPARATION / ADMINISTRATION

The source text states to prepare the ingredients as a decoction. Today, the decoction may be prepared using the doses suggested in brackets.

CHINESE THERAPEUTIC ACTIONS

1. Activates blood circulation and dispels blood stagnation
2. Warms and regulates menstruation to relieve pain

CLINICAL MANIFESTATIONS

Blood stagnation in the lower abdomen: pain and fullness in the lower abdominal region; formation of mass in the lower abdomen; irregular estrus; menstrual pain, low back pain and lower abdominal fullness during estrus; excess menstrual bleeding that is black and/or purplish with blood clots (in primates); and *beng lou* (flooding and spotting) with lower abdominal pain.

VETERINARY CLINICAL APPLICATIONS

Female and male infertility, menstrual abnormalities in primates, uterine bleeding, endometriosis, oophoritic cyst, ovarian cyst, pelvic inflammatory disease, and idiopathic colic pain in horses.

EXPLANATION

Shao Fu Zhu Yu Tang (Drive Out Blood Stasis in the Lower Abdomen Decoction) is designed specifically for blood stagnation in the lower abdomen. It activates blood circulation to dispel blood stagnation, activates qi circulation to relieve pain, and warms the lower *jiao* to restore normal menstruation. This formula can be applied to primates and used to treat infertility in these species. Clinically, the animal may show pain and fullness in the lower abdominal region, menstrual pain, excess menstrual bleeding that is black and/or purplish with blood clots, and multiple cycles of bleeding (between 3-5 times) within one cycle. Abdominal surgery often results in blood stagnation, and in horses this often involves the large colon and may result in persistent pain even after the problem is surgically corrected, necessitating the use of this formula to resolve blood stagnation.

In this formula, *Dang Gui* (Radix Angelicae Sinensis), *Chuan Xiong* (Rhizoma Chuanxiong), and *Chi Shao* (Radix Paeoniae Rubra) nourish the blood, activate blood circulation, and eliminate blood stasis. *Wu Ling Zhi* (Faeces Trogopteri) disperses blood stasis to relieve pain. *Pu Huang* (Pollen Typhae) regulates blood circulation. *Yan Hu Suo* (Rhizoma Corydalis) and *Mo Yao* (Myrrha) activate qi and blood circulation to relieve pain. *Gan Jiang* (Rhizoma Zingiberis) warms the menses and dispels cold. *Xiao Hui Xiang* (Fructus Foeniculi) and *Rou Gui* (Cortex Cinnamomi) warm the lower *jiao* to relieve pain.

Shào Fù Zhú Yū Tāng

(Drive Out Blood Stasis in the Lower Abdomen Decoction)

***Shao Fu Zhu Yu Tang* (Drive Out Blood Stasis in the Lower Abdomen Decoction)**

Diagnosis	Clinical Signs	Treatment	Herbs
Blood stagnation in the lower abdomen	• Pain and fullness in the lower abdominal region and formation of a mass in the lower abdomen: blood stagnation in the lower *jiao* area • Menstrual pain, multiple cycles of bleeding (between 3-5 times) within one period, excess menstrual bleeding that is black and purplish with blood clots: blood stagnation affecting menstruation	• Activates blood circulation and dispels blood stagnation • Warms and regulates menstruation to relieve pain	• *Dang Gui* (Radix Angelicae Sinensis), *Chuan Xiong* (Rhizoma Chuanxiong), and *Chi Shao* (Radix Paeoniae Rubra) nourish the blood, activate blood circulation, and eliminate blood stasis. • *Wu Ling Zhi* (Faeces Trogopteri) disperses blood stasis to relieve pain. • *Pu Huang* (Pollen Typhae) regulates blood circulation. • *Yan Hu Suo* (Rhizoma Corydalis) and *Mo Yao* (Myrrha) activate qi and blood circulation to relieve pain. • *Gan Jiang* (Rhizoma Zingiberis) warms the menses and dispels cold. • *Xiao Hui Xiang* (Fructus Foeniculi) and *Rou Gui* (Cortex Cinnamomi) warm the lower *jiao* to relieve pain.

VETERINARY MODIFICATIONS

- For amenorrhea or dysmenorrhea (in primates) with blood stagnation accompanied by constipation, add *Da Huang* (Radix et Rhizoma Rhei) and *Mang Xiao* (Natrii Sulfas).
- For infertility due to the absence of ovulation, add *Shan Yao* (Rhizoma Dioscoreae) or *Zi He Che* (Placenta Hominis).
- With early menstruation (in primates), add *Huang Qin* (Radix Scutellariae).
- With continuous and incessant menstrual bleeding (in primates) due to heat, add *Huang Qin* (Radix Scutellariae) and *Huang Lian* (Rhizoma Coptidis).
- For cysts and fibroids in the lower abdominal area with pain and dark menstrual discharge (in primates), add *Hai Zao* (Sargassum), *Hai Dai* (Thallus Laminariae), *Kun Bu* (Thallus Eckloniae), *Xia Ku Cao* (Spica Prunellae), *Jin Yin Hua* (Flos Lonicerae Japonicae), *Zi Cao* (Radix Arnebiae), *Mu Li* (Concha Ostreae), *E Zhu* (Rhizoma Curcumae), *San Leng* (Rhizoma Sparganii), *Bie Jia* (Carapax Trionycis), and *Sang Ji Sheng* (Herba Taxilli).
- For chronic hepatitis, liver cirrhosis, and ascites, add *Chai Hu* (Radix Bupleuri), *Ban Lan Gen* (Radix Isatidis), *Huang Jing* (Rhizoma Polygonati), *Huang Qi* (Radix Astragali), *Gou Qi Zi* (Fructus Lycii), and *Ren Shen* (Radix et Rhizoma Ginseng).

CAUTIONS / CONTRAINDICATIONS

Shao Fu Zhu Yu Tang is contraindicated during pregnancy.

PHARMACOLOGICAL EFFECTS

Anti-inflammatory: According to one *in vitro* study, administration of *Shao Fu Zhu Yu Tang* at doses of 8g/kg or 16g/kg was associated with a marked anti-inflammatory effect in rats. The study noted that while *Shao Fu Zhu Yu Tang* and hydrocortisone both have marked anti-inflammatory effects, their mechanisms and side effects are quite different. The use of hydrocortisone was associated with the various side effects of the corticosteroid drugs, while *Shao Fu Zhu Yu Tang* did not have such side effects.[1]

HUMAN CLINICAL STUDIES AND RESEARCH

1. **Female infertility**: According to one study, 45 of 46 patients successfully became pregnant after taking 3-5 packs of herbs per month starting at the beginning of the period, for 1-4 months. The causes of infertility included inflammation of the fallopian tubes, chronic pelvic inflammatory diseases, and anovulation. The standard herbal treatment was *Shao Fu Zhu Yu Tang*. Modifications included the addition of *Li Zhi He* (Semen Litchi), *Che Qian Zi* (Semen Plantaginis), *Jin Yin Hua* (Flos Lonicerae Japonicae), *Chuan Lian Zi* (Fructus Toosendan), *Pu Gong Ying* (Herba Taraxaci), and others specifically for inflammation of the fallopian tubes.[2] According to another study of 50 women with infertility (3-11 years) due to obstructed fallopian tubes, use of modified *Shao Fu Zhu Yu Tang* was associated with successful gestation in 51% of patients.[3]
2. **Male infertility**: One study reported successful treatment of male infertility in 17 of 20 patients using modified *Shao Fu Zhu Yu Tang*. The duration of treatment ranged from 20-40 days. In addition to the base formula, *Huang Jing*

Shào Fù Zhú Yū Tāng

(Drive Out Blood Stasis in the Lower Abdomen Decoction)

(Rhizoma Polygonati) was added for yang deficiency; *Fen Bi Xie* (Rhizoma Dioscoreae Hypoglaucae), *Shi Chang Pu* (Rhizoma Acori Tatarinowii), *Shi Wei* (Folium Pyrrosiae), and *Che Qian Zi* (Semen Plantaginis) were added for presence of pus in the sperm; *Huang Qi* (Radix Astragali) and *Yin Yang Huo* (Herba Epimedii) were added for poor sperm motility; and Kidney tonics for low sperm count.[4]

3. **Male infertility from sperm disorders**: Use of *Shao Fu Zhu Yu Tang* was associated with improvement in sperm mobility, quantity, and quality in 36 patients with chronic prostatitis after treatment for 60 days. The increase in sperm mobility was evaluated by computer-assisted semen analysis, and sperm quantity and quality with a high-powered intravital microscope. The mechanisms of this effect were attributed to increased sperm acrosin activity levels.[5]
4. **Ectopic gestation**: Use of modified *Shao Fu Zhu Yu Tang* successfully terminated gestation in all of 12 women with ectopic gestation. The herbal formula contained *Dan Shen* (Radix et Rhizoma Salviae Miltiorrhizae) 15g, dry-fried *Lai Fu Zi* (Semen Raphani) 15g, *Yi Mu Cao* (Herba Leonuri) 15g, *Chi Shao* (Radix Paeoniae Rubra) 10g, *Chuan Niu Xi* (Radix Cyathulae) 10g, *Hong Hua* (Flos Carthami) 6g, *Xiao Hui Xiang* (Fructus Foeniculi) 6g, *Tian Hua Fen* (Radix Trichosanthis) 15-30g, *Yi Yi Ren* (Semen Coicis) 20g, *Pu Huang* (Pollen Typhae) 17g, and *Gan Cao* (Radix et Rhizoma Glycyrrhizae) 5g. The treatment protocol was to cook the herbs in water, and administer the decoction in two to three equally-divided doses 1 hour before meals. In addition, anti-inflammatory drugs were given as adjunct therapy as needed. The duration of treatment ranged from 3 to 21 days.[6]
5. **Hysteromyoma**: Use of modified *Shao Fu Zhu Yu Tang* in 14 patients with hysteromyoma was associated with complete recovery in 8 cases, significant improvement in 4 cases, slight improvement in 1 case, and no effect in 1 case. The base formula was *Shao Fu Zhu Yu Tang* with the removal of *Gan Jiang* (Rhizoma Zingiberis) and *Chi Shao* (Radix Paeoniae Rubra), and addition of *Hong Hua* (Flos Carthami), *Tao Ren* (Semen Persicae), *San Leng* (Rhizoma Sparganii), *E Zhu* (Rhizoma Curcumae), *Juan Bai* (Herba Selaginellae), and *Yi Mu Cao* (Herba Leonuri). *Xiang Fu* (Rhizoma Cyperi), *Chuan Lian Zi* (Fructus Toosendan), and *Li Zhi He* (Semen Litchi) were added for severe qi stagnation; *Shui Zhi* (Hirudo), *Dan Shen* (Radix et Rhizoma Salviae Miltiorrhizae), and *Yi Mu Cao* (Herba Leonuri) were added for severe blood stagnation; and *Ba Zhen Tang* (Eight-Treasure Decoction) was given during the recovery period.[7]
6. **Endometriosis**: One study reported 97.5% effectiveness using modified *Shao Fu Zhu Yu Tang* to treat 40 women with endometriosis. For those with endometriosis characterized by cold obstruction and blood stagnation, unmodified *Shao Fu Zhu Yu Tang* was used for treatment. For those with endometriosis characterized by qi deficiency and blood stagnation, *Shao Fu Zhu Yu Tang* was modified by eliminating *Wu Ling Zhi* (Faeces Trogopteri) and adding *Huang Qi* (Radix Astragali), *Dang Shen* (Radix Codonopsis), *Sheng Ma* (Rhizoma Cimicifugae), and *Mu Xiang* (Radix Aucklandiae).[8]
7. **Oophoritic cyst**: Use of modified *Shao Fu Zhu Yu Tang* was associated with complete recovery in 46 of 50 patients. In addition to *Shao Fu Zhu Yu Tang*, modifications included the addition of *Nu Zhen Zi* (Fructus Ligustri Lucidi) and *Mo Han Lian* (Herba Ecliptae) for prolonged bleeding and increased menstrual discharge; *Huang Qi* (Radix Astragali) and *Dang Shen* (Radix Codonopsis) for qi deficiency; *Liu Wei Di Huang Wan* (Six-Ingredient Pill with Rehmannia) for yin deficiency; *San Qi* (Radix et Rhizoma Notoginseng) and *Yi Mu Cao* (Herba Leonuri) for severe abdominal pain caused by blood stagnation; and general tonic herbs when swelling and inflammation subsided. The duration of treatment ranged from 30-60 packs of herbs.[9]
8. **Dysmenorrhea**: Numerous studies have shown that *Shao Fu Zhu Yu Tang* treats dysmenorrhea. According to one study of 100 patients with dysmenorrhea characterized by cold and blood stagnation, administration of *Shao Fu Zhu Yu Tang* (starting 1 week before the period for 7-10 days) followed by *Wen Jing Tang* (Warm the Channels Decoction) (starting after the period for 2-3 months total) was associated with 100% effectiveness.[10] According to another study, use of modified *Shao Fu Zhu Yu Tang* for 1-8 packs was associated with marked success in 54 patients with dysmenorrhea. Of 46 patients who had complete recovery, no recurrences were reported within one year. Of 4 patients who had moderate improvement, no recurrences were reported within 3 months. Three had only symptomatic relief and 1 had no effect.[11]
9. **Uterine bleeding**: *Shao Fu Zhu Yu Tang* was shown to be effective in treating 32 women with uterine bleeding associated with functional disorder. In addition to this formula, modifications were made by adding *Bai Zhu* (Rhizoma Atractylodis Macrocephalae), *Dang Shen* (Radix Codonopsis), and *Huang Qi* (Radix Astragali) for qi deficiency; *Mu Dan Pi* (Cortex Moutan), *Ce Bai Ye* (Cacumen Platycladi), and *Di Huang* (Radix Rehmanniae) for heat in the blood; *Shu Di Huang* (Radix Rehmanniae Praeparata), *Xu Duan* (Radix Dipsaci), and *Tu Si Zi* (Semen Cuscutae) for Kidney deficiency. The treatment protocol was to administer the herbs in decoction starting on the first day of the period, for a total of 4 packs of herbs.[12]

Shào Fù Zhú Yū Tāng

(Drive Out Blood Stasis in the Lower Abdomen Decoction)

10. **Pelvic inflammatory disease**: Forty-two women with pelvic inflammatory disease due to various causes (ligation, abortion, miscarriage, etc.) were treated with complete recovery in 26 cases, marked improvement in 9 cases, slight improvement in 4 cases, and no effect in 3 cases. The overall effectiveness was 92%. The herbal treatment contained *Shao Fu Zhu Yu Tang,* minus *Gan Jiang* (Rhizoma Zingiberis), plus *Bai Jiang Cao* (Herba cum Radice Patriniae) and *Huang Qi* (Radix Astragali). *Pu Gong Ying* (Herba Taraxaci), *Huang Bo* (Cortex Phellodendri Chinensis) and liquor-processed *Da Huang* (Radix et Rhizoma Rhei) were added for damp-heat; *Wu Zhu Yu* (Fructus Evodiae), *Wu Yao* (Radix Linderae), *Gan Jiang* (Rhizoma Zingiberis), and larger doses of *Xiao Hui Xiang* (Fructus Foeniculi) and *Rou Gui* (Cortex Cinnamomi) for qi stagnation with cold; and *San Leng* (Rhizoma Sparganii), and *E Zhu* (Rhizoma Curcumae) for qi and blood stagnation.[13]
11. **Ulcerative colitis**: One study reported 88.7% effectiveness using modified *Shao Fu Zhu Yu Tang* to treat 44 patients with ulcerative colitis.[14]
12. **Urinary stones**: One-hundred patients with urinary stones (16 in the kidneys, 81 in the ureters, and 3 in the bladder) treated with modified *Shao Fu Zhu Yu Tang* showed complete recovery in 65 cases, marked improvement in 22 cases, and no benefit in 13 cases. The overall effectiveness was 87%. In addition to the base formula, the herbal treatment was modified as follows: *Bai Shao* (Radix Paeoniae Alba) and *Gan Cao* (Radix et Rhizoma Glycyrrhizae) for soreness and pain of the lower back; *Bai Mao Gen* (Rhizoma Imperatae) and *Hu Po* (Succinum) for hematuria; *Huang Qi* (Radix Astragali) and *Dang Shen* (Radix Codonopsis) for qi deficiency; *Di Huang* (Radix Rehmanniae) and *Mo Han Lian* (Herba Ecliptae) for yin deficiency; *Jin Qian Cao* (Herba Lysimachiae) and *Shi Wei* (Folium Pyrrosiae) for painful urination; and removal of *Gan Jiang* (Rhizoma Zingiberis) and *Gui Zhi* (Ramulus Cinnamomi) for damp-heat.[15]

SUGGESTED ACUPUNCTURE TREATMENT

Xinshu (BL 15), *Geshu* (BL 17), *Xuehai* (SP 10), *Zhongji* (CV 3), *Tianshu* (ST 25), and *Diji* (SP 8) relieve blood stagnation in the lower abdomen.

AUTHORS' COMMENTS

Shao Fu Zhu Yu Tang is used to treat conditions of blood stasis located in the lower abdomen and palpable, fixed abdominal masses. This formula is warming, as it contains *Rou Gui* (Cortex Cinnamomi), *Sheng Jiang* (Rhizoma Zingiberis Recens) and *Xiao Hui Xiang* (Fructus Foeniculi) and should not be used in animals with yin deficiency and heat unless modified. The clinical applications of this formula in veterinary medicine have been expanded to include the treatment of infertility in primates in addition to domestic animals. It can be combined with *Xiao Yao San* (Rambling Powder) or *Chai Hu Shu Gan San* (Bupleurum Powder to Spread the Liver), depending on the case. In mares with painful estrus cycles, it can be combined with *Tao Hong Si Wu Tang* (Four-Substance Decoction with Safflower and Peach Pit) with excellent results.

Blood stasis can occur in the abdomen following surgery, which can lead to chronic, unidentifiable episodes of pain. This formula can be very effective in cases of post-surgical colic when the practitioner is confident that the patient is not in need of emergency medical or surgical intervention.

This formula can be given to male dogs with chronic prostatitis and poor sperm counts to increase conception rates. Successful treatment can take up to 90 days. It should not be used in males with yin deficiency and heat as a cause of infertility.

References

1. *Zhong Yao Yao Li Yu Lin* Chuang (Pharmacology and Clinical Applications of Chinese Herbs), 1987; 37.
2. *Zhong Yi Za Zhi* (Journal of Chinese Medicine), 1985; 1:36.
3. *Hu Nan Yi Yao Za Zhi* (Hunan Journal of Medicine and Herbology), 1983; 3:52.
4. *He Nan Zhong Yi* (Henan Chinese Medicine), 1985; 3:29.
5. Yang CC, Chen JC, Chen GW, Chen YS, Chung JG. Effects of Shao-Fu-Zhu-Yu-Tang on motility of human sperm. American Journal of Chinese Medicine. 2003; 31(4):573-9.
6. *Hu Bei Zhong Yi Za Zhi* (Hubei Journal of Chinese Medicine), 1991; 7(5)17.
7. *Bei Jing Zhong Yi* (Beijing Chinese Medicine), 1987; 5:34.
8. *Zhong Xi Yi Jie He Za Zhi* (Journal of Integrated Chinese and Western Medicine), 1988; 10:639.
9. *Xin Zhong Yi* (New Chinese Medicine), 1995; 8:40.
10. *He Nan Zhong Yi* (Henan Chinese Medicine), 1981; 9:39.
11. *Zhe Jiang Zhong Yi Za Zhi* (Zhejiang Journal of Chinese Medicine), 1964; 11:17.
12. *Shi Yong Zhong Xi Yi Jie He Za Zhi* (Practical Journal of Integrated Chinese and Western Medicines), 1993; 6(6):380.
13. *Hu Bei Zhong Yi Za Zhi* (Hubei Journal of Chinese Medicine), 1993; 15(3):23.
14. *Zhong Yi Yao Xin Xi* (Information on Chinese Medicine and Herbology), 1990; 7(6):37.
15. *Zhong Xi Yi Jie He Za Zhi* (Journal of Integrated Chinese and Western Medicine), 1985; 5:271.

Shēn Tòng Zhú Yū Tāng

(Drive Out Blood Stasis from a Painful Body Decoction)

身痛逐瘀湯
身痛逐瘀汤

Pinyin Name: *Shen Tong Zhu Yu Tang*
Literal Name: Drive Out Blood Stasis from a Painful Body Decoction
Alternate Name: Cnidium and Notopterygium Combination
Original Source: *Yi Lin Gai Cuo* (Corrections of Errors Among Physicians) by Wang Qing-Ren in 1830

COMPOSITION

Tao Ren (Semen Persicae)	9g
Hong Hua (Flos Carthami)	9g
Dang Gui (Radix Angelicae Sinensis)	9g
Chuan Xiong (Rhizoma Chuanxiong)	6g
Mo Yao (Myrrha)	6g
Wu Ling Zhi (Faeces Trogopteri), *chao* (dry-fried)	6g
Di Long (Pheretima)	6g
Qin Jiao (Radix Gentianae Macrophyllae)	3g
Qiang Huo (Rhizoma et Radix Notopterygii)	3g
Xiang Fu (Rhizoma Cyperi)	3g
Niu Xi (Radix Achyranthis Bidentatae)	9g
Gan Cao (Radix et Rhizoma Glycyrrhizae)	6g

DOSAGE / PREPARATION / ADMINISTRATION

Prepare as a decoction.

CHINESE THERAPEUTIC ACTIONS

1. Activates qi and blood circulation
2. Dispels blood stagnation and opens the channels and collaterals
3. Unblocks *bi zheng* (painful obstruction syndrome) and relieves pain

CLINICAL MANIFESTATIONS

Pain due to qi and blood stagnation blocking the channels and collaterals: pain in the shoulder, elbow, waist and/or hind limb; and persistent, generalized pain throughout the whole body that does not respond to treatment.

VETERINARY CLINICAL APPLICATIONS

Osteoarthritis, rheumatoid arthritis, immune mediated polyarthritis, sciatica, painful hindquarters, cranial cruciate rupture, back pain, intervertebral disk disease, cervical pain and neuralgia, temporomandibular joint dysplasia, panosteitis, craniomandibular osteopathy (CMO), hypertrophic osteodystrophy (HOD) and eosinophilic myositis.

EXPLANATION

Shen Tong Zhu Yu Tang (Drive Out Blood Stasis from a Painful Body Decoction) activates qi and blood circulation, dispels blood stagnation, opens the channels and collaterals, and relieves pain. Clinically, it is often used for pain due to stagnation of qi and blood. The pain may be located in the shoulder, elbow, waist, leg, or throughout the whole body.

In this formula, *Tao Ren* (Semen Persicae) and *Hong Hua* (Flos Carthami) activate blood circulation and eliminate blood stasis. *Dang Gui* (Radix Angelicae Sinensis) and *Chuan Xiong* (Rhizoma Chuanxiong) nourish the blood and promote blood circulation. *Mo Yao* (Myrrha) relieves pain by invigorating blood circulation. *Wu Ling Zhi* (Faeces Trogopteri) and *Di Long* (Pheretima) dispel blood stasis and open the channels and collaterals. *Qin Jiao* (Radix Gentianae Macrophyllae) and *Qiang Huo* (Rhizoma et Radix Notopterygii) dispel wind-dampness to relieve pain. *Xiang Fu* (Rhizoma Cyperi) activates qi to relieve pain. *Niu Xi* (Radix Achyranthis Bidentatae) strengthens the bones, tendons, and soft tissues. *Gan Cao* (Radix et Rhizoma Glycyrrhizae) harmonizes the herbs in the formula.

Shēn Tòng Zhú Yū Tāng

(Drive Out Blood Stasis from a Painful Body Decoction)

***Shen Tong Zhu Yu Tang* (Drive Out Blood Stasis from a Painful Body Decoction)**

Diagnosis	Clinical Signs	Treatment	Herbs
Pain due to qi and blood stagnation	Pain in the shoulder, elbow, waist, leg, and/or the whole body: qi and blood stagnation blocking the channels and collaterals	• Activates qi and blood circulation • Dispels blood stagnation and opens the channels and collaterals • Unblocks *bi zheng* (painful obstruction syndrome) and relieves pain	• *Tao Ren* (Semen Persicae) and *Hong Hua* (Flos Carthami) activate blood circulation and eliminate blood stasis. • *Dang Gui* (Radix Angelicae Sinensis) and *Chuan Xiong* (Rhizoma Chuanxiong) nourish the blood and promote blood circulation. • *Mo Yao* (Myrrha) invigorates blood circulation and relieves pain. • *Wu Ling Zhi* (Faeces Trogopteri) and *Di Long* (Pheretima) dispel blood stasis and open the channels and collaterals. • *Qin Jiao* (Radix Gentianae Macrophyllae) and *Qiang Huo* (Rhizoma et Radix Notopterygii) dispel wind-dampness to relieve pain. • *Xiang Fu* (Rhizoma Cyperi) activates qi circulation to relieve pain. • *Niu Xi* (Radix Achyranthis Bidentatae) strengthens the bones, tendons, and soft tissues. • *Gan Cao* (Radix et Rhizoma Glycyrrhizae) harmonizes the herbs.

VETERINARY MODIFICATIONS

- With pain in the upper body, add *Ge Gen* (Radix Puerariae Lobatae) and *Sang Zhi* (Ramulus Mori).
- With pain in the lower body, add *Du Huo* (Radix Angelicae Pubescentis), *Gou Ji* (Rhizoma Cibotii), *Xu Duan* (Radix Dipsaci) and *Sang Ji Sheng* (Herba Taxilli).
- With pain in the extremities, add *Sang Zhi* (Ramulus Mori) and *Gui Zhi* (Ramulus Cinnamomi).

CAUTIONS / CONTRAINDICATIONS

Use of *Shen Tong Zhu Yu Tang* is contraindicated during pregnancy.[1]

PHARMACOLOGICAL EFFECTS

Analgesic and anti-inflammatory: According to *in vitro* studies, administration of *Shen Tong Zhu Yu Tang* in tincture form was effective in relieving pain and reducing inflammation.[2]

HUMAN CLINICAL STUDIES AND RESEARCH

1. ***Bi zheng* (painful obstruction syndrome)**: Administration of *Shen Tong Zhu Yu Tang* in 32 patients with *bi zheng* (painful obstruction syndrome) was associated with complete recovery in 12 cases, significant improvement in 10 cases, moderate improvement in 7 cases, and no improvement in 3 cases. The overall effectiveness was 90.6%. The herbal formula used *Shen Tong Zhu Yu Tang* as the base, with the addition of *Huang Qi* (Radix Astragali) and *Dang Shen* (Radix Codonopsis) for qi deficiency; *Fang Feng* (Radix Saposhnikoviae) and *Wei Ling Xian* (Radix et Rhizoma Clematidis) for wind; *Zhi Chuan Wu* (Radix Aconiti Praeparata) and *Xi Xin* (Radix et Rhizoma Asari) for cold; *Fu Ling* (Poria) and *Yi Yi Ren* (Semen Coicis) for damp; *Gui Zhi* (Ramulus Cinnamomi) and *Sang Zhi* (Ramulus Mori) for pain in the upper limbs; *Sang Ji Sheng* (Herba Taxilli), *Xu Duan* (Radix Dipsaci), and *Gou Ji* (Rhizoma Cibotii) for pain in the lower limbs; *Ge Gen* (Radix Puerariae Lobatae) for pain in the neck; and *Feng Fang* (Nidus Vespae), *Wu Shao She* (Zaocys), *Quan Xie* (Scorpio), and dry-fried *Chuan Shan Jia* (Squama Manis) for stiff joints with deformation. For *re bi* (heat painful obstruction), *Jin Yin Hua* (Flos Lonicerae Japonicae), *Cang Zhu* (Rhizoma Atractylodis), and *Huang Bo* (Cortex Phellodendri Chinensis) were added, and *Qin Jiao* (Radix Gentianae Macrophyllae), *Qiang Huo* (Rhizoma et Radix Notopterygii), and *Chuan Xiong* (Rhizoma Chuanxiong) were removed. For *shi-re bi* (damp-heat painful obstruction), *Huang Lian* (Rhizoma Coptidis), *Jin Yin Hua* (Flos Lonicerae Japonicae), and *Yu Jin* (Radix Curcumae) were added, and *Niu Xi* (Radix Achyranthis Bidentatae), *Qin Jiao* (Radix Gentianae Macrophyllae), *Qiang Huo* (Rhizoma et Radix Notopterygii), and *Chuan Xiong* (Rhizoma Chuanxiong) were removed.[3]

Shēn Tòng Zhú Yū Tāng

(Drive Out Blood Stasis from a Painful Body Decoction)

2. **Arthritis**: Use of modified *Shen Tong Zhu Yu Tang* in 67 patients with arthritis was associated with complete recovery in 50 patients, significant improvement in 14 cases, and no effect in 3 cases. Modifications included the addition of *Fu Zi* (Radix Aconiti Lateralis Praeparata), *Xi Xin* (Radix et Rhizoma Asari), and *Wei Ling Xian* (Radix et Rhizoma Clematidis) for arthritis due to cold; *Ren Dong Teng* (Caulis Lonicerae Japonicae), *Shi Gao* (Gypsum Fibrosum), *Huang Bo* (Cortex Phellodendri Chinensis), and *Yi Yi Ren* (Semen Coicis), and removal of *Qiang Huo* (Rhizoma et Radix Notopterygii), for arthritis due to heat; *Bai Shao* (Radix Paeoniae Alba) for stiffness of the tendons and ligaments; and *Jin Qian Bai Hua She* (Bungarus Parvus) and *Wu Shao She* (Zaocys) for "mobile" arthritis that affects multiple joints.[4]
3. **Rheumatoid arthritis**: One study of 46 patients with rheumatoid arthritis reported marked success using modified *Shen Tong Zhu Yu Tang*. Of 46 patients, the study reported recovery in 12 cases, improvement in 25 cases, slight improvement in 7 cases, and no effect in 2 cases. The duration of treatment was 2 months per course of treatment, for 3 courses total. The study also noted that the effect of the herbs was comparable to or better than that in the control group that received aspirin. The herbal formula contained *Shen Tong Zhu Yu Tang* as the base formula, and added *Gui Zhi* (Ramulus Cinnamomi), *Fang Feng* (Radix Saposhnikoviae), and *Wei Ling Xian* (Radix et Rhizoma Clematidis) for wind-dampness; *Gui Zhi* (Ramulus Cinnamomi), *Gan Jiang* (Rhizoma Zingiberis), and *Fu Ling* (Poria) for damp-cold; addition of *Cang Zhu* (Rhizoma Atractylodis), *Huang Bo* (Cortex Phellodendri Chinensis), and *Fang Feng* (Radix Saposhnikoviae), and removal of *Qiang Huo* (Rhizoma et Radix Notopterygii), for damp-heat; the addition of *Di Huang* (Radix Rehmanniae), *Gou Qi Zi* (Fructus Lycii), and *Nu Zhen Zi* (Fructus Ligustri Lucidi), and removal of *Qiang Huo* (Rhizoma et Radix Notopterygii) and *Qin Jiao* (Radix Gentianae Macrophyllae), for Kidney yin deficiency; and the addition of *Rou Gui* (Cortex Cinnamomi) and *Shan Zhu Yu* (Fructus Corni), and removal of *Qiang Huo* (Rhizoma et Radix Notopterygii) and *Qin Jiao* (Radix Gentianae Macrophyllae), for Kidney yang deficiency.[5]
4. **Sciatica**: Administration of *Shen Tong Zhu Yu Tang* for 7-45 days (average of 17.4 days) in 36 patients with sciatica was associated with complete recovery in 29 cases, significant improvement in 6 cases, and no effect in 1 case. The overall effectiveness was 97.2%. Furthermore, of 24 patients who returned for follow-up one year later, only 1 had recurrence.[6]
5. **Pain in the lower back and legs**: Administration of *Shen Tong Zhu Yu Tang* has been shown in 2 studies to effectively treat pain in the lower back and legs. Of 67 patients, the first study reported complete recovery in 53 cases, improvement in 9 cases, and no effect in 5 cases.[7] Of 52 patients in the second study, 12 had complete recovery, 26 had significant improvement, 9 had moderate improvement, and 5 had no effect.[8]
6. **Lumbago**: One study reported good results using modified *Shen Tong Zhu Yu Tang* to treat acute low back pain. Modifications included the addition of *Dang Shen* (Radix Codonopsis) and *Huang Qi* (Radix Astragali) for qi deficiency; and *Yan Hu Suo* (Rhizoma Corydalis) and *Qi Ye Lian* (Radix Schefflerae) for severe pain. The herbal treatment also was applied topically to the affected area. Of 15 patients, the study reported complete recovery in 8 cases, significant improvement in 3 cases, moderate improvement in 3 cases, and no benefit in 1 case.[9]
7. **Hyperosteogeny**: Hyperosteogeny of the lumbar spine was treated with modified *Shen Tong Zhu Yu Tang* with good results. Of 25 patients, the study reported complete relief in 18 cases, significant relief in 4 cases, and no effect in 3 cases.[10]

SUGGESTED ACUPUNCTURE TREATMENT

Xinshu (BL 15), *Geshu* (BL 17), *Xuehai* (SP 10), *Ganshu* (BL 18), *Fengmen* (BL 12), *Pishu* (BL 20), *Yanglingquan* (GB 34), and other applicable local points may be used to activate the blood circulation and relieve pain throughout the body.

AUTHORS' COMMENTS

Shen Tong Zhu Yu Tang is used to treat conditions of pain and *bi zheng* (painful obstruction syndrome) due to blood stagnation and stasis in the channels, collaterals, and the whole body. It is extremely useful in horses, in particular for "cold backed" animals and in navicular disease. The clinical applications in veterinary medicine are numerous, and it is one of the most commonly used formulas to treat pain of the musculoskeletal system in animals.

In general, the pain-relieving properties of this formula can be augmented by the addition of *Ji Xue Teng* (Caulis Spatholobi), *Yan Hu Suo* (Rhizoma Corydalis), *Ru Xiang* (Gummi Olibanum), and *Du Huo* (Radix Angelicae Pubescentis).

- For eosinophilic myositis, add *Si Miao San* (Four-Marvel Powder).
- For craniomandibular osteopathy due to Kidney and Liver yin deficiencies, add *Liu Wei Di Huang Wan* (Six-Ingredient Pill with Rehmannia); with fever, add *Zhi Bai Di Huang Wan* (Anemarrhena, Phellodendron, and

Shēn Tòng Zhú Yū Tāng

(Drive Out Blood Stasis from a Painful Body Decoction)

Rehmannia Pill); with qi deficiency, add *Si Jun Zi Tang* (Four-Gentlemen Decoction).

- With acute intervertebral disk disease, combine with *Xiao Huo Luo Dan* (Minor Invigorate the Collaterals Special Pill).

References

1. *Zhong Yao Ming Fang Yao Li Yu Ying Yong* (Pharmacology and Applications of Famous Herbal Formulas), 1989; 466-468.
2. *Zhong Yao Yan Jiu* (Research of Chinese Herbology), 1993; 6(4):15.
3. *Xin Zhong Yi* (New Chinese Medicine), 1995; 9:42.
4. *Yun Nan Zhong Yao Zhi* (Yunan Journal of Chinese Herbal Medicine), 1989; 3:46.
5. *Bei Jing Zhong Yi Za Zhi* (Beijing Journal of Chinese Medicine), 1988; 6:35.
6. *Si Chuan Zhong Yi* (Sichuan Chinese Medicine), 1985; 11:50.
7. *Hu Nan Zhong Yi Za Zhi* (Hunan Journal of Chinese Medicine), 1987; 1:12.
8. *Zhe Jiang Zhong Yi Za Zhi* (Zhejiang Journal of Chinese Medicine), 1987; 10:452.
9. *Guang Xi Zhong Yi Yao* (Guangxi Chinese Medicine and Herbology), 1987; 2:47.
10. *Gan Su Zhong Yi* (Gansu Chinese Medicine), 1993; 9:46.

Fù Yuán Huó Xuè Tāng

(Revive Health by Invigorating the Blood Decoction)

復元活血湯
复元活血汤

Pinyin Name: *Fu Yuan Huo Xue Tang*
Literal Name: Revive Health by Invigorating the Blood Decoction
Alternate Names: *Shang Ke Fu Yuan Huo Xue Tang* (Revive Health by Invigorating the Blood Decoction from the Trauma Department), *Fu Yuan Huo Hsieh Tang*, *Fu Yuan Huo Xieh Tang*, Recovery and Blood Activating Decoction, Recovery Blood Activating Decoction, Tangkuei and Persica Combination
Original Source: *Yi Xue Fa Ming* (Medical Innovations) by Li Gao in the Jin Dynasty

COMPOSITION

Da Huang (Radix et Rhizoma Rhei), *jin* (soaked) in liquor	30g
Chai Hu (Radix Bupleuri)	15g
Dang Gui (Radix Angelicae Sinensis)	9g
Tao Ren (Semen Persicae), *jin* (soaked) in liquor and *yan* (ground) till muddy	50 pieces [9g]
Hong Hua (Flos Carthami)	6g
Tian Hua Fen (Radix Trichosanthis)	9g
Chuan Shan Jia (Squama Manis), *pao* (blast-fried)	6g
Gan Cao (Radix et Rhizoma Glycyrrhizae)	6g

Fù Yuán Huó Xuè Tāng

(Revive Health by Invigorating the Blood Decoction)

Note: *Chuan Shan Jia* (Squama Manis) is derived from an endangered animal and is rarely used as a medicinal substance today. Its discussion here is included primarily for academic purposes, to reflect the historical use of this substance in its original formulation. Most herbal products today have removed it completely or replaced it with substitutes with similar functions.

DOSAGE / PREPARATION / ADMINISTRATION

Grind all of the ingredients into a coarse powder except for *Tao Ren* (Semen Persicae), which should be ground until muddy. Cook 30g of the herbs in 1.5 bowls of water and 0.5 bowl of grain-based liquor until the liquid is reduced to 70%. Take the warm, strained decoction before meals. Discontinue the formula once the pain is relieved.

CHINESE THERAPEUTIC ACTIONS

1. Activates blood circulation and dispels blood stasis
2. Soothes the Liver and opens the channels and collaterals

CLINICAL MANIFESTATIONS

Traumatic injuries with stagnation of qi and blood: traumatic or performance injuries, pain and swelling in the chest and hypochondriac region, musculoskeletal or soft tissue injuries, and severe, excruciating pain.

VETERINARY CLINICAL APPLICATIONS

Traumatic injuries, musculoskeletal or soft tissue injuries, bone fractures, hypochondriac pain, and intercostal neuralgia.

EXPLANATION

Fu Yuan Huo Xue Tang (Revive Health by Invigorating the Blood Decoction) was originally designed to treat traumatic and external injuries with blood stasis under the hypochondrium. All traumatic and external injuries are characterized in part by qi and blood stagnation, regardless of the severity or area of injury. When there is an injury, the blood leaves the vessels and forms obstruction along the channels and collaterals. These obstructions block the smooth flow of qi, induce pain and numbness, and cause local swelling and inflammation. Moreover, since the Liver is the organ that stores blood, stagnation of blood in the peripheral parts of the body affects the normal functions of the Liver. If Liver qi becomes stagnant, the animal may experience hypochondriac pain. Although this formula is designed to treat injuries to the chest and hypochondriac regions, it is also effective for various other types of musculoskeletal and soft tissue injuries.

In this formula, *Da Huang* (Radix et Rhizoma Rhei) drains heat and blood stasis to reduce pain and swelling. *Chai Hu* (Radix Bupleuri) smoothes Liver qi stagnation and relieves hypochondriac fullness and pain. It also guides *Da Huang* (Radix et Rhizoma Rhei) to the hypochondriac region to enhance its effect. *Dang Gui* (Radix Angelicae Sinensis), *Tao Ren* (Semen Persicae), and *Hong Hua* (Flos Carthami) activate blood circulation, remove blood stasis, reduce swelling, and relieve pain. These herbs have a synergistic effect and are frequently used together. *Tian Hua Fen* (Radix Trichosanthis) clears heat and reduces swelling. It also promotes the generation of muscle tissues.

***Fu Yuan Huo Xue Tang* (Revive Health by Invigorating the Blood Decoction)**

Diagnosis	Clinical Signs	Treatment	Herbs
Traumatic injuries with stagnation of qi and blood	• Swelling, inflammation, numbness, and pain: qi stagnation from traumatic injuries • Severe pain and bruises: blood stagnation from traumatic injuries • Chest and hypochondriac pain: Liver qi stagnation	• Activates blood circulation and dispels blood stasis • Soothes the Liver and opens the channels and collaterals	• *Da Huang* (Radix et Rhizoma Rhei) drains heat and blood stasis to reduce pain and swelling. • *Chai Hu* (Radix Bupleuri) regulates qi circulation and smoothes Liver qi stagnation. • *Dang Gui* (Radix Angelicae Sinensis), *Tao Ren* (Semen Persicae), and *Hong Hua* (Flos Carthami) activate blood circulation, remove blood stasis, reduce swelling, and relieve pain. • *Tian Hua Fen* (Radix Trichosanthis) clears heat, reduces swelling, and promotes the generation of muscle tissue. • *Chuan Shan Jia* (Squama Manis) breaks up blood stasis and opens the channels and collaterals. • *Gan Cao* (Radix et Rhizoma Glycyrrhizae) relieves spasms and cramps and harmonizes the herbs.

Fù Yuán Huó Xuè Tāng

(Revive Health by Invigorating the Blood Decoction)

Chuan Shan Jia (Squama Manis) is one of the most effective herbs for breaking up blood stasis and opening the channels and collaterals. Lastly, *Gan Cao* (Radix et Rhizoma Glycyrrhizae) not only relieves muscle spasms and cramps, but also harmonizes all of the herbs.

VETERINARY MODIFICATIONS

- With more qi stagnation, add *Mu Xiang* (Radix Aucklandiae), *Xiang Fu* (Rhizoma Cyperi), *Qing Pi* (Pericarpium Citri Reticulatae Viride), and *Zhi Qiao* (Fructus Aurantii).
- With more severe blood stasis, add *San Qi* (Radix et Rhizoma Notoginseng), *Ru Xiang* (Gummi Olibanum), *Mo Yao* (Myrrha) and *Yu Jin* (Radix Curcumae).
- With severe pain, add *Yan Hu Suo* (Rhizoma Corydalis).
- With distention and pain in the chest and hypochondriac region, add *Qing Pi* (Pericarpium Citri Reticulatae Viride) and *Chuan Lian Zi* (Fructus Toosendan).
- With abdominal bloating, add *Hou Po* (Cortex Magnoliae Officinalis) and *Zhi Qiao* (Fructus Aurantii).
- With upper back pain, add *Gui Zhi* (Ramulus Cinnamomi) and *Jiang Huang* (Rhizoma Curcumae Longae).
- With pain in the lower extremities, add *Chuan Niu Xi* (Radix Cyathulae) and *Mu Gua* (Fructus Chaenomelis).
- For traumatic injuries to the extremities, remove *Chai Hu* (Radix Bupleuri); and add *Gui Zhi* (Ramulus Cinnamomi) and *Sang Zhi* (Ramulus Mori).

CAUTIONS / CONTRAINDICATIONS

- *Fu Yuan Huo Xue Tang* is contraindicated during pregnancy, and in weak and deficient animals.
- This formula should be used with caution in patients with Spleen qi deficiency, as this formula may cause loose stools or diarrhea.

HUMAN CLINICAL STUDIES AND RESEARCH

1. **Hepatic abscess**: Thirty-eight patients with hepatic abscess were divided into 5 diagnostic groups and treated accordingly with modified *Fu Yuan Huo Xue Tang*. Those diagnosed with liver abscess with qi and blood stagnation were treated with this formula without modification. Those with damp-heat in the Liver and Gallbladder accompanied by blood stagnation received this formula plus 10g each of *Long Dan* (Radix et Rhizoma Gentianae), *Chai Hu* (Radix Bupleuri), *Huang Qin* (Radix Scutellariae), *Zhi Zi* (Fructus Gardeniae), *Che Qian Zi* (Semen Plantaginis), *Mu Tong* (Caulis Akebiae), *Lian Qiao* (Fructus Forsythiae), *Shi Chang Pu* (Rhizoma Acori Tatarinowii), *Bai Bian Dou* (Semen Lablab Album), and *Huo Xiang* (Herba Agastaches). Those diagnosed with heat and toxins accompanied by qi and blood stagnation received this formula plus 15g each of *Ye Ju Hua* (Flos Chrysanthemi Indici), *Jin Yin Hua* (Flos Lonicerae Japonicae), *Zi Hua Di Ding* (Herba Violae), *Tu Fu Ling* (Rhizoma Smilacis Glabrae), *Pu Gong Ying* (Herba Taraxaci), and 10g of *Huang Qin* (Radix Scutellariae). Those diagnosed with cold accompanied by obstruction of the channels and collaterals received this formula plus 10g each of *Fu Zi* (Radix Aconiti Lateralis Praeparata), *Chuan Xiong* (Rhizoma Chuanxiong), and *Xiang Fu* (Rhizoma Cyperi), and 12g each of *Yi Yi Ren* (Semen Coicis), *Bai Jiang Cao* (Herba cum Radice Patriniae), and *Zao Jiao* (Fructus Gleditsiae). Lastly, those diagnosed with *zheng* (upright) *qi* deficiency with stagnation and toxins received this formula plus *Bai Zhu* (Rhizoma Atractylodis Macrocephalae) 10g, *Chuan Xiong* (Rhizoma Chuanxiong) 10g, *Shu Di Huang* (Radix Rehmanniae Praeparata) 12g, *Bai Shao* (Radix Paeoniae Alba) 12g, *Dang Shen* (Radix Codonopsis) 15g, and *Fu Ling* (Poria) 15g. The treatment protocol was to administer the herbs in decoction daily, with the duration of treatment ranging from 13-145 days (average of 34.7 days). Of 38 patients, the study reported complete recovery in 14 cases, near-complete recovery in 17 cases, and moderate improvement in 7 cases.[1]
2. **Hypochondriac pain**: Use of modified *Fu Yuan Huo Xue Tang* in 82 patients with hypochondriac pain characterized by Liver and blood stagnation was associated with remission in 25 cases, near-remission in 40 cases, improvement in 8 cases, and no effect in 9 cases.[2]
3. **Costal chondritis**: One study reported marked effectiveness using modified *Fu Yuan Huo Xue Tang* in treating 100 patients with costal chondritis with a history of illness between 15 days to 3.5 years. The herbs were given in decoction daily, for an average duration of 65 days of treatment.[3]
4. **Ocular hemorrhage**: One study reported 95.2% effectiveness using modified *Fu Yuan Huo Xue Tang* to treat 21 cases of internal eye bleeding associated with external trauma. The average duration of treatment was 6 days.[4]
5. ***Xiong bi* (painful obstruction of the chest)**: One study reported 82% effectiveness using *Fu Yuan Huo Xue Tang* to treat *xiong bi* (painful obstruction of the chest) in 48 patients. In addition to the original formula, the treatment was modified by adding *Yu Jin* (Radix Curcumae) and *Ge Gen* (Radix Puerariae Lobatae) for feeling of chest oppression and shortness of breath; *Gua Lou* (Fructus Trichosanthis) and *Zhi Zi* (Fructus Gardeniae) for irritability and dry mouth; *Yan Hu Suo* (Rhizoma Corydalis), *Xiang Fu* (Rhizoma Cyperi), and *Jiang Xiang* (Lignum Dalbergiae Odoriferae) for severe chest pain; *Dou Kou* (Fructus Amomi Rotundus) and *Shan Zha* (Fructus Crataegi) for food stagnation and poor appetite;

Fù Yuán Huó Xuè Tāng

(Revive Health by Invigorating the Blood Decoction)

Fu Ling (Poria), *Di Long* (Pheretima), and *Sheng Jiang* (Rhizoma Zingiberis Recens) for palpitations accompanied by edema in the lower legs; and *Fu Zi* (Radix Aconiti Lateralis Praeparata), *Gui Zhi* (Ramulus Cinnamomi), and *Ren Shen* (Radix et Rhizoma Ginseng) for sweating accompanied by cold extremities.[5]

6. **Scapulocostal syndrome**: Use of *Fu Yuan Huo Xue Tang* was effective in treating 280 patients with stiffness and pain in the shoulder and scapula regions.[6]
7. **Bone fractures**: Concurrent use of *Fu Yuan Huo Xue Tang* plus *Qi Li San* (Seven-Thousandths of a Tael Powder) within the first 2 weeks of injury was shown to have a marked effect in reducing swelling and relieving pain in over 10,000 patients with bone fractures.[7]
8. **Concussion**: Use of modified *Fu Yuan Huo Xue Tang* was associated with 100% effectiveness in treating 53 patients with concussion. Modifications to the original formula included the addition of *Shi Chang Pu* (Rhizoma Acori Tatarinowii) and *Yuan Zhi* (Radix Polygalae) for unconsciousness; *Chuan Xiong* (Rhizoma Chuanxiong) and *Man Jing Zi* (Fructus Viticis) for dizziness; *Zhe Shi* (Haematitum) and *Zhu Ru* (Caulis Bambusae in Taenia) for nausea and vomiting; *Ge Gen* (Radix Puerariae Lobatae) for neck stiffness; and *Suan Zao Ren* (Semen Ziziphi Spinosae) and *Yuan Zhi* (Radix Polygalae) for insomnia. Of 53 patients, the study reported complete recovery in 48 cases within 3-30 days, and improvement in 5 cases.[8]
9. **Intestinal adhesion**: Use of modified *Fu Yuan Huo Xue Tang* was associated with complete recovery in all 17 patients with intestinal adhesion, without recurrence for 6 months. The herbal treatment contained this formula with modifications such as the addition of *San Leng* (Rhizoma Sparganii), *E Zhu* (Rhizoma Curcumae), *Chi Shao* (Radix Paeoniae Rubra), and *Bai Shao* (Radix Paeoniae Alba) for severe abdominal pain; *Mu Xiang* (Radix Aucklandiae) and *Da Fu Pi* (Pericarpium Arecae) for severe abdominal distention; *Ban Xia* (Rhizoma Pinelliae) and *Zhe Shi* (Haematitum) for severe nausea and vomiting; *Zhi Shi* (Fructus Aurantii Immaturus) and *Xuan Ming Fen* (Natrii Sulfas Exsiccatus) for constipation accompanied by dry mouth and tongue.[9]

SUGGESTED ACUPUNCTURE TREATMENT

1. Points: *Geshu* (BL 17), *Xuehai* (SP 10), *Qimen* (LR 14), and *Yanglingquan* (GB 34).
2. Technique: sedation.

Geshu (BL 17) and *Xuehai* (SP 10) activate the blood and remove blood stagnation. *Qimen* (LR 14) regulates Liver qi flow to activate the blood. *Yanglingquan* (GB 34), the *he* (uniting) point of the Gallbladder, relieves pain in the hypochondriac region.

AUTHORS' COMMENTS

Fu Yuan Huo Xue Tang is one of the best formulas for treating physical injuries (trauma, sports, and external injuries) with pain, swelling, inflammation, bruising, and damage to the soft tissues. This formula originally was designed for trauma in the hypochondriac (rib cage) region, but is equally effective for injuries in the rest of the body. Animals with rib fractures, chest pain and injury to the diaphragm secondary to vehicular trauma, bite wounds, poor saddle fit, or surgery can especially benefit from the use of this formula. *Chuan Shan Jia* (Squama Manis), commonly known as anteater or pangolin scales, is responsible for the strong blood-moving properties of this formula; if this substance is removed from the formula, its ability to resolve blood stasis will be significantly diminished. In this case, replace *Chuan Shan Jia* (Squama Manis) with *Ru Xiang* (Gummi Olibanum) and *Mo Yao* (Myrrha) to improve the effects of pain relief and resolution of blood stasis.

References

1. *Zhong Guo Zhong Xi Yi Jie He Za Zhi* (Chinese Journal of Integrative Chinese and Western Medicine), 1993; 8:491.
2. *Fu Jian Zhong Yi Yao* (Fujian Chinese Medicine and Herbology), 1994; 1:33.
3. *Shan Dong Zhong Yi Za Zhi* (Shandong Journal of Chinese Medicine), 1994; 1:42.
4. *Shi Yong Zhong Yi Yao Za Zhi* (Journal of Practical Chinese Medicine and Medicinals), 1999; 8:11.
5. *Zhong Yi Yao Xin Xi* (Information on Chinese Medicine and Herbology), 1995; 1:45.
6. *Yun Nan Zhong Yi Zhong Yao Za Zhi* (Yunan Journal of Chinese Medicine and Medicinals), 1997; 1:23.
7. *Zhong Yi Fang Ji Xian Dai Yan Jiu* (Modern Study of Medical Formulas in Traditional Chinese Medicine), 1997; 999.
8. *Zhe Jiang Zhong Yi Za Zhi* (Zhejiang Journal of Chinese Medicine), 1996; 5:301.
9. *Jiang Su Zhong Yi* (Jiangsu Chinese Medicine), 1999; 3:31.

Zhèng Gǔ Zǐ Jīn Dān (Purple and Gold Pill for Righteous Bones)

正骨紫金丹

Pinyin Name: *Zheng Gu Zi Jin Dan*
Literal Name: Purple and Gold Pill for Righteous Bones
Alternate Names: *Cheng Ku Tzu Chin Tan*, Rhubarb and Carthamus Formula
Original Source: *Yi Zong Jin Jian* (Golden Mirror of the Medical Tradition) by Wu Qian in 1742

COMPOSITION

Dang Gui (Radix Angelicae Sinensis)	60g
Bai Shao (Radix Paeoniae Alba)	60g
Xue Jie (Sanguis Draconis)	30g
Hong Hua (Flos Carthami)	30g
Er Cha (Catechu)	30g
Mu Dan Pi (Cortex Moutan)	15g
Da Huang (Radix et Rhizoma Rhei), prepared	30g
Mu Xiang (Radix Aucklandiae)	30g
Ding Xiang (Flos Caryophylli)	30g
Lian Zi (Semen Nelumbinis)	60g
Fu Ling (Poria)	60g
Gan Cao (Radix et Rhizoma Glycyrrhizae)	9g

Note: It is important to emphasize that prepared *Da Huang* (Radix et Rhizoma Rhei) is specifically used to clear heat and drain bruises. The use of unprepared *Da Huang* (Radix et Rhizoma Rhei) is inappropriate, as it will likely cause diarrhea due to its strong purgative and laxative effects.

DOSAGE / PREPARATION / ADMINISTRATION

The source text states to grind all of the ingredients into a fine powder, then mix the powder with honey to form pills. Take 9g of the pills with a grain-based liquor or *Tong Bian* (Infantis Urina).

CHINESE THERAPEUTIC ACTIONS

1. Activates blood circulation and dispels blood stasis
2. Opens the channels and collaterals
3. Reduces swelling and bruising

CLINICAL MANIFESTATIONS

Traumatic injuries: various types of physical injuries with pain, swelling, inflammation, bruising, and damage to both soft tissues and bone.

VETERINARY CLINICAL APPLICATIONS

Various types of physical injuries with pain, swelling, inflammation, bruising, and damage to both soft tissue and bone.

EXPLANATION

Zheng Gu Zi Jin Dan (Purple and Gold Pill for Righteous Bones) contains herbs to relieve pain, reduce swelling and bruises, and facilitate recovery of injuries to both soft tissues and bone. *Dang Gui* (Radix Angelicae Sinensis) and *Bai Shao* (Radix Paeoniae Alba) activate blood circulation, nourish the blood, and replenish blood lost through injury. *Xue Jie* (Sanguis Draconis) and *Hong Hua* (Flos Carthami) break up blood stagnation and facilitate the generation of new blood. *Er Cha* (Catechu) and *Mu Dan Pi* (Cortex Moutan) cool the blood and clear heat. *Da Huang* (Radix et Rhizoma Rhei) eliminates heat and drains blood stasis. *Mu Xiang* (Radix Aucklandiae) and *Ding Xiang* (Flos Caryophylli) activate qi circulation and relieve pain. *Lian Zi* (Semen Nelumbinis) and *Fu Ling* (Poria) tonify the Spleen and reduce swelling via urination. *Gan Cao* (Radix et Rhizoma Glycyrrhizae) harmonizes the herbs in the formula. In short, this is an excellent formula and is commonly the first choice for treating traumatic injuries to the exterior parts of the body.

Zhèng Gŭ Zĭ Jīn Dān (Purple and Gold Pill for Righteous Bones)

***Zheng Gu Zi Jin Dan* (Purple and Gold Pill for Righteous Bones)**

Diagnosis	Clinical Signs	Treatment	Herbs
Traumatic injuries	Physical injuries with pain, swelling, inflammation, and bruising: qi and blood stagnation with damage to the soft tissues and bone	• Activates blood circulation and dispels blood stasis • Opens the channels and collaterals • Reduces swelling and bruising	• *Dang Gui* (Radix Angelicae Sinensis) and *Bai Shao* (Radix Paeoniae Alba) activate blood circulation, nourish the blood, and replenish blood lost through injury. • *Xue Jie* (Sanguis Draconis) and *Hong Hua* (Flos Carthami) break up blood stagnation and facilitate the generation of new blood. • *Er Cha* (Catechu) and *Mu Dan Pi* (Cortex Moutan) cool the blood and clear heat. • *Da Huang* (Radix et Rhizoma Rhei) eliminates heat and drains blood stasis. • *Mu Xiang* (Radix Aucklandiae) and *Ding Xiang* (Flos Caryophylli) activate qi circulation and relieve pain. • *Lian Zi* (Semen Nelumbinis) and *Fu Ling* (Poria) tonify the Spleen and reduce swelling via urination. • *Gan Cao* (Radix et Rhizoma Glycyrrhizae) harmonizes the herbs.

VETERINARY MODIFICATIONS

- With severe pain, add *Ru Xiang* (Gummi Olibanum) and *Mo Yao* (Myrrha).
- With prominent redness and swelling in bone fractures, add *You Gui Wan* (Restore the Right [Kidney] Pill) and *Huang Bo* (Cortex Phellodendri Chinensis).

SUGGESTED ACUPUNCTURE TREATMENT

1. Points: *Xuehai* (SP 10), *Sanyinjiao* (SP 6), *Taichong* (LR 3), *Neiguan* (PC 6), *Housanli* (ST 36), and *ah shi* points.
2. Technique: sedation and bleeding.

The acupuncture points can be divided into two parts: treating the cause and treating the particular clinical signs. *Xuehai* (SP 10), together with *Sanyinjiao* (SP 6), invigorates the blood and removes stagnation, and when combined with *Taichong* (LR 3), clears heat in the blood. *Neiguan* (PC 6) and *Housanli* (ST 36) regulate qi, relieve pain, and tonify the Spleen. Symptomatically, needling *ah shi* points and bleeding the local areas regulate qi, clear heat, remove stagnation, and reduce swelling.

AUTHORS' COMMENTS

Zheng Gu Zi Jin Dan and *Fu Yuan Huo Xue Tang* (Revive Health by Invigorating the Blood Decoction) both activate blood circulation and remove blood stasis in the treatment of musculoskeletal injuries from trauma.

- *Zheng Gu Zi Jin Dan* has a more generalized action and is more effective in opening the channels and collaterals to treat swelling and bruising.
- *Fu Yuan Huo Xue Tang* is directed more at treating the hypochondriac region and contains herbs that soothe Liver qi and dredge the channels.

Bŭ Yáng Huán Wŭ Tāng (Tonify the Yang to Restore Five Decoction)

補陽還五湯
补阳还五汤

Pinyin Name: *Bu Yang Huan Wu Tang*
Literal Name: Tonify the Yang to Restore Five Decoction
Alternate Names: *Pu Yang Huan Wu Tang*, Yang Nourishing Five Returning Decoction, Invigorating Recuperation Decoction, Astragalus and Peony Combination
Original Source: *Yi Lin Gai Cuo* (Corrections of Errors Among Physicians) by Wang Qing-Ren in 1830

COMPOSITION

Huang Qi (Radix Astragali)	120g
Dang Gui Wei (Extremitas Radix Angelicae Sinensis)	6g
Chuan Xiong (Rhizoma Chuanxiong)	3g
Chi Shao (Radix Paeoniae Rubra)	4.5g
Hong Hua (Flos Carthami)	3g
Tao Ren (Semen Persicae)	3g
Di Long (Pheretima)	3g

DOSAGE / PREPARATION / ADMINISTRATION

Prepare as a decoction.

CHINESE THERAPEUTIC ACTIONS

1. Tonifies qi
2. Activates blood circulation
3. Opens the channels and collaterals

CLINICAL MANIFESTATIONS

Post-stroke sequelae: hemiplegia, deviation of the mouth and eyes, involuntary salivation, atrophy of the hind limbs, frequent urination or urinary incontinence, a pale tongue, and a weak, wiry pulse.

VETERINARY CLINICAL APPLICATIONS

Degenerative myelopathy, muscle atrophy, paralysis, chronic intervertebral disk disease, post-laminectomy, fecal incontinence, urinary incontinence, fibrocartilaginous emboli (FCE), facial paralysis, weak hindquarters, post-concussion, polyneuritis, Horner's syndrome, polymyositis, diabetes mellitus, Cushing's disease, Addison's disease, chronic nephritis, epilepsy, and progressive retinal atrophy (PRA).

EXPLANATION

Bu Yang Huan Wu Tang (Tonify the Yang to Restore Five Decoction) is designed to treat various post-stroke clinical signs. After a stroke, the qi may become deficient, the blood stagnant, and the channels and collaterals obstructed. As a result, the muscles and tendons become malnourished, and the body cannot carry out normal physical functions, resulting in clinical signs such as hemiplegia, deviation of the mouth and eyes, involuntary salivation, and urinary incontinence. Hemiplegia and deviation of the mouth and eyes indicate blood stagnation obstructing the channels and collaterals. Involuntary salivation and urinary incontinence indicate qi deficiency with the inability to control bodily functions.

This formula uses a large dose of *Huang Qi* (Radix Astragali) to greatly tonify *zheng* (upright) and *yuan* (source) *qi*. Abundance of qi promotes blood circulation and allows

***Bu Yang Huan Wu Tang* (Tonify the Yang to Restore Five Decoction)**

Diagnosis	Clinical Signs	Treatment	Herbs
Post-stroke sequelae	• Hemiplegia and deviation of the mouth and eyes: blood stagnation obstructing the channels and collaterals • Involuntary salivation and urinary incontinence: qi deficiency with the inability to control body functions	• Tonifies qi • Activates blood circulation • Opens the channels and collaterals	• *Huang Qi* (Radix Astragali) greatly tonifies *zheng* (upright) and *yuan* (source) *qi*. • *Dang Gui Wei* (Extremitas Radix Angelicae Sinensis), *Chuan Xiong* (Rhizoma Chuanxiong), *Chi Shao* (Radix Paeoniae Rubra), *Tao Ren* (Semen Persicae), and *Hong Hua* (Flos Carthami) activate the blood and eliminate blood stasis. • *Di Long* (Pheretima) unblocks the channels and collaterals to restore normal physical functions.

Bŭ Yáng Huán Wŭ Tāng (Tonify the Yang to Restore Five Decoction)

elimination of blood stasis without damaging the body. *Dang Gui Wei* (Extremitas Radix Angelicae Sinensis), *Chuan Xiong* (Rhizoma Chuanxiong), *Chi Shao* (Radix Paeoniae Rubra), *Tao Ren* (Semen Persicae), and *Hong Hua* (Flos Carthami) activate the blood and eliminate blood stasis. *Di Long* (Pheretima) unblocks the channels and collaterals to restore normal physical functions. With sufficient qi, normal blood circulation, and unobstructed channels and collaterals, the body will gradually recover from all of the clinical signs of the previous injury or blockage.

VETERINARY MODIFICATIONS

- With urinary incontinence, add *Yi Zhi* (Fructus Alpiniae Oxyphyllae), *Wu Yao* (Radix Linderae) and *Sang Piao Xiao* (Ootheca Mantidis).
- For progressive retinal atrophy, add *Ji Xue Teng* (Caulis Spatholobi), *Gou Qi Zi* (Fructus Lycii) and *Bai Shao* (Radix Paeoniae Alba).
- With facial paralysis and deviation of the eyes and mouth, add *Bai Fu Zi* (Rhizoma Typhonii), *Jiang Can* (Bombyx Batryticatus), and *Quan Xie* (Scorpio).
- For initial onset of hemiplegia, add *Fang Feng* (Radix Saposhnikoviae).
- For chronic hemiplegia without improvement, add *Shui Zhi* (Hirudo) and *Meng Chong* (Tabanus).
- With paralysis of the hind limbs, add *Du Zhong* (Cortex Eucommiae) and *Niu Xi* (Radix Achyranthis Bidentatae).
- With impaired mental functions, add *Shi Chang Pu* (Rhizoma Acori Tatarinowii), *Yin Xing Ye* (Folium Ginkgo), and *Jiu Ceng Ta* (Herba Ocimi Basilici).
- With cold conditions, add *Fu Zi* (Radix Aconiti Lateralis Praeparata), *Rou Gui* (Cortex Cinnamomi), and *Ba Ji Tian* (Radix Morindae Officinalis).
- With Spleen and Stomach deficiencies, add *Dang Shen* (Radix Codonopsis) and *Bai Zhu* (Rhizoma Atractylodis Macrocephalae).
- With profuse phlegm, add *Ban Xia* (Rhizoma Pinelliae) and *Tian Zhu Huang* (Concretio Silicea Bambusae).
- With irritability and a wiry, deficient, rapid pulse, add *Zhi Zi* (Fructus Gardeniae) and *Suan Zao Ren* (Semen Ziziphi Spinosae).
- With congestive heart failure, add *San Qi* (Radix et Rhizoma Notoginseng) and *Dan Shen* (Radix et Rhizoma Salviae Miltiorrhizae).

CAUTIONS / CONTRAINDICATIONS

- *Bu Yang Huan Wu Tang* is contraindicated in animals with Liver wind rising, yin-deficient heat, or stagnation of phlegm.
- Because this formula contains strong blood-activating and blood-stasis removing herbs, it should not be used immediately after trauma with cerebral hemorrhage.
- This formula is contraindicated in animals that have a forceful pulse, which indicates an excess condition. This formula contains a large dose of *Huang Qi* (Radix Astragali), a tonic herb with ascending properties, and may exacerbate excess conditions.

PHARMACOLOGICAL EFFECTS

1. **Effects on the central nervous system**: According to various *in vitro* studies, administration of *Bu Yang Huan Wu Tang* was associated with dilating blood vessels in the brain and improving blood perfusion to the brain.[1] The effect lasted for up to 1 hour following intravenous injection of this formula at 0.25-0.5 g/kg.[2] Furthermore, it was shown that use of *Bu Yang Huan Wu Tang* facilitated the healing and recovery of subjects who suffered from nervous system damage to the brain and spine.[3]
2. **Antiplatelet, anticoagulant and thrombolytic**: *Bu Yang Huan Wu Tang* has been shown to have antiplatelet, anticoagulant, and thrombolytic effects in both *in vitro* and *in vivo* studies.[4,5,6]
3. **Antihyperlipidemic**: According to various *in vitro* studies, administration of *Bu Yang Huan Wu Tang* was associated with a reduction in total cholesterol levels and triglyceride levels. No significant changes were noted in HDL.[7,8]
4. **Cardiovascular**: In one study of anesthetized rabbits, administration of *Bu Yang Huan Wu Tang* showed different effects at different doses. At 0.5 g/kg given via intravenous injection, no significant changes were noted to blood pressure and heart rate. At 1.0 to 2.0 g/kg given via intravenous injection, blood pressure was reduced for up to 20 minutes with no changes to heart rate.[9]

HUMAN CLINICAL STUDIES AND RESEARCH

1. **Cerebrovascular disease**: Use of *Bu Yang Huan Wu Tang* plus *Gui Zhi* (Ramulus Cinnamomi) and *Fu Zi* (Radix Aconiti Lateralis Praeparata) in 32 patients with cerebrovascular disease was associated with recovery in 12 cases, significant improvement in 17 cases, moderate improvement in 2 cases, and no effect in 1 case.[10]
2. **Cerebral infarction**: Fifty patients with cerebral infarction due to stenosis of the artery were treated with *Bu Yang Huan Wu Tang* with complete recovery in 31 cases, significant recovery in 9 cases, moderate improvement in 5 cases, and no effect in 5 cases.[11]
3. **Stroke**: According to one study, 150 patients with stroke characterized by qi deficiency and blood stagnation were treated with complete recovery in 64 cases, marked improvement in 40 cases, moderate improvement in 45 cases, and fatality in 1 case. Treatment included herbs,

Bǔ Yáng Huán Wǔ Tāng (Tonify the Yang to Restore Five Decoction)

acupuncture, and *tui-na*. The herbal formula contained *Bu Yang Huan Wu Tang* plus *Dan Shen* (Radix et Rhizoma Salviae Miltiorrhizae) and *Ji Xue Teng* (Caulis Spatholobi).[12]

4. **Ischemic cerebrovascular disorder**: Administration of *Bu Yang Huan Wu Tang* has been shown in many studies to treat patients with ischemic stroke. According to one study, use of this formula plus *Chuan Shan Jia* (Squama Manis) and *Ji Xue Teng* (Caulis Spatholobi) for 2-3 months in 103 patients was associated with 96.3% effectiveness.[13] According to another study, concurrent treatment of herbs (*Bu Yang Huan Wu Tang* daily for 10 days per course of treatment) and acupuncture (every other day for 5 treatments per course) was associated with 97.7% effectiveness among 45 patients with ischemic cerebrovascular disorder.[14]
5. **Post-stroke sequelae**: Many studies of *Bu Yang Huan Wu Tang* have shown it to be one of the most effective herbal formulas for post-stroke sequelae. One study of 35 post-stroke patients reported 94% effectiveness when treated with modified *Bu Yang Huan Wu Tang*. The herbal formula contained *Huang Qi* (Radix Astragali) 30-120g, *Dang Gui* (Radix Angelicae Sinensis) 10g, *Chi Shao* (Radix Paeoniae Rubra) 10g, *Tao Ren* (Semen Persicae) 10g, *Hong Hua* (Flos Carthami) 10g, *Di Long* (Pheretima) 10g, *Dan Shen* (Radix et Rhizoma Salviae Miltiorrhizae) 30g, and *Chuan Xiong* (Rhizoma Chuanxiong) 6g. *Ban Xia* (Rhizoma Pinelliae) and *Chen Pi* (Pericarpium Citri Reticulatae) were added for phlegm and dampness; *Tian Ma* (Rhizoma Gastrodiae) and *Gou Teng* (Ramulus Uncariae cum Uncis) for Liver yang rising; *Dang Shen* (Radix Codonopsis) for qi and blood deficiencies; and *Da Huang* (Radix et Rhizoma Rhei) and *Huo Ma Ren* (Fructus Cannabis) for constipation. The herbs were cooked in water, and the decoction was taken in two equally-divided doses in the afternoon and evening.[15]
6. **Paralysis**: Ninety-three patients with paralysis due to stroke were treated with *Bu Yang Huan Wu Tang* plus *Ji Xue Teng* (Caulis Spatholobi), *Niu Xi* (Radix Achyranthis Bidentatae), *Qian Nian Jian* (Rhizoma Homalomenae), and other herbs with good results (complete recovery in 40 cases, significant improvement in 31 cases, moderate improvement in 20 cases, and no effect in 2 cases).[16]
7. **Facial paralysis**: One study reported complete recovery in 18 of 20 patients with facial paralysis using *Bu Yang Huan Wu Tang* plus *Qian Zheng San* (Lead to Symmetry Powder).[17] Another study reported complete recovery in all 15 patients with facial paralysis using *Bu Yang Huan Wu Tang* plus *Wu Gong* (Scolopendra), *Fang Feng* (Radix Saposhnikoviae), *Jiang Can* (Bombyx Batryticatus), and others.[18]
8. **Brain trauma**: One study reported 97.2% effectiveness using *Bu Yang Huan Wu Tang* to treat brain trauma in 36 patients (between 8-62 years of age, 17 days to 11 years history of illness). Clinical improvements included relief of, dizziness, insomnia, excessive dreams, poor memory, speech difficulties, and paralysis. Of 36 patients, the study reported complete recovery in 26 cases, marked improvement in 9 cases, and no effect in 1 case. Each course of treatment was 30 days.[19]
9. **Coronary heart disease**: *Bu Yang Huan Wu Tang* was reported in several studies to treat coronary heart disease. According to one study, use of modified *Bu Yang Huan Wu Tang* in decoction daily for 30 days per course of treatment was associated with 96.3% effectiveness for 82 patients.[20] According to another study, coronary heart disease characterized by qi deficiency and blood stagnation was treated with 83.7% effectiveness using *Bu Yang Huan Wu Tang* plus *Yu Jin* (Radix Curcumae) 10g, *Yi Mu Cao* (Herba Leonuri) 10g, *Gua Lou* (Fructus Trichosanthis) 10g, *Xie Bai* (Bulbus Allii Macrostemonis) 10g, and *Ban Xia* (Rhizoma Pinelliae) 10g. The herbs were given in decoction daily, for 10 days per course of treatment.[21]
10. **Poliomyelitis**: One study reported good results in treating poliomyelitis in young children using *Bu Yang Huan Wu Tang* plus *Yin Yang Huo* (Herba Epimedii) as the base formula, with modifications as needed. *Quan Xie* (Scorpio) and *Wu Gong* (Scolopendra) were added for treating the early stage of illness. *Qian Zheng San* (Lead to Symmetry Powder) was added for deviation of the eyes and mouth. *Sang Zhi* (Ramulus Mori) was added for paralysis of the arms, and *Niu Xi* (Radix Achyranthis Bidentatae) for paralysis of the legs. The study reported complete recovery in 37 of 42 patients.[22]
11. **Polyneuritis**: Use of herbs topically as an herbal wash proved beneficial for treating polyneuritis. The warm herbal formula contained *Bu Yang Huan Wu Tang* plus *Dang Shen* (Radix Codonopsis), *Fu Ling* (Poria), *Bai Zhu* (Rhizoma Atractylodis Macrocephalae), and others as needed. The treatment protocol was to cook the herbs in 1500 mL of water to yield 1000 mL of solution. (50g of ethanol was added to the final solution.) The herbal solution was applied topically to the affected area as an herbal wash. Of 19 patients, 13 had significant improvement and 6 had moderate improvement.[23]
12. **Chronic nephritis**: Use of *Bu Yang Huan Wu Tang* plus *Da Huang* (Radix et Rhizoma Rhei), *Ji Nei Jin* (Endothelium Corneum Gigeriae Galli), *Cang Zhu* (Rhizoma Atractylodis), and *Sang Ji Sheng* (Herba Taxilli) in 108 patients with chronic nephritis was associated with 96.3% effectiveness (73 with complete recovery, 16 with marked improvement, 15 with moderate improvement, and 4 with no effect).[24]

Bŭ Yáng Huán Wŭ Tāng (Tonify the Yang to Restore Five Decoction)

13. **Sciatica**: Administration of *Bu Yang Huan Wu Tang* has been shown to be effective in treating sciatica. In one study of 100 patients with sciatica, 98% effectiveness was reported using *Bu Yang Huan Wu Tang* plus *Gui Zhi* (Ramulus Cinnamomi), *Gan Cao* (Radix et Rhizoma Glycyrrhizae), *Dang Shen* (Radix Codonopsis), and *Ji Xue Teng* (Caulis Spatholobi) for 8-25 packs of herbs.[25] Another study reported 92% effectiveness among 53 patients with sciatica using *Bu Yang Huan Wu Tang* plus *Fu Zi* (Radix Aconiti Lateralis Praeparata), *Rou Gui* (Cortex Cinnamomi), *Wu Gong* (Scolopendra), and *Quan Xie* (Scorpio).[26]
14. **Numbness**: Administration of *Bu Yang Huan Wu Tang* was associated with 98% effectiveness in treating 56 patients with numbness from various causes such as hyperlipidemia, post-stroke sequelae, or hypertension. The herbal formula contained *Huang Qi* (Radix Astragali) 60g, *Dang Gui* (Radix Angelicae Sinensis) 12g, *Chi Shao* (Radix Paeoniae Rubra) 12g, *Wu Gong* (Scolopendra) 12g, *Quan Xie* (Scorpio) 12g, *Hai Feng Teng* (Caulis Piperis Kadsurae) 12g, *Tao Ren* (Semen Persicae) 10g, *Hong Hua* (Flos Carthami) 10g, *Chuan Xiong* (Rhizoma Chuanxiong) 10g, *Di Long* (Pheretima) 10g, and *Fu Zi* (Radix Aconiti Lateralis Praeparata) 3g. Modifications were made by: adding *Dan Shen* (Radix et Rhizoma Salviae Miltiorrhizae) for blood stagnation; *He Shou Wu* (Radix Polygoni Multiflori) for blood deficiency; *Ban Xia* (Rhizoma Pinelliae) and *Fu Ling* (Poria) for dampness; and *Niu Xi* (Radix Achyranthis Bidentatae) and *Long Gu* (Os Draconis) for Liver yang rising. The herbs were given daily in decoction. Of 56 patients, the study reported complete recovery in 25 cases, improvement in 30 cases, and no effect in 1 case.[27]

TOXICOLOGY

Bu Yang Huan Wu Tang has very little toxicity. According to one acute toxicology study, the LD_{50} in mice via injection is equivalent to 149 g/kg of dried herbs.[28]

SUGGESTED ACUPUNCTURE TREATMENT

1. Points: *Jianyu* (LI 15), *Quchi* (LI 11), *Waiguan* (TH 5), *Hegu* (LI 4), *Huantiao* (GB 30), *Yanglingquan* (GB 34), *Housanli* (ST 36), *Jiexi* (ST 41), *Kunlun* (BL 60), and additional points listed below for specific clinical signs.
2. Technique: tonification.

Since the yang is damaged after a stroke, it is important to tonify the major points of the yang channels. The *yangming* channel is the channel with the most qi and blood, therefore it should be the focus of the treatment. Besides the above points, others may be added to treat severe paralysis of the fore or hind limbs.

- *Jianjing* (LI 15), *Yangchi* (TH 4), and *Houxi* (SI 3) are effective in treating paralysis of the front limbs.
- *Fengmen* (BL 12), *Yinshi* (ST 33), and *Tianping* (GV 5) should be added in case of paralysis of the hind limbs.
- For deviation of the mouth and eyes, *Dicang* (ST 4), *Daying* (ST 5), *Chengqi* (ST 1), *Yangbai* (GB 14), *Zanzhu* (BL 2), *Yingxiang* (LI 20), *Tongziliao* (GB 1), and *Hegu* (LI 4) should be used.
- For spasms of the elbow, add *Quchi* (LI 11).
- For spasms of the carpus, add *Daling* (PC 7).
- For spasms of the front foot, add *Baxie* (extra point).
- For spasms of the stifle, add *Ququan* (LR 8).
- For spasms of the hock, add *Taixi* (KI 3).
- For spasms of the hind foot, add *Bafeng* (extra point).

AUTHORS' COMMENTS

Bu Yang Huan Wu Tang is a formula commonly used for treating dogs with degenerative myelopathy characterized by qi deficiency and blood stasis. It can take several months to see results with this formula regardless of the condition treated, and it is important to continue taking the formula for a sufficient period of time to see clinical improvement. Although the formula may not appear to be beneficial to many owners that have dogs with degenerative myelopathy, discontinuing the herbs in many cases has swiftly led to significant decline. In cases of facial paralysis, add *Quan Xie* (Scorpio), *Jiang Can* (Bombyx Batryticatus), and *Ji Xue Teng* (Caulis Spatholobi). For the treatment of fibrocartilaginous emboli (FCE), add *Ban Xia* (Rhizoma Pinelliae), *Ji Xue Teng* (Caulis Spatholobi), *Dan Shen* (Radix et Rhizoma Salviae Miltiorrhizae), *Wu Gong* (Scolopendra), *Quan Xie* (Scorpio), and *Niu Xi* (Radix Achyranthis Bidentatae).

This formula was formulated by Dr. Wang Qing-Ren, who believed that when the qi is normal and healthy, it is 100% functional, with an equal 50% bilateral distribution. Since severe qi deficiency is the primary imbalance in this syndrome, *Huang Qi* (Radix Astragali) is used as the chief herb at a very large dose to strongly tonify *zheng* (upright) *qi* and *yuan* (source) *qi*, generate flesh, and improve atrophy. This herb also tonifies qi to move the blood and transform blood stasis. Qi deficiency leads to blood deficiency, which in turn impedes the circulation of *yuan* (source) *qi* and aggravates the muscle atrophy. Therefore, small doses of invigorating herbs, such as *Chuan Xiong* (Rhizoma Chuanxiong), *Tao Ren* (Semen Persicae), *Hong Hua* (Flos Carthami), *Dang Gui* (Radix Angelicae Sinensis), *Chi Shao* (Radix Paeoniae Rubra), and *Di Long* (Pheretima), are added to enhance the blood-transforming function of this formula. In short, this formula aims at tonifying yang qi and nourishing the blood, muscles and sinews to restore bodily functions.

References

1. *Zhong Cheng Yao Yan Jiu* (Research of Chinese Patent Medicine), 1982; (7):34.
2. *Zhong Cheng Yao Yan Jiu* (Research of Chinese Patent Medicine), 1986; (12):29.
3. *Zhong Xi Yi Jie He Za Zhi* (Journal of Integrated Chinese and Western Medicine), 1984; 8:491.
4. *Zhong Cheng Yao Yan Jiu* (Research of Chinese Patent Medicine), 1983; 8:31.
5. *Hu Nan Zhong Yi Xue Yuan Xue Bao* (Journal of Hunan University of Traditional Chinese Medicine), 1989; 9:545.
6. *Yun Nan Zhong Yi Za Zhi* (Yunan Journal of Chinese Medicine), 1992; 13(1):23.
7. *Xin Zhong Yi* (New Chinese Medicine), 1984; 1:46.
8. *Zhong Guo Zhong Yao Za Zhi* (People's Republic of China Journal of Chinese Herbology), 1995; 20(11):685.
9. *Zhong Cheng Yao Yan Jiu* (Research of Chinese Patent Medicine), 1986; 3:28.
10. *Gui Yang Zhong Yi Xue Yuan Xue Bao* (Journal of Guiyang University of Traditional Chinese Medicine), 1992; 1:32.
11. *Zhe Jiang Zhong Yi Za Zhi* (Zhejiang Journal of Chinese Medicine), 1997; 7:317.
12. *Liao Ning Zhong Yi Za Zhi* (Liaoning Journal of Chinese Medicine), 1984; 9:26.
13. *Zhong Yi Za Zhi* (Journal of Chinese Medicine), 1984; 9:45.
14. *Guang Xi Zhong Yi Yao* (Guangxi Chinese Medicine and Herbology), 1993; 16(4):9.
15. *Guang Dong Yi Xue* (Guangdong Medicine), 1992; 13(1):39.
16. *He Bei Zhong Yi Za Zhi* (Hebei Journal of Chinese Medicine), 1986; 6:17.
17. *Yun Nan Zhong Yi Za Zhi* (Yunan Journal of Chinese Medicine), 1985; 5:64.
18. *Nei Meng Gu Zhong Yi Yao* (Traditional Chinese Medicine and Medicinals of Inner Mongolia), 1987; 2:24.
19. *Shan Dong Zhong Yi Za Zhi* (Shandong Journal of Chinese Medicine), 1993; 12(3):21.
20. *Hu Bei Zhong Yi Za Zhi* (Hubei Journal of Chinese Medicine), 1994; 16(1):17.
21. *Tian Jin Zhong Yi* (Tianjin Chinese Medicine), 1993; 5:22.
22. *Cheng Du Zhong Yi Xue Yuan Xue Bao* (Journal of Chengdu University of Traditional Chinese Medicine), 1991; 2:27.
23. *Si Chuan Zhong Yi* (Sichuan Chinese Medicine), 1996; 2:22.
24. *Shi Yong Zhong Yi Nei Ke Za Zhi* (Journal of Practical Chinese Internal Medicine), 1990; 4(3):123.
25. *Guang Xi Zhong Yi Yao* (Guangxi Chinese Medicine and Herbology), 1980; 2:6.
26. *Zhong Yi Fang Ji Xian Dai Yan Jiu* (Modern Study of Medical Formulas in Traditional Chinese Medicine), 1997; 1012.
27. *Shan Xi Zhong Yi* (Shanxi Chinese Medicine), 1995; 16(9):394.
28. *Xin Yi Yao Xue Za Zhi* (New Journal of Medicine and Herbology), 1977; 9:40.

Shī Xiào Săn (Sudden Smile Powder)

失笑散

Pinyin Name: *Shi Xiao San*
Literal Name: Sudden Smile Powder
Alternate Name: Sudden Smile Formula
Original Source: *Tai Ping Hui Min He Ji Ju Fang* (Imperial Grace Formulary of the Tai Ping Era) by the Imperial Medical Department in 1078-85

COMPOSITION

Wu Ling Zhi (Faeces Trogopteri), *yan* (ground) to small particles with liquor	[6g]
Pu Huang (Pollen Typhae), *chao* (dry-fried) until aromatic	[6g]

Shī Xiào Săn (Sudden Smile Powder)

DOSAGE / PREPARATION / ADMINISTRATION

The source text states to grind equal amount of both ingredients into a fine powder. Cook 6g of the powder with vinegar and condense it into a paste. Add 1 bowl of water and cook it again until the liquid is reduced to 70%. Take the warm decoction before meals. Today, this formula is prepared by grinding the ingredients into a fine powder. Take 6g of the powder with a grain-based liquor or vinegar. This formula may also be prepared as a decoction with the doses suggested in brackets.

CHINESE THERAPEUTIC ACTIONS

1. Activates blood circulation and removes blood stasis
2. Disperses stagnation and stops pain

CLINICAL MANIFESTATIONS

Blood stasis in the body: sharp pain in the chest or abdomen, postpartum bleeding due to retention of placenta, and acute onset of pain in the lower abdomen.

VETERINARY CLINICAL APPLICATIONS

Infertility, uterine bleeding caused by abortion or miscarriage, postpartum abdominal pain, and pain due to liver cancer.

EXPLANATION

Shi Xiao San (Sudden Smile Powder) is a commonly used formula for treating various presentations of pain caused by blood stasis and obstruction of blood circulation. It is especially useful for treating blood stagnation in the Liver channel.

This formula combines *Wu Ling Zhi* (Faeces Trogopteri) with *Pu Huang* (Pollen Typhae) to activate blood circulation, remove blood stagnation, and relieve pain. This formula is prepared with grain-based liquor to enhance the effect to warm the channels and invigorate blood circulation. Furthermore, this formula is taken with vinegar to improve the function to disperse blood stasis and relieve pain.

VETERINARY MODIFICATIONS

- With more severe qi stagnation, add *Chuan Lian Zi* (Fructus Toosendan) and *Xiang Fu* (Rhizoma Cyperi).
- With more cold, add *Pao Jiang* (Rhizoma Zingiberis Praeparatum) and *Xiao Hui Xiang* (Fructus Foeniculi).
- With irregular menstruation due to blood stasis and blood deficiency in primates, add *Si Wu Tang* (Four-Substance Decoction).

CAUTIONS / CONTRAINDICATIONS

- *Shi Xiao San* is contraindicated during pregnancy.
- This formula should be used with caution in patients with a weak or sensitive stomach.

PHARMACOLOGICAL EFFECTS

1. **Cardiovascular**: According to *in vitro* studies, use of *Shi Xiao San* was associated with reduced blood pressure and heart rate in both frogs and rabbits.[1,2]
2. **Antiplatelet**: According to an *in vitro* study in rats, administration of *Shi Xiao San* was associated with marked antiplatelet effect 4 hours after oral ingestion. The researchers noted that this formula has an antiplatelet effect comparable to aspirin.[3]
3. **Effect on the uterus**: According to clinical studies, *Shi Xiao San* has a marked regulatory effect on the uterus. It may stimulate contraction of the uterus to facilitate passage of placental remnants in postpartum women, or relax smooth muscle to relieve menstrual cramps in women with dysmenorrhea or premenstrual syndrome.[4]

HUMAN CLINICAL STUDIES AND RESEARCH

1. **Dysmenorrhea**: Many studies have reported success using *Shi Xiao San* to treat painful menstruation. According to one study, use of the formula in 108 women with dysmenorrhea was associated with significant relief in 72 cases, moderate improvement in 34 cases, and no effect in 2 cases. The treatment started herbal therapy 2-3 days prior to the period, for 5-7 packs of herbs per course of treatment.[5] Another study reported 97.5% effectiveness using this formula to treat 80 patients with dysmenorrhea. The treatment protocol was to administer one pack of herbs in decoction daily, starting 3 days before the period, for

***Shi Xiao San* (Sudden Smile Powder)**

Diagnosis	Clinical Signs	Treatment	Herbs
Blood stasis in the body	Abdominal pain, postpartum bleeding due to retention of lochia, irregular menstruation, and sharp pain in the lower abdomen: blood stasis with obstructed blood circulation	• Activates blood circulation and removes blood stasis • Disperses stagnation and stops pain	• *Wu Ling Zhi* (Faeces Trogopteri) activates blood circulation, removes blood stagnation, and relieves pain. • *Pu Huang* (Pollen Typhae) activates blood circulation, stops bleeding, and relieves pain.

Shī Xiào Săn (Sudden Smile Powder)

6 packs of herbs per course of treatment, for a total of 3 menstrual cycles.[6]

2. **Endometriosis**: Thirty patients with endometriosis were treated with herbs, with complete recovery in 12 cases, marked improvement in 16 cases, and no effect in 2 cases. The herbal treatment contained dry-fried *Pu Huang* (Pollen Typhae) 8g, *Wu Ling Zhi* (Faeces Trogopteri) 12g, *Xue Jie* (Sanguis Draconis) 1.5g, and *San Qi* (Radix et Rhizoma Notoginseng) 1.5g.[7]
3. **Uterine bleeding**: According to one study, women with excessive uterine bleeding (in volume or duration) were treated with 84.7% effectiveness using *Dang Gui* (Radix Angelicae Sinensis) 9-12g, *Chuan Xiong* (Rhizoma Chuanxiong) 6-9g, *Pu Huang* (Pollen Typhae) 6-9g, dry-fried *Wu Ling Zhi* (Faeces Trogopteri) 10g, and *Tao Ren* (Semen Persicae) 10g. Of 59 patients, the study reported marked improvement in 43 cases, moderate improvement in 7 cases, and no effect in 9 cases.[8]
4. **Uterine bleeding caused by abortion or miscarriage**: *Shi Xiao San* has been shown to be effective in stopping bleeding in women with profuse bleeding following miscarriage. Most treatment protocols use *Shi Xiao San* as the base formula, with the addition of *Gui Zhi Fu Ling Wan* (Cinnamon Twig and Poria Pill) to discharge placental remnants, *Bu Zhong Yi Qi Tang* (Tonify the Middle and Augment the Qi Decoction) and/or *Gui Pi Tang* (Restore the Spleen Decoction) for qi and blood deficiencies, and heat-clearing herbs for infection.[9,10]
5. **Angina pectoris and coronary artery disease**: One study reported good results using *Shi Xiao San* to treat 46 patients with angina and coronary artery disease. The herbal formula contained 15g each of *Wu Ling Zhi* (Faeces Trogopteri), *Pu Huang* (Pollen Typhae), *Chuan Xiong* (Rhizoma Chuanxiong), *Tao Ren* (Semen Persicae), and *Hong Hua* (Flos Carthami). The treatment protocol was to administer the herbs in decoction daily, for 1 month per course of treatment, for 1-5 courses total. Of 44 patients, the study reported 88.6% effectiveness based on symptomatic evaluation, and 28.1% effectiveness based on EKG readings.[11]
6. **Viral hepatitis**: One study of 200 patients with viral hepatitis reported a 70% recovery rate using *Shi Xiao San* plus *Yin Chen Hao Tang* (Artemisia Scoparia Decoction). The base formula contained *Wu Ling Zhi* (Faeces Trogopteri) 10-15g, dry-fried *Pu Huang* (Pollen Typhae) 10-15g, *Yin Chen* (Herba Artemisiae Scopariae) 30-60g, *Zhi Zi* (Fructus Gardeniae) 10g, and *Da Huang* (Radix et Rhizoma Rhei) 10-30g. Other herbs were added depending on the condition of the individual. For acute hepatitis with jaundice, *Huang Bo* (Cortex Phellodendri Chinensis), *Yi Yi Ren* (Semen Coicis), *Fu Ling* (Poria), *Yu Jin* (Radix Curcumae), *Pu Gong Ying* (Herba Taraxaci), and *Jin Qian Cao* (Herba Lysimachiae) were added. For acute hepatitis without jaundice, *Long Dan* (Radix et Rhizoma Gentianae), *Mu Dan Pi* (Cortex Moutan), *Ze Xie* (Rhizoma Alismatis), *Fu Ling* (Poria), *Yi Yi Ren* (Semen Coicis), *Che Qian Zi* (Semen Plantaginis), *Mu Tong* (Caulis Akebiae), and *Chi Shao* (Radix Paeoniae Rubra) were added. For chronic infectious hepatitis, *Yu Jin* (Radix Curcumae), *Yan Hu Suo* (Rhizoma Corydalis), *Bai Shao* (Radix Paeoniae Alba), *Dang Gui* (Radix Angelicae Sinensis), *Chuan Xiong* (Rhizoma Chuanxiong), *Bai Zhu* (Rhizoma Atractylodis Macrocephalae), *Ji Nei Jin* (Endothelium Corneum Gigeriae Galli), and *Yi Yi Ren* (Semen Coicis) were added. For chronic active hepatitis, *Chi Shao* (Radix Paeoniae Rubra), *Mu Dan Pi* (Cortex Moutan), *Long Dan* (Radix et Rhizoma Gentianae), vinegar-processed *Chai Hu* (Radix Bupleuri), *Yu Jin* (Radix Curcumae), *Pu Gong Ying* (Herba Taraxaci), *Zhi Qiao* (Fructus Aurantii), *Yan Hu Suo* (Rhizoma Corydalis), and *Bai Hua She She Cao* (Herba Hedyotis) were added. With hepatomegaly or splenomegaly, *Dang Gui* (Radix Angelicae Sinensis), *Bai Shao* (Radix Paeoniae Alba), *Chuan Xiong* (Rhizoma Chuanxiong), *Yu Jin* (Radix Curcumae), *Yan Hu Suo* (Rhizoma Corydalis), *Zhi Qiao* (Fructus Aurantii), processed *Bie Jia* (Carapax Trionycis), *San Leng* (Rhizoma Sparganii), *E Zhu* (Rhizoma Curcumae), and *Bai Hua She She Cao* (Herba Hedyotis) were added. Of 139 patients with acute viral hepatitis, 112 experienced complete recovery. Of 61 patients with chronic viral hepatitis, 28 had recovered completely.[12]

SUGGESTED ACUPUNCTURE TREATMENT

1. Points: *Geshu* (BL 17) and *Xuehai* (SP 10).
2. Technique: sedation.

Geshu (BL 17) is one of the *ba hui* (eight meeting) points dominating the blood. It can be used for various types of blood disorders. Here, it is used to activate and regulate blood circulation. *Xuehai* (SP 10), literally "sea of blood," activates blood and dispels blood stagnation.

AUTHORS' COMMENTS

The literal translation of *Shi Xiao San* on a word-for-word basis is *shi* (lose) *xiao* (smile) *san* (powder). However, this literal translation is misleading and does not convey the true meaning of the formula. When *Shi Xiao San* is prescribed to treat severe pain associated with dysmenorrhea, the formula has such a strong and immediate effect to relieve pain that the patients break into a "sudden smile." They are often at a loss as to why the pain disappeared so quickly. So, while the literal translation of *Shi Xiao San* is "lose a smile powder," the actual meaning is "at-a-loss and smile powder."

Shī Xiào Sǎn (Sudden Smile Powder)

References

1. *Shan Xi Yi Yao Za Zhi* (Shanxi Journal of Medicine and Herbology), 1974; 8:11.
2. *Shan Xi Yi Yao Za Zhi* (Shanxi Journal of Medicine and Herbology), 1974; 8:17.
3. *Zhong Yao Xian Dai Yan Jiu Yu Ying Yong* (Modern Study of Traditional Chinese Medicine), 1997; 1087.
4. *Shang Hai Zhong Yi Yao Za Zhi* (Shanghai Journal of Chinese Medicine and Herbology), 1963; 9:1.
5. *Xin Jiang Zhong Yi Yao* (Xinjiang Chinese Medicine and Herbology), 1986; 1:32.
6. *He Bei Zhong Yi* (Hebei Chinese Medicine), 1991; 3:16.
7. *Jiang Su Zhong Yi* (Jiangsu Chinese Medicine), 1990; 8:14.
8. *Hu Bei Zhong Yi Za Zhi* (Hubei Journal of Chinese Medicine), 1990; 4:17.
9. *Zhe Jiang Zhong Yi Xue Yuan Xue Bao* (Journal of Zhejiang University of Chinese Medicine), 1985; 2:20.
10. *Hu Bei Zhong Yi Za Zhi* (Hubei Journal of Chinese Medicine), 1986; 2:42.
11. *Xin Yi Yao Xue Za Zhi* (New Journal of Medicine and Herbology), 1976; 5:41.
12. *Hu Bei Zhong Yi Za Zhi* (Hubei Journal of Chinese Medicine), 1985; 5:17.

Huó Luò Xiào Líng Dān

(Fantastically Effective Pill to Invigorate the Collaterals)

活絡效靈丹

活络效灵丹

Pinyin Name: *Huo Luo Xiao Ling Dan*

Literal Name: Fantastically Effective Pill to Invigorate the Collaterals

Original Source: *Yi Xue Zhong Zhong Can Xi Lu* (Records of Heart-Felt Experiences in Medicine With Reference to the West) by Zhang Xi-Chun in 1918-34

COMPOSITION

Dan Shen (Radix et Rhizoma Salviae Miltiorrhizae)	15g
Ru Xiang (Gummi Olibanum), fresh	15g
Mo Yao (Myrrha), fresh	15g
Dang Gui (Radix Angelicae Sinensis)	15g

DOSAGE / PREPARATION / ADMINISTRATION

Prepare as a decoction. This formula may also be administered in powder form. Grind the ingredients into powder, using the doses given above. Take the powder in four equally divided doses with a warm, grain-based liquor.

CHINESE THERAPEUTIC ACTIONS

1. Activates blood circulation and dispels blood stasis
2. Unblocks the collaterals and relieves pain

Huó Luò Xiào Líng Dān

(Fantastically Effective Pill to Invigorate the Collaterals)

CLINICAL MANIFESTATIONS

Qi and blood stagnation: chest and abdominal pain, pain of the limbs, bruises and swelling due to trauma, and other external disorders such as skin abscesses, scrofulae, and ulcers.

VETERINARY CLINICAL APPLICATIONS

Bi zheng (painful obstruction syndrome), degenerative joint disease, canine hip dysplasia, elbow and shoulder dysplasia, intervertebral disk disease, sciatica, fibrocartilaginous emboli, spondylosis, cerebrovascular accident, and cervical spondylosis.

EXPLANATION

Huo Luo Xiao Ling Dan (Fantastically Effective Pill to Invigorate the Collaterals) treats various types of pain and disorders, both external and internal, due to qi and blood stagnation. The formula uses *Dan Shen* (Radix et Rhizoma Salviae Miltiorrhizae) to invigorate blood circulation and remove blood stasis. *Ru Xiang* (Gummi Olibanum) and *Mo Yao* (Myrrha) activate qi and blood circulation to relieve pain. *Dang Gui* (Radix Angelicae Sinensis) nourishes the blood and activates blood circulation.

VETERINARY MODIFICATIONS

- With leg pain, add *Niu Xi* (Radix Achyranthis Bidentatae).
- With arm pain, add *Lian Qiao* (Fructus Forsythiae).
- With painful abdomen due to pancreatitis, add *Tao Ren* (Semen Persicae) and *Wu Ling Zhi* (Faeces Trogopteri).
- With yang-type sores with redness and swelling, add *Jin Yin Hua* (Flos Lonicerae Japonicae), *Lian Qiao* (Fructus Forsythiae), and *Zhi Mu* (Rhizoma Anemarrhenae).
- With yin-type sores that are hard, add *Rou Gui* (Cortex Cinnamomi) and *Lu Jiao Jiao* (Colla Cornus Cervi).
- With chronic sores that are slow to heal, add *Huang Qi* (Radix Astragali), *Zhi Mu* (Rhizoma Anemarrhenae), and *Gan Cao* (Radix et Rhizoma Glycyrrhizae).
- With abscesses of the internal organs, add *San Qi* (Radix et Rhizoma Notoginseng) and *Niu Bang Zi* (Fructus Arctii).

CAUTIONS / CONTRAINDICATIONS

- *Huo Luo Xiao Ling Dan* is contraindicated during pregnancy and in the absence of blood stasis.[1]
- The use of this formula is sometimes associated with nausea, vomiting, and gastrointestinal discomfort. Under these circumstances, the doses of *Ru Xiang* (Gummi Olibanum) and *Mo Yao* (Myrrha) should be reduced to 6g to 9g from 15g.[2,3]

HUMAN CLINICAL STUDIES AND RESEARCH

1. ***Bi zheng* (painful obstruction syndrome)**: Administration of customized *Huo Luo Xiao Ling Dan* in 123 patients with *bi zheng* (painful obstruction syndrome) was associated with complete recovery in 102 cases, improvement in 17 cases, and no effect in 4 cases. The study stated that most patients began to notice an effect after 5 packs of herbs, improvement after 10 packs of herbs, and recovery between 20-40 packs of herbs.[4]
2. **Heel pain**: One study reported good results using modified *Huo Luo Xiao Ling Dan* to treat 60 patients with heel pain. Modifications to the formula included the addition of *Shi Hu* (Caulis Dendrobii) 15g, *Di Huang* (Radix Rehmanniae) 15g, and *Huang Bo* (Cortex Phellodendri Chinensis) 12g for yin deficiency; and *Dang Shen* (Radix Codonopsis) 12-15g and *Huang Qi* (Radix Astragali) 12-15g for qi deficiency. Of 60 patients, 45 recovered completely (able to resume normal physical activities without any restrictions), 14 experienced significant improvement (slight pain only after prolonged physical activities), and 1 had no benefit.[5]
3. **Sciatica**: *Huo Luo Xiao Ling Dan* has been shown in several studies to effectively treat sciatica. According to one study, 61 patients with sciatica were treated with good results using modified *Huo Luo Xiao Ling Dan*. Modifications to the formula included addition of *Du Huo* (Radix Angelicae Pubescentis) 10g, *Qin Jiao* (Radix Gentianae Macrophyllae) 10g, and *Fang Feng* (Radix Saposhnikoviae) 10g for wind-cold; *Du Huo* (Radix Angelicae Pubescentis) 10g, *Ze Lan* (Herba Lycopi) 10g, and *Shen Jin Cao* (Herba Lycopodii) 20g for damp-cold;

***Huo Luo Xiao Ling Dan* (Fantastically Effective Pill to Invigorate the Collaterals)**

Diagnosis	Clinical Signs	Treatment	Herbs
Qi and blood stagnation	Heart and abdominal pain, pain of the arms and legs, and bruises and swelling due to trauma: qi and blood stagnation	• Activates the blood and dispels blood stasis • Unblocks the collaterals and relieves pain	• *Dan Shen* (Radix et Rhizoma Salviae Miltiorrhizae) invigorates blood circulation and removes blood stasis. • *Ru Xiang* (Gummi Olibanum) and *Mo Yao* (Myrrha) activate the blood and qi to relieve pain. • *Dang Gui* (Radix Angelicae Sinensis) nourishes the blood and activates blood circulation.

Huó Luò Xiào Líng Dān

(Fantastically Effective Pill to Invigorate the Collaterals)

Huang Bo (Cortex Phellodendri Chinensis) 15g, *Zhi Mu* (Rhizoma Anemarrhenae) 10g, and *Mu Fang Ji* (Radix Cocculi Trilobi) 12g for damp-heat; and *Ma Qian Zi* (Semen Strychni) 0.3-0.9g and *Bai Zhi* (Radix Angelicae Dahuricae) 10g for severe pain. The treatment protocol was to cook the herbs in water, and administer the decoction in two equally-divided doses with a small amount of grain-based liquor daily, for 5 days per course of treatment, for 3-4 courses total. Of 61 patients, the study reported recovery in 43 cases, significant improvement in 12 cases, moderate improvement in 4 cases, and no effect in 2 cases.[6]

Another study reported 98% effectiveness using modified formulas to treat 119 patients with sciatica. The herbal treatment contained *Huo Luo Xiao Ling Dan* and *Shao Yao Gan Cao Tang* (Peony and Licorice Decoction) as the base formulas. Modifications included the addition of *Tao Ren* (Semen Persicae) and *Hong Hua* (Flos Carthami) for severe pain; *Zhi Chuan Wu* (Radix Aconiti Praeparata), *Zhi Cao Wu* (Radix Aconiti Kusnezoffii Praeparata), and *Cang Zhu* (Rhizoma Atractylodis) for severe pain during cold, rainy days; and *Wei Ling Xian* (Radix et Rhizoma Clematidis) and *Si Gua Luo* (Retinervus Luffae Fructus) for pain in the limbs. Of 119 patients, the study reported complete recovery in 89 cases, improvement in 29 cases, and no effect in 1 case.[7]

4. **Ischemic stroke**: One study reported good results when 77 patients with ischemic stroke were treated with large doses of modified *Huo Luo Xiao Ling Dan*. The herbal treatment contained 24 grams each of *Ru Xiang* (Gummi Olibanum), *Mo Yao* (Myrrha), *Dan Shen* (Radix et Rhizoma Salviae Miltiorrhizae), and *Dang Gui* (Radix Angelicae Sinensis). The duration of treatment was 10 days per course, for 3-5 courses total. Of 77 patients, the study reported near-complete recovery in 40 cases, significant improvement in 22 cases, moderate improvement in 12 cases, no effect in 2 cases, and fatality in 1 case.[8]
5. **Thromboangiitis obliterans**: Use of *Huo Luo Xiao Ling Dan* plus *Si Miao Yong An Tang* (Four-Valiant Decoction for Well-Being) in 17 patients with thromboangiitis obliterans was associated with complete recovery in 11 cases, significant improvement in 2 cases, and no effect in 4 cases. The treatment protocol was to cook the herbs in decoction, and administer the decoction in three to four equally-divided doses daily.[9]
6. **Cervical spondylosis**: One study reported good results treating cervical spondylosis using both oral and topical applications of herbs. For oral use, the herbal treatment contained *Huo Luo Xiao Ling Dan*, with the addition of *Gui Zhi* (Ramulus Cinnamomi) 5g, *Qiang Huo* (Rhizoma et Radix Notopterygii) 10g, and *Xi Xin* (Radix et Rhizoma Asari) 5g for cold; *Di Long* (Pheretima) 10g, *Ju Hua* (Flos Chrysanthemi) 10g, and *Sheng Ma* (Rhizoma Cimicifugae) 10g for heat; *Bai Jie Zi* (Semen Sinapis) 10g and *Fu Ling* (Poria) 10g for damp and phlegm; and *Qiang Huo* (Rhizoma et Radix Notopterygii) 10g and *Sang Zhi* (Ramulus Mori) 10g for numbness. The herbs were cooked in water, and the decoction was administered in three equally-divided doses, with a small amount of grain-based liquor. The herb residue (from the decoction) was combined with 50g of *Tou Gu Cao* (Caulis Impatientis) and a small amount of *Hua Jiao* (Pericarpium Zanthoxyli), cooked in water, and the resultant solution applied topically to the affected area. The duration was 5 packs of herbs per course of treatment, for 4-7 courses total. Of 50 patients, the study reported complete recovery in 23 cases, significant improvement in 17 cases, moderate improvement in 8 cases, and no effect in 2 cases.[10]

SUGGESTED ACUPUNCTURE TREATMENT

1. Points: *Geshu* (BL 17), *Xuehai* (SP 10), and special points listed below.
2. Techniques: even method and sedation.

Geshu (BL 17) and *Xuehai* (SP 10) are general points for activating blood circulation and removing blood stagnation. Depending on the location of the blood stasis and pain, the following points may be used:

- *Xinshu* (BL 15), *Juque* (CV 14), *Yinxi* (HT 6), and *Shanzhong* (CV 17) for pain in the chest
- *Zhongwan* (CV 12), *Housanli* (ST 36), *Daheng* (SP 15), and *Gongsun* (SP 4) for abdominal pain
- Local points may be selected for localized trauma

AUTHORS' COMMENTS

Huo Luo Xiao Ling Dan is not typically used as a sole formula for the treatment of neuromuscular and musculoskeletal diseases in veterinary medicine. Instead, it is combined with various formulas to comprehensively treat the condition and/or constitutional weakness.

- For chronic arthritis, spondylosis or intervertebral disk disease, combine with *Du Huo Ji Sheng Tang* (Angelica Pubescens and Taxillus Decoction).
- For chronic arthritis, spondylosis or intervertebral disk disease that is accompanied by Kidney qi and yang deficiencies, combine with *Jin Gui Shen Qi Wan* (Kidney Qi Pill from the Golden Cabinet).
- For cervical pain or intervertebral disk disease, combine with *Juan Bi Tang* (Remove Painful Obstruction Decoction).
- For acute *bi zheng* (painful obstruction syndrome) caused by wind-cold-dampness, combine with *Shu Jing Huo*

Huó Luò Xiào Líng Dān
(Fantastically Effective Pill to Invigorate the Collaterals)

Xue Tang (Relax the Channels and Invigorate the Blood Decoction).

Huo Luo Xiao Ling Dan, Xiao Huo Luo Dan (Minor Invigorate the Collaterals Special Pill) and *Da Huo Luo Dan* (Major Invigorate the Collaterals Special Pill) are three formulas that have similar names and contain the herbs *Mo Yao* (Myrrha) and *Ru Xiang* (Gummi Olibanum). While all three formulas function to unblock the channels and collaterals, they are quite different in their other actions.

- *Huo Luo Xiao Ling Dan* activates blood circulation, dispels blood stasis, and dredges the collaterals to relieve pain. This formula is effective for various types of pain and disorders due to qi and blood stagnation, such as chest and abdominal pain, pain of the limbs, and bruises and swelling due to trauma. It is categorized as a blood-regulating formula.
- *Xiao Huo Luo Dan* is more suitable for treating obstruction of wind, cold, and dampness, accumulation of phlegm, and stagnation of blood in the channels and collaterals in animals that are otherwise healthy. All of the herbs in this formula focus on the treatment of excess conditions. This formula is categorized as a wind-damp-dispelling formula.
- *Da Huo Luo Dan* treats obstruction of the collaterals in animals with underlying qi and blood deficiencies. This formula uses qi- and blood-tonifying herbs to support the underlying deficiencies, along with herbs to dispel wind and open the channels and collaterals. This formula is categorized as a wind-damp-dispelling formula.

References

1. *Zhong Yao Ming Fang Yao Li Yu Ying Yong* (Pharmacology and Applications of Famous Herbal Formulas), 1989; 470-472.
2. *Shan Xi Xin Yi Yao* (New Medicine and Herbology of Shanxi), 1979; (11):47.
3. *Yun Nan Zhong Yi Za Zhi* (Yunan Journal of Chinese Medicine), 1983; (2):20.
4. *Hu Bei Zhong Yi Za Zhi* (Hubei Journal of Chinese Medicine), 1986; 5:21.
5. *Zhe Jiang Zhong Yi Za Zhi* (Zhejiang Journal of Chinese Medicine), 1993; 8:349.
6. *Si Chuan Zhong Yi* (Sichuan Chinese Medicine), 1993; 9:23.
7. *Ji Lin Zhong Yi Yao* (Jilin Chinese Medicine and Herbology), 1997; 2:10.
8. *Shan Xi Zhong Yi* (Shanxi Chinese Medicine), 1986; (6):152.
9. *Shan Dong Zhong Yi Za Zhi* (Shandong Journal of Chinese Medicine), 1991; 5:24.
10. *Hu Bei Zhong Yi Za Zhi* (Hubei Journal of Chinese Medicine), 1993; 5:14.

Dān Shēn Yǐn (Salvia Decoction)

丹參飲

Pinyin Name: *Dan Shen Yin*
Literal Name: Salvia Decoction
Original Source: *Shi Fang Ge Kuo* (Collected Songs about Contemporary Formulas) by Chen Nian-Zi in 1801

COMPOSITION

Dan Shen (Radix et Rhizoma Salviae Miltiorrhizae)	30g
Tan Xiang (Lignum Santali Albi)	3-4.5g
Sha Ren (Fructus Amomi)	3-4.5g

DOSAGE / PREPARATION / ADMINISTRATION

The source text states to cook the herbs with one cup of water until the combination is reduced to 70% of its original volume. Take the strained decoction while it is warm.

CHINESE THERAPEUTIC ACTIONS

1. Activates blood circulation and removes blood stasis
2. Activates qi circulation and stops pain

CLINICAL MANIFESTATIONS

Heart [epigastric] and stomach pain due to qi and blood stagnation.

VETERINARY CLINICAL APPLICATIONS

Pain secondary to pancreatitis, stomach pain and ulceration, and cardiovascular disease.

EXPLANATION

Dan Shen Yin (Salvia Decoction) is designed to treat heart [epigastric] and stomach pain due to qi and blood stagnation. The actual location of the pain is in the epigastrium, the area slightly below the heart. The pain is in a fixed location, and is worse with pressure upon palpation. Since this formula is slightly on the cold side, it is more suitable for epigastric pain caused by blood stagnation and heat.

In this formula, a large dose of *Dan Shen* (Radix et Rhizoma Salviae Miltiorrhizae) is used to activate blood circulation and remove blood stagnation. *Tan Xiang* (Lignum Santali Albi) and *Sha Ren* (Fructus Amomi) activate qi circulation and relieve pain. Together, these three herbs activate qi and blood circulation and relieve pain.

VETERINARY MODIFICATIONS

- With nausea and vomiting, add *Ban Xia* (Rhizoma Pinelliae) and *Zhu Ru* (Caulis Bambusae in Taenia).
- With pain characterized by heat, add *Mu Dan Pi* (Cortex Moutan) and *Huang Qin* (Radix Scutellariae).

CAUTIONS / CONTRAINDICATIONS

Dan Shen Yin should be used with caution in animals that have bleeding disorders, because it contains a large dose of *Dan Shen* (Radix et Rhizoma Salviae Miltiorrhizae), which may prolong bleeding.

PHARMACOLOGICAL EFFECTS

1. **Cardiovascular**: *Dan Shen Yin* has been shown to affect the cardiovascular system by dilating the coronary artery, increasing blood perfusion to the cardiac muscles, and reducing blood pressure.[1]
2. **Antiplatelet**: According to an *in vitro* study, administration of *Dan Shen Yin* was associated with a marked antiplatelet effect. Researchers noted the effect to be comparable to aspirin.[2]

HUMAN CLINICAL STUDIES AND RESEARCH

1. **Ulceration**: According to one study, 106 patients with various types of ulcerations were treated with complete recovery in 70 cases, improvement in 31 cases, and no effect in 5 cases. The overall effectiveness was 95.3%. The herbal treatment included *Dan Shen Yin* plus *Chuan Lian Zi* (Fructus Toosendan) and *Yan Hu Suo* (Rhizoma Corydalis).[3]
2. **Chronic atrophic gastritis**: Continuous administration of modified *Dan Shen Yin* for 1-3 months was associated

***Dan Shen Yin* (Salvia Decoction)**

Diagnosis	Clinical Signs	Treatment	Herbs
Heart [epigastric] and stomach pain due to qi and blood stagnation	Epigastric pain at a fixed location: qi and blood stagnation	• Activates blood circulation and removes blood stasis • Activates qi circulation and stops pain	• *Dan Shen* (Radix et Rhizoma Salviae Miltiorrhizae) activates blood circulation and removes blood stagnation. • *Tan Xiang* (Lignum Santali Albi) and *Sha Ren* (Fructus Amomi) activate qi circulation and relieve pain.

Dān Shēn Yǐn (Salvia Decoction)

with a 92.7% success rate among 102 patients with chronic atrophic gastritis characterized by blood stagnation with deficiency and cold.[4]

3. **Chronic gastritis**: Two studies reported marked effects using *Dan Shen Yin* to treat gastritis. One study reported 88.7% effectiveness in 106 patients with chronic gastritis using *Dan Shen Yin* plus *Dang Shen* (Radix Codonopsis), *Hong Hua* (Flos Carthami), and others as necessary.[5] Another study of 42 patients reported complete recovery in 20 cases and improvement in 22 cases using *Dan Shen Yin* plus *Pu Huang* (Pollen Typhae), vinegar-processed *Yan Hu Suo* (Rhizoma Corydalis), *Pu Gong Ying* (Herba Taraxaci), and others.[6]
4. **Epigastric pain**: One study of 58 patients with epigastric pain reported 98.3% effectiveness using modified *Dan Shen Yin*. The herbal treatment contained *Dan Shen Yin* plus *Fo Shou* (Fructus Citri Sarcodactylis), *Qian Nian Jian* (Rhizoma Homalomenae), *Zhi Gan Cao* (Radix et Rhizoma Glycyrrhizae Praeparata cum Melle), *Xiang Fu* (Rhizoma Cyperi), *Zi Wan* (Radix et Rhizoma Asteris), dry-fried *Bai Shao* (Radix Paeoniae Alba), processed *Da Huang* (Radix et Rhizoma Rhei), and others, depending on the pattern of disharmony. For severe qi stagnation with hypochondriac fullness and pain, *Yu Jin* (Radix Curcumae) and *Qing Pi* (Pericarpium Citri Reticulatae Viride) were added. For blood stagnation with chronic pain, *Yan Hu Suo* (Rhizoma Corydalis) and *E Zhu* (Rhizoma Curcumae) were added. For acid reflux and belching, *Zuo Jin Wan* (Left Metal Pill) and *Hai Piao Xiao* (Endoconcha Sepiae) were added. For food stagnation, charred *Shan Zha* (Fructus Crataegi), charred *Shen Qu* (Massa Fermentata), and charred *Mai Ya* (Fructus Hordei Germinatus) were added. For loose stools due to Spleen deficiency, *Dang Shen* (Radix Codonopsis) was added and *Da Huang* (Radix et Rhizoma Rhei) was removed.[7]

SUGGESTED ACUPUNCTURE TREATMENT

1. Points: *Geshu* (BL 17), *Xuehai* (SP 10), *Zhongwan* (CV 12), *Housanli* (ST 36), and *Neiguan* (PC 6).
2. Technique: sedation.

Geshu (BL 17) and *Xuehai* (SP 10) activate the blood and remove blood stagnation. *Zhongwan* (CV 12) is the *mu* (collecting) point of the Stomach. *Housanli* (ST 36) is the *he* (uniting) point of the Stomach. Along with *Neiguan* (PC 6), they regulate the Stomach qi flow and harmonize the Stomach to relieve pain.

AUTHORS' COMMENTS

Dan Shen Yin (Salvia Decoction) can be used to treat gastric ulcers and hematemesis in dogs and horses, following excessive use of aspirin and/or non-steroidal anti-inflammatory drugs (NSAIDs). To improve clinical efficacy, combine with *Xiao Yao San* (Rambling Powder), *Er Chen Tang* (Two-Cured Decoction) or *Yu Nu Jian* (Jade Woman Decoction), depending on the condition. It can also be used to treat post-surgical pain in animals that have had gastric surgery and pain secondary to pancreatitis; the addition of *Yan Hu Suo* (Rhizoma Corydalis) improves pain relief and the combination should be administered initially at the lowest therapeutic dose. This formula is also beneficial in animals with congestive heart failure, depending on the clinical signs.

References

1. *Zhong Yi Ming Fang Lin Chuang Xin Yong* (Contemporary Clinical Applications of Classic Chinese Formulas), 2001; 144.
2. *Zhong Yi Ming Fang Lin Chuang Xin Yong* (Contemporary Clinical Applications of Classic Chinese Formulas), 2001; 144.
3. *Shan Dong Zhong Yi Za Zhi* (Shandong Journal of Chinese Medicine), 1986; 2:21.
4. *Zhong Yi Za Zhi* (Journal of Chinese Medicine), 1986; 4:20.
5. *Zhong Xi Yi Jie He Za Zhi* (Journal of Integrated Chinese and Western Medicine), 1985; 5:267.
6. *Guang Ming Zhong Yi* (Guangming Chinese Medicine), 1998; 13(2):27.
7. *Zhe Jiang Zhong Yi Za Zhi* (Zhejiang Journal of Chinese Medicine), 1997; 3:101.

Wēn Jīng Tāng (Warm the Channels Decoction)

温經湯
温经汤

Pinyin Name: *Wen Jing Tang*
Literal Name: Warm the Channels Decoction
Alternate Names: *Wen Ching Tang*, Warm the Menses Decoction, Channel-Warming Decoction, Meridians-Warming Decoction, Tangkuei and Evodia Combination
Original Source: *Jin Gui Yao Lue* (Essentials from the Golden Cabinet) by Zhang Zhong-Jing in the Eastern Han Dynasty

COMPOSITION

Wu Zhu Yu (Fructus Evodiae)	9g
Gui Zhi (Ramulus Cinnamomi)	6g
Dang Gui (Radix Angelicae Sinensis)	6g
Chuan Xiong (Rhizoma Chuanxiong)	6g
Bai Shao (Radix Paeoniae Alba)	6g
Mu Dan Pi (Cortex Moutan)	6g
E Jiao (Colla Corii Asini)	6g
Mai Dong (Radix Ophiopogonis)	1 cup [9g]
Ren Shen (Radix et Rhizoma Ginseng)	6g
Gan Cao (Radix et Rhizoma Glycyrrhizae)	6g
Ban Xia (Rhizoma Pinelliae)	0.5 cup [6g]
Sheng Jiang (Rhizoma Zingiberis Recens)	6g

DOSAGE / PREPARATION / ADMINISTRATION

The source text states to cook the herbs in 10 cups [2,000 mL] of water until the liquid is reduced to 3 cups [600 mL]. Take the warm, strained decoction in three equally divided doses.

CHINESE THERAPEUTIC ACTIONS

1. Warms the menses and disperses cold
2. Nourishes the blood and dispels blood stasis

CLINICAL MANIFESTATIONS

Deficiency and cold of the *chong* (thoroughfare) and *ren* (conception) channels with blood stagnation: irregular estrus, afternoon fever, irritability, dry mouth and lips, lower abdominal pain, and infertility.

VETERINARY CLINICAL APPLICATIONS

Irregular estrus, dysmenorrhea, amenorrhea, anovulation, uterine bleeding, luteal phase defects, and infertility.

EXPLANATION

Wen Jing Tang (Warm the Channels Decoction) treats deficiency and cold of the *chong* (thoroughfare) and *ren* (conception) channels, accompanied by blood stagnation. The *chong* channel is the "sea of blood," and the *ren* channel dominates the uterus. Both of these channels originate in the lower abdomen, and are closely related to menstruation. Deficiency and cold of the *chong* and *ren* channels lead to qi and blood stagnation, causing irregular menstruation, continuous bleeding, coldness and pain in the lower abdomen, and infertility. Irritability and dry mouth and lips may occur as a result of blood deficiency and deficiency heat.

This is a rather complicated syndrome characterized by deficiency and excess, and by heat and cold. Therefore, optimal treatment requires the use of herbs to warm the channels, dispel cold, nourish the blood, and dispel blood stasis. This formula uses *Wu Zhu Yu* (Fructus Evodiae) and *Gui Zhi* (Ramulus Cinnamomi) to warm the channels, disperse cold, and open the blood vessels. *Dang Gui* (Radix Angelicae Sinensis), *Chuan Xiong* (Rhizoma Chuanxiong), and *Bai Shao* (Radix Paeoniae Alba) nourish and activate the blood, dispel blood stasis, and regulate menstruation. *Mu Dan Pi* (Cortex Moutan) activates blood circulation and relieves the clinical signs of deficiency heat, such as afternoon fever and hot plantar/palmar surfaces of the feet. *E Jiao* (Colla Corii Asini) and *Mai Dong* (Radix Ophiopogonis) nourish yin, moisten dryness, and clear deficiency heat. *Ren Shen* (Radix et Rhizoma Ginseng) and *Gan Cao* (Radix et Rhizoma Glycyrrhizae) tonify qi and strengthen the Spleen, which in turn produces blood and controls blood circulation. *Ban Xia* (Rhizoma Pinelliae) disperses any hardness in the body to help remove blood stasis. *Sheng Jiang* (Rhizoma Zingiberis Recens), besides harmonizing the herbs in this formula, also warms

Wēn Jīng Tāng (Warm the Channels Decoction)

Wen Jing Tang **(Warm the Channels Decoction)**

Diagnosis	Clinical Signs	Treatment	Herbs
Deficiency and cold of the *chong* (thoroughfare) and *ren* (conception) channels with blood stagnation	• Irregular menstruation, continuous bleeding, coldness and pain in the lower abdomen and infertility: deficiency and cold of the *chong* (thoroughfare) and *ren* (conception) channels with qi and blood stagnation • Irritability and dry mouth and lips: blood deficiency with deficiency heat • Lower abdominal pain: qi and blood stagnation	• Warms the menses and disperses cold • Nourishes the blood and dispels blood stasis	• *Wu Zhu Yu* (Fructus Evodiae) and *Gui Zhi* (Ramulus Cinnamomi) warm the channels, disperse cold, and open the blood vessels. • *Dang Gui* (Radix Angelicae Sinensis), *Chuan Xiong* (Rhizoma Chuanxiong), and *Bai Shao* (Radix Paeoniae Alba) nourish and activate the blood, dispel blood stasis, and regulate menstruation. • *Mu Dan Pi* (Cortex Moutan) activates blood circulation and relieves deficiency heat clinical signs. • *E Jiao* (Colla Corii Asini) and *Mai Dong* (Radix Ophiopogonis) nourish yin, moisten dryness, and clear deficiency heat. • *Ren Shen* (Radix et Rhizoma Ginseng) and *Gan Cao* (Radix et Rhizoma Glycyrrhizae) tonify qi and strengthen the Spleen. • *Ban Xia* (Rhizoma Pinelliae) disperses hardness in the body to help remove blood stasis. • *Sheng Jiang* (Rhizoma Zingiberis Recens) harmonizes the herbs, warms the Stomach, and promotes the digestion of food and the absorption of nutrients.

the Stomach to promote the digestion of food and the absorption of nutrients.

VETERINARY MODIFICATIONS

- With qi stagnation, add *Xiang Fu* (Rhizoma Cyperi) and *Wu Yao* (Radix Linderae).
- With qi deficiency, remove *Mu Dan Pi* (Cortex Moutan), *Chuan Xiong* (Rhizoma Chuanxiong), and *Wu Zhu Yu* (Fructus Evodiae), and add *Huang Qi* (Radix Astragali).
- With continuous, light-colored uterine bleeding, remove *Mu Dan Pi* (Cortex Moutan), and add *Ai Ye* (Folium Artemisiae Argyi) and *Shu Di Huang* (Radix Rehmanniae Praeparata).
- With *beng lou* (flooding and spotting), add *Ai Ye* (Folium Artemisiae Argyi) and increase the dose of *E Jiao* (Colla Corii Asini).
- With vaginal discharge accompanied by itching, add *Jin Yin Hua* (Flos Lonicerae Japonicae), *Lian Qiao* (Fructus Forsythiae), and *Che Qian Zi* (Semen Plantaginis).

CAUTIONS / CONTRAINDICATIONS

Wen Jing Tang is contraindicated in cases characterized by excess, heat, and blood stasis.

PHARMACOLOGICAL EFFECTS

1. **Anti-inflammatory**: One study reported that *Wen Jing Tang* had an anti-inflammatory effect in treating dysmenorrhea, a common gynecological complaint. A preparation of *Wen Jing Tang* in rat uterine smooth muscle *in vitro* suppressed spontaneous contractions and prostaglandins F2alpha-induced contractions. *Wen Jing Tang* used in this study was extracted from a 50% alcohol solution and subsequently freeze-dried.[1]
2. **Endocrine**: According to an *in vivo* study in women with first- and second-grade amenorrhea, 8 weeks treatment with *Wen Jing Tang* induced a significant increase in plasma follicle-stimulating hormone, luteinizing hormone, and estradiol levels in both hyper- and hypo-functioning patients. The study reported that ovulation occurred in 61.3% and 66.7% of patients with first-grade amenorrhea, and in 27.3% and 22.4% of patients with second-grade amenorrhea, respectively. Based on these results, the study concluded that *Wen Jing Tang* was effective in improving gonadotropin and estradiol secretion in the treatment of either hyper- or hypo-functioning anovulatory women.[2] According to an *in vitro* study of female rats, administration of *Wen Jing Tang* at 5 or 500 mcg/mL increased luteinizing hormone release (60-95% increase) from the pituitary through hypothalamic LH-RH.[3] The study noted that *Wen Jing Tang* stimulated ovarian steroidogenesis and was attributed to stimulation of the hypothalamus-pituitary axis; increased secretion of sex steroid hormones (17-beta-estradiol and progesterone);

Wēn Jīng Tāng (Warm the Channels Decoction)

cytokine-induced neutrophil chemoattractant with interleukin-1beta; and tumor necrosis factor alpha.[4]

3. **Effect on bone density**: According to one study on the prevention and treatment of osteoporosis, *Wen Jing Tang*, *Ba Wei Di Huang Wan* (Eight-Ingredient Pill with Rehmannia), and *Shi Quan Da Bu Tang* (All-Inclusive Great Tonifying Decoction) were administered for 49 days to rats with ovariectomy. In comparison with sham-operated rats, bone mineral density (BMD) of the tibias decreased by 20% in ovariectomized rats, but the BMD was unaffected in rats treated with herbs or 17-beta-estradiol. The study concluded that these three formulas are as effective as 17-beta-estradiol in preventing bone loss induced by ovariectomy by preserving the fine particle surface of the bone.[5]

HUMAN CLINICAL STUDIES AND RESEARCH

1. **Uterine bleeding**: One study reported 96.2% effectiveness using modified *Wen Jing Tang* to treat 104 patients with uterine bleeding. The duration of treatment varied between 2-6 menstrual cycles. Of 104 patients, the study reported complete recovery in 38 cases, significant improvement in 40 cases, moderate improvement in 22 cases, and no effect in 4 cases.[6]
2. **Infertility**: Administration of modified *Wen Jing Tang* was associated with 88% effectiveness in treating 292 women with infertility. Modifications to the formula were made as follows: for early menstruation, *Tao Ren* (Semen Persicae) and *Hong Hua* (Flos Carthami) were added, and *Gui Zhi* (Ramulus Cinnamomi) and *Wu Zhu Yu* (Fructus Evodiae) were removed; for late menstruation, *Bu Gu Zhi* (Fructus Psoraleae), *Du Zhong* (Cortex Eucommiae), *Tao Ren* (Semen Persicae), and *Hong Hua* (Flos Carthami) were added, and *Mu Dan Pi* (Cortex Moutan) and *Mai Dong* (Radix Ophiopogonis) were removed; and for irregular menstruation (early or late), *Chai Hu* (Radix Bupleuri), *Yu Jin* (Radix Curcumae), and *Xiang Fu* (Rhizoma Cyperi) were added. For hypermenorrhea, *Xu Duan* (Radix Dipsaci), *Sang Ji Sheng* (Herba Taxilli), and *Lu Jiao Jiao* (Colla Cornus Cervi) were added; and for hypomenorrhea, *San Leng* (Rhizoma Sparganii), *Chuan Shan Jia* (Squama Manis), and *Yi Mu Cao* (Herba Leonuri) were added. The treatment protocol was to administer the herbs in decoction, starting on the first day of the period, continuously for 5 days.[7]
3. **Amenorrhea**: According to one study, use of *Wen Jing Tang* in 10 women between 20-28 years of age with amenorrhea was associated with complete recovery in 3 cases, improvement in 5 cases, and no effect in 2 cases. The treatment protocol was to administer the herbs starting at 5g/day. The dosage was increased by 2.5g/day for 4 weeks, to reach a final dosage of 15g/day.[8] The mechanism of *Wen Jing Tang* to treat amenorrhea in anovulatory cycles in young women is attributed either to enhanced pituitary response to Gn-RH, or to improved pulsatile secretion of Gn-RH, which induces normalization of the diencephalon-pituitary-ovarian endocrine system in anovulatory patients.[9]
4. **Anovulation**: One study evaluated the efficacy of *Wen Jing Tang* for treating anovulation in women with high basal levels of luteinizing hormone. The study randomly divided 100 patients (38 with polycystic ovarian syndrome, and 62 with non-polycystic ovarian syndrome) into two groups: 52 were treated with *Wen Jing Tang* and 48 with placebo. The results showed that *Wen Jing Tang* induced significant decreases in plasma luteinizing hormone and significant increases in plasma estradiol levels (43.5%), in 8 weeks of herbal treatment. The rate of menstrual cycle improvement (including successful ovulation) was 50% in the polycystic ovarian syndrome group and 60% in the non-polycystic ovarian syndrome group.[10]
5. **Luteal phase defects**: One study evaluated the efficacy of *Wen Jing Tang* in treating luteal phase defects by comparing 103 subjects treated with herbs (7.5 g/day) and 94 control subjects. The study reported a 79.6% rate of correction of luteal phase defects in patients treated with *Wen Jing Tang*, with clinical improvements such as decreased plasma luteinizing hormone, increased 17-beta-estradiol concentration in the follicular phase, increased progesterone (66.7%) in the mid-luteal phase ($P < .05$), development of the dominant follicle ($P < .01$) and endometrium ($P < .001$), and prolongation of the luteal phase (43%, $P < .001$) as measured by basal body temperature. Furthermore, the gestation rate in patients desiring gestation was 49.5% (41/83). The study concluded *Wen Jing Tang* to be an effective treatment for luteal phase defects.[11]
6. **Vaginitis**: According to one study, administration of *Wen Jing Tang* at 2.5g, three times daily for 2 weeks, was effective in treating 45 women with vaginitis due to various causes. Improvements included relief of sensations of burning, itching, discomfort, and pain. The study also noted that this formula may be used topically as an herbal wash or vaginal suppository.[12]

HERB-DRUG INTERACTION

Clomiphene citrate: According to one study, 16 infertile women who did not respond to clomiphene citrate alone were successfully treated with a combination of *Wen Jing Tang* and clomiphene citrate. The treatment protocol involved administration of *Wen Jing Tang* at a dose of 5 g/day every day from day 2 of the menstrual cycle, and clomiphene citrate at 150mg a day for 5 days from day 5 of the cycle. The study reported that ovulation occurred in

Wēn Jīng Tāng (Warm the Channels Decoction)

43.8% of the patients, and 48.6% of the cycles. No cases of ovarian hyperstimulation syndrome were observed. The researchers concluded that the combination of *Wen Jing Tang* and clomiphene citrate is an effective treatment for infertility due to anovulation, and should be used first before therapy with human menopausal gonadotropin.[13]

SUGGESTED ACUPUNCTURE TREATMENT

1. Points: *Qihai* (CV 6), *Qixue* (KI 13), *Sanyinjiao* (SP 6), *Mingmen* (GV 4), *Taixi* (KI 3), *Geshu* (BL 17), *Xuehai* (SP 10), *Pishu* (BL 20), and *Housanli* (ST 36).
2. Technique: tonification and moxibustion.

Qihai (CV 6) enters the uterus, while *Qixue* (KI 13) is the intersecting point of the Kidney and *chong* (thoroughfare) channels. Combining both points regulates the *chong* (thoroughfare) and *ren* (conception) channels. *Sanyinjiao* (SP 6) nourishes yin, blood, and the *chong* and *ren* channels. *Mingmen* (GV 4) and *Taixi* (KI 3) warm and nourish the Kidney to dispel cold. *Geshu* (BL 17) and *Xuehai* (SP 10) activate blood and remove blood stagnation. *Housanli* (ST 36) and *Pishu* (BL 20) tonify the Spleen to strengthen the body's qi.

AUTHORS' COMMENTS

Wen Jing Tang is literally known as "Warm the Channels Decoction" because it warms and tonifies cold and deficiency in the *chong* (thoroughfare) and *ren* (conception) channels to treat disorders such as irregular menstruation, dysmenorrhea, and *beng lou* (flooding and spotting) in primates.

Wen Jing Tang is commonly used to treat *beng lou* (flooding and spotting). In this case, it is normal for patients to experience more bleeding initially. However, after the blood stasis is resolved, the bleeding gradually will cease.

References

1. Hsu CS, Yang JK, Yang LL. Effect of a dysmenorrhea Chinese medicinal prescription on uterus contractility in vitro. Phytother Res. 2003 Aug; 17(7):778-83.
2. Ushiroyama T, Hosotani T, Yamashita Y, Yamashita H, Ueki M. Effects of Unkei-to on FSH, LH and estradiol in anovulatory young women with hyper- or hypo-functioning conditions. Am J Chin Med. 2003; 31(5):763-71.
3. Miyake A, Lee JW, Tasaka K, Ohtsuka S, Aono T. Wen-jing-tang, a traditional Chinese herbal medicine increases luteinizing hormone release in vitro. Am J Chin Med. 1986; 14(3-4):157-60.
4. Yasui T, Matsuzaki T, Ogata R, Kiyokawa M, Ushigoe K, Uemura H, Kuwahara A, Ikawa H, Maegawa M, Furumoto H, Aono T, Irahara M. The herbal medicine Unkei-to stimulates the secretion of a cytokine-induced neutrophil chemoattractant, CINC/gro, in the rat ovarian cell culture. Am J Reprod Immunol. 2003 Jan;49(1):14-20.
5. Hidaka S, Okamoto Y, Nakajima K, Suekawa M, Liu SY. Preventive effects of traditional Chinese (Kampo) medicines on experimental osteoporosis induced by ovariectomy in rats. Calcif Tissue Int. 1997 Sep;61(3):239-46.
6. *Zhe Jiang Zhong Yi Za Zhi* (Zhejiang Journal of Chinese Medicine), 1993; 28(7):299.
7. *Shan Xi Zhong Yi* (Shanxi Chinese Medicine), 1996; 6:250.
8. *He Han Yi Yao Xue Hui Zhi* (Hehan Journal of Medicine and Herbology), 1986; 3(3):233.
9. Ushiroyama T, Tsubokura S, Ikeda A, Ueki M. The effect of unkei-to on pituitary gonadotropin secretion and ovulation in anovulatory cycles of young women. Am J Chin Med. 1995;23(3-4):223-30.
10. Ushiroyama T, Ikeda A, Sakai M, Hosotani T, Suzuki Y, Tsubokura S, Ueki M. Effects of unkei-to, an herbal medicine, on endocrine function and ovulation in women with high basal levels of luteinizing hormone secretion. Journal of Reproductive Medicine. 2001 May; 46(5):451-6.
11. Ushiroyama T, Ikeda A, Higashio S, Hosotani T, Yamashita H, Yamashita Y, Suzuki Y, Ueki M. Unkei-to for correcting luteal phase defects. Journal of Reproductive Medicine. 2003 Sep; 48(9):729-34.
12. *Zhong Cheng Yao* (Study of Chinese Patent Medicine), 1990; 12(1):44.
13. Yoshimoto Y, Miyake A, Tasaka K, Aono T, Tanizawa O. Ovulation following combined therapy with wen-jing-tang and clomiphene citrate therapy in anovulatory women. Am J Chin Med. 1989;17 (3-4):243-4.

Ài Fù Nuǎn Gōng Wán

(Mugwort and Cyperus Pill for Warming the Womb)

艾附暖宫丸
艾附暖宮丸

Pinyin Name: *Ai Fu Nuan Gong Wan*
Literal Name: Mugwort and Cyperus Pill for Warming the Womb
Alternate Name: Mugwort and Cyperus Combination
Original Source: *Ren Zhai Zhi Zhi* (Straight Directions of Benevolent Aid) by Yang Tu-Ying in 1264

COMPOSITION

Ai Ye (Folium Artemisiae Argyi), large leaves without twigs	90g [6g]
Xiang Fu (Rhizoma Cyperi), *zhu* (boiled) with vinegar, *dao* (pounded) into paste, and *bei* (stone baked) till dry in low heat	180g [12g]
Wu Zhu Yu (Fructus Evodiae), without twigs	90g [6g]
Rou Gui (Cortex Cinnamomi)	15g [5g]
Huang Qi (Radix Astragali)	90g [6g]
Dang Gui (Radix Angelicae Sinensis), *xi* (washed) with liquor	90g [6g]
Chuan Xiong (Rhizoma Chuanxiong)	90g [6g]
Bai Shao (Radix Paeoniae Alba), *chao* (dry-fried) with liquor	90g [6g]
Xu Duan (Radix Dipsaci)	45g [5g]
Di Huang (Radix Rehmanniae), *xi* (washed) with liquor and *bei* (stone baked) till dry	30g [6g]

DOSAGE / PREPARATION / ADMINISTRATION

The source text states to grind all of the ingredients into a fine powder and form into small pills with rice vinegar. The pills should resemble the size of *Wu Tong Zi* (Semen Firmianae), a small seed approximately 5 mm in diameter. Take 50-70 pills [6g] between meals with water that has been mixed with a small amount of vinegar. Today, this formula may be prepared as a decoction with the doses suggested in brackets.

CHINESE THERAPEUTIC ACTIONS

1. Warms the uterus and the channels
2. Nourishes the blood and activates blood circulation

CLINICAL MANIFESTATIONS

Deficiency and cold of the uterus: vaginal discharge, painful limbs, lethargy, low energy, decreased food intake, irregular estrus, occasional lower abdominal pain, and infertility.

VETERINARY CLINICAL APPLICATIONS

Irregular estrus (or menstruation in primates) and female infertility.

EXPLANATION

Ai Fu Nuan Gong Wan (Mugwort and Cyperus Pill for Warming the Womb) warms the uterus and the *chong* (thoroughfare) and *ren* (conception) channels, nourishes the blood, and activates blood circulation.

In this formula, *Ai Ye* (Folium Artemisiae Argyi) and *Xiang Fu* (Rhizoma Cyperi) are the chief herbs. *Ai Ye* (Folium Artemisiae Argyi) warms the channels, dispels cold, and relieves pain. *Xiang Fu* (Rhizoma Cyperi) regulates qi and relieves menstrual pain. *Wu Zhu Yu* (Fructus Evodiae) and *Rou Gui* (Cortex Cinnamomi) warm the channels, dispel cold, and activate the blood. *Huang Qi* (Radix Astragali) tonifies qi and lifts yang. *Dang Gui* (Radix Angelicae Sinensis), *Chuan Xiong* (Rhizoma Chuanxiong), and *Bai Shao* (Radix Paeoniae Alba) regulate menstruation by activating and nourishing the blood. *Xu Duan* (Radix Dipsaci) stops bleeding with its hemostatic action. *Di Huang* (Radix Rehmanniae) nourishes yin and promotes the secretion of body fluids.

Ài Fù Nuǎn Gōng Wán

(Mugwort and Cyperus Pill for Warming the Womb)

***Ai Fu Nuan Gong Wan* (Mugwort and Cyperus Pill for Warming the Womb)**

Diagnosis	Clinical Signs	Treatment	Herbs
Deficiency and cold of the uterus	• Vaginal discharge, sallow and yellowish facial complexion, irregular menstruation and infertility: deficiency and cold of the uterus • Lethargy, lack of energy, decreased food intake, and painful limbs: deficiency and cold	• Warms the uterus and channels • Nourishes and activates the blood	• *Ai Ye* (Folium Artemisiae Argyi) warms the channels, dispels cold, and relieves pain. • *Xiang Fu* (Rhizoma Cyperi) regulates qi and relieves menstrual pain. • *Wu Zhu Yu* (Fructus Evodiae) and *Rou Gui* (Cortex Cinnamomi) warm the channels, dispel cold, and activate the blood. • *Huang Qi* (Radix Astragali) tonifies qi and lifts yang. • *Dang Gui* (Radix Angelicae Sinensis), *Chuan Xiong* (Rhizoma Chuanxiong), and *Bai Shao* (Radix Paeoniae Alba) regulate menstruation and activate and nourish the blood. • *Xu Duan* (Radix Dipsaci) stops bleeding. • *Di Huang* (Radix Rehmanniae) nourishes yin and promotes the secretion of body fluids.

CAUTIONS / CONTRAINDICATIONS

- The source text recommends avoiding raw or cold foods while taking *Ai Fu Nuan Gong Wan.*

HUMAN CLINICAL STUDIES AND RESEARCH

Infertility: Use of modified *Ai Fu Nuan Gong Wan* was shown to have some effectiveness in treating 50 women with infertility. The herbal formula contained the original formula plus *Pu Huang* (Pollen Typhae), *Tu Si Zi* (Semen Cuscutae), and *Yi Mu Cao* (Herba Leonuri). The treatment protocol was to cook the herbs in water, and administer the decoction in three equally-divided doses daily. After six months of treatment, the study reported gestation in 25 cases, improved regularity of menstrual cycles (but not yet pregnant) in 19 cases, and no effect in 6 cases.[1] In another study, use of modified *Ai Fu Nuan Gong Wan* was effective in treating infertility due to such causes as irregular menstruation, blocked fallopian tubes, and abnormal development of the uterus. Of 72 patients, 65 successfully became pregnant, 4 had marked improvement of lower abdominal pain, and 3 had no benefit. The duration of treatment ranged from 1-12 months.[2]

SUGGESTED ACUPUNCTURE TREATMENT

1. Points: *Qihai* (CV 6), *Guanyuan* (CV 4), *Qixue* (KI 13), *Sanyinjiao* (SP 6), *Mingmen* (GV 4), *Taixi* (KI 3), *Xuehai* (SP 10), *Pishu* (BL 20), and *Housanli* (ST 36).
2. Techniques: tonification and moxibustion.

Guanyuan (CV 4) and *Qihai* (CV 6) enter the uterus. *Qixue* (KI 13) is the intersecting point of the Kidney and *chong* (thoroughfare) channels. Combining these points regulates the *chong* (thoroughfare) and *ren* (conception) channels. *Sanyinjiao* (SP 6) nourishes yin and blood in the *chong* and *ren* channels. *Mingmen* (GV 4) and *Taixi* (KI 3) warm and nourish the Kidney to dispel cold. *Xuehai* (SP 10) activates blood circulation and removes blood stagnation. *Housanli* (ST 36) and *Pishu* (BL 20) tonify the Spleen to strengthen qi.

AUTHORS' COMMENTS

Ai Fu Nuan Gong Wan and *Wen Jing Tang* (Warm the Channels Decoction) have similar functions in treating deficiency and cold of the uterus:

- *Ai Fu Nuan Gong Wan* more strongly nourishes the blood and warms the uterus. It treats conditions characterized by deficiency and cold of the uterus, with more blood deficiency.
- *Wen Jing Tang* more strongly removes blood stagnation. It treats conditions characterized by deficiency and cold of the uterus, with both blood deficiency and blood stagnation.

References

1. *Jiang Xi Zhong Yi Yao* (Jiangxi Chinese Medicine and Herbology), 1993; 6:45.
2. *Shan Xi Zhong Yi* (Shanxi Chinese Medicine), 1995; 11(5):20.

Shēng Huà Tāng (Generation and Transformation Decoction)

生化湯
生化汤

Pinyin Name: *Sheng Hua Tang*
Literal Name: Generation and Transformation Decoction
Alternate Names: Blood-Producing and Clotting-Cleaning Decoction, Blood-Regenerating and Stasis-Resolving Decoction, Tangkuei and Ginger Combination
Original Source: *Fu Qing Zhu Nu Ke* (Women's Diseases According to Fu Qing-Zhu) by Fu Shan in 1827

COMPOSITION

Dang Gui (Radix Angelicae Sinensis)	24g
Chuan Xiong (Rhizoma Chuanxiong)	9g
Tao Ren (Semen Persicae)	14 pieces [6g]
Pao Jiang (Rhizoma Zingiberis Praeparatum), *pao* (blast-fried) till black	1.5g
Zhi Gan Cao (Radix et Rhizoma Glycyrrhizae Praeparata cum Melle)	1.5g

DOSAGE / PREPARATION / ADMINISTRATION

The source text states to prepare the ingredients as a decoction by cooking the herbs in a liquid made of equal amounts of grain-based liquor and *Tong Bian* (Infantis Urina). Today, the herbs are usually decocted with water, with or without the addition of a grain-based liquor.

CHINESE THERAPEUTIC ACTIONS

1. Activates blood circulation and dispels blood stasis
2. Warms the channels and relieves pain

CLINICAL MANIFESTATIONS

Postpartum blood deficiency with cold: retention of the placenta causing bleeding and pain in the lower abdomen.

VETERINARY CLINICAL APPLICATIONS

Postpartum care to relieve pain and stop bleeding, resolve retained placenta, resolve lower abdominal pain caused by blood stasis, and uterine bleeding caused by abortion or miscarriage.

EXPLANATION

Sheng Hua Tang (Generation and Transformation Decoction) is designed to treat postpartum blood deficiency complicated by cold invasion and blood stasis. After delivery, the mother's body is naturally blood deficient. Consequently, the deficient state of the body enables the cold pathogenic factor to invade the body and cause cold stagnation and blood stasis, producing clinical manifestations of continuous bleeding with a cold sensation and pain in the lower abdomen.

To successfully treat this syndrome, herbs need to be prescribed to tonify postpartum blood deficiency and eliminate blood stagnation. These two methods cannot be used separately because the use of only blood tonics may create more blood stasis, and the use of only blood-invigorating herbs will exacerbate the blood deficiency. Therefore, the optimal treatment is to incorporate both methods to generate blood production and transform blood stasis.

***Sheng Hua Tang* (Generation and Transformation Decoction)**

Diagnosis	Clinical Signs	Treatment	Herbs
Postpartum blood deficiency with cold	• Postpartum bleeding: retention of placenta • Cold sensation and pain in the lower abdomen: cold accumulation and blood stagnation	• Activates blood circulation and dispels blood stasis • Warms the channels and stops pain	• *Dang Gui* (Radix Angelicae Sinensis) nourishes the blood and activates blood circulation. • *Chuan Xiong* (Rhizoma Chuanxiong) activates qi and blood circulation. • *Tao Ren* (Semen Persicae) activates the blood and breaks up blood stagnation. • *Pao Jiang* (Rhizoma Zingiberis Praeparatum) warms the channels, disperses cold, and relieves pain. • *Zhi Gan Cao* (Radix et Rhizoma Glycyrrhizae Praeparata cum Melle) harmonizes the herbs.

Shēng Huà Tāng (Generation and Transformation Decoction)

This formula uses *Dang Gui* (Radix Angelicae Sinensis) to nourish the blood and activate blood circulation. *Chuan Xiong* (Rhizoma Chuanxiong) activates qi and blood circulation. *Tao Ren* (Semen Persicae) activates blood circulation and breaks up blood stagnation. *Pao Jiang* (Rhizoma Zingiberis Praeparatum) warms the channels, disperses cold, and relieves pain. *Zhi Gan Cao* (Radix et Rhizoma Glycyrrhizae Praeparata cum Melle) harmonizes the herbs in this formula. Lastly, the grain-based alcohol warms and opens the channels and blood vessels; it also potentiates the effects of the herbs. *Tong Bian* (Infantis Urina) benefits the yang and dissolves blood stasis. Overall, this formula tonifies the blood, activates blood circulation, removes blood stasis, warms the channels, and relieves pain.

VETERINARY MODIFICATIONS

- With postpartum abdominal pain due to blood stagnation, add *Hong Hua* (Flos Carthami) and *Bai Shao* (Radix Paeoniae Alba).
- With severe postpartum abdominal pain due to blood stagnation, add *Pu Huang* (Pollen Typhae), *Wu Ling Zhi* (Faeces Trogopteri), and *Yan Hu Suo* (Rhizoma Corydalis).
- With postpartum lower abdominal coldness and pain, add *Rou Gui* (Cortex Cinnamomi) and *Xiao Hui Xiang* (Fructus Foeniculi).
- With postpartum fever, add *Chai Hu* (Radix Bupleuri) and *Huang Qin* (Radix Scutellariae).
- With postpartum qi deficiency and increased risk of qi collapse, wait until after all the placental remains have been fully discharged, then add *Ren Shen* (Radix et Rhizoma Ginseng) and *Huang Qi* (Radix Astragali).
- For postpartum constipation, add *Rou Cong Rong* (Herba Cistanches) and *Zhi Qiao* (Fructus Aurantii).

CAUTIONS / CONTRAINDICATIONS

- *Sheng Hua Tang* is not suitable for animals with blood stagnation accompanied by interior heat because this formula contains many herbs that are warm in nature.
- Use of this formula is contraindicated during pregnancy.
- Although this formula effectively treats retained placenta, it should be used only when needed, in cases of retained placenta characterized by cold and blood stasis.[1]

PHARMACOLOGICAL EFFECTS

1. **Effect on the uterus**: According to an *in vitro* study, administration of *Sheng Hua Tang* was associated with increased uterine contractions in mice, especially pregnant ones.[2]
2. **Anticoagulant**: An *in vitro* study showed *Sheng Hua Tang* to have a marked anticoagulant effect.[3]

HUMAN CLINICAL STUDIES AND RESEARCH

1. **Postpartum care**: *Sheng Hua Tang* has been used as the standard herbal therapy for postpartum care in traditional Chinese medicine, with its actions well-documented by clinical studies. It has been shown to effectively treat retention of lochia,[4] to facilitate return of the uterus to its normal position,[5] to relieve pain associated with uterine contractions,[6] and to address many postpartum complications.[7]
2. **Retention of lochia**: Retention of lochia was successfully treated in 32 of 34 patients using *Sheng Hua Tang* plus *Zhi Qiao* (Fructus Aurantii), and others as needed.[8]
3. **Hysteromyoma or metrypertrophia**: Hysteromyoma or metrypertrophia were treated successfully using *Sheng Hua Tang* plus dry-fried *Jing Jie* (Herba Schizonepetae) and *Yi Mu Cao* (Herba Leonuri) as the base formula, and the addition of *San Leng* (Rhizoma Sparganii), *E Zhu* (Rhizoma Curcumae), and *Rou Gui* (Cortex Cinnamomi) for hardness and nodules. Of 24 patients with hysteromyoma, the study reported complete recovery in 8 cases, improvement in 13 cases, and no effect in 3 cases, after 30 packs of herbs. Of 46 patients with metrypertrophia, the study reported complete recovery in 25 cases, improvement in 18 cases, and no effect in 3 cases, after 30 packs of herbs.[9]
4. **Ectopic pregnancy**: One study reported successful treatment in all 21 cases of ectopic pregnancy using modified *Sheng Hua Tang*, with the removal of *Gan Cao* (Radix et Rhizoma Glycyrrhizae) and *Pao Jiang* (Rhizoma Zingiberis Praeparatum), and the addition of *Gui Zhi* (Ramulus Cinnamomi), *Fu Ling* (Poria), *Chi Shao* (Radix Paeoniae Rubra), *Mu Dan Pi* (Cortex Moutan), and others as needed.[10]
5. **Uterine bleeding caused by abortion or miscarriage**: Many studies have reported a marked effect using modified *Sheng Hua Tang* to treat uterine bleeding due to various causes. In one study, use of *Sheng Hua Tang* and *Shi Xiao San* (Sudden Smile Powder) in 80 patients with uterine bleeding was associated with complete recovery in 72 cases, improvement in 6 cases, and no effect in 2 cases.[11] According to another report, 90 patients with uterine bleeding associated with abortion, miscarriage, or labor were treated with *Sheng Hua Tang* plus *Yi Mu Cao* (Herba Leonuri), *Pu Huang* (Pollen Typhae), and *Xue Yu Tan* (Crinis Carbonisatus) with good results. The duration of treatment was 5 packs of herbs per course of treatment, with most patients needing only one course of treatment.[12] Lastly, use of *Sheng Hua Tang* plus *Pu Gong Ying* (Herba Taraxaci), *Yi Mu Cao* (Herba Leonuri), and *E Jiao* (Colla Corii Asini) was associated with complete recovery in 31 of 36 patients with uterine bleeding caused

Shēng Huà Tāng (Generation and Transformation Decoction)

by abortion. The duration of treatment ranged from 3-6 packs of herbs.[13]

SUGGESTED ACUPUNCTURE TREATMENT

1. Points: *Zhongji* (CV 3), *Qichong* (ST 30), *Diji* (SP 8), and *Guanyuan* (CV 4).
2. Techniques: tonification, sedation, and moxibustion.

Zhongji (CV 3) enters the uterus. *Qichong* (ST 30) is an intersecting point of the Stomach and *chong* (thoroughfare) channels. Together, these two points regulate the *chong* and *ren* (conception) channels. *Diji* (SP 8), the *xi* (cleft) point of the Spleen channel, activates blood circulation and relieves pain. Moxibustion on *Guanyuan* (CV 4) disperses cold and relieves pain.

AUTHORS' COMMENTS

Sheng Hua Tang dispels blood stasis and treats retained placenta with lower abdominal coldness and pain. This widely used formula is one of the most popular postpartum formulas in China today for clearing blood stasis. In certain parts of China, it is customary to give this formula immediately after delivery to ensure successful discharge of placental remnants and should be considered in postpartum mares, especially if quick return of uterine tone and breeding on the foal heat is desired.

References

1. *Zhong Yao Ming Fang Yao Li Yu Ying Yong* (Pharmacology and Applications of Famous Herbal Formulas), 1989.
2. *Shan Xi Yi Yao Za Zhi* (Shanxi Journal of Medicine and Herbology), 1980; 9(3):6.
3. *Zhong Cheng Yao* (Study of Chinese Patent Medicine), 1993; 15(1):44.
4. *Guang Dong Zhong Yi* (Guangdong Chinese Medicine), 1962; 9:17.
5. *Xin Zhong Yi* (New Chinese Medicine), 1977; 4:38.
6. *Zhong Yi Fang Ji Xian Dai Yan Jiu* (Modern Study of Medical Formulas in Traditional Chinese Medicine), 1997; 1093-1094.
7. *Jiang Xi Zhong Yi Yao* (Jiangxi Chinese Medicine and Herbology), 1960; 6:25.
8. *He Nan Zhong Yi* (Henan Chinese Medicine), 1993; 4:35.
9. *Shan Xi Yi Yao Za Zhi* (Shanxi Journal of Medicine and Herbology), 1980; 6:21.
10. *Xin Zhong Yi* (New Chinese Medicine), 1984; 11:33.
11. *Yun Nan Zhong Yi Za Zhi* (Yunan Journal of Chinese Medicine), 1988; 3:43.
12. *Jiang Xi Zhong Yi Yao* (Jiangxi Chinese Medicine and Herbology), 1988; 3:21.
13. *Shan Dong Zhong Yi Za Zhi* (Shandong Journal of Chinese Medicine), 1995; 14(6):253.

Guì Zhī Fú Líng Wán (Cinnamon Twig and Poria Pill)

桂枝茯苓丸

Pinyin Name: *Gui Zhi Fu Ling Wan*
Literal Name: Cinnamon Twig and Poria Pill
Alternate Names: *Kuei Chih Fu Ling Wan*, *Qui Zhi Fu Ling Wang*, *Duo Ming Wan*, *Cui Sheng Tang*, Cinnamon Twig and Hoelen Pill, Cinnamon and Hoelen Formula
Original Source: *Jin Gui Yao Lue* (Essentials from the Golden Cabinet) by Zhang Zhong-Jing in the Eastern Han Dynasty

COMPOSITION

Gui Zhi (Ramulus Cinnamomi)	[6g]
Fu Ling (Poria)	[6g]
Tao Ren (Semen Persicae)	[6g]
Mu Dan Pi (Cortex Moutan)	[6g]
Chi Shao (Radix Paeoniae Rubra)	[6g]

BLOOD-REGULATING FORMULAS 13

Guì Zhī Fú Líng Wán (Cinnamon Twig and Poria Pill)

Note: The source text states the use of *Shao Yao* (Radix Paeoniae) in this formula, without specifying whether it is *Chi Shao* (Radix Paeoniae Rubra) or *Bai Shao* (Radix Paeoniae Alba). Today, *Chi Shao* (Radix Paeoniae Rubra) is usually used, as it has a better effect than *Bai Shao* (Radix Paeoniae Alba) to invigorate blood circulation and clear heat.

DOSAGE / PREPARATION / ADMINISTRATION

The source text states to grind equal amounts of the ingredients into powder and mix with honey to form into pills. The pills should resemble rabbit droppings in size. Take 1 pill before meals. If there is no response, increase to 3 pills per dose. Today this formula may be given in decoction with the doses suggested in brackets.

CHINESE THERAPEUTIC ACTIONS

1. Activates blood circulation and breaks up blood stasis
2. Disperses the formation of abnormal masses in the abdomen

CLINICAL MANIFESTATIONS

Blood stasis in the uterus (during gestation): instability of the fetus, continuous dripping of purplish-black blood, and abdominal pain that is worse with pressure.

VETERINARY CLINICAL APPLICATIONS

Endometriosis, ovarian cysts, pelvic inflammatory disease, placentitis, dysmenorrhea, amenorrhea, irregular menstruation in primates, instability of the fetus and stillbirth.

EXPLANATION

Gui Zhi Fu Ling Wan (Cinnamon Twig and Poria Pill) treats blood stasis in the womb during gestation. In such circumstances, blood stasis causes dripping of blood and instability of the fetus. If the blood stasis is not cleared, then the dripping of blood continues and the gestation will be adversely affected. However, blood-invigorating herbs must be used with extreme caution as they increase the risks of miscarriage. This formula is designed to gently and safely eliminate blood stasis and abdominal masses, without injuring the fetus or the mother.

In this formula, *Gui Zhi* (Ramulus Cinnamomi) warms the blood and opens the vessels to facilitate the smooth flow of blood. *Fu Ling* (Poria) has a draining effect, which guides blood stasis downward and eliminates it. *Fu Ling* (Poria) also tonifies the Heart and Spleen, which helps to stabilize gestation and calm the fetus. *Tao Ren* (Semen Persicae) treats the underlying cause of the disorder by activating blood circulation and breaking up blood stasis. Blood stasis or masses in the abdomen may produce heat after an extended period; therefore, *Mu Dan Pi* (Cortex Moutan) and *Chi Shao* (Radix Paeoniae Rubra) are used to both activate blood circulation and clear the heat. The herbs are mixed with honey and administered as pills to moderate their potency and provide a gradual, gentle, and sustained effect over a long period of time.

VETERINARY MODIFICATIONS

- With amenorrhea, add *Zhi Shi* (Fructus Aurantii Immaturus) and *Hong Hua* (Flos Carthami).
- With severe blood stasis, add *San Leng* (Rhizoma Sparganii) and *E Zhu* (Rhizoma Curcumae).

CAUTIONS / CONTRAINDICATIONS

- *Gui Zhi Fu Ling Wan* gently treats blood stasis accompanied by minor presentation of heat. This formula is not suitable for serious conditions of blood stagnation, excess heat in the blood, and the absence of blood stasis.
- Animals with blood stasis and a deficient constitution should use *Dang Gui Shao Yao San* (Tangkuei and Peony Powder) instead of *Gui Zhi Fu Ling Wan*.
- Use of this formula has occasionally been associated with side effects such as abdominal distention and mild constipation.[1]

***Gui Zhi Fu Ling Wan* (Cinnamon Twig and Poria Pill)**

Diagnosis	Clinical Signs	Treatment	Herbs
Blood stasis in the uterus (during gestation)	Instability of the fetus, continuous uterine bleeding, and abdominal pain that worsens with pressure: blood stasis in the womb during gestation	• Activates blood circulation and breaks up blood stasis • Disperses abnormal masses in the abdomen	• *Gui Zhi* (Ramulus Cinnamomi) warms the blood and opens the vessels to facilitate blood circulation. • *Fu Ling* (Poria) eliminates and guides blood stasis downward. It also strengthens the Heart and Spleen to calm the fetus and stabilize gestation. • *Tao Ren* (Semen Persicae) activates blood circulation and breaks up blood stasis. • *Mu Dan Pi* (Cortex Moutan) and *Chi Shao* (Radix Paeoniae Rubra) activate blood circulation and clear heat.

Guì Zhī Fú Líng Wán (Cinnamon Twig and Poria Pill)

PHARMACOLOGICAL EFFECTS

1. **Antiplatelet**: According to clinical studies, administration of *Gui Zhi Fu Ling Wan* was associated with a marked antiplatelet effect, with potency similar to or greater than aspirin.[2] In addition, use of *Gui Zhi Fu Ling Wan* was associated with reduced blood viscosity. The onset of therapeutic action began 30 minutes after oral ingestion, and lasted up to 180 minutes.[3] This formula, however, does not seem to have a significant effect on prothrombin time (PT).[4]
2. **Anti-inflammatory**: A bolus dose of *Gui Zhi Fu Ling Wan* (60 g/kg via oral ingestion or 10 g/kg via intraperitoneal injection) was associated with a marked anti-inflammatory effect in mice. The onset of action began approximately 30 minutes after administration, and lasted for up to 72 hours. It was proposed that the mechanism of this anti-inflammatory action is not related to the adrenal glands or glucocorticoids, because long-term use of this formula did not contribute to increased adrenal glands weight. Furthermore, in subjects whose adrenal glands had been surgically removed, *Gui Zhi Fu Ling Wan* had marked anti-inflammatory effect.[5]
3. **Endocrine**: Administration of *Gui Zhi Fu Ling Wan* to rats at 300mg/kg for 14 days was associated with a marked reduction of LH and FSH.[6] *Gui Zhi Fu Ling Wan* has been shown to act as an LH-RH antagonist and/or as a weak anti-estrogen.[7]
4. **Nephroprotective**: One study reported a marked effect in retarding the progression of renal damage by administering *Gui Zhi Fu Ling Wan* to rats with diabetic nephropathy. The mechanism of this nephroprotective effect was attributed to its ability to improve metabolic abnormalities associated with diabetes.[8]
5. **Antioxidative**: Two studies reported that *Gui Zhi Fu Ling Wan* has a dose-dependent antioxidative effect to prevent the progression of atherosclerosis in cholesterol-fed rabbits.[9,10]
6. **Effect on uterine adenomyosis**: One study reported marked effects using *Gui Zhi Fu Ling Wan* to prevent and treat mice with uterine adenomyosis, a condition characterized by the abnormal growth of glands and stroma into and beyond the smooth muscle layers of the uterus. The study suggested *Gui Zhi Fu Ling Wan* to be a useful tool for the treatment of uterine adenomyosis in humans as well.[11]

HUMAN CLINICAL STUDIES AND RESEARCH

1. **Pelvic inflammatory disease**: Administration of modified *Gui Zhi Fu Ling Wan* was associated with marked effectiveness in treating 200 patients with pelvic inflammatory disease. The herbal treatment contained this formula plus *Xiang Fu* (Rhizoma Cyperi), *Yan Hu Suo* (Rhizoma Corydalis), and *Dang Gui* (Radix Angelicae Sinensis). [12]
2. **Oophoritic cysts**: Use of herbs in 300 patients with oophoritic cysts was associated with a 95% rate of effectiveness. The herbal treatment contained *Gui Zhi Fu Ling Wan*, *Huang Yao Zi* (Herba Dioscoreae Bulbiferae), *Ji Nei Jin* (Endothelium Corneum Gigeriae Galli), *Shui Zhi* (Hirudo), *Li Zhi He* (Semen Litchi), and *Wu Yao* (Radix Linderae). The herbs were cooked in water, and the decoction was taken in four equally-divided doses daily. Also, *Da Huang Zhe Chong Wan* (Rhubarb and Eupolyphaga Pill) was given twice daily, morning and night. The duration of treatment ranged from 3-6 months. Of 300 patients, the study reported complete recovery in 225 cases, improvement in 30 cases, and no effect in 15 cases. Information was unavailable on 30 patients who did not complete the study.[13]
3. **Endometriosis**: One study reported marked success in treating endometriosis in 38 patients using *Gui Zhi Fu Ling Wan* plus *Da Huang* (Radix et Rhizoma Rhei) and *Gan Cao* (Radix et Rhizoma Glycyrrhizae). Modifications were made by adding *San Leng* (Rhizoma Sparganii), *E Zhu* (Rhizoma Curcumae), and *Chuan Shan Jia* (Squama Manis) in severe cases; *Ru Xiang* (Gummi Olibanum), *Mo Yao* (Myrrha) and *Lu Lu Tong* (Fructus Liquidambaris) for severe pain; large doses of *Da Huang* (Radix et Rhizoma Rhei) and *Tao Ren* (Semen Persicae) for constipation; *Huang Qi* (Radix Astragali) and *Dang Shen* (Radix Codonopsis) for generalized weakness and qi deficiency; and *Dang Gui* (Radix Angelicae Sinensis), *Xiang Fu* (Rhizoma Cyperi), and *Yi Mu Cao* (Herba Leonuri) for irregular menstruation.[14] According to a case report, use of *Gui Zhi Fu Ling Wan* in treating one endometriotic patient controlled the disorder and kept the patient symptom-free for more than 7 months. Furthermore, the study reported a decrease in specific IgM antibody titer without any suppression of serum CA-125 and estradiol levels.[15]
4. **Amenorrhea**: According to one study, administration of *Gui Zhi Fu Ling Wan* was associated with a marked effect in treating amenorrhea in 20 patients with 2 months to 3 years history of illness. The study reported menstruation in 8 cases after 1-3 packs of herbs, in 7 cases after 4-6 packs of herbs, and no change in 5 cases.[16]

HERB-DRUG INTERACTION

Drug-induced menopause: One study evaluated the therapeutic effects of herbal medicines on menopausal clinical signs induced by gonadotropin-releasing hormone-agonist therapy in Japanese women with endometriosis, adenomyosis, or leiomyoma. According to this study, menopausal clinical signs induced by gonadotropin-releasing hormone-agonist therapy in 13 patients were successfully treated with *Gui Zhi Fu Ling Wan*, *Dang Gui*

Guì Zhī Fú Líng Wán (Cinnamon Twig and Poria Pill)

Shao Yao San (Tangkuei and Peony Powder), *Shao Yao Gan Cao Tang* (Peony and Licorice Decoction), *Jia Wei Xiao Yao San* (Augmented Rambling Powder), *Tao He Cheng Qi Tang* (Peach Pit Decoction to Order the Qi), or *Gui Zhi Tang* (Cinnamon Twig Decoction). Most importantly, there were no significant changes in serum estradiol levels after treatment with these herbal medicines. The researchers concluded that these herbal medicines can be recommended for menopausal clinical signs induced by gonadotropin-releasing hormone agonists without a negative effect on serum estradiol levels.[17]

TOXICOLOGY

Gui Zhi Fu Ling Wan has very little toxicity. Oral ingestion of this formula at 250g/kg (maximum capacity of the stomach) in mice for one week did not cause any fatalities or abnormal reactions.[18]

SUGGESTED ACUPUNCTURE TREATMENT

Acupuncture treatment should be avoided in those pregnancies where the fetus tends to be unstable.

AUTHORS' COMMENTS

Gui Zhi Fu Ling Wan is commonly used to treat blood stasis in the uterus or lochia that manifests in dark black blood and low abdominal pain that worsens with pressure. The veterinary application of this formula is in the treatment of primates. Classic textbooks suggest that the dosage must be strictly followed, starting at one pill per dose. If there is no response, the dosage may be increased up to three pills per dose. The dosage must never be drastically increased in an attempt to achieve an immediate effect. This condition can only be treated with low doses of herbs to gently dissolve and disperse blood stasis. Furthermore, this formula is prepared in honey pill form, as this dosage form slowly releases the ingredients for absorption to provide a gradual, gentle, and sustained effect over a long period of time.

Gui Zhi Fu Ling Wan treats blood stagnation in the womb, yet it is named after *Gui Zhi* (Ramulus Cinnamomi) and *Fu Ling* (Poria), but not any of the blood-invigorating herbs in this formula, such as *Tao Ren* (Semen Persicae), *Chi Shao* (Radix Paeoniae Rubra) or *Mu Dan Pi* (Cortex Moutan). This signifies that blood stagnation in the womb is a delicate situation that cannot simply be treated with herbs that activate blood circulation. Instead, *Gui Zhi* (Ramulus Cinnamomi) must be used to warm and open the blood vessels to create an "entry" for the blood-invigorating herbs to reach the affected area, and *Fu Ling* (Poria) needs to be used to provide an "exit" to guide and eliminate blood stasis downward. Furthermore, *Gui Zhi* (Ramulus Cinnamomi) and *Fu Ling* (Poria) are very gentle herbs and will not harm either the mother or the fetus.

Gui Zhi Fu Ling Wan can be used to treat persistent postpartum bleeding in primiparous dogs secondary to subinvolution of placental sites (SIPS) and/or retention of placenta. In these cases, the formula helps to remove stagnant blood, stop bleeding, and cleanse the uterus. Sub-fertile mares with intrauterine cysts can be treated with this formula, though treatment should start long before the breeding season, as this condition needs a long time to resolve. In addition, it can be used in dogs to cleanse the postpartum uterus. The formula can be useful in mares that exhibit back pain during estrus, though in mares with severe, stabbing pain, a formula that tonifies and moves the blood is a better option, such as *Tao Hong Si Wu Tang* (Four-Substance Decoction with Safflower and Peach Pit).

In addition to the original clinical application (blood stasis during gestation), *Gui Zhi Fu Ling Wan* is now used to treat various disorders characterized by blood stasis:

- This formula can also be used for irregular menstruation, post-menstrual abdominal pain, or continuous spotting of blood after delivery, with abdominal pain that is worse with pressure.
- It is also effective for amenorrhea due to blood stasis, in which the patient experiences abdominal fullness and pain that increase with palpation and pressure. Immobile masses in the lower abdomen are indicative of blood stasis, with dark and purplish blood reflecting the same diagnosis. Furthermore, blood stasis is often accompanied by clinical signs such as flushed face, abdominal fullness and pain (the pain increases with palpation or pressure), shoulder stiffness, dizziness, and cold feet.
- This formula also treats dysmenorrhea due to blood stasis in the uterus, with clinical signs such as blood stasis, uterine bleeding of dark purplish blood, abdominal fullness and pain (pain increases with pressure or palpation), immobile masses in the lower abdomen with pain and tenderness, and abdominal pain caused by abnormal abdominal masses or previous blood stasis in the uterus.

References

1. *Zhong Yao Ming Fang Yao Li Yu Ying Yong* (Pharmacology and Applications of Famous Herbal Formulas), 1989; 455-457.
2. *Guo Wai Yi Xue* (Foreign Medicine), 1987; 9(2):32.
3. *Zhong Yi Fang Ji Xian Dai Yan Jiu* (Modern Study of Medical Formulas in Traditional Chinese Medicine), 1997; 1119.
4. *Guo Wai Yi Xue* (Foreign Medicine), 1983; 4:206.
5. *Zhong Yao Yao Li Yu Lin Chuang* (Pharmacology and Clinical Applications of Chinese Herbs), 1985; 13.
6. *Guo Wai Yi Xue* (Foreign Medicine), 1988; 10(4):45.

Guì Zhī Fú Líng Wán (Cinnamon Twig and Poria Pill)

7. Sakamoto S, Kudo H, Kawasaki T, Kuwa K, Kasahara N, Sassa S, Okamoto R. Effects of a Chinese herbal medicine, keishi-bukuryo-gan, on the gonadal system of rats. J Ethnopharmacol. 1988 Jul-Aug;23 (2-3):151-8.
8. Nakagawa T, Yokozawa T, Terasawa K, Nakanishi K. Therapeutic usefulness of Keishi-bukuryo-gan for diabetic nephropathy. J Pharm Pharmacol. 2003 Feb;55(2):219-27.
9. Sekiya N, Goto H, Shimada Y, Terasawa K. Inhibitory effects of Keishi-bukuryo-gan on free radical induced lysis of rat red blood cells. Phytother Res. 2002 Jun;16(4):373-6.
10. Tanaka T, Umesaki N, Mizuno K, Fujino Y, Ogita S. Anti-endometrial IgM autoantibodies in endometriotic patients: a preliminary study. Clin Exp Obstet Gynecol. 2000;27(2):133-7.
11. Mori T, Sakamoto S, Singtripop T, Park MK, Kato T, Kawashima S, Nagasawa H. Suppression of spontaneous development of uterine adenomyosis by a Chinese herbal medicine, keishi-bukuryo-gan, in mice. Planta Med. 1993 Aug;59(4):308-11.
12. *Xin Zhong Yi* (New Chinese Medicine), 1975; 6:33.
13. *Zhong Yi Za Zhi* (Journal of Chinese Medicine), 1994; 35(6):355.
14. *Shang Hai Zhong Yi Yao Za Zhi* (Shanghai Journal of Chinese Medicine and Herbology), 1996; 6:32.
15. Tanaka T, Mizuno K, Umesaki N, Ogita S. A preliminary immunopharmacological study of an antiendometriotic herbal medicine, Keishi-bukuryo-gan. Osaka City Med J. 1998 Jun; 44(1):117-24.
16. *Gui Yang Zhong Yi Xue Yuan Xue Bao* (Journal of Guiyang Chinese Medical University), 1992; 14(2):9.
17. Tanaka T. Effects of herbal medicines on menopausal symptoms induced by gonadotropin-releasing hormone agonist therapy. Clin Exp Obstet Gynecol. 2001;28(1):20-3.
18. *Zhong Yao Yao Li Yu Lin Chuang* (Pharmacology and Clinical Applications of Chinese Herbs), 1985; 13.

Zhé Chōng Yǐn (Break the Conflict Decoction)

折衝飲
折冲饮

Pinyin Name: *Zhe Chong Yin*
Literal Name: Break the Conflict Decoction
Alternate Name: Cinnamon and Persica Combination
Original Source: *Fu Ke Chan Lun Fang* (Discussion of Formulas for Obstetrics and Gynecology)

COMPOSITION

Gui Zhi (Ramulus Cinnamomi)	3g
Tao Ren (Semen Persicae)	3g
Hong Hua (Flos Carthami)	1.5g
Mu Dan Pi (Cortex Moutan)	1.5g
Dang Gui (Radix Angelicae Sinensis)	2.4g
Bai Shao (Radix Paeoniae Alba)	3g
Chuan Xiong (Rhizoma Chuanxiong)	2.4g
Yan Hu Suo (Rhizoma Corydalis)	1.5g
Chuan Niu Xi (Radix Cyathulae)	2.4g
Gan Cao (Radix et Rhizoma Glycyrrhizae)	0.3g

BLOOD-REGULATING FORMULAS 13

Zhé Chōng Yǐn (Break the Conflict Decoction)

DOSAGE / PREPARATION / ADMINISTRATION

The source text states to cook all of the ingredients in 2.5 bowls of water until the liquid is reduced to 1.5 bowls. Take the strained decoction while warm.

CLINICAL MANIFESTATIONS

Blood stagnation in the lower *jiao*: acute or chronic pain in the lower abdominal region and lower back, irregular estrus, dysmenorrhea, and amenorrhea.

VETERINARY CLINICAL APPLICATIONS

Irregular estrus, dysmenorrhea, and pelvic inflammatory disease in primates.

EXPLANATION

Zhe Chong Yin (Break the Conflict Decoction) treats blood stagnation in the lower *jiao* that interferes with normal menstruation and causes severe pain. Because of blood stagnation, patients may experience sharp, stabbing pain in a fixed location. In addition, blood stagnation impairs the normal flow of blood, leading to irregular menstruation, dysmenorrhea, and amenorrhea. This formula also can be used to treat blood stagnation in the lower *jiao* following a miscarriage.

This formula contains many herbs that activate blood circulation, eliminate blood stasis, and disperse obstruction. *Gui Zhi* (Ramulus Cinnamomi) promotes the circulation of yang qi and dispels stagnation in the lower *jiao*. *Tao Ren* (Semen Persicae) and *Hong Hua* (Flos Carthami) activate blood circulation, dispel blood stasis, and relieve pain. *Mu Dan Pi* (Cortex Moutan) promotes both qi and blood circulation to disperse stagnation. *Dang Gui* (Radix Angelicae Sinensis), *Bai Shao* (Radix Paeoniae Alba), and *Chuan Xiong* (Rhizoma Chuanxiong) tonify the blood, move blood circulation, and relieve pain. *Yan Hu Suo* (Rhizoma Corydalis) and *Chuan Niu Xi* (Radix Cyathulae), in addition to activating qi and blood circulation, also relieve pain. Lastly, *Gan Cao* (Radix et Rhizoma Glycyrrhizae) harmonizes the herbs. Overall, this is one of the best formulas for treating various obstetric and gynecological disorders characterized by blood stagnation in the lower *jiao*.

VETERINARY MODIFICATIONS

- With blood stagnation during menstruation, add *San Leng* (Rhizoma Sparganii) and *E Zhu* (Rhizoma Curcumae).
- With painful menstruation, add *Xiang Fu* (Rhizoma Cyperi) and *Ai Ye* (Folium Artemisiae Argyi).
- With painful menstruation due to wind and cold, add *Xiao Chai Hu Tang* (Minor Bupleurum Decoction).
- With abdominal pain after delivery, add *Sheng Hua Tang* (Generation and Transformation Decoction).

SUGGESTED ACUPUNCTURE TREATMENT

1. Points: *Guanyuan* (CV 4), *Geshu* (BL 17), *Xuehai* (SP 10), *Sanyinjiao* (SP 6), *Zigong* (CV 19), *Zhongji* (CV 3), and *Diji* (SP 8).
2. Technique: tonification.

Geshu (BL 17), *Xuehai* (SP 10), and *Sanyinjiao* (SP 6) promote the circulation of qi and blood to remove stagnation. *Guanyuan* (CV 4), *Zigong* (CV 19), *Zhongji* (CV 3), and *Diji* (SP 8) warm the lower *jiao*, unblock the channels, and relieve pain.

AUTHORS' COMMENTS

The primary application of *Zhe Chong Yin* in veterinary medicine is in the treatment of infertility in primates.

***Zhe Chong Yin* (Break the Conflict Decoction)**

Diagnosis	Clinical Signs	Treatment	Herbs
Blood stagnation in the lower *jiao*	• Sharp, stabbing pain in a fixed location: blood stagnation in the lower *jiao* • Irregular menstruation, dysmenorrhea, and amenorrhea: blood stagnation affecting menstruation	• Activates blood circulation and dispels blood stasis • Disperses stagnation and clears obstruction	• *Gui Zhi* (Ramulus Cinnamomi) promotes circulation of yang qi and dispels stagnation in the lower *jiao*. • *Tao Ren* (Semen Persicae) and *Hong Hua* (Flos Carthami) activate blood, dispel blood stasis, and relieve pain. • *Mu Dan Pi* (Cortex Moutan) promotes both qi and blood circulation to disperse stagnation. • *Dang Gui* (Radix Angelicae Sinensis), *Bai Shao* (Radix Paeoniae Alba), and *Chuan Xiong* (Rhizoma Chuanxiong) tonify the blood, move blood circulation, and relieve pain. • *Yan Hu Suo* (Rhizoma Corydalis) and *Chuan Niu Xi* (Radix Cyathulae) activate qi and blood circulation and relieve pain. • *Gan Cao* (Radix et Rhizoma Glycyrrhizae) harmonizes the herbs.

Biē Jiǎ Jiān Wán (Soft-Shelled Turtle Shell Pill)

鱉甲煎丸
鳖甲煎丸

Pinyin Name: *Bie Jia Jian Wan*
Literal Name: Soft-Shelled Turtle Shell Pill
Original Source: *Jin Gui Yao Lue* (Essentials from the Golden Cabinet) by Zhang Zhong-Jing in the Eastern Han Dynasty

COMPOSITION

Bie Jia (Carapax Trionycis), *zhi* (fried with liquid)	90g
Da Huang (Radix et Rhizoma Rhei)	22.5g
Mang Xiao (Natrii Sulfas)	90g
Tu Bie Chong (Eupolyphaga seu Steleophaga), *ao* (simmered)	37g
Qiang Lang (Catharsium Molossus), *ao* (simmered)	45g
Shu Fu (Armadillidium), *ao* (simmered)	22.5g
Chai Hu (Radix Bupleuri)	45g
Huang Qin (Radix Scutellariae)	22.5g
Bai Shao (Radix Paeoniae Alba)	37g
Hou Po (Cortex Magnoliae Officinalis)	22.5g
She Gan (Rhizoma Belamcandae), *pao* (blast-fried)	22.5g
Ting Li Zi (Semen Descurainiae seu Lepidii)	7.5g
Ban Xia (Rhizoma Pinelliae)	7.5g
Gan Jiang (Rhizoma Zingiberis)	22.5g
Gui Zhi (Ramulus Cinnamomi)	22.5g
Ren Shen (Radix et Rhizoma Ginseng)	7.5g
E Jiao (Colla Corii Asini)	22.5g
Tao Ren (Semen Persicae)	15g
Mu Dan Pi (Cortex Moutan)	37g
Ling Xiao Hua (Flos Campsis)	22.5g
Feng Fang (Nidus Vespae), *zhi* (fried with liquid)	30g
Qu Mai (Herba Dianthi)	22.5g
Shi Wei (Folium Pyrrosiae)	22.5g

DOSAGE / PREPARATION / ADMINISTRATION

The source text states to first mix 3kg of burnt ash with 10kg of grain-based liquor. Then filter out and discard the burnt ash. Add *Bie Jia* (Carapax Trionycis) to the strained liquid and cook it until the mixture becomes a thick paste. The remaining 22 herbs are ground into a fine powder, then mixed with this herbal paste and *Feng Mi* (Mel) to make small pills. Take 3g of pills three times daily.

CHINESE THERAPEUTIC ACTIONS

1. Activates qi and blood circulation
2. Dispels dampness and dissolves phlegm
3. Softens hardness and resolves masses

CLINICAL MANIFESTATIONS

Splenomegaly, hepatomegaly, abdominal pain, muscle wasting and poor appetite.

VETERINARY CLINICAL APPLICATIONS

Splenomegaly, hepatomegaly, hepatitis, liver cirrhosis and liver cancer.

EXPLANATION

Bie Jia Jian Wan (Soft-Shelled Turtle Shell Pill) historically was used to treat malaria with splenomegaly. Today, it is used to treat abdominal masses. Because of the chronic nature of this illness, there will be signs of qi and yang deficiencies, qi and blood stagnation, and damp and phlegm accumulation. The formation of masses may occur in the abdomen, hypochondrium, or in the form of splenomegaly.

In this formula, *Bie Jia* (Carapax Trionycis) softens nodules and resolves masses. The burnt ash and grain-based liquor help *Bie Jia* (Carapax Trionycis) activate blood circulation, remove blood stasis, soften nodules, and resolve masses. *Da Huang* (Radix et Rhizoma Rhei), *Mang*

Biē Jiă Jiān Wán (Soft-Shelled Turtle Shell Pill)

***Bie Jia Jian Wan* (Soft-Shelled Turtle Shell Pill)**

Diagnosis	Clinical Signs	Treatment	Herbs
Malaria with splenomegaly	• Immobile masses in the hypochondrium and abdominal pain: damp and phlegm accumulation • Muscle wasting and decreased food intake: underlying qi and blood deficiencies	• Activates qi and blood circulation • Dispels dampness and dissolves phlegm • Softens hardness and resolves masses	• *Bie Jia* (Carapax Trionycis) softens nodules and resolves masses. • *Da Huang* (Radix et Rhizoma Rhei), *Mang Xiao* (Natrii Sulfas), *Tu Bie Chong* (Eupolyphaga seu Steleophaga), *Qiang Lang* (Catharsium Molossus), and *Shu Fu* (Armadillidium) break up blood stasis and resolve masses. • *Chai Hu* (Radix Bupleuri), *Huang Qin* (Radix Scutellariae), and *Bai Shao* (Radix Paeoniae Alba) harmonize the *shaoyang* and regulate Liver qi circulation. • *Hou Po* (Cortex Magnoliae Officinalis), *She Gan* (Rhizoma Belamcandae), *Ting Li Zi* (Semen Descurainiae seu Lepidii), and *Ban Xia* (Rhizoma Pinelliae) regulate qi and dispel phlegm. • *Gan Jiang* (Rhizoma Zingiberis) and *Gui Zhi* (Ramulus Cinnamomi) warm the body. • *Ren Shen* (Radix et Rhizoma Ginseng) and *E Jiao* (Colla Corii Asini) tonify qi and nourish the blood. • *Tao Ren* (Semen Persicae), *Mu Dan Pi* (Cortex Moutan), *Ling Xiao Hua* (Flos Campsis) and *Feng Fang* (Nidus Vespae) activate blood circulation and remove blood stasis. • *Qu Mai* (Herba Dianthi) and *Shi Wei* (Folium Pyrrosiae) regulate water circulation and dispel dampness.

Xiao (Natrii Sulfas), *Tu Bie Chong* (Eupolyphaga seu Steleophaga), *Qiang Lang* (Catharsium Molossus), and *Shu Fu* (Armadillidium) break up blood stasis and resolve masses. *Chai Hu* (Radix Bupleuri), *Huang Qin* (Radix Scutellariae), and *Bai Shao* (Radix Paeoniae Alba) harmonize the *shaoyang* and regulate Liver qi circulation. *Hou Po* (Cortex Magnoliae Officinalis), *She Gan* (Rhizoma Belamcandae), *Ting Li Zi* (Semen Descurainiae seu Lepidii), and *Ban Xia* (Rhizoma Pinelliae) regulate qi and dispel phlegm. *Gan Jiang* (Rhizoma Zingiberis) and *Gui Zhi* (Ramulus Cinnamomi) warm the body. *Ren Shen* (Radix et Rhizoma Ginseng) and *E Jiao* (Colla Corii Asini) tonify qi and nourish the blood. *Tao Ren* (Semen Persicae), *Mu Dan Pi* (Cortex Moutan), *Ling Xiao Hua* (Flos Campsis), and *Feng Fang* (Nidus Vespae) activate blood circulation and remove blood stasis. *Qu Mai* (Herba Dianthi) and *Shi Wei* (Folium Pyrrosiae) regulate water circulation and dispel dampness. Overall, this formula has a good balance of warm and cold, tonifying and sedating, and qi- and blood-activating herbs.

VETERINARY MODIFICATIONS

- With general weakness and deficiency, add *Huang Qi* (Radix Astragali), *Bai Zhu* (Rhizoma Atractylodis Macrocephalae), *Shu Di Huang* (Radix Rehmanniae Praeparata), and *Dang Gui* (Radix Angelicae Sinensis).
- With decreased food intake and indigestion, add *Shan Zha* (Fructus Crataegi), *Shen Qu* (Massa Fermentata), and *Ji Nei Jin* (Endothelium Corneum Gigeriae Galli).
- To improve clinical efficacy and relieve pain, add *Ji Xue Teng* (Caulis Spatholobi), *Hong Hua* (Flos Carthami) and *Yan Hu Suo* (Rhizoma Corydalis).

CAUTIONS / CONTRAINDICATIONS

Bie Jia Jian Wan contains many herbs that strongly activate qi and blood circulation, dispel dampness, and dissolve phlegm. It should be used with caution in patients with *zheng* (upright) *qi* deficiency.

Biē Jiă Jiān Wán (Soft-Shelled Turtle Shell Pill)

SUGGESTED ACUPUNCTURE TREATMENT

1. Points: *Zhangmen* (LR 13), *Qimen* (LR 14), *Geshu* (BL 17), *Taichong* (LR 3), *Waiguan* (TH 5), *Fenglong* (ST 40), *Shenque* (CV 8), *Housanli* (ST 36), *Sanyinjiao* (SP 6), *Pishu* (BL 20), *Xuehai* (SP 10), *Ganshu* (BL 18), and *Yinlingquan* (SP 9).
2. Technique: even method and moxibustion.

Zhangmen (LR 13) softens nodules and activates qi circulation in the local area. *Qimen* (LR 14), *Xuehai* (SP 10), *Ganshu* (BL 18), and *Geshu* (BL 17) activate blood circulation to break stagnation. *Taichong* (LR 3) and *Waiguan* (TH 5) regulate qi. *Fenglong* (ST 40) and *Yinlingquan* (SP 9) dispel dampness. Moxibustion on *Shenque* (CV 8), *Housanli* (ST 36), *Sanyinjiao* (SP 6), and *Pishu* (BL 20) tonifies qi and yin.

Section 2

止血剂 — Stop-Bleeding Formulas

Shí Huī Sǎn (Ten Partially-Charred Substances Powder) 十灰散

Pinyin Name: *Shi Hui San*
Literal Name: Ten Partially-Charred Substances Powder
Original Source: *Shi Yao Shen Shu* (Miraculous Book of Ten Remedies) by Ge Qian-Sun in 1348

COMPOSITION

Da Ji (Radix Euphorbiae seu Knoxiae)	[9g]
Xiao Ji (Herba Cirsii)	[9g]
He Ye (Folium Nelumbinis)	[9g]
Qian Cao (Radix et Rhizoma Rubiae)	[9g]
Ce Bai Ye (Cacumen Platycladi)	[9g]
Bai Mao Gen (Rhizoma Imperatae)	[9g]
Zong Lu (Petiolus Trachycarpi)	[9g]
Zhi Zi (Fructus Gardeniae)	[9g]
Da Huang (Radix et Rhizoma Rhei)	[9g]
Mu Dan Pi (Cortex Moutan)	[9g]

DOSAGE / PREPARATION / ADMINISTRATION

The source text instructs to char to ashes equal amounts of the ingredients and grind into a fine powder. Separately pound *Ou Jie* (Nodus Nelumbinis Rhizomatis) or *Lai Fu Zi* (Semen Raphani) to obtain their juice. Take 15g of the powder per dose after meals with half a bowl of juice. Today, this formula may be prepared as a decoction with the doses suggested in brackets.

CHINESE THERAPEUTIC ACTIONS

Cools the blood and stops bleeding

CLINICAL MANIFESTATIONS

Bleeding caused by heat in the *xue* (blood) level: hematemesis, hemoptysis, and other sudden onset bleeding symptoms.

VETERINARY CLINICAL APPLICATIONS

Hematemesis, hyphema, and gastrointestinal bleeding.

EXPLANATION

Shi Hui San (Ten Partially-Charred Substances Powder) treats bleeding caused by heat in the *xue* (blood) level. Interior heat can invade the blood and force it out of the blood vessels, resulting in the reckless movement of blood in various types of bleeding. Because of heat, the bleeding is accompanied by bright red blood and a red or deep red tongue.

In this formula, *Da Ji* (Radix Euphorbiae seu Knoxiae), *Xiao Ji* (Herba Cirsii), *He Ye* (Folium Nelumbinis), *Qian Cao* (Radix et Rhizoma Rubiae), *Ce Bai Ye* (Cacumen Platycladi), and *Bai Mao Gen* (Rhizoma Imperatae) cool the blood and stop bleeding. *Zong Lu* (Petiolus Trachycarpi) astringes the blood and provides immediate effect to stop bleeding. *Zhi Zi* (Fructus Gardeniae) clears heat and purges fire, while *Da Huang* (Radix et Rhizoma Rhei) drains the heat and fire downward. *Mu Dan Pi* (Cortex Moutan) has two functions in this formula: it clears heat to stop bleeding, and it activates blood circulation to prevent blood stasis. Blood activation is vital, because the sole use of stop-bleeding herbs in this case may lead to blood stagnation. The juice of *Ou Jie* (Nodus Nelumbinis Rhizomatis) or *Lai Fu Zi* (Semen Raphani) may be added to enhance the actions of clearing heat, cooling the blood, and stopping the bleeding.

Shí Huī Sǎn (Ten Partially-Charred Substances Powder)

***Shi Hui San* (Ten Partially-Charred Substances Powder)**

Diagnosis	Clinical Signs	Treatment	Herbs
Bleeding due to heat in the *xue* (blood) level	Sudden onset bleeding: heat in the interior forcing blood out of the vessels	Cools the blood and stops bleeding	• *Da Ji* (Radix Euphorbiae seu Knoxiae), *Xiao Ji* (Herba Cirsii), *He Ye* (Folium Nelumbinis), *Qian Cao* (Radix et Rhizoma Rubiae), *Ce Bai Ye* (Cacumen Platycladi), and *Bai Mao Gen* (Rhizoma Imperatae) cool the blood and stop bleeding. • *Zong Lu* (Petiolus Trachycarpi) astringes the blood to stop bleeding immediately. • *Zhi Zi* (Fructus Gardeniae) clears heat and purges fire. • *Da Huang* (Radix et Rhizoma Rhei) drains heat and fire downwards. • *Mu Dan Pi* (Cortex Moutan) clears heat to stop bleeding and activates blood circulation to prevent blood stasis. • *Ou Jie* (Nodus Nelumbinis Rhizomatis) or *Lai Fu Zi* (Semen Raphani) enhances the actions of clearing heat, cooling the blood, and stopping bleeding.

All of the herbs are charred to ashes to enhance their hemostatic effect. The formula is prepared and stored in powder form so that it can be administered immediately when needed.

VETERINARY MODIFICATION

With acute bleeding due to heat flaring up, add *Niu Xi* (Radix Achyranthis Bidentatae) and *Zhe Shi* (Haematitum), and increase the doses of *Da Huang* (Radix et Rhizoma Rhei) and *Zhi Zi* (Fructus Gardeniae). Administer the formula in decoction form for faster results.

CAUTIONS / CONTRAINDICATIONS

- *Shi Hui San* should be used only as a short-term therapy to stop bleeding. Once the bleeding has stopped, the cause of bleeding must be identified and treated accordingly.
- This formula is designed for bleeding caused by an excess condition of heat in the *xue* (blood) level. It is contraindicated in bleeding conditions caused by deficiency and cold.

PHARMACOLOGICAL EFFECTS

Hemostatic: One study evaluated the hemostatic effect of *Shi Hui San* prepared by various methods. Method I was to char the herbs until the smoke turned from white to yellow in color, with the herbs appearing black on the outside and dark brown on the inside. Loss of herb weight on charring was 20%. Method II was to char the herbs until the smoke turned from white to yellow to bluegreen in color, with the herbs appearing black on the outside and inside. Loss of herb weight on charring was 40%. Method III was to char the herbs until the smoke turned from white to yellow to bluegreen to clear in color, with the herbs appearing burnt on the outside and black on the inside. Loss of herb weight on charring was 60%. Method IV was to char the herbs until the smoke turned from white to yellow to bluegreen to clear in color, with the herbs appearing completely burnt throughout. Loss of herb weight on charring was 80%. These four preparations were then given to rabbits and their hemostatic effects were evaluated. Of the four preparations, the study concluded that the hemostatic effect was most potent in method I, followed by method II and method III. Method IV had no significant impact.[1]

HUMAN CLINICAL STUDIES AND RESEARCH

1. **Hematemesis in pulmonary tuberculosis**: *Shi Hui San* was used to stop bleeding in pulmonary tuberculosis patients who were coughing blood. Herbal treatment effectively stopped bleeding in most patients within 4-6 days. Overall, the treatment was effective in 22 out of 27 patients.[2]
2. **Hematemesis in bronchiectasis**: Modified *Shi Hui San* given in decoction was effective in 8 bronchiectasis patients coughing blood. The treatment protocol was to combine *Shi Hui San* with *San Qi* (Radix et Rhizoma Notoginseng), *Chuan Bei Mu* (Bulbus Fritillariae Cirrhosae), and powdered *Bai Ji* (Rhizoma Bletillae). The herbs were cooked in water, and the decoction given in three equally-divided doses daily. Bleeding stopped in most patients within 1-2 days, with complete recovery between 6-20 days. No recurrence was reported by patients in follow-up evaluations one year after treatment.[3]

Shí Huī Sǎn (Ten Partially-Charred Substances Powder)

3. **Hyphema**: Modified *Shi Hui San* was used to treat 10 patients with bleeding caused by external injuries to the anterior chamber of the eye. The treatment protocol was to administer *Shi Hui San* with 10g of *Hong Hua* (Flos Carthami) one time daily until the bleeding stopped. The patients were also treated with 1% atropine ophthalmic paste one time daily. The study reported that the bleeding stopped within 3-9 days. Upon discharge, 9 of 10 patients had restored normal visual acuity and all 10 had normal ocular pressure.[4]
4. **Gastrointestinal bleeding**: Administration of *Shi Hui San* and *Zuo Jin Wan* (Left Metal Pill) was shown to effectively treat upper gastrointestinal bleeding resulting from gastric or duodenal ulcers.[5]

SUGGESTED ACUPUNCTURE TREATMENT

1. Points: *Feishu* (BL 13), *Yuji* (LU 10), *Laogong* (PC 8), and *Xingjian* (LR 2).
2. Technique: sedation.

Feishu (BL 13) and *Yuji* (LU 10) sedate Lung heat to stop bleeding. *Laogong* (PC 8) clears heat to stop it from forcing blood out of the vessels. *Xingjian* (LR 2) sedates Liver fire and reverses ascending qi to normalize blood circulation.

AUTHORS' COMMENTS

Shi Hui San is designed to be an emergency herbal formula that quickly stops bleeding. It focuses primarily on treating the symptom (bleeding), and not the cause. Therefore, once the bleeding has stopped, the cause of bleeding should be determined and treated accordingly. *Shi Hui San* should not be taken for a prolonged period of time or in high doses.

In *Shi Hui San*, all ten herbs are partially charred to ash to enhance the astringent and hemostatic effects of the formula. Because of this unique processing, the formula is named appropriately "Ten Partially-Charred Substances Powder."

References

1. *Nei Meng Gu Zhong Yi Yao* (Traditional Chinese Medicine and Medicinals of Inner Mongolia), 1984; 3:46.
2. *Fu Jian Zhong Yi Yao* (Fujian Chinese Medicine and Herbology), 1960; 4:27.
3. *Shi Zhen Guo Yao Yan Jiu* (Research of Shizhen Herbs), 1997; 4:301.
4. *Zhong Guo Zhong Xi Yi Jie He Za Zhi* (Chinese Journal of Integrative Chinese and Western Medicine), 1987; 3:175.
5. *Zhe Jiang Zhong Yi Yao* (Zhejiang Chinese Medicine and Herbology), 1963; 7:4.

Sì Shēng Wán (Four-Fresh Pill)

四生丸

Pinyin Name: *Si Sheng Wan*
Literal Name: Four-Fresh Pill
Alternate Name: Rehmannia Four Formula
Original Source: *Fu Ren Liang Fang* (Fine Formulas for Women) by Chen Zi-Ming in 1237

COMPOSITION

Ce Bai Ye (Cacumen Platycladi), fresh	[12g]
Di Huang (Radix Rehmanniae), fresh	[15g]
He Ye (Folium Nelumbinis), fresh	[9g]
Ai Ye (Folium Artemisiae Argyi), fresh	[9g]

Si Shēng Wán (Four-Fresh Pill)

DOSAGE / PREPARATION / ADMINISTRATION

The source text states to grind equal amounts of the ingredients into powder and form into pills the size of egg yolks. Cook one pill with water and take the decoction. Today, this formula may be prepared as a decoction with the doses suggested in brackets.

CHINESE THERAPEUTIC ACTIONS

Cools the blood and stops bleeding

CLINICAL MANIFESTATIONS

Bleeding caused by heat in the *xue* (blood) level: hematemesis and epistaxis with bright red blood, a dry mouth and throat, a red or deep red tongue, and a wiry, rapid pulse.

VETERINARY CLINICAL APPLICATIONS

Hemoptysis, hematemesis, hematochezia, epistaxis, tuberculosis, and bronchiectasis.

EXPLANATION

Si Sheng Wan (Four-Fresh Pill) treats hematemesis or epistaxis caused by heat in the *xue* (blood) level. If the heat factor invades the *xue* (blood) level and forces the blood out of their vessels, then clinical signs of bleeding, such as hematemesis or epistaxis with bright red blood, may occur. The dry mouth and throat are the result of heat damaging yin and body fluids. A red tongue and a wiry, rapid pulse indicate excess heat in the interior.

This formula uses *Ce Bai Ye* (Cacumen Platycladi) to cool the blood and stop bleeding. *Di Huang* (Radix Rehmanniae) clears heat, cools the blood, and nourishes yin and body fluids. *He Ye* (Folium Nelumbinis) and *Ai Ye* (Folium Artemisiae Argyi) stop bleeding and disperse blood stagnation.

VETERINARY MODIFICATIONS

- With severe bleeding, add *Qian Cao* (Radix et Rhizoma Rubiae), *Mo Han Lian* (Herba Ecliptae), and *Ou Jie* (Nodus Nelumbinis Rhizomatis).
- With excessive uterine bleeding, add *Jiao Ai Tang* (Ass-Hide Gelatin and Mugwort Decoction).
- With bleeding ulcers, add *Huang Qin* (Radix Scutellariae), *Bai Zhu* (Rhizoma Atractylodis Macrocephalae), *Fu Zi* (Radix Aconiti Lateralis Praeparata), *E Jiao* (Colla Corii Asini), and *Gan Cao* (Radix et Rhizoma Glycyrrhizae).
- With hemoptysis, add *Bai Mao Gen* (Rhizoma Imperatae).
- With hematochezia, add *Di Yu* (Radix Sanguisorbae).
- With constipation due to excess and heat, add *Qian Niu Zi* (Semen Pharbitidis), *Da Huang* (Radix et Rhizoma Rhei), *Zao Jiao* (Fructus Gleditsiae), and *Mang Xiao* (Natrii Sulfas).

CAUTIONS / CONTRAINDICATIONS

Si Sheng Wan should be discontinued when the desired effect is achieved. Prolonged use or overdosing will result in cold accumulation, which may further aggravate the blood stasis.

SUGGESTED ACUPUNCTURE TREATMENT

1. Points: *Laogong* (PC 8), *Weizhong* (BL 40), *Diwuhui* (GB 42), *Ximen* (PC 4), *Kongzui* (LU 6), *Duanxue* and *Tianping*
2. Technique: sedation.

Laogong (PC 8) clears blood heat and stops heat from forcing blood out of the vessels. *Weizhong* (BL 40) clears heat in the blood. *Diwuhui* (GB 42) sedates Liver heat and stops the bleeding. *Ximen* (PC 4), the *xi* (cleft) point of the Pericardium channel, and *Kongzui* (LU 6), the *xi* (cleft) point of the Lung, stop bleeding. If vomiting of blood occurs, add *Shangwan* (CV 13), *Burong* (ST 19), and *Liangqiu* (ST 34) to harmonize the Stomach and stop the bleeding. For nosebleed, add *Shenting* (GV 24), *Fengfu* (GV 16), and *Yixi* (BL 45) to sedate heat and stop the bleeding. *Duanxue* and *Tianping* are classical veterinary points used to stop hemorrhage in horses and dogs, respectively.

AUTHORS' COMMENTS

Si Sheng Wan is a formula that treats bleeding caused by heat in the blood; however, it focuses on the branch

***Si Sheng Wan* (Four-Fresh Pill)**

Diagnosis	Clinical Signs	Treatment	Herbs
Bleeding due to heat in the *xue* (blood) level	• Hematemesis or epistaxis with bright red blood: heat in the *xue* (blood) level forcing blood out of the vessels • Dry mouth and throat: heat damaging yin and body fluids • Red tongue and a wiry, rapid pulse: excess heat in the interior	Cools the blood and stops bleeding	• *Ce Bai Ye* (Cacumen Platycladi) cools the blood and stops bleeding. • *Di Huang* (Radix Rehmanniae) clears heat, cools the blood, and nourishes yin and body fluids. • *He Ye* (Folium Nelumbinis) and *Ai Ye* (Folium Artemisiae Argyi) stop bleeding and disperse blood stagnation.

Sì Shēng Wán (Four-Fresh Pill)

or clinical signs and not on the underlying cause of the bleeding. Once the bleeding is under control, this formula should be discontinued, and a formula that addresses the root cause of the bleeding should be used. Although it was originally formulated to treat blood-heat disorders in the upper *jiao*, it can be used to treat blood-heat disorders affecting other parts of the body as well.

For *Si Sheng Wan*, the original text specifically emphasized using the fresh, unprocessed form of all four herbs to maximize the heat-clearing and blood-cooling effects. Thus, this formula is appropriately named "Four-Fresh Pill." However, the fresh, unprocessed form of these four herbs may not be readily available. In that case, to enhance the hemostatic effect, herbs such as *Xiao Ji* (Herba Cirsii), *Bai Mao Gen* (Rhizoma Imperatae), *Ou Jie* (Nodus Nelumbinis Rhizomatis), and *Xian He Cao* (Herba Agrimoniae) can be added.

Huái Huā Sǎn (Sophora Japonica Flower Powder)
槐花散

Pinyin Name: *Huai Hua San*
Literal Name: Sophora Japonica Flower Powder
Alternate Names: Sophora Flower Powder, Sophora Flower Formula
Original Source: *Pu Ji Ben Shi Fang* (Formulas of Universal Benefit from My Practice) by Xu Shu-Wei in 1132

COMPOSITION

Huai Hua (Flos Sophorae), *chao* (dry-fried)	[12g]
Ce Bai Ye (Cacumen Platycladi), *chu* (pestled) and *bei* (stone baked)	[12g]
Jing Jie Sui (Spica Schizonepetae)	[6g]
Zhi Qiao (Fructus Citri Aurantii), *chao* (dry-fried) with bran till yellow	[6g]

DOSAGE / PREPARATION / ADMINISTRATION

The source text states to grind equal amounts of the ingredients into a fine powder and take 6g with rice soup on an empty stomach before meals. Today, this formula may be prepared as a decoction with the doses suggested in brackets. Note: The original doses of herbs are unavailable from the source text.

CHINESE THERAPEUTIC ACTIONS

1. Clears the Intestines and stops bleeding
2. Dispels wind and redirects qi

CLINICAL MANIFESTATIONS

Hematochezia due to *chang feng* (intestinal wind) and *zang du* (solid organ toxins): bleeding before or after defecation, blood in the stools, bleeding from rectal polyps, and frank blood that is bright red or dark black in color.

VETERINARY CLINICAL APPLICATIONS

Rectal or intestinal bleeding, rectal polyps, acute episodes or relapse of inflammatory bowel disease, ulcerative colitis, perianal fistula, anal gland sacculitis, and perianal and perivulvar dermatitis.

EXPLANATION

Huai Hua San (Sophora Japonica Flower Powder) treats *chang feng* (intestinal wind) and *zang du* (solid organ toxins). *Chang feng* is caused by wind attacking the Intestines, leading to the discharge of bright red blood before defecation or in the stools. *Zang du* is caused by toxins

Huái Huā Săn (Sophora Japonica Flower Powder)

Huai Hua San **(Sophora Japonica Flower Powder)**

Diagnosis	Clinical Signs	Treatment	Herbs
Hematochezia due to *chang feng* (intestinal wind) and *zang du* (solid organ toxins)	• Bright red blood in the stools: *chang feng* (intestinal wind) due to wind attacking the Intestines • Dysentery with dark black blood in the stools: *zang du* (solid organ toxins)	• Clears the Intestines and stops bleeding • Dispels wind and descends qi	• *Huai Hua* (Flos Sophorae) clears damp-heat in the Intestines, cools the blood, and stops bleeding. • *Ce Bai Ye* (Cacumen Platycladi) cools the blood and stops bleeding. • *Jing Jie Sui* (Spica Schizonepetae) disperses wind and stops bleeding. • *Zhi Qiao* (Fructus Aurantii) activates qi circulation in the Intestines to dispel toxins.

attacking the *zang* (solid organs), leading to dysentery with dark black blood in the stools. Both conditions are characterized by wind, heat and toxins attacking the Intestines.

In this formula, *Huai Hua* (Flos Sophorae) clears damp-heat in the Intestines, cools the blood, and stops bleeding. *Ce Bai Ye* (Cacumen Platycladi) helps *Huai Hua* (Flos Sophorae) cool the blood and stop bleeding. *Jing Jie Sui* (Spica Schizonepetae) disperses wind from the Intestines. It also enters the *xue* (blood) level and stops bleeding. *Zhi Qiao* (Fructus Aurantii) activates qi circulation in the Intestines to dispel toxins.

VETERINARY MODIFICATIONS

- With excessive bleeding, add *Di Yu* (Radix Sanguisorbae) and *Xiao Ji* (Herba Cirsii).
- With blood in the stools accompanied by abdominal pain and tenesmus, add *Mu Xiang* (Radix Aucklandiae) and *Hou Po* (Cortex Magnoliae Officinalis).
- With dry, hard stools accompanied by bleeding, add *Mang Xiao* (Natrii Sulfas) and *Huo Ma Ren* (Fructus Cannabis).
- With blood deficiency due to excessive bleeding, add *Dang Gui* (Radix Angelicae Sinensis) and *E Jiao* (Colla Corii Asini).
- With qi deficiency due to chronic bleeding, add *Huang Qi* (Radix Astragali), *Dang Shen* (Radix Codonopsis), and *Sheng Ma* (Rhizoma Cimicifugae).
- For bleeding rectal polyps and prolapsed rectum, remove *Ce Bai Ye* (Cacumen Platycladi) and *Jing Jie* (Herba Schizonepetae), and add *Dang Gui* (Radix Angelicae Sinensis), *Huang Qin* (Radix Scutellariae), *Fang Feng* (Radix Saposhnikoviae), and *Di Yu* (Radix Sanguisorbae).
- With excess heat in the Intestines, add *Huang Lian* (Rhizoma Coptidis) and *Huang Bo* (Cortex Phellodendri Chinensis).

CAUTIONS / CONTRAINDICATIONS

- *Huai Hua San* is cold and thus is not suitable for long-term use.
- This formula is not suitable for chronic rectal bleeding or for hematochezia with clinical signs of qi or yin deficiency.

SUGGESTED ACUPUNCTURE TREATMENT

1. Points: *Changqiang* (GV 1), *Ciliao* (BL 32), *Chengshan* (BL 57), and *Shangjuxu* (ST 37).
2. Technique: sedation.

Changqiang (GV 1) is an empirical point for treating wind in the Intestines. *Ciliao* (BL 32) clears damp-heat from the lower *jiao*. *Chengshan* (BL 57) is an essential point for treating damp-heat disorders of the anus and rectum. *Shangjuxu* (ST 37), the lower *he* (uniting) point of the Large Intestine, clears damp-heat from the Large Intestine.

AUTHORS' COMMENTS

Originally formulated to treat *chang feng* (intestinal wind) and *zang du* (solid organ toxins) in humans, *Huai Hua San* is used today to treat many disorders in animals:

- For acute episodes of inflammatory bowel disease with intestinal bleeding, use it with *Xiang Lian Wan* (Aucklandia and Coptis Pill).
- For the treatment of anal sacculitis and perivulvar and perianal dermatitis, combine it with *Long Dan Xie Gan Tang* (Gentiana Decoction to Drain the Liver).
- For the treatment of perianal fistula, combine with *Si Miao San* (Four-Marvel Powder) and *Tu Fu Ling* (Rhizoma Smilacis Glabrae), *Huang Bo* (Cortex Phellodendri Chinensis), *Che Qian Zi* (Semen Plantaginis), *Yi Yi Ren* (Semen Coicis), *Ji Xue Teng* (Caulis Spatholobi), and *Dan Shen* (Radix et Rhizoma Salviae Miltiorrhizae).
- For canine parvovirus and equine clostridial dysentery, combine with *Bai Tou Weng Tang* (Pulsatilla Decoction).

Xiăo Jì Yĭn Zĭ (Cirsium Decoction)

小薊飲子
小蓟饮子

Pinyin Name: *Xiao Ji Yin Zi*
Literal Name: Cirsium Decoction
Alternate Name: Cephalanoplos Decoction
Original Source: *Dan Xi Xin Fa* (Teachings of [Zhu] Dan-Xi) by Zhu Zhen-Heng in 1481

COMPOSITION

Xiao Ji (Herba Cirsii)	15g
Ou Jie (Nodus Nelumbinis Rhizomatis)	15g [9g]
Pu Huang (Pollen Typhae), *chao* (dry-fried)	15g [9g]
Hua Shi (Talcum)	15g
Mu Tong (Caulis Akebiae)	15g [9g]
Dan Zhu Ye (Herba Lophatheri)	15g [9g]
Zhi Zi (Fructus Gardeniae)	15g [9g]
Di Huang (Radix Rehmanniae), *xi* (washed)	120g [30g]
Dang Gui (Radix Angelicae Sinensis), *jin* (soaked) in liquor	15g [6g]
Zhi Gan Cao (Radix et Rhizoma Glycyrrhizae Praeparata cum Melle)	15g [6g]

DOSAGE / PREPARATION / ADMINISTRATION

The source text states to coarsely grind all of the ingredients. Cook 12g of the powder with 1.5 bowls of water until the liquid is reduced to 80%. Take the warm, strained decoction on an empty stomach before meals. Today, this formula may be prepared as a decoction with the doses suggested in brackets.

CHINESE THERAPEUTIC ACTIONS

1. Cools the blood and stops bleeding
2. Promotes urination and treats *lin zheng* (dysuria syndrome)

CLINICAL MANIFESTATIONS

Xue lin (bloody dysuria) caused by heat in the lower *jiao*: hematuria, frequent urination with a burning sensation and pain, a red tongue, and a rapid pulse.

VETERINARY CLINICAL APPLICATIONS

Acute urinary tract infection, feline lower urinary tract disease, proteinuria, hematuria, and acute glomerulonephritis.

EXPLANATION

Xiao Ji Yin Zi (Cirsium Decoction) treats *xue lin* (bloody dysuria) caused by heat in the lower *jiao*. In this

***Xiao Ji Yin Zi* (Cirsium Decoction)**

Diagnosis	Clinical Signs	Treatment	Herbs
Xue lin (bloody dysuria) caused by heat in the lower *jiao*	• Hematuria and frequent urination with burning pain: heat stagnating in the Urinary Bladder • Red tongue and a rapid pulse: heat condition	• Cools the blood and stops bleeding • Promotes urination and treats *lin zheng* (dysuria syndrome)	• *Xiao Ji* (Herba Cirsii) cools the blood and stops the bleeding. • *Ou Jie* (Nodus Nelumbinis Rhizomatis) and *Pu Huang* (Pollen Typhae) cool the blood, stop bleeding, and resolve blood stasis. • *Hua Shi* (Talcum) clears heat and promotes urination to relieve pain. • *Mu Tong* (Caulis Akebiae), *Dan Zhu Ye* (Herba Lophatheri), and *Zhi Zi* (Fructus Gardeniae) drain fire from the Heart, Lung, and *San Jiao*. • *Di Huang* (Radix Rehmanniae) nourishes yin, cools the blood, and clears heat. • *Dang Gui* (Radix Angelicae Sinensis) nourishes the blood and prevents the cold herbs in this formula from injuring the body. • *Zhi Gan Cao* (Radix et Rhizoma Glycyrrhizae Praeparata cum Melle) harmonizes the herbs.

Xiǎo Jì Yǐn Zǐ (Cirsium Decoction)

syndrome, heat stagnates in the Urinary Bladder and damages the vessels, causing various urinary disorders such as hematuria and frequent urination with burning pain. A red tongue body and a rapid pulse indicate heat.

The treatment plan for this syndrome is to cool the blood, stop bleeding, promote urination, and relieve pain. This formula uses *Xiao Ji* (Herba Cirsii) as the chief herb to cool the blood and stop bleeding. *Ou Jie* (Nodus Nelumbinis Rhizomatis) and *Pu Huang* (Pollen Typhae) cool the blood, stop bleeding, and resolve blood stasis. These two herbs effectively stop bleeding without creating blood stasis. *Hua Shi* (Talcum) clears heat and promotes urination. *Mu Tong* (Caulis Akebiae), *Dan Zhu Ye* (Herba Lophatheri), and *Zhi Zi* (Fructus Gardeniae) drain fire from the Heart, Lung, and *San Jiao*. Since the presence of heat may damage yin and blood, *Di Huang* (Radix Rehmanniae) and *Dang Gui* (Radix Angelicae Sinensis) are added to clear heat, cool the blood, nourish yin, and tonify the blood. *Dang Gui* (Radix Angelicae Sinensis) also prevents the cold herbs in this formula from injuring the body. *Zhi Gan Cao* (Radix et Rhizoma Glycyrrhizae Praeparata cum Melle) harmonizes the herbs.

VETERINARY MODIFICATIONS

- With significant bleeding, add *Bai Mao Gen* (Rhizoma Imperatae) and *Mu Dan Pi* (Cortex Moutan).
- With severe pain during urination, add *Hu Po* (Succinum).
- With dysuria characterized by blood stagnation and heat, add *Shi Wei* (Folium Pyrrosiae), *Pu Gong Ying* (Herba Taraxaci) and *Huang Bo* (Cortex Phellodendri Chinensis).
- For chronic *xue lin* (bloody dysuria) with qi and blood deficiencies, reduce the doses of *Hua Shi* (Talcum) and *Mu Tong* (Caulis Akebiae), and add *Dang Shen* (Radix Codonopsis), *Huang Qi* (Radix Astragali), and *E Jiao* (Colla Corii Asini).
- With more heat, replace *Zhi Gan Cao* (Radix et Rhizoma Glycyrrhizae Praeparata cum Melle) with *Gan Cao* (Radix et Rhizoma Glycyrrhizae).

CAUTIONS / CONTRAINDICATIONS

- *Xiao Ji Yin Zi* should only be used to treat excess types of *xue lin* (bloody dysuria), as it contains mostly cold and draining herbs.
- Chronic cases of *xue lin* (bloody dysuria) are often accompanied by underlying deficiencies, and must also be treated with tonifying herbs.

HUMAN CLINICAL STUDIES AND RESEARCH

1. **Proteinuria**: Use of *Xiao Ji Yin Zi* plus *He Di* (Calyx Nelumbinis) in 35 patients with proteinuria was associated with 97% effectiveness (complete recovery in 19 cases, marked improvement in 9 cases, moderate improvement in 6 cases, and no improvement in 1 case). Patients were instructed to take the herbs daily, maintain a low-sodium diet, avoid exposure to wind and cold, and refrain from sexual activity during the treatment period.[1]
2. **Hematuria in urinary infection**: *Xiao Ji Yin Zi* and *Ba Zheng San* (Eight-Herb Powder for Rectification) were used to treat hematuria due to acute urinary infection. The treatment strategy was to use *Xiao Ji Yin Zi* as the main formula for *xue lin* (bloody dysuria), and *Ba Zheng San* (Eight-Herb Powder for Rectification) for *re lin* (heat dysuria). Furthermore, modifications were made by adding *Mu Dan Pi* (Cortex Moutan) and *Bai Mao Gen* (Rhizoma Imperatae) for excessive blood in the urine; and *Qu Mai* (Herba Dianthi) and *Che Qian Zi* (Semen Plantaginis) for burning sensations and pain in the urethra. Of 48 patients, the study reported complete recovery in 28 cases, significant improvement in 4 cases, moderate improvement in 10 cases, and no effect in 6 cases. The overall effectiveness was 87.5%. The duration of treatment ranged from 2-9 days.[2]

SUGGESTED ACUPUNCTURE TREATMENT

1. Points: *Guanyuan* (CV 4), *Laogong* (PC 8), *Rangu* (KI 2), and *Waiguan* (TH 5).
2. Technique: sedation.

Guanyuan (CV 4), as the *mu* (collecting) point of the Small Intestine, sedates heat in the Small Intestine and relieves dysuria. *Laogong* (PC 8) sedates heat in the Heart and Pericardium by helping to cool the blood. *Rangu* (KI 2) nourishes yin and clears heat. *Waiguan* (TH 5) clears heat from all three *jiaos*.

AUTHORS' COMMENTS

Hematuria corresponds to *xue lin* (bloody dysuria) in Chinese medicine. *Xiao Ji Yin Zi* is used to treat hematuria caused by heat that stagnates in the Urinary Bladder and damages the vessels to cause hematuria. Of all the formulas that treat hematuria, this is the strongest to cool the blood, stop bleeding, and resolve moderate to severe hematuria. It can be used to treat hematuria secondary to transitional cell carcinoma of the bladder. It also can be combined with *Ba Zheng San* (Eight-Herb Powder for Rectification) to treat cystitis with moderate to severe hematuria.

References

1. *Hu Nan Yi Yao Za Zhi* (Hunan Journal of Medicine and Herbology), 1984; 6:14.
2. *Hei Long Jiang Zhong Yi Yao* (Heilongjiang Journal of Chinese Medicine and Herbology), 1985; 3:43.

BLOOD-REGULATING FORMULAS 13

Jiāo Ài Tāng (Ass-Hide Gelatin and Mugwort Decoction)

膠艾湯
胶艾汤

Pinyin Name: *Jiao Ai Tang*

Literal Name: Ass-Hide Gelatin and Mugwort Decoction

Alternate Names: *Chiung Kuei Jiao Ai Tang, Qiong Gui Jiao Ai Tang, Xiong Gui Jiao Ai Tang*, Cnidium, Tang-kuei, Gelatin, and Mugwort Leaf Decoction; Cnidium, Tangkuei, Gelatin and Artemisia Decoction

Original Source: *Jin Gui Yao Lue* (Essentials from the Golden Cabinet) by Zhang Zhong-Jing in the Eastern Han Dynasty

COMPOSITION

E Jiao (Colla Corii Asini)	6g [6-9g]
Ai Ye (Folium Artemisiae Argyi)	9g
Dang Gui (Radix Angelicae Sinensis)	9g
Di Huang (Radix Rehmanniae)	18g [12-15g]
Bai Shao (Radix Paeoniae Alba)	12g
Chuan Xiong (Rhizoma Chuanxiong)	6g
Gan Cao (Radix et Rhizoma Glycyrrhizae)	6g

DOSAGE / PREPARATION / ADMINISTRATION

The source text states to cook the ingredients, except *E Jiao* (Colla Corii Asini), with 5 cups [1,000 mL] of water and 3 cups [600 mL] of grain-based liquor until the liquid is reduced to 3 cups [600 mL]. Discard the herbal residue. Dissolve *E Jiao* (Colla Corii Asini) into the warm, strained decoction until it melts completely. Take 1 cup [200 mL] of the warm decoction, three times daily. The source text recommends taking the formula until the clinical signs are resolved. Today, it is prepared as a decoction by cooking the herbs in water using the doses suggested in brackets, with or without a grain-based liquor. *E Jiao* (Colla Corii Asini) is dissolved into the warm, strained decoction immediately before serving.

CHINESE THERAPEUTIC ACTIONS

1. Tonifies the blood and stops bleeding
2. Regulates estrus and calms the fetus

CLINICAL MANIFESTATIONS

Beng lou (flooding and spotting) caused by deficiency and damage to the *chong* (thoroughfare) and *ren* (conception) channels: irregular estrus, menorrhagia, and pale, thin, bloody vaginal discharge without clots. It is also effective for unstable pregnancy with uterine pain and/or bleeding, and continuous bleeding after premature delivery or abortion.

VETERINARY CLINICAL APPLICATIONS

Prevention of spontaneous abortion, excessive menstrual bleeding, excessive bleeding during gestation, excessive postpartum bleeding in primates.

EXPLANATION

Jiao Ai Tang (Ass-Hide Gelatin and Mugwort Decoction) treats *beng lou* (flooding and spotting) caused by deficiency and damage to the *chong* (thoroughfare) and *ren* (conception) channels. The *chong* channel is the sea of blood, and the *ren* channel dominates the uterus and fetus. If the *chong* and *ren* channels are damaged and become deficient, excessive and prolonged bleeding may occur. For pregnant animals, this condition is characterized by unstable gestation, restless fetus, uterine bleeding, and abdominal pain.

The treatment plan for this syndrome is to tonify the blood, stop bleeding, regulate menstruation, and stabilize the fetus. In this formula, *E Jiao* (Colla Corii Asini) nourishes the blood and stops bleeding. *Ai Ye* (Folium Artemisiae Argyi) warms the menses and stops bleeding. Combined, these two herbs regulate menstruation, treat *beng lou* (flooding and spotting), and stabilize the fetus. To tonify and move the blood and regulate menstruation, this formula uses *Dang Gui* (Radix Angelicae Sinensis), *Di Huang* (Radix Rehmanniae), *Bai Shao* (Radix Paeoniae Alba), and *Chuan Xiong* (Rhizoma Chuanxiong), the four herbs in the blood-tonifying formula *Si Wu Tang* (Four-Substance Decoction). *Gan Cao* (Radix et Rhizoma Glycyrrhizae) also tonifies qi and harmonizes all of the herbs in the formula. In addition, the combination of *Gan Cao* (Radix et Rhizoma Glycyrrhizae) and *E Jiao* (Colla Corii Asini) stops bleeding; and the combination of *Gan Cao* (Radix et Rhizoma Glycyrrhizae) and *Bai Shao* (Radix Paeoniae Alba) relieves pain. Lastly, the grain-based liquor increases the impact of the herbs and prevents the development of blood stasis.

Jiāo Ài Tāng (Ass-Hide Gelatin and Mugwort Decoction)

Jiao Ai Tang **(Ass-Hide Gelatin and Mugwort Decoction)**

Diagnosis	Clinical Signs	Treatment	Herbs
Beng lou (flooding and spotting)	Excessive and prolonged menstrual bleeding with thin blood without clots: deficiency of the *chong* (thoroughfare) and *ren* (conception) channels	• Tonifies the blood and stops bleeding • Regulates menstruation and calms the fetus	• *E Jiao* (Colla Corii Asini) nourishes the blood and stops bleeding. • *Ai Ye* (Folium Artemisiae Argyi) warms the menses and stops bleeding. • *Dang Gui* (Radix Angelicae Sinensis), *Di Huang* (Radix Rehmanniae), *Bai Shao* (Radix Paeoniae Alba), and *Chuan Xiong* (Rhizoma Chuanxiong) tonify the blood and regulate blood circulation. • *Gan Cao* (Radix et Rhizoma Glycyrrhizae) tonifies qi and harmonizes the herbs.

VETERINARY MODIFICATIONS

- With qi deficiency, add *Ren Shen* (Radix et Rhizoma Ginseng) and *Huang Qi* (Radix Astragali).
- With pain in the abdomen and lower back, add *Zhi Shi* (Fructus Aurantii Immaturus) and *Hou Po* (Cortex Magnoliae Officinalis).
- With excessive bleeding, add *Xian He Cao* (Herba Agrimoniae) and *Di Yu* (Radix Sanguisorbae).
- With profuse bleeding, add charred *Di Yu* (Radix Sanguisorbae) and charred *Ai Ye* (Folium Artemisiae Argyi).
- With abdominal pain due to blood stagnation, add *Yan Hu Suo* (Rhizoma Corydalis) and *San Qi* (Radix et Rhizoma Notoginseng).
- With unstable gestation, add *Bao Chan Wu You Fang* (Preserve Pregnancy and Care-Free Decoction).
- With constant and restless movement of the fetus due to deficiency, add *Du Zhong* (Cortex Eucommiae), *Xu Duan* (Radix Dipsaci), and *Sang Ji Sheng* (Herba Taxilli).

CAUTIONS / CONTRAINDICATIONS

Jiao Ai Tang is contraindicated in cases of hypermenorrhea, or *beng lou* (flooding and spotting) caused by heat.

HUMAN CLINICAL STUDIES AND RESEARCH

1. **Uterine bleeding**: Administration of *Jiao Ai Tang* effectively treated 25 patients with uterine bleeding due to functional disorders. The herbs were given in decoction once a day, with treatment duration varying from 4 to 8 packs of herbs.[1]
2. **Thrombocytopenic purpura**: Administration of modified *Jiao Ai Tang* was associated with 94% effectiveness in treating 17 patients with thrombocytopenic purpura. The herbal treatment contained this formula plus *Xuan Shen* (Radix Scrophulariae), *Mai Dong* (Radix Ophiopogonis), *Dan Shen* (Radix et Rhizoma Salviae Miltiorrhizae), and *Ren Shen* (Radix et Rhizoma Ginseng). Of 17 patients, the study reported significant improvement in 12 cases, moderate improvement in 4 cases, and no benefit in 1 case.[2]
3. **Duodenal ulcers and bleeding**: One study reported recovery in 49 of 50 patients with gastrointestinal bleeding caused by duodenal ulcers when treated with modified *Jiao Ai Tang* for 3-7 days. Recovery was confirmed by absence of blood in the stools and resolution of all clinical signs.[3]

SUGGESTED ACUPUNCTURE TREATMENT

1. Points: *Guanyuan* (CV 4), *Siman* (KI 14), *Pishu* (BL 20), *Housanli* (ST 36), *Geshu* (BL 17), *Shenshu* (BL 23), and *Jiaoxin* (KI 8).
2. Technique: tonification.

Guanyuan (CV 4) is an essential point for tonifying the body. *Siman* (KI 14) is an intersecting point of the Kidney and *chong* (thoroughfare) channels. They are combined to nourish and regulate the *chong* (thoroughfare) and *ren* (conception) channels. *Pishu* (BL 20), *Housanli* (ST 36), and *Geshu* (BL 17) nourish qi and regulate the blood. *Shenshu* (BL 23) and *Jiaoxin* (KI 8) consolidate Kidney qi to stop bleeding.

AUTHORS' COMMENTS

Jiao Ai Tang (Ass-Hide Gelatin and Mugwort Decoction) has application in veterinary medicine to treat unstable gestation with uterine pain and/or bleeding, and continuous bleeding after premature delivery or abortion; it helps to prevent miscarriages in domestic animals and primates.

References

1. *Zhong Hua Fu Chan Ke Za Zhi* (Chinese Journal of Obstetrics and Gynecology), 1959; 5:413.
2. *Hei Long Jiang Zhong Yi Yao* (Heilongjiang Journal of Chinese Medicine and Herbology), 1990; 6:15.
3. *Zhong Yi Fang Ji Xian Dai Yan Jiu* (Modern Study of Medical Formulas in Traditional Chinese Medicine), 1997; 1145.

Chapter 13 — Summary — Blood-Regulating Formulas

SECTION 1: BLOOD-INVIGORATING AND STASIS-REMOVING FORMULAS

Name	Similarities	Differences
Tao He Cheng Qi Tang (Peach Pit Decoction to Order the Qi)	Breaks up blood stasis and drains it downward	Treats blood stagnation in the lower *jiao*
Tong Qiao Huo Xue Tang (Unblock the Orifices and Invigorate the Blood Decoction)	Activate blood circulation, dispel blood stagnation	Opens the sensory orifices in the head and face
Xue Fu Zhu Yu Tang (Drive Out Stasis in the Mansion of Blood Decoction)		Treats blood stagnation in the chest (upper *jiao*)
Ge Xia Zhu Yu Tang (Drive Out Blood Stasis Below the Diaphragm Decoction)		Treats blood stagnation below the diaphragm (middle *jiao*)
Shao Fu Zhu Yu Tang (Drive Out Blood Stasis in the Lower Abdomen Decoction)		Treats blood stagnation in the lower abdomen (lower *jiao*)
Shen Tong Zhu Yu Tang (Drive Out Blood Stasis from a Painful Body Decoction)		Treats qi and blood stagnation throughout the body (extremities)
Fu Yuan Huo Xue Tang (Revive Health by Invigorating the Blood Decoction)	Activate blood circulation, dispel blood stasis, treat traumatic injuries	Traumatic injuries with pain and swelling in the chest and hypochondriac region
Zheng Gu Zi Jin Dan (Purple and Gold Pill for Righteous Bones)		Traumatic injuries of the soft tissues and bones
Bu Yang Huan Wu Tang (Tonify the Yang to Restore Five Decoction)	Activates blood circulation, opens the channels and collaterals	Tonifies qi, treats post-stroke sequelae
Shi Xiao San (Sudden Smile Powder)	Activate blood circulation, remove blood stasis, relieve chest and abdominal pain	Treats pain due to blood stagnation in the Liver channel
Huo Luo Xiao Ling Dan (Fantastically Effective Pill to Invigorate the Collaterals)		Treats swelling and pain due to blood stagnation from trauma
Dan Shen Yin (Salvia Decoction)		Treats pain in the epigastric and abdominal regions due to qi and blood stagnation
Wen Jing Tang (Warm the Channels Decoction)	Activate blood circulation, warm the channels/uterus, treat gynecological disorders	Warms the *chong* (thoroughfare) and *ren* (conception) channels, disperses cold, nourishes the blood
Ai Fu Nuan Gong Wan (Mugwort and Cyperus Pill for Warming the Womb)		Warms the uterus, nourishes the blood
Sheng Hua Tang (Generation and Transformation Decoction)		Warms the channels, stops pain
Gui Zhi Fu Ling Wan (Cinnamon Twig and Poria Pill)	Activate blood circulation, remove blood stasis, treat gynecological disorders	Gently activates blood circulation, gradually dissolves blood stagnation
Zhe Chong Yin (Break the Conflict Decoction)		Strongly activates blood circulation, dispels blood stasis, disperses stagnation
Bie Jia Jian Wan (Soft-Shelled Turtle Shell Pill)	Breaks up and eliminates stagnation, softens hardness and resolves masses	Activates qi and blood circulation, dispels dampness and phlegm

Chapter 13 — Summary

Tao He Cheng Qi Tang (Peach Pit Decoction to Order the Qi) clears heat and breaks up and dispels blood stasis. It is especially indicated for blood stagnation with heat in the lower *jiao* causing acute lower abdominal pain, irritability, thirst, fever at night, and, in severe cases, mania.

There are five formulas that have similar functions to activate blood circulation and dispel blood stagnation. The difference between each of the five formulas is that they treat blood stagnation in different parts of the body.

- ***Tong Qiao Huo Xue Tang*** (Unblock the Orifices and Invigorate the Blood Decoction) activates blood circulation and opens the sensory orifices. It treats blood stagnation in the head and face, with signs and symptoms such as dry eyes, head and face pain, impaired vision and poor hearing.
- ***Xue Fu Zhu Yu Tang*** (Drive Out Stasis in the Mansion of Blood Decoction) activates qi and blood circulation, removes blood stagnation, and relieves pain. It is used to treat qi and blood stagnation in the chest, with prolonged and fixed stabbing pain in the chest.
- ***Ge Xia Zhu Yu Tang*** (Drive Out Blood Stasis Below the Diaphragm Decoction) activates qi and blood circulation, dispels blood stagnation, and relieves pain. It is most effective for blood stagnation below the diaphragm that is characterized by symptoms such as fixed abdominal pain, and bloating and pain in the hypochondriac and abdominal regions.
- ***Shao Fu Zhu Yu Tang*** (Drive Out Blood Stasis in the Lower Abdomen Decoction) activates blood circulation and dispels blood stagnation. This formula is commonly used to treat blood stagnation in the lower abdomen, with signs and symptoms such as pain and bloating in the lower abdominal region and formation of masses in the lower abdominal region.
- ***Shen Tong Zhu Yu Tang*** (Drive Out Blood Stasis from a Painful Body Decoction) activates qi and blood circulation, dispels blood stagnation, and opens the channels and collaterals. It is excellent in treating *bi zheng* (painful obstruction syndrome) due to qi and blood stagnation blocking the channels and collaterals. Clinical manifestations include pain in the shoulder, elbow, extremities or in the whole body.

Fu Yuan Huo Xue Tang (Revive Health by Invigorating the Blood Decoction) and ***Zheng Gu Zi Jin Dan*** (Purple and Gold Pill for Righteous Bones) have excellent functions to treat traumatic injuries by activating blood circulation and dispelling blood stasis.

- *Fu Yuan Huo Xue Tang* treats severe, stabbing pain in the hypochondriac (ribcage, chest, sternum, and diaphragm) region due to trauma. This formula activates blood circulation, removes blood stasis, soothes Liver qi, and dredges the collaterals.
- *Zheng Gu Zi Jin Dan* treats many different types of soft tissue and bone injuries, with symptoms such as pain, swelling, inflammation, and bruising. The main actions of this formula are to activate blood circulation, dispel blood stasis, open the channels and collaterals, and reduce swelling and bruises.

Bu Yang Huan Wu Tang (Tonify the Yang to Restore Five Decoction) tonifies qi, activates blood circulation, and invigorates the functions of the channels and collaterals. It is designed for post-stroke sequelae characterized by qi deficiency and blood stagnation, with symptoms such as hemiplegia, deviation of the mouth and eyes, involuntary leakage of saliva, atrophy of the lower extremities, and frequent urination or urinary incontinence. In veterinary medicine, it has found application to treat degenerative myelopathy.

Shi Xiao San (Sudden Smile Powder), ***Huo Luo Xiao Ling Dan*** (Fantastically Effective Pill to Invigorate the Collaterals), and ***Dan Shen Yin*** (Salvia Decoction) are formulas with similar functions to activate blood circulation, remove blood stasis, and relieve chest and abdominal pain. However, their clinical applications are rather different.

- *Shi Xiao San* activates blood circulation, removes blood stasis, disperses nodules, and stops pain. It is used mainly for sharp abdominal pain due to blood stagnation; it is also effective for post-parturition bleeding due to retained placenta in the uterus.

Chapter 13 — Summary

- *Huo Luo Xiao Ling Dan* activates blood circulation, dispels blood stasis, and dredges the collaterals to relieve pain. This formula is effective for various types of pain and disorders due to qi and blood stagnation, such as chest and abdominal pain, pain of the extremities, and bruises and swelling due to trauma.
- *Dan Shen Yin* activates qi and blood circulation, removes blood stasis, and stops pain. It is used for heart (epigastric region) and stomach (upper abdominal area) pain due to qi and blood stagnation. The pain is fixed and is intensified by pressure.

Wen Jing Tang (Warm the Channels Decoction), ***Ai Fu Nuan Gong Wan*** (Mugwort and Cyperus Pill for Warming the Womb), and ***Sheng Hua Tang*** (Generation and Transformation Decoction) are three formulas specifically designed for the treatment of gynecological disorders and can be used to treat primates. All three have similar functions to activate blood circulation, remove blood stasis, and warm the channels/uterus.

- *Wen Jing Tang* treats blood stagnation due to deficiency cold in the *ren* (conception) and *chong* (thoroughfare) channels. This formula warms the channels, disperses cold, nourishes the blood, and removes blood stasis. Clinical manifestations include irregular menstruation, afternoon fever, irritability, dry mouth and lips, abdominal fullness, lower abdominal pain, and possible infertility.
- *Ai Fu Nuan Gong Wan* treats deficiency and cold of the uterus. It warms the uterus, nourishes the blood, and activates blood circulation. Clinical manifestations include leukorrhea, painful extremities, lethargy, lack of energy, low appetite, irregular menstruation, lower abdominal pain, and infertility.
- *Sheng Hua Tang* treats blood stagnation with interior cold and blood deficiency after delivery. It can activate blood circulation, remove blood stasis, warm the channels, and stop pain. Clinical manifestations include continuous bleeding due to retained placenta in the uterus, and cold sensations with pain in the lower abdomen.

Gui Zhi Fu Ling Wan (Cinnamon Twig and Poria Pill) and ***Zhe Chong Yin*** (Break the Conflict Decoction) exert similar actions to activate blood circulation and remove blood stasis.

- *Gui Zhi Fu Ling Wan* is used traditionally during pregnancy to treat blood stagnation in the uterus. Clinical manifestations of this condition include instability of the fetus, continuous dripping of purplish black blood, and abdominal pain that is aggravated by pressure. Due to the delicate condition of pregnancy, this formula is composed carefully of herbs that gently activate blood circulation and gradually dissolve blood stagnation.
- *Zhe Chong Yin* treats irregular menstruation, dysmenorrhea, and amenorrhea due to blood stagnation in the lower *jiao* with severe pain in the lower abdominal region. It is potent in activating blood circulation, dispelling blood stasis, dissolving stagnation, and dispersing obstruction.

Bie Jia Jian Wan (Soft-Shelled Turtle Shell Pill) functions strongly to activate qi and blood circulation, dispel dampness and phlegm, and resolve hardness and masses. It is used primarily to treat chronic malaria with an enlarged spleen. Today, this formula may be used for splenomegaly, hepatomegaly, hepatitis, and liver cirrhosis.

Chapter 13 — Summary

SECTION 2: STOP-BLEEDING FORMULAS

Name	Similarities	Differences
Shi Hui San (Ten Partially-Charred Substances Powder)	Cool the blood, stop bleeding	Stops bleeding from the upper parts of the body, such as hematemesis, hemoptysis, and gastrointestinal bleeding
Si Sheng Wan (Four-Fresh Pill)		Stops bleeding from the upper parts of the body, such as hematemesis and epistaxis
Huai Hua San (Sophora Japonica Flower Powder)		Stops bleeding from the lower parts of the body, such as hematochezia
Xiao Ji Yin Zi (Cirsium Decoction)		Stops bleeding from the lower parts of the body, such as hematuria
Jiao Ai Tang (Ass-Hide Gelatin and Mugwort Decoction)	Tonifies the blood, stops bleeding	Regulates menstruation and calms the fetus

Shi Hui San (Ten Partially-Charred Substances Powder) cools the blood and stops bleeding. It is used for hematemesis, hemoptysis, and other bleeding symptoms due to blood heat affecting the upper parts of the body. This is the most commonly used hemostatic formula for emergency cases of bleeding. Cease administration of this formula once the desired effect is achieved.

Si Sheng Wan (Four-Fresh Pill) cools the blood and stops bleeding. It is used for hematemesis and epistaxis with bright red blood, and a dry mouth and throat due to blood heat affecting the upper parts of the body. Administration of this formula should be stopped once the desired effect is achieved.

Huai Hua San (Sophora Japonica Flower Powder) stops rectal bleeding and clears wind, heat, and/or damp toxins in the Intestines. It is used for hematochezia and dysentery, with bleeding prior to, or after, defecation; rectal fissures and polyps; and bright or dark red blood in the stools.

Xiao Ji Yin Zi (Cirsium Decoction) cools the blood, stops bleeding, and promotes urination. It is used for *xue lin* (bloody dysuria) with heat causing hematuria, frequent urination with burning sensations and pain, a red tongue, and a rapid pulse.

Jiao Ai Tang (Ass-Hide Gelatin and Mugwort Decoction) tonifies the blood, stops bleeding, regulates menstruation, and stabilizes pregnancy. It is used to treat deficiency and damage to the *ren* (conception) and *chong* (thoroughfare) channels, with clinical manifestations such as menorrhagia, excessive menstrual bleeding, or excessive bleeding during pregnancy or post-parturition.

Chapter 14

— Wind-Expelling Formulas

治风剂

王焘 Wāng Táo

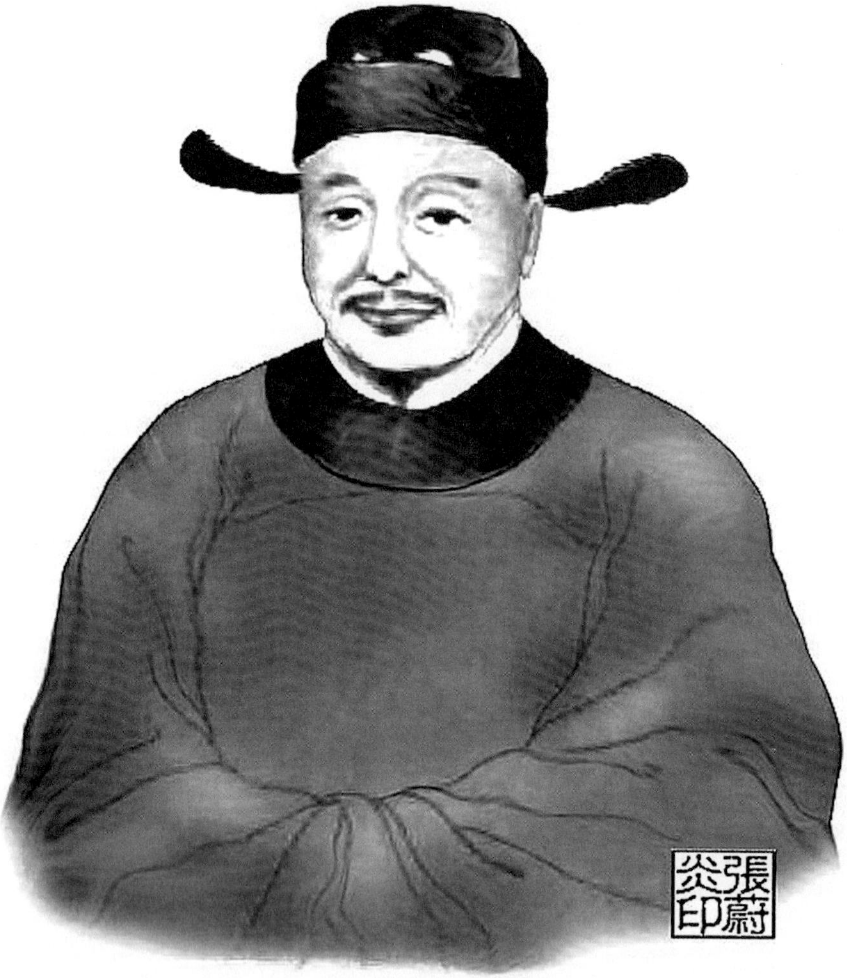

王焘 Wāng Táo, 670 – 755.

王燾 Wāng Táo

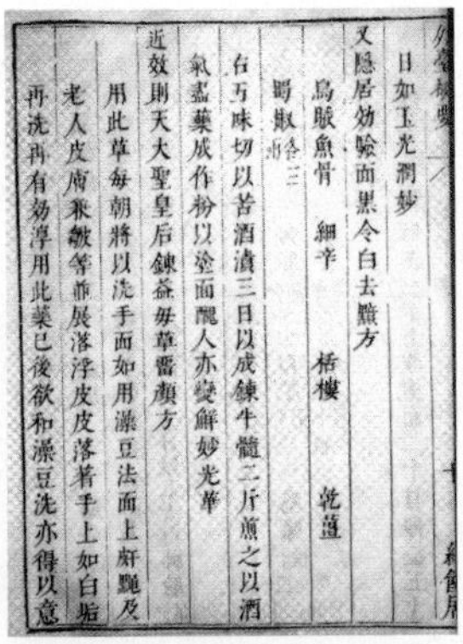

日如玉光潤妙
又隱居効驗面黑令白去䵟方
烏賊魚骨　細辛　栝樓　乾薑
蜀椒各三兩
右五味切以苦酒漬三日以成鍊牛髓二斤煎之以酒
氣盡藥成作粉以塗面醜人亦變鮮妙光華
近效則天大聖皇后鍊益母草留顏方
用此草每朝將以洗手面如用澡豆法面上䵟䵳及
老人皮膚兼皺等並展落浮皮皮落著手上如白垢
再洗再有効淳用此藥已後欲和澡豆洗亦得以意

外台秘要 *Wai Tai Mi Yao* (Arcane Essentials from the Imperial Library) in 752.

Wang Tao was born into the Imperial family. Wang was the grandson of 唐太宗 Tang Tai-Zong, one of the most famous emperors in the Tang dynasty. Although Wang and his mother were privileged members of the Imperial family, they were always ill. Because of frequent contact with the best doctors in the entire country, Wang gradually developed an interest in medicine. With easy access to the best physicians in the Imperial Palace and the most comprehensive library in the country, the young scholar was in an excellent position to gain an overview of the field, and a discerning eye for the patterns and details in published work. Wang spend more than 20 years integrating all of the existing medical texts, filling in any omissions, and correcting errors. Published in 752 CE, *Wai Tai Mi Yao* (Arcane Essentials from the Imperial Library) was the most comprehensive text compiled during that era. It documented over 1,000 medical problems and over 6,900 herbal formulas for use in gynecology, obstetrics, pediatrics, psychiatry, dermatology, opthalmology, dentistry, and osteopathy. Carefully written and referenced in great detail, this text gave ordinary people an unique opportunity to gain deeper insight and understanding of medicine. Wang was credited as a great scholar of Traditional Chinese Medicine. *Wai Tai Mi Yao* (Arcane Essentials from the Imperial Library) was regarded by many as 世宝 a World Treasure.

Representative formulas from *Wai Tai Mi Yao* (Arcane Essentials from the Imperial Library) include:

- *Cong Bai Qi Wei Yin* (Scallion Decoction with Seven Ingredients)
- *Shi Gao Tang* (Gypsum Decoction)
- *Huang Lian Jie Du Tang* (Coptis Decoction to Relieve Toxicity)
- *Zi Xue Dan* (Purple Snow Pill)
- *Shen Mi Tang* (Mysterious Decoction)
- *Xu Ming Tang* (Prolong Life Decoction)

Dynasties & Kingdoms	Year
Xia Dynasty 夏	2100-1600 BCE
Shang Dynasty 商	1600-1100 BCE
Zhou Dynasty 周	1100-221 BCE
Qin Dynasty 秦	221-207 BCE
Han Dynasty 漢	206 BCE-220
Three Kingdoms 三國	220-280
Western Jin Dynasty 西晉	265-316
Eastern Jin Dynasty 東晉	317-420
Northern and Southern Dynasties 北南朝	420-581
Sui Dynasty 隋	581-618
Tang Dynasty 唐	**618-907**
Five Dynasties 五代	907-960
Song Dynasty 宋	960-1279
Liao Dynasty 潦	916-1125
Jin Dynasty 金	1115-1234
Yuan Dynasty 元	1271-1368
Ming Dynasty 明	1368-1644
Qing Dynasty 清	1644-1911
Republic of China 中華民國	1912-Present Day
People's Republic of China 中華人民共和國	1949-Present Day

WIND-EXPELLING FORMULAS 14

Table of Contents

Chapter 14 — Overview

治风剂 — Wind-Expelling Formulas

Definition: Wind-expelling formulas treat both external and internal wind. They disperse and release external wind with acrid herbs, while they calm and extinguish internal wind with cold herbs.

Wind is the source of a wide variety of diseases with a large number of clinical manifestations, which students of Chinese medicine are trained to recognize. Wind readily combines with other pathogenic factors, which use wind as a vehicle for penetrating into the body. For this reason, wind is considered to be the master pathogen. Pathogenic wind possesses the same qualities as natural, or elemental, wind. Disorders of this nature have acute or sudden onset; and the clinical signs involved come and go quickly, change rapidly, and move from one part of the body to another part. An acute flare-up of chronic disease is often due to wind, which tends to injure both the blood and yin. Due to its violent and blustery nature, wind can cause a large amount of damage to the body in a relatively short period of time and can be quite serious or life threatening. Wind disorders are classified as exterior (externally contracted) or interior (internally generated). The etiology and pathophysiology of external and internal wind are quite different and must be clearly differentiated in order to choose the appropriate wind-expelling formulas. External wind is dispersed and released to the exterior using acrid herbs, while internal wind is calmed and extinguished through the use of cold herbs.

External wind rarely enters the body alone and is often accompanied by one or more pathogenic factors, such as cold, heat and dampness, giving rise to syndromes known as wind-cold, wind-heat, and wind-dampness. It should be noted that the term "wind" describes clinical signs and may be represented by many different disease agents that all produce similar effects in the animals. Wind is a yang pathogenic factor, and, as such, its movement is upward and outward. It attacks the upper and exterior (yang) parts of the body, such as the face and head, eyes, skin, muscles, joints, tendons, ligaments, bones, channels and collaterals. The main clinical signs of external wind syndromes are aversion to wind, nasal discharge, sneezing, sore throat, cough, neck stiffness and pain, numbness of the extremities, painful joints, itching and eczema of the skin, a thin, white tongue coating, and a superficial, floating pulse.

Internal wind disorders produce abnormal or involuntary movement and are caused by an imbalance or dysfunction of the Liver, which is often described as Liver wind. The Liver controls the smooth, harmonious movement of qi and blood in the body, and imbalance impairs this function and results in abnormal movement. In nature, wind can gently rustle the most delicate flower or bluster violently and uproot even the largest trees. In patients, this can be expressed in mild tremors or violent seizures. Disorders of internal wind manifest in clinical signs such as spasms, trembling of the extremities, rigidity of the neck, hemiplegia, sudden unconsciousness, facial asymmetry, paralysis, and seizures. Both excess and deficient conditions can contribute to internal wind; these conditions include extreme heat, ascendant Liver yang, Kidney and Liver yin deficiency, and blood deficiency.

The greatest application of wind-dispelling formulas in veterinary medicine is in the treatment of dermatological conditions, canine idiopathic vestibular syndrome, equine photosensitive head shaking, facial paralysis and seizure disorders. Facial paralysis, common in middle-aged to geriatric

Chapter 14 — Overview

dogs, is considered idiopathic by western medicine and has no specific treatment. Affected dogs typically have hemiplegia of the face, lack of sensation in the affected area, drooping or inability to move the lip and ear that results in drooling and dysphagia, and an eyelid unable to close or blink. Chinese medicine names this condition *zhong feng* (wind stroke), and it can be caused by either external or internal wind. Facial paralysis in dogs is thought to be due to a combination of internal wind and phlegm that obstructs the channels and collaterals of the face and results in paralysis and the associated clinical signs. Many dogs with this condition have concurrent Spleen qi deficiency and Kidney and Liver yin deficiency, leading to Liver yang rising. Without treatment, the paralysis is often permanent, and early clinical signs (drooling, dropping of food, and a drooping lip and eyelid) become chronic signs, such as facial musculature contraction and atrophy. The use of appropriate wind-dispelling formulas early in the disease (the first two weeks) can often lead to resolution of the paralysis and a return to normal function.

One of the cardinal signs of wind is itching. Wind disorders associated with itching can originate outside the body and are called external wind. Skin disease typically develops from the presence of more than one pathogenic factor in combination with wind, such as dampness, heat or dryness. It should be noted that the term "external wind" can include factors not directly related to climate, such as external parasites, inhalant and contact allergens, and drug and vaccine reactions. External wind invades the body when Lung and *wei* (defensive) *qi* are deficient and unable to protect the surface from invasion, when there is a pre-existing internal damp and heat accumulation, and when yin and blood are deficient. The pruritis seen in early cases of external wind is typically acute, seasonal, and excess in nature. Itching can also be generated internally from a deficiency of yin and blood, deficiency and stagnation of qi and blood, and from accumulation of pathogenic factors, such as dampness, phlegm, blood heat, and toxic heat. Imbalance or dysfunction of one or more of the *zang fu* organs can also lead to the development of these pathogenic factors. For example, chronic Liver qi stagnation, Liver fire, Liver yin and blood deficiencies, Liver and Gallbladder damp-heat, Spleen and Stomach damp-heat, and Kidney yin and *jing* (essence) deficiencies can all lead to itching. These cases are usually chronic and non-seasonal in nature and characterized by signs of both excess and deficiency, with deficiency being the root cause of the problem that leads to the development of excess signs.

Animals with deficiency or dysfunction of the internal organs and internally generated wind are highly susceptible to seasonal attack by external wind. Invasion of both internal and external wind results in cases of itching that are both acute and severe. There are six common Chinese veterinary medicine skin patterns corresponding to itching and canine atopy. These are: external wind, wind-heat, damp-heat, yin deficiency, blood deficiency, and blood stagnation. These six patterns can be further complicated by the presence of blood heat. Blood heat, often caused by external toxic heat pathogens like allergens, is often the primary factor in severe immune-mediated skin diseases and is a common component of mild cases. Multiple patterns that overlap make skin conditions a challenge to treat, as both excess and deficiency can be present in the same animal. The complexity of dermatological disease usually requires the use of multiple herbal formulas and extended treatment times, especially to resolve chronic and severe cases. The use of herbal medications alone or in combination with conventional medications is a highly effective method for treating itching in the veterinary patient, provided a correct diagnosis has been made and client compliance is good.

Proper treatment of wind disorders must begin with an accurate differential diagnosis to determine the main characteristics of the disorder: external or internal wind, deficiency or excess, and cold or hot. External wind must be treated with <u>acrid</u> and <u>dispersing</u> herbs that dispel external wind, and internal wind must be treated with <u>cold</u> herbs that extinguish internal wind. Furthermore, wind is often complicated by heat, cold, dampness, or phlegm, which must be addressed with the addition of appropriate herbs. External and internal wind may engender each other, or occur at the same

Chapter 14 — Overview

time, leading to more complications. All these potential complications must be considered to ensure successful treatment.

SUBCATEGORIES OF ACTION

Wind-expelling formulas are thus divided into external wind-releasing formulas and internal wind-extinguishing formulas.

1. External Wind-Releasing Formulas

These formulas are suitable for treating various illnesses caused by external wind attacking the body. The external wind-releasing formulas are suitable for treating the invasion of external wind past the skin layer into the muscles, tendons, ligaments, bones, joints, channels, and collaterals. Commonly seen clinical manifestations include skin rash, itching, facial paralysis and asymmetry, dysphasia, joint pain, numbness, and limited movement. Furthermore, tetanus is considered an external wind disorder, in which external wind enters the body via open wounds on the skin to cause clinical signs such as lockjaw, spasms and cramps, and, in severe cases, kyphosis.

Herbs frequently used to disperse wind from the exterior include *Qiang Huo* (Rhizoma et Radix Notopterygii), *Du Huo* (Radix Angelicae Pubescentis), *Fang Feng* (Radix Saposhnikoviae), *Chuan Xiong* (Rhizoma Chuanxiong), *Bai Zhi* (Radix Angelicae Dahuricae), *Jing Jie* (Herba Schizonepetae), and *Bai Fu Zi* (Rhizoma Typhonii). Exemplar formulas include *Chuan Xiong Cha Tiao San* (Ligusticum Chuanxiong Powder to be Taken with Green Tea), *Qian Zheng San* (Lead to Symmetry Powder), and *Da Qin Jiao Tang* (Major Gentiana Macrophylla Decoction).

Note: Two other chapters of this text discuss formulas that treat external wind. Chapter 1: Exterior-Releasing Formulas discusses the use of herbs that treat external wind invading only the superficial parts of the body (e.g., the skin) causing various exterior clinical signs, such as fever and aversion to cold. Chapter 17: Wind-Damp Dispelling Formulas discusses the use of herbs to address external wind-dampness attacking the muscles and joints, such as that found in *bi zheng* (painful obstruction syndrome).

2. Internal Wind-Extinguishing Formulas

These formulas are suitable for treating internal Liver wind rising associated with excess or deficiency conditions. Excess is characterized by extreme heat or hyperactive Liver yang causing the wind to rise upward. Deficiency is characterized by wind rising due to underlying yin and blood deficiencies.

Internal wind may rise upward as a result of extreme heat or hyperactive Liver yang. If the rising wind is caused by extreme heat, there may be persistent high fever, unconsciousness, and spasms and cramps of the four extremities. If the rising wind is caused by hyperactivity of Liver yang, there may be red eyes, irritability, restlessness, seizures, trembling and shaking, facial paralysis, and hemiplegia.

Rising of wind caused by extreme heat or hyperactive Liver yang is considered an excess syndrome; therefore, the proper treatment plan is to sedate the Liver and extinguish wind. Herbs and formulas that sedate the Liver and calm wind include *Gou Teng* (Ramulus Uncariae cum Uncis), *Shi Jue Ming* (Concha Haliotidis), *Tian Ma* (Rhizoma Gastrodiae), *Ju Hua* (Flos Chrysanthemi), *Mu Li* (Concha Ostreae), and *Ji Li* (Fructus Tribuli). Exemplar formulas include *Tian Ma Gou Teng Yin* (Gastrodia and Uncaria Decoction) and *Zhen Gan Xi Feng Tang* (Sedate the Liver and Extinguish Wind Decoction).

Internal wind may develop when there are underlying deficiencies. In cases of chronic *wen bing* (warm disease) damaging yin and/or blood, the rise of internal wind may lead to clinical signs such as muscle spasms and cramps with peristalsis-like involuntary movements of the extremities. The proper treatment plan in this case would be to nourish yin and blood and extinguish internal wind. Herbs that nourish yin and blood to subdue rising wind include *Di Huang* (Radix Rehmanniae), *Bai Shao* (Radix Paeoniae Alba), *E Jiao* (Colla Corii Asini), and *Ji Zi Huang* (Galli Vitellus). An exemplar formula is *Da Ding Feng Zhu* (Major Arrest Wind Pearl).

Chapter 14 — Overview

CAUTION / CONTRAINDICATION

- Proper diagnosis is crucial in the treatment of wind disorders. External wind must be released or dispersed outward, while internal Liver wind should be calmed and extinguished. Incorrect treatment of internal wind using external wind-releasing formulas that are acrid and dispersing in nature will worsen the condition by stimulating Liver yang and stirring Liver wind. Similarly, incorrect treatment of external wind internal wind-extinguishing formulas will complicate the disorder by deepening the injury.
- Herbs that disperse external wind are often acrid, warm and drying. Therefore, they should be used with caution in animals with underlying deficiency of yin and/or body fluids.
- External wind is often accompanied by other pathogenic factors, such as heat, cold, dampness, or phlegm, which should also be addressed. This is especially true in the treatment of seizure disorders where phlegm is a major component.
- External wind also may trigger the rise of internal Liver wind, leading to a complicated exterior and interior condition. In this case, both external and internal wind must be addressed at the same time.
- Internal wind may be complicated by excess (extreme heat or Liver yang hyperactivity) or deficiency (yin and/or blood deficiencies) and must be diagnosed and treated accordingly.

PHARMACOLOGICAL EFFECTS & CLINICAL APPLICATIONS

Wind is responsible for a wide variety of disorders. Accordingly, wind-expelling formulas are used to treat a broad spectrum of diseases and illnesses.

1. **External Wind-Releasing Formulas** generally treat conditions affecting the exterior parts of the body, such as the skin, muscles, tendons, ligaments, bones, joints, channels, and collaterals. Common clinical applications include:
   - **Skin disorders**: Pharmacologically, external wind-releasing formulas have mast cell stabilizing and antiallergic effects,[1,2] and are used to treat skin disorders such as itching,[3] urticaria,[4,5] eczema,[6] psoriasis,[7] and neurodermatitis.[8] *Xiao Feng San* (Eliminate Wind Powder) and *Dang Gui Yin Zi* (Tangkuei Decoction) are two representative external wind-releasing formulas that treat dermatological disorders.
   - **Facial paralysis**: *Qian Zheng San* (Lead to Symmetry Powder) and *Yu Zhen San* (True Jade Powder) are two external wind-releasing formulas frequently used to treat facial paralysis.[9,10,11,12]
   - **Pain**: Analgesic and anti-inflammatory effects are well documented among external wind-releasing formulas.[13,14] Clinically, these formulas are used to treat trigeminal pain,[15] and numbness and paralysis of the peripheral nerves.[16] An exemplar formula is *Qian Zheng San* (Lead to Symmetry Powder).

2. **Internal Wind-Extinguishing Formulas** usually treat cardiovascular disorders, such as hypertension, stroke, and post-stroke sequelae.
   - **Hypertension**: Internal wind-extinguishing formulas are well-documented for their antihypertensive effects to lower blood pressure.[17,18,19] Formulas that effectively treat hypertension include *Gou Teng San* (Uncaria Powder),[20] *Zhen Gan Xi Feng Tang* (Sedate the Liver and Extinguish Wind Decoction),[21] and *Tian Ma Gou Teng Yin* (Gastrodia and Uncaria Decoction).[22]
   - **Stroke and post-stroke sequelae**: Internal wind-extinguishing formulas have been shown to be effective in the prevention and treatment of stroke, and in the management of post-stroke sequelae. The mechanisms of action have been attributed in part to antiplatelet effects,[23] antihypertensive effects,[24] and the activation of nitric oxide synthase to improve cerebral circulation.[25] Formulas commonly used in the prevention and treatment of stroke include *Gou Teng San* (Uncaria Powder),[26] *Zhen Gan Xi Feng Tang* (Sedate the Liver and Extinguish Wind Decoction),[27] *Tian Ma Gou Teng Yin* (Gastrodia and Uncaria Decoction),[28] and *Di Huang Yin Zi* (Rehmannia Decoction).[29] Formulas frequently used to treat post-stroke sequelae include *Da Ding Feng Zhu* (Major Arrest Wind Pearl) and *Di Huang Yin Zi* (Rehmannia Decoction).[30,31]

Chapter 14 — Overview

- **Others**: Internal wind-extinguishing formulas may also treat other cardiovascular or circulatory disorders, including but not limited to dizziness,[32] tinnitus,[33] Alzheimer's disease,[34] vascular dementia,[35] and concussion.[36] Exemplar formulas include *Gou Teng San* (Uncaria Powder) and *Tian Ma Gou Teng Yin* (Gastrodia and Uncaria Decoction).

References

1. *Zhong Guo Yao Li Xue Bao* (Chinese Herbal Pharmacology Journal), 1990; 5:34.
2. Shichijo K, Saito H. Effect of Chinese herbal medicines and disodium cromoglycate on IgE-dependent histamine release from mouse cultured mast cells. Int J Immunopharmacol. 1997 Nov-Dec; 19(11-12):677-82.
3. *Zhong Yi Yao Xue Bao* (Report of Chinese Medicine and Herbology), 1986; 5:50.
4. *Ji Lin Zhong Yi Yao* (Jilin Chinese Medicine and Herbology), 1985; 1:29.
5. *Tie Dao Yi Xue* (Tiedao Medicine), 1988; 4:230.
6. *Xin Yi Yao Xue Za Zhi* (New Journal of Medicine and Herbology), 1976; 8:15.
7. *Nei Meng Gu Zhong Yi Za Zi* (Inner Mongolia Journal of Traditional Chinese Medicine), 1992; 1:14.
8. *Zhong Guo Zhong Xi Yi Jie He Za Zhi* (Chinese Journal of Integrative Chinese and Western Medicine), 1992; 181.
9. *Nei Meng Gu Zhong Yi Yao* (Traditional Chinese Medicine and Medicinals of Inner Mongolia), 1990; 9(4):18.
10. *He Bei Zhong Yi* (Hebei Chinese Medicine), 1985; 4:30.
11. *Shi Zhen Guo Yao Yan Jiu* (Research of Shizhen Herbs), 1996; 7(1):13.
12. *Shan Xi Zhong Yi* (Shanxi Chinese Medicine), 1991; 12(10):465.
13. *Zhong Yi Fang Ji Xian Dai Yan Jiu* (Modern Study of Medical Formulas in Traditional Chinese Medicine), 1997; 1206.
14. *Zhong Yi Fang Ji Xian Dai Yan Jiu* (Modern Study of Medical Formulas in Traditional Chinese Medicine), 1997; 1206.
15. *Shan Dong Yi Yao* (Shandong Medicine and Herbology), 1994; 12:55.
16. *Zhe Jiang Zhong Yi Za Zhi* (Zhejiang Journal of Chinese Medicine), 1989; 6:255.
17. *Guo Wai Yi Xue* (Foreign Medicine), 1988; 8:53.
18. *Xin Zhong Yi* (New Chinese Medicine), 1980; 12:45.
19. *Zhong Yi Yao Yan Jiu Can Kao* (Research and Discussion of Chinese Medicine and Herbology), 1979; 9:25.
20. *Guo Wai Yi Xue* (Foreign Medicine), 1979; 2:35.
21. *Shi Yong Zhong Yi Nei Ke Za Zhi* (Journal of Practical Chinese Internal Medicine), 1990; 1:26.
22. *Shi Yong Zhong Yi Nei Ke Za Zhi* (Journal of Practical Chinese Internal Medicine), 1990; 1:26.
23. *Guo Wai Yi Xue* (Foreign Medicine), 1992; 5:48.
24. *Guo Wai Yi Xue* (Foreign Medicine), 1988; 8:53.
25. Sugimoto A, Goto K, Ishige A, Komatsu Y, Miyamoto KI. Effect of Choto-san, a Kampo medicine, on the cerebral blood flow autoregulation in spontaneously hypertensive rats. Jpn J Pharmacol. 2000 Jun; 83(2):135-42.
26. Goto H, Yang Q, Kita T, Hikiami H, Shimada Y, Terasawa K. Effects of Choto-san on microcirculation, serum nitric oxide and lipid peroxides in patients with asymptomatic cerebral infarction. Am J Chin Med. 2001; 29(1):83-9.
27. *Zhe Jiang Zhong Yi Xue Yuan Xue Bao* (Journal of Zhejiang University of Chinese Medicine), 1988; 5:18.
28. *Liao Ning Zhong Yi Za Zhi* (Liaoning Journal of Chinese Medicine), 1984; 9:26.
29. *Zhe Jiang Zhong Yi Xue Yuan Xue Bao* (Journal of Zhejiang University of Chinese Medicine), 1995; 4:8.
30. *Zhong Yi Han Shou Tong Xun* (Reports of Chinese Medicine), 1993; 5:43.
31. *Hei Long Jiang Zhong Yi Yao* (Heilongjiang Chinese Medicine and Herbology), 1995; 2:14.
32. *Shan Xi Zhong Yi Xue Yuan Xue Bao* (Journal of Shanxi University School of Chinese Medicine), 1996; 19(4):28.
33. *Guo Wai Yi Xue* (Foreign Medicine), 1982; 1:51.
34. *He Han Yi Yao Xue Hui Zhi* (Hehan Journal of Medicine and Herbology), 1989; 3:454.
35. Itoh T, Shimada Y, Terasawa K. Efficacy of Choto-san on vascular dementia and the protective effect of the hooks and stems of Uncaria sinensis on glutamate-induced neuronal death. Mech Ageing Dev. 1999 Nov; 111(2-3):155-73.
36. *Nei Meng Gu Zhong Yi Yao* (Traditional Chinese Medicine and Medicinals of Inner Mongolia), 1990; 1:2.

Section 1

疏散外风剂
— External Wind-Releasing Formulas

Xiāo Fēng Sǎn (Eliminate Wind Powder)
消風散
消风散

Pinyin Name: *Xiao Feng San*
Literal Name: Eliminate Wind Powder
Alternate Names: *Hsiao Feng San*, Wind-Dispelling Formula, Wind-Dispelling Powder, Tangkuei and Arctium Formula
Original Source: *Wai Ke Zheng Zong* (True Lineage of External Medicine) by Chen Shi-Gong in 1617

COMPOSITION

Jing Jie (Herba Schizonepetae)	3g [6g]
Fang Feng (Radix Saposhnikoviae)	3g [6g]
Chan Tui (Periostracum Cicadae)	3g [6g]
Niu Bang Zi (Fructus Arctii)	3g [6g]
Cang Zhu (Rhizoma Atractylodis)	3g [6g]
Ku Shen (Radix Sophorae Flavescentis)	3g [6g]
Mu Tong (Caulis Akebiae)	1.5g [3g]
Shi Gao (Gypsum Fibrosum)	3g [6g]
Zhi Mu (Rhizoma Anemarrhenae)	3g [6g]
Di Huang (Radix Rehmanniae)	3g [6g]
Dang Gui (Radix Angelicae Sinensis)	3g [6g]
Hei Zhi Ma (Semen Sesami Nigrum)	3g [6g]
Gan Cao (Radix et Rhizoma Glycyrrhizae)	1.5g [3g]

DOSAGE / PREPARATION / ADMINISTRATION

The source text recommends cooking the ingredients with 2 bowls of water until the liquid is reduced to 80% (1.6 bowls). Take the strained decoction while warm. Today, the decoction can be prepared using the doses given in brackets above.

CHINESE THERAPEUTIC ACTIONS

1. Expels wind and nourishes the blood
2. Clears heat and dispels dampness

CLINICAL MANIFESTATIONS

Rashes: eczema and skin rashes with red discoloration affecting a large part of the body, severe itching and leakage of fluids upon scratching, a dark pink to red tongue, and a superficial, rapid and forceful pulse.

VETERINARY CLINICAL APPLICATIONS

Dermatitis, atopic dermatitis, urticaria and folliculitis (furunculosis).

EXPLANATION

Xiao Feng San (Eliminate Wind Powder) treats wind-dampness and wind-heat attacking the skin and muscle layers of the body, giving rise to skin rashes, dermatitis, severe itching, and leakage of fluids. The treatment approach for this syndrome is to dispel wind and dampness, clear heat, and cool the blood.

Jing Jie (Herba Schizonepetae), *Fang Feng* (Radix Saposhnikoviae), *Chan Tui* (Periostracum Cicadae), and *Niu Bang Zi* (Fructus Arctii) are the chief herbs that dispel wind from the exterior. *Cang Zhu* (Rhizoma Atractylodis) strengthens the Spleen and dries dampness. *Ku Shen* (Radix Sophorae

Xiāo Fēng Săn (Eliminate Wind Powder)

Xiao Feng San (Eliminate Wind Powder)

Diagnosis	Clinical Signs	Treatment	Herbs
Rashes	• Skin rashes or dermatitis with red discoloration, and severe itching and discharge of fluids: wind-dampness and wind-heat attacking the skin and muscle layers of the body • Dark pink to red tongue, and a superficial, rapid and forceful pulse: wind-damp or wind-heat condition	• Expels wind and nourishes the blood • Clears heat and dispels dampness	• *Jing Jie* (Herba Schizonepetae), *Fang Feng* (Radix Saposhnikoviae), *Chan Tui* (Periostracum Cicadae), and *Niu Bang Zi* (Fructus Arctii) dispel wind from the exterior. • *Cang Zhu* (Rhizoma Atractylodis) strengthens the Spleen and dries dampness. • *Ku Shen* (Radix Sophorae Flavescentis) clears heat and dries dampness. • *Mu Tong* (Caulis Akebiae) eliminates damp-heat through diuresis. • *Shi Gao* (Gypsum Fibrosum) and *Zhi Mu* (Rhizoma Anemarrhenae) clear heat and sedate fire. • *Di Huang* (Radix Rehmanniae), *Dang Gui* (Radix Angelicae Sinensis), and *Hei Zhi Ma* (Semen Sesami Nigrum) tonify the blood, nourish yin, and moisten dryness. • *Gan Cao* (Radix et Rhizoma Glycyrrhizae) clears heat, eliminates toxins, and harmonizes the herbs.

Flavescentis) clears heat and dries dampness. *Mu Tong* (Caulis Akebiae) eliminates damp-heat through diuresis. *Shi Gao* (Gypsum Fibrosum) and *Zhi Mu* (Rhizoma Anemarrhenae) clear heat and sedate fire. Since wind-dampness and wind-heat may injure yin and blood, *Di Huang* (Radix Rehmanniae), *Dang Gui* (Radix Angelicae Sinensis), and *Hei Zhi Ma* (Semen Sesami Nigrum) are added to tonify the blood, nourish yin, and moisten dryness. *Gan Cao* (Radix et Rhizoma Glycyrrhizae) clears heat, eliminates toxins, and harmonizes the formula.

VETERINARY MODIFICATIONS

- With more wind-heat, add *Jin Yin Hua* (Flos Lonicerae Japonicae) and *Lian Qiao* (Fructus Forsythiae).
- With more damp-heat, add *Di Fu Zi* (Fructus Kochiae), *Che Qian Zi* (Semen Plantaginis) and *Tu Fu Ling* (Rhizoma Smilacis Glabrae).
- With heat in the *xue* (blood) level, add *Chi Shao* (Radix Paeoniae Rubra), *Mu Dan Pi* (Cortex Moutan) and *Zi Cao* (Radix Arnebiae).
- With more infection add, *Lian Qiao* (Fructus Forsythiae), *Zhi Zi* (Fructus Gardeniae) and *Ban Lan Gen* (Radix Isatidis).
- For moist, oozing dermatitis with fluids in the lesions, add *Yi Yi Ren* (Semen Coicis).
- With significant dampness and yeast, double the amount of *Ku Shen* (Radix Sophorae Flavescentis).
- With more itching add, *Bai Xian Pi* (Cortex Dictamni), *Chan Tui* (Periostracum Cicadae), *Jiang Can* (Bombyx Batryticatus) and *Zi Cao* (Radix Arnebiae).

CAUTIONS / CONTRAINDICATIONS

- While taking *Xiao Feng San*, the following are contraindicated in the diet: spicy or greasy foods and seafood.
- Many herbs in this formula are acrid (exterior-releasing herbs) and drying (damp-dispelling herbs) and may damage yin and blood. Therefore, this formula should be used with caution in patients with yin and blood deficiencies.[1]

PHARMACOLOGICAL EFFECTS

1. **Antiallergic and immunosuppressive**: Administration of *Xiao Feng San* was associated with marked action to treat allergy and suppress the immune systems of mice.[2]
2. **Mast cell stabilizer**: Administration of *Xiao Feng San* and *Ma Huang Xing Ren Gan Cao Shi Gao Tang* (Ephedra, Apricot Kernel, Licorice, and Gypsum Decoction) at 4-40 mcg/mL was found to inhibit IgE-dependent histamine released from mouse-cultured mast cells.[3]

HUMAN CLINICAL STUDIES AND RESEARCH

1. **Urticaria**: One study reported 97.6% effectiveness using modified *Xiao Feng San* to treat 124 patients with urticaria. Modifications to the formula included the addition of *Jin Yin Hua* (Flos Lonicerae Japonicae), *Wu Gong* (Scolopendra), *Zhi Zi* (Fructus Gardeniae), and *Huang Lian* (Rhizoma Coptidis) for wind-heat; *Ma Huang* (Herba Ephedrae) and *Gui Zhi* (Ramulus Cinnamomi) for wind-cold; and *He Shou Wu* (Radix Polygoni Multiflori), *Wu Wei Zi* (Fructus Schisandrae Chinensis), and *Wu Mei* (Fructus Mume) for yin deficiency. The herbs were given one time daily in decoction. Of 124 patients, the

WIND-EXPELLING FORMULAS 14

Xiāo Fēng Sǎn (Eliminate Wind Powder)

study reported complete recovery in 85 cases, significant improvement in 36 cases, and no effect in 3 cases.[4]

2. **Eczema**: Use of *Xiao Feng San* in 44 patients with eczema was associated with complete recovery in 38 cases and near-complete recovery in 6 cases. The herbs were given on a daily basis, for an average of 20 days (ranging between 5 and 23 days). Those with severe eczema also received topical application of herbs, made by grinding fresh *Ma Chi Xian* (Herba Portulacae) into an herbal paste. In addition to herbal treatment, all patients were instructed to maintain a bland diet and avoid spicy and pungent foods.[5]
3. **Psoriasis**: One study reported satisfactory results using modified *Xiao Feng San* to treat psoriasis. The herbal treatment contained *Jin Yin Hua* (Flos Lonicerae Japonicae) 15g, *Lian Qiao* (Fructus Forsythiae) 15g, *Fang Feng* (Radix Saposhnikoviae) 15g, *Dang Gui* (Radix Angelicae Sinensis) 8g, *Qing Dai* (Indigo Naturalis) 12g, *Jing Jie* (Herba Schizonepetae) 10g, *Di Huang* (Radix Rehmanniae) 12g, *Niu Bang Zi* (Fructus Arctii) 10g, *Di Fu Zi* (Fructus Kochiae) 10g, *Bai Xian Pi* (Cortex Dictamni) 12g, *Cang Zhu* (Rhizoma Atractylodis) 8g, *Chan Tui* (Periostracum Cicadae) 10g, *Zi Cao* (Radix Arnebiae) 10g, *Shi Gao* (Gypsum Fibrosum) 12g, and *Gan Cao* (Radix et Rhizoma Glycyrrhizae) 3g. The herbs were given in decoction daily.[6]

HERB-DRUG INTERACTION

Ampicillin-induced rash: Ampicillin-induced allergic rash in 68 patients was treated with herbs with 96% effectiveness, as reported in one study. The herbal treatment contained *Dang Gui* (Radix Angelicae Sinensis) 9g, *Di Huang* (Radix Rehmanniae) 9g, *Hei Zhi Ma* (Semen Sesami Nigrum) 9g, *Jing Jie* (Herba Schizonepetae) 9g, *Fang Feng* (Radix Saposhnikoviae) 9g, *Niu Bang Zi* (Fructus Arctii) 9g, *Chan Tui* (Periostracum Cicadae) 9g, *Cang Zhu* (Rhizoma Atractylodis) 9g, *Ku Shen* (Radix Sophorae Flavescentis) 9g, *Duan Shi Gao* (Gypsum Fibrosum Praeparatum) 9g, *Zhi Mu* (Rhizoma Anemarrhenae) 9g, *Gan Cao* (Radix et Rhizoma Glycyrrhizae) 4g, and *Mu Tong* (Caulis Akebiae) 4g as the base formula. Modifications were made when necessary, with the addition of *Lian Qiao* (Fructus Forsythiae) 6g for wind-heat; *Chi Shao* (Radix Paeoniae Rubra) 9g for heat in the blood; *Da Huang* (Radix et Rhizoma Rhei) 6g for heat and toxins; and the addition of *Che Qian Zi* (Semen Plantaginis) 6g and elimination of *Cang Zhu* (Rhizoma Atractylodis) for damp-heat. The study reported complete recovery in 65 of 68 patients within 1-4 packs of herbs given via herbal decoction.[7]

SUGGESTED ACUPUNCTURE TREATMENT

1. Points: *Fengchi* (GB 20), *Tianzhu* (BL 10), *Fengmen* (BL 12), *Jianyu* (LI 15), *Yangxi* (LI 5), *Dazhui* (GV 14), *Quchi* (LI 11), *Yinlingquan* (SP 9), *Sanyinjiao* (SP 6), and *Shenmen* (HT 7).
2. Technique: sedation and tonification.

This acupuncture treatment is designed to dispel wind, nourish the blood, clear heat, and eliminate dampness. *Fengchi* (GB 20), *Tianzhu* (BL 10), and *Fengmen* (BL 12) clear wind to stop the itch. *Jianyu* (LI 15), *Yangxi* (LI 5), and *Dazhui* (GV 14) are combined to dispel wind and clear heat. *Quchi* (LI 11) clears heat from the *yangming* level. *Yinlingquan* (SP 9) strengthens the Spleen and dispels dampness. *Sanyinjiao* (SP 6) nourishes the blood and promotes blood circulation. *Shenmen* (HT 7) relieves itching.

AUTHORS' COMMENTS

From a traditional Chinese medical perspective, *Xiao Feng San* treats dermatological disorders caused by wind-dampness and wind-heat attacking the skin. In terms of anatomy and physiology, such dermatological disorders are similar in location and manifestation to allergic or hypersensitivity reactions. Clinical applications include skin rashes and hives, itching and dermatitis secondary to environmental allergens, fleas, drugs, chemicals, or food. *Xiao Feng San* can also be combined with other formulas for additional clinical applications:

- In cases of wind-heat that has progressed to pyoderma, *Xiao Feng San* can be combined with *Yin Qiao San* (Honeysuckle and Forsythia Powder).
- For pyoderma caused by internally generated heat in the Liver, it can be combined with *Long Dan Xie Gan Tang* (Gentiana Decoction to Drain the Liver).
- It can be combined with *Dang Gui Yin Zi* (Tangkuei Decoction) to treat chronic dermatitis cases in which the underlying chronic yin and blood deficiencies have predisposed the animal to external wind invasion, especially during seasonal allergy times in the spring and fall.

In addition to using *Xiao Feng San* internally to relieve itching, *Ku Shen* (Radix Sophorae Flavescentis) and *She Chuang Zi* (Fructus Cnidii) can be used as an external wash to enhance the overall effects. Furthermore, administration of a topical application of *Ma Chi Xian* (Herba Portulacae) as an herbal paste also increases the overall effectiveness of *Xiao Feng San*.

Xiāo Fēng Sǎn (Eliminate Wind Powder)

References

1. *Zhong Yao Ming Fang Yao Li Yu Ying Yong* (Pharmacology and Applications of Famous Herbal Formulas), 1989; 529-531.
2. *Zhong Guo Yao Li Xue Bao* (Chinese Herbal Pharmacology Journal), 1990; 5:34.
3. Shichijo K, Saito H. Effect of Chinese herbal medicines and disodium cromoglycate on IgE-dependent histamine release from mouse cultured mast cells. Int J Immunopharmacol. 1997 Nov-Dec; 19(11-12):677-82.
4. *Ji Lin Zhong Yi Yao* (Jilin Chinese Medicine and Herbology), 1985; 1:29.
5. *Xin Yi Yao Xue Za Zhi* (New Journal of Medicine and Herbology), 1976; 8:15.
6. *Nei Meng Gu Zhong Yi Za Zi* (Inner Mongolia Journal of Traditional Chinese Medicine), 1992; 1:14.
7. *Si Chuan Zhong Yi* (Sichuan Chinese Medicine), 1993; 11(4):34.

Dāng Guī Yǐn Zǐ (Tangkuei Decoction)

當歸飲子

当归饮子

Pinyin Name: *Dang Gui Yin Zi*

Literal Name: Tangkuei Decoction

Alternate Names: *Tang Kuei Yin Tzu*, Tang-kuei Drink, Tangkuei and Tribulus Combination

Original Source: *Chong Ding Yan Shi Ji Sheng Fang* (Revised Formulas to Aid the Living from the Yan Family)

COMPOSITION

Di Huang (Radix Rehmanniae)	30g [9g]
Dang Gui (Radix Angelicae Sinensis)	30g [9g]
Bai Shao (Radix Paeoniae Alba)	30g [9g]
Chuan Xiong (Rhizoma Chuanxiong)	30g [9g]
Ji Li (Fructus Tribuli), *chao* (dry-fried)	30g [9g]
Jing Jie (Herba Schizonepetae)	30g [9g]
Fang Feng (Radix Saposhnikoviae)	30g [9g]
Huang Qi (Radix Astragali)	15g [6g]
He Shou Wu (Radix Polygoni Multiflori)	15g [6g]
Gan Cao (Radix et Rhizoma Glycyrrhizae)	15g [3g]

DOSAGE / PREPARATION / ADMINISTRATION

The source text recommends grinding the ingredients into a coarse powder. Cook 12g of the powder with 5 slices of *Sheng Jiang* (Rhizoma Zingiberis Recens) in 1.5 large bowls of water until the liquid is reduced to 80% (1.2 large bowls). Take the warm, strained decoction any time during the day. Today, this formula may be prepared as a decoction using the doses suggested in brackets above.

CHINESE THERAPEUTIC ACTIONS

1. Tonifies the blood and moistens dryness
2. Dispels wind and relieves itching

CLINICAL MANIFESTATIONS

Skin disorders caused by blood deficiency and external wind: hives, anemia, alopecia, dull, dry hair coat, hair that is easily depilated, dry skin, dandruff, dryness, itch-

Dāng Guī Yǐn Zǐ (Tangkuei Decoction)

ing and dandruff at the mane and tail, cracked paw pads and claws, dry and cracked hooves, hyperpigmentation and lichenification, itching (especially at night), generalized chronic itching, a pale, dry tongue, and a rapid, thin, deep, weak pulse.

VETERINARY CLINICAL APPLICATIONS

Pruritis, atopic dermatitis, urticaria, alopecia, persistent lick-granulomas, dandruff and poor hair coat, dry skin with chronic itching, cracked and bleeding nails and paw pads, and poor hoof quality.

EXPLANATION

Dang Gui Yin Zi (Tangkuei Decoction) treats skin disorders caused by blood deficiency and external wind. Blood deficiency can lead to malnourishment of the skin and hair coat, characterized by dryness, dandruff, lack of moisture, and lack of skin tone. Animals with chronic blood deficiency accompanied by external wind and heat usually show more serious clinical signs of dermatological disorders, such as chronic atopic dermatitis with hyperpigmentation and lichenification, self-mutilation from itching and scratching with or without abscesses, and ulceration. Horses will be particularly prone to severe dandruff and itching of the mane and tail.

Dang Gui Yin Zi follows the principles of *Si Wu Tang* (Four-Substance Decoction) to tonify the blood, with the addition of herbs that treat wind and heat. *Di Huang* (Radix Rehmanniae) nourishes the blood and tonifies the Kidney. *Dang Gui* (Radix Angelicae Sinensis) both tonifies and activates blood circulation. *Bai Shao* (Radix Paeoniae Alba) nourishes the blood and consolidates yin. *Chuan Xiong* (Rhizoma Chuanxiong) activates and regulates blood circulation. *Ji Li* (Fructus Tribuli) dispels both internal and external wind to relieve itching, while *Jing Jie* (Herba Schizonepetae) and *Fang Feng* (Radix Saposhnikoviae) dispel External wind and treat various skin disorders. *Huang Qi* (Radix Astragali) tonifies *wei* (defensive) *qi* and strengthens the exterior. *He Shou Wu* (Radix Polygoni Multiflori) nourishes *jing* (essence) and blood. Lastly, *Gan Cao* (Radix et Rhizoma Glycyrrhizae) harmonizes the formula.

VETERINARY MODIFICATIONS

- For alopecia due to severe yin and blood deficiencies, add *Gou Qi Zi* (Fructus Lycii), *Huo Ma Ren* (Fructus Cannabis), *Ji Xue Teng* (Caulis Spatholobi) and *E Jiao* (Colla Corii Asini).
- For qi deficiency, add *Dang Shen* (Radix Codonopsis).
- With constipation, combine with *Ma Zi Ren Wan* (Hemp Seed Pill).
- With dry, scaly skin, lichenification and hyperpigmentation due to blood stasis, add *Dan Shen* (Radix et Rhizoma Salviae Miltiorrhizae), *Hong Hua* (Flos Carthami) and *E Jiao* (Colla Corii Asini).

***Dang Gui Yin Zi* (Tangkuei Decoction)**

Diagnosis	Clinical Signs	Treatment	Herbs
Skin disorders caused by blood deficiency and wind	• Dry skin and hair coat, lack of moisture, and a lack of skin tone: blood unable to nourish the skin • Pruritis, dermatitis, and urticaria, with or without abscesses and ulceration: exterior wind and heat affecting the skin	• Tonifies the blood and moistens dryness • Dispels wind and relieves itching	• *Di Huang* (Radix Rehmanniae) nourishes the blood and tonifies the Kidney. • *Dang Gui* (Radix Angelicae Sinensis) tonifies the blood and regulates blood circulation. • *Bai Shao* (Radix Paeoniae Alba) nourishes the blood and consolidates yin. • *Chuan Xiong* (Rhizoma Chuanxiong) activates and regulates blood circulation. • *Ji Li* (Fructus Tribuli) dispels both internal and external wind to relieve itching. • *Jing Jie* (Herba Schizonepetae) and *Fang Feng* (Radix Saposhnikoviae) dispel exterior wind. • *Huang Qi* (Radix Astragali) tonifies *wei* (defensive) *qi* and strengthens the exterior. • *He Shou Wu* (Radix Polygoni Multiflori) nourishes *jing* (essence) and blood. • *Gan Cao* (Radix et Rhizoma Glycyrrhizae) harmonizes the herbs.

Dāng Guī Yǐn Zǐ (Tangkuei Decoction)

- With severe itchy skin, combine with *Chan Tui* (Periostracum Cicadae), *Gou Teng* (Ramulus Uncariae cum Uncis), *Shou Wu Teng* (Caulis Polygoni Multiflori), and *He Huan Pi* (Cortex Albiziae).
- With dryness and atrophy of the skin due to lack of secretion from sebaceous and sweat glands, add *Shan Zhu Yu* (Fructus Corni) and *Huo Ma Ren* (Fructus Cannabis).
- To nourish the skin and improve poor hair coat quality, combine with *Liu Wei Di Huang Wan* (Six-Ingredient Pill with Rehmannia) or *Ba Wei Di Huang Wan* (Eight-Ingredient Pill with Rehmannia).

CAUTIONS / CONTRAINDICATIONS

While taking *Dang Gui Yin Zi*, patients should not be given foods that are greasy and fatty, as well as foods that are spicy, pungent, or stimulating in nature.

HUMAN CLINICAL STUDIES AND RESEARCH

1. **Itching**: Administration of a modified *Dang Gui Yin Zi* formula was 96.15% effective in treating 78 geriatric patients with constant itching of the skin. The formula contained 12-15g of *Dang Gui* (Radix Angelicae Sinensis); 10-12 g each of *Shu Di Huang* (Radix Rehmanniae Praeparata), *Huang Qi* (Radix Astragali), *Ji Li* (Fructus Tribuli), *Chuan Xiong* (Rhizoma Chuanxiong), *Jing Jie* (Herba Schizonepetae), and *Bai Shao* (Radix Paeoniae Alba); 30g of *He Shou Wu* (Radix Polygoni Multiflori); and 6g each of *Fang Feng* (Radix Saposhnikoviae) and *Gan Cao* (Radix et Rhizoma Glycyrrhizae). The treatment protocol was to cook the herbs in water, and drink the decoction in two to three equally-divided doses daily. The average duration of treatment was 26.5 packs of herbs. Out of 78 patients, the study reported complete recovery in 36 cases and improvement in 39 cases. Complete recovery was defined as relief of symptoms, with no recurrence 1-2 months after the termination of herbal treatment.[1]
2. **Urticaria**: Administration of *Dang Gui Yin Zi* had marked effectiveness in treating 56 patients with chronic urticaria that did not respond to drug treatment. The herbal treatment used *Dang Gui Yin Zi* as the base, and added *Dang Shen* (Radix Codonopsis) and *Bai Zhu* (Rhizoma Atractylodis Macrocephalae) for qi deficiency; *Mu Dan Pi* (Cortex Moutan) and *Xuan Shen* (Radix Scrophulariae) for yin deficiency; *Huang Qin* (Radix Scutellariae) and *Tu Fu Ling* (Rhizoma Smilacis Glabrae) for damp-heat; *Wu Zhu Yu* (Fructus Evodiae) and *Rou Gui* (Cortex Cinnamomi) for damp-cold; and *Chi Shao* (Radix Paeoniae Rubra) and *Dan Shen* (Radix et Rhizoma Salviae Miltiorrhizae) for blood stagnation. The treatment protocol was to cook the herbs in water, and drink the decoction in two to three equally-divided doses daily. The patients were instructed to discontinue the use of drugs during herbal treatment. Of 56 patients, the study reported complete recovery in 29 cases and moderate improvement in 16 cases after the first 5-day course of treatment. After the second course of treatment, the study reported complete recovery in 40 cases and moderate improvement in 12 cases. The rate of effectiveness was 80% after the first course, and 92.8% after the second course. The study also noted that the group with qi and blood deficiencies was most responsive to the herbal treatment.[2]
3. **Neurodermatitis**: One report stated that administration of modified *Dang Gui Yin Zi*, plus topical application of steroids, was more effective (96.5% effectiveness in 86 patients) than topical application of steroids alone (65.4% effectiveness in 52 patients). The herbal formula contained 10g each of *Dang Gui* (Radix Angelicae Sinensis), *Chi Shao* (Radix Paeoniae Rubra), *Fang Feng* (Radix Saposhnikoviae), *Ji Li* (Fructus Tribuli), *Huang Qi* (Radix Astragali), *Hong Hua* (Flos Carthami), *Chan Tui* (Periostracum Cicadae), and *Di Fu Zi* (Fructus Kochiae); 15g of *Di Huang* (Radix Rehmanniae); 6g of *Chuan Xiong* (Rhizoma Chuanxiong); 30g of *He Shou Wu* (Radix Polygoni Multiflori), and others as deemed necessary.[3]
4. **Ichthyosis**: In one case report, a patient with a 10-year history of noninflammatory scaling of the skin was treated successfully with 50 doses of *Dang Gui Yin Zi*, without recurrence during the 3 years of follow-up.[4] According to another report, a modified *Dang Gui Yin Zi* formula was found to have good effect in treating ichthyosis with rough, scale-like appearance of the skin all over the extremities, back, and chest. The herbal treatment contained *Dang Gui* (Radix Angelicae Sinensis) 10g, *Chuan Xiong* (Rhizoma Chuanxiong) 10g, *Bai Shao* (Radix Paeoniae Alba) 10g, *Gou Qi Zi* (Fructus Lycii) 10g, *Huang Qi* (Radix Astragali) 10g, *Bai Zhu* (Rhizoma Atractylodis Macrocephalae) 10g, *Di Fu Zi* (Fructus Kochiae) 10g, *Zi Cao* (Radix Arnebiae) 10g, *Ji Li* (Fructus Tribuli) 10g, *Chi Shao* (Radix Paeoniae Rubra) 6g, *He Shou Wu* (Radix Polygoni Multiflori) 10g, dry-fried *Jing Jie* (Herba Schizonepetae) 5g, *Fang Feng* (Radix Saposhnikoviae) 6g, and *Gan Cao* (Radix et Rhizoma Glycyrrhizae) 3g. The herbs were cooked in water, and the decoction administered in two equally-divided doses daily. The average duration of treatment was slightly over 6 months.[5]
5. **Alopecia**: Continuous administration of *Dang Gui Yin Zi* for 2-4 months was effective in treating 6 of 7 patients with alopecia. The hair was restored to normal quantity and color. In addition, no further hair loss was reported in these 6 patients upon follow-up, one year after the discontinuation of herbal treatment.[6]

Dāng Guī Yǐn Zǐ (Tangkuei Decoction)

SUGGESTED ACUPUNCTURE TREATMENT

1. Points: *Sanyinjiao* (SP 6), *Geshu* (BL 17), *Xuehai* (SP 10), *Quchi* (LI 11), *Fengchi* (GB 20), *Tianzhu* (BL 10), *Fengmen* (BL 12), *Housanli* (ST 36), and *Fuliu* (KI 7).
2. Technique: tonification and even method.

Sanyinjiao (SP 6), *Geshu* (BL 17), and *Xuehai* (SP 10) tonify the blood; *Housanli* (ST 36) tonifies qi; and *Fuliu* (KI 7) tonifies yin. Needling *Quchi* (LI 11) with even method dispels wind; *Fengchi* (GB 20), *Tianzhu* (BL 10), and *Fengmen* (BL 12) dispel wind and relieve the itch.

AUTHORS' COMMENTS

From a traditional Chinese medical perspective, *Dang Gui Yin Zi* treats dermatological disorders caused by blood deficiency and external wind. In terms of anatomy and physiology, such dermatological disorders are similar to atrophy of the skin tissue, hair follicles, sebaceous glands, and sweat glands. *Dang Gui Yin Zi* is a derivative of *Si Wu Tang* (Four-Substance Decoction) and in general is used more commonly to treat chronic skin disorders in geriatric animals or younger animals that suffer from yin and blood deficiencies secondary to chronic administration of antimicrobial and steroidal medications and overwork. Clinically, it can be used for any dry, scaly, red, pruritic skin rash. For severe, chronic skin rashes with alopecia and dry, red, scaly skin with lichenification and hyperpigmentation, *Dang Gui Yin Zi* (Tangkuei Decoction) is much more effective when combined with additional herbs that move the blood.

Xiao Feng San (Eliminate Wind Powder) and *Dang Gui Yin Zi* both treat skin disorders characterized by wind at the exterior and blood deficiency in the interior.

- *Xiao Feng San* clears wind-dampness and wind-heat and nourishes and cools the blood. It mainly treats dermatitis, hives, urticaria and other skin disorders primarily caused by dampness and heat invading the exterior. It is used more commonly for acute, seasonal skin disorders.
- *Dang Gui Yin Zi* tonifies the blood, moistens dryness, and releases wind. It is more effective for pruritis, dermatitis, urticaria, and other skin conditions complicated by both exterior (wind) and interior (dryness with blood deficiency) factors. It is typically used for skin disorders of a chronic nature. However, in acute cases, it can be combined with *Xiao Feng San* (Eliminate Wind Powder), and the dose then is decreased when the acute signs resolve.

References

1. *Zhong Yi Yao Xue Bao* (Report of Chinese Medicine and Herbology), 1986; 5:50.
2. *Tie Dao Yi Xue* (Tiedao Medicine), 1988; 4:230.
3. *Zhong Guo Zhong Xi Yi Jie He Za Zhi* (Chinese Journal of Integrative Chinese and Western Medicine), 1992; 181.
4. *Zhong Yi Za Zhi* (Journal of Chinese Medicine), 1985; 6:442.
5. *Hu Nan Zhong Yi Za Zhi* (Hunan Journal of Chinese Medicine), 1989; 5:33.
6. *Si Chuan Zhong Yi* (Sichuan Chinese Medicine), 1989; 8:47.

Qīān Zhèng Sǎn (Lead to Symmetry Powder)

牽正散
牵正散

Pinyin Name: *Qian Zheng San*
Literal Name: Lead to Symmetry Powder
Alternate Name: Lead to Symmetry Formula
Original Source: *Yang Shi Jia Zang Fang* (Collected Formulas of the Yang Family) by Yang Tan in 1178

COMPOSITION

Bai Fu Zi (Rhizoma Typhonii)	[6g]
Jiang Can (Bombyx Batryticatus)	[6g]
Quan Xie (Scorpio), remove toxins	[3g]

DOSAGE / PREPARATION / ADMINISTRATION

The source text recommends grinding equal amounts of the fresh ingredients into powder. Take 3g per dose with a warm, grain-based liquor. Today, this formula may be prepared as a decoction with the doses suggested in brackets.

CHINESE THERAPEUTIC ACTIONS

1. Dispels wind
2. Resolves phlegm
3. Stops spasms

CLINICAL MANIFESTATIONS

Zhong feng (wind stroke): deviation of the eyes and mouth, facial spasms, hemiplegia, paresis and paralysis.

VETERINARY CLINICAL APPLICATIONS

Facial paralysis, paresis, paralysis, hemiplegia, Horner's syndrome, equine photic head shaking, temporohyoid osteopathy, seizure disorder, and fibrocartilaginous emboli (FCE) in dogs.

EXPLANATION

According to traditional Chinese medicine, *zhong feng* (wind stroke) can affect either the channels and collaterals, or the *zang fu* organs. *Zhong feng* (wind stroke) affecting the channels and collaterals is characterized by deviation of the face and paralysis of the limbs. *Zhong feng* (wind stroke) affecting the *zang fu* organs involves loss of consciousness, hemiplegia, distortion of the face, dysphagia, and absence of urination and defecation during the attack.

Qian Zheng San (Lead to Symmetry Powder) is designed specifically for *zhong feng* (wind stroke) affecting the channels and collaterals, with obstruction of wind and phlegm in the face. The channels affected are foot *yangming* [Stomach], which encircles the mouth and lips, and foot *taiyang* [Urinary Bladder], which reaches the inner canthus of the eyes. When these two channels are attacked by wind and obstructed by phlegm, the wind and phlegm factors block the qi and blood circulation and cause malnourishment of the muscles and tendons, producing clinical signs such as deviation of the eyes and mouth. Facial spasms may also occur.

To effectively treat this syndrome, wind and phlegm must be dispelled. At the same time, qi and blood circulation in the channels and collaterals have to be restored, and the spasms stopped. This formula uses *Bai Fu Zi* (Rhizoma Typhonii) to dispel wind and clear phlegm in the head. *Jiang Can* (Bombyx Batryticatus) and *Quan Xie* (Scorpio) dispel wind and stop spasms. In addition, *Jiang Can* (Bombyx Batryticatus) resolves phlegm, while *Quan Xie* (Scorpio) opens the channels and collaterals. These three herbs synergistically address the cause of *zhong feng* (wind stroke). Lastly, grain-based liquor enhances the blood circulation and the distribution of the herbs to the affected areas.

***Qian Zheng San* (Lead to Symmetry Powder)**

Diagnosis	Clinical Signs	Treatment	Herbs
Zhong feng (wind stroke)	Deviation of the eyes and mouth and facial spasms: obstruction of wind and phlegm in the channels and collaterals	• Dispels wind • Resolves phlegm • Stops spasms	• *Bai Fu Zi* (Rhizoma Typhonii) dispels wind and clears phlegm in the head and face. • *Jiang Can* (Bombyx Batryticatus) and *Quan Xie* (Scorpio) dispel wind and stop spasms.

Qiān Zhèng Săn (Lead to Symmetry Powder)

VETERINARY MODIFICATIONS

- For facial paralysis caused by wind-cold, add *Qiang Huo* (Rhizoma et Radix Notopterygii) and *Fang Feng* (Radix Saposhnikoviae).
- For facial paralysis caused by wind-dampness, add *Wu Gong* (Scolopendra).
- For facial twitching, add *Wu Gong* (Scolopendra), *Tian Ma* (Rhizoma Gastrodiae), and *Di Long* (Pheretima).

CAUTIONS / CONTRAINDICATIONS

- *Qian Zheng San* is acrid, warm, and drying in nature and should be reserved for *zhong feng* (wind stroke) characterized by cold, wind and phlegm.
- Because *Bai Fu Zi* (Rhizoma Typhonii) is acrid, warm, and drying in nature, this formula is not recommended for treating deviation of the mouth or hemiplegia due to internal Liver wind rising, or due to qi deficiency and blood stagnation. Modifications (such as listed above) are necessary to address the complications and associated conditions.
- Because *Bai Fu Zi* (Rhizoma Typhonii) and *Quan Xie* (Scorpio) are toxic, doses of these herbs should not exceed 6g when used in decoction.
- Use of this formula is contraindicated during pregnancy.[1]

PHARMACOLOGICAL EFFECTS

1. **Cardiovascular**: According to *in vitro* studies, administration of *Qian Zheng San* was associated with reduced peripheral vascular resistance in both rabbits and rats. The onset of action began approximately 10-20 minutes after administration, and reached maximal effect after 30 minutes.[2]
2. **Effect on the central nervous system**: Administration of *Qian Zheng San* has been shown to have both sedative and antiepileptic effects. Intraperitoneal injection, intravenous injection, and oral ingestion of this formula were associated with sedation in rabbits. Use of a *Qian Zheng San* preparation was effective in treating mice with artificially-induced seizures.[3]

HUMAN CLINICAL STUDIES AND RESEARCH

1. **Facial paralysis**: *Qian Zheng San* has been shown in many studies to effectively treat facial paralysis. According to one study, 60 patients with facial paralysis were treated with integrative TCM treatments (herbs and acupuncture) with complete recovery in 50 cases and significant improvement in 2 cases. The herbal treatment included *Qian Zheng San* plus *Wu Gong* (Scolopendra), *Tian Ma* (Rhizoma Gastrodiae), *Di Long* (Pheretima), and *Fang Feng* (Radix Saposhnikoviae). The treatment protocol consisted of grinding all the substances into a fine powder, and administering 5g of the powder two times daily with grain-based liquor. The patients also received electro-acupuncture treatments. The average duration of treatment to achieve recovery was 2 weeks, ranging from 3 to 30 days.[4]

   According to another study, use of modified *Qian Zheng San* in 50 patients with facial paralysis was associated with 98% effectiveness (complete recovery in 44 cases, significant improvement in 3 cases, moderate improvement in 2 cases, and no effect in 1 case). The treatment protocol was to cook the herbs in water and administer the decoction in three equally-divided doses daily. The herbal treatment contained *Qian Zheng San* plus *Fang Feng* (Radix Saposhnikoviae), *Wu Gong* (Scolopendra), *Qiang Huo* (Rhizoma et Radix Notopterygii), *Ge Gen* (Radix Puerariae Lobatae), and *Gou Teng* (Ramulus Uncariae cum Uncis) as the base formula. Modifications included the addition of *Dan Nan Xing* (Arisaema cum Bile), *Shi Chang Pu* (Rhizoma Acori Tatarinowii), *Zhu Ru* (Caulis Bambusae in Taenia), and *Ban Xia* (Rhizoma Pinelliae) for excess conditions characterized by tongue stiffness and tremors with a yellow, greasy tongue coating; *Di Huang Yin Zi* (Rehmannia Decoction) for deficiency conditions characterized by weakness of the tongue with white tongue coating; *Huang Qi* (Radix Astragali), *Dang Shen* (Radix Codonopsis), *Tai Zi Shen* (Radix Pseudostellariae), and *Huang Jing* (Rhizoma Polygonati) for qi deficiency with shortness of breath; *Tao Ren* (Semen Persicae), *Hong Hua* (Flos Carthami), and *Chi Shao* (Radix Paeoniae Rubra) for blood stagnation with purplish discoloration of the lips; *Bai Zhu* (Rhizoma Atractylodis Macrocephalae) and *Fu Ling* (Poria) for excessive salivation; *Shi Gao* (Gypsum Fibrosum), *Jin Yin Hua* (Flos Lonicerae Japonicae), and *Lian Qiao* (Fructus Forsythiae) for red face and yellow tongue coating; and *Ju Hua* (Flos Chrysanthemi), *Bai Zhi* (Radix Angelicae Dahuricae), *Chai Hu* (Radix Bupleuri), and *Chuan Xiong* (Rhizoma Chuanxiong) for headache.[5]

   Lastly, 88 patients with facial paralysis were treated with great success using herbs and/or acupuncture. The herbal treatment contained *Qian Zheng San* plus *Fang Feng* (Radix Saposhnikoviae), *Jin Yin Hua* (Flos Lonicerae Japonicae), *Tao Ren* (Semen Persicae), *Chuan Xiong* (Rhizoma Chuanxiong), *Huang Qin* (Radix Scutellariae), *Dan Shen* (Radix et Rhizoma Salviae Miltiorrhizae), *Chan Tui* (Periostracum Cicadae), *Bai Ji* (Rhizoma Bletillae), *Di Huang* (Radix Rehmanniae), *Wu Gong* (Scolopendra), and others as needed. *Ma Huang* (Herba Ephedrae) and *Xi Xin* (Radix et Rhizoma Asari) were added for external wind-cold; *Sang Ye* (Folium Mori) and *Bo He* (Herba Menthae) were added for external wind-heat; *Xi Yang Shen* (Radix Panacis Quinquefolii) for qi deficiency; *Dang Gui* (Radix Angelicae Sinensis) and *Bai Shao* (Radix Paeoniae Alba) for blood deficiency; *Tian Ma* (Rhizoma Gastrodiae) and

Qiān Zhèng Săn (Lead to Symmetry Powder)

Meng Shi (Lapis Micae seu Chloriti) for chronic illness with phlegm obstructing the channels and collaterals; and *Gou Teng* (Ramulus Uncariae cum Uncis), *Di Huang* (Radix Rehmanniae), and *Zhi Chuan Wu* (Radix Aconiti Praeparata) for wind and phlegm obstructing the channels and collaterals. Of 88 patients, 68 received concurrent herbs and acupuncture treatment, and 20 received acupuncture treatment only. The duration of treatment ranged from 2 days to 1 year. The study reported a 95% rate of recovery.[6]

2. **Trigeminal neuralgia**: Use of modified *Qian Zheng San* in 52 patients was associated with 94.2% effectiveness. The herbal treatment contained this formula plus *Dang Gui* (Radix Angelicae Sinensis), *Chan Tui* (Periostracum Cicadae), and others as the base formula. Furthermore, modifications included the addition of *Huang Qin* (Radix Scutellariae), *Gou Teng* (Ramulus Uncariae cum Uncis), and *Shi Gao* (Gypsum Fibrosum) for wind-heat; *Bai Fu Zi* (Rhizoma Typhonii), *Xi Xin* (Radix et Rhizoma Asari), and *Ma Huang* (Herba Ephedrae) for wind-cold; *Tao Ren* (Semen Persicae), *Hong Hua* (Flos Carthami), *Ban Xia* (Rhizoma Pinelliae), and *Dan Nan Xing* (Arisaema cum Bile) for blood stagnation and phlegm obstruction; and *Di Huang* (Radix Rehmanniae), *Mu Dan Pi* (Cortex Moutan), *Gui Ban* (Plastrum Testudinis), and *Nu Zhen Zi* (Fructus Ligustri Lucidi) for yin deficiency with blood heat. Of 52 patients, the study reported significant relief of pain in 32 cases, moderate improvement in 17 cases, and no benefit in 3 cases.[7]

SUGGESTED ACUPUNCTURE TREATMENT

1. Points: *Fengchi* (GB 20), *Hegu* (LI 4), *Fenglong* (ST 40), *Dicang* (ST 4), *Yangbai* (GB 14), *Sibai* (ST 2), *Jiache* (ST 6), and other special points listed below.
2. Technique: sedation or mild electrostimulation.

Fengchi (GB 20) and *Hegu* (LI 4) dispel wind and heat, especially in the head and face. *Fenglong* (ST 40) dispels phlegm. *Yangbai* (GB 14), *Sibai* (ST 2), *Dicang* (ST 4), and *Jiache* (ST 6), as local points in the affected areas, promote qi and blood circulation, relieve muscle spasms, and correct facial deviation due to stroke.

This treatment may be modified as follows: *Zanzhu* (BL 2), *Tongziliao* (GB 1), and *Sizhukong* (TH 23) to correct drooping of the eyelids and ear; *Lianquan* (CV 23) to treat tongue flaccidity; *Chengjiang* (CV 24) and *Renzhong* (GV 26) to restore deviation of the lips; and *Yingxiang* (LI 20) for deviation of the nose.

RELATED FORMULA

Zhĭ Jīng Săn (Stop Spasms Powder)
止痙散
止痉散
Pinyin Name: *Zhi Jing San*
Literal Name: Stop Spasms Powder
Original Source: *Shang Hai Zhong Yi Xue Yuan* (Shanghai University of Chinese Medicine)

Quan Xie (Scorpio)	
Wu Gong (Scolopendra)	

The source text states to grind equal amounts of the ingredients into a fine powder. Take 1-1.5g of powder with boiled water two to four times daily.

The main actions of this formula are to dispel wind and stop muscle spasms. Clinically, *Zhi Jing San* (Stop Spasms Powder) can treat muscle spasms, cramps, and seizure disorder. This formula also relieves pain and is especially effective for intractable joint pain.

Quan Xie (Scorpio) and *Wu Gong* (Scolopendra) are substances derived from insects that can be used in veterinary medicine to help control seizures. *Zhi Jing San* (Stop Spasms Powder) is comprised of these two herbs in a 50:50 ratio. These two substances can be toxic, and the utmost care must be used in determining dosage and duration of herbal formulas that contain these herbs. The use of potentially toxic animal- and/or insect-based substances is warranted in cases where the life of the animal is threatened from their disease or if the owner is considering euthanasia. These herbal formulas can be made in-house and/or made-to-order from any reputable herbal company.

AUTHORS' COMMENTS

Qian Zheng San is the representative formula for treating *zhong feng* (wind stroke) characterized by deviation of the eyes and mouth and facial spasms. This formula and other related formulas are rarely used alone in the treatment of dogs and cats; instead, they are combined with formulas that tonify underlying deficiencies of qi, yin and blood and that resolve stagnation. The herbs in these formulas are typically used in an aggressive manner to stop seizures, relieve severe joint pain, clear obstruction of the channels and collaterals, and activate qi and blood circulation in cases in which other therapies have proven ineffective.

Qian Zheng San can be used in combination with *Zhi Jing San* (Stop Spasms Powder) or other formulas to treat biomedical disorders with intractable seizures, such as idiopathic epilepsy, meningitis, brain tumors in dogs or cats, intractable joint pain, paresis and paralysis secondary to intervertebral disk disease and fibrocartilaginous emboli (FCE) in dogs. In horses, facial paralysis often occurs after direct injury to the meridians and can be seen in post-anesthesia cases in which excessive pressure had been applied to the facial nerve for an extended time period. In these patients, *Qian Zheng San* can be combined with *Xue Fu Zhu Yu Tang* (Drive Out Stasis in the Mansion of Blood Decoction) for good effects. In cases of photic head shaking, in which trigeminal nerve neuropathy may be a cause of the behavior, combining *Qian Zheng San* and *Xiao Feng San* (Eliminate Wind Powder) to both dredge the meridians and remove excess wind is helpful.

References

1. *Zhong Yao Ming Fang Yao Li Yu Ying Yong* (Pharmacology and Applications of Famous Herbal Formulas), 1989; 532-533.
2. *Zhong Yao Yao Li Yu Lin Chuang* (Pharmacology and Clinical Applications of Chinese Herbs), 1987; 3:332.
3. *Zhong Yi Fang Ji Xian Dai Yan Jiu* (Modern Study of Medical Formulas in Traditional Chinese Medicine), 1997; 1170.
4. *Nei Meng Gu Zhong Yi Yao* (Traditional Chinese Medicine and Medicinals of Inner Mongolia), 1990; 9(4):18.
5. *He Bei Zhong Yi* (Hebei Chinese Medicine), 1985; 4:30.
6. *Shi Zhen Guo Yao Yan Jiu* (Research of Shizhen Herbs), 1996; 7(1):13.
7. *Si Chuan Zhong Yi* (Sichuan Chinese Medicine), 1998; 2:25.

Wū Yào Shùn Qì Săn (Lindera Powder to Smooth the Flow of Qi)

烏藥順氣散

乌药顺气散

Pinyin Name: *Wu Yao Shun Qi San*

Literal Name: Lindera Powder to Smooth the Flow of Qi

Alternate Names: *Wu Yao Chun Chi San, Wu Yao Shun Chi San*, Lindera Chi-Regulating Formula, Lindera Chi-Regulating Powder, Lindera Formula

Original Source: *Tai Ping Hui Min He Ji Ju Fang* (Imperial Grace Formulary of the Tai Ping Era) by the Imperial Medical Department in 1078-85

COMPOSITION

Wu Yao (Radix Linderae)	60g
Chen Pi (Pericarpium Citri Reticulatae)	60g
Jiang Can (Bombyx Batryticatus), *chao* (dry-fried)	30g
Ma Huang (Herba Ephedrae)	60g
Chuan Xiong (Rhizoma Chuanxiong)	30g
Jie Geng (Radix Platycodonis)	30g
Pao Jiang (Rhizoma Zingiberis Praeparatum), *pao* (blast-fried)	15g
Zhi Qiao (Fructus Citri Aurantii), *chao* (dry-fried) with bran	30g
Bai Zhi (Radix Angelicae Dahuricae)	30g
Gan Cao (Radix et Rhizoma Glycyrrhizae), *chao* (dry-fried)	30g

Wū Yào Shùn Qì Săn (Lindera Powder to Smooth the Flow of Qi)

DOSAGE / PREPARATION / ADMINISTRATION

The source text recommends grinding the ingredients into a fine powder. Cook 9g of the powder with 3 slices of *Sheng Jiang* (Rhizoma Zingiberis Recens) and 1 piece of *Da Zao* (Fructus Jujubae) in 1 bowl of water until the liquid is reduced to 70%. Take the strained decoction while it is warm.

CHINESE THERAPEUTIC ACTIONS

1. Dispels wind
2. Activates qi circulation and relieves pain
3. Eliminates phlegm

CLINICAL MANIFESTATIONS

1. *Zhong feng* (wind stroke): arthralgia, numbness and pain throughout the body, dysphasia, muscle and tendon stiffness, and paralysis.
2. Leg *qi* with leg weakness and difficulty in walking.
3. Internal wind with cold or blood deficiency: pain in the hypochondrium, epigastric and abdominal fullness, vomiting, diarrhea, and borborygmus.

VETERINARY CLINICAL APPLICATIONS

Cerebrovascular accident, cerebral hemorrhage, paresis, paralysis, hemiplegia, facial paralysis, wind-cold *bi zheng* (painful obstruction syndrome), and canine idiopathic vestibular disease.

EXPLANATION

Wu Yao Shun Qi San (Lindera Powder to Smooth the Flow of Qi) treats *zhong feng* (wind stroke) and its subsequent complications, such as muscle paralysis and limited mobility. In this case, the wind attacks the channels and collaterals in the extremities, causing numbness, stiffness, and pain throughout the body. This formula can also treat animals with weak legs and difficulty in walking. This formula is useful in the treatment of geriatric patients with internal wind and cold, or animals with internal wind and blood deficiency. Clinical presentations include hypochondriac pain, epigastric and abdominal fullness, vomiting, diarrhea, and borborygmus.

Wu Yao (Radix Linderae) dispels wind, promotes qi circulation, and relieves pain. *Chen Pi* (Pericarpium Citri Reticulatae) regulates qi flow. *Jiang Can* (Bombyx Batryticatus) subdues wind and dispels phlegm. *Ma Huang* (Herba Ephedrae) dispels external wind-cold and regulates qi circulation. *Chuan Xiong* (Rhizoma Chuanxiong) dispels wind and activates blood circulation to relieve pain. *Jie Geng* (Radix Platycodonis) opens inhibited Lung qi and eliminates phlegm. *Pao Jiang* (Rhizoma Zingiberis Praeparatum) warms the Spleen and Lung to dissolve phlegm. *Zhi Qiao* (Fructus Aurantii) activates qi flow and eliminates phlegm. *Bai Zhi* (Radix Angelicae Dahuricae)

Wu Yao Shun Qi San (Lindera Powder to Smooth the Flow of Qi)

Diagnosis	Clinical Signs	Treatment	Herbs
Zhong feng (wind stroke)	Numbness, stiffness and pain throughout the body, arthralgia, dysphasia, and paralysis: wind attacking the channels and collaterals	• Dispels wind • Activates qi and relieves pain • Eliminates phlegm	• *Wu Yao* (Radix Linderae) dispels wind, promotes qi circulation, and relieves pain. • *Chen Pi* (Pericarpium Citri Reticulatae) regulates qi flow. • *Jiang Can* (Bombyx Batryticatus) subdues wind and dispels phlegm. • *Ma Huang* (Herba Ephedrae) dispels external wind-cold and regulates qi circulation. • *Chuan Xiong* (Rhizoma Chuanxiong) dispels wind and activates blood circulation to relieve pain. • *Jie Geng* (Radix Platycodonis) opens inhibited Lung qi and eliminates phlegm. • *Pao Jiang* (Rhizoma Zingiberis Praeparatum) warms the Spleen and Lung to dissolve phlegm. • *Zhi Qiao* (Fructus Aurantii) activates qi flow and eliminates phlegm. • *Bai Zhi* (Radix Angelicae Dahuricae) dispels wind and activates qi flow to relieve pain. • *Gan Cao* (Radix et Rhizoma Glycyrrhizae), *Sheng Jiang* (Rhizoma Zingiberis Recens) and *Da Zao* (Fructus Jujubae) harmonize the herbs.

dispels wind and activates qi flow to relieve pain. *Gan Cao* (Radix et Rhizoma Glycyrrhizae), *Sheng Jiang* (Rhizoma Zingiberis Recens), and *Da Zao* (Fructus Jujubae) harmonize the formula.

VETERINARY MODIFICATIONS

- For paralysis characterized by qi and blood deficiencies, add *Ren Shen* (Radix et Rhizoma Ginseng), *Bai Zhu* (Rhizoma Atractylodis Macrocephalae), *Dang Gui* (Radix Angelicae Sinensis), *Chuan Xiong* (Rhizoma Chuanxiong), and *Mai Dong* (Radix Ophiopogonis).
- If there is pain throughout the entire body, add *Dang Gui* (Radix Angelicae Sinensis), *Rou Gui* (Cortex Cinnamomi), *Ru Xiang* (Gummi Olibanum), and *Mo Yao* (Myrrha).
- With coldness and pain in the extremities, add *Fu Zi* (Radix Aconiti Lateralis Praeparata), *Rou Gui* (Cortex Cinnamomi), and *Wei Ling Xian* (Radix et Rhizoma Clematidis).
- With swelling and edema in the legs, add *Niu Xi* (Radix Achyranthis Bidentatae), *Du Huo* (Radix Angelicae Pubescentis), and *Wu Jia Pi* (Cortex Acanthopanacis).
- With soreness and pain in the lower back, add *Du Zhong* (Cortex Eucommiae) and *Niu Xi* (Radix Achyranthis Bidentatae).
- With body aches and bone pain, add *Niu Xi* (Radix Achyranthis Bidentatae) and *Sang Ji Sheng* (Herba Taxilli).
- If accompanied by spasms and cramps, add *Mu Gua* (Fructus Chaenomelis) and *Bai Shao* (Radix Paeoniae Alba).
- With numbness and pain in the body, add *Xiao Xu Ming Tang* (Minor Prolong Life Decoction).

CAUTIONS / CONTRAINDICATIONS

Use of *Wu Yao Shun Qi San* is contraindicated during pregnancy.

SUGGESTED ACUPUNCTURE TREATMENT

1. Points: *Zhizheng* (SI 7), *Fengmen* (BL 12), *Diji* (SP 8), *Shanzhong* (CV 17), *Hegu* (LI 4), *Fenglong* (ST 40), and *Housanli* (ST 36).
2. Technique: sedation.

These points aim to treat stroke due to wind attacking the channels. Because external wind always attacks the *taiyang* channel first, *Zhizheng* (SI 7) is chosen from the hand *taiyang* channel to regulate qi. *Zhizheng* (SI 7) is combined with *Fengmen* (BL 12) to dispel wind and disperse cold from the exterior. *Diji* (SP 8), the *xi* (cleft) point of the Spleen channel, *Shanzhong* (CV 17), and *Hegu* (LI 4) activate qi and blood and remove blood stagnation. Finally, *Fenglong* (ST 40) dispels dampness, and *Housanli* (ST 36) harmonizes the middle *jiao*.

AUTHORS' COMMENTS

Wu Yao Shun Qi San can be used in cases of acute wind-cold *bi zheng* (painful obstruction syndrome) and intervertebral disk disease in all species, as well as fibrocartilaginous emboli in dogs, where cold and phlegm are major pathogenic factors. After the acute signs of wind-cold *bi zheng* (painful obstruction syndrome) have resolved, it is best to discontinue *Wu Yao Shun Qi San*, since this formula is not suitable for long-term use. Formulas that contain tonic herbs are most suitable for chronic wind-cold *bi zheng* (painful obstruction syndrome), such as *Du Huo Ji Sheng Tang* (Angelica Pubescens and Taxillus Decoction), *San Bi Tang* (Three-Painful Obstruction Decoction), and *Juan Bi Tang* (Remove Painful Obstruction Decoction).

Xiao Huo Luo Dan (Minor Invigorate the Collaterals Special Pill) and *Wu Yao Shun Qi San* are both used to treat acute intervertebral disk disease with presenting signs of paresis and paralysis or pain.

- *Xiao Huo Luo Dan* is a stronger formula and is better at warming the channels and dispersing cold than *Wu Yao Shun Qi San*. *Xiao Huo Luo Dan* is a harsh formula that contains no tonifying herbs and is often combined with another formula to tonify underlying deficiencies of qi, blood, and Liver and Kidney yin.
- *Wu Yao Shun Qi San* is a better choice to use in the weak, geriatric, debilitated and yin-deficient animals. A good example is canine idiopathic vestibular disease, or as it is commonly called, "old dog vestibular disease." Animals for which this formula is appropriate have a thick, white tongue coating and a slippery pulse, both of which indicate the presence of phlegm. *Wu Yao Shun Qi San* can be combined with *Shi Quan Da Bu Tang* (All-Inclusive Great Tonifying Decoction) for animals with qi deficiency, or with *Tian Ma Gou Teng Yin* (Gastrodia and Uncaria Decoction) for animals with deficiency of Liver and Kidney yin. Acupuncture, in combination with herbal medications, is essential to resolve the condition quickly and prevent residual head tilt and weakness.

Section 2

平熄内风剂 — Internal Wind-Extinguishing Formulas

Gōu Téng Săn (Uncaria Powder)

鈎藤散
钩藤散

Pinyin Name: *Gou Teng San*
Literal Name: Uncaria Powder
Alternate Names: *Kou Teng San*, Gambir Formula
Original Source: *Pu Ji Ben Shi Fang* (Formulas of Universal Benefit from My Practice) by Xu Shu-Wei in 1132

COMPOSITION

Gou Teng (Ramulus Uncariae cum Uncis)	15g
Ren Shen (Radix et Rhizoma Ginseng)	15g
Fu Ling (Poria)	15g
Fu Shen (Poria Pararadicis)	15g
Mai Dong (Radix Ophiopogonis)	15g
Chen Pi (Pericarpium Citri Reticulatae)	15g
Ban Xia (Rhizoma Pinelliae), *jin* (soaked) in and *xi* (washed) with liquid	15g
Fang Feng (Radix Saposhnikoviae)	15g
Ju Hua (Flos Chrysanthemi)	15g
Shi Gao (Gypsum Fibrosum)	30g
Zhi Gan Cao (Radix et Rhizoma Glycyrrhizae Praeparata cum Melle)	3g

DOSAGE / PREPARATION / ADMINISTRATION

The source text recommends grinding the ingredients into powder and cooking 12g of the powder with 7 slices of *Sheng Jiang* (Rhizoma Zingiberis Recens) in water. Take the strained decoction while it is warm.

CHINESE THERAPEUTIC ACTIONS

1. Clears heat from the Liver channel
2. Directs Liver yang downward and extinguishes Liver wind

CLINICAL MANIFESTATIONS

Liver excess: marked changes in emotions and behavior, irritability, muscle spasms in the shoulders and back, red eyes, and restlessness at night.

VETERINARY CLINICAL APPLICATIONS

Hypertension, vestibular disease, dizziness, seizure disorder, idiopathic epilepsy, and cognitive dysfunction.

EXPLANATION

Gou Teng San (Uncaria Powder) treats Liver excess. Clinically, the animals mainly show excess heat in the Liver channel, Liver qi stagnation, and heat affecting the Heart. As heat travels upward along the Liver channel, the animals experience clinical signs of irritability, aggressiveness, ataxia, head tilt, and nystagmus. Heat in the Liver channel is often complicated by Liver qi stagnation, leading to clinical signs such as marked changes in emotions and behavior. When heat travels upward and affects the Heart, animals may experience palpitations and insomnia. Moreover, animals with heat in the Liver channel may have Liver yin deficiency because heat damages yin. This condition is seen in middle-aged animals that are fed a high carbohydrate diet and those confined to small spaces for large parts of the day. This results in Liver qi stagnation and subsequent Liver and Heart fire.

Gōu Téng Săn (Uncaria Powder)

***Gou Teng San* (Uncaria Powder)**

Diagnosis	Clinical Signs	Treatment	Herbs
Liver excess	• Irritability and dizziness: heat traveling upwards along the Liver channel • Marked changes in emotions and behavior: Liver qi stagnation with heat in the Liver channel • Palpitations and insomnia: Liver heat affecting the Heart	• Clears heat from the Liver channel • Directs Liver yang downward and extinguishes Liver wind	• *Gou Teng* (Ramulus Uncariae cum Uncis) regulates Liver qi, clears heat from the Liver channel, and calms Liver wind. • *Ren Shen* (Radix et Rhizoma Ginseng), *Fu Ling* (Poria), and *Fu Shen* (Poria Paradicis) tonify qi and tranquilize the *shen* (spirit). • *Mai Dong* (Radix Ophiopogonis) nourishes yin. • *Chen Pi* (Pericarpium Citri Reticulatae) and *Ban Xia* (Rhizoma Pinelliae) smooth the qi flow and direct qi downward. • *Fang Feng* (Radix Saposhnikoviae) and *Ju Hua* (Flos Chrysanthemi) clear wind and heat from the eyes and head. • *Shi Gao* (Gypsum Fibrosum) clears excess heat. • *Sheng Jiang* (Rhizoma Zingiberis Recens) and *Gan Cao* (Radix et Rhizoma Glycyrrhizae) harmonize all of the herbs.

Gou Teng (Ramulus Uncariae cum Uncis), the chief herb, regulates Liver qi, clears heat from the Liver channel, calms Liver wind, and relieves spasms. It effectively addresses all of the clinical excess signs in this condition. *Ren Shen* (Radix et Rhizoma Ginseng), *Fu Ling* (Poria) and *Fu Shen* (Poria Paradicis) tonify qi and tranquilize the *shen* (spirit). *Mai Dong* (Radix Ophiopogonis) nourishes yin. *Chen Pi* (Pericarpium Citri Reticulatae) and *Ban Xia* (Rhizoma Pinelliae) smooth the qi flow and direct qi downward. *Fang Feng* (Radix Saposhnikoviae) and *Ju Hua* (Flos Chrysanthemi) clear wind and heat from the eyes and head. *Shi Gao* (Gypsum Fibrosum) clears excess heat. *Sheng Jiang* (Rhizoma Zingiberis Recens) and *Gan Cao* (Radix et Rhizoma Glycyrrhizae) harmonize the herbs.

VETERINARY MODIFICATIONS

- With Liver yin deficiency, add *Bai Shao* (Radix Paeoniae Alba) and *He Shou Wu* (Radix Polygoni Multiflori).
- With cognitive dysfunction, add *Tian Zhu Huang* (Concretio Silicea Bambusae) and *Yin Xing Ye* (Folium Ginkgo).
- With renal hypertension, add *Tian Ma* (Rhizoma Gastrodiae) and *Sang Ji Sheng* (Herba Taxilli).

PHARMACOLOGICAL EFFECTS

1. **Cardiovascular**: Administration of *Gou Teng San* in rats was associated with a dose-dependant reduction of blood pressure and heartbeat.[1] It prevented stroke and prolonged life span in stroke-prone hypertensive rats.[2] The mechanisms for lowering blood pressure and preventing stroke were attributed to activation of nitric oxide synthase and improvement in cerebral circulation.[3]
2. **Antiplatelet**: According to *in vitro* studies in rats, *Gou Teng San* was shown to have marked antiplatelet effects. It improved blood circulation to the peripheral parts of the body and reduced mortality caused by embolism.[4]
3. **Neuroprotective**: Administration of *Gou Teng San* was associated with significantly delaying neuronal cell death in the hippocampal CA1 region after ischemia. The mechanism was attributed to its free-radical-scavenging activity.[5]
4. **Antioxidant**: *Gou Teng San* has been shown in several studies to have marked antioxidant and free-radical-scavenging effects, and may be used to treat radical-mediated diseases.[6,7]
5. **Anticonvulsant**: Administration of *Gou Teng San* was associated with a dose-dependent effect in treating mice with convulsions induced by picrotoxine, strychinine, and electroshock. *Gou Teng* (Ramulus Uncariae cum Uncis) is believed to be the main active ingredient in this mechanism, as the formula was ineffective without this herb. The active constituents of *Gou Teng* (Ramulus Uncariae cum Uncis) have been isolated and identified as geissoschizine methylether, hirsuteine, hirsutine, and isocorynoxeine.[8]
6. **Antidementia**: One study reported *Gou Teng San* to be effective in treating patients with vascular dementia. The antidementia effects were attributed to the anti-hypertensive, free-radical-scavenging, and anti-excitotoxic activities of this formula.[9] Furthermore, another study in mice reported that long-term administration of *Gou Teng San* could improve, to some extent, the impairment of memory caused by aging.[10]

Gōu Téng Sǎn (Uncaria Powder)

7. **Antiamnestic**: According to one study in mice, administration of *Gou Teng San* was associated with antiamnestic effects based on the stimulation of serotonin 1A receptors.[11]

HUMAN CLINICAL STUDIES AND RESEARCH

1. **Hypertension**: One study reported 91.7% effectiveness using modified *Gou Teng San* to treat high blood pressure in 182 patients (64 males, 118 females, mostly over 40 years of age). The herbal formula contained *Gou Teng* (Ramulus Uncariae cum Uncis) 3g, *Shi Gao* (Gypsum Fibrosum) 8g, *Chen Pi* (Pericarpium Citri Reticulatae) 3g, *Ban Xia* (Rhizoma Pinelliae) 4g, *Fu Ling* (Poria) 3.5g, *Ren Shen* (Radix et Rhizoma Ginseng) 2g, *Ju Hua* (Flos Chrysanthemi) 2g, *Gan Cao* (Radix et Rhizoma Glycyrrhizae) 1g, *Sheng Jiang* (Rhizoma Zingiberis Recens) 1.5g, *Mai Dong* (Radix Ophiopogonis) 4g, and *Fang Feng* (Radix Saposhnikoviae) 4g. The treatment protocol was to give the herbs in decoction, for an average of 7.4 months. Of 182 patients, the study reported a marked effect in 32 patients, moderate improvement in 60 patients, slight improvement in 75 patients, and no effect in 15 patients.[12]
2. **Cerebral infarction**: One study reported beneficial effects using *Gou Teng San* to treat 15 patients with asymptomatic cerebral infarction. Therapeutic benefits included improved microcirculation and decreased serum nitric oxide and lipid peroxides.[13]
3. **Alzheimer's disease**: One hundred and eighty patients with Alzheimer's disease were treated with beneficial effect using *Gou Teng San*. The treatment protocol was to use this formula in powder, at 7.5 g/day, for 8-12 weeks. Improvements included improved cognitive and physical activities, such as short-term memory, sleeping patterns, and speech patterns.[14]
4. **Dementia**: *Gou Teng San* was effective in the treatment of vascular dementia in two studies. According to one well-controlled but non-double blind study (60 patients), use of herbs was effective in global improvement rating, utility rating, and improvement of subjective clinical signs, psychiatric clinical signs, and disturbance in daily living activities. In the other study, a double-blind controlled study (139 patients), use of herbs was effective in global improvement rating, utility rating, and improvement of subjective clinical signs, psychiatric clinical signs, and disturbance in daily living activities.[15]

SUGGESTED ACUPUNCTURE TREATMENT

1. Points: *Ququan* (LR 8), *Taichong* (LR 3), *Ganshu* (BL 18), *Housanli* (ST 36), *Fenglong* (ST 40), *Fengchi* (GB 20), and *Quchi* (LI 11).
2. Technique: sedation.

Taichong (LR 3), *Ququan* (LR 8), and *Ganshu* (BL 18) regulate Liver qi and clear Liver heat. *Housanli* (ST 36) tonifies qi and *Fenglong* (ST 40) disperses phlegm. *Fengchi* (GB 20) and *Quchi* (LI 11) clear heat and dispel wind.

AUTHORS' COMMENTS

Gou Teng San (Uncaria Powder) and *Gou Teng Yin* (Uncaria Decoction) have similar names, but are different formulas.

- *Gou Teng San* treats Liver excess, with Liver heat, Liver yang, and Liver fire rising. It can be used to treat seizure disorders characterized by heat and excess, hypertension, vestibular disease, and cognitive dysfunction in the dog.
- *Gou Teng Yin* treats Liver heat and wind rising, with underlying deficiency. It is commonly used to treat animals with seizure disorder due to Kidney and Liver yin deficiencies.

References

1. *Guo Wai Yi Xue* (Foreign Medicine), 1988; 8:53.
2. Shimada Y, Yang Q, Yokoyama K, Goto H, Kasahara Y, Sekiya N, Hikiami H, Terasawa K. Choto-san prevents occurrence of stroke and prolongs life span in stroke-prone spontaneously hypertensive rats. Am J Chin Med. 2003; 31(1):79-85.
3. Sugimoto A, Goto K, Ishige A, Komatsu Y, Miyamoto KI. Effect of Choto-san, a Kampo medicine, on the cerebral blood flow autoregulation in spontaneously hypertensive rats. Jpn J Pharmacol. 2000 Jun; 83(2):135-42.
4. *Guo Wai Yi Xue* (Foreign Medicine), 1992; 5:48.
5. Dohi K, Satoh K, Ikeda Y, Ohtaki H, Shioda S, Aruga T. Neuroprotective effect from ischemia and direct free radical scavenging activity of Choto-san (kampo medicine). Acta Neurochir Suppl. 2003; 86:123-7.
6. Okayasu H, Suzuki F, Satoh K, Shioda S, Dohi K, Ikeda Y, Nakashima H, Komatsu N, Fujimaki M, Hashimoto K, Maki J, Sakagami H. Comparison of cytotoxicity and radical scavenging activity between tea extracts and Chinese medicines. In Vivo. 2003 Nov-Dec; 17(6):577-81.
7. Sekiya N, Shimada Y, Shibahara N, Takagi S, Yokoyama K, Kasahara Y, Sakakibara I, Terasawa K. Inhibitory effects of Choto-san (Diao-teng-san), and hooks and stems of Uncaria sinensis on free radical-induced lysis of rat red blood cells. Phytomedicine. 2002 Oct; 9(7):636-40.
8. Mimaki Y, Toshimizu N, Yamada K, Sashida Y. Anti-convulsion effects of choto-san and chotoko (Uncariae Uncis cam Ramlus) in mice, and identification of the active principles. Yakugaku Zasshi. 1997 Dec; 117(12):1011-21.
9. Watanabe H, Zhao Q, Matsumoto K, Tohda M, Murakami Y, Zhang SH, Kang TH, Mahakunakorn P, Maruyama Y, Sakakibara I, Aimi N, Takayama H. Pharmacological evidence for antidementia effect of Choto-san (Gouteng-san), a traditional Kampo medicine. Pharmacol Biochem Behav. 2003 Jun; 75(3):635-43.
10. Mizushima Y, Kan S, Yoshida S, Irie Y, Urata Y. Effect of Choto-san, a Kampo medicine, on impairment of passive avoidance performance in senescence accelerated mouse (SAM). Phytother Res. 2003 May; 17(5):542-5.
11. Yuzurihara M, Goto K, Sugimoto A, Ishige A, Komatsu Y, Shimada Y, Terasawa K. Effect of Choto-san, a kampo medicine, on impairment of passive avoidance performance in mice. Phytother Res. 1999 May; 13(3):233-5.
12. *Guo Wai Yi Xue* (Foreign Medicine), 1979; 2:35.

13. Goto H, Yang Q, Kita T, Hikiami H, Shimada Y, Terasawa K. Effects of Choto-san on microcirculation, serum nitric oxide and lipid peroxides in patients with asymptomatic cerebral infarction. Am J Chin Med. 2001; 29(1):83-9.
14. *He Han Yi Yao Xue Hui Zhi* (Hehan Journal of Medicine and Herbology), 1989; 3:454.
15. Itoh T, Shimada Y, Terasawa K. Efficacy of Choto-san on vascular dementia and the protective effect of the hooks and stems of Uncaria sinensis on glutamate-induced neuronal death. Mech Ageing Dev. 1999 Nov; 111(2-3):155-73.

Zhèn Gān Xí Fēng Tāng

(Sedate the Liver and Extinguish Wind Decoction)

鎮肝熄風湯
镇肝熄风汤

Pinyin Name: *Zhen Gan Xi Feng Tang*
Literal Name: Sedate the Liver and Extinguish Wind Decoction
Alternate Name: Hematite and Scrophularia Combination
Original Source: *Yi Xue Zhong Zhong Can Xi Lu* (Records of Heart-Felt Experiences in Medicine with Reference to the West) by Zhang Xi-Chun in 1918-34

COMPOSITION

Niu Xi (Radix Achyranthis Bidentatae)	30g
Zhe Shi (Haematitum), *ya* (pressed) into fine particles	30g
Long Gu (Os Draconis), *dao* (pounded) into small particles	15g
Mu Li (Concha Ostreae), *dao* (pounded) into small particles	15g
Gui Ban (Plastrum Testudinis), *dao* (pounded) into small particles	15g
Xuan Shen (Radix Scrophulariae)	15g
Tian Dong (Radix Asparagi)	15g
Bai Shao (Radix Paeoniae Alba)	15g
Yin Chen (Herba Artemisiae Scopariae)	6g
Chuan Lian Zi (Fructus Toosendan), *dao* (pounded) into small particles	6g
Mai Ya (Fructus Hordei Germinatus)	6g
Gan Cao (Radix et Rhizoma Glycyrrhizae)	4.5g

Zhèn Gān Xí Fēng Tāng

(Sedate the Liver and Extinguish Wind Decoction)

DOSAGE / PREPARATION / ADMINISTRATION

Prepare the ingredients as a decoction.

CHINESE THERAPEUTIC ACTIONS

1. Sedates the Liver and extinguishes Liver wind
2. Nourishes yin and anchors yang

CLINICAL MANIFESTATIONS

Liver yang and wind rising due to Liver and Kidney yin deficiencies, with disrupted or reversed flow of qi and blood: ataxia, swelling of the eyes, irritability, red swollen eyes, belching, seizures in some animals, a red tongue, and a wiry, forceful pulse.

VETERINARY CLINICAL APPLICATIONS

Seizure disorder, epilepsy, systemic hypertension, treatment of cerebral hemorrhage secondary to hypertension and/or head trauma secondary to vehicular or blunt trauma, ischemic stroke, and glaucoma in dogs.

EXPLANATION

Zhen Gan Xi Feng Tang (Sedate the Liver and Extinguish Wind Decoction) treats the various symptoms of Liver yang and wind rising, with underlying Kidney and Liver yin deficiencies. When Liver and Kidney yin are deficient, Liver yang and wind may rise uncontrollably. The hyperactive Liver yang and wind ascend and invade the head, causing dizziness. Because the Liver and Kidney open to the eyes and ears respectively, hyperactive Liver yang and deficient Kidney yin may lead to swelling and redness of the eyes and poor hearing. Irritability and red eyes are due to hyperactivity of Liver yang, while seizures and convulsions are due to hyperactivity of Liver wind. When the Liver is in a state of excess, it may overact on the Stomach, causing belching. In severe cases, Liver yang may disturb qi and blood circulation and cause hypertension. A red tongue and a wiry, forceful pulse are indications of Liver yang excess.

Niu Xi (Radix Achyranthis Bidentatae) is used as the chief herb in this formula. Bitter and sour, it enters the Liver and Kidney channels and nourishes these two organs. It also directs the blood downward to quickly correct the reversed flow of qi and blood. *Zhe Shi* (Haematitum), *Long Gu* (Os Draconis), and *Mu Li* (Concha Ostreae) sedate hyperactive Liver yang and calm Liver wind. *Gui Ban* (Plastrum Testudinis), *Xuan Shen* (Radix Scrophulariae), *Tian Dong* (Radix Asparagi), and *Bai Shao* (Radix Paeoniae Alba) nourish yin and body fluids to restrain hyperactive yang. *Yin Chen* (Herba Artemisiae Scopariae), *Chuan Lian Zi* (Fructus Toosendan), and *Mai Ya* (Fructus Hordei Germinatus) smooth Liver qi circulation and prevent Liver qi stagnation. *Gan Cao* (Radix et Rhizoma Glycyrrhizae) harmonizes the herbs. The combination of *Mai Ya* (Fructus Hordei Germinatus) and *Gan Cao* (Radix et Rhizoma Glycyrrhizae) regulates Stomach qi and protects the stomach from the harsh mineral substances.

VETERINARY MODIFICATIONS

- If there is severe heat, add *Shi Gao* (Gypsum Fibrosum).
- If there is severe phlegm, add *Dan Nan Xing* (Arisaema cum Bile).
- With Liver yang and Liver wind rising, add *Bai Zi Ren* (Semen Platycladi).

***Zhen Gan Xi Feng Tang* (Sedate the Liver and Extinguish Wind Decoction)**

Diagnosis	Clinical Signs	Treatment	Herbs
Liver yang and wind rising due to Liver and Kidney yin deficiencies	• Dizziness, poor hearing, and redness and swelling of the eyes: Liver yang rising and Kidney yin deficiency • Irritability, hypertension, and red eyes: Liver yang rising • Seizures and convulsions: Liver wind rising • Red tongue and a wiry, forceful pulse: Liver yang excess	• Sedates the Liver and extinguishes Liver wind • Nourishes yin and anchors yang	• *Niu Xi* (Radix Achyranthis Bidentatae) nourishes the Liver and Kidney and guides the blood downward. • *Zhe Shi* (Haematitum), *Long Gu* (Os Draconis), and *Mu Li* (Concha Ostreae) sedate hyperactive Liver yang and calm Liver wind. • *Gui Ban* (Plastrum Testudinis), *Xuan Shen* (Radix Scrophulariae), *Tian Dong* (Radix Asparagi), and *Bai Shao* (Radix Paeoniae Alba) nourish yin and body fluids to restrain hyperactive yang. • *Yin Chen* (Herba Artemisiae Scopariae), *Chuan Lian Zi* (Fructus Toosendan), and *Mai Ya* (Fructus Hordei Germinatus) smooth Liver qi circulation. • *Gan Cao* (Radix et Rhizoma Glycyrrhizae) harmonizes the herbs.

Zhèn Gān Xí Fēng Tāng

(Sedate the Liver and Extinguish Wind Decoction)

- For treatment of aggression, add *Zhen Zhu* (Margarita) and *Hu Po* (Succinum).
- For hypertension, add *Gou Teng* (Ramulus Uncariae cum Uncis), *Xia Ku Cao* (Spica Prunellae), and *Ju Hua* (Flos Chrysanthemi).
- For glaucoma, add *Ju Hua* (Flos Chrysanthemi), *Xia Ku Cao* (Spica Prunellae), *Gou Qi Zi* (Fructus Lycii), *Mu Tong* (Caulis Akebiae), *Dan Shen* (Radix et Rhizoma Salviae Miltiorrhizae), and *Ze Xie* (Rhizoma Alismatis).

CAUTIONS / CONTRAINDICATIONS

- *Zhen Gan Xi Feng Tang* is not recommended for dizziness caused by blood deficiency, qi deficiency, Kidney deficiency, or accumulation of dampness and phlegm.[1]
- This formula contains many rich, heavy and cloying substances and can easily damage the middle *jiao*; it is not for long-term use without modification in the treatment of seizure disorders.
- This formula is not suitable for hypertension characterized by Kidney yin and yang deficiencies.[2]
- Occasional skin rashes have been reported following the use of *Zhen Gan Xi Feng Tang*.[3]

PHARMACOLOGICAL EFFECTS

Antihypertensive: Administration of *Zhen Gan Xi Feng Tang* was associated with a marked reduction in blood pressure in anesthetized cats. The initial onset of action began 20 minutes after oral ingestion, and reduced the blood pressure by 29 mmHg for 40-100 minutes. Moreover, a greater antihypertensive effect was noted when *Zhen Gan Xi Feng Tang* was modified by eliminating *Gui Ban* (Plastrum Testudinis), *Mai Ya* (Fructus Hordei Germinatus), *Yin Chen* (Herba Artemisiae Scopariae), and *Gan Cao* (Radix et Rhizoma Glycyrrhizae); and adding *Xia Ku Cao* (Spica Prunellae), *Gou Teng* (Ramulus Uncariae cum Uncis), *He Shou Wu* (Radix Polygoni Multiflori), and *Shou Wu Teng* (Caulis Polygoni Multiflori). This modified *Zhen Gan Xi Feng Tang* was determined to have a more potent effect and a longer duration of action, reducing blood pressure by 43.5 mmHg for 80-110 minutes.[4]

HUMAN CLINICAL STUDIES AND RESEARCH

1. **Hypertension**: One study reported good results for treatment of primary hypertension characterized by Liver yang rising, using modified *Zhen Gan Xi Feng Tang* or *Tian Ma Gou Teng Yin* (Gastrodia and Uncaria Decoction).[5]
2. **Concussion**: Use of *Zhen Gan Xi Feng Tang* in 23 patients with concussion was associated with complete recovery in 18 patients, improvement in 4 patients, and discontinuation of treatment in 1 patient (reason unknown). In addition to this formula, *Shi Di* (Calyx Kaki) and *Zhu Ru* (Caulis Bambusae in Taenia) were added for nausea and vomiting; *San Qi* (Radix et Rhizoma Notoginseng) was added for subdermal bleeding and bruises; and *Suan Zao Ren* (Semen Ziziphi Spinosae) and *Zhen Zhu Mu* (Concha Margaritiferae) for insomnia and palpitations.[6]

SUGGESTED ACUPUNCTURE TREATMENT

1. Points: *Taichong* (LR 3), *Baihui* (GV 20), *Fengfu* (GV 16), *Taixi* (KI 3), and *Renzhong* (GV 26).
2. Technique: sedation.

Taichong (LR 3), the *yuan* (source) point of the Liver channel, is used in combination with *Baihui* (GV 20) and *Fengfu* (GV 16) to sedate Liver yang and calm Liver wind. *Renzhong* (GV 26) promotes qi and blood circulation. *Taixi* (KI 3) nourishes yin and yang.

If the animal is unconscious, prick and bleed the *jing* (well) points of all twelve channels to release heat and help return consciousness.

AUTHORS' COMMENTS

Zhen Gan Xi Feng Tang is commonly used to treat aggression and seizure disorder characterized by both excess (Liver yang and wind rising) and deficiency (Kidney and Liver yin deficiencies) in dogs. This formula, in combination with *Suan Zao Ren Tang* (Sour Jujube Decoction), has shown excellent application in the treatment of aggression.

Zhen Gan Xi Feng Tang is often combined with herbs or formulas that resolve phlegm, as phlegm is a common pathological factor in the pathophysiology of epilepsy. For instance, combining this formula in a 50/50 ratio with *Ban Xia Bai Zhu Tian Ma Tang* (Pinellia, Atractylodes Macrocephala, and Gastrodia Decoction) can help control both the Liver wind and phlegm aspects of idiopathic epilepsy.

Zhen Gan Xi Feng Tang can be combined with *Qi Ju Di Huang Wan* (Lycium Fruit, Chrysanthemum, and Rehmannia Pill) or modified with single herbs to treat acute and chronic glaucoma and hypertension characterized by Kidney and Liver yin deficiencies, Liver yang rising, and Liver wind in dogs. In addition to herbal treatment, acupuncture is essential for obtaining the fastest results in the treatment of acute glaucoma.

Zhèn Gān Xí Fēng Tāng

(Sedate the Liver and Extinguish Wind Decoction)

References

1. *Zhong Yao Ming Fang Yao Li Yu Ying Yong* (Pharmacology and Applications of Famous Herbal Formulas), 1989; 560-561.
2. *Zhong Yao Ming Fang Yao Li Yu Ying Yong* (Pharmacology and Applications of Famous Herbal Formulas), 1989; 560-561.
3. *Zhong Yao Ming Fang Yao Li Yu Ying Yong* (Pharmacology and Applications of Famous Herbal Formulas), 1989; 560-561.
4. *Xin Zhong Yi* (New Chinese Medicine), 1980; 12:45.
5. *Shi Yong Zhong Yi Nei Ke Za Zhi* (Journal of Practical Chinese Internal Medicine), 1990; 1:26.
6. *Nei Meng Gu Zhong Yi Yao* (Traditional Chinese Medicine and Medicinals of Inner Mongolia), 1990; 1:2.

Jiàn Líng Tāng (Construct Roof Tiles Decoction)

建瓴湯

建瓴汤

Pinyin Name: *Jian Ling Tang*
Literal Name: Construct Roof Tiles Decoction
Alternate Name: Dioscorea and Achyranthes Combination
Original Source: *Yi Xue Zhong Zhong Can Xi Lu* (Records of Heart-Felt Experiences in Medicine with Reference to the West) by Zhang Xi-Chun in 1918-34

COMPOSITION

Niu Xi (Radix Achyranthis Bidentatae)	30g
Zhe Shi (Haematitum), *ya* (pressed) into fine particles	24g
Long Gu (Os Draconis), *dao* (pounded) into fine particles	18g
Mu Li (Concha Ostreae), *dao* (pounded) into fine particles	18g
Shan Yao (Rhizoma Dioscoreae)	30g
Di Huang (Radix Rehmanniae)	18g
Bai Shao (Radix Paeoniae Alba)	12g
Bai Zi Ren (Semen Platycladi)	12g

DOSAGE / PREPARATION / ADMINISTRATION

The source text advises to prepare the ingredients as a decoction using water filled with iron rust.

CHINESE THERAPEUTIC ACTIONS

1. Sedates the Liver and extinguishes Liver wind
2. Nourishes yin and calms the *shen* (spirit)

CLINICAL MANIFESTATIONS

Liver yang rising: ataxia, palpitations, forgetfulness, irritability, restlessness, a red to purple tongue, and a wiry pulse.

VETERINARY CLINICAL APPLICATIONS

Seizure disorder, epilepsy, behavioral disorder, systemic hypertension, prevention of cerebral hemorrhage secondary to hypertension, and ischemic stroke.

Jiàn Líng Tāng (Construct Roof Tiles Decoction)

EXPLANATION

When Liver yang ascends, it affects the Heart and head. Disturbance of the Heart leads to disturbance of the *shen* (spirit); thus, animals usually experience palpitations, irritability, anxiety and restlessness at night. When Liver yang ascends to the head, animals exhibit clinical signs of red eyes, dizziness, and seizures. Liver yang excess leads to restlessness and irritability because the Liver controls the emotions. A red to purple tongue and a wiry pulse are indicative of Liver yang excess.

Therapeutic functions of *Jian Ling Tang* (Construct Roof Tiles Decoction) include calming Liver yang, extinguishing Liver wind, tranquilizing the *shen* (spirit), and nourishing yin. *Niu Xi* (Radix Achyranthis Bidentatae) enters the Liver and Kidney and leads the blood downward to calm hyperactive yang and wind. Moreover, *Niu Xi* (Radix Achyranthis Bidentatae) nourishes the Liver and Kidney to calm the wind and yang. *Zhe Shi* (Haematitum), *Long Gu* (Os Draconis), and *Mu Li* (Concha Ostreae) sedate hyperactive Liver yang and calm Liver wind. *Shan Yao* (Rhizoma Dioscoreae) nourishes yin and strengthens the Spleen and Kidney, which are easily damaged by excess Liver yang. *Di Huang* (Radix Rehmanniae) clears heat, nourishes yin, and promotes the generation of body fluids. *Bai Shao* (Radix Paeoniae Alba) nourishes yin and body fluids to restrain hyperactive yang. *Bai Zi Ren* (Semen Platycladi) nourishes the Heart and calms the *shen* to relieve palpitations, restless sleep, restlessness and irritability.

VETERINARY MODIFICATIONS

With excessive phlegm, add *Dan Nan Xing* (Arisaema cum Bile).

HUMAN CLINICAL STUDIES AND RESEARCH

Hypertension: Numerous studies have shown *Jian Ling Tang* to be effective in treating hypertension. According to one study, use of modified *Jian Ling Tang* was associated with 88.9% effectiveness in treating 90 patients with primary hypertension.[1] In another study, use of *Jian Ling Tang* was associated with 93.7% effectiveness in treating 66 patients with hypertension.[2]

SUGGESTED ACUPUNCTURE TREATMENT

1. Points: *Taichong* (LR 3), *Baihui* (GV 20), *Fengfu* (GV 16), *Taixi* (KI 3), *Renzhong* (GV 26), and *Shenmen* (HT 7).
2. Technique: sedation.

Taichong (LR 3), the *yuan* (source) point of the Liver channel, is used in combination with *Baihui* (GV 20) and *Fengfu* (GV 16) to sedate Liver yang and calm Liver wind. *Renzhong* (GV 26) promotes qi and blood circulation. *Taixi* (KI 3) nourishes yin and yang. *Shenmen* (HT 7) tranquilizes the mind, and relieves irritability and restlessness at night.

AUTHORS' COMMENTS

Zhen Gan Xi Feng Tang (Sedate the Liver and Extinguish Wind Decoction) and *Jian Ling Tang* both treat Liver wind rising and yin deficiency with secondary hypertension. Both formulas contain rich, cloying, heavy herbs; it is recommended that Spleen tonic herbs or formulas be used in conjunction with these formulas in animals with weak gastrointestinal function.

- *Zhen Gan Xi Feng Tang* is stronger at extinguishing wind to treat excess conditions, but weaker at nourishing yin. Clinically, this formula is more effective in ***treating*** retinal and/or cerebral hemorrhage secondary to hypertension in cats and dogs.
- *Jian Ling Tang* moderately sedates Liver yang, but strongly nourishes yin and tranquilizes the mind. Clinically, this formula is more effective in ***preventing*** retinal and cerebral hemorrhage; it is also more effective in the treatment of *shen* (spirit) disturbance. As it contains more yin tonics,

***Jian Ling Tang* (Construct Roof Tiles Decoction)**

Diagnosis	Clinical Signs	Treatment	Herbs
Liver yang rising	• Restless sleep, restlessness, fidgeting and irritability: Liver yang affecting the Heart and disturbing the *shen* (spirit) • Dizziness and seizures: Liver yang rising to the head • Red tongue and a wiry pulse: Liver yang excess	• Sedates the Liver and extinguishes Liver wind • Nourishes yin and calms the *shen*	• *Niu Xi* (Radix Achyranthis Bidentatae) nourishes the Liver and Kidney to calm wind and yang. • *Zhe Shi* (Haematitum), *Long Gu* (Os Draconis), and *Mu Li* (Concha Ostreae) sedate hyperactive Liver yang and calm Liver wind. • *Shan Yao* (Rhizoma Dioscoreae), *Di Huang* (Radix Rehmanniae), and *Bai Shao* (Radix Paeoniae Alba) nourish yin and generate fluids. • *Bai Zi Ren* (Semen Platycladi) nourishes the Heart and calms the *shen* to relieve palpitations, restless sleep, and excessive dreams.

Jiàn Líng Tāng (Construct Roof Tiles Decoction)

it can be used for a longer period of time than *Zhen Gan Xi Feng Tang* (Sedate the Liver and Extinguish Wind Decoction).

References

1. *Liao Ning Zhong Ji Yi Kan* (Liaoning Journal of Medium Medicine), 1994; 7:312.
2. *Xin Zhong Yi* (New Chinese Medicine), 1981; 12:46.

Tiān Má Gōu Téng Yǐn (Gastrodia and Uncaria Decoction)

天麻鈎藤飲
天麻钩藤饮

Pinyin Name: *Tian Ma Gou Teng Yin*
Literal Name: Gastrodia and Uncaria Decoction
Alternate Name: Gambir Combination
Original Source: *Za Bing Zheng Zhi Xin Yi* (New Significance of Patterns and Treatment in Miscellaneous Diseases)

COMPOSITION

Tian Ma (Rhizoma Gastrodiae)	9g
Gou Teng (Ramulus Uncariae cum Uncis), post-decocted	12g
Zhi Zi (Fructus Gardeniae)	9g
Huang Qin (Radix Scutellariae)	9g
Shi Jue Ming (Concha Haliotidis), pre-decocted	18g
Yi Mu Cao (Herba Leonuri)	9g
Chuan Niu Xi (Radix Cyathulae)	12g
Du Zhong (Cortex Eucommiae)	9g
Sang Ji Sheng (Herba Taxilli)	9g
Shou Wu Teng (Caulis Polygoni Multiflori)	9g
Fu Shen (Poria Pararadicis), processed with *Zhu Sha* (Cinnabaris)	9g

Note: The source text directs the herbalist to process *Fu Shen* (Poria Paradicis) with *Zhu Sha* (Cinnabaris) to enhance the effects of calming the *shen* (spirit) and relieving restless sleep. However, *Zhu Sha* (Cinnabaris) is rarely used as a medicinal substance today. Its discussion here is included primarily for academic purposes, to reflect the historical use of this substance in its original formulation. Most herbal products today have removed it completely, or replaced it with substitutes with similar functions. For additional information on the toxicity, please refer to *Chinese Medical Herbology and Pharmacology* by John Chen and Tina Chen.

Tiān Má Gōu Téng Yǐn (Gastrodia and Uncaria Decoction)

DOSAGE / PREPARATION / ADMINISTRATION

Prepare the ingredients as a decoction.

CHINESE THERAPEUTIC ACTIONS

1. Calms Liver yang and extinguishes Liver wind
2. Clears heat
3. Activates blood circulation
4. Tonifies the Liver and Kidney

CLINICAL MANIFESTATIONS

Hyperactivity of Liver yang and Liver wind: red eyes, irritability, anxiety, restlessness at night, trembling, shaking of the legs, and seizures.

VETERINARY CLINICAL APPLICATIONS

Systemic hypertension, prevention and treatment of seizures and epilepsy, canine and equine idiopathic vestibular disease, behavioral disorder, trembling and shaking of the extremities, muscle spasms, and facial paralysis.

EXPLANATION

Tian Ma Gou Teng Yin (Gastrodia and Uncaria Decoction) treats Liver yang hyperactivity and Liver wind rising. Excess Liver yang may lead to the rising of Liver wind, which then invades the head to cause trembling and shaking of the legs, and seizures. Excess Liver yang may also affect the *shen* (spirit), causing restless sleep, irritability, anxiety, and restlessness at night.

This formula contains *Tian Ma* (Rhizoma Gastrodiae) and *Gou Teng* (Ramulus Uncariae cum Uncis) to calm Liver yang and extinguish Liver wind. *Zhi Zi* (Fructus Gardeniae) and *Huang Qin* (Radix Scutellariae) clear heat, sedate fire and prevent Liver yang from rising. *Shi Jue Ming* (Concha Haliotidis) clears heat and calms Liver yang. *Yi Mu Cao* (Herba Leonuri) activates blood circulation and regulates water circulation. *Chuan Niu Xi* (Radix Cyathulae) leads the blood downward to calm the Liver. *Du Zhong* (Cortex Eucommiae) and *Sang Ji Sheng* (Herba Taxilli) tonify the Liver and Kidney. *Shou Wu Teng* (Caulis Polygoni Multiflori) and *Fu Shen* (Poria Paradicis) calm the *shen* and relieve restless sleep and restlessness.

VETERINARY MODIFICATIONS

- With severe Liver yang rising, add *Zhe Shi* (Haematitum), *Long Gu* (Os Draconis), and *Mu Li* (Concha Ostreae).
- With Liver yin deficiency, add *Bai Shao* (Radix Paeoniae Alba) and *Gui Ban* (Plastrum Testudinis).
- For trembling legs, add *Jiang Can* (Bombyx Batryticatus).
- For cluster seizures, add *Xie Cao* (Radix et Rhizoma Valerianae).
- When there are post-stroke complications, add *Chi Shao* (Radix Paeoniae Rubra), *Tao Ren* (Semen Persicae), and *Hong Hua* (Flos Carthami).
- With thirst and phlegm accumulation, add *Bei Mu* (Bulbus Fritillariae) and *Zhu Ru* (Caulis Bambusae in Taenia).
- For hypertension, add *Huai Hua* (Flos Sophorae), *Hai Zao* (Sargassum), *Xia Ku Cao* (Spica Prunellae), *Jue Ming Zi* (Semen Cassiae) and *Zhen Zhu Mu* (Concha Margaritiferae).

Tian Ma Gou Teng Yin **(Gastrodia and Uncaria Decoction)**

Diagnosis	Clinical Signs	Treatment	Herbs
Hyperactivity of Liver yang and Liver wind	• Seizures and trembling and shaking of the limbs: Liver yang and Liver wind rising • Restless sleep and sleep disturbances: *shen* (spirit) disturbance	• Calms Liver yang and extinguishes Liver wind • Clears heat • Activates blood circulation • Tonifies the Liver and Kidney	• *Tian Ma* (Rhizoma Gastrodiae) and *Gou Teng* (Ramulus Uncariae cum Uncis) calm Liver yang and extinguish Liver wind. • *Zhi Zi* (Fructus Gardeniae) and *Huang Qin* (Radix Scutellariae) clear heat, sedate fire, and prevent Liver yang from rising. • *Shi Jue Ming* (Concha Haliotidis) clears heat and calms Liver yang. • *Yi Mu Cao* (Herba Leonuri) activates blood circulation and regulates water circulation. • *Chuan Niu Xi* (Radix Cyathulae) leads blood downward to calm the Liver. • *Du Zhong* (Cortex Eucommiae) and *Sang Ji Sheng* (Herba Taxilli) tonify the Liver and Kidney. • *Shou Wu Teng* (Caulis Polygoni Multiflori) and *Fu Shen* (Poria Paradicis) calm the *shen* and relieve restless sleep.

Tiān Má Gōu Téng Yǐn (Gastrodia and Uncaria Decoction)

CAUTIONS / CONTRAINDICATIONS

Tian Ma Gou Teng Yin is contraindicated in conditions characterized by Liver wind rising resulting from yin deficiency, with clinical signs such as a red tongue body and a scanty or mirror-like tongue coating.[1]

PHARMACOLOGICAL EFFECTS

Antihypertensive: Use of *Tian Ma Gou Teng Yin* markedly reduced blood pressure in dogs. However, it did not affect subjects with normal blood pressure. Based on this finding, the researchers suggest that this formula has a regulating effect on blood pressure.[2]

HUMAN CLINICAL STUDIES AND RESEARCH

1. **Hypertension**: Administration of *Tian Ma Gou Teng Yin* was effective in treating hypertension. In one study with 213 patients with primary hypertension, use of modified *Tian Ma Gou Teng Yin* or *Zhen Gan Xi Feng Tang* (Sedate the Liver and Extinguish Wind Decoction) was associated with marked effectiveness in reducing blood pressure in 156 patients, moderately reducing blood pressure in 19 patients, and no effect in 6 patients. The overall rate of effectiveness was 97.18%. Note: Information was unavailable on patients that did not complete the study.[3]
2. **Epilepsy**: In one study, 15 children with epilepsy were treated with good results using modified *Tian Ma Gou Teng Yin*. The herbal formula contained *Tian Ma* (Rhizoma Gastrodiae) 9g, *Gou Teng* (Ramulus Uncariae cum Uncis) 12g, *Shi Jue Ming* (Concha Haliotidis) 18g, *Huang Qin* (Radix Scutellariae) 9g, *Fu Ling* (Poria) 12g, *Shi Chang Pu* (Rhizoma Acori Tatarinowii) 8g, *Bai Shao* (Radix Paeoniae Alba) 12g, *Ju Hua* (Flos Chrysanthemi) 12g, *Nu Zhen Zi* (Fructus Ligustri Lucidi) 12g, *Dan Nan Xing* (Arisaema cum Bile) 9g, and others as needed. The herbs were given in decoction daily, for one month per course of treatment, for 1 to 6 courses total (average of 3 courses). Of 15 patients, the study reported significant improvement in 8 patients, moderate improvement in 4 patients, and no effect in 3 patients.[4]
3. **Ischemic stroke**: Use of modified *Tian Ma Gou Teng Yin* was associated with good success treating ischemic stroke in 243 patients. The study reported 68.42% effectiveness in 76 patients with stroke due to Liver fire and obstruction of channels and collaterals using this formula; 70% effectiveness in 150 patients with stroke due to qi deficiency and blood stagnation using this formula plus *Bu Yang Huan Wu Tang* (Tonify the Yang to Restore Five Decoction); and 53% effectiveness in 17 patients with stroke due to rising of yang and wind using this formula plus *Zhen Gan Xi Feng Tang* (Sedate the Liver and Extinguish Wind Decoction).[5]
4. **Dizziness**: Concurrent use of *Tian Ma Gou Teng Yin* and *Wen Dan Tang* (Warm the Gallbladder Decoction) was effective in treating all 24 patients with dizziness due to inner ear imbalance. The herbs were given in decoction daily.[6] According to another study, use of modified *Tian Ma Gou Teng Yin* was associated with 84.6% effectiveness in treating 78 patients with dizziness and vertigo. The herbal formula was based on *Tian Ma Gou Teng Yin*, with the addition of *Zhi Mu* (Rhizoma Anemarrhenae) and *Ju Hua* (Flos Chrysanthemi), and the elimination of *Yi Mu Cao* (Herba Leonuri). Additional modifications were made as needed.[7]
5. **Facial spasms**: Use of modified *Tian Ma Gou Teng Yin* in decoction daily for 7 to 14 days effectively treated 46 patients with facial spasms (32 with complete recovery, 8 with marked improvement, and 6 with slight improvement). The herbal formula was modified by removing *Shi Jue Ming* (Concha Haliotidis), *Zhi Zi* (Fructus Gardeniae), and *Shou Wu Teng* (Caulis Polygoni Multiflori), and adding *Bai Shao* (Radix Paeoniae Alba), *Dang Gui* (Radix Angelicae Sinensis), and *Gui Zhi* (Ramulus Cinnamomi). Furthermore, *Dang Shen* (Radix Codonopsis) was added for chronic deficiency; *Di Huang* (Radix Rehmanniae) and *Mai Dong* (Radix Ophiopogonis) were added for fluid deficiency; *Jue Ming Zi* (Semen Cassiae) and *Ju Hua* (Flos Chrysanthemi) were added for tinnitus and stuffy head due to Liver yang rising; *Mu Tong* (Caulis Akebiae) and *Che Qian Cao* (Herba Plantaginis) were added for dysuria; and *Da Huang* (Radix et Rhizoma Rhei) and *Feng Mi* (Mel) were added for constipation.[8]

TOXICOLOGY

According to one study, administration of *Tian Ma Gou Teng Yin* in 168 adults was associated with thirst in 5 patients. No other abnormalities were noted.[9]

SUGGESTED ACUPUNCTURE TREATMENT

1. Points: *Taichong* (LR 3), *Longhui*, *Fengchi* (GB 20), *Zuqiaoyin* (GB 44), *Anshen* and *Dafengmen*.
2. Technique: sedation.

Taichong (LR 3) sedates Liver yang and calms Liver wind. *Longhui* and *Fengchi* (GB 20) relieve dizziness. *Zuqiaoyin* (GB 44) clears heat from the Gallbladder channel. *Anshen* and *Dafengmen* are classical points that are particularly helpful in the treatment of seizure disorders.

AUTHORS' COMMENTS

Tian Ma Gou Teng Yin is commonly used to treat seizure disorders characterized by Liver wind, yin deficiency,

Tiān Má Gōu Téng Yǐn (Gastrodia and Uncaria Decoction)

Spleen qi deficiency, and phlegm in dogs. It can be used in young or middle-aged animals. Because phlegm is found in seizure disorders of dogs, this formula is very commonly combined with *Ban Xia Bai Zhu Tian Ma Tang* (Pinellia, Atractylodes Macrocephala, and Gastrodia Decoction). Together, these formulas calm the Liver, extinguish Liver wind, nourish yin, tonify the Spleen, dry dampness, and transform phlegm. It has been the authors' experience that this combination is highly effective in the control and/or complete elimination of seizures in dogs. The earlier the formulas are used in young animals (two years of age or younger), the greater the probability of complete resolution of the seizures. Occasionally, toxic heat becomes a factor in the development of seizure disorders. This most often occurs when the seizures start shortly after vaccination. In these cases, combining with *Huang Lian Jie Du Tang* (Coptis Decoction to Relieve Toxicity) may be more effective. When the seizures are controlled and the toxins are cleared, practitioners can transition to *Tian Ma Gou Teng Yin* alone.

Tian Ma Gou Teng Yin, *Zhen Gan Xi Feng Tang* (Sedate the Liver and Extinguish Wind Decoction) and *Jian Ling Tang* (Construct Roof Tiles Decoction) all treat Liver yang rising, Liver wind, and yin deficiency.

- *Tian Ma Gou Teng Yin* calms the Liver, extinguishes Liver wind, clears heat and nourishes the Liver and Kidney yin and is better at clearing Liver heat and sedating Liver fire. Clinically, this formula would be chosen for animals that have restlessness and irritability. This formula can be used longer term than the other formulas and is one of the first herbal formulas of choice to use in the treatment of idiopathic epilepsy in young or middle-aged dogs.
- *Zhen Gan Xi Feng Tang* contains many strong, heavy sedating herbals and is stronger at extinguishing wind to treat excess conditions, and weaker at nourishing yin. Clinically, this formula is more effective than the others in sedating and calming Liver yang and treating acute glaucoma, hypertension, and subsequent cerebral and retinal hemorrhage.
- *Jian Ling Tang* moderately sedates Liver yang, nourishes yin, and tranquilizes the mind. Clinically, this formula is more effective in calming the *shen* (spirit), particularly in animals that have anxiety, are irritable or aggressive, wake up frequently, and whine or pace during the night. It is stronger than *Tian Ma Gou Teng Yin* in treating hypertension.

All three formulas are used to treat seizures and systemic hypertension in dogs and cats; the formula chosen depends on the amount of heat, Liver wind, and *shen* (spirit) disturbance present in addition to constitution. *Zhen Gan Xi Feng Tang* (Sedate the Liver and Extinguish Wind Decoction) and *Jian Ling Tang* (Construct Roof Tiles Decoction) both contain heavy sedating herbals which can disturb the function of the Spleen and Stomach. It is advised to use single herbs and/or another formula that protects the middle *jiao*, when using these formulas for more than a few weeks.

The authors have used all of these formulas in combination with conventional antihypertensive medications, such as amlodipine besylate (Norvasc), without adverse effects. In acute cases, *Zhen Gan Xi Feng Tang* (Sedate the Liver and Extinguish Wind Decoction) is used as a first choice, followed by *Jian Ling Tang* (Construct Roof Tiles Decoction). *Tian Ma Gou Teng Yin* is used most often as a long-term maintenance formula. All of the formulas may require modification, depending on the animal's underlying condition, for best effects. The dose of the herbal formula is added to the conventional drug at a low dose. The dose of the herbal is gradually increased and the conventional drug decreased, with close monitoring of the blood pressure on a weekly basis. In many animals, the use of conventional medications may be discontinued once the underlying deficiencies and/or excess have resolved. These formulas can be used as the primary antihypertensive in place of conventional drugs, and their effects may be seen within 3-7 days, with full effect taking up to 2 weeks or more, depending on the formula chosen and the modifications made to the original formula.

References

1. *Zhong Yi Lin Chuan Fang Ji Xue* (Clinical Study of Chinese Herbal Formulas), 1995; 262-263.
2. *Zhong Yi Yao Yan Jiu Can Kao* (Research and Discussion of Chinese Medicine and Herbology), 1979; 9:25.
3. *Shi Yong Zhong Yi Nei Ke Za Zhi* (Journal of Practical Chinese Internal Medicine), 1990; 1:26.
4. *Tian Jin Zhong Yi* (Tianjin Chinese Medicine), 1995; 6:25.
5. *Liao Ning Zhong Yi Za Zhi* (Liaoning Journal of Chinese Medicine), 1984; 9:26.
6. *Si Chuan Zhong Yi* (Sichuan Chinese Medicine), 1988; 3:29.
7. *Shan Xi Zhong Yi Xue Yuan Xue Bao* (Journal of Shanxi University School of Chinese Medicine), 1996; 19(4):28.
8. *Xin Zhong Yi* (New Chinese Medicine), 1993; 10:28.
9. *Zhong Cheng Yao Yan Jiu* (Research of Chinese Patent Medicine), 1987; 3:17.

Dà Dìng Fēng Zhū (Major Arrest Wind Pearl)

大定風珠
大定风珠

Pinyin Name: *Da Ding Feng Zhu*
Literal Name: Major Arrest Wind Pearl
Original Source: *Wen Bing Tiao Bian* (Systematic Differentiation of Warm Diseases) by Wu Ju-Tong in 1798

COMPOSITION

Ji Zi Huang (Galli Vitellus)	2 yolks
E Jiao (Colla Corii Asini)	9g
Di Huang (Radix Rehmanniae)	18g
Mai Dong (Radix Ophiopogonis)	18g
Bai Shao (Radix Paeoniae Alba)	18g
Gui Ban (Plastrum Testudinis)	12g
Bie Jia (Carapax Trionycis)	12g
Mu Li (Concha Ostreae)	12g
Huo Ma Ren (Fructus Cannabis)	6g
Wu Wei Zi (Fructus Schisandrae Chinensis)	6g
Zhi Gan Cao (Radix et Rhizoma Glycyrrhizae Praeparata cum Melle)	12g

DOSAGE / PREPARATION / ADMINISTRATION

The source text states to cook the ingredients with 8 cups of water until the decoction is reduced to 3 cups. Discard the residue. Blend *Ji Zi Huang* (Galli Vitellus) into the strained decoction and take the resulting mixture in three equally divided doses daily.

CHINESE THERAPEUTIC ACTIONS

1. Nourishes yin
2. Extinguishes Liver wind

CLINICAL MANIFESTATIONS

Severe yin deficiency with Liver wind rising: extreme lack of energy, clonic convulsions, a deep red tongue body with a scanty tongue coating, and a deficient pulse.

VETERINARY CLINICAL APPLICATIONS

Stroke, spasms and cramps, seizures, trembling and shaking of the extremities, post-stroke insomnia, post-stroke paralysis, and encephalitis.

EXPLANATION

Da Ding Feng Zhu (Major Arrest Wind Pearl) treats severe yin deficiency with Liver wind rising. This condition may

***Da Ding Feng Zhu* (Major Arrest Wind Pearl)**

Diagnosis	Clinical Signs	Treatment	Herbs
Severe yin deficiency with Liver wind rising	• Depletion of energy and a deep red tongue with little coating: severe yin deficiency • Seizures, trembling, and shaking: Liver wind rising • Deficient pulse: deficiency condition	• Nourishes yin • Extinguishes Liver wind	• *Ji Zi Huang* (Galli Vitellus) and *E Jiao* (Colla Corii Asini) nourish yin and body fluids to extinguish Liver wind. • *Di Huang* (Radix Rehmanniae), *Mai Dong* (Radix Ophiopogonis) and *Bai Shao* (Radix Paeoniae Alba) nourish yin and soften the Liver. • *Gui Ban* (Plastrum Testudinis), *Bie Jia* (Carapax Trionycis) and *Mu Li* (Concha Ostreae) nourish yin and anchor the yang. • *Huo Ma Ren* (Fructus Cannabis) nourishes yin and moistens dryness. • *Wu Wei Zi* (Fructus Schisandrae Chinensis) and *Zhi Gan Cao* (Radix et Rhizoma Glycyrrhizae Praeparata cum Melle) enhance the yin-tonifying action of the other herbs.

Dà Dìng Fēng Zhū (Major Arrest Wind Pearl)

be caused by chronic *wen bing* (warm disease) disorders with heat consuming yin and fluids, or the inappropriate use of herbs leading to damage of yin and loss of fluids. Severe yin deficiency may lead to depletion of energy and a deep red tongue with little coating. Severe yin deficiency also contributes to Liver wind rising, which may cause clonic convulsions. A deficient pulse suggests severe yin deficiency. Animals with this condition are typically geriatric or greatly debilitated and have a strong tendency to go into shock. Animals for whom this formula is appropriate fall into two categories: those with chronic systemic disease, such as diabetes mellitus, hyperadrenocorticism, and chronic renal disease; and young animals with severe seizure disorders and deficiencies of Kidney yin and *jing* (essence). This pattern is common in animals that have been heavily and chronically medicated, and in multiparous females, particularly bitches, that have had multiple back-to-back pregnancies and poor nutrition.

This formula uses *Ji Zi Huang* (Galli Vitellus) and *E Jiao* (Colla Corii Asini) to nourish yin and body fluids to extinguish Liver wind. *Di Huang* (Radix Rehmanniae), *Mai Dong* (Radix Ophiopogonis), and *Bai Shao* (Radix Paeoniae Alba) nourish yin and soften the Liver. *Gui Ban* (Plastrum Testudinis), *Bie Jia* (Carapax Trionycis), and *Mu Li* (Concha Ostreae) nourish yin and anchor the yang. *Huo Ma Ren* (Fructus Cannabis) nourishes yin and moistens dryness. *Wu Wei Zi* (Fructus Schisandrae Chinensis) and *Zhi Gan Cao* (Radix et Rhizoma Glycyrrhizae Praeparata cum Melle) are sour and sweet herbs that enhance the yin-tonifying action of the other herbs in this formula.

VETERINARY MODIFICATIONS

- With dyspnea due to qi deficiency, add *Ren Shen* (Radix et Rhizoma Ginseng).
- With palpitations, add *Fu Shen* (Poria Paradicis), *Ren Shen* (Radix et Rhizoma Ginseng), and *Xiao Mai* (Fructus Tritici).
- With phlegm, add *Tian Zhu Huang* (Concretio Silicea Bambusae) and *Bei Mu* (Bulbus Fritillariae).
- With low-grade fever, add *Bai Wei* (Radix et Rhizoma Cynanchi Atrati) and *Di Gu Pi* (Cortex Lycii).

CAUTIONS / CONTRAINDICATIONS

Da Ding Feng Zhu should be used only for severe yin deficiency with no excess heat. It is not suitable for animals that have both severe yin deficiency and excess interior heat.

HUMAN CLINICAL STUDIES AND RESEARCH

1. **Post-stroke insomnia**: Thirty-six patients with post-stroke insomnia (an average of 3 months history of illness) were treated with marked effect using *Da Ding Feng Zhu*. The study reported an overall effectiveness of 94.4% (with at least 3 to 4 hours of sleep per night without the use of pharmaceutical drugs).[1]
2. **Post-stroke paralysis**: One hundred patients with post-stroke paralysis were treated with 98% effectiveness using both herbs and acupuncture. Herbal treatment varied depending on the diagnosis: modified *Da Ding Feng Zhu* was used for yin deficiency and yang excess; modified *Dao Tan Tang* (Guide Out Phlegm Decoction) was used for phlegm accumulation; modified *Bu Yang Huan Wu Tang* (Tonify the Yang to Restore Five Decoction) was used for qi deficiency and blood stagnation; and modified *Di Huang Yin Zi* (Rehmannia Decoction) was used for deficiency of *yuan* (source) *qi*. Acupuncture treatment included scalp or body acupuncture. The study noted that patients who received scalp acupuncture responded better than those who received body acupuncture.[2]
3. **Liver fibrosis**: One study reported beneficial effects using *Da Ding Feng Zhu* to treat liver fibrosis. Of 56 patients, 30 were treated with herbs and 26 were treated with colchicine. After 3 months of treatment, the study reported that the herb group had significantly lowered levels of hyaluronic acid (HA), procollagen III (PC-III), IV collagen (IV-C), and laminin (LN), while the drug group only had lowered levels of HA. The study concluded that *Da Ding Feng Zhu* is effective in lowering serum indices in liver fibrosis.[3]
4. **Encephalitis**: Administration of *Da Ding Feng Zhu* was beneficial in treating complications of encephalitis during recovery in 8 children. Complications of encephalitis included cognitive and speech impairment. The average duration of treatment was approximately one month.[4]

SUGGESTED ACUPUNCTURE TREATMENT

1. Points: *Ganshu* (BL 18), *Shenshu* (BL 23), *Taixi* (KI 3), *Zhaohai* (KI 6), *Sanyinjiao* (SP 6), *Taichong* (LR 3), *Baihui* (GV 20), and *Longhui*.
2. Technique: tonification.

Ganshu (BL 18), *Shenshu* (BL 23), *Taixi* (KI 3), *Zhaohai* (KI 6), and *Sanyinjiao* (SP 6) tonify Liver and Kidney yin to treat the underlying yin deficiency. *Taichong* (LR 3), *Baihui* (GV 20), and *Longhui*, on the other hand, calm Liver wind that arises as a result of yin deficiency.

Dà Dìng Fēng Zhū (Major Arrest Wind Pearl)

AUTHORS' COMMENTS

Da Ding Feng Zhu contains herbs to nourish yin and extinguish wind. It extinguishes Liver wind by treating the root (deficiency of yin). This formula is not readily available commercially, but it can be formulated via special order from many major herbal companies. It is valuable to use in animals that have intractable seizures, weakness and constant trembling of the rear legs, and in patients debilitated from chemotherapy or chronic febrile disease.

References

1. *Zhong Yi Han Shou Tong Xun* (Reports of Chinese Medicine), 1993; 5:43.
2. *Shan Xi Zhong Yi* (Shanxi Chinese Medicine), 1987; 1:19.
3. Li W, Wang C, Zhang J. Effects of da ding feng zhu decoction in 30 cases of liver fibrosis. Journal of Traditional Chinese Medicine. 2003 Dec; 23(4):251-4.
4. *Hu Bei Zhong Yi Za Zhi* (Hubei Journal of Chinese Medicine), 1982; 6:51.

Chapter 14 — Summary

— Wind-Expelling Formulas

SECTION 1: EXTERNAL WIND-RELEASING FORMULAS

Name	Similarities	Differences
Xiao Feng San (Eliminate Wind Powder)	Expel wind, nourish the blood	Clears wind-dampness, dispels wind-heat
Dang Gui Yin Zi (Tangkuei Decoction)		Tonifies the blood, moistens dryness
Qian Zheng San (Lead to Symmetry Powder)	Dispels wind, resolves phlegm	Dispels wind from the face, treats spasms, cramps, and deviation of the eyes and mouth
Wu Yao Shun Qi San (Lindera Powder to Smooth the Flow of Qi)	Dispels wind, treats *zhong feng* (wind stroke)	Dispels wind from the body, activates qi circulation, relieves pain

Xiao Feng San (Eliminate Wind Powder) and ***Dang Gui Yin Zi*** (Tangkuei Decoction) treat skin disorders characterized by wind at the exterior and blood deficiency in the interior.

- *Xiao Feng San* treats rashes, atopic dermatitis, and other skin disorders arising from wind, dampness, and heat invasion. It clears wind-dampness and wind-heat, and nourishes and cools the blood.
- *Dang Gui Yin Zi* treats atopic dermatitis, rash, urticaria, and other skin conditions due to wind at the exterior and blood deficiency and dryness in the interior. It tonifies the blood, moistens dryness, and releases wind.

Qian Zheng San (Lead to Symmetry Powder) dispels wind and dissolves phlegm. It treats wind attacking the face, characterized by facial spasms and deviation of the eyes and mouth. The cause is blockage of the channels and collaterals by wind and phlegm.

Wu Yao Shun Qi San (Lindera Powder to Smooth the Flow of Qi) dispels wind to treat *zhong feng* (wind stroke). It activates qi circulation and opens the channels and collaterals. It treats wind attacking the body, with complications such as joint pain, numbness and pain throughout the body, dysphasia, stiffness of the muscles and tendons, and paralysis.

Chapter 14 — Summary

SECTION 2: INTERNAL WIND-EXTINGUISHING FORMULAS

Name	Similarities	Differences
Gou Teng San (Uncaria Powder)	Calm the Liver, extinguish Liver wind	Clears Liver heat, sedates Liver yang, extinguishes Liver wind
Zhen Gan Xi Feng Tang (Sedate the Liver and Extinguish Wind Decoction)		Nourishes Liver and Kidney yin
Jian Ling Tang (Construct Roof Tiles Decoction)		Nourishes yin, calms the *shen* (spirit)
Tian Ma Gou Teng Yin (Gastrodia and Uncaria Decoction)		Tonifies the Liver and Kidney
Da Ding Feng Zhu (Major Arrest Wind Pearl)	Extinguishes Liver wind, nourishes yin	Strongly nourishes yin and tonifies the blood

Gou Teng San (Uncaria Powder) primarily treats Liver excess conditions characterized by Liver heat, Liver yang, and Liver wind rising. Clinical manifestations include seizures, trembling, palpitations, and marked changes in emotions and behavior.

Zhen Gan Xi Feng Tang (Sedate the Liver and Extinguish Wind Decoction) can be used for Liver yang and wind rising due to Liver and Kidney yin deficiencies. Clinical manifestations include hypertension, redness and swelling of the eyes, itching of the skin, irritability, a red face, belching, a wiry, forceful pulse, and, in severe cases, seizures.

Jian Ling Tang (Construct Roof Tiles Decoction) treats mild to moderate cases of Liver yang rising with *shen* (spirit) disturbance. Clinical manifestations include hypertension, palpitations, poor concentration and performance, irritability, restlessness, night restlessness and a wiry, pulse.

Tian Ma Gou Teng Yin (Gastrodia and Uncaria Decoction) clears heat, activates the blood, and calms the *shen* (spirit). It is used for Liver yang and wind rising, with signs such as trembling and shaking of the extremities and seizure disorders.

Da Ding Feng Zhu (Major Arrest Wind Pearl) calms Liver wind and strongly tonifies yin and blood. It is used for severe yin deficiency with Liver wind. Clinical signs include intractable seizures, lack of energy, a deep red tongue with a scanty tongue coating, and a deficient pulse.

Chapter 15

— Dryness-Relieving Formulas

治燥剂

陶弘景 Tăo Hóng-Jĭng

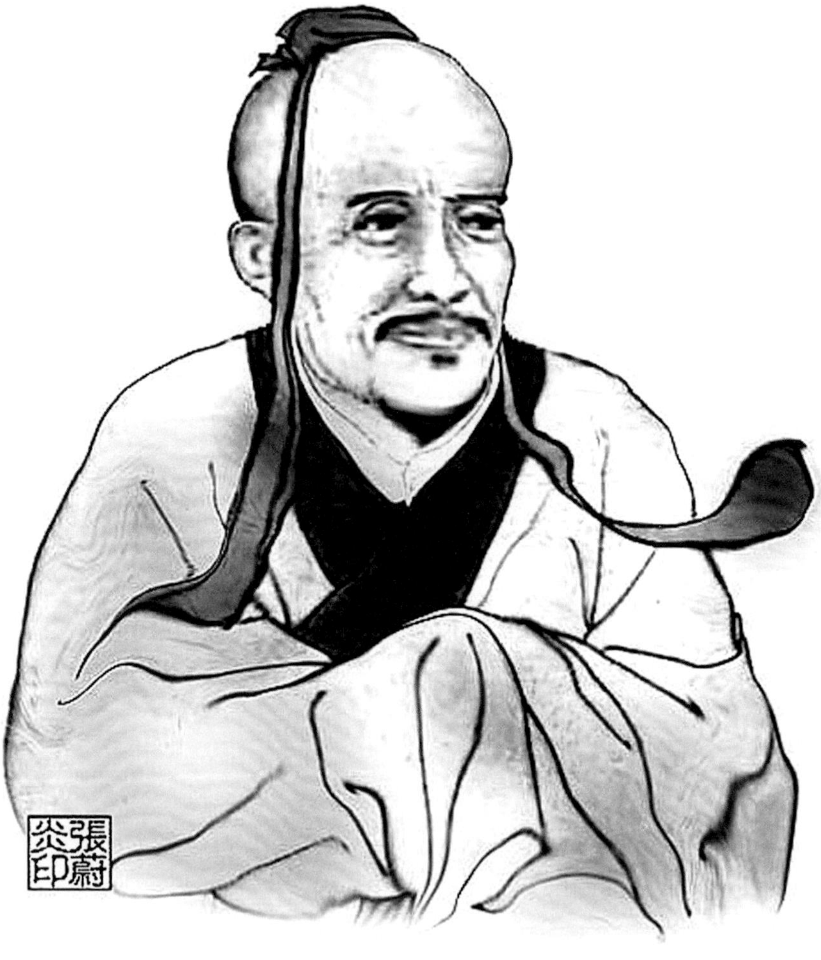

陶弘景 Tăo Hóng-Jĭng, 456 – 536.

陶弘景 Tăo Hóng-Jĭng

The greatest contribution of Tao Hong-Jing to medicine was his revision of the 神农本草经 *Shen Nong Ben Cao Jing* (Divine Husbandman's Classic of the Materia Medica). A few hundred years after its publication in the second century CE, many parts of this text were missing. While many physicians attempted to restore the text to its original state, some filled the gaps with erroneous information, others inadvertently deleted original text, and none differentiated their personal input from the materials of the source text. As a result, this classic text became marred by errors, duplications and missing parts.

Tao embarked on a mission to restore and expand upon this classic text. In addition to the 365 medicinal substances listed in the original text, he added another 365 of the most useful medicinal substances of his time. He also expanded the contents to include subjects such as the processing of herbs, treatment of diseases, herbal antidotes for poisoning, cautions and contraindications, and herb-herb interactions. Furthermore, to distinguish the original work from his personal input, he marked the original work in red, and his own in black. Published in 480-498, 本草经集注 *Ben Cao Jing Ji Zhu* (Collection of Commentaries on the Classic of the Materia Medica) is a text of great historical importance. Not only did it restore and preserve one of the most important works in traditional Chinese medicine, it expanded the clinical usefulness of the work and had an incredible influence on later generations of practitioners.

Dynasties & Kingdoms	Year
Xia Dynasty 夏	2100-1600 BCE
Shang Dynasty 商	1600-1100 BCE
Zhou Dynasty 周	1100-221 BCE
Qin Dynasty 秦	221-207 BCE
Han Dynasty 漢	206 BCE-220
Three Kingdoms 三國	220-280
Western Jin Dynasty 西晉	265-316
Eastern Jin Dynasty 東晉	317-420
Northern and Southern Dynasties 北南朝	**420-581**
Sui Dynasty 隋	581-618
Tang Dynasty 唐	618-907
Five Dynasties 五代	907-960
Song Dynasty 宋	960-1279
Liao Dynasty 遼	916-1125
Jin Dynasty 金	1115-1234
Yuan Dynasty 元	1271-1368
Ming Dynasty 明	1368-1644
Qing Dynasty 清	1644-1911
Republic of China 中華民國	1912-Present Day
People's Republic of China 中華人民共和國	1949-Present Day

Table of Contents

Chapter 15 — Overview

治燥剂 — Dryness-Relieving Formulas

Definition: Dryness-relieving formulas disperse and moisten external dryness and nourish and moisten internal dryness.

Dryness is one of the *liu yin* (six exogenous factors) or climatic factors; it consumes and depletes body fluids and has a tendency to injure yin and blood. It is a yang pathogenic factor that may be contracted externally or develop internally. These two presentations—external and internal dryness—have many similarities. Due to the inter-relationships among the different *zang fu* organs and regions of the body, differentiation between external and internal dryness is not always straightforward. In general, dryness-relieving formulas disperse and moisten external dryness and nourish and moisten internal dryness. Conversely, if formulas that enrich yin and moisten dryness (appropriate for internal dryness) are used when the external pathogenic influence is still present, it will cause that influence to linger and may exacerbate the condition. It is important to properly distinguish between external and internal dryness, because if herbs that disperse dryness at the exterior are mistakenly used in cases of internal dryness with yin deficiency, they will aggravate injury to qi and yin.

External dryness is often associated with the environment to which a patient is exposed. It often appears during the autumn months, as summer dampness vanishes and autumn dryness appears. It follows that dryness is a common pathogenic factor in arid or desert climates and can also be artificially produced by central heating and air conditioning, irrespective of the season or location. Dryness usually enters the body through the nose and mouth, and the organ most affected by external dryness is the Lung. External dryness may affect the body and cause the following clinical signs: fever, aversion to cold, dry mouth, sore throat, dry coughing, or coughing with scanty sputum. External dryness may combine with coolness (which usually appears in the late fall and early winter when the environment starts to turn cold) or warmth (which usually is present in the late summer and early fall when the environment is still warm). The treatment approach for external dryness is to ventilate and disperse the dryness. In cases of dryness complicated by coolness or warmth, add herbs accordingly to treat the associated conditions.

Internal dryness is the most common cause of pathological dryness seen in veterinary medicine. Internal dryness may occur as a result of chronic illness, febrile disease, chronic medication, prolonged vomiting or diarrhea, overfeeding of hot, dry foods, blood deficiency, chronic over-training, over-breeding, and the inappropriate use of acrid and warm herbs. All of these conditions result in consumption of body fluids and damage to *jing* (essence) and yin of the *zang fu* organs. The organs most often affected are the Stomach, Lung, Spleen, Kidney and Large Intestine. Depending on which of these *zang fu* organs are most affected, internal dryness is classified into three groups: upper, middle, or lower *jiao* dryness syndromes. Upper *jiao* dryness affects the Lung and leads to dry coughing. Middle *jiao* dryness affects the Spleen and Stomach and leads to vomiting and lack of appetite, or dry heat with ravenous appetite and constant hunger. Lower *jiao* dryness may affect the Kidney and lead to *xiao ke* (wasting and thirsting) syndrome. Lower *jiao* dryness may also affect the Large Intestine, causing dry stool, constipation and impaction. One of the most common reasons for dryness in cats and dogs is the consumption of hot, damp or hot, dry foods. These foods deplete Stomach yin and eventually result in Kidney yin deficiency and the development of *xiao ke*

Chapter 15 — Overview

(wasting and thirsting) syndrome, such as diabetes and hyperadrenocorticism. Overtraining is the most common pattern of dryness in the horse and most commonly affects the Lung and leads to chronic, dry cough, mild cases of heaves, and skin disorders.

The treatment plan for internal dryness is to moisten the dryness and nourish yin of the affected *zang fu* organ(s) in the affected *jiao*(s). However, dryness-relieving formulas contain rich, cloying herbs, which may obstruct the qi flow and lead to gastrointestinal upset. They promote dampness and should not be used without modification in animals with dampness and deficiency of the middle *jiao*. Common conditions for which dryness-relieving formulas are used in veterinary medicine include: acute and chronic bronchitis, bronchiectasis, emphysema, upper respiratory tract infection, recovery from pneumonia, spontaneous pneumothorax, neoplasia of the nose, throat and lungs, gastritis, gastric ulcers, habitual constipation, recovery from infectious diseases, and endocrinopathies (diabetes mellitus, diabetes insipidus, hyperadrenocorticism).

SUBCATEGORIES OF ACTION

Dryness may affect the exterior and interior parts of the body. Similarly, dryness-relieving formulas are divided into dispersing and moistening formulas to treat external dryness, and nourishing and moistening formulas to treat internal dryness.

1. **Dispersing and Moistening Formulas**

   These formulas are designed to treat external dryness, which may be complicated by other *liu yin* (six exogenous factors) and become cool-dryness or warmth-dryness.

   - External cool-dryness is the result of the combination of cold and dry pathogenic factors that usually occur in the late fall and early winter as the environment becomes increasing cold and dry. As cool-dryness dominates the environment, it may attack the Lung and lead to such clinical signs as aversion to cold, coughing, nasal congestion, dry mouth, and dry throat. Thus, external cool-dryness should be treated with warm herbs that gently disperse and moisten dryness, such as *Zi Su Ye* (Folium Perillae), *Jie Geng* (Radix Platycodonis), *Qian Hu* (Radix Peucedani), and *Xing Ren* (Semen Armeniacae Amarum). One exemplar formula is *Xing Su San* (Apricot Kernel and Perilla Leaf Powder).
   - External warmth-dryness is the result of the combination of heat and dryness pathogenic factors that usually occur in the late summer and early fall when the environment is still relatively warm and dry. When these pathogens attack the Lung, they cause clinical signs such as fever, dry coughing, dyspnea, irritability, and thirst. This condition of warmth-dryness should be treated with cold herbs that gently disperse and moisten dryness, such as *Sang Ye* (Folium Mori), *Xing Ren* (Semen Armeniacae Amarum), *Nan Sha Shen* (Radix Adenophorae), *Bei Sha Shen* (Radix Glehniae), and *Mai Dong* (Radix Ophiopogonis). Exemplar formulas include *Sang Xing Tang* (Mulberry Leaf and Apricot Kernel Decoction) and *Qing Zao Jiu Fei Tang* (Eliminate Dryness and Rescue the Lung Decoction).

2. **Nourishing and Moistening Formulas**

   These formulas treat internal dryness syndromes characterized by lack of yin and body fluids in the *zang fu* organs. Clinical manifestations and treatment vary, depending on the affected area.

   - Upper *jiao* dryness affects the Lung and may cause dry coughing with scanty or no sputum, dry mouth and throat, and wheezing. This condition usually is treated with herbs and formulas that nourish and moisten the dryness in the Lung, such as *Nan Sha Shen* (Radix Adenophorae), *Bei Sha Shen* (Radix Glehniae), *Tian Dong* (Radix Asparagi), *Mai Dong* (Radix Ophiopogonis), and *Bai He Gu Jin Tang* (Lily Bulb Decoction to Preserve the Metal).
   - Middle *jiao* dryness affects the Stomach and leads to vomiting, lack of appetite or ravenous appetite, thirst, and a dry mouth and throat. This condition usually is treated with herbs and formulas that nourish and moisten the dryness in the Spleen and Stomach, such as *Shi Hu* (Caulis Dendrobii),

Chapter 15 — Overview

Yu Zhu (Rhizoma Polygonati Odorati), *Mai Dong* (Radix Ophiopogonis), and *Mai Men Dong Tang* (Ophiopogonis Decoction).

- Lower *jiao* dryness affects the Kidney and leads to *xiao ke* (wasting and thirsting) syndrome. This condition is usually treated with herbs and formulas that nourish and moisten dryness in the Kidney, such as *Di Huang* (Radix Rehmanniae), *Shu Di Huang* (Radix Rehmanniae Praeparata), *Nu Zhen Zi* (Fructus Ligustri Lucidi), and *Yu Ye Tang* (Jade Fluid Decoction).
- Lower *jiao* dryness may also affect the Large Intestine and cause dry stool, constipation and impaction. This condition is usually treated with herbs and formulas that nourish and moisten the dryness in the Large Intestine, such as *Xuan Shen* (Radix Scrophulariae) and *Zeng Ye Tang* (Increase the Fluids Decoction).

CAUTIONS / CONTRAINDICATIONS

- When treating dryness disorders, it is important to note that dryness can easily transform into heat and begin to damage yin and consume qi. Therefore, in addition to using dryness-relieving herbs, it is often necessary to add herbs to clear heat, purge fire, tonify qi, and promote the generation of body fluids.
- Animals with dryness disorders should not be treated with acrid and aromatic herbs that consume qi, or bitter and drying herbs that injure yin, as the use of these herbs will only deplete more qi and yin.
- Dryness-relieving formulas have nourishing and moistening effects and, as such, are often heavy and greasy in nature. Prolonged or excessive use of these formulas will create internal dampness and stagnation of qi. Therefore, these formulas should be used with caution in animals with Spleen qi deficiency and loose stools, qi stagnation, phlegm stagnation, and damp accumulation. It is often necessary to combine these formulas with herbs that tonify the Spleen and Stomach to promote their digestion and absorption by the body.

PHARMACOLOGICAL EFFECTS & CLINICAL APPLICATIONS

In traditional Chinese medicine, dryness-relieving formulas are generally used to treat imbalances of the Lung, Stomach, Kidney, and Large Intestine. From a biomedical perspective, these formulas are most effective in treating chronic respiratory disorders, gastrointestinal (stomach and intestines) disorders, and metabolic disorders.

- **Respiratory disorders**: Dryness-relieving formulas are very effective for treating chronic cases of respiratory disorders. Clinical indications include cough,[1,2,3,4] postinfectious cough,[5,6] dyspnea,[7] pneumonia,[8] chronic bronchitis,[9] bronchiectasis,[10] pneumothorax,[11] pulmonary tuberculosis,[12] and lung cancer.[13] The mechanisms of action for dryness-relieving formulas have been attributed in part to antitussive,[14] mucoactive,[15] and antibiotic effects of the herbs.[16] Exemplar formulas include *Xing Su San* (Apricot Kernel and Perilla Leaf Powder), *Qing Zao Jiu Fei Tang* (Eliminate Dryness and Rescue the Lung Decoction), *Sha Shen Mai Dong Tang* (Glehnia and Ophiopogonis Decoction), *Bai He Gu Jin Tang* (Lily Bulb Decoction to Preserve the Metal), and *Mai Men Dong Tang* (Ophiopogonis Decoction),
- **Gastrointestinal disorders**: Dryness-relieving formulas are effective in treating chronic cases of gastrointestinal disorders. Indications include, but are not limited to, atrophic gastritis,[17,18] chronic gastritis,[19] chronic atrophic gastritis,[20] chronic peptic ulcer disease,[21] and constipation.[22] Representative formulas include *Sha Shen Mai Dong Tang* (Glehnia and Ophiopogonis Decoction) and *Mai Men Dong Tang* (Ophiopogonis Decoction).
- **Diabetes mellitus**: Administration of certain dryness-relieving herbs and formulas has been shown to have hypoglycemic effect to lower plasma glucose levels.[23,24,25,26] Formulas that have been shown to be effective in treating diabetes mellitus include *Sha Shen Mai Dong Tang* (Glehnia and Ophiopogonis Decoction),[27] *Bai He Gu Jin Tang* (Lily Bulb Decoction to Preserve the Metal),[28] *Yu Ye Tang* (Jade Fluid Decoction),[29] and *Zeng Ye Tang* (Increase the Fluids Decoction).[30]
- **Bleeding**: Dryness-relieving formulas do not have direct or potent action to stop bleeding. Rather, they are generally used to treat chronic cases of lung and stomach disorders accompanied by

Chapter 15 — Overview

nosebleeds and coughing or vomiting of blood. *Qing Zao Jiu Fei Tang* (Eliminate Dryness and Rescue the Lung Decoction) is commonly used to treat epistaxis, hemoptysis, and hematemesis.[31,32,33]

- **Infection and inflammation**: Some dryness-relieving formulas have antibiotic and anti-inflammatory effects[34,35] and have been used for such conditions as sore throat,[36] laryngitis,[37,38] tonsillitis,[39] pharyngitis,[40] and cheilitis.[41] One exemplar formula is *Zeng Ye Tang* (Increase the Fluids Decoction).

References

1. *Guang Xi Zhong Yi Yao* (Guangxi Chinese Medicine and Herbology), 1985, 6:37.
2. *Shan Xi Zhong Yi* (Shanxi Chinese Medicine), 1992, 11:492.
3. *Shan Xi Zhong Yi* (Shanxi Chinese *Medicine*), 1993, 9:413.
4. Watanabe N, Gang C, Fukuda T. The effects of bakumondo-to (Mai-Men-Dong-Tang) on asthmatic and non-asthmatic patients with increased cough sensitivity. Nihon Kokyuki Gakkai Zasshi. 2004 Jan;42(1):49-55.
5. Isohama Y, Kai H, Miyata T. Bakumondo-to, a traditional herbal medicine, stimulates phosphatidylcholine secretion, through the synergistic cross-talk between different signal transduction systems in alveolar type II cells. Nippon Yakurigaku Zasshi. 1997 Oct;110 Suppl 1:120P-125P.
6. Fujimori K, Suzuki E, Arakawa M. Clinical features of postinfectious chronic cough. Arerugi. 1997 May;46(5):420-5.
7. *Si Chuan Zhong Yi* (Sichuan Chinese Medicine), 1989, 2:19.
8. *He Bei Zhong Yi* (Hebei Chinese Medicine), 1998, 1:40.
9. *Guo Wai Yi Xue* (Foreign Medicine), 1993, 6:29.
10. *Hu Bei Zhong Yi Za Zhi* (Hubei Journal of Chinese Medicine), 1995, 5:14.
11. *Xin Yi Xue* (New Medicine), 1977, 4-5:197.
12. *Zhong Guo Zhong Xi Yi Jie He Za Zhi* (Chinese Journal of Integrative Chinese and Western Medicine), 1991, 2:119.
13. *Hei Long Jiang Zhong Yi Yao* (Heilongjiang Chinese Medicine and Herbology), 1982, 4:25.
14. Kamei J, Nakamura R, Ichiki H, Kubo M. Antitussive principles of Glycyrrhizae radix, a main component of the Kampo preparations Bakumondo-to (Mai-men-dong-tang). Eur J Pharmacol. 2003 May 23;469(1-3):159-63.
15. Miyata T. Novel approach to respiratory pharmacology--pharmacological basis of cough, sputum and airway clearance. Yakugaku Zasshi. 2003 Dec;123(12):987-1006.
16. *Fu Jian Zhong Yi Yao* (Fujian Chinese Medicine and Herbology), 1964, 9:1.
17. *Zhong Xi Yi Jie He Za Zhi* (Journal of Integrated Chinese and Western Medicine), 1986, 6:342.
18. *Zhe Jiang Zhong Yi Za Zhi* (Zhejiang Journal of Chinese Medicine), 1990, 10:437.
19. *An Hui Zhong Yi Xue Yuan Xue Bao* (Journal of Anhui University School of Medicine), 1994, 2:25.
20. *Shi Yong Zhong Xi Yi Jie He Za Zhi* (Practical Journal of Integrated Chinese and Western Medicines), 1998, 7:631.
21. *Zhong Yi Za Zhi* (Journal of Chinese Medicine), 1964, 11:11.
22. *Zhong Yi Ming Fang Lin Chuang Xin Yong* (Contemporary Clinical Applications of Classic Chinese Formulas), 2001, 723.
23. Miyata T. Novel approach to respiratory pharmacology--pharmacological basis of cough, sputum and airway clearance. Yakugaku Zasshi. 2003 Dec;123(12):987-1006.
24. *Zhong Yao Tong Bao* (Journal of Chinese Herbology), 1994, 4:33.
25. *Zhong Yao Yao Li Yu Lin Chuang* (Pharmacology and Clinical Applications of Chinese Herbs), 1992: 21.
26. *Zhong Yao Tong Bao* (Journal of Chinese Herbology), 1982, 6:32.
27. *Shan Xi Zhong Yi* (Shanxi Chinese Medicine), 1995, 11:482.
28. *Yun Nan Zhong Yi Za Zhi* (Yunan Journal of Chinese Medicine), 1995, 4:22.
29. *Shan Xi Zhong Yi* (Shanxi Chinese Medicine), 1991, 2:51.
30. *Zhong Yi Za Zhi* (Journal of Chinese Medicine), 1985, 6:31.
31. *Gui Yang Zhong Yi Xue Yuan Xue Bao* (Journal of Guiyang Chinese Medical University), 1992, 4:47.
32. *Bei Jing Zhong Yi* (Beijing Chinese Medicine), 1996, 1:22.
33. *Nan Jing Zhong Yi Xue Yuan Xue Bao* (Journal of Nanjing University of Traditional Chinese Medicine), 1989, 4:25.
34. *Zhong Guo Zhong Xi Yi Jie He Za Zhi* (Chinese Journal of Integrative Chinese and Western Medicine), 1982, 2:153.
35. *Fu Jian Zhong Yi Yao* (Fujian Chinese Medicine and Herbology), 1964, 9:1.
36. *Shi Yong Zhong Xi Yi Jie He Za Zhi* (Practical Journal of Integrated Chinese and Western Medicines), 1992, 5(9):533.
37. *Zhong Yi Za Zhi* (Journal of Chinese Medicine), 1984, 4:50.
38. *Shan Xi Zhong Yi* (Shanxi Chinese Medicine), 1995, 5:203.
39. *Zhong Hua Er Bi Hou Ke Za Zhi* (Chinese Journal of Otolaryngology), 1958, 6:445.
40. *Shan Xi Zhong Yi* (Shanxi Chinese Medicine), 1992, 6:248.
41. *Si Chuan Zhong Yi* (Sichuan Chinese Medicine), 1986, 12:48.

Section 1

轻宣润燥剂
— Dispersing and Moistening Formulas

Xing Sū Sǎn (Apricot Kernel and Perilla Leaf Powder)
杏蘇散
杏苏散

Pinyin Name: *Xing Su San*
Literal Name: Apricot Kernel and Perilla Leaf Powder
Alternate Names: *Hsing Su San*, Apricot and Perilla Powder, Apricot Seed and Perilla Formula
Original Source: *Wen Bing Tiao Bian* (Systematic Differentiation of Warm Diseases) by Wu Ju-Tong in 1798

COMPOSITION

Zi Su Ye (Folium Perillae)	[6-9g]
Qian Hu (Radix Peucedani)	[6-9g]
Ku Xing Ren (Semen Armeniacae Amarum)	[6-9g]
Jie Geng (Radix Platycodonis)	[6g]
Ban Xia (Rhizoma Pinelliae)	[6-9g]
Fu Ling (Poria)	[6-9g]
Zhi Qiao (Fructus Citri Aurantii)	[6g]
Chen Pi (Pericarpium Citri Reticulatae)	[6g]
Sheng Jiang (Rhizoma Zingiberis Recens)	[6g]
Da Zao (Fructus Jujubae)	[6g]
Gan Cao (Radix et Rhizoma Glycyrrhizae)	[3-6g]

DOSAGE / PREPARATION / ADMINISTRATION

The source text lists the ingredients of this formula, but does not specify the doses and preparation. Today, this formula may be prepared as a decoction with the doses suggested in brackets.

CHINESE THERAPEUTIC ACTIONS

1. Dispels cool-dryness
2. Ventilates the Lung and dissolves phlegm

CLINICAL MANIFESTATIONS

Exterior syndrome of cool-dryness: aversion to cold, sneezing, coughing with thin sputum, stuffy nose, a dry mouth, and a wiry pulse.

VETERINARY CLINICAL APPLICATIONS

Acute feline and equine upper respiratory tract infection, canine infectious tracheobronchitis, nasal congestion, tracheitis, cough, and dyspnea.

EXPLANATION

Xing Su San (Apricot Kernel and Perilla Leaf Powder) dispels exterior cool-dryness and ventilates Lung qi. If the cool-dryness factors invade the exterior parts of the body, then clinical signs such as aversion to cold will occur, without sweating. The cool-dryness factors also may invade the Lung, compromising its function of distributing water. As a result, water accumulates and turns into phlegm and causes clinical signs such as coughing, stuffy nose, and a dry mouth.

In this formula, *Zi Su Ye* (Folium Perillae) and *Qian Hu* (Radix Peucedani) gently induce sweating to release the exterior cool-dryness factors. *Ku Xing Ren* (Semen Armeniacae Amarum) and *Jie Geng* (Radix Platycodonis) ventilate the Lung and regulate Lung qi to relieve coughing. *Ban Xia* (Rhizoma Pinelliae) and *Fu Ling* (Poria) eliminate dampness and dissolve phlegm. *Zhi Qiao* (Fructus Aurantii) and *Chen Pi* (Pericarpium Citri Reticulatae)

Xìng Sū Sǎn (Apricot Kernel and Perilla Leaf Powder)

***Xing Su San* (Apricot Kernel and Perilla Leaf Powder)**

Diagnosis	Clinical Signs	Treatment	Herbs
Exterior cool-dryness	• Aversion to cold and absence of sweating: exterior cool-dryness • Sneezing, coughing with thin sputum, and a stuffy nose: obstructed Lung qi circulation • Wiry pulse: interior phlegm	• Dispels cool-dryness • Ventilates the Lung and regulates Lung qi circulation • Dissolves phlegm	• *Zi Su Ye* (Folium Perillae) and *Qian Hu* (Radix Peucedani) release the exterior cool-dryness. • *Ku Xing Ren* (Semen Armeniacae Amarum) and *Jie Geng* (Radix Platycodonis) ventilate the Lung and regulate Lung qi. • *Zhi Qiao* (Fructus Aurantii) and *Chen Pi* (Pericarpium Citri Reticulatae) regulate the Lung qi. • *Ban Xia* (Rhizoma Pinelliae) and *Fu Ling* (Poria) eliminate dampness and dissolve phlegm. • *Sheng Jiang* (Rhizoma Zingiberis Recens) and *Da Zao* (Fructus Jujubae) harmonize the *ying* (nutritive) and *wei* (defensive) levels. • *Gan Cao* (Radix et Rhizoma Glycyrrhizae) harmonizes all of the herbs.

regulate Lung qi and expand the chest. *Sheng Jiang* (Rhizoma Zingiberis Recens), *Da Zao* (Fructus Jujubae), and *Gan Cao* (Radix et Rhizoma Glycyrrhizae) harmonize the *ying* (nutritive) and *wei* (defensive) levels.

VETERINARY MODIFICATIONS

- With more heat or fever, add *Chai Hu* (Radix Bupleuri) and *Huang Qin* (Radix Scutellariae).
- With thirst and dry mouth, add *Huang Qin* (Radix Scutellariae) and *Shi Gao* (Gypsum Fibrosum).
- With wind-cold at the exterior, add *Fang Feng* (Radix Saposhnikoviae) and *Jing Jie* (Herba Schizonepetae).
- For severe cough, add *Zi Wan* (Radix et Rhizoma Asteris) and *Kuan Dong Hua* (Flos Farfarae).
- For productive cough with phlegm, add *Er Chen Tang* (Two-Cured Decoction).
- For cough and dyspnea due to wind-cold invasion, add *Ding Chuan Tang* (Arrest Wheezing Decoction).
- In the absence of sweating, with a wiry or tight pulse, add *Qiang Huo* (Rhizoma et Radix Notopterygii).

CAUTIONS/CONTRAINDICTIONS

- *Xing Su San* is an acrid and warm formula that treats exterior cool-dryness or wind-cold. It should not be used if the condition is characterized by warm-dryness or wind-heat.
- This formula is gentle in nature and potency. It should only be used for mild-to-moderate cases of exterior cool-dryness or wind-cold conditions. Those with severe exterior conditions may require stronger acrid and warm exterior-releasing herbs, such as *Ma Huang* (Herba Ephedrae), *Gui Zhi* (Ramulus Cinnamomi) and *Qiang Huo* (Rhizoma et Radix Notopterygii).

HUMAN CLINICAL STUDIES AND RESEARCH

1. **Cough**: Administration of modified *Xing Su San* was shown in numerous studies to effectively treat various types of cough. One study of 560 patients with cough due to an exterior condition reported complete recovery in 478 patients, significant improvement in 47 patients, moderate improvement in 16 patients, and no effect in 19 patients. The herbal formula contained *Ku Xing Ren* (Semen Armeniacae Amarum) 9g, *Zi Su Ye* (Folium Perillae) 9g, *Qian Hu* (Radix Peucedani) 12g, *Ban Xia* (Rhizoma Pinelliae) 9g, *Chen Pi* (Pericarpium Citri Reticulatae) 9g, *Sha Shen* (Radix Glehniae seu Adenophorae) 15g, *Gua Lou* (Fructus Trichosanthis) 12g, *Sang Bai Pi* (Cortex Mori) 12g, *Bei Mu* (Bulbus Fritillariae) 9g, *Jie Geng* (Radix Platycodonis) 9g, and *Gan Cao* (Radix et Rhizoma Glycyrrhizae) 6g. The herbs were cooked in water, and decoction taken in two equally-divided doses daily.[1]
2. **Coughing and dyspnea**: Use of modified *Xing Su San* was associated with a 95% rate of effectiveness in treating 57 children with coughing and dyspnea. The herbal formula contained *Ku Xing Ren* (Semen Armeniacae Amarum) 9g, *Qian Hu* (Radix Peucedani) 9g, *Fu Ling* (Poria) 9g, *Huang Qin* (Radix Scutellariae) 9g, *Jie Geng* (Radix Platycodonis) 6g, *Ban Xia* (Rhizoma Pinelliae) 6g, *Gan Cao* (Radix et Rhizoma Glycyrrhizae) 6g, *Chen Pi* (Pericarpium Citri Reticulatae) 6g, *Sang Bai Pi* (Cortex Mori) 6g, and *Bai Bu* (Radix Stemonae) 10g. The herbs were cooked in water, and decoction taken in three equally-divided doses daily. Of 57 patients, the study reported complete recovery in 38 patients, improvement in 16 patients, and no benefit in 3 patients. The duration of treatment ranged from 3 to 9 packs of herbs.[2]

Xìng Sū Sǎn (Apricot Kernel and Perilla Leaf Powder)

SUGGESTED ACUPUNCTURE TREATMENT

1. Points: *Fengchi* (GB 20), *Lieque* (LU 7), *Hegu* (LI 4), *Yinlingquan* (SP 9), *Fenglong* (ST 40), *Neiguan* (PC 6) and *Dingchuan*.
2. Technique: sedation.

Fengchi (GB 20) relieves exterior clinical signs through its wind-dispersing action. *Lieque* (LU 7), the *luo* (connecting) point of the Lung channel, and *Hegu* (LI 4), the *yuan* (source) point of the Large Intestine channel, ventilate the Lung, regulate qi, and stop coughing. *Yinlingquan* (SP 9) and *Fenglong* (ST 40) dissolve dampness and dispel phlegm. *Neiguan* (PC 6) regulates qi and relieves chest congestion. *Dingchuan* is a classical point used for cough and to support the Lung.

AUTHORS' COMMENTS

Xing Su San can be used to treat early cases of upper respiratory tract infection and infectious tracheobronchitis caused by wind, cold and dryness in veterinary patients. This formula is particularly effective for those conditions contracted during the change of season in autumn. This formula is not appropriate for use when heat signs (fever and yellow ocular or nasal discharge) are present. For significant nasal congestion, it can be combined with *Qing Bi Tang* (Clear the Nose Decoction) or *Cang Er Zi San* (Xanthium Powder).

Xing Su San is the representative formula for treating cough due to cool-dryness affecting the Lung. This type of cough occurs commonly in areas where the weather is cold and dry.

Xing Su San, *Sang Xing Tang* (Mulberry Leaf and Apricot Kernel Decoction), and *Qing Zao Jiu Fei Tang* (Eliminate Dryness and Rescue the Lungs Decoction) all treat dryness attacking the Lung.

- *Xing Su San* has a mild action to treat cool-dryness attacking the Lung, when the chief complaints are sneezing, coughing with thin, white sputum, and nasal obstruction.
- *Sang Xing Tang* has a moderate action to treat warmth-dryness attacking the Lung. It is used mainly for mild to moderate cases of warmth-dryness, with clinical sign of cough with scanty or no sputum.
- *Qing Zao Jiu Fei Tang* has potent function to treat warmth-dryness attacking the Lung. It is used for severe cases of warmth-dryness attacking the Lung, with chief manifestations of fever, thirst, cough, dyspnea, and chest and hypochondriac pain.[3]

References

1. *Guang Xi Zhong Yi Yao* (Guangxi Chinese Medicine and Herbology), 1985; 6:37.
2. *Si Chuan Zhong Yi* (Sichuan Chinese Medicine), 1989; 2:19.
3. Wang MZ, et al. *Zhong Yi Xue Wen Da Ti Ku* (Questions and Answers on Traditional Chinese Medicine: Herbal Formulas).

Sāng Xìng Tāng (Mulberry Leaf and Apricot Kernel Decoction)

桑杏湯
桑杏汤

Pinyin Name: *Sang Xing Tang*
Literal Name: Mulberry Leaf and Apricot Kernel Decoction
Original Source: *Wen Bing Tiao Bian* (Systematic Differentiation of Warm Diseases) by Wu Ju-Tong in 1798

COMPOSITION

Sang Ye (Folium Mori)	3g
Dan Dou Chi (Semen Sojae Praeparatum)	3g
Ku Xing Ren (Semen Armeniacae Amarum)	4.5g
Sha Shen (Radix Glehniae seu Adenophorae)	6g
Zhe Bei Mu (Bulbus Fritillariae Thunbergii)	3g
Li Pi (Pericarpium Pyri)	3g
Zhi Zi Pi (Pericarpium Gardeniae)	3g

DOSAGE / PREPARATION / ADMINISTRATION

The source text states to cook the ingredients with two cups of water until the decoction is reduced to one cup. Take the strained decoction while it is warm. Repeat this process if the condition is severe. The original text advises to cook *Sang Xing Tang* for only a short period of time. The rationale is that since this is a mild case of warmth-dryness, a light decoction will be sufficient for treatment.

CHINESE THERAPEUTIC ACTIONS

Dispels and ventilates warmth-dryness

CLINICAL MANIFESTATIONS

Exterior warmth-dryness affecting the Lung: dry coughing without sputum, or with scanty, sticky sputum, thirst, dry throat, a red tongue and a rapid, big pulse especially on the right.

VETERINARY CLINICAL APPLICATIONS

Bronchitis, coughing in diabetic patients with chronic respiratory disease and hemoptysis.

EXPLANATION

Sang Xing Tang (Mulberry Leaf and Apricot Kernel Decoction) is designed to treat mild cases of exterior warmth-dryness invading the Lung. Warmth-dryness is mild in nature and invades only the exterior of the body. Therefore, the animal does not have a high fever. Also, the warmth-dryness may invade the Lung to disrupt qi circulation, dry up fluids, and cause clinical signs such as dry coughing (with or without sputum), thirst, dry throat, a red tongue, and a big, rapid pulse.

This formula uses *Sang Ye* (Folium Mori) and *Dan Dou Chi* (Semen Sojae Praeparatum) to ventilate the Lung and dispel warmth-dryness. *Ku Xing Ren* (Semen Armeniacae

***Sang Xing Tang* (Mulberry Leaf and Apricot Kernel Decoction)**

Diagnosis	Clinical Signs	Treatment	Herbs
Exterior warmth-dryness affecting the Lung	• Thirst, dry throat, and dry coughing: warmth-dryness damaging body fluids • A red tongue and a rapid, big pulse: warmth-dryness	• Dispels and ventilates warmth-dryness • Clears Lung heat	• *Sang Ye* (Folium Mori) and *Dan Dou Chi* (Semen Sojae Praeparatum) ventilate the Lung and dispel the warmth-dryness. • *Ku Xing Ren* (Semen Armeniacae Amarum) ventilates the Lung and regulates Lung qi. • *Sha Shen* (Radix Glehniae seu Adenophorae) nourishes yin and moistens the Lung. • *Zhe Bei Mu* (Bulbus Fritillariae Thunbergii) clears the Lung and dissolves phlegm. • *Li Pi* (Pericarpium Pyri) moistens the Lung, generates fluids, and stops coughing. • *Zhi Zi Pi* (Pericarpium Gardeniae) clears heat in the Lung and diaphragm.

Sāng Xìng Tāng (Mulberry Leaf and Apricot Kernel Decoction)

Amarum) ventilates the Lung and regulates Lung qi. *Sha Shen* (Radix Glehniae seu Adenophorae) nourishes yin and moistens the Lung. *Zhe Bei Mu* (Bulbus Fritillariae Thunbergii) clears the Lung and dissolves phlegm. *Li Pi* (Pericarpium Pyri) moistens the Lung, generates fluids, and stops coughing. *Zhi Zi Pi* (Pericarpium Gardeniae) clears heat in the Lung and the diaphragm.

VETERINARY MODIFICATIONS

- With cough accompanied by thick, yellow sputum, add *Tian Hua Fen* (Radix Trichosanthis) and *Gua Lou* (Fructus Trichosanthis).
- With heat and dryness injuring the Lung collaterals, leading to coughing of blood, add *Lu Gen* (Rhizoma Phragmitis), *Bai Mao Gen* (Rhizoma Imperatae), *Qing Dai* (Indigo Naturalis), and *Gua Lou* (Fructus Trichosanthis).
- With swollen lymph nodes and difficulty swallowing, add *Xuan Shen* (Radix Scrophulariae) and *Ma Bo* (Lasiosphaera seu Calvatia).
- For severe thirst, add *Shi Gao* (Gypsum Fibrosum) and *Tian Hua Fen* (Radix Trichosanthis).
- With epistaxis, add *Mo Han Lian* (Herba Ecliptae) and *Bai Mao Gen* (Rhizoma Imperatae).
- With severe epistaxis due to heat, add *Qing Dai* (Indigo Naturalis), *Qing Hao* (Herba Artemisiae Annuae), *Mu Dan Pi* (Cortex Moutan), *Di Huang* (Radix Rehmanniae), and *Ce Bai Ye* (Cacumen Platycladi).
- With hemoptysis due to bronchiectasis, remove *Dan Dou Chi* (Semen Sojae Praeparatum), and add *Qing Dai* (Indigo Naturalis), *Gua Lou Pi* (Pericarpium Trichosanthis), and *He Zi* (Fructus Chebulae).

CAUTIONS / CONTRAINDICATIONS

- *Sang Xing Tang* should only be cooked for a short period of time to preserve its efficacy, as many herbs in this formula are aromatic.
- This formula is moderate in potency and should only be used to treat lung disorders of mild to moderate severity.

SUGGESTED ACUPUNCTURE TREATMENT

1. Points: *Dazhui* (GV 14), *Feishu* (BL 13), *Chize* (LU 5), *Lieque* (LU 7), *Taixi* (KI 3), *Taiyuan* (LU 9), *Tiantu* (CV 22), *Shaoshang* (LU 11) and *Dingchuan*.
2. Technique: even method and bleeding.

Bleed *Shaoshang* (LU 11) to clear Lung heat. *Dazhui* (GV 14) clears heat. *Feishu* (BL 13) and *Chize* (LU 5) ventilate the Lung. *Lieque* (LU 7) regulates Lung qi. *Taixi* (KI 3) and *Taiyuan* (LU 9) tonify yin and moisten the Lung. *Tiantu* (CV 22) and the classical point *Dingchuan* control cough

AUTHORS' COMMENTS

Sang Xing Tang can be combined with *Zi Wan Tang* (Aster Decoction) for animals that have deficiency of Lung qi and yin, hemoptysis, phlegm and heat. This pattern can be seen in chronically ill or geriatric animals recovering from respiratory disease and cancer. It treats mild to moderate diseases; for more severe diseases, please refer to *Qing Zao Jiu Fei Tang* (Eliminate Dryness and Rescue the Lung Decoction).

Xing Su San (Apricot Kernel and Perilla Leaf Powder) and *Sang Xing Tang* both treat cough caused by Lung dryness.

- *Xing Su San* treats cold-dryness attacking the Lung. Chief complaints include aversion to cold, absence of sweating, and cough with thin, white sputum.
- *Sang Xing Tang* treats warmth-dryness attacking the Lung. Chief complaints include dry cough with absence of sputum, thirst, and dry mouth and throat.[1]

Sang Xing Tang and *Sang Ju Yin* (Mulberry Leaf and Chrysanthemum Decoction) both contain *Ku Xing Ren* (Semen Armeniacae Amarum) and *Sang Ye* (Folium Mori) to clear the Lung, relieve cough, and expel exterior factor.

- *Sang Xing Tang* treats dryness with heat attacking the Lung. This formula contains moistening herbs, such as *Sha Shen* (Radix Glehniae seu Adenophorae) and *Bei Mu* (Bulbus Fritillariae), to treat the clinical signs of dryness.
- *Sang Ju Yin* treats wind-heat attacking the Lung. It contains heat-clearing herbs, such as *Bo He* (Herba Menthae), *Lu Gen* (Rhizoma Phragmitis), and *Lian Qiao* (Fructus Forsythiae).[2]

References

1. Wang MZ, et al. *Zhong Yi Xue Wen Da Ti Ku* (Questions and Answers on Traditional Chinese Medicine: Herbal Formulas).
2. Wang MZ, et al. *Zhong Yi Xue Wen Da Ti Ku* (Questions and Answers on Traditional Chinese Medicine: Herbal Formulas).

DRYNESS-RELIEVING FORMULAS 15

Qīng Zào Jiù Fèi Tāng

(Eliminate Dryness and Rescue the Lung Decoction)

清燥救肺湯
清燥救肺汤

Pinyin Name: *Qing Zao Jiu Fei Tang*

Literal Name: Eliminate Dryness and Rescue the Lung Decoction

Alternate Names: *Ching Tsao Chiu Fei Tang, Ching Zao Jiu Fei Tang*, Dryness-Clearing and Lung-Rescuing Decoction, Eriobotrya and Ophiopogon Combination

Original Source: *Yi Men Fa Lu* (Precepts for Physicians) by Yu Chang in 1658

COMPOSITION

Sang Ye (Folium Mori)	9g
Shi Gao (Gypsum Fibrosum), *duan* (calcined)	7.5g
Mai Dong (Radix Ophiopogonis)	3.6g
Ku Xing Ren (Semen Armeniacae Amarum), *chao* (dry-fried) to yellow	2.1g
Pi Pa Ye (Folium Eriobotryae), *zhi* (fried with honey) to yellow	3g
E Jiao (Colla Corii Asini)	2.4g
Hu Ma Ren (Semen Sesami Indici), *chao* (dry-fried) and *yan* (ground) to small particles	3g
Ren Shen (Radix et Rhizoma Ginseng)	2.1g
Gan Cao (Radix et Rhizoma Glycyrrhizae)	3g

DOSAGE / PREPARATION / ADMINISTRATION

Cook the ingredients with 1 bowl of water until the liquid is reduced to 60% of the original volume. Take the warm, strained decoction two to three times daily.

CHINESE THERAPEUTIC ACTIONS

1. Clears dryness
2. Moistens and nourishes Lung yin
3. Tonifies qi

CLINICAL MANIFESTATIONS

Warmth-dryness injuring the Lung: fever, thirst, dry cough with no sputum; exercise intolerance, dyspnea, chest and hypochondriac pain, irritability; dryness of the nose, mouth and throat, dry skin and dandruff; a red, dry tongue with no coating, and a big, rapid, but deficient pulse.

VETERINARY CLINICAL APPLICATIONS

Persistent, non-productive cough, pneumonia, bronchitis, epistaxis and hemoptysis secondary to lung cancer, cough and hemoptysis post heartworm treatment, and itching.

EXPLANATION

Qing Zao Jiu Fei Tang (Eliminate Dryness and Rescue the Lung Decoction) is designed to treat severe cases of warmth-dryness injuring the Lung. Warmth-dryness may invade the exterior, causing fever. If the warmth-dryness invades the Lung and reverses the normal flow of Lung qi, then coughing, exercise intolerance, dyspnea, chest and hypochondriac pain may occur. Because warmth-dryness may easily damage Lung yin and body fluids, clinical signs such as coughing with no sputum, dry nose and mouth, and thirst may be expected. A red, dry tongue with no coating and a big, rapid, but deficient pulse indicate the presence of dryness and heat, and damage of qi and yin.

This formula contains *Sang Ye* (Folium Mori) to ventilate and moisten dryness and release the pathogenic factors from the Lung. *Shi Gao* (Gypsum Fibrosum) and *Mai Dong* (Radix Ophiopogonis) clear Lung heat and moisten the dryness. These three herbs form a good balance, as they function to release the exterior, clear the warmth, and moisten the dryness. Furthermore, though *Shi Gao* (Gypsum Fibrosum) is heavy, sinking and cold in nature, prescribing it at a lower dose will not interfere with the releasing effect of *Sang Ye* (Folium Mori). *Ku Xing Ren* (Semen Armeniacae Amarum) and *Pi Pa Ye* (Folium Eriobotryae) benefit the Lung and regulate the flow of Lung qi. *E Jiao* (Colla Corii Asini) and *Hu Ma Ren* (Semen Sesami Indici) moisten the Lung and nourish Lung yin. *Ren Shen* (Radix et Rhizoma Ginseng) and *Gan Cao* (Radix et Rhizoma Glycyrrhizae) tonify qi and the middle *jiao*, which, in turn, enhances the production of Lung qi.

Qīng Zào Jiù Fèi Tāng

(Eliminate Dryness and Rescue the Lung Decoction)

Qing Zao Jiu Fei Tang **(Eliminate Dryness and Rescue the Lung Decoction)**

Diagnosis	Clinical Signs	Treatment	Herbs
Warmth-dryness injuring the Lung	• Fever: warmth-dryness at the exterior • Coughing, exercise intolerance, dyspnea, and chest and hypochondriac pain: reversed qi flow due to warmth-dryness invading the Lung • Coughing with no sputum, dry nose and mouth, and thirst: warmth-dryness damaging yin and body fluids • A red, dry tongue with no coating and a big, rapid, but deficient pulse: warmth-dryness damaging qi and yin	• Clears dryness • Moistens the Lung	• *Sang Ye* (Folium Mori) moistens dryness and releases pathogenic factors from the Lung. • *Shi Gao* (Gypsum Fibrosum) and *Mai Dong* (Radix Ophiopogonis) clear Lung heat and moisten dryness. • *Ku Xing Ren* (Semen Armeniacae Amarum) and *Pi Pa Ye* (Folium Eriobotryae) benefit the Lung and regulate the flow of Lung qi. • *E Jiao* (Colla Corii Asini) and *Hu Ma Ren* (Semen Sesami Indici) moisten the Lung and nourish Lung yin. • *Ren Shen* (Radix et Rhizoma Ginseng) and *Gan Cao* (Radix et Rhizoma Glycyrrhizae) tonify qi.

VETERINARY MODIFICATIONS

- With profuse, difficult to expectorate sputum, add *Chuan Bei Mu* (Bulbus Fritillariae Cirrhosae) and *Gua Lou Pi* (Pericarpium Trichosanthis).
- With thirst and high fever due to excess heat, add *Shui Niu Jiao* (Cornu Bubali).
- With hemoptysis, add *Ce Bai Ye* (Cacumen Platycladi), *Xian He Cao* (Herba Agrimoniae), *Bai Ji* (Rhizoma Bletillae) and *Bai Mao Gen* (Rhizoma Imperatae).
- For constipation, add *Huo Ma Ren* (Fructus Cannabis), *Rou Cong Rong* (Herba Cistanches), and *Tao Ren* (Semen Persicae).
- For itchy, dry and hot skin, add *Bai Xian Pi* (Cortex Dictamni), *Chi Shao* (Radix Paeoniae Rubra), *Di Huang* (Radix Rehmanniae) and *Ji Xue Teng* (Caulis Spatholobi).
- For cough that is worse at night, add *Zhi Mu* (Rhizoma Anemarrhenae) and *Huang Bo* (Cortex Phellodendri Chinensis).

CAUTIONS / CONTRAINDICATIONS

- *Qing Zao Jiu Fei Tang* contains many tonic herbs that are cloying; they should be used with Spleen and Stomach tonic herbs or formulas in cases of middle *jiao* deficiency.
- Patients with warmth-dryness injuring the Lung often have underlying deficiencies. Therefore, foods and herbs that are acrid, aromatic, bitter and drying should be avoided, as they will further damage qi and yin.

HUMAN CLINICAL STUDIES AND RESEARCH

1. **Cough**: Administration of *Qing Zao Jiu Fei Tang* in 100 patients with cough due to Lung heat was associated with complete recovery in 50 patients, significant improvement in 40 patients, and moderate improvement in 10 patients. The patients were instructed to discontinue antibiotic drugs during herbal treatment.[1] In another study, 67 patients with a dry, non-productive cough refractory to antibiotic drug therapy were treated with good results using modified *Qing Zao Jiu Fei Tang*. The study reported that most patients began to feel improvement after 4 days of herbal therapy.[2]
2. **Sore throat**: One study reported good effect for treatment of sore throat using *Qing Zao Jiu Fei Tang* plus *Chan Tui* (Periostracum Cicadae), *Zi Wan* (Radix et Rhizoma Asteris), and *Bai Bu* (Radix Stemonae). Of 73 patients, the study reported complete recovery in 59 patients, improvement in 12 patients, and no improvement in 2 patients. The overall rate of effectiveness was 97.25%.[3]
3. **Laryngitis**: Administration of modified *Qing Zao Jiu Fei Tang* was reported in one study to be effective in treating 84 of 85 patients with loss of voice due to laryngitis. Modifications to the base formula included addition of *Jing Jie* (Herba Schizonepetae) and *Fang Feng* (Radix Saposhnikoviae) for wind-cold; *Chuan Bei Mu* (Bulbus Fritillariae Cirrhosae) and *Jie Geng* (Radix Platycodonis) for phlegm and heat; *Shi Gao* (Gypsum Fibrosum) for excess heat; and *Da Huang* (Radix et Rhizoma Rhei) for constipation. For individuals with Lung and Kidney deficiencies, *He Zi* (Fructus Chebulae) and *Huang Qi* (Radix Astragali) were added, *Sha Shen* (Radix Glehniae seu Adenophorae) was used in place of *Ren Shen* (Radix et Rhizoma Ginseng), and *Shi Hu* (Caulis Dendrobii) was used in place of *Shi Gao* (Gypsum Fibrosum).[4]
4. **Pneumonia**: Administration of modified *Qing Zao Jiu Fei Tang* was associated with 85% effectiveness in treating

Qīng Zào Jiù Fèi Tāng

(Eliminate Dryness and Rescue the Lung Decoction)

26 patients with pneumonia with clinical signs such as frequent coughing, and scant sticky sputum that is difficult to expectorate. Modifications to the base formula included addition of *Wu Wei Zi* (Fructus Schisandrae Chinensis) and *Su Zi* (Fructus Perillae) for severe cough and dyspnea; *Di Huang* (Radix Rehmanniae) and charred *Zhi Zi* (Fructus Gardeniae) for constipation; and *Bai Shao* (Radix Paeoniae Alba) and *Yan Hu Suo* (Rhizoma Corydalis) for chest pain caused by cough. Of 26 patients, the study reported significant effects in 5 patients, moderate improvement in 17 patients, and no help in 4 patients.[5]

5. **Epistaxis**: One study reported successful termination of nosebleeds within 3 days in all of 24 patients using *Qing Zao Jiu Fei Tang* plus *Bai Mao Gen* (Rhizoma Imperatae), *Qian Cao* (Radix et Rhizoma Rubiae), and charred *Ou Jie* (Nodus Nelumbinis Rhizomatis).[6]
6. **Hemoptysis**: According to one study, use of modified *Qing Zao Jiu Fei Tang* was associated with good results to treat 38 patients with coughing of blood.[7]
7. **Itching**: Administration of modified *Qing Zao Jiu Fei Tang* was found to be effective in treating 18 geriatric patients with simple itching skin without other complications. Of 18 patients, the study reported complete recovery in 9 patients, improvement in 7 patients, and no benefit in 2 patients.[8]

SUGGESTED ACUPUNCTURE TREATMENT

1. Points: *Waiguan* (TH 5), *Hegu* (LI 4), *Feishu* (BL 13), *Jingqu* (LU 8), *Lieque* (LU 7), *Shanzhong* (CV 17), *Zhaohai* (KI 6), *Taixi* (KI 3), and *Housanli* (ST 36).
2. Techniques: tonification and sedation.

Waiguan (TH 5) and *Hegu* (LI 4) moisten and ventilate the Lung. *Feishu* (BL 13) and *Jingqu* (LU 8) clear heat from the Lung channel. *Lieque* (LU 7) and *Shanzhong* (CV 17) regulate the Lung qi. *Zhaohai* (KI 6) and *Taixi* (KI 3) nourish the yin. *Housanli* (ST 36) tonifies all three *jiaos*, which in turn strengthens Lung qi.

AUTHORS' COMMENTS

Qing Zao Jiu Fei Tang is a formula that is generally used to treat chronic respiratory conditions with cough and/or epistaxis caused by heat and dryness in animals that have underlying deficiencies and that also have accompanying attack by wind warmth. Many of these animals have developed a dry cough following an infection or chronic illness, and while most of the Lung heat has been cleared, the patient is left with a nagging non-productive cough that is often worse at night. In cases in which there is excessive dryness, it can be combined with *Sha Shen Mai Dong Tang* (Glehnia and Ophiopogonis Decoction). It should not be used to treat excess conditions with productive cough, as it contains many rich and cloying herbs that can ultimately worsen the animal's condition.

This formula can be used to treat hemoptysis due to lung cancer and concurrent chemotherapy, or for hemoptysis post heartworm treatment. In these cases, it should be combined with *Ce Bai Ye* (Cacumen Platycladi), *Xian He Cao* (Herba Agrimoniae) and *Bai Ji* (Rhizoma Bletillae) to improve clinical results. *Qing Zao Jiu Fei Tang* contains *Shi Gao* (Gypsum Fibrosum) and is not for prolonged use or for animals without obvious heat (fever). In mild cases, use *Sang Xing Tang* (Mulberry Leaf and Apricot Kernel Decoction). Treatment should not exceed 5-7 days without re-assessment, especially if the formula is combined with antimicrobial drugs. For animals that have coughing with more heat and phlegm, it can be combined with *Zi Wan Tang* (Aster Decoction). For hemoptysis due to more heat than dryness, *Ma Huang Xing Ren Gan Cao Shi Gao Tang* (Ephedra, Apricot Kernel, Licorice, and Gypsum Decoction) should be used.

Qing Zao Jiu Fei Tang can also be used for fever and dry, non-productive cough in chronically ill or geriatric patients with pneumonia or post-pneumonia and are unresponsive to antibiotic therapy. It can be modified by adding *Chuan Bei Mu* (Bulbus Fritillariae Cirrhosae) and *Tao Ren* (Semen Persicae) to hasten and improve results. These animals typically have untreated pre-existing qi and yin deficiencies that are responsible for the persistent fever, cough, and lack of response to conventional drugs. *Qing Zao Jiu Fei Tang* can be combined with antimicrobial drugs; however, it is often necessary to give herbs or another formula to tonify the middle *jiao* to prevent gastrointestinal upset.

Qing Zao Jiu Fei Tang can also be used to treat hot, dry skin disorders when the primary pathology involves dryness of the Lung. For dermatological diseases, combine with *Xue Fu Zhu Yu Tang* (Drive Out Stasis in the Mansion of Blood Decoction) to improve clinical results. This combination can be used for 2-4 weeks and should not be used in animals with Spleen qi deficiency without adding herbs or another formula to protect and tonify the middle *jiao*.

Warmth-dryness attacking the Lung is often accompanied by underlying deficiencies of qi, yin, and body fluids. Thus, to properly treat this syndrome, the warmth-dryness must be cleared and the Lung must be moistened.

Qīng Zào Jiù Fèi Tāng

(Eliminate Dryness and Rescue the Lung Decoction)

It is important to note that this formula achieves this goal with the use of sweet and cold heat-clearing herbs, such as *Shi Gao* (Gypsum Fibrosum), and not with bitter, cold and drying heat-clearing herbs, such as *Huang Qin* (Radix Scutellariae).

Sang Xing Tang and *Qing Zao Jiu Fei Tang* (Mulberry Leaf and Apricot Kernel Decoction) both effectively treat warmth-dryness affecting the Lung.

- *Sang Xing Tang* is typically used for mild cases of warmth-dryness affecting the Lung, with such clinical signs as mild fever and mild cough.
- *Qing Zao Jiu Fei Tang* is generally reserved for severe cases of warmth-dryness injuring the Lung, with such clinical signs as high fever, cough, dyspnea, chest and hypochondriac pain, irritability, thirst, and dry mouth and throat.

References

1. *Zhong Yi Han Shou Tong Xun* (Reports of Chinese Medicine), 1989, 1:37.
2. *Shan Xi Zhong Yi* (Shanxi Chinese Medicine), 1992, 11:492.
3. *Shi Yong Zhong Xi Yi Jie He Za Zhi* (Practical Journal of Integrated Chinese and Western Medicines), 1992, 5(9):533.
4. *Zhong Yi Za Zhi* (Journal of Chinese Medicine), 1984, 4:50.
5. *Shi Yong Zhong Xi Yi Jie He Za Zhi* (Practical Journal of Integrated Chinese and Western Medicines), 1998, 12:1065.
6. *Gui Yang Zhong Yi Xue Yuan Xue Bao* (Journal of Guiyang Chinese Medical University), 1992, 4:47.
7. *Bei Jing Zhong Yi* (Beijing Chinese Medicine), 1996, 1:22.
8. *Shang Hai Yi Yao Za Zhi* (Shanghai Journal of Medicine and Herbology), 1996, 10:19.

Section 2

滋阴润燥剂
— Nourishing and Moistening Formulas

Bǎi Hé Gù Jīn Tāng (Lily Bulb Decoction to Preserve the Metal)
百合固金湯
百合固金汤

Pinyin Name: *Bai He Gu Jin Tang*
Literal Name: Lily Bulb Decoction to Preserve the Metal
Alternate Names: *Pai Ho Ku Chin Tang (Wan)*, *Bei Ho Gu Jin Tang (Wan)*, Lily Gold-Firming Decoction (Pill), Lily Metal-Consolidation Decoction (Pill), Lily Combination
Original Source: *Yi Fang Ji Jie* (Analytical Collection of Medical Formulas) by Wang Ang in 1682

COMPOSITION

Di Huang (Radix Rehmanniae)	6g
Shu Di Huang (Radix Rehmanniae Praeparata)	9g
Mai Dong (Radix Ophiopogonis)	4.5g
Bai He (Bulbus Lilii)	3g
Zhe Bei Mu (Bulbus Fritillariae Thunbergii)	3g
Xuan Shen (Radix Scrophulariae)	2.4g
Dang Gui (Radix Angelicae Sinensis)	3g
Bai Shao (Radix Paeoniae Alba), *chao* (dry-fried)	3g
Jie Geng (Radix Platycodonis)	2.4g
Gan Cao (Radix et Rhizoma Glycyrrhizae)	3g

DOSAGE / PREPARATION / ADMINISTRATION
Prepare the ingredients as a decoction.

CHINESE THERAPEUTIC ACTIONS
1. Nourishes yin and moistens the Lung
2. Dissolves phlegm and stops coughing

CLINICAL MANIFESTATIONS
Yin deficiency of the Lung and Kidney: coughing, hemoptysis, low-grade fever in the evenings, general weakness, irritability, dryness, insomnia, restlessness, excessive panting (especially at night), constipation, short urination, heat aversion, a preference for cool surfaces/places, increased to ravenous appetite, increased thirst, trembling and jerking during sleep, poor hearing or deafness, hypersensitivity to acupuncture, a red tongue body with little to no coating, and a rapid, fine pulse.

VETERINARY CLINICAL APPLICATIONS
Cough, hemoptysis, bronchiectasis, chronic bronchitis, chronic obstructive pulmonary disease (COPD) or recurrent airway obstruction (RAO), pneumothorax, lung cancer and asthma.

EXPLANATION
Bai He Gu Jin Tang (Lily Bulb Decoction to Preserve the Metal) is designed to treat Lung and Kidney yin deficiencies. Yin deficiency of the Lung and Kidney may lead to deficiency heat and injury of the blood vessels. Injury of the lung capillaries may lead to bleeding and coughing with streaks of blood. Constipation and a dry, sore throat are due to deficiency heat drying up the body fluids. A low-grade fever in the evenings, general weakness, irritability, dryness, insomnia, restlessness, excessive panting (especially at night), short urination, heat aversion, a preference for cool surfaces/places, increased to ravenous appetite, increased thirst, trembling and jerking during sleep, poor

Bǎi Hé Gù Jīn Tāng (Lily Bulb Decoction to Preserve the Metal)

***Bai He Gu Jin Tang* (Lily Bulb Decoction to Preserve the Metal)**

Diagnosis	Clinical Signs	Treatment	Herbs
Lung and Kidney yin deficiencies	• Coughing, with streaks of blood in the sputum: deficiency heat injuring the blood vessels • Dry, sore throat and constipation: deficiency heat consuming body fluids • Low-grade fever in the evenings, restlessness, excessive panting (especially at night): yin-deficient heat rising upward • Red tongue body with little coating and a rapid, fine pulse: yin-deficient heat	• Nourishes yin and moistens the Lung • Dissolves phlegm and stops coughing	• *Di Huang* (Radix Rehmanniae) and *Shu Di Huang* (Radix Rehmanniae Praeparata) nourish yin and clear deficiency fire. • *Di Huang* (Radix Rehmanniae) and *Xuan Shen* (Radix Scrophulariae) cool the blood, clear deficiency fire, and stops bleeding. • *Mai Dong* (Radix Ophiopogonis), *Bai He* (Bulbus Lilii) and *Zhe Bei Mu* (Bulbus Fritillariae Thunbergii) nourish yin, moisten the Lung, dissolve phlegm, and stop coughing. • *Dang Gui* (Radix Angelicae Sinensis) and *Bai Shao* (Radix Paeoniae Alba) nourish yin and tonify the blood. • *Jie Geng* (Radix Platycodonis) smoothes the Lung qi, relieves coughing, and dissolves phlegm. • *Gan Cao* (Radix et Rhizoma Glycyrrhizae) harmonizes all of the herbs.

hearing or deafness, hypersensitivity to acupuncture, a red tongue body with little to no coating, and a rapid, fine pulse are all typical signs of yin-deficient heat.

Di Huang (Radix Rehmanniae) and *Shu Di Huang* (Radix Rehmanniae Praeparata) nourish yin and clear deficiency fire. *Di Huang* (Radix Rehmanniae) further cools the blood and stops bleeding. *Mai Dong* (Radix Ophiopogonis), *Bai He* (Bulbus Lilii), and *Zhe Bei Mu* (Bulbus Fritillariae Thunbergii) nourish yin, moisten the Lung, dissolve phlegm, and stop coughing. *Xuan Shen* (Radix Scrophulariae) cools the blood, clears the deficiency fire, and moistens dryness. *Dang Gui* (Radix Angelicae Sinensis) and *Bai Shao* (Radix Paeoniae Alba) nourish yin and blood. *Jie Geng* (Radix Platycodonis) smoothes the Lung qi, relieves coughing, and dissolves phlegm. *Gan Cao* (Radix et Rhizoma Glycyrrhizae) harmonizes all of the herbs in the formula. Lastly, the combination of *Gan Cao* (Radix et Rhizoma Glycyrrhizae) and *Jie Geng* (Radix Platycodonis) helps to relieve the sore throat.

VETERINARY MODIFICATIONS

- With more severe cough and dyspnea, add *Ku Xing Ren* (Semen Armeniacae Amarum), *Wu Wei Zi* (Fructus Schisandrae Chinensis), and *Kuan Dong Hua* (Flos Farfarae).
- With thick, yellow sputum, add *Gua Lou* (Fructus Trichosanthis) and *Zhu Ru* (Caulis Bambusae in Taenia).
- With coughing of blood, remove *Jie Geng* (Radix Platycodonis), and add *Bai Mao Gen* (Rhizoma Imperatae), *Ce Bai Ye* (Cacumen Platycladi) and *Xian He Cao* (Herba Agrimoniae).
- With wheezing and dyspnea due to profuse phlegm, add *Xie Bai San* (Drain the White Powder).
- With wheezing and dyspnea due to heat, add *San Huang Xie Xin Tang* (Three-Yellow Decoction to Sedate the Epigastrium).
- If there are more heat signs, add *Zhi Mu* (Rhizoma Anemarrhenae) and *Yu Xing Cao* (Herba Houttuyniae).

CAUTIONS / CONTRAINDICATIONS

- *Bai He Gu Jin Tang* is contraindicated in patients in whom coughing is characterized by excess conditions.
- Many herbs in this formula are hard to digest since they are cold, sweet, and heavy in nature. Therefore, patients with Spleen deficiency, characterized by loose stools, abdominal fullness and pain, and poor appetite, should use this formula with caution. Using a formula such as *Liu Jun Zi Tang* (Six-Gentlemen Decoction) concurrently with this formula in Spleen deficient patients is often advisable.

HUMAN CLINICAL STUDIES AND RESEARCH

1. **Cough**: One study reported 90% effectiveness using modified *Bai He Gu Jin Tang* to treat 30 patients with cough characterized by dryness and heat. Modifications included addition of *Jin Yin Hua* (Flos Lonicerae Japonicae), *Ban Lan Gen* (Radix Isatidis), and *Niu Bang Zi* (Fructus Arctii) for sore throat; *Zi Su Ye* (Folium Perillae), *Huang Lian* (Rhizoma Coptidis), and *Gua Lou* (Fructus

DRYNESS-RELIEVING FORMULAS 15

Băi Hé Gù Jīn Tāng (Lily Bulb Decoction to Preserve the Metal)

Trichosanthis) for feelings of oppression and pain in the chest; *Tian Zhu Huang* (Concretio Silicea Bambusae) for insomnia; and *Gua Lou Zi* (Semen Trichosanthis) for constipation.[1] Another study reported 97.6% effectiveness using *Bai He Gu Jin Tang* to treat 42 children with chronic cough.[2]

2. **Bronchiectasis**: One study reported good results using herbs to treat 50 patients with hemoptysis associated with bronchiectasis. The herbal formula contained *Di Huang* (Radix Rehmanniae) 15g, *Mai Dong* (Radix Ophiopogonis) 15g, *Bai He* (Bulbus Lilii) 15g, *Xian He Cao* (Herba Agrimoniae) 15g, *Bai Shao* (Radix Paeoniae Alba) 12g, *Dang Gui* (Radix Angelicae Sinensis) 12g, *Xuan Shen* (Radix Scrophulariae) 12g, *Bai Mao Gen* (Rhizoma Imperatae) 30g, *Bei Mu* (Bulbus Fritillariae) 6g, and *Gan Cao* (Radix et Rhizoma Glycyrrhizae) 6g. Additional modifications were made as needed. The treatment protocol was to administer one pack of herbs daily, for 15 to 20 packs continuously. The study reported marked improvements in most patients, with relief of clinical signs such as cough and hemoptysis, and reduction of phlegm.[3]
3. **Pneumothorax**: In one study, 30 patients with pneumothorax were divided into two groups and treated accordingly. Group one received *Bai He Gu Jin Tang*, one pack of herbs per day via decoction for 10 days per course, for a total of 3 to 4 courses of treatment. Group two received standard allopathic medical treatment (details of treatment were unavailable at the time of publication). The study noted that both treatments were effective. However, the average length of hospitalization was only 18.93 days for patients in the herb group, while the average was 27.85 days for the allopathic medicine group.[d] Another study reported marked success using the following formula to treat pneumothorax: *Bai He Gu Jin Tang* with the removal of *Dang Gui* (Radix Angelicae Sinensis) and *Shu Di Huang* (Radix Rehmanniae Praeparata) and the addition of *Sha Shen* (Radix Glehniae seu Adenophorae), *Pi Pa Ye* (Folium Eriobotryae), and *Gua Lou Pi* (Pericarpium Trichosanthis). Pneumothorax was resolved after an average of 11 days, with a range of 2 to 20 days.[5]
4. **Lung cancer**: According to one study, administration of *Bai He Gu Jin Tang* was associated with symptomatic improvement in 22 of 38 patients with lung cancer characterized by Lung yin deficiency.[6]
5. **Diabetes mellitus**: Diabetes mellitus was treated effectively using modified *Bai He Gu Jin Tang* daily in decoction, for 20 days per course of treatment, for 4 courses total. Of 46 patients, the study reported improvement in 38 cases and no effect in 8 cases.[7]

SUGGESTED ACUPUNCTURE TREATMENT

1. Points: *Shenshu* (BL 23), *Taixi* (KI 3), *Zhaohai* (KI 6), *Taiyuan* (LU 9), *Sanyinjiao* (SP 6), *Feishu* (BL 13), *Lieque* (LU 7), *Chize* (LU 5), *Kongzui* (LU 6), *Tiantu* (CV 22) *Yinxi* (HT 6) and *Dingchuan*.
2. Techniques: tonify *Shenshu* (BL 23), *Taixi* (KI 3), and *Zhaohai* (KI 6); even method for all other points.

To tonify yin, *Taixi* (KI 3), *shu* (stream) point and *yuan* (source) point of the Kidney channel, *Zhaohai* (KI 6), and *Shenshu* (BL 23), *shu* (transport) point of the Kidney, are chosen. *Taiyuan* (LU 9) and *Sanyinjiao* (SP 6) can be used to nourish yin. In addition, select other points to treat the patient's individual clinical manifestations. *Feishu* (BL 13), *Lieque* (LU 7), *Tiantu* (CV 22), *Dingchuan*, a classical point, and *Chize* (LU 5) stop coughing and dissolve phlegm. *Kongzui* (LU 6) clears heat and stops bleeding. *Yinxi* (HT 6) stops night sweats and panting.

AUTHORS' COMMENTS

Bai He Gu Jin Tang is one of the most commonly used formulas to treat cough from Lung and Kidney yin deficiencies, with deficiency heat rising. Deficiency of these two organs can develop from internal causes (chronic disease, chronic medication) or from external causes (exogenous heat pathogen, dry, hot environment). This formula is effective for both conditions. For example, a dry, unproductive cough that follows an upper respiratory infection in cats or infectious tracheobronchitis in dogs can be treated with this formula. Likewise, a dry, unproductive cough secondary to chronic renal insufficiency or lung cancer in dogs can be treated with this formula. *Bai He Gu Jin Tang* contains many rich and cloying herbs and will cause gastrointestinal upset in animals that are Spleen deficient. This is often the case in chronically ill or aged animals. It is recommended to use herbs that tonify the middle *jiao* when using this formula in these animals. In dogs with nasal or lung cancer that are undergoing radiation or chemotherapy and are Spleen deficient, this formula can be combined with *Bu Zhong Yi Qi Tang* (Tonify the Middle and Augment the Qi Decoction), as many of these animals have significant qi and yin deficiencies. For animals that have more phlegm than yin deficiency, it is more appropriate to use *Bei Mu Gua Lou San* (Fritillaria and Trichosanthes Fruit Powder), or use a 1:1 ratio of the two formulas.

This is also a very common formula for treating RAO (heaves) in horses. Yin deficiency can occur from many of the reasons, both interior and external, mentioned above, as well as from deficiency that occurs from overwork. This

Bǎi Hé Gù Jīn Tāng (Lily Bulb Decoction to Preserve the Metal)

will lead to dryness of both the upper and lower respiratory tract, yin-deficient heat, and damage to Lung qi, all of which contribute to the cough and dyspnea associated with RAO. Often, the corresponding qi deficiency in RAO patients can be treated by combining *Bai He Gu Jin Tang* with *Ren Shen Ge Jie San* (Ginseng and Gecko Powder) in ratios proportional to the more prominent deficiency. Additionally, deficiencies of both yin and qi can make patients more susceptible to pathogens. This situation can be further complicated by invasions of wind-heat and wind-cold, making it necessary to treat these excess factors as well.

Bai He Gu Jin Tang treats cough with blood-streaked sputum, yet it purposely excludes herbs that stop bleeding in its formulation. Bleeding in this case is caused by Kidney and Lung yin deficiencies, with deficiency fire flaring upward and injuring the channels and collaterals. The herbs used in this formula focus on nourishing yin and cooling deficiency fire. By treating the cause of the bleeding, there is no need to add additional herbs to stop bleeding. When yin is nourished, the bleeding will stop automatically.[8]

Qing Zao Jiu Fei Tang (Eliminate Dryness and Rescue the Lung Decoction) and *Bai He Gu Jin Tang* both nourish yin and moisten dryness to treat dry cough with scanty sputum.

- *Qing Zao Jiu Fei Tang* treats dry cough due to exterior warmth-dryness attacking the body, with concurrent yin deficiency and clinical signs of fever and a dry throat and mouth. It contains herbs that regulate the flow of Lung qi, tonify qi, and clear heat from excess. Since it contains *Shi Gao* (Gypsum Fibrosum), it is not for long-term use without modification. Animals for which this formula is appropriate have cough, a red, dry tongue with no coating, and a big, rapid, deficient pulse.
- *Bai He Gu Jin Tang* treats dry cough from Kidney and Lung yin deficiencies, with deficiency heat rising. Besides the dry cough, there are other yin-deficient clinical signs, such as restlessness, dry nose and throat, a red tongue with little coating, and a weak, thin, rapid pulse. This formula is better at nourishing yin.

Bai He Gu Jin Tang and *Mai Men Dong Tang* (Ophiopogonis Decoction) have similar effects to nourish yin and moisten the Lung. Their differences are as follows:

- *Bai He Gu Jin Tang* tonifies Lung and Kidney yin and clears deficiency heat. It is most effective for asthma, RAO, and dry, nonproductive cough in animals with chronic respiratory disease and/or in post-recovery from respiratory infection.
- *Mai Men Dong Tang* tonifies Lung and Stomach yin and redirects abnormally rising qi. It is used to treat cough with difficult-to-expectorate sputum and vomiting with lack of appetite. Moreover, it is one of the major formulas used in veterinary medicine to treat pituitary hyperadrenocorticism (Cushing's disease) and diabetes mellitus, both of which are categorized as *xiao ke* (wasting and thirsting) syndrome in Chinese medicine.

References

1. *Fu Jian Zhong Yi Yao* (Fujian Chinese Medicine and Herbology), 1995; 1:46.
2. *Shan Xi Zhong Yi* (Shanxi Chinese *Medicine*), 1993; 9:413.
3. *Hu Bei Zhong Yi Za Zhi* (Hubei Journal of Chinese Medicine), 1995; 5:14.
4. *Zhong Xi Yi Jie He Za Zhi* (Journal of Integrated Chinese and Western Medicine), 1986; 5:280.
5. *Xin Yi Xue* (New Medicine), 1977; 4-5:197.
6. *Hei Long Jiang Zhong Yi Yao* (Heilongjiang Chinese Medicine and Herbology), 1982; 4:25.
7. *Yun Nan Zhong Yi Za Zhi* (Yunan Journal of Chinese Medicine), 1995; 4:22.
8. Wang MZ, et al. *Zhong Yi Xue Wen Da Ti Ku* (Questions and Answers on Traditional Chinese Medicine: Herbal Formulas).

Mài Mén Dōng Tāng (Ophiopogonis Decoction)

麥門冬湯
麦门冬汤

Pinyin Name: *Mai Men Dong Tang*
Literal Name: Ophiopogonis Decoction
Alternate Name: Ophiopogon Combination
Original Source: *Jin Gui Yao Lue* (Essentials from the Golden Cabinet) by Zhang Zhong-Jing in the Eastern Han Dynasty

COMPOSITION

Mai Dong (Radix Ophiopogonis)	7 cups [60-70g]
Ban Xia (Rhizoma Pinelliae)	1 cup [10-18g]
Ren Shen (Radix et Rhizoma Ginseng)	9g [6-9g]
Geng Mi (Semen Oryzae)	0.3 cup [6g]
Da Zao (Fructus Jujubae)	12 pieces [3-4 pieces]
Gan Cao (Radix et Rhizoma Glycyrrhizae)	6g [6g]

DOSAGE / PREPARATION / ADMINISTRATION

The source text states to cook the ingredients with 12 cups [2,400 mL] of water until the liquid is reduced to 6 cups [1,200 mL]. Take 1 cup [200 mL] of the warm, strained decoction three times during the day and once at night. Today, this formula may be prepared as a decoction with the doses suggested in brackets.

CHINESE THERAPEUTIC ACTIONS

1. Nourishes Lung and Stomach yin
2. Redirects the reversed flow of qi and harmonizes the middle *jiao*

CLINICAL MANIFESTATIONS

1. Lung yin deficiency: coughing with difficult-to-expectorate sputum, coughing or spitting of saliva, dry mouth and throat, a red tongue body with a scanty tongue coating, and a thready, rapid pulse.
2. Stomach yin deficiency: nausea, gastric ulcers, vomiting, thirst, dry throat, a red tongue with little coating, and a thready, rapid pulse.

VETERINARY CLINICAL APPLICATIONS

Canine hyperadrenocorticism, diabetes mellitus, nausea, vomiting, dry mouth and throat, gastritis, bronchitis, cough secondary to interstitial pneumonia and post-infection cough.

EXPLANATION

Mai Men Dong Tang (Ophiopogonis Decoction) is designed to treat Lung and/or Stomach yin deficiencies with deficiency fire rising. The deficiency fire disrupts the normal flow of Lung qi, and causes it to move upward instead of downward, which produces cough. Moreover, deficiency fire damages body fluids, and, as a result, patients experience sputum that cannot be easily expectorated, thirst, and a dry mouth and throat. Stomach yin deficiency may lead to reversed flow of qi upward, causing nausea and vomiting. A red tongue with little coating and a thready, rapid pulse are typical signs of yin-deficient fire.

This formula contains *Mai Dong* (Radix Ophiopogonis) to nourish Lung and Stomach yin and clear deficiency fire.

***Mai Men Dong Tang* (Ophiopogonis Decoction)**

Diagnosis	Clinical Signs	Treatment	Herbs
Lung and/or Stomach yin deficiencies	• Coughing: reversed flow of Lung qi • Nausea and vomiting: reversed flow of Stomach qi • Difficult-to-expectorate sputum, thirst, and a dry mouth and throat: deficiency fire • Red tongue with little coating and a thready, rapid pulse: yin-deficient fire	• Nourishes Lung and Stomach yin • Corrects the reversed flow of qi and harmonizes the middle *jiao*	• *Mai Dong* (Radix Ophiopogonis) nourishes yin and clears deficiency fire. • *Ban Xia* (Rhizoma Pinelliae) corrects the reversed flow of qi and dissolves phlegm. • *Ren Shen* (Radix et Rhizoma Ginseng) tonifies qi and generates body fluids. • *Geng Mi* (Semen Oryzae), *Da Zao* (Fructus Jujubae), and *Gan Cao* (Radix et Rhizoma Glycyrrhizae) nourish the Spleen and Stomach.

Mài Mén Dōng Tāng (Ophiopogonis Decoction)

Ban Xia (Rhizoma Pinelliae) corrects the reversed flow of qi and dissolves phlegm. These two herbs also provide mutual checks and balances, as *Mai Dong* (Radix Ophiopogonis) controls the drying nature of *Ban Xia* (Rhizoma Pinelliae), while *Ban Xia* (Rhizoma Pinelliae) balances the cloying nature of *Mai Dong* (Radix Ophiopogonis). *Ren Shen* (Radix et Rhizoma Ginseng) combines with *Mai Dong* (Radix Ophiopogonis) to tonify qi and generate body fluids. *Geng Mi* (Semen Oryzae), *Da Zao* (Fructus Jujubae), and *Gan Cao* (Radix et Rhizoma Glycyrrhizae) nourish the Spleen and Stomach and tonify *zhong* (central) *qi*.

VETERINARY MODIFICATIONS

- With low-grade fever, add *Yin Chai Hu* (Radix Stellariae) and *Di Gu Pi* (Cortex Lycii).
- When there is severe damage to the body fluids, add *Bei Sha Shen* (Radix Glehniae) and *Yu Zhu* (Rhizoma Polygonati Odorati).
- With thirst and irritability, add *Shi Gao* (Gypsum Fibrosum) and *Zhi Mu* (Rhizoma Anemarrhenae).
- If there is severe injury to yin and fluids, add *Bei Sha Shen* (Radix Glehniae) and *Yu Zhu* (Rhizoma Polygonati Odorati).
- With burning epigastric pain or dry heaves caused by Stomach yin deficiency, add *Bai He* (Bulbus Lilii).
- With extreme dryness, add *Tian Dong* (Radix Asparagi), *Bei Sha Shen* (Radix Glehniae) and *Nan Sha Shen* (Radix Adenophorae).
- With qi deficiency, combine with *Bu Zhong Yi Qi Tang* (Tonify the Middle and Augment the Qi Decoction).
- With Kidney yin deficiency, combine with *Liu Wei Di Huang Wan* (Six-Ingredient Pill with Rehmannia).
- With Kidney yin-deficient heat, combine with *Zhi Bai Di Huang Wan* (Anemarrhena, Phellodendron, and Rehmannia Pill).

CAUTIONS / CONTRAINDICATIONS

Mai Men Dong Tang is not suitable for atrophy of the Lung characterized by deficiency and cold.[1]

PHARMACOLOGICAL EFFECTS

1. **Antitussive**: According to various *in vitro* studies, administration of *Mai Men Dong Tang* was associated with antitussive effects to stop cough.[2] The mechanism of this antitussive effect was attributed in part to *Gan Cao* (Radix et Rhizoma Glycyrrhizae), which contain a potent antitussive compound, liquilitin apioside.[3]
2. **Respiratory**: *Mai Men Dong Tang* has been shown to have mucoactive effect on the production or composition of airway secretions, resulting in increased effectiveness of mucociliary clearance. In addition, *Mai Men Dong Tang* also reduced airway hyper-responsiveness by inhibiting the release of acetylcholine from vagus nerve terminals. Clinically, it has been used successfully to treat bronchitis and pharyngitis accompanying severe dry cough.[4,5]
3. **Hypoglycemic**: Administration of a water extract of *Mai Men Dong Tang* at 500 mg/kg given via intraperitoneal injection was shown to decrease blood glucose in mice with hereditary diabetes mellitus.[6]
4. **Beta-adrenergic**: According to a study in canines, administration of *Mai Men Dong Tang* potentiated beta-adrenergic functioning in airway smooth muscle, which reflects the efficacy of this formula to treat asthma and airway hyperresponsiveness.[7]

HUMAN CLINICAL STUDIES AND RESEARCH

1. **Nausea and vomiting**: One study reported 92.8% effectiveness using modified *Mai Men Dong Tang* to treat stubborn nausea and vomiting characterized by Stomach yin deficiency. The duration of treatment ranged from 3 to 9 packs of herbs. The herbal formula contained *Mai Dong* (Radix Ophiopogonis), *Ban Xia* (Rhizoma Pinelliae), *Ren Shen* (Radix et Rhizoma Ginseng), *Zhi Gan Cao* (Radix et Rhizoma Glycyrrhizae Praeparata cum Melle), *Geng Mi* (Semen Oryzae), *Da Zao* (Fructus Jujubae), *Zhu Ru* (Caulis Bambusae in Taenia), *Shi Hu* (Caulis Dendrobii), and *Pi Pa Ye* (Folium Eriobotryae). Of 42 patients, the study reported complete recovery in 20 cases, significant improvement in 15 cases, moderate improvement in 4 cases, and no effect in 3 cases.[8]
2. **Dry mouth and throat**: Administration of *Mai Men Dong Tang* was associated with marked success in 258 patients with dry mouth and throat due to various causes (radiation treatment, pharyngitis, and others). The formula was given in extract form, at 9g per day, for 1 to 4 weeks.[9]
3. **Stomach cramps**: One study reported success using *Mai Men Dong Tang* to treat gastrointestinal cramps with nausea, vomiting, poor appetite, and other clinical signs. A total of 3 packs of herbs were given in decoction.[10]
4. **Gastritis**: One study reported 78.57% effectiveness using modified *Mai Men Dong Tang* to treat 70 cases of chronic gastritis. Modifications to the base formula included the addition of *Si Ni San* (Frigid Extremities Powder) for Liver and Stomach disharmony; *Ban Xia Xie Xin Tang* (Pinellia Decoction to Drain the Epigastrium) for the presence of both cold and heat; *Li Zhong Tang* (Regulate the Middle Decoction) or *Xiao Jian Zhong Tang* (Minor Construct the Middle Decoction) for deficiency and cold of the Spleen and Stomach; and modifications of *Mai Men Dong Tang* for Stomach yin deficiency. The treatment protocol was to administer one pack of herbs in decoction daily, for each 1 month course of treatment.[11]

Mài Mén Dōng Tāng (Ophiopogonis Decoction)

5. **Chronic atrophic gastritis**: In one study, 30 patients with chronic atrophic gastritis were treated with good results using *Mai Men Dong Tang*. Clinical results include relief of clinical signs, such as bloating, distention, and abdominal pain.[12]
6. **Peptic ulcer disease**: One study reported a 95% effectiveness using modified *Mai Men Dong Tang* to treat 19 patients with peptic ulcer with a history of 1-5 years of illness. Most patients reported relief of clinical signs within an average of 9 packs of herbs.[13]
7. **Bronchitis**: According to one study, use of 9 grams per day of extract of *Mai Men Dong Tang* was associated with marked improvement for treatment of chronic bronchitis in 20 patients (5 males and 15 females). The study noted that 17 of 20 patients had a dry non-productive cough.[14]
8. **Cough**: According to one study, administration of *Mai Men Dong Tang* was associated with marked antitussive effects in both asthmatic and non-asthmatic patients. *Mai Men Dong Tang* was found to significantly improve the cough threshold value in 76% of patients with bronchial asthma, and in 82% without bronchial asthma. The study stated that *Mai Men Dong Tang* is an effective therapeutic preparation for cough hypersensitivity accompanying chronic diseases involving coughing, especially in cases of severe allergic inflammation.[15]
9. **Cough from interstitial pneumonia**: According to one case report, use of *Mai Men Dong Tang* was associated with dramatic relief of intractable dry cough within 10 days in a 50 year-old woman with progressive systemic sclerosis accompanied by interstitial pneumonia. Prior to herbal treatment, she was given a variety of antitussive agents over a one year period without success. The researchers stated that *Mai Men Dong Tang* may be a good antitussive agent for interstitial pneumonia associated with a dry cough that is resistant to other antitussives.[16]
10. **Postinfectious cough**: *Mai Men Dong Tang* was shown in many studies to be effective in the management of postinfectious cough.[17,18] According to one case study, use of *Mai Men Dong Tang* was associated with marked effects to suppress cough in a 63-year-old woman with interstitial lung disease and increased sensitivity of the cough reflex. Clinical improvements included subjective relief of cough, decreased cough scores, improved quality of life scores, and improved sensitivity of the cough reflex measured by inhalation of capsaicin.[19]

HERB-DRUG INTERACTION

- **Enalapril-induced cough**: Administration of *Mai Men Dong Tang* was found to be effective in treating 5 patients with dry cough induced by use of enalapril for 12 to 65 weeks. The treatment protocol was to administer the herbs in extract form, 9 grams per day in three equally-divided doses. Of 5 patients, the study reported significant improvement in 2 cases, moderate improvement in 2 cases, and no benefit in 1 case. Most patients responded within 2 to 4 days of herbal therapy, with no side effects noted.[20] The mechanisms were attributed to antitussive and mucoactive effects of *Mai Men Dong Tang*.[21]
- **Capsaicin-induced cough**: According to one study of 21 bronchial asthmatics with cough sensitivity to capsaicin, administration of 9 g/day of *Mai Men Dong Tang* significantly increased the cough threshold. The study noted that *Mai Men Dong Tang* was most effective in women, in asthmatic subjects with severe airway inflammation, and in patients having a disease duration of less than 1 year.[22]

TOXICOLOGY

Administration of *Mai Men Dong Tang* was associated with one case report of Stevens-Johnson syndrome. According to the report, after ingestion of this herbal formula, a 66-year-old female started to develop bullous and eroded lesions on the skin of her entire body and the mucous membranes of her oral cavity, conjunctiva, and cornea. A challenge test was done with a one hundredth dose, and it was positive at 72 hours. She was treated with methylprednisolone for a total of 5 days.[23]

SUGGESTED ACUPUNCTURE TREATMENT

1. Points: *Feishu* (BL 13), *Weishu* (BL 21), *Fuliu* (KI 7), *Taixi* (KI 3), and *Sanyinjiao* (SP 6).
2. Technique: tonification.

The underlying cause of this syndrome is Lung and Stomach yin deficiencies, leading to secondary problems such as reversed flow of qi, exuberance of fire, and body fluid damage. Therefore, *Feishu* (BL 13), *Weishu* (BL 21), *Fuliu* (KI 7), *Taixi* (KI 3), and *Sanyinjiao* (SP 6) are used together to nourish Lung and Stomach yin. However, if the patient shows coughing with dyspnea, *Shanzhong* (CV 17) and *Taiyuan* (LU 9) should be added. If the patient has nausea and vomiting as well, add *Zhongwan* (CV 12) and *Housanli* (ST 36).

AUTHORS' COMMENTS

Mai Men Dong Tang is one of the most common formulas for the treatment of early to moderate cases of pituitary dependent hyperadrenocorticism (Cushing's disease) in dogs. The cause of this disease is considered to be multifactorial and due to a combination of patterns. The most common patterns include chronic Liver qi stagnation with Spleen and Stomach damp-heat and phlegm, which eventually lead to deficiencies of the Lung and Stomach and the development of a pituitary mass. It is much more common for horses suffering from Cushing's disease to

Mài Mén Dōng Tāng (Ophiopogonis Decoction)

have a yang deficiency pattern; proper identification of an animal's deficiencies is crucial in these cases.

Mai Men Dong Tang should be administered in concentrated granule or powdered herb form for best results. A high dose (1-2 grams) is needed even for small dogs (less than 10 kg). Large dogs can take up to 4-5 grams per dose. It is best to initially administer the formula three times daily for the first 1-2 weeks of treatment. Response time is generally short and a decrease in polyphagia, polydipsia, polyuria and panting is typically reported by dog owners within this period. Dogs can take this formula long term (5 years) with modifications over time. The most commonly seen problem during progression of the disease is the development of qi deficiency. Kidney and Liver yin deficiencies and Liver qi stagnation and/or heat must also be addressed to effectively manage Cushing's disease; this formula can be combined with *Chai Hu Shu Gan San* (Bupleurum Powder to Spread the Liver), *Jia Wei Xiao Yao San* (Augmented Rambling Powder), *Tian Ma Gou Teng Yin* (Gastrodia and Uncaria Decoction) or *Yi Guan Jian* (Linking Decoction), depending on the clinical signs, to achieve this goal. In early cases the alkaline phosphatase level can be returned to normal and/or existing hypertension resolved using a combination of these formulas. Many dogs can be treated with herbal medications alone for up to 4 years before instituting conventional medical therapy. The authors have used *Mai Men Dong Tang* concurrently with the conventional medications trilostane and mitotane (lysodren), without adverse effects. The combination of trilostane and herbal medications has been found to be the treatment of choice in advanced cases of canine Cushing's disease, based on resolution of clinical signs and fewer number of adverse effects, as compared to lysodren therapy. Advanced cases of the disease will require administration of herbal formulas that moisten dryness, nourish yin, tonify qi, and control and resolve qi and blood stagnation.

Lung and/or Stomach yin deficiency with deficiency fire rising is a delicate condition that needs to be treated carefully. Strong heat-clearing herbs such as *Huang Lian* (Rhizoma Coptidis) and *Huang Qin* (Radix Scutellariae) are not appropriate, as they will consume yin and worsen the condition. Therefore, herbs such as *Mai Dong* (Radix Ophiopogonis) are used since they have gentle effects to nourish yin and clear deficiency fire. Because *Mai Dong* (Radix Ophiopogonis) is mild in potency, a large amount (60-70g) is needed or else the effects will not be realized.

Mai Men Dong Tang, Qing Zao Jiu Fei Tang (Eliminate Dryness and Rescue the Lungs Decoction) and *Bai He Gu Jin Tang* (Lily Bulb Decoction to Preserve the Metal) all treat cough and dyspnea caused by Lung yin deficiency.

- *Mai Men Dong Tang* treats Lung and Stomach yin deficiencies and has minimal ability to clear deficiency heat; it has the ability to address middle *jiao* weakness, with signs of nausea and vomiting.
- *Qing Zao Jiu Fei Tang* treats cough, Lung dryness and Lung qi reversal caused by warmth-dryness attacking from the exterior and injuring Lung yin. It is the least nourishing of the three formulas and contains herbs that tonify qi in addition to yin. For early recovery from external heat pathogen invasion, this formula is the most appropriate.
- *Bai He Gu Jin Tang* treats Lung and Kidney yin deficiencies with deficiency heat. This formula is the best at nourishing yin overall; if severe signs of yin deficiency are present, this formula would be the most appropriate to use.

References

1. *Zhong Yao Ming Fang Yao Li Yu Ying Yong* (Pharmacology and Applications of Famous Herbal Formulas), 1989; 614-615.
2. *Guo Wai Yi Xue* (Foreign Medicine), 1993; 6:29.
3. Kamei J, Nakamura R, Ichiki H, Kubo M. Antitussive principles of Glycyrrhizae radix, a main component of the Kampo preparations Bakumondo-to (Mai-men-dong-tang). Eur J Pharmacol. 2003 May 23; 469(1-3):159-63.
4. Miyata T. Novel approach to respiratory pharmacology--pharmacological basis of cough, sputum and airway clearance. Yakugaku Zasshi. 2003 Dec; 123(12):987-1006.
5. Aizawa H, Yoshida M, Inoue H, Hara N. Traditional oriental herbal medicine, Bakumondo-to, suppresses vagal neuro-effector transmission in guinea pig trachea. J Asthma. 2003; 40(5):497-503.
6. *Guo Wai Yi Xue* (Foreign Medicine), 1981; 6:10.
7. Tamaoki J, Chiyotani A, Takeyama K, Kanemura T, Sakai N, Konno K. Potentiation of beta-adrenergic function by saiboku-to and bakumondo-to in canine bronchial smooth muscle. Jpn J Pharmacol. 1993 Jun; 62(2):155-9.
8. *He Nan Zhong Yi* (Henan Chinese Medicine), 1990; 1:21.
9. *Guo Wai Yi Xue* (Foreign Medicine), 1995; 3:30.
10. *Si Chuan Zhong Yi* (Sichuan Chinese Medicine), 1991; 9:29.
11. *An Hui Zhong Yi Xue Yuan Xue Bao* (Journal of Anhui University School of Medicine), 1994; 2:25.
12. *Shi Yong Zhong Xi Yi Jie He Za Zhi* (Practical Journal of Integrated Chinese and Western Medicines), 1998; 7:631.
13. *Zhong Yi Za Zhi* (Journal of Chinese Medicine), 1964; 11:11.
14. *Guo Wai Yi Xue* (Foreign Medicine), 1993; 6:29.
15. Watanabe N, Gang C, Fukuda T. The effects of bakumondo-to (Mai-Men-Dong-Tang) on asthmatic and non-asthmatic patients with increased cough sensitivity. Nihon Kokyuki Gakkai Zasshi. 2004 Jan; 42(1):49-55.
16. Mizushima Y, Hirata A, Hori T, Sawazaki S, Sugiyama E, Kobayashi M. Antitussive effect of herbal medicine bakumondo-to: a case report. American Journal of Chinese Medicine. 1996; 24(3-4):321-5.
17. Isohama Y, Kai H, Miyata T. Bakumondo-to, a traditional herbal medicine, stimulates phosphatidylcholine secretion, through the synergistic cross-talk between different signal transduction systems in alveolar type II cells. Nippon Yakurigaku Zasshi. 1997 Oct; 110 Suppl 1:120P-125P.

Mài Mén Dōng Tāng (Ophiopogonis Decoction)

18. Fujimori K, Suzuki E, Arakawa M. Clinical features of postinfectious chronic cough. Arerugi. 1997 May; 46(5):420-5.
19. Fujimori K, Suzuki E, Gejyo F. Effect of Bakumondo-to on increased sensitivity of the cough reflex in a Sjogren syndrome patient with interstitial lung disease. Arerugi. 2001 Apr; 50(4):407-13.
20. *Guo Wai Yi Xue* (Foreign Medicine), 1993; 1:29.
21. Miyata T. Novel approach to respiratory pharmacology--pharmacological basis of cough, sputum and airway clearance. Yakugaku Zasshi. 2003 Dec; 123(12):987-1006.
22. Watanabe N, Cheng G, Fukuda T. Effects of Bakumondo-to (Mai-Men-Dong-Tang) on cough sensitivity to capsaicin in asthmatic patients with cough hypersensitivity. Arerugi. 2003 May; 52(5):485-91.
23. Mochitomi Y, Inoue A, Kawabata H, Ishida S, Kanzaki T. Stevens-Johnson syndrome caused by a health drink (Eberu) containing ophiopogonis tuber. Journal of Dermatology. 1998 Oct; 25(10):662-5.

Shā Shēn Mài Dōng Tāng (Glehnia and Ophiopogonis Decoction)

沙參麥冬湯

沙参麦冬汤

Pinyin Name: *Sha Shen Mai Dong Tang*
Literal Name: Glehnia and Ophiopogonis Decoction
Alternate Name: Glehnia and Ophiopogon Combination
Original Source: *Wen Bing Tiao Bian* (Systematic Differentiation of Warm Diseases) by Wu Ju-Tong in 1798

COMPOSITION

Sha Shen (Radix Glehniae seu Adenophorae)	9g
Mai Dong (Radix Ophiopogonis)	9g
Yu Zhu (Rhizoma Polygonati Odorati)	6g
Tian Hua Fen (Radix Trichosanthis)	4.5g
Sang Ye (Folium Mori)	4.5g
Bai Bian Dou (Semen Lablab Album)	4.5g
Gan Cao (Radix et Rhizoma Glycyrrhizae)	3g

Note: The source text uses *Sha Shen* (Radix Glehniae seu Adenophorae) as the chief herb but does not specify whether it is *Bei Sha Shen* (Radix Glehniae) or *Nan Sha Shen* (Radix Adenophorae). Both herbs have similar functions to moisten Lung yin, nourish the Stomach, and generate body fluids. However, *Bei Sha Shen* (Radix Glehniae) is stronger in nourishing yin and clearing heat, while *Nan Sha Shen* (Radix Adenophorae) is better at nourishing yin and dispelling phlegm. Therefore, *Bei Sha Shen* (Radix Glehniae) is generally considered more suitable for this formula.

DOSAGE / PREPARATION / ADMINISTRATION

Cook the ingredients with 5 cups of water until the liquid is reduced to 2 cups. Take the decoction one time daily.

Shā Shēn Mài Dōng Tāng (Glehnia and Ophiopogonis Decoction)

CHINESE THERAPEUTIC ACTIONS

1. Clears and nourishes the Lung and Stomach
2. Promotes secretion of body fluids and moistens dryness

CLINICAL MANIFESTATIONS

Dryness damaging Lung and Stomach yin: dry throat, thirst, fever, dry coughing, and dry, sticky sputum.

VETERINARY CLINICAL APPLICATIONS

Atrophic gastritis, epigastric pain, lung cancer, pneumonia, bronchitis, dry cough and diabetes mellitus.

EXPLANATION

Sha Shen Mai Dong Tang (Glehnia and Ophiopogonis Decoction) nourishes Lung and Stomach yin, promotes secretion of body fluids, and moistens dryness. It utilizes *Sha Shen* (Radix Glehniae seu Adenophorae) and *Mai Dong* (Radix Ophiopogonis) to promote the generation of fluids, moisten dryness, and nourish Lung and Stomach yin. These two herbs also help to clear heat and dryness. *Yu Zhu* (Rhizoma Polygonati Odorati) and *Tian Hua Fen* (Radix Trichosanthis) promote the generation of fluids and relieve thirst. *Sang Ye* (Folium Mori) releases warmth and dryness from the Lung. *Bai Bian Dou* (Semen Lablab Album) and *Gan Cao* (Radix et Rhizoma Glycyrrhizae) benefit qi, strengthen the middle *jiao,* and harmonize all of the herbs.

VETERINARY MODIFICATIONS

- With dry coughing and scanty sputum, add *Chuan Bei Mu* (Bulbus Fritillariae Cirrhosae) and *Gua Lou* (Fructus Trichosanthis).
- With chronic cough due to heat, add *Di Gu Pi* (Cortex Lycii) and *Jie Geng* (Radix Platycodonis).
- With constipation, add *Xuan Shen* (Radix Scrophulariae) and *Di Huang* (Radix Rehmanniae).

PHARMACOLOGICAL EFFECTS

Gastrointestinal: *Sha Shen Mai Dong Tang* has been shown to have various effects on the gastrointestinal system. It has protective effects against ethanol-induced stomach ulcers and bleeding in rats. It has a marked protective effect against drug-induced damage to the stomach and its mucous membrane. The mechanism of action is attributed in part to the increased generation of stomach mucous membrane and decreased production of stomach acid. Lastly, the formula is deemed to be more effective at higher dose (20 g/kg) than lower dose (10 g/kg).[1,2]

HUMAN CLINICAL STUDIES AND RESEARCH

1. **Atrophic gastritis**: Administration of *Sha Shen Mai Dong Tang* was shown to effectively treat chronic atrophic gastritis. According to one study of 88 patients, improvement was seen in 97.7% of the patients, based on symptomatic evaluation, and improvement in 47.7% based on gastroscope evaluation.[3]
2. **Epigastric pain**: *Sha Shen Mai Dong Tang* was used in 40 patients to treat epigastric pain characterized by yin deficiency. Most patients had a history of between 7 and 20 years of illness. Clinical manifestations included dull or burning pain, especially on an empty stomach, a red tongue with little moisture and few fissures, and a fine, rapid pulse. The herbal formula contained *Bei Sha Shen* (Radix Glehniae) 20g, *Mai Dong* (Radix Ophiopogonis) 12g, *Yu Zhu* (Rhizoma Polygonati Odorati) 10g, *Shi Hu* (Caulis Dendrobii) 15g, *Bai He* (Bulbus Lilii) 10g, *Shan Yao* (Rhizoma Dioscoreae) 15g, *Dan Shen* (Radix et Rhizoma Salviae Miltiorrhizae) 15g, and *Zhi Gan Cao* (Radix et Rhizoma Glycyrrhizae Praeparata cum Melle) 10g. The treatment protocol was to cook the herbs in water and administer the decoction in two to three equally-divided doses. Of 40 patients, the study reported complete recovery in 21 patients, marked improvement

***Sha Shen Mai Dong Tang* (Glehnia and Ophiopogonis Decoction)**

Diagnosis	Clinical Signs	Treatment	Herbs
Dryness damaging Lung and Stomach yin	• Dry coughing and dry, sticky sputum: dryness damaging Lung yin • Dry throat and thirst: dryness damaging Stomach yin	• Clears and nourishes the Lung and Stomach • Generates body fluids and moistens dryness	• *Sha Shen* (Radix Glehniae seu Adenophorae) and *Mai Dong* (Radix Ophiopogonis) promote the generation of fluids, moisten dryness, and nourish Lung and Stomach. • *Yu Zhu* (Rhizoma Polygonati Odorati) and *Tian Hua Fen* (Radix Trichosanthis) promote the generation of fluids and relieve thirst. • *Sang Ye* (Folium Mori) releases warmth and dryness from the Lung. • *Bai Bian Dou* (Semen Lablab Album) and *Gan Cao* (Radix et Rhizoma Glycyrrhizae) benefit qi, strengthen the middle *jiao,* and harmonize all of the herbs.

Shā Shēn Mài Dōng Tāng (Glehnia and Ophiopogonis Decoction)

in 15 patients, moderate improvement in 3 patients, and no benefit in 1 patient. The overall effectiveness was 97.5%.[4]

3. **Lung cancer**: According to one study, administration of *Sha Shen Mai Dong Tang* plus a 10% *Ya Dan Zi* (Fructus Bruceae) preparation in 23 patients with lung cancer was associated with partial relief in 21.74%, stabilization in 39.13%, and no benefit in 39.13% of patients.[5]
4. **Pneumonia**: One study of 25 children with pneumonia reported complete recovery in 22 patients, significant improvement in 2 patients, and no benefit in 1 patient, after treatment with modified *Sha Shen Mai Dong Tang*.[6]
5. **Dry cough**: One study reported 96% effectiveness using modified *Sha Shen Mai Dong Tang* to treat 154 patients with dry cough. The herbal formula contained *Sha Shen* (Radix Glehniae seu Adenophorae), *Mai Dong* (Radix Ophiopogonis), *Yu Zhu* (Rhizoma Polygonati Odorati), *Tian Hua Fen* (Radix Trichosanthis), *Gan Cao* (Radix et Rhizoma Glycyrrhizae), *Sang Ye* (Folium Mori), *Bai Bian Dou* (Semen Lablab Album), and others. Furthermore, *Ge Gen* (Radix Puerariae Lobatae), *Bai Zhi* (Radix Angelicae Dahuricae), *Lian Qiao* (Fructus Forsythiae), *Chai Hu* (Radix Bupleuri), and *Ban Lan Gen* (Radix Isatidis) were added for cough with an exterior condition; and *Ku Xing Ren* (Semen Armeniacae Amarum), *Zhe Bei Mu* (Bulbus Fritillariae Thunbergii), *Chuan Bei Mu* (Bulbus Fritillariae Cirrhosae), *Yu Xing Cao* (Herba Houttuyniae), and others were added for severe cough. The treatment protocol was to administer the herbs in decoction, for 2 to 5 days per treatment course. Of 154 patients, the study reported complete recovery in 76 patients, significant improvement in 54 patients, moderate improvement in 18 patients, and no benefit in 6 patients.[7]
6. **Cough and wheezing in children**: According to one study, 40 children with cough and wheezing were treated with good results using modified *Sha Shen Mai Dong Tang*. The herbal formula contained *Sha Shen* (Radix Glehniae seu Adenophorae), *Mai Dong* (Radix Ophiopogonis), *Tian Hua Fen* (Radix Trichosanthis), *Yu Zhu* (Rhizoma Polygonati Odorati), *Bai Bian Dou* (Semen Lablab Album), *Sang Ye* (Folium Mori), *Di Long* (Pheretima), *Jie Geng* (Radix Platycodonis), *Pi Pa Ye* (Folium Eriobotryae), and *Gan Cao* (Radix et Rhizoma Glycyrrhizae). Additional modifications were made by adding *Huang Qin* (Radix Scutellariae), and *Shi Gao* (Gypsum Fibrosum) for fever; and *Ma Huang* (Herba Ephedrae) and *Ku Xing Ren* (Semen Armeniacae Amarum) for severe wheezing. The dose of herbs varied depending on the age of the children. Of 40 patients, the study reported complete recovery in 29 patients, improvement in 9 patients, and no benefit in 2 patients.[8]
7. **Diabetes mellitus**: Administration of *Sha Shen Mai Dong Tang* in 186 patients with diabetes mellitus was associated with marked benefit in 106 patients, moderate effectiveness in 60 patients, and no benefit in 20 patients. The overall rate of effectiveness was 89.2%.[9]

SUGGESTED ACUPUNCTURE TREATMENT

1. Points: *Hegu* (LI 4), *Feishu* (BL 13), *Lieque* (LU 7), *Zhaohai* (KI 6), *Housanli* (ST 36), and *Weishu* (BL 21).
2. Technique: tonification.

Hegu (LI 4) moistens and ventilates the Lung. *Feishu* (BL 13) clears heat from the Lung channel. *Lieque* (LU 7) regulates Lung qi. *Zhaohai* (KI 6) nourishes the yin. *Housanli* (ST 36) tonifies all three *jiaos*, which in turn strengthens Lung qi. *Weishu* (BL 21) tonifies Lung and Stomach yin.

AUTHORS' COMMENTS

Sha Shen Mai Dong Tang was originally developed to treat Lung and Stomach dryness and damage to yin from an attack by external dryness, one of the *liu yin* (six exogenous factors). Today it can be used to treat fluid damage and dryness that results from chronic medication, chemotherapy or radiation, and following a febrile disease. Animals for whom this formula is appropriate have a dry, hacking cough, dry nose and mouth, and a dry, red tongue with little coating.

Clinically, practitioners may find that performance horses will suffer combined damage to the yin of both the Lung and Stomach from overwork, poor diet, and the administration of NSAIDs. This can lead to a presentation of a dry cough, along with clinical signs consistent with gastritis or gastric ulcer: epigastric and upper thoracic pain, a sour stomach or reflux, and poor performance. *Sha Shen Mai Dong Tang* may be used alone or in combination with *Xiao Yao San* (Rambling Powder) in such cases.

This formula can be used to treat diabetes mellitus from qi and yin deficiencies in dogs and cats, with appropriate clinical signs. It should be combined with *Huang Qi* (Radix Astragali), *Bai Zhu* (Rhizoma Atractylodis Macrocephalae), *Cang Zhu* (Rhizoma Atractylodis), *Xi Yang Shen* (Radix Panacis Quinquefolii), *Shan Yao* (Rhizoma Dioscoreae), *Shu Di Huang* (Radix Rehmanniae Praeparata), *Wu Wei Zi* (Fructus Schisandrae Chinensis) and *Ge Gen* (Radix Puerariae Lobatae) for best results.

Qing Zao Jiu Fei Tang (Eliminate Dryness and Rescue the Lungs Decoction) and *Sha Shen Mai Dong Tang* both contain *Sang Ye* (Folium Mori), *Mai Dong* (Radix

Shā Shēn Mài Dōng Tāng (Glehnia and Ophiopogonis Decoction)

Ophiopogonis), and *Gan Cao* (Radix et Rhizoma Glycyrrhizae) to moisten dryness.

- *Qing Zao Jiu Fei Tang* also contains *Shi Gao* (Gypsum Fibrosum), *Ren Shen* (Radix et Rhizoma Ginseng), *Hei Zhi Ma* (Semen Sesami Nigrum), *E Jiao* (Colla Corii Asini), *Ku Xing Ren* (Semen Armeniacae Amarum), and *Pi Pa Ye* (Folium Eriobotryae). *Qing Zao Jiu Fei Tang* has a stronger effect to ventilate the Lung, dispel exterior dryness, and clear heat. It nourishes yin and benefits qi.
- *Sha Shen Mai Dong Tang* also contains *Sha Shen* (Radix Glehniae seu Adenophorae), *Yu Zhu* (Rhizoma Polygonati Odorati), *Bai Bian Dou* (Semen Lablab Album), and *Tian Hua Fen* (Radix Trichosanthis). *Sha Shen Mai Dong Tang* has a weaker action to ventilate exterior heat-dryness, as its main effect is to moisten the Lung and Stomach and treat dryness with less exterior clinical signs.[10]

Sang Xing Tang (Mulberry Leaf and Apricot Kernel Decoction) and *Sha Shen Mai Dong Tang* both treat heat and dryness.

- *Sang Xing Tang* treats heat and dryness injuring the Lung at the exterior level, with a mild cough and slight thirst.
- *Sha Shen Mai Dong Tang* treats heat and dryness injuring yin, manifesting in Lung and Stomach yin-deficient clinical signs of more severe thirst, dry cough with scanty sputum, nausea, and poor appetite.[11]

References

1. *Zhong Yi Fang Ji Xian Dai Yan Jiu* (Modern Study of Medical Formulas in Traditional Chinese Medicine), 1997.
2. *Bei Jing Zhong Yi Xue Yuan Xue Bao* (Journal of Beijing University School of Medicine), 1994, 4:50.
3. *Zhong Xi Yi Jie He Za Zhi* (Journal of Integrated Chinese and Western Medicine), 1986, 6:342.
4. *Hu Nan Zhong Yi Za Zhi* (Hunan Journal of Chinese Medicine), 1987, 5:22.
5. *Ji Lin Zhong Yi Yao* (Jilin Chinese Medicine and Herbology), 1989, 3:19.
6. *He Bei Zhong Yi* (Hebei Chinese Medicine), 1998, 1:40.
7. *Si Chuan Zhong Yi* (Sichuan Chinese Medicine), 1987, 4:25.
8. *Shang Hai Zhong Yi Yao Za Zhi* (Shanghai Journal of Chinese Medicine and Herbology), 1990, 7:29.
9. *Shan Xi Zhong Yi* (Shanxi Chinese Medicine), 1995, 11:482.
10. Wang MZ, et al. *Zhong Yi Xue Wen Da Ti Ku* (Questions and Answers on Traditional Chinese Medicine: Herbal Formulas).
11. Wang MZ, et al. *Zhong Yi Xue Wen Da Ti Ku* (Questions and Answers on Traditional Chinese Medicine: Herbal Formulas).

Yù Yè Tāng (Jade Fluid Decoction)

玉液湯

玉液汤

Pinyin Name: *Yu Ye Tang*
Literal Name: Jade Fluid Decoction
Original Source: *Yi Xue Zhong Zhong Can Xi Lu* (Records of Heart-Felt Experiences in Medicine with Reference to the West) by Zhang Xi-Chun in 1918-34

COMPOSITION

Huang Qi (Radix Astragali)	15g
Shan Yao (Rhizoma Dioscoreae)	30g
Ge Gen (Radix Puerariae Lobatae)	4.5g
Zhi Mu (Rhizoma Anemarrhenae)	18g
Tian Hua Fen (Radix Trichosanthis)	9g
Ji Nei Jin (Endothelium Corneum Gigeriae Galli)	6g
Wu Wei Zi (Fructus Schisandrae Chinensis)	9g

Yù Yè Tāng (Jade Fluid Decoction)

DOSAGE / PREPARATION / ADMINISTRATION

Prepare the ingredients as a decoction.

CHINESE THERAPEUTIC ACTIONS

1. Tonifies qi, nourishes yin, and generates body fluids
2. Moistens dryness and relieves thirst

CLINICAL MANIFESTATIONS

Xiao ke (wasting and thirsting) syndrome: polydipsia with constant thirst, polyuria with increased volume and frequency of urination, turbid urine, lethargy, shortness of breath, and a weak, thin and forceless pulse.

VETERINARY CLINICAL APPLICATIONS

Diabetes mellitus, chronic gastritis, and epigastric pain.

EXPLANATION

Yu Ye Tang (Jade Fluid Decoction) treats chronic *xiao ke* (wasting and thirsting) syndrome characterized by qi and yin deficiencies with dryness and Kidney deficiency. When qi is deficient, water cannot be distributed properly to various parts of the body. With Lung and Stomach dryness, yin and body fluids become damaged. As a result, there is constant thirst and increased intake of water. Because of Kidney deficiency and abnormal water fluid distribution, there may be polyuria with an increase in both volume and frequency of urination, and turbid urine. Lastly, because of qi deficiency, there may be lethargy and shortness of breath. A pulse that is weak, thin and forceless indicates exhaustion of qi and body fluids.

Huang Qi (Radix Astragali) and *Shan Yao* (Rhizoma Dioscoreae), the two chief herbs, tonify qi and yin respectively. *Huang Qi* (Radix Astragali) tonifies Spleen qi, which in turn helps to regulate water circulation to relieve thirst. *Shan Yao* (Rhizoma Dioscoreae) relieves polyuria by tonifying the Spleen and consolidating the Kidney and stops polydipsia by moistening the Lung and generating body fluids. *Ge Gen* (Radix Puerariae Lobatae) causes qi to ascend, which helps to distribute the fluids to the *zang* (solid organs). *Zhi Mu* (Rhizoma Anemarrhenae) and *Tian Hua Fen* (Radix Trichosanthis) nourish yin and moisten dryness to relieve thirst. *Ji Nei Jin* (Endothelium Corneum Gigeriae Galli) assists the Spleen in properly distributing the fluids; its enzymes especially help the Spleen and Stomach in digestion. *Wu Wei Zi* (Fructus Schisandrae Chinensis) astringes yin and consolidates Kidney *jing* (essence).

VETERINARY MODIFICATIONS

- With more qi deficiency, add *Ren Shen* (Radix et Rhizoma Ginseng) or *Xi Yang Shen* (Radix Panacis Quinquefolii).
- With severe polydipsia, increase the dosage of *Tian Hua Fen* (Radix Trichosanthis) and *Ge Gen* (Radix Puerariae Lobatae) and add *Mai Dong* (Radix Ophiopogonis).
- With severe polyphagia, add *Huang Lian* (Rhizoma Coptidis) and *Cang Zhu* (Rhizoma Atractylodis).
- With severe polyuria, add *Shan Zhu Yu* (Fructus Corni).

PHARMACOLOGICAL EFFECTS

Hypoglycemic: *Yu Ye Tang* has been shown in many studies to effectively reduce plasma glucose levels in rabbits and mice. The onset of the hypoglycemic action was observed after approximately 2 to 3 hours, and lasted until 6 to 7.5 hours after oral ingestion of this formula.[1,2,3]

***Yu Ye Tang* (Jade Fluid Decoction)**

Diagnosis	Clinical Signs	Treatment	Herbs
Xiao ke (wasting and thirsting) syndrome	• Thirst and increased intake of water: dryness damaging yin and body fluids • Polyuria with an increase in both volume and frequency of urination, and turbid urine: Kidney deficiency and abnormal water fluid distribution • Lethargy and shortness of breath: qi deficiency • A deficient, fine and forceless pulse: exhaustion of qi and body fluids.	• Tonifies qi and generates body fluids • Moistens dryness and relieves thirst	• *Huang Qi* (Radix Astragali) tonifies Spleen qi. • *Shan Yao* (Rhizoma Dioscoreae) tonifies the Spleen and Kidney to relieve polyuria and polydipsia. • *Ge Gen* (Radix Puerariae Lobatae) causes qi to ascend and helps to distribute the fluids. • *Zhi Mu* (Rhizoma Anemarrhenae) and *Tian Hua Fen* (Radix Trichosanthis) nourish yin and moisten dryness to relieve the thirst. • *Ji Nei Jin* (Endothelium Corneum Gigeriae Galli) benefits the Spleen to improve distribution of water and digestion of food. • *Wu Wei Zi* (Fructus Schisandrae Chinensis) astringes yin and consolidates Kidney *jing* (essence).

Yù Yè Tāng (Jade Fluid Decoction)

HUMAN CLINICAL STUDIES AND RESEARCH

1. **Diabetes mellitus**: *Yu Ye Tang* was shown in many studies to effectively treat diabetes mellitus. According to one study of 60 diabetic patients treated with modified *Yu Ye Tang*, 29 had marked improvement, 25 showed moderate improvement, and 6 had no effect. The herbal formula contained *Shan Yao* (Rhizoma Dioscoreae) 30g, *Tian Hua Fen* (Radix Trichosanthis) 30g, *Huang Qi* (Radix Astragali) 25g, *Zhi Mu* (Rhizoma Anemarrhenae) 15g, *Ji Nei Jin* (Endothelium Corneum Gigeriae Galli) 15g, *Ge Gen* (Radix Puerariae Lobatae) 15g, and *Wu Wei Zi* (Fructus Schisandrae Chinensis) 12g. Modifications included addition of *Shan Zhu Yu* (Fructus Corni) 15g, *Yi Zhi* (Fructus Alpiniae Oxyphyllae) 15g, *Fu Pen Zi* (Fructus Rubi) 20g, and *Sang Piao Xiao* (Ootheca Mantidis) 30g for soreness of the lower back and knees, fatigue, frequent urination, and cloudy urine.[4]

   Another study reported 94.1% effectiveness using modified *Yu Ye Tang* to treat 51 patients with diabetes characterized by qi and yin deficiencies. The herbal formula was based on the modification of *Yu Ye Tang*, and contained *Ren Shen* (Radix et Rhizoma Ginseng), *Zhi Mu* (Rhizoma Anemarrhenae), *Ji Nei Jin* (Endothelium Corneum Gigeriae Galli), *Wu Wei Zi* (Fructus Schisandrae Chinensis), *Shan Yao* (Rhizoma Dioscoreae), *Huang Qi* (Radix Astragali), *Ge Gen* (Radix Puerariae Lobatae), and *Tian Hua Fen* (Radix Trichosanthis). The treatment protocol was to administer the formula in decoction daily, for 60 days per course of treatment, for a total of 3 to 6 courses. Of 51 patients, the study reported significant improvement in 22 cases, moderate improvement in 26 cases, and no effect in 3 cases.[5]
2. **Chronic gastritis**: One study reported a 69% success rate using modified *Yu Ye Tang* to treat chronic gastritis. Of 127 patients, the study reported complete recovery in 87 cases, improvement in 39 cases, and no effect in 1 case.[6]
3. **Epigastric pain**: Use of *Yu Ye Tang* was beneficial in treating 126 patients with epigastric pain characterized by Stomach yin deficiency. Western medical diagnoses included hypertrophic gastritis, gastric ulcer, duodenal ulcer, superficial gastritis, atrophic gastritis, and others. The herbal formula contained *Shan Yao* (Rhizoma Dioscoreae) 30g, *Huang Qi* (Radix Astragali) 15g, *Zhi Mu* (Rhizoma Anemarrhenae) 18g, *Ji Nei Jin* (Endothelium Corneum Gigeriae Galli) 6g, *Ge Gen* (Radix Puerariae Lobatae) 5g, *Wu Wei Zi* (Fructus Schisandrae Chinensis) 10g, and *Tian Hua Fen* (Radix Trichosanthis) 10g. Other modifications were made as needed. The herbs were cooked in water, and the decoction was administered in two to three equally-divided doses. Of 126 patients, the study reported complete recovery in 87 cases and improvement in 39 cases. The duration of treatment ranged from 30 to 100 packs of herbs.[7]

SUGGESTED ACUPUNCTURE TREATMENT

1. Points: *Shenshu* (BL 23), *Taixi* (KI 3), *Pishu* (BL 20), *Sanyinjiao* (SP 6), *Yinlingquan* (SP 9), *Weishu* (BL 21), *Zhongwan* (CV 12), and *Neiting* (ST 44).
2. Technique: tonification.

Patients with *xiao ke* (wasting and thirsting) syndrome usually have constant thirst, hunger, and frequent urination. The treatment plan must focus on tonifying qi and body fluids, as well as clearing heat. *Shenshu* (BL 23) and *Taixi* (KI 3) tonify Kidney yin and reduce polyuria. *Pishu* (BL 20), *Yinlingquan* (SP 9), and *Sanyinjiao* (SP 6) tonify Spleen qi to promote body fluids. *Weishu* (BL 21), *Zhongwan* (CV 12), and *Neiting* (ST 44) clear Stomach heat and stop thirst.

AUTHORS' COMMENTS

Yu Ye Tang is best for chronic *xiao ke* (wasting and thirsting) syndrome with damage to qi and yin. Chief complaints include constant polyphagia, polydipsia and polyuria. This formula is not commercially available but can easily be prepared in-house.

Yu Ye Tang and *Liu Wei Di Huang Wan* (Six-Ingredient Pill with Rehmannia) both treat *xiao ke* (wasting and thirsting) syndrome. However, there are some differences:

- *Yu Ye Tang* treats *xiao ke* (wasting and thirsting) syndrome caused by dryness secondary to Kidney deficiency and the inability of the qi to properly disseminate fluids throughout the body. Besides thirst and desire to drink, other clinical signs include frequent and profuse urination, fatigue, shortness of breath, and a weak, thin and forceless pulse.
- *Liu Wei Di Huang Wan* treats *xiao ke* (wasting and thirsting) syndrome caused by Kidney and Liver yin deficiencies. Associated clinical signs include soreness and weakness of the lower back and knees, dizziness, tinnitus, dry throat and mouth, a red tongue with a scanty coating, and a thin, rapid pulse.[8]
- In many cases of chronic diabetes, these two formula are combined and additional herbs or other formulas are added, such as *Bu Yang Huan Wu Tang* (Tonify the Yang to Restore Five Decoction) and *Xue Fu Zhu Yu Tang* (Drive Out Stasis in the Mansion of Blood Decoction) to treat blood stagnation.

Yù Yè Tāng (Jade Fluid Decoction)

References

1. *Zhong Yao Tong Bao* (Journal of Chinese Herbology), 1994; 4:33.
2. *Zhong Yao Yao Li Yu Lin Chuang* (Pharmacology and Clinical Applications of Chinese Herbs), 1992; 21.
3. *Zhong Yao Tong Bao* (Journal of Chinese Herbology), 1982; 6:32.
4. *He Nan Zhong Yi* (Henan Chinese Medicine), 1990; 6:22.
5. *Shan Xi Zhong Yi* (Shanxi Chinese Medicine), 1991; 2:51.
6. *Zhe Jiang Zhong Yi Za Zhi* (Zhejiang Journal of Chinese Medicine), 1990; 10:437.
7. *Hu Bei Zhong Yi Za Zhi* (Hubei Journal of Chinese Medicine), 1990; 6:8.
8. Wang MZ, et al. *Zhong Yi Xue Wen Da Ti Ku* (Questions and Answers on Traditional Chinese Medicine: Herbal Formulas).

Yù Quán Wán (Jade Spring Pill)

玉泉丸

Pinyin Name: *Yu Quan Wan*
Literal Name: Jade Spring Pill
Alternate Names: *Yu Chuan Wan,* Jade-Spring Pill, Jade Source Combination
Original Source: *Za Bing Yuan Liu Xi Zhu* (Wondrous Lantern for Peering into Origin and Development of Miscellaneous Diseases) by Shen Jin-Ao in 1773

COMPOSITION

Tian Hua Fen (Radix Trichosanthis)	45g
Di Huang (Radix Rehmanniae)	30g
Ge Gen (Radix Puerariae Lobatae)	45g
Fu Ling (Poria)	30g
Mai Dong (Radix Ophiopogonis)	30g
Ren Shen (Radix et Rhizoma Ginseng)	30g
Huang Qi (Radix Astragali)	15g
Huang Qi (Radix Astragali), *mi zhi* (fried with honey)	15g
Wu Mei (Fructus Mume), *bei* (stone-baked)	30g
Wu Wei Zi (Fructus Schisandrae Chinensis)	30g
Gan Cao (Radix et Rhizoma Glycyrrhizae)	30g

DOSAGE / PREPARATION / ADMINISTRATION

The source text instructs to stone-bake *Wu Mei* (Fructus Mume) and fry 15g (which represents half of the total amount) of *Huang Qi* (Radix Astragali) with honey. Grind all of the ingredients into powder and form into pills with honey. The pills should resemble large bullets in size. Chew and swallow one pill per dose with warm water.

CHINESE THERAPEUTIC ACTIONS

1. Generates body fluids to relieve thirst
2. Nourishes yin to moisten dryness
3. Tonifies qi

CLINICAL MANIFESTATIONS

Xiao ke (wasting and thirsting) syndrome: irritability, thirst, polyphagia, polydipsia and polyuria, a red, dry tongue, and a weak, thin pulse.

Yù Quán Wán (Jade Spring Pill)

VETERINARY CLINICAL APPLICATIONS

Diabetes mellitus and diabetes insipidus.

EXPLANATION

Yu Quan Wan (Jade Spring Pill) treats *xiao ke* (wasting and thirsting) syndrome due to yin and qi deficiencies, a condition characterized by increased thirst and water intake (polydipsia), increased hunger with food intake (polyphagia), increased urination (polyuria), and decreased body weight. The underlying etiology of advanced or established *xiao ke* syndrome is yin and/or qi deficiency with heat, especially of the Lung, Stomach, and Kidney. In addition to polydipsia, polyphagia, and polyuria, patients may also have classic signs of yin deficiency with heat: generalized weakness, irritability, insomnia, restlessness, excessive panting (especially at night), dry cough, constipation or dry feces, short urination, heat aversion, a preference for cool surfaces/places, trembling and jerking during sleep, poor hearing or deafness, hypersensitivity to acupuncture, a red tongue body with little to no coating, and a rapid, weak, thin pulse. Sometimes chronic deficiency heat patients may experience chronic low-grade fever.

In this formula, *Tian Hua Fen* (Radix Trichosanthis) and *Di Huang* (Radix Rehmanniae) promote the generation of body fluids and clear heat. *Ge Gen* (Radix Puerariae Lobatae) has an ascending function and disperses fluids to various parts of the body. These three herbs work synergistically to promote and disperse fluids and treat *xiao ke* (wasting and thirsting) syndrome. *Fu Ling* (Poria) strengthens the Spleen and Stomach and promotes normal urination. *Mai Dong* (Radix Ophiopogonis) nourishes the Lung and Stomach and addresses the underlying yin deficiency. *Ren Shen* (Radix et Rhizoma Ginseng) and *Huang Qi* (Radix Astragali) tonify qi. *Wu Mei* (Fructus Mume) and *Wu Wei Zi* (Fructus Schisandrae Chinensis) relieve thirst. *Gan Cao* (Radix et Rhizoma Glycyrrhizae) harmonizes all of the herbs in the formula.

VETERINARY MODIFICATIONS

- With more yin deficiency and interior heat, add *Bie Jia* (Carapax Trionycis) and *Mu Dan Pi* (Cortex Moutan).
- With phlegm, add *Chen Pi* (Pericarpium Citri Reticulatae) and *Ban Xia* (Rhizoma Pinelliae).
- With Kidney yang deficiency, add *Tu Si Zi* (Semen Cuscutae), *Fu Zi* (Radix Aconiti Lateralis Praeparata), *Rou Gui* (Cortex Cinnamomi), and *Xian Mao* (Rhizoma Curculiginis).
- With Kidney yin deficiency, add *Xuan Shen* (Radix Scrophulariae), *Gou Qi Zi* (Fructus Lycii), and *Gui Ban* (Plastrum Testudinis).
- With excessive hunger, increase the dosage of *Di Huang* (Radix Rehmanniae) and add *Shu Di Huang* (Radix Rehmanniae Praeparata).
- For the treatment of blood stasis, it can be combined with *Dan Shen* (Radix et Rhizoma Salviae Miltiorrhizae), *Hong Hua* (Flos Carthami) and *Mao Dong Qing* (Radix Ilicis Pubescentis).

CAUTIONS / CONTRAINDICATIONS

Avoid acrid and spicy foods while taking *Yu Quan Wan*.[1]

***Yu Quan Wan* (Jade Spring Pill)**

Diagnosis	Clinical Signs	Treatment	Herbs
Xiao ke (wasting and thirsting) syndrome	• Increased thirst and water intake with a dry mouth and tongue: yin deficiency with Lung heat • Increased hunger and food intake: yin deficiency with Stomach heat • Increased urination: Kidney deficiency	• Generates body fluids to relieve thirst • Nourishes yin to moisten dryness	• *Tian Hua Fen* (Radix Trichosanthis) and *Di Huang* (Radix Rehmanniae) promote the generation of body fluids and clear heat. • *Ge Gen* (Radix Puerariae Lobatae) has an ascending function and disperses fluids to various parts of the body. • *Fu Ling* (Poria) strengthens the Spleen and Stomach and promotes normal urination. • *Mai Dong* (Radix Ophiopogonis) nourishes Lung and Stomach yin. • *Ren Shen* (Radix et Rhizoma Ginseng) and *Huang Qi* (Radix Astragali) tonify qi. • *Wu Mei* (Fructus Mume) and *Wu Wei Zi* (Fructus Schisandrae Chinensis) relieve thirst. • *Gan Cao* (Radix et Rhizoma Glycyrrhizae) harmonizes all of the herbs.

Yù Quán Wán (Jade Spring Pill)

PHARMACOLOGICAL EFFECTS

Hypoglycemic: Administration of *Yu Quan Wan* in capsules or pills was associated with a reduction in plasma glucose levels in rabbits, with the action beginning approximately 3 hours after oral ingestion, and continuing for approximately 9 to 12 hours.[2]

HUMAN CLINICAL STUDIES AND RESEARCH

Diabetes mellitus: Administration of *Yu Quan Wan* four times daily was associated with 86.35% effectiveness in treating 30 patients with type II diabetes.[3] Another study also reported good results using modified *Yu Quan Wan* four times daily to treat 18 patients with diabetes mellitus characterized by polydipsia, polyphagia, polyuria, and weight loss.[4]

TOXICOLOGY

In one acute toxicology study, administration of *Yu Quan Wan* in powder form at 12.5 g/kg/day in two equally-divided doses for two days did not cause any abnormal reactions within a 72 hour period of observation.[5]

SUGGESTED ACUPUNCTURE TREATMENT

1. Points: *Chize* (LU 5), *Jiexi* (ST 41), *Fuliu* (KI 7), *Yemen* (TH 2), *Housanli* (ST 36), *Guanyuan* (CV 4), *Yinlingquan* (SP 9), *Taiyuan* (LU 9), and *Taichong* (LR 3).
2. Technique: even method.

Chize (LU 5), *Jiexi* (ST 41), *Fuliu* (KI 7), and *Yemen* (TH 2) generate body fluids. *Housanli* (ST 36) and *Guanyuan* (CV 4) tonify qi. *Yinlingquan* (SP 9), *Taiyuan* (LU 9), and *Taichong* (LR 3) nourish yin to moisten dryness.

AUTHORS' COMMENTS

Yu Quan Wan is one of the most common formulas used to treat diabetes in dogs and cats due to qi and yin deficiencies. This formula tonifies qi and yin and promotes the production of body fluids. It can be used to treat any pattern of diabetes, including Type I diabetes (IDDM: insulin dependent diabetes mellitus) and Type II diabetes (NIDDM: non-insulin dependent diabetes mellitus). The cause of IDDM is poorly characterized and is considered to be multi-factorial in nature; the end result is a destruction of the islets of Langerhans and the subsequent inability to produce insulin or "insulin deficiency." NIDDM is largely associated with obesity and cellular insulin insensitivity. Initially, insulin production can be much higher than normal in this condition with "insulin excess." When given early in the disease and with appropriate dietary therapy, *Yu Quan Wan* has shown the ability to reverse NIDDM in cats. In early cases, this formula can be used to reverse diabetes, stop the destruction of pancreatic beta cells, and preserve their remaining function.

The goal of using herbal formula in an integrative approach to diabetes is to promote or enhance the effectiveness of insulin and/or drug therapy to treat insulin resistance, improve glucose tolerance, normalize blood sugar levels, and reduce unwanted side effects. Human studies have shown that tight control of blood glucose in diabetic patients dramatically decreases the risks of the side effects of uncontrolled hyperglycemia and the development of ocular, renal, and neurovascular diseases. In light of these statistics, it would seem prudent to use whatever safe and reasonable therapies that are currently available to maintain precise blood glucose control in pets, just as is done in humans. The authors have used herbal medications in combination with insulin for ten years for the treatment of diabetes in dogs and cats. An integrative approach helps prevent secondary complications of diabetes, promotes a high quality of life, and improves longevity in chronic diabetic patients.

There are many patent formulas sold under the name "*Yu Quan Wan*," and each contains different herbs that are modifications of the original formula and may vary in action. It is important to read each formula's herbal composition so that accurate prescribing and modification can be made. Another reason for the formula's popularity is that it can easily be combined with many other formulas to achieve good results. *Yu Quan Wan* should initially be given three times daily and can be combined with oral hypoglycemics and insulin without adverse effects. The combination of *Yu Quan Wan*, oral hypoglycemic drugs and insulin is synergistic; however, the onset of action of this formula is gradual, and the dosage of insulin can be safely and easily adjusted through monitoring of clinical signs, weekly blood glucose evaluations in the short term, and via fructosamine levels or blood glucose curve every 3-4 weeks in the long term.

Yu Quan Wan is often combined with other formulas to treat diabetes and its complications:

- To further nourish yin in chronic disease, combine with *Liu Wei Di Huang Wan* (Six-Ingredient Pill with Rehmannia).
- To nourish yin and clear deficiency heat, combine with *Zhi Bai Di Huang Wan* (Anemarrhena, Phellodendron, and Rehmannia Pill).
- For animals with qi and/or yang deficiency, combine with *Ba Wei Di Huang Wan* (Eight-Ingredient Pill with Rehmannia).

Yù Quán Wán (Jade Spring Pill)

- In chronic cases with blood stasis and neuropathy or wounds that are slow to heal, it can be combined with *Xue Fu Zhu Yu Tang* (Drive Out Stasis in the Mansion of Blood Decoction), *Tao Hong Si Wu Tang* (Four-Substance Decoction with Safflower and Peach Pit), or *Bu Yang Huan Wu Tang* (Tonify the Yang to Restore Five Decoction) with appropriate clinical signs.

Yu Ye Tang (Jade Fluid Decoction) and *Yu Quan Wan* are two formulas that treat *xiao ke* (wasting and thirsting) syndrome with therapeutic effects to tonify qi, nourish yin, generate body fluids, and moisten dryness.

- *Yu Ye Tang* uses *Huang Qi* (Radix Astragali) and *Shan Yao* (Rhizoma Dioscoreae) as chief herbs and has a stronger function to tonify qi in addition to yin.
- *Yu Quan Wan* uses *Tian Hua Fen* (Radix Trichosanthis) and *Di Huang* (Radix Rehmanniae) as chief herbs and has a more potent effect to nourish yin, clear deficiency heat, and generate body fluids.
- These two formulas can be combined together in a 1:1 ratio to more strongly tonify qi and yin to improve clinical results.

References

1. *Zhong Yao Ming Fang Yao Li Yu Ying Yong* (Pharmacology and Applications of Famous Herbal Formulas), 1989; 316-317.
2. *Zhong Cheng Yao* (Study of Chinese Patent Medicine), 1992; 1:29.
3. *He Bei Zhong Yi* (Hebei Chinese Medicine), 1993; 4:5.
4. *Zhong Yi Za Zhi* (Journal of Chinese Medicine), 1984; 2:71.
5. *Zhong Cheng Yao Yan Jiu* (Research of Chinese Patent Medicine), 1982; 4:27.

Zēng Yè Tāng (Increase the Fluids Decoction)

增液湯

增液汤

Pinyin Name: *Zeng Ye Tang*

Literal Name: Increase the Fluids Decoction

Original Source: *Wen Bing Tiao Bian* (Systematic Differentiation of Warm Diseases) by Wu Ju-Tong in 1798

COMPOSITION

Xuan Shen (Radix Scrophulariae)	30g
Mai Dong (Radix Ophiopogonis)	24g
Di Huang (Radix Rehmanniae)	24g

DOSAGE / PREPARATION / ADMINISTRATION

Cook the ingredients with 8 cups of water and reduce it to 3 cups. For patients with dry mouth, take the entire decoction at once. Repeat this process if the patient does not have a bowel movement.

CHINESE THERAPEUTIC ACTIONS

1. Nourishes yin and clears heat
2. Moistens dryness and facilitates defecation

Zēng Yè Tāng (Increase the Fluids Decoction)

CLINICAL MANIFESTATIONS

Yangming fu (hollow organs) syndrome with yin and body fluids damage: lack of body fluids characterized by constipation, dry throat, thirst, and a deep, forceless pulse.

VETERINARY CLINICAL APPLICATIONS

Constipation and diabetes mellitus.

EXPLANATION

Zeng Ye Tang (Increase the Fluids Decoction) treats *yangming fu* (hollow organs) syndrome with severe damage to yin and body fluids. Normally, *yangming fu* syndrome should be treated with downward draining herbs to quickly move the stools in constipation. However, if yin and body fluids are already severely damaged due to heat and dryness, downward draining herbs could further damage yin and body fluids. For this reason, yin-nourishing and dryness-moistening methods are employed in this condition, rather than downward draining herbs, to facilitate defecation.

Xuan Shen (Radix Scrophulariae), which is salty, bitter and cold, softens hardness, moistens dryness, and clears heat. *Mai Dong* (Radix Ophiopogonis) nourishes yin and body fluids. *Di Huang* (Radix Rehmanniae) nourishes yin and moistens dryness. All three herbs work synergistically to promote bowel movements by nourishing yin, moistening dryness, and clearing heat.

VETERINARY MODIFICATIONS

- For constipation that is unresolved after taking this formula, add a small amount of *Da Huang* (Radix et Rhizoma Rhei) and *Mang Xiao* (Natrii Sulfas) to soften and purge the stool.
- For Stomach yin deficiency with mirror-like tongue coating, and dry lips and throat, add *Sha Shen* (Radix Glehniae seu Adenophorae), *Yu Zhu* (Rhizoma Polygonati Odorati), and *Shi Hu* (Caulis Dendrobii).

CAUTIONS / CONTRAINDICATIONS

- *Zeng Ye Tang* should only be used for constipation caused by heat and dryness severely damaging yin and body fluids. It should not be used indiscriminately to treat constipation, since it does not have any direct purgative or laxative effects.
- This formula is intended to promote defecation by nourishing yin and body fluids. Therefore, the dosage of this formula may be adjusted according to the severity of the constipation.

PHARMACOLOGICAL EFFECTS

1. **Effect on body fluids**: Administration of *Zeng Ye Tang* in mice effectively minimized the loss of body fluids and electrolytes by relieving diarrhea induced by *Fan Xie Ye* (Folium Sennae).[1]
2. **Anti-inflammatory**: One study reported marked effectiveness in reducing inflammation in mice and rats using a preparation of *Zeng Ye Tang* given via intravenous injection at 25-30 mL/kg for 2 to 3 days.[2]
3. **Antipyretic**: One study reported that *Zeng Ye Tang* had a marked effect to reduce body temperature in rabbits with artificially-induced fever.[3]

HUMAN CLINICAL STUDIES AND RESEARCH

1. **Pharyngitis**: One study reported 90.7% effectiveness using modified *Zeng Ye Tang* to treat 97 patients with chronic pharyngitis. The herbal formula contained *Xuan Shen* (Radix Scrophulariae), *Mai Dong* (Radix Ophiopogonis), *Jie Geng* (Radix Platycodonis), and *Gan Cao* (Radix et Rhizoma Glycyrrhizae). Of 97 patients, 63 had complete recovery, 25 had moderate improvement, and 9 received no benefit.[4]
2. **Cheilitis**: One study reported that use of modified *Zeng Ye Tang* was effective to treat inflammation of the lips. The herbal formula contained *Xuan Shen* (Radix Scrophulariae), *Di Huang* (Radix Rehmanniae), *Mai Dong* (Radix Ophiopogonis), *Jin Yin Hua* (Flos Lonicerae Japonicae), *Shi Hu* (Caulis Dendrobii), *Mu Dan Pi* (Cortex Moutan), and *Gan Cao* (Radix et Rhizoma Glycyrrhizae). Of 15 patients, the study reported complete recovery in 12 cases, significant improvement in 2 cases, and slight improvement in 1 case.[5]
3. **Rhinitis**: One study reported improvement in 54 of 65 patients with atrophic rhinitis when treated with *Zeng*

***Zeng Ye Tang* (Increase the Fluids Decoction)**

Diagnosis	Clinical Signs	Treatment	Herbs
Yangming fu (hollow organs) syndrome	• Constipation with dry throat and thirst: heat severely damaging yin and body fluids in the Intestines • Deep, forceless pulse: deficiency condition	• Nourishes yin and clears heat • Moistens dryness and facilitates defecation	• *Xuan Shen* (Radix Scrophulariae) softens hardness, moistens dryness, and clears heat. • *Mai Dong* (Radix Ophiopogonis) nourishes yin and body fluids. • *Di Huang* (Radix Rehmanniae) nourishes yin and moistens dryness.

Zēng Yè Tāng (Increase the Fluids Decoction)

Ye Tang plus *Ba Zhen Tang* (Eight-Treasure Decoction). In addition to these two formulas, modifications were made by using *Shi Hu* (Caulis Dendrobii) and *Yu Zhu* (Rhizoma Polygonati Odorati) for Stomach yin deficiency; *Mo Han Lian* (Herba Ecliptae) and *Xian He Cao* (Herba Agrimoniae) for nosebleeds; and *Huang Bo* (Cortex Phellodendri Chinensis) and *Zhi Mu* (Rhizoma Anemarrhenae) for foul smells in the nose. Lastly for individuals who suffer from severe rhinitis in fall and winter, *Chi Shao* (Radix Paeoniae Rubra) and larger doses of *Chuan Xiong* (Rhizoma Chuanxiong) and *Dang Gui* (Radix Angelicae Sinensis) were added to the formula.[6]

4. **Stomatitis caused by radiation treatment**: Use of *Zeng Ye Tang* was beneficial among 120 patients with nose cancer to alleviate stomatitis associated with radiation treatment. Clinical manifestations included thirst, dry mouth, thickened saliva, feeling of stickiness in the mouth, redness and swelling of gums, and ulcerations of the oral cavity with severe pain. The herbal formula contained *Di Huang* (Radix Rehmanniae) 12-25g, *Xuan Shen* (Radix Scrophulariae) 18g, *Mai Dong* (Radix Ophiopogonis) 15g, and others as needed. The herbs were cooked in water, and the decoction was administered in three to four equally-divided doses daily. The study reported that the herbs were effective in alleviating side effects associated with radiation treatment such as thirst, thickened saliva, red and swollen gums, ulcerations of the mouth, and pain. Of 120 patients, the study reported complete recovery in 41 cases, significant improvement in 65 cases, moderate improvement in 13 cases, and no effect in 1 case.[7]
5. **Constipation**: One study reported great success using *Zeng Ye Tang* to treat constipation. Of 50 patients, 41 had normal bowel movement within 3 days and 9 within 6 days.[8]
6. **Diabetes mellitus**: Administration of *Zeng Ye Tang* plus *Dang Shen* (Radix Codonopsis), *Shan Zhu Yu* (Fructus Corni) and others was shown in one study to reduce blood glucose levels in 102 patients with type II diabetes mellitus. Of 102 patients, the study reported significant effects in 30 cases, moderate effect in 57 cases, and no effect in 15 cases. The overall rate of effectiveness was 85.3%.[9]
7. **Morning sickness**: Intravenous infusion of 500-1000 mL of *Zeng Ye Tang* was effective in treating nausea and vomiting in 44 of 45 pregnant women.[10]
8. **Post-surgical recovery**: One study reported good results using *Zeng Ye Tang* for 20 post-surgical patients. Improvements noted included faster recovery of intestinal peristalsis.[11]
9. **Varicose vein**: One study reported complete recovery in all 16 patients with varicose veins and associated sores of the legs, when treated with modified *Zeng Ye Tang*. Modifications included the addition of *Hai Zao* (Sargassum), *Kun Bu* (Thallus Eckloniae), and *Bie Jia* (Carapax Trionycis) for the presence of hardness and nodules in the legs; *Ze Xie* (Rhizoma Alismatis), *Fang Ji* (Radix Stephaniae Tetrandrae), and *Yi Yi Ren* (Semen Coicis) for sores and ulcerations with profuse discharge; *Chuan Lian Zi* (Fructus Toosendan) and *Yan Hu Suo* (Rhizoma Corydalis) for severe pain; and *Ji Xue Teng* (Caulis Spatholobi) and *Hong Hua* (Flos Carthami) for the presence of noticeable dark, purple spots on the legs. Herbs were also applied topically to treat sores and ulcerations.[12]

TOXICOLOGY

According to an acute toxicology study, the LD_{50} of *Zeng Ye Tang* given via intravenous injection is 84.1 g/kg in mice. In a chronic toxicology study in rabbits, administration of a 10% *Zeng Ye Tang* preparation given via intravenous injection daily for 30 days did not contribute to any significant changes in body weight, blood exam, or abnormalities of liver, kidney or heart.[13]

SUGGESTED ACUPUNCTURE TREATMENT

1. Points: *Shenshu* (BL 23), *Taixi* (KI 3), *Sanyinjiao* (SP 6), *Dachangshu* (BL 25), *Fujie* (SP 14), and *Neiting* (ST 44).
2. Technique: tonification.

The chief complaint of *yangming fu* (hollow organs) syndrome is constipation. To treat constipation with acupuncture, the selection of points must include points to nourish the yin, clear heat, and eliminate dryness. *Shenshu* (BL 23), *Taixi* (KI 3), and *Sanyinjiao* (SP 6) nourish yin and eliminate dryness. *Neiting* (ST 44) clears heat from the *yangming* stage. *Dachangshu* (BL 25) and *Fujie* (SP 14) are commonly combined together to regulate the bowel movement.

AUTHORS' COMMENTS

In classic texts, constipation characterized by yin and fluid deficiencies is compared to a boat stuck in the riverbed due to low water flow. In such cases, forcefully pushing the boat down the river will only further damage the boat. Instead, the ideal solution is to direct the boat to deeper water, so that it may float and flow smoothly. Similarly, constipation marked by yin and fluid deficiencies cannot be forcefully treated with drastic purgatives and laxatives, which will only further damage yin and consume fluids. Instead, herbs that nourish yin and moisten dryness must be used to treat the underlying cause of this condition.

In veterinary medicine, *Zeng Ye Tang* is primarily used to treat constipation in elderly dogs and cats, The herbs

Zēng Yè Tāng (Increase the Fluids Decoction)

are easily mixed into food, and the addition of a small amount of *Fan Xie Ye* (Folium Sennae) in the first few doses is helpful for initial stool production.

References

1. *Zhong Yi Fang Ji Xian Dai Yan Jiu* (Modern Study of Medical Formulas in Traditional Chinese Medicine),1997; 1306.
2. *Zhong Guo Zhong Xi Yi Jie He Za Zhi* (Chinese Journal of Integrative Chinese and Western Medicine), 1982; 2:153.
3. *Zhong Yi Fang Ji Xian Dai Yan Jiu* (Modern Study of Medical Formulas in Traditional Chinese Medicine),1997; 1306-1307.
4. *Shan Xi Zhong Yi* (Shanxi Chinese Medicine), 1992; 6:248.
5. *Si Chuan Zhong Yi* (Sichuan Chinese Medicine), 1986; 12:48.
6. *Zhe Jiang Zhong Yi Za Zhi* (Zhejiang Journal of Chinese Medicine), 1980; 5:220.
7. *Guang Xi Zhong Yi Yao* (Guangxi Chinese Medicine and Herbology), 1981; 5:25.
8. *Zhong Yi Ming Fang Lin Chuang Xin Yong* (Contemporary Clinical Applications of Classic Chinese Formulas), 2001; 723.
9. *Zhong Yi Za Zhi* (Journal of Chinese Medicine), 1985; 6:31.
10. *Zhong Yi Za Zhi* (Journal of Chinese Medicine), 1986; 12:5.
11. *Zhong Xi Yi Jie He Za Zhi* (Journal of Integrated Chinese and Western Medicine), 1988; 7:423.
12. *Xin Zhong Yi* (New Chinese Medicine), 1998; 9:45.
13. *Zhong Yi Fang Ji Xian Dai Yan Jiu* (Modern Study of Medical Formulas in Traditional Chinese Medicine), 1997; 1312.

Chapter 15 — Summary

— Dryness-Relieving Formulas

SECTION 1: DISPERSING AND MOISTENING FORMULAS

Name	Similarities	Differences
Xing Su San (Apricot Kernel and Perilla Leaf Powder)	Relieves cool-dryness	Dispels cool-dryness, ventilates the Lung, dissolves phlegm
Sang Xing Tang (Mulberry Leaf and Apricot Kernel Decoction)	Relieve warmth-dryness	Gently clears warmth-dryness
Qing Zao Jiu Fei Tang (Eliminate Dryness and Rescue the Lung Decoction)		Strongly clears warmth-dryness, nourishes yin, moistens dryness

Xing Su San (Apricot Kernel and Perilla Leaf Powder) dispels exterior cool-dryness, ventilates the Lung, and dissolves phlegm. It is used for exterior cool-dryness characterized by aversion to cold, absence of sweating, coughing with thin and watery sputum, and stuffy nose.

Sang Xing Tang (Mulberry Leaf and Apricot Kernel Decoction) and ***Qing Zao Jiu Fei Tang*** (Eliminate Dryness and Rescue the Lung Decoction) both treat warmth-dryness affecting the Lung.

- *Sang Xing Tang* is used for mild cases of exterior warmth-dryness attacking the Lung. It ventilates the Lung and dispels warmth-dryness from the Lung. Clinical manifestations include slight fever, dry cough with little or no sputum, thirst, and dry throat.
- *Qing Zao Jiu Fei Tang* is employed for severe warmth-dryness attacking the Lung. It strongly moistens dryness and nourishes the Lung. The main clinical manifestations include fever, thirst, coughing with no sputum, dyspnea, and pain in the chest and hypochondriac region.

SECTION 2: NOURISHING AND MOISTENING FORMULAS

Name	Similarities	Differences
Bai He Gu Jin Tang (Lily Bulb Decoction to Preserve the Metal)	Nourishes and tonifies Lung and Kidney yin	Dissolves phlegm, stops coughing
Mai Men Dong Tang (Ophiopogonis Decoction)	Nourish and tonify Lung and Stomach yin	Redirects the reversed flow of qi, harmonizes the middle *jiao*
Sha Shen Mai Dong Tang (Glehnia and Ophiopogonis Decoction)		Promotes secretion of body fluids, moistens dryness
Yu Ye Tang (Jade Fluid Decoction)	Nourish yin, generate body fluids, and moisten dryness	Strongly tonifies qi and nourishes yin
Yu Quan Wan (Jade Spring Pill)		Strongly clears deficiency heat and generates body fluids
Zeng Ye Tang (Increase the Fluids Decoction)	Generates body fluids in the Large Intestine, moistens dryness	Clears heat

Bai He Gu Jin Tang (Lily Bulb Decoction to Preserve the Metal) nourishes Lung and Kidney yin, dissolves phlegm, and stops coughing. Due to Lung and Kidney yin-deficient fire, a sore throat and coughing with streaks of blood in the sputum may occur.

Mai Men Dong Tang (Ophiopogonis Decoction) nourishes Lung and Stomach yin, corrects the reversed flow of qi, and harmonizes the middle *jiao*. It is used for Lung and Stomach yin deficiencies with manifestations of coughing, sputum that cannot be expectorated easily, vomiting, thirst, a dry

Chapter 15 — Summary

throat and mouth, and Cushing's disease, a form of *xiao ke* (wasting and thirsting) syndrome with excessive panting, hunger, thirst and urination in dogs.

Sha Shen Mai Dong Tang (Glehnia and Ophiopogonis Decoction) nourishes Lung and Stomach yin, promotes the secretion of body fluids, and moistens dryness. It is most effective for dryness damaging Lung and Stomach yin, with clinical signs such as dry throat, thirst, fever, dry cough, and dry, sticky sputum.

Yu Ye Tang (Jade Fluid Decoction) tonifies qi, nourishes yin, and generates body fluids. It is used for *xiao ke* (wasting and thirsting) syndrome with constant thirst, polyuria, turbid urine, lethargy, and shortness of breath.

Yu Quan Wan (Jade Spring Pill) generates body fluids to relieve thirst and nourishes yin to moisten dryness. It treats *xiao ke* (wasting and thirsting) syndrome with yin-deficient heat affecting the Lung, Stomach, and Kidney. Clinical manifestations include irritability, thirst, increased intake of water, dry mouth and tongue, and increased frequency of urination.

Zeng Ye Tang (Increase the Fluids Decoction) nourishes yin, clears heat, moistens dryness, and promotes defecation. It is indicated for *yangming fu* (hollow organs) syndrome, in which yin has been damaged, resulting in constipation with dry stools.

Chapter 16

— Damp-Dispelling Formulas

祛湿剂

王肯堂 Wāng Kĕn-Tāng

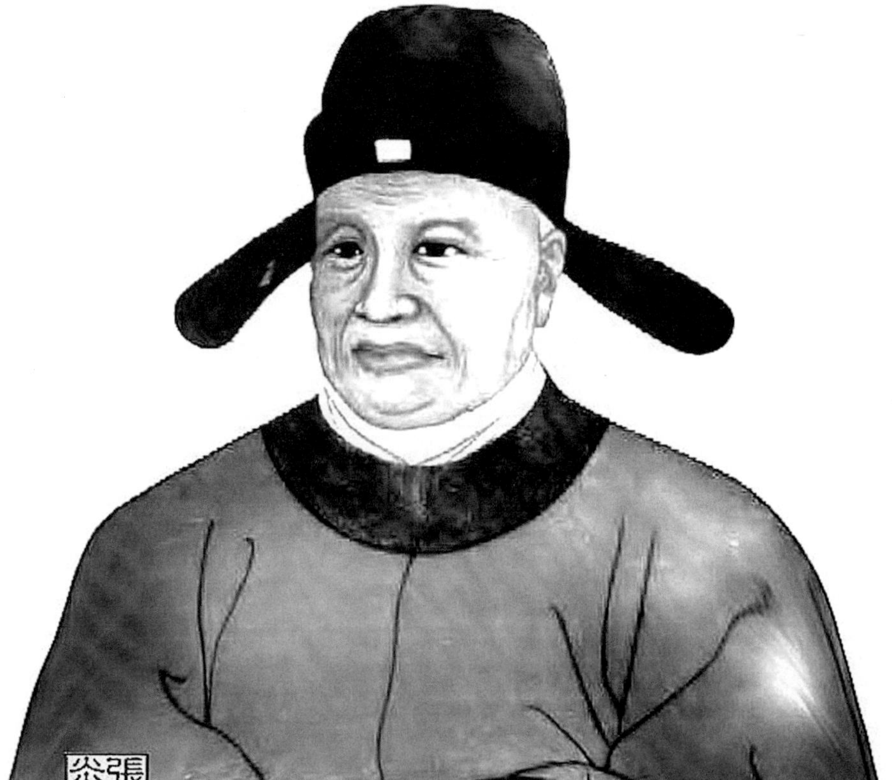

王肯堂 Wāng Kĕn-Tāng, 1549 – 1613.

王肯堂 Wāng Kĕn-Tāng

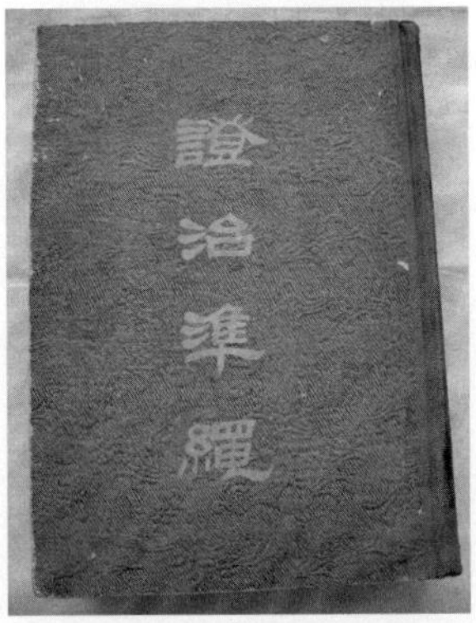

症治准绳 *Zheng Zhi Zhun Sheng*
(Standards of Patterns and Treatments)
in 1602.

Wang Ken-Tang was born during the Ming dynasty. When he was 17 years old, his mother became seriously ill. She was treated by many famous doctors who made differing diagnoses and prescribed various, sometimes conflicting, treatments. In the end, no one was able to cure her. Her condition slowly deteriorated, and she eventually passed away. Wang Ken-Tang was inspired to study medicine because of this tragic loss.

In his pursuit of medicine, Wang studied many texts and integrated the knowledge of all of the schools of thought that he encountered. In addition to being an excellent clinician, he dedicated the last ten years of his life to documenting his clinical experiences. Wang wrote many books to detail the pathology and treatment of many disorders, including internal medicine, gynecology, pediatrics, external medicine, the treatment of sores and abscesses, and other miscellaneous illnesses. Among his most famous works are:

- 症治准绳 *Zheng Zhi Zhun Sheng* (Standards of Patterns and Treatments),
- 妇症治准绳 *Fu Ke Zheng Zhi Zhun Sheng* (Standards of Patterns and Treatments in Gynecology)
- 儿科症治准绳 *Er Ke Zheng Zhi Zhun Sheng* (Standards of Patterns and Treatments in Pediatrics)
- 外科症治准绳 *Wai Ke Zheng Zhi Zhun Sheng* (Standards of Patterns and Treatments in External Medicine)
- 痈科症治准绳 *Yong Ke Zheng Zhi Zhun Sheng* (Standards of Patterns and Treatments in Sores and Abscesses)

Formulas written by Wang Ken-Tang include:

- *Shao Yao Tang* (Peony Decoction)
- *Qing Xin Li Ge Tang* (Clear the Epigastrium and Benefit the Diaphragm Decoction)
- *San Huang Shi Gao Tang* (Three-Yellow and Gypsum Decoction)
- *Qing Liang Yin* (Clearing and Cooling Decoction)
- *Qing Gu San* (Cool the Bones Powder)
- *Si Shen Wan* (Four-Miracle Pill)
- *Dao Shui Fu Ling Tang* (Poria Decoction to Drain Water)
- *Jian Pi Wan* (Strengthen the Spleen Pill)

Dynasties & Kingdoms	Year
Xia Dynasty 夏	2100-1600 BCE
Shang Dynasty 商	1600-1100 BCE
Zhou Dynasty 周	1100-221 BCE
Qin Dynasty 秦	221-207 BCE
Han Dynasty 漢	206 BCE-220
Three Kingdoms 三國	220-280
Western Jin Dynasty 西晉	265-316
Eastern Jin Dynasty 東晉	317-420
Northern and Southern Dynasties 北南朝	420-581
Sui Dynasty 隋	581-618
Tang Dynasty 唐	618-907
Five Dynasties 五代	907-960
Song Dynasty 宋	960-1279
Liao Dynasty 遼	916-1125
Jin Dynasty 金	1115-1234
Yuan Dynasty 元	1271-1368
Ming Dynasty 明	**1368-1644**
Qing Dynasty 清	1644-1911
Republic of China 中華民國	1912-Present Day
People's Republic of China 中華人民共和國	1949-Present Day

Table of Contents

Chapter 16 — Overview

祛湿剂 — Damp-Dispelling Formulas

Definition: Damp-dispelling formulas dry dampness, resolve turbidity, promote urination, and relieve dysuria. Damp-dispelling formulas are used primarily to treat disorders characterized by the accumulation of dampness and water.

Dampness is a yin pathogen that is heavy (turbid), thick, greasy, and stagnating in nature; it disrupts the normal flow of qi. Damp disorders typically develop slowly over time and once established become chronic, difficult to resolve, and recur frequently. Treatment is generally prolonged and improvements are gradual, requiring time, patience and consistent re-evaluation to be successful.

Dampness can be contracted via the environment (exogenous dampness) or generated from internal imbalance (endogenous dampness). It often affects the exterior (skin, muscles, joints, channels and collaterals) level of the body and the internal organs at the same time because of the normal communication between the superficial channels of the body, the muscles, and the *zang fu* organs. Exogenous dampness can occur as a result of trauma or surgery, from toxic heat or from prolonged exposure to wet environmental conditions, such as rain or humid weather, and thus develops in animals that sleep outdoors at night without appropriate shelter. Animals that work, swim or hunt repeatedly in rainy or humid weather are also at risk. Animals that sustain trauma or undergo surgery with excessive scarring can develop obstruction of the channels and vessels that leads to poor circulation of blood and qi, with stasis and accumulation of fluids and edema. Toxic heat particularly affecting the skin can cause accumulation of dampness. Once skin lesions develop, they obstruct the flow of qi and blood, causing the development of edema, abscesses and sores. Clinical signs of exogenous dampness include: fever, aversion to cold, edema (especially of the head and face), dermatitis, cellulitis, elbow hygroma, and stiff, swollen, and painful joints. Dampness is the primary exogenous factor associated with late summer and early autumn (the actual time of this season is variable, depending on the geographical location), and many patients will have flare-ups of chronic conditions during this time of year.

Endogenous dampness can be internally generated as a result of inappropriate diet and feeding practices and lack of exercise. This type of dampness is very common in dogs and cats fed commercial dry pet food that contains large amounts of grains such as corn, wheat and soybean, or fed dairy products; it is also common in horses fed high levels of concentrates, especially those containing molasses. Such diets promote the development of dampness and impair the transformation and transportation functions of the Spleen. In Chinese medicine, there is an important saying: "the Spleen dislikes cold and dampness." In order to have normal digestive and fluid metabolic functions, the Spleen must be kept warm and free of dampness. Obese animals, regardless of their diet, also exhibit this pattern. Obesity in Chinese medicine is associated with the chronic generation and retention of dampness and heat. The Spleen (this term also includes the pancreas) is the organ that deals with ingested food and water on a daily basis and so plays a central role in normal fluid metabolism. For this reason, Chinese herbal formulas used to treat damp conditions typically include herbs that strengthen the Spleen. Internally generated dampness can also result from regular feeding of refrigerated and/or raw foods to young maturing animals, while in geriatric animals internally generated dampness is caused by the age-related decline of Spleen function.

Chapter 16 — Overview

Damp-cold conditions can also develop from chronic use of antibiotics (energetically cold substances) and secondary to abdominal surgery (cold exposure).

The Spleen is inherently weak in immature animals and dislikes cold and dampness. A raw food diet should not be fed to immature dogs until the Spleen has fully developed at approximately one year of age. Depending on the animal, food should be warmed to body temperature prior to feeding and/or mixed with digestive enzymes as needed. The vomiting of warm, body temperature, macerated, partially digested food by non-domestic canines to feed their offspring achieves this purpose. The cold Spleen is unable to process food and water appropriately, and dampness accumulates with signs of cold damp disorders. Once dampness is established in the body, it can be very difficult to resolve; the weakened Spleen self-perpetuates a cycle of dysfunction and damp production that often becomes chronic. Chronic dampness may eventually generate heat, leading to a variety of damp-heat disorders. If dietary management is not included as part of the treatment, it is likely that the damp condition will persist and recurrences will be frequent. Clinical signs of endogenous dampness include: poor appetite, nausea, cough, vomiting, diarrhea, jaundice, edema of the lower limbs and dysuria, ascites, hydrothorax and pulmonary edema. The Spleen is weakened by inactivity ("prolonged sitting injures the Spleen"), and it is recommended that all animals have regular daily exercise to maintain normal transportation and transformation functions.

The distinction between exogenous and endogenous dampness is not always clear. Exogenous dampness manifests acutely, after prolonged environmental exposure. Endogenous damp disorders usually involve the Lung, Spleen and Kidney, which act as a team to maintain normal water metabolism in the body. The Lung disperses water, the Spleen absorbs water, and the Kidney eliminates water. If the teamwork among these three organs is disrupted with abnormal metabolism and circulation of body fluids, then water and dampness accumulate. The *San Jiao* can also play a role in the development of damp disorders. As it is the water pathway of the body and coordinates the flow of body fluids, obstruction of any of the three *jiao*s can result in damp accumulation. Similar obstruction and disorder of the Urinary Bladder will result in dysuria and retention of water.

The causes of dampness are often interwoven and frequently involve dysfunction of one or more *zang fu* organs. Accurate diagnosis of whether dampness is exogenous or endogenous is essential for the successful treatment of damp disorders. Following diagnosis, damp-dispelling herbal formulas are chosen based on their abilities to release the exterior and disperse dampness, dry dampness and harmonize the Spleen and Stomach, regulate and dispel the blockage of the water pathways, promote urination (diuresis), dispel dampness and clear heat in the lower *jiao*, or transform water by the tonification of yang. Dampness frequently combines with other pathogenic factors such as heat, cold, wind, and summer-heat and/or other disorders to produce more complicated patterns. It is the nature of dampness to create stagnation, which in turn generates heat, which over time condenses into phlegm and leads to the development of urinary, renal or gallstones.

Dampness is an equal opportunity pathogen. It will invade any part of the body and affect individuals with either deficient or excess constitutions. If dampness is located in the upper part of the body, exterior-releasing herbs are used to disperse the dampness. If dampness accumulates internally and/or in the lower part of the body, herbs that are aromatic, bitter, and drying are used to resolve dampness, or alternatively, sweet and bland diuretic herbs are used to dispel dampness. If dampness develops secondary to deficient yang and cold, then herbs that warm yang and dispel cold should be used. If dampness combines with heat or causes qi stagnation, then herbs that clear heat or promote qi flow are added. Spleen deficiency is a common component of nearly all damp disorders in animals, and herbal formulas to tonify the Spleen are often added to the treatment protocols. [Note: Formulas that dispel wind-dampness to treat *bi zheng* (painful obstruction syndrome) are discussed in Chapter 17: Wind-Damp Dispelling Formulas.]

Chapter 16 — Overview

Western biomedical diseases commonly associated with dampness in veterinary medicine for which the use of damp-dispelling formulas may be appropriate include: peripheral edema, pulmonary edema, ascites, pleural effusion, pericardial effusion, anorexia, vomiting, diarrhea, gastric ulcer, gastroenteritis, gastric dilation, pancreatitis, jaundice, hepatitis, feline cholangitis, hepatic lipidosis, gallstones, feline lower urinary tract inflammation, chronic urinary tract infection, urolithiasis, hematuria, sterile cystitis, renal cyst, polycystic kidney, pyelonephritis, renal failure, nephrotic syndrome, anuria, prostatitis, vaginal discharge, anal gland sacculitis, and damp-heat dermatitis conditions.

SUBCATEGORIES OF ACTION

Because of the complexity of damp disorders, damp-dispelling formulas are divided into four sub-categories to reflect the nature of the disorders and the corresponding characteristics of the formulas.

1. **Damp-Drying and Stomach-Harmonizing Formulas**

   These formulas treat damp stagnation and turbidity that is accompanied by disharmony of the Spleen and Stomach. Typical clinical manifestations include epigastric and abdominal distention and fullness, belching, nausea, vomiting, acid regurgitation, diarrhea, decreased appetite, and fatigue.

   Patterns of disharmony of the Spleen and Stomach characterized by dampness are usually treated with bitter and warm herbs to dry dampness, or with aromatic herbs to resolve dampness, such as *Cang Zhu* (Rhizoma Atractylodis), *Bai Bian Dou* (Semen Lablab Album), *Huo Xiang* (Herba Agastaches), and *Hou Po* (Cortex Magnoliae Officinalis). Exemplar formulas include *Ping Wei San* (Calm the Stomach Powder) and *Huo Xiang Zheng Qi San* (Agastache Powder to Rectify the Qi).

2. **Heat-Clearing and Damp-Dispelling Formulas**

   These formulas address exterior damp-heat, interior damp-heat, or damp-heat in the lower *jiao*. Clinical applications include summer-heat, jaundice, and *re lin* (heat dysuria).

   Herbs commonly used to clear heat and resolve dampness include *Yin Chen* (Herba Artemisiae Scopariae), *Yi Yi Ren* (Semen Coicis), and *Hua Shi* (Talcum). Herbs that clear heat and dry dampness include *Huang Lian* (Rhizoma Coptidis), *Huang Bo* (Cortex Phellodendri Chinensis), *Huang Qin* (Radix Scutellariae), and *Zhi Zi* (Fructus Gardeniae). Representative formulas are *Yin Chen Hao Tang* (Artemisia Scoparia Decoction), *San Ren Tang* (Three-Nut Decoction), and *Ba Zheng San* (Eight-Herb Powder for Rectification).

3. **Water-Regulating and Damp-Resolving Formulas**

   These formulas treat excess damp accumulation blocking the water pathways, with clinical manifestations of edema, uroschesis, retention of urine, turbid urine, and diarrhea. In these cases, herbs are used to dispel dampness and resolve water accumulation through urination.

   Commonly used herbs include *Fu Ling* (Poria), *Ze Xie* (Rhizoma Alismatis), and *Zhu Ling* (Polyporus). Exemplar formulas that regulate water and resolve dampness include *Wu Ling San* (Five-Ingredient Powder with Poria) and *Wu Pi San* (Five-Peel Powder).

4. **Warm Formulas that Dissolve Dampness**

   These formulas treat cold-type of damp disorders, in which yang fails to transform water. Clinical manifestations include edema of the body and legs, urinary difficulty, *tan yin* (phlegm retention), *bi zheng* (painful obstruction syndrome), and leg *qi* caused by damp-cold accumulation.

   These disorders are treated with herbs that warm yang and regulate water, such as *Gui Zhi* (Ramulus Cinnamomi), *Bai Zhu* (Rhizoma Atractylodis Macrocephalae), *Fu Zi* (Radix Aconiti Lateralis Praeparata), and *Fu Ling* (Poria). Two representative formulas are *Ling Gui Zhu Gan Tang* (Poria, Cinnamon Twig, Atractylodes Macrocephala, and Licorice Decoction) and *Zhen Wu Tang* (True Warrior Decoction).

Chapter 16 — Overview

CAUTIONS / CONTRAINDICATIONS

Damp-dispelling formulas often incorporate two general categories of herbs: aromatic, acrid, and warm herbs that dry dampness; and sweet and bland herbs that resolve dampness. Although effective, both types of herbs easily damage yin and body fluids. Therefore, these formulas should be used with caution during pregnancy, in patients with constitutional yin or body fluid deficiencies, and in animals with general weakness after chronic illness.

PHARMACOLOGICAL EFFECTS & CLINICAL APPLICATIONS

From the traditional Chinese medical perspective, dampness is a complex disorder that may be complicated by other factors and affect different parts of the body. Correspondingly, damp-dispelling formulas have a wide range of pharmacological effects and clinical applications.

1. **Damp-drying and Stomach-harmonizing formulas** are primarily used to treat gastrointestinal disorders.
   - **Gastrointestinal disorders**: *Ping Wei San* (Calm the Stomach Powder) and *Huo Xiang Zheng Qi San* (Agastache Powder to Rectify the Qi) are two of the most commonly used and researched formulas for treating gastrointestinal disorders. *Ping Wei San* has been used to treat gastritis,[1] ulcerative colitis,[2] epigastric pain from gastritis,[3] peptic ulcer disease,[4] and anorexia.[5] *Huo Xiang Zheng Qi San* has been used to treat diarrhea,[6] gastroenteritis,[7] food poisoning,[8] and enteritis.[9]

2. **Heat-clearing and damp-dispelling formulas** clear damp-heat from the Liver, Gallbladder, and lower *jiao*. Pharmacologically, these formulas have antibiotic and anti-inflammatory effects and have been used successfully to treat infections, as well as liver, gallbladder, kidney, and urinary disorders.
   - **Infection**: Many heat-clearing and damp-dispelling formulas have antibiotic effects, and have been successfully used to treat various types of infections. For example, *San Ren Tang* (Three-Nut Decoction) has been shown to treat pneumonia and otitis media,[10,11] *Gan Lu Xiao Du Dan* (Sweet Dew Special Pill to Eliminate Toxins) has been used to address encephalitis and laryngopharyngitis,[12,13] and *Ba Zheng San* (Eight-Herb Powder for Rectification) is effective for urethritis and urinary tract infection.[14,15]
   - **Liver disorders**: These formulas have hepatoprotective and antifibrotic effects.[16,17,18] Clinical applications include acute viral hepatitis,[19] acute icteric hepatitis,[20] acute infectious icteric hepatitis,[21] and hepatitis with hepatomegaly.[22] Exemplar formulas include *Yin Chen Hao Tang* (Artemisia Scoparia Decoction), *San Ren Tang* (Three-Nut Decoction), and *Gan Lu Xiao Du Dan* (Sweet Dew Special Pill to Eliminate Toxins).
   - **Gallbladder disorders**: These formulas have cholagogic and choleretic effects to stimulate and increase the production and release of bile acids to treat jaundice and cholestatic liver diseases.[23,24,25] Additional clinical applications include biliary atresia,[26] cholecystitis,[27] and icteric hepatitis.[28,29] Exemplar formulas include *Yin Chen Hao Tang* (Artemisia Scoparia Decoction) and *San Ren Tang* (Three-Nut Decoction).
   - **Kidney and urinary disorders**: These formulas have been used successfully to treat various kidney disorders (glomerulonephritis,[30] nephritis,[31] pyelonephritis,[32] and urinary stones [33]) and urinary disorders (urethritis and urinary tract infection [34,35]). Exemplar formulas include *San Ren Tang* (Three-Nut Decoction) and *Ba Zheng San* (Eight-Herb Powder for Rectification).

3. **Water-regulating and damp-resolving formulas** are used for excess damp accumulation that blocks the water pathways. From the perspectives of conventional medicine, these formulas have a marked diuretic function and are effective in treating various conditions characterized by water retention, such as cardiovascular, kidney, and urinary disorders.
   - **Edema**: Many of these formulas have a marked diuretic effect to increase the elimination of urine, sodium, chloride, potassium, and other electrolytes.[36] Clinically, *Wu Ling San* (Five-Ingredient

Chapter 16 — Overview

Powder with Poria), *Zhu Ling Tang* (Polyporus Decoction), and *Wu Pi San* (Five-Peel Powder) are three commonly used formulas for treating edema.[37,38,39]

- **Cardiovascular disorders**: Many of these formulas have a direct or indirect effect in treating cardiovascular disorders. Some formulas have a diuretic effect to eliminate water and reduce cardiovascular stress.[40,41,42,43] Other formulas have vasodilative actions to reduce blood pressure.[44] Lastly, some formulas have positive chronotropic and inotropic effects on the heart.[45] Exemplar formulas include *Wu Ling San* (Five-Ingredient Powder with Poria) and *Fang Ji Huang Qi Tang* (Stephania and Astragalus Decoction).
- **Kidney and urinary disorders**: Water-regulating and damp-resolving formulas have been successfully used to treat urinary disorders, such as nephritis,[46] acute nephritis,[47] renal failure,[48] urinary stones,[49,50] hydrocephalus,[51] uroschesis,[52] and hydronephrosis.[53,54] They can also be used for conditions such as hematuria,[55] galacturia,[56] and general urinary tract disorders.[57] The mechanisms of action are attributed in part to the diuretic effect of eliminating excess water retention,[58,59] and protecting the kidneys by decreasing plasma levels of blood urea nitrogen and creatinine.[60] Exemplar formulas include *Wu Ling San* (Five-Ingredient Powder with Poria), *Wei Ling Tang* (Calm the Stomach and Poria Decoction), *Zhu Ling Tang* (Polyporus Decoction), and *Fang Ji Huang Qi Tang* (Stephania and Astragalus Decoction).

4. **Warm formulas that resolve dampness** are commonly used to treat cardiovascular, kidney, and urinary disorders.
   - **Cardiovascular disorders**: These formulas have been successfully used to treat cardiovascular disorders such as hypertension,[61] coronary artery disease,[62] and cardiac failure.[63,64] The pharmacological effects are attributed in part to circulatory improvements, such as decreased resistance of blood flow, reduced blood viscosity, increased blood perfusion to internal organs, and decreased workload for the heart.[65] Exemplar formulas include *Ling Gui Zhu Gan Tang* (Poria, Cinnamon Twig, Atractylodes Macrocephala, and Licorice Decoction) and *Zhen Wu Tang* (True Warrior Decoction).
   - **Kidney disorders**: These formulas have been effectively used to treat nephritis,[66] hydronephrosis,[67] nephrotic syndrome,[68] and chronic renal failure.[69] The mechanism of action is attributed to the nephroprotective effect which reduces the amount of protein and cells in the urine.[70] Exemplar formulas include *Ling Gui Zhu Gan Tang* (Poria, Cinnamon Twig, Atractylodes Macrocephala, and Licorice Decoction) and *Zhen Wu Tang* (True Warrior Decoction).
   - **Urinary disorders**: Certain warm formulas that dispel dampness, such as *Bi Xie Fen Qing Yin* (Dioscorea Hypoglauca Decoction to Separate the Clear), have been successfully used to treat such urinary disorders as urethritis,[71] galacturia,[72] and *lin zheng* (dysuria syndrome).[73]

References

1. *Nan Jing Zhong Yi Yao Da Xue Xue Bao* (Journal of Nanjing University of Traditional Chinese Medicine and Medicinals), 1995; 2:29.
2. *Shi Yong Zhong Yi Nei Ke Za Zhi* (Journal of Practical Chinese Internal Medicine), 1994; 8(1):32.
3. *Xin Zhong Yi* (New Chinese Medicine), 1994; 26(8):54.
4. *Liao Ning Zhong Yi Za Zhi* (Liaoning Journal of Chinese Medicine), 1990; 14(11):20.
5. *Zhong Yi Yao Yan Jiu* (Research of Chinese Medicine and Herbology), 1994; 1:20.
6. *Shan Dong Zhong Yi Xue Yuan Xue Bao* (Journal of Shandong University School of Chinese Medicine), 1993; 1:39.
7. *Zhong Cao Yao* (Chinese Herbal Medicine), 1992; 9:479.
8. *Shan Xi Zhong Yi* (Shanxi Chinese Medicine), 1990; 5:224.
9. *Zhe Jiang Zhong Yi Xue Yuan Xue Bao* (Journal of Zhejiang University of Chinese Medicine), 1994; 3:8.
10. *Hu Nan Zhong Yi Za Zhi* (Hunan Journal of Chinese Medicine), 1998; 3:50.
11. *Zhe Jiang Zhong Yi Za Zhi* (Zhejiang Journal of Chinese Medicine), 1991; 6:255.
12. *Jiang Su Zhong Yi* (Jiangsu Chinese Medicine), 1997; 7:12.
13. *Xin Zhong Yi* (New Chinese Medicine), 1997; 7:57.
14. *Guang Xi Zhong Yi Yao* (Guangxi Chinese Medicine and Herbology), 1992; 4:9.
15. *Shan Xi Zhong Yi* (Shanxi Chinese Medicine), 1998; 10:448.
16. Yamashiki M, Mase A, Arai I, Huang XX, Nobori T, Nishimura A, Sakaguchi S, Inoue K. Effects of the Japanese herbal medicine 'Inchinkoto' (TJ-135) on concanavalin A-induced hepatitis in mice. Clin Sci (Lond). 2000 Nov; 99(5):421-31.

Chapter 16 — Overview

17. Iinuma Y, Kubota M, Yagi M, Kanada S, Yamazaki S, Kinoshita Y. Effects of the herbal medicine Inchinko-to on liver function in postoperative patients with biliary atresia--a pilot study. J Pediatr Surg. 2003 Nov; 38(11):1607-11.
18. Sakaida I, Tsuchiya M, Kawaguchi K, Kimura T, Terai S, Okita K. Herbal medicine Inchin-ko-to (TJ-135) prevents liver fibrosis and enzyme- altered lesions in rat liver cirrhosis induced by a choline-deficient L-amino acid-defined diet. J Hepatol. 2003 Jun; 38(6):762-9.
19. *Shan Xi Zhong Yi* (Shanxi Chinese Medicine), 1993; 4:17.
20. *Zhong Yi Za Zhi* (Journal of Chinese Medicine), 1982; 7:46.
21. *Shan Xi Zhong Yi* (Shanxi Chinese Medicine), 1998; 3:19.
22. *Zhe Jiang Zhong Yi Za Zhi* (Zhejiang Journal of Chinese Medicine), 1980; 10:462.
23. *Zhong Yi Za Zhi* (Journal of Chinese Medicine), 1982; 7:72.
24. *Zhong Yi Ming Fang Lin Chuang Xin Yong* (Contemporary Clinical Applications of Classic Chinese Formulas), 2001; 508
25. Shoda J, Miura T, Utsunomiya H, Oda K, Yamamoto M, Kano M, Ikegami T, Tanaka N, Akita H, Ito K, Suzuki H, Sugiyama Y. Genipin enhances Mrp2 (Abcc2)-mediated bile formation and organic anion transport in rat liver. Hepatology. 2004 Jan; 39(1):167-78.
26. Kobayashi H, Horikoshi K, Yamataka A, Lane GJ, Yamamoto M, Miyano T. Beneficial effect of a traditional herbal medicine (inchin-ko-to) in postoperative biliary atresia patients. Pediatric Surgery International. 17(5-6):386-9, 2001 Jul.
27. *Si Chuan Zhong Yi* (Sichuan Chinese Medicine), 1988; 9:27.
28. *Zhong Yi Za Zhi* (Journal of Chinese Medicine), 1982; 7:46.
29. *Shan Xi Zhong Yi* (Shanxi Chinese Medicine), 1998; 3:19.
30. *Zhong Yi Fang Ji Xian Dai Yan Jiu* (Modern Study of Medical Formulas in Traditional Chinese Medicine), 1997, 1355.
31. *Ha Er Bing Zhong Yi* (Haerbing Chinese Medicine), 1960; 9:15.
32. *Liao Ning Zhong Yi Za Zhi* (Liaoning Journal of Chinese Medicine), 1986; 1:19.
33. *Ji Lin Zhong Yi Yao* (Jilin Chinese Medicine and Herbology), 1983; 5:19.
34. *Guang Xi Zhong Yi Yao* (Guangxi Chinese Medicine and Herbology), 1992; 4:9.
35. *Shan Xi Zhong Yi* (Shanxi Chinese Medicine), 1998; 10:448.
36. *Guo Wai Yi Xue Zhong Yi Zhong Yao Fen Ce* (Monograph of Chinese Herbology from Foreign Medicine), 1981; 2:121.
37. *Zhong Yi Fang Ji Xian Dai Yan Jiu* (Modern Study of Medical Formulas in Traditional Chinese Medicine), 1997; 1407.
38. *Guo Wai Yi Xue* (Foreign Medicine), 1983; 5:292.
39. *Shan Xi Zhong Yi* (Shanxi Chinese Medicine), 1991; 12(2):89.
40. *Zhong Hua Yi Xue Za Zhi* (Chinese Journal of Medicine), 1961; 17(1):7.
41. *Guo Wai Yi Xue Zhong Yi Zhong Yao Fen Ce* (Monograph of Chinese Herbology from Foreign Medicine), 1983; 6:24.
42. *Guo Wai Yi Xue Zhong Yi Zhong Yao Fen Ce* (Monograph of Chinese Herbology from Foreign Medicine), 1981; 3:173.
43. *Guo Wai Yi Xue Zhong Yi Zhong Yao Fen Ce* (Monograph of Chinese Herbology from Foreign Medicine), 1984; 5:78.
44. *Tian Jin Zhong Yi* (Tianjin Chinese Medicine), 1994; 4:29.

Chapter 16 — Overview

45. Sugiyama A, Takahara A, Satoh Y, Yoneyama M, Saegusa Y, Hashimoto K. Cardiac effects of clinically available Kampo medicine assessed with canine isolated, blood-perfused heart preparations. Jpn J Pharmacol. 2002 Mar; 88(3):307-13.
46. *Guang Xi Zhong Yi Yao* (Guangxi Chinese Medicine and Herbology), 1984; 4(10):16.
47. *Si Chuan Zhong Yi* (Sichuan Chinese Medicine), 1985; 9:19.
48. *Zhong Yi Za Zhi* (Journal of Chinese Medicine), 1993; 1:42.
49. *Zhong Yi Ming Fang Lin Chuang Xin Yong* (Contemporary Clinical Applications of Classic Chinese Formulas), 2001; 133.
50. Takada M, Yano H, Kanbara N, Kurita T, Kohri K, Kato Y, Iguchi M. Effect of Chorei-to on spontaneous discharge of urinary stones after extracorporeal shock wave lithotripsy (ESWL). Hinyokika Kiyo. 1997 Apr; 43(4):311-4.
51. *Xin Yi Yao Xue Za Zhi* (New Journal of Medicine and Herbology), 1978; 8:45.
52. *Si Chuan Zhong Yi* (Sichuan Chinese Medicine), 1997; 4:26.
53. *Shan Xi Zhong Yi* (Shanxi Chinese Medicine), 1989; 10(8):352.
54. *Shan Dong Zhong Yi Za Zhi* (Shandong Journal of Chinese Medicine), 1995; 8:345.
55. *Zhong Yi Ming Fang Lin Chuang Xin Yong* (Contemporary Clinical Applications of Classic Chinese Formulas), 2001; 636.
56. *Zhong Guo Nong Cun Yi Xue* (Chinese Agricultural Medicine), 1990; 3:33.
57. Horii A, Maekawa M. Clinical evaluation of chorei-to and chorei-to-go-shimotsu-to in patients with lower urinary tract symptoms. Hinyokika Kiyo. 1988 Dec; 34(12):2237-41.
58. *Zhong Yi Fang Ji Xian Dai Yan Jiu* (Modern Study of Medical Formulas in Traditional Chinese Medicine), 1997; 1407.
59. *Zhong Hua Yi Xue Za Zhi* (Chinese Journal of Medicine), 1961; 17(1):7.
60. *Guo Wai Yi Xue Zhong Yi Zhong Yao Fen Ce* (Monograph of Chinese Herbology from Foreign Medicine), 1983; 3:43.
61. *Shan Xi Zhong Yi* (Shanxi Chinese Medicine), 1983; 2:6.
62. *Zhong Yi Han Shou Tong Xun* (Reports of Chinese Medicine), 1992; 2:41.
63. *Tian Jin Yi Yao Za Zhi* (Journal of Tianjin Medicine and Herbology), 1967; 8:503.
64. *Zhong Ji Yi Kan* (Medium Medical Journal), 1990; 3:30.
65. *Zhong Xi Yi Jie He Za Zhi* (Journal of Integrated Chinese and Western Medicine), 1988; 8(8):457.
66. *Zhong Yi Za Zhi* (Journal of Chinese Medicine), 1981; 11:835.
67. *Shi Yong Zhong Yi Yao Za Zhi* (Journal of Practical Chinese Medicine and Medicinals), 1999; 6:11.
68. *Shan Xi Zhong Yi* (Shanxi Chinese Medicine), 1987; 2:70.
69. *Zhong Yi Ming Fang Lin Chuang Xin Yong* (Contemporary Clinical Applications of Classic Chinese Formulas), 2001; 1995, 4:46.
70. *Zhong Yi Fang Ji Xian Dai Yan Jiu* (Modern Study of Medical Formulas in Traditional Chinese Medicine), 1997; 1453.
71. *Xin Zhong Yi* (New Chinese Medicine), 1995; 7:43.
72. *Shan Xi Zhong Yi* (Shanxi Chinese Medicine), 1994; 6:273.
73. *Ji Lin Zhong Yi* (Jilin Chinese Medicine), 1990; 2:16.

Section 1

燥湿和胃剂
— Damp-Drying and Stomach-Harmonizing Formulas

Píng Wèi Sǎn (Calm the Stomach Powder)
平胃散

Pinyin Name: *Ping Wei San*
Literal Name: Calm the Stomach Powder
Alternate Names: *Ping Wei San (Wan)*, Stomach-Comforting Formula (Pill), Stomach-Calming Powder, Magnolia and Ginger Formula
Original Source: *Tai Ping Hui Min He Ji Ju Fang* (Imperial Grace Formulary of the Tai Ping Era) by the Imperial Medical Department in 1078-85

COMPOSITION

Cang Zhu (Rhizoma Atractylodis), *jin* (soaked) in rice water for 2 days	2,400g [15g]
Hou Po (Cortex Magnoliae Officinalis), *chao* (dry-fried) with ginger juice till aromatic	1,500g [9g]
Chen Pi (Pericarpium Citri Reticulatae)	1,500g [9g]
Gan Cao (Radix et Rhizoma Glycyrrhizae), *cuo* (grated) and *chao* (dry-fried)	900g [4g]

DOSAGE / PREPARATION / ADMINISTRATION

The source text instructions are to grind the ingredients into a fine powder. Cook 6g of the powder with 2 slices of *Sheng Jiang* (Rhizoma Zingiberis Recens) and 2 pieces of *Da Zao* (Fructus Jujubae) in 1 bowl of water until it is reduced to 70% volume. Take the hot, strained decoction on an empty stomach before meals, with the optional addition of a pinch of salt. The source text states that the frequent use of this formula regulates qi, harmonizes the Stomach, removes chronic food stagnation, dissolves phlegm, and prevents invasion of wind, cold, and dampness.

Today, this formula is commonly prepared and administered in powder or decoction form. For powder, grind the herbs into a fine powder and take 3-5g per dose with a decoction made from *Sheng Jiang* (Rhizoma Zingiberis Recens) and *Da Zao* (Fructus Jujubae). For decoction, use the doses suggested in brackets.

CHINESE THERAPEUTIC ACTIONS

1. Dries dampness and strengthens the Spleen
2. Activates qi circulation and harmonizes the Stomach

CLINICAL MANIFESTATIONS

Damp accumulation in the Spleen and Stomach: distention of the epigastrium and abdomen, poor appetite, anorexia, vomiting, loose to watery stool, belching, borborygmus, lethargy, exercise intolerance, poor performance, possibly a white greasy tongue coating, and a slippery pulse.

VETERINARY CLINICAL APPLICATIONS

Poor appetite, anorexia, acute and chronic vomiting, peri-prandial colic, duodenitis, diarrhea, acute and chronic gastritis, idiopathic gastric hypomotility syndrome, acute and chronic indigestion, bilious vomiting syndrome, gastric ulcer, post-operative indigestion and poor appetite, acute and chronic indigestion post-antibiotic therapy, poor appetite with vomiting and/or watery stools in juvenile and geriatric animals fed raw and refrigerated diets.

EXPLANATION

Ping Wei San (Calm the Stomach Powder) is the basic formula for treating damp accumulation in the Spleen and Stomach. The Spleen is responsible for the transportation and transformation of food and water and prefers a dry environment. If dampness accumulates and stagnates in the Spleen and impairs its functions, then loss of appetite and diarrhea may occur. Damp accumulation also causes qi stagnation, resulting in fullness and distention of the abdomen and borborygmus. If dampness impairs the descending functions of Stomach qi and causes disharmony, then nausea, vomiting, belching and abdominal bloating

Píng Wèi Sǎn (Calm the Stomach Powder)

***Ping Wei San* (Calm the Stomach Powder)**

Diagnosis	Clinical Signs	Treatment	Herbs
Damp accumulation in the Spleen and Stomach	• Poor appetite, anorexia and diarrhea: damp accumulation affecting the Spleen and Stomach • Distention of the epigastrium and abdomen and borborygmus: qi stagnation and damp accumulation • Vomiting and belching: reversed flow of Stomach qi • Exercise intolerance, poor performance and lethargy: damp accumulation • Greasy tongue coating and a slippery pulse: damp accumulation	• Dries dampness and strengthens the Spleen • Activates qi circulation and harmonizes the Stomach	• *Cang Zhu* (Rhizoma Atractylodis) dries dampness and strengthens the Spleen. • *Hou Po* (Cortex Magnoliae Officinalis) activates qi, dispels dampness, and relieves fullness and distention. • *Chen Pi* (Pericarpium Citri Reticulatae) regulates qi and relieves stagnation. • *Sheng Jiang* (Rhizoma Zingiberis Recens) and *Da Zao* (Fructus Jujubae) harmonize the Spleen and Stomach. • *Gan Cao* (Radix et Rhizoma Glycyrrhizae) harmonizes the middle *jiao* and the rest of the herbs.

may occur. Exercise intolerance, poor performance, and lethargy are signs of damp accumulation. A white, greasy tongue coating and a slippery pulse indicate more severe dampness.

This formula's chief herb, *Cang Zhu* (Rhizoma Atractylodis), is bitter, dry, and warm. It dries dampness and strengthens the Spleen. The deputy herb, *Hou Po* (Cortex Magnoliae Officinalis), activates qi, dispels dampness, and relieves fullness and distention in the epigastrium and abdomen. *Chen Pi* (Pericarpium Citri Reticulatae) helps *Hou Po* (Cortex Magnoliae Officinalis) to regulate qi and relieve stagnation. *Sheng Jiang* (Rhizoma Zingiberis Recens) and *Da Zao* (Fructus Jujubae) harmonize the Spleen and Stomach. *Gan Cao* (Radix et Rhizoma Glycyrrhizae) harmonizes the middle *jiao* and all of the herbs in the formula.

VETERINARY MODIFICATIONS

- With damp-cold accumulation, add *Gan Jiang* (Rhizoma Zingiberis), *Cao Dou Kou* (Semen Alpiniae Katsumadai) and *Rou Gui* (Cortex Cinnamomi).
- With bloating of the abdomen, add *Mu Xiang* (Radix Aucklandiae) and *Zhi Qiao* (Fructus Aurantii).
- With gastric and abdominal pain, add *Yan Hu Suo* (Rhizoma Corydalis) and *Xiang Fu* (Rhizoma Cyperi).
- With indigestion and poor appetite, add *Shan Zha* (Fructus Crataegi), *Mai Ya* (Fructus Hordei Germinatus), and *Shen Qu* (Massa Fermentata).
- With poor appetite due to Spleen deficiency, add *Ren Shen* (Radix et Rhizoma Ginseng) and *Huang Qi* (Radix Astragali).
- For diarrhea, add *Bai Zhu* (Rhizoma Atractylodis Macrocephalae), *Yi Yi Ren* (Semen Coicis), and *Bai Bian Dou* (Semen Lablab Album).
- For diarrhea with mucus due to cold, add *Wu Zhu Yu* (Fructus Evodiae).
- For constipation, add *Da Huang* (Radix et Rhizoma Rhei) and *Mang Xiao* (Natrii Sulfas).

CAUTIONS / CONTRAINDICATIONS

Ping Wei San contains many bitter, acrid, warm and drying herbs that consume yin and blood. The use of this formula is contraindicated in pregnancy and should be used with caution in cases with significant yin or blood deficiency.[1]

HUMAN CLINICAL STUDIES AND RESEARCH

1. **Gastritis**: According to one study of 46 patients (12 with chronic superficial gastritis, 26 with superficial atrophic gastritis, and 8 with atrophic gastritis), administration of modified *Ping Wei San* for one month per course of treatment was associated with complete recovery in 8 cases, significant improvement in 18 cases, moderate improvement in 16 cases, and no effect in 4 cases (all four had atrophic gastritis). The herbal formula contained *Ping Wei San* as the base formula, with the addition of *Ban Xia* (Rhizoma Pinelliae) and *Cao Guo* (Fructus Tsaoko) for more dampness; *Huang Lian* (Rhizoma Coptidis) and *Zhu Ru* (Caulis Bambusae in Taenia) for more damp-heat; dry-fried *Chai Hu* (Radix Bupleuri) and processed *Xiang Fu* (Rhizoma Cyperi) for qi stagnation; *Gao Liang Jiang* (Rhizoma Alpiniae Officinarum) for interior cold; and *Dang Shen* (Radix Codonopsis) and *Bai Zhu* (Rhizoma Atractylodis Macrocephalae) for deficiency of the middle *jiao*.[2]

Píng Wèi Săn (Calm the Stomach Powder)

2. **Ulcerative colitis**: Administration of modified *Ping Wei San* was associated with approximately 80% effectiveness in treating ulcerative colitis. The herbal formula contained *Cang Zhu* (Rhizoma Atractylodis), *Hou Po* (Cortex Magnoliae Officinalis), *Fang Feng* (Radix Saposhnikoviae), *Sheng Ma* (Rhizoma Cimicifugae), *Dang Shen* (Radix Codonopsis), and *Huang Qi* (Radix Astragali). In addition, charred *Da Huang* (Radix et Rhizoma Rhei), charred *Jin Yin Hua* (Flos Lonicerae Japonicae), and charred *Di Yu* (Radix Sanguisorbae) were added for hematochezia.[3]
3. **Epigastric pain caused by gastritis**: Use of modified *Ping Wei San* was effective in treating epigastric pain caused by gastritis (other causes were ruled out). The herbal formula contained *Xiang Fu* (Rhizoma Cyperi) 12-15g, *Gao Liang Jiang* (Rhizoma Alpiniae Officinarum) 4-8g, *Tan Xiang* (Lignum Santali Albi) 4-6g, *Dan Shen* (Radix et Rhizoma Salviae Miltiorrhizae) 15-30g, *Fo Shou* (Fructus Citri Sarcodactylis) 10g, *Wu Yao* (Radix Linderae) 10g, *Bai He* (Bulbus Lilii) 15-30g, *Huang Lian* (Rhizoma Coptidis) 3-4g, *Pu Gong Ying* (Herba Taraxaci) 30g, and *Gan Cao* (Radix et Rhizoma Glycyrrhizae) 6g. Furthermore, *Huang Qi* (Radix Astragali) and *Ren Shen* (Radix et Rhizoma Ginseng) were added for qi deficiency; *Gui Zhi* (Ramulus Cinnamomi) and *Bai Shao* (Radix Paeoniae Alba) were added, and *Huang Lian* (Rhizoma Coptidis) was removed, for the presence of cold; *Zi Su Geng* (Caulis Perillae) and *Xiang Yuan* (Fructus Citri) were added for epigastric fullness; *E Zhu* (Rhizoma Curcumae) or *Shi Xiao San* (Sudden Smile Powder) was added for blood stagnation; *Shi Hu* (Caulis Dendrobii) and a larger dose of *Bai Shao* (Radix Paeoniae Alba) were added and *Gao Liang Jiang* (Rhizoma Alpiniae Officinarum) removed, for yin deficiency. The treatment protocol was to give 1 pack of herbs in decoction daily, for 1 month per course of treatment, for 1-3 courses total. Of 56 patients, the study reported complete recovery in 33 cases, improvement in 20 cases, and no effect in 3 cases. The overall rate of effectiveness was approximately 95%.[4]
4. **Peptic ulcer disease**: One study reported complete recovery in 22 of 35 patients using modified *Ping Wei San* to treat gastric and/or duodenal ulcers. The herbal formula contained *Bai Shao* (Radix Paeoniae Alba) 25g, *Gan Cao* (Radix et Rhizoma Glycyrrhizae) 15g, *Chen Pi* (Pericarpium Citri Reticulatae) 15g, *Hou Po* (Cortex Magnoliae Officinalis) 15g, *Cang Zhu* (Rhizoma Atractylodis) 15g, *Huang Lian* (Rhizoma Coptidis) 5g, and *Wu Zhu Yu* (Fructus Evodiae) 5g. The duration of treatment ranged from 15-65 days, with an average of 45 days.[5]
5. **Anorexia**: One study reported success using modified *Ping Wei San* to treat 80 children with anorexia. The herbal formula contained *Cang Zhu* (Rhizoma Atractylodis) 7.5g, *Hou Po* (Cortex Magnoliae Officinalis) 6g, *Chen Pi* (Pericarpium Citri Reticulatae) 6g, *Fu Ling* (Poria) 6g, *Zhi Qiao* (Fructus Aurantii) 6g, *Ji Nei Jin* (Endothelium Corneum Gigeriae Galli) 9g, and *Gan Cao* (Radix et Rhizoma Glycyrrhizae) 5g. Additional modifications were made as needed. The duration of treatment ranged from 2-12 packs of herbs, with an average of 8 packs. The study reported improvement in appetite in all 80 children.[6]

SUGGESTED ACUPUNCTURE TREATMENT

1. Points: *Zhangmen* (LR 13), *Gongsun* (SP 4), *Pishu* (BL 20), *Weishu* (BL 21), *Housanli* (ST 36), and *Sanyinjiao* (SP 6). In addition, use *Qihaishu* and *Mijiaogan* for horses, and *Shagen* for dogs and cats.
2. Technique: even method.

The objectives of these points are to dry dampness in the Spleen and Stomach and activate qi circulation. *Zhangmen* (LR 13), the *mu* (collecting) point of the Spleen, is combined with *Gongsun* (SP 4) to strengthen the Spleen. *Pishu* (BL 20) and *Weishu* (BL 21) are the *shu* (transport) points on the back for Spleen and Stomach and can be used to strengthen the Spleen and Stomach and regulate the middle *jiao*. *Housanli* (ST 36) alone relieves nausea, but when it is used with *Sanyinjiao* (SP 6), there is a synergistic effect of activating qi and drying dampness. *Qihaishu* is the classical point for tonifying the Spleen in horses. *Mijiaogan* and *Shagen* are classical points for stimulating appetite.

AUTHORS' COMMENTS

Ping Wei San serves as a base formula for many gastrointestinal formulas and is used to treat dampness stagnating in the middle *jiao* and Intestines. In veterinary medicine, this formula has found application to treat poor appetite and chronic indigestion following surgery or antibiotic therapy and secondary to dry and raw foods and refrigerated diets. It can be used alone, but is often combined with another formula to treat gastrointestinal diseases. The focus of *Ping Wei San* is on resolving dampness and not on tonifying the Spleen and Stomach. In cases with deficiency, a tonic herbal formula should be used concurrently. A course of treatment using *Ping Wei San* as a sole therapy should not exceed 10 days without re-evaluation and/or modification. Following treatment with *Ping Wei San* or for animals that have chronic disease and Spleen deficiency, this formula may be combined with *Liu Jun Zi Tang* (Six-Gentlemen Decoction) in a 1:1 ratio.

References

1. *Zhong Yi Lin Chuan Fang Ji Xue* (Clinical Study of Chinese Herbal Formulas), 1995; 217-218.
2. *Nan Jing Zhong Yi Yao Da Xue Xue Bao* (Journal of Nanjing University of Traditional Chinese Medicine and Medicinals), 1995; 2:29.

Píng Wèi Săn (Calm the Stomach Powder)

3. *Shi Yong Zhong Yi Nei Ke Za Zhi* (Journal of Practical Chinese Internal Medicine), 1994; 8(1):32.
4. *Xin Zhong Yi* (New Chinese Medicine), 1994; 26(8):54.
5. *Liao Ning Zhong Yi Za Zhi* (Liaoning Journal of Chinese Medicine), 1990; 14(11):20.
6. *Zhong Yi Yao Yan Jiu* (Research Journal of Chinese Medicine and Herbology), 1994; 1:20.

Xiāng Shā Píng Wèi Săn

(Cyperus and Amomum Powder to Calm the Stomach)

香砂平胃散

Pinyin Name: *Xiang Sha Ping Wei San*
Literal Name: Cyperus and Amomum Powder to Calm the Stomach
Alternate Name: Cyperus Cardamon and Atractylodes Formula
Original Source: *Wan Bing Hui Chun* (Restoration of Health from the Myriad Diseases) by Gong Ting-Xian in 1587

COMPOSITION

Cang Zhu (Rhizoma Atractylodis), *zhi* (prepared) with rice water	6g
Hou Po (Cortex Magnoliae Officinalis), *chao* (dry-fried) with ginger juice	6g
Zhi Qiao (Fructus Citri Aurantii), *chao* (dry-fried) with bran	0.9g
Chen Pi (Pericarpium Citri Reticulatae)	6g
Sha Ren (Fructus Amomi)	1.5g
Xiang Fu (Rhizoma Cyperi), *chao* (dry-fried) with *Tong Bian* (Infantis Urina)	3g
Mu Xiang (Radix Aucklandiae)	1.5g
Shan Zha (Fructus Crataegi)	0.9g
Mai Ya (Fructus Hordei Germinatus), *chao* (dry-fried)	0.9g
Shen Qu (Massa Fermentata), *chao* (dry-fried)	0.9g
Gan Jiang (Rhizoma Zingiberis)	0.9g
Gan Cao (Radix et Rhizoma Glycyrrhizae)	0.9g

Xiāng Shā Píng Wèi Săn

(Cyperus and Amomum Powder to Calm the Stomach)

DOSAGE / PREPARATION / ADMINISTRATION

The source text states to grind all of the ingredients except *Mu Xiang* (Radix Aucklandiae) into a fine powder, cook the powder with 3 slices of *Sheng Jiang* (Rhizoma Zingiberis Recens) and 1 snatch of *Lai Fu Zi* (Semen Raphani) in water. Take the warm, strained decoction with separately powdered *Mu Xiang* (Radix Aucklandiae).

CHINESE THERAPEUTIC ACTIONS

1. Harmonizes the middle *jiao* and resolves dampness
2. Regulates qi and reduces food stagnation

CLINICAL MANIFESTATIONS

Spleen and Stomach disharmony: nausea, vomiting, belching, abdominal bloating, abdominal pain, diarrhea, and indigestion.

VETERINARY CLINICAL APPLICATIONS

Food stagnation, grain overload, colic with bloating, chronic vomiting of food, indigestion, poor appetite and diarrhea.

EXPLANATION

Xiang Sha Ping Wei San (Cyperus and Amomum Powder to Calm the Stomach) treats disharmony of the Spleen and Stomach manifesting as impaired digestive functions. As a result, dampness accumulates in the middle *jiao*, causing reversed flow of qi upward. The resultant symptoms include nausea, vomiting, and belching. Stagnation in the middle *jiao* causes indigestion, abdominal pain, distention, and fullness. Lastly, there may be diarrhea, as food cannot be digested and absorbed properly.

To properly address this condition, this formula uses herbs that are aromatic, bitter, and warm to dry dampness, strengthen the Spleen, and harmonize the middle *jiao*. *Cang Zhu* (Rhizoma Atractylodis) dries dampness and strengthens the Spleen to relieve fullness and distention, treat poor appetite, and stop diarrhea. *Hou Po* (Cortex Magnoliae Officinalis) and *Zhi Qiao* (Fructus Aurantii) activate qi circulation to disperse stagnation. *Chen Pi* (Pericarpium Citri Reticulatae) and *Sha Ren* (Fructus Amomi) move qi, dry dampness, and eliminate phlegm. *Xiang Fu* (Rhizoma Cyperi) and *Mu Xiang* (Radix Aucklandiae) soothe Liver qi and relieve pain. *Shan Zha* (Fructus Crataegi), *Mai Ya* (Fructus Hordei Germinatus), and *Shen Qu* (Massa Fermentata) promote digestion and alleviate food stagnation. *Gan Jiang* (Rhizoma Zingiberis) warms the middle *jiao* and relieves nausea. *Gan Cao* (Radix et Rhizoma Glycyrrhizae) relieves abdominal pain and harmonizes all of the herbs in the formula.

VETERINARY MODIFICATIONS

- With Spleen deficiency, add *Bai Zhu* (Rhizoma Atractylodis Macrocephalae) and *Dang Shen* (Radix Codonopsis).
- With Spleen and Stomach deficiencies, add *Huang Qi* (Radix Astragali) and *Shan Yao* (Rhizoma Dioscoreae).
- To nourish yin and relieve spasms and cramping of the gastrointestinal tract, add *Bai Shao* (Radix Paeoniae Alba).

***Xiang Sha Ping Wei San* (Cyperus and Amomum Powder to Calm the Stomach)**

Diagnosis	Clinical Signs	Treatment	Herbs
Disharmony of the Spleen and Stomach	• Nausea, vomiting and belching: reversed flow of qi due to stagnation in the middle *jiao* • Indigestion, abdominal bloating, abdominal pain and diarrhea: stagnation in the middle *jiao* with disharmony of the Spleen and Stomach	• Harmonizes the middle *jiao* and resolves dampness • Regulates qi and reduces food stagnation	• *Cang Zhu* (Rhizoma Atractylodis) dries dampness and strengthens the Spleen. • *Hou Po* (Cortex Magnoliae Officinalis) and *Zhi Qiao* (Fructus Aurantii) activate qi circulation to disperse stagnation. • *Chen Pi* (Pericarpium Citri Reticulatae) and *Sha Ren* (Fructus Amomi) move the qi, dry dampness, and eliminate phlegm. • *Xiang Fu* (Rhizoma Cyperi) and *Mu Xiang* (Radix Aucklandiae) soothe Liver qi circulation and relieve pain. • *Shan Zha* (Fructus Crataegi), *Mai Ya* (Fructus Hordei Germinatus), and *Shen Qu* (Massa Fermentata) promote digestion and alleviate food stagnation. • *Gan Jiang* (Rhizoma Zingiberis) warms and harmonizes the middle *jiao*. • *Gan Cao* (Radix et Rhizoma Glycyrrhizae) relieves abdominal pain and harmonizes all of the herbs.

Xiāng Shā Píng Wèi Săn

(Cyperus and Amomum Powder to Calm the Stomach)

- For nausea and vomiting caused by food stagnation, add *Huo Xiang* (Herba Agastaches) and *Zhu Ru* (Caulis Bambusae in Taenia).
- With long-term food stagnation, remove *Gan Jiang* (Rhizoma Zingiberis), and add *Da Huang* (Radix et Rhizoma Rhei).

SUGGESTED ACUPUNCTURE TREATMENT

1. Points: *Yinlingquan* (SP 9), *Zhongwan* (CV 12), *Housanli* (ST 36), *Weishu* (BL 21), *Fenglong* (ST 40), *Taichong* (LR 3), *Tianshu* (ST 25), *Jianli* (CV 11) and *Jiangya*.
2. Technique: moxibustion and sedation.

Taichong (LR 3), *Tianshu* (ST 25), and *Housanli* (ST 36) promote qi circulation and disperse stagnation. *Weishu* (BL 21) regulates normal qi flow of the Stomach. *Yinlingquan* (SP 9), *Fenglong* (ST 40), and *Jianli* (CV 11) promote digestion and reduce dampness. Apply moxibustion on *Zhongwan* (CV 12) to strengthen the middle *jiao*. *Jiangya*, a classical point, helps treat colic pain in horses.

AUTHORS' COMMENTS

Xiang Sha Ping Wei San dries dampness, relieves food stagnation, mildly strengthens the Spleen, and promotes digestion. It is commonly used to treat food stagnation due to overfeeding and/or feeding species inappropriate diets. As such, it can be very helpful in horses that are experiencing bloating after grain overload or overeating spring grass. Dogs and cats are commonly fed exclusive dry food diets with high grain content that predispose them to food stagnation and the development of damp accumulation and qi stagnation in the middle *jiao*. This is particularly true for cats (which are obligatory carnivores) fed dry cat foods with little natural fiber. Clinical manifestations include abdominal pain with food ingestion, poor appetite (or good appetite with vomiting immediately after eating), belching, diarrhea, abdominal bloating and discomfort, and preference for cold water.

Xiang Sha Ping Wei San is formulated by adding *Mu Xiang* (Radix Aucklandiae) and *Sha Ren* (Fructus Amomi) to *Ping Wei San* (Calm the Stomach Powder). The addition of *Mu Xiang* (Radix Aucklandiae) and *Sha Ren* (Fructus Amomi) gives *Xiang Sha Ping Wei San* a greater effect to relieve qi stagnation in the middle *jiao* and stop vomiting than *Ping Wei San* (Calm the Stomach Powder). However, the ability of *Xiang Sha Ping Wei San* to tonify the Spleen is weak, and if significant Spleen deficiency is present, this formula will need to be modified.

Bù Huàn Jīn Zhèng Qì Săn

(Rectify the Qi Powder Worth More than Gold)

不換金正氣散
不换金正气散

Pinyin Name: *Bu Huan Jin Zheng Qi San*
Literal Name: Rectify the Qi Powder Worth More than Gold
Alternate Names: *Pu Huan Chin Cheng Chi San*, Priceless Chi-Regulating Formula, Pinellia Atractylodes and Agastache Formula
Original Source: *Tai Ping Hui Min He Ji Ju Fang* (Imperial Grace Formulary of the Tai Ping Era) by the Imperial Medical Department in 1078-85

COMPOSITION

Cang Zhu (Rhizoma Atractylodis)
Hou Po (Cortex Magnoliae Officinalis)
Chen Pi (Pericarpium Citri Reticulatae)
Gan Cao (Radix et Rhizoma Glycyrrhizae)
Huo Xiang (Herba Agastaches)
Ban Xia (Rhizoma Pinelliae)

DOSAGE / PREPARATION / ADMINISTRATION

The source text states to grind equal amounts of the ingredients into a fine powder. Cook 9g of the powder with 3 slices of *Sheng Jiang* (Rhizoma Zingiberis Recens) and 2 pieces of *Da Zao* (Fructus Jujubae) in 1.5 bowls of water until it is reduced to 80% volume. Take the hot, strained decoction before meals. Today, this formula is prepared by grinding all of the ingredients into a fine powder. Take 3-6g of the powder with a decoction made from *Sheng Jiang* (Rhizoma Zingiberis Recens) and *Da Zao* (Fructus Jujubae).

CHINESE THERAPEUTIC ACTIONS

1. Activates qi and resolves dampness
2. Harmonizes the Stomach and stops vomiting

CLINICAL MANIFESTATIONS

Damp accumulation in the middle *jiao*: vomiting, diarrhea, fever and trembling, abdominal distention, and other urgent conditions such as sudden turmoil disorder, a red to purple tongue, and a rapid, slippery pulse.

VETERINARY CLINICAL APPLICATIONS

Acute vomiting or gastric reflux, colic, ileus, acute or chronic gastroenteritis, food poisoning with anorexia, vomiting, diarrhea, belching, and acid reflux.

EXPLANATION

Bu Huan Jin Zheng Qi San (Rectify the Qi Powder Worth More than Gold) is often used in cases in which there are excessive damp accumulation symptoms, such as fever and trembling, vomiting, diarrhea, abdominal distention, and other urgent symptoms associated with diseases, such as dysentery and sudden turmoil disorder.

The chief herb, *Cang Zhu* (Rhizoma Atractylodis), is bitter, drying, and warm and strongly dries dampness and strengthens the Spleen. The deputy herb, *Hou Po* (Cortex Magnoliae Officinalis), activates qi, dispels dampness, and relieves fullness and distention in the epigastrium and abdomen. The assistant herb, *Chen Pi* (Pericarpium Citri Reticulatae), regulates qi and relieves stagnation. Together, these three herbs dry dampness, strengthen the Spleen, and harmonize the Stomach. *Huo Xiang* (Herba Agastaches), being strongly aromatic, activates qi, dispels dampness, harmonizes the Stomach to relieve nausea and vomiting, and eliminates exterior damp-heat. *Ban Xia* (Rhizoma Pinelliae) dries dampness and corrects the reversed Stomach qi to relieve nausea and vomiting. *Gan Cao* (Radix et Rhizoma Glycyrrhizae) harmonizes all of the herbs in the formula.

Bu Huan Jin Zheng Qi San is a modification of *Ping Wei San* (Calm the Stomach Powder), with the addition of *Huo Xiang* (Herba Agastaches) and *Ban Xia* (Rhizoma Pinelliae). The addition of these two herbs gives this formula a stronger ability to dispel dampness and regulate qi.

Bù Huàn Jīn Zhèng Qì Săn

(Rectify the Qi Powder Worth More than Gold)

***Bu Huan Jin Zheng Qi San* (Rectify the Qi Powder Worth More than Gold)**

Diagnosis	Clinical Signs	Treatment	Herbs
Accumulation of dampness in the middle *jiao*	Fever, anorexia, vomiting, reflux, diarrhea, and abdominal bloating: dampness accumulation	• Activates qi and resolves dampness • Harmonizes the Stomach and stops vomiting	• *Cang Zhu* (Rhizoma Atractylodis) strongly dries dampness and strengthens the Spleen. • *Hou Po* (Cortex Magnoliae Officinalis) activates qi, dispels dampness, and relieves fullness and distention in the epigastrium and abdomen. • *Chen Pi* (Pericarpium Citri Reticulatae) regulates qi and relieves stagnation. • *Huo Xiang* (Herba Agastaches) activates qi, dispels dampness, and harmonizes the Stomach. • *Ban Xia* (Rhizoma Pinelliae) dries dampness and redirects Stomach qi. • *Gan Cao* (Radix et Rhizoma Glycyrrhizae) harmonizes the herbs.

VETERINARY MODIFICATIONS

- With vomiting accompanied by excessive amount of sputum and saliva, add *Fu Ling* (Poria) and *Jie Geng* (Radix Platycodonis).
- With wind-cold invasion, add *Fang Feng* (Radix Saposhnikoviae) and *Cong Bai* (Bulbus Allii Fistulosi).
- With severe diarrhea and vomiting, combine with *Huang Lian Tang* (Coptis Decoction).

CAUTIONS / CONTRAINDICATIONS

- Since many herbs in this formula are warm and drying in nature, patients with significant yin or blood deficiencies should use this formula with caution.
- Avoid foods that are raw, cold, oily, or greasy while taking *Bu Huan Jin Zheng Qi San*.

SUGGESTED ACUPUNCTURE TREATMENT

1. Points: *Zhangmen* (LR 13), *Gongsun* (SP 4), *Pishu* (BL 20), *Weishu* (BL 21), *Housanli* (ST 36), *Yanglingquan* (GB 34), *Sanyinjiao* (SP 6), *Dazhui* (GV 14), *Zhongwan* (CV 12), *Tianshu* (ST 25) and *Qihaishu*.
2. Technique: even method.

The selection of acupuncture points here is similar to that for *Ping Wei San* (Calm the Stomach Powder), because the underlying problem is the same in both cases. *Bu Huan Jin Zheng Qi San*, however, focuses more on drying dampness. Accordingly, *Dazhui* (GV 14), *Zhongwan* (CV 12), and *Tianshu* (ST 25) are used to activate qi circulation, dry dampness, and to stop nausea and diarrhea. The combination of *Housanli* (ST 36) and *Yanglingquan* (GB 34) is useful to stop vomiting. *Qihaishu*, a classical point, strengthens the Spleen in horses.

AUTHORS' COMMENTS

Bu Huan Jin Zheng Qi San was originally designed to treat urgent conditions such as dysentery and sudden turmoil disorder. Today, this formula is used to address acute gastrointestinal conditions from invasion of damp-heat pathogens, with vomiting, diarrhea, and abdominal distention in dogs from eating spoiled or rotten food. It can also be used to treat acute vomiting and diarrhea following kenneling. Common uses in horses include colic associated with the eating of moldy hay and post-surgical ileus. In horses with severe reflux, the stomach should be emptied as much as possibly prior to the administration of the formula, which will likely have to be given via nasogastic tube and in conjunction with acupuncture treatment. *Bu Huan Jin Zheng Qi San* is not for long-term use, and the formula should be discontinued as soon as the clinical signs resolve, typically in 24-48 hours.

Fú Líng Yǐn (Poria Decoction)

茯苓飲
茯苓饮

Pinyin Name: *Fu Ling Yin*
Literal Name: Poria Decoction
Alternate Name: Hoelen Combination
Original Source: *Jin Gui Yao Lue* (Essentials from the Golden Cabinet) by Zhang Zhong-Jing in the Eastern Han Dynasty

COMPOSITION

Fu Ling (Poria)	9g
Bai Zhu (Rhizoma Atractylodis Macrocephalae)	9g
Ren Shen (Radix et Rhizoma Ginseng)	6g
Chen Pi (Pericarpium Citri Reticulatae)	4.5g
Zhi Shi (Fructus Aurantii Immaturus)	6g
Sheng Jiang (Rhizoma Zingiberis Recens)	12g

DOSAGE / PREPARATION / ADMINISTRATION

The source text instructions are to cut the ingredients into small pieces and cook them in 6 cups [1,200 mL] of water until the liquid is reduced to 1.8 cups [360 mL]. Take the strained decoction in three equally divided doses.

CHINESE THERAPEUTIC ACTIONS

1. Strengthens the Spleen
2. Harmonizes the middle *jiao*
3. Resolves phlegm and dampness

CLINICAL MANIFESTATIONS

Damp-phlegm accumulation in the chest and Stomach: excessive gas and bloating, colic, lack of appetite or poor appetite due to excessive gas in the stomach, belching, nausea, and mild resistance in the epigastric region upon palpation.

VETERINARY CLINICAL APPLICATIONS

Anorexia, gastritis, gastric dilation and bilious vomiting.

EXPLANATION

Fu Ling Yin (Poria Decoction) treats damp-phlegm accumulation in the chest and Stomach that develops secondary to Spleen deficiency. Animals may cough up or vomit clear, watery fluid and experience symptoms such as excess gas in the stomach, bloating, and the inability to eat. Some animals may also have clinical signs of standing with the head down with belching, borborygmus and/or nausea. Horses may have little to no reflux but large quantities of sour-smelling gas that is evident on passing a nasogastric tube.

In this formula, *Fu Ling* (Poria) and *Bai Zhu* (Rhizoma Atractylodis Macrocephalae) strengthen the Spleen and Stomach to dispel water stagnation in the middle *jiao. Ren Shen* (Radix et Rhizoma Ginseng) tonifies qi and restores the normal functions of the Stomach. *Chen Pi* (Pericarpium Citri Reticulatae) and *Zhi Shi* (Fructus Aurantii Immaturus) regulate qi circulation to relieve feelings of fullness and bloating. These two herbs also strengthen the Spleen

***Fu Ling Yin* (Poria Decoction)**

Diagnosis	Clinical Signs	Treatment	Herbs
Damp-phlegm in the chest and Stomach	Excessive gas and bloating, lack of appetite, belching, and nausea: stagnation of phlegm and dampness	• Strengthens the Spleen • Harmonizes the middle *jiao* • Resolves phlegm and dampness	• *Fu Ling* (Poria) and *Bai Zhu* (Rhizoma Atractylodis Macrocephalae) strengthen the Spleen and Stomach to dispel dampness in the middle *jiao*. • *Ren Shen* (Radix et Rhizoma Ginseng) tonifies qi and restores the normal function of the Stomach. • *Chen Pi* (Pericarpium Citri Reticulatae) and *Zhi Shi* (Fructus Aurantii Immaturus) regulate qi circulation and strengthen the Spleen and Stomach. • *Sheng Jiang* (Rhizoma Zingiberis Recens) harmonizes the herbs.

Fú Líng Yǐn (Poria Decoction)

and Stomach to increase appetite. *Sheng Jiang* (Rhizoma Zingiberis Recens) harmonizes the formula.

VETERINARY MODIFICATIONS

- With nausea and belching, add *Ban Xia* (Rhizoma Pinelliae).
- With indigestion, add *Mai Ya* (Fructus Hordei Germinatus) and *Shan Zha* (Fructus Crataegi).
- With stagnation of phlegm and water, add *Ban Xia* (Rhizoma Pinelliae) and *Jie Geng* (Radix Platycodonis).
- With inability to eat, add *Sha Ren* (Fructus Amomi) and *Shen Qu* (Massa Fermentata).

SUGGESTED ACUPUNCTURE TREATMENT

1. Points: *Fenglong* (ST 40), *Yinlingquan* (SP 9), *Housanli* (ST 36), *Pishu* (BL 20), *Weishu* (BL 21), *Tianshu* (ST 25), *Guanyuan* (CV 4), and *Qihaishu*, *Mijiaogan*, and *Shangen*.
2. Technique: even method and moxibustion.

Fenglong (ST 40), *Yinlingquan* (SP 9), and *Housanli* (ST 36) strengthen the Spleen and Stomach and dispel phlegm. *Pishu* (BL 20) and *Weishu* (BL 21) are the *shu* (transport) points on the back for Spleen and Stomach and help to strengthen and regulate Spleen and Stomach qi. *Tianshu* (ST 25), together with *Housanli* (ST 36), regulates qi and relieves fullness. Moxibustion on *Guanyuan* (CV 4) tonifies Spleen and Stomach qi. *Qihaishu* is the classical point for tonifying the Spleen in the horse. To increase appetite, use *Mijiaogan* in horses and *Shangen* in dogs and cats.

AUTHORS' COMMENTS

Fu Ling Yin can be used to treat gastric dilation in dogs. From a Chinese medicine perspective, gastric dilation can occur due to consumption of dry food diets with high carbohydrate content that leads to the production of dampness. Once gastric dilation has been diagnosed, it is recommended that this formula be given for a minimum of two to four weeks to prevent recurrence and progression to life-threatening gastric dilation with volvulus. *Fu Ling Yin* focuses on resolving Spleen deficiency and not on draining dampness. If profuse dampness is present, it may be best to use a short course (5-7 days) of *Ping Wei San* (Calm the Stomach Powder) or *Xiang Sha Ping Wei San* (Cyperus and Amomum Powder to Calm the Stomach) prior to the use of this formula. A change to a Spleen-tonifying diet is recommended for treatment to be effective while using *Fu Ling Yin*. All of the aforementioned formulas should not be used in the presence of damp-heat, as they all contain warm, drying herbs.

Fu Ling Yin is commonly used in horses in acute episodes of gas colic. Although feed changes may be necessary, the most likely cause of this problem is an underlying weakness of the Spleen. Therefore, prevention of further incidents will center on concurrent administration of formulas such as *Liu Jun Zi Tang* (Six-Gentlemen Decoction) or *Bu Zhong Yi Qi Tang* (Tonify the Middle and Augment the Qi Decoction).

This formula is also effective in the treatment of anorexia and poor appetite post-surgery and post-chemotherapy due to damp accumulation. It can be combined with *Ping Wei San* (Calm the Stomach Powder) to achieve a greater effect to regulate qi, relieve gastric bloating, and dry dampness. Both formulas contain *Chen Pi* (Pericarpium Citri Reticulatae) and *Sheng Jiang* (Rhizoma Zingiberis Recens), and this should be taken into consideration when determining the dosage of the combined formula.

Huò Xiāng Zhèng Qì Săn (Agastache Powder to Rectify the Qi)

藿香正氣散
藿香正气散

Pinyin Name: *Huo Xiang Zheng Qi San*
Literal Name: Agastache Powder to Rectify the Qi
Alternate Names: *Huo Hsiang Cheng Qi San* (*Wan*), *Huo Xiang Zheng Qi San* (*Wan*), Agastache Qi-Regulating Formula (Pill), Agastache Genuine-Qi Powder (Pill), Agastache Formula
Original Source: *Tai Ping Hui Min He Ji Ju Fang* (Imperial Grace Formulary of the Tai Ping Era) by the Imperial Medical Department in 1078-85

COMPOSITION

Huo Xiang (Herba Agastaches)	90g [15g]
Zi Su Ye (Folium Perillae)	30g [5g]
Bai Zhi (Radix Angelicae Dahuricae)	30g [5g]
Ban Xia Qu (Rhizoma Pinelliae Massa Fermentata)	60g [10g]
Chen Pi (Pericarpium Citri Reticulatae)	60g [10g]
Bai Zhu (Rhizoma Atractylodis Macrocephalae)	60g [10g]
Fu Ling (Poria)	30g [5g]
Hou Po (Cortex Magnoliae Officinalis), *zhi* (fried with ginger juice)	60g [10g]
Da Fu Pi (Pericarpium Arecae)	30g [5g]
Jie Geng (Radix Platycodonis)	60g [10g]
Zhi Gan Cao (Radix et Rhizoma Glycyrrhizae Praeparata cum Melle)	75g [12g]

DOSAGE / PREPARATION / ADMINISTRATION

The source text instructions are to grind the ingredients into a fine powder. Cook 6g of the powder with 3 slices of *Sheng Jiang* (Rhizoma Zingiberis Recens) and 1 piece of *Da Zao* (Fructus Jujubae) in 1 large bowl of water until it is reduced to 70%. Take the strained decoction while it is hot. Additionally, the source text recommends covering the body with blankets to promote sweating.

Today, this formula is generally prepared by grinding the herbs into a fine powder. Take 6g of the powder per dose with a decoction made from *Sheng Jiang* (Rhizoma Zingiberis Recens) and *Da Zao* (Fructus Jujubae). This formula may also be prepared as a decoction with the doses suggested in brackets.

CHINESE THERAPEUTIC ACTIONS

1. Releases the exterior and dispels dampness
2. Regulates qi and harmonizes the middle *jiao*

CLINICAL MANIFESTATIONS

Exterior wind-cold invasion accompanied by interior dampness: vomiting and diarrhea, gastric reflux, fever, aversion to cold, epigastric or abdominal pain, and a rapid, superficial and slippery pulse.

VETERINARY CLINICAL APPLICATIONS

Acute viral or bacterial gastroenteritis, acute vomiting and diarrhea from dietary indiscretion or food poisoning.

EXPLANATION

Huo Xiang Zheng Qi San (Agastache Powder to Rectify the Qi) is commonly used to treat vomiting and diarrhea caused by an exterior wind-cold attack accompanied by interior dampness. Because of wind-cold at the exterior, fever, and aversion to cold may be present. Damp stagnation and turbidity in the interior cause qi obstruction, leading to epigastric or abdominal pain. Diarrhea and vomiting occur as dampness and turbidity accumulate in the Stomach and Intestines, which block clear qi from moving upward and turbid qi from moving downward. In severe cases, there may be a white, greasy tongue coating and a rapid, superficial and slippery pulse, both of which are signs of dampness in the interior.

To treat this syndrome, not only must the exterior wind-cold be expelled, but the interior dampness and turbidity must be eliminated. Moreover, the qi should be regulated and the middle *jiao* harmonized. This formula uses a large dose of *Huo Xiang* (Herba Agastaches) to release exterior wind-cold and dispel dampness. In addition, *Huo Xiang* (Herba Agastaches) treats nausea and vomiting by enabling the clear qi to ascend and turbid qi to descend. *Zi Su Ye* (Folium Perillae) and *Bai Zhi* (Radix Angelicae Dahuricae) help *Huo Xiang* (Herba Agastaches) release the exterior wind-cold and dispel interior dampness and turbidity. *Ban Xia Qu* (Rhizoma Pinelliae Massa Fermentata) and *Chen Pi* (Pericarpium Citri Reticulatae) dry dampness, harmonize the Stomach, redirect the reversed

Huò Xiāng Zhèng Qì Săn (Agastache Powder to Rectify the Qi)

Huo Xiang Zheng Qi San (Agastache Powder to Rectify the Qi)

Diagnosis	Clinical Signs	Treatment	Herbs
Exterior wind-cold accompanied by interior dampness	• Fever and aversion to cold: exterior wind-cold • Epigastric or abdominal pain: damp accumulation in the interior • Diarrhea and vomiting: dampness and turbidity affecting the Spleen and Stomach • White, greasy tongue coating and a rapid, slippery pulse: interior dampness	• Releases the exterior and dispels dampness • Regulates qi and harmonizes the middle *jiao*	• *Huo Xiang* (Herba Agastaches) releases exterior wind-cold and dispels dampness. • *Zi Su Ye* (Folium Perillae) and *Bai Zhi* (Radix Angelicae Dahuricae) release the exterior wind-cold and dispel interior dampness and turbidity. • *Ban Xia Qu* (Rhizoma Pinelliae Massa Fermentata) and *Chen Pi* (Pericarpium Citri Reticulatae) dry dampness, harmonize the Stomach, and redirect the reversed flow of qi. • *Bai Zhu* (Rhizoma Atractylodis Macrocephalae) and *Fu Ling* (Poria) strengthen the Spleen, dispel dampness, and harmonize the middle *jiao*. • *Hou Po* (Cortex Magnoliae Officinalis) and *Da Fu Pi* (Pericarpium Arecae) activate qi and dispel dampness. • *Jie Geng* (Radix Platycodonis) ventilates the Lung and resolves dampness. • *Sheng Jiang* (Rhizoma Zingiberis Recens), *Da Zao* (Fructus Jujubae), and *Zhi Gan Cao* (Radix et Rhizoma Glycyrrhizae Praeparata cum Melle) regulate the Spleen and Stomach and harmonize the herbs.

flow of qi, and relieve vomiting. *Bai Zhu* (Rhizoma Atractylodis Macrocephalae) and *Fu Ling* (Poria) strengthen the Spleen, dispel dampness, harmonize the middle *jiao*, and stop diarrhea. *Hou Po* (Cortex Magnoliae Officinalis) and *Da Fu Pi* (Pericarpium Arecae) activate qi to dispel dampness and relieve fullness. *Jie Geng* (Radix Platycodonis) ventilates the Lung to release exterior wind-cold and resolve dampness. *Sheng Jiang* (Rhizoma Zingiberis Recens), *Da Zao* (Fructus Jujubae), and *Zhi Gan Cao* (Radix et Rhizoma Glycyrrhizae Praeparata cum Melle) regulate the Spleen and Stomach and harmonize all of the herbs in this formula.

The emphasis of this formula is on dispelling dampness and harmonizing the Stomach. It has only a minor focus on expelling exterior wind-cold. It is best suited for treating exterior syndromes accompanied by internal dampness, causing disharmony in the middle *jiao* during the summer months. Historically, this formula has also been used to treat malaria and sudden turmoil disorder.

VETERINARY MODIFICATIONS

- With more heat, add *Huang Lian* (Rhizoma Coptidis) and *Huang Qin* (Radix Scutellariae).
- With more cold, add *Fu Zi* (Radix Aconiti Lateralis Praeparata) and *Gan Jiang* (Rhizoma Zingiberis).
- With more dampness, add *Yi Yi Ren* (Semen Coicis) and *Cang Zhu* (Rhizoma Atractylodis).
- With abdominal pain and diarrhea, add *Cang Zhu* (Rhizoma Atractylodis) and *Huang Lian* (Rhizoma Coptidis).
- With tenesmus, add *Zhi Shi* (Fructus Aurantii Immaturus).
- With indigestion, add *Shen Qu* (Massa Fermentata) and *Shan Zha* (Fructus Crataegi).
- With epigastric and abdominal distention caused by qi stagnation, add *Mu Xiang* (Radix Aucklandiae) and *Yan Hu Suo* (Rhizoma Corydalis).

CAUTIONS / CONTRAINDICATIONS

- Most of the herbs in this formula are acrid and drying. Therefore, *Huo Xiang Zheng Qi San* is contraindicated in patients with yin and blood deficiencies.

PHARMACOLOGICAL EFFECTS

1. **Antispasmodic**: *Huo Xiang Zheng Qi San* was shown in many studies to effectively relax the smooth muscles of the gastrointestinal tract to relieve spasms and cramps.[1,2]
2. **Antiemetic**: One study reported that *Huo Xiang Zheng Qi San* was effective in relieving nausea and vomiting in pigeons with artificially-induced vomiting. The formula was given in liquid form, 11.64% concentration, at 20 mL/kg.[3]
3. **Antibacterial**: According to *in vitro* studies, administration of *Huo Xiang Zheng Qi San* was associated with an inhibitory effect against *Staphylococcus aureus*, *Salmonella typhi*, *Bacillus dysenteriae*, and *Bacillus proteus*.[4,5]

Huò Xiāng Zhèng Qì Sǎn (Agastache Powder to Rectify the Qi)

HUMAN CLINICAL STUDIES AND RESEARCH

1. **Diarrhea**: Use of *Huo Xiang Zheng Qi San* effectively treated diarrhea in infants between 6 months and 3 years of age. Of 96 patients, the study reported complete recovery in 85 cases, improvement in 6 cases, and no improvement in 5 cases. The diarrhea generally stopped within 12-72 hours.[6]
2. **Gastroenteritis**: Administration of *Huo Xiang Zheng Qi San* was associated with effective treatment of acute gastroenteritis. Of 150 patients treated with this formula in powder form, 95 had complete recovery and 55 had improvement. Of 40 patients treated with this formula in decoction form, 39 had complete recovery.[7]
3. **Enteritis**: One study reported 95% effectiveness using *Huo Xiang Zheng Qi San* to treat 50 patients with acute enteritis during the summer and fall seasons.[8]
4. **Food poisoning**: Administration of modified *Huo Xiang Zheng Qi San* was associated with complete recovery within 52 hours in all 33 patients with acute food poisoning. Clinical improvements included resolution of symptoms such as body aches and pains, and abdominal distention.[9]

TOXICOLOGY

No toxicity was reported in one acute toxicology study in laboratory animal subjects using *Huo Xiang Zheng Qi San* in powder extract form.[10] According to another study, oral administration of a 53.2% *Huo Xiang Zheng Qi San* solution at 25 mL/kg twice daily (approximately 583 times the normal human dose) for 7 days did not cause any abnormal reactions or fatality.[11]

SUGGESTED ACUPUNCTURE TREATMENT

1. Points: *Fengchi* (GB 20), *Hegu* (LI 4), *Zhangmen* (LR 13), *Gongsun* (SP 4), *Yinlingquan* (SP 9), *Neiguan* (PC 6), *Housanli* (ST 36), *Zhongwan* (CV 12), *Tianshu* (ST 25), and *Yemen* (TH 2).
2. Technique: sedation.

The goal of this acupuncture treatment is to relieve the exterior symptoms while harmonizing the middle *jiao*. *Fengchi* (GB 20) and *Hegu* (LI 4) dispel the exterior wind-cold factor. *Zhangmen* (LR 13), *Gongsun* (SP 4), and *Yinlingquan* (SP 9) strengthen the Spleen and resolve dampness. *Neiguan* (PC 6) and *Housanli* (ST 36) harmonize the middle *jiao* and dissolve dampness. *Zhongwan* (CV 12) regulates qi to relieve nausea. *Tianshu* (ST 25) regulates qi to stop epigastric and abdominal pain. *Yemen* (TH 2), a common point for treating malaria, is used to harmonize the *shaoyang* and restore normal Stomach qi.

AUTHORS' COMMENTS

Huo Xiang Zheng Qi San strongly transforms dampness and harmonizes the Stomach. Its action of releasing exterior wind-cold, however, is not as strong as other exterior-releasing formulas. *Huo Xiang Zheng Qi San* is effective to treat dampness caused by invasion of exogenous pathogenic toxins, such as bacteria or viruses. In equine patients, this may present as mild colic or loose stool accompanied by some muscle trembling. In such cases, moldy hay or a mild viral infection are often suspected. This formula is appropriate for acute gastroenteritis in dogs from dietary discretion, especially food poisoning from eating spoiled or rotten food. It contains *Huo Xiang* (Herba Agastaches) and *Zi Su Ye* (Folium Perillae), which are useful in treating salmonella infection.

Huo Xiang Zheng Qi San, *Liu He Tang* (Harmonize the Six Decoction), and *Bu Huan Jin Zheng Qi San* (Rectify the Qi Powder Worth More than Gold) are three formulas that have been used to treat sudden turmoil disorder. Sudden turmoil disorders are defined as those conditions that produce acute onset of simultaneous vomiting and diarrhea with or without abdominal pain.

- *Huo Xiang Zheng Qi San* contains *Huo Xiang* (Herba Agastaches) as the chief herb; it focuses on releasing exterior wind-cold in addition to dispelling interior dampness.
- *Liu He Tang* contains *Ren Shen* (Radix et Rhizoma Ginseng) as the chief herb. It is the most tonifying of the three formulas and has the greatest ability to strengthen the Spleen and harmonize the middle *jiao*.
- *Bu Huan Jin Zheng Qi San* contains *Cang Zhu* (Rhizoma Atractylodis), which is bitter and warm, as the chief herb. This formula has the strongest ability to dry dampness compared to the other two formulas.
- These three formulas are very effective and often resolve the clinical signs within 24-72 hours; once signs have resolved, the formula should be stopped. However, these formulas focus on treating cold and damp pathogenic factors and have little ability to clear heat or eliminate toxins. They are contraindicated in acute gastroenteritis when signs of heat predominate.

References

1. *Zhong Cheng Yao Yan Jiu* (Research of Chinese Patent Medicine), 1984; 6(5):15.
2. *Zhong Cao Yao* (Chinese Herbal Medicine), 1984; 12:15.
3. *Zhong Cheng Yao* (Study of Chinese Patent Medicine), 1990; 12(4):31.
4. *Zhong Cao Yao* (Chinese Herbal Medicine), 1984; 12:15.
5. *Zhong Cheng Yao* (Study of Chinese Patent Medicine), 1990; 12(4):31.

Huò Xiāng Zhèng Qì Sǎn (Agastache Powder to Rectify the Qi)

6. *Shan Dong Zhong Yi Xue Yuan Xue Bao* (Journal of Shandong University School of Chinese Medicine), 1993; 1:39.
7. *Zhong Cao Yao* (Chinese Herbal Medicine), 1992; 9:479.
8. *Zhe Jiang Zhong Yi Xue Yuan Xue Bao* (Journal of Zhejiang University of Chinese Medicine), 1994; 3:8.
9. *Shan Xi Zhong Yi* (Shanxi Chinese Medicine), 1990; 5:224.
10. *Zhong Cao Yao* (Chinese Herbal Medicine), 1992; 23(9):479.
11. *Zhong Cheng Yao* (Study of Chinese Patent Medicine), 1990; 12(4):31.

Liù Hé Tāng (Harmonize the Six Decoction)

六和湯

六和汤

Pinyin Name: *Liu He Tang*

Literal Name: Harmonize the Six Decoction

Alternate Name: Cardamon Combination

Original Source: *Tai Ping Hui Min He Ji Ju Fang* (Imperial Grace Formulary of the Tai Ping Era) by the Imperial Medical Department in 1078-85

COMPOSITION

Ren Shen (Radix et Rhizoma Ginseng)	30g [3-5g]
Zhi Gan Cao (Radix et Rhizoma Glycyrrhizae Praeparata cum Melle)	30g [3-5g]
Huo Xiang (Herba Agastaches)	60g [6-10g]
Sha Ren (Fructus Amomi)	30g [3-5g]
Ban Xia (Rhizoma Pinelliae), *pao* (blast-fried) in liquid 7 times	30g [3-5g]
Hou Po (Cortex Magnoliae Officinalis), *zhi* (fried) with ginger juice	120g [12-15g]
Ku Xing Ren (Semen Armeniacae Amarum)	30g [3-5g]
Xiang Ru (Herba Moslae)	120g [12-15g]
Bai Bian Dou (Semen Lablab Album), *chao* (dry-fried) with ginger juice	60g [6-10g]
Mu Gua (Fructus Chaenomelis)	60g [6-10g]
Chi Fu Ling (Poria Rubra)	60g [6-10g]

DOSAGE / PREPARATION / ADMINISTRATION

The source text instructions are to grind the ingredients into powder. Cook 12g of the powder with 3 slices of *Sheng Jiang* (Rhizoma Zingiberis Recens) and 1 piece of *Da Zao* (Fructus Jujubae) in 1.5 bowls of water until it is reduced to 80% volume. Take the warm, strained decoction any time during the day. Today, this formula may be prepared as a decoction with the doses suggested in brackets.

CHINESE THERAPEUTIC ACTIONS

1. Strengthens the Spleen and harmonizes the Stomach
2. Resolves dampness and dispels summer-heat

Liù Hé Tāng (Harmonize the Six Decoction)

CLINICAL MANIFESTATIONS

Damp accumulation caused by an inappropriate diet, leading to Spleen and Stomach dysfunction: vomiting, diarrhea, distention in the chest and diaphragm, and possibly a white, greasy tongue coating.

VETERINARY CLINICAL APPLICATIONS

Heat stroke, disturbance of the gastrointestinal system characterized by decreased appetite, vomiting, and diarrhea. Cats and dogs may develop these clinical signs from eating cold, raw and/or damp foods, especially during hot and humid weather. Similarly, horses given cold water too soon after being worked may develop an acute colic or similar clinical signs that begin shortly after the insult.

EXPLANATION

Liu He Tang (Harmonize the Six Decoction) is indicated for patients with dampness attacking and damaging the Spleen and Stomach caused by an inappropriate diet. This condition often arises on hot and humid summer days after eating raw, cold, or uncooked foods. Damp accumulation creates disharmony of the Spleen and Stomach, which causes such clinical signs as nausea and vomiting. Obstructed qi from dampness results in distention in the chest and diaphragm. Diarrhea is caused by dampness affecting the Spleen. Historically, this formula has been used to treat sudden turmoil disorder with vomiting and diarrhea.

The treatment plan for this syndrome is to dispel dampness, harmonize the Stomach, and strengthen the Spleen. In this formula, *Ren Shen* (Radix et Rhizoma Ginseng) and *Zhi Gan Cao* (Radix et Rhizoma Glycyrrhizae Praeparata cum Melle) strengthen the Spleen and dispel dampness. *Huo Xiang* (Herba Agastaches) and *Sha Ren* (Fructus Amomi) dispel dampness from the exterior and dry dampness in the interior. *Ban Xia* (Rhizoma Pinelliae), *Hou Po* (Cortex Magnoliae Officinalis), and *Ku Xing Ren* (Semen Armeniacae Amarum) regulate the qi flow and dispel dampness. *Xiang Ru* (Herba Moslae) and *Bai Bian Dou* (Semen Lablab Album) strengthen the Spleen and dispel dampness. *Mu Gua* (Fructus Chaenomelis) and *Chi Fu Ling* (Poria Rubra) dispel dampness, smooth the qi flow, and harmonize the middle *jiao*. *Zhi Gan Cao* (Radix et Rhizoma Glycyrrhizae Praeparata cum Melle), *Sheng Jiang* (Rhizoma Zingiberis Recens), and *Da Zao* (Fructus Jujubae) harmonize the Spleen and Stomach as well as harmonize the rest of the herbs in this formula.

VETERINARY MODIFICATIONS

- With exterior cold, add *Zi Su Ye* (Folium Perillae) and *Xiang Fu* (Rhizoma Cyperi).
- With severe exterior summer-dampness, increase the doses of *Xiang Ru* (Herba Moslae) and *Huo Xiang* (Herba Agastaches).
- With severe damp-heat accumulation, add *Yi Yi Ren* (Semen Coicis), *Hua Shi* (Talcum), *Che Qian Cao* (Herba Plantaginis), and *Huang Lian* (Rhizoma Coptidis).

CAUTIONS / CONTRAINDICATIONS

Liu He Tang is dry and aromatic; therefore, it is not suitable for patients who have yin or body fluid deficiencies.

***Liu He Tang* (Harmonize the Six Decoction)**

Diagnosis	Clinical Signs	Treatment	Herbs
Spleen and Stomach dysfunction with damp accumulation	• Nausea and vomiting: disharmony of the Spleen and Stomach caused by damp accumulation • Distention in the chest and diaphragm: dampness obstructing qi flow • Diarrhea: dampness affecting the Spleen	• Strengthens the Spleen and harmonizes the Stomach • Resolves dampness and dispels summer-heat	• *Ren Shen* (Radix et Rhizoma Ginseng) and *Zhi Gan Cao* (Radix et Rhizoma Glycyrrhizae Praeparata cum Melle) strengthen the Spleen and dispel dampness. • *Huo Xiang* (Herba Agastaches) and *Sha Ren* (Fructus Amomi) dispel dampness from the exterior and dry dampness in the interior. • *Ban Xia* (Rhizoma Pinelliae), *Hou Po* (Cortex Magnoliae Officinalis), and *Ku Xing Ren* (Semen Armeniacae Amarum) regulate the qi flow and dispel dampness. • *Xiang Ru* (Herba Moslae) and *Bai Bian Dou* (Semen Lablab Album) strengthen the Spleen and dispel dampness. • *Mu Gua* (Fructus Chaenomelis) and *Chi Fu Ling* (Poria Rubra) dispel dampness, regulate the qi flow, and harmonize the middle *jiao*. • *Sheng Jiang* (Rhizoma Zingiberis Recens) and *Da Zao* (Fructus Jujubae) harmonize the herbs.

Liù Hé Tāng (Harmonize the Six Decoction)

SUGGESTED ACUPUNCTURE TREATMENT

1. Points: *Zhangmen* (LR 13), *Gongsun* (SP 4), *Yinlingquan* (SP 9), *Neiguan* (PC 6), *Housanli* (ST 36), *Zhongwan* (CV 12), *Tianshu* (ST 25), and *Pishu* (BL 20).
2. Technique: sedation.

This acupuncture point selection is similar to that for *Huo Xiang Zheng Qi San* (Agastache Powder to Rectify the Qi), except that *Fengchi* (GB 20), *Hegu* (LI 4), and *Yemen* (TH 2) are omitted since there are no clinical signs of an exterior invasion, such as fever and trembling. *Zhangmen* (LR 13), *Gongsun* (SP 4), and *Yinlingquan* (SP 9) strengthen the Spleen and resolve dampness. *Neiguan* (PC 6) and *Housanli* (ST 36) harmonize the middle *jiao* and resolve dampness. *Zhongwan* (CV 12) relieves nausea, while *Tianshu* (ST 25) stops epigastric or abdominal pain. Finally, *Pishu* (BL 20), the *shu* (transport) point of the Spleen, tonifies the Spleen and resolves dampness.

AUTHORS' COMMENTS

Liu He Tang, literally "Harmonize the Six Decoction," refers to the goal of harmonizing the Spleen and Stomach to ensure optimal absorption of the nutrients and proper nourishment of the "six" *fu* (hollow organs). It can be used to treat poor appetite, episodic vomiting, and lack of weight gain in juvenile dogs fed a refrigerated and/or raw food diet. The Spleen is inherently weak in immature animals and dislikes cold and dampness. A raw food diet should not be fed to immature dogs until the Spleen has fully developed at approximately one year of age. It would seem prudent to warm foods to body temperature prior to feeding and/or mix with digestive enzymes as needed. The vomiting of warm, macerated, partially digested food by non-domestic canines to feed their offspring achieves this purpose. This formula is effective in treating damp accumulation and disharmony of the Spleen and Stomach in dogs and cats secondary to feeding ice cream and ice water during the summer months.

Section 2

清热祛湿剂
— Heat-Clearing and Damp-Dispelling Formulas

Yīn Chén Hāo Tāng (Artemisia Scoparia Decoction)
茵陳蒿湯
茵陈蒿汤

Pinyin Name: *Yin Chen Hao Tang*
Literal Name: Artemisia Scoparia Decoction
Alternate Name: Artemisia Combination
Original Source: *Shang Han Lun* (Discussion of Cold-Induced Disorders) by Zhang Zhong-Jing in the Eastern Han Dynasty

COMPOSITION

Yin Chen (Herba Artemisiae Scopariae)	18g
Zhi Zi (Fructus Gardeniae)	14 pieces [9g]
Da Huang (Radix et Rhizoma Rhei)	6g

DOSAGE / PREPARATION / ADMINISTRATION

The source text instructions are to first cook *Yin Chen* (Herba Artemisiae Scopariae) in 12 cups [2,400 mL] of water until the liquid is reduced to 6 cups [1,200 mL]. Add the other two herbs and cook the decoction until the liquid is reduced to 3 cups [600 mL]. Take the strained decoction in three equally divided doses.

The source text states that use of the formula will induce normal urine that resembles the juice of *Zao Jiao* (Fructus Gleditsiae), which is pure red in color. After one night, the abdominal fullness will be relieved and the yellow discoloration of the eyes and skin will come out with the urine. Today, this formula is generally prepared as a decoction by cooking all three herbs at the same time.

CHINESE THERAPEUTIC ACTIONS

1. Clears heat
2. Resolves dampness
3. Relieves jaundice

CLINICAL MANIFESTATIONS

Acute damp-heat jaundice: bright yellow discoloration of the skin and sclera, fever, trembling, vomiting, diarrhea, lethargy, dysuria, thirst, a yellow, greasy tongue coating, and a deep, rapid and wiry pulse.

VETERINARY CLINICAL APPLICATIONS

Acute jaundice, acute hepatitis, acute toxic hepatopathy, acute pancreatitis, acute feline cholangiohepatitis, hepatomegaly, splenomegaly, feline cholangitis, hepatic lipidosis, acute cholelithiasis, liver cancer, liver cirrhosis, leptospirosis, hyperlipidemia, lymphadenopathy, and abdominal effusion.

EXPLANATION

Yin Chen Hao Tang (Artemisia Scoparia Decoction) is the formula of choice to treat damp-heat jaundice, a condition caused by stagnation of dampness and heat in the interior. This type of damp-heat jaundice, commonly referred to as yang jaundice, is characterized by a bright discoloration of the skin that resembles the color of fresh orange peel. The damp-heat can manifest outward to the muscles and skin, causing bright yellow discoloration of the skin and sclera. The damp-heat can also affect the lower *jiao*, producing abdominal effusion and dysuria. The heat may consume body fluids, causing thirst. A yellow, greasy tongue coating and a deep, rapid and wiry pulse both suggest damp-heat in the interior.

This formula contains *Yin Chen* (Herba Artemisiae Scopariae), the premier herb choice for clearing damp-heat jaundice. *Zhi Zi* (Fructus Gardeniae) clears damp-heat

Yīn Chén Hāo Tāng (Artemisia Scoparia Decoction)

***Yin Chen Hao Tang* (Artemisia Scoparia Decoction)**

Diagnosis	Clinical Signs	Treatment	Herbs
Damp-heat jaundice	• Bright yellow discoloration of the skin and sclera: damp-heat manifesting outward • Abdominal effusion and dysuria: damp-heat traveling downward • Thirst: damp-heat consuming body fluids • Yellow, greasy tongue coating and a deep, rapid pulse: damp-heat in the interior	• Clears heat • Resolves dampness • Relieves jaundice	• *Yin Chen* (Herba Artemisiae Scopariae) clears damp-heat from the Liver and Gallbladder. • *Zhi Zi* (Fructus Gardeniae) clears damp-heat in all three *jiaos* and drains it out of the body through urination. • *Da Huang* (Radix et Rhizoma Rhei) purges damp-heat through defecation.

in the three *jiaos* and drains damp-heat out of the body through urination. *Da Huang* (Radix et Rhizoma Rhei) drains damp-heat through defecation. These three herbs have a synergistic effect to maximize the treatment result.

VETERINARY MODIFICATIONS

- For jaundice with more dampness, add *Fu Ling* (Poria), *Ze Xie* (Rhizoma Alismatis), and *Zhu Ling* (Polyporus).
- For jaundice with more heat, add *Huang Bo* (Cortex Phellodendri Chinensis) and *Long Dan* (Radix et Rhizoma Gentianae).
- For severe jaundice, add *Hu Zhang* (Rhizoma et Radix Polygoni Cuspidati) and *Pu Gong Ying* (Herba Taraxaci).
- With gallbladder inflammation or infection, add *Jin Qian Cao* (Herba Lysimachiae), *Long Dan* (Radix et Rhizoma Gentianae), *Ji Nei Jin* (Endothelium Corneum Gigeriae Galli), *Li Zhi He* (Semen Litchi), *Zhi Qiao* (Fructus Aurantii), and *Wei Ling Xian* (Radix et Rhizoma Clematidis).
- With oliguria, add *Fu Ling* (Poria), *Ze Xie* (Rhizoma Alismatis), and *Hua Shi* (Talcum).
- With dysuria, add *Mu Tong* (Caulis Akebiae), *Hua Shi* (Talcum), and *Jin Qian Cao* (Herba Lysimachiae).
- With thirst, add *Huang Lian* (Rhizoma Coptidis) and *Huang Qin* (Radix Scutellariae).
- With fever and trembling, add *Chai Hu* (Radix Bupleuri) and *Huang Qin* (Radix Scutellariae).
- With scanty, yellow urine, add *Jin Qian Cao* (Herba Lysimachiae) and *Ze Xie* (Rhizoma Alismatis).
- With hypochondriac pain, add *Chai Hu* (Radix Bupleuri), *Chuan Lian Zi* (Fructus Toosendan), *Yu Jin* (Radix Curcumae), and *Xiang Fu* (Rhizoma Cyperi).
- With hypochondriac pain and abdominal distention, add *Yu Jin* (Radix Curcumae), *Zhi Qiao* (Fructus Aurantii), and *Chuan Lian Zi* (Fructus Toosendan).
- With poor appetite, add *Shan Zha* (Fructus Crataegi) and *Mai Ya* (Fructus Hordei Germinatus).
- With nausea and vomiting, add *Huang Lian* (Rhizoma Coptidis), *Bai Shao* (Radix Paeoniae Alba), and *Ban Xia* (Rhizoma Pinelliae).

CAUTIONS / CONTRAINDICATIONS

- *Yin Chen Hao Tang* should be used only for acute damp-heat (yang) jaundice and not damp-cold (yin) jaundice.
- This formula contains *Da Huang* (Radix et Rhizoma Rhei) and therefore is not for long-term use.
- The use of this formula is contraindicated during pregnancy.[1]

PHARMACOLOGICAL EFFECTS

1. **Cholagogic**: *Yin Chen Hao Tang* was associated with stimulating an increased production and release of bile acids. The alcohol extract of the formula was determined to be more effective than the water extract. In comparison with the control group that did not receive any herbs, administration of the alcohol extract increased the production of bile by 51.28%, while administration of the water extract increased the production of bile by 45.85%.[2] Some researchers have noted that to obtain the maximum cholagogic effect, a larger dose of *Da Huang* (Radix et Rhizoma Rhei) should be used in its fresh form or should be post-decocted. *Yin Chen* (Herba Artemisiae Scopariae) should also be post-decocted. This study also suggested that *Zhi Zi* (Fructus Gardeniae) did not enhance the cholagogic effect of the formula, and that it may be omitted.[3]
2. **Choleretic**: One study reported *Yin Chen Hao Tang* to be a potent therapeutic agent for a number of cholestatic liver diseases by enhancing the bile acid-independent secretory capacity of hepatocytes. This therapeutic effect was attributed in part to genipin, an active compound of *Zhi Zi* (Fructus Gardeniae).[4]
3. **Hepatoprotective**: *Yin Chen Hao Tang* has been shown in many studies to effectively protect the liver from various drug- or chemical-induced hepatitis, including

acetaminophen, carbon tetrachloride, alpha-naphthylisothiocyanate (ANIT), and concanavalin A.[5,6,7] This action was attributed to inhibited production of inflammatory cytokines and enhanced production of anti-inflammatory cytokines. The researchers also stated that administration of *Yin Chen Hao Tang* may be useful for treating severe acute hepatitis accompanying cholestasis in cases of autoimmune hepatitis.[8]

4. **Hepatoprotective and antifibrotic**: In 6 postoperative patients with biliary atresia, administration of *Yin Chen Hao Tang* was found to have a long-term protective and antifibrotic effect on the liver in patients with abnormal levels of liver enzyme and hyaluronic acid.[9] Another study showed that use of *Yin Chen Hao Tang* prevented artificially-induced liver fibrosis in rats.[10]
5. **Antihyperlipidemic**: Use of *Yin Chen Hao Tang* in mice was associated with a decrease in total cholesterol, LDL, and triglycerides levels, and an increase in HDL levels.[11]

HUMAN CLINICAL STUDIES AND RESEARCH

1. **Hepatitis**: *Yin Chen Hao Tang* has been shown in many studies to be beneficial in treating hepatitis. Administration of modified *Yin Chen Hao Tang* to 247 patients with acute infectious icteric hepatitis was associated with recovery in 83 cases within 7 days, 158 cases within 15 days, and 6 cases within 20 days. The herbal treatment consisted of this formula plus *Bai Jiang Cao* (Herba cum Radice Patriniae), *Huang Bo* (Cortex Phellodendri Chinensis), *Long Dan* (Radix et Rhizoma Gentianae), *Yu Jin* (Radix Curcumae), and others.[12] Another study of 50 patients with acute icteric hepatitis who were treated with modified *Yin Chen Hao Tang* showed recovery in 47 cases, improvement in 2 cases, and no effect in 1 case (98% overall effectiveness). The herbal treatment contained this formula with the following modifications: *Huang Qin* (Radix Scutellariae), *Huang Lian* (Rhizoma Coptidis), and *Long Dan* (Radix et Rhizoma Gentianae) for more heat than dampness; *Cang Zhu* (Rhizoma Atractylodis), *Fu Ling* (Poria) and *Pei Lan* (Herba Eupatorii) for more dampness than heat; *Hou Po* (Cortex Magnoliae Officinalis) and *Lai Fu Zi* (Semen Raphani) for abdominal distention; *Zhu Ru* (Caulis Bambusae in Taenia), *Ban Xia* (Rhizoma Pinelliae) and *Sheng Jiang* (Rhizoma Zingiberis Recens) for nausea and vomiting; and *Yan Hu Suo* (Rhizoma Corydalis) and *Chuan Lian Zi* (Fructus Toosendan) for hypochondriac pain.[13] Lastly, one study reported good results using *Yin Chen Hao Tang* plus *Che Qian Zi* (Semen Plantaginis) and *Mu Tong* (Caulis Akebiae) to treat infants with acute viral hepatitis.[14]
2. **Jaundice**: It has been confirmed via numerous studies that *Yin Chen Hao Tang* is beneficial in treating jaundice. One study reported 90% effectiveness using modified *Yin Chen Hao Tang* to treat jaundice in 20 patients (16 with complete recovery, 2 with improvement, and 2 with no effect). The herbal treatment contained this formula plus *Bai Hua She She Cao* (Herba Hedyotis), *Da Qing Ye* (Folium Isatidis), *Ji Gu Cao* (Herba Abri), and others.[15] According to another study, use of modified *Yin Chen Hao Tang* was associated with 91% effectiveness to treat patients with persistent jaundice even after surgical removal of the gallbladder. The herbal treatment contained this formula, plus *Huang Qin* (Radix Scutellariae), *Yu Jin* (Radix Curcumae), *Jin Qian Cao* (Herba Lysimachiae), and others. Of 12 patients in this study, 5 had significant improvement, 6 had moderate improvement, and 1 had no effect.[16] Lastly, 32 patients with jaundice associated with viral hepatitis were treated with large doses of *Yin Chen Hao Tang* with good results. In addition to the base formula, modifications included the addition of *Ban Xia* (Rhizoma Pinelliae) and *Zhu Ru* (Caulis Bambusae in Taenia) for nausea and vomiting; *Zhu Ling* (Polyporus), *Fu Ling* (Poria), and *Da Fu Pi* (Pericarpium Arecae) for accumulation of water; *Dan Shen* (Radix et Rhizoma Salviae Miltiorrhizae) and *Yu Jin* (Radix Curcumae) for hepatomegaly or splenomegaly; *Qin Jiao* (Radix Gentianae Macrophyllae) and *Qin Pi* (Cortex Fraxini) for itchy skin; and *Chai Hu* (Radix Bupleuri) and *Huang Qin* (Radix Scutellariae) for chills and fever. Of 32 patients, the study reported significant improvement in 23 cases and moderate improvement in 9 cases.[17]
3. **Hyperlipidemia**: Use of *Yin Chen Hao Tang* plus *Long Dan Xie Gan Tang* (Gentiana Decoction to Drain the Liver) to treat hyperlipidemia was associated with a reduction of cholesterol levels in 77 of 88 patients. The patients were instructed to discontinue all other herbal and drug treatment for hyperlipidemia throughout the study.[18]

SUGGESTED ACUPUNCTURE TREATMENT

1. Points: *Zhiyang* (GV 9), *Wangu* (SI 4), *Ganshu* (BL 18), *Danshu* (BL 19), *Yanglingquan* (GB 34), *Taichong* (LR 3), and *Shaochong* (HT 9).
2. Technique: sedation.

This acupuncture treatment aims to resolve dampness and relieve jaundice. *Zhiyang* (GV 9) and *Wangu* (SI 4) are used together to dispel dampness and clear heat. *Ganshu* (BL 18) and *Danshu* (BL 19) are the *shu* (transport) points on the back for Liver and Gallbladder and help to regulate their function. *Yanglingquan* (GB 34), *Taichong* (LR 3), and *Shaochong* (HT 9) harmonize the Liver and Gallbladder to relieve jaundice. In addition, if the patient shows

Yīn Chén Hāo Tāng (Artemisia Scoparia Decoction)

severe signs and symptoms of heat, *Dazhui* (GV 14) can be added to clear heat. If there is severe dampness, add *Yinlingquan* (SP 9) and *Fenglong* (ST 40).

AUTHORS' COMMENTS

Jaundice is always associated with dampness and can develop from external or internal causes; it is classified as either acute or chronic in nature.

- Externally generated damp-heat is often caused by invasion of external pathogenic factors (infectious disease) that lodge in the Liver and Gallbladder and produce toxic-heat. This type of jaundice is also called yang-type jaundice, characterize by its acute nature with bright yellow discoloration of the skin and sclera. Exogenous pathogenic factors that can cause acute jaundice include leptospirosis, liver flukes, and systemic viral and rickettsial diseases. Alternatively, ingested toxins like tansy ragwort and reactions to blood or plasma transfusions can also produce cases of yang jaundice. Acute jaundice that goes untreated or improperly treated becomes chronic, is usually a combination of excess and deficiency, and is associated with damp-cold and Spleen deficiency. *Yin Chen Hao Tang* can be used alone to treat acute (yang-type) jaundice with more heat than dampness caused by liver cancer, acute hepatitis, acute cholangitis, liver cirrhosis, infectious diseases and drug-induced hepatic necrosis. In the treatment of acute leptospirosis with severe heat signs, combine with *Long Dan Xie Gan Tang* (Gentiana Decoction to Drain the Liver) and add herbs to tonify the Spleen. Many dogs are Spleen deficient due to eating commercial dry food diets and will require Spleen support if given both of these cold bitter formulas.
- Internally generated damp-heat often develops from improper diet, Spleen deficiency, and chronic antibiotic use. This type of jaundice is usually slow to develop and is called yin-type jaundice, which is typified by a duller yellow color, cold accumulation, and stagnation. It may, however, have acute exacerbations, such as cases of anorexic hyperlipidemia in horses and cats, which are more typical of yang jaundice, where there is more heat and the jaundice is brighter and may have an orange tint. *Yin Chen Hao Tang* (Artemisia Scoparia Decoction) is not typically used alone for cases of yin jaundice. For chronic disease, it is usually combined with other herbs or formulas to further drain dampness, clear heat, stop pain, relieve stagnation, and support the middle *jiao*.

Yin Chen Hao Tang is for short-term use only, as it contains *Da Huang* (Radix et Rhizoma Rhei), which is cold and can easily injure qi. This formula is very effective and works quickly if dosed appropriately; the jaundice can resolve in as little as 5-7 days. Once the jaundice has resolved, this formula should be stopped and another chosen to treat the root cause of the disease and prevent damage to the Spleen. A course of treatment should not exceed 5-7 days without re-evaluation.

References

1. *Zhong Yao Ming Fang Yao Li Yu Ying Yong* (Pharmacology and Applications of Famous Herbal Formulas), 1989; 423-425.
2. *Zhong Yao Yao Li Yu Lin Chuang* (Pharmacology and Clinical Applications of Chinese Herbs), 1987; 3:52.
3. *Zhong Yi Za Zhi* (Journal of Chinese Medicine), 1982; 7:72.
4. Shoda J, Miura T, Utsunomiya H, Oda K, Yamamoto M, Kano M, Ikegami T, Tanaka N, Akita H, Ito K, Suzuki H, Sugiyama Y. Genipin enhances Mrp2 (Abcc2)-mediated bile formation and organic anion transport in rat liver. Hepatology. 2004 Jan; 39(1):167-78.
5. *Zhong Yao Yao Li Yu Lin Chuang* (Pharmacology and Clinical Applications of Chinese Herbs), 1992; 8:40.
6. *Shan Xi Yi Yao Za Zhi* (Shanxi Journal of Medicine and Herbology), 1975; 3:79.
7. *Zhong Xi Yi Jie He Za Zhi* (Journal of Integrated Chinese and Western Medicine), 1985; 6:56.
8. Yamashiki M, Mase A, Arai I, Huang XX, Nobori T, Nishimura A, Sakaguchi S, Inoue K. Effects of the Japanese herbal medicine 'Inchinko-to' (TJ-135) on concanavalin A-induced hepatitis in mice. Clin Sci (Lond). 2000 Nov; 99(5):421-31.
9. Iinuma Y, Kubota M, Yagi M, Kanada S, Yamazaki S, Kinoshita Y. Effects of the herbal medicine Inchinko-to on liver function in postoperative patients with biliary atresia--a pilot study. J Pediatr Surg. 2003 Nov; 38(11):1607-11.
10. Sakaida I, Tsuchiya M, Kawaguchi K, Kimura T, Terai S, Okita K. Herbal medicine Inchin-ko-to (TJ-135) prevents liver fibrosis and enzyme-altered lesions in rat liver cirrhosis induced by a choline-deficient L-amino acid-defined diet. J Hepatol. 2003 Jun; 38(6): 762-9.
11. *Zhong Cheng Yao* (Study of Chinese Patent Medicine), 1992; 7:34.
12. *Zhong Yi Ming Fang Lin Chuang Xin Yong* (Contemporary Clinical Applications of Classic Chinese Formulas), 2001; 507.
13. *Shan Xi Zhong Yi* (Shanxi Chinese Medicine), 1998; 3:19.
14. *Shan Xi Zhong Yi* (Shanxi Chinese Medicine), 1993; 4:17.
15. *Tian Jin Zhong Yi* (Tianjin Chinese Medicine), 1986; 2:34.
16. *Jiang Su Zhong Yi* (Jiangsu Chinese Medicine), 1996; 5:17.
17. *Zhong Yi Ming Fang Lin Chuang Xin Yong* (Contemporary Clinical Applications of Classic Chinese Formulas), 2001; 508.
18. *Shan Xi Zhong Yi* (Shanxi Chinese Medicine), 1997; 5:220.

Yīn Chén Wǔ Líng Sǎn

(Artemisia Scoparia and Five-Ingredient Powder with Poria)

茵陳五苓散
茵陈五苓散

Pinyin Name: *Yin Chen Wu Ling San*
Literal Name: Artemisia Scoparia and Five-Ingredient Powder with Poria
Alternate Names: Capillaries and Hoelen Five Formula, Artemisia and Hoelen Five Formula
Original Source: *Jin Gui Yao Lue* (Essentials from the Golden Cabinet) by Zhang Zhong-Jing in the Eastern Han Dynasty

COMPOSITION

Yin Chen (Herba Artemisiae Scopariae)	7.5g
Wu Ling San (Five-Ingredient Powder with Poria)	3.75g

DOSAGE / PREPARATION / ADMINISTRATION

The source text instructs to grind the ingredients into powder. Take one spoonful [6g] of the powder, three times daily after meals.

CHINESE THERAPEUTIC ACTIONS

Dispels dampness and treats jaundice

CLINICAL MANIFESTATIONS

Damp-heat jaundice (more dampness than heat): anorexia, vomiting, loose stools, abdominal bloating, scanty concentrated urine and dysuria.

VETERINARY CLINICAL APPLICATIONS

Jaundice, acute hepatitis, acute infectious disease, liver cirrhosis, drug-induced hepatitis, nephritis and pancreatitis.

EXPLANATION

Yin Chen Wu Ling San (Artemisia Scoparia and Five-Ingredient Powder with Poria) is comprised of *Yin Chen* (Herba Artemisiae Scopariae) plus *Wu Ling San* (Five-Ingredient Powder with Poria). *Yin Chen* (Herba Artemisiae Scopariae) clears damp-heat and relieves jaundice. *Wu Ling San* (Five-Ingredient Powder with Poria) regulates water circulation, promotes urination, and relieves dysuria. Clinically, this formula may be used to treat damp-heat jaundice (more damp than heat) with dysuria.

Please refer to *Wu Ling San* (Five-Ingredient Powder with Poria) for a detailed explanation of this formula.

VETERINARY MODIFICATIONS

- With fever and thirst, add *Shi Gao* (Gypsum Fibrosum) and *Zhi Mu* (Rhizoma Anemarrhenae).
- With dysuria, add *Mu Tong* (Caulis Akebiae) and *Di Huang* (Radix Rehmanniae).

PHARMACOLOGICAL EFFECTS

1. **Diuretic**: Administration of *Yin Chen Wu Ling San* at normal doses in adults did not significantly affect the urine output or concentration of electrolytes. However, at higher doses, it did increase the urine output without changing the concentration of the electrolytes.[1]
2. **Hepatoprotective**: One study reported that *Yin Chen Wu Ling San* had a protective effect against alcohol-induced liver damage in mice.[2]

HUMAN CLINICAL STUDIES AND RESEARCH

1. **Yellow discoloration of the palms and soles**: Use of *Yin Chen Wu Ling San* plus *Bai Mao Gen* (Rhizoma Imperatae), *Dan Shen* (Radix et Rhizoma Salviae Miltiorrhizae) and *Hua Shi* (Talcum) was associated with a 100% success rate in treating 6 patients with yellow discoloration of the palms and soles. The cause of this illness was unrelated to jaundice, as confirmed by Western medicine. The traditional Chinese medical diagnosis was Spleen and blood deficiencies, with damp-heat accumulation.[3]

Yin Chen Wu Ling San **(Artemisia Scoparia and Five-Ingredient Powder with Poria)**

Diagnosis	Clinical Signs	Treatment	Herbs
Damp-heat jaundice	Jaundice, anorexia, vomiting, loose stools, abdominal bloating, and dysuria: damp-heat	Dispels dampness and treats jaundice	• *Yin Chen* (Herba Artemisiae Scopariae) clears damp-heat and relieves jaundice. • *Wu Ling San* (Five-Ingredient Powder with Poria) regulates water circulation, dispels dampness, and relieves dysuria.

Yīn Chén Wǔ Líng Sǎn

(Artemisia Scoparia and Five-Ingredient Powder with Poria)

2. **Hyperlipoproteinemia**: Sixty patients with hyperlipoproteinemia were divided into two groups of 30 patients each and treated with herbs. Group one received *Yin Chen Wu Ling San*, and group two received a preparation of *Jiao Gu Lan* (Rhizoma seu Herba Gynostemmatis). In group one, the study reported significant improvement in 19 cases, moderate improvement in 9 cases, and no effect in 2 cases (93% effectiveness). In group two, the study reported significant improvement in 6 cases, moderate improvement in 20 cases, and no effect in 4 cases (86.7% effectiveness).[4]
3. **Hepatitis and jaundice**: It has been shown in many studies that use of *Yin Chen Wu Ling San* with pharmaceuticals was associated with marked success in treating individuals with hepatitis and/or jaundice. One formula that successfully treated jaundice contained the following ingredients: *Yin Chen* (Herba Artemisiae Scopariae) 30g, dry-fried *Bai Zhu* (Rhizoma Atractylodis Macrocephalae) 30g, *Chi Fu Ling* (Poria Rubra) 30g, *Dan Shen* (Radix et Rhizoma Salviae Miltiorrhizae) 30g, *Fu Zi* (Radix Aconiti Lateralis Praeparata) 10-30g, *Ting Li Zi* (Semen Descurainiae seu Lepidii) 10-20g, *Ze Xie* (Rhizoma Alismatis) 15g, *Dang Shen* (Radix Codonopsis) 10g, *Gui Zhi* (Ramulus Cinnamomi) 10g, and *Zhi Gan Cao* (Radix et Rhizoma Glycyrrhizae Praeparata cum Melle) 10g.[5] For icteric hepatitis, one successful formula contained the following ingredients: *Yin Chen Wu Ling San* plus *Chuan Xiong* (Rhizoma Chuanxiong), *Dang Gui* (Radix Angelicae Sinensis), and *Da Huang* (Radix et Rhizoma Rhei).[6]

SUGGESTED ACUPUNCTURE TREATMENT

1. Points: *Pangguangshu* (BL 28), *Zhongji* (CV 3), *Yinlingquan* (SP 9), *Shuifen* (CV 9), *Waiguan* (TH 5), *Yanglingquan* (GB 34), and *Taichong* (LR 3).
2. Technique: sedation.

Pangguangshu (BL 28) and *Zhongji* (CV 3) regulate Urinary Bladder qi. When combined with *Yinlingquan* (SP 9), these three points dispel dampness and promote diuresis. In addition, *Shuifen* (CV 9) regulates the water passages to promote urination. *Waiguan* (TH 5), which connects with the *yangwei* (linking) channel, relieves exterior pathogenic factors, and regulates water in all three *jiaos*. *Yanglingquan* (GB 34) and *Taichong* (LR 3) sedate Liver heat and relieve jaundice.

AUTHORS' COMMENTS

Yin Chen Hao Tang (Artemisia Scoparia Decoction) and *Yin Chen Wu Ling San* both treat damp-heat jaundice.

- *Yin Chen Hao Tang* is the most effective formula to clear heat. It contains *Zhi Zi* (Fructus Gardeniae), which clears heat in all three *jiaos*. This formula is generally considered the first choice for damp-heat jaundice with more heat than dampness. This formula is for short-term use.
- *Yin Chen Wu Ling San* is more appropriate for jaundice characterized by more dampness than heat. It has excellent ability to drain dampness but lacks heat-clearing herbs. In addition to jaundice, the presence of dysuria is a prominent indicator for the use of this formula. This formula is usually administered for a longer period of time than *Yin Chen Hao Tang* in order to achieve a therapeutic effect, as damp conditions are generally more difficult to resolve. It is also more suitable for long-term use since it does not contains *Da Huang* (Radix et Rhizoma Rhei).

References

1. *Guo Wai Yi Xue Zhong Yi Zhong Yao Fen Ce* (Monograph of Chinese Herbology from Foreign Medicine), 1983; 6:24.
2. *Guo Wai Yi Xue Zhong Yi Zhong Yao Fen Ce* (Monograph of Chinese Herbology from Foreign Medicine), 1986; 8(1):22.
3. *Bei Jing Zhong Yi* (Beijing Chinese Medicine), 1987; 5:33.
4. *Zhong Guo Zhong Xi Yi Jie He Za Zhi* (Chinese Journal of Integrative Chinese and Western Medicine), 1996; 8:470.
5. *Hu Bei Zhong Yi Za Zhi* (Hubei Journal of Chinese Medicine), 1986; 3:50.
6. *Shang Hai Zhong Yi Yao Za Zhi* (Shanghai Journal of Chinese Medicine and Herbology), 1984; 8:20.

Sān Rén Tāng (Three-Nut Decoction)

三仁湯
三仁汤

Pinyin Name: *San Ren Tang*
Literal Name: Three-Nut Decoction
Alternate Name: Triple Nut Combination
Original Source: *Wen Bing Tiao Bian* (Systematic Differentiation of Warm Diseases) by Wu Ju-Tong in 1798

COMPOSITION

Ku Xing Ren (Semen Armeniacae Amarum)	15g [12g]
Dou Kou (Fructus Amomi Rotundus)	6g
Yi Yi Ren (Semen Coicis)	18g
Hua Shi (Talcum), *shui fei* (refined with water)	18g
Tong Cao (Medulla Tetrapanacis)	6g
Zhu Ye (Herba Phyllostachys)	6g
Ban Xia (Rhizoma Pinelliae)	15g [10g]
Hou Po (Cortex Magnoliae Officinalis)	6g

DOSAGE / PREPARATION / ADMINISTRATION

The source text instructs to cook the ingredients with 8 bowls of fresh spring water until it is reduced to 3 bowls. Take 1 bowl three times daily. Today, this formula may be prepared as a decoction with the doses suggested in brackets.

CHINESE THERAPEUTIC ACTIONS

1. Ventilates and smoothes the qi
2. Clears damp-heat

CLINICAL MANIFESTATIONS

Early stage of damp-warmth affecting the *qi* (energy) level: aversion to cold, painful body, absence of hunger and thirst, a pink to pale tongue, and a thin, wiry pulse or slippery pulse.

VETERINARY CLINICAL APPLICATIONS

Pneumonia, fever of unknown origin, urinary tract infection, gastroenteritis, damp-heat dermatitis and chronic otitis.

EXPLANATION

San Ren Tang (Three-Nut Decoction) treats early stage damp-warmth (more dampness than heat) affecting the *qi* (energy) level. This condition usually occurs in late summer when there is an abundance of damp-warmth in the environment, and in animals with pre-existing Spleen deficiency. Damp-warmth in the environment may affect the exterior of the body, causing headache and aversion to cold. Spleen deficiency may lead to damp production and subsequent formation of heat. The dampness and heat can obstruct qi flow in the muscles, causing generalized body

***San Ren Tang* (Three-Nut Decoction)**

Diagnosis	Clinical Signs	Treatment	Herbs
Early stage of damp-warmth affecting the *qi* (energy) level	• Generalized pain of the body: accumulation of dampness in the flesh and muscles obstructing qi circulation • Thin, wiry pulse or slippery pulse: Spleen deficiency with damp accumulation • Pale tongue: qi deficiency	• Ventilates and smoothes qi • Clears damp-heat	• *Ku Xing Ren* (Semen Armeniacae Amarum) ventilates and regulates Lung qi and relieves chest oppression. • *Dou Kou* (Fructus Amomi Rotundus) dries dampness and activates the qi flow. • *Yi Yi Ren* (Semen Coicis) drains dampness through urination and strengthens the Spleen. • *Hua Shi* (Talcum), *Tong Cao* (Medulla Tetrapanacis) and *Zhu Ye* (Herba Phyllostachys) clear heat, drain dampness, and clear heat via urination. • *Ban Xia* (Rhizoma Pinelliae) and *Hou Po* (Cortex Magnoliae Officinalis) activate qi circulation, drain dampness, and relieve distention.

Sān Rén Tāng (Three-Nut Decoction)

pain. A pale tongue is commonly seen in qi-deficient animals. A wiry, thin pulse may be present in patients suffering from pain and qi deficiency, while a slippery pulse may be present with severe damp accumulation.

This formula contains the acrid herb *Ku Xing Ren* (Semen Armeniacae Amarum) to regulate Lung qi and allow it to descend. The Lung is one of the organs that regulate water metabolism; restoring the normal flow of Lung qi helps resolve dampness in the entire body. *Dou Kou* (Fructus Amomi Rotundus) is an aromatic herb that dries dampness, awakens the Spleen, and activates qi flow. *Yi Yi Ren* (Semen Coicis) drains dampness through urination and strengthens the Spleen. *Hua Shi* (Talcum), *Tong Cao* (Medulla Tetrapanacis), and *Zhu Ye* (Herba Phyllostachys) clear heat, drain dampness, and clear heat via urination, respectively. *Ban Xia* (Rhizoma Pinelliae) and *Hou Po* (Cortex Magnoliae Officinalis) activate qi circulation, dispel dampness, and relieve distention.

VETERINARY MODIFICATIONS

- For the initial stages of *wen bing* (warm diseases) with dampness affecting the *wei* (defensive) level, add *Huo Xiang* (Herba Agastaches) and *Xiang Ru* (Herba Moslae).
- With heat, add *Huang Lian* (Rhizoma Coptidis) and *Huang Qin* (Radix Scutellariae).
- With severe damp and heat, combine with *Gan Lu Xiao Du Dan* (Sweet Dew Special Pill to Eliminate Toxins).
- With epigastric and abdominal bloating, add *Lai Fu Zi* (Semen Raphani) and *Shen Qu* (Massa Fermentata).

CAUTIONS / CONTRAINDICATIONS

San Ren Tang treats conditions characterized by more dampness than heat. It is not suitable in cases characterized by more heat than dampness, or with the presence of dryness and heat.

HUMAN CLINICAL STUDIES AND RESEARCH

1. **Pneumonia**: Forty patients with pneumonia were treated with *San Ren Tang* with complete recovery in 36 cases and improvement in 4 cases. The average duration of treatment was 4.8 days. The treatment used *San Ren Tang* as the base formula with the addition of *Da Qing Ye* (Folium Isatidis) for heat, *Sang Bai Pi* (Cortex Mori) for excessive perspiration, *Tai Zi Shen* (Radix Pseudostellariae) for weakness and deficiency, *Sha Shen* (Radix Glehniae seu Adenophorae) for damaged body fluids, and *Gua Lou Zi* (Semen Trichosanthis) for constipation.[1]
2. **Hepatitis**: Use of modified *San Ren Tang* was associated with beneficially treating acute icteric hepatitis characterized by damp-heat affecting all three *jiaos*. The herbal treatment contained the following ingredients: *Yin Chen* (Herba Artemisiae Scopariae) 30g, *Tu Yin Chen* (Herba Origani), *Ku Xing Ren* (Semen Armeniacae Amarum) 5g, *Dou Kou* (Fructus Amomi Rotundus) 5g, *Yi Yi Ren* (Semen Coicis) 12g, *Hou Po* (Cortex Magnoliae Officinalis) 9g, *Dan Zhu Ye* (Herba Lophatheri) 6g, *Ban Xia* (Rhizoma Pinelliae) 9g, *Tong Cao* (Medulla Tetrapanacis) 5g, *Hua Shi* (Talcum) 18g, and *Zhi Zi* (Fructus Gardeniae) 12g. The herbs were administered in decoction form daily for 12 days.[2]
3. **Cholecystitis**: *San Ren Tang* was used to treat 38 patients with cholecystitis with complete recovery in 15 cases and improvement in 23 cases. The herbal formula used *San Ren Tang* as the base formula. *Chai Hu* (Radix Bupleuri) and *Huang Qin* (Radix Scutellariae) were added for aversion to cold and bitter taste in the mouth; *Yan Hu Suo* (Rhizoma Corydalis) and *Yu Jin* (Radix Curcumae) were added for hypochondriac pain; *Huo Xiang* (Herba Agastaches) and *Pei Lan* (Herba Eupatorii) were added for nausea, vomiting and abdominal distention; *Yin Chen* (Herba Artemisiae Scopariae) for jaundice; *Shan Zha* (Fructus Crataegi), *Mai Ya* (Fructus Hordei Germinatus), and *Shen Qu* (Massa Fermentata) were added for aversion to greasy, oily foods; and *Zhi Shi* (Fructus Aurantii Immaturus) was added for constipation.[3]
4. **Glomerulonephritis**: One hundred and twenty patients with glomerulonephritis (78 males and 42 females; between 6-45 years of age) were treated with complete recovery in 103 cases, significant improvement in 11 cases, and no effect in 6 cases. The herbal formula contained *Ku Xing Ren* (Semen Armeniacae Amarum) 15g, *Dou Kou* (Fructus Amomi Rotundus) 15g, *Yi Yi Ren* (Semen Coicis) 20g, *Hou Po* (Cortex Magnoliae Officinalis) 15g, *Ban Xia* (Rhizoma Pinelliae) 15g, *Tong Cao* (Medulla Tetrapanacis) 10g, *Hua Shi* (Talcum) 15g, *Zhu Ye* (Herba Phyllostachys) 20g, *Shi Wei* (Folium Pyrrosiae) 30g, *Bai Mao Gen* (Rhizoma Imperatae) 30g, and others as needed. The duration of treatment ranged from 6-30 days, with an average of 12 days.[4]
5. **Gastroenteritis**: One study reported marked success using modified *San Ren Tang* to treat 300 patients with acute gastroenteritis. Clinical manifestations included edema, decreased urination, hematuria, proteinuria, elevated blood pressure, chest congestion with shortness of breath, cough with a small amount of foamy sputum, epigastric fullness, poor appetite, and nausea. The herbal formula contained *Ku Xing Ren* (Semen Armeniacae Amarum) 10g, *Dou Kou* (Fructus Amomi Rotundus) 10g, *Yi Yi Ren* (Semen Coicis) 30g, *Hua Shi* (Talcum) 15g, *Zhu Ye* (Herba Phyllostachys) 10g, *Hou Po* (Cortex Magnoliae Officinalis) 15g, *Tong Cao* (Medulla Tetrapanacis) 15g, *Ban Xia* (Rhizoma Pinelliae) 10g, charred *Shan Zha* (Fructus Crataegi) 15g, and *Gan Cao* (Radix et Rhizoma

Sān Rén Tāng (Three-Nut Decoction)

Glycyrrhizae) 5g. Additional modifications were made as needed. The herbs were cooked in water, and administered via decoction daily. The duration of treatment ranged from 2 to 8 packs of herbs. The study reported complete recovery or improvement in all 300 patients.[5]

SUGGESTED ACUPUNCTURE TREATMENT

1. Points: *Kongzui* (LU 6), *Hegu* (LI 4), *Zhongwan* (CV 12), *Housanli* (ST 36), *Neiguan* (PC 6), *Sanyinjiao* (SP 6), *Yinlingquan* (SP 9), and *Zhigou* (TH 6).
2. Technique: sedation.

Kongzui (LU 6) and *Hegu* (LI 4) ventilate the Lung, relieve exterior symptoms, clear heat, and dispel dampness. *Zhongwan* (CV 12), *Housanli* (ST 36), and *Neiguan* (PC 6) harmonize the middle *jiao*, strengthen the Stomach, regulate qi, and dispel dampness. *Sanyinjiao* (SP 6) and *Yinlingquan* (SP 9) will dispel dampness and also help to strengthen the Spleen, which is often deficient in these patients. *Zhigou* (TH 6) harmonizes all three *jiaos*, clears heat, and dispels dampness. Altogether, these points treat summer febrile syndrome by clearing heat and dispelling dampness.

AUTHORS' COMMENTS

San Ren Tang, literally "Three-Nut Decoction," is so named because this formula contains three *ren* (seeds, nuts or fruits): *Ku Xing Ren* (Semen Armeniacae Amarum), *Yi Yi Ren* (Semen Coicis), and *Dou Kou* (Fructus Amomi Rotundus), which is also known as *Bai Dou Ren*.

This formula is used to address the problem of chronic dampness in veterinary medicine. If significant heat signs are present, additional herbs or formulas that clear heat must be used to address this complaint. It can be used to help consolidate the treatment of damp-heat conditions, after the major clinical signs have resolved, by dispelling the remaining dampness from the body.

References

1. *Hu Nan Zhong Yi Za Zhi* (Hunan Journal of Chinese Medicine), 1998; 3:50.
2. *Zhong Yi Za Zhi* (Journal of Chinese Medicine), 1982; 7:46.
3. *Si Chuan Zhong Yi* (Sichuan Chinese Medicine), 1988; 9:27.
4. *Zhong Yi Fang Ji Xian Dai Yan Jiu* (Modern Study of Medical Formulas in Traditional Chinese Medicine), 1997; 1355.
5. *Shi Yong Zhong Yi Nei Ke Za Zhi* (Journal of Practical Chinese Internal Medicine), 1995; 1:12.

Gān Lù Xiāo Dú Dān (Sweet Dew Special Pill to Eliminate Toxin)

甘露消毒丹

Pinyin Name: *Gan Lu Xiao Du Dan*
Literal Name: Sweet Dew Special Pill to Eliminate Toxin
Alternate Names: *Kan Lu Hsiao Tu Tan, Pu Ji Xiao Du Dan*, Talc and Scute Formula, Sweet Dew Detoxication Pellet, Universal Benefit Special Pill to Eliminate Toxin, Forsythia and Acorus Formula
Original Source: *Xu Ming Yi Lei An* (Continuation of Famous Physicians' Cases Organized by Categories) by Wei Zhi-Xiu in 1770

COMPOSITION

Hua Shi (Talcum), *shui fei* (refined with water)	450g [15g]
Yin Chen (Herba Artemisiae Scopariae)	330g [11g]
Huang Qin (Radix Scutellariae)	300g [10g]
Shi Chang Pu (Rhizoma Acori Tatarinowii)	180g [6g]
Dou Kou (Fructus Amomi Rotundus)	120g [4g]
Huo Xiang (Herba Agastaches)	120g [4g]
She Gan (Rhizoma Belamcandae)	120g [4g]
Bo He (Herba Menthae)	120g [4g]
Chuan Bei Mu (Bulbus Fritillariae Cirrhosae)	150g [5g]
Mu Tong (Caulis Akebiae)	150g [5g]
Lian Qiao (Fructus Forsythiae)	120g [4g]

DOSAGE / PREPARATION / ADMINISTRATION

The source text instructs to sun-dry the ingredients and grind them into a fine powder. Take 9g of the powder per dose with boiled water. This formula is also given in pill form and is prepared by mixing the powdered herbs with *Shen Qu* (Massa Fermentata) to form pills. Take 1 pill [9g] per dose with boiled water. Today, this formula may be prepared as a decoction with the doses suggested in brackets.

CHINESE THERAPEUTIC ACTIONS

1. Resolves dampness and dissolves turbidity
2. Clears heat and eliminates toxins

CLINICAL MANIFESTATIONS

Damp-warmth febrile disorders or epidemic diseases (infectious diseases) affecting the *qi* (energy) level: fever, lethargy, pain of the extremities, swelling of the lower cheeks, yellow discoloration of the skin, vomiting, diarrhea, thirst, scanty, dark, turbid urine, a red tongue, and a rapid, wiry pulse or a slippery pulse.

VETERINARY CLINICAL APPLICATIONS

Pneumonia, hepatitis, jaundice, pyelonephritis, fever of unknown origin, encephalitis, stomatitis, mandibular lymphadenopathy, laryngopharyngitis, acute gastroenteritis, and leptospirosis.

EXPLANATION

Gan Lu Xiao Du Dan (Sweet Dew Special Pill to Eliminate Toxins) treats febrile disorder or epidemic diseases affecting the *qi* (energy) level. Warmth and dampness (equal amounts of each) may each intensify the severity of the other, causing fever, lethargy, and pain of the extremities. Damp-warmth can cause qi stagnation, leading to vomiting or diarrhea. Furthermore, damp-warmth may rise upward and cause sore throat and mandibular lymphadenopathy. It may also travel downward to produce scanty, dark, turbid urine; it may travel outward to the skin to cause jaundice. In severe cases, a pale and white tongue coating may be present if the animal is weak and the qi is severely deficient; a thick and greasy tongue coating may be present if the animal has severe damp accumulation; and a dry and yellow tongue coating indicates excess heat.

This formula contains *Hua Shi* (Talcum) to clear damp-heat, *Yin Chen* (Herba Artemisiae Scopariae) to dispel damp-heat and drain the yellow discoloration of the skin, and *Huang Qin* (Radix Scutellariae) to dry dampness and eliminate heat-toxins. *Shi Chang Pu* (Rhizoma Acori Tatarinowii), *Dou Kou* (Fructus Amomi Rotundus), and *Huo Xiang* (Herba Agastaches) are acrid and aromatic herbs that resolve dampness and turbidity and activate qi circulation. *She Gan* (Rhizoma Belamcandae), *Bo He* (Herba Menthae) and *Chuan Bei Mu* (Bulbus Fritillariae Cirrhosae) cause the Lung qi to descend and relieve sore throat. *Mu Tong* (Caulis Akebiae) helps *Hua Shi* (Talcum)

Gān Lù Xiāo Dú Dān (Sweet Dew Special Pill to Eliminate Toxin)

Gan Lu Xiao Du Dan (Sweet Dew Special Pill to Eliminate Toxin)

Diagnosis	Clinical Signs	Treatment	Herbs
Damp-warmth febrile disorders or epidemic diseases affecting the *qi* (energy) level	• Fever, lethargy, and pain of the extremities: presence of damp-warmth • Vomiting or diarrhea: qi stagnation due to damp-warmth accumulation • Sore throat and swelling of the lymph nodes: damp-warmth traveling upward • Scanty, dark, turbid urine: damp-warmth traveling downward • Jaundice: damp-warmth traveling outward	• Resolves dampness and turbidity • Clears heat and eliminates toxins	• *Hua Shi* (Talcum), *Yin Chen* (Herba Artemisiae Scopariae), and *Huang Qin* (Radix Scutellariae) clear heat, dry dampness, and eliminate toxins. • *Shi Chang Pu* (Rhizoma Acori Tatarinowii), *Dou Kou* (Fructus Amomi Rotundus), and *Huo Xiang* (Herba Agastaches) resolve dampness and turbidity and activate qi circulation. • *She Gan* (Rhizoma Belamcandae), *Bo He* (Herba Menthae) and *Chuan Bei Mu* (Bulbus Fritillariae Cirrhosae) cause the Lung qi to descend and relieve soreness and swelling. • *Mu Tong* (Caulis Akebiae) clears damp-heat through diuresis. • *Lian Qiao* (Fructus Forsythiae) clears heat and eliminates toxins.

and *Yin Chen* (Herba Artemisiae Scopariae) clear damp-heat through diuresis; and *Lian Qiao* (Fructus Forsythiae) helps *Huang Qin* (Radix Scutellariae) clear heat and eliminate toxins.

VETERINARY MODIFICATIONS

- With prominent signs of jaundice, add *Zhi Zi* (Fructus Gardeniae) and *Da Huang* (Radix et Rhizoma Rhei).
- With severe lymph node enlargement, add *Shan Dou Gen* (Radix et Rhizoma Sophorae Tonkinensis) and *Ban Lan Gen* (Radix Isatidis).
- With fever, add *Ku Shen* (Radix Sophorae Flavescentis) and *Huang Lian* (Rhizoma Coptidis).
- For cholecystitis, add *Jin Qian Cao* (Herba Lysimachiae).
- For pyelonephritis, add *Qu Mai* (Herba Dianthi), *Bian Xu* (Herba Polygoni Avicularis), *Bai Mao Gen* (Rhizoma Imperatae), *Da Ji* (Herba Cirsii Japonici), *Xiao Ji* (Herba Cirsii), and *Shi Wei* (Folium Pyrrosiae).
- For leptospirosis, add *Zhi Zi* (Fructus Gardeniae), *Huang Lian* (Rhizoma Coptidis), *Jin Yin Hua* (Flos Lonicerae Japonicae), *Long Dan* (Radix et Rhizoma Gentianae) and *Ban Lan Gen* (Radix Isatidis).

CAUTIONS / CONTRAINDICATIONS

- *Gan Lu Xiao Du Dan* should be used with caution in cases of damp-heat with underlying yin and body fluid deficiencies.[1]
- Avoid eating foods that are raw, cold, oily, or greasy while taking this formula.[2]

PHARMACOLOGICAL EFFECTS

1. **Antipyretic**: Administration of *Gan Lu Xiao Du Dan* via oral ingestion in rats was associated with reduced body temperature in both normal subjects and those with artificially-induced fever. The duration of action was approximately 2 hours.[3]
2. **Hepatoprotective**: Use of *Gan Lu Xiao Du Dan* had protective effects against liver damage induced by carbon tetrachloride. The formula was administered as an oral decoction for a total of 12 days.[4]

HUMAN CLINICAL STUDIES AND RESEARCH

1. **Laryngopharyngitis**: One study reported marked success using *Gan Lu Xiao Du Dan* to treat both acute and chronic laryngopharyngitis. Of 58 patients, the study reported complete recovery in 30 cases and significant improvement in 28 cases.[5]
2. **Stomatitis**: One study reported complete recovery from recurrent stomatitis using *Gan Lu Xiao Du Dan* to treat ulcers, and upon healing, using *Yu Ping Feng San* (Jade Windscreen Powder) to prevent recurrence.[6]
3. **Hepatitis**: According to one study, 26 infants with acute infectious hepatitis were treated with modified *Gan Lu Xiao Du Dan* with marked effects. The treatment protocol was to administer the herbs in decoction, with duration of treatment up to 5 weeks. Clinical improvement included relief of jaundice, decrease of liver enzyme levels, reduction of hepatomegaly, and improved appetite.[7] Another study reported marked success treating 182 cases of acute icteric jaundice in children using *Gan Lu Xiao Du Dan* plus *Chai Hu* (Radix Bupleuri), *Fo Shou* (Fructus Citri Sarcodactylis), and *Yu Jin* (Radix Curcumae).[8]

Gān Lù Xiāo Dú Dān (Sweet Dew Special Pill to Eliminate Toxin)

4. **Fever**: One study reported 94.8% effectiveness using modified *Gan Lu Xiao Du Dan* to treat 78 patients with fever due to infectious disorders. Clinical manifestations included chills, fever, resolution of chills but not fever after perspiration, headache, feeling of heaviness in the head, fatigue, and loose stools. In addition to *Gan Lu Xiao Du Dan*, modifications included addition of *Yi Yi Ren* (Semen Coicis) and *Ban Xia* (Rhizoma Pinelliae) for excess dampness; and *Shi Gao* (Gypsum Fibrosum) for high fever. Of 78 patients, the study reported significant improvement in 31 cases, improvement in 43 cases, and no effect in 4 cases.[9]
5. **Encephalitis**: One study reported complete recovery from encephalitis in 13 of 16 patients using modified *Gan Lu Xiao Du Dan*. Modifications were made based on the individual condition of the patients. For early stage of encephalitis with fever, gradual onset of symptoms, presence of dampness, and greasy tongue coating, *She Gan* (Rhizoma Belamcandae) and *Lian Qiao* (Fructus Forsythiae) were removed, and *Dan Dou Chi* (Semen Sojae Praeparatum) and *Ku Xing Ren* (Semen Armeniacae Amarum) were added to the herbal formula. For middle stage of encephalitis with the disease migrating to the interior, and dampness turning into heat, with symptoms such as a bitter taste in the mouth, restlessness, and a red tongue body with yellow tongue coating, *Bo He* (Herba Menthae), *She Gan* (Rhizoma Belamcandae) and *Bei Mu* (Bulbus Fritillariae) were removed, and *Huang Lian* (Rhizoma Coptidis), *Zhi Zi* (Fructus Gardeniae) and a larger dose of *Huang Qin* (Radix Scutellariae) were added. For late stage of encephalitis, with restlessness and muscle spasms, *She Gan* (Rhizoma Belamcandae), *Bo He* (Herba Menthae) and *Mu Tong* (Caulis Akebiae) were removed, and *Yu Jin* (Radix Curcumae) was added. Lastly, drugs such as dexamethasone were given if necessary.[10]

SUGGESTED ACUPUNCTURE TREATMENT

1. Points: *Dazhui* (GV 14), *Zhiyang* (GV 9), *Wangu* (SI 4), *Hegu* (LI 4), *Weiyang* (BL 39), *Tiantu* (CV 22), *Yuji* (LU 10), *Weijian* and *Erjian*.
2. Technique: sedation.

The objective of this acupuncture treatment is to clear heat, eliminate toxins, and dispel dampness. *Dazhui* (GV 14) and *Zhiyang* (GV 9) regulate qi within the *du* (governing) channel. *Wangu* (SI 4) and *Hegu* (LI 4) clear heat and eliminate toxins from the *taiyang* and *yangming* channels. *Weiyang* (BL 39) dispels dampness, regulates water, and promotes diuresis. *Tiantu* (CV 22), the intersecting point of the *yangwei* (linking) and *ren* (conception) channels, regulates Lung qi, and relieves sore throat. Lastly, *Yuji* (LU 10), as the *ying* (spring) point of the Lung channel, clears Lung heat and relieves sore throat. *Weijian* and *Erjian* are classical points that clear heat.

AUTHORS' COMMENTS

Gan Lu Xiao Du Dan treats warmth and dampness (equal amounts of each) with the presence of heat-toxins. *Gan Lu Xiao Du Dan* was developed to treat seasonal epidemic disorders which occur during the late autumn or summer months. The invasion of the body by epidemic pathogenic factors corresponds to the contraction of infectious diseases in Western medicine. The modern application of this formula includes any disorder with clinical signs affecting the *qi* (energy) level. Epidemiologic studies of leptospirosis show that clinical cases of the disease are diagnosed most often in the early fall and summer months. *Gan Lu Xiao Du Dan* is appropriate to treat the peracute and subacute stages of the disease within the first one to three weeks of the disease. Following treatment of the initial infection, another formula must be chosen to prevent subsequent development of chronic hepatitis or chronic nephritis. Similarly, this formula can be used in the early stages of epidemic equine diseases, particularly those that are associated with signs of both heat and dampness, such as rhinopneumonitis, *Streptococcus equi*, and equine viral arteritis. For the treatment of feline infectious diseases, add *Bai Hua She She Cao* (Herba Hedyotis) and *Da Qing Ye* (Folium Isatidis).

References

1. *Zhong Yao Ming Fang Yao Li Yu Ying Yong* (Pharmacology and Applications of Famous Herbal Formulas), 1989; 425-426.
2. *Zhong Yao Ming Fang Yao Li Yu Ying Yong* (Pharmacology and Applications of Famous Herbal Formulas), 1989; 425-426.
3. *Zhong Guo Zhong Yao Za Zhi* (People's Republic of China Journal of Chinese Herbology), 1989; 14(5):50.
4. *Zhong Guo Zhong Yao Za Zhi* (People's Republic of China Journal of Chinese Herbology), 1993; 18(10):625.
5. *Xin Zhong Yi* (New Chinese Medicine), 1997; 7:57.
6. *Zhong Cheng Yao* (Study of Chinese Patent Medicine), 1991; 5:46.
7. *Zhe Jiang Zhong Yi Za Zhi* (Zhejiang Journal of Chinese Medicine), 1980; 10:462.
8. *Si Chuan Zhong Yi* (Sichuan Chinese Medicine), 1986; 3:31.
9. *Gan Su Zhong Yi* (Gansu Chinese Medicine), 1995; 8(4):21.
10. *Jiang Su Zhong Yi* (Jiangsu Chinese Medicine), 1997; 7:12.

Bā Zhèng Sǎn (Eight-Herb Powder for Rectification)

八正散

Pinyin Name: *Ba Zheng San*
Literal Name: Eight-Herb Powder for Rectification
Alternate Names: *Pa Cheng San*, Dianthus Formula, Eight Corrections Powder
Original Source: *Tai Ping Hui Min He Ji Ju Fang* (Imperial Grace Formulary of the Tai Ping Era) by the Imperial Medical Department in 1078-85

COMPOSITION

Mu Tong (Caulis Akebiae)	480g [9g]
Qu Mai (Herba Dianthi)	480g [9g]
Bian Xu (Herba Polygoni Avicularis)	480g [9g]
Hua Shi (Talcum)	480g [9g]
Che Qian Zi (Semen Plantaginis)	480g [9g]
Zhi Zi (Fructus Gardeniae)	480g [9g]
Da Huang (Radix et Rhizoma Rhei), *wei* (roasted), *qie* (sliced) and *bei* (stone-baked)	480g [9g]
Zhi Gan Cao (Radix et Rhizoma Glycyrrhizae Praeparata cum Melle)	480g [9g]

DOSAGE / PREPARATION / ADMINISTRATION

The source text advises to grind equal amounts of the ingredients into a fine powder. Cook 6g of the powder with *Deng Xin Cao* (Medulla Junci) in 1 bowl of water until the liquid is reduced to 70% volume. Take the warm, strained decoction after meals and before bedtime. For children, reduce the dose according to age and/or body weight. Today, it is ground into powder and taken 6-9g per dose. This formula may be prepared as a decoction with the doses suggested in brackets.

CHINESE THERAPEUTIC ACTIONS

1. Clears heat and sedates fire
2. Regulates water circulation and relieves *lin zheng* (dysuria syndrome)

CLINICAL MANIFESTATIONS

Downward flow of damp-heat to the lower *jiao*: *re lin* (heat dysuria) syndrome, *xue lin* (bloody dysuria) syndrome, hematuria, pollakiuria, strangury, crystalluria, incontinence, scanty drips of urine, lower abdominal pain, fever in severe cases, lethargy, poor appetite, a red tongue, and a slippery, rapid pulse.

VETERINARY CLINICAL APPLICATIONS

Urinary tract infection, urethritis, pyelonephritis, urolithiasis and prostatitis.

EXPLANATION

Ba Zheng San (Eight-Herb Powder for Rectification) treats the downward flow of damp-heat to the lower *jiao*. Stagnant damp-heat in the Urinary Bladder causes various urinary disorders, such as *re lin* (heat dysuria), *xue lin*

***Ba Zheng San* (Eight-Herb Powder for Rectification)**

Diagnosis	Clinical Signs	Treatment	Herbs
Downward flow of damp-heat to the lower *jiao*	• Dysuria, hematuria, pollakiuria, strangury, crystalluria, incontinence, scanty drips of urine, pain: damp-heat in the Urinary Bladder • Fever, poor appetite, lethargy, a red tongue and a slippery, rapid pulse: damp-heat in the interior	• Clears heat and sedates fire • Regulates water circulation and relieves *lin zheng* (dysuria syndrome)	• *Mu Tong* (Caulis Akebiae), *Qu Mai* (Herba Dianthi), *Bian Xu* (Herba Polygoni Avicularis), *Hua Shi* (Talcum), and *Che Qian Zi* (Semen Plantaginis) induce urination, relieve dysuria, and clear damp-heat. • *Zhi Zi* (Fructus Gardeniae) sedates damp-heat in all three *jiaos*. • *Da Huang* (Radix et Rhizoma Rhei) purges heat and sedates fire. • *Deng Xin Cao* (Medulla Junci) leads the heat down and out through urination. • *Zhi Gan Cao* (Radix et Rhizoma Glycyrrhizae Praeparata cum Melle) harmonizes the herbs and relieves pain.

Bā Zhèng Săn (Eight-Herb Powder for Rectification)

(bloody dysuria), and many others as listed above. The tongue and pulse parameters indicate damp-heat in the body.

In this formula, *Mu Tong* (Caulis Akebiae), *Qu Mai* (Herba Dianthi), *Bian Xu* (Herba Polygoni Avicularis), *Hua Shi* (Talcum), and *Che Qian Zi* (Semen Plantaginis) induce urination, relieve dysuria, and clear damp-heat. *Zhi Zi* (Fructus Gardeniae) sedates damp-heat in all three *jiaos*. *Da Huang* (Radix et Rhizoma Rhei) purges heat and sedates fire. *Deng Xin Cao* (Medulla Junci) leads the heat down and out through urination. *Zhi Gan Cao* (Radix et Rhizoma Glycyrrhizae Praeparata cum Melle) harmonizes the herbs and relieves pain.

VETERINARY MODIFICATIONS

- For *xue lin* (bloody dysuria), add *Xiao Ji* (Herba Cirsii) and *Bai Mao Gen* (Rhizoma Imperatae).
- For *shi lin* (stone dysuria), add *Jin Qian Cao* (Herba Lysimachiae) and *Hai Jin Sha* (Spora Lygodii).
- For *shi-re lin* (damp-heat dysuria) with severe burning sensations and dark yellow urine, add *Huang Bo* (Cortex Phellodendri Chinensis), *Jin Yin Hua* (Flos Lonicerae Japonicae), *Pu Gong Ying* (Herba Taraxaci), *Bai Hua She She Cao* (Herba Hedyotis), and *Zi Hua Di Ding* (Herba Violae).
- With more painful urination and distention of the lower abdomen, add *Yan Hu Suo* (Rhizoma Corydalis), *Huang Lian* (Rhizoma Coptidis) and *Di Huang* (Radix Rehmanniae), *Wu Yao* (Radix Linderae) and *Chuan Lian Zi* (Fructus Toosendan).
- With edema, add *Wu Ling San* (Five-Ingredient Powder with Poria).

CAUTIONS / CONTRAINDICATIONS

- *Ba Zheng San* contains many strong herbs that are bitter and cold. It is not suitable for patients with weakness or generalized deficiencies since these herbs can easily damage the Spleen and yin causing a decline in the overall constitution of the patient. This formula should be discontinued when the desired effects are achieved. Long-term use of this formula is contraindicated.
- Patients with a sensitive gastrointestinal tract may wish to take *Ba Zheng San* without *Da Huang* (Radix et Rhizoma Rhei) since *Da Huang* may cause loose stools and discomfort.
- *Ba Zheng San* is designed for *re lin* (heat dysuria) and *xue lin* (bloody dysuria). This formula should be modified accordingly (see above modifications) prior to its use for other types of *lin zheng* (dysuria syndrome). It is contraindicated in *gao lin* (cloudy dysuria), *qi lin* (qi dysuria), and *lao lin* (fatigue dysuria) unless modified accordingly.
- This formula is contraindicated during pregnancy.

PHARMACOLOGICAL EFFECTS

Antibacterial: *Ba Zheng San* has been shown in *in vitro* studies to have an inhibitory effect against *E. coli*, *Bacillus proteus*, *Bacillus paratyphosus*, *Bacillus dysenteriae*, *Staphylococcus aureus,* and others.[1]

HUMAN CLINICAL STUDIES AND RESEARCH

1. ***Lin zheng* (dysuria syndrome)**: Modified *Ba Zheng San* was used successfully to treat *lin zheng* (dysuria syndrome) infections transmitted via sexual intercourse. The herbal treatment included *Tu Fu Ling* (Rhizoma Smilacis Glabrae) 30g, *Hua Shi* (Talcum) 30g, *Fen Bi Xie* (Rhizoma Dioscoreae Hypoglaucae) 20g, *Cang Zhu* (Rhizoma Atractylodis) 15g, *Huang Bo* (Cortex Phellodendri Chinensis) 15g, *Che Qian Zi* (Semen Plantaginis) 15g, *Mu Tong* (Caulis Akebiae) 10g, *Bian Xu* (Herba Polygoni Avicularis) 10g, *Zhi Zi* (Fructus Gardeniae) 10g, *Da Huang* (Radix et Rhizoma Rhei) 10g, and *Gan Cao* (Radix et Rhizoma Glycyrrhizae) 3g. Additional modifications were made as needed. The treatment protocol was to administer the decoction in three equally-divided doses, for 3 days per course of treatment. Out of 32 patients, the study reported complete recovery in 18 cases, marked improvement in 13 cases, and no effect in 1 case.[2]
2. **Urethritis**: Administration of *Ba Zheng San* has been associated with marked effect in numerous studies. In one study, use of modified *Ba Zheng San* in 36 patients showed complete recovery in 20 cases, marked effect in 15 cases, and no effect in 1 case.[3] In another study, oral administration of modified *Ba Zheng San* in 48 patients resulted in complete recovery in 26 cases, marked improvement in 21 cases, and no effect in one case.[4]
3. **Urinary tract infection**: Ninety-seven patients with urinary tract infection were treated with good results using *Ba Zheng San*. Clinical presentations included frequent urination, urinary urgency, dysuria, low back pain, and fever. The study reported 96.91% success, with complete recovery in 76 cases, moderate improvement in 18 cases, and no effect in 3 cases. [5]
4. **Pyelonephritis**: Administration of modified *Ba Zheng San* was associated with a 88.5% success in female patients with pyelonephritis. Out of 67 cases, the study reported complete recovery in 54 cases, improvement in 5 cases, and no effect in 8 cases.[6]
5. **Nephritis**: Administration of *Ba Zheng San* was shown to have therapeutic results when used to treat acute nephritis. Out of 11 cases, there was complete recovery in 4 cases, marked improvement in 5 cases, and slight improvement in 2 cases. Immediate improvements included alleviation of edema and proteinuria. Kidney function was restored to normal in most cases.[7]

Bā Zhèng Săn (Eight-Herb Powder for Rectification)

6. **Urinary stones**: Administration of *Ba Zheng San* contributed to successful passage of urinary stones in 21 of 34 patients. The treatment protocol was to use a large dose of *Ba Zheng San* plus *Di Long* (Pheretima), *Ji Nei Jin* (Endothelium Corneum Gigeriae Galli), and *Hu Po* (Succinum). The patients were instructed to continue taking the herbs until the successful passage of stones. The duration of treatment varied from 3 to 108 days, with an average of 42.2 days.[8]
7. **Prostatic hypertrophy**: Administration of *Ba Zheng San* was associated with 89.3% effectiveness in treating geriatric men with prostatic hypertrophy. Out of 28 patients, the study showed recovery in 8 cases, marked effect in 12 cases, improvement in 5 cases, and no results in 3 cases.[9]

SUGGESTED ACUPUNCTURE TREATMENT

1. Points: *Pangguangshu* (BL 28), *Zhongji* (CV 3), *Dazhui* (GV 14), *Zutonggu* (BL 66), *Yinlingquan* (SP 9), *Xingjian* (LR 2), *Waiguan* (TH 5), *Hegu* (LI 4), and *Taixi* (KI 3).
2. Technique: sedation.

The objectives of treating damp-heat dysuria are to induce diuresis, dispel dampness, and clear heat. *Pangguangshu* (BL 28) and *Zhongji* (CV 3) regulate qi and dispel dampness from the Urinary Bladder. *Yinlingquan* (SP 9), the *he* (uniting) point of the Spleen channel, can induce diuresis when combined with *Pangguangshu* (BL 28) and *Zhongji* (CV 3). *Dazhui* (GV 14) and *Zutonggu* (BL 66) clear hear in the lower *jiao*. Because the Liver channel passes through the inguinal region, *Xingjian* (LR 2) is selected to clear heat. *Waiguan* (TH 5) and *Hegu* (LI 4) also help *Xingjian* (LR 2) clear heat. *Taixi* (KI 3), the *yuan* (source) point of the Kidney channel, can tonify the Kidney and regulate the water passages.

RELATED FORMULA

Sān Jín Pái Shí Tāng

(Three Gold Decoction to Expel Stone)

三金排石湯

三金排石汤

Pinyin Name: *San Jin Pai Shi Tang*

Literal Name: Three Gold Decoction to Expel Stone

Original Source: *An Hui Zhong Yi Xue Yuan* (Anhui University School of Medicine) in 1990

Hai Jin Sha (Spora Lygodii)	10-20g
Jin Qian Cao (Herba Lysimachiae)	20-30g
Ji Nei Jin (Endothelium Corneum Gigeriae Galli)	10-20g
Chuan Lian Zi (Fructus Toosendan)	5g
Yan Hu Suo (Rhizoma Corydalis)	5g
Wei Ling Xian (Radix et Rhizoma Clematidis)	20-30g
Zhi Qiao (Fructus Aurantii)	10-20g
Fu Ling (Poria)	15-20g
Zhu Ling (Polyporus)	15-20g
Ze Xie (Rhizoma Alismatis)	15-20g

San Jin Pai Shi Tang (Three Gold Decoction to Expel Stone) clears heat and promotes normal urination. It is most effective in treating *shi lin* (stone dysuria) with painful urination. This formula is very effective in the treatment of urinary stones in veterinary patients. To increase the therapeutic effect and for the treatment of difficult cases, the following modifications can be made:

- To increase ability to dissolve stones or crystals, add *Shi Wei* (Folium Pyrrosiae) and increase the dose of *Jin Qian Cao* (Herba Lysimachiae) and *Ji Nei Jin* (Endothelium Corneum Gigeriae Galli).
- To promote urination and relieve dysuria, add *Hua Shi* (Talcum) and *Che Qian Zi* (Semen Plantaginis).
- To clear heat, add *Zhi Zi* (Fructus Gardeniae), *Qu Mai* (Herba Dianthi), *Mu Tong* (Caulis Akebiae), *Tu Fu Ling* (Rhizoma Smilacis Glabrae), and *Pu Gong Ying* (Herba Taraxaci).
- For hematuria, add *Xiao Ji* (Herba Cirsii) and *Bai Mao Gen* (Rhizoma Imperatae).
- For blood stagnation and lower back pain, add *Wu Yao* (Radix Linderae) and *Chuan Lian Zi* (Fructus Toosendan).
- With pain, add *Yan Hu Suo* (Rhizoma Corydalis) and *Gan Cao* (Radix et Rhizoma Glycyrrhizae).
- With anxiety, pacing and vocalizing, add *Hu Po* (Succinum).

San Jin Pai Shi Tang is not available as a ready-made formula. It can be easily formulated in-house or prepared by any major herbal company. It may also be directly combined without modification with *Ba Zheng San* (Eight-Herb Powder for Rectification) for cystitis with bladder stones and pyelonephritis with renal stones.

AUTHORS' COMMENTS

Ba Zheng San is the most commonly used herbal formula for the treatment of damp-heat in the lower *jiao* (urinary tract infection) in veterinary medicine. It is cold and bitter in nature and is not recommended for longer than 7-10 days without re-evaluation or modification. Weak, geriatric and Spleen-deficient animals will not be able to take this formula without modification, as it can scatter the qi and cause further weakness. It is highly recommended to administer a Spleen tonic formula while using *Ba Zheng San* in conjunction with antibiotic therapy to prevent damage to the middle *jiao*. This formula has been successfully used with modification in dogs for the treatment

Bā Zhèng Săn (Eight-Herb Powder for Rectification)

of chronic, recurrent urinary tract infection in order to avoid administration of lifelong antimicrobial therapy. For acute pyelonephritis, it may be combined with *Long Dan Xie Gan Tang* (Gentiana Decoction to Drain the Liver), *Shui Ding Xiang* (Herba Ludwigiae Prostratae), and *Xian Feng Cao* (Herba Bidentis). A course of treatment should not exceed 7 days without re-examination. The addition of herbs to tonify the Spleen and protect the middle *jiao* is also advised while using these two formulas.

Ba Zheng San is not recommended in powder or granular form for oral administration in dogs and cats due to its strong taste. Many animals will refuse to take it on a regular basis if it is mixed into their food. The use of tea pills, tablets or capsules will meet with the highest compliance from animals. Horses and ruminants will readily eat both powdered and granular formulas mixed into feed.

Ba Zheng San, *Wu Lin San* (Five-Ingredient Powder for Painful Urinary Dysfunction) and *Zhu Ling Tang* (Polyporus Decoction) are all used to treat urinary tract infection (UTI) in dogs and cats. Though more common in ruminants, especially goats, these formulas are also very effective in treating cattle and horses with UTI, crystalluria, and urolithiasis.

- *Ba Zheng San*, largely composed of heat- and damp-clearing herbs, is more suitable for treating *re lin* (heat dysuria) syndrome. It is the formula of choice for UTI characterized by damp-heat and a positive bacterial urine culture.
- *Wu Lin San*, containing herbs that cool the blood to control hematuria, is more suitable for *xue lin* (bloody dysuria) syndrome. Its heat-clearing ability is not as strong as *Ba Zheng San*, but it is stronger than *Zhu Ling Tang*. *Wu Lin San* can be used to treat UTI with crystals and small stones present, and herbs to further clear heat are usually needed in severe cases with documented UTI. It can be combined with *Ba Zheng San* for cases with significant heat in addition to bloody urine.
- *Zhu Ling Tang* contains *E Jiao* (Colla Corii Asini) and is the most tonifying of the three formulas. It has good efficacy to drain dampness but weak ability to clear heat. Its yin- and blood-nourishing properties make it more appropriate for the treatment of chronic urinary tract infection, which typically involves a mixture of excess and deficiency. This is often the formula of choice to use concurrently with antibiotics in weak patients and older dogs and cats with UTI, as it is less cold than the other two formulas. Its ability to drain dampness complements antibiotic therapy to help clear infection and prevent recurrence. Antibiotics are very effective in clearing heat but not dampness; many cases of UTI become chronic because the heat is cleared, but the damp persists.

References

1. *Zhong Yi Yao Xin Xi* (Information on Chinese Medicine and Herbology), 1987; 6:31.
2. *Guang Xi Zhong Yi Yao* (Guangxi Chinese Medicine and Herbology), 1992; 4:9.
3. *An Hui Zhong Yi Xue Yuan Xue Bao* (Journal of Anhui University School of Medicine), 1994; 4:30.
4. *Guang Xi Zhong Yi Yao* (Guangxi Chinese Medicine and Herbology), 1992; 4:9.
5. *Shan Xi Zhong Yi* (Shanxi Chinese Medicine), 1998; 10:448.
6. *Liao Ning Zhong Yi Za Zhi* (Liaoning Journal of Chinese Medicine), 1986; 1:19.
7. *Ha Er Bing Zhong Yi* (Haerbing Chinese Medicine), 1960; 9:15.
8. *Ji Lin Zhong Yi Yao* (Jilin Chinese Medicine and Herbology), 1983; 5:19.
9. *Jiang Xi Zhong Yi Yao* (Jiangxi Chinese Medicine and Herbology), 1990; 2:15.

Wǔ Lín Sǎn (Five-Ingredient Powder for Painful Urinary Dysfunction)

五淋散

Pinyin Name: *Wu Lin San*
Literal Name: Five-Ingredient Powder for Painful Urinary Dysfunction
Alternate Names: Five-Strangury Formula, Gardenia and Hoelen Formula
Original Source: *Tai Ping Hui Min He Ji Ju Fang* (Imperial Grace Formulary of the Tai Ping Era) by the Imperial Medical Department in 1078-85

COMPOSITION

Chi Fu Ling (Poria Rubra)	180g [9g]
Dang Gui (Radix Angelicae Sinensis)	150g [7g]
Chi Shao (Radix Paeoniae Rubra)	600g [15g]
Zhi Zi (Fructus Gardeniae)	600g [15g]
Gan Cao (Radix et Rhizoma Glycyrrhizae)	150g [7g]

DOSAGE / PREPARATION / ADMINISTRATION

The source text instructs to grind the ingredients into a fine powder. Cook 6g of the powder with 1 bowl of water until the liquid is reduced to 80% volume. Take the decoction on an empty stomach before meals. Today, this formula may be prepared as a decoction with the doses suggested in brackets.

CHINESE THERAPEUTIC ACTIONS

1. Clears heat and cools the blood
2. Regulates water circulation and relieves *lin zheng* (dysuria syndrome)

CLINICAL MANIFESTATIONS

Heat in the Urinary Bladder: *xue lin* (bloody dysuria) with blood in the urine and severe pain upon urination, with crystals or small stones in the urine.

VETERINARY CLINICAL APPLICATIONS

Urinary tract infection, hematuria, feline lower urinary tract disease, and urolithiasis.

EXPLANATION

Wu Lin San (Five-Ingredient Powder for Painful Urinary Dysfunction) clears heat, cools the blood, and promotes normal urination. It treats *xue lin* (bloody dysuria) and *re lin* (heat dysuria) syndromes characterized by heat in the Urinary Bladder, with symptoms such as hematuria, dysuria, or cloudy urine.

In this formula, *Chi Fu Ling* (Poria Rubra) clears heat and promotes urination. *Dang Gui* (Radix Angelicae Sinensis) and *Chi Shao* (Radix Paeoniae Rubra) nourish the blood and moisten dryness. *Zhi Zi* (Fructus Gardeniae) clears heat and cools the blood. *Gan Cao* (Radix et Rhizoma Glycyrrhizae) relieves pain and harmonizes the formula.

VETERINARY MODIFICATIONS

- For *shi lin* (stone dysuria), add *Hai Jin Sha* (Spora Lygodii), *Jin Qian Cao* (Herba Lysimachiae), and *Shi Wei* (Folium Pyrrosiae).
- For *xue lin* (bloody dysuria), add *Xiao Ji* (Herba Cirsii), *Mo Han Lian* (Herba Ecliptae), and *Bai Mao Gen* (Rhizoma Imperatae).
- For *re lin* (heat dysuria), add *Huang Lian* (Rhizoma Coptidis).
- For *lin zheng* (dysuria syndrome) with qi deficiency in elderly patients, add *Ren Shen* (Radix et Rhizoma Ginseng), *Huang Qi* (Radix Astragali), and *Sheng Ma* (Rhizoma Cimicifugae).
- For *lin zheng* (dysuria syndrome) with blood stagnation, add *Tao Ren* (Semen Persicae), *Mu Dan Pi* (Cortex

***Wu Lin San* (Five-Ingredient Powder for Painful Urinary Dysfunction)**

Diagnosis	Clinical Signs	Treatment	Herbs
Heat in the Urinary Bladder	Hematuria, dysuria, and cloudy urine: heat in the Urinary Bladder	• Clears heat and cools the blood • Regulates water circulation and relieves *lin zheng* (dysuria syndrome)	• *Chi Fu Ling* (Poria Rubra) clears heat and promotes urination. • *Dang Gui* (Radix Angelicae Sinensis) and *Chi Shao* (Radix Paeoniae Rubra) nourish the blood and moisten dryness. • *Zhi Zi* (Fructus Gardeniae) clears heat and cools the blood. • *Gan Cao* (Radix et Rhizoma Glycyrrhizae) relieves pain and harmonizes all of the herbs.

Wŭ Lín Săn (Five-Ingredient Powder for Painful Urinary Dysfunction)

Moutan), *Yan Hu Suo* (Rhizoma Corydalis), and *Hu Po* (Succinum).

- With thirst due to heat and fire, add *Hua Shi* (Talcum) and *Shi Gao* (Gypsum Fibrosum).
- With jaundice, add *Yin Chen* (Herba Artemisiae Scopariae) and *Huang Qin* (Radix Scutellariae).

SUGGESTED ACUPUNCTURE TREATMENT

1. Points: *Pangguangshu* (BL 28), *Zhongji* (CV 3), *Yinlingquan* (SP 9), *Xingjian* (LR 2), *Waiguan* (TH 5), *Taixi* (KI 3), *Xuehai* (SP 10), *Geshu* (BL 17), *Weizhong* (BL 40), and *Duanxue*.
2. Technique: sedation.

The objectives of treating damp-heat dysuria are to induce diuresis, dispel dampness, and clear heat. *Pangguangshu* (BL 28) and *Zhongji* (CV 3) regulate qi and dispel dampness from the Urinary Bladder. *Yinlingquan* (SP 9), the *he* (uniting) point of the Spleen channel, induces diuresis when combined with *Pangguangshu* (BL 28) and *Zhongji* (CV 3). Because the Liver channel passes through the inguinal region, *Xingjian* (LR 2) is selected to clear heat. *Waiguan* (TH 5) helps *Xingjian* (LR 2) clear heat. *Taixi* (KI 3), the *yuan* (source) point of the Kidney channel, tonifies the Kidney and regulates the water passages. *Xuehai* (SP 10), *Geshu* (BL 17), and *Weizhong* (BL 40) enhances the treatment by cooling the blood and promoting diuresis. *Duanxue* is a classical equine point for stopping hemorrhage and can be helpful in cases where there is a great deal of blood in the urine.

AUTHORS' COMMENTS

Wu Lin San, *Ba Zheng San* (Eight-Herb Powder for Rectification), *Zhu Ling Tang* (Polyporus Decoction), *Dao Chi San* (Guide Out the Red Powder), and *Xiao Ji Yin Zi* (Cirsium Decoction) are all used in veterinary medicine to treat hematuria, with or without a documented urinary tract infection (UTI). Hematuria corresponds to *xue lin* (bloody dysuria) in Chinese medicine. The conditions for the use of each of these formulas are quite different, and close attention to the clinical history and tongue and pulse diagnosis is needed in order to choose the appropriate formula.

- *Wu Lin San* contains herbs that cool the blood in addition to clearing heat and is more suitable for *xue lin* (bloody dysuria) syndrome than *Ba Zheng San*. The hematuria seen in this case may be associated with crystals or small stones with obvious pain on urination. A documented UTI may not always be present. This formula works well for cats diagnosed with feline lower urinary tract disease with bloody urine, mucus and crystals without bacterial infection. This condition is promoted and exacerbated by feeding a dry, high starch, species inappropriate diet to cats, which are obligatory carnivores.
- *Ba Zheng San*, with its heat-clearing and damp-dispelling actions, is suitable for treating hematuria due to heat and dampness. The hematuria in this case is usually associated with a positive bacterial culture, a red tongue with a yellow coating, and a forceful, wiry to slippery pulse. This formula has the greatest ability to clear heat, which causes damage to the vessels of the bladder and leads to mild to moderate hematuria.
- *Zhu Ling Tang* nourishes yin and blood and is the most tonifying of the four formulas. It has minimal ability to stop bleeding, has limited ability to clear heat, but has an excellent ability to drain dampness and is used to treat mild cases of hematuria, or intermittent hematuria, especially in cats. The tongue and pulse indicate yin deficiency, and there may or may not be an active UTI present.
- *Dao Chi San* is used to treat hematuria caused by Heart fire. The Heart fire empties into the Small Intestine and then into the Bladder, resulting in hematuria. This condition can be seen in cats with a fire constitution and that are under stress. One of the most common causes of stress in cats is being one of a multiple cat household and complete indoor confinement. Chronic stress leads to Liver qi stagnation, which eventually turns to fire. The fire then invades the Heart. The fire flares upward to cause ulceration of the tongue and mouth and can also pour downward through the channels to the Heart's associated organ—the Small Intestine. The fire is transmitted to the Urinary Bladder, scorching the bladder walls and vasculature and causing bleeding with hematuria. This condition will not resolve unless the root cause is treated. These cats are often fractious and demonstrate significant anxiety; the tongue may be dark red to purple. The urine is often sterile and no crystals are seen. However, chronic Heart fire can lead to a weakness of the Urinary Bladder and Kidney, and over time, promote development of UTI. This formula will require modification to improve its heat-clearing ability to treat UTI. It may also be combined with *Ba Zheng San* for the treatment of UTI. This condition is promoted and exacerbated by feeding a species inappropriate diet to cats, which are obligatory carnivores.
- *Xiao Ji Yin Zi* is used to treat hematuria caused by heat that stagnates in the Urinary Bladder, damaging the vessels and leading to hematuria. This formula is the strongest of the four to cool the blood, stop bleeding and resolve moderate to severe hematuria; its heat-clearing ability is second to that of *Ba Zheng San*. It can be used to treat hematuria secondary to transitional cell carcinoma of the bladder. This formula can be combined with *Ba Zheng San* to treat mixed bacterial UTI with moderate to severe hematuria.

Section 3

利水渗湿剂 — Water-Regulating and Damp-Resolving Formulas

Wŭ Líng Săn (Five-Ingredient Powder with Poria) 五苓散

Pinyin Name: *Wu Ling San*
Literal Name: Five-Ingredient Powder with Poria
Alternate Names: Five-Ling Formula, Poria Powder with Five Herbs, Hoelen Five Herb Formula
Original Source: *Shang Han Lun* (Discussion of Cold-Induced Disorders) by Zhang Zhong-Jing in the Eastern Han Dynasty

COMPOSITION

Ze Xie (Rhizoma Alismatis)	3.75g [15g]
Zhu Ling (Polyporus)	2.25g [9g]
Fu Ling (Poria)	2.25g [9g]
Bai Zhu (Rhizoma Atractylodis Macrocephalae)	2.25g [9g]
Gui Zhi (Ramulus Cinnamomi)	1.5g [6g]

DOSAGE / PREPARATION / ADMINISTRATION

The source text instructs to grind the ingredients into powder and take 1 spoonful [6g] with boiled water three times daily. The source text recommends drinking plenty of warm water to promote sweating. Today, it is normally taken in powder form, 3-6g per dose. This formula may also be prepared as a decoction with the doses suggested in brackets.

CHINESE THERAPEUTIC ACTIONS

1. Regulates water circulation, strengthens the Spleen, promotes urination and drains dampness
2. Warms yang, disperses water accumulation and resolves edema

CLINICAL MANIFESTATIONS

1. Exterior syndrome accompanied by accumulation of water and dampness in the interior: fever, irritability, thirst with a strong desire to drink but vomiting immediately after drinking, urinary difficulty, a white tongue coating, and a superficial pulse.
2. Accumulation of water and dampness in the interior: fluid in the abdomen, fluid in the chest cavity, edema of the limbs and ventrum, loose stools, dysuria, dyspnea, coughing, and a slippery pulse.

VETERINARY CLINICAL APPLICATIONS

Peripheral edema, edema from traumatic injury, glomerulonephritis, renal cyst, chronic renal failure, urolithiasis, urinary tract infection, ascites, hydrothorax and pulmonary edema secondary to congestive heart failure.

EXPLANATION

Wu Ling San (Five-Ingredient Powder with Poria) is originally used in *Shang Han Lun* (Discussion of Cold-Induced Disorders) to treat water accumulation syndrome caused by exterior disorders. This syndrome begins with *taiyang* exterior (channel) syndrome, and, if left untreated, the pathogen may travel via the *taiyang* channel to affect the *taiyang* organ of the Urinary Bladder. Today, this formula has application in veterinary medicine as a general diuretic for the accumulation of dampness and subsequent edema of the limbs and body cavities secondary to weak transportation and transformation functions of the Spleen. It has only a mild ability to tonify the Spleen and should be combined with a Spleen tonic formula for animals that have significant Spleen qi deficiency.

Ze Xie (Rhizoma Alismatis), the chief herb, directly enters the Urinary Bladder to induce urination and eliminate water accumulation. *Zhu Ling* (Polyporus) and *Fu Ling* (Poria)

Wŭ Líng Săn (Five-Ingredient Powder with Poria)

***Wu Ling San* (Five-Ingredient Powder with Poria)**

Diagnosis	Clinical Signs	Treatment	Herbs
Exterior syndrome accompanied by accumulation of water and dampness in the interior	• Fever: exterior condition • Fluid in the abdomen and thorax, cough, dyspnea, edema, loose stools, and dysuria: accumulation of water and dampness in the interior • Slippery pulse: damp accumulation	• Regulates water circulation and dispels dampness • Warms yang and disperses water accumulation	• *Ze Xie* (Rhizoma Alismatis) induces urination and eliminates water accumulation. • *Zhu Ling* (Polyporus) and *Fu Ling* (Poria) strengthen the Spleen, resolve dampness, and eliminate water accumulation. • *Bai Zhu* (Rhizoma Atractylodis Macrocephalae) strengthens the Spleen to dispel water and dampness. • *Gui Zhi* (Ramulus Cinnamomi) releases the exterior and promotes the flow of yang qi in the interior.

act as deputy herbs to strengthen the diuretic function of *Ze Xie* (Rhizoma Alismatis). *Bai Zhu* (Rhizoma Atractylodis Macrocephalae) strengthens the Spleen to dispel water and dampness. *Gui Zhi* (Ramulus Cinnamomi) relieves the *taiyang* syndrome with its exterior-releasing action and promotes the flow of yang qi in the interior to help invigorate the function of the Urinary Bladder. This formula can also be used to treat edema or urinary difficulty. In addition, since this formula can help the body excrete water through urination, it can also treat the type of diarrhea caused by excessive water or dampness traveling with the feces. The diarrhea stops once the water is separated from the feces and is directed out of the body through urination.

VETERINARY MODIFICATIONS

- With damp-heat jaundice, add *Yin Chen* (Herba Artemisiae Scopariae); or use *Yin Chen Wu Ling San* (Artemisia Scoparia and Five-Ingredient Powder with Poria).
- With edema due to Spleen deficiency, add *Wu Pi San* (Five-Peel Powder), *Dang Shen* (Radix Codonopsis) and *Huang Qi* (Radix Astragali).
- With edema due to Kidney yang deficiency, add *Wu Pi San* (Five-Peel Powder) and *Fu Zi* (Radix Aconiti Lateralis Praeparata).

CAUTIONS / CONTRAINDICATIONS

- *Wu Ling San* contains warm, pungent, diuretic herbs that can damage yin and fluids; it should be modified for use in yin-deficient animals.
- Because *Wu Ling San* eliminates excess body fluids through the urine, it should not be used for a prolonged period of time. Close monitoring of electrolytes is indicated when combined with conventional diuretic therapy.
- This formula is contraindicated in horses that have depleted body fluids from profuse sweating or excessive vomiting or diarrhea, as its use could lead to further loss of body fluids
- In order to restore normal water metabolism, the Spleen and Kidney must be tonified if they are deficient, as these two organs regulate water circulation. *Wu Ling San* is not for long-term use without modification.
- In horses, stool should be monitored to avoid impaction colic when being used to treat edema. Prophylactic administration of a bran mash or mineral oil may be indicated in some cases.

PHARMACOLOGICAL EFFECTS

1. **Diuretic**: *Wu Ling San* had a marked diuretic effect in rats 1-2 hours after oral ingestion.[1] Another study reported that intravenous injection of *Wu Ling San* in dogs was associated with increased elimination of urine, sodium, chloride, potassium, and other electrolytes.[2] Lastly, administration of *Wu Ling San* in healthy adults was associated with 112% increase in urine output without any side effects.[3]
2. **Antihypertensive**: One study reported a significant and prolonged reduction in blood pressure using a *Wu Ling San* preparation in rats. The mechanism of this antihypertensive effect was attributed to the diuretic and vasodilative actions of the formula. The herbal formula contained the following ingredients: *Zhu Ling* (Polyporus) 9g, *Ze Xie* (Rhizoma Alismatis) 15g, *Bai Zhu* (Rhizoma Atractylodis Macrocephalae) 9g, *Fu Ling* (Poria) 9g, and *Gui Zhi* (Ramulus Cinnamomi) 6g.[4]
3. **Nephroprotective**: Administration of *Wu Ling San* was associated with protecting the kidneys by decreasing plasma levels of blood urea nitrogen (BUN) and creatinine (Cr). This formula was found to also increase urine output, as well as elimination of electrolytes such as sodium, chloride, potassium, calcium, and magnesium.[5]

Wǔ Líng Sǎn (Five-Ingredient Powder with Poria)

4. **Hepatoprotective**: *Wu Ling San* has been shown to have a remarkable hepatoprotective effect in mice, especially against alcohol-induced liver damage.[6]

HUMAN CLINICAL STUDIES AND RESEARCH

1. **Acute nephritis**: According to one study, 36 of 38 patients with acute nephritis had complete recovery using herbs in decoction. The herbal formula contained *Wu Ling San*, *Bai Mao Gen* (Rhizoma Imperatae) and other herbs as deemed necessary. The study reported resolution of edema in 25 cases within 1-5 days, and 13 cases within 6-10 days. The duration of treatment was 15 days or less in 27 cases, 16-30 days in 9 cases, and over 1 month in 2 cases.[7]
2. **Renal failure**: Modified *Wu Ling San* had good results in treating early stages of renal failure. Out of 20 patients, one study reported a marked improvement in 6 cases and slight improvement in 14 cases.[8] Another study reported 87.5% effectiveness using modified *Wu Ling San* to treat 24 patients with acute renal failure caused by chemotherapy treatments.[9]
3. **Urolithiasis**: One study reported marked effect using modified *Wu Ling San* to treat urinary stones. Of 53 patients, 33 successfully passed stones. The duration of treatment varied between 2-50 packs of herbs.[10]
4. **Liver cirrhosis and ascites**: Use of modified *Wu Ling San* was associated with 89% effectiveness for treatment of 43 patients with liver cirrhosis and ascites. The herbal formula contained *Wu Ling San* plus *Dan Shen* (Radix et Rhizoma Salviae Miltiorrhizae), *Che Qian Zi* (Semen Plantaginis), *Bai Mao Gen* (Rhizoma Imperatae), *Da Fu Pi* (Pericarpium Arecae), *Dang Gui* (Radix Angelicae Sinensis), and *Chi Shao* (Radix Paeoniae Rubra) given in decoction. 30g of *Da Huang* (Radix et Rhizoma Rhei) were given via rectal enema. Of 43 patients, the study reported complete recovery in 23 cases, improvement in 13 cases, and no effect in 4 cases. The average duration of treatment was 31 days. Information was unavailable on 3 individuals who did not complete the study.[11]
5. **Hydrocephalus**: Use of modified *Wu Ling San* was beneficial in 4 patients with hydrocephalus. The herbal formula was given in decoction, and contained *Fu Ling* (Poria) 15g, *Da Fu Pi* (Pericarpium Arecae) 15g, *Zhu Ling* (Polyporus) 10g, *Ze Xie* (Rhizoma Alismatis) 10g, *Niu Xi* (Radix Achyranthis Bidentatae) 10g, *Che Qian Zi* (Semen Plantaginis) 10g, *Bai Zhu* (Rhizoma Atractylodis Macrocephalae) 5g, and *Gui Zhi* (Ramulus Cinnamomi) 2g.[12]

HERB-DRUG INTERACTION

Selective serotonin reuptake inhibitors (SSRIs): Use of *Wu Ling San* was beneficial in relieving adverse gastrointestinal events such as nausea and dyspepsia associated with the use of SSRIs in 20 patients (17 females and 3 males, between 21 to 74 years of age). After adding this formula to the previous drug regimen, the study reported complete disappearance of nausea and dyspepsia in 9 cases, improvement in 4 cases, slight improvement in 2 cases, and no change in 5 cases. Addition of *Wu Ling San* to SSRIs did not cause any adverse events in the 20 patients.[13]

SUGGESTED ACUPUNCTURE TREATMENT

1. Points: *Pangguangshu* (BL 28), *Zhongji* (CV 3), *Yinlingquan* (SP 9), *Pianli* (LI 6), *Weiyang* (BL 39), *Pishu* (BL 20), *Weishu* (BL 21), *Shuifen* (CV 9), and *Waiguan* (TH 5).
2. Technique: sedation.

Pangguangshu (BL 28) and *Zhongji* (CV 3) regulate Urinary Bladder qi; when these two points are combined with *Yinlingquan* (SP 9), they dispel dampness and promote diuresis. *Pianli* (LI 6) and *Weiyang* (BL 39) also promote diuresis. *Pishu* (BL 20) and *Weishu* (BL 21) tonify the Spleen and help disperse edema. *Shuifen* (CV 9) also regulates the water passages to promote urination. *Waiguan* (TH 5), which connects with the *yangwei* (linking) channel, relieves exterior pathogenic factors and regulates water in all three *jiaos*. Together, these five points regulate qi and water and induce diuresis.

AUTHORS' COMMENTS

Wu Ling San may be used for any condition arising from an accumulation and retention of dampness that obstructs the water pathways and affects the primary organs of water metabolism in the body. If the Urinary Bladder qi is unable to transform and eliminate fluids, then edema, urinary obstruction and painful dysuria can occur. Accumulated fluids can disrupt the Lung's dispersing and descending function, causing coughing and wheezing; it can also adversely affect the Spleen's transportation and transformation functions. *Wu Ling San* promotes urination and drains dampness, strengthens the Spleen, warms yang, and strengthens the transforming functions of qi, making it useful to treat edema and fluid accumulation that develop secondary to renal, cardiac and hepatic disease. This formula works wonderfully in horses for the treatment of primary limb edema; it is also a very good choice for postpartum ventral edema and edema secondary to abdominal surgery. The use of herbal treatment in these cases is often a better alternative than the corticosteroids, which are often given for such conditions. During the use of this formula, patients should be monitored for proper hydration to avoid impaction.

Wŭ Líng Săn (Five-Ingredient Powder with Poria)

To effectively treat fluid accumulation in the body cavities, *Wu Ling San* requires modification and/or combination with other formulas to achieve a satisfactory therapeutic effect. It can be combined with *Wu Pi San* (Five-Peel Powder) or *Zhen Wu Tang* (True Warrior Decoction) to treat pulmonary edema secondary to congestive heart failure. In the treatment of ascites, it can be combined with *Shi Pi San* (Bolster the Spleen Powder) or *Wu Pi San* (Five-Peel Powder).

Herbal diuretic formulas can be given with conventional diuretic drugs, such as furosemide or spironolactone. The concurrent use of herbal and conventional diuretics is often necessary if the animal experiences adverse reactions, electrolyte disturbance or depletion and azotemia from high doses of conventional diuretic drugs. Integrative use of the two therapeutic agents may also be required in cases of refractory edema, in particular refractory pulmonary edema. It is best to begin by giving the lowest therapeutic dose of the diuretic herbal formula while monitoring the fluid and electrolyte status of the animal. Initially, the dosage of conventional medication is left the same and the herbal diuretic added. The effect of combined therapies on the resolution of edema and/or fluid accumulation is regularly evaluated over a period of two weeks. The dosage of the herbal diuretic may be increased and/or the dosage of the conventional diuretic can be gradually decreased during this time period. In general, it will take several weeks to find the optimal dosing regimen for each individual animal. Many animals can be taken off conventional diuretic therapy altogether in mild to moderate cases. If edema or fluid accumulation recurs, conventional diuretic medications can simply be administered again in small increments and/or the dosage and formulation of the herbal formulas are re-evaluated and adjusted. For chronic cases of edema or fluid accumulation, all basic herbal diuretic formulas used initially will require modification and/or the addition of another formula to address the root problem in the long term. This typically means further support and tonification of the Spleen and Kidney, and/or resolution of blood stagnation affecting the water pathways. In some cases, normalization and promotion of the dispersing and descending functions of the Lung is required.

Wu Ling San is helpful in the treatment of urinary tract infection and urolithiasis by promoting diuresis to flush out and detoxify the Kidney and Urinary Bladder. It can be combined with *Ba Zheng San* (Eight-Herb Powder for Rectification) or *Wu Lin San* (Five-Ingredient Powder for Painful Urinary Dysfunction). For animals with ascites secondary to liver failure, Cushing's disease, or neoplasia characterized by poor appetite, cold limbs, chronic diarrhea and Spleen yang deficiency, combine with *Fu Zi Li Zhong Wan* (Prepared Aconite Pill to Regulate the Middle).

There are three formulas with similar compositions that regulate water, promote urination, and dispel dampness:

- *Wu Ling San* (Five-Ingredient Powder with Poria) is considered to be a general standard diuretic formula. It has the dual functions of releasing the exterior syndrome and dispelling accumulation of water and dampness in the interior.
- *Wei Ling Tang* (Calm the Stomach and Poria Decoction) combines *Ping Wei San* (Calm the Stomach Powder) and *Wu Ling San*. It warms cold and dispels dampness affecting the middle *jiao*. It strengthens the Spleen and harmonizes the Stomach to treat accumulation of water and dampness in the interior causing abdominal distention and edema.
- *Yin Chen Wu Ling San* (Artemisia Scoparia and Five-Ingredient Powder with Poria) is formulated by adding *Yin Chen* (Herba Artemisiae Scopariae) to *Wu Ling San* to treat damp-heat jaundice (more dampness than heat) with urinary difficulty.

References

1. *Zhong Yi Fang Ji Xian Dai Yan Jiu* (Modern Study of Medical Formulas in Traditional Chinese Medicine), 1997; 1407.
2. *Guo Wai Yi Xue Zhong Yi Zhong Yao Fen Ce* (Monograph of Chinese Herbology from Foreign Medicine), 1981; 2:121.
3. *Zhong Hua Yi Xue Za Zhi* (Chinese Journal of Medicine), 1961; 17(1):7.
4. *Tian Jin Zhong Yi* (Tianjin Chinese Medicine), 1994; 4:29.
5. *Guo Wai Yi Xue Zhong Yi Zhong Yao Fen Ce* (Monograph of Chinese Herbology from Foreign Medicine), 1983; 3:43.
6. *Guo Wai Yi Xue Zhong Yi Zhong Yao Fen Ce* (Monograph of Chinese Herbology from Foreign Medicine), 1986; 1:22.
7. *Si Chuan Zhong Yi* (Sichuan Chinese Medicine), 1985; 9:19.
8. *Xin Zhong Yi* (New Chinese Medicine), 1987; 7:44.
9. *Zhong Yi Za Zhi* (Journal of Chinese Medicine), 1993; 1:42.
10. *Zhong Yi Ming Fang Lin Chuang Xin Yong* (Contemporary Clinical Applications of Classic Chinese Formulas), 2001; 133.
11. *Shan Xi Zhong Yi* (Shanxi Chinese Medicine), 1989; 7:295.
12. *Xin Yi Yao Xue Za Zhi* (New Journal of Medicine and Herbology), 1978; 8:45.
13. Yamada K, Yagi G, Kanba S. Effectiveness of Gorei-san (TJ-17) for treatment of SSRI-induced nausea and dyspepsia: preliminary observations. Clinical Neuropharmacology. 26(3):112-4, 2003 May-Jun.

Wèi Líng Tāng (Calm the Stomach and Poria Decoction)

胃苓湯
胃苓汤

Pinyin Name: *Wei Ling Tang*
Literal Name: Calm the Stomach and Poria Decoction
Alternate Names: Weiling Decoction, Stomach-Comforting with Five-Ling Decoction, Magnolia and Hoelen Combination
Original Source: *Dan Xi Xin Fa* (Teachings of [Zhu] Dan-Xi) by Zhu Zhen-Heng in 1481

COMPOSITION

Ping Wei San (Calm the Stomach Powder)	3g
Wu Ling San (Five-Ingredient Powder with Poria)	3g

DOSAGE / PREPARATION / ADMINISTRATION

The source text instructs to cook the ingredients with *Sheng Jiang* (Rhizoma Zingiberis Recens) and *Da Zao* (Fructus Jujubae). Take the decoction on an empty stomach.

CHINESE THERAPEUTIC ACTIONS

Dispels dampness, strengthens the Spleen, and harmonizes the Stomach

CLINICAL MANIFESTATIONS

External cold damaging the Stomach and Spleen during the late summer and early fall, causing dysfunction in water metabolism with the inability of the Spleen to transform and transport fluids: poor appetite, anorexia, vomiting, loose stools containing undigested food, chronic, watery diarrhea, edema, fullness of the abdomen, and dysuria.

VETERINARY CLINICAL APPLICATIONS

Acute and chronic gastroenteritis, post-surgical vomiting, diarrhea, poor appetite and abdominal distention, gastroenteritis secondary to raw or refrigerated diet, pulmonary edema, ascites secondary to nephrotic syndrome, ascites secondary to acute toxic hepatopathy. This formula is useful in horses with anorexia and concurrent damp signs, such as peripheral edema, ascites, and mild diarrhea.

EXPLANATION

Wei Ling Tang (Calm the Stomach and Poria Decoction) is composed of *Ping Wei San* (Calm the Stomach Powder) plus *Wu Ling San* (Five-Ingredient Powder with Poria). Thus, this formula can both harmonize the Stomach and dispel dampness. Clinically, it is often used for external cold damaging the Stomach and Spleen during the late summer and early fall. Animals in this case may have loose stools containing undigested food, chronic diarrhea, edema, abdominal fullness, and dysuria. The use of this formula is indicated for animals with signs of cold and dampness affecting the middle *jiao*; animals may have a greasy, white tongue coating and a slippery pulse.

Please refer to *Ping Wei San* (Calm the Stomach Powder) and *Wu Ling San* (Five-Ingredient Powder with Poria) for additional and detailed explanations of these two formulas.

VETERINARY MODIFICATIONS

- With exterior wind-cold, add *Bai Shao* (Radix Paeoniae Alba) and *Chai Hu* (Radix Bupleuri).
- With diarrhea, dysentery, and abdominal pain, add *Xiang Fu* (Rhizoma Cyperi) and *Sha Ren* (Fructus Amomi).
- With vomiting of phlegm and saliva, add *Jie Geng* (Radix Platycodonis) and *Ban Xia* (Rhizoma Pinelliae).

***Wei Ling Tang* (Calm the Stomach and Poria Decoction)**

Diagnosis	Clinical Signs	Treatment	Herbs
External cold damaging the Stomach and Spleen	• Poor appetite, vomiting, loose stools containing undigested food, thirst, and diarrhea: dampness affecting the Spleen and Stomach • Edema, ascites and dysuria: obstructed water circulation	• Dispels dampness • Harmonizes the Stomach	• *Ping Wei San* (Calm the Stomach Powder) dries dampness, activates qi circulation, strengthens the Spleen, and harmonizes the Stomach. • *Wu Ling San* (Five-Ingredient Powder with Poria) warms yang, dispels dampness, and disperses water accumulation

Wèi Líng Tāng (Calm the Stomach and Poria Decoction)

HUMAN CLINICAL STUDIES AND RESEARCH

1. **Nephritis**: Twenty children with acute nephritis (duration of illness ranged from 5 to 63 days) were treated with marked improvement using modified *Wei Ling Tang*. Clinical presentation of the patients included edema and presence of red blood cells, white blood cells, and protein in the urine. The herbal formula contained *Cang Zhu* (Rhizoma Atractylodis) 6g, *Hou Po* (Cortex Magnoliae Officinalis) 9g, *Zhi Qiao* (Fructus Aurantii) 9g, *Zhu Ling* (Polyporus) 9g, *Ze Xie* (Rhizoma Alismatis) 9g, *Mu Tong* (Caulis Akebiae) 9g, *Che Qian Zi* (Semen Plantaginis) 9g, *Mu Xiang* (Radix Aucklandiae) 1g, *Chen Pi* (Pericarpium Citri Reticulatae) 3g, *Gan Cao* (Radix et Rhizoma Glycyrrhizae) 3g, and others as deemed necessary. The study reported satisfactory results in all 20 cases.[1]
2. **Diarrhea**: *Wei Ling Tang* has been shown in various studies to effectively treat diarrhea. According to one study, use of this formula was associated with 90% effectiveness in 31 children with acute diarrhea.[2] In another study, diarrhea due to acute enteritis in 125 patients was treated with complete recovery in 105 cases, significant improvement in 6 cases, moderate improvement in 4 cases, and no effect in 10 cases.[3]

SUGGESTED ACUPUNCTURE TREATMENT

1. Points: *Pangguangshu* (BL 28), *Zhongji* (CV 3), *Yinlingquan* (SP 9), *Shuifen* (CV 9), *Waiguan* (TH 5), *Zhangmen* (LR 13), *Gongsun* (SP 4), *Housanli* (ST 36), *Tongguan*, *Shangen*, and *Jianwei*.
2. Technique: sedation.

Pangguangshu (BL 28) and *Zhongji* (CV 3) regulate the qi of the Urinary Bladder; when combined with *Yinlingquan* (SP 9), these three points dispel dampness and promote diuresis. *Shuifen* (CV 9) also regulates the water passages to promote urination. *Waiguan* (TH 5), which connects with the *yangwei* (linking) channel, relieves exterior pathogenic factors and regulates water in all three *jiaos*. Together, these five points regulate qi and water and induce diuresis. *Zhangmen* (LR 13), *Gongsun* (SP 4), *Housanli* (ST 36), and *Yinlingquan* (SP 9) assist in dispelling dampness and harmonizing the Stomach. *Tongguan* is a classical equine point to promote appetite and treat gastrointestinal disorders. *Shangen* and *Jianwei* are classical canine points for appetite stimulation and to treat gastric orders, respectively.

AUTHORS' COMMENTS

Wei Ling Tang treats chronic, watery diarrhea due to damp-cold in dogs and horses. Damp-cold conditions can develop from chronic antibiotic use, post-surgery, and by regular consumption of refrigerated food in dogs and cats. The animals for which this formula is indicated have a pale purple tongue and a weak and deep pulse.

References

1. *Guang Xi Zhong Yi Yao* (Guangxi Chinese Medicine and Herbology), 1984; 4(10):16.
2. *Hu Nan Zhong Yi Za Zhi* (Hunan Journal of Chinese Medicine), 1990; 2:48.
3. *Shan Xi Zhong Yi* (Shanxi Chinese Medicine), 1989; 10(6):28.

Zhū Líng Tāng (Polyporus Decoction)

豬苓湯
猪苓汤

Pinyin Name: *Zhu Ling Tang*
Literal Name: Polyporus Decoction
Alternate Names: *Chu Ling Tang*, Polyporus Combination
Original Source: *Shang Han Lun* (Discussion of Cold-Induced Disorders) by Zhang Zhong-Jing in the Eastern Han Dynasty

COMPOSITION

Zhu Ling (Polyporus)	3g [9g]
Fu Ling (Poria)	3g [9g]
Ze Xie (Rhizoma Alismatis)	3g [9g]
Hua Shi (Talcum), *fen sui* (pulverized)	3g [9g]
E Jiao (Colla Corii Asini)	3g [9g]

DOSAGE / PREPARATION / ADMINISTRATION

The source text instructs to cook all of the ingredients, except *E Jiao* (Colla Corii Asini), with 4 cups [800 mL] of water until the liquid is reduced to 2 cups [400 mL]. Discard the residue and completely dissolve *E Jiao* (Colla Corii Asini) in the strained decoction. Take 0.7 cup [140 mL] of the warm decoction three times daily. Today, this formula may be prepared as a decoction with the doses suggested in brackets.

CHINESE THERAPEUTIC ACTIONS

1. Regulates water circulation
2. Clears heat and nourishes yin

CLINICAL MANIFESTATIONS

1. Interlocking of water and heat: dysuria, fever, thirst with a strong desire to drink, irritability, insomnia, with or without coughing, vomiting and diarrhea.
2. *Xue lin* (bloody dysuria) syndrome: painful urination, difficult urination with dripping of urine, and fullness and pain in the lower abdomen.

VETERINARY CLINICAL APPLICATIONS

Urinary tract infection, hematuria, hemoglobinuria, urethritis, dysuria, edema, glomerulonephritis, urolithiasis, retention of urine, hydronephrosis and prostatitis.

EXPLANATION

Zhu Ling Tang (Polyporus Decoction) was first introduced in *Shang Han Lun* (Discussion of Cold-Induced Disorders) for treating the condition of interlocking of water and heat. This condition starts as a *taiyang* syndrome at the exterior, and then transforms into a *yangming* or *shaoyang* syndrome with resultant heat formation. The heat, when interlocked with water inside the body, impairs the proper distribution of water. Clinical presentations include

***Zhu Ling Tang* (Polyporus Decoction)**

Diagnosis	Clinical Signs	Treatment	Herbs
Interlocking of water and heat	• Dysuria, difficult urination with dribbling of urine, painful urination, and blood in the urine: impaired distribution of water due to interlocking of water and heat • Desire to drink: heat consuming body fluids • Irritability and restlessness: heat disturbing the *shen* (spirit) • Coughing: interlocking of water and heat affecting the Lung • Vomiting: interlocking of water and heat affecting the Stomach • Diarrhea: interlocking of water and heat affecting the Large Intestine	• Regulates water circulation • Clears heat and nourishes yin	• *Zhu Ling* (Polyporus), *Fu Ling* (Poria) and *Ze Xie* (Rhizoma Alismatis) dispel water accumulation and dampness through urination. • *Hua Shi* (Talcum) clears heat and relieves dysuria. • *E Jiao* (Colla Corii Asini) nourishes yin and moistens dryness.

Zhū Líng Tāng (Polyporus Decoction)

dysuria, difficult urination with dribbling of urine, painful urination, and blood in the urine. The interlocking of heat and water also injures the yin and causes thirst with a strong desire to drink, irritability, and insomnia. Lastly, interlocking of water and heat also affects the Lung to cause coughing, the Stomach to cause nausea and vomiting, and the Large Intestine to cause diarrhea.

The treatment plan is to regulate water circulation and dispel dampness through urination, as well as to clear heat and nourish yin. *Zhu Ling* (Polyporus), *Fu Ling* (Poria), and *Ze Xie* (Rhizoma Alismatis) dispel water accumulation and dampness through urination. *Hua Shi* (Talcum) clears heat and relieves dysuria. *E Jiao* (Colla Corii Asini) nourishes yin and moistens dryness. These five herbs have a proper balance to drain water without injuring yin and to nourish yin without creating more stagnation.

VETERINARY MODIFICATIONS

- For *re lin* (heat dysuria), add *Zhi Zi* (Fructus Gardeniae) and *Che Qian Zi* (Semen Plantaginis); or combine with *Ba Zheng San* (Eight-Herb Powder for Rectification).
- For *xue lin* (bloody dysuria), add *Bai Mao Gen* (Rhizoma Imperatae) and *Xiao Ji* (Herba Cirsii); or combine with *Xiao Ji Yin Zi* (Cirsium Decoction).
- For *shi lin* (stone dysuria), add *Hai Jin Sha* (Spora Lygodii) and *Jin Qian Cao* (Herba Lysimachiae).
- For severe dysuria, add *Mu Tong* (Caulis Akebiae) and *Di Huang* (Radix Rehmanniae).
- With frequent urination, add *Cang Zhu* (Rhizoma Atractylodis) and *Bai Zhu* (Rhizoma Atractylodis Macrocephalae).
- With irritability, add *Hu Po* (Succinum) and *Zhi Zi* (Fructus Gardeniae); or combine with *Qing Xin Lian Zi Yin* (Lotus Seed Decoction to Clear the Heart).
- With restlessness, irritability, and thirst, add *Shi Gao* (Gypsum Fibrosum) and *Zhi Mu* (Rhizoma Anemarrhenae).

CAUTIONS / CONTRAINDICATIONS

Zhu Ling Tang primarily regulates water circulation and dispels water accumulation. Although it has a minor effect to nourish yin and moisten dryness, it should not be used in cases of extreme thirst due to severe damage of body fluids, such as from profuse sweating.[1]

PHARMACOLOGICAL EFFECTS

1. **Diuretic**: Administration of *Zhu Ling Tang* at 10 times the normal dose for 1 month was associated with a marked diuretic effect in rats. The study noted that there were no noticeable changes to the electrolyte levels, such as calcium, magnesium, and potassium.[2,3]
2. **Nephroprotective**: One study reported that *Zhu Ling Tang* given via oral ingestion at 1 g/kg for 12 months was associated with protective and healing effects on the kidneys, and with prolonged life.[4]
3. **Effect on urinary stones**: One study reported that *in vitro* and *in vivo* administrations of *Zhu Ling Tang* corresponded with prevention of urinary stones by reducing struvite crystal formation and increasing the spontaneous discharge of stones in the urine.[5]

HUMAN CLINICAL STUDIES AND RESEARCH

1. **Edema**: Administration of an herbal extract of *Zhu Ling Tang* to 11 patients at 2.5g per dose, twice daily for 1 month, was associated with marked increase in urination and reduction of edema. There were no significant changes to the blood levels of sodium and potassium.[6]
2. **Hematuria**: Use of modified *Zhu Ling Tang* was associated with 88.2% effectiveness in treating patients with blood in the urine due to various causes. Of 68 patients, the study reported complete recovery in 46 cases, improvement in 14 cases, and no effect in 8 cases.[7]
3. **Urolithiasis**: One study reported 97.1% effectiveness using modified *Zhu Ling Tang* to treat 35 patients with urinary stones. In addition to the base formula, modifications were made by adding *Pu Huang* (Pollen Typhae), *Da Ji* (Herba Cirsii Japonici), *Xiao Ji* (Herba Cirsii), and *Di Long* (Pheretima) for hematuria; and *Bai Shao* (Radix Paeoniae Alba) and *Mu Gua* (Fructus Chaenomelis) for severe colicky pain. The study reported relief of colicky pain within 20 minutes to 7 days. Stones were successfully expelled within 3 to 28 days in 31 of 35 patients.[8] According to another study, administration of *Zhu Ling Tang* was helpful in reducing the number of days (from an average of 21.5 days to 16.0 days) to successfully eliminate urinary stones.[9]
4. **Uroschesis**: One study reported a marked effect in treating 60 geriatric patients with uroschesis using modified *Zhu Ling Tang*. Modifications included addition of *Rou Gui* (Cortex Cinnamomi) and *Fu Zi* (Radix Aconiti Lateralis Praeparata) for aversion to cold, and soreness and weakness of the lower back and knees; *Ren Shen* (Radix et Rhizoma Ginseng) and *Huang Qi* (Radix Astragali) for soft, weak voice; *Chuan Shan Jia* (Squama Manis) and *Jin Qian Cao* (Herba Lysimachiae) for dysuria with lower abdominal fullness and distention; and *Ji Nei Jin* (Endothelium Corneum Gigeriae Galli) and *Jian Shen Qu* (Massa Fermentata Praeparata) for poor appetite. Most patients were able to resume normal urination within 3-6 packs of herbal treatment. Of 60 patients, the study reported complete recovery in 56 cases, improvement in 3 cases, and no effect in 1 case.[10]

Zhū Líng Tāng (Polyporus Decoction)

5. **Hydronephrosis**: One study reported 91.1% effectiveness using modified *Zhu Ling Tang* to treat 45 patients with hydronephrosis. Modifications to the base formula included the addition of *Jin Qian Cao* (Herba Lysimachiae), *Hai Jin Sha* (Spora Lygodii), *Shi Wei* (Folium Pyrrosiae), *Wang Bu Liu Xing* (Semen Vaccariae), *Niu Xi* (Radix Achyranthis Bidentatae), and *Ji Nei Jin* (Endothelium Corneum Gigeriae Galli) for urinary stones; *Mu Tong* (Caulis Akebiae) and *Bian Xu* (Herba Polygoni Avicularis) for frequent, urgent, and painful urination; *Da Huang* (Radix et Rhizoma Rhei) for constipation; *Qian Cao* (Radix et Rhizoma Rubiae), *Mo Han Lian* (Herba Ecliptae), and *Bai Mao Gen* (Rhizoma Imperatae) for hematuria; and *Ze Lan* (Herba Lycopi), *Yi Mu Cao* (Herba Leonuri), *Gui Zhi* (Ramulus Cinnamomi), and others for prostatic hypertrophy. Of 45 patients, the study reported complete recovery in 38 cases, improvement in 3 cases, and no effect in 4 cases.[11]
6. **Cystitis**: One study reported marked success in treating 107 patients with acute cystitis using 1-6 packs of modified *Zhu Ling Tang*.[12]
7. **Urinary tract disorder**: According to one study of 30 patients who complained of lower urinary tract clinical signs without pyuria, administration of *Zhu Ling Tang* was associated with an efficacy rate of 92.9% for pollakisuria, 85.8% for miction pain, 85.7% for voiding discomfort, and 76.0% for total efficacy rate. No side effects were reported.[13]

SUGGESTED ACUPUNCTURE TREATMENT

1. Points: *Pangguangshu* (BL 28), *Zhongji* (CV 3), *Shuifen* (CV 9), *Xingjian* (LR 2), and *Taixi* (KI 3).
2. Technique: sedation.

These points induce diuresis, clear heat, and nourish yin. *Pangguangshu* (BL 28) and *Zhongji* (CV 3) regulate Kidney qi. *Shuifen* (CV 9) promotes diuresis. *Xingjian* (LR 2) clears heat. *Taixi* (KI 3) nourishes yin to moisten dryness.

AUTHORS' COMMENTS

The primary use of *Zhu Ling Tang* (Polyporus Decoction) in veterinary medicine is for the treatment of urinary tract infection accompanied by yin deficiency. It has very weak ability to clear heat and requires modification to effectively treat urinary tract infections. For further discussion, please refer to the Authors' Comments section of *Ba Zheng San* (Eight-Herb Powder for Rectification).

Wu Ling San (Five-Ingredient Powder with Poria) and *Zhu Ling Tang* both promote urination, drain dampness, and treat dysuria.

- *Wu Ling San* treats accumulation of water and dampness in the interior accompanied by exterior clinical signs. It warms yang and promotes the qi transforming function of the Bladder. *Wu Ling San* is contraindicated in animals with significant yin deficiency.
- *Zhu Ling Tang* treats accumulation of water and dampness with heat in the interior. It treats urinary tract infection with yin deficiency. It can dispel dampness without injuring body fluids, nourish yin without entrapment of heat pathogens, stop bleeding, and clear heat. These properties make this formula useful in the treatment of dysuria and hemoglobinuria from exertional rhabdomyolysis in horses.

References

1. *Zhong Yi Lin Chuan Fang Ji Xue* (Clinical Study of Chinese Herbal Formulas), 1995; 228-229.
2. *Guo Wai Yi Xue Zhong Yi Zhong Yao Fen Ce* (Monograph of Chinese Herbology from Foreign Medicine), 1981; 3:173.
3. *Guo Wai Yi Xue Zhong Yi Zhong Yao Fen Ce* (Monograph of Chinese Herbology from Foreign Medicine), 1984; 5:78.
4. *Guo Wai Yi Xue Zhong Yi Zhong Yao Fen Ce* (Monograph of Chinese Herbology from Foreign Medicine), 1984; 5:78.
5. Koide T, Yamaguchi S, Utsunomiya M, Yoshioka T, Sugiyama K. The inhibitory effect of kampou extracts on in vitro calcium oxalate crystallization and in vivo stone formation in an animal model. Int J Urol. 1995 May; 2(2):81-6.
6. *Guo Wai Yi Xue* (Foreign Medicine), 1983; 5:292.
7. *Zhong Yi Ming Fang Lin Chuang Xin Yong* (Contemporary Clinical Applications of Classic Chinese Formulas), 2001; 636.
8. *Zhe Jiang Zhong Yi Xue Yuan Xue Bao* (Journal of Zhejiang University of Chinese Medicine), 1997; 4:35.
9. Takada M, Yano H, Kanbara N, Kurita T, Kohri K, Kato Y, Iguchi M. Effect of Chorei-to on spontaneous discharge of urinary stones after extracorporeal shock wave lithotripsy (ESWL). Hinyokika Kiyo. 1997 Apr; 43(4):311-4.
10. *Si Chuan Zhong Yi* (Sichuan Chinese Medicine), 1997; 4:26.
11. *Shan Dong Zhong Yi Za Zhi* (Shandong Journal of Chinese Medicine), 1995; 8:345.
12. *Zhe Jiang Zhong Yi Za Zhi* (Zhejiang Journal of Chinese Medicine), 1982; 10:448.
13. Horii A, Maekawa M. Clinical evaluation of chorei-to and chorei-to-go-shimotsu-to in patients with lower urinary tract symptoms. Hinyokika Kiyo. 1988 Dec; 34(12):2237-41.

Wǔ Pí Sǎn (Five-Peel Powder)

五皮散

Pinyin Name: *Wu Pi San*
Literal Name: Five-Peel Powder
Alternate Names: *Wu Pi Yin*, Five-Pi Drink, Five Kinds of Peels Drink, Hoelen and Areca Combination
Original Source: *Zhong Zang Jing* (Treasury Classic) by Hua-Tuo in the Han Dynasty

COMPOSITION

Fu Ling Pi (Cortex Poria)	[9g]
Sheng Jiang Pi (Pericarpium Zingiberis Recens)	[9g]
Sang Bai Pi (Cortex Mori)	[9g]
Da Fu Pi (Pericarpium Arecae)	[9g]
Chen Pi (Pericarpium Citri Reticulatae)	[9g]

DOSAGE / PREPARATION / ADMINISTRATION

The source text instructs to grind equal amounts of the ingredients into a coarse powder. Cook 9g of the powder with 1.5 bowls of water until the liquid is reduced to 80% volume. Take the warm, strained decoction any time during the day. Today, this formula may be prepared as a decoction with the doses suggested in brackets.

CHINESE THERAPEUTIC ACTIONS

1. Drains dampness and reduces swelling and edema
2. Regulates qi and strengthens the Spleen

CLINICAL MANIFESTATIONS

Pi shui (skin water) due to Spleen deficiency and damp accumulation: generalized edema of the whole body, fluid accumulation in the body cavities, heaviness of the body and extremities, epigastric and abdominal distention, shortness of breath, rapid breathing, urinary difficulty, and edema during gestation. There may be a white, greasy tongue coating and a deep, moderate pulse.

VETERINARY CLINICAL APPLICATIONS

Edema secondary to renal and cardiac disease, chronic glomerulonephritis, pulmonary edema secondary to congestive heart failure, chronic liver failure or neoplasia with ascites, edema of purpura hemorrhagica, edema during gestation, and edema from traumatic injury.

EXPLANATION

When the Spleen is deficient, dampness accumulates in the interior and then overflows to the skin and muscles, causing generalized edema and swelling throughout the body and extremities. Damp accumulation can obstruct the flow of qi and cause epigastric and abdominal distention. If the damp accumulation affects the Lung, shortness of breath and rapid breathing may occur. Because water circulation is impaired, urinary difficulty may also occur.

Wu Pi San (Five-Peel Powder) uses *Fu Ling Pi* (Cortex Poria) to dispel dampness and relieve edema through diuresis. This herb also strengthens the Spleen and

***Wu Pi San* (Five-Peel Powder)**

Diagnosis	Clinical Signs	Treatment	Herbs
Pi shui (skin water) due to Spleen deficiency and damp accumulation	• Edema and swelling throughout the body and extremities: damp accumulation with Spleen deficiency • Epigastric and abdominal distention: damp accumulation obstructing qi circulation • Shortness of breath and rapid breathing: damp accumulation affecting the Lung • Urinary difficulty: damp accumulation affecting the Urinary Bladder	• Eliminates dampness and reduces swelling and edema • Regulates qi and strengthens the Spleen	• *Fu Ling Pi* (Cortex Poria) dispels dampness and relieves edema through diuresis. • *Sheng Jiang Pi* (Pericarpium Zingiberis Recens) disperses accumulation of water and dampness. • *Sang Bai Pi* (Cortex Mori) redirects the rising Lung qi and restores normal water metabolism. • *Da Fu Pi* (Pericarpium Arecae) activates qi circulation and relieves distention. • *Chen Pi* (Pericarpium Citri Reticulatae) harmonizes Stomach qi and disperses dampness.

Wŭ Pí Săn (Five-Peel Powder)

improves its transformation and transportation functions. *Sheng Jiang Pi* (Pericarpium Zingiberis Recens) disperses accumulation of water and dampness. *Sang Bai Pi* (Cortex Mori) redirects the rising Lung qi and restores normal water metabolism. *Da Fu Pi* (Pericarpium Arecae) activates qi circulation to disperse fluids and relieve distention. *Chen Pi* (Pericarpium Citri Reticulatae) harmonizes Stomach qi and disperses turbid dampness.

VETERINARY MODIFICATIONS

- With water accumulation in the face, head and neck, add *Zi Su Ye* (Folium Perillae), *Jing Jie* (Herba Schizonepetae), *Fang Feng* (Radix Saposhnikoviae), and *Qin Jiao* (Radix Gentianae Macrophyllae).
- With water accumulation of the distal extremities, add *Chi Xiao Dou* (Semen Phaseoli), *Fu Ling* (Poria), *Ze Xie* (Rhizoma Alismatis), *Fang Ji* (Radix Stephaniae Tetrandrae), and *Che Qian Zi* (Semen Plantaginis).
- With severe edema, add *Wu Ling San* (Five-Ingredient Powder with Poria).
- With edema during gestation, remove *Sang Bai Pi* (Cortex Mori), and add *Bai Zhu* (Rhizoma Atractylodis Macrocephalae).
- With facial edema, add *Chen Pi* (Pericarpium Citri Reticulatae) and *Sang Bai Pi* (Cortex Mori).
- With generalized weakness and deficiency, add *Dang Shen* (Radix Codonopsis), *Huang Qi* (Radix Astragali), and *Bai Zhu* (Rhizoma Atractylodis Macrocephalae).
- With coldness, add *Gan Jiang* (Rhizoma Zingiberis) and *Rou Gui* (Cortex Cinnamomi).
- With abdominal distention, add *Bai Zhu* (Rhizoma Atractylodis Macrocephalae) and *Cang Zhu* (Rhizoma Atractylodis).

CAUTIONS / CONTRAINDICATIONS

Avoid foods that are raw, cold, oily, greasy or hard to digest while taking *Wu Pi San*.

HUMAN CLINICAL STUDIES AND RESEARCH

1. **Edema**: *Wu Pi San* was shown in two studies to have satisfactory results in treating edema.[1]
2. **Traumatic injuries with swelling and inflammation**: Sixty-three patients with swelling and inflammation due to external trauma were effectively treated using *Wu Pi San* plus *Bai Zhu* (Rhizoma Atractylodis Macrocephalae) and *San Qi* (Radix et Rhizoma Notoginseng). *Gui Zhi* (Ramulus Cinnamomi) and *Sang Zhi* (Ramulus Mori) were added if the upper extremities were affected, and *Chuan Niu Xi* (Radix Cyathulae) was added for the lower extremities. The study reported marked effectiveness in all 63 patients, with swelling reduced in 18 cases after 2 days, 30 cases after 3 days, and 15 cases after 7 days.[2]

SUGGESTED ACUPUNCTURE TREATMENT

1. Points: *Pishu* (BL 20), *Yinlingquan* (SP 9), *Housanli* (ST 36), *Zhongfu* (LU 1), *Shuifen* (CV 9) and *Qihaishu*.
2. Technique: both tonification and sedation.

The main focus is to relieve edema by tonifying the Spleen and dispelling dampness. Both *Pishu* (BL 20), the *shu* (transport) point of the Spleen channel, and *Yinlingquan* (SP 9), the *he* (uniting) point of the Spleen channel, tonify the Spleen to dispel dampness and promote diuresis. *Housanli* (ST 36) harmonizes the middle *jiao* and strengthens qi. *Zhongfu* (LU 1) regulates Lung qi, which in turn controls the water passages inside the body. *Shuifen* (CV 9) regulates the water passages and induces diuresis. *Qihaishu* is a classical equine point for Spleen tonification.

RELATED FORMULA

Wŭ Pí Săn (Five-Peel Powder)
五皮散
Pinyin Name: *Wu Pi San*
Literal Name: Five-Peel Powder
Original Source: *Tai Ping Hui Min He Ji Ju Fang* (Imperial Grace Formulary of the Tai Ping Era) by the Imperial Medical Department in 1078-85

Sheng Jiang Pi (Pericarpium Zingiberis Recens)
Wu Jia Pi (Cortex Acanthopanacis)
Di Gu Pi (Cortex Lycii)
Da Fu Pi (Pericarpium Arecae)
Fu Ling Pi (Cortex Poria)

Wu Pi San (Five-Peel Powder) treats edema by eliminating dampness, reducing swelling, dispelling wind-dampness, and opening the channels and collaterals.

Wu Pi San is the identical name of the main formula and the related formula; both have the same name, similar compositions, and essentially the same functions. Both formulas contain *Fu Ling Pi* (Cortex Poria), *Sheng Jiang Pi* (Pericarpium Zingiberis Recens), and *Da Fu Pi* (Pericarpium Arecae).

- *Wu Pi San*, from *Zhong Zang Jing* (Treasury Classic) by Hua-Tuo, contains *Sang Bai Pi* (Cortex Mori) and *Chen Pi* (Pericarpium Citri Reticulatae) and is better at regulating qi circulation.
- *Wu Pi San*, from *Tai Ping Hui Min He Ji Ju Fang* (Imperial Grace Formulary of the Tai Ping Era) by the Imperial Medical Department, contains *Wu Jia Pi* (Cortex Acanthopanacis) and *Di Gu Pi* (Cortex Lycii) and has strong functions to dispel wind-dampness and open the channels and collaterals.

Wŭ Pí Săn (Five-Peel Powder)

AUTHORS' COMMENTS

Wu Pi San (Five-Peel Powder) is used for edema caused by Spleen qi deficiency and accumulation of water. It is made up of five peels, or "skins," of herbal medicines to treat superficial or skin edema. It promotes urination, drains dampness, and regulates qi to resolve edema; it has only a mild ability to tonify the Spleen. In chronic or severe disease, it must be combined with other herbs or formulas to further tonify the Spleen and to increase its therapeutic effects. It treats pitting edema and can be used to reduce swelling and edema of the face and head from hypersensitivity reactions. For the treatment of ascites, it can be combined with *Si Jun Zi Tang* (Four-Gentlemen Decoction), *Bu Zhong Yi Qi Tang* (Tonify the Middle and Augment the Qi Decoction), or *Xiang Sha Liu Jun Zi Tang* (Six-Gentlemen Decoction with Aucklandia and Amomum). It has been used long term to treat pulmonary edema in combination with furosemide and enalapril without ill effects in the canine. These animals were also taking other herbal medications in addition to *Wu Pi San* to treat their primary disease of congestive heart failure and to tonify the Spleen. For oliguria secondary to renal failure with severe ascites, it can be combined with *Wu Ling San* (Five-Ingredient Powder with Poria). Once the clinical signs resolve, the dose should be decreased and a formula that addresses the underlying deficiencies should be added.

The key factor to choosing *Wu Pi San* over *Wu Ling San* (Five-Ingredient Powder with Poria) to treat edema in horses is the presence of Spleen deficiency. In otherwise healthy animals that develop damp accumulation and edema, *Wu Ling San* is an excellent choice. In patients that are debilitated, such as geriatric horses with chronic protein-losing enteropathy or liver failure, *Wu Pi San* is the better choice. It can be helpful to combine this formula with a stronger Spleen tonic, such as *Shen Ling Bai Zhu San* (Ginseng, Poria, and Atractylodes Macrocephala Powder) in a 1:1 ratio for better effect.

References

1. *Shan Xi Zhong Yi* (Shanxi Chinese Medicine), 1991; 12(2):89.
2. *Zhe Jiang Zhong Yi Za Zhi* (Zhejiang Journal of Chinese Medicine), 1994; 11:511.

Jiǔ Wèi Bīng Láng Jiā Wú Fú Tāng

(Areca Nine Decoction plus Evodia and Poria)

九味檳榔加吳茯湯
九味槟榔加吴茯汤

Pinyin Name: *Jiu Wei Bing Lang Jia Wu Fu Tang*
Literal Name: Areca Nine Decoction plus Evodia and Poria
Alternate Name: Areca Seed Combination
Original Source: *Qian Tian Jia Fang* (Family Formulas of Qian Tian-Jia)

COMPOSITION

Bing Lang (Semen Arecae)
Chen Pi (Pericarpium Citri Reticulatae)
Hou Po (Cortex Magnoliae Officinalis)
Mu Xiang (Radix Aucklandiae)
Zi Su Ye (Folium Perillae)
Wu Zhu Yu (Fructus Evodiae)
Gui Zhi (Ramulus Cinnamomi)
Fu Ling (Poria)
Da Huang (Radix et Rhizoma Rhei)
Sheng Jiang (Rhizoma Zingiberis Recens)
Gan Cao (Radix et Rhizoma Glycyrrhizae)

DOSAGE / PREPARATION / ADMINISTRATION

The source text instructs to prepare the ingredients as a decoction.

CHINESE THERAPEUTIC ACTIONS

1. Dispels water accumulation
2. Disperses qi and blood stagnation
3. Warms yang

CLINICAL MANIFESTATION

Water accumulation in the limbs with qi and blood stagnation: pitting edema, fatigue and weakness of the limbs.

VETERINARY CLINICAL APPLICATIONS

Acute or chronic edema of the limbs, edema secondary to traumatic injury or bite wounds, post-surgical edema, snakebite or spider bite edema, edema secondary to neoplasia of the limbs, edema secondary to chronic renal disease.

EXPLANATION

Jiu Wei Bing Lang Jia Wu Fu Tang (Areca Nine Decoction plus Evodia and Poria) treats water accumulation in the legs accompanied by qi and blood stagnation. Pitting edema in the legs is diagnostic of water accumulation. As water accumulation affects the upper and middle *jiaos*, patients may experience shortness of breath and cough. Water accumulation may also contribute to damp stagnation, leading to lethargy and poor appetite. Furthermore, chronic water accumulation leads to qi and blood stagnation, which is characterized by fatigue and weakness of the legs.

In this formula, *Bing Lang* (Semen Arecae) breaks up qi stagnation, eliminates water accumulation, and dispels phlegm. *Chen Pi* (Pericarpium Citri Reticulatae) regulates qi and dries dampness. *Hou Po* (Cortex Magnoliae Officinalis) dispels dampness, removes stagnation, and disperses distention. *Mu Xiang* (Radix Aucklandiae) promotes qi circulation and relieves pain and distention. *Zi Su Ye* (Folium Perillae), with its light and acrid properties, regulates qi circulation and harmonizes the middle *jiao*. *Wu Zhu Yu* (Fructus Evodiae) and *Gui Zhi* (Ramulus Cinnamomi) warm the yang to eliminate water and phlegm stagnation. *Fu Ling* (Poria) strengthens the Spleen, dispels dampness, and eliminates water accumulation. *Da Huang* (Radix et Rhizoma Rhei) clears heat and relieves constipation. *Sheng Jiang* (Rhizoma Zingiberis Recens) and *Gan Cao* (Radix et Rhizoma Glycyrrhizae) harmonize all of the herbs in this formula.

Jiŭ Wèi Bīng Láng Jiā Wú Fú Tāng

(Areca Nine Decoction plus Evodia and Poria)

***Jiu Wei Bing Lang Jia Wu Fu Tang* (Areca Nine Decoction plus Evodia and Poria)**

Diagnosis	Clinical Signs	Treatment	Herbs
Water accumulation in the legs with qi and blood stagnation	• Pitting edema in the limbs: water accumulation in the extremities • Poor appetite, shortness of breath, and cough: water accumulation in the upper and middle *jiaos* • Weakness of the legs: qi and blood stagnation secondary to water accumulation	• Dispels water accumulation • Disperses qi and blood stagnation • Relieves constipation	• *Bing Lang* (Semen Arecae) breaks up qi stagnation, eliminates water accumulation, and dispels phlegm. • *Chen Pi* (Pericarpium Citri Reticulatae) regulates qi and dries dampness. • *Hou Po* (Cortex Magnoliae Officinalis) dispels dampness, removes stagnation, and disperses distention. • *Mu Xiang* (Radix Aucklandiae) promotes qi circulation and relieves pain and distention. • *Zi Su Ye* (Folium Perillae) regulates qi circulation and harmonizes the middle *jiao*. • *Wu Zhu Yu* (Fructus Evodiae) and *Gui Zhi* (Ramulus Cinnamomi) warm the yang to eliminate water and phlegm stagnation. • *Fu Ling* (Poria) strengthens the Spleen, dispels dampness, and eliminates water accumulation. • *Da Huang* (Radix et Rhizoma Rhei) clears heat and relieves constipation. • *Sheng Jiang* (Rhizoma Zingiberis Recens) and *Gan Cao* (Radix et Rhizoma Glycyrrhizae) harmonize the herbs in this formula.

SUGGESTED ACUPUNCTURE TREATMENT

1. Points: *Shanzhong* (CV 17), *Qihai* (CV 6), *Neiguan* (PC 6), *Zhongwan* (CV 12), *Yinlingquan* (SP 9), *Guanyuan* (CV 4), *Tianshu* (ST 25), and *Xiajuxu* (ST 39).
2. Technique: moxibustion and even method.

Shanzhong (CV 17) and *Qihai* (CV 6) regulate qi and disperse stagnation. Needle *Neiguan* (PC 6) and *Zhongwan* (CV 12) to harmonize the middle *jiao*. To eliminate water accumulation, apply moxibustion on *Guanyuan* (CV 4) to warm yang, and needle *Yinlingquan* (SP 9) to regulate the water passages. *Tianshu* (ST 25) and *Xiajuxu* (ST 39) relieve constipation.

AUTHORS' COMMENTS

The primary application of *Jiu Wei Bing Lang Jia Wu Fu Tang* in veterinary medicine is in the treatment of limb edema with stagnation of qi and blood. In acute cases of edema due to injury, surgery or bite wounds, the formula should be discontinued as soon as the edema resolves, and another formula that promotes and accelerates healing should be given.

Jiu Wei Bing Lang Jia Wu Fu Tang contains herbs to warm yang to transform accumulated fluids; it has little ability to tonify the Spleen. This formula also contains *Da Huang* (Radix et Rhizoma Rhei) and should not be used long term without modification. For long-term use in chronic renal disease, cancer, or Cushing's disease, this formula will require modification or should be combined with another formula to address the underlying problem.

In cases of stubborn edema without underlying deficiency, this formula can be combined with herbs that invigorate blood, like *Dan Shen* (Radix et Rhizoma Salviae Miltiorrhizae) or *Dang Gui* (Radix Angelicae Sinensis), or it can be combined with formulas with similar action, such as *Huo Luo Xiao Ling Dan* (Fantastically Effective Pill to Invigorate the Collaterals).

Fēn Xiāo Tāng (Separate and Reduce Decoction)

分消湯
分消汤

Pinyin Name: *Fen Xiao Tang*
Literal Name: Separate and Reduce Decoction
Alternate Name: Hoelen and Alisma Combination
Original Source: *Wan Bing Hui Chun* (Restoration of Health from the Myriad Diseases) by Gong Ting-Xian in 1587

COMPOSITION

Cang Zhu (Rhizoma Atractylodis), *jin* (soaked) in rice water and *chao* (dry-fried)	3g
Bai Zhu (Rhizoma Atractylodis Macrocephalae)	3g
Hou Po (Cortex Magnoliae Officinalis), *chao* (dry-fried) with ginger juice	3g
Chen Pi (Pericarpium Citri Reticulatae)	3g
Mu Xiang (Radix Aucklandiae)	0.9g
Xiang Fu (Rhizoma Cyperi)	2.4g
Zhi Shi (Fructus Aurantii Immaturus), *chao* (dry-fried) with bran	3g
Da Fu Pi (Pericarpium Arecae)	2.4g
Sha Ren (Fructus Amomi)	2.1g
Zhu Ling (Polyporus)	2.4g
Ze Xie (Rhizoma Alismatis)	2.4g
Fu Ling (Poria)	3g

DOSAGE / PREPARATION / ADMINISTRATION

The source text instructs to cook the ingredients with 1 slice of *Sheng Jiang* (Rhizoma Zingiberis Recens) and 1 piece of *Deng Xin Cao* (Medulla Junci) in water to make a decoction.

CHINESE THERAPEUTIC ACTIONS

1. Strengthens the Spleen
2. Regulates qi circulation to relieve fullness and distention
3. Regulates the water passages to eliminate water stagnation

CLINICAL MANIFESTATIONS

1. Severe abdominal fullness and distention due to Spleen deficiency: severe fullness and drum-like distention in the abdomen, anorexia, poor appetite, lethargy and vomiting.
2. Water stagnation due to Spleen deficiency: abdominal distention, dyspnea, ascites, limb edema, belching, vomiting, dysuria, oliguria and constipation.

VETERINARY CLINICAL APPLICATIONS

Peripheral edema, ascites secondary to nephrotic syndrome, chronic liver failure, protein-losing enteropathy, ascites secondary to severe parasite infections, liver or abdominal cancer and heart failure.

EXPLANATION

Fen Xiao Tang (Separate and Reduce Decoction) treats severe abdominal fullness with drum-like distention characterized by Spleen deficiency and damp accumulation. Spleen deficiency, besides giving rise to damp accumulation, may cause inadequate transportation and transformation of nutrients. The dampness and untransformed nutrients usually accumulate in the abdomen, causing abdominal distention and dyspnea due to pressure on the diaphragm. Poor appetite and anorexia are the results of Spleen deficiency, and vomiting arises from Stomach disharmony. Dysuria and oliguria are the results of dampness and fluids not unable to pass out of the body through urination.

There are two major categories of herbs employed in this treatment strategy: herbs to strengthen the Spleen and Stomach, and herbs to eliminate dampness and water stagnation. *Cang Zhu* (Rhizoma Atractylodis) and *Bai Zhu* (Rhizoma Atractylodis Macrocephalae), both bitter, dry, and warm, resolve dampness and strengthen the Spleen. *Hou Po* (Cortex Magnoliae Officinalis) activates qi circulation, dispels dampness, and relieves fullness and distention in the epigastrium and abdomen. *Chen Pi* (Pericarpium Citri Reticulatae), *Mu Xiang* (Radix Aucklandiae), and *Xiang Fu* (Rhizoma Cyperi) regulate qi and relieve stagnation. *Zhi Shi* (Fructus Aurantii Immaturus), *Da Fu Pi* (Pericarpium Arecae), and *Sha Ren* (Fructus Amomi) strengthen the Spleen and Stomach to restore the normal food transformation and transportation. *Sheng Jiang* (Rhizoma Zingiberis Recens) harmonizes the Spleen and Stomach. *Zhu Ling* (Polyporus), *Ze Xie* (Rhizoma Alismatis), and *Fu Ling* (Poria) dispel water and dampness through diuresis. *Deng Xin Cao* (Medulla

Fēn Xiāo Tāng (Separate and Reduce Decoction)

***Fen Xiao Tang* (Separate and Reduce Decoction)**

Diagnosis	Clinical Signs	Treatment	Herbs
Severe abdominal fullness and distention due to Spleen deficiency and damp accumulation	• Abdominal distention and dyspnea: accumulation of dampness in the abdomen • Loss of appetite: Spleen deficiency • Vomiting: disharmony in the Stomach	• Strengthens the Spleen • Regulates qi circulation to relieve fullness and distention • Regulates water passages to eliminate water stagnation	• *Cang Zhu* (Rhizoma Atractylodis) and *Bai Zhu* (Rhizoma Atractylodis Macrocephalae) dry dampness and strengthen the Spleen. • *Hou Po* (Cortex Magnoliae Officinalis) activates qi circulation, dispels dampness, and relieves fullness and distention. • *Chen Pi* (Pericarpium Citri Reticulatae), *Mu Xiang* (Radix Aucklandiae), and *Xiang Fu* (Rhizoma Cyperi) regulate qi and relieve stagnation. • *Zhi Shi* (Fructus Aurantii Immaturus), *Da Fu Pi* (Pericarpium Arecae), and *Sha Ren* (Fructus Amomi) strengthen the Spleen and Stomach to restore the normal food transformation and transportation. • *Sheng Jiang* (Rhizoma Zingiberis Recens) harmonizes the Spleen and Stomach. • *Zhu Ling* (Polyporus), *Ze Xie* (Rhizoma Alismatis), and *Fu Ling* (Poria) dispel water and dampness through diuresis. • *Deng Xin Cao* (Medulla Junci) regulates qi, harmonizes the Spleen, induces diuresis, and clears heat.

Junci) has a wide variety of clinical functions, including regulating qi, harmonizing the Spleen, inducing diuresis, and clearing heat.

VETERINARY MODIFICATIONS

With increased respiration rate, add *Chen Xiang* (Lignum Aquilariae Resinatum).

SUGGESTED ACUPUNCTURE TREATMENT

1. Points: *Pangguangshu* (BL 28), *Zhongji* (CV 3), *Yinlingquan* (SP 9), *Zhangmen* (LR 13), *Gongsun* (SP 4), *Housanli* (ST 36), *Sanyinjiao* (SP 6), *Pishu* (BL 20), *Weishu* (BL 21), *Zhongwan* (CV 12) and *Qihaishu*.
2. Technique: tonification and sedation.

This point selection aims to relieve severe abdominal fullness and distention due to Spleen deficiency. *Pangguangshu* (BL 28) and *Zhongji* (CV 3) regulate qi in the Urinary Bladder and restore its normal function. *Yinlingquan* (SP 9), the *he* (uniting) point of the Spleen channel, *Zhangmen* (LR 13), the *mu* (collecting) point of the Spleen, and *Gongsun* (SP 4) are used together to strengthen the Spleen, regulate water passages, and dispel dampness. *Zhongwan* (CV 12), *Pishu* (BL 20), *Weishu* (BL 21), *Housanli* (ST 36), and *Sanyinjiao* (SP 6) tonify the Spleen and Stomach, and relieve abdominal fullness and distention. *Qihaishu* is a classical equine point helpful for qi deficiency and gaseous bowel.

AUTHORS' COMMENTS

Fen Xiao Tang is used to treat severe cases of water accumulation (such as ascites and edema) caused by Spleen deficiency. Ascites is generally described as a drum-like distention in the abdomen, while pits that remain in the skin tissue after pressure is applied are characterized as edema. Ascites and pitting edema are two diagnostic signs for prescribing this formula. This formula addresses the branch (i.e., fluid accumulation) and typically is combined with other herbs or formulas to address the root problem of kidney, heart or liver disease. The animals for which this formula is appropriate have no signs of cold or yang deficiency. Older animals with edema or ascites and chronic disease usually have some degree of Spleen or Kidney yang deficiency and require herbs to support and warm yang in order to move fluids and control or resolve ascites.

Dǎo Shŭi Fú Líng Tāng (Poria Decoction to Drain Water)

導水茯苓湯
导水茯苓汤

Pinyin Name: *Dao Shui Fu Ling Tang*
Literal Name: Poria Decoction to Drain Water
Alternate Names: *Tao Shui Fu Ling Tang*, Hoelen, Atractylodes, and Areca Decoction
Original Source: *Zheng Zhi Zhun Sheng* (Standards of Patterns and Treatments) by Wang Ken-Tang in 1602

COMPOSITION

Chi Fu Ling (Poria Rubra)	90g
Ze Xie (Rhizoma Alismatis)	90g
Bai Zhu (Rhizoma Atractylodis Macrocephalae)	90g
Mu Gua (Fructus Chaenomelis)	30g
Bing Lang (Semen Arecae)	30g
Mai Dong (Radix Ophiopogonis)	90g
Zi Su Ye (Folium Perillae)	30g
Deng Xin Cao (Medulla Junci)	22.5g
Chen Pi (Pericarpium Citri Reticulatae)	22.5g
Mu Xiang (Radix Aucklandiae)	22.5g
Sha Ren (Fructus Amomi)	22.5g
Sang Bai Pi (Cortex Mori)	30g
Da Fu Pi (Pericarpium Arecae)	22.5g

DOSAGE / PREPARATION / ADMINISTRATION

The source text instructs to prepare the ingredients as a decoction.

CHINESE THERAPEUTIC ACTIONS

1. Dispels stagnant water and dries dampness
2. Eliminates water from the Lung
3. Harmonizes the Spleen

CLINICAL MANIFESTATIONS

Severe water accumulation: general edema of the body and extremities, dysuria, oliguria, dyspnea and coughing.

VETERINARY CLINICAL APPLICATIONS

Edema secondary to chronic renal failure, nephrotic syndrome, amyloidosis, refractory pulmonary edema, pulmonary edema and dyspnea secondary to congestive heart failure, dilated cardiomyopathy, hypertrophic cardiomyopathy, hydrothorax, pericardial effusion and ascites secondary to hepatic and cardiac failure or disease.

EXPLANATION

Dao Shui Fu Ling Tang (Poria Decoction to Drain Water) treats severe fluid accumulation affecting both urination and breathing. With severe fluid accumulation, animals often develop pitting edema, dysuria, and oliguria. This kind of edema, in which the tissue shows prolonged pits produced by pressure, is commonly described as "rotten melon." Because the Lung regulates the water passages, excess water retention will affect its normal functions. The animal will experience wheezing, dyspnea and coughing, especially at night and when lying in a horizontal position.

To effectively treat this condition, this formula uses herbs that dispel stagnant water from the body. *Chi Fu Ling* (Poria Rubra) and *Ze Xie* (Rhizoma Alismatis) are diuretic herbs that eliminate water accumulation through diuresis. *Chi Fu Ling* (Poria Rubra) and *Bai Zhu* (Rhizoma Atractylodis Macrocephalae) strengthen the Spleen and dry dampness. *Mu Gua* (Fructus Chaenomelis) dispels dampness from the lower body and is especially effective in treating beriberi. *Bing Lang* (Semen Arecae) eliminates water and disperses stagnant qi in the chest. *Mai Dong* (Radix Ophiopogonis) nourishes the Lung, suppresses cough, and eliminates phlegm. *Zi Su Ye* (Folium Perillae) directs qi downward and relieves chest fullness. *Deng Xin Cao* (Medulla Junci) promotes normal urination and eliminates dampness and swelling. *Chen Pi* (Pericarpium Citri Reticulatae), *Mu Xiang* (Radix Aucklandiae), and *Sha Ren* (Fructus Amomi) regulate qi and reduce qi stagnation. *Sang Bai Pi* (Cortex Mori) regulates Lung qi to relieve wheezing and dyspnea. *Da Fu Pi* (Pericarpium Arecae) regulates water circulation and treats edema and abdominal fullness and distention.

Dǎo Shǔi Fú Líng Tāng (Poria Decoction to Drain Water)

Dao Shui Fu Ling Tang (Poria Decoction to Drain Water)

Diagnosis	Clinical Signs	Treatment	Herbs
Severe water accumulation	• Pitting edema: severe water accumulation • Dysuria and oliguria: water accumulation affecting urination • Wheezing and dyspnea: water accumulation affecting the Lung	• Dispels stagnant water and dries dampness • Eliminates water from the Lung	• *Chi Fu Ling* (Poria Rubra) and *Ze Xie* (Rhizoma Alismatis) eliminate water accumulation through diuresis. • *Chi Fu Ling* (Poria Rubra) and *Bai Zhu* (Rhizoma Atractylodis Macrocephalae) strengthen the Spleen and dry dampness. • *Mu Gua* (Fructus Chaenomelis) dispels dampness from the lower body. • *Bing Lang* (Semen Arecae) eliminates water and disperses stagnant qi in the chest. • *Mai Dong* (Radix Ophiopogonis) nourishes the Lung, suppresses cough, and eliminates phlegm. • *Zi Su Ye* (Folium Perillae) guides qi downward and relieves chest fullness. • *Deng Xin Cao* (Medulla Junci) promotes normal urination and eliminates dampness and swelling. • *Chen Pi* (Pericarpium Citri Reticulatae), *Mu Xiang* (Radix Aucklandiae), and *Sha Ren* (Fructus Amomi) regulate qi and reduce qi stagnation. • *Sang Bai Pi* (Cortex Mori) regulates Lung qi to relieve wheezing and dyspnea. • *Da Fu Pi* (Pericarpium Arecae) regulates water circulation and treats edema and abdominal fullness and distention.

VETERINARY MODIFICATIONS

- With oliguria, add *Mu Tong* (Caulis Akebiae), *Che Qian Zi* (Semen Plantaginis), and *Di Huang* (Radix Rehmanniae).
- With cough and dyspnea, add *Hou Po* (Cortex Magnoliae Officinalis) and *Ku Xing Ren* (Semen Armeniacae Amarum).

SUGGESTED ACUPUNCTURE TREATMENT

1. Points: *Yinlingquan* (SP 9), *Shuidao* (ST 28), *Zhongji* (CV 3), *Fenglong* (ST 40), *Shanzhong* (CV 17), *Neiguan* (PC 6), *Chize* (LU 5), and *Lieque* (LU 7).
2. Technique: sedation.

Yinlingquan (SP 9) and *Shuidao* (ST 28) regulate the water passages. *Zhongji* (CV 3) promotes urination. *Fenglong* (ST 40) transforms phlegm and dampness. *Shanzhong* (CV 17) and *Neiguan* (PC 6) regulate qi and promote qi circulation by eliminating water accumulation. *Chize* (LU 5) and *Lieque* (LU 7) clear the Lung to relieve wheezing and dyspnea.

AUTHORS' COMMENTS

The literal name of *Dao Shui Fu Ling Tang* is "poria decoction to drain water," and this formula is used to drain stagnant water from the body. It has a strong ability to treat edema that develops secondary to renal and cardiac disease and can be safely administered to cats for the treatment of pulmonary edema. It does not have great ability to warm Spleen or Kidney yang to regulate water; thus it can be combined with *Zhen Wu Tang* (True Warrior Decoction) in cases of severe edema due to nephrotic syndrome with yang deficiency. Once the edema is controlled, *Zhen Wu Tang* should be discontinued, but *Dao Shui Fu Ling Tang* may be continued for a longer period of time to control the edema, as it is less warming and fairly well-balanced. Diuretic herbal formulas that treat the branch are nearly always combined with other herbs or formulas to treat the underlying or root disorder responsible for the edema or fluid accumulation.

Dao Shui Fu Ling Tang, *Fen Xiao Tang* (Separate and Reduce Decoction), and *Jiu Wei Bing Lang Jia Wu Fu Tang* (Areca Nine Decoction plus Evodia and Poria) all treat peripheral and pulmonary edema and fluid accumulation in the chest and abdominal cavities.

Dǎo Shǔi Fú Líng Tāng (Poria Decoction to Drain Water)

- *Dao Shui Fu Ling Tang* dispels stagnant water, dries dampness, eliminates water from the Lung, and harmonizes the Spleen. It is better at treating pulmonary edema and hydrothorax from congestive heart failure.
- *Fen Xiao Tang* strengthens the Spleen, activates qi circulation, and regulates water circulation. It is mainly used to treat Spleen deficiency accompanied by severe cases of water accumulation in the abdomen (ascites with drum-like distention in the abdomen) and lower legs (pitting edema with prolonged presence of pits produced by pressure).
- *Jiu Wei Bing Lang Jia Wu Fu Tang* drains water accumulation, regulates qi, and breaks up qi and blood stagnation. It primarily treats qi and blood stagnation accompanied by water accumulation in the legs (pitting edema) and in the chest. It is best for treating limb edema from a variety of acute and chronic disorders or injury.
- It should be noted that these three formulas treat edema by dispelling dampness and regulating water circulation; however, they do not contain herbs that warm Kidney or Spleen yang to transform dampness. In cases with cold signs and deficiencies of Kidney, Spleen or Heart yang, these formulas will require modification or additional formulas added to warm yang in order to facilitate normal fluid metabolism.

Section 4

温化水湿剂
— Warm Formulas that Dissolve Dampness

Líng Guì Zhú Gān Tāng

(Poria, Cinnamon Twig, Atractylodes Macrocephala, and Licorice Decoction)

苓桂朮甘湯
苓桂术甘汤

Pinyin Name: *Ling Gui Zhu Gan Tang*
Literal Name: Poria, Cinnamon Twig, Atractylodes Macrocephala, and Licorice Decoction
Alternate Names: *Fu Ling Gui Zhi Bai Zhu Gan Cao Tang, Ling Kuei Shu Kan Tang, Ling Gui Shu Gan Tang*, Hoelen, Cinnamon Twig, Atractylodes and Licorice Decoction; Poria, Cinnamon, Bighead Atractylodes and Licorice Decoction; Hoelen and Atractylodes Combination
Original Source: *Jin Gui Yao Lue* (Essentials from the Golden Cabinet) by Zhang Zhong-Jing in the Eastern Han Dynasty

COMPOSITION

Fu Ling (Poria)	12g
Gui Zhi (Ramulus Cinnamomi)	9g
Bai Zhu (Rhizoma Atractylodis Macrocephalae)	6g
Zhi Gan Cao (Radix et Rhizoma Glycyrrhizae Praeparata cum Melle)	6g

DOSAGE / PREPARATION / ADMINISTRATION

The source text instructions are to cook the ingredients with 6 cups [1,200 mL] of water until the liquid is reduced to 3 cups [600 mL]. Take the warm, strained decoction in three equally divided doses.

CHINESE THERAPEUTIC ACTIONS

1. Warms and dissolves *tan yin* (phlegm retention)
2. Strengthens the Spleen and dispels dampness

CLINICAL MANIFESTATIONS

Tan yin (phlegm retention) syndrome caused by yang deficiency of the middle *jiao*: hypochondriac and epigastric bloating, nystagmus, shortness of breath, coughing. There may be a white, slippery tongue coating and a wiry, slippery pulse.

VETERINARY CLINICAL APPLICATIONS

Edema secondary to chronic renal failure, nephrotic syndrome, amyloidosis, hydronephrosis, pulmonary edema secondary to heart failure, hydrothorax, pericardial effusion and ascites secondary to hepatic, cardiac or renal disease.

EXPLANATION

According to the source text, *Ling Gui Zhu Gan Tang* (Poria, Cinnamon Twig, Atractylodes Macrocephala, and Licorice Decoction) was originally used to treat individuals who developed yang deficiency in the middle *jiao* after being incorrectly treated with emetic or downward draining methods for an exterior syndrome. As yang becomes deficient, the Spleen loses its ability to transform and transport food, resulting in water and dampness turning into *tan yin* (phlegm retention). If the phlegm blocks the passage of the ascending yang qi, nystagmus may occur. If it affects the Lung and disrupts the circulation of qi, coughing and shortness of breath occur. If it affects the circulation of qi around the Heart, palpitations occur.

In this formula, *Fu Ling* (Poria) acts as the chief herb to strengthen the Spleen, dispel dampness, and disperse phlegm. *Gui Zhi* (Ramulus Cinnamomi) disperses

Líng Guì Zhú Gān Tāng

(Poria, Cinnamon Twig, Atractylodes Macrocephala, and Licorice Decoction)

***Ling Gui Zhu Gan Tang* (Poria, Cinnamon Twig, Atractylodes Macrocephala, and Licorice Decoction)**

Diagnosis	Clinical Signs	Treatment	Herbs
Tan yin (phlegm retention) syndrome with yang deficiency of the middle *jiao*	• Hypochondriac and epigastric bloating: phlegm accumulation in the chest • Palpitations: phlegm accumulation affecting the Heart • Dyspnea and coughing: fluid accumulation affecting the Lung • White, slippery tongue coating and a wiry, slippery pulse: damp accumulation	• Warms and dissolves *tan yin* (phlegm retention) • Strengthens the Spleen and dispels dampness	• *Fu Ling* (Poria) strengthens the Spleen, dispels dampness, and disperses phlegm. • *Gui Zhi* (Ramulus Cinnamomi) disperses accumulated fluids and warms the body to dissolve phlegm. • *Bai Zhu* (Rhizoma Atractylodis Macrocephalae) strengthens the Spleen and dries dampness. • *Zhi Gan Cao* (Radix et Rhizoma Glycyrrhizae Praeparata cum Melle) tonifies qi and harmonizes the herbs.

accumulated fluids and warms the body to dissolve phlegm. *Bai Zhu* (Rhizoma Atractylodis Macrocephalae) strengthens the Spleen and dries dampness. *Zhi Gan Cao* (Radix et Rhizoma Glycyrrhizae Praeparata cum Melle) tonifies the qi and harmonizes the herbs.

VETERINARY MODIFICATIONS

- With nausea or vomiting from profuse phlegm accumulation, add *Er Chen Tang* (Two-Cured Decoction).
- With abdominal pain due to deficiency and cold, combine with *Li Zhong Tang* (Regulate the Middle Decoction).
- With diarrhea caused by Spleen qi deficiency and damp accumulation, add *Ping Wei San* (Calm the Stomach Powder).
- With generalized weakness and fatigue, combine with *Xiao Jian Zhong Tang* (Minor Construct the Middle Decoction).
- With epigastric distention or borborygmus, add *Zhi Shi* (Fructus Aurantii Immaturus).
- With early congestive heart failure and pulmonary edema, combine with *Sheng Mai San* (Generate the Pulse Powder) or *Zhi Gan Cao Tang* (Honey-Fried Licorice Decoction).
- With cough and pulmonary edema, add *Ting Li Da Zao Xie Fei Tang* (Descurainia and Jujube Decoction to Drain the Lung) or *Wu Ling San* (Five-Ingredient Powder with Poria).
- With edema of the limbs and decreased urination, add *Zhu Ling* (Polyporus) and *Ze Xie* (Rhizoma Alismatis).

CAUTIONS / CONTRAINDICATIONS

Ling Gui Zhu Gan Tang contains warm and drying herbs which may consume or injure body fluids. Therefore, it is contraindicated in cases of significant yin and/or body fluid deficiencies.

PHARMACOLOGICAL EFFECTS

1. **Cardiovascular**: Administration of *Ling Gui Zhu Gan Tang* via intraperitoneal injection at 20 mL/kg in mice was effective in preventing irregular heartbeat and increasing resistance against ischemia.[1]
2. **Sedative and hypnotic**: Administration of *Ling Gui Zhu Gan Tang* was associated with a sedative and hypnotic effect. It prolonged sleeping time induced by barbiturates and reduced spontaneous activities in mice.[2]

HUMAN CLINICAL STUDIES AND RESEARCH

1. **Coronary artery disease**: Use of modified *Ling Gui Zhu Gan Tang* in 16 patients with coronary artery disease and angina was associated with marked improvement in 10 cases, moderate improvement in 5 cases, and no effect in 1 case.[3]
2. **Cardiac failure**: Ninety-six patients who were unresponsive to digitalis after long-term use or intolerant because of side effects were treated with *Ling Gui Zhu Gan Tang* plus *Sheng Mai San* (Generate the Pulse Powder) or *Zhi Gan Cao Tang* (Honey-Fried Licorice Decoction) with good results. Of 96 patients, the study reported significant improvement in 39 cases, moderate improvement in 36 cases, and no effect in 21 cases. The overall effectiveness was 77%.[4]
3. **Nephrotic syndrome**: One study reported good results using both herbs and drugs to treat 17 patients with severe nephrotic syndrome. The herbal treatment contained *Ling Gui Zhu Gan Tang* plus *Yi Mu Cao* (Herba Leonuri), *Qian Shi* (Semen Euryales), *Ze Xie* (Rhizoma Alismatis), *Bai Mao Gen* (Rhizoma Imperatae), and others as needed. Hormonal drug treatment was given as needed. After 3 months of treatment, the study reported complete remission in 9 cases, near-complete remission in 5 cases, partial remission in 2 cases, and no effect in 1 case.[5]

Líng Guì Zhú Gān Tāng

(Poria, Cinnamon Twig, Atractylodes Macrocephala, and Licorice Decoction)

4. **Hydronephrosis**: Use of modified *Ling Gui Zhu Gan Tang* in 33 patients with hydronephrosis was associated with significant improvement in 21 cases, moderate improvement in 9 cases, and no effect in 3 cases. Additions to the original formula included *Chuan Lian Zi* (Fructus Toosendan) and *Chi Shao* (Radix Paeoniae Rubra) for low back pain; *Shi Wei* (Folium Pyrrosiae) for painful urination; *Bai Mao Gen* (Rhizoma Imperatae) and *Hu Po* (Succinum) for hematuria; and *Ban Xia* (Rhizoma Pinelliae) for nausea and vomiting.[6]

SUGGESTED ACUPUNCTURE TREATMENT

1. Points: *Housanli* (ST 36), *Yinlingquan* (SP 9), *Shuifen* (CV 9), and *Waiguan* (TH 5).
2. Technique: tonification and moxibustion.

Housanli (ST 36) and *Yinlingquan* (SP 9) tonify the Spleen, harmonize the middle *jiao*, and dispel dampness. *Shuifen* (CV 9) and *Waiguan* (TH 5) induce diuresis, but through differing mechanisms. *Shuifen* (CV 9) regulates the water passages, while *Waiguan* (TH 5) activates yang to move water. Moxibustion is used to tonify yang.

AUTHORS' COMMENTS

Ling Gui Zhu Gan Tang and *Zhen Wu Tang* (True Warrior Decoction) have similar herbal composition and are used for similar diseases. However, *Ling Gui Zhu Gan Tang*, which contains *Gui Zhi* (Ramulus Cinnamomi), does not warm yang to transform fluids as well as *Zhen Wu Tang*, which contains *Fu Zi* (Radix Aconiti Lateralis Praeparata) and *Sheng Jiang* (Rhizoma Zingiberis Recens). *Ling Gui Zhu Gan Tang* is used to treat moderate cases of edema or fluid accumulation from Spleen yang deficiency, while *Zhen Wu Tang* (True Warrior Decoction) is for more severe cases. *Ling Gui Zhu Gan Tang* is typically modified for long-term use in the treatment of cardiac and renal diseases with persistent edema.

References

1. *Bei Jing Zhong Yi Xue Yuan Xue Bao* (Journal of Beijing University School of Medicine), 1990; 13(4):47.
2. *Guo Wai Yi Xue Zhong Yi Zhong Yao Fen Ce* (Monograph of Chinese Herbology from Foreign Medicine), 1987; 9(20:40).
3. *Zhong Yi Han Shou Tong Xun* (Reports of Chinese Medicine), 1992; 2:41.
4. *Tian Jin Yi Yao Za Zhi* (Journal of Tianjin Medicine and Herbology), 1967; 8:503.
5. *Shan Xi Zhong Yi* (Shanxi Chinese Medicine), 1987; 2:70.
6. *Shi Yong Zhong Yi Yao Za Zhi* (Journal of Practical Chinese Medicine and Medicinals), 1999; 6:11.

Zhēn Wǔ Tāng (True Warrior Decoction)

真武湯
真武汤

Pinyin Name: *Zhen Wu Tang*
Literal Name: True Warrior Decoction
Alternate Names: *Chen Wu Tang*, Divine Black Bird Decoction, Ginger Aconite Hoelen and Peony Combination
Original Source: *Shang Han Lun* (Discussion of Cold-Induced Disorders) by Zhang Zhong-Jing in the Eastern Han Dynasty

COMPOSITION

Fu Zi (Radix Aconiti Lateralis Praeparata), *pao* (blast-fried)	1 piece [9g]
Fu Ling (Poria)	9g
Sheng Jiang (Rhizoma Zingiberis Recens)	9g
Bai Zhu (Rhizoma Atractylodis Macrocephalae)	6g
Bai Shao (Radix Paeoniae Alba)	9g

DOSAGE / PREPARATION / ADMINISTRATION

The source text instructs to cook the ingredients with 8 cups [1,600 mL] of water until the liquid is reduced to 3 cups [600 mL]. Take 0.7 cup [140 mL] of the warm, strained decoction three times daily.

CHINESE THERAPEUTIC ACTIONS

Warms yang and regulates water metabolism

CLINICAL MANIFESTATIONS

1. Spleen and Kidney yang deficiencies with water accumulation: cyanosis, dysuria, oliguria, coughing, dyspnea, abdominal distention, abdominal pain, diarrhea, swelling and edema of the limbs, pulmonary edema, hydrothorax, absence of thirst, a pale to purple tongue, and a deep, weak pulse.
2. *Taiyang* disorder: presence of exterior condition and fever unresolved after sweating, and muscle twitching.

VETERINARY CLINICAL APPLICATIONS

Edema secondary to chronic renal failure, nephrotic syndrome, amyloidosis, refractory pulmonary edema, pulmonary edema secondary to congestive heart failure, equine Cushing's disease, dilated cardiomyopathy, hypertrophic cardiomyopathy, hydrothorax, pericardial effusion and ascites secondary to hepatic and cardiac failure or disease.

EXPLANATION

Zhen Wu Tang (True Warrior Decoction) is one of the main formulas for treating water accumulation caused by Spleen and Kidney yang deficiencies. The Spleen and Kidney are two very important organs involved in water metabolism. The Spleen is responsible for transforming and transporting water, while the Kidney is responsible for eliminating water. If the yang of these two organs is deficient, the body cannot maintain normal water

***Zhen Wu Tang* (True Warrior Decoction)**

Diagnosis	Clinical Signs	Treatment	Herbs
Spleen and Kidney yang deficiencies with water accumulation	• Dysuria, oliguria: stagnant water circulation • Cyanosis, edema of the limbs, coughing, dyspnea, and abdominal distention: accumulation of dampness and water • Abdominal pain, loose stools or diarrhea: Spleen and Kidney yang deficiencies • Pale to purple tongue and a deep, weak pulse: damp and cold condition	• Warms the yang and regulates water	• *Fu Zi* (Radix Aconiti Lateralis Praeparata) warms Spleen and Kidney yang. • *Fu Ling* (Poria) strengthens the Spleen, induces urination, and dispels water accumulation. • *Sheng Jiang* (Rhizoma Zingiberis Recens) warms the body, dispels cold, and disperses water accumulation. • *Bai Zhu* (Rhizoma Atractylodis Macrocephalae) strengthens the Spleen and dries dampness. • *Bai Shao* (Radix Paeoniae Alba) relieves pain, and balances and prevents the warm herbs from injuring yin.

Zhēn Wǔ Tāng (True Warrior Decoction)

metabolism. If water and dampness accumulate in the body, they will overflow to the skin and muscles causing swelling, pain, and heavy sensations in the limbs. If water and dampness block the normal rising of yang qi, lethargy and mental dullness can manifest. If water and dampness travel downward, loose stools or diarrhea may occur. Since the water circulation is stagnant, urinary difficulty may also occur.

Fu Zi (Radix Aconiti Lateralis Praeparata), the chief herb in this formula, warms the Spleen and Kidney to raise the yang. *Fu Ling* (Poria), the deputy herb, strengthens the Spleen, induces urination, and dispels water accumulation. *Sheng Jiang* (Rhizoma Zingiberis Recens) has two main functions: it helps *Fu Zi* (Radix Aconiti Lateralis Praeparata) warm the body to dispel cold, and it assists *Fu Ling* (Poria) to disperse and dispel water. *Bai Zhu* (Rhizoma Atractylodis Macrocephalae), the assistant herb, strengthens the Spleen and dries dampness to promote the Spleen's transformation functions. *Bai Shao* (Radix Paeoniae Alba), in addition to preventing the acrid, warm herbs in this formula from injuring yin, also relieves abdominal pain.

This formula may also be used to treat *taiyang* disorder in which the exterior condition remains after sweating. As a result of sweating, yin and body fluids are both damaged, leading to palpitations, vertigo, and muscle twitching.

VETERINARY MODIFICATIONS

- With cough due to cold and water affecting the Lung, add *Gan Jiang* (Rhizoma Zingiberis), *Xi Xin* (Radix et Rhizoma Asari), and *Wu Wei Zi* (Fructus Schisandrae Chinensis).
- With diarrhea, remove *Bai Shao* (Radix Paeoniae Alba), and add *Gan Jiang* (Rhizoma Zingiberis).
- With vomiting, remove *Fu Zi* (Radix Aconiti Lateralis Praeparata) and add a larger dose of *Sheng Jiang* (Rhizoma Zingiberis Recens).

CAUTIONS / CONTRAINDICATIONS

Zhen Wu Tang treats water accumulation caused by Spleen and Kidney yang deficiencies. Use of this formula is inappropriate if the water accumulation is caused only by excess condition.

PHARMACOLOGICAL EFFECTS

1. **Circulatory**: Administration of this formula for 22 days was associated with decreased resistance of blood flow, reduced blood viscosity, increased blood perfusion to internal organs, and decreased workload for the heart.[1]
2. **Nephroprotective**: Administration of *Zhen Wu Tang* was associated with beneficial effects in rats with chronic renal failure.[2] In one study of 18 patients with compromised renal functions, use of modified *Zhen Wu Tang* was associated with a reduction of IgA, IgG, IgM, and TF in the urine.[3]

HUMAN CLINICAL STUDIES AND RESEARCH

1. **Cardiac failure**: Administration of modified *Zhen Wu Tang* has been shown to have a beneficial effect in treating cardiac failure. One study used *Zhen Wu Tang* plus *Wu Jia Pi* (Cortex Acanthopanacis), *Dan Shen* (Radix et Rhizoma Salviae Miltiorrhizae), and *Yi Mu Cao* (Herba Leonuri) as the base formula for treating heart failure.[4] Another study used *Zhen Wu Tang* plus *Tao Ren* (Semen Persicae) and *Hong Hua* (Flos Carthami) as the base formula to treat cardiopulmonary disorder with heart failure.[5]
2. **Hypertension**: One study reported 93% effectiveness using *Zhen Wu Tang* with *Fang Ji Fu Ling Tang* (Stephania and Poria Decoction) to treat 63 patients with hypertension characterized by yang deficiency.[6]
3. **Nephritis**: One study reported 80% effectiveness using modified *Zhen Wu Tang* to treat 30 patients with nephritis with edema. The study reported increased urination after an average of 17 days, and relief of edema after an average of 57 days.[7]
4. **Chronic renal failure**: *Zhen Wu Tang* has been reported in several studies to have beneficial effects in treating chronic renal failure. According to one study, use of modified *Zhen Wu Tang* in 12 patients with chronic renal failure was associated with remission in 3 cases, marked improvement in 5 cases, moderate improvement in 2 cases, and no effect in 2 cases.[8] In another study, use of modified *Zhen Wu Tang* was associated with 94.4% success in treating chronic renal disorder characterized by Kidney yang deficiency. Of 18 patients, the study reported remission of all symptoms in 8 cases, partial remission of symptoms in 9 cases, and no effect in 1 case.[9]

SUGGESTED ACUPUNCTURE TREATMENT

1. Points: *Shenshu* (BL 23), *Mingmen* (GV 4), *Guanyuan* (CV 4), *Pishu* (BL 20), *Housanli* (ST 36), *Zhangmen* (LR 13), and *Shuifen* (CV 9).
2. Technique: tonification with moxibustion.

Because yang deficiency is the underlying problem, the priority is to tonify Spleen and Kidney yang. In addition, supportive treatment is needed to relieve water accumulation. *Shenshu* (BL 23), *Mingmen* (GV 4), and *Guanyuan* (CV 4) tonify Kidney yang, while *Pishu* (BL 20) and *Housanli* (ST 36) tonify Spleen yang. *Zhangmen* (LR 13), the *mu* (collecting) point of the Spleen, tonifies Spleen qi and relieves abdominal pain. *Shuifen* (CV 9) regulates the water passages to promote diuresis. Finally, moxibustion

Zhēn Wǔ Tāng (True Warrior Decoction)

may be used to tonify yang and reinforce the acupuncture treatment.

AUTHORS' COMMENTS

Zhen Wu Tang is one of the best formulas for treating edema or excess water retention due to Spleen and Kidney yang deficiencies. This is one of the most commonly used formulas in veterinary medicine for the treatment of pulmonary edema associated with heart failure due to Spleen, Kidney and Heart yang deficiencies. This is also true for concurrent renal and cardiac failure. *Zhen Wu Tang* is effective and can be safely used with conventional diuretics. Therapy with this formula should begin at the lowest therapeutic dose, especially if used in combination with conventional diuretics, and gradually increased as needed. It should be noted that the sole use of Chinese herbal medicine to treat advanced or complicated cases of pulmonary edema and cardiac disease is neither common nor recommended. In general, the integrated management of cardiac disease using conventional and Chinese medicine has been found to be superior to using one system of medicine alone.

In the treatment of refractory pulmonary edema, *Zhen Wu Tang* must be modified and/or combined with other formulas to effectively treat the edema. It may be combined with *Ting Li Da Zao Xie Fei Tang* (Descurainia and Jujube Decoction to Drain the Lung) or *Dao Shui Fu Ling Tang* (Poria Decoction to Drain Water). Use modified *Zhen Wu Tang* by replacing *Sheng Jiang* (Rhizoma Zingiberis Recens) with *Gan Jiang* (Rhizoma Zingiberis) and adding *Rou Gui* (Cortex Cinnamomi), *Ren Shen* (Radix et Rhizoma Ginseng), *Ting Li Zi* (Semen Descurainiae seu Lepidii), *Huang Qi* (Radix Astragali), *Zhu Ling* (Polyporus), *Ze Xie* (Rhizoma Alismatis), *Yi Mu Cao* (Herba Leonuri) and *Dan Shen* (Radix et Rhizoma Salviae Miltiorrhizae). Once the edema is under control, the warming herbs may be discontinued and the remainder of the formula can be modified and given longer term. *Zhen Wu Tang* is a branch (edema, fluid accumulation) formula; it is not suitable for long-term use without appropriate modification.

Zhen Wu Tang is the formula of choice for dogs with pulmonary edema due to Heart and Kidney and/or Spleen yang deficiency; however, it is not the first choice for cats. The control and resolution of pulmonary edema in cats should first be attempted using herbal diuretic formulas that do not contain *Fu Zi* (Radix Aconiti Lateralis Praeparata) before using one that does. This is because cats are more sensitive to the effects of *Fu Zi* (Radix Aconiti Lateralis Praeparata) than dogs. *Fu Zi* (Radix Aconiti Lateralis Praeparata) is a medicinal herb with hot property. It is speculated that the feline sensitivity to this herb may be in part be due to the cat's overall fire constitution as a species as well as due to differences in the metabolism of aconite by cats compared to other animals. For pulmonary edema in cats, it is recommended to use *Ling Gui Zhu Gan Tang* (Poria, Cinnamon Twig, Atractylodes Macrocephala, and Licorice Decoction), which is similar to *Zhen Wu Tang*. It is not as strong in warming yang and moving water as *Zhen Wu Tang*, as it contains only *Gui Zhi* (Ramulus Cinnamomi) instead of *Fu Zi* (Radix Aconiti Lateralis Praeparata), but it is a safer choice initially to begin therapy of pulmonary edema in cats. Other choices to treat pulmonary edema and hydrothorax in cats include the combination of *Wu Ling San* and *Wu Pi San* (Five-Peel Powder) or *Dao Shui Fu Ling Tang* (Poria Decoction to Drain Water). For the treatment of severe edema or refractory edema in the feline, it may be necessary to use *Zhen Wu Tang* at a low dose in combination with other herbal formula just as in dogs. For the treatment of cardiomyopathy (dilated cardiomyopathy in dogs and hypertrophic cardiomyopathy in cats), *Zhen Wu Tang* will need to be further modified or additional formulas added to treat yin deficiency, arrhythmias and blood stagnation that are typically present in this disease.

Zhen Wu Tang can be an effective formula in the treatment of equine Cushing's disease. A common pattern in these animals is a primary Kidney yang deficiency that leads to a cold invasion, subsequent Spleen yang deficiency, and the common presentation is fat accumulation in the neck and suborbital space, pendulous belly, long hair coat, and pain in the front feet. Though this formula would need to be used primarily as an adjunct for dysfunctions of water metabolism, it can be successfully combined with formulas such as *You Gui Wan* (Restore the Right [Kidney] Pill) and *Si Ni Tang* (Frigid Extremities Decoction) for herbal treatment.

References

1. *Zhong Xi Yi Jie He Za Zhi* (Journal of Integrated Chinese and Western Medicine), 1988; 8(8):457.
2. *Zhong Guo Yi Yao Bao* (Chinese Journal of Medicine and Medicinals), 1991; 6(4):46.
3. *Zhong Yi Fang Ji Xian Dai Yan Jiu* (Modern Study of Medical Formulas in Traditional Chinese Medicine), 1997; 1453.
4. *Shi Yong Zhong Xi Yi Jie He Za Zhi* (Practical Journal of Integrated Chinese and Western Medicines), 1995; 7:443.
5. *Zhong Ji Yi Kan* (Medium Medical Journal), 1990; 3:30.
6. *Shan Xi Zhong Yi* (Shanxi Chinese Medicine), 1983; 2:6.
7. *Zhong Yi Za Zhi* (Journal of Chinese Medicine), 1981; 11:835
8. *Zhong Guo Zhong Yi Yao Xue Bao* (Chinese Journal of Chinese Medicine and Herbology), 1991; 4:10.
9. *Zhong Yi Ming Fang Lin Chuang Xin Yong* (Contemporary Clinical Applications of Classic Chinese Formulas), 2001; 4:46.

Shí Pí Săn (Bolster the Spleen Powder)

實脾散
实脾散

Pinyin Name: *Shi Pi San*
Literal Name: Bolster the Spleen Decoction
Original Source: *Chong Ding Ji Sheng Fang* (Revised Formulas to Aid the Living)

COMPOSITION

Fu Zi (Radix Aconiti Lateralis Praeparata), *pao* (blast-fried)	30g [6g]
Gan Jiang (Rhizoma Zingiberis), *pao* (blast-fried)	30g [6g]
Fu Ling (Poria)	30g [6g]
Bai Zhu (Rhizoma Atractylodis Macrocephalae)	30g [6g]
Mu Gua (Fructus Chaenomelis)	30g [6g]
Hou Po (Cortex Magnoliae Officinalis), *chao* (dry-fried) with ginger	30g [6g]
Mu Xiang (Radix Aucklandiae), do not expose to heat	30g [6g]
Bing Lang (Semen Arecae)	30g [6g]
Cao Guo (Fructus Tsaoko)	30g [6g]
Zhi Gan Cao (Radix et Rhizoma Glycyrrhizae Praeparata cum Melle)	15g [3g]

DOSAGE / PREPARATION / ADMINISTRATION

The source text instructs to grind the ingredients into a coarse powder. Cook 12g of the powder with 5 slices of *Sheng Jiang* (Rhizoma Zingiberis Recens) and 1 piece of *Da Zao* (Fructus Jujubae) in 1.5 bowls of water until the liquid is reduced to 70% volume. Take the warm, strained decoction any time during the day. Today, this formula may be prepared as a decoction with the doses suggested in brackets.

CHINESE THERAPEUTIC ACTIONS

1. Warms yang and strengthens the Spleen
2. Activates qi and promotes water circulation

CLINICAL MANIFESTATIONS

Yin shui (yin edema) due to Spleen and Kidney yang deficiencies: severe pitting edema of the lower limbs, cold ears, extremities and paws, absence of thirst, chest and abdominal fullness and distention, borborygmus, loose stools with undigested food, and chronic diarrhea. There may be a thick, greasy tongue coating and a deep, slow pulse.

VETERINARY CLINICAL APPLICATIONS

Peripheral edema, edema and fluid accumulation secondary to renal disease, chronic renal failure, glomerulonephritis, congestive heart failure, and ascites from liver failure, cirrhosis or cancer.

EXPLANATION

Shi Pi San (Bolster the Spleen Powder) is commonly used to treat *yin shui* (yin edema) due to Spleen and Kidney yang deficiencies. According to traditional Chinese medicine theory, the Spleen transforms and transports water. If Spleen yang becomes deficient and cannot carry out its normal functions, water and dampness accumulates, leading to edema in the lower limbs. Accumulation of water and dampness will affect qi circulation, leading to chest and abdominal fullness and distention. Moreover, the deficient Spleen yang will not be able to warm the body, causing cold ears, lumbar region, extremities and paws. Loose stools or diarrhea reflects Spleen and Kidney yang deficiencies and failure of yang to disperse the water upward. A thick, greasy tongue coating indicates damp accumulation. A deep, slow pulse indicates Spleen and Kidney yang deficiencies.

This formula uses *Fu Zi* (Radix Aconiti Lateralis Praeparata) and *Gan Jiang* (Rhizoma Zingiberis) to warm Spleen and Kidney yang, activate water circulation, and relieve edema. *Fu Ling* (Poria) and *Bai Zhu* (Rhizoma Atractylodis Macrocephalae) tonify the Spleen and dispel dampness via urination. *Mu Gua* (Fructus Chaenomelis) awakens the Spleen, dissolves dampness, and eliminates water accumulation. *Hou Po* (Cortex Magnoliae Officinalis), *Mu Xiang* (Radix Aucklandiae), *Bing Lang* (Semen Arecae), and *Cao Guo* (Fructus Tsaoko) activate qi, regulate water circulation, and dissolve dampness. *Zhi Gan Cao* (Radix et Rhizoma Glycyrrhizae Praeparata cum Melle), *Sheng Jiang* (Rhizoma Zingiberis Recens), and *Da Zao* (Fructus Jujubae) tonify the Spleen and harmonize the herbs in this formula.

Shí Pí Săn (Bolster the Spleen Powder)

***Shi Pi San* (Bolster the Spleen Powder)**

Diagnosis	Clinical Signs	Treatment	Herbs
Yin shui (yin edema) due to Spleen and Kidney yang deficiencies	• Severe edema in the lower half of the body: yang deficiency unable to regulate water circulation • Loose stools or chronic diarrhea: yang deficiency unable to disperse the water upward • Cold ears, extremities and paws: yang deficiency unable to warm • Thick, greasy tongue coating: damp accumulation • Deep, slow pulse: Spleen and Kidney yang deficiencies	• Warms yang and strengthens the Spleen • Activates qi and promotes water circulation	• *Fu Zi* (Radix Aconiti Lateralis Praeparata) and *Gan Jiang* (Rhizoma Zingiberis) warm Spleen and Kidney yang. • *Fu Ling* (Poria) and *Bai Zhu* (Rhizoma Atractylodis Macrocephalae) tonify the Spleen and dispel dampness. • *Mu Gua* (Fructus Chaenomelis) awakens the Spleen, dissolves dampness, and eliminates water accumulation. • *Hou Po* (Cortex Magnoliae Officinalis), *Mu Xiang* (Radix Aucklandiae), *Bing Lang* (Semen Arecae), and *Cao Guo* (Fructus Tsaoko) activate qi, regulate water circulation, and dissolve dampness. • *Zhi Gan Cao* (Radix et Rhizoma Glycyrrhizae Praeparata cum Melle), *Sheng Jiang* (Rhizoma Zingiberis Recens), and *Da Zao* (Fructus Jujubae) tonify the Spleen and harmonize the herbs.

VETERINARY MODIFICATIONS

- With loose stools, add *Da Fu Pi* (Pericarpium Arecae).
- With lethargy due to qi deficiency, add *Dang Shen* (Radix Codonopsis), *Bai Zhu* (Rhizoma Atractylodis Macrocephalae), and *Huang Qi* (Radix Astragali).
- With severe swelling and edema, and decreased urinary output, add *Zhu Ling* (Polyporus), *Ze Xie* (Rhizoma Alismatis) and *Gui Zhi* (Ramulus Cinnamomi).

CAUTIONS / CONTRAINDICATIONS

Shi Pi San treats edema due to deficiency. It is inappropriate for edema characterized by an excess condition.

HUMAN CLINICAL STUDIES AND RESEARCH

Hydramnios: Use of *Shi Pi San* was associated with 93% effectiveness in treating hydramnios. Of 18 patients, the study reported complete recovery in 16 cases and no effect in 2 cases.[1]

SUGGESTED ACUPUNCTURE TREATMENT

1. Points: *Pishu* (BL 20), *Housanli* (ST 36), *Yinlingquan* (SP 9), *Shenshu* (BL 23), *Taixi* (KI 3), *Qihai* (CV 6), *Shuifen* (CV 9), *Neiguan* (PC 6), *Tianshu* (ST 25) and *Qihaishu*.
2. Technique: tonification and moxibustion.

The main treatment objectives are to tonify Spleen and Kidney yang and strengthen Spleen qi. Supportive treatments are required as well, such as inducing diuresis and regulating qi circulation. *Pishu* (BL 20), *Housanli* (ST 36), and *Yinlingquan* (SP 9) strengthen the Spleen, harmonize the middle *jiao*, and promote diuresis. *Shenshu* (BL 23) and *Taixi* (KI 3) nourish Kidney yin and warm Kidney yang. Moxibustion on *Qihai* (CV 6) tonifies yang to activate qi. *Shuifen* (CV 9) regulates the water passages, which in turn promotes diuresis and relieves edema. *Neiguan* (PC 6) and *Tianshu* (ST 25) regulate qi to relieve fullness of the chest and abdomen. *Qihaishu* is a classical equine point used to tonify the Spleen.

AUTHORS' COMMENTS

Because the main emphasis of *Shi Pi San* is to strengthen the Spleen to activate qi and regulate water metabolism, it is translated as "Bolster the Spleen Powder."

Zhen Wu Tang (True Warrior Decoction) and *Shi Pi San* have similar functions and compositions. Both formulas contain herbs that warm Spleen and Kidney yang to facilitate water circulation and elimination.

- *Zhen Wu Tang* is best at warming and strengthening Kidney yang and is used primarily to treat water accumulation due to Kidney and Heart yang deficiencies. It is better at treating pulmonary edema and hydrothorax from cardiac disease than *Shi Pi San*.
- *Shi Pi San* focuses on tonifying Spleen yang and is used mainly to treat water accumulation with clinical signs of poor appetite, chronic diarrhea with undigested food, pitting edema of the lower extremities, and ascites.

Reference

1. *Si Chuan Zhong Yi* (Sichuan Chinese Medicine), 1995; 7:36.

Chapter 16 — Summary

— Damp-Dispelling Formulas

SECTION 1: DAMP-DRYING AND STOMACH-HARMONIZING FORMULAS

Name	Similarities	Differences
Ping Wei San (Calm the Stomach Powder)	Dry dampness, strengthen the Spleen and Stomach	Base formula that dries dampness in the middle *jiao*
Xiang Sha Ping Wei San (Cyperus and Amomum Powder to Calm the Stomach)		Stronger effect to activate qi circulation and unblock qi stagnation
Bu Huan Jin Zheng Qi San (Rectify the Qi Powder Worth More than Gold)		Stronger effect to dispel dampness and regulate qi
Fu Ling Yin (Poria Decoction)		Dispels dampness and phlegm
Huo Xiang Zheng Qi San (Agastache Powder to Rectify the Qi)	Dispel interior dampness, relieve acute onset of nausea and vomiting	Releases exterior wind-cold
Liu He Tang (Harmonize the Six Decoction)		Strengthens the Spleen and Stomach, harmonizes the middle *jiao*

Ping Wei San (Calm the Stomach Powder) dries dampness, strengthens the Spleen, activates qi circulation, and harmonizes the Stomach. This is the main formula for treating damp accumulation in the Spleen and Stomach. Epigastric and abdominal bloating is the main clinical manifestation. Animals may present with a thin, white, greasy tongue coating.

Xiang Sha Ping Wei San (Cyperus and Amomum Powder to Calm the Stomach) and ***Bu Huan Jin Zheng Qi San*** (Rectify the Qi Powder Worth More than Gold) are both modifications of *Ping Wei San* (Calm the Stomach Powder). These three formulas have similar functions to dry dampness, strengthen the Spleen and Stomach, activate qi and blood circulation, and promote digestion. All have excellent functions to treat damp accumulation in the Spleen and Stomach with clinical signs such as indigestion, abdominal pain, nausea, vomiting, and diarrhea.

- *Xiang Sha Ping Wei San* has a stronger function to activate qi circulation and unblock qi stagnation.
- *Bu Huan Jin Zheng Qi San* has a stronger effect to dispel dampness and regulate qi.

Fu Ling Yin (Poria Decoction) strengthens the Spleen and Stomach, harmonizes the middle *jiao*, and dispels phlegm and dampness. It treats damp-phlegm accumulation with excessive gas and bloating, no appetite, inability to eat due to excessive gas in the stomach, belching, nausea, and mild resistance in the epigastric region upon palpation.

Huo Xiang Zheng Qi San (Agastache Powder to Rectify the Qi) and ***Liu He Tang*** (Harmonize the Six Decoction) have similar functions of treating acute cases of dampness affecting the interior, with acute onset of nausea and vomiting.

- *Huo Xiang Zheng Qi San* releases exterior wind-cold, dispels dampness, regulates qi, and harmonizes the middle *jiao*. It treats exterior wind-cold with interior dampness, causing clinical signs such as fever, vomiting, diarrhea, and epigastric or abdominal pain.
- *Liu He Tang* dissolves summer-dampness, strengthens the Spleen, and harmonizes the middle *jiao*. It mainly treats improper diet consumed during the summertime, leading to damp accumulation in the middle *jiao* affecting the normal transportation and transformation functions of the Spleen and Stomach. Clinical manifestations include fever, nausea, vomiting, borborygmus, and diarrhea.

Chapter 16 — Summary

SECTION 2: HEAT-CLEARING AND DAMP-DISPELLING FORMULAS

Name	Similarities	Differences
Yin Chen Hao Tang (Artemisia Scoparia Decoction)	Clear damp-heat, relieve jaundice	Principal formula for damp-heat jaundice
Yin Chen Wu Ling San (Artemisia Scoparia and Five-Ingredient Powder with Poria)		Relieves urinary difficulty
San Ren Tang (Three-Nut Decoction)	Clear damp-heat	Stronger effect to dispel dampness
Gan Lu Xiao Du Dan (Sweet Dew Special Pill to Eliminate Toxins)		Stronger effect to clear heat and eliminate toxins
Ba Zheng San (Eight-Herb Powder for Rectification)	Clear damp-heat in the lower *jiao*	Clears heat and sedates fire
Wu Lin San (Five-Ingredient Powder for Painful Urinary Dysfunction)		Clears heat and cools the blood

Yin Chen Hao Tang (Artemisia Scoparia Decoction) is the principal formula for treating yang-type jaundice caused by damp-heat. It clears heat, dissolves dampness, and relieves jaundice. Clinical manifestations include yellow discoloration of the skin and sclera, slight abdominal fullness, dysuria, thirst. Animals may present with a yellow, greasy tongue coating, and a deep, rapid pulse.

Yin Chen Wu Ling San (Artemisia Scoparia and Five-Ingredient Powder with Poria) is formulated by adding *Yin Chen* (Herba Artemisiae Scopariae) to *Wu Ling San* (Five-Ingredient Powder with Poria). This formula treats damp-heat jaundice (more heat than dampness) with dysuria.

San Ren Tang (Three-Nut Decoction) and ***Gan Lu Xiao Du Dan*** (Sweet Dew Special Pill to Eliminate Toxins) have similar functions to treat damp-warmth affecting the *qi* (energy) level.

- *San Ren Tang* has a stronger action to dispel dampness than to clear heat. It is mainly used in the beginning stage (*qi* [energy] level) of summer febrile syndrome, with dampness being more predominant than heat. Clinical manifestations include stiffness and pain of the body, reduced appetite, and no thirst.
- *Gan Lu Xiao Du Dan* has more potent effects to dissolve dampness and turbidity, clear heat, and eliminate toxins. This formula treats damp-warmth febrile disorders or epidemic diseases in the beginning stage (*qi* [energy] level) with equal amounts of dampness and heat. Clinical manifestations include fever, lethargy, thirst, scanty, turbid urine, sore throat, yellow discoloration of the skin, vomiting, and diarrhea.

Ba Zheng San (Eight-Herb Powder for Rectification) and ***Wu Lin San*** (Five-Ingredient Powder for Painful Urinary Dysfunction) are two formulas that clear damp-heat in the lower *jiao* to treat *lin zheng* (dysuria syndrome).

- *Ba Zheng San* clears heat, sedates fire, induces urination, and relieves *re lin* (heat dysuria). This is the main formula for *re lin* (heat dysuria) with damp-heat entangling in the lower *jiao,* causing clinical signs of turbid and dark urine, painful urination, lower abdominal pain and distention, dry mouth and throat, scanty drips of urine, or anuria in severe cases.
- *Wu Lin San* clears heat, cools the blood, induces urination, and relieves *xue lin* (bloody dysuria). It is commonly used to treat heat in the Urinary Bladder, leading to urinary difficulty, the presence of blood in the urine, severe pain upon urination, and cloudy urine with possible sandy particles in the urine.

Chapter 16 — Summary

SECTION 3: WATER-REGULATING AND DAMP-RESOLVING FORMULAS

Name	Similarities	Differences
Wu Ling San (Five-Ingredient Powder with Poria)	Regulate water circulation, dispel dampness	Warms yang, releases the exterior
Wei Ling Tang (Calm the Stomach and Poria Decoction)		Harmonizes the Stomach
Zhu Ling Tang (Polyporus Decoction)		Clears heat, nourishes yin
Wu Pi San (Five-Peel Powder)	Regulates water circulation, reduces edema	Strengthens the Spleen, regulates qi circulation
Jiu Wei Bing Lang Jia Wu Fu Tang (Areca Nine Decoction plus Evodia and Poria)	Regulate water circulation, eliminate water accumulation	Disperses qi and blood stagnation, treats water accumulation in the extremities
Fen Xiao Tang (Separate and Reduce Decoction)		Strengthens the Spleen, treats water accumulation in the abdomen and lower extremities
Dao Shui Fu Ling Tang (Poria Decoction to Drain Water)		Strongly drains water accumulation, treats severe water accumulation throughout the body

Wu Ling San (Five-Ingredient Powder with Poria) dispels dampness through diuresis, warms yang, and disperses water fluids. This formula is used in veterinary medicine as a general diuretic for the accumulation of damp and subsequent edema of the limbs and body cavities secondary to weak transportation and transformation function of the Spleen.

Wei Ling Tang (Calm the Stomach and Poria Decoction) combines *Ping Wei San* (Calm the Stomach Powder) with *Wu Ling San* (Five-Ingredient Powder with Poria). It dispels dampness and harmonizes the Stomach to treat accumulation of water and dampness in the interior causing abdominal bloating and edema.

Zhu Ling Tang (Polyporus Decoction) induces diuresis, clears heat, and nourishes yin. It is used for yin deficiency with interlocking of water and heat in the Urinary Bladder with clinical signs such as dysuria, fever, thirst with a strong desire to drink, irritability, and insomnia. This formula can also be used for *xue lin* (bloody dysuria) with characteristics of extremely painful urination with blood, and fullness and pain in the lower abdomen.

Wu Pi San (Five-Peel Powder) is the principal formula used to treat edema of the whole body caused by Spleen deficiency and damp accumulation. This formula eliminates dampness and water, regulates qi, and strengthens the Spleen. Clinical manifestations include edema of the whole body, heaviness of the limbs, no aversion to wind, epigastric and abdominal bloating, shortness of breath, rapid breathing, and dysuria.

Jiu Wei Bing Lang Jia Wu Fu Tang (Areca Nine Decoction plus Evodia and Poria) dispels water accumulation and disperses qi and blood stagnation. It primarily treats qi and blood stagnation accompanied by water accumulation in the extremities (beriberi and pitting edema) and in the chest (congestive heart failure). Clinical manifestations include edema, numbness and weakness of the extremities, fatigue and palpitations.

Fen Xiao Tang (Separate and Reduce Decoction) strengthens the Spleen, activates qi circulation, and regulates water circulation. It is mainly used to treat Spleen deficiency accompanied by severe cases of water accumulation in the abdomen (ascites with drum-like distention in the abdomen) and lower extremities (pitting edema with prolonged presence of pits produced by pressure).

Chapter 16 — Summary

Dao Shui Fu Ling Tang (Poria Decoction to Drain Water) dispels stagnant water, dries dampness, eliminates water from the Lung, and harmonizes the Spleen. It treats severe water accumulation, as seen in cases of nephritis, ascites, edema, congestive heart failure, and dysuria.

SECTION 4: WARM FORMULAS THAT DISSOLVE DAMPNESS

Name	Similarities	Differences
Ling Gui Zhu Gan Tang (Poria, Cinnamon Twig, Atractylodes Macrocephala, and Licorice Decoction)	Warms yang in the middle *jiao*, dispels dampness and phlegm	Warms yang, dispels dampness, resolves *tan yin* (phlegm retention)
Zhen Wu Tang (True Warrior Decoction)	Invigorate the yang, regulate water circulation	Strongly tonifies Kidney yang
Shi Pi San (Bolster the Spleen Powder)		Strongly tonifies Spleen yang

Ling Gui Zhu Gan Tang (Poria, Cinnamon Twig, Atractylodes Macrocephala, and Licorice Decoction) is the main formula for treating *tan yin* (phlegm retention) syndrome. It invigorates yang to disperse phlegm retention, strengthens the Spleen, and dispels dampness. The main clinical manifestations include hypochondriac discomfort, shortness of breath, coughing and palpitations.

Zhen Wu Tang (True Warrior Decoction) and ***Shi Pi San*** (Bolster the Spleen Powder) warm the Spleen, Kidney and Heart, invigorate yang qi, and regulate water circulation. Both formulas treat edema due to yang deficiency.

- *Zhen Wu Tang* is more effective at tonifying Kidney yang with water accumulation. It warms Spleen and Kidney yang to treat stiffness, heaviness and pain of the limbs, abdominal pain, diarrhea, edema of the limbs, urinary difficulty, no thirst. Animals may present with a thin, white tongue coating and a deep pulse. It is frequently used in veterinary medicine to treat congestive heart failure and pulmonary edema due to Kidney and Heart yang deficiencies.
- *Shi Pi San* is stronger at warming the Spleen and activating qi circulation. It can be used for *yin shui* (yin edema) and ascites caused by Spleen yang deficiency.

Chapter 17

— Wind-Damp Dispelling Formulas

祛风湿剂

孙思邈 Sún Sí-Miǎo

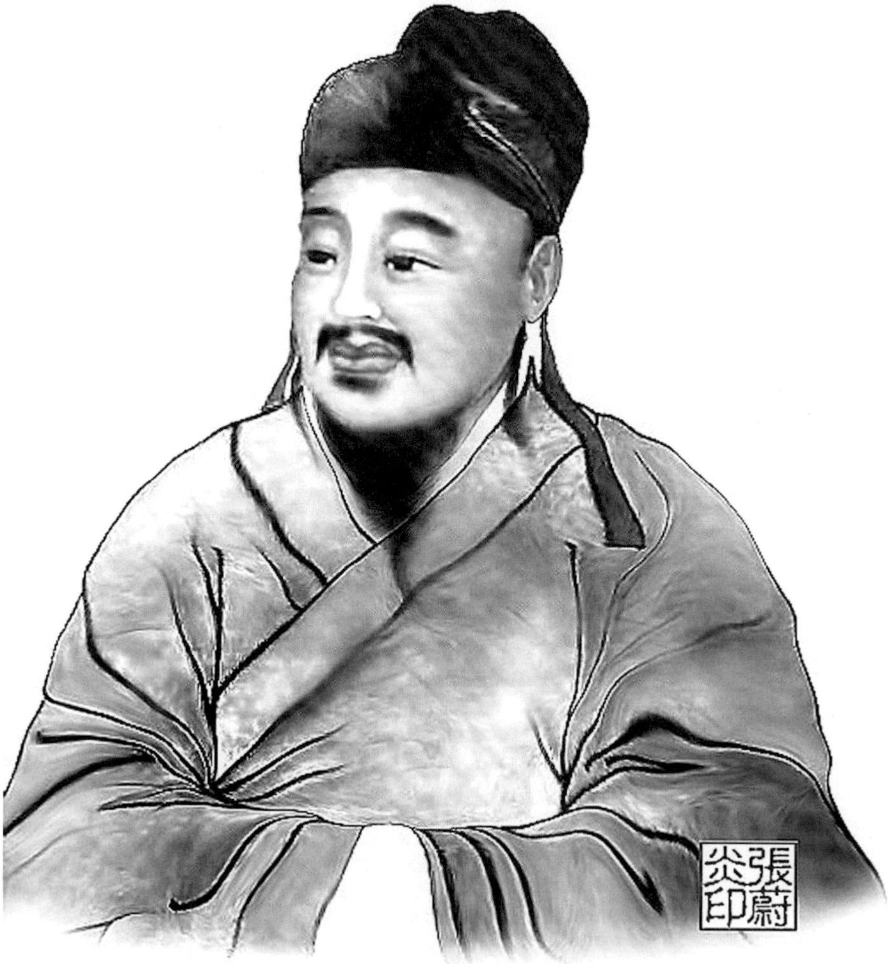

孙思邈 Sún Sí-Miǎo, 581 – 682.

孙思邈 Sún Sī-Miăo

Born into a family mired in poverty and growing up as a chronically ill child, Sun Si-Miao realized the importance of health. He spent over 80 years of his life studying and practicing Traditional Chinese Medicine. Because Sun grew up as a peasant, he treated every patient equally, without regard for or inquiry into their background (whether they were royalty or peasants). Due to his own childhood illness, Sun strongly emphasized the importance of prevention, stating that "superior medicine ***prevents*** disease, and inferior medicine ***treats*** disease." Most importantly, Sun believed that every human life is worth more than a thousand pieces of gold, and expressed his dedication to this concept by incorporating it in naming all his publications.

备急千金要方 *Bei Ji Qian Jin Yao Fang* (Thousands of Golden Prescriptions for Emergencies) is considered to be the first encyclopedia of Traditional Chinese Medicine. It addresses a wide variety of topics, such as internal and external medicine, gynecology, pediatrics, toxicology, diet, *tui-na*, pulse diagnosis, acupuncture, and more. Examples of his remedies are the use of oxen or sheep liver to treat night blindness, and sheep or deer thyroid glands and seaweed to treat goiter. 千金要方 *Qian Jin Yao Fang* (Thousand Ducat Prescriptions) and 千金翼方 *Qian Jin Yi Fang* (Supplement to the Thousand Ducat Formulas) elaborated upon and discussed in great detail all aspects of herbs and herbal formulas, including growing, harvesting, processing and storage of herbs and their uses in treatment. These two texts not only discussed herbal medicine in great detail, but offered great insights in acupuncture as well. Sun documented over 200 extraordinary points, including the discovery of *Shixuan* points and the naming of the *ah shi* point.[1] Sun strongly emphasized the importance of integrating acupuncture and herbs, and stated "[use of] acupuncture without herbs, or herbs without acupuncture, is not an act of a fine physician."

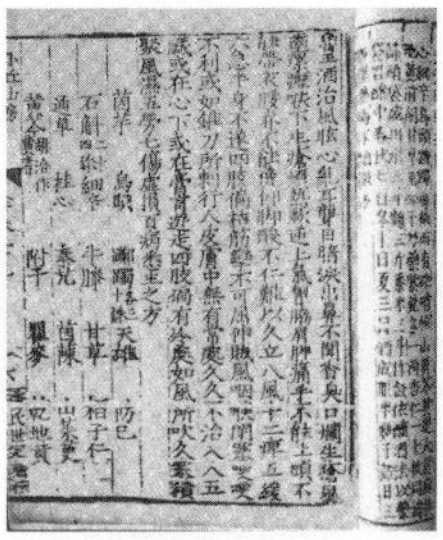

备急千金要方
Bei Ji Qian Jin Yao Fang
(Thousands of Golden Prescriptions for Emergencies) in the middle of the 7th century.

Sun treated many patients in his lifetime, and was most famous for one incident, a story known as "opening the casket to revive the dead." According to legend, Sun encountered a funeral when he was traveling one day. As the family prepared to bury the deceased, Sun looked on and suddenly shouted: "Stop! Stop! This person may still be alive!" The family answered: "She is dead. Do not speak nonsense." Sun replied: "If she is really dead, her blood will clot. However, if you look carefully, there are drops of blood slowly seeping out from the casket. How can you be certain she is dead?" Upon inquiry with the husband, Sun found out that the presumed deceased was a middle-aged woman who was having a difficult labor trying to deliver her first child. Sun immediately lifted the casket lid to treat her with both acupuncture and herbs. After Sun inserted three needles, in *Renzhong* (GV 26), *Zhongwan* (CV 12) and *Zhongji* (CV 3), the woman promptly awakened. After taking an herbal decoction, she safely delivered a healthy baby.

Sun Si-Miao has made enormous contributions to all aspects of medicine and medicinal substances, and is remembered as 药王 the King of Medicine.

Exemplar formulas by Sun Si-Miao include:

- *Wei Rui Tang* (Polygonatum Odoratum Decoction)
- *Wen Pi Tang* (Warm the Spleen Decoction)
- *Dang Gui Jian Zhong Tang* (Tangkuei Decoction to Construct the Middle)
- *Ci Zhu Wan* (Magnetite and Cinnabar Pill)
- *Zhen Zhong Dan* (Pillow Special Pill)
- *Xiao Xu Ming Tang* (Minor Prolong Life Decoction)
- *Du Huo Ji Sheng Tang* (Angelica Pubescens and Taxillus Decoction)
- *Yan Tang Tan Tu Fang* (Salt Decoction to Induce Vomiting)
- *Wei Jing Tang* (Reed Decoction)

Dynasties & Kingdoms	Year
Xia Dynasty 夏	2100-1600 BCE
Shang Dynasty 商	1600-1100 BCE
Zhou Dynasty 周	1100-221 BCE
Qin Dynasty 秦	221-207 BCE
Han Dynasty 漢	206 BCE-220
Three Kingdoms 三國	220-280
Western Jin Dynasty 西晉	265-316
Eastern Jin Dynasty 東晉	317-420
Northern and Southern Dynasties 北南朝	420-581
Sui Dynasty 隋	**581-618**
Tang Dynasty 唐	618-907
Five Dynasties 五代	907-960
Song Dynasty 宋	960-1279
Liao Dynasty 潦	916-1125
Jin Dynasty 金	1115-1234
Yuan Dynasty 元	1271-1368
Ming Dynasty 明	1368-1644
Qing Dynasty 清	1644-1911
Republic of China 中華民國	1912-Present Day
People's Republic of China 中華人民共和國	1949-Present Day

1. When the practitioner palpates a point and the patient exclaims 'ah' in pain, the "*ah shi* point" has been located.

Table of Contents

Chapter 17 — Overview

祛风湿剂 — Wind-Damp Dispelling Formulas

Definition: Wind-damp dispelling formulas target exterior factors (wind-dampness, damp-heat, damp-cold, or damp-phlegm) that attack the superficial parts of the body, block the channels and collaterals, and cause swelling, inflammation, and pain. In addition to dispelling exterior factors, these formulas open the channels and collaterals, relax the tendons and ligaments, and relieve pain. Wind-damp disorders are characterized by clinical signs such as body aches, pain and numbness in the back and stifles, and edema of the extremities.

Wind-damp dispelling formulas are some of the most frequently used in veterinary medicine, as they are commonly used to treat wind-damp disorders characterized by joint pain, pain in the back, neck and stifles and edema of the limbs. Horses are consistently exposed to the environment and often travel from one climate to another. These situations can leave them susceptible to pathogenic invasion of the exterior, which produces the subsequent aches and pains. The environment will also affect dogs, though their coats offer a greater degree of protection. However, outdoor kennels with concrete floors can lead to damp and cold accumulation, as can situations of working in cold weather, as hunting and herding dogs often do. More commonly, older animals present with chronic pain and internal deficiencies that allow pathogens to accumulate. These patients often have been on multiple non-steroidal anti-inflammatory drugs, switching from one to another as the side-effects cause gastrointestinal, liver, or kidney problems. A comprehensive understanding of wind-damp dispelling formulas allows Chinese medicine veterinary practitioners to offer clients and patients solutions for pain management that can help the performance of young animals and the quality of life of geriatrics.

Wind-damp dispelling formulas are frequently used to treat *bi zheng* (painful obstruction syndrome), a condition characterized by stagnation and obstruction that may affect any tissue or organ, causing pain in the muscles, tendons, ligaments, or bones. In addition to affecting any part of the body, exterior wind-damp disorders may be complicated by cold or heat, leading to damp-cold or damp-heat disorders at the exterior. Since exterior wind-damp disorders are frequently associated with stagnation in the channels and collaterals, this condition should be treated by adding blood-activating herbs to wind-damp dispelling formulas. There is a common saying in traditional Chinese medicine: "to treat wind, one must first treat the blood; when the blood moves, the wind will extinguish itself." Chronic, exterior wind-damp disorders may cause animals to become deficient; thus, adding qi-tonifying herbs to these formulas may be necessary in these situations. Furthermore, different types of *bi zheng* do not necessarily occur singularly; rather, several types may occur together. Because there are multiple causes and complications, accurate diagnosis of *bi zheng* is essential for successful treatment.

- *Xing bi* (mobile painful obstruction) is caused by <u>wind</u> attacking the body. Like wind, which is light and mobile, *xing bi* is characterized by pain in the upper body; more specifically, it is characterized by pain that travels from one area to another, or pain that changes in degree and character.
- *Tong bi* (extremely painful obstruction) is characterized by <u>cold</u>. Like cold, which is stationary and constricting, *tong bi* is distinguished by severe pain at a fixed location. This type of pain intensifies with exposure to cold and is relieved by exposure to warmth.
- *Zhuo bi* (fixed painful obstruction) often occurs when <u>dampness</u> affects specific, fixed areas. Like dampness, which is heavy and sinking, *zhuo bi* is characterized by pain and swelling in the lower

Chapter 17 — Overview

extremities. The joint movement is stiff, and this type of pain is not as sharp as that of *tong bi* (extremely painful obstruction).

- *Re bi* (heat painful obstruction) is characterized by local redness, swelling, burning, and pain. The heat is often caused by prolonged obstruction of the channels and collaterals by wind, cold, or dampness. In other cases, patients with a great deal of internal heat, which often arises as a result of a poor diet, are attacked by wind, cold, and dampness.
- *Wan bi* (stubborn painful obstruction) generally occurs after chronic or repetitive injuries to the same area, leading to stiffness, numbness, joint deformity, and reduced mobility.
- *Wei bi* (atrophic painful obstruction) is caused by Liver and Kidney deficiencies, characterized by atrophy, weakness and pain of the muscles and bones.
- *Xue bi* (blood painful obstruction) involves blood disorders, characterized by dull or sharp pain. Dull pain may be caused by a lack of blood to nourish the tendons and bones. Sharp pain, on the other hand, is often related to blood stagnation blocking the channels and collaterals.
- *Zhou bi* (generalized painful obstruction) is characterized by generalized pain in the bones and joints.

SUBCATEGORIES OF ACTION

Wind-damp disorders have multiple causes and complications. Therefore, wind-damp dispelling formulas are divided into four subcategories to delineate the nature of the disorders and the characteristics of the formulas.

1. Wind-Damp Dispelling Formulas

These formulas primarily dispel wind, cold, and dampness at the exterior parts of the body, causing clinical signs such as back pain, stiffness and heaviness of movement, and pain in the extremities.

Commonly used herbs that dispel wind-dampness include *Qiang Huo* (Rhizoma et Radix Notopterygii), *Du Huo* (Radix Angelicae Pubescentis), and *Fang Feng* (Radix Saposhnikoviae). Exemplar formulas are *Qiang Huo Sheng Shi Tang* (Notopterygium Decoction to Overcome Dampness) and *Du Huo Ji Sheng Tang* (Angelica Pubescens and Taxillus Decoction).

2. Damp-Cold Dispelling Formulas

These formulas mainly warm yang and dispel cold and dampness from the exterior parts of the body to treat *bi zheng* (painful obstruction syndrome) characterized by cold, dampness, and pain.

Commonly used herbs include *Zhi Chuan Wu* (Radix Aconiti Praeparata), *Zhi Cao Wu* (Radix Aconiti Kusnezoffii Praeparata), *Fu Zi* (Radix Aconiti Lateralis Praeparata), *Gui Zhi* (Ramulus Cinnamomi), *Ma Huang* (Herba Ephedrae), *Cang Zhu* (Rhizoma Atractylodis), and *Bai Zhu* (Rhizoma Atractylodis Macrocephalae). Exemplar formulas include *Xiao Huo Luo Dan* (Minor Invigorate the Collaterals Special Pill) and *San Bi Tang* (Three-Painful Obstruction Decoction).

3. Damp-Heat Dispelling Formulas

These formulas treat *bi zheng* (painful obstruction syndrome) characterized by heat and dampness, by clearing heat and dispelling dampness at the exterior parts of the body.

Commonly used herbs include *Cang Zhu* (Rhizoma Atractylodis), *Yi Yi Ren* (Semen Coicis), *Zhi Mu* (Rhizoma Anemarrhenae), and *Huang Bo* (Cortex Phellodendri Chinensis). Representative formulas include *Gui Zhi Shao Yao Zhi Mu Tang* (Cinnamon Twig, Peony, and Anemarrhena Decoction) and *Er Miao San* (Two-Marvel Powder).

4. Damp-Phlegm Dispelling Formulas

Formulas in this category dry dampness and eliminate phlegm obstructing the channels and collaterals. Commonly used herbs include *Cang Zhu* (Rhizoma Atractylodis), *Bai Zhu* (Rhizoma Atractylodis Macrocephalae), *Ban Xia* (Rhizoma Pinelliae), and *Tian Nan Xing* (Rhizoma Arisaematis). The sole formula in this category is *Er Zhu Tang* (Two-Atractylodes Decoction).

Chapter 17 — Overview

CAUTIONS / CONTRAINDICATIONS

- Many wind-damp dispelling herbs and formulas are acrid, warm, and drying in nature and may consume yin and blood. Therefore, they should be used with caution in animals with yin and/or blood deficiency.
- Wind-damp dispelling formulas are contraindicated in cases of interior Liver wind rising. The use of wind-damp dispelling formulas that are acrid, warm, and drying will only exacerbate Liver wind conditions.
- Some herbs used in wind-damp dispelling formulas, such as *Zhi Chuan Wu* (Radix Aconiti Praeparata) and *Zhi Cao Wu* (Radix Aconiti Kusnezoffii Praeparata), are extremely hot and potentially toxic and must be used with caution to avoid unwanted adverse effects.

PHARMACOLOGICAL EFFECTS & CLINICAL APPLICATIONS

Wind-damp dispelling formulas primarily treat musculoskeletal disorders. Pharmacologically, these formulas demonstrate remarkable analgesic and anti-inflammatory effects.[1,2,3] Clinical applications include presentations of swelling, inflammation, and pain at various locations throughout the body.

- **Arthritis**: Wind-damp dispelling formulas have been used successfully to treat many different types of arthritis, including, but not limited to osteoarthritis,[4] rheumatic arthritis,[5] gout,[6,7] periarthritis of the shoulders,[8] and many others.[9,10] Exemplar formulas include *Du Huo Ji Sheng Tang* (Angelica Pubescens and Taxillus Decoction), *Xiao Huo Luo Dan* (Minor Invigorate the Collaterals Special Pill), *Er Miao San* (Two-Marvel Powder), and *Juan Bi Tang* (Remove Painful Obstruction Decoction).
- **Neck pain**: According to clinical studies, neck pain can be treated effectively with *Qiang Huo Sheng Shi Tang* (Notopterygium Decoction to Overcome Dampness),[11] *Du Huo Ji Sheng Tang* (Angelica Pubescens and Taxillus Decoction),[12] and *Juan Bi Tang* (Remove Painful Obstruction Decoction).[13]
- **Sciatica**: *Du Huo Ji Sheng Tang* (Angelica Pubescens and Taxillus Decoction) and *Xiao Huo Luo Dan* (Minor Invigorate the Collaterals Special Pill) have been shown to successfully treat sciatica in several clinical studies.[14,15,16]
- **Neurodermatitis:** *Er Miao San* (Two-Marvel Powder) and *Dang Gui Nian Tong Tang* (Tangkuei Decoction to Lift the Pain) have been shown to effectively treat neurodermatitis.[17,18]
- **Musculoskeletal disorders**: Wind-damp dispelling formulas may also be used to treat other conditions characterized by swelling, inflammation, and pain. Clinical applications include hyperosteogeny,[19] prolapse of lumbar intervertebral disk,[20] ankylosing spondylitis,[21,22] and soft-tissue injuries.[23]

References

1. *Zhong Yi Fang Ji Xian Dai Yan Jiu* (Modern Study of Medical Formulas in Traditional Chinese Medicine), 1997; 1466.
2. Lin CC, Chen MF, Chen CF. The anti-inflammatory effects of Chinese crude drug prescriptions on experimental arthritis. Am J Chin Med. 1995; 23(2):145-52.
3. *Zhong Guo Zhong Yao Za Zhi* (People's Republic of China Journal of Chinese Herbology), 1995; 3:159.
4. *Ji Lin Zhong Yi Yao* (Jilin Chinese Medicine and Herbology), 1998; 4:15.
5. *Si Chuan Zhong Yi* (Sichuan Chinese Medicine), 1996; 14(10):38.
6. Chou CT, Kuo SC. The anti-inflammatory and anti-hyperuricemic effects of Chinese herbal formula danggui-nian-tong-tang on acute gouty arthritis: a comparative study with indomethacin and allopurinol. American Journal of Chinese Medicine. 1995; 23(3-4):261-71.
7. *Si Chuan Zhong Yi* (Sichuan Chinese Medicine), 1997; 11:47.
8. *Yun Nan Zhong Yi Za Zhi* (Yunan Journal of Chinese Medicine), 1984; 5(6):63.
9. *Hu Bei Zhong Yi Xue Yuan Xue Bao* (Journal of Hubei University of Medicine), 1993; 2:56.
10. *Shi Yong Zhong Yi Nei Ke Za Zhi* (Journal of Practical Chinese Internal Medicine), 1997; 2:36.
11. *Hu Nan Zhong Yi Za Zhi* (Hunan Journal of Chinese Medicine), 1997; 2:13.
12. *An Hui Zhong Yi Xue Yuan Xue Bao* (Journal of Anhui University School of Medicine), 1995; 14(1):37.
13. *Xin Zhong Yi* (New Chinese Medicine), 1994; 26(10):51.
14. *Zhong Yi Han Shou Tong Xun* (Reports of Chinese Medicine), 1989; 2:42.
15. *Shi Yong Zhong Yi Yao Za Zhi* (Journal of Practical Chinese Medicine and Medicinals), 1996; 2:18.

Chapter 17 — Overview

16. *Nei Meng Gu Zhong Yi Yao* (Traditional Chinese Medicine and Medicinals of Inner Mongolia), 1992; 3:24.
17. *Zhong Yuan Yi Kan* (Resource Journal of Chinese Medicine), 1990; 4:12.
18. *Hu Nan Zhong Yi Za Zhi* (Hunan Journal of Chinese Medicine), 1992; 8(4):42.
19. *Guang Xi Zhong Yi Yao* (Guangxi Chinese Medicine and Herbology), 1990; 13(3):38.
20. *Yun Nan Zhong Yi Za Zhi* (Yunan Journal of Chinese Medicine), 1997; 18(6):7.
21. *Shi Yong Zhong Yi Yao Za Zhi* (Journal of Practical Chinese Medicine and Medicinals), 1996; 1:6.
22. *Xin Zhong Yi* (New Chinese Medicine), 1994; 7:24.
23. *Hu Bei Zhong Yi Za Zhi* (Hubei Journal of Chinese Medicine), 1990; 4:44.

Section 1

祛风胜湿剂
— Wind-Damp Dispelling Formulas

Qiāng Huó Shèng Shī Tāng
(Notopterygium Decoction to Overcome Dampness)
羌活勝濕湯
羌活胜湿汤

Pinyin Name: *Qiang Huo Sheng Shi Tang*
Literal Name: Notopterygium Decoction to Overcome Dampness
Alternate Names: *Chiang Huo Sheng Shih Tang*, Chiang-huo Dampness-Overcoming Decoction, Notopterygium Damp-Expelling Decoction, Notopterygium and Tuhuo Combination
Original Source: *Nei Wai Shang Bian Huo Lun* (Clarifying Doubts about Injury from Internal and External Causes) by Li Gao in 1247

COMPOSITION

Qiang Huo (Rhizoma et Radix Notopterygii)	3g [6g]
Du Huo (Radix Angelicae Pubescentis)	3g [6g]
Fang Feng (Radix Saposhnikoviae)	1.5g [3g]
Gao Ben (Rhizoma et Radix Ligustici)	1.5g [3g]
Chuan Xiong (Rhizoma Chuanxiong)	1.5g [3g]
Man Jing Zi (Fructus Viticis)	0.9g [2g]
Zhi Gan Cao (Radix et Rhizoma Glycyrrhizae Praeparata cum Melle)	1.5g [3g]

DOSAGE / PREPARATION / ADMINISTRATION
The source text instructions are to grind the ingredients into a coarse powder and cook it with 2 bowls of water until the liquid is reduced to 1 bowl. Take the hot, strained decoction before meals on an empty stomach. Today, this formula may be prepared as a decoction with the doses suggested in brackets.

CHINESE THERAPEUTIC ACTIONS
Dispels wind and eliminates dampness

CLINICAL MANIFESTATIONS
Wind-dampness at the exterior: pain, stiffness and immobility of the shoulders and back, low back pain with difficulty of movement, heaviness of the body, a white tongue coating, and a superficial pulse.

VETERINARY CLINICAL APPLICATIONS
Acute cervical and lower back pain, acute cervical intervertebral disk disease, acute generalized stiffness and joint pain, generalized body pain, limb edema, and acute upper respiratory infection.

EXPLANATION
Qiang Huo Sheng Shi Tang (Notopterygium Decoction to Overcome Dampness) treats wind-dampness at the exterior affecting the muscles. This syndrome may occur when an animal has lived in a damp and humid environment for a long period of time. The wind-damp factor may attack the *taiyang* channels and cause immobility and pain of the shoulders and back. Wind-dampness blocks the circulation and causes qi and blood stagnation, which, in turn, leads to neck pain, heaviness of the body, and low back pain.

This formula uses *Qiang Huo* (Rhizoma et Radix Notopterygii) and *Du Huo* (Radix Angelicae Pubescentis) to dispel wind-dampness from both the upper and lower body, respectively. *Fang Feng* (Radix Saposhnikoviae) and *Gao Ben* (Rhizoma et Radix Ligustici) dispel wind-dampness from

Qiāng Huó Shèng Shī Tāng

(Notopterygium Decoction to Overcome Dampness)

***Qiang Huo Sheng Shi Tang* (Notopterygium Decoction to Overcome Dampness)**

Diagnosis	Clinical Signs	Treatment	Herbs
Wind-dampness at the exterior	• Stiffness and pain in the neck, shoulders and back: wind-damp factor attacking the *taiyang* channels • Cervical pain, body stiffness, and low back pain: wind-dampness obstructing qi and blood circulation	Dispels wind and eliminates dampness	• *Qiang Huo* (Rhizoma et Radix Notopterygii) and *Du Huo* (Radix Angelicae Pubescentis) dispel wind-dampness from both the upper and lower body. • *Fang Feng* (Radix Saposhnikoviae) and *Gao Ben* (Rhizoma et Radix Ligustici) dispel wind-dampness from the *taiyang* channels. • *Chuan Xiong* (Rhizoma Chuanxiong) activates blood circulation and relieves pain. • *Man Jing Zi* (Fructus Viticis) dispels wind and relieves pain. • *Zhi Gan Cao* (Radix et Rhizoma Glycyrrhizae Praeparata cum Melle) harmonizes the herbs.

the *taiyang* channels. *Chuan Xiong* (Rhizoma Chuanxiong) activates blood circulation and relieves pain. *Man Jing Zi* (Fructus Viticis) dispels wind and relieves pain. *Zhi Gan Cao* (Radix et Rhizoma Glycyrrhizae Praeparata cum Melle) harmonizes the herbs in the formula.

VETERINARY MODIFICATIONS

- With stiffness and pain in the head, neck and shoulders, add *Ge Gen* (Radix Puerariae Lobatae) and *Chi Shao* (Radix Paeoniae Rubra).
- With stiffness of the extremities and low back, add *Fang Ji* (Radix Stephaniae Tetrandrae) and *Fu Zi* (Radix Aconiti Lateralis Praeparata).
- With joint inflammation and pain, add *Cang Zhu* (Rhizoma Atractylodis), *Huang Bo* (Cortex Phellodendri Chinensis), and *Yi Yi Ren* (Semen Coicis).
- For arthritis pain, add *Chuan Xiong* (Rhizoma Chuanxiong), *Wei Ling Xian* (Radix et Rhizoma Clematidis), and *Wu Shao She* (Zaocys).

CAUTIONS / CONTRAINDICATIONS

- *Qiang Huo Sheng Shi Tang* contains exterior-releasing herbs to dispel wind-dampness from the exterior. While it is normal to experience mild sweating when taking this formula, profuse sweating should be avoided because it will damage both yin and yang.
- *Qiang Huo Sheng Shi Tang* contains many acrid and warm herbs; thus, it is for acute use only without modification. It should be modified for use long term, or to treat animals with chronic disorders or underlying yin deficiency.
- This formula is contraindicated for aches and pains due to *re bi* (heat painful obstruction), or in animals with underlying yin deficiency.

PHARMACOLOGICAL EFFECTS

1. **Anti-inflammatory**: *Qiang Huo Sheng Shi Tang* given at doses of 2.5 g/kg had marked effect to reduce inflammation.[1]
2. **Antipyretic**: Essential oils of *Qiang Huo Sheng Shi Tang* were shown to have antipyretic effects in mice.[2]

HUMAN CLINICAL STUDIES AND RESEARCH

1. **Edema**: One study reported good results using *Qiang Huo Sheng Shi Tang* to treat edema, with modifications as follows: *Dang Shen* (Radix Codonopsis) and dry-fried *Bai Zhu* (Rhizoma Atractylodis Macrocephalae) for qi deficiency; *Fu Ling Pi* (Cortex Poria), *Ze Xie* (Rhizoma Alismatis), *Che Qian Zi* (Semen Plantaginis), and *Mu Tong* (Caulis Akebiae) for decreased volume and frequency of urination; *Gu Ya* (Fructus Setariae Germinatus), *Mai Ya* (Fructus Hordei Germinatus), dry-fried *Lai Fu Zi* (Semen Raphani), and *Shan Zha* (Fructus Crataegi) for food stagnation; and *Ba Ji Tian* (Radix Morindae Officinalis) and *Yin Yang Huo* (Herba Epimedii) for Kidney yang deficiency. Of 25 patients, urination was increased in all 25 cases within 2 packs of herbs. The edema was resolved in 4 cases within 6 packs of herbs, and in 6 cases within 10-15 packs.[3]
2. **Cervical disorders**: Use of *Qiang Huo Sheng Shi Tang* effectively treated 28 patients with cervical disorders with various clinical presentations. Modifications included the addition of *Gou Qi Zi* (Fructus Lycii) and *Sha Yuan Zi* (Semen Astragali Complanati) for blurred vision; *Qin Jiao* (Radix Gentianae Macrophyllae), *Quan Xie* (Scorpio), and *Wu Gong* (Scolopendra) for muscle stiffness in the face; *Hou Po* (Cortex Magnoliae Officinalis) and *Zi Su Geng* (Caulis Perillae) for difficulties with swallowing; *Dan Shen* (Radix et Rhizoma Salviae Miltiorrhizae), *Jiang Can* (Bombyx Batryticatus), and *Quan Xie* (Scorpio) for numbness of the tongue; *Ren Shen* (Radix et Rhizoma

Qiāng Huó Shèng Shī Tāng

(Notopterygium Decoction to Overcome Dampness)

Ginseng), *Huang Qi* (Radix Astragali), and *Sheng Ma* (Rhizoma Cimicifugae) with hypotension; and *Fu Ling* (Poria), *Ze Xie* (Rhizoma Alismatis), *Che Qian Zi* (Semen Plantaginis), and *Niu Xi* (Radix Achyranthis Bidentatae) with hypertension. Of 28 patients, the study reported complete recovery in 19 cases, marked effect in 5 cases, and no effect in 4 cases.[4]

SUGGESTED ACUPUNCTURE TREATMENT

1. Points: *Fengmen* (BL 12), *Fengchi* (GB 20), *Yaoyangguan* (GV 3), *Yanglingquan* (GB 34), *Sanyinjiao* (SP 6), and *Weizhong* (BL 40).
2. Technique: sedation with moxibustion.

These acupuncture points focus on dispelling wind and dampness from the exterior. *Fengmen* (BL 12) and *Fengchi* (GB 20) are two classic points that dispel wind and expel external pathogenic factors. *Yaoyangguan* (GV 3) warms yang to dispel dampness. *Yanglingquan* (GB 34), the *ba hui* (eight meeting) point dominating the tendons, relieves muscle stiffness and pain. *Sanyinjiao* (SP 6) tonifies blood and regulates blood circulation. *Weizhong* (BL 40) specifically treats lower back pain. Depending on the area of the pain, local points may be selected as well.

AUTHORS' COMMENTS

Qiang Huo Sheng Shi Tang is typically used for healthy young, robust animals that have been outdoors for extended periods of time and prolonged exposure to wind and dampness, without adequate rest. This formula has found application in herding, hunting, dock and other performance and working dogs that by necessity spend long hours in windy and damp conditions. Similar conditions apply for performance horses. These animals are often body clipped for competition, which exposes their exterior to the elements. Blankets can counteract this to some extent, but even these do not cover all the clipped areas and are certainly not used during training. Horses managed this way in cold and damp climates will suffer acute bouts of the various wind-damp etiologies. Animals for which this formula is appropriate will have a white tongue coating and a floating or superficial pulse, as well as a history of recent environmental exposure to wind and dampness.

Qiang Huo Sheng Shi Tang and *Jiu Wei Qiang Huo Tang* (Nine-Herb Decoction with Notopterygium) both contain *Qiang Huo* (Rhizoma et Radix Notopterygii) as the main ingredient, and both treat the presence of wind-dampness at the exterior. Their differences are as follows:

- *Qiang Huo Sheng Shi Tang* dispels wind-dampness and primarily treats stiffness, immobility, and pain in the neck, shoulder and back. It has a greater ability to clear dampness, but does not clear interior heat, when compared to *Jiu Wei Qiang Huo Tang* (Nine-Herb Decoction with Notopterygium).
- *Jiu Wei Qiang Huo Tang* dispels wind, cold, and dampness from the exterior and clears heat from the interior. It mainly treats animals with both exterior and interior conditions, with such clinical signs as fever, chills, mild aches and pains, and thirst.

References

1. *Zhong Yi Fang Ji Xian Dai Yan Jiu* (Modern Study of Medical Formulas in Traditional Chinese Medicine), 1997; 1466.
2. *Zhong Yao Yao Li Yu Lin Chuang* (Pharmacology and Clinical Applications of Chinese Herbs), 1995; 11(4):1.
3. *Zhe Jiang Zhong Yi Za Zhi* (Zhejiang Journal of Chinese Medicine), 1997; 5:206.
4. *Hu Nan Zhong Yi Za Zhi* (Hunan Journal of Chinese Medicine), 1997; 2:13.

Juān Bì Tāng (Remove Painful Obstruction Decoction)

蠲痹湯
蠲痹汤

Pinyin Name: *Juan Bi Tang*
Literal Name: Remove Painful Obstruction Decoction
Alternate Names: *Chuan Pi Tang*, Impediment-Alleviating Decoction, Blockage-Relieving Decoction, Notopterygium and Turmeric Combination
Original Source: *Bai Yi Xuan Fang* (Selected Formulas)

COMPOSITION

Qiang Huo (Rhizoma et Radix Notopterygii)	45g [9g]
Fang Feng (Radix Saposhnikoviae)	45g [9g]
Chi Shao (Radix Paeoniae Rubra)	45g [9g]
Jiang Huang (Rhizoma Curcumae Longae)	45g [9g]
Huang Qi (Radix Astragali), *mi zhi* (fried with honey)	45g [9g]
Dang Gui (Radix Angelicae Sinensis)	45g [9g]
Zhi Gan Cao (Radix et Rhizoma Glycyrrhizae Praeparata cum Melle)	15g [3g]

DOSAGE / PREPARATION / ADMINISTRATION

The source text instructs to grind the ingredients into a coarse powder. Cook 15g of the powder with 5 slices of *Sheng Jiang* (Rhizoma Zingiberis Recens) in 2 bowls of water until the liquid is reduced to 1 bowl. Take the strained decoction while warm. Today, this formula may be prepared as a decoction with the doses suggested in brackets.

CHINESE THERAPEUTIC ACTIONS

1. Tonifies qi
2. Harmonizes the *ying* (nutritive) and *wei* (defensive) levels
3. Dispels wind and dampness

CLINICAL MANIFESTATIONS

Bi zheng (painful obstruction syndrome) caused by wind-dampness and accompanied by deficiencies of *ying* (nutritive) and *wei* (defensive) *qi*: pain in the neck, shoulder, and arm, and numbness of the extremities.

VETERINARY CLINICAL APPLICATIONS

Osteoarthritis, bursitis, periarthritis of the shoulders, elbows and carpus, lower back pain, elbow dysplasia, shoulder dysplasia, cervical intervertebral disk disease, cervical and thoracic spondylosis and neck pain.

EXPLANATION

Juan Bi Tang (Remove Painful Obstruction Decoction) treats *bi zheng* (painful obstruction syndrome) due to deficiencies of *ying* (nutritive) and *wei* (defensive) *qi* with concurrent attack by wind-dampness. It is most effective for pain located in the upper parts of the body, such as the neck, shoulders, front limbs, and elbows. As a result of the underlying deficiency in *ying* (nutritive) and

***Juan Bi Tang* (Remove Painful Obstruction Decoction)**

Diagnosis	Clinical Signs	Treatment	Herbs
Bi zheng (painful obstruction syndrome) caused by wind-dampness at the exterior and deficiencies of *ying* (nutritive) and *wei* (defensive) *qi* in the interior	• Pain in the neck, shoulder, and front limb, and heaviness of the body and extremities: wind-dampness at the exterior • Numbness and weakness: deficiencies of *ying* (nutritive) and *wei* (defensive) *qi*	• Tonifies qi and harmonizes the *ying* (nutritive) and *wei* (defensive) levels • Dispels wind and dampness	• *Qiang Huo* (Rhizoma et Radix Notopterygii) and *Fang Feng* (Radix Saposhnikoviae) dispel wind-dampness and relieve pain. • *Chi Shao* (Radix Paeoniae Rubra) and *Jiang Huang* (Rhizoma Curcumae Longae) activate qi and blood circulation. • *Huang Qi* (Radix Astragali) and *Dang Gui* (Radix Angelicae Sinensis) tonify qi and blood and harmonize the *ying* (nutritive) and *wei* (defensive) levels. • *Zhi Gan Cao* (Radix et Rhizoma Glycyrrhizae Praeparata cum Melle) and *Sheng Jiang* (Rhizoma Zingiberis Recens) harmonize the herbs in the formula.

Juān Bì Tāng (Remove Painful Obstruction Decoction)

wei (defensive) *qi*, patients experience numbness in the extremities, general weakness, and stiffness of the body. Moreover, deficiency of *ying* (nutritive) and *wei* (defensive) *qi* leaves the animal more vulnerable to attack by wind-dampness, a condition characterized by muscle stiffness, aches and pains, muscle spasms and cramps, and difficulty in moving.

In this formula, *Qiang Huo* (Rhizoma et Radix Notopterygii) and *Fang Feng* (Radix Saposhnikoviae) dispel wind-dampness and relieve pain. *Chi Shao* (Radix Paeoniae Rubra) and *Jiang Huang* (Rhizoma Curcumae Longae) activate qi and blood circulation. *Huang Qi* (Radix Astragali) and *Dang Gui* (Radix Angelicae Sinensis) tonify qi and blood and harmonize the *ying* (nutritive) and *wei* (defensive) levels. *Zhi Gan Cao* (Radix et Rhizoma Glycyrrhizae Praeparata cum Melle) and *Sheng Jiang* (Rhizoma Zingiberis Recens) harmonize the herbs in the formula.

VETERINARY MODIFICATIONS

- With muscle aches and pains in the front limbs due to wind-cold-dampness, add *Gui Zhi* (Ramulus Cinnamomi), *Sang Zhi* (Ramulus Mori) and *Wei Ling Xian* (Radix et Rhizoma Clematidis).
- With muscle aches and pains in the hind limbs and lumbar spine, add *Du Zhong* (Cortex Eucommiae), *Niu Xi* (Radix Achyranthis Bidentatae), and *Du Huo* (Radix Angelicae Pubescentis).
- With excessive dampness, add *Cang Zhu* (Rhizoma Atractylodis), *Fang Ji* (Radix Stephaniae Tetrandrae), and *Yi Yi Ren* (Semen Coicis).
- With severe pain due to cold, add *Fu Zi* (Radix Aconiti Lateralis Praeparata).

PHARMACOLOGICAL EFFECTS

Anti-inflammatory: One study reported marked effect using *Juan Bi Tang* at 4-8 g/kg to reduce swelling and inflammation. *Juan Bi Tang*, however, did not show analgesic effect at doses of 4, 8 and 16 g/kg.[1]

HUMAN CLINICAL STUDIES AND RESEARCH

1. **Periarthritis of the shoulders**: In one study of 50 patients with periarthritis of the shoulders, the use of herbs was associated with complete recovery in 34 cases, significant improvement in 10 cases, and moderate improvement in 6 cases. The base formula contained *Juan Bi Tang* plus *Gui Zhi* (Ramulus Cinnamomi) and *Tou Gu Cao* (Caulis Impatientis) as guiding herbs. Modifications were made by adding a larger dose of *Huang Qi* (Radix Astragali) or *Si Jun Zi Tang* (Four-Gentlemen Decoction) for pain affecting the right shoulder; *Dang Gui* (Radix Angelicae Sinensis) or *Si Wu Tang* (Four-Substance Decoction) for pain affecting the left shoulder; *Ge Gen Tang* (Kudzu Decoction) for pain in both the neck and shoulders; *Xiao Chai Hu Tang* (Minor Bupleurum Decoction) for concurrent neck pain; *Huang Qi Gui Zhi Wu Wu Tang* (Astragalus and Cinnamon Twig Five-Substance Decoction) for numbness and weakness of the arms; *Ban Xia Bai Zhu Tian Ma Tang* (Pinellia, Atractylodes Macrocephala, and Gastrodia Decoction) for headaches; and others. The herbs were given in decoction, and most patients had complete recovery after approximately 10-20 packs of herbs.[2]
2. **Neck pain**: Forty-eight patients with neck pain were treated successfully using modified *Juan Bi Tang*. The herbal formula contained *Qiang Huo* (Rhizoma et Radix Notopterygii) 12g, *Fang Feng* (Radix Saposhnikoviae) 12g, *Jiang Huang* (Rhizoma Curcumae Longae) 12g, *Dang Gui* (Radix Angelicae Sinensis) 10g, *Chi Shao* (Radix Paeoniae Rubra) 15g, honey-processed *Huang Qi* (Radix Astragali), and *Zhi Gan Cao* (Radix et Rhizoma Glycyrrhizae Praeparata cum Melle) 8g. Additional modifications were made as needed. The treatment protocol was to cook the herbs in water, and administer the decoction in three equally-divided doses for 20 days per course of treatment. Of 48 patients, the study reported complete recovery in 36 cases, significant improvement in 11 cases, and no effect in 1 case.[3]

SUGGESTED ACUPUNCTURE TREATMENT

1. Points: *Fengmen* (BL 12), *Fengchi* (GB 20), *Waiguan* (TH 5), *Yanglingquan* (GB 34), *Sanyinjiao* (SP 6), *Hegu* (LI 4) and *Housanli* (ST 36).
2. Technique: sedation with moxibustion.

The selection of acupuncture points focuses on dispelling wind and dampness from the exterior. *Fengmen* (BL 12) and *Fengchi* (GB 20) are two classic points to dispel wind and expel external pathogenic factors. *Waiguan* (TH 5) stops pain in the front limbs and can dispel wind and cold. *Yanglingquan* (GB 34), one of the *ba hui* (eight meeting) points dominating the tendons, relieves stiffness and pain. *Sanyinjiao* (SP 6) tonifies blood and regulates blood circulation, and *Housanli* (ST 36) tonifies qi. *Housanli* (ST 36) and *Hegu* (LI 4) used together can disperse pathogens and stop pain, especially when moxa is employed. Depending on the area of the pain, local points may be selected as well.

AUTHORS' COMMENTS

Juan Bi Tang is commonly used to treat elbow and shoulder osteoarthritis and cervical pain due to arthritis, spondylosis and intervertebral disk disease in dogs and cats. In horses, this formula is effective at treating neck pain from

Juān Bì Tāng (Remove Painful Obstruction Decoction)

osteoarthritis or strain, pain of the mid-back and withers area, and mild degenerative joint disease of the front limbs. This formula can be used to treat both acute and chronic disease depending on the formulation used, and it is a good first choice as a pain-management formula if the exact nature of the *bi zheng* (painful obstruction syndrome) involved is difficult to assess.

For geriatric animals with significant Kidney and Liver yin deficiencies and multiple joint osteoarthritis affecting the forequarters and rear quarters, or with generalized spondylosis of the spine or cervical and lumbar intervertebral disk disease, combine this formula with *Du Huo Ji Sheng Tang* (Angelica Pubescens and Taxillus Decoction) to comprehensively treat the upper and lower body. These two formulas can be further modified to improve their analgesic properties by the addition of the single herb *Yan Hu Suo* (Rhizoma Corydalis). This herb can be added to the formula and given in combination with the formulas or put into the animal's food. In cases where the condition is stubborn and the cervical pain is extreme, combine with *Shen Tong Zhu Yu Tang* (Drive Out Blood Stasis from a Painful Body Decoction).

Note: There are several different formulas on the market labeled "*Juan Bi Tang,*" so it important to read what individual herbs are included in each formula in order to determine its appropriate use.

References

1. *Zhong Yao Yao Li Yu Lin Chuang* (Pharmacology and Clinical Applications of Chinese Herbs), 1995; 11:20.
2. *Yun Nan Zhong Yi Za Zhi* (Yunan Journal of Chinese Medicine), 1984; 5(6):63.
3. *Xin Zhong Yi* (New Chinese Medicine), 1994; 26(10):51.

Dú Huó Jì Shēng Tāng (Angelica Pubescens and Taxillus Decoction)

獨活寄生湯
独活寄生汤

Pinyin Name: *Du Huo Ji Sheng Tang*
Literal Name: Angelica Pubescens and Taxillus Decoction
Alternate Names: *Tu Huo Chi Sheng Tang*, Tu-huo and Loranthus Decoction, Pubescent Angelica and Loranthus Decoction, Tuhuo and Taxillus Combination
Original Source: *Bei Ji Qian Jin Yao Fang* (Thousands of Golden Prescriptions for Emergencies) by Sun Si-Miao in the Tang Dynasty

COMPOSITION

Du Huo (Radix Angelicae Pubescentis)	9g
Xi Xin (Radix et Rhizoma Asari)	6g
Fang Feng (Radix Saposhnikoviae)	6g
Qin Jiao (Radix Gentianae Macrophyllae)	6g
Sang Ji Sheng (Herba Taxilli)	6g
Du Zhong (Cortex Eucommiae)	6g
Chuan Niu Xi (Radix Cyathulae)	6g
Dang Gui (Radix Angelicae Sinensis)	6g
Chuan Xiong (Rhizoma Chuanxiong)	6g
Di Huang (Radix Rehmanniae)	6g
Bai Shao (Radix Paeoniae Alba)	6g
Ren Shen (Radix et Rhizoma Ginseng)	6g
Fu Ling (Poria)	6g
Gui Xin (Cortex Rasus Cinnamomi)	6g
Gan Cao (Radix et Rhizoma Glycyrrhizae)	6g

DOSAGE / PREPARATION / ADMINISTRATION

The source text instructs to grind the ingredients into a coarse powder and cook it in 10 cups of water until the liquid is reduced to 3 cups. Take the warm, strained decoction in three equally divided doses. The source text also advises to keep the body warm and to avoid exposure to cold.

CHINESE THERAPEUTIC ACTIONS

1. Dispels wind-dampness
2. Relieves *bi zheng* (painful obstruction syndrome)
3. Nourishes the Liver and Kidney
4. Tonifies qi and blood

CLINICAL MANIFESTATIONS

Chronic *bi zheng* (painful obstruction syndrome) with Liver and Kidney insufficiencies and qi and blood deficiencies: soreness and pain in the lower back and stifles, stiffness with difficult and limited range of motion in the limbs and extremities, aversion to cold and a preference for warmth, a pale tongue with a white tongue coating, and a thin, weak pulse.

VETERINARY CLINICAL APPLICATIONS

Chronic cervical and back pain, osteoarthritis of the spine, hips, stifles, and hocks; spondylosis, thoracic-lumbar intervertebral disk disease, lumbosacral disease, canine hip dysplasia, tears of the anterior cruciate ligament, patellar luxation pain and orthopedic post-surgical recovery.

EXPLANATION

Du Huo Ji Sheng Tang (Angelica Pubescens and Taxillus Decoction) treats *bi zheng* (painful obstruction syndrome) characterized by chronic accumulation of wind, cold, and dampness with Liver and Kidney insufficiencies and qi and blood deficiencies. This syndrome begins with accumulation of wind, cold, and dampness in the channels and collaterals. As they obstruct qi and blood circulation, malnourishment of the Liver and Kidney occurs. If this condition becomes chronic, qi, blood, Liver, and Kidney all become deficient. Thus, besides having aches and pains, the patient may also experience weakness of the knees and lower back, as well as difficulty in moving the limbs and extremities.

Since this condition is complicated by both excess (accumulation of wind, cold, and dampness) and deficiency (of the Liver, Kidney, qi, and blood), optimal treatment

Dú Huó Jì Shēng Tāng (Angelica Pubescens and Taxillus Decoction)

***Du Huo Ji Sheng Tang* (Angelica Pubescens and Taxillus Decoction)**

Diagnosis	Clinical Signs	Treatment	Herbs
Chronic *bi zheng* (painful obstruction syndrome) with excess and deficiency	• Soreness and pain in the lower back and stifles: wind-dampness affecting the muscles • Stiffness with difficult, limited range of motion in the limbs and extremities, aversion to cold and a preference for warmth: qi, blood, Liver and Kidney deficiencies	• Dispels wind-dampness and stops pain • Nourishes the Liver and Kidney • Tonifies qi and blood	• *Du Huo* (Radix Angelicae Pubescentis) and *Xi Xin* (Radix et Rhizoma Asari) dispel wind, cold, and dampness. • *Fang Feng* (Radix Saposhnikoviae) and *Qin Jiao* (Radix Gentianae Macrophyllae) dispel wind-dampness. • *Sang Ji Sheng* (Herba Taxilli), *Du Zhong* (Cortex Eucommiae), and *Chuan Niu Xi* (Radix Cyathulae) dispel wind and dampness and tonify the Liver and Kidney. • *Dang Gui* (Radix Angelicae Sinensis), *Chuan Xiong* (Rhizoma Chuanxiong), *Di Huang* (Radix Rehmanniae), and *Bai Shao* (Radix Paeoniae Alba) tonify and activate blood circulation. • *Ren Shen* (Radix et Rhizoma Ginseng) and *Fu Ling* (Poria) strengthen the Spleen and tonify qi. • *Gui Xin* (Cortex Rasus Cinnamomi) warms the channels and opens the blood vessels. • *Gan Cao* (Radix et Rhizoma Glycyrrhizae) harmonizes the herbs.

requires the use of herbs that concurrently dispel wind, cold, and dampness, as well as herbs that nourish the Liver and Kidney, tonify qi and blood, and relieve pain.

In this formula, a large dose of *Du Huo* (Radix Angelicae Pubescentis) is used to dispel wind, cold, and dampness in the lower parts of the body. *Xi Xin* (Radix et Rhizoma Asari) disperses wind, cold, and dampness and relieves pain. *Fang Feng* (Radix Saposhnikoviae) dispels wind and dampness. *Qin Jiao* (Radix Gentianae Macrophyllae) dispels wind and dampness and soothes the tendons. *Sang Ji Sheng* (Herba Taxilli), *Du Zhong* (Cortex Eucommiae), and *Chuan Niu Xi* (Radix Cyathulae) dispel wind and dampness and also tonify the Liver and Kidney. *Dang Gui* (Radix Angelicae Sinensis), *Chuan Xiong* (Rhizoma Chuanxiong), *Di Huang* (Radix Rehmanniae), and *Bai Shao* (Radix Paeoniae Alba) tonify blood and activate blood circulation. *Ren Shen* (Radix et Rhizoma Ginseng) and *Fu Ling* (Poria) strengthen the Spleen and tonify qi. *Gui Xin* (Cortex Rasus Cinnamomi) warms the channels and opens the blood vessels. *Gan Cao* (Radix et Rhizoma Glycyrrhizae) harmonizes the herbs in the formula.

VETERINARY MODIFICATIONS

- For *tong bi* (extremely painful obstruction) with more cold, add *Fu Zi* (Radix Aconiti Lateralis Praeparata) and *Gan Jiang* (Rhizoma Zingiberis).
- For *zhuo bi* (fixed painful obstruction) with more dampness, remove *Shu Di Huang* (Radix Rehmanniae Praeparata), and add *Fang Ji* (Radix Stephaniae Tetrandrae), *Yi Yi Ren* (Semen Coicis), and *Cang Zhu* (Rhizoma Atractylodis).
- For *xue bi* (blood painful obstruction) with blood stagnation, add *Hong Hua* (Flos Carthami) and *Tao Ren* (Semen Persicae).
- With sore back and painful stifles, add *Qiang Huo* (Rhizoma et Radix Notopterygii) and *Xu Duan* (Radix Dipsaci).
- With severe pain, add *Zhi Chuan Wu* (Radix Aconiti Praeparata), *Zhi Cao Wu* (Radix Aconiti Kusnezoffii Praeparata), *Yan Hu Suo* (Rhizoma Corydalis), *Jin Qian Bai Hua She* (Bungarus Parvus), *Di Long* (Pheretima), and *Hong Hua* (Flos Carthami).
- With muscle weakness, add *Huang Qi* (Radix Astragali) and *Bai Zhu* (Rhizoma Atractylodis Macrocephalae).

CAUTIONS / CONTRAINDICATIONS

- *Du Huo Ji Sheng Tang* should be used with caution during pregnancy.
- This formula is contraindicated in *bi zheng* (painful obstruction syndrome) caused by excess heat or damp-heat.

PHARMACOLOGICAL EFFECTS

1. **Analgesic and anti-inflammatory**: *Du Huo Ji Sheng Tang* has been shown to relieve pain and reduce inflammation in both rats and mice.[1,2]
2. **Anti-inflammatory**: Administration of *Du Huo Ji Sheng Tang* or *Dang Gui Nian Tong Tang* (Tangkuei Decoction to Lift the Pain) was associated with marked anti-inflammatory effects in suppressing the development of chronic

arthritis induced by carrageenan or complete Freund's adjuvant. The researchers suggested that these herbal formulas may be considered as alternatives for non-steroid anti-inflammatory drugs (NSAID).[3]

3. **Circulatory**: One study reported decreased vascular resistance and increased blood perfusion to the brain using *Du Huo Ji Sheng Tang* administered orally or via injection.[4]
4. **Antiplatelet**: *Du Huo Ji Sheng Tang* was shown to have a significant antiplatelet effect in rabbits.[5]

HUMAN CLINICAL STUDIES AND RESEARCH

1. **Neck pain**: Use of modified *Du Huo Ji Sheng Tang* in one study for 1-4 courses of treatment was associated with 97% effectiveness. Of 69 patients, the study reported complete recovery in 41 cases, significant improvement in 20 cases, moderate improvement in 6 cases, and no effect in 2 cases.[6] In another neck pain study, modified *Du Huo Ji Sheng Tang* in 43 patients was associated with significant improvement in 31 cases, improvement in 8 cases, and slight improvement in 4 cases. The herbal treatment contained *Du Huo* (Radix Angelicae Pubescentis), *Dang Shen* (Radix Codonopsis), *Du Zhong* (Cortex Eucommiae), *Sang Ji Sheng* (Herba Taxilli), *Shu Di Huang* (Radix Rehmanniae Praeparata), *Fu Ling* (Poria), *Bai Shao* (Radix Paeoniae Alba), *Qin Jiao* (Radix Gentianae Macrophyllae), *Fang Feng* (Radix Saposhnikoviae), *Gui Zhi* (Ramulus Cinnamomi), *Chuan Niu Xi* (Radix Cyathulae), *Niu Xi* (Radix Achyranthis Bidentatae), *Dang Gui* (Radix Angelicae Sinensis), *Chuan Xiong* (Rhizoma Chuanxiong), *Hong Hua* (Flos Carthami), *Tao Ren* (Semen Persicae), *Yan Hu Suo* (Rhizoma Corydalis), *Xi Xin* (Radix et Rhizoma Asari), and *Gan Cao* (Radix et Rhizoma Glycyrrhizae). In addition, 16 mL of a *Dan Shen* (Radix et Rhizoma Salviae Miltiorrhizae) preparation was given via injection one time daily.[7]
2. **Sciatica**: In one study, use of modified *Du Huo Ji Sheng Tang* in 100 patients with sciatica was associated with recovery in 87 cases, significant improvement in 7 cases, moderate improvement in 3 cases, and no effect in 3 cases.[8] Another study reported significant relief of numbness and pain within 5 packs of modified *Du Huo Ji Sheng Tang* in 65 of 80 patients.[9] Additionally, use of modified *Du Huo Ji Sheng Tang* was associated with complete recovery in 85 of 105 patients who suffered from sciatica due to various causes. The herbal treatment contained this formula plus *Fang Ji* (Radix Stephaniae Tetrandrae), *Hai Tong Pi* (Cortex Erythrinae), *Ru Xiang* (Gummi Olibanum), *Mo Yao* (Myrrha), and others as needed.[10]
3. **Hyperosteogeny**: Thirty patients with hyperosteogeny of the knees were treated with complete recovery in 14 cases, significant improvement in 9 cases, moderate improvement in 4 cases, and no effect in 3 cases. The herbal treatment used *Du Huo Ji Sheng Tang* as the base formula, with the addition of *Fu Zi* (Radix Aconiti Lateralis Praeparata) 10g for increased severity of pain with exposure to cold; and *Jin Qian Bai Hua She* (Bungarus Parvus) 15g and *Wu Shao She* (Zaocys) 15g for chronic illness with limited mobility and altered physical appearance of the joints. The duration of treatment ranged from 2 months to 10 years.[11]
4. **Osteoarthritis**: Use of modified *Du Huo Ji Sheng Tang* in 24 patients with osteoarthritis for 1 week to 3 months was associated with complete recovery in 14 cases, significant improvement in 4 cases, moderate improvement in 3 cases, and no effect in 3 cases. The overall effectiveness was 87.5%.[12] Another study of 262 patients with osteoarthritis of the knees reported 94.7% effectiveness when treated with modified *Du Huo Ji Sheng Tang*. The clinical presentations included swelling, inflammation, and pain of the knees, with occasional deformation of the joint. The herbal treatment contained this formula plus *Wu Gong* (Scolopendra), *Mu Li* (Concha Ostreae), and others. In addition, an herbal paste was also applied topically to the affected areas. Of 262 patients, the study reported significant improvement in 77 cases, moderate improvement in 118 cases, moderate improvement in 55 cases, and no effect in 12 cases.[13]
5. **Rheumatic arthritis**: One study reported a marked effect using *Du Huo Ji Sheng Tang* plus *Si Miao San* (Four-Marvel Powder) to treat rheumatic arthritis of the knees characterized by pain, swelling, inflammation, numbness, decreased range of motion, and difficulty in walking. Of 104 patients, the study reported complete recovery in 84 cases, improvement in 11 cases, and no effect in 9 cases. The overall effectiveness was 91.3%.[14]
6. **Ankylosing spondylitis**: Use of modified *Du Huo Ji Sheng Tang* showed good results in treating 22 patients with a history of 3 months or more of ankylosing spondylitis characterized by stiffness and pain of the lower back. Modifications included the addition of *Gou Ji* (Rhizoma Cibotii) 10g, *Tu Si Zi* (Semen Cuscutae) 10g, and larger doses for *Sang Ji Sheng* (Herba Taxilli), *Du Zhong* (Cortex Eucommiae), and *Xu Duan* (Radix Dipsaci) for severe low back pain; *Bai Jie Zi* (Semen Sinapis) 6g, *San Leng* (Rhizoma Sparganii) 10g, and *E Zhu* (Rhizoma Curcumae) 10g were added for chronic illness with phlegm accumulation. The duration of treatment was 2 months per course of treatment. Of 22 patients, the study reported significant improvement in 6 cases, moderate improvement in 14 cases, and no effect in 2 cases. The overall effectiveness was 90.9%.[15]
7. ***Bi zheng* (painful obstruction syndrome)**: Administration of *Du Huo Ji Sheng Tang* three times daily for 60-90 days

in 52 patients was associated with significant improvement in 35 cases, moderate improvement in 15 cases, and no effect in 2 cases.[16] Another study reported marked effect using modified *Du Huo Ji Sheng Tang* to treat various types of *bi zheng*. The herbal treatment used this formula as the base formula, with the following modifications: *Qiang Huo* (Rhizoma et Radix Notopterygii), *Sang Zhi* (Ramulus Mori), and *Ge Gen* (Radix Puerariae Lobatae) for wind; *Ma Huang* (Herba Ephedrae) and *Xi Xin* (Radix et Rhizoma Asari) for cold; *Yi Yi Ren* (Semen Coicis), *Cang Zhu* (Rhizoma Atractylodis), and *Mu Gua* (Fructus Chaenomelis) for dampness; *Quan Xie* (Scorpio), *Wu Gong* (Scolopendra), and *Jin Qian Bai Hua She* (Bungarus Parvus) for stubborn pain; *Chuan Shan Jia* (Squama Manis), *Tao Ren* (Semen Persicae), and *Hong Hua* (Flos Carthami) for blood stagnation; and *Ren Shen* (Radix et Rhizoma Ginseng) for generalized deficiency due to chronic illness. Of 55 patients, the study reported recovery in 22 cases, improvement in 30 cases, and no effect in 3 cases.[17]

8. **Prolapse of lumbar intervertebral disk**: Use of modified *Du Huo Ji Sheng Tang* was associated with improvement in 46 of 50 patients with prolapse of lumbar intervertebral disk confirmed by physical exam and CT scan. The herbal treatment contained this formula with modifications based on clinical presentations. For dampness and cold, *Fu Zi* (Radix Aconiti Lateralis Praeparata) 20g was added. For damp-heat, *Huang Bo* (Cortex Phellodendri Chinensis) 15g, *Huang Qin* (Radix Scutellariae) 12g, and *Cang Zhu* (Rhizoma Atractylodis) 15g were added, while *Gui Zhi* (Ramulus Cinnamomi), *Xi Xin* (Radix et Rhizoma Asari), and *Di Huang* (Radix Rehmanniae) were removed. For chronic pain with blood stagnation, *Dan Shen* (Radix et Rhizoma Salviae Miltiorrhizae) 20g was added.[18]
9. **Postpartum aches and pains**: One study reported marked results using modified *Du Huo Ji Sheng Tang* to treat 80 women with aches and pains after labor. In addition to this formula, modifications were made by adding *Fu Zi* (Radix Aconiti Lateralis Praeparata), larger doses of *Gui Zhi* (Ramulus Cinnamomi) and *Fang Ji* (Radix Stephaniae Tetrandrae) for wind-cold; *Mu Gua* (Fructus Chaenomelis) and *Cang Zhu* (Rhizoma Atractylodis) for dampness; *Sang Zhi* (Ramulus Mori) and *Jiang Huang* (Rhizoma Curcumae Longae) for pain in the arms and shoulders; and *Niu Xi* (Radix Achyranthis Bidentatae) for pain in the lower body. Of 80 patients, the study reported complete recovery in 58 cases, significant improvement in 14 cases, moderate improvement in 6 cases, and no effect in 2 cases.[19] Note: Information is unavailable regarding whether these individuals were nursing while on the herbal treatment. Please consult additional information on the safety status of each individual herb prior to using them for nursing mothers.

SUGGESTED ACUPUNCTURE TREATMENT

1. Points: *Fengchi* (GB 20), *Dazhui* (GV 14), *Ganshu* (BL 18), *Shenshu* (BL 23), *Zhishi* (BL 52), *Taixi* (KI 3), *Housanli* (ST 36), *Sanyinjiao* (SP 6), *Yaoyangguan* (GV 3), *Weizhong* (BL 40), *Yanglingquan* (GB 34), *Kunlun* (BL 60), and local points. Classical points such as *Shenshu* and *Shenpeng* are also beneficial.
2. Technique: tonification and moxibustion.

Dazhui (GV 14) and *Fengchi* (GB 20) are two classic points that dispel wind and expel external pathogenic factors. *Ganshu* (BL 18), *Shenshu* (BL 23), *Zhishi* (BL 52) and *Taixi* (KI 3) nourish the Liver and Kidney. *Housanli* (ST 36) and *Sanyinjiao* (SP 6) tonify qi, strengthen the Spleen, nourish the blood, and activate blood circulation. *Yaoyangguan* (GV 3) warms yang to dispel cold and dampness. *Weizhong* (BL 40) relieves lower back pain, while *Yanglingquan* (GB 34) relieves muscle stiffness and cramps. *Kunlun* (BL 60) relieves generalized pain and is considered an "aspirin point." *Shenshu* and *Shenpeng* are classical equine points that eliminate cold and warm yang. Local points may be selected to activate qi and blood circulation to relieve pain.

AUTHORS' COMMENTS

Du Huo Ji Sheng Tang is one of the most commonly used formulas in veterinary medicine to treat muscle, joint and spinal pain due to both excess and deficiency. It has found application as a preventative, recovery and direct therapeutic formula with emphasis on the back and rear quarters in veterinary patients. This formula is indicated for chronic *bi zheng* (painful obstruction syndrome) with obstruction of wind, cold, and dampness, accompanied by Liver and Kidney insufficiencies and qi and blood deficiencies; thus, it is a vital formula in the treatment of aging animals. On balance, the formula is more effective at dispersing cold than others in the category and is useful in those *bi zheng* (painful obstruction syndrome) that can be further classified as *tong bi* (extremely painful obstruction). *Du Huo Ji Sheng Tang* can be used as a preventative measure against rupture of the anterior cruciate ligament due to the degeneration of joints, tendons, and ligaments resulting from aging in middle age and geriatric animals or secondary to Kidney deficiencies (yin and *jing* [essence]) in younger animals. *Du Huo Ji Sheng Tang* is an important recovery formula to use in post-surgical spinal and coxofemoral joint patients to improve healing times and prevent further degeneration of the hips, spine and inter-vertebral disks. It is also one of the most effective

Dú Huó Jì Shēng Tāng (Angelica Pubescens and Taxillus Decoction)

formulas for treating non-surgical, chronic back pain in overweight, middle-aged pets, and can be combined with *Shu Jing Huo Xue Tang* (Relax the Channels and Invigorate the Blood Decoction) to increase the analgesic effects. For severe back pain in horses, so called "cold-backed" individuals, the formula can be combined with *Shen Tong Zhu Yu Tang* (Drive Out Blood Stasis from a Painful Body Decoction). *Du Huo Ji Sheng Tang* can also be combined with *Juan Bi Tang* (Remove Painful Obstruction Decoction) to treat generalized multiple joint pain from chronic osteoarthritis.

References

1. *Zhong Cheng Yao Yan Jiu* (Research of Chinese Patent Medicine), 1988; 5:28.
2. *Zhong Cao Yao* (Chinese Herbal Medicine), 1992; 23(3):133.
3. Lin CC, Chen MF, Chen CF. The anti-inflammatory effects of Chinese crude drug prescriptions on experimental arthritis. Am J Chin Med. 1995; 23(2):145-52.
4. *Zhong Yi Fang Ji Xian Dai Yan Jiu* (Modern Study of Medical Formulas in Traditional Chinese Medicine), 1997; 1469.
5. *Zhong Yao Yao Li Yu Lin Chuang* (Pharmacology and Clinical Applications of Chinese Herbs), 1990; 6(6):7.
6. *Zhe Jiang Zhong Yi Za Zhi* (Zhejiang Journal of Chinese Medicine), 1993; 3:134.
7. *An Hui Zhong Yi Xue Yuan Xue Bao* (Journal of Anhui University School of Medicine), 1995; 14(1):37.
8. *Zhong Yi Han Shou Tong Xun* (Reports of Chinese Medicine), 1989; 2:42.
9. *Gui Yang Yi Xue Yuan Xue Bao* (Journal of Guiyang Medical University), 1987; 4:31.
10. *Shi Yong Zhong Yi Yao Za Zhi* (Journal of Practical Chinese Medicine and Medicinals), 1996; 2:18.
11. *Guang Xi Zhong Yi Yao* (Guangxi Chinese Medicine and Herbology), 1990; 13(3):38.
12. *Jiang Su Zhong Yi* (Jiangsu Chinese Medicine), 1993; 3:11.
13. *Ji Lin Zhong Yi Yao* (Jilin Chinese Medicine and Herbology), 1998; 4:15.
14. *Si Chuan Zhong Yi* (Sichuan Chinese Medicine), 1996; 14(10):38.
15. *Shi Yong Zhong Yi Yao Za Zhi* (Journal of Practical Chinese Medicine and Medicinals), 1996; 1:6.
16. *Shan Xi Zhong Yi* (Shanxi Chinese Medicine), 1989; 3:10.
17. *Zhe Jiang Zhong Yi Za Zhi* (Zhejiang Journal of Chinese Medicine), 1998; 4:165.
18. *Yun Nan Zhong Yi Za Zhi* (Yunan Journal of Chinese Medicine), 1997; 18(6):7.
19. *Shi Yong Zhong Yi Yao Za Zhi* (Journal of Practical Chinese Medicine and Medicinals), 1998; 14(4):11.

Sān Bì Tāng (Three-Painful Obstruction Decoction)

三痹湯
三痹汤

Pinyin Name: *San Bi Tang*
Literal Name: Three-Painful Obstruction Decoction
Alternate Names: *San Pi Tang*, Chin-chiu and Tu-huo Decoction, Three Blockage Syndrome Decoction, Tuhuo and Astragalus Combination
Original Source: *Fu Ren Liang Fang* (Fine Formulas for Women) by Chen Zi-Ming in 1237

COMPOSITION

Du Huo (Radix Angelicae Pubescentis)	15g [3g]
Xi Xin (Radix et Rhizoma Asari)	30g [6g]
Qin Jiao (Radix Gentianae Macrophyllae)	15g [3g]
Fang Feng (Radix Saposhnikoviae)	30g [6g]
Gui Xin (Cortex Rasus Cinnamomi)	30g [6g]
Du Zhong (Cortex Eucommiae), *chao* (dry-fried) with ginger juice	30g [6g]
Xu Duan (Radix Dipsaci)	30g [6g]
Niu Xi (Radix Achyranthis Bidentatae)	30g [6g]
Dang Gui (Radix Angelicae Sinensis)	30g [6g]
Chuan Xiong (Rhizoma Chuanxiong)	15g [3g]
Bai Shao (Radix Paeoniae Alba)	30g [6g]
Di Huang (Radix Rehmanniae)	15g [3g]
Huang Qi (Radix Astragali)	30g [6g]
Ren Shen (Radix et Rhizoma Ginseng)	30g [6g]
Fu Ling (Poria)	30g [6g]
Gan Cao (Radix et Rhizoma Glycyrrhizae)	30g [6g]

DOSAGE / PREPARATION / ADMINISTRATION

The source text instructs to grind the ingredients into powder. Cook 15g of the powder with 3 slices of *Sheng Jiang* (Rhizoma Zingiberis Recens) and 1 piece of *Da Zao* (Fructus Jujubae) in 2 bowls of water until it is reduced to 1 bowl. Take the strained decoction while it is warm on an empty stomach. Today, this formula may be prepared as a decoction with the doses suggested in brackets.

CHINESE THERAPEUTIC ACTIONS

1. Tonifies qi and nourishes the blood
2. Dispels wind, cold, and dampness

CLINICAL MANIFESTATIONS

Joint pain due to stagnation of wind, cold, and dampness with underlying qi and blood deficiencies: stiffness, pain, trembling and shaking of the muscles and joints, decreased range of motion, pain that worsens with exposure to cold and damp weather.

VETERINARY CLINICAL APPLICATIONS

Osteoarthritis, general aches and pains in the muscles and joints, aches and pains from viral infection, and trembling and shaking of the legs.

EXPLANATION

San Bi Tang (Three-Painful Obstruction Decoction) treats *bi zheng* (painful obstruction syndrome) characterized by accumulation of wind, cold, and dampness with qi and blood deficiencies. This condition begins with accumulation of wind, cold, and dampness in the channels and collaterals. As these pathogens block qi and blood circulation, they cause malnourishment of the muscles and tendons in the limbs, resulting in stiffness and pain with decreased range of motion. The pain is intensified with exposure to cold and damp weather.

This formula contains *Du Huo* (Radix Angelicae Pubescentis) and *Xi Xin* (Radix et Rhizoma Asari) to dispel wind, eliminate dampness, relieve pain, and alleviate *bi zheng* (painful obstruction syndrome). *Qin Jiao* (Radix Gentianae Macrophyllae) and *Fang Feng* (Radix Saposhnikoviae) dispel wind and eliminate dampness. *Gui Xin* (Cortex Rasus Cinnamomi) warms the body and dispels cold. *Du Zhong* (Cortex Eucommiae), *Xu Duan* (Radix Dipsaci), and *Niu Xi* (Radix Achyranthis Bidentatae) tonify the Kidney and strengthen bones and tendons. *Dang Gui* (Radix Angelicae Sinensis), *Chuan Xiong* (Rhizoma

Sān Bì Tāng (Three-Painful Obstruction Decoction)

***San Bi Tang* (Three-Painful Obstruction Decoction)**

Diagnosis	Clinical Signs	Treatment	Herbs
Joint pain due to stagnation of wind, cold, and dampness with underlying qi and blood deficiencies	• Stiffness and pain of the muscles and joints, and decreased range of motion: qi and blood deficiencies • Pain that worsens with exposure to cold and damp weather: accumulation of wind, cold, and dampness	• Tonifies qi and nourishes the blood • Dispels wind, cold, and dampness	• *Du Huo* (Radix Angelicae Pubescentis) and *Xi Xin* (Radix et Rhizoma Asari) dispel wind, eliminate dampness, relieve pain, and alleviate *bi zheng* (painful obstruction syndrome). • *Qin Jiao* (Radix Gentianae Macrophyllae) and *Fang Feng* (Radix Saposhnikoviae) dispel wind and eliminate dampness. • *Du Zhong* (Cortex Eucommiae), *Xu Duan* (Radix Dipsaci) and *Niu Xi* (Radix Achyranthis Bidentatae) tonify the Kidney and strengthen bones and tendons. • *Gui Xin* (Cortex Rasus Cinnamomi) warms the body and dispels cold. • *Dang Gui* (Radix Angelicae Sinensis), *Chuan Xiong* (Rhizoma Chuanxiong), *Bai Shao* (Radix Paeoniae Alba), and *Di Huang* (Radix Rehmanniae) nourish yin, tonify the blood, and activate blood circulation. • *Huang Qi* (Radix Astragali), *Ren Shen* (Radix et Rhizoma Ginseng), *Fu Ling* (Poria), and *Gan Cao* (Radix et Rhizoma Glycyrrhizae) tonify qi and strengthen the Spleen.

Chuanxiong), *Bai Shao* (Radix Paeoniae Alba) and *Di Huang* (Radix Rehmanniae) nourish yin, tonify the blood, and activate blood circulation. *Huang Qi* (Radix Astragali), *Ren Shen* (Radix et Rhizoma Ginseng), *Fu Ling* (Poria), and *Gan Cao* (Radix et Rhizoma Glycyrrhizae) tonify qi and strengthen the Spleen.

VETERINARY MODIFICATIONS

- For *bi zheng* (painful obstruction syndrome) with more wind, add *Qiang Huo* (Rhizoma et Radix Notopterygii) and *Gui Zhi* (Ramulus Cinnamomi).
- For *bi zheng* (painful obstruction syndrome) with more cold, add *Ma Huang* (Herba Ephedrae) and *Fu Zi* (Radix Aconiti Lateralis Praeparata).
- For *bi zheng* (painful obstruction syndrome) with more dampness, add *Cang Zhu* (Rhizoma Atractylodis) and *Yin Chen* (Herba Artemisiae Scopariae).
- For chronic, stubborn, recalcitrant pain, add *Wu Gong* (Scolopendra), *Wu Shao She* (Zaocys), *Yan Hu Suo* (Rhizoma Corydalis), *Hong Hua* (Flos Carthami), and *Tao Ren* (Semen Persicae).
- For qi deficiency and hindquarter weakness in addition to pain, add *Ren Shen* (Radix et Rhizoma Ginseng), *Bai Zhu* (Rhizoma Atractylodis Macrocephalae), and *Gui Ban* (Plastrum Testudinis).

SUGGESTED ACUPUNCTURE TREATMENT

1. Points: *Fengchi* (GB 20), *Dazhui* (GV 14), *Ganshu* (BL 18), *Shenshu* (BL 23), *Zhishi* (BL 52), *Taixi* (KI 3), *Housanli* (ST 36), *Sanyinjiao* (SP 6), *Yaoyangguan* (GV 3), *Weizhong* (BL 40), *Yanglingquan* (GB 34), *Qihai* (CV 6), *Xuehai* (SP 10), and other local points.
2. Technique: tonification and moxibustion.

Dazhui (GV 14) and *Fengchi* (GB 20) dispel wind and expel external pathogenic factors. *Ganshu* (BL 18), *Shenshu* (BL 23), *Zhishi* (BL 52), and *Taixi* (KI 3) nourish Liver and Kidney yin. *Housanli* (ST 36) and *Sanyinjiao* (SP 6) tonify qi, strengthen the Spleen, nourish the blood, and activate blood circulation. *Yaoyangguan* (GV 3) warms yang to dispel cold and dampness. *Weizhong* (BL 40) relieves lower back pain, while *Yanglingquan* (GB 34) relieves muscle stiffness and cramps. *Qihai* (CV 6) and *Xuehai* (SP 10) tonify qi and blood. Local points may be selected to activate qi and blood circulation to relieve pain.

AUTHORS' COMMENTS

San Bi Tang, literally "Three-Painful Obstruction Decoction," is so named because it has an excellent effect to dispel wind, cold, and dampness, the three most common factors leading to *bi zheng* (painful obstruction syndrome). It can be combined with *Shu Jing Huo Xue Tang* (Relax the Channels and Invigorate the Blood Decoction) to treat acute non-surgical injury to the stifle joint with mild laxity or partial tear of the anterior cruciate ligament and to treat chronic back pain due to spondylosis and intervertebral disk disease. This formula is also indicated in animals that have trembling and shaking of the rear legs due to Kidney and Liver yin deficiencies and qi and blood stagnation.

Sān Bì Tāng (Three-Painful Obstruction Decoction)

Du Huo Ji Sheng Tang (Angelica Pubescens and Taxillus Decoction) and *San Bi Tang* have similar effects to treat *bi zheng* (painful obstruction syndrome) with exterior excess and interior deficiency.

- *Du Huo Ji Sheng Tang* focuses on *bi zheng* (painful obstruction syndrome) with exterior excess (wind-cold-damp) and interior deficiency (of the Liver and Kidney). It is most effective for *bi zheng* (painful obstruction syndrome) affecting the lower body, including the back and stifles, and in cases where cold predominates.
- *San Bi Tang* targets *bi zheng* (painful obstruction syndrome) with exterior excess (wind-cold-dampness) and interior deficiency (of qi and blood). It is most suitable for *bi zheng* (painful obstruction syndrome) characterized by stiffness, pain, and decreased range of motion in the spine and the extremities.

Shū Jīng Huó Xuè Tāng

(Relax the Channels and Invigorate the Blood Decoction)

疏經活血湯

疏经活血汤

Pinyin Name: *Shu Jing Huo Xue Tang*
Literal Name: Relax the Channels and Invigorate the Blood Decoction
Alternate Names: *Shu Ching Huo Hsieh Tang*, Clematis and Stephania Blood-Activating Decoction, Clematis and Stephania Combination
Original Source: *Wan Bing Hui Chun* (Restoration of Health from the Myriad Diseases) by Gong Ting-Xian in 1587

COMPOSITION

Dang Gui (Radix Angelicae Sinensis), *xi* (washed) with liquor	3.6g
Bai Shao (Radix Paeoniae Alba), *chao* (dry-fried) with liquor	4.5g
Di Huang (Radix Rehmanniae), *xi* (washed) with liquor	3g
Chuan Xiong (Rhizoma Chuanxiong)	1.8g
Tao Ren (Semen Persicae), *jian* (decocted) and *chao* (dry-fried)	3g
Fu Ling (Poria)	2.1g
Cang Zhu (Rhizoma Atractylodis), *jin* (soaked) in rice water	3g
Chen Pi (Pericarpium Citri Reticulatae)	3g
Qiang Huo (Rhizoma et Radix Notopterygii)	1.8g
Bai Zhi (Radix Angelicae Dahuricae)	1.8g
Wei Ling Xian (Radix et Rhizoma Clematidis), *xi* (washed) in liquor	3g
Fang Ji (Radix Stephaniae Tetrandrae), *xi* (washed) with liquor	1.8g
Fang Feng (Radix Saposhnikoviae)	1.8g
Long Dan (Radix et Rhizoma Gentianae)	1.8g
Chuan Niu Xi (Radix Cyathulae), *xi* (washed) with liquor	3g
Gan Cao (Radix et Rhizoma Glycyrrhizae)	1.2g

Shū Jīng Huó Xuè Tāng

(Relax the Channels and Invigorate the Blood Decoction)

DOSAGE / PREPARATION / ADMINISTRATION

The source text instructs to cook the ingredients with 3 slices of *Sheng Jiang* (Rhizoma Zingiberis Recens) in water. Take the warm, strained decoction on an empty stomach. The source text recommends avoiding foods that are raw, cold, or damp in nature.

CHINESE THERAPEUTIC ACTIONS

1. Dredges the channels and collaterals
2. Invigorates blood circulation
3. Dispels dampness

CLINICAL MANIFESTATIONS

Body pain caused by exterior pathogens attacking the body with underlying deficiency: severe muscle pain, painful joints, radiating pain and stiffness in the extremities and pain in the trunk.

VETERINARY CLINICAL APPLICATIONS

Osteoarthritis, neuralgia, poor performance, navicular disease, intervertebral disk disease, acute non-surgical back pain, soft tissue injuries, hemiplegia, stiffness and pain of the limbs.

EXPLANATION

Shu Jing Huo Xue Tang (Relax the Channels and Invigorate the Blood Decoction) treats *bi zheng* (painful obstruction syndrome) characterized by deficiency in the interior and excess at the exterior. The deficiency arises as a result of chronic disease, overwork, excessive activity, over breeding, improper nutrition, and aging, all of which lead to emptiness of the channels and collaterals. As a result, wind, cold, and dampness can more easily attack the exterior, cause qi and blood stagnation, and produce pain all over the body.

The first four herbs in this formula, *Dang Gui* (Radix Angelicae Sinensis), *Bai Shao* (Radix Paeoniae Alba), *Di Huang* (Radix Rehmanniae), and *Chuan Xiong* (Rhizoma Chuanxiong), tonify the blood and activate blood circulation. *Tao Ren* (Semen Persicae) breaks up blood stagnation. *Fu Ling* (Poria) dispels dampness through diuresis, while *Cang Zhu* (Rhizoma Atractylodis) dries dampness. *Chen Pi* (Pericarpium Citri Reticulatae) regulates qi flow and dries dampness. *Qiang Huo* (Rhizoma et Radix Notopterygii), *Bai Zhi* (Radix Angelicae Dahuricae), *Wei Ling Xian* (Radix et Rhizoma Clematidis), *Fang Ji* (Radix Stephaniae

***Shu Jing Huo Xue Tang* (Relax the Channels and Invigorate the Blood Decoction)**

Diagnosis	Clinical Signs	Treatment	Herbs
Body aches due to exterior pathogen invasion with underlying deficiency	Stiffness and pain of the muscles and joints: deficiency of the channels and collaterals leading to invasion of wind, cold and dampness	• Dredges the channels and collaterals • Invigorates blood circulation • Dispels dampness	• *Dang Gui* (Radix Angelicae Sinensis), *Bai Shao* (Radix Paeoniae Alba), *Di Huang* (Radix Rehmanniae), and *Chuan Xiong* (Rhizoma Chuanxiong) tonify blood and activate blood circulation. • *Tao Ren* (Semen Persicae) breaks up blood stagnation. • *Fu Ling* (Poria) dispels dampness through diuresis. • *Cang Zhu* (Rhizoma Atractylodis) dries dampness. • *Chen Pi* (Pericarpium Citri Reticulatae) regulates qi flow and dries dampness. • *Qiang Huo* (Rhizoma et Radix Notopterygii), *Bai Zhi* (Radix Angelicae Dahuricae), *Wei Ling Xian* (Radix et Rhizoma Clematidis), *Fang Ji* (Radix Stephaniae Tetrandrae), and *Fang Feng* (Radix Saposhnikoviae) activate qi circulation, dispel wind and dampness, and relieve pain. • *Long Dan* (Radix et Rhizoma Gentianae) drains heat and dampness. • *Chuan Niu Xi* (Radix Cyathulae) activates blood circulation and tonifies the body. • *Gan Cao* (Radix et Rhizoma Glycyrrhizae) harmonizes the herbs.

Shū Jīng Huó Xuè Tāng

(Relax the Channels and Invigorate the Blood Decoction)

Tetrandrae), and *Fang Feng* (Radix Saposhnikoviae) activate qi circulation, dispel wind and dampness, and relieve pain. *Long Dan* (Radix et Rhizoma Gentianae) drains heat and dampness. *Chuan Niu Xi* (Radix Cyathulae) activates blood circulation and tonifies the body. *Gan Cao* (Radix et Rhizoma Glycyrrhizae) harmonizes the herbs.

VETERINARY MODIFICATIONS

- With pain in the upper body, add *Bo He* (Herba Menthae) and *Gui Zhi* (Ramulus Cinnamomi).
- With pain in the lower body, add *Mu Gua* (Fructus Chaenomelis), *Mu Tong* (Caulis Akebiae), *Du Huo* (Radix Angelicae Pubescentis), *Huang Bo* (Cortex Phellodendri Chinensis), and *Yi Yi Ren* (Semen Coicis).
- With qi deficiency, add *Ren Shen* (Radix et Rhizoma Ginseng) and *Bai Zhu* (Rhizoma Atractylodis Macrocephalae).
- With blood deficiency, increase the doses of *Dang Gui* (Radix Angelicae Sinensis), *Bai Shao* (Radix Paeoniae Alba), *Shu Di Huang* (Radix Rehmanniae Praeparata), and *Chuan Xiong* (Rhizoma Chuanxiong).
- With phlegm, add *Tian Nan Xing* (Rhizoma Arisaematis) and *Ban Xia* (Rhizoma Pinelliae).
- With weakness and pain of the muscles and tendons, add *Huang Qi* (Radix Astragali) and *Bai Zhu* (Rhizoma Atractylodis Macrocephalae).
- With soreness and pain of the lower back and legs, add *Xu Duan* (Radix Dipsaci) and *Hong Hua* (Flos Carthami).
- With severe pain or paralysis of the legs, add *Mu Gua* (Fructus Chaenomelis), *Mu Tong* (Caulis Akebiae), *Huang Bo* (Cortex Phellodendri Chinensis), and *Yi Yi Ren* (Semen Coicis).

CAUTIONS / CONTRAINDICATIONS

Avoid foods that are raw, cold or damp in nature while taking *Shu Jing Huo Xue Tang*.

PHARMACOLOGICAL EFFECTS

Analgesic and anti-inflammatory: Administration of *Shu Jing Huo Xue Tang* was associated with reduction of pain and inflammation in adjuvant arthritic rats. The mechanism of action was attributed primarily to increased blood circulation.[1]

SUGGESTED ACUPUNCTURE TREATMENT

1. Points: *Xinshu* (BL 15), *Ganshu* (BL 18), *Pishu* (BL 20), *Weishu* (BL 21), *Taichong* (LR 3), *Fenglong* (ST 40), *Fengmen* (BL 12), *Guanyuan* (CV 4), *Yinlingquan* (SP 9), *Geshu* (BL 17), *Ligou* (LR 5), and local *ah shi* points.
2. Technique: tonification; avoid sedation; electroacupuncture and/or aquapuncture may be helpful.

Because the Heart controls the blood and the Liver stores the blood, *Xinshu* (BL 15), the *shu* (transport) point of Heart, and *Ganshu* (BL 18), the *shu* point of Liver, are used to tonify blood and body fluids. *Pishu* (BL 20), the *shu* point of Spleen, and *Weishu* (BL 21), the *shu* point of Stomach, strengthen the middle *jiao* and promote the production of qi and blood. *Taichong* (LR 3) and *Fenglong* (ST 40) move blood and relieve stagnation. *Fengmen* (BL 12), *Guanyuan* (CV 4), and *Yinlingquan* (SP 9) dispel wind, cold, and dampness. *Geshu* (BL 17) activates blood circulation, and *Ligou* (LR 5) regulates qi circulation. In addition, local *ah shi* points may be used to relieve pain.

AUTHORS' COMMENTS

The primary action of *Shu Jing Huo Xue Tang* is to invigorate the blood and resolve blood stasis to relieve acute muscle, joint and spinal pain; it is not for long-term use unless modified. This is a useful formula in performance animals that experience joint and muscle pain over the course of a competition or show season. Weeks or months of work will deplete blood and qi and weaken *wei* (defensive) *qi*, which makes it easier for pathogens to invade. This can lead to non-specific joint and muscle pain and the development of *ah shi* points in the muscles of the back and hind limbs. It can be used for acute intervertebral disk disease in dogs. This formula is indicated in animals that display a dark red to purple tongue and a wiry pulse. *Shu Jing Huo Xue Tang* is often combined with *Du Huo Ji Sheng Tang* (Angelica Pubescens and Taxillus Decoction) to treat animals with spondylosis, chronic, non-surgical back and stifle pain with underlying deficiencies.

Reference

1. Kanai S, Taniguchi N, Higashino H. Study of sokei-kakketu-to (shu-jing-huo-xue-tang) in adjuvant arthritis rats. Am J Chin Med. 2003; 31(6):879-84.

Yì Yǐ Rén Tāng (Coicis Decoction)

薏苡仁湯
薏苡仁汤

Pinyin Name: *Yi Yi Ren Tang*
Literal Name: Coicis Decoction
Alternate Name: Coix Combination
Original Source: *Zhang Shi Yi Tong* (Comprehensive Medicine According to Master Zhang) by Zhang Lu-Xuan in 1695

COMPOSITION

Ma Huang (Herba Ephedrae)	2.4g
Gui Zhi (Ramulus Cinnamomi)	2.4g
Dang Gui (Radix Angelicae Sinensis)	4.5g
Bai Shao (Radix Paeoniae Alba), *xi* (washed) with liquor	4.5g
Cang Zhu (Rhizoma Atractylodis), *ban* (blended) and *chao* (dry-fried) with *Hei Zhi Ma* (Semen Sesami Nigrum)	3g
Yi Yi Ren (Semen Coicis), *pao* (blast-fried) with ginger	30g
Zhi Gan Cao (Radix et Rhizoma Glycyrrhizae Praeparata cum Melle)	2.1g
Sheng Jiang (Rhizoma Zingiberis Recens)	7 slices [4.5g]

DOSAGE / PREPARATION / ADMINISTRATION

The source text instructs to prepare the formula as a decoction.

CHINESE THERAPEUTIC ACTIONS

1. Dispels wind and dampness
2. Benefits qi
3. Activates blood circulation

CLINICAL MANIFESTATIONS

Bi zheng (painful obstruction syndrome) caused by wind-dampness: stiffness and pain of the extremities, heaviness of movement, edema of the limbs, swelling of the joints, decreased mobility and limited range of motion in the joints.

VETERINARY CLINICAL APPLICATIONS

Chronic *bi zheng* (painful obstruction syndrome) with wind, cold, and dampness (dampness being dominant); chronic osteoarthritis that worsens with weather changes, chronic joint pain, canine hip dysplasia, intervertebral disk disease, immune-mediated polyarthritis, limb edema and pain without heat, canine rheumatoid arthritis and masticatory myositis.

EXPLANATION

Yi Yi Ren Tang (Coicis Decoction) was originally designed to treat *bi zheng* (painful obstruction syndrome) caused by wind-dampness. This condition, however, often occurs with complications, as wind-dampness may combine with cold and attack the muscles and joints, leading to such

***Yi Yi Ren Tang* (Coicis Decoction)**

Diagnosis	Clinical Signs	Treatment	Herbs
Bi zheng (painful obstruction syndrome) due to wind, cold, and dampness	Stiffness and pain of the extremities, painful, swollen joints and inflammation, decreased mobility, and limited range of motion in the joints: wind, cold, and dampness attacking the muscles and joints	• Dispels wind and dampness • Benefits qi • Activates blood circulation	• *Ma Huang* (Herba Ephedrae) and *Gui Zhi* (Ramulus Cinnamomi) dispel wind-cold from the exterior and drain dampness through urination. • *Gui Zhi* (Ramulus Cinnamomi) opens the channels and collaterals in the extremities to relieve pain. • *Dang Gui* (Radix Angelicae Sinensis) and *Bai Shao* (Radix Paeoniae Alba) activate blood circulation, harmonize the *ying* (nutritive) and *wei* (defensive) levels, and relieve pain. • *Cang Zhu* (Rhizoma Atractylodis) and *Yi Yi Ren* (Semen Coicis) drain dampness. • *Zhi Gan Cao* (Radix et Rhizoma Glycyrrhizae Praeparata cum Melle) harmonizes the herbs.

Yì Yǐ Rén Tāng (Coicis Decoction)

clinical signs as stiffness, painful, swollen joints and inflammation.

The primary goals of this formula are to dispel wind, cold, and dampness, activate qi and blood circulation, and relieve pain. *Ma Huang* (Herba Ephedrae) and *Gui Zhi* (Ramulus Cinnamomi) are two of the strongest herbs for dispelling wind-cold from the exterior. They both also have a diuretic effect to drain dampness through urination. *Gui Zhi* (Ramulus Cinnamomi) also opens the channels and collaterals in the extremities to relieve pain. *Dang Gui* (Radix Angelicae Sinensis) and *Bai Shao* (Radix Paeoniae Alba) activate blood circulation, harmonize the *ying* (nutritive) and *wei* (defensive) levels, and relieve pain. *Cang Zhu* (Rhizoma Atractylodis) and *Yi Yi Ren* (Semen Coicis) drain dampness through urination. *Zhi Gan Cao* (Radix et Rhizoma Glycyrrhizae Praeparata cum Melle) harmonizes the herbs in the formula.

VETERINARY MODIFICATIONS

- With cold, add *Fu Zi* (Radix Aconiti Lateralis Praeparata).
- With heat, add *Huang Bo* (Cortex Phellodendri Chinensis) and *Shi Gao* (Gypsum Fibrosum).
- For stronger pain relief, add *Du Huo* (Radix Angelicae Pubescentis), *Yan Hu Suo* (Rhizoma Corydalis) and *Fang Ji* (Radix Stephaniae Tetrandrae).

SUGGESTED ACUPUNCTURE TREATMENT

1. Points: *Fengshi* (GB 31), *Hegu* (LI 4), *Taichong* (LR 3), *Pishu* (BL 20), *Weishu* (BL 21), *Housanli* (ST 36), *Sanyinjiao* (SP 6), *Yinlingquan* (SP 9), *Yanglingquan* (GB 34), and *ah shi* points.
2. Technique: moxibustion and even method.

Fengshi (GB 31), *Hegu* (LI 4), and *Taichong* (LR 3) dispel wind-cold and the combination is especially effective with moxa. *Pishu* (BL 20), *Weishu* (BL 21) and *Housanli* (ST 36) help to resolve damp by strengthening the Spleen. *Sanyinjiao* (SP 6) activates blood circulation. Use electro-stimulation across needles at *Yinlingquan* (SP 9) and *Yanglingquan* (GB 34) to dispel dampness and benefit the tendons. Apply moxibustion on *ah shi* points and local areas to relieve pain.

AUTHORS' COMMENTS

Yi Yi Ren Tang (Coicis Decoction) is used to treat a variety of musculoskeletal disorders caused by the invasion of wind-cold-dampness. It is frequently used to treat *bi zheng* (painful obstruction syndrome) characterized by swollen, painful joints, with a predominance of stiffness and decreased range of motion. Animals for which this formula is appropriate often have a slippery pulse. *Yi Yi Ren Tang* is not typically used alone, but instead it is combined with other herbs or another formula to improve pain relief, clear heat, and resolve dampness, depending on the case. It can be used to treat canine immune-mediated polyarthritis (IPA) with hot, swollen painful joints by adding *Shi Gao* (Gypsum Fibrosum), *Huang Bo* (Cortex Phellodendri Chinensis), and *Yan Hu Suo* (Rhizoma Corydalis).

Shàng Zhōng Xià Tōng Yòng Tòng Fēng Wán

(Upper, Middle, and Lower General-Use Pill for Wind-Pain)

上中下通用痛風丸

上中下通用痛风丸

Pinyin Name: *Shang Zhong Xia Tong Yong Tong Feng Wan*

Literal Name: Upper, Middle, and Lower General-Use Pill for Wind-Pain

Alternate Names: *Shang Chung Hsia Tung Yung Tung Feng Wan*, Cinnamon and Angelica Pill, Cinnamon and Angelica Formula

Original Source: *Dan Xi Xin Fa* (Teachings of [Zhu] Dan-Xi) by Zhu Zhen-Heng in 1481

COMPOSITION

Gui Zhi (Ramulus Cinnamomi)	[3g]
Qiang Huo (Rhizoma et Radix Notopterygii)	[3g]
Fang Ji (Radix Stephaniae Tetrandrae)	[9g]
Wei Ling Xian (Radix et Rhizoma Clematidis)	[3g]
Chuan Xiong (Rhizoma Chuanxiong)	[9g]
Tao Ren (Semen Persicae)	[9g]
Hong Hua (Flos Carthami)	[3g]
Bai Zhi (Radix Angelicae Dahuricae)	[9g]
Long Dan (Radix et Rhizoma Gentianae)	[9g]
Huang Bo (Cortex Phellodendri Chinensis)	[21g]
Cang Zhu (Rhizoma Atractylodis)	[21g]
Tian Nan Xing (Rhizoma Arisaematis)	[21g]
Shen Qu (Massa Fermentata)	[9g]

DOSAGE / PREPARATION / ADMINISTRATION

This formula is prepared using the doses suggested in brackets and administered as pills with warm water.

CHINESE THERAPEUTIC ACTIONS

1. Dispels wind and dissolves dampness
2. Activates blood circulation and eliminates bruising

CLINICAL MANIFESTATIONS

Generalized *bi zheng* (painful obstruction syndrome): aches and pains in the limbs and throughout the body.

VETERINARY CLINICAL APPLICATIONS

Generalized body and joint pain, arthritis, osteoarthritis, degenerative joint disease, cervical and lumbar intervertebral disk disease, canine hip dysplasia, elbow dysplasia, shoulder dysplasia and polymyositis.

EXPLANATION

Shang Zhong Xia Tong Yong Tong Feng Wan (Upper, Middle, and Lower General-Use Pill for Wind-Pain) is a generalized formula that treats aches and pains due to various causes in varied locations in the body. *Bi zheng* (painful obstruction syndrome) can be a complicated disorder because the causes include cold, heat, dampness, phlegm, and stagnation. This formula simplifies the diagnostic procedure by focusing on relieving pain. Therefore, it can be used for aches and pains throughout the body (upper, middle, and lower) due to various causes.

This formula contains herbs with numerous functions to reduce swelling, relieve pain, disperse stagnation, and open the channels and collaterals. *Gui Zhi* (Ramulus Cinnamomi), *Qiang Huo* (Rhizoma et Radix Notopterygii), *Fang Ji* (Radix Stephaniae Tetrandrae), and *Wei Ling Xian* (Radix et Rhizoma Clematidis) reduce swelling and relieve pain. *Chuan Xiong* (Rhizoma Chuanxiong), *Tao Ren* (Semen Persicae), and *Hong Hua* (Flos Carthami) activate blood circulation and relieve pain. *Bai Zhi* (Radix Angelicae Dahuricae) dispels wind from the exterior and relieves pain in the head region. *Long Dan* (Radix et Rhizoma Gentianae) and *Huang Bo* (Cortex Phellodendri Chinensis) clear heat and reduce swelling and inflammation. *Cang Zhu* (Rhizoma Atractylodis) dries dampness, while *Tian Nan Xing* (Rhizoma Arisaematis) eliminates phlegm. *Shen Qu* (Massa Fermentata) harmonizes and protects the middle *jiao*.

Shàng Zhōng Xià Tōng Yòng Tòng Fēng Wán
(Upper, Middle, and Lower General-Use Pill for Wind-Pain)

***Shang Zhong Xia Tong Yong Tong Feng Wan* (Upper, Middle and Lower General-Use Pill for Wind-Pain)**

Diagnosis	Clinical Signs	Treatment	Herbs
Generalized *bi zheng* (painful obstruction syndrome)	Aches and pains in the arms, legs, and throughout the body: stagnation of cold, heat, dampness, and phlegm	• Dispels wind and dissolves dampness • Activates blood circulation and eliminates bruising	• *Gui Zhi* (Ramulus Cinnamomi), *Qiang Huo* (Rhizoma et Radix Notopterygii), *Fang Ji* (Radix Stephaniae Tetrandrae), and *Wei Ling Xian* (Radix et Rhizoma Clematidis) reduce swelling and relieve pain. • *Chuan Xiong* (Rhizoma Chuanxiong), *Tao Ren* (Semen Persicae), and *Hong Hua* (Flos Carthami) activate blood circulation and relieve pain. • *Bai Zhi* (Radix Angelicae Dahuricae) dispels wind from the exterior and relieves pain in the head region. • *Long Dan* (Radix et Rhizoma Gentianae) and *Huang Bo* (Cortex Phellodendri Chinensis) clear heat and reduce swelling and inflammation. • *Cang Zhu* (Rhizoma Atractylodis) dries dampness, and *Tian Nan Xing* (Rhizoma Arisaematis) eliminates phlegm. • *Shen Qu* (Massa Fermentata) harmonizes and protects the middle *jiao*.

VETERINARY MODIFICATIONS

- For *bi zheng* (painful obstruction syndrome) caused by wind, cold, and dampness, add *Fang Feng* (Radix Saposhnikoviae) and *Du Huo* (Radix Angelicae Pubescentis).
- For *bi zheng* (painful obstruction syndrome) caused by blood deficiency, add *Dang Gui* (Radix Angelicae Sinensis) and *Bai Shao* (Radix Paeoniae Alba).
- For *bi zheng* (painful obstruction syndrome) caused by qi deficiency, add *Ren Shen* (Radix et Rhizoma Ginseng) and *Huang Qi* (Radix Astragali).
- For *bi zheng* (painful obstruction syndrome) caused by dampness and phlegm, add *Er Chen Tang* (Two-Cured Decoction).

SUGGESTED ACUPUNCTURE TREATMENT

1. Points: *Waiguan* (TH 5), *Yinlingquan* (SP 9), and *ah shi* points.
2. Technique: bleeding and even method.

To treat the cause, needle *Waiguan* (TH 5) to dispel wind and *Yinlingquan* (SP 9) to dissolve dampness; to treat the clinical signs, needle the *ah shi* points and general "aspirin points" such as *Kunlun* (BL 60) and *Hegu* (LI 4) and bleed any red, swollen, or painful areas.

AUTHORS' COMMENTS

Shang Zhong Xia Tong Yong Tong Feng Wan is an all-purpose pain-relieving formula used to treat *bi zheng* (painful obstruction syndrome) with wind-cold-dampness. The focus of this formula is on pain relief, and it lacks tonic herbs and should be combined with constitutional formulas for long-term use. It is a valuable formula to have, as it can relieve pain from *bi zheng* (painful obstruction syndrome) anywhere in the body and can be easily modified or combined with another formula to treat underlying deficiencies and hot or cold musculoskeletal conditions.

Section 2

温散寒湿剂
— Damp-Cold Dispelling Formulas

Xiǎo Huó Luò Dān (Minor Invigorate the Collaterals Special Pill)
小活絡丹
小活络丹

Pinyin Name: *Xiao Huo Luo Dan*
Literal Name: Minor Invigorate the Collaterals Special Pill
Alternate Names: *Huo Luo Dan* (Invigorate the Collaterals Special Pill), Myrrh and Aconite Formula
Original Source: *Tai Ping Hui Min He Ji Ju Fang* (Imperial Grace Formulary of the Tai Ping Era) by the Imperial Medical Department in 1078-85

COMPOSITION

Zhi Chuan Wu (Radix Aconiti Praeparata), *pao* (blast-fried)	180g [6g]
Zhi Cao Wu (Radix Aconiti Kusnezoffii Praeparata), *pao* (blast-fried)	180g [6g]
Tian Nan Xing (Rhizoma Arisaematis), *pao* (blast-fried)	180g [6g]
Ru Xiang (Gummi Olibanum), *yan* (ground) to small particles	66g [5g]
Mo Yao (Myrrha), *yan* (ground) to small particles	66g [5g]
Di Long (Pheretima)	180g [6g]

DOSAGE / PREPARATION / ADMINISTRATION

The source text instructs to first blast-fry *Zhi Cao Wu* (Radix Aconiti Kusnezoffii Praeparata), *Zhi Chuan Wu* (Radix Aconiti Praeparata), and *Tian Nan Xing* (Rhizoma Arisaematis) to eliminate their toxicity. Then, grind the ingredients into a fine powder and mix with grain-based liquor to form into small pills. The pills should resemble the size of *Wu Tong Zi* (Semen Firmianae), a small seed approximately 5 mm in diameter. Take 20 pills on an empty stomach at noon with cold, grain-based liquor or tea made from *Jing Jie* (Herba Schizonepetae).

Today, the ingredients are ground into a fine powder, sifted together, and formed into pills with honey. Take 1 pill [3g] twice daily, with aged, grain-based liquor or warm, boiled water. This formula may also be prepared as a decoction with the doses suggested in brackets.

CHINESE THERAPEUTIC ACTIONS

1. Dispels wind and dampness
2. Resolves phlegm and dredges the channels
3. Activates blood circulation and stops pain

CLINICAL MANIFESTATIONS

1. Obstruction of wind, cold, and dampness in the channels and collaterals: muscle spasms and cramps, limited mobility and difficult movement of the joints, painful extremities, and migratory pain.
2. *Zhong feng* (wind stroke) with dampness and phlegm obstruction, and blood stasis in the channels and collaterals: numbness and pain in the extremities, and heaviness and pain in the lower back and legs.

VETERINARY CLINICAL APPLICATIONS

Acute arthritis, acute soft tissue injuries, navicular disease, exertional rhabdomyolysis, spondylosis, lumbosacral disease, acute intervertebral disk disease (IVDD) with paresis and paralysis, fibrocartilaginous emboli (FCE), hemiplegia, and post-surgical intervertebral disk disease recovery.

EXPLANATION

Xiao Huo Luo Dan (Minor Invigorate the Collaterals Special Pill) treats blocked qi and blood circulation caused by obstruction of wind, cold, and dampness in the channels and collaterals. The formula may be used for muscle

Xiǎo Huó Luò Dān (Minor Invigorate the Collaterals Special Pill)

***Xiao Huo Luo Dan* (Minor Invigorate the Collaterals Special Pill)**

Diagnosis	Clinical Signs	Treatment	Herbs
Obstruction of wind, cold, and dampness in the channels and collaterals	• Spasms and cramps, limited mobility, difficult movement and painful extremities, paresis and paralysis: obstruction of wind, cold, and dampness in the channels and collaterals • Pain and decreased sensations in the extremities: dampness and phlegm obstruction with blood stasis in the channels and collaterals	• Dispels wind, cold, and dampness • Resolves phlegm and dredges the channels • Activates blood circulation and stops pain	• *Zhi Chuan Wu* (Radix Aconiti Praeparata) and *Zhi Cao Wu* (Radix Aconiti Kusnezoffii Praeparata) dispel wind-cold, warm and dredge the collaterals, and relieve pain. • *Tian Nan Xing* (Rhizoma Arisaematis) dries dampness and resolves phlegm. • *Ru Xiang* (Gummi Olibanum) and *Mo Yao* (Myrrha) activate qi and blood circulation and remove blood stasis. • *Di Long* (Pheretima) opens the channels and collaterals.

and joint disorders with symptoms such as spasms and cramps, limited mobility, difficult movement, and painful extremities. It may also be used for *zhong feng* (wind stroke) caused by obstruction of dampness, phlegm, and blood stasis in the channels and collaterals, leading to numbness and pain of the extremities.

In this formula, *Zhi Chuan Wu* (Radix Aconiti Praeparata) and *Zhi Cao Wu* (Radix Aconiti Kusnezoffii Praeparata) dispel wind and dampness and warm and dredge the channels and collaterals. These two herbs also have a strong effect to dispel cold and relieve pain. *Tian Nan Xing* (Rhizoma Arisaematis) dries dampness and resolves phlegm in the channels and collaterals to relieve pain. *Ru Xiang* (Gummi Olibanum) and *Mo Yao* (Myrrha) activate qi and blood circulation and remove blood stasis. *Di Long* (Pheretima) opens the channels and collaterals. When taken with grain-based liquor, the herbs have a more powerful effect to dispel wind and cold, resolve dampness and phlegm, eliminate qi and blood stagnation, and open the channels and collaterals.

VETERINARY MODIFICATIONS

- For neuralgia, add *Chi Shao* (Radix Paeoniae Rubra), *Wei Ling Xian* (Radix et Rhizoma Clematidis), and *Chuan Xiong* (Rhizoma Chuanxiong).
- For post-surgical recovery, add *Dan Shen* (Radix et Rhizoma Salviae Miltiorrhizae) and *San Qi* (Radix et Rhizoma Notoginseng).
- For arthritis, add *Qiang Huo* (Rhizoma et Radix Notopterygii) and *Yi Tiao Gen* (Radix Moghaniae).
- If there is more wind, add *Da Qin Jiao Tang* (Major Gentiana Macrophylla Decoction).
- With Liver and Kidney yin deficiencies manifesting in weakness of the joints, add *Du Huo Ji Sheng Tang* (Angelica Pubescens and Taxillus Decoction).
- With severe pain, add *Yan Hu Suo* (Rhizoma Corydalis) and increase the doses of *Ru Xiang* (Gummi Olibanum) and *Mo Yao* (Myrrha).

CAUTIONS / CONTRAINDICATIONS

- *Xiao Huo Luo Dan* is a potent formula designed for individuals who have a strong constitution and who are generally healthy. It should be used with caution in animals with blood deficiency or yin-deficient heat.
- The use of this formula is contraindicated during pregnancy.

PHARMACOLOGICAL EFFECTS

1. **Analgesic**: Administration of *Xiao Huo Luo Dan* at 20-100 mg/kg was associated with a marked analgesic effect in mice.[1]
2. **Sedative**: One study reported a dose-dependant sedative effect in mice.[2]
3. **Pharmacokinetic**: One study reported *Xiao Huo Luo Dan* to have a two-compartment model of distribution, with an average half-life of 13.16 hours.[3]

HUMAN CLINICAL STUDIES AND RESEARCH

1. **Soft-tissue injuries**: Topical application of *Xiao Huo Luo Dan* was associated with excellent results in treating 50 patients with soft-tissue injuries. The topical preparation was made by soaking the pills in 75% ethanol then crushing the pills into paste. The herbal paste was applied to the affected area every other day for intact skin. If the wound was open, it was thoroughly cleaned and disinfected prior to application of the herbal paste. The study reported complete recovery in 49 of 50 patients within 3-5 applications of the herbal paste.[4]
2. **Sciatica**: Concurrent use of modified *Xiao Huo Luo Dan* via oral ingestion and topical application was associated with marked relief of sciatica. The treatment protocol was

Xiǎo Huó Luò Dān (Minor Invigorate the Collaterals Special Pill)

to cook the herbs in water and drink the decoction in two equally-divided doses daily. The herb residue was applied topically to the affected area. Each course of treatment was 20 days. Out of 32 patients, 20 had complete recovery, 7 had significant improvement, 3 had slight improvement, and 2 had no change. The overall effectiveness was 93.75%.[5]

3. **Arthritis**: Topical application of modified *Xiao Huo Luo Dan* was effective in relieving pain in all 50 patients. The herbal formula contained unprocessed *Chuan Wu* (Radix Aconiti), unprocessed *Cao Wu* (Radix Aconiti Kusnezoffii), *Di Long* (Pheretima), unprocessed *Tian Nan Xing* (Rhizoma Arisaematis), *Ru Xiang* (Gummi Olibanum), *Mo Yao* (Myrrha), *Ma Qian Zi* (Semen Strychni), *Hong Hua* (Flos Carthami), *Shui Zhi* (Hirudo), and *Mu Gua* (Fructus Chaenomelis), all in equal portions. The herbs were ground into a fine powder, mixed with water to make a paste, and applied topically to the affected area. Of 50 patients, the study reported complete relief in 8 cases, significant improvement in 27 cases, and moderate improvement in 5 cases.[6] Note: The treatment protocol for this study was to apply the herbs *topically* since unprocessed *Chuan Wu* (Radix Aconiti), *Cao Wu* (Radix Aconiti Kusnezoffii), and *Tian Nan Xing* (Rhizoma Arisaematis) can be extremely toxic if ingested orally.

TOXICOLOGY

Overdose of *Xiao Huo Luo Dan* (Minor Invigorate the Collaterals Special Pill) has been associated with occasional toxicity. Reported side effects in humans include numbness in the hands and feet, stiff tongue, dizziness, pale face, cold extremities, sweating, nausea, vomiting, diarrhea, palpitations, arrhythmia, and loss of consciousness. Allergy and acute gastrointestinal bleeding have been reported as well. The toxicity is attributed to *Zhi Chuan Wu* (Radix Aconiti Praeparata), *Zhi Cao Wu* (Radix Aconiti Kusnezoffii Praeparata), and *Tian Nan Xing* (Rhizoma Arisaematis).[7,8,9]

Toxicity associated with the use of this formula may be treated initially with gastric lavage. Administration of intravenous fluids with dexamethasone (10mg twice daily) is also helpful. Use of an herbal decoction with *Gan Cao* (Radix et Rhizoma Glycyrrhizae) and *Lu Dou* (Semen Phaseoli Radiati) has also shown beneficial effects.[10]

SUGGESTED ACUPUNCTURE TREATMENT

1. Selection of points depends on the affected area(s):
   - Shoulder: *Jianjing* (LI 15), *Jianliao* (TH 14), and *Naoshu* (SI 10)
   - Elbow: *Qiansanli* (LI 10), *Quchi* (LI 11), *Hegu* (LI 4), *Tianjing* (TH 10), *Waiguan* (TH 5), and *Chize* (LU 5)
   - Carpus: *Yangchi* (TH 4), *Yangxi* (LI 5), *Wangu* (SI 4), and *Waiguan* (TH 5)
   - Back: *Renzhong* (GV 26), *Shenzhu* (GV 12), *Yaoyangguan* (GV 3) and *Huatuojiaji* points.
   - Hip: *Huantiao* (GB 30), *Juliao* (GB 29), and *Xuanzhong* (GB 39)
   - Thigh: *Bashan* (BL 54), *Chengfu* (BL 36), and *Yinlingquan* (SP 9)
   - Stifle: *Dubi* (ST 35), *Liangqiu* (ST 34), *Yanglingquan* (GB 34), and *Xiguan* (LR 7)
   - Hock: *Shenmai* (BL 62), *Zhaohai* (KI 6), *Kunlun* (BL 60), and *Qiuxu* (GB 40)
2. Technique: even method and moxibustion or aquapuncture.

Because pathogenic factors attack different regions of the body, selection of acupuncture points varies depending on the area affected. Despite the wide variation in point selection, the main objectives are to dispel wind, cold, and dampness, harmonize qi and blood, and promote the smooth circulation of qi and blood in the channels and collaterals.

In addition, if the pain is migratory, add *Fengmen* (BL 12), *Geshu* (BL 17), and *Ganshu* (BL 18); if the pain is fixed, add *Pishu* (BL 20), *Housanli* (ST 36), and *Yinlingquan* (SP 9); and if the pain is severe, add *Shenshu* (BL 23) and *Mingmen* (GV 4).

AUTHORS' COMMENTS

Xiao Huo Luo Dan is one of the most commonly used herbal formulas for the treatment of acute intervertebral disk disease (IVDD) with paresis and paralysis in dogs due to wind, cold and phlegm. Horses with back pain also respond favorably to this formula. It can also be given for chronic *bi zheng* (painful obstruction syndrome) and IVDD cases when wind, cold and dampness have abruptly aggravated the condition. It contains many warm and acrid herbs, and it is not for long-term use without modification, especially in yin-deficient animals. It is often combined with *Du Huo Ji Sheng Tang* (Angelica Pubescens and Taxillus Decoction) for animals with chronic, non-surgical back pain and post-surgical IVDD patients. Many IVDD patients are qi deficient with weak middle *jiao* function, and it is common to combine *Xiao Huo Luo Dan* with a formula such as *Shen Ling Bai Zhu San* (Ginseng, Poria, and Atractylodes Macrocephala Powder), *Bu Zhong Yi Qi Tang* (Tonify the Middle and Augment the Qi Decoction), or *Liu Wei Di Huang Wan* (Six-Ingredient Pill with Rehmannia).

Xiao Huo Luo Dan can be used to resolve hemiplegia secondary to fibrocartilaginous emboli (FCE) in dogs.

Xiǎo Huó Luò Dān (Minor Invigorate the Collaterals Special Pill)

It is typically combined with a nourishing formula to tonify qi, yin and blood deficiencies that typically underlie this condition. It can take up to six months of treatment to restore adequate function or resolve this condition. If treatment is started immediately after the onset of the disease, the chances of return to normal function are much greater than treatment started weeks after the initial onset. Acupuncture is essential to combine with herbal therapy in these cases, as the combination is superior to the use of herbs alone.

Although wind and dampness are the pathogens that initially invade the muscles and joints, they often create other complications, such as qi, blood and phlegm stagnation. Therefore, treatment of *bi zheng* (painful obstruction syndrome) requires the use of herbs that treat these associated conditions and complications. In this formula, strong herbs such as *Zhi Chuan Wu* (Radix Aconiti Praeparata) and *Zhi Cao Wu* (Radix Aconiti Kusnezoffii Praeparata) warm and dredge the collaterals, dispel cold and relieve pain. *Tian Nan Xing* (Rhizoma Arisaematis) dries dampness and resolves phlegm. *Ru Xiang* (Gummi Olibanum) and *Mo Yao* (Myrrha) are aromatic substances that activate qi and blood circulation and remove blood stasis. Lastly, *Di Long* (Pheretima) is used as a guiding herb to open the channels and collaterals.

References

1. *Zhong Guo Zhong Yao Za Zhi* (People's Republic of China Journal of Chinese Herbology), 1995; 3:159.
2. *Zhong Yi Yao Xue Bao* (Report of Chinese Medicine and Herbology), 1995; 6:13.
3. *Zhong Cheng Yao* (Study of Chinese Patent Medicine), 1994; 3:34.
4. *Hu Bei Zhong Yi Za Zhi* (Hubei Journal of Chinese Medicine), 1990; 4:44.
5. *Nei Meng Gu Zhong Yi Yao* (Traditional Chinese Medicine and Medicinals of Inner Mongolia), 1992; 3:24.
6. *Hu Bei Zhong Yi Xue Yuan Xue Bao* (Journal of Hubei University of Medicine), 1993; 2:56.
7. *Zhong Yuan Yi Kan* (Resource Journal of Chinese Medicine), 1986; 5:43.
8. *Zhong Hua Yi Xue Za Zhi* (Chinese Journal of Medicine), 1979; 2:123.
9. *Zhong Yao Ming Fang Yao Li Yu Ying Yong* (Pharmacology and Applications of Famous Herbal Formulas), 1989; 539-541.
10. *Zhong Guo Zhong Yao Za Zhi* (People's Republic of China Journal of Chinese Herbology), 1995; 6:375.

Dà Fáng Fēng Tāng (Major Saposhnikovia Decoction)

大防風湯
大防风汤

Pinyin Name: *Da Fang Feng Tang*
Literal Name: Major Saposhnikovia Decoction
Alternate Name: Major Siler Combination
Original Source: *Tai Ping Hui Min He Ji Ju Fang* (Imperial Grace Formulary of the Tai Ping Era) by the Imperial Medical Department in 1078-85

COMPOSITION

Dang Gui (Radix Angelicae Sinensis), *xi* (washed), *jin* (soaked) in liquor, and *chao* (dry-fried)	60g
Shu Di Huang (Radix Rehmanniae Praeparata), *xi* (washed)	60g
Bai Shao (Radix Paeoniae Alba)	60g
Chuan Xiong (Rhizoma Chuanxiong)	45g
Ren Shen (Radix et Rhizoma Ginseng)	30g
Bai Zhu (Rhizoma Atractylodis Macrocephalae)	60g
Huang Qi (Radix Astragali), *chao* (dry-fried)	60g
Niu Xi (Radix Achyranthis Bidentatae), *jin* (soaked) in liquor and *chao* (dry-fried)	30g
Du Zhong (Cortex Eucommiae), *chao* (dry-fried)	60g
Fang Feng (Radix Saposhnikoviae)	60g
Qiang Huo (Rhizoma et Radix Notopterygii)	30g
Fu Zi (Radix Aconiti Lateralis Praeparata), *pao* (blast-fried)	45g
Zhi Gan Cao (Radix et Rhizoma Glycyrrhizae Praeparata cum Melle)	30g

DOSAGE / PREPARATION / ADMINISTRATION

The source text instructs to grind the ingredients into powder. Cook 15g of the powder with 7 slices of *Sheng Jiang* (Rhizoma Zingiberis Recens) and 1 piece of *Da Zao* (Fructus Jujubae) in 1.5 bowls of water until the liquid is reduced to 80% volume. Take the warm, strained decoction on an empty stomach before meals.

CHINESE THERAPEUTIC ACTIONS

1. Tonifies qi and blood
2. Strengthens the muscles and tendons
3. Dispels wind, cold, and dampness

CLINICAL MANIFESTATIONS

Weakness and paralysis of the lower extremities caused by deficiency of qi and blood: generalized pain and decreased sensations in the limbs, weak stifles, muscle atrophy of the extremities, difficult movement, hemiplegia, neuralgia and *wei zheng* (atrophy syndrome).

VETERINARY CLINICAL APPLICATIONS

Chronic osteoarthritis, chronic founder, paralysis of the lower extremities, hemiplegia, weak hindquarters, muscle atrophy, and neuralgia.

EXPLANATION

Da Fang Feng Tang (Major Saposhnikovia Decoction) was designed originally to treat conditions called *li feng* (dysenteric wind) and *he xi feng* (crane's knee wind). Both conditions are characterized by severe qi and blood deficiencies with wind, cold, and dampness at the exterior. *Li feng* is a condition that occurs after dysentery, in which patients have trouble walking due to severe pain and atrophy of the leg muscles. *He xi feng* is a condition in which there is such severe atrophy of the leg muscles that the legs appear to be covered only by skin, resembling the knees of a crane. Animals with *he xi feng* suffer from severe pain and swelling of the stifles, and they have difficulty in flexion and extension.

This formula contains herbs that tonify qi and blood, nourish the muscles and tendons, and dispel wind, cold, and dampness. *Dang Gui* (Radix Angelicae Sinensis), *Shu Di Huang* (Radix Rehmanniae Praeparata), *Bai Shao* (Radix Paeoniae Alba), and *Chuan Xiong* (Rhizoma Chuanxiong) tonify the blood and activate blood circulation. *Ren Shen* (Radix et Rhizoma Ginseng), *Bai Zhu* (Rhizoma Atractylodis Macrocephalae), and *Huang Qi* (Radix Astragali) tonify qi and strengthen the Spleen. *Niu Xi* (Radix Achyranthis Bidentatae) and *Du Zhong* (Cortex Eucommiae) tonify the Kidney, nourish the tendons and muscles, and relieve pain. *Fang Feng* (Radix Saposhnikoviae) and *Qiang Huo* (Rhizoma et Radix Notopterygii) dispel wind and relieve numbness and joint pain. *Fu Zi* (Radix Aconiti

Dà Fáng Fēng Tāng (Major Saposhnikovia Decoction)

Da Fang Feng Tang (Major Saposhnikovia Decoction)

Diagnosis	Clinical Signs	Treatment	Herbs
Li feng (dysenteric wind) and *he xi feng* (crane's knee wind)	• Trouble walking due to severe pain and atrophy of the leg muscles: *li feng* (dysenteric wind) characterized by severe deficiency of qi and blood • Severe atrophy of the leg muscles, severe pain, and swelling of the knees with difficulty in knee flexion and extension: *he xi feng* (crane's knee wind) characterized by severe deficiency of qi and blood	• Tonifies qi and blood • Strengthens muscles and tendons • Dispels wind, cold, and dampness	• *Dang Gui* (Radix Angelicae Sinensis), *Shu Di Huang* (Radix Rehmanniae Praeparata), *Bai Shao* (Radix Paeoniae Alba), and *Chuan Xiong* (Rhizoma Chuanxiong) tonify the blood and activate blood circulation. • *Ren Shen* (Radix et Rhizoma Ginseng), *Bai Zhu* (Rhizoma Atractylodis Macrocephalae), and *Huang Qi* (Radix Astragali) tonify qi and strengthen the Spleen. • *Niu Xi* (Radix Achyranthis Bidentatae) and *Du Zhong* (Cortex Eucommiae) tonify the Kidney, nourish the tendons and muscles, and relieve pain. • *Fang Feng* (Radix Saposhnikoviae) and *Qiang Huo* (Rhizoma et Radix Notopterygii) dispel wind and relieve numbness and joint pain. • *Fu Zi* (Radix Aconiti Lateralis Praeparata) dispels cold and dampness. • *Zhi Gan Cao* (Radix et Rhizoma Glycyrrhizae Praeparata cum Melle) and *Sheng Jiang* (Rhizoma Zingiberis Recens) harmonize the herbs.

Lateralis Praeparata), a hot herb, dispels cold and dampness. *Zhi Gan Cao* (Radix et Rhizoma Glycyrrhizae Praeparata cum Melle) and *Sheng Jiang* (Rhizoma Zingiberis Recens) harmonize the herbs in this formula. Overall, this formula effectively treats *bi zheng* (painful obstruction syndrome) with a constitutional deficiency of qi and blood, wind attacking the muscles and joints, and atrophy and impairment of the skeletal muscles.

VETERINARY MODIFICATIONS

For pain with blood stagnation, add *Tao Ren* (Semen Persicae) and *Hong Hua* (Flos Carthami).

CAUTIONS / CONTRAINDICATIONS

Da Fang Feng Tang is designed for musculoskeletal disorders caused by severe qi and blood deficiencies. Arthritis or musculoskeletal disorders characterized by excess without deficiency should not be treated with this formula as the warm and hot herbs may worsen the excessive condition.

PHARMACOLOGICAL EFFECTS

Antirheumatic: According to studies in mice, administration of *Da Fang Feng Tang* was associated with inhibiting iNOS expression and decreasing anti-collagen IgG antibody. The researchers suggested that *Da Fang Feng Tang* may be effective in treating rheumatoid arthritis in humans.[1,2]

SUGGESTED ACUPUNCTURE TREATMENT

1. Points: *Sanyinjiao* (SP 6), *Xuehai* (SP 10), *Geshu* (BL 17), *Housanli* (ST 36), *Shenshu* (BL 23), *Pishu* (BL 20), *Yanglingquan* (GB 34), *Hegu* (LI 4), *Fengchi* (GB 20), *Houxi* (SI 3), local points and points for pain such as *Kunlun* (BL 60).
2. Technique: moxibustion and tonification.

Sanyinjiao (SP 6), *Xuehai* (SP 10), and *Geshu* (BL 17) tonify the blood. *Housanli* (ST 36), *Shenshu* (BL 23), and *Pishu* (BL 20) tonify qi. *Shenshu* (BL 23) and *Yanglingquan* (GB 34) strengthen bones and tendons. *Hegu* (LI 4) and *Fengchi* (GB 20) dispel wind and cold. *Houxi* (SI 3) opens the channels to relieve stagnation and pain. Apply moxibustion on the joints and local areas to warm the channels and relieve pain.

AUTHORS' COMMENTS

The animals for which this formula is indicated are typically weak, debilitated and geriatric, with severe underlying qi and blood deficiencies. These deficiencies weaken the exterior significantly and allow for the development of chronic *bi zheng* (painful obstruction syndrome) due to wind-cold-dampness. Old dogs with bilateral anterior cruciate ligament rupture (surgically repaired or not) and those with chronic, moderate to

Dà Fáng Fēng Tāng (Major Saposhnikovia Decoction)

severe patellar luxation are in this category. Older horses commonly lose significant muscle mass over their topline and hindquarters, leaving them both weak and stiff. Both species are persistently lame with stifles and hocks that are thickened and enlarged on examination, with greatly decreased range of motion and significant bony changes on radiographic evaluation.

References

1. Wang LR, Ishiguro N, Yamada E, Nishida Y, Sato K, Iwata H. The effect of da-fang-feng-tang on treatment of type II collagen-induced arthritis in DBA/1 mice. Am J Chin Med. 1999; 27(2):205-15.
2. Joe SM, Lee IS, Lee YT, Lee JH, Choi BT. Suppression of collagen-induced arthritis in rats by continuous administration of dae-bang-poong-tang (da-fang-feng-tang). Am J Chin Med. 2001; 29(2):355-65.

Section 3

燥湿清热剂
— Damp-Heat Dispelling Formulas

Guì Zhī Sháo Yào Zhī Mǔ Tāng

(Cinnamon Twig, Peony, and Anemarrhena Decoction)

桂枝芍藥知母湯
桂枝芍药知母汤

Pinyin Name: *Gui Zhi Shao Yao Zhi Mu Tang*
Literal Name: Cinnamon Twig, Peony, and Anemarrhena Decoction
Alternate Names: *Kuei Chih Shao Yao Chih Mu Tang*, Cinnamon and Anemarrhena Combination
Original Source: *Jin Gui Yao Lue* (Essentials from the Golden Cabinet) by Zhang Zhong-Jing in the Eastern Han Dynasty

COMPOSITION

Gui Zhi (Ramulus Cinnamomi)	12g
Ma Huang (Herba Ephedrae)	6g
Fang Feng (Radix Saposhnikoviae)	12g
Fu Zi (Radix Aconiti Lateralis Praeparata), *pao* (blast-fried)	6g
Bai Shao (Radix Paeoniae Alba)	9g
Zhi Mu (Rhizoma Anemarrhenae)	12g
Gan Cao (Radix et Rhizoma Glycyrrhizae)	6g
Bai Zhu (Rhizoma Atractylodis Macrocephalae)	15g
Sheng Jiang (Rhizoma Zingiberis Recens)	15g

DOSAGE / PREPARATION / ADMINISTRATION

The source text instructs to cook the ingredients in 7 cups [1,400 mL] of water until the liquid is reduced to 2 cups [400 mL]. Take 0.7 cup [210 mL] of the warm, strained decoction three times daily.

CHINESE THERAPEUTIC ACTIONS

1. Dispels wind-dampness
2. Clears heat from obstruction
3. Unblocks the channels and collaterals

CLINICAL MANIFESTATIONS

Bi zheng (painful obstruction syndrome) caused by obstruction of wind-dampness and formation of heat: swollen and painful joints that are warm to the touch, poor appetite, emaciation, lethargy, atrophy of the muscle, decreased sensations in the extremities, and difficulty in walking and moving.

VETERINARY CLINICAL APPLICATIONS

Acute and chronic immune-mediated polyarthritis (IPA), chronic arthritis, founder associated with equine Cushing's disease, chronic intervertebral disc disease (IVDD), canine rheumatoid arthritis, polymyositis, masticatory myositis.

EXPLANATION

Gui Zhi Shao Yao Zhi Mu Tang (Cinnamon Twig, Peony, and Anemarrhena Decoction) treats *bi zheng* (painful obstruction syndrome) caused by accumulation of wind-dampness. Obstruction of wind-dampness in the joints leads to the formation of heat, manifesting as joint swelling and pain. In these cases, the heat generated is caused solely by the obstruction, so the heat remains localized in those specific areas without producing systemic signs (fever) of excessive heat. The obstruction also blocks the supply of blood and nutrients to the area, thus contributing to the

Guì Zhī Sháo Yào Zhī Mǔ Tāng

(Cinnamon Twig, Peony, and Anemarrhena Decoction)

Gui Zhi Shao Yao Zhi Mu Tang **(Cinnamon Twig, Peony, and Anemarrhena Decoction)**

Diagnosis	Clinical Signs	Treatment	Herbs
Bi zheng (painful obstruction syndrome) caused by wind-dampness and heat	• Joint swelling, joints warm to the touch and pain: obstruction of wind-dampness with formation of heat • Atrophy of the muscles and decreased sensations in the extremities with difficulty in walking and moving: lack of nourishment due to obstructions • Edema, decreased appetite, weight loss, emaciation, and lethargy: accumulation of dampness in various parts of the body	• Dispels wind-dampness • Clears heat • Unblocks the channels and collaterals	• *Gui Zhi* (Ramulus Cinnamomi), *Ma Huang* (Herba Ephedrae) and *Fang Feng* (Radix Saposhnikoviae) dispel wind from the exterior. • *Fu Zi* (Radix Aconiti Lateralis Praeparata) warms the body and joints and relieves pain. • *Zhi Mu* (Rhizoma Anemarrhenae) clears heat and reduces swelling. • *Bai Shao* (Radix Paeoniae Alba) and *Gan Cao* (Radix et Rhizoma Glycyrrhizae) relieve muscle spasms and cramps. • *Bai Zhu* (Rhizoma Atractylodis Macrocephalae) strengthens the Spleen, dries dampness, and relieves edema. • *Sheng Jiang* (Rhizoma Zingiberis Recens) warms the middle *jiao* to improve appetite and increase food intake.

gradual atrophy of the muscles and numbness of the extremities. The muscle atrophy is sometimes so severe that *he xi feng* (crane's knee wind) is used to describe the condition in which the joint appears to be covered by nothing but the skin. Swelling, pain, and muscle atrophy all contribute to difficulty in walking and moving. In patients with chronic *bi zheng* (painful obstruction syndrome), dampness may affect other parts of the body. Damp accumulation in the lower extremities leads to edema; damp stagnation in the middle *jiao* leads to decreased appetite, weight loss and emaciation; and dampness obstructing the normal flow of qi leads to lethargy and dizziness.

In this formula, *Gui Zhi* (Ramulus Cinnamomi) and *Ma Huang* (Herba Ephedrae) warm and unblock the channels and collaterals. These two herbs, along with *Fang Feng* (Radix Saposhnikoviae), also dispel wind from the exterior parts of the body. *Fu Zi* (Radix Aconiti Lateralis Praeparata) warms the body and joints and relieves pain. Because *Fu Zi* (Radix Aconiti Lateralis Praeparata) is an extremely hot herb, cold herbs such as *Bai Shao* (Radix Paeoniae Alba) and *Zhi Mu* (Rhizoma Anemarrhenae) are used to balance the temperature of the formula and reduce any side effects that might be caused by *Fu Zi* (Radix Aconiti Lateralis Praeparata). Additionally, *Zhi Mu* (Rhizoma Anemarrhenae) clears heat and reduces swelling. *Bai Shao* (Radix Paeoniae Alba) and *Gan Cao* (Radix et Rhizoma Glycyrrhizae) synergistically relieve pain and treat muscle spasms and cramps. *Bai Zhu* (Rhizoma Atractylodis Macrocephalae) strengthens the Spleen, dries dampness, and relieves edema. *Sheng Jiang* (Rhizoma Zingiberis Recens) warms the middle *jiao* to improve appetite and increase food intake.

VETERINARY MODIFICATIONS

- With stiffness and pain of the joints that lessen with heat, increase the dose of *Gui Zhi* (Ramulus Cinnamomi), *Ma Huang* (Herba Ephedrae), and *Fu Zi* (Radix Aconiti Lateralis Praeparata).
- With body aches, numbness, and joint swelling that worsen in rainy, cold weather, add more *Bai Zhu* (Rhizoma Atractylodis Macrocephalae) and *Fu Zi* (Radix Aconiti Lateralis Praeparata).
- With joint pain that lessens during the day and worsens at night, add more *Zhi Mu* (Rhizoma Anemarrhenae), *Bai Shao* (Radix Paeoniae Alba), and *Gan Cao* (Radix et Rhizoma Glycyrrhizae).
- For *bi zheng* (painful obstruction syndrome) with more damp accumulation, add *Fu Ling* (Poria), *Yi Yi Ren* (Semen Coicis), and *Cang Zhu* (Rhizoma Atractylodis).
- With frequent recurrence of pain due to qi deficiency, add *Huang Qi* (Radix Astragali).
- For hot joints, add *Cang Zhu* (Rhizoma Atractylodis), *Sang Zhi* (Ramulus Mori), *Huang Bo* (Cortex Phellodendri Chinensis) and *Ren Dong Teng* (Caulis Lonicerae Japonicae).
- For animals with fever, add *Shi Gao* (Gypsum Fibrosum) and *Chi Shao* (Radix Paeoniae Rubra).

Guì Zhī Sháo Yào Zhī Mǔ Tāng

(Cinnamon Twig, Peony, and Anemarrhena Decoction)

- To improve pain relief, add *Yan Hu Suo* (Rhizoma Corydalis), *Mo Yao* (Myrrha), *Hong Hua* (Flos Carthami) and *Ru Xiang* (Gummi Olibanum).

SUGGESTED ACUPUNCTURE TREATMENT

1. Points: local points.
2. Technique: moxibustion, bleeding, or sedation.

Sedate with moxibustion on the local acupuncture points, or bleed locally along with moxibustion.

AUTHORS' COMMENTS

Gui Zhi Shao Yao Zhi Mu Tang can be used to treat the biomedically defined condition of immune-mediated polyarthritis (IPA) in dogs. In most cases of IPA, the joints are nearly always warm or hot to the touch and therefore could easily be classified into the category of hot *bi zheng* (painful obstruction syndrome). There are multiple Chinese medicine patterns that correspond to a diagnosis of IPA in dogs. One of the most common patterns for which this formula is indicated is constitutional Kidney and Liver yin deficiencies, which invite the invasion of wind-cold-dampness. The situation is often further complicated by feeding a poor or species inappropriate diet, which promotes the production of dampness. In this type of pattern, the exogenous pathogenic factors of wind, cold and dampness cause local stagnation and pain of the joints. In many cases, especially chronic conditions, the cold and damp factors (the root cause) have transformed into heat, and the excess signs obscure the underlying deficiencies. The situation is made even more challenging if the animal is on chronic steroidal medication; the longer the animal has been medicated, the more difficult it will be to treat the animal. A careful history and physical examination is essential in making the correct Chinese medicine diagnosis and thus choosing the appropriate formula. This formula is too warming for cases when signs of systemic (fever) heat are present. *Bai Hu Jia Gui Zhi Tang* (White Tiger plus Cinnamon Twig Decoction) should be used in acute cases of IPA with fever and hot swollen joints. Most cases of immune-mediated polyarthritis will initially require the concurrent use of conventional (corticosteroids) and Chinese herbal medications. The dosage of steroidal drugs can be gradually reduced when acupuncture and herbs resolve the excess and underlying deficiencies. Weaning an animal off of conventional medications too quickly can result in an abrupt relapse, and it is recommended that the animal be evaluated on a weekly basis after initial herbal therapy has begun. It can take 3-6 weeks to see noticeable improvement. To improve clinical results and pain relief in severe cases, *Gui Zhi Shao Yao Zhi Mu Tang* can be combined with *Shen Tong Zhu Yu Tang* (Drive Out Blood Stasis from a Painful Body Decoction).

Gui Zhi Shao Yao Zhi Mu Tang and *Dang Gui Nian Tong Tang* (Tangkuei Decoction to Lift the Pain) can both be used to treat acute and chronic IPA without signs of systemic heat. *Gui Zhi Shao Yao Zhi Mu Tang* dispels wind-dampness, mildly clears heat, and nourishes yin. It is used to treat IPA with heat in the joints caused by obstruction from wind-cold-dampness. It is warming and should not be used in cases in which there is systemic heat. For cases with severely hot joints, add *Yan Hu Suo* (Rhizoma Corydalis), *Ren Dong Teng* (Caulis Lonicerae Japonicae) and *Xi Xian Cao* (Herba Siegesbeckiae). *Dang Gui Nian Tong Tang* (Tangkuei Decoction to Lift the Pain) dispels wind-dampness, has stronger heat-clearing properties, is better at dispelling dampness, and is more nourishing. It contains herbs to nourish qi and blood and can be used long term for patients that are weak and debilitated.

Equine Cushing's disease is another condition in which the use of *Gui Zhi Shao Yao Zhi Mu Tang* can be very effective. In many of these cases, a deficiency of Kidney yang leads to the accumulation of cold and dampness throughout the patient. Both of these pathogens lead to obstruction in the channels, which results in muscle atrophy, lethargy, inappetence, and, most importantly for this formula, the development of heat in the hooves and laminitic pain. It is important for the practitioner to understand that while this formula will help with the pain associated with laminitis, a formula such as *You Gui Wan* (Restore the Right [Kidney] Pill) needs to be given to address the underlying deficiency.

Èr Miào Săn (Two-Marvel Powder)

二妙散

Pinyin Name: *Er Miao San*
Literal Name: Two-Marvel Powder
Original Source: *Dan Xi Xin Fa* (Teachings of [Zhu] Dan-Xi) by Zhu Zhen-Heng in 1481

COMPOSITION

Huang Bo (Cortex Phellodendri Chinensis), *chao* (dry-fried)	15g
Cang Zhu (Rhizoma Atractylodis), *jin* (soaked) in rice water and *chao* (dry-fried)	15g

DOSAGE / PREPARATION / ADMINISTRATION

The source text instructions are to soak *Cang Zhu* (Rhizoma Atractylodis) in rice water first. Dry-fry equal amounts of both herbs and then grind them into powder. Take the powder with boiled water and the fresh juice of *Sheng Jiang* (Rhizoma Zingiberis Recens). Today, this formula is prepared by grinding equal amounts of the ingredients into powder. Take 6g per dose two to three times daily. It may also be prepared as a decoction with the doses suggested in brackets.

CHINESE THERAPEUTIC ACTIONS

Clears heat and dries dampness

CLINICAL MANIFESTATIONS

Damp-heat attacking the lower half of the body: aches and pains in the bones and tendons, leg weakness and atrophy, redness, swelling, and pain of the stifles with burning sensations, vaginal discharge characterized by damp-heat, sores in the lower body characterized by damp-heat, infections of the lower limbs of horses (e.g., scratches, mud fever, greasy heel), scanty, yellow urine, and a yellow, greasy tongue coating.

VETERINARY CLINICAL APPLICATIONS

Osteoarthritis, polyarthritis, cellulitis, canine rheumatoid arthritis, polymyositis, and spondylosis.

EXPLANATION

Er Miao San (Two-Marvel Powder) treats *bi zheng* (painful obstruction syndrome) in the lower half of the body due to damp-heat. Damp-heat may attack the bones and tendons, causing aches and pains with redness, swelling, and burning sensations. Chronic cases of damp-heat may contribute to weakness and atrophy of the leg muscles. Damp-heat may also affect the *dai* (girdle) channel and genital region, causing vaginal discharge and perivulvar and perianal dermatitis. Lastly, damp-heat may also interfere with the urinary system, causing scanty, yellow urine. A yellow, greasy tongue coating is a sign of damp-heat in the body.

Huang Bo (Cortex Phellodendri Chinensis), with its tendency to travel to the lower body, clears heat and dries dampness. *Cang Zhu* (Rhizoma Atractylodis), bitter and warm, also dries dampness. *Er Miao San* contains only two herbs, yet it achieves marvelous results, which is why it is named "Two-Marvel Powder."

VETERINARY MODIFICATIONS

- For *wei zheng* (atrophy syndrome) caused by damp-heat, add *Xi Xian Cao* (Herba Siegesbeckiae), *Wu Jia Pi* (Cortex Acanthopanacis), and *Lu Xian Cao* (Herba Pyrolae).
- For leg *qi* caused by damp-heat, add *Yi Yi Ren* (Semen Coicis), *Mu Gua* (Fructus Chaenomelis), and *Bing Lang* (Semen Arecae).

***Er Miao San* (Two-Marvel Powder)**

Diagnosis	Clinical Signs	Treatment	Herbs
Damp-heat attacking the lower body	• Aches and pains with redness, swelling, and burning sensations: damp-heat attacking the bones and tendons • Weakness and atrophy of the leg muscles: damp-heat accumulation blocking nourishment to the muscles • Vaginal discharge and scanty, yellow urine: damp-heat affecting the lower body • Yellow, greasy tongue coating: damp-heat in the body	Clears heat and dries dampness	• *Huang Bo* (Cortex Phellodendri Chinensis) clears heat and dries dampness in the lower *jiao* • *Cang Zhu* (Rhizoma Atractylodis) strengthens the Spleen and dries dampness.

Èr Miào Săn (Two-Marvel Powder)

- With redness and swelling of the joints, add *Ren Dong Teng* (Caulis Lonicerae Japonicae), *Mu Gua* (Fructus Chaenomelis), and *Qin Jiao* (Radix Gentianae Macrophyllae).
- For *bi zheng* (painful obstruction syndrome) with more heat than dampness, add *Huang Lian* (Rhizoma Coptidis), *Long Dan* (Radix et Rhizoma Gentianae), and *Ku Shen* (Radix Sophorae Flavescentis).
- For *bi zheng* (painful obstruction syndrome) with more dampness than heat, add *Hua Shi* (Talcum), *Fang Ji* (Radix Stephaniae Tetrandrae), and *Tong Cao* (Medulla Tetrapanacis).

CAUTIONS / CONTRAINDICATIONS

- *Er Miao San* is indicated for *bi zheng* (painful obstruction syndrome) with equal amounts of heat and dampness. Modification is needed if the amount of heat and dampness are not the same.
- This formula is contraindicated in patients with Liver and Kidney yin deficiencies, or with body fluids consumed by Lung heat.
- Avoid foods that are sweet, fatty, or greasy.[1]

HUMAN CLINICAL STUDIES AND RESEARCH

1. **Arthritis**: Modified *Er Miao San* was used to treat 278 patients with various types of arthritis. Modifications included: *Jin Yin Hua* (Flos Lonicerae Japonicae), *Pu Gong Ying* (Herba Taraxaci), *Zi Hua Di Ding* (Herba Violae), and *Tu Fu Ling* (Rhizoma Smilacis Glabrae) were added for arthritis with heat characterized by redness, inflammation, swelling, and pain; *Yi Yi Ren* (Semen Coicis), *Bai Hua She She Cao* (Herba Hedyotis), and larger doses of *Tu Fu Ling* (Rhizoma Smilacis Glabrae) and *Huang Bo* (Cortex Phellodendri Chinensis) were added for arthritis with damp-heat and toxins characterized by red spots; *Di Huang* (Radix Rehmanniae) and *Mu Dan Pi* (Cortex Moutan) were added for arthritis with yin-deficient heat characterized by a red tongue and a fine, rapid pulse; *Che Qian Cao* (Herba Plantaginis), *Fang Ji* (Radix Stephaniae Tetrandrae), and *Yi Yi Ren* (Semen Coicis) were added for accumulation of fluids in the joints. Out of 278 patients, the study reported complete recovery in 160 cases, significant improvement in 62 cases, moderate improvement in 44 cases, and no effect in 12 cases.[2]
2. **Gouty arthritis**: Use of modified *Er Miao San* topically and *San Miao Wan* (Three-Marvel Pill) orally was effective in treating acute gouty arthritis. The treatment protocol was to apply *Er Miao San* plus *Du Huo* (Radix Angelicae Pubescentis) and *Fu Rong Ye* (Folium Hibisci) topically to the affected area, and ingest *San Miao Wan* (Three-Marvel Pill) orally. The study reported that most people experienced a reduction of the clinical signs (redness, swelling, and pain of the joints) within 1-2 days, and complete recovery within 5 days.[3]
3. **Ankylosing spondylitis**: Sixteen patients with ankylosing spondylitis characterized by damp-heat were effectively treated with an integrative approach using non-steroidal anti-inflammatory drugs, acupuncture, massage, and modified *Er Miao San*. The herbal formula contained *Cang Zhu* (Rhizoma Atractylodis), *Huang Bo* (Cortex Phellodendri Chinensis), *Sang Ji Sheng* (Herba Taxilli), *Gan Cao* (Radix et Rhizoma Glycyrrhizae), *Qin Jiao* (Radix Gentianae Macrophyllae), *Fang Ji* (Radix Stephaniae Tetrandrae), *Gou Ji* (Rhizoma Cibotii), *Shi Nan Teng* (Ramulus Piper), and *Xu Chang Qing* (Radix et Rhizoma Cynanchi Paniculati). The researchers noted that the integrative treatment was better than any one treatment alone.[4] Note: Details of the integrative treatment were not available at the time of publication.
4. **Neurodermatitis**: An integrative treatment effectively treated 65 patients with neurodermatitis within an average of 7 days. The treatment protocol used modified *Er Miao San* as a topical herbal wash, followed by topical application of a mixture of dexamethasone, chloramphenicol, and rubbing alcohol. This treatment was repeated every other day.[5]
5. **Eczema**: In one study of 68 eczema patients, the use of *Er Miao San* was associated with a 47.06% rate of complete recovery and a 33.8% rate of improvement. The overall effectiveness was 80.86%.[6]
6. **Erythromelalgia**: Use of modified *Er Miao San* for 6 days was associated with 92.67% effectiveness in treating 176 patients with paroxysmal vasodilation with burning pain, increased skin temperature, and redness of the feet and hands. The herbal formula contained *Huang Bo* (Cortex Phellodendri Chinensis), *Cang Zhu* (Rhizoma Atractylodis), *Chuan Niu Xi* (Radix Cyathulae), *Fang Ji* (Radix Stephaniae Tetrandrae), and *Bai Zhi* (Radix Angelicae Dahuricae).[7]
7. **Fungal infection**: One study reported satisfactory results using modified *Er Miao San* topically to treat fungal infection on the feet. The herbal formula contained *Ku Shen* (Radix Sophorae Flavescentis), *Bai Fan* (Alumen), *Zi Cao* (Radix Arnebiae), and *Xu Chang Qing* (Radix et Rhizoma Cynanchi Paniculati). The herbs were cooked in water, and the resultant solution was used as an herbal soak. The patients were instructed to soak the affected area in the herbal solution for 20-30 minutes twice daily in the morning and at night.[8]

SUGGESTED ACUPUNCTURE TREATMENT

1. Points: *Neiting* (ST 44), *Gongsun* (SP 4), *Yinlingquan* (SP 9), and other special points listed below.
2. Technique: sedation.

Èr Miào Săn (Two-Marvel Powder)

Selection of acupuncture points can be divided into two parts: treating the cause and treating the particular clinical signs. In treating the cause, dispelling damp-heat and promoting diuresis are the main objectives. *Neiting* (ST 44), the *ying* (spring) point of the Stomach channel, clears heat from the *yangming* channel. *Gongsun* (SP 4), the *luo* (connecting) point of the Spleen channel, and *Yinlingquan* (SP 9), the *he* (uniting) point of the Spleen channel, clear damp-heat and promote diuresis.

Symptomatically, if patients have painful joints, add *Fengmen* (BL 12), *Geshu* (BL 17), *Ganshu* (BL 18), and other local points; for weakness of the legs, add *Pishu* (BL 20), *Biguan* (ST 31), *Liangqiu* (ST 34), *Housanli* (ST 36), and *Jiexi* (ST 41); for redness, swelling, and pain of the stifles, add *Hegu* (LI 4), *Housanli* (ST 36), and *Xuehai* (SP 10); for leukorrhea due to damp-heat, add *Fengchi* (GB 20), *Zhongji* (CV 3), and *Xialiao* (BL 34); and for skin abscess and ulceration, add *Taodao* (GV 13) and *Feishu* (BL 13).

RELATED FORMULAS

Sān Miào Wán (Three-Marvel Pill)

三妙丸

Pinyin Name: *San Miao Wan*

Literal Name: Three-Marvel Pill

Alternate Name: *San Miao San* (Three-Marvel Powder), Atractylodes and Phellodendron Formula

Original Source: *Yi Xue Zheng Zhuan* (True Lineage of Medicine) by Yu Tian-Min in 1515

Huang Bo (Cortex Phellodendri Chinensis), *ban* (blended) with liquor and *chao* (dry-fried)	120g [12g]
Cang Zhu (Rhizoma Atractylodis), *jin* (soaked) in rice water for 1-2 nights and *bei* (stone-baked) to dry	180g [18g]
Chuan Niu Xi (Radix Cyathulae)	60g [6g]

The source text instructs to grind the ingredients into powder and form into small pills with flour. The pills should resemble the size of *Wu Tong Zi* (Semen Firmianae), a small seed approximately 5 mm in diameter. Take 50-70 pills on an empty stomach with a decoction made from salt and *Sheng Jiang* (Rhizoma Zingiberis Recens). Today, this formula may be prepared as a decoction with the doses suggested in brackets.

San Miao Wan (Three-Marvel Pill) clears heat and dries dampness and is indicated for damp-heat affecting the lower half of the body. Patients may have joint pain, leg numbness, and burning sensations. Clinical applications include arthritis, spondylosis, myositis, dermatitis with rashes, and canine atopy.

Sì Miào Wán (Four-Marvel Pill)

四妙丸

Pinyin Name: *Si Miao Wan*

Literal Name: Four-Marvel Pill

Alternate Name: *Si Miao San* (Four-Marvel Powder)

Original Source: *Cheng Fang Bian Du* (Convenient Reader of Established Formulas) by Zhang Bing-Cheng in 1904

Huang Bo (Cortex Phellodendri Chinensis)	[12g]
Yi Yi Ren (Semen Coicis)	[12g]
Cang Zhu (Rhizoma Atractylodis)	[12g]
Niu Xi (Radix Achyranthis Bidentatae)	[12g]

The source text instructs to grind the ingredients into powder and form into small pills with water. Take 6-9g of pills per dose with warm water. Today, this formula may be prepared as a decoction with the doses suggested in brackets.

Si Miao Wan (Four-Marvel Pill) clears heat and dissolves dampness; it is good for treating damp-heat affecting the lower half of the body. Animals may show signs of inflammation, pain and swelling of the joints, muscle atrophy, weakness of the hindquarters, and dermatitis.

Si Miao Wan is one of the most commonly used formulas in veterinary medicine to treat acute and chronic damp-heat disorders. It has been effectively used to treat immune-mediated polyarthritis with hot, swollen joints, infectious arthritis, canine rheumatoid arthritis, canine atopy, feline miliary dermatitis, perianal and perivulvar dermatitis, anal gland sacculitis, acute and chronic otitis, uveitis, recurrent pyoderma, equine scratches, pododermatitis, interdigital cysts, folliculitis, seborrhea, malassezia dermatitis, masticatory myositis, polymyositis, chronic urinary tract infection, feline lower urinary tract disease, vaginitis and pancreatitis.

Si Miao Wan can be used to treat infectious arthritis (bacterial, Lyme disease) and immune-mediated polyarthritis. These conditions are characterized by a red tongue with white to yellow coating; a rapid, forceful, and slippery to wiry pulse; fever; and red, hot, swollen and painful joints. For this purpose, it is combined with *Bai Hu Tang* (White Tiger Decoction), and together these two formulas dispel wind, drain dampness, clear heat and eliminate toxins. In the treatment of infectious arthritis, it can be additionally combined with *Yin Qiao San* (Honeysuckle and Forsythia Powder) to improve its ability to eliminate toxic heat. These formulas can upset the middle *jiao*, and it is recommended that Spleen tonic herbs be used

Èr Miào Săn (Two-Marvel Powder)

concurrently, especially in animals that have taken or are currently being treated with antimicrobial drugs.

For the treatment of skin disorders, *Si Miao Wan* is commonly combined with other formulas, such as *Long Dan Xie Gan Tang* (Gentiana Decoction to Drain the Liver), *Xiao Feng San* (Eliminate Wind Powder), or *Dang Gui Yin Zi* (Tangkuei Decoction). In the treatment of chronic urinary tract infections (UTI), it is often used in combination with antimicrobial drugs to treat damp-heat in the Urinary Bladder. In these cases, while antibiotics clear heat, they do not typically drain dampness, and *Si Miao Wan* is indispensable for this purpose. It can be combined with *Ba Zheng San* (Eight-Herb Powder for Rectification), *Xiao Ji Yin Zi* (Cirsium Decoction) and *Wu Lin San* (Five-Ingredient Powder for Painful Urinary Dysfunction) in the treatment of antimicrobial resistant chronic UTI.

AUTHORS' COMMENTS

Er Miao San (Two-Marvel Powder), *San Miao Wan* (Three-Marvel Pill), and *Si Miao Wan* (Four-Marvel Pill) all treat musculoskeletal disorders characterized by damp-heat attacking the lower half of the body. Of these three formulas, *Si Miao Wan* is the most commonly used in veterinary medicine.

- *Er Miao San* is the original formula that contains two herbs with equal emphasis on eliminating both dampness and heat.
- *San Miao Wan* is formulated with the addition of *Chuan Niu Xi* (Radix Cyathulae), which guides the formula to the lower parts of the body and tonifies the Liver and Kidney.
- *Si Miao Wan* is formulated with the addition of *Niu Xi* (Radix Achyranthis Bidentatae) and *Yi Yi Ren* (Semen Coicis) to tonify the Liver and Kidney and dry dampness. Of the three, this formula is most suitable for chronic cases of damp-heat affecting the lower half of the body, causing decreased sensations and atrophy.

References

1. *Zhong Yao Ming Fang Yao Li Yu Ying Yong* (Pharmacology and Applications of Famous Herbal Formulas), 1989; 416-417.
2. *Shi Yong Zhong Yi Nei Ke Za Zhi* (Journal of Practical Chinese Internal Medicine), 1997; 2:36.
3. *Si Chuan Zhong Yi* (Sichuan Chinese Medicine), 1997; 11:47.
4. *Xin Zhong Yi* (New Chinese Medicine), 1994; 7:24.
5. *Zhong Yuan Yi Kan* (Resource Journal of Chinese Medicine), 1990; 4:12.
6. *Zhe Jiang Zhong Yi Za Zhi* (Zhejiang Journal of Chinese Medicine), 1983; 10:468.
7. *Hu Nan Zhong Yi Za Zhi* (Hunan Journal of Chinese Medicine), 1987; 5:24.
8. *Shan Dong Zhong Yi Za Zhi* (Shandong Journal of Chinese Medicine), 1989; 8(4):50.

Dāng Guī Niǎn Tòng Tāng (Tangkuei Decoction to Lift the Pain)

當歸拈痛湯
当归拈痛汤

Pinyin Name: *Dang Gui Nian Tong Tang*
Literal Name: Tangkuei Decoction to Lift the Pain
Alternate Names: *Tang Kuei Nien Tung Tang*, Tang-kuei and Pain-Assuaging Decoction, Tangkuei and Anemarrhena Combination
Original Source: *Lan Shi Mi Cang* (Secrets from the Orchid Chamber) by Li Gao in 1336

COMPOSITION

Qiang Huo (Rhizoma et Radix Notopterygii)	15g
Ge Gen (Radix Puerariae Lobatae)	6g
Fang Feng (Radix Saposhnikoviae)	9g
Sheng Ma (Rhizoma Cimicifugae)	6g
Huang Qin (Radix Scutellariae), *xi* (washed) with liquor	9g
Ku Shen (Radix Sophorae Flavescentis), *chao* (dry-fried) in liquor	6g
Zhi Mu (Rhizoma Anemarrhenae), *xi* (washed) with liquor	9g
Yin Chen (Herba Artemisiae Scopariae), *xi* (washed) with liquor	15g
Ze Xie (Rhizoma Alismatis)	9g
Zhu Ling (Polyporus)	9g
Bai Zhu (Rhizoma Atractylodis Macrocephalae)	4.5g
Cang Zhu (Rhizoma Atractylodis)	6g
Ren Shen (Radix et Rhizoma Ginseng)	6g
Dang Gui (Radix Angelicae Sinensis)	9g
Zhi Gan Cao (Radix et Rhizoma Glycyrrhizae Praeparata cum Melle)	15g

DOSAGE / PREPARATION / ADMINISTRATION

The source text instructs to grind the ingredients into a coarse powder. Cook 30g of the powder in 2.5 bowls of water until the liquid is reduced to 1 bowl. Take the strained decoction while it is warm.

CHINESE THERAPEUTIC ACTIONS

1. Dispels wind and dampness
2. Clears heat and relieves pain

CLINICAL MANIFESTATIONS

Dampness and heat affecting the joints and extremities: joint or musculoskeletal pain with redness, mild fever, swelling, and inflammation, stiffness in the shoulders and back, dermatological disorders of the lower extremities with itching and pain, skin ulceration and abscess, a red tongue with a white to yellow coating, and a rapid, slippery to wiry pulse.

VETERINARY CLINICAL APPLICATIONS

Arthritis and arthralgia with inflammation and joint swelling, generalized joint and musculoskeletal pain, pododermatitis, interdigital cyst, dermatitis of the lower extremities, anal and vulvar itching, dysuria, hematuria, trigeminal nerve pain, neuritis, polyneuritis, neuralgia, cellulitis, canine rheumatoid arthritis and immune-mediated polyarthritis.

EXPLANATION

Dang Gui Nian Tong Tang (Tangkuei Decoction to Lift the Pain) is one of the most effective formulas for treating joint and musculoskeletal disorders caused by damp-heat, with signs of mild fever, pain, redness, swelling, and inflammation. Due to the damp nature of the illness, animals may experience stiffness throughout the shoulders and back. Due to the presence of heat, patients may experience redness, swelling, and inflammation in the joints and muscles. Moreover, as dampness and heat travel downward, animals may feel itching and pain in the lower extremities. In severe cases, there may also be ulceration and abscess of the skin.

In this formula, *Qiang Huo* (Rhizoma et Radix Notopterygii), *Ge Gen* (Radix Puerariae Lobatae), *Fang Feng* (Radix Saposhnikoviae), and *Sheng Ma* (Rhizoma Cimicifugae) dispel wind and dampness to relieve pain. *Huang Qin* (Radix Scutellariae), *Ku Shen* (Radix Sophorae Flavescentis), *Zhi Mu* (Rhizoma Anemarrhenae), and *Yin Chen* (Herba Artemisiae Scopariae) eliminate damp-heat from the body. *Ze Xie* (Rhizoma Alismatis) and *Zhu Ling*

Dāng Guī Niǎn Tòng Tāng (Tangkuei Decoction to Lift the Pain)

***Dang Gui Nian Tong Tang* (Tangkuei Decoction to Lift the Pain)**

Diagnosis	Clinical Signs	Treatment	Herbs
Dampness and heat affecting the joints and extremities	• Lethargy and stiffness: damp accumulation in the body • Redness, swelling, and inflammation in the joints and muscles, mild fever: heat affecting the joints and muscles • Itching and pain in the lower extremities: damp-heat traveling downward • Skin ulceration and abscess: damp-heat traveling outward • Rapid, slippery to wiry pulse: damp-heat condition	• Dispels wind and dampness • Clears heat and relieves pain	• *Qiang Huo* (Rhizoma et Radix Notopterygii), *Ge Gen* (Radix Puerariae Lobatae), *Fang Feng* (Radix Saposhnikoviae), and *Sheng Ma* (Rhizoma Cimicifugae) dispel wind and dampness to relieve pain. • *Huang Qin* (Radix Scutellariae), *Ku Shen* (Radix Sophorae Flavescentis), *Zhi Mu* (Rhizoma Anemarrhenae), and *Yin Chen* (Herba Artemisiae Scopariae) eliminate damp-heat from the body. • *Ze Xie* (Rhizoma Alismatis) and *Zhu Ling* (Polyporus) resolve dampness. • *Bai Zhu* (Rhizoma Atractylodis Macrocephalae) and *Cang Zhu* (Rhizoma Atractylodis) strengthen the Spleen and dry dampness. • *Ren Shen* (Radix et Rhizoma Ginseng) and *Dang Gui* (Radix Angelicae Sinensis) tonify qi and blood. • *Zhi Gan Cao* (Radix et Rhizoma Glycyrrhizae Praeparata cum Melle) harmonizes the herbs.

(Polyporus) resolve dampness and promote diuresis. *Bai Zhu* (Rhizoma Atractylodis Macrocephalae) and *Cang Zhu* (Rhizoma Atractylodis) strengthen the Spleen and dry dampness. *Ren Shen* (Radix et Rhizoma Ginseng) and *Dang Gui* (Radix Angelicae Sinensis) tonify qi and blood to facilitate recovery. *Zhi Gan Cao* (Radix et Rhizoma Glycyrrhizae Praeparata cum Melle) harmonizes the herbs in this formula.

VETERINARY MODIFICATIONS

- With severe pain with redness, swelling and inflammation, add *Huang Lian* (Rhizoma Coptidis) and *Shi Gao* (Gypsum Fibrosum).
- With severe pain in the joints and extremities, add *Gui Zhi* (Ramulus Cinnamomi) and *Bai Shao* (Radix Paeoniae Alba).
- With itching and pain of the skin, add *Jin Yin Hua* (Flos Lonicerae Japonicae) and *Lian Qiao* (Fructus Forsythiae).
- With severe swelling of the stifles and legs, add *Fang Ji* (Radix Stephaniae Tetrandrae) and *Mu Gua* (Fructus Chaenomelis).
- With body aches, add *Jiang Huang* (Rhizoma Curcumae Longae) and *Hai Tong Pi* (Cortex Erythrinae).
- With severe swelling and pain due to damp-heat, combine with *Huang Lian Jie Du Tang* (Coptis Decoction to Relieve Toxicity).
- With skin ulceration and abscess, combine with *Tuo Li Xiao Du Yin* (Drain the Interior and Detoxify Decoction).
- With damp-heat dermatitis, combine with *Yi Yi Ren* (Semen Coicis), *Tu Fu Ling* (Rhizoma Smilacis Glabrae) and *Lian Qiao* (Fructus Forsythiae).

CAUTIONS / CONTRAINDICATIONS

Avoid foods that are spicy, pungent, oily, or greasy.[1]

PHARMACOLOGICAL EFFECTS

Anti-inflammatory: Administration of *Dang Gui Nian Tong Tang* or *Du Huo Ji Sheng Tang* (Angelica Pubescens and Taxillus Decoction) was associated with a marked anti-inflammatory effect to suppress the development of chronic arthritis induced by carrageenan or complete Freund's adjuvant. The researchers suggested that these herbal formulas may be considered as alternatives for non-steroid anti-inflammatory drugs (NSAIDS).[2]

HUMAN CLINICAL STUDIES AND RESEARCH

1. **Neurodermatitis**: Use of modified *Dang Gui Nian Tong Tang* in 30 patients was associated with complete recovery in 22 cases, improvement in 7 cases, and no effect in 1 case.[3]
2. **Impetigo herpetiformis**: One study of 86 patients with impetigo herpetiformis reported good results using modified *Dang Gui Nian Tong Tang* both internally and topically. The herbal treatment had the following modifications: for early-stage, during the eruption of lesions, *Bai Zhi* (Radix Angelicae Dahuricae) and *Dang Shen* (Radix Codonopsis) were removed, and *Tu Fu Ling* (Rhizoma

Dāng Guī Niǎn Tòng Tāng (Tangkuei Decoction to Lift the Pain)

Smilacis Glabrae), *Zi Hua Di Ding* (Herba Violae), *Ye Ju Hua* (Flos Chrysanthemi Indici), and *Jin Yin Hua* (Flos Lonicerae Japonicae) were added; during healing, *Di Fu Zi* (Fructus Kochiae) and *Chan Tui* (Periostracum Cicadae) were added to relieve itching. The treatment protocol was to cook the herbs in water two separate times and drink the decoction orally. The herb residue was cooked in water a third time and the resultant solution used as an herbal wash to the affected area. The study reported complete recovery in all 86 patients within 12 packs of herbs.[4]

3. **Rash**: Use of modified *Dang Gui Nian Tong Tang* in 47 patients with rash was associated with complete recovery in 38 cases, significant improvement in 5 cases, moderate improvement in 2 cases, and no effect in 2 cases. The duration of treatment ranged from 5 to 32 packs of herbs.[5]
4. **Gout**: One study reported 90% effectiveness using modified *Dang Gui Nian Tong Tang* to treat gout in 40 patients. The herbal formula contained *Dang Gui Nian Tong Tang* plus *Hu Zhang* (Rhizoma et Radix Polygoni Cuspidati), *Song Jie* (Lignum Pini Nodi), *Mu Gua* (Fructus Chaenomelis), and *Ren Dong Teng* (Caulis Lonicerae Japonicae). The duration of treatment ranged from 20-98 days, with most showing symptomatic improvements after 33-40 days and normalization of plasma uric acid levels after 90 days. Of 40 patients, the study reported complete recovery in 7 cases, improvement in 29 cases, and no response in 4 cases.[6]
5. ***Bi zheng* (painful obstruction syndrome)**: *Dang Gui Nian Tong Tang* has been shown to effectively treat musculoskeletal pain affecting various parts of the body, including shoulders, arms, and legs.[7,8,9,10]

SUGGESTED ACUPUNCTURE TREATMENT

1. Points: *Fengmen* (BL 12), *Hegu* (LI 4), *Yinlingquan* (SP 9), *Fenglong* (ST 40), *Quchi* (LI 11), *Xuehai* (SP 10), *Weizhong* (BL 40), *Quze* (PC 3), *Housanli* (ST 36), *Sanyinjiao* (SP 6), and *ah shi* points.
2. Technique: sedation and bleeding.

Fengmen (BL 12) and *Hegu* (LI 4) dispel wind. *Yinlingquan* (SP 9) and *Fenglong* (ST 40) eliminate dampness. To remove damp-heat, sedate *Quchi* (LI 11) and *Xuehai* (SP 10), and bleed *Weizhong* (BL 40) for the lower part of the body, and *Quze* (PC 3) for the upper part. *Housanli* (ST 36) and *Sanyinjiao* (SP 6) activate the circulation of qi and blood. *Ah shi* points relieve heat, redness, swelling, and pain in the affected area.

AUTHORS' COMMENTS

Dang Gui Nian Tong Tang is effective for the treatment of acute and chronic immune-mediated polyarthritis (IPA) in dogs characterized by hot, swollen and painful joints. This formula contains more tonifying herbs than *Bai Hu Tang* (White Tiger Decoction) and *Si Miao Wan* (Four-Marvel Pill) for the treatment of polyarthritis, and thus it can be given for a longer period of time. It can be combined with *Shang Zhong Xia Tong Yong Tong Feng Wan* (Upper, Middle, and Lower General-Use Pill for Wind-Pain) to relieve pain and improve and hasten therapeutic results. *Dang Gui Nian Tong Tang* is a good formula to use in dogs when there is concurrent musculoskeletal and arthritis pain and damp-heat skin conditions affecting the ventral surface of the body and the lower extremities. This condition commonly occurs in middle-aged and geriatric dogs that are obese. It is particularly useful in treating damp-heat skin conditions affecting the lower limbs in dogs.

Dang Gui Nian Tong Tang can be combined with *Si Miao Wan* (Four-Marvel Pill) to more effectively treat severe and stubborn cases of dermatitis and damp-heat skin disorders affecting the lower body, such as cellulitis, perianal and vulvar dermatitis, equine scratches, pododermatitis and interdigital cysts. To treat severe cases of interdigital cyst and pododermatitis, it can be combined with *Long Dan Xie Gan Tang* (Gentiana Decoction to Drain the Liver) to achieve rapid resolution of the acute stage of the condition. A course of treatment should not exceed 7-10 days without re-evaluation. At that point, it is best to use herbs that drain chronic dampness, such as *Si Miao Wan* (Four-Marvel Pill) in combination with *Dang Gui Nian Tong Tang*.

References

1. *Zhong Yao Ming Fang Yao Li Yu Ying Yong* (Pharmacology and Applications of Famous Herbal Formulas), 1989; 426-428.
2. Lin CC, Chen MF, Chen CF. The anti-inflammatory effects of Chinese crude drug prescriptions on experimental arthritis. Am J Chin Med. 1995; 23(2):145-52.
3. *Hu Nan Zhong Yi Za Zhi* (Hunan Journal of Chinese Medicine), 1992; 8(4):42.
4. *Hu Nan Zhong Yi Za Zhi* (Hunan Journal of Chinese Medicine), 1990; 6(6):42.
5. *Hu Bei Zhong Yi Za Zhi* (Hubei Journal of Chinese Medicine), 1986; 1:21.
6. *Zhong Yi Za Zhi* (Journal of Chinese Medicine), 1987; 28(2):60.
7. *Si Chuan Zhong Yi* (Sichuan Chinese Medicine), 1986; 4(1):44.
8. *Ji Lin Zhong Yi Yao* (Jilin Chinese Medicine and Herbology), 1989; 2:33.
9. *Hei Long Jiang Zhong Yi Yao* (Heilongjiang Chinese Medicine and Herbology), 1986; 6:43.
10. *He Bei Zhong Yi* (Hebei Chinese Medicine), 1993; 15(5):33.

Section 4

燥湿祛痰剂
— Damp-Phlegm Dispelling Formula

Èr Zhú Tāng (Two-Atractylodes Decoction)

二朮湯
二术汤

Pinyin Name: *Er Zhu Tang*
Literal Name: Two-Atractylodes Decoction
Alternate Name: Atractylodes and Arisaema Combination
Original Source: *Wan Bing Hui Chun* (Restoration of Health from the Myriad Diseases) by Gong Ting-Xian in 1587

COMPOSITION

Ban Xia (Rhizoma Pinelliae), *zhi* (prepared) with ginger	6g
Tian Nan Xing (Rhizoma Arisaematis)	3g
Bai Zhu (Rhizoma Atractylodis Macrocephalae)	3g
Cang Zhu (Rhizoma Atractylodis), *xi* (washed) in rice water and *chao* (dry-fried)	4.5g
Fu Ling (Poria)	3g
Qiang Huo (Rhizoma et Radix Notopterygii)	3g
Xiang Fu (Rhizoma Cyperi)	3g
Wei Ling Xian (Radix et Rhizoma Clematidis)	3g
Chen Pi (Pericarpium Citri Reticulatae)	3g
Huang Qin (Radix Scutellariae), *zhi* (prepared) with liquor	3g
Gan Cao (Radix et Rhizoma Glycyrrhizae)	3g

DOSAGE / PREPARATION / ADMINISTRATION

The source text instructs to cook the ingredients with *Sheng Jiang* (Rhizoma Zingiberis Recens). Take the strained decoction while it is warm.

CHINESE THERAPEUTIC ACTIONS

1. Dispels dampness and eliminates phlegm
2. Opens the channels and collaterals to relieve pain

CLINICAL MANIFESTATIONS

Musculoskeletal disorders of the front limbs due to phlegm stagnation: aches and pains in the carpus, elbow, and shoulder, bursitis, and tendonitis.

VETERINARY CLINICAL APPLICATIONS

Pain of the forelimb, particularly on extension, bicipital bursitis, chronic suspensory ligament inflammation, cervical disc neuralgia.

EXPLANATION

Er Zhu Tang (Two-Atractylodes Decoction) treats musculoskeletal aches and pains due to damp and phlegm accumulation in the upper body. Dampness initially arises as a result of the inability of the Spleen to transport and transform water and food. Thus, patients may experience gastrointestinal weakness as a result of Spleen deficiency. Over time, dampness turns into phlegm, and the phlegm accumulates in the muscles, causing aches and pains and other musculoskeletal disorders.

In this formula, *Ban Xia* (Rhizoma Pinelliae) and *Tian Nan Xing* (Rhizoma Arisaematis) dry dampness and eliminate phlegm. *Bai Zhu* (Rhizoma Atractylodis Macrocephalae), *Cang Zhu* (Rhizoma Atractylodis), and *Fu Ling* (Poria) strengthen the Spleen and Stomach and dry dampness. *Qiang Huo* (Rhizoma et Radix Notopterygii) dispels wind and dries dampness. Together with *Xiang Fu* (Rhizoma Cyperi) and *Wei Ling Xian* (Radix et Rhizoma Clematidis),

Èr Zhú Tāng (Two-Atractylodes Decoction)

***Er Zhu Tang* (Two-Atractylodes Decoction)**

Diagnosis	Clinical Signs	Treatment	Herbs
Aches and pains due to damp and phlegm accumulation	Aches and pains in the carpus, forearm, elbow, and shoulders: damp and phlegm accumulation in the upper body	• Dispels dampness and eliminates phlegm • Opens the channels and collaterals to relieve pain	• *Ban Xia* (Rhizoma Pinelliae) and *Tian Nan Xing* (Rhizoma Arisaematis) dry dampness and eliminate phlegm. • *Bai Zhu* (Rhizoma Atractylodis Macrocephalae), *Cang Zhu* (Rhizoma Atractylodis), and *Fu Ling* (Poria) strengthen the Spleen and Stomach and dry dampness. • *Qiang Huo* (Rhizoma et Radix Notopterygii) dispels wind and dries dampness. • *Xiang Fu* (Rhizoma Cyperi), *Wei Ling Xian* (Radix et Rhizoma Clematidis), and *Chen Pi* (Pericarpium Citri Reticulatae) regulate qi circulation. • *Huang Qin* (Radix Scutellariae) clears damp-heat and reduces swelling and inflammation. • *Sheng Jiang* (Rhizoma Zingiberis Recens) relieves nausea and vomiting by redirecting Stomach qi downward. • *Gan Cao* (Radix et Rhizoma Glycyrrhizae) harmonizes the herbs.

these three herbs regulate qi circulation, open up the peripheral channels and collaterals, benefit the joints, and relieve muscle aches and pains. *Chen Pi* (Pericarpium Citri Reticulatae) activates and regulates the qi flow to remove the residual phlegm and dampness. *Huang Qin* (Radix Scutellariae) clears damp-heat and reduces swelling and inflammation. *Sheng Jiang* (Rhizoma Zingiberis Recens) relieves nausea and vomiting by redirecting Stomach qi downward; it also reduces the toxicity of *Ban Xia* (Rhizoma Pinelliae). *Gan Cao* (Radix et Rhizoma Glycyrrhizae) harmonizes the herbs in this formula.

VETERINARY MODIFICATIONS

- With neck stiffness, add *Ge Gen* (Radix Puerariae Lobatae) and *Gan Cao* (Radix et Rhizoma Glycyrrhizae).
- With edema, add *Wu Ling San* (Five-Ingredient Powder with Poria).
- With soreness and pain of the joints, add *Niu Xi* (Radix Achyranthis Bidentatae), *Xu Duan* (Radix Dipsaci), and *Mu Fang Ji* (Radix Cocculi Trilobi).
- With phlegm in the Lung, add *Jie Geng* (Radix Platycodonis) and *Chai Hu* (Radix Bupleuri).
- For sciatica, add *Shu Jing Huo Xue Tang* (Relax the Channels and Invigorate the Blood Decoction).

SUGGESTED ACUPUNCTURE TREATMENT

1. Points: *Jianjing* (LI 15), *Qianfeng* (SI 9), *Bozhong* (GB 21), *Fenglong* (ST 40), and *Chengshan* (BL 57).
2. Technique: even method.

Needle *Jianjing* (LI 15), *Qianfeng* (SI 9), and *Bozhong* (GB 21) on the affected side of the body to relieve the pain. Apply electrostimulation across needles at *Fenglong* (ST 40) and *Chengshan* (BL 57) to dissolve phlegm, remove stagnation, and relieve pain in the front limbs and shoulders. Local points should also be used.

AUTHORS' COMMENTS

The primary function of *Er Zhu Tang* is to dry dampness, resolve phlegm, open the channels and relieve pain. This formula should be prescribed in cases where more commonly used formulas have failed to relieve the pain and arthralgia. In these cases, unless the phlegm is resolved, it will continue to obstruct the channels and cause pain.

Er Zhu Tang can be combined with *Du Huo Ji Sheng Tang* (Angelica Pubescens and Taxillus Decoction) to treat non-responsive, stubborn, chronic back pain. It can be combined with *Shu Jing Huo Xue Tang* (Relax the Channels and Invigorate the Blood Decoction) to improve pain relief. For unresponsive neck, shoulder and elbow pain in dogs and horses, it can be combined with *Ge Gen Tang* (Kudzu Decoction) to help resolve the problem.

Chapter 17 — Summary

— Wind-Damp Dispelling Formulas

SECTION 1: WIND-DAMP DISPELLING FORMULAS

Name	Similarities	Differences
Qiang Huo Sheng Shi Tang (Notopterygium Decoction to Overcome Dampness)	Dispel wind and dampness, treat *bi zheng* (painful obstruction syndrome)	Treats soreness and pain of the neck, shoulders, and back
Juan Bi Tang (Remove Painful Obstruction Decoction)		Treats soreness and pain of the upper body with underlying *ying* (nutritive) and *wei* (defensive) *qi* deficiencies
Du Huo Ji Sheng Tang (Angelica Pubescens and Taxillus Decoction)		Treats soreness and pain of the lower back and knees with qi, blood, and yin deficiencies
San Bi Tang (Three-Painful Obstruction Decoction)		Treats soreness and pain with qi and blood deficiencies
Shu Jing Huo Xue Tang (Relax the Channels and Invigorate the Blood Decoction)		Treats aches and pains due to damp accumulation and blood stagnation with underlying deficiencies
Yi Yi Ren Tang (Coicis Decoction)		Treats numbness, swelling, and pain of the extremities due to wind-dampness
Shang Zhong Xia Tong Yong Tong Feng Wan (Upper, Middle, and Lower General-Use Pill for Wind-Pain)		Treats aches and pains throughout the entire body

Qiang Huo Sheng Shi Tang (Notopterygium Decoction to Overcome Dampness) dispels wind and eliminates dampness. It is most effective for wind-dampness at the exterior affecting the shoulder and back. Clinical manifestations include signs such as stiffness and immobility of the neck and shoulders, heaviness of the body, back pain with difficulty of movement, a white tongue coating, and a superficial pulse.

Juan Bi Tang (Remove Painful Obstruction Decoction) dispels wind-dampness, tonifies qi, and harmonizes *ying* (nutritive) and *wei* (defensive) levels. This formula is most effective for *bi zheng* (painful obstruction syndrome) due to wind-dampness with underlying *ying* (nutritive) and *wei* (defensive) *qi* deficiencies. Clinical manifestations include shoulder pain, neck pain, and decreased sensations of the extremities.

Du Huo Ji Sheng Tang (Angelica Pubescens and Taxillus Decoction) dispels wind-dampness, nourishes the Liver and Kidney, and tonifies qi and blood. It is generally used to treat chronic *bi zheng* (painful obstruction syndrome) with qi, blood, Liver and Kidney deficiencies. Clinical manifestations include low back pain, knee pain, painful joints, difficult movement of the extremities, aversion to cold, a preference for warmth, and lethargy.

Chapter 17 — Summary

San Bi Tang (Three-Painful Obstruction Decoction) dispels wind-cold-dampness, tonifies qi, and nourishes blood. It treats *bi zheng* (painful obstruction syndrome) due to stagnation of wind-cold-dampness with underlying qi and blood deficiencies. Clinical manifestations include decreased sensations and pain of the muscles and joints, decreased range of motion, and pain aggravated by exposure to cold and damp weather.

Shu Jing Huo Xue Tang (Relax the Channels and Invigorate the Blood Decoction) dispels dampness, activates blood circulation, and opens the channels and collaterals. It is an excellent formula to treat *bi zheng* (painful obstruction syndrome) characterized by damp accumulation and blood stagnation blocking the channels and collaterals. Clinical signs include severe muscle ache, painful joints, radiating pain in the leg, decreased sensations in the lower extremities, and pain in the trunk and extremities.

Yi Yi Ren Tang (Coicis Decoction) dispels wind-dampness, activates blood circulation, and tonifies qi. It treats *bi zheng* (painful obstruction syndrome) characterized by wind-dampness with decreased sensations and pain of the extremities and decreased mobility and range of motion of the joints with swelling and inflammation.

Shang Zhong Xia Tong Yong Tong Feng Wan (Upper, Middle, and Lower General-Use Pill for Wind-Pain) dispels wind, dissolves dampness, activates blood circulation, and eliminates blood stasis. It is designed to treat generalized *bi zheng* (painful obstruction syndrome) that affects the entire body (upper, middle, and lower).

SECTION 2: DAMP-COLD DISPELLING FORMULAS

Name	Similarities	Differences
Xiao Huo Luo Dan (Minor Invigorate the Collaterals Special Pill)	Dispel damp-cold, treat *bi zheng* (painful obstruction syndrome)	Opens the channels and collaterals, dispels dampness and phlegm
Da Fang Feng Tang (Major Saposhnikovia Decoction)		Tonifies qi and blood, strengthens the muscles and tendons

Xiao Huo Luo Dan (Minor Invigorate the Collaterals Special Pill) dispels wind-cold-dampness, dissolves phlegm, dredges the channels, activates blood circulation, and stops pain. Stagnation of wind, cold, dampness, phlegm, and blood may produce clinical manifestations of difficult movement of the joints, pain and numbness in the extremities, paralysis, hemiplegia and weakness of the hindquarters.

Da Fang Feng Tang (Major Saposhnikovia Decoction) dispels wind, cold and dampness, tonifies qi and blood, and strengthens muscles and tendons. It is used to treat weakness and paralysis of the lower extremities due to deficiencies of qi and blood. Clinical manifestations include generalized pain and numbness in the legs, weak knees, atrophy of the leg muscles, and difficulty of movement, hemiplegia, and neuralgia.

Chapter 17 — Summary

SECTION 3: DAMP-HEAT DISPELLING FORMULAS

Name	Similarities	Differences
Gui Zhi Shao Yao Zhi Mu Tang (Cinnamon Twig, Peony, and Anemarrhena Decoction)	Dispels wind-dampness, clears heat	Reduces swelling, inflammation, and pain in the joints
Er Miao San (Two-Marvel Powder)	Dispel damp-heat, treat *bi zheng* (painful obstruction syndrome)	Clears damp-heat affecting the lower body
Dang Gui Nian Tong Tang (Tangkuei Decoction to Lift the Pain)		Treats damp-heat affecting the joints and extremities

Gui Zhi Shao Yao Zhi Mu Tang (Cinnamon Twig, Peony, and Anemarrhena Decoction) dispels wind-dampness, clears heat, and unblocks the channels and collaterals. It is primarily used to treat *bi zheng* (painful obstruction syndrome) characterized by invasion of wind-dampness and accumulation of heat, with clinical signs such as warm, swollen and painful joints, emaciation, atrophy of the muscle, numbness of the extremities, and difficulty with walking and movement.

Er Miao San (Two-Marvel Powder) clears heat and dries dampness. It is used for mild damp-heat attacking the lower half of the body. Clinical manifestations include pain in the lower body, redness, swelling, weakness of the hind quarters, scanty, yellow urine, and vaginal discharge. *Si Miao San* (Four-Marvel Powder), an associated formula, is frequently used in veterinary medicine for damp-heat joint disease, chronic urinary damp-heat, damp-heat vaginitis, and damp-heat skin diseases affecting the ventral and lower body.

Dang Gui Nian Tong Tang (Tangkuei Decoction to Lift the Pain) dispels wind, resolves dampness, clears heat, and relieves pain. It is one of the most effective formulas for treating damp-heat type of joint and musculoskeletal disorders with pain, redness, swelling and inflammation. Clinical manifestations include joint or musculoskeletal pain with redness, mild fever, swelling and inflammation, stiffness of the neck, shoulders and back, dermatological disorders in the lower extremities with itching and pain, ulceration and abscess of the skin, and a deep, rapid, slippery to wiry pulse.

SECTION 4: DAMP-PHLEGM DISPELLING FORMULA

Name	Similarities	Differences
Er Zhu Tang (Two-Atractylodes Decoction)	Dispels dampness, eliminates phlegm	Opens up the channels and collaterals

Er Zhu Tang (Two-Atractylodes Decoction) dispels dampness, eliminates phlegm, opens up the channels and collaterals, and relieves pain. It treats stubborn musculoskeletal disorders of the arms and shoulders due to damp and phlegm stagnation. Clinical manifestations include aches and pains in the carpus, elbow, shoulder and neck, bursitis, tendinitis, and frozen shoulder.

Chapter 18

— Phlegm-Dispelling Formulas

祛痰剂

朱震亨 Zhú Zhèn-Héng

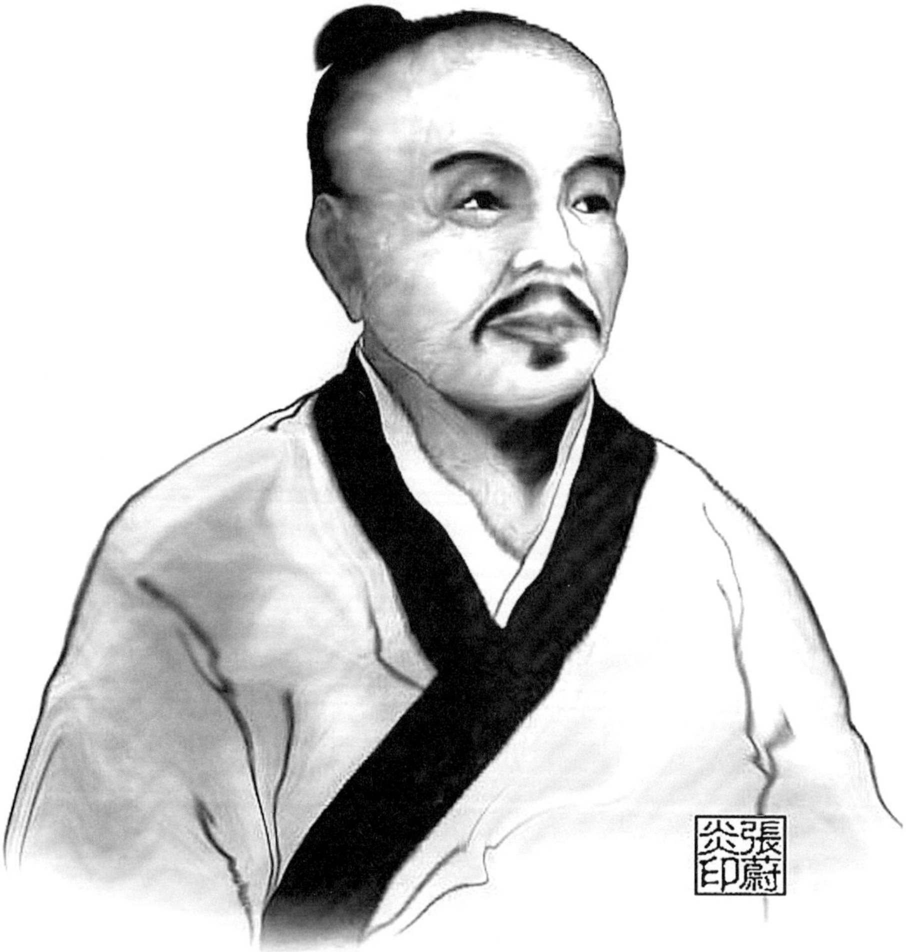

朱震亨 Zhú Zhèn-Héng, also known as
朱丹溪 Zhú Dán-Xí, 1281 – 1358.

朱震亨 Zhú Zhèn-Héng

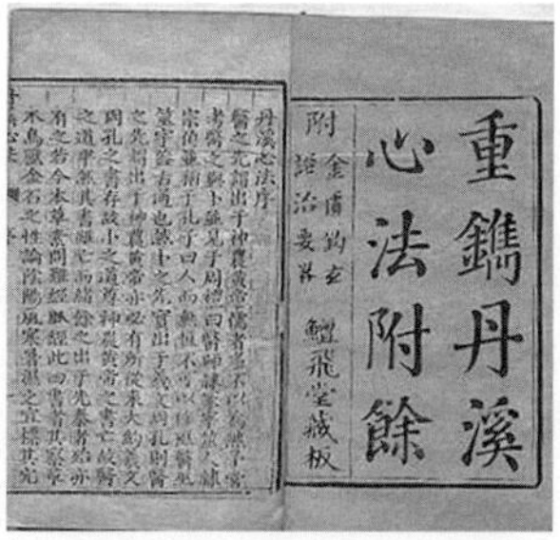

丹溪心法 *Dan Xi Xin Fa* (Teachings of [Zhu] Dan-Xi), published in 1481.

Known as a wonder child, Zhu Zhen-Heng excelled in academia, rapidly passing his peers. He was able to recite thousands of verses by the time he was six years old. Because of his outstanding achievements at such a young age, Zhu's family had great hopes for him. Unfortunately, Zhu's father died when the boy was 15, and his mother was forced to raise three children on her own. With three young children and no man in the family, Zhu's family was repeatedly harassed and robbed by local bandits. Nonetheless, Zhu's mother maintained high spirits, and successfully raised all three children.

When Zhu was 30 years old, his mother became chronically ill and did not respond to treatment by any of the local physicians. Having been heavily influenced by her throughout his life, Zhu decided to undertake her treatment himself. He began to study medicine on his own, and five years later, successfully cured his mother's condition. This success ignited his interest, and he continued his pursuit of medicine. However, he improved little in the next ten years of studying on his own. Finally, at age 44, he bid farewell to his family, to go in search of a teacher. After a cross-country journey, he learned of 罗知梯 Luo Zhi-Ti, one of the best physicians of the time. However, Luo refused to accept any apprentices. To show his dedication, Zhu waited outside Luo's residence every day, without exception, for three months. Finally, touched by Zhu's dedication and sincerity, Luo accepted him as an apprentice. In the next three years, Zhu studied diligently, tirelessly. According to his biography, one of the most important lessons Zhu learned was to not rigidly follow only one school of thought, but to master and integrate all of them.

Zhu is most famous for one of his adages: "阳常有余, 阴常不足. Yang is often in excess, yin is often insufficient." He observed this problem because many physicians during this era prescribed formulas from *Tai Ping Hui Min He Ji Ju Fang* (Imperial Grace Formulary of the Tai Ping Era). These formulas were warm and drying and often damaged yin and created fire. To correct this problem, he proposed many theories and formulas to nourish yin and purge fire. Today, he is credited as the founder of 滋阴派 the Yin-Nourishing Style.

Though Zhu did not begin his formal training in medicine until 44 years of age, he excelled in his later years as he did in his youth, and became known as one of the best physicians of his time. When he died at 77, he left volumes of drafts of his clinical experiences. His writings were later organized and published by his apprentices. Among the most famous of his works was the 丹溪心法 *Dan Xi Xin Fa* (Teachings of [Zhu] Dan-Xi) 1481.

Zhu Zhen-Heng is remembered by many as "one-dose Zhu," for his outstanding ability to cure disease with just one dose of herbs.

Some of the formulas written by Zhu Zhen-Heng are:

- *Dang Gui Long Hui Wan* (Tangkuei, Gentiana, and Aloe Pill)
- *Zuo Jin Wan* (Left Metal Pill)
- *Da Bu Yin Wan* (Great Tonify the Yin Pill)
- *Hu Qian Wan* (Hidden Tiger Pill)
- *Yu Ping Feng San* (Jade Windscreen Powder)
- *Yue Ju Wan* (Escape Restraint Pill)
- *Wei Ling Tang* (Calm the Stomach and Poria Decoction)
- *Bi Xie Fen Qing Yin* (Dioscorea Hypoglauca Decoction to Separate the Clear)
- *Er Miao San* (Two-Marvel Powder)
- *Gun Tan Wan* (Vaporize Phlegm Pill)
- *Bao He Wan* (Preserve Harmony Pill)

Dynasties & Kingdoms	Year
Xia Dynasty 夏	2100-1600 BCE
Shang Dynasty 商	1600-1100 BCE
Zhou Dynasty 周	1100-221 BCE
Qin Dynasty 秦	221-207 BCE
Han Dynasty 漢	206 BCE-220
Three Kingdoms 三國	220-280
Western Jin Dynasty 西晉	265-316
Eastern Jin Dynasty 東晉	317-420
Northern and Southern Dynasties 北南朝	420-581
Sui Dynasty 隋	581-618
Tang Dynasty 唐	618-907
Five Dynasties 五代	907-960
Song Dynasty 宋	960-1279
Liao Dynasty 遼	916-1125
Jin Dynasty 金	1115-1234
Yuan Dynasty 元	**1271-1368**
Ming Dynasty 明	1368-1644
Qing Dynasty 清	1644-1911
Republic of China 中華民國	1912-Present Day
People's Republic of China 中華人民共和國	1949-Present Day

Table of Contents

Chapter 18 — Overview — Phlegm-Dispelling Formulas

Definition: Phlegm-dispelling formulas dissolve and dispel phlegm.

Phlegm is a pathological factor that develops from the disruption of normal water metabolism. Traditional Chinese medicine describes two types of phlegm: *tan* (visible phlegm) and *yin* (invisible phlegm).

- *Tan* is the thick phlegm that travels in the channel and collateral pathways and affects different parts of the body. As thick phlegm, *tan* may form rubbery nodules, tumors or masses, or it can be a mucus-type substance vomited, spat out, or coughed up. *Tan* can affect every part of the body because it travels in the channel and collateral pathways and follows the ascending and descending flow of qi.
- *Yin* is thin, watery phlegm that generally remains in the area where it was formed, and because it is not readily observable, it is called internal or invisible phlegm.

In clinical practice, the differences between *tan* (visible phlegm) and *yin* (invisible phlegm) are not clearly demarcated, but rather often indistinct; visible phlegm may be an indicator of invisible phlegm and vice versa. Phlegm-dispelling formulas dissolve and dispel phlegm and treat the symptoms and the causes of illnesses. Phlegm forms because of a dysfunction of the *zang fu* organs that control water metabolism: the Spleen (which transforms and transports water), the Kidney (which eliminates water), and the Lung (which distributes water). Though there may be other contributing factors, the basis of all phlegm disorders is disruption of the transformation and transportation function of the Spleen. If the Spleen's functions are impaired, water accumulates and stagnates, causing dampness and phlegm. For this reason, nearly all herbal formulas that treat phlegm contain herbs which strengthen the Spleen.

Obstruction of qi flow is a critical component of phlegm diseases: it is both a cause of, and an effect from, phlegm. If the flow of qi slows, dampness will accumulate and, given enough time, transform into phlegm. Conversely, once phlegm is present in large enough quantities, it obstructs the flow of qi, preventing it from ascending, descending, exiting and entering, leading to dysfunction of the *zang fu* organs. In Chinese medicine it is said that the Spleen *produces* phlegm, while the Lung *stores* phlegm. In practice, the Lung is often the organ most affected by phlegm disorders. When phlegm affects the Liver, it causes phlegm-wind, or seizure, disorders. When obstructing the Heart and the sensory orifices, *shen* (spirit) disturbance (behavioral disorders) with anxiety and manic behavior occurs. Though phlegm interferes with the smooth flow of qi, it also moves with qi, which is why the *zang fu* organs are not the only parts of the body affected; all four limbs as well as the channels and collaterals can become involved, making diagnosis and treatment a challenge. All of these factors must be taken into consideration when formulating a treatment plan, as strategies will vary depending on the pathophysiology. As is so often the case in Chinese medicine, accurate determination of the cause is crucial to success.

Damp-phlegm is caused by Spleen deficiency, which leads to an accumulation of dampness that transforms into phlegm. The treatment strategy in these cases is to dry dampness, dispel phlegm, and strengthen the Spleen's transporting function. Common clinical signs include a swollen tongue with a sticky or greasy coating, cough with copious, clear or white sputum, vomiting, nausea, and

Chapter 18 — Overview

a slippery to wiry pulse. Herbal formulas that dry dampness and expel phlegm may be used to treat veterinary biomedical diseases such as upper respiratory tract infection, chronic bronchitis, pneumonia, chronic vomiting and gastritis.

Heat-phlegm develops when fire scorches body fluids and transforms or "cooks" them into phlegm. As heat is the source of this type of phlegm disorder, it is necessary to use herbs that clear heat and dispel phlegm. Animals with heat-phlegm can present with fever, anxiety, restlessness, pacing, inability to lay down and rest, panting, open-mouth breathing, dyspnea, increased respiratory rate, gagging, productive cough with thick, yellow sputum, hemoptysis, and constipation. Some animals may have chest pain on palpation and have a greasy, yellow tongue and a slippery, rapid pulse. Heat-phlegm formulas may be used to treat acute and chronic canine and feline bronchitis, bronchitis secondary to canine heartworm disease, canine infectious tracheobronchitis, acute and chronic bacterial pneumonia, aspiration pneumonia, lung cancer, lung abscess and behavioral disorders.

Dry-phlegm is caused by dryness of the Lung, which injures fluids and creates phlegm that obstructs the flow of Lung qi; effective treatment requires herbs which regulate qi, moisten the Lung and dispel phlegm at the same time. A common mistake in treatment is to prescribe heavy, rich, stagnating tonic herbs, which produce even more phlegm, or acrid, dispersing herbs, which further damage Lung fluids. Clinical signs of this disorder include cough with hard-to-expectorate sticky sputum, a red, dry tongue with little coating, and a rapid, thin, wiry to slippery but strong pulse. A dry, sore throat may result in hoarse vocalization. This pattern is often mis-diagnosed as Lung yin deficiency; however, if it were a case of Lung yin deficiency, there would be additional signs of yin deficiency and heat and a rapid, thin, *weak* pulse. Cough from yin deficiency should not be treated with these formulas.

Cold-phlegm can develop from coldness in the Lung or from Spleen and/or Kidney yang deficiency. Cold invasion impairs fluid metabolism and results in accumulation and stagnation of fluids. The basic strategy in all cases of cold-phlegm is to warm yang while dispelling phlegm. Clinical signs include wheezing, poor appetite, vomiting, gagging, coughing up of clear to white, thick, copious sputum, a pale, swollen tongue with a greasy coating, and a wiry, slippery pulse. With appropriate clinical signs, cold-phlegm formulas may be used to treat chronic gastritis and vomiting from chronic antimicrobial administration, chronic vomiting and food stagnation in cats, chronic nephritis, and acute and chronic bronchitis.

Wind-phlegm can be externally contracted or internally generated. The internal type occurs when an animal has pre-existing phlegm and suffers internal movement of Liver wind. Phlegm follows wind upward, obstructing the channels and collaterals of the head and sensory orifices, with clinical signs such as vertigo, dizziness, and, in severe cases, seizures or loss of consciousness. Externally contracted wind interferes with the Lung's function of dispersing and descending body fluids and causes accumulation of dampness and production of phlegm. External wind-phlegm presents with wheezing, gagging, coughing with copious sputum, and treatment is directed at ventilating the Lung and calming and dispelling wind. Other clinical signs of wind-phlegm include: loss of appetite, poor digestion, a swollen tongue with a white, slippery to greasy coating, and a slippery or wiry pulse. Veterinary conditions that can be treated with wind-phlegm formulas include poor athletic performance with easy fatigue, facial paralysis, upper respiratory disease, bronchitis, hypertension, glaucoma, seizure disorder, epilepsy and geriatric vestibular disease.

Phlegm can stagnate in the channels and collaterals of the body and become subcutaneous nodules that are soft and rubbery (lipomas) or firm to hard (benign or malignant tumors) and that may progressively enlarge. This process can also take place internally with the enlargement of organs and other tissues to produce masses in the chest or abdominal cavity. Lymph nodes throughout the body can be affected by phlegm, with local or generalized enlargement as well. In veterinary medicine the pathogenesis of masses and tumors commonly involves Spleen qi deficiency and the production of dampness and phlegm; Liver qi stagnation and Liver fire arising from an inappropriate diet; chronic stress and lack of exercise; Kidney and Liver yin deficiencies and deficiency fire from Kidney *jing* (essence) deficiency; or chronic disease and overwork. In the latter two cases, the heat consumes body fluids, thus producing phlegm. Appropriate herbs must be used to open the channels and collaterals, soften hardness, clear heat, resolve dampness, tonify yin, and disperse stagnation of qi, blood and phlegm. In many of these cases the tongue is often red and swollen with a thick, greasy, white to yellow coating, and the pulse is wiry, slippery, and rapid. From a veterinary perspective, phlegm is one of the key disease factors in the development of cancer and an area of great interest and study among veterinarians who practice Chinese medicine. In Chinese medicine it is said, "phlegm is the mother of hundreds of disorders." Because phlegm disorders are complex in nature, optimal treatment requires accurate differential diagnosis as to the source of the phlegm and the use of herbs to concurrently treat both the cause and the symptoms. If an unusual disorder proves difficult to treat, the doctor should always consider phlegm as a likely etiology and realize that phlegm is difficult to clear or eliminate once formed, and the duration of treatment is often prolonged. Herbs that transform dampness and phlegm often do so through the feces and urine; it is not unusual to see loose or odiferous stools following the administration of these formulas.

SUBCATEGORIES OF ACTION

Phlegm-dispelling formulas are divided into five subcategories to accurately differentiate the nature of the disorders and the characteristics of the corresponding formulas.

1. Damp-Drying and Phlegm-Dissolving Formulas

These formulas are designed to treat damp-phlegm. The main signs and symptoms include coughing with profuse sputum that can be easily expectorated, distention of the epigastrium, nausea, vomiting, and lethargy. The tongue coating is usually white and greasy, or sticky. The pulse is wiry or slippery.

Herbs commonly used to dry dampness and dissolve phlegm include *Ban Xia* (Rhizoma Pinelliae) and *Tian Nan Xing* (Rhizoma Arisaematis). Furthermore, to prevent accumulation of dampness and phlegm, herbs are commonly used to strengthen the Spleen and regulate qi, such as *Chen Pi* (Pericarpium Citri Reticulatae) and *Bai Zhu* (Rhizoma Atractylodis Macrocephalae). Exemplar formulas that dry dampness and dissolve phlegm include *Er Chen Tang* (Two-Cured Decoction) and *Wen Dan Tang* (Warm the Gallbladder Decoction).

2. Heat-Clearing and Phlegm-Dissolving Formulas

These formulas treat heat-phlegm syndromes, with common manifestations of fever, dyspnea, increased respiratory rate, restlessness and a reluctance to lie down, gagging, wheezing, coughing, chest pain, thick, yellow mucus that is difficult to expectorate, a red tongue body with a greasy, yellow coating, and a slippery, rapid pulse.

Herbs that clear heat and dissolve phlegm include *Gua Lou* (Fructus Trichosanthis) and *Dan Nan Xing* (Arisaema cum Bile). Representative formulas include *Qing Qi Hua Tan Wan* (Clear the Qi and Transform Phlegm Pill) and *Xiao Xian Xiong Tang* (Minor Sinking into the Chest Decoction).

In severe cases of heat-phlegm syndromes, the sensory orifices may be blocked, leading to unconsciousness, seizures, epilepsy and convulsions. Such critical conditions must be treated with strong formulas that clear heat and open the sensory orifices, such as *An Gong Niu Huang Wan* (Calm the Palace Pill with Cattle Gallstone) and *Zi Xue* (Purple Snow) [*see* Chapter 10: Orifice-Opening Formulas].

3. Dryness-Moistening and Phlegm-Dissolving Formula

This formula treats dry-phlegm that manifests as thick, sticky sputum that cannot be easily expectorated, dryness and soreness of the throat, and hoarse and raspy vocalization.

Herbs commonly used to moisten dryness and dissolve phlegm are *Chuan Bei Mu* (Bulbus Fritillariae Cirrhosae), *Zhe Bei Mu* (Bulbus Fritillariae Thunbergii), and *Gua Lou* (Fructus

Chapter 18 — Overview

Trichosanthis). One exemplar formula is *Bei Mu Gua Lou San* (Fritillaria and Trichosanthes Fruit Powder).

4. **Warm Formulas that Dissolve Cold-Phlegm**
These formulas treat cold-phlegm syndromes with common clinical manifestations of wheezing, gagging, coughing with white, watery sputum, and a greasy, white tongue coating.
Herbs that warm and dissolve phlegm include *Xi Xin* (Radix et Rhizoma Asari) and *Gan Jiang* (Rhizoma Zingiberis). Exemplar formulas include *San Zi Yang Qin Tang* (Three-Seed Decoction to Nourish One's Parents) and *Ling Gan Wu Wei Jiang Xin Tang* (Poria, Licorice, Schisandra, Ginger, and Asarum Decoction).

5. **Wind-Expelling and Phlegm-Dissolving Formulas**
These formulas treat wind-phlegm in the interior, which arises when internal phlegm is accompanied by Liver wind rising, causing symptoms of dizziness, vertigo, seizures, epilepsy, and loss of consciousness. In this case, herbs that dispel phlegm should be combined with herbs that extinguish Liver wind. Representative formulas include *Ban Xia Bai Zhu Tian Ma Tang* (Pinellia, Atractylodes Macrocephala, and Gastrodia Decoction) and *Ding Xian Wan* (Arrest Seizures Pill).
Note: External wind-phlegm is a condition in which the pathogenic wind attacks the Lung and impairs its descending and dispersing functions. Consequently, turbid phlegm is created. Clinically, the signs and symptoms of this condition include aversion to wind, fever, and cough with profuse sputum. This condition is treated with herbs that release wind from the exterior and dispel phlegm from the interior; *Zhi Sou San* (Stop Coughing Powder) is one exemplar formula. For additional information, please refer to Chapter 1: Exterior-Releasing Formulas.

CAUTIONS / CONTRAINDICATIONS

- Phlegm-dispelling formulas should be used with caution in patients with hemoptysis, as many of these formulas are very drying in nature and may promote more coughing and bleeding.
- Phlegm-dispelling formulas generally have strong moving and dispersing effects; they will consume qi over time. They should be used as needed and discontinued when the desired effects are achieved.

PHARMACOLOGICAL EFFECTS & CLINICAL APPLICATIONS

Phlegm-dispelling formulas can treat a wide variety of diseases. From a biomedical perspective, phlegm-dispelling formulas have an extremely wide range of pharmacological effects and clinical applications. The most commonly used indications include respiratory disorders, gastrointestinal disorders, seizures, epilepsy, stroke, and others.

- **Respiratory disorders**: Phlegm-dispelling formulas have a marked influence on the respiratory tract, and have been used to treat a wide variety of respiratory tract disorders. Pharmacologically, these formulas have demonstrated expectorant,[1] antitussive,[2] and antiasthmatic effects.[3] Clinically, these formulas have been used successfully to treat diseases such as acute bronchitis,[4,5] chronic bronchitis,[6] aspiration pneumonia,[7] interstitial pneumonia,[8] tuberculous pleurisy,[9] exudative pleurisy,[10] bronchial asthma,[11] cough,[12] and silicosis.[13] Exemplar formulas that treat bronchitis include *Er Chen Tang* (Two-Cured Decoction), *Xiao Xian Xiong Tang* (Minor Sinking into the Chest Decoction), and *San Zi Yang Qin Tang* (Three-Seed Decoction to Nourish One's Parents). Exemplar formulas that treat pneumonia include *Qing Fei Tang* (Clear the Lung Decoction) and *Qing Qi Hua Tan Wan* (Clear the Qi and Transform Phlegm Pill). *Xiao Xian Xiong Tang* (Minor Sinking into the Chest Decoction) may be used to treat pleurisy and silicosis. *Zhi Sou San* (Stop Coughing Powder) may be used for cough.
- **Gastrointestinal disorders**: Phlegm-dispelling formulas have a marked effect on the gastrointestinal tract, and may be used to treat many gastrointestinal disorders, such as gastritis,[14] epigastric pain,[15] erosive gastritis,[16] and reflux esophagitis.[17] The pharmacological effects are attributed in part to the inhibition of gastric acid production.[18,19] Exemplar formulas include *Er Chen Tang*

Chapter 18 — Overview

(Two-Cured Decoction), *Wen Dan Tang* (Warm the Gallbladder Decoction), and *Xiao Xian Xiong Tang* (Minor Sinking into the Chest Decoction).

- **Seizures and epilepsy**: *Er Chen Tang* (Two-Cured Decoction) and *Gun Tan Wan* (Vaporize Phlegm Pill) are two phlegm-dispelling formulas that have demonstrated effectiveness in treating seizures and epilepsy.[20,21]
- **Stroke**: *Wen Dan Tang* (Warm the Gallbladder Decoction) and *Gun Tan Wan* (Vaporize Phlegm Pill) are two formulas that have been used effectively to treat stroke.[22,23] *Ban Xia Bai Zhu Tian Ma Tang* (Pinellia, Atractylodes Macrocephala, and Gastrodia Decoction) may be used to treat facial paralysis that follows as a post-stroke sequelae.[24]
- **Meniere's syndrome**: *Wen Dan Tang* (Warm the Gallbladder Decoction) and *Ban Xia Bai Zhu Tian Ma Tang* (Pinellia, Atractylodes Macrocephala, and Gastrodia Decoction) are two formulas that have shown marked success in treating Meniere's syndrome.[25,26]

References

1. *Zhong Yi Fang Ji Xian Dai Yan Jiu* (Modern Study of Medical Formulas in Traditional Chinese Medicine), 1997.
2. *Zhong Cheng Yao* (Study of Chinese Patent Medicine), 1988; 9:27.
3. *Zhong Yao Yao Li Yu Lin Chuang* (Pharmacology and Clinical Applications of Chinese Herbs), 1992; 8(3):15.
4. *Zhong Ji Yi Kan* (Medium Medical Journal), 1994; 12:45.
5. *Zhong Yi Ming Fang Lin Chuang Xin Yong* (Contemporary Clinical Applications of Classic Chinese Formulas), 2001; 138.
6. *Zhong Yuan Yi Kan* (Resource Journal of Chinese Medicine), 1994; 5:44.
7. Mantani N, Kasahara Y, Kamata T, Sekiya N, Shimada Y, Usuda K, Sakakibara I, Hattori N, Terasawa K. Effect of Seihai-to, a Kampo medicine, in relapsing aspiration pneumonia--an open-label pilot study. Phytomedicine. 2002 Apr; 9(3):195-201.
8. *Shi Yong Zhong Xi Yi Jie He Za Zhi* (Practical Journal of Integrated Chinese and Western Medicines), 1995; 3:152.
9. *Shang Hai Yi Yao Za Zhi* (Shanghai Journal of Medicine and Herbology), 1986; 1:36.
10. *Shan Xi Zhong Yi* (Shanxi Chinese Medicine), 1994; 15(8):368.
11. *Shan Xi Zhong Yi* (Shanxi Chinese Medicine), 1995; 4:148.
12. *Yun Nan Zhong Yi Zhong Yao Za Zhi* (Yunnan Journal of Traditional Chinese Medicine and Herbal Medicine), 1999; 4:15.
13. *Bei Jing Zhong Yi Yao Da Xue Xue Bao* (Journal of Beijing University of Medicine and Medicinals), 1994; 17(1):37.
14. *Bei Jing Zhong Yi* (Beijing Chinese Medicine), 1990; 1:5.
15. *Nei Meng Gu Zhong Yi Yao* (Traditional Chinese Medicine and Medicinals of Inner Mongolia), 1998; 3:19.
16. *Jiang Xi Zhong Yi Yao* (Jiangxi Chinese Medicine and Herbology), 1998; 6:22.
17. *Hu Bei Zhong Yi Za Zhi* (Hubei Journal of Chinese Medicine), 1997; 3:20.
18. *Zhong Yao Xian Dai Yan Jiu Yu Ying Yong* (Modern Study of Traditional Chinese Medicine), 1993; 165, 199, 388, 490.
19. *Zhong Cheng Yao Yan Jiu* (Research of Chinese Patent Medicine), 1985; 8:23.
20. *Shi Yong Zhong Yi Nei Ke Za Zhi* (Journal of Practical Chinese Internal Medicine), 1994; 2:17.
21. *An Hui Zhong Yi Xue Yuan Xue Bao* (Journal of Anhui University School of Medicine), 1988; 3:33.
22. *Shan Xi Zhong Yi* (Shanxi Chinese Medicine), 1995; 16(9):393.
23. *Si Chuan Zhong Yi* (Sichuan Chinese Medicine), 1995; 2:20.
24. *Bei Jing Zhong Yi* (Beijing Chinese Medicine), 1991; 6:31.
25. *Zhe Jiang Zhong Yi Xue Yuan Xue Bao* (Journal of Zhejiang University of Chinese Medicine), 1998; 3:25.
26. *Shi Yong Zhong Yi Za Zhi* (Journal of Practical Chinese Medicine), 1998; 7:22.

Section 1

燥湿化痰剂

— Damp-Drying and Phlegm-Dissolving Formulas

Èr Chén Tāng (Two-Cured Decoction)

二陳湯

二陈汤

Pinyin Name: *Er Chen Tang*

Literal Name: Two-Cured Decoction

Alternate Names: *Er Chen Wan, Erh Chen Tang* (*Wan*), Two-Chen Decoction (Pill), Two Vintage Herbs Decoction, Citrus and Pinellia Combination

Original Source: *Tai Ping Hui Min He Ji Ju Fang* (Imperial Grace Formulary of the Tai Ping Era) by the Imperial Medical Department in 1078-85

COMPOSITION

Ban Xia (Rhizoma Pinelliae), *xi* (washed) with liquid 7 times	15g
Ju Hong (Exocarpium Citri Rubrum)	15g
Fu Ling (Poria)	9g
Zhi Gan Cao (Radix et Rhizoma Glycyrrhizae Praeparata cum Melle)	4.5g

DOSAGE / PREPARATION / ADMINISTRATION

The source text states to grind all of the ingredients into a coarse powder. Cook 12g of the powder with 7 slices of *Sheng Jiang* (Rhizoma Zingiberis Recens) and 1 piece of *Wu Mei* (Fructus Mume) in one large bowl of water until the liquid is reduced to 60%. Take the hot, strained decoction any time during the day. Today, this formula may be prepared as a decoction with 3g of *Sheng Jiang* (Rhizoma Zingiberis Recens) and 1 piece of *Wu Mei* (Fructus Mume).

CHINESE THERAPEUTIC ACTIONS

1. Dries dampness and dissolves phlegm
2. Regulates qi and harmonizes the middle *jiao*

CLINICAL MANIFESTATIONS

Damp-phlegm accumulation: profuse, white sputum, nausea, vomiting of thin phlegm, borborygmus, lethargy, weak extremities, ataxia, a greasy, swollen tongue, and a slippery pulse.

VETERINARY CLINICAL APPLICATIONS

Acute and chronic bronchitis, tracheitis, gastritis, peptic ulcer disease, nausea, excessive salivation, vomiting and goiter.

EXPLANATION

Er Chen Tang (Two-Cured Decoction) is the basic formula for treating damp-phlegm. According to traditional Chinese medicine theory, the Spleen sends up clear fluids to the upper *jiao*. If this function is impaired, dampness may accumulate in the Spleen and create phlegm. Thus, damp-phlegm syndromes usually result from Spleen deficiency or dysfunction. If the Spleen is deficient and full of dampness, its functions of transportation and transformation will be impaired, which will lead to insufficient supply of nutrients to the body and the extremities. The result will be lethargy and weak extremities. The Lung, on the other hand, stores phlegm. Phlegm accumulation in the Lung manifests as coughing with profuse sputum. Nausea and vomiting are due to damp-phlegm obstructing Stomach qi and causing it to rise abnormally.

Èr Chén Tāng (Two-Cured Decoction)

Er Chen Tang (Two-Cured Decoction)

Diagnosis	Clinical Signs	Treatment	Herbs
Damp-phlegm accumulation	• Coughing and gagging with profuse sputum: damp-phlegm affecting the Lung • Nausea and vomiting: reversed flow of Stomach qi due to damp-phlegm accumulation • Lethargy and weak extremities: damp-phlegm affecting the Spleen • Vertigo: yang qi unable to ascend due to damp-phlegm accumulation • Greasy, swollen tongue and a slippery pulse: damp-phlegm condition	• Dries dampness and dissolves phlegm • Regulates qi and harmonizes the middle *jiao*	• *Ban Xia* (Rhizoma Pinelliae) breaks up and dissolves phlegm and dries dampness. • *Ju Hong* (Exocarpium Citri Rubrum) activates and regulates qi. • *Fu Ling* (Poria) strengthens the Spleen and dispels dampness. • *Sheng Jiang* (Rhizoma Zingiberis Recens) relieves nausea and vomiting by guiding Stomach qi downward. • *Wu Mei* (Fructus Mume) astringes the Lung to prevent qi loss. • *Zhi Gan Cao* (Radix et Rhizoma Glycyrrhizae Praeparata cum Melle) harmonizes all of the herbs.

Ban Xia (Rhizoma Pinelliae) acts as the chief herb in this formula because it is the best herb to break up and dissolve phlegm stagnation. Its acrid and warm properties can dry dampness, dissolve phlegm, and open pathways for the qi to flow. In addition, it corrects the reversed flow of Stomach qi to relieve nausea and vomiting. *Ju Hong* (Exocarpium Citri Rubrum) activates and regulates qi to remove residual phlegm and dampness. *Fu Ling* (Poria) strengthens the Spleen and dispels dampness. *Sheng Jiang* (Rhizoma Zingiberis Recens) relieves nausea and vomiting by guiding Stomach qi downward, and helps to detoxify *Ban Xia* (Rhizoma Pinelliae). Since animals with this syndrome already have qi deficiency, a very small amount of *Wu Mei* (Fructus Mume) is used to astringe the Lung to prevent qi loss. The restraining effect of *Wu Mei* (Fructus Mume) also balances the dispersing nature of *Ban Xia* (Rhizoma Pinelliae), thereby minimizing the potential side effects of both herbs. *Zhi Gan Cao* (Radix et Rhizoma Glycyrrhizae Praeparata cum Melle) harmonizes all of the herbs and regulates the Lung and Spleen.

VETERINARY MODIFICATIONS

- For cold-phlegm characterized by clear sputum, add the juice of *Sheng Jiang* (Rhizoma Zingiberis Recens) and increase the dose of *Ban Xia* (Rhizoma Pinelliae).
- For heat-phlegm characterized by yellow sputum, add *Huang Qin* (Radix Scutellariae), *Gua Lou* (Fructus Trichosanthis), *Huang Lian* (Rhizoma Coptidis), *Zhu Ru* (Caulis Bambusae in Taenia), and *Dan Nan Xing* (Arisaema cum Bile).
- For damp-phlegm characterized by white sputum, add *Cang Zhu* (Rhizoma Atractylodis), *Bai Zhu* (Rhizoma Atractylodis Macrocephalae), and *Hou Po* (Cortex Magnoliae Officinalis).
- For dry-phlegm characterized by sputum that is yellow, thick and difficult to expectorate, add *Gua Lou* (Fructus Trichosanthis), *Ku Xing Ren* (Semen Armeniacae Amarum), and *Bei Mu* (Bulbus Fritillariae).
- For qi stagnation and phlegm accumulation, add *Hou Po* (Cortex Magnoliae Officinalis) and *Zhi Shi* (Fructus Aurantii Immaturus).
- For phlegm produced by food stagnation, add *Shan Zha* (Fructus Crataegi), *Mai Ya* (Fructus Hordei Germinatus), and *Shen Qu* (Massa Fermentata).
- For stubborn phlegm (chronic), add *Zhi Shi* (Fructus Aurantii Immaturus), *Dan Nan Xing* (Arisaema cum Bile), *Fu Hai Shi* (Pumice), and *Mang Xiao* (Natrii Sulfas).
- For nausea and vomiting due to cold in the Stomach and a deficient body constitution, add *Mu Xiang* (Radix Aucklandiae) and *Sha Ren* (Fructus Amomi).
- For vomiting with abdominal pain due to heat, combine with *Huang Lian Tang* (Coptis Decoction).
- With indigestion or food stagnation, combine with *Ping Wei San* (Calm the Stomach Powder).
- If accompanied by depression, add *Yue Ju Wan* (Escape Restraint Pill).
- For pulmonary emphysema, add *Kuan Dong Hua* (Flos Farfarae), *Zi Wan* (Radix et Rhizoma Asteris), and *Sha Ren* (Fructus Amomi).
- For asthma caused by heat, add *Ma Huang* (Herba Ephedrae), *Ku Xing Ren* (Semen Armeniacae Amarum), *Shi Gao* (Gypsum Fibrosum), and *Sang Bai Pi* (Cortex Mori).

Èr Chén Tāng (Two-Cured Decoction)

CAUTIONS / CONTRAINDICATIONS

- *Er Chen Tang* is acrid and drying and is not suitable for cough caused by Lung yin deficiency or Lung dryness. Similarly, this formula should not be used if the animal has scanty sputum, blood-streaked sputum, or coughing with blood.
- This formula is acrid, warm, and drying. Short-term use of this formula may be associated with dry mouth and thirst. Long-term use may cause consumption of yin and body fluids.[1]

PHARMACOLOGICAL EFFECTS

1. **Respiratory**: Ingredients of *Er Chen Tang* have been shown to have antitussive, expectorant, and antiasthmatic effects.[2]
2. **Gastrointestinal**: Ingredients of *Er Chen Tang* may inhibit the production of gastric acid.[3]

HUMAN CLINICAL STUDIES AND RESEARCH

1. **Bronchitis**: Use of modified *Er Chen Tang* showed marked effectiveness in treating bronchitis. Out of 109 patients who had uncomplicated bronchitis, marked improvement was reported in 105 cases; and out of 66 who had bronchitis with wheezing and dyspnea, marked improvement was reported in 59 cases.[4]
2. **Bronchiolitis**: According to one study, 80 patients with bronchiolitis were treated with marked improvement in 48 cases, moderate improvement in 31 cases, and no effect in 1 case. The herbal treatment contained *Er Chen Tang* plus *Zi Su Zi* (Fructus Perillae), *Wu Wei Zi* (Fructus Schisandrae Chinensis), and *Jie Geng* (Radix Platycodonis).[5]
3. **Gastritis**: Use of modified *Er Chen Tang* was associated with 71% effectiveness in treating 128 patients with chronic atrophic gastritis. The herbal treatment included *Er Chen Tang* with *Bai Zhu* (Rhizoma Atractylodis Macrocephalae), *Sha Ren* (Fructus Amomi), and others as deemed necessary.[6]
4. **Diabetes mellitus**: Use of modified *Er Chen Tang* was effective in treating diabetes mellitus characterized by damp-heat. The herbal treatment included *Er Chen Tang* with *Cang Zhu* (Rhizoma Atractylodis), *Bai Zhu* (Rhizoma Atractylodis Macrocephalae), *Jue Ming Zi* (Semen Cassiae), *Dan Shen* (Radix et Rhizoma Salviae Miltiorrhizae), and *Ge Gen* (Radix Puerariae Lobatae) as the base formula. Out of 32 patients, the study reported complete recovery in 4 cases, marked effectiveness in 16 cases, slight improvement in 10 cases, and no effect in 2 cases. The overall effectiveness was 93.8%.[7]
5. **Seizures**: Use of modified *Er Chen Tang* was associated with 76.92% effectiveness in treating seizures. Out of 52 patients, the study reported marked effect in 12 cases, moderate effect in 28 cases, and no effect in 12 cases. Modifications were made on an individual basis.[8]
6. **Goiter**: In one report, use of *Er Chen Tang* effectively reduced the size of thyroid enlargement in 5 out of 7 patients. All patients received the classic formula without modifications or any other treatments.[9]

SUGGESTED ACUPUNCTURE TREATMENT

1. Points: *Pishu* (BL 20), *Feishu* (BL 13), *Taiyuan* (LU 9), *Fenglong* (ST 40), *Hegu* (LI 4), and *Chengjiang* (CV 24).
2. Technique: sedation.

In treating cough caused by dampness and phlegm, the selection of acupuncture points should aim to eliminate phlegm, dispel dampness, regulate qi, and harmonize the middle *jiao*. Since the Spleen produces phlegm and the Lung stores phlegm, select *Pishu* (BL 20), the *shu* (transport) point of the Spleen, and *Feishu* (BL 13), the *shu* (transport) point of the Lung, to reduce production of pathogenic fluids and dispel phlegm and dampness. *Taiyuan* (LU 9) strengthens the Spleen, dispels dampness, and eliminates phlegm. *Fenglong* (ST 40) and *Hegu* (LI 4) lower the reversed flow of qi, harmonize the Stomach, and eliminate phlegm. *Chengjiang* (CV 24) helps to disperse phlegm and dampness.

RELATED FORMULAS

Dǎo Tán Tāng (Guide Out Phlegm Decoction)
導痰湯
导痰汤
Pinyin Name: *Dao Tan Tang*
Literal Name: Guide Out Phlegm Decoction
Original Source: *Ji Sheng Fang* (Formulas to Aid the Living) by Yan Yong-He in 1253

Ban Xia (Rhizoma Pinelliae), *xi* (washed) with liquid 7 times	120g [12g]
Tian Nan Xing (Rhizoma Arisaematis), *pao* (blast-fried)	30g [6g]
Ju Hong (Exocarpium Citri Rubrum)	30g [6g]
Zhi Shi (Fructus Aurantii Immaturus), *chao* (dry-fried) with bran	30g [6g]
Chi Fu Ling (Poria Rubra)	30g [6g]
Zhi Gan Cao (Radix et Rhizoma Glycyrrhizae Praeparata cum Melle)	15g [3g]

The source text states to grind the herbs into powder. Cook 12g of the powder with 10 slices of *Sheng Jiang* (Rhizoma Zingiberis Recens) in 2 bowls of water until it is reduced to 80%. Take the warm, strained decoction after meals.

Èr Chén Tāng (Two-Cured Decoction)

Today, this formula may be prepared as a decoction with the doses suggested in brackets.

Dao Tan Tang (Guide Out Phlegm Decoction) dries dampness, dispels phlegm, activates qi circulation, and unblocks stagnation. Clinically, it treats phlegm stagnation in the chest and diaphragm with clinical signs of coughing, nausea, and poor appetite. This formula also can be used for Liver wind rising with phlegm, with symptoms such as inability to eat due to nausea and vomiting and vertigo.

This formula is not available in ready made form and can be made in house and used to treat geriatric vestibular disease. It should be modified for use in animals with yin deficiency and/or Spleen qi deficiency.

Dí Tán Tāng (Scour Phlegm Decoction)
滌痰湯
涤痰汤
Pinyin Name: *Di Tan Tang*
Literal Name: Scour Phlegm Decoction
Original Source: *Zheng Zhi Zhun Sheng* (Standards of Patterns and Treatments) by Wang Ken-Tang in 1602

Dan Nan Xing (Arisaema cum Bile), *zhi* (prepared) with ginger	7.5g [12g]
Ban Xia (Rhizoma Pinelliae), *xi* (washed) with liquid 7 times	7.5g [12g]
Zhi Shi (Fructus Aurantii Immaturus), *chao* (dry-fried) with bran	6g [10g]
Fu Ling (Poria)	6g [10g]
Ju Hong (Exocarpium Citri Rubrum)	4.5g [7.5g]
Shi Chang Pu (Rhizoma Acori Tatarinowii)	3g [5g]
Ren Shen (Radix et Rhizoma Ginseng)	3g [5g]
Zhu Ru (Caulis Bambusae in Taenia)	2.1g [3.5g]
Gan Cao (Radix et Rhizoma Glycyrrhizae)	1.5g [2.5g]

The source text states to prepare the ingredients as a decoction by cooking the herbs with 5 slices of *Sheng Jiang* (Rhizoma Zingiberis Recens) in 2 bowls of water until it is reduced to 1 bowl. Take the warm, strained decoction after meals.

Di Tan Tang (Scour Phlegm Decoction) eliminates phlegm and opens the sensory orifices. Clinically, this formula is indicated for animals with *zhongfeng* (wind stroke) caused by phlegm obstruction with facial paralysis, fibrocartilaginous emboli (FCE), and intervertebral disk disease (IVDD) with paresis and paralysis. With the appropriate clinical signs, it can be used to treat seizure disorders and epilepsy in dogs; it can be combined with *Tian Ma Gou Teng Yin* (Gastrodia and Uncaria Decoction) if there are signs of more heat and wind, or with *Zhen Gan Xi Feng Tang* (Sedate the Liver and Extinguish Wind Decoction) if there is more deficiency of Liver and Kidney yin.

AUTHORS' COMMENTS

Er Chen Tang, literally "Two-Cured Decoction," is so named because its two main ingredients—*Ban Xia* (Rhizoma Pinelliae) and *Ju Hong* (Exocarpium Citri Rubrum)—are more effective when cured and aged. *Er Chen Tang* is the fundamental formula for treating damp and phlegm accumulation. Depending on the other pathogenic factors involved, additional herbs should be added for maximum effect. Please refer to the Modifications section for details.

Er Chen Tang can be combined with *Xiao Yao San* (Rambling Powder) to treat gastric ulcers in dogs or horses due to stress and for the prevention of ulcers. For the treatment of lipomas caused by phlegm obstructing the channels in dogs, *Er Chen Tang* can be combined with *Mu Li* (Concha Ostreae), *Xuan Shen* (Radix Scrophulariae), *Ge Qiao* (Concha Meretricis seu Cyclinae), *Mang Xiao* (Natrii Sulfas), *Hai Zao* (Sargassum), and *Kun Bu* (Thallus Ecklonae).

Er Chen Tang, *Dao Tan Tang* (Guide Out Phlegm Decoction), and *Di Tan Tang* (Scour Phlegm Decoction) all dry dampness and dissolve phlegm.

- *Er Chen Tang* is the standard formula and first choice for treating damp and phlegm accumulation. It treats a wide variety of disorders characterized by dampness and phlegm. It can be used alone, but it is more often combined with additional herbs or formulas to specifically tailor the therapy to the individual animal.
- *Dao Tan Tang* is a much stronger formula for eliminating phlegm. Not only can it eliminate phlegm from the chest, but it also resolves phlegm that is accompanied by Liver wind.
- *Di Tan Tang* eliminates phlegm and opens the sensory orifices. It is used mostly for dogs with epilepsy, seizure disorders, and facial paralysis. With the appropriate clinical signs, it can also be used for post-fibrocartilaginous emboli (FCE) animals and those with intervertebral disk disease (IVDD) with paresis and paralysis

References

1. *Zhong Yao Ming Fang Yao Li Yu Ying Yong* (Pharmacology and Applications of Famous Herbal Formulas), 1989; 567-570.
2. *Zhong Yao Xian Dai Yan Jiu Yu Ying Yong* (Modern Study of Traditional Chinese Medicine), 1993; 165, 199, 388, 490.
3. *Zhong Yao Xian Dai Yan Jiu Yu Ying Yong* (Modern Study of Traditional Chinese Medicine), 1993; 165, 199, 388, 490.

4. *Jiang Xi Zhong Yi Yao* (Jiangxi Chinese Medicine and Herbology), 1988; 1:16.
5. *Zhong Ji Yi Kan* (Medium Medical Journal), 1994; 12:45.
6. *Bei Jing Zhong Yi* (Beijing Chinese Medicine), 1990; 1:5.
7. *Zhe Jiang Zhong Yi Za Zhi* (Zhejiang Journal of Chinese Medicine), 1994; 1:9.
8. *Shi Yong Zhong Yi Nei Ke Za Zhi* (Journal of Practical Chinese Internal Medicine), 1994; 2:17.
9. *Zhe Jiang Zhong Yi Za Zhi* (Zhejiang Journal of Chinese Medicine), 1966; 1:17.

Wēn Dǎn Tāng (Warm the Gallbladder Decoction)

溫膽湯

温胆汤

Pinyin Name: *Wen Dan Tang*

Literal Name: Warm the Gallbladder Decoction

Alternate Names: *Wen Tan Tang,* Gallbladder Warming Decoction, Gallbladder-Warming Decoction, Hoelen and Bamboo Combination

Original Source: *San Yin Ji Yi Bing Zheng Fang Lun* (Discussion of Illnesses, Patterns, and Formulas Related to the Unification of the Three Etiologies) by Chen Yan in 1174

COMPOSITION

Ban Xia (Rhizoma Pinelliae), *xi* (washed) with liquid 7 times	6g
Zhu Ru (Caulis Bambusae in Taenia)	6g
Zhi Shi (Fructus Aurantii Immaturus), *chao* (dry-fried) with bran	6g
Chen Pi (Pericarpium Citri Reticulatae)	9g
Fu Ling (Poria)	4.5g
Zhi Gan Cao (Radix et Rhizoma Glycyrrhizae Praeparata cum Melle)	3g

DOSAGE / PREPARATION / ADMINISTRATION

The source text states to grind the ingredients into powder. Cook 12g of the powder with 5 slices of *Sheng Jiang* (Rhizoma Zingiberis Recens) and 1 piece of *Da Zao* (Fructus Jujubae) in 1.5 large bowls of water until the liquid is reduced to 70%. Take the strained decoction before meals.

CHINESE THERAPEUTIC ACTIONS

1. Regulates qi and dissolves phlegm
2. Clears heat in the Gallbladder
3. Harmonizes the Gallbladder and Stomach

CLINICAL MANIFESTATIONS

Gallbladder and Stomach disharmony accompanied by heat-phlegm: irritability, restlessness at night, tachycardia and/or arrhythmia, seizures, nausea, vomiting, mild thirst, and a greasy tongue, and a rapid, slippery or wiry pulse.

Wēn Dǎn Tāng (Warm the Gallbladder Decoction)

VETERINARY CLINICAL APPLICATIONS

Ataxia, circling, behavioral disorders (anxiety, fearfulness), eating disorders (wood chewing, dirt licking, grass eating, fecal eating), seizure disorders, and epilepsy.

EXPLANATION

Wen Dan Tang (Warm the Gallbladder Decoction) treats disharmony of the Gallbladder and Stomach, accompanied by heat-phlegm in the interior. The Gallbladder, which belongs to the wood element, has a dispersing and discharging characteristic. Stagnation inhibits the dispersing and discharging nature of the Gallbladder, which in turn may cause it to overact on the Stomach and produce disharmony between the two organs. This disharmony eventually creates heat-phlegm, which manifests in symptoms such as irritability, insomnia, and palpitations. Nausea and vomiting arise when heat-phlegm blocks the normal descent of Stomach qi, forcing it to move adversely upward. In severe cases, heat-phlegm may obstruct the sensory orifices and cause seizures and epilepsy. Mild thirst may occur as a result of interior heat consuming body fluids.

This formula uses *Ban Xia* (Rhizoma Pinelliae) to dry dampness, dissolve phlegm, harmonize the Stomach, and redirect the reversed flow of Stomach qi downward. *Zhu Ru* (Caulis Bambusae in Taenia) clears heat, dissolves phlegm, and relieves irritability. *Zhi Shi* (Fructus Aurantii Immaturus) breaks up qi stagnation and dispels phlegm. *Chen Pi* (Pericarpium Citri Reticulatae) regulates qi flow and dries dampness. *Fu Ling* (Poria) strengthens the Spleen to eliminate dampness and phlegm. *Sheng Jiang* (Rhizoma Zingiberis Recens), *Da Zao* (Fructus Jujubae), and *Zhi Gan Cao* (Radix et Rhizoma Glycyrrhizae Praeparata cum Melle) strengthen the Spleen and harmonize the Stomach.

VETERINARY MODIFICATIONS

- With vomiting, add *Zi Su Ye* (Folium Perillae) and *Huang Lian* (Rhizoma Coptidis).
- With nausea, vomiting, and chest oppression, add *Huo Xiang* (Herba Agastaches) and *Shi Chang Pu* (Rhizoma Acori Tatarinowii).
- With irritability due to interior heat, add *Zhi Zi* (Fructus Gardeniae).
- With behavioral disorder, insomnia and palpitations due to fear and fright, add *Suan Zao Ren* (Semen Ziziphi Spinosae).
- With heart palpitations, add *Yuan Zhi* (Radix Polygalae) and *Shi Chang Pu* (Rhizoma Acori Tatarinowii).
- For epilepsy, add *Yu Jin* (Radix Curcumae), *Shi Chang Pu* (Rhizoma Acori Tatarinowii), *Dan Nan Xing* (Arisaema cum Bile), *Gou Teng* (Ramulus Uncariae cum Uncis), and *Quan Xie* (Scorpio).

CAUTIONS / CONTRAINDICATIONS

Wen Dan Tang is contraindicated in the following cases: insomnia caused by Heart deficiency, palpitations caused by blood deficiency, and vomiting or nausea caused by Stomach cold.

HUMAN CLINICAL STUDIES AND RESEARCH

1. **Vertigo**: Administration of *Wen Dan Tang* was reported in one study to effectively treat vertigo. Of 53 patients, 35 had complete recovery, 13 had improvement, and 5 had no effect. Modifications to the original formula

Wen Dan Tang (Warm the Gallbladder Decoction)

Diagnosis	Clinical Signs	Treatment	Herbs
Disharmony of the Gallbladder and Stomach accompanied by heat-phlegm	• Irritability, insomnia, and palpitations: heat-phlegm rising upward • Seizures and epilepsy: heat-phlegm obstructing the sensory orifices • Nausea and vomiting: reversed flow of Stomach qi • Thirst: interior heat consuming body fluids	• Regulates qi and dissolves phlegm • Clears heat in the Gallbladder • Harmonizes the Gallbladder and Stomach	• *Ban Xia* (Rhizoma Pinelliae) dries dampness, dissolves phlegm, and harmonizes the Stomach. • *Zhu Ru* (Caulis Bambusae in Taenia) clears heat, dissolves phlegm, and relieves irritability. • *Zhi Shi* (Fructus Aurantii Immaturus) breaks up qi stagnation and dispels phlegm. • *Chen Pi* (Pericarpium Citri Reticulatae) regulates qi flow and dries dampness. • *Fu Ling* (Poria) strengthens the Spleen to eliminate dampness and phlegm. • *Sheng Jiang* (Rhizoma Zingiberis Recens), *Da Zao* (Fructus Jujubae), and *Zhi Gan Cao* (Radix et Rhizoma Glycyrrhizae Praeparata cum Melle) strengthen the Spleen and harmonize the Stomach.

Wēn Dǎn Tāng (Warm the Gallbladder Decoction)

included the addition of *Xuan Fu Hua* (Flos Inulae) and *Zhe Shi* (Haematitum) for nausea and vomiting; *Shi Chang Pu* (Rhizoma Acori Tatarinowii) and *Ju Hua* (Flos Chrysanthemi) for tinnitus; *Chuan Xiong* (Rhizoma Chuanxiong) and *Man Jing Zi* (Fructus Viticis) for headache; *Long Dan* (Radix et Rhizoma Gentianae) and *Huang Qin* (Radix Scutellariae) for a bitter taste in the mouth; *Suan Zao Ren* (Semen Ziziphi Spinosae) and *He Huan Pi* (Cortex Albiziae) for insomnia; *Gui Ban* (Plastrum Testudinis) and *Du Zhong* (Cortex Eucommiae) for soreness and weakness of the lower back and knees; and *Gou Teng* (Ramulus Uncariae cum Uncis), *Shi Jue Ming* (Concha Haliotidis), and *Niu Xi* (Radix Achyranthis Bidentatae) for hypertension.[1]

2. **Psychiatric disorders**: *Wen Dan Tang* has been shown in several clinical studies to have a beneficial effect in treating various psychiatric disorders. According to one study, it has a 96% effectiveness in treating 149 patients with severe psychiatric disorders such as schizophrenia, bipolar disorders, reactive psychosis, and others. The duration of treatment ranged from 3 to 12 packs of herbs in most cases.[2]
3. ***Dian kuang* (mania and withdrawal)**: Thirty patients with *dian kuang* (mania and withdrawal) were treated with 87% effectiveness using *Wen Dan Tang* plus *Mu Li* (Concha Ostreae), *Zhen Zhu Mu* (Concha Margaritiferae), and *Mai Dong* (Radix Ophiopogonis). Of 30 patients, the study reported recovery in 13 cases, significant improvement in 5 cases, moderate improvement in 8 cases, and no effect in 4 cases. The average duration of treatment was 78.7 days, with a range of 16-224 days.[3]
4. **Epigastric pain**: One study reported good results using modified *Wen Dan Tang* to treat epigastric pain characterized by damp-heat. Modifications to this formula included the addition of *Cang Zhu* (Rhizoma Atractylodis) and *Pei Lan* (Herba Eupatorii) for more damp than heat; and *Lian Qiao* (Fructus Forsythiae), *Pu Gong Ying* (Herba Taraxaci), and *Zhe Bei Mu* (Bulbus Fritillariae Thunbergii) for more heat than damp; *Huang Lian* (Rhizoma Coptidis) and *Wu Zhu Yu* (Fructus Evodiae) for acid reflux; *Dan Shen* (Radix et Rhizoma Salviae Miltiorrhizae) and charred *Shan Zha* (Fructus Crataegi) for blood stagnation; and *Tai Zi Shen* (Radix Pseudostellariae) and *Sha Shen* (Radix Glehniae seu Adenophorae) for qi and yin deficiencies due to damp-heat. Of 42 patients, the study reported complete recovery in 33 cases, improvement in 7 cases, and no effect in 2 cases.[4]
5. **Stroke**: *Wen Dan Tang* has been used successfully to treat both acute episodes and sequelae of stroke. According to one study on treatment of acute stroke in 35 patients, use of herbs was associated with complete recovery in 15 cases, improvement in 17 cases, and no effect in 3 cases. The herbal formula contained *Chen Pi* (Pericarpium Citri Reticulatae), *Fu Ling* (Poria), *Ban Xia* (Rhizoma Pinelliae), *Zhi Shi* (Fructus Aurantii Immaturus), *Zhu Ru* (Caulis Bambusae in Taenia), *Shi Chang Pu* (Rhizoma Acori Tatarinowii), and *Gan Cao* (Radix et Rhizoma Glycyrrhizae). Additional modifications were made as needed.[5] According to another study, 34 patients with sequelae of stroke were treated with significant improvement in 10 cases, improvement in 22 cases, and no effect in 2 cases. The herbal formula contained *Wen Dan Tang* plus *San Qi* (Radix et Rhizoma Notoginseng), *Huang Qi* (Radix Astragali), and *Di Long* (Pheretima).[6]
6. **Diabetic microvascular complications**: Administration of modified *Wen Dan Tang* was effective in treating diabetic retinopathy, diabetic nephropathy, and "diabetic foot," which are three diabetic microvascular complications characterized by qi and phlegm stagnation.[7]
7. **Organophosphorus poisoning**: Use of modified *Wen Dan Tang* was associated with marked success in treating organophosphorus poisoning with symptoms such as headache, irritability, insomnia, excessive dreaming, chest oppression, fatigue, nausea, vomiting, depression, inability to concentrate, memory impairment, and others. Of 42 patients, the study reported complete recovery in 34 cases and improvement in 8 cases. The duration of treatment ranged from 3 to 32 days, with an average of 14.5 days.[8]

SUGGESTED ACUPUNCTURE TREATMENT

1. Points: *Pishu* (BL 20), *Feishu* (BL 13), *Taiyuan* (LU 9), *Zhongwan* (CV 12), *Fenglong* (ST 40), *Hegu* (LI 4), *Xiaxi* (GB 43), *Shaochong* (HT 9), and other special points listed below.
2. Technique: sedation.

This selection of acupuncture points aims to harmonize the Gallbladder and Stomach, clear heat, and eliminate phlegm. *Pishu* (BL 20), *Feishu* (BL 13), and *Taiyuan* (LU 9) strengthen the Spleen, dispel dampness, and eliminate phlegm. *Zhongwan* (CV 12) clears phlegm-heat and harmonizes the Stomach. *Fenglong* (ST 40) and *Hegu* (LI 4) correct the reversed flow of qi, harmonize the Stomach, and eliminate phlegm. *Xiaxi* (GB 43) and *Shaochong* (HT 9) clear heat from the Gallbladder and Liver.

Clinically, the patient may show various signs and symptoms associated with Gallbladder and Stomach disharmony with heat and phlegm. If the patient has insomnia with excessive dreams, add *Lidui* (ST 45) and *Yinbai* (SP 1); for palpitations due to fright, add *Lingdao* (HT 4) and *Ximen* (PC 4); for nausea and vomiting, add

Wēn Dǎn Tāng (Warm the Gallbladder Decoction)

Housanli (ST 36) and *Neiguan* (PC 6); and for epilepsy, add *Benshen* (GB 13), *Shenzhu* (GV 12), and *Jiuwei* (CV 15).

References

1. *Zhong Yi Ming Fang Lin Chuang Xin Yong* (Contemporary Clinical Applications of Classic Chinese Formulas), 2001; 696.
2. *Zhe Jiang Zhong Yi Za Zhi* (Zhejiang Journal of Chinese Medicine), 1958; 5:5.
3. *Zhong Yi Za Zhi* (Journal of Chinese Medicine), 1984; 11:831.
4. *Nei Meng Gu Zhong Yi Yao* (Traditional Chinese Medicine and Medicinals of Inner Mongolia), 1998; 3:19.
5. *Xin Zhong Yi* (New Chinese Medicine), 1994; 26(8):45.
6. *Shan Xi Zhong Yi* (Shanxi Chinese Medicine), 1995; 16(9):393.
7. g Gao L. Qi-promoting and phlegm-resolving method for treatment of diabetic microvascular complications. Journal of Traditional Chinese Medicine. 2000 Jun; 20(2):104-9.
8. *Hu Nan Zhong Yi* (Hunan Journal of Traditional Chinese Medicine), 1976; 3(3):46.

Fú Líng Wán (Poria Pill)

茯苓丸

茯苓丸

Pinyin Name: *Fu Ling Wan*
Literal Name: Poria Pill
Original Source: *Fu Ren Da Quan Liang Fang* (Complete Fine Formulas for Women) by Chen Zi-Ming in 1237

COMPOSITION

Ban Xia (Rhizoma Pinelliae)	60g [9g]
Fu Ling (Poria)	30g [6g]
Zhi Qiao (Fructus Citri Aurantii), *chao* (dry-fried) with bran	15g [3g]
Po Xiao (Sal Glauberis)	0.3g [3g]

DOSAGE / PREPARATION / ADMINISTRATION

The source text states to grind the ingredients into powder and form into small pills using the juice of *Sheng Jiang* (Rhizoma Zingiberis Recens). The pills should resemble the size of *Wu Tong Zi* (Semen Firmianae), a small seed approximately 5 mm in diameter. Take 20 pills (6g) after meals with a decoction made from *Sheng Jiang* (Rhizoma Zingiberis Recens). Today, this formula may be prepared as a decoction with the doses suggested in brackets.

CHINESE THERAPEUTIC ACTIONS

1. Dries dampness and activates qi
2. Softens nodules and dissolves phlegm

CLINICAL MANIFESTATIONS

Phlegm stagnation in the epigastrium: pain in both front limbs, edema of the extremities, a greasy tongue, and a wiry, slippery pulse.

Fú Líng Wán (Poria Pill)

VETERINARY CLINICAL APPLICATIONS

Muscle pain, edema, cervical pain and stiffness, poor appetite, abdominal bloating, vomiting of thick, white mucus, and cough.

EXPLANATION

Fu Ling Wan (Poria Pill) treats damp and phlegm stagnation in the epigastrium, which arises from an underlying Spleen deficiency. Spleen deficiency leads to damp accumulation and, ultimately, to phlegm stagnation in the chest and epigastrium. Dampness and phlegm may travel via the channels and collaterals to cause pain in the front limbs or edema of the extremities. A greasy tongue and a wiry, slippery pulse indicate damp and phlegm accumulation.

This formula uses *Ban Xia* (Rhizoma Pinelliae) to dry dampness and dispel phlegm. *Fu Ling* (Poria) strengthens the Spleen and dispels dampness. *Zhi Qiao* (Fructus Aurantii) activates qi to dispel phlegm. *Po Xiao* (Sal Glauberis) softens nodules and facilitates the elimination of phlegm. The juice of *Sheng Jiang* (Rhizoma Zingiberis Recens) dissolves phlegm and detoxifies *Ban Xia* (Rhizoma Pinelliae).

VETERINARY MODIFICATIONS

- With swelling and pain of the limbs, add *Sang Zhi* (Ramulus Mori) and *Di Long* (Pheretima).
- For cough with thick sputum, add *Ge Qiao* (Concha Meretricis seu Cyclinae) and *Gua Lou* (Fructus Trichosanthis).

CAUTIONS / CONTRAINDICATIONS

- *Fu Ling Wan* should be used with caution in patients with generalized deficiencies.
- This formula is contraindicated for prolonged use. It should be discontinued as soon as the desired effect is achieved.

SUGGESTED ACUPUNCTURE TREATMENT

1. Points: *Pishu* (BL 20), *Yinlingquan* (SP 9), *Fenglong* (ST 40), *Neiguan* (PC 6), and *Shangjuxu* (ST 37).
2. Technique: sedation.

Since the main problem in this presentation is phlegm stagnation, the selected acupuncture points focus on elimination of phlegm. Because the Spleen produces phlegm, *Pishu* (BL 20) and *Yinlingquan* (SP 9) are used to strengthen the Spleen and reduce phlegm production. *Fenglong* (ST 40) dissolves dampness and phlegm. *Neiguan* (PC 6) regulates qi to dissolve phlegm. Finally, *Shangjuxu* (ST 37) eliminates dampness and phlegm from the lower *jiao*.

AUTHORS' COMMENTS

Fu Ling Wan can be used to treat animals with stiffness and pain of the forelegs and neck, in the absence of obvious musculoskeletal abnormalities. Radiographs and other imaging are unable to identify a structural lesion; however, the animal behaves as if they do. These animals have a white, greasy tongue and a slippery pulse, and herbs given for pain relief do not resolve the pain and stiffness. This formula can be combined with *Chai Hu Shu Gan San* (Bupleurum Powder to Spread the Liver) to help further regulate the qi and resolve nodules of the soft tissues and relieve pain in the upper body.

Fu Ling Wan also treats cough with profuse sputum, accompanied by distention of the epigastrium. These animals will have a productive cough accompanied by mild abdominal bloating. They may also have intermittent gagging and vomiting of thick, white mucus and poor appetite. To relieve vomiting and food stagnation caused by phlegm and water accumulation in the epigastrium, *Fu Ling Wan* can be modified with herbs such as *Chen Pi*

***Fu Ling Wan* (Poria Pill)**

Diagnosis	Clinical Signs	Treatment	Herbs
Phlegm stagnation in the epigastrium	• Pain in both arms and edema of the extremities: phlegm stagnation in the channels and collaterals • Abdominal bloating, vomiting of thick, white mucus, a greasy tongue, and a wiry, slippery pulse: damp and phlegm accumulation	• Dries dampness and activates qi • Softens nodules and dissolves phlegm	• *Ban Xia* (Rhizoma Pinelliae) dries dampness and dispels phlegm. • *Fu Ling* (Poria) strengthens the Spleen and dispels dampness. • *Zhi Qiao* (Fructus Aurantii) activates qi to dispel phlegm. • *Po Xiao* (Sal Glauberis) softens nodules and facilitates the elimination of phlegm. • *Sheng Jiang* (Rhizoma Zingiberis Recens) dissolves phlegm and detoxifies *Ban Xia* (Rhizoma Pinelliae).

Fú Líng Wán (Poria Pill)

(Pericarpium Citri Reticulatae), *Shen Qu* (Massa Fermentata), and *Mai Ya* (Fructus Hordei Germinatus). Many animals will readily eat these additional herbs in their food.

It is important to note that the front limb pain in this syndrome is caused by damp and phlegm stagnation in the epigastrium. From the epigastrium, dampness and phlegm travel via the channels and collaterals to the extremities to cause pain and edema. Optimal treatment requires the use of herbs to dry dampness and dispel phlegm. Since wind-damp-cold factors are ***not*** the cause of this syndrome, herbs that dispel wind-damp-cold should not be used, as they will only consume qi and complicate the illness.

Section 2

清热化痰剂
— Heat-Clearing and Phlegm-Dissolving Formulas

Qīng Qì Huà Tán Wán (Clear the Qi and Transform Phlegm Pill)
清氣化痰丸
清气化痰丸

Pinyin Name: *Qing Qi Hua Tan Wan*
Literal Name: Clear the Qi and Transform Phlegm Pill
Alternate Name: Pinellia and Scute Formula
Original Source: *Yi Fang Kao* (Investigation of Medical Formulas) by Wu Kun in 1584

COMPOSITION

Dan Nan Xing (Arisaema cum Bile)	45g [9g]
Huang Qin (Radix Scutellariae), *chao* (dry-fried) with liquor	30g [6g]
Gua Lou Zi (Semen Trichosanthis), oil removed	30g [6g]
Zhi Shi (Fructus Aurantii Immaturus), *chao* (dry-fried) with bran	30g [6g]
Chen Pi (Pericarpium Citri Reticulatae)	30g [6g]
Fu Ling (Poria)	30g [6g]
Ku Xing Ren (Semen Armeniacae Amarum)	30g [6g]
Ban Xia (Rhizoma Pinelliae), *zhi* (prepared)	45g [9g]

DOSAGE / PREPARATION / ADMINISTRATION

The source text states to grind the ingredients into powder and form into pills with fresh juice from *Sheng Jiang* (Rhizoma Zingiberis Recens). Take 6g of pills per dose with warm, boiled water. Today, this formula may be prepared as a decoction with the doses suggested in brackets.

CHINESE THERAPEUTIC ACTIONS

1. Clears heat and dissolves phlegm
2. Regulates qi and stops coughing

CLINICAL MANIFESTATIONS

Phlegm-heat stagnation in the Lung: loud cough that is worse at night and early morning with thick, yellow phlegm that cannot be completely expectorated; gagging, choking, dyspnea, chest congestion, restlessness; scanty, dark urine; a red tongue and a slippery, rapid pulse.

VETERINARY CLINICAL APPLICATIONS

Hemoptysis, coughing, acute bacterial pneumonia, aspiration pneumonia, acute bronchitis, feline upper respiratory tract infections, equine rhinopneumonitis, canine infectious tracheobronchitis and secondary bacterial infections, acute bronchial asthma.

EXPLANATION

Qing Qi Hua Tan Wan (Clear the Qi and Transform Phlegm Pill) treats phlegm-heat syndromes accompanied by thick, yellow sputum and a slippery, rapid pulse. The origin of these syndromes can be traced to the presence of internal fire, which dries and thickens the body fluids, turning them into phlegm. When phlegm accumulates in the Lung, it produces Lung qi stagnation and cough. The sputum is thick and yellowish because of the internal fire. Scanty, dark urine results when the internal fire affects the lower *jiao*. A red tongue and a slippery, rapid pulse suggest phlegm and heat accumulation in the interior.

This formula uses *Dan Nan Xing* (Arisaema cum Bile) to clear heat and dissolve phlegm. *Huang Qin* (Radix Scutellariae) and *Gua Lou Zi* (Semen Trichosanthis) clear Lung heat and eliminate phlegm. Since phlegm obstructs the flow of qi, *Zhi Shi* (Fructus Aurantii Immaturus) and *Chen*

Qīng Qì Huà Tán Wán (Clear the Qi and Transform Phlegm Pill)

Qing Qi Hua Tan Wan **(Clear the Qi and Transform Phlegm Pill)**

Diagnosis	Clinical Signs	Treatment	Herbs
Phlegm-heat in the Lung	• Cough with thick, yellow sputum that cannot be completely expectorated: phlegm-heat stagnation in the Lung • Scanty, dark urine: internal fire affecting the lower *jiao* • Red tongue and a slippery, rapid pulse: phlegm-heat accumulation in the interior	• Clears heat and dissolves phlegm • Regulates qi and stops cough	• *Dan Nan Xing* (Arisaema cum Bile) clears heat and dissolves phlegm. • *Huang Qin* (Radix Scutellariae) and *Gua Lou Zi* (Semen Trichosanthis) clear Lung heat and eliminate phlegm. • *Zhi Shi* (Fructus Aurantii Immaturus) and *Chen Pi* (Pericarpium Citri Reticulatae) remove qi stagnation and dissolve phlegm. • *Fu Ling* (Poria) strengthens the Spleen and drains dampness to prevent the formation of more phlegm. • *Ku Xing Ren* (Semen Armeniacae Amarum) causes the Lung qi to descend and relieves cough. • *Ban Xia* (Rhizoma Pinelliae) breaks up phlegm stagnation and dries dampness.

Pi (Pericarpium Citri Reticulatae) remove qi stagnation and dissolve phlegm. Because the Spleen is the organ that produces dampness and phlegm, *Fu Ling* (Poria) is used to strengthen the Spleen and drain dampness, preventing the formation of more phlegm. *Ku Xing Ren* (Semen Armeniacae Amarum) causes the Lung qi to descend and relieves cough, and *Ban Xia* (Rhizoma Pinelliae) breaks up phlegm stagnation and dries dampness. Lastly, the fresh juice from *Sheng Jiang* (Rhizoma Zingiberis Recens) has a strong dispersing property, which helps transform phlegm; therefore, it is added to the herbs to form pills.

VETERINARY MODIFICATIONS

- With fever, add *Shi Gao* (Gypsum Fibrosum) and *Huang Qin* (Radix Scutellariae).
- With cough and thirst due to severe Lung heat, add *Shi Gao* (Gypsum Fibrosum) and *Zhi Mu* (Rhizoma Anemarrhenae); or combine with *Ma Huang Xing Ren Gan Cao Shi Gao Tang* (Ephedra, Apricot Kernel, Licorice, and Gypsum Decoction).
- With profuse sputum and rapid respiration, add *Yu Xing Cao* (Herba Houttuyniae) and *Sang Bai Pi* (Cortex Mori).
- If there is constipation, add *Mang Xiao* (Natrii Sulfas).

CAUTIONS / CONTRAINDICATIONS

Use of this formula is contraindicated during pregnancy.[1]

SUGGESTED ACUPUNCTURE TREATMENT

1. Points: *Jingqu* (LU 8), *Feishu* (BL 13), *Fenglong* (ST 40), *Zhiyang* (GV 9), *Hegu* (LI 4), *Shanzhong* (CV 17), *Pishu* (BL 20), and *Yinlingquan* (SP 9).
2. Technique: sedation.

The objectives of acupuncture treatment are to clear heat, dissolve phlegm, regulate qi, and stop coughing. *Jingqu* (LU 8) and *Feishu* (BL 13) clear Lung heat and dispel phlegm. *Fenglong* (ST 40) eliminates dampness and phlegm. *Zhiyang* (GV 9) and *Hegu* (LI 4) clear heat and relieve exterior factors. *Shanzhong* (CV 17) regulates qi circulation and relieves chest stuffiness. *Pishu* (BL 20) and *Yinlingquan* (SP 9) strengthen the Spleen and eliminate dampness.

AUTHORS' COMMENTS

Qing Qi Hua Tan Wan is commonly used in veterinary medicine to treat acute cough, respiratory disease and bacterial infection with yellow phlegm and heat signs. The animals for which this formula is appropriate typically have pre-existing phlegm from eating a poor diet and then contract a wind-cold or wind-heat pathogen which invades the Lung, resulting in cough with thick, yellow mucus. To improve its ability to treat heat (infection) and/or treat cough, this formula can be combined with *Yin Qiao San* (Honeysuckle and Forsythia Powder) if there is more heat; *Sang Ju Yin* (Mulberry Leaf and Chrysanthemum Decoction) with mild cough; or *Ma Huang Xing Ren Gan Cao Shi Gao Tang* (Ephedra, Apricot Kernel, Licorice, and Gypsum Decoction) with severe cough. If deficiency of the middle *jiao* is present, these formulas must be combined with herbs and/or formulas that tonify the middle *jiao* to prevent nausea and vomiting, especially in weak animals. In order to improve clinical results, this formula or formula combinations may need to be given for a minimum of 1-2 weeks. Administration of the formula should be discontinued 2-3 days after the cough and yellow mucus have cleared, and a more tonifying formula given as needed. It is often the case that after the acute respiratory condition has resolved, there can be residual thick, clear to white phlegm and even a mild cough. After treatment with *Qing Qi Hua Tan Wan*, the animals should be switched over to *Er Chen Tang* (Two-Cured Decoction) or another appropriate formula that clears phlegm-damp at a low dose, and any deficiencies of the Lung and Spleen should be tonified to consolidate treatment and prevent relapse. As a pathogenic factor, phlegm is notoriously difficult to clear or eliminate, and stopping treatment too early can result in relapse; however, giving a phlegm formula for too long can dry the animal out and damage yin. Phlegm-clearing formulas are quite drying in nature and should not be used in animals with significant yin and body fluid deficiencies. In animals that are yin deficient, the formula *Zi Wan Tang* (Aster Decoction) can be given, following treatment with *Qing Qi Hua Tan Wan*.

Reference

1. *Zhong Yao Ming Fang Yao Li Yu Ying Yong* (Pharmacology and Applications of Famous Herbal Formulas), 1989; 591-592.

Qīng Fèi Yǐn (Clear the Lung Drink)

清肺飲
清肺饮

Pinyin Name: *Qing Fei Yin*
Literal Name: Clear the Lung Drink
Alternate Names: *Ching Fai Yin, Qing Fai Yin*, Lung-Clearing Drink, Platycodon and Apricot Seed Formula
Original Source: *Yi Fang Ji Jie* (Analytical Collection of Medical Formulas) by Wang Ang in 1682

COMPOSITION

Ku Xing Ren (Semen Armeniacae Amarum)	3g
Zhe Bei Mu (Bulbus Fritillariae Thunbergii)	3g
Wu Wei Zi (Fructus Schisandrae Chinensis)	1.5g
Fu Ling (Poria)	3g
Ju Hong (Exocarpium Citri Rubrum)	1.5g
Jie Geng (Radix Platycodonis)	1.5g
Gan Cao (Radix et Rhizoma Glycyrrhizae)	1.5g

DOSAGE / PREPARATION / ADMINISTRATION

The source text states to cook the herbs with *Sheng Jiang* (Rhizoma Zingiberis Recens). Take the warm, strained decoction between meals.

CHINESE THERAPEUTIC ACTIONS

Clears the Lung and dissolves phlegm

Qīng Fèi Yǐn (Clear the Lung Drink)

CLINICAL MANIFESTATIONS

Cough caused by phlegm and damp accumulation: cough with sputum, thoracic discomfort, lethargy and poor performance, a red tongue, and a slippery pulse.

VETERINARY CLINICAL APPLICATIONS

Cough due to upper respiratory disease, bronchitis and bronchial asthma.

EXPLANATION

Qing Fei Yin (Clear the Lung Drink) treats cough caused by phlegm and damp accumulation. As a result of the accumulation, the Lung qi cannot descend, causing qi reversal and cough. The presence of sputum indicates dampness and phlegm.

This formula contains herbs to clear the Lung, dissolve phlegm, and moisten the Lung. *Ku Xing Ren* (Semen Armeniacae Amarum) causes Lung qi to descend, and it is commonly used to treat cough and dyspnea. *Zhe Bei Mu* (Bulbus Fritillariae Thunbergii) clears fire, dissolves phlegm, and moistens the Lung. *Wu Wei Zi* (Fructus Schisandrae Chinensis) stabilizes and binds to preserve the Lung from further loss of qi. *Fu Ling* (Poria) strengthens the Spleen and dissolves dampness. *Ju Hong* (Exocarpium Citri Rubrum) activates qi and relieves stagnation. *Jie Geng* (Radix Platycodonis) clears the Lung and eliminates phlegm. *Gan Cao* (Radix et Rhizoma Glycyrrhizae) and *Sheng Jiang* (Rhizoma Zingiberis Recens) harmonize the formula. In short, this formula treats mild to moderate cases of cough caused by phlegm and damp accumulation.

VETERINARY MODIFICATIONS

- If there is clear nasal discharge due to wind, add *Bo He* (Herba Menthae), *Fang Feng* (Radix Saposhnikoviae), and *Zi Su Ye* (Folium Perillae).
- With more heat, add *Shi Gao* (Gypsum Fibrosum) and *Zhi Mu* (Rhizoma Anemarrhenae).
- For chronic cough caused by Lung deficiency, add *Ren Shen* (Radix et Rhizoma Ginseng) and *Huang Qi* (Radix Astragali).
- For cough and dyspnea accompanied by profuse phlegm, add *Sang Bai Pi* (Cortex Mori) and *Di Gu Pi* (Cortex Lycii).
- With phlegm due to food stagnation, add *Shan Zha* (Fructus Crataegi), *Xiang Fu* (Rhizoma Cyperi), and *Zhi Shi* (Fructus Aurantii Immaturus).

SUGGESTED ACUPUNCTURE TREATMENT

1. Points: *Tiantu* (CV 22), *Chize* (LU 5), *Taiyuan* (LU 9), *Yinlingquan* (SP 9), and *Zhongwan* (CV 12).
2. Technique: even method.

Tiantu (CV 22), *Chize* (LU 5), and *Taiyuan* (LU 9) cleanse the Lung, promote qi circulation, and dissolve phlegm. *Yinlingquan* (SP 9) regulates the water passages. *Zhongwan* (CV 12) strengthens the middle *jiao* to eliminate dampness.

AUTHORS' COMMENTS

Qing Fei Yin is a basic formula that is used to treat coughing from nearly every type of Lung damp-phlegm condition. In dogs and cats, it is most often used to treat geriatric

Qing Fei Yin (Clear the Lung Drink)

Diagnosis	Clinical Signs	Treatment	Herbs
Cough due to accumulation of phlegm and dampness	Cough with sputum, chest discomfort and fatigue: reversed qi flow due to accumulation of phlegm and dampness	Clears the Lung and dissolves phlegm	• *Ku Xing Ren* (Semen Armeniacae Amarum) causes qi to descend to treat cough and dyspnea. • *Zhe Bei Mu* (Bulbus Fritillariae Thunbergii) clears fire, dissolves phlegm, and moistens the Lung. • *Wu Wei Zi* (Fructus Schisandrae Chinensis) stabilizes and binds Lung qi. • *Fu Ling* (Poria) strengthens the Spleen and dissolves dampness. • *Ju Hong* (Exocarpium Citri Rubrum) activates qi and relieves stagnation. • *Jie Geng* (Radix Platycodonis) clears the Lung and eliminates phlegm. • *Gan Cao* (Radix et Rhizoma Glycyrrhizae) and *Sheng Jiang* (Rhizoma Zingiberis Recens) harmonize the formula.

Qīng Fèi Yǐn (Clear the Lung Drink)

animals with chronic cough, especially in the late afternoon and evening. The cough is productive and often clear to white mucus is coughed up, or the animal is seen to repeatedly gag and choke with expectoration of mucus. Geriatric animals are often significantly yin deficient, and many have developed phlegm from Spleen qi deficiency due to poor diet, chronic medications and aging. In horses, deficiency from travel and performance can create similar deficiencies and similar symptoms. Often horses will cough while being worked, sometimes to the point where it is necessary to stop training. Horses that have recovered from a more severe infection and now have a persistent cough, or those that suffer from mild cases of heaves, may also be treated with this formula.

This formula can be used to treat Lung yin deficiency with damp-phlegm cough (productive cough) with minimal signs of heat by adding *Ban Xia* (Rhizoma Pinelliae), *Tian Nan Xing* (Rhizoma Arisaematis), *Mai Dong* (Radix Ophiopogonis), *Tian Dong* (Radix Asparagi), *Zhi Mu* (Rhizoma Anemarrhenae), *Di Huang* (Radix Rehmanniae), *Huang Bo* (Cortex Phellodendri Chinensis), *Bai Shao* (Radix Paeoniae Alba), *Chuan Xiong* (Rhizoma Chuanxiong), and *Dang Gui* (Radix Angelicae Sinensis). To treat dry phlegm and a non-productive cough that is hacking and harsh with little expectoration, add *Gua Lou* (Fructus Trichosanthis), *Tian Dong* (Radix Asparagi) and *Zhi Mu* (Rhizoma Anemarrhenae). *Qing Fei Yin* is a mild formula for clearing heat and dissolving phlegm in the Lung. The animals for which this formula is appropriate have mild signs of heat and phlegm and are typically in good health; they just have a cough for which no structural etiology can be found.

Qing Fei Yin and *Qing Qi Hua Tan Wan* (Clear the Qi and Transform Phlegm Pill) both clear heat and dissolve phlegm in the Lung. However, *Qing Fei Yin* has only mild heat-clearing capabilities. If significant heat in the Lung is present, *Qing Qi Hua Tan Wan* (Clear the Qi and Transform Phlegm Pill) should be chosen, especially when yellow sputum is present. These two formulas treat excess conditions and have little ability to tonify qi, yin or body fluid deficiencies without modification. If a ready-made formula is desired for animals with significant qi, yin and body fluid deficiencies, it is best to use formulas such as *Qing Fei Tang* (Clear the Lung Decoction), *Zi Wan Tang* (Aster Decoction), or *Ren Shen Xie Fei Tang* (Ginseng Decoction to Sedate the Lung).

Qīng Fèi Tāng (Clear the Lung Decoction)

清肺湯
清肺汤

Pinyin Name: *Qing Fei Tang*
Literal Name: Clear the Lung Decoction
Alternate Names: *Ching Fei Tang*, Lung-Clearing Decoction, Platycodon and Fritillaria Decoction, Platycodon and Fritillaria Combination
Original Source: *Wan Bing Hui Chun* (Restoration of Health from the Myriad Diseases) by Gong Ting-Xian in 1587

COMPOSITION

Huang Qin (Radix Scutellariae)	4.5g
Zhi Zi (Fructus Gardeniae)	2.1g
Ku Xing Ren (Semen Armeniacae Amarum)	2.1g
Zhe Bei Mu (Bulbus Fritillariae Thunbergii)	3g
Zhu Ru (Caulis Bambusae in Taenia)	3g
Sang Bai Pi (Cortex Mori)	3g
Jie Geng (Radix Platycodonis)	3g
Mai Dong (Radix Ophiopogonis)	2.1g
Tian Dong (Radix Asparagi)	2.1g
Dang Gui (Radix Angelicae Sinensis)	2.1g
Gan Cao (Radix et Rhizoma Glycyrrhizae)	0.9g
Chen Pi (Pericarpium Citri Reticulatae)	3g
Fu Ling (Poria)	3g
Wu Wei Zi (Fructus Schisandrae Chinensis)	7 pieces

DOSAGE / PREPARATION / ADMINISTRATION

The source text states to grate and cook the herbs with *Sheng Jiang* (Rhizoma Zingiberis Recens) and *Da Zao* (Fructus Jujubae). Take the warm, strained decoction after meals.

CHINESE THERAPEUTIC ACTIONS

1. Dispels heat and phlegm from the chest
2. Moistens the Lung and relieves cough

CLINICAL MANIFESTATIONS

Chronic cough caused by heat and phlegm in the Lung: severe cough, thick and sticky phlegm varying from white to yellow to green in color, hoarse or abnormal vocalization, a red tongue and a rapid, slippery pulse.

VETERINARY CLINICAL APPLICATIONS

Chronic bronchitis, pneumonia, aspiration pneumonia, bronchiectasis, laryngitis and tuberculosis.

EXPLANATION

Qing Fei Tang (Clear the Lung Decoction) addresses chronic cases of heat and phlegm attacking the Lung, leading to phlegm accumulation with underlying deficiency. When heat and phlegm obstruct the Lung, the flow of qi is reversed, resulting in severe cough. In addition, phlegm accumulation can cause thick, sticky sputum, with color varying from white to yellow to green. The chronic nature of this illness also contributes to yin and fluid deficiencies, leading to sore, itchy throat, hoarseness and abnormal vocalization.

This formula contains herbs to dispel heat and phlegm, moisten the Lung, and relieve cough. *Huang Qin* (Radix Scutellariae) and *Zhi Zi* (Fructus Gardeniae) clear damp-heat from the upper *jiao*, thereby addressing the heat and phlegm condition in the Lung. *Ku Xing Ren* (Semen Armeniacae Amarum), *Zhe Bei Mu* (Bulbus Fritillariae Thunbergii), *Zhu Ru* (Caulis Bambusae in Taenia), and *Sang Bai Pi* (Cortex Mori) clear the Lung and cause qi to descend. *Jie Geng* (Radix Platycodonis) eliminates the accumulation of sputum and phlegm. *Mai Dong* (Radix Ophiopogonis) and *Tian Dong* (Radix Asparagi) have a synergistic effect to moisten the Lung and nourish yin. *Dang Gui* (Radix Angelicae Sinensis) and *Gan Cao* (Radix et Rhizoma Glycyrrhizae) nourish the blood and balance the bitter and cold nature of *Huang Qin* (Radix Scutellariae) and *Zhi Zi* (Fructus Gardeniae). *Chen Pi* (Pericarpium Citri Reticulatae) regulates the proper flow of qi. *Fu Ling* (Poria) strengthens the Spleen to dry dampness and reduce phlegm production. *Wu Wei Zi* (Fructus Schisandrae Chinensis) stabilizes and binds the Lung to prevent further

Qīng Fèi Tāng (Clear the Lung Decoction)

***Qing Fei Tang* (Clear the Lung Decoction)**

Diagnosis	Clinical Signs	Treatment	Herbs
Chronic cough due to heat and phlegm in the Lung	• Cough with thick, sticky, white to yellow green sputum: reversed qi flow due to heat and phlegm obstructing the Lung • Sore, itchy throat and hoarseness: yin and fluid deficiencies	• Dispels heat and phlegm from the chest • Moistens the Lung and relieves cough	• *Huang Qin* (Radix Scutellariae) and *Zhi Zi* (Fructus Gardeniae) clear damp-heat from the Lung in the upper *jiao*. • *Ku Xing Ren* (Semen Armeniacae Amarum), *Zhe Bei Mu* (Bulbus Fritillariae Thunbergii), *Zhu Ru* (Caulis Bambusae in Taenia) and *Sang Bai Pi* (Cortex Mori) clear the Lung and cause Lung qi to descend. • *Jie Geng* (Radix Platycodonis) eliminates the accumulation of sputum and phlegm. • *Mai Dong* (Radix Ophiopogonis) and *Tian Dong* (Radix Asparagi) moisten the Lung and nourish yin. • *Dang Gui* (Radix Angelicae Sinensis) and *Gan Cao* (Radix et Rhizoma Glycyrrhizae) nourish the blood. • *Chen Pi* (Pericarpium Citri Reticulatae) regulates the proper flow of qi. • *Fu Ling* (Poria) strengthens the Spleen to dry dampness and reduce phlegm production. • *Wu Wei Zi* (Fructus Schisandrae Chinensis) stabilizes and binds the Lung to prevent further loss of Lung qi. • *Sheng Jiang* (Rhizoma Zingiberis Recens) and *Da Zao* (Fructus Jujubae) harmonize the formula.

loss of Lung qi. *Sheng Jiang* (Rhizoma Zingiberis Recens) and *Da Zao* (Fructus Jujubae) harmonize the formula.

VETERINARY MODIFICATIONS

- With more heat, swelling and pain, add *Shi Gao* (Gypsum Fibrosum), *Jin Yin Hua* (Flos Lonicerae Japonicae) and *Lian Qiao* (Fructus Forsythiae).
- With stubborn phlegm that is difficult to expectorate, add *Gua Lou* (Fructus Trichosanthis), *Zhi Shi* (Fructus Aurantii Immaturus), and *Zhu Li* (Succus Bambusae); and remove *Wu Wei Zi* (Fructus Schisandrae Chinensis).
- With cough, asthma, and increased respiration, add *Zi Su Zi* (Fructus Perillae) and *Zhu Li* (Succus Bambusae). Remove *Jie Geng* (Radix Platycodonis).
- With chronic cough, add *Bai Zhu* (Rhizoma Atractylodis Macrocephalae), *Bai Shao* (Radix Paeoniae Alba), and *Di Huang* (Radix Rehmanniae); and remove *Jie Geng* (Radix Platycodonis), *Zhe Bei Mu* (Bulbus Fritillariae Thunbergii), and *Ku Xing Ren* (Semen Armeniacae Amarum).
- With high fever and blood in the sputum, add *Bai Shao* (Radix Paeoniae Alba), *Di Huang* (Radix Rehmanniae), *Zi Wan* (Radix et Rhizoma Asteris), *E Jiao* (Colla Corii Asini), and *Zhu Li* (Succus Bambusae); and remove *Wu Wei Zi* (Fructus Schisandrae Chinensis), *Ku Xing Ren* (Semen Armeniacae Amarum), *Zhe Bei Mu* (Bulbus Fritillariae Thunbergii), and *Jie Geng* (Radix Platycodonis).

PHARMACOLOGICAL EFFECTS

1. **Expectorant**: According to one study, administration of 500 mg/kg of *Qing Fei Tang* in powder extract via oral ingestion was associated with a marked expectorant effect, with the onset of action beginning after 3 hours. No expectorant effect was observed when the formula was given at lower doses, such as 50 and 100 mg/kg.[1,2]
2. **Antiallergic**: This formula has an inhibitory effect on leukotriene (LT) B4 synthesis of human alveolar macrophages. In one study, two-week cultured basophil levels identified by alcian blue-safranin staining and those histamine contents assayed fluorometrically were inhibited by this formula in a dose-dependent manner. Since *Qing Fei Tang* modulates basophil growth and differentiation *in vitro* and/or *in vivo*, the study suggested that the formula has an antiallergic effect and may be useful for controlling allergic diseases including bronchial asthma.[3]
3. **Respiratory**: Administration of *Qing Fei Tang* was associated with various effects on the respiratory system, including but not limited to inhibited release of slow reacting substance of anaphylaxis from the lung, suppressed chemiluminescence of oxygen radicals, increased output volume and fatty acid contents in respiratory tract fluid,

Qīng Fèi Tāng (Clear the Lung Decoction)

and facilitated tracheal mucociliary transport.[4] According to one study in mice, use of *Qing Fei Tang* was associated with reduced mortality for aspiration pneumonia artificially-induced with *Streptococcus pneumoniae* and gastric juice. The mechanism of this effect was attributed to the decreased activity of xanthine oxidase and reduction of oxygen radical production in inflamed lungs.[5]

4. **Anti-inflammatory**: *Qing Fei Tang* can be used to treat inflammatory lung diseases through its anti-inflammatory action to inhibit the oxidative and arachidonate metabolism of local inflammatory lung cells.[6]

HUMAN CLINICAL STUDIES AND RESEARCH

Aspiration pneumonia: According to a randomized, controlled clinical trial, 15 patients with relapsing aspiration pneumonia were divided into two groups. Eight patients were treated with conventional Western medicine, and 7 were treated with *Qing Fei Tang*. After a study period of 16 weeks, the study reported a significant reduction of relapse of aspiration pneumonia and reduction in antibiotic use in patients treated with *Qing Fei Tang*, in comparison with drug therapy group. Swallowing reflex, however, did not change in patients treated with *Qing Fei Tang*. No adverse reactions were reported in either group. The study concluded that *Qing Fei Tang* is an effective therapy for treatment of aspiration pneumonia. It improved the defense mechanism or excessive inflammation caused by pneumonia in the lower airway, but did not improve the swallowing reflex.[7]

SUGGESTED ACUPUNCTURE TREATMENT

1. Points: *Quchi* (LI 11), *Feishu* (BL 13), *Kongzui* (LU 6), *Chize* (LU 5), *Tiantu* (CV 22), *Fenglong* (ST 40), *Taixi* (KI 3), *Sanyinjiao* (SP 6), *Zhongwan* (CV 12), *Yinlingquan* (SP 9), *Taiyuan* (LU 9) and *Dingchuan*.
2. Technique: even method.

Quchi (LI 11) clears Lung heat. *Feishu* (BL 13), *Kongzui* (LU 6), *Chize* (LU 5), and *Tiantu* (CV 22) descend qi and arrest cough. *Fenglong* (ST 40) dissolves phlegm. *Taixi* (KI 3), *Sanyinjiao* (SP 6), and *Yinlingquan* (SP 9) regulate body fluids and preserve yin. *Zhongwan* (CV 12) regulates qi in the *San Jiao*. *Taiyuan* (LU 9) tonifies Lung qi. *Dingchuan* is a classical point to stop cough.

RELATED FORMULA

Qīng Fèi Tāng (Clear the Lung Decoction)

清肺湯
清肺汤

Pinyin Name: *Qing Fei Tang*
Literal Name: Clear the Lung Decoction
Original Source: *Han Fang Yi Xue* (Kampo Medicine)

Huang Qin (Radix Scutellariae)	
Jie Geng (Radix Platycodonis)	
Fu Ling (Poria)	
Chen Pi (Pericarpium Citri Reticulatae)	
Bei Mu (Bulbus Fritillariae)	
Sang Bai Pi (Cortex Mori)	
Dang Gui (Radix Angelicae Sinensis)	
Tian Dong (Radix Asparagi)	
Zhi Zi (Fructus Gardeniae)	
Ku Xing Ren (Semen Armeniacae Amarum)	
Mai Dong (Radix Ophiopogonis)	
Wu Wei Zi (Fructus Schisandrae Chinensis)	
Gan Cao (Radix et Rhizoma Glycyrrhizae)	
Zhu Ru (Caulis Bambusae in Taenia)	

These two formulas have essentially the same ingredients and functions. *Qing Fei Tang* (Clear the Lung Decoction), which appeared in *Wan Bing Hui Chun* (Restoration of Health from the Myriad Diseases), is the original formulation. *Qing Fei Tang* (Clear the Lung Decoction) from *Han Fang Yi Xue* (Kampo Medicine) is the revised formulation, which clears heat and dissolves thick, yellow phlegm.

AUTHORS' COMMENTS

Qing Fei Tang (Clear the Lung Decoction) is often combined with *Yin Qiao San* (Honeysuckle and Forsythia Powder) to clear heat and treat infection, especially in animals with pneumonia. The combination of these two formulas is particularly helpful in older dogs that have repeated bouts of chronic aspiration pneumonia from laryngeal tie back surgery for laryngeal paralysis. The chronic nature of these attacks eventually leads to deficiencies of the Lung, yin and body fluids. This combination of formulas can also be used for dogs with chronic megaesophagus with aspiration pneumonia as well.

For animals that have yin deficiency and chronic aspiration pneumonia which suddenly exacerbates into an acute crisis with high fever, dyspnea and copious amounts of thick, yellow to green sputum and nasal discharge, this formula can be combined with *Huang Lian Jie Du Tang* (Coptis Decoction to Relieve Toxicity) at the lowest possible dose. *Huang Lian Jie Du Tang* (Coptis Decoction to Relieve Toxicity) is very cold and bitter and can easily injure yin and the middle *jiao*; however, with proper use it is invaluable for acute situations such as outlined above. Additional herbs or another formula to protect the middle *jiao* should be added as needed. This combination can be used for 3-5 days (or 3-6 doses) until the fever has subsided, at which time, another formula can be chosen, depending on the clinical signs.

Qīng Fèi Tāng (Clear the Lung Decoction)

Qing Fei Tang (Clear the Lung Decoction) and *Qing Fei Yin* (Clear the Lung Drink) are two formulas with similar names, but have different functions and indications.

- *Qing Fei Tang* is a potent formula that treats chronic cough with both excess (heat and phlegm) and deficiency (underlying yin and fluid deficiencies). It clears heat, dispels phlegm, moistens the Lung, and relieves cough.
- *Qing Fei Yin* is a mild to moderate formula that treats cough characterized by only excess (phlegm and dampness). It dissolves dampness, dispels phlegm, and relieves coughing.

References

1. *Guo Wai Yi Xue Zhong Yi Zhong Yao Fen Ce* (Monograph of Chinese Herbology from Foreign Medicine), 1986; 4:18.
2. *Zhong Yi Fang Ji Xian Dai Yan Jiu* (Modern Study of Medical Formulas in Traditional Chinese Medicine), 1997; 1496.
3. Tanno Y, Shindoh Y, Takishima T. Modulation of human basophil growth in vitro by xiao-qing-long-tang (syo-seiryu-to), chai-pu-tang (saiboku-to), qing-fei-tang (seihai-to), baicalein and ketotifen., American Journal of Chinese Medicine. 1989; 17(1-2):45-50.
4. Miyamoto K, Furusawa K, Kuroiwa A, Saito M, Miyata T, Furukawa T. Effects of qing-fei-tang on the airway inflammation and clearance. Am J Chin Med. 1990; 18(1-2):5-18.
5. Iwasaki K, Wang Q, Satoh N, Yoshida S, Akaike T, Sekizawa K, Maeda H, Sasaki H. Effects of qing fei tang (TJ-90) on aspiration pneumonia in mice. Phytomedicine. 1999 May; 6(2):95-101.
6. Tanno Y, Kakuta Y, Aikawa T, Shindoh Y, Ohno I, Takishima T.Effects of Qing-Fei-Tang (seihai-to) and baicalein, its main component flavonoid, on lucigenin-dependent chemiluminescence and leukotriene B4 synthesis of human alveolar macrophages. Am J Chin Med. 1988; 16(3-4):145-54.
7. Mantani N, Kasahara Y, Kamata T, Sekiya N, Shimada Y, Usuda K, Sakakibara I, Hattori N, Terasawa K. Effect of Seihai-to, a Kampo medicine, in relapsing aspiration pneumonia--an open-label pilot study. Phytomedicine. 2002 Apr; 9(3):195-201.

Zǐ Wǎn Tāng (Aster Decoction)

紫菀湯
紫菀汤

Pinyin Name: *Zi Wan Tang*
Literal Name: Aster Decoction
Alternate Names: *Tzu Wan Tang*, Aster Combination
Original Source: *Yi Fang Ji Jie* (Analytical Collection of Medical Formulas) by Wang Ang in 1682

COMPOSITION

Zhi Mu (Rhizoma Anemarrhenae)
Zi Wan (Radix et Rhizoma Asteris)
Zhe Bei Mu (Bulbus Fritillariae Thunbergii)
Jie Geng (Radix Platycodonis)
Ren Shen (Radix et Rhizoma Ginseng)
Fu Ling (Poria)
Wu Wei Zi (Fructus Schisandrae Chinensis)
E Jiao (Colla Corii Asini)
Gan Cao (Radix et Rhizoma Glycyrrhizae)

Zǐ Wǎn Tāng (Aster Decoction)

DOSAGE / PREPARATION / ADMINISTRATION

The source text states to grind all of the ingredients into a coarse powder and cook it with *Sheng Jiang* (Rhizoma Zingiberis Recens) in water to make a decoction, which then should be strained and taken while warm. Note: The source text did not specify the doses for the ingredients.

CHINESE THERAPEUTIC ACTIONS

1. Clears heat and dissolves phlegm
2. Relieves cough
3. Protects the Lung

CLINICAL MANIFESTATIONS

Chronic cough caused by Lung heat and yin deficiency: chronic cough with clear to yellow phlegm, bloody sputum, lung abscesses, a red, dry tongue, and a weak, rapid pulse.

VETERINARY CLINICAL APPLICATIONS

Pulmonary parenchymal disease and eosinophilic granulomatosis secondary to canine heartworm disease, pulmonary tuberculosis, asthma, emphysema, cough in cancer patients, cough in animals undergoing chemotherapy or radiation, hemoptysis and cough due to chronic pulmonary disorders.

EXPLANATION

Zi Wan Tang (Aster Decoction) treats chronic Lung disorders characterized by heat and underlying yin deficiency. When chronic heat attacks the Lung, it causes cough, profuse phlegm and sputum, dyspnea, and fever. Furthermore, as heat consumes yin and body fluids, patients may experience chest tightness, discomfort, abscess, and blood in the sputum; they may also develop a red, dry tongue and a weak, rapid pulse.

This formula uses herbs that treat both the cause and the symptoms. *Zhi Mu* (Rhizoma Anemarrhenae) clears heat while preserving the integrity of yin and body fluids. *Zi Wan* (Radix et Rhizoma Asteris) regulates Lung qi and relieves cough. *Zhe Bei Mu* (Bulbus Fritillariae Thunbergii) and *Jie Geng* (Radix Platycodonis) dissolve phlegm, relieve cough, and drain pus. *Ren Shen* (Radix et Rhizoma Ginseng) tonifies Lung qi, while *Fu Ling* (Poria) tonifies Spleen qi. *Wu Wei Zi* (Fructus Schisandrae Chinensis) stabilizes and binds the Lung to prevent further loss of qi through coughing. *E Jiao* (Colla Corii Asini) tonifies the blood and stops bleeding. Lastly, *Gan Cao* (Radix et Rhizoma Glycyrrhizae) harmonizes the formula.

VETERINARY MODIFICATIONS

- With more sputum and blood, add *Ting Li Zi* (Semen Descurainiae seu Lepidii), *Da Zao* (Fructus Jujubae), *Zhu Ru* (Caulis Bambusae in Taenia) and *Di Huang* (Radix Rehmanniae).
- For chronic non-productive cough, add *Mai Dong* (Radix Ophiopogonis) and *Zhi Shi* (Fructus Aurantii Immaturus).
- For cough and dyspnea caused by qi deficiency, increase the dosage of *Ren Shen* (Radix et Rhizoma Ginseng) and add *Chen Pi* (Pericarpium Citri Reticulatae) and *Ku Xing Ren* (Semen Armeniacae Amarum).
- With hemoptysis due to lung abscess, add *San Huang Xie Xin Tang* (Three-Yellow Decoction to Sedate the Epigastrium).

***Zi Wan Tang* (Aster Decoction)**

Diagnosis	Clinical Signs	Treatment	Herbs
Chronic cough caused by Lung heat and yin deficiency	• Cough and dyspnea with profuse phlegm and sputum and fever: Lung heat • Chest tightness and discomfort with abscess and blood in the sputum: Lung heat consuming yin and body fluids	• Clears heat and dissolves phlegm • Relieves cough • Protects the Lung	• *Zhi Mu* (Rhizoma Anemarrhenae) clears heat while preserving yin and body fluids. • *Zi Wan* (Radix et Rhizoma Asteris) regulates Lung qi and relieves cough. • *Zhe Bei Mu* (Bulbus Fritillariae Thunbergii) and *Jie Geng* (Radix Platycodonis) dissolve phlegm, relieve cough, and drain pus. • *Ren Shen* (Radix et Rhizoma Ginseng) tonifies Lung qi and *Fu Ling* (Poria) tonifies Spleen qi. • *Wu Wei Zi* (Fructus Schisandrae Chinensis) stabilizes and binds the Lung. • *E Jiao* (Colla Corii Asini) tonifies the blood and stops bleeding. • *Gan Cao* (Radix et Rhizoma Glycyrrhizae) harmonizes all of the herbs.

Zǐ Wǎn Tāng (Aster Decoction)

- If the heat and toxins are severe, and for animals who are unresponsive to antimicrobial drugs or have a stubborn infection, consider adding one or more of the following: *Feng Wei Cao* (Herba Pteris), *Zi Hua Di Ding* (Herba Violae), *Hu Yao Huang* (Herba Leucas Mollissimae), *Da Ding Huang* (Caulis Euonymi), *Jin Yin Hua* (Flos Lonicerae Japonicae), *Pu Gong Ying* (Herba Taraxaci), *Qing Dai* (Indigo Naturalis), *Shi Gao* (Gypsum Fibrosum) and *Huang Bo* (Cortex Phellodendri Chinensis).

SUGGESTED ACUPUNCTURE TREATMENT

1. Points: *Chize* (LU 5), *Fuliu* (KI 7), *Lieque* (LU 7), *Fenglong* (ST 40), *Feishu* (BL 13), *Pishu* (BL 20), *Taiyuan* (LU 9), *Yixi* (BL 45), and *Xuehai* (SP 10).
2. Technique: sedation and tonification.

Sedate *Chize* (LU 5) and *Fuliu* (KI 7) to clear heat in order to regulate body fluids. Sedate *Lieque* (LU 7) to regulate Lung qi and *Fenglong* (ST 40) to dissolves phlegm. Tonify *Feishu* (BL 13), *Pishu* (BL 20), and *Taiyuan* (LU 9) to strengthen Lung and Spleen qi. Tonify *Yixi* (BL 45) and *Xuehai* (SP 10) to nourish the blood.

AUTHORS' COMMENTS

Zi Wan Tang can be used to treat chronic respiratory diseases of dogs and cats. It is used most frequently in animals with lung cancer, emphysema, and in animals undergoing treatment for systemic fungal infection (blastomycosis, histoplasmosis and coccidioidomycosis). This formula can be used to treat chronic cough in cats and dogs recovering from heartworm disease with pulmonary parenchymal disease and pulmonary eosinophilic granulomatosis. Long-term respiratory disease causes significant qi and yin deficiencies, and the chronic use of medications (for months) further damages qi, yin and body fluids. This formula is appropriate for dogs and cats with chronic pulmonary diseases characterized by lethargy, exercise intolerance, hemoptysis, dry hacking or productive cough, chest pain, fever, dyspnea, and lung abscess or masses. *Zi Wan Tang* can be combined with *Ren Shen Xie Fei Tang* (Ginseng Decoction to Sedate the Lung); this combination tonifies qi, yin and body fluids and is more effective in clearing heat and infection than either formula alone. In young, debilitated and geriatric animals, it can also be combined with *Xie Bai San* (Drain the White Powder) to further clear Lung heat and control cough and dyspnea.

Jié Gěng Tāng (Platycodon Decoction)
桔梗湯
桔梗汤

Pinyin Name: *Jie Geng Tang*
Literal Name: Platycodon Decoction
Alternate Names: *Chieh Keng Tang*, Platycodon Combination
Original Source: *Shang Han Lun* (Discussion of Cold-Induced Disorders) by Zhang Zhong-Jing in the Eastern Han Dynasty

COMPOSITION

Jie Geng (Radix Platycodonis)	3g
Gan Cao (Radix et Rhizoma Glycyrrhizae)	6g

Jié Gĕng Tāng (Platycodon Decoction)

DOSAGE / PREPARATION / ADMINISTRATION

The source text states to cook the herbs in 3 cups of water until the liquid is reduced to 1 cup. Strain and take the decoction while warm.

CHINESE THERAPEUTIC ACTIONS

1. Eliminates phlegm and pus
2. Clears deficiency fire and toxins

CLINICAL MANIFESTATIONS

Phlegm stagnation: coughing, swelling and pain of the throat, and thick, sticky sputum with mucus and blood. Animals may also experience congestion in the chest, a dry mouth without thirst, and thick, sticky sputum with a foul odor.

VETERINARY CLINICAL APPLICATIONS

Pulmonary gangrene, pulmonary abscess, bronchitis and laryngeal lymphosarcoma in cats.

EXPLANATION

Jie Geng Tang (Platycodon Decoction) treats phlegm stagnation in the chest with deficiency fire rising. When phlegm stagnation is complicated by fire that dries body fluids, the sputum becomes thick and sticky. In addition, if deficiency fire dries the fluids and damages the internal organs, there may be blood and mucus in the sputum. As deficiency fire travels upward, it may cause cough and sore throat with swelling and pain.

Jie Geng Tang is a simple formula with only two ingredients: *Jie Geng* (Radix Platycodonis), a bitter and acrid herb that opens and disperses phlegm stagnation; and *Gan Cao* (Radix et Rhizoma Glycyrrhizae), a sweet and neutral herb that resolves phlegm stagnation. The combination of these two herbs has a synergistic effect to eliminate phlegm stagnation in the chest. Furthermore, *Jie Geng* (Radix Platycodonis) regulates qi and relieves cough, while *Gan Cao* (Radix et Rhizoma Glycyrrhizae) tonifies Lung qi and enhances overall recovery.

VETERINARY MODIFICATIONS

For severe conditions, heat-clearing and toxin-eliminating herbs should be added, since *Jie Geng Tang* simply treats phlegm stagnation.

SUGGESTED ACUPUNCTURE TREATMENT

1. Points: *Tiantu* (CV 22) and *Yuji* (LU 10).
2. Technique: sedation.

Sedate *Tiantu* (CV 22) and *Yuji* (LU 10) to clear Lung heat, dissolve phlegm, and benefit the throat.

AUTHORS' COMMENTS

Jie Geng Tang is typically not used as a sole formula in veterinary medicine. Instead, it is used as an adjunctive formula to improve the efficacy of other formulas to treat phlegm stagnation in the larynx and chest. It can be used to reduce pain and swelling in the treatment of laryngeal lymphosarcoma in cats.

Jie Geng Tang (Platycodon Decoction)

Diagnosis	Clinical Signs	Treatment	Herbs
Phlegm stagnation in the chest with deficiency fire rising	• Chest congestion: phlegm stagnation in the chest • Thick, sticky sputum with blood and mucus: deficiency fire consuming body fluids and damaging the internal organs • Cough and sore throat with swelling and pain: deficiency fire traveling upward	• Eliminates phlegm and pus • Clears deficiency fire and toxins	• *Jie Geng* (Radix Platycodonis) disperses phlegm stagnation and regulates Lung qi circulation. • *Gan Cao* (Radix et Rhizoma Glycyrrhizae) resolves phlegm stagnation and tonifies Lung qi.

Rén Shēn Xiè Fèi Tāng (Ginseng Decoction to Sedate the Lung)

人參瀉肺湯
人参泻肺汤

Pinyin Name: *Ren Shen Xie Fei Tang*
Literal Name: Ginseng Decoction to Sedate the Lung
Alternate Name: Ginseng and Scute Combination
Original Source: *Tai Ping Hui Min He Ji Ju Fang* (Imperial Grace Formulary of the Tai Ping Era) by the Imperial Medical Department in 1078-85

COMPOSITION

Huang Qin (Radix Scutellariae)
Zhi Zi (Fructus Gardeniae)
Bo He (Herba Menthae)
Zhi Qiao (Fructus Citri Aurantii)
Ku Xing Ren (Semen Armeniacae Amarum)
Lian Qiao (Fructus Forsythiae)
Sang Bai Pi (Cortex Mori)
Jie Geng (Radix Platycodonis)
Da Huang (Radix et Rhizoma Rhei)
Ren Shen (Radix et Rhizoma Ginseng)
Gan Cao (Radix et Rhizoma Glycyrrhizae)

DOSAGE / PREPARATION / ADMINISTRATION

The source text states to grind equal amounts of all of the ingredients into a coarse powder. Cook 30g of the powder in 2 cups of water until the liquid is reduced to 1 cup. Take the warm, strained decoction after meals.

CHINESE THERAPEUTIC ACTIONS

1. Clears heat and sedates the Lung
2. Eliminates phlegm and regulates qi

CLINICAL MANIFESTATIONS

Lung heat with phlegm accumulation: wheezing, dyspnea, cough with profuse sputum, constipation, a red tongue, and a rapid, slippery pulse.

VETERINARY CLINICAL APPLICATIONS

Upper respiratory tract infection, bronchitis, pneumonia, bronchial asthma, and pulmonary abscess.

EXPLANATION

Ren Shen Xie Fei Tang (Ginseng Decoction to Sedate the Lung) treats Lung heat accompanied by phlegm accumulation and qi flow obstruction. The presence of phlegm is evident in the yellow sputum discharge. Heat and phlegm create discomfort and distention in the chest; they also obstruct the normal qi flow, causing wheezing, dyspnea, and cough.

In this formula, *Huang Qin* (Radix Scutellariae), *Zhi Zi* (Fructus Gardeniae), and *Bo He* (Herba Menthae) clear heat in the Lung and address the excess condition. *Zhi Qiao* (Fructus Aurantii) regulates qi, while *Ku Xing Ren* (Semen Armeniacae Amarum) guides Lung qi downward. Together, these two herbs restore the normal flow of Lung qi to relieve wheezing, dyspnea, and cough. *Lian Qiao* (Fructus Forsythiae), *Sang Bai Pi* (Cortex Mori), and *Jie Geng* (Radix Platycodonis) clear heat and phlegm to dispel sputum and relieve congestion and fullness. *Da Huang* (Radix et Rhizoma Rhei) purges downward and enables the elimination of heat via defecation. *Ren Shen* (Radix et Rhizoma Ginseng) strengthens the Lung and Spleen and prevents the bitter and cold herbs in the formula from damaging these two organs. Lastly, *Gan Cao* (Radix et Rhizoma Glycyrrhizae) reduces inflammation in the Lung and harmonizes the herbs within the formula.

Rén Shēn Xiè Fèi Tāng (Ginseng Decoction to Sedate the Lung)

***Ren Shen Xie Fei Tang* (Ginseng Decoction to Sedate the Lung)**

Diagnosis	Clinical Signs	Treatment	Herbs
Lung heat with phlegm accumulation	• Wheezing, dyspnea and cough with a feeling of discomfort and distention in the chest: heat and phlegm affecting Lung qi circulation • Yellow sputum: heat and phlegm condition	• Clears heat and sedates the Lung • Eliminates phlegm and regulates qi	• *Huang Qin* (Radix Scutellariae), *Zhi Zi* (Fructus Gardeniae), and *Bo He* (Herba Menthae) clear heat in the Lung and address the excess condition. • *Zhi Qiao* (Fructus Aurantii) regulates qi, while *Ku Xing Ren* (Semen Armeniacae Amarum) causes Lung qi to descend. • *Lian Qiao* (Fructus Forsythiae), *Sang Bai Pi* (Cortex Mori), and *Jie Geng* (Radix Platycodonis) clear heat and phlegm to dispel sputum and relieve congestion and fullness. • *Da Huang* (Radix et Rhizoma Rhei) purges heat downward. • *Ren Shen* (Radix et Rhizoma Ginseng) strengthens the Lung and Spleen and prevents the bitter and cold herbs from damaging these two organs. • *Gan Cao* (Radix et Rhizoma Glycyrrhizae) harmonizes the herbs.

VETERINARY MODIFICATIONS

- For cough with profuse sputum, add *Fu Ling* (Poria) and *Chen Pi* (Pericarpium Citri Reticulatae).
- With bloating in the chest and epigastrium, add *Huang Lian* (Rhizoma Coptidis) and *Hou Po* (Cortex Magnoliae Officinalis).
- For acute recurrent bronchitis and heat, add *Shi Gao* (Gypsum Fibrosum) and *Zhi Mu* (Rhizoma Anemarrhenae).

SUGGESTED ACUPUNCTURE TREATMENT

1. Points: *Fengmen* (BL 12), *Quchi* (LI 11), *Tiantu* (CV 22), *Lieque* (LU 7), *Fenglong* (ST 40), *Housanli* (ST 36), and *Feishu* (BL 13).
2. Technique: sedation and tonification.

Sedate *Fengmen* (BL 12) and *Quchi* (LI 11) to clear Lung heat. Sedate *Tiantu* (CV 22) to guide Lung qi downward, and *Lieque* (LU 7) and *Fenglong* (ST 40) to clear damp-heat from the Lung. Tonify *Housanli* (ST 36) and *Feishu* (BL 13) to regulate qi circulation.

AUTHORS' COMMENTS

Ren Shen Xie Fei Tang is used in cases in which there is cough with more heat than phlegm and qi deficiency. For cough with more copious phlegm, it can be combined with *Er Chen Tang* (Two-Cured Decoction). For animals with chronic cough and respiratory disease, it can be combined with *Zi Wan Tang* (Aster Decoction) or *Qing Fei Tang* (Clear the Lung Decoction) to treat qi, yin and body fluid deficiencies, clear heat, and resolve phlegm.

Section 3

润燥化痰剂
— Dryness-Moistening and Phlegm-Dissolving Formula

Bèi Mǔ Guā Lóu Sǎn (Fritillaria and Trichosanthes Fruit Powder)

貝母瓜蔞散
贝母瓜蒌散

Pinyin Name: *Bei Mu Gua Lou San*
Literal Name: Fritillaria and Trichosanthes Fruit Powder
Alternate Name: Fritillaria and Trichosanthes Fruit Formula
Original Source: *Yi Xue Xin Wu* (Medical Revelations) by Cheng Guo-Peng in 1732

COMPOSITION

Zhe Bei Mu (Bulbus Fritillariae Thunbergii)	4.5g
Gua Lou (Fructus Trichosanthis)	3g
Tian Hua Fen (Radix Trichosanthis)	2.4g
Fu Ling (Poria)	2.4g
Ju Hong (Exocarpium Citri Rubrum)	2.4g
Jie Geng (Radix Platycodonis)	2.4g

DOSAGE / PREPARATION / ADMINISTRATION

The source text states to prepare the ingredients as a decoction.

CHINESE THERAPEUTIC ACTIONS

1. Moistens the Lung and clears heat
2. Regulates qi and dissolves phlegm

CLINICAL MANIFESTATIONS

Lung dryness with phlegm accumulation: coughing, dry throat, and thick, sticky sputum.

VETERINARY CLINICAL APPLICATIONS

Bronchitis, sore throat, and dry cough.

EXPLANATION

Bei Mu Gua Lou San (Fritillaria and Trichosanthes Fruit Powder) treats Lung dryness with phlegm accumulation. Lung dryness may consume fluids and create phlegm. Because the pathogenic factor in this syndrome is dryness, the phlegm is thick and sticky. Dryness of the throat is due to injury of the body fluids.

This formula uses *Zhe Bei Mu* (Bulbus Fritillariae Thunbergii) to clear heat, moisten the Lung, dispel phlegm, and stop coughing. *Gua Lou* (Fructus Trichosanthis) clears heat, moistens dryness, regulates qi, and breaks up phlegm stagnation. *Tian Hua Fen* (Radix Trichosanthis) clears heat, dissolves phlegm, promotes the generation of body fluids, and moistens dryness. *Fu Ling* (Poria) strengthens the Spleen and removes dampness. *Ju Hong* (Exocarpium Citri Rubrum) activates qi circulation and dissolves phlegm. *Jie Geng* (Radix Platycodonis) ventilates the Lung to stop cough and eliminate phlegm.

Bèi Mŭ Guā Lóu Săn (Fritillaria and Trichosanthes Fruit Powder)

***Bei Mu Gua Lou San* (Fritillaria and Trichosanthes Fruit Powder)**

Diagnosis	Clinical Signs	Treatment	Herbs
Lung dryness with phlegm accumulation	• Coughing with thick, sticky sputum: dryness consuming and turning fluids into phlegm • Dry throat: dryness injuring body fluids	• Moistens the Lung and clears heat • Regulates qi and dissolves phlegm	• *Zhe Bei Mu* (Bulbus Fritillariae Thunbergii) clears heat, moistens the Lung, dispels phlegm, and stops coughing. • *Gua Lou* (Fructus Trichosanthis) clears heat, moistens dryness, regulates qi, and breaks up phlegm stagnation. • *Tian Hua Fen* (Radix Trichosanthis) clears heat, dissolves phlegm, promotes the generation of body fluids, and moistens dryness. • *Fu Ling* (Poria) strengthens the Spleen and removes dampness. • *Ju Hong* (Exocarpium Citri Rubrum) activates qi to dissolve phlegm. • *Jie Geng* (Radix Platycodonis) ventilates the Lung to stop cough and eliminate phlegm.

VETERINARY MODIFICATIONS

- With exterior wind invasion, add *Sang Ye* (Folium Mori), *Ku Xing Ren* (Semen Armeniacae Amarum), *Qian Hu* (Radix Peucedani), and *Niu Bang Zi* (Fructus Arctii).
- With blood-streaked sputum due to yin deficiency, add *Sha Shen* (Radix Glehniae seu Adenophorae), *Mai Dong* (Radix Ophiopogonis), *Lu Gen* (Rhizoma Phragmitis), *Xian He Cao* (Herba Agrimoniae), *Mu Hu Die* (Semen Oroxyli), and *Qian Cao* (Radix et Rhizoma Rubiae); and remove *Ju Hong* (Exocarpium Citri Rubrum).
- For cough with thick, yellow sputum, add *Huang Lian* (Rhizoma Coptidis), *Zhi Zi* (Fructus Gardeniae), *Dan Nan Xing* (Arisaema cum Bile), and *Gan Cao* (Radix et Rhizoma Glycyrrhizae); and remove *Tian Hua Fen* (Radix Trichosanthis), *Fu Ling* (Poria), and *Jie Geng* (Radix Platycodonis).
- With dry mouth, add *Xuan Shen* (Radix Scrophulariae), *Di Huang* (Radix Rehmanniae), *Mai Dong* (Radix Ophiopogonis), and *Lu Gen* (Rhizoma Phragmitis).

CAUTIONS / CONTRAINDICATIONS

Bei Mu Gua Lou San is contraindicated for cough due to Kidney yin deficiency or due to deficiency heat rising, unless properly modified.

SUGGESTED ACUPUNCTURE TREATMENT

1. Points: *Yuji* (LU 10), *Feishu* (BL 13), *Taixi* (KI 3), *Zhaohai* (KI 6), *Yinlingquan* (SP 9), *Pishu* (BL 20), *Lieque* (LU 7), and *Neiguan* (PC 6).
2. Technique: sedation.

The treatment objectives are to moisten the Lung, clear heat, regulate qi, and dissolve phlegm. *Yuji* (LU 10) and *Feishu* (BL 13) clear heat and moisten dryness. *Taixi* (KI 3) and *Zhaohai* (KI 6) tonify Kidney yin. *Yinlingquan* (SP 9) and *Pishu* (BL 20) strengthen the Spleen to dispel dampness and eliminate phlegm. Lastly, *Lieque* (LU 7) and *Neiguan* (PC 6) regulate Lung qi and eliminate phlegm.

AUTHORS' COMMENTS

A common use for this formula in veterinary medicine is in geriatric animals with yin deficiency accompanied by a gagging, choking cough that produces a small amount of thick, viscous phlegm. For this use, it must be combined with *Mai Men Dong Tang* (Ophiopogonis Decoction) or *Bai He Gu Jin Tang* (Lily Bulb Decoction to Preserve the Metal). The combination of each in a 1:1 ratio is recommended to begin treatment and should be adjusted over time. Care should be taken in animals with Spleen deficiency, and herbs or formulas that strengthen Spleen functions are recommended as needed.

Section 4

温化寒痰剂
— Warm Formulas that Dissolve Cold-Phlegm

Líng Gān Wǔ Wèi Jiāng Xīn Tāng
(Poria, Licorice, Schisandra, Ginger, and Asarum Decoction)

苓甘五味姜辛湯
苓甘五味姜辛汤

Pinyin Name: *Ling Gan Wu Wei Jiang Xin Tang*
Literal Name: Poria, Licorice, Schisandra, Ginger, and Asarum Decoction
Original Source: *Jin Gui Yao Lue* (Essentials from the Golden Cabinet) by Zhang Zhong-Jing in the Eastern Han Dynasty

COMPOSITION

Gan Jiang (Rhizoma Zingiberis)	9g
Xi Xin (Radix et Rhizoma Asari)	9g [3g]
Fu Ling (Poria)	12g
Wu Wei Zi (Fructus Schisandrae Chinensis)	0.5 cup [3-6g]
Gan Cao (Radix et Rhizoma Glycyrrhizae)	9g

DOSAGE / PREPARATION / ADMINISTRATION

The source text states to cook the ingredients with 8 cups [1,600 mL] of water until the liquid is reduced to 3 cups [600 mL]. Take 0.5 cup [100 mL] of the warm, strained decoction three times daily. Today, this formula may be prepared as a decoction with the doses suggested in brackets.

CHINESE THERAPEUTIC ACTIONS

Warms the Lung and resolves *yin* (invisible phlegm)

CLINICAL MANIFESTATIONS

Retention of cold-type *yin* (invisible phlegm): coughing with profuse, white, watery sputum, discomfort in the chest and diaphragm regions, a greasy tongue and a wiry, slippery pulse.

VETERINARY CLINICAL APPLICATIONS

Bronchitis and cough

EXPLANATION

Ling Gan Wu Wei Jiang Xin Tang (Poria, Licorice, Schisandra, Ginger, and Asarum Decoction) treats retention of cold-type *yin* (invisible phlegm) due to yang deficiency and yin excess, with accumulation of water and dampness. Spleen yang deficiency compromises the Spleen's normal functioning and may lead to interior cold formation and damp accumulation, which precipitate retention of cold-type *yin* (invisible phlegm). This phlegm may be stored in the Lung and affect the Lung's qi flow. Consequently, coughing with profuse, white, watery sputum occurs. A greasy tongue and a wiry, slippery pulse are signs of interior cold and phlegm.

Gan Jiang (Rhizoma Zingiberis), the chief herb in this formula, warms the Lung, dispels cold, dissolves dampness, and resolves *yin* (invisible phlegm). *Xi Xin* (Radix et Rhizoma Asari), an acrid and warm herb, warms the Lung, disperses cold, and assists *Gan Jiang* (Rhizoma Zingiberis) in resolving *yin* (invisible phlegm). *Fu Ling* (Poria) strengthens the Spleen and resolves dampness. *Wu Wei Zi* (Fructus Schisandrae Chinensis) astringes Lung qi to stop coughing. Moreover, the astringent effect of *Wu Wei Zi* (Fructus Schisandrae Chinensis) moderates the dispersing function of *Xi Xin* (Radix et Rhizoma Asari) to effectively relieve cough. *Gan Cao* (Radix et Rhizoma Glycyrrhizae) harmonizes all of the herbs in the formula.

Líng Gān Wǔ Wèi Jiāng Xīn Tāng

(Poria, Licorice, Schisandra, Ginger, and Asarum Decoction)

Ling Gan Wu Wei Jiang Xin Tang **(Poria, Licorice, Schisandra, Ginger, and Asarum Decoction)**

Diagnosis	Clinical Signs	Treatment	Herbs
Retention of cold-type *yin* (invisible phlegm)	• Coughing with profuse, white, watery sputum: accumulation of phlegm obstructing Lung qi circulation • Greasy tongue and a wiry, slippery pulse: interior cold and phlegm	Warms the Lung and resolves *yin* (invisible phlegm)	• *Gan Jiang* (Rhizoma Zingiberis) warms the Lung, dispels cold, dissolves dampness, and resolves *yin* (invisible phlegm). • *Xi Xin* (Radix et Rhizoma Asari) warms the Lung and disperses cold. • *Fu Ling* (Poria) strengthens the Spleen and resolves dampness. • *Wu Wei Zi* (Fructus Schisandrae Chinensis) astringes Lung qi to stop coughing. • *Gan Cao* (Radix et Rhizoma Glycyrrhizae) harmonizes all of the herbs.

VETERINARY MODIFICATIONS

- With profuse phlegm and nausea or vomiting, add *Ban Xia* (Rhizoma Pinelliae).
- With severe coughing, add *Ku Xing Ren* (Semen Armeniacae Amarum).
- If there are signs of exterior wind condition, add *Zi Su Ye* (Folium Perillae), and replace *Gan Jiang* (Rhizoma Zingiberis) with *Sheng Jiang* (Rhizoma Zingiberis Recens).
- With Spleen deficiency and decreased food intake, add *Dang Shen* (Radix Codonopsis), *Bai Zhu* (Rhizoma Atractylodis Macrocephalae), and *Chen Pi* (Pericarpium Citri Reticulatae).
- With epigastric bloating, add *Chen Pi* (Pericarpium Citri Reticulatae) and *Zhi Qiao* (Fructus Aurantii).

CAUTIONS / CONTRAINDICATIONS

Ling Gan Wu Wei Jiang Xin Tang contains many warm and drying herbs, and is contraindicated in cases of cough or dyspnea caused by Lung heat, dryness, yin deficiency, or phlegm-fire accumulation.

SUGGESTED ACUPUNCTURE TREATMENT

1. Points: *Feishu* (BL 13), *Pishu* (BL 20), *Yinlingquan* (SP 9), *Taiyuan* (LU 9), and *Fenglong* (ST 40).
2. Techniques: tonification and moxibustion.

Because retention of cold and phlegm is at the center of this syndrome, the treatment strategy focuses on warming the Lung to resolve phlegm. *Feishu* (BL 13), the *shu* (transport) point of the Lung, and *Pishu* (BL 20), the *shu* (transport) point of the Spleen, are selected because the Spleen produces phlegm and the Lung stores phlegm. *Yinlingquan* (SP 9) strengthens the Spleen and dispels dampness, while *Taiyuan* (LU 9) tonifies the Lung. *Fenglong* (ST 40) harmonizes the Stomach and eliminates phlegm. Finally, moxibustion can be used to warm yang and dispel cold.

Sān Zǐ Yǎng Qīn Tāng

(Three-Seed Decoction to Nourish One's Parents)

三子養親湯
三子养亲汤

Pinyin Name: *San Zi Yang Qin Tang*
Literal Name: Three-Seed Decoction to Nourish One's Parents
Alternate Name: Three-Seed Combination
Original Source: *Han Shi Yi Tong* (Comprehensive Medicine According to Master Han) by Han Mao in 1522

COMPOSITION

Bai Jie Zi (Semen Sinapis)	[6g]
Zi Su Zi (Fructus Perillae)	[9g]
Lai Fu Zi (Semen Raphani)	[9g]

DOSAGE / PREPARATION / ADMINISTRATION

The source text states to dry-fry the ingredients and crush open the seeds. Place a maximum of 9g of the herbs in a silk sack and cook it with a large amount of water. Do not overcook.* Take the decoction in small sips frequently throughout the day. The source text recommends adding honey for patients with constipation, and to include 3 slices of *Sheng Jiang* (Rhizoma Zingiberis Recens) in the winter. Today, this formula is prepared by crushing the seeds (using the suggested doses in brackets), placing them all in a cheesecloth bag, and cooking them in water. Take the decoction frequently in small amounts throughout the day. [*Please see Authors' Comments for explanation.]

CHINESE THERAPEUTIC ACTIONS

1. Redirects Lung qi and soothes the diaphragm
2. Dissolves phlegm and promotes food digestion

CLINICAL MANIFESTATIONS

Phlegm retention with qi stagnation: coughing with profuse sputum, wheezing, dyspnea, indigestion even with decreased intake of food, a white, greasy tongue coating, and a slippery pulse.

VETERINARY CLINICAL APPLICATIONS

Chronic bronchitis, pulmonary emphysema, asthma, bronchial asthma, cardiopulmonary disease, and cough.

EXPLANATION

San Zi Yang Qin Tang (Three-Seed Decoction to Nourish One's Parents) was originally designed to treat geriatric patients with phlegm retention and qi stagnation. Because geriatric patients often have qi deficiency, overeating or consumption of cold or raw food easily leads to stagnation of food and qi. If the qi becomes stagnated, the fluids will not be distributed properly, and dampness and phlegm may accumulate as a result. Phlegm retention may cause reversed flow of Lung qi, resulting in coughing, dyspnea, and chest oppression. Stagnation of food and Stomach qi may lead to lack of appetite and indigestion. The white, greasy tongue coating and the slippery pulse suggest qi deficiency and phlegm retention.

This formula uses *Bai Jie Zi* (Semen Sinapis) to warm the Lung, dissolve phlegm, and soothe the diaphragm. *Zi Su Zi* (Fructus Perillae) disperses phlegm and guides the reversed flow of Lung qi downward to relieve coughing and wheezing. *Lai Fu Zi* (Semen Raphani) activates Stomach qi, resolves food stagnation, and eliminates phlegm.

PHARMACOLOGICAL EFFECTS

1. **Antiasthmatic**: *San Zi Yang Qin Tang* has been shown in many studies to effectively reverse airway obstruction. The mechanism of this action is attributed to its ability to relax the smooth muscles and reverse bronchial constriction.[1]
2. **Antitussive**: According to one study, administration of *San Zi Yang Qin Tang* was associated with a marked antitussive effect in mice with artificially-induced cough. The antitussive effect began approximately 1 hour after oral ingestion.[2]
3. **Expectorant**: One study reported marked expectorant and antitussive effects using *San Zi Yang Qin Tang* at 20 g/kg given in decoction via oral ingestion.[3]

HUMAN CLINICAL STUDIES AND RESEARCH

1. **Cough**: One study used *San Zi Yang Qin Tang* to treat 40 patients with chronic and stubborn cough. Out of 40 patients, 14 had cough for more than 10 years, and 15 were geriatric persons 60 years of age and older. The study reported successful treatment of cough in 25 cases within 3-5 days, and 15 cases within 14 days.[4]

Sān Zǐ Yǎng Qīn Tāng
(Three-Seed Decoction to Nourish One's Parents)

San Zi Yang Qin Tang (Three-Seed Decoction to Nourish One's Parents)

Diagnosis	Clinical Signs	Treatment	Herbs
Phlegm retention with qi stagnation	• Coughing, dyspnea and chest oppression: phlegm retention in the Lung causing reversed qi flow and qi stagnation • Lack of appetite and indigestion: phlegm retention in the Stomach affecting digestive functions • White, greasy tongue coating and slippery pulse: qi deficiency and phlegm retention	• Descends Lung qi and soothes the diaphragm • Dissolves phlegm and promotes digestion of food	• *Bai Jie Zi* (Semen Sinapis) dissolves phlegm. • *Zi Su Zi* (Fructus Perillae) redirects qi to relieve coughing and wheezing. • *Lai Fu Zi* (Semen Raphani) resolves food stagnation and eliminates phlegm.

2. **Pediatric cough**: Daily usage of modified *San Zi Yang Qin Tang* successfully treated 25 children with chronic cough. The herbal treatment included *Lai Fu Zi* (Semen Raphani), *Zi Su Zi* (Fructus Perillae), *Ting Li Zi* (Semen Descurainiae seu Lepidii), *Zi Wan* (Radix et Rhizoma Asteris), *Jing Jie* (Herba Schizonepetae), *Qian Hu* (Radix Peucedani), *Ku Xing Ren* (Semen Armeniacae Amarum), *Wu Wei Zi* (Fructus Schisandrae Chinensis), and *Gan Cao* (Radix et Rhizoma Glycyrrhizae) as the base formula. Modifications were made by adding *Dang Shen* (Radix Codonopsis), *Fu Ling* (Poria), and *Bai Zhu* (Rhizoma Atractylodis Macrocephalae) for Spleen and Lung qi deficiencies; *Sha Shen* (Radix Glehniae seu Adenophorae), *Mai Dong* (Radix Ophiopogonis), and *Chuan Bei Mu* (Bulbus Fritillariae Cirrhosae) for qi and yin deficiencies; *Mao Dong Qing* (Radix Ilicis Pubescentis), *Dan Shen* (Radix et Rhizoma Salviae Miltiorrhizae), *Chi Shao* (Radix Paeoniae Rubra), and *Jiang Can* (Bombyx Batryticatus) for phlegm and blood stagnation. The herbs were given in decoction daily. The study reported successful treatment in all 25 patients.[5]
3. **Bronchial asthma**: Administration of modified *San Zi Yang Qin Tang* via oral inhalation was successful in treating 53 patients with bronchial asthma. Improvements included relief of wheezing, dyspnea, lowered heartbeat, and resolution of 3 concave signs. Out of 53 patients, 39 had complete recovery within 1-2 days and 14 within 3-4 days. The average time required to achieve complete recovery was 2.08 days.[6]
4. **Bronchitis**: Eighty-eight children with acute bronchitis were treated successfully using *San Zi Yang Qin Tang* plus *San Ao Tang* (Three-Unbinding Decoction). Improvement was noted in most cases within 3 packs of herbs. The study reported a 65.9% rate of recovery, 86.4% rate of significant improvement, and 96.6% effectiveness. Those who did not respond to the treatment also had Spleen and Lung qi deficiencies with a suppressed immune system.[7]
5. ***Mei he qi* (plum-pit *qi*)**: Modified *San Zi Yang Qin Tang* was used to treat 32 patients with plum-pit *qi* with complete recovery in 15 cases, marked improvement in 13 cases, and no effect in 4 cases. The overall effectiveness was 87.5%.[8,9]

TOXICOLOGY

San Zi Yang Qin Tang has very little toxicity. According to one study, the LD_{50} for oral administration of this formula in mice cannot be measured. Oral administration of up to 120 g/kg (maximum capacity of the stomach) of this formula did not cause any fatality.[10]

SUGGESTED ACUPUNCTURE TREATMENT

1. Points: *Zhongfu* (LU 1), *Kongzui* (LU 6), *Fenglong* (ST 40), *Shanzhong* (CV 17), *Housanli* (ST 36), and *Gongsun* (SP 4).
2. Technique: sedation.

The selection of acupuncture points focuses on redirecting Lung qi downward, eliminating phlegm, activating Stomach qi, and removing food stagnation. *Zhongfu* (LU 1) and *Kongzui* (LU 6) regulate Lung qi to dissolve phlegm. *Shanzhong* (CV 17) descends Lung qi to relieve coughing and wheezing. The combination of *Zhongfu* (LU 1), *Kongzui* (LU 6), and *Shanzhong* (CV 17) effectively corrects the qi flow of the Lung. *Fenglong* (ST 40) eliminates phlegm, while *Housanli* (ST 36) and *Gongsun* (SP 4) tonify and regulate the Spleen and Stomach to promote digestion and remove phlegm.

AUTHORS' COMMENTS

San Zi Yang Qin Tang treats the symptoms (phlegm retention with qi stagnation), not the cause (qi deficiency) of the illness. Thus, once the acute clinical manifestations are relieved, some qi-tonic herbs should be added to strengthen the qi. Moreover, the doses of the three herbs in the formula are frequently adjusted, depending on the

Sān Zǐ Yǎng Qīn Tāng

(Three-Seed Decoction to Nourish One's Parents)

symptoms presented by the patient. Because this formula is relatively strong and is aimed at treating the symptoms, it is cooked with a large amount of water for only a short period of time to ensure that the potency of the decoction is not too strong. Furthermore, the decoction is not to be taken all at once, but in small amounts throughout the day for sustained symptomatic relief.

References

1. *Zhong Yao Yao Li Yu Lin Chuang* (Pharmacology and Clinical Applications of Chinese Herbs), 1992, 8(3):15.
2. *Zhong Yao Yao Li Yu Lin Chuang* (Pharmacology and Clinical Applications of Chinese Herbs), 1992, 8(3):15.
3. *Si Chuan Zhong Yi* (Sichuan Chinese Medicine), 1989, 7(11):10.
4. *Zhong Yao Tong Bao* (Journal of Chinese Herbology), 1986, 8:56.
5. *Xin Zhong Yi* (New Chinese Medicine), 1995, 9:50.
6. *Shan Xi Zhong Yi* (Shanxi Chinese Medicine), 1995, 4:148.
7. *Shang Hai Yi Yao Za Zhi* (Shanghai Journal of Medicine and Herbology), 1991, 10:22.
8. *Hei Long Jiang Zhong Yi Yao* (Heilongjiang Chinese Medicine and Herbology), 1992, 6:31.
9. *Guang Xi Zhong Yi Yao* (Guangxi Chinese Medicine and Herbology), 1988, 11(3):43.
10. *Zhong Yao Yao Li Yu Lin Chuang* (Pharmacology and Clinical Applications of Chinese Herbs), 1992, 8(3):15.

Section 5

治风化痰剂
— Wind-Expelling and Phlegm-Dissolving Formulas

Bàn Xià Bái Zhú Tiān Má Tāng

(Pinellia, Atractylodes Macrocephala, and Gastrodia Decoction)

半夏白朮天麻湯
半夏白术天麻汤

Pinyin Name: *Ban Xia Bai Zhu Tian Ma Tang*

Literal Name: Pinellia, Atractylodes Macrocephala, and Gastrodia Decoction

Alternate Names: *Pan Hsia Tien Ma Pai Shu Tang, Ban Xia Tian Ma Bai Shu Tang*, Pinellia, Gastrodia, and Atractylodes Decoction; Pinellia, Gastrodia and Bighead Atractylodes Decoction; Pinellia and Gastrodia Combination

Original Source: *Yi Xue Xin Wu* (Medical Revelations) by Cheng Guo-Peng in 1732

COMPOSITION

Ban Xia (Rhizoma Pinelliae)	4.5g [9g]
Tian Ma (Rhizoma Gastrodiae)	3g [6g]
Bai Zhu (Rhizoma Atractylodis Macrocephalae)	9g [15g]
Fu Ling (Poria)	3g [6g]
Ju Hong (Exocarpium Citri Rubrum)	3g [6g]
Gan Cao (Radix et Rhizoma Glycyrrhizae)	1.5g [3g]

DOSAGE / PREPARATION / ADMINISTRATION

The source text states to prepare the ingredients as a decoction with 1 slice of *Sheng Jiang* (Rhizoma Zingiberis Recens) and 2 pieces of *Da Zao* (Fructus Jujubae). Today, this formula may be prepared as a decoction with the doses suggested in brackets.

CHINESE THERAPEUTIC ACTIONS

1. Dries dampness and dissolves phlegm
2. Soothes the Liver and subdues Liver wind

CLINICAL MANIFESTATIONS

Wind and phlegm rising upward: ataxia, nausea, vomiting, copious sputum, a pale pink tongue, and a wiry, slippery pulse.

VETERINARY CLINICAL APPLICATIONS

Seizures, epilepsy, dizziness, ataxia, circling, chronic vomiting, facial paralysis, and nasosinusitis.

EXPLANATION

Ban Xia Bai Zhu Tian Ma Tang (Pinellia, Atractylodes Macrocephala, and Gastrodia Decoction) treats rising of wind and phlegm with key symptoms such as cough, nausea and vomiting, and a sticky tongue coating in severe cases. Wind and phlegm syndrome occurs as a result of a combination of Spleen and Liver disorders. Spleen deficiency results in the formation of dampness and phlegm. The phlegm can be accompanied by Liver wind rising. Together, these factors rise and disturb many parts of the upper body. In severe cases, seizures can develop due to the combination of turbid dampness, phlegm, and Liver wind traveling to the head. The biomedical disease of epilepsy corresponds to this pathomechanism. Nausea and vomiting are caused by damp-phlegm obstruction in the middle *jiao*.

The treatment plan is to dissolve phlegm, subdue Liver wind, strengthen the Spleen, and dispel dampness. *Ban Xia* (Rhizoma Pinelliae) dries dampness, dissolves phlegm, and

Bàn Xià Bái Zhú Tiān Má Tāng

(Pinellia, Atractylodes Macrocephala, and Gastrodia Decoction)

***Ban Xia Bai Zhu Tian Ma Tang* (Pinellia, Atractylodes Macrocephala, and Gastrodia Decoction)**

Diagnosis	Clinical Signs	Treatment	Herbs
Wind and phlegm rising	• Dizziness, vertigo and heaviness of the head: phlegm and Liver wind rising to the head • Nausea and vomiting: damp-phlegm obstruction in the middle *jiao* • Pale pink tongue and a wiry, slippery pulse: damp-phlegm in the interior	• Dries dampness and dissolves phlegm • Soothes the Liver and subdues Liver wind	• *Ban Xia* (Rhizoma Pinelliae) dries dampness and dissolves phlegm. • *Tian Ma* (Rhizoma Gastrodiae) subdues Liver wind. • *Bai Zhu* (Rhizoma Atractylodis Macrocephalae) and *Fu Ling* (Poria) strengthen the Spleen and dispel dampness. • *Ju Hong* (Exocarpium Citri Rubrum) regulates qi and dissolves phlegm. • *Sheng Jiang* (Rhizoma Zingiberis Recens) and *Da Zao* (Fructus Jujubae) harmonize the Spleen and Stomach. • *Gan Cao* (Radix et Rhizoma Glycyrrhizae) harmonizes all of the herbs.

redirects the reversed flow of Stomach qi downward to stop nausea and vomiting. *Tian Ma* (Rhizoma Gastrodiae) subdues Liver wind and alleviates dizziness and vertigo. These two chief herbs are essential in treating dizziness, vertigo, headache, and other symptoms caused by wind and phlegm. *Bai Zhu* (Rhizoma Atractylodis Macrocephalae) strengthens the Spleen and dries dampness, while *Fu Ling* (Poria) strengthens the Spleen and dispels dampness. *Ju Hong* (Exocarpium Citri Rubrum) regulates qi and dissolves phlegm. *Sheng Jiang* (Rhizoma Zingiberis Recens) and *Da Zao* (Fructus Jujubae) harmonize the Spleen and Stomach, while *Gan Cao* (Radix et Rhizoma Glycyrrhizae) harmonizes all of the herbs.

VETERINARY MODIFICATIONS

- To improve efficacy of seizure control due to Liver excess, add *Jiang Can* (Bombyx Batryticatus), *Gou Teng* (Ramulus Uncariae cum Uncis), *Dan Nan Xing* (Arisaema cum Bile) and *Quan Xie* (Scorpio).
- With profuse phlegm and damp accumulation, add *Ze Xie* (Rhizoma Alismatis) and *Gui Zhi* (Ramulus Cinnamomi).
- With Liver yang rising, add *Gou Teng* (Ramulus Uncariae cum Uncis) and *Zhe Shi* (Haematitum).
- With qi deficiency, add *Dang Shen* (Radix Codonopsis) and *Huang Qi* (Radix Astragali).
- With sinusitis or rhinitis, add *Xin Yi Hua* (Flos Magnoliae).

CAUTIONS / CONTRAINDICATIONS

Ban Xia Bai Zhu Tian Ma Tang should not be used for dizziness caused by Liver and Kidney yin deficiencies, or dizziness or vertigo caused by Liver yang rising.

HUMAN CLINICAL STUDIES AND RESEARCH

1. **Dizziness and vertigo**: *Ban Xia Bai Zhu Tian Ma Tang* has been shown in many studies to effectively treat dizziness and vertigo due to various causes. According to one study, use of the formula plus *Zi Su Ye* (Folium Perillae) and *Ze Xie* (Rhizoma Alismatis) in decoction daily was very effective in treating acute onset of dizziness and vertigo accompanied by nausea, vomiting, and tinnitus.[1]

   Another study reported 98% effectiveness using modified *Ban Xia Bai Zhu Tian Ma Tang* to treat dizziness and vertigo due to inner ear imbalance. Of 50 patients, 28 had complete recovery (resolution of all symptoms without recurrence within 1 year of follow-ups), significant improvement in 21 cases (resolution of all symptoms with recurrence associated with stress, fatigue, and other causes) and no effect in 1 case.[2]

   Lastly, one study combined *Ban Xia Bai Zhu Tian Ma Tang* and *Wen Dan Tang* (Warm the Gallbladder Decoction) to treat dizziness in 80 patients with complete recovery in 51 cases, improvement in 20 cases, and no effect in 9 cases. The composition of the herbal treatment included these two formulas without *Bai Zhu* (Rhizoma Atractylodis Macrocephalae) and *Gan Cao* (Radix et Rhizoma Glycyrrhizae), and with the addition of *Gou Teng* (Ramulus Uncariae cum Uncis), *Zhu Ru* (Caulis Bambusae in Taenia), *Ci Shi* (Magnetitum), and others as deemed necessary.[3]
2. **Facial paralysis**: According to one study, 17 patients with facial paralysis characterized by deviation of the eyes and mouth were treated with modified *Ban Xia Bai Zhu Tian Ma Tang* with complete recovery in 10 cases, significant results in 4 cases, moderate results in 2 cases, and no effect in 1 case. The overall effectiveness was 94%.

Bàn Xià Bái Zhú Tiān Má Tāng

(Pinellia, Atractylodes Macrocephala, and Gastrodia Decoction)

The herbal treatment contained this formula plus *Qiang Huo* (Rhizoma et Radix Notopterygii), *Bai Jie Zi* (Semen Sinapis), *Hong Hua* (Flos Carthami), *Quan Xie* (Scorpio), and *Wu Gong* (Scolopendra). The treatment protocol was to grind all herbs into a fine powder, and administer with a small amount of warm grain-based alcohol.[4]

3. **Nasosinusitis**: Administration of modified *Ban Xia Bai Zhu Tian Ma Tang* was associated with marked success in treating 50 patients with nasosinusitis. The herbal formula contained *Ban Xia* (Rhizoma Pinelliae) 10g, *Tian Ma* (Rhizoma Gastrodiae) 10g, *Cang Er Zi* (Fructus Xanthii) 10g, *Bai Zhi* (Radix Angelicae Dahuricae) 10g, *Yan Hu Suo* (Rhizoma Corydalis) 10g, *Gan Cao* (Radix et Rhizoma Glycyrrhizae) 10g, *Bai Zhu* (Rhizoma Atractylodis Macrocephalae) 15-30g, *Huang Qi* (Radix Astragali) 15-30g, *Xi Xin* (Radix et Rhizoma Asari) 4g, *Huang Qin* (Radix Scutellariae) 12g, *Yu Xing Cao* (Herba Houttuyniae) 30g, *Chuan Xiong* (Rhizoma Chuanxiong) 15g, *Lian Qiao* (Fructus Forsythiae) 15g, *Dan Shen* (Radix et Rhizoma Salviae Miltiorrhizae) 15g, *Niu Xi* (Radix Achyranthis Bidentatae) 15g, *Bai Shao* (Radix Paeoniae Alba) 15g, and *Huo Xiang* (Herba Agastaches) 6g. The herbal formula was given in decoction daily. Of 50 patients, the study reported complete recovery in 35 cases and improvement in 15 cases. The duration of treatment ranged from 10-30 days.[5]

SUGGESTED ACUPUNCTURE TREATMENT

1. Points: *Xingjian* (LR 2), *Shuiquan* (KI 5), *Zhongwan* (CV 12), *Yinlingquan* (SP 9), and *Longhui*.
2. Technique: sedation.

The treatment objectives are to dry dampness, dissolve phlegm, and dispel Liver wind. *Xingjian* (LR 2) calms Liver wind to relieve vertigo and dizziness. *Shuiquan* (KI 5) nourishes Kidney yin and indirectly controls Liver wind. *Zhongwan* (CV 12), the *mu* (collecting) point of the Stomach, harmonizes the Stomach to relieve nausea. *Yinlingquan* (SP 9), the *he* (uniting) point of the Spleen channel, strengthens the Spleen and dispels dampness. Finally, *Longhui* is specifically selected to relieve headache, dizziness, and vertigo.

RELATED FORMULA

***Bàn Xià Bái Zhú Tiān Má Tāng* (Pinellia, Atractylodes Macrocephala, and Gastrodia Decoction)**

半夏白朮天麻湯
半夏白术天麻汤

Pinyin Name: *Ban Xia Bai Zhu Tian Ma Tang*

Literal Name: Pinellia, Atractylodes Macrocephala, and Gastrodia Decoction

Original Source: *Pi Wei Lun* (Discussion of the Spleen and Stomach) by Li Gao in 1249

Huang Bo (Cortex Phellodendri Chinensis)	0.6g [1g]
Gan Jiang (Rhizoma Zingiberis)	0.6g [1g]
Tian Ma (Rhizoma Gastrodiae)	1.5g [2.5g]
Cang Zhu (Rhizoma Atractylodis)	1.5g [2.5g]
Fu Ling (Poria)	1.5g [2.5g]
Huang Qi (Radix Astragali)	1.5g [2.5g]
Ze Xie (Rhizoma Alismatis)	1.5g [2.5g]
Ren Shen (Radix et Rhizoma Ginseng)	1.5g [2.5g]
Bai Zhu (Rhizoma Atractylodis Macrocephalae)	3g [5g]
Shen Qu (Massa Fermentata), *chao* (dry-fried)	3g [5g]
Ban Xia (Rhizoma Pinelliae), *xi* (washed) in liquid 7 times	4.5g [7.5g]
Mai Ya (Fructus Hordei Germinatus)	4.5g [7.5g]
Chen Pi (Pericarpium Citri Reticulatae)	4.5g [7.5g]

The source text states to cook the herbs in 2 bowls of water until it is reduced down to 1 bowl. Take the warm, strained decoction after meals. Today, this formula may be prepared as a decoction with the doses suggested in brackets.

This formula has functions to dry dampness, dissolve phlegm, benefit qi, and harmonize the Stomach. It is designed to treat headache due to phlegm retention with signs and symptoms such as nausea, vomiting, thick, sticky saliva and sputum, dizziness and vertigo, irritability, a stifling sensation in the chest, shortness of breath, severe headache, heavy sensations in the body, cold extremities, and restless sleep.

AUTHORS' COMMENTS

Ban Xia Bai Zhu Tian Ma Tang is one of the most common formulas for treating seizure disorder and epilepsy caused by Spleen qi deficiency, Liver wind, and phlegm rising in dogs. It is most often combined with the herbal formula *Tian Ma Gou Teng Yin* (Gastrodia and Uncaria Decoction). The use of the combination of *Ban Xia Bai Zhu Tian Ma Tang* and *Tian Ma Gou Teng Yin* (Gastrodia and Uncaria Decoction) has proven effective in the treatment of the biomedical disease epilepsy. The authors have used this combination to treat dogs with variable clinical results. Some dogs were able to discontinue anticonvulsant medications altogether, while in others, the dose and number of conventional medications (phenobarbitol, potassium bromide, diazepam, gabapentin, levetiracetam, felbatol, zonisamide) were significantly decreased. The combination of herbal formula with conventional medications is

Bàn Xià Bái Zhú Tiān Má Tāng
(Pinellia, Atractylodes Macrocephala, and Gastrodia Decoction)

considered to be synergistic and resulted in no adverse effects over many months of concurrent use.

In the authors' clinical experience, the average duration of herbal formula use until discontinuation of conventional medications is 6-10 months. The decrease in conventional medication should always be made slowly with not more than a 20 percent decrease per month or breakthrough seizure activity can occur. The greatest success was observed in younger animals (2 years of age and younger) immediately after diagnosis. However, this herbal combination has been used successfully in dogs that are 6-8 years of age as well. The dogs for which this treatment protocol is most appropriate are typically purebred, have deficiencies of the Kidney, Liver and Spleen, as well as show signs of Liver wind and phlegm. Without appropriate dietary management to strengthen the Spleen's transportation and transformation functions and prevent the continued damp and phlegm formation, treatment results will be less than optimal.

Some cases will be non-responsive to this herbal combination and require modification or a different formula altogether. However, for seizures and epilepsy with a strong component of phlegm and underlying Spleen qi deficiency, the combination of these two herbal formulas would make a good first choice.

References

1. *Shi Yong Zhong Yi Nei Ke Za Zhi* (Journal of Practical Chinese Internal Medicine), 1993, 4:190.
2. *Tian Jin Zhong Yi* (Tianjin Chinese Medicine), 1995, 2:16.
3. *Bei Jing Zhong Yi* (Beijing Chinese Medicine), 1997, 5:50.
4. *Bei Jing Zhong Yi* (Beijing Chinese Medicine), 1991, 6:31.
5. *Shan Xi Zhong Yi* (Shanxi Chinese Medicine), 1995, 16(2):63.

Dìng Xiān Wán (Arrest Seizures Pill)

定癇丸
定痫丸

Pinyin Name: *Ding Xian Wan*
Literal Name: Arrest Seizures Pill
Alternate Name: Succinum Combination
Original Source: *Yi Xue Xin Wu* (Medical Revelations) by Cheng Guo-Peng in 1732

COMPOSITION

Dan Nan Xing (Arisaema cum Bile), *zhi* (prepared) 9 times	15g [3g]
Ban Xia (Rhizoma Pinelliae), *chao* (dry-fried) with ginger juice	30g [6g]
Chen Pi (Pericarpium Citri Reticulatae), *xi* (washed)	21g [4.5g]
Chuan Bei Mu (Bulbus Fritillariae Cirrhosae)	30g [6g]
Fu Ling (Poria), *zheng* (steamed)	30g [6g]
Mai Dong (Radix Ophiopogonis)	60g [12g]
Dan Shen (Radix et Rhizoma Salviae Miltiorrhizae), *zheng* (steamed) with liquor	60g [12g]
Shi Chang Pu (Rhizoma Acori Tatarinowii), *chu* (pestled) to powder	15g [3g]
Quan Xie (Scorpio), remove the tails and *xi* (washed) with licorice water	15g [3g]
Jiang Can (Bombyx Batryticatus), *xi* (washed) with licorice water and *chao* (dry-fried)	15g [3g]
Tian Ma (Rhizoma Gastrodiae)	30g [6g]
Zhu Sha (Cinnabaris), *shui fei* (refined with water) and *yan* (ground) into thin particles	9g [2g]
Hu Po (Succinum), *zhu* (boiled) till soft and *yan* (ground) with *Deng Xin Cao* (Medulla Junci)	15g [3g]
Yuan Zhi (Radix Polygalae), *pao* (blast-fried) with licorice water	21g [4.5g]
Fu Shen (Poria Pararadicis), *zheng* (steamed)	30g [6g]

Note: *Zhu Sha* (Cinnabaris) is a potentially toxic heavy metal and is rarely used as a medicinal substance today. Its discussion here is included primarily for academic purposes, to reflect the historical use of this substance in its original formulation. Most herbal products today have removed it completely, or replaced it with substitutes with similar functions. For additional information on the toxicity, please refer to *Chinese Medical Herbology and Pharmacology* by John Chen and Tina Chen.

DOSAGE / PREPARATION / ADMINISTRATION

The source text states to grind the ingredients into powder and form into pills using the resultant mixture of the following liquids: a small bowl [100 mL] of *Zhu Li* (Succus Bambusae), a small cup [50 mL] of fresh juice of *Sheng Jiang* (Rhizoma Zingiberis Recens), and a thick herbal paste made from condensing 120g of *Gan Cao* (Radix et Rhizoma Glycyrrhizae). The pills are coated with *Zhu Sha* (Cinnabaris) and should resemble a large bullet in size [approximately 6g]. Take one pill per dose with warm, boiled water in the morning and at night.

CHINESE THERAPEUTIC ACTIONS

Eliminates phlegm and subdues Liver wind

CLINICAL MANIFESTATIONS

Phlegm and heat rising: sudden onset of seizures and epilepsy, loss of balance, semi-unconsciousness or complete loss of consciousness, falling down, tonic-clonic seizures, deviation of the mouth or tongue, involuntary salivation, hypersalivation, involuntary urination and defecation, sudden vocalization, a red to purple tongue, and a wiry to slippery pulse.

VETERINARY CLINICAL APPLICATIONS

Acute seizure disorder, acute epilepsy in dogs, seizures secondary to brain tumors in dogs and cats and seizures secondary to granulomatous meningoencephalitis (GME) in dogs.

EXPLANATION

Ding Xian Wan (Arrest Seizures Pill) treats seizures and epilepsy caused by Liver wind rising and phlegm obstructing the sensory orifices. According to traditional Chinese medicine, seizures and epilepsy can be caused by many factors, such as excess heat, yin deficiency, poor genetics (i.e., *jing* [essence] deficiency), phlegm stagnation, blood stagnation, emotional imbalance, injury, poor diet, overexertion or overwork. Most commonly, seizures and epilepsy occur when Liver wind and phlegm rise

Dìng Xián Wán (Arrest Seizures Pill)

Ding Xian Wan (Arrest Seizures Pill)

Diagnosis	Clinical Signs	Treatment	Herbs
Rising of phlegm and heat	• Seizures and epilepsy, a red to purple tongue, and a wiry to slippery pulse: Liver wind and phlegm rising together to the head • Sudden loss of consciousness and loss of balance: phlegm blocking the sensory orifices • Convulsions: phlegm obstructing the channels and collaterals	Eliminates phlegm and subdues Liver wind	• *Zhu Li* (Succus Bambusae) clears heat, dissolves phlegm, and opens the sensory orifices. • *Dan Nan Xing* (Arisaema cum Bile) clears heat and dissolves phlegm. • *Ban Xia* (Rhizoma Pinelliae), *Chen Pi* (Pericarpium Citri Reticulatae), *Chuan Bei Mu* (Bulbus Fritillariae Cirrhosae), *Fu Ling* (Poria) and *Mai Dong* (Radix Ophiopogonis) dispel phlegm, direct qi downwards, and prevent yin damage. • *Dan Shen* (Radix et Rhizoma Salviae Miltiorrhizae) eliminates blood stagnation. • *Shi Chang Pu* (Rhizoma Acori Tatarinowii) warms and opens the sensory orifices. • *Quan Xie* (Scorpio), *Jiang Can* (Bombyx Batryticatus) and *Tian Ma* (Rhizoma Gastrodiae) subdue Liver wind and stop muscle convulsions. • *Zhu Sha* (Cinnabaris), *Hu Po* (Succinum), *Yuan Zhi* (Radix Polygalae), *Deng Xin Cao* (Medulla Junci) and *Fu Shen* (Poria Paradicis) calm the *shen* (spirit) and enhance the treatment of seizures and epilepsy. • *Sheng Jiang* (Rhizoma Zingiberis Recens) and *Gan Cao* (Radix et Rhizoma Glycyrrhizae) harmonize all of the herbs.

together to the head. As phlegm rises, it blocks the sensory orifices, causing sudden loss of consciousness, loss of balance, deviation of the mouth, hypersalivation, and involuntary urination and defecation. If Liver wind and phlegm block the channels and collaterals, patients will have tonic-clonic type of convulsions.

Zhu Li (Succus Bambusae) clears heat, dissolves phlegm, and opens the sensory orifices. *Dan Nan Xing* (Arisaema cum Bile) clears heat and dissolves phlegm. Together, these two herbs treat all types of seizures, convulsions, and stroke disorders. *Ban Xia* (Rhizoma Pinelliae), *Chen Pi* (Pericarpium Citri Reticulatae), *Chuan Bei Mu* (Bulbus Fritillariae Cirrhosae), *Fu Ling* (Poria), and *Mai Dong* (Radix Ophiopogonis) dispel phlegm and direct qi downward. They also prevent the warm and drying herbs from damaging yin. *Dan Shen* (Radix et Rhizoma Salviae Miltiorrhizae) eliminates blood stagnation. *Shi Chang Pu* (Rhizoma Acori Tatarinowii) warms and opens the sensory orifices. *Quan Xie* (Scorpio) and *Jiang Can* (Bombyx Batryticatus) subdue Liver wind and stop muscle convulsions. *Tian Ma* (Rhizoma Gastrodiae) subdues Liver wind and dissolves phlegm. *Zhu Sha* (Cinnabaris), *Hu Po* (Succinum), *Deng Xin Cao* (Medulla Junci), *Yuan Zhi* (Radix Polygalae), and *Fu Shen* (Poria Paradicis) calm the *shen* (spirit) and enhance the overall function of treating seizures and epilepsy. Lastly, *Sheng Jiang* (Rhizoma Zingiberis Recens) and *Gan Cao* (Radix et Rhizoma Glycyrrhizae) harmonize all of the herbs.

VETERINARY MODIFICATIONS

- With more heat present, add *Zhi Zi* (Fructus Gardeniae) and *Long Dan* (Radix et Rhizoma Gentianae).
- With chronic and frequent seizure attacks due to deficiency of *zheng* (upright) *qi*, add *Ren Shen* (Radix et Rhizoma Ginseng).
- With constipation, add *Da Huang* (Radix et Rhizoma Rhei) and *Mang Xiao* (Natrii Sulfas).
- With continuous twitching and spasms, add *Gou Teng* (Ramulus Uncariae cum Uncis).

CAUTIONS / CONTRAINDICATIONS

- *Ding Xian Wan* treats seizures and epilepsy caused by Liver wind rising and phlegm. It should not be used indiscriminately to treat seizures and epilepsy caused by other factors, such as Liver fire, Liver and Kidney yin deficiencies, and Spleen and Stomach deficiencies.
- This formula treats acute cases of seizures and epilepsy. Once the condition is stabilized, this formula should be discontinued, and additional supportive therapy started.

Dìng Xián Wán (Arrest Seizures Pill)

AUTHORS' COMMENTS

Ding Xian Wan is designed to treat acute onset of seizures characterized by rising of phlegm, heat, and Liver wind. Although effective, the use of this formula alone is insufficient for the overall management of seizures and epilepsy. Optimal treatment of seizures and epilepsy must focus on treating both the symptoms and the cause. During acute seizures, the emphasis is on treating the symptoms; this entails eliminating phlegm and extinguishing Liver wind. During remission, the emphasis is on treating the root cause, such as strengthening the Spleen, tonifying Kidney and Liver yin and blood, nourishing the Heart, resolving blood stagnation, and regulating qi and blood circulation. Long-term care of animals with seizures and epilepsy must also include dietary management and lifestyle adjustments; otherwise, the results of treatment will be marginal to ineffective. Chronic seizure activity leads to progressive qi and yin deficiencies over time. Without herbal therapy, acupuncture and dietary management, the deficiencies worsen, and development and accumulation of phlegm continues, leading to more frequent and severe seizures.

Ding Xian Wan is typically used for frequent and difficult to control seizures and is not for long-term use without modification. It is a harsh formula and has no nourishing capabilities. It is recommended that the dose be decreased incrementally over time, as soon as the condition allows. It is often appropriate to decrease the dosage when there have been no seizures for 1-3 months (depending on the seizure frequency initially). It is considered prudent to perform initial blood chemistry evaluations and then regularly monitor these values during the use of this formula; the same applies for conventional anticonvulsant therapy.

Ding Xian Wan can be combined with *Xue Fu Zhu Yu Tang* (Drive Out Stasis in the Mansion of Blood Decoction) for the treatment of seizures secondary to brain tumors in dogs and cats and granulomatous meningoencephalitis (GME) in dogs. This combination of herbal formulas has been used in conjunction with conventional anticonvulsant drugs without adverse effect.

Chapter 18 — Summary

— Phlegm-Dispelling Formulas

SECTION 1: DAMP-DRYING AND PHLEGM-DISSOLVING FORMULAS

Name	Similarities	Differences
Er Chen Tang (Two-Cured Decoction)	Dry dampness, dissolve phlegm	Regulates qi, harmonizes the middle *jiao*
Wen Dan Tang (Warm the Gallbladder Decoction)		Clears Gallbladder heat, harmonizes the Stomach
Fu Ling Wan (Poria Pill)		Activates qi, softens nodules

Er Chen Tang (Two-Cured Decoction) is the most basic formula to dry dampness and dissolve phlegm. Internal dampness and phlegm stagnation due to Spleen deficiency produce coughing with profuse sputum, chest congestion, nausea, and vomiting.

Wen Dan Tang (Warm the Gallbladder Decoction) treats Gallbladder and Stomach disharmony with phlegm heat. The main clinical manifestations include irritability, palpitations, insomnia, nausea and vomiting, seizures and epilepsy.

Fu Ling Wan (Poria Pill) dispels phlegm, regulates qi, and softens nodules. Due to phlegm stagnation in the middle *jiao* that travels via the channels and collaterals, manifestations of painful arms and edema of the extremities can be seen.

SECTION 2: HEAT-CLEARING AND PHLEGM-DISSOLVING FORMULAS

Name	Similarities	Differences
Qing Qi Hua Tan Wan (Clear the Qi and Transform Phlegm Pill)	Clear heat, dissolve phlegm in the Lung	Regulates qi circulation, relieves cough
Qing Fei Yin (Clear the Lung Drink)		Resolves dampness and phlegm
Qing Fei Tang (Clear the Lung Decoction)	Clear heat, dissolve phlegm in the Lung, treat deficiencies	Nourishes yin and body fluids
Zi Wan Tang (Aster Decoction)		Nourishes yin and body fluids, stops bleeding
Jie Geng Tang (Platycodon Decoction)		Tonifies Lung qi
Ren Shen Xie Fei Tang (Ginseng Decoction to Sedate the Lung)		Tonifies qi, regulates qi circulation

Qing Qi Hua Tan Wan (Clear the Qi and Transform Phlegm Pill) and ***Qing Fei Yin*** (Clear the Lung Drink) both clear heat and dissolve phlegm in the Lung.

- *Qing Qi Hua Tan Wan* clears heat, eliminates phlegm, regulates qi and arrests cough. It treats phlegm-heat congestion in the chest, accompanied by coughing with copious, yellow sputum that cannot be easily expectorated.
- *Qing Fei Yin* dissolves dampness and phlegm and clears the Lung. It treats cough caused by accumulation of phlegm and dampness, with clinical signs such as coughing with sputum, and fatigue.

Chapter 18 — Summary

Qing Fei Tang (Clear the Lung Decoction), ***Zi Wan Tang*** (Aster Decoction), ***Jie Geng Tang*** (Platycodon Decoction), and ***Ren Shen Xie Fei Tang*** (Ginseng Decoction to Sedate the Lung) have similar functions to clear heat, dissolve phlegm, and support underlying deficiencies. They are used frequently to address Lung phlegm-heat, accompanied by qi, yin and/or body fluid deficiencies.

- *Qing Fei Tang* dispels phlegm-heat from the chest, moistens the Lung, and relieves cough. It treats chronic cough due to phlegm-heat in the Lung with yin and body fluid deficiencies. Clinical manifestations include severe cough, thick and sticky phlegm, a red tongue and a rapid, slippery to wiry pulse.
- *Zi Wan Tang* clears heat, dissolves phlegm, and nourishes yin and body fluids. It treats chronic cough due to Lung heat and yin deficiency, with clinical signs such as chronic cough, excess phlegm, fever due to over-exertion, the presence of lung abscesses, and blood in the sputum.
- *Jie Geng Tang* eliminates pus and phlegm, dispels toxins, and clears deficiency fire. It is commonly used to treat Lung phlegm stagnation, with clinical signs such as cough, and swelling and pain of the throat. Because the phlegm consumes yin and body fluids, deficiency fire arises and leads to clinical signs such as thick, sticky sputum with mucous and blood or foul odor.
- *Ren Shen Xie Fei Tang* clears heat, sedates the Lung, eliminates phlegm, and regulates qi circulation. It treats Lung heat with wheezing, dyspnea, bloating of the epigastrium, cough with profuse sputum, and constipation. This formula contains *Ren Shen* (Radix et Rhizoma Ginseng) to tonify qi, strengthen the Lung and Spleen, and prevent the draining herbs from consuming body fluids.

SECTION 3: DRYNESS-MOISTENING AND PHLEGM-DISSOLVING FORMULA

Name	Similarities	Differences
Bei Mu Gua Lou San (Fritillaria and Trichosanthes Fruit Powder)	Moistens the Lung, dissolves phlegm	Clears Lung heat, regulates Lung qi

Bei Mu Gua Lou San (Fritillaria and Trichosanthes Fruit Powder) moistens the Lung, dissolves phlegm, clears heat, and regulates qi circulation. It is indicated for coughing with thick, sticky sputum that cannot be expectorated easily.

SECTION 4: WARM FORMULAS THAT DISSOLVE COLD-PHLEGM

Name	Similarities	Differences
Ling Gan Wu Wei Jiang Xin Tang (Poria, Licorice, Schisandra, Ginger, and Asarum Decoction)	Dissolve cold phlegm	Warms and tonifies the Lung and Spleen
San Zi Yang Qin Tang (Three-Seed Decoction to Nourish One's Parents)		Guides Lung qi downward, resolves food stagnation

Ling Gan Wu Wei Jiang Xin Tang (Poria, Licorice, Schisandra, Ginger, and Asarum Decoction) warms the Lung and dispels cold-phlegm accumulation. Key clinical manifestations include coughing with profuse, white, watery sputum, and a wiry, slippery pulse.

San Zi Yang Qin Tang (Three-Seed Decoction to Nourish One's Parents) dispels phlegm retention, unblocks qi stagnation, and resolves food stagnation. Clinical manifestations include coughing with profuse sputum, lack of appetite with indigestion, and a slippery pulse.

Chapter 18 — Summary

SECTION 5: WIND-EXPELLING AND PHLEGM-DISSOLVING FORMULAS

Name	Similarities	Differences
Ban Xia Bai Zhu Tian Ma Tang (Pinellia, Atractylodes Macrocephala, and Gastrodia Decoction)	Calm Liver wind, dissolve phlegm	Treats headache, dizziness, and vertigo
Ding Xian Wan (Arrest Seizures Pill)		Treats seizures and epilepsy

Ban Xia Bai Zhu Tian Ma Tang (Pinellia, Atractylodes Macrocephala, and Gastrodia Decoction) dries dampness, dissolves phlegm, smoothes the Liver, and subdues Liver wind. In addition to the usual phlegm manifestations, seizures and tremors caused by Liver wind rising can also be seen.

Ding Xian Wan (Arrest Seizures Pill) eliminates phlegm and subdues Liver wind. It primarily treats rising of Liver wind and phlegm. Clinical manifestations include sudden onset of seizures and epilepsy, semi-unconsciousness or complete loss of consciousness, tonic-clonic seizures, deviation of the mouth, hypersalivation, and involuntary urination and defecation.

Chapter 19

— Reducing, Guiding, and Dissolving Formulas

消导化积剂

李杲 Lǐ Gǎo

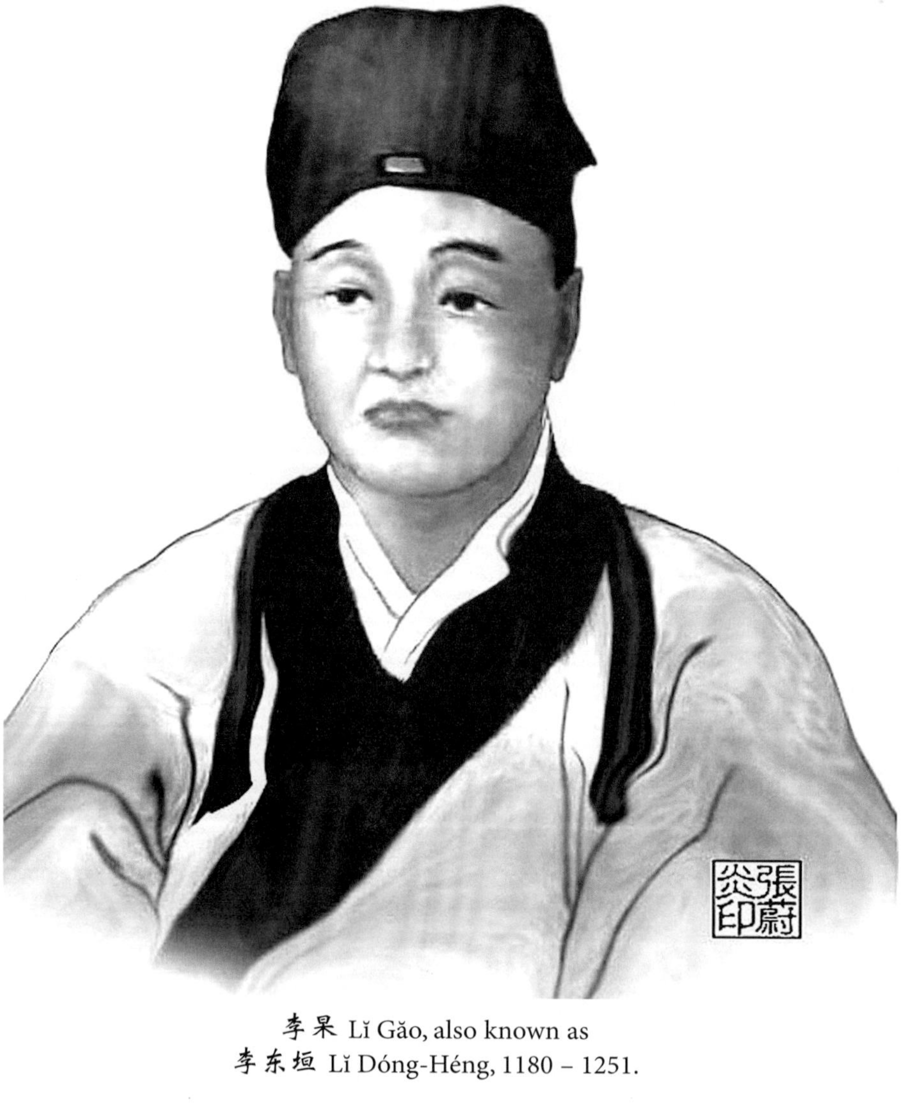

李杲 Lǐ Gǎo, also known as
李东垣 Lǐ Dóng-Héng, 1180 – 1251.

李杲 Lǐ Gǎo

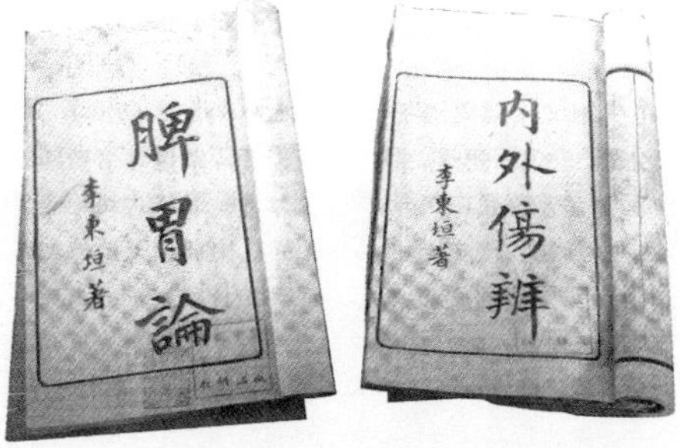

脾胃论 *Pi Wei Lun* (Discussion of the Spleen and Stomach) and 内外伤辨惑论 *Nei Wai Shang Bian Huo Lun* (Clarifying Doubts about Injury from Internal and External Causes).

Li Gao, also known as Li Dong-Heng, was born into a very wealthy family. Yet unlike many of the very rich, he never hesitated to share his wealth to help those who were less fortunate during times of famine from drought or flood. However, no amount of money helped his mother when she was seriously ill. She was seen by numerous physicians, all of whom made conflicting diagnoses, and prescribed differing treatments. Li blamed himself for not knowing medicine, and watched helplessly as his mother's health continued to deteriorate and she eventually died. Li vowed to study and practice medicine, so no others would ever have to die from inadequate care.

Li Gao is best known for treating disorders of the Spleen and Stomach. He believed that the Spleen and Stomach are the source of *yuan* (source) *qi*, and adequate *yuan* (source) *qi* is the key to health. Conversely, when the Spleen and Stomach are deficient, *yuan* (source) *qi* is weakened and diseases begin to surface. He proposed that three main factors damage the Spleen and Stomach: 1) inappropriate diet, 2) excessive physical labor, and 3) unbalanced emotions. From this base of understanding, Li could demonstrate that damage to the Spleen and Stomach contributes to the rise of hundreds of different disorders. Li specialized in using tonic herbs to selectively supplement the Spleen and Stomach, and developed the famous formula *Bu Zhong Yi Qi Tang* (Tonify the Middle and Augment the Qi Decoction).

Li Gao wrote many books throughout his life. The three most well-known are 脾胃论 *Pi Wei Lun* (Discussion of the Spleen and Stomach), 兰室秘藏 *Lan Shi Mi Cang* (Secrets from the Orchid Chamber) and 内外伤辨惑论 *Nei Wai Shang Bian Huo Lun* (Clarifying Doubts about Injury from Internal and External Causes). Many formulas from these references are still used today, such as:

- *Run Chang Wan* (Moisten the Intestines Pill)
- *Qing Wei San* (Clear the Stomach Powder)
- *Sheng Mai San* (Generate the Pulse Powder)
- *Bu Zhong Yi Qi Tang* (Tonify the Middle and Augment the Qi Decoction)
- *Dang Gui Bu Xue Tang* (Tangkuei Decoction to Tonify the Blood)
- *Hou Po Wen Zhong Tang* (Magnolia Bark Decoction for Warming the Middle)
- *Tian Tai Wu Yao San* (Top-Quality Lindera Powder)
- *Qiang Huo Sheng Shi Tang* (Notopterygium Decoction to Overcome Dampness)
- *Dang Gui Nian Tong Tang* (Tangkuei Decoction to Lift the Pain)
- *Zhi Shi Dao Zhi Wan* (Immature Bitter Orange Pill to Guide Out Stagnation)
- *Zhi Shi Xiao Pi Wan* (Immature Bitter Orange Pill to Reduce Focal Distention)
- *Zhi Zhu Wan* (Immature Bitter Orange and Atractylodes Macrocephala Pill)

Dynasties & Kingdoms	Year
Xia Dynasty 夏	2100-1600 BCE
Shang Dynasty 商	1600-1100 BCE
Zhou Dynasty 周	1100-221 BCE
Qin Dynasty 秦	221-207 BCE
Han Dynasty 漢	206 BCE-220
Three Kingdoms 三國	220-280
Western Jin Dynasty 西晉	265-316
Eastern Jin Dynasty 東晉	317-420
Northern and Southern Dynasties 北南朝	420-581
Sui Dynasty 隋	581-618
Tang Dynasty 唐	618-907
Five Dynasties 五代	907-960
Song Dynasty 宋	960-1279
Liao Dynasty 遼	916-1125
Jin Dynasty 金	**1115-1234**
Yuan Dynasty 元	1271-1368
Ming Dynasty 明	1368-1644
Qing Dynasty 清	1644-1911
Republic of China 中華民國	1912-Present Day
People's Republic of China 中華人民共和國	1949-Present Day

Table of Contents

Chapter 19 — Overview

— Reducing, Guiding, and Dissolving Formulas

Definition: Reducing, guiding, and dissolving formulas consist of herbs that reduce (digest) foods, guide out stagnation, and dissolve accumulations. This method of treatment is known as *xiao fa* (reducing), one of the *ba fa* (eight treatment methods) described in the *Huang Di Nei Jing* (Yellow Emperor's Inner Classic) in the first or second century A.D.

Reducing, guiding, and dissolving formulas generally treat food stagnation, abdominal rigidity, ileus, and various types of stagnation, accumulation, and masses. From a biomedical perspective, the herbs in these formulas stimulate production of gastric acid, increase intestinal peristalsis, reduce gas formation, relieve bloating, contain digestive enzymes (lipase, amylase, protease, pancreatin), control hyperlipidemia, and have antibiotic properties.

Reducing, guiding, and dissolving formulas treat two main types of disorders: food stagnation and food accumulation.

- Food stagnation refers to the accumulation of food in the digestive system, primarily the middle *jiao*. In domestic animals this occurs from feeding poor diets comprised of difficult-to-digest and damp-heat producing foods, acute episodes of overeating, or consumption of contaminated food. This damages the Spleen and Stomach and inhibits the proper receiving, transforming, and transporting of food. The qi mechanisms become clogged and produce damp-heat, further complicating treatment. Food stagnation may also be caused by constitutional deficiencies of the Spleen and Stomach, leading to difficulties in digesting food. Both conditions require additional herbs to promote digestion and strengthen the Spleen and Stomach. Food stagnation patterns are characterized by epigastric and abdominal bloating accompanied by pain, poor appetite, foul-smelling belching, flatulence, vomiting, diarrhea, or constipation. Patients usually present with a red tongue that has a white to yellow, greasy coating and a slippery to wiry pulse.
- Food accumulation, in contrast to simple food stagnation, is a more chronic condition caused by long-term overeating or feeding of a species inappropriate diet. For these reasons, both food accumulation and stagnation, as well as obesity, are common in dogs and cats. Cats fed a commercial kibble diet high in grains are especially prone to chronic food stagnation. Dry food diets with high amounts of carbohydrate produce dampness, phlegm and heat in the Stomach, which lead to stagnation of food and qi and eventually weaken the Spleen, Stomach and Intestines. Abdominal bloating, vomiting, intermittent constipation and diarrhea, and anorexia may occur due to prolonged accumulation and stagnation of qi, blood, cold, heat, food, or phlegm. In these cases, herbs that activate qi and blood circulation, dispel dampness and phlegm, soften masses, and relieve distention must be included in the treatment strategy. Clinical signs of food accumulation include poor appetite, bloating or distension of the epigastrium and abdomen, vomiting, palpable fecal mass, constipation, loose and watery diarrhea, a red tongue with a greasy, white to yellow tongue coating, and a weak, deficient pulse. Horses tend to be fed more species appropriate diets, with high amounts of forage and only supplemental concentrates. However, it is becoming more common for horses to have prolonged periods of stall confinement, less grazing, and increased levels of concentrated feed. These factors alone can lead to chronic food stagnation or accumulation, but this pattern occurs to a greater degree when foods high in molasses or overly processed are the concentrate of choice. Even pasture horses given free access to lush pasture can chronically overeat and develop these patterns.

Chapter 19 — Overview

Common veterinary biomedical conditions treated with reducing, guiding and dissolving formulas include poor appetite, acute and chronic vomiting syndromes, diarrhea, constipation or impaction, acute and chronic gastroenteritis, chronic bloating, acute pancreatitis, acute or chronic cholecystitis, peptic ulcer, inflammatory bowel disease, and motion sickness. Reducing, guiding and resolving formulas are also commonly used as an adjunct to cancer therapy in animals undergoing chemotherapy or radiation treatments and that have gastroenteritis and poor appetite.

Reducing formulas are similar to purging or downward-draining formulas in that both are used to dispel abnormal accumulation in the interior. However, reducing, guiding, and dissolving formulas are gentler in nature than downward-draining formulas; they are suitable for treating chronic syndromes with mild clinical signs and are appropriate for weaker patients. Furthermore, these formulas are most effective for dissolving hardness and nodules that cannot be quickly eliminated, but require long-term use of herbs to gradually soften and eliminate the masses. In contrast, downward-draining or purging formulas (*see* Chapter 2), are harsh in nature and should be reserved only for acute syndromes with severe clinical signs (i.e., acute constipation or intestinal obstruction). These formulas are most useful in treating accumulations that can and must be purged immediately and quickly, such as acute constipation or intestinal obstruction. Another distinction of reducing formulas is the transforming capabilities not found in downward-draining formulas. Even though reducing and dissolving formulas are milder in action than downward-draining formulas, they are still dispersing in nature. When treating animals with deficiency of the middle *jiao*, or those that have sustained injury to *zheng* (upright) *qi* from chronic food stagnation and accumulation, the treatment must include herbs that support qi and strengthen the Spleen.

SUBCATEGORIES OF ACTION

Reducing, guiding, and dissolving formulas are divided into two subcategories to differentiate accurately the nature of the disorders and the characteristics of the corresponding formulas.

1. **Reducing, Guiding, and Dissolving Formulas that Treat Food Stagnation**
These formulas commonly treat food stagnation with clinical manifestations of chest and epigastric bloating, belching, flatulence, acid regurgitation with a foul smell, abdominal pain, nausea, vomiting, and diarrhea. Herbs commonly used to treat food stagnation include *Shan Zha* (Fructus Crataegi), *Shen Qu* (Massa Fermentata), and *Lai Fu Zi* (Semen Raphani). Exemplar formulas include *Bao He Wan* (Preserve Harmony Pill) and *Zhi Shi Dao Zhi Wan* (Immature Bitter Orange Pill to Guide Out Stagnation).
Spleen and Stomach deficiencies and food stagnation often occur together, because either pre-existing deficiencies of the Spleen and Stomach contribute to food stagnation, or prolonged food stagnation damages the Spleen and Stomach. In these cases, it is necessary to use simultaneously qi-tonifying herbs to strengthen the Spleen and Stomach and reducing herbs to treat food stagnation. The emphasis on tonifying or reducing may be adjusted according to the constitution of the animal and the severity of the food stagnation. Commonly used herbs that strengthen the Spleen and Stomach include *Ren Shen* (Radix et Rhizoma Ginseng), *Bai Zhu* (Rhizoma Atractylodis Macrocephalae), and *Fu Ling* (Poria). An exemplar formula is *Jian Pi Wan* (Strengthen the Spleen Pill).

2. **Reducing, Guiding, and Dissolving Formulas that Relieve Distention**
These formulas are used mainly for distention, accompanied by clinical signs of general accumulation and stagnation, such as abdominal bloating, immobile mass in the abdomen and hypochondrium, poor appetite, decreased intake of food, and wasting of muscles. Optimal treatment for this condition includes the use of herbs that activate qi circulation, invigorate blood circulation, resolve dampness, dissolve phlegm, and soften hardness. A representative formula is *Zhi Shi Xiao Pi Wan* (Immature Bitter Orange Pill to Reduce Focal Distention).

Chapter 19 — Overview

CAUTIONS / CONTRAINDICATIONS

- Reducing, guiding, and dissolving formulas are generally given in pill form to gradually treat food stagnation and relieve distention. The use of decoction is not appropriate because the stagnation and accumulation in these cases can only be slowly reduced, guided out, or dissolved, not quickly purged out by the immediate and potent actions of a decoction.
- Reducing, guiding, and dissolving formulas are relatively mild, but they nonetheless consume qi and may cause weakness and deficiency with long-term use. Therefore, these formulas should be used with caution in animals that have underlying weakness and deficiency.

PHARMACOLOGICAL EFFECTS & CLINICAL APPLICATIONS

While reducing, guiding, and dissolving formulas commonly treat gastrointestinal disorders, they also have effect to treat gastrolithiasis and cholelithiasis.

- **Gastrointestinal disorders**: Pharmacological effects demonstrated by these herbs and formulas include increased production of gastric acid,[1] increased production of bile acid,[2] and increased intestinal peristalsis.[3] Clinically, these formulas have been used successfully to treat digestive disorders such as indigestion,[4,5] anorexia,[6] intestinal obstruction,[7] stenosis of colon and rectum,[8] chronic gastritis,[9] atrophic gastritis,[10] constipation,[11] and acute abdomen.[12] Exemplar formulas that treat gastrointestinal disorders include *Bao He Wan* (Preserve Harmony Pill) and *Zhi Shi Dao Zhi Wan* (Immature Bitter Orange Pill to Guide Out Stagnation).
- **Gastrolithiasis and cholelithiasis**: Reducing, guiding, and dissolving formulas can also be used to treat stomach and gallbladder stones.[13,14] The exact mechanisms of action are unclear, but can probably be attributed to the ability of these herbs and formulas to stimulate the production and release of gastric and bile acids, increase gastric emptying time, and increase intestinal peristalsis.[15,16] Exemplar formulas that treat stomach and gallbladder stones include *Bao He Wan* (Preserve Harmony Pill) and *Zhi Shi Xiao Pi Wan* (Immature Bitter Orange Pill to Reduce Focal Distention).

References

1. *Ying Yang Xue Bao* (Report of Nutrition), 1984; 6(2):109.
2. *Zhong Yao Yao Li Yu Lin Chuang* (Pharmacology and Clinical Applications of Chinese Herbs), 1991; 7(4):1.
3. *Zhong Hua Yi Xue Za Zhi* (Chinese Journal of Medicine), 1956; 42:946.
4. *Fu Jian Zhong Yi Yao* (Fujian Chinese Medicine and Herbology), 1985; 3(8):18.
5. *Zhong Yi Za Zhi* (Journal of Chinese Medicine), 1959; 9:630.
6. *Liao Ning Zhong Yi Za Zhi* (Liaoning Journal of Chinese Medicine), 1996; 12:550.
7. *Zhong Yi Ming Fang Lin Chuang Xin Yong* (Contemporary Clinical Applications of Classic Chinese Formulas), 2001; 502.
8. *Guang Xi Zhong Yi Yao* (Guangxi Chinese Medicine and Herbology), 1999; 2:33.
9. *Zhong Yi Yao Xue Bao* (Report of Chinese Medicine and Herbology), 1991; 3:39.
10. *Shan Xi Zhong Yi* (Shanxi Chinese Medicine), 1997; 7:304.
11. *Zhe Jiang Zhong Yi Xue Yuan Xue Bao* (Journal of Zhejiang University of Chinese Medicine), 1996; 2:28.
12. *Jiang Su Zhong Yi* (Jiangsu Chinese Medicine), 1982; 6:3.
13. *Shan Dong Zhong Yi Za Zhi* (Shandong Journal of Chinese Medicine), 1993; 4:21.
14. *Hu Bei Zhong Yi Za Zhi* (Hubei Journal of Chinese Medicine), 1998; 5:38.
15. *Zhong Yao Yao Li Yu Lin Chuang* (Pharmacology and Clinical Applications of Chinese Herbs), 1991; 7(1):8.
16. *Hu Bei Zhong Yi Za Zhi* (Hubei Journal of Chinese Medicine), 1998; 5:38.

Section 1

消食化积剂 — Reducing, Guiding, and Dissolving Formulas that Treat Food Stagnation

Bǎo Hé Wán (Preserve Harmony Pill) 保和丸

Pinyin Name: *Bao He Wan*
Literal Name: Preserve Harmony Pill
Alternate Names: Harmony-Preserving Pill, Citrus and Crataegus Formula
Original Source: *Dan Xi Xin Fa* (Teachings of [Zhu] Dan-Xi) by Zhu Zhen-Heng in 1481

COMPOSITION

Shan Zha (Fructus Crataegi)	180g [18g]
Shen Qu (Massa Fermentata)	60g [6g]
Lai Fu Zi (Semen Raphani)	30g [6g]
Ban Xia (Rhizoma Pinelliae)	90g [9g]
Chen Pi (Pericarpium Citri Reticulatae)	30g [6g]
Fu Ling (Poria)	90g [9g]
Lian Qiao (Fructus Forsythiae)	30g [6g]

DOSAGE / PREPARATION / ADMINISTRATION

The source text states to grind the ingredients into powder and form into small pills. The pills should resemble the size of *Wu Tong Zi* (Semen Firmianae), a small seed approximately 5 mm in diameter. Take 70-80 pills between meals with warm, boiled water. Today, this formula may be taken as pills or decoction. For pills, grind the herbs into powder and form into pills with water. Take 6-9g of pills per dose with warm, boiled water. For decoction, use the suggested doses in brackets.

CHINESE THERAPEUTIC ACTIONS

Reduces food stagnation and harmonizes the Stomach

CLINICAL MANIFESTATIONS

Food stagnation and indigestion: epigastric and abdominal bloating and pain; halitosis, acid regurgitation, belching and/or flatulence with a rotten smell, nausea, vomiting, possible diarrhea, poor appetite, a red tongue. In severe cases, there may be a greasy, white to yellow coating and a rapid, slippery pulse.

VETERINARY CLINICAL APPLICATIONS

Acute and chronic gastroenteritis from poor diet or dietary indiscretion, acute exacerbation of chronic gastroenteritis, poor appetite, vomiting, adjunct to chemotherapy or radiation treatment, motion sickness, diarrhea, and abdominal bloating or colic after eating.

EXPLANATION

Bao He Wan (Preserve Harmony Pill) is one of the most commonly used formulas to treat all types of food stagnation. This condition is usually caused by an inappropriate diet or overeating. Excessive intake of food that remains undigested and stagnates in the stomach will impair the digestive function. Food stagnation causes qi stagnation, which may result in bloating and pain in the epigastrium and abdomen. When Stomach qi stagnates and cannot descend, acid regurgitation, nausea, and vomiting occur. When Spleen qi stagnates and cannot ascend, diarrhea results.

Shan Zha (Fructus Crataegi) functions as the chief herb to digest any kind of food stagnation; it is especially effective in helping to digest meat (protein) and fatty, greasy foods. *Shen Qu* (Massa Fermentata) resolves food stagnation and

Bǎo Hé Wán (Preserve Harmony Pill)

Bao He Wan **(Preserve Harmony Pill)**

Diagnosis	Clinical Signs	Treatment	Herbs
Food stagnation	• Indigestion with epigastric and abdominal bloating and pain: food stagnation • Acid regurgitation, belching, poor appetite, nausea, and vomiting: reversed flow of Stomach qi • Red tongue that may have a yellow, greasy coating in severe cases and a rapid, slippery pulse: food stagnation	• Reduces food stagnation • Harmonizes the Stomach	• *Shan Zha* (Fructus Crataegi) promotes the digestion of foods (meat and fatty, greasy foods). • *Shen Qu* (Massa Fermentata) strengthens the Spleen and promotes the digestion of foods (alcohol and spoiled or rotten foods). • *Lai Fu Zi* (Semen Raphani) guides qi downward and promotes the digestion of foods (starch and carbohydrates). • *Ban Xia* (Rhizoma Pinelliae) and *Chen Pi* (Pericarpium Citri Reticulatae) activate qi circulation and harmonize the Stomach. • *Fu Ling* (Poria) strengthens the Spleen and dispels dampness. • *Lian Qiao* (Fructus Forsythiae) clears heat associated with food stagnation.

strengthens the Spleen; it is effective for the digestion of alcohol and spoiled or rotten foods that arise from chronic food stagnation. *Lai Fu Zi* (Semen Raphani) guides qi downward; it is best for digesting starch and carbohydrates. Combined together, these three herbs can treat any type of food stagnation. *Ban Xia* (Rhizoma Pinelliae) and *Chen Pi* (Pericarpium Citri Reticulatae) activate qi circulation and harmonize the Stomach to relieve nausea and vomiting. *Fu Ling* (Poria) dispels dampness, strengthens the Spleen, and stops diarrhea. Food stagnation is often accompanied by heat, which is cleared by *Lian Qiao* (Fructus Forsythiae).

VETERINARY MODIFICATIONS

- For severe food stagnation and constipation, add *Bing Lang* (Semen Arecae), *Zhi Shi* (Fructus Aurantii Immaturus), *Da Fu Pi* (Pericarpium Arecae) and *Da Huang* (Radix et Rhizoma Rhei).
- For food stagnation turning into heat, evident by a red tongue body and a yellow tongue coating, and a rapid pulse, add *Huang Lian* (Rhizoma Coptidis) and *Huang Qin* (Radix Scutellariae).
- For severe nausea, such as that found in cancer patients or motion sickness, add *Sheng Jiang* (Rhizoma Zingiberis Recens).
- For severe bloating and colic, add *E Zhu* (Rhizoma Curcumae), *San Leng* (Rhizoma Sparganii), and *Mu Xiang* (Radix Aucklandiae).
- For indigestion accompanied by an exterior condition (e.g., a superficial, rapid pulse and a white, greasy tongue coating), add *Huo Xiang* (Herba Agastaches), *Zi Su Ye* (Folium Perillae), and *Jin Yin Hua* (Flos Lonicerae Japonicae).
- With severe nausea and vomiting, add *Sha Ren* (Fructus Amomi) and *Huo Xiang* (Herba Agastaches).
- With vomiting and diarrhea, add *Huo Xiang* (Herba Agastaches) and *Pei Lan* (Herba Eupatorii).
- To enhance the overall digestive function, add *Mai Ya* (Fructus Hordei Germinatus), *Gu Ya* (Fructus Setariae Germinatus), and *Ji Nei Jin* (Endothelium Corneum Gigeriae Galli).

CAUTIONS / CONTRAINDICATIONS

- *Bao He Wan* is not suitable for food stagnation due to Spleen deficiency.
- Avoid oily, greasy, or fatty foods while taking this formula.
- This formula should be used with caution during pregnancy.[1]

HUMAN CLINICAL STUDIES AND RESEARCH

1. **Indigestion**: According to one study, *Bao He Wan* effectively treated indigestion in 69 children. Those with indigestion characterized by food stagnation were treated with only *Bao He Wan*. Additions to this base formula included *Bai Zhu* (Rhizoma Atractylodis Macrocephalae) for chronic diarrhea with deficiency; and *Ji Nei Jin* (Endothelium Corneum Gigeriae Galli) and *He Ye* (Folium Nelumbinis) for poor appetite associated with diarrhea and/or nausea. Of 69 patients, the study reported complete recovery in 61 cases, improvement in 5 cases, and no effect in 3 cases. The overall effectiveness was 95.65%.[2]

Bǎo Hé Wán (Preserve Harmony Pill)

2. **Atrophic gastritis**: One study reported a marked effect using modified *Bao He Wan* to treat 34 patients with chronic atrophic gastritis. In addition to this formula, modifications were made by adding *Huang Qi* (Radix Astragali) and *Tai Zi Shen* (Radix Pseudostellariae) for qi deficiency; *Gui Zhi* (Ramulus Cinnamomi) and *Gao Liang Jiang* (Rhizoma Alpiniae Officinarum) for presence of cold; *Dan Shen* (Radix et Rhizoma Salviae Miltiorrhizae) and *Tan Xiang* (Lignum Santali Albi) for blood stagnation; and *Zhe Shi* (Haematitum) for belching. The herbs were cooked in water, and the decoction given in two equally-divided doses, for 3 months per course of treatment. The study reported significant improvement in 25 of 34 cases.[3]
3. **Gastrolithiasis**: One study reported that the combination of *Bao He Wan* and *Xiao Cheng Qi Tang* (Minor Order the Qi Decoction) was effective in treating stomach stones in 29 of 33 patients (18 males and 15 females). The herbal formula contained charred *Shan Zha* (Fructus Crataegi), charred *Shen Qu* (Massa Fermentata), charred *Mai Ya* (Fructus Hordei Germinatus), *Ji Nei Jin* (Endothelium Corneum Gigeriae Galli), *Ban Xia* (Rhizoma Pinelliae), *Chen Pi* (Pericarpium Citri Reticulatae), *Hou Po* (Cortex Magnoliae Officinalis), *Zhi Shi* (Fructus Aurantii Immaturus), and *Da Huang* (Radix et Rhizoma Rhei). In addition, *San Leng* (Rhizoma Sparganii), *E Zhu* (Rhizoma Curcumae), and *Bing Lang* (Semen Arecae) were added for individuals who were otherwise healthy, as they are too strong for individuals with deficiencies. The duration of treatment ranged from 20-30 days. The largest stone identified was 12 x 20 cm.[4]

HERB-DRUG INTERACTION

Chemotherapy-induced gastrointestinal side-effects: Use of modified *Bao He Wan* relieved gastrointestinal side effects associated with chemotherapy in cancer patients in one study. In addition to *Bao He Wan*, modifications were made by adding *Huang Qi* (Radix Astragali) and *Bai Zhu* (Rhizoma Atractylodis Macrocephalae) for fatigue and poor appetite; *Da Huang* (Radix et Rhizoma Rhei) [processed with grain-based liquor] for yellow tongue coating with constipation; *Sha Shen* (Radix Glehniae seu Adenophorae), *Mai Dong* (Radix Ophiopogonis), and *Shi Hu* (Caulis Dendrobii) for thirst and red tongue body with dry tongue coating. The treatment protocol was to administer the herbs in decoction for 10 days. Of 110 patients, 105 had complete recovery and 5 had improvement.[5]

TOXICOLOGY

According to one study on acute toxicology, administration of *Bao He Wan* at 120 g/kg via oral ingestion twice daily for 7 days did not contribute to any abnormal reactions in mice. Similarly, administration of this formula in adults at 650 times the normal dose did not contribute to any abnormal reactions. Furthermore, in one study on chronic toxicology, daily administration of this formula at 8, 16 and 32 g/kg one time daily for 4 weeks caused no abnormalities in blood tests or internal organs such as liver, kidneys, heart, stomach, and intestines.[6]

SUGGESTED ACUPUNCTURE TREATMENT

1. Points: *Xiawan* (CV 10), *Liangmen* (ST 21), *Xuanji* (CV 21), *Housanli* (ST 36), *Tianshu* (ST 25), *Qihai* (CV 6), *Zhongwan* (CV 12), *Neiguan* (PC 6), *Fengchi* (GB 20), *Shangen* and *Mijiaogan*.
2. Technique: sedation.

When treating indigestion, the goals are to promote digestion and harmonize the Stomach. *Xiawan* (CV 10), *Liangmen* (ST 21), and *Xuanji* (CV 21) activate qi to promote digestion. *Housanli* (ST 36) harmonizes the Stomach and stops nausea. *Tianshu* (ST 25) relieves epigastric and abdominal problems such as fullness, rigidity, distention, pain, and diarrhea. *Qihai* (CV 6) and *Zhongwan* (CV 12) relieve stagnation in the Stomach and distention in the abdomen. *Neiguan* (PC 6) alleviates nausea. *Fengchi* (GB 20) is used as a preventive measure to clear heat, which generally occurs as a result of food stagnation. To stimulate appetite, needle *Shangen* and *Mijiaogan*, which are classical points in dogs and horses, respectively.

AUTHORS' COMMENTS

Bao He Wan is designed for mild to moderate cases of food stagnation and indigestion, in which *zheng* (upright) *qi* is not yet damaged. The idea that overeating injures the middle *jiao* was first discussed in the *Huang Di Nei Jing* (Yellow Emperor's Inner Classic) in the first or second century A.D. Key clinical signs include abdominal bloating and pain, acid regurgitation, belching and/or flatulence with a rotten smell, nausea, vomiting, poor appetite, a red tongue with a greasy, white to yellow coating in severe cases, and a slippery pulse. The primary pathology involves stagnation of qi and food, which causes Stomach qi to rebel and rise upward. This formula is not appropriate for animals with food stagnation arising from underlying Spleen deficiency. It has minimal heat-clearing abilities, and if damp-heat is a concern, then other herbs or another formula must be added to address these pathogenic factors.

Acute food stagnation is often seen in dogs and horses that gorge. After the immediate situation has resolved from treatment with *Bao He Wan*, it is often recommended to follow the treatment with the formula *Xiang Sha Liu Jun*

Bǎo Hé Wán (Preserve Harmony Pill)

Zi Tang (Six-Gentlemen Decoction with Aucklandia and Amomum) to strengthen the Spleen. In cases in which there is obvious damp-heat, it can be combined with *Zhi Shi Dao Zhi Wan* (Immature Bitter Orange Pill to Guide Out Stagnation).

Chronic cases of food accumulation and stagnation with underlying Spleen qi deficiency and poor digestion commonly develop in dogs and cats fed poor-quality, commercial dry food diets and horses fed excessive quantities of concentrated feeds. In mild cases, it is best to add *Bai Zhu* (Rhizoma Atractylodis Macrocephalae) and *Huang Qi* (Radix Astragali) to enhance the overall function of the formula to tonify and strengthen the Spleen. Clinically, it may also be used in geriatric and cancer patients that are chronically medicated and have food stagnation with qi deficiency and poor digestion.

Classic texts use the term "dissolve" to describe herbs that treat indigestion and food stagnation. However, these herbs do not literally "dissolve" foods; rather, they stimulate the gastrointestinal tract and facilitate food digestion, thereby reducing accumulation and stagnation.

References

1. *Zhong Yao Ming Fang Yao Li Yu Ying Yong* (Pharmacology and Applications of Famous Herbal Formulas), 1989; 619-620.
2. *Fu Jian Zhong Yi Yao* (Fujian Chinese Medicine and Herbology), 1985; 3(8):18.
3. *Hu Bei Zhong Yi Za Zhi* (Hubei Journal of Chinese Medicine), 1992; 6:10.
4. *Shan Dong Zhong Yi Za Zhi* (Shandong Journal of Chinese Medicine), 1993; 4:21.
5. *Zhong Yi Yao Xin Xi* (Information on Chinese Medicine and Herbology), 1995; 12(6):45.
6. *Zhong Yi Yao Xin Xi* (Information on Chinese Medicine and Herbology), 1995; 11:25.

Zhǐ Shí Dǎo Zhì Wán

(Immature Bitter Orange Pill to Guide Out Stagnation)

枳實導滯丸
枳实导滞丸

Pinyin Name: *Zhi Shi Dao Zhi Wan*
Literal Name: Immature Bitter Orange Pill to Guide Out Stagnation
Original Source: *Nei Wai Shang Bian Huo Lun* (Clarifying Doubts about Injury from Internal and External Causes) by Li Gao in 1247

COMPOSITION

Da Huang (Radix et Rhizoma Rhei)	30g [9g]
Zhi Shi (Fructus Aurantii Immaturus), *chao* (dry-fried) with bran	15g [9g]
Huang Lian (Rhizoma Coptidis)	9g [6g]
Huang Qin (Radix Scutellariae)	9g [6g]
Fu Ling (Poria)	9g [6g]
Ze Xie (Rhizoma Alismatis)	6g [6g]
Bai Zhu (Rhizoma Atractylodis Macrocephalae)	9g [6g]
Shen Qu (Massa Fermentata), *chao* (dry-fried)	15g [9g]

DOSAGE / PREPARATION / ADMINISTRATION

The source text states to grind the ingredients into a fine powder and form into small pills with water. The pills should resemble the size of *Wu Tong Zi* (Semen Firmianae), a small seed approximately 5 mm in diameter. Take 50-70 pills per dose, between meals with warm water. Adjust the dose depending on the severity of the condition. Today, this formula may be taken as pills or decoction. For pills,

Zhǐ Shí Dǎo Zhì Wán

(Immature Bitter Orange Pill to Guide Out Stagnation)

grind the herbs into powder and form into small pills with water. Take 6-9g of pills per dose with warm, boiled water twice daily. For decoction, use the suggested doses in brackets.

CHINESE THERAPEUTIC ACTIONS

1. Reduces, guides out, and dissolves stagnation
2. Clears heat and dispels dampness

CLINICAL MANIFESTATIONS

Food stagnation and damp-heat accumulation in the Stomach and Intestines: bloating and pain in the epigastric and abdominal regions, diarrhea or constipation, scanty, dark urine, a red tongue that in severe cases may have a white to yellow, greasy coating, and a deep, forceful and/or slippery pulse.

VETERINARY CLINICAL APPLICATIONS

Acute or chronic gastroenteritis, food poisoning, diarrhea, inflammatory bowel disease, and chronic constipation.

EXPLANATION

Zhi Shi Dao Zhi Wan (Immature Bitter Orange Pill to Guide Out Stagnation) treats food stagnation and damp-heat accumulation in the Stomach and Intestines. Stagnation of food and damp-heat may lead to qi stagnation, which may result in abdominal bloating and pain in the epigastric and abdominal regions. Diarrhea may occur as a result of indigestion and formation of damp-heat in the Intestines, while constipation may occur as a result of interior heat drying body fluids. Scanty, dark urine results when interior heat consumes body fluids. A red, greasy tongue and a deep, slippery and/or forceful pulse indicate stagnation of food and damp-heat.

This formula uses *Da Huang* (Radix et Rhizoma Rhei) to purge stagnant food and damp-heat, as well as to remove any harmful retention through defecation. *Zhi Shi* (Fructus Aurantii Immaturus) breaks up qi and food stagnation to reduce epigastric and abdominal fullness and pain. *Huang Lian* (Rhizoma Coptidis) and *Huang Qin* (Radix Scutellariae) clear heat, dry dampness, and relieve diarrhea. *Fu Ling* (Poria) and *Ze Xie* (Rhizoma Alismatis) regulate water circulation and dispel dampness. *Bai Zhu* (Rhizoma Atractylodis Macrocephalae) strengthens the Spleen and dries dampness. In addition, *Bai Zhu* (Rhizoma Atractylodis Macrocephalae) prevents the bitter and cold herbs from damaging the body. *Shen Qu* (Massa Fermentata) helps digest stagnant food and harmonizes the middle *jiao*.

VETERINARY MODIFICATIONS

- For more severe fullness, distention and rectal tenesmus due to qi stagnation, add *Mu Xiang* (Radix Aucklandiae) and *Bing Lang* (Semen Arecae).
- With diarrhea and dysentery due to toxic heat, add *Jin Yin Hua* (Flos Lonicerae Japonicae) and *Bai Tou Weng* (Radix Pulsatillae).
- With nausea and vomiting or reflux, add *Zhu Ru* (Caulis Bambusae in Taenia).

***Zhi Shi Dao Zhi Wan* (Immature Bitter Orange Pill to Guide Out Stagnation)**

Diagnosis	Clinical Signs	Treatment	Herbs
Food stagnation and damp-heat accumulation in the Stomach and Intestines	• Bloating and pain in the epigastric and abdominal regions: food and qi stagnation • Diarrhea: damp-heat in the Intestines • Constipation: interior heat drying body fluids • Scanty, dark urine: interior heat consuming body fluids • Red tongue with a white to yellow, greasy coating and a deep, slippery and/or forceful pulse: damp-heat in the interior	• Reduces, guides out, and dissolves stagnation • Clears heat and dispels dampness	• *Da Huang* (Radix et Rhizoma Rhei) purges the stagnant food and clears excess heat. • *Zhi Shi* (Fructus Aurantii Immaturus) breaks up qi and food stagnation. • *Huang Lian* (Rhizoma Coptidis) and *Huang Qin* (Radix Scutellariae) clear heat and dry dampness. • *Fu Ling* (Poria) and *Ze Xie* (Rhizoma Alismatis) regulate water circulation and dispel dampness. • *Bai Zhu* (Rhizoma Atractylodis Macrocephalae) strengthens the Spleen and dries dampness. • *Shen Qu* (Massa Fermentata) helps digest stagnant food and harmonizes the middle *jiao*.

Zhǐ Shí Dǎo Zhì Wán

(Immature Bitter Orange Pill to Guide Out Stagnation)

CAUTIONS / CONTRAINDICATIONS

- *Zhi Shi Dao Zhi Wan* is contraindicated in patients with loose stools or diarrhea that do not have food stagnation. Such patients have deficient conditions without excess, and the use of formulas that contain *Da Huang* (Radix et Rhizoma Rhei) is not appropriate, as it may cause damages to the body.
- This formula should be used with caution in animals with food stagnation and indigestion due to Spleen deficiency, as many herbs in this formula are bitter and cold and may further injure the Spleen.
- Use of this formula is contraindicated in pregnancy.
- Avoid feeding of raw and cold foods while taking this formula.[1]

HUMAN CLINICAL STUDIES AND RESEARCH

Chronic constipation: One study evaluated the effectiveness of treating chronic constipation in 60 patients (mostly women, with history of chronic constipation for up to 20 years) via herbs and control group. The herb group had 31 patients, and the control group had 29 patients. The patients in the herb group were given *Zhi Shi Dao Zhi Wan* for 5 days. Of 31 patients in the herb group, 25 had significant improvement, 3 had moderate improvement, and 3 had no effect (90% effectiveness). Of 29 patients in the control group, 12 had significant improvement, 8 had moderate improvement, and 9 had no effect (70% effectiveness). The difference between the two groups was statistically significant ($p<0.05$).[2] The treatment protocol for the control group was unavailable at the time of publication.

SUGGESTED ACUPUNCTURE TREATMENT

1. Points: *Tianshu* (ST 25), *Shangjuxu* (ST 37), *Xiawan* (CV 10), *Xuanji* (CV 21), *Neiting* (ST 44), *Pangguangshu* (BL 28), *Zhongji* (CV 3), and *Yinlingquan* (SP 9).
2. Technique: sedation.

Tianshu (ST 25), the *mu* (collecting) point of the Stomach, and *Shangjuxu* (ST 37), the lower *he* (uniting) point of the Large Intestine, harmonize the Stomach and Large Intestine and dispel damp-heat through the Intestines. *Xiawan* (CV 10) and *Xuanji* (CV 21) activate qi and relieve food stagnation. *Neiting* (ST 44) clears heat and dries dampness. *Pangguangshu* (BL 28) and *Zhongji* (CV 3) regulate the Urinary Bladder to restore its normal functions. Finally, *Yinlingquan* (SP 9) strengthens the Spleen and dries dampness.

AUTHORS' COMMENTS

Zhi Shi Dao Zhi Wan is designed for acute or chronic, moderate to severe cases of food stagnation with damp-heat in the Stomach and Intestines. Patients usually present with a red tongue that may have a white to yellow, greasy coating in severe cases and a slippery and/or deep, forceful pulse. This formula is not commercially available, but can easily be made in house. It is can be used for the treatment of inflammatory bowel disease in dogs and cats. It can be used in combination with *Bao He Wan* (Preserve Harmony Pill) in the treatment of acute pancreatitis and cholecystitis, with the appropriate clinical signs.

Zhi Shi Dao Zhi Wan, *Mu Xiang Bing Lang Wan* (Aucklandia and Betel Nut Pill), *Jian Pi Wan* (Strengthen the Spleen Pill), and *Zhi Shi Xiao Pi Wan* (Immature Bitter Orange Pill to Reduce Focal Distention) all treat food stagnation and poor digestion:

- *Zhi Shi Dao Zhi Wan* removes stagnation. It focuses more on relieving constipation or diarrhea and abdominal bloating than on strengthening the Spleen and Stomach. It has a better ability to tonify the Spleen and clear dampness and a milder action to resolve food stagnation and bloating than *Mu Xiang Bing Lang Wan*.
- *Mu Xiang Bing Lang Wan* has a stronger action to activate qi and treat qi stagnation. It is used for more serious cases of stagnation and accumulation, with severe abdominal bloating, diarrhea or constipation, distention, and pain. Once the clinical signs have resolved, it should be discontinued and a milder formula given to consolidate the effects of the treatment.
- *Jian Pi Wan* primarily tonifies the Spleen and resolves diarrhea; it secondarily relieves food stagnation. It has the weakest ability of the four formulas to relieve food stagnation, but it has more tonic properties, which make it a better choice for weak, chronically ill and geriatric patients. It can be given longer term.
- *Zhi Shi Xiao Pi Wan* primarily removes stagnation and relieves fullness and distention; it secondarily strengthens the Spleen and Stomach.

References

1. *Zhong Yao Ming Fang Yao Li Yu Ying Yong* (Pharmacology and Applications of Famous Herbal Formulas), 1989; 623.
2. *Zhe Jiang Zhong Yi Xue Yuan Xue Bao* (Journal of Zhejiang University of Chinese Medicine), 1996; 2:28.

Mù Xiāng Bīng Láng Wán (Aucklandia and Betel Nut Pill)

木香檳榔丸
木香槟榔丸

Pinyin Name: *Mu Xiang Bing Lang Wan*
Literal Name: Aucklandia and Betel Nut Pill
Alternate Name: Saussurea and Areca Seed Formula
Original Source: *Ru Men Shi Qin* (Confucians' Duties to their Parents) by Zhang Cong-Zheng in 1228

COMPOSITION

Mu Xiang (Radix Aucklandiae)	30g [3g]
Bing Lang (Semen Arecae)	30g [3g]
Qian Niu Zi (Semen Pharbitidis)	120g [10g]
Da Huang (Radix et Rhizoma Rhei)	90g [5g]
Qing Pi (Pericarpium Citri Reticulatae Viride)	30g [3g]
Chen Pi (Pericarpium Citri Reticulatae)	30g [3g]
Xiang Fu (Rhizoma Cyperi), *chao* (dry-fried)	120g [10g]
E Zhu (Rhizoma Curcumae), *shao* (burned)	30g [3g]
Huang Lian (Rhizoma Coptidis), *chao* (dry-fried) with bran	30g [3g]
Huang Bo (Cortex Phellodendri Chinensis)	90g [5g]

DOSAGE / PREPARATION / ADMINISTRATION

The source text states to grind the ingredients into a fine powder and form into small pills with water. The pills should resemble small beans in size. Take 30 pills [6g] after meals with a decoction made from *Sheng Jiang* (Rhizoma Zingiberis Recens). Today, this formula may be taken as pills or decoction. For pills, grind the herbs into powder and form into small pills with water. Take 3-6g of pills per dose with warm, boiled water twice daily. For decoction, use the suggested doses in brackets.

CHINESE THERAPEUTIC ACTIONS

1. Activates qi circulation and guides out stagnation
2. Attacks accumulation and purges heat

CLINICAL MANIFESTATIONS

Food stagnation and damp-heat accumulation: fullness, bloating and pain in the epigastric and abdominal regions, dysentery with red (blood) or white (mucus) stools, tenesmus, constipation, a red tongue that in severe cases may have a white to yellow, greasy coating, and a rapid, deep, excess pulse.

VETERINARY CLINICAL APPLICATIONS

Acute gastroenteritis, dietary indiscretion, acute impaction and constipation, diarrhea.

EXPLANATION

Mu Xiang Bing Lang Wan (Aucklandia and Betel Nut Pill) treats qi stagnation and damp-heat accumulation due to food stagnation. Food stagnation can cause qi stagnation, which may lead to fullness, bloating, and pain in the epigastric and abdominal regions, as well as constipation. Food stagnation may also lead to damp-heat accumulation, which often descends to the lower *jiao* to cause dysentery and tenesmus. A red tongue with a yellow, greasy tongue coating suggests damp-heat in the interior, and the rapid, deep, excess pulse is a sign of constipation and food stagnation.

In this formula, *Mu Xiang* (Radix Aucklandiae) and *Bing Lang* (Semen Arecae) activate qi circulation and break up stagnation to relieve epigastric and abdominal fullness, distention, and pain. *Qian Niu Zi* (Semen Pharbitidis) and *Da Huang* (Radix et Rhizoma Rhei) purge damp-heat and reduce stagnation and accumulation. *Qing Pi* (Pericarpium Citri Reticulatae Viride) and *Chen Pi* (Pericarpium Citri Reticulatae) activate qi circulation to relieve qi stagnation. *Xiang Fu* (Rhizoma Cyperi) and *E Zhu* (Rhizoma Curcumae) smooth the qi flow to relieve pain. *Huang Lian* (Rhizoma Coptidis) and *Huang Bo* (Cortex Phellodendri Chinensis) clear heat and dry dampness to stop dysentery.

VETERINARY MODIFICATIONS

- With qi stagnation in the chest and food retention in the abdomen, add *Zhi Qiao* (Fructus Aurantii).
- For severe constipation, add *Mang Xiao* (Natrii Sulfas) and *Zhi Qiao* (Fructus Aurantii).
- For severe bloating, add *Zhi Qiao* (Fructus Aurantii).
- For damp-heat dysentery, remove *Chen Pi* (Pericarpium Citri Reticulatae), *E Zhu* (Rhizoma Curcumae), *Qian Niu*

Mù Xiāng Bīng Láng Wán (Aucklandia and Betel Nut Pill)

***Mu Xiang Bing Lang Wan* (Aucklandia and Betel Nut Pill)**

Diagnosis	Clinical Signs	Treatment	Herbs
Food stagnation and damp-heat accumulation	• Bloating and pain in the epigastric and abdominal regions: food and qi stagnation • Dysentery and tenesmus with red [blood] or white [mucus] stools: damp-heat accumulation in the lower *jiao* • Constipation: food stagnation • A red tongue with a yellow, greasy tongue coating: damp-heat in the interior	• Activates qi circulation and guides out stagnation • Attacks accumulation • Sedates heat	• *Mu Xiang* (Radix Aucklandiae) and *Bing Lang* (Semen Arecae) activate qi circulation and break up stagnation. • *Qian Niu Zi* (Semen Pharbitidis) and *Da Huang* (Radix et Rhizoma Rhei) purge damp-heat and reduce stagnation and accumulation. • *Qing Pi* (Pericarpium Citri Reticulatae Viride) and *Chen Pi* (Pericarpium Citri Reticulatae) activate qi circulation to relieve qi stagnation. • *Xiang Fu* (Rhizoma Cyperi) and *E Zhu* (Rhizoma Curcumae) smooth the qi flow to relieve pain. • *Huang Lian* (Rhizoma Coptidis) and *Huang Bo* (Cortex Phellodendri Chinensis) clear heat and dry dampness.

Zi (Semen Pharbitidis), and add *Qin Pi* (Cortex Fraxini) and *Bai Tou Weng* (Radix Pulsatillae).

- With phlegm accumulation, add *Ban Xia* (Rhizoma Pinelliae) and *Fu Ling* (Poria).
- With damp-heat accumulation, add *Yin Chen* (Herba Artemisiae Scopariae) and *Zhi Zi* (Fructus Gardeniae).
- With significant pain, add *Yan Hu Suo* (Rhizome Corydalis).

CAUTIONS / CONTRAINDICATIONS

- *Mu Xiang Bing Lang Wan* contains potent herbs to activate qi circulation, clear heat, and eliminate stagnation and accumulation. It should be reserved for animals with excess conditions without underlying deficiencies. The use of this formula is contraindicated in deficient patients (especially those with Spleen and Stomach deficiencies), as this formula will injure *zheng* (upright) *qi* and complicate the illness.
- This formula is contraindicated during pregnancy. It should be used with caution in geriatric individuals with generalized weakness and deficiencies.[1]

HUMAN CLINICAL STUDIES AND RESEARCH

1. **Stenosis of colon and rectum**: Administration of 10g of *Mu Xiang Bing Lang Wan* twice daily in 23 patients with stenosis of colon and rectum was associated with good results. Depending on the severity of the condition, the duration of treatment ranged from 3 months to 1 year. Of 23 patients, 13 had complete recovery, 7 had improvement, and 3 had no response. The overall effectiveness was 87%.[2]
2. **Acute abdomen**: Administration of *Mu Xiang Bing Lang Wan* was reported in 2 case studies to be effective for treatment of acute abdomen.[3]

SUGGESTED ACUPUNCTURE TREATMENT

1. Points: *Hegu* (LI 4), *Tianshu* (ST 25), *Shangjuxu* (ST 37), *Weishu* (BL 21), *Zhongwan* (CV 12), and *Neiting* (ST 44).
2. Technique: sedation.

The objectives of this acupuncture treatment are to dispel damp-heat and promote digestion. *Hegu* (LI 4), the *yuan* (source) point of the Large Intestine, *Tianshu* (ST 25), the *mu* (collecting) point of the Large Intestine, and *Shangjuxu* (ST 37), the lower *he* (uniting) point of the Large Intestine, all dispel damp-heat, regulate qi and blood, and promote digestion. *Weishu* (BL 21) and *Zhongwan* (CV 12) help to regulate Stomach qi. *Neiting* (ST 44), the *ying* (spring) point of the Stomach, supplements *Hegu* (LI 4) in clearing heat from the *yangming* channel.

AUTHORS' COMMENTS

Mu Xiang Bing Lang Wan is one of the strongest formulas for dispelling food stagnation; it treats cases involving epigastric and abdominal bloating and pain. It should be discontinued when the excess has been cleared, and a milder formula, such as *Bao He Wan,* should be given to consolidate the effects of the treatment.

Zhi Shi Dao Zhi Wan (Immature Bitter Orange Pill to Guide Out Stagnation) and *Mu Xiang Bing Lang Wan* both treat food stagnation with damp-heat accumulation.

Mù Xiāng Bīng Láng Wán (Aucklandia and Betel Nut Pill)

- *Zhi Shi Dao Zhi Wan* has a stronger action to dispel dampness and relieve constipation or diarrhea; it is more tonic in nature. It is used for mild to moderate cases of stagnation and accumulation, with abdominal bloating.
- *Mu Xiang Bing Lang Wan* has a stronger action to activate qi and treat qi stagnation. It is used for more serious cases of stagnation and accumulation, with severe abdominal bloating, pain, and constipation or diarrhea.

References

1. *Zhong Yao Ming Fang Yao Li Yu Ying Yong* (Pharmacology and Applications of Famous Herbal Formulas), 1989; 624.
2. *Guang Xi Zhong Yi Yao* (Guangxi Chinese Medicine and Herbology), 1999; 2:33.
3. *Jiang Su Zhong Yi* (Jiangsu Chinese Medicine), 1982; 6:3.

Jiàn Pí Wán (Strengthen the Spleen Pill)
健脾丸

Pinyin Name: *Jian Pi Wan*
Literal Name: Strengthen the Spleen Pill
Alternate Names: *Chian Pi Wan*, Spleen-Strengthening Pill
Original Source: *Zheng Zhi Zhun Sheng* (Standards of Patterns and Treatments) by Wang Ken-Tang in 1602

COMPOSITION

Ren Shen (Radix et Rhizoma Ginseng)	45g [9g]
Bai Zhu (Rhizoma Atractylodis Macrocephalae), *chao* (dry-fried)	75g [15g]
Fu Ling (Poria)	60g [10g]
Gan Cao (Radix et Rhizoma Glycyrrhizae)	22.5g [6g]
Shan Yao (Rhizoma Dioscoreae)	30g [6g]
Rou Dou Kou (Semen Myristicae), oil removed	30g [6g]
Shan Zha (Fructus Crataegi)	30g [6g]
Shen Qu (Massa Fermentata), *chao* (dry-fried)	30g [6g]
Mai Ya (Fructus Hordei Germinatus), *chao* (dry-fried)	30g [6g]
Mu Xiang (Radix Aucklandiae), *yan* (ground) to small particles	22.5g [6g]
Sha Ren (Fructus Amomi)	30g [6g]
Chen Pi (Pericarpium Citri Reticulatae)	30g [6g]
Huang Lian (Rhizoma Coptidis), *chao* (dry-fried) with liquor	22.5g [6g]

DOSAGE / PREPARATION / ADMINISTRATION

The source text states to grind the ingredients into a fine powder. Steam the powder and form it into pills, which should resemble *Lu Dou* (Semen Phaseoli Radiati) in size. Take 50 pills per dose, twice daily with rice soup on an empty stomach. Today, this formula may be taken as pills or decoction. For pills, grind the herbs into powder and form into pills with water. Take 6-9g of pills per dose with warm, boiled water twice daily. For decoction, use the suggested doses in brackets.

CHINESE THERAPEUTIC ACTIONS

1. Strengthens the Spleen and harmonizes the Stomach
2. Reduces food stagnation and stops diarrhea

Jiàn Pí Wán (Strengthen the Spleen Pill)

CLINICAL MANIFESTATIONS

Food stagnation and interior heat accumulation due to Spleen and Stomach deficiencies: nausea, lethargy, decreased food intake, chronic indigestion and food stagnation, abdominal and epigastric bloating, borborygmus, loose stools and diarrhea, a greasy tongue coating, and a deficient, weak pulse.

VETERINARY CLINICAL APPLICATIONS

Poor digestion, poor appetite and gastroenteritis secondary to organ failure, chemotherapy and cancer, inflammatory bowel disease and diarrhea.

EXPLANATION

When the Spleen and Stomach are deficient, food cannot be digested properly. The undigested food may accumulate and stagnate in the middle *jiao*. As a result of food stagnation, there will be poor appetite and abdominal bloating. Food stagnation creates damp accumulation, which may travel downward and cause loose stools and diarrhea with undigested food. Food stagnation may also create interior heat, which may cause the tongue coating to appear slightly yellow. A greasy tongue coating suggests dampness and food accumulation, and a deficient, weak pulse reflects Spleen and Stomach deficiencies.

Jian Pi Wan (Strengthen the Spleen Pill) is formulated following the principles of *Si Jun Zi Tang* (Four-Gentlemen Decoction): *Ren Shen* (Radix et Rhizoma Ginseng), *Bai Zhu* (Rhizoma Atractylodis Macrocephalae), *Fu Ling* (Poria), and *Gan Cao* (Radix et Rhizoma Glycyrrhizae) tonify qi, strengthen the Spleen and Stomach, dispel dampness, and relieve diarrhea. *Shan Yao* (Rhizoma Dioscoreae) and *Rou Dou Kou* (Semen Myristicae) strengthen the Spleen and stop diarrhea. *Shan Zha* (Fructus Crataegi), *Shen Qu* (Massa Fermentata), and *Mai Ya* (Fructus Hordei Germinatus) promote digestion and reduce food stagnation. *Mu Xiang* (Radix Aucklandiae), *Sha Ren* (Fructus Amomi), and *Chen Pi* (Pericarpium Citri Reticulatae) activate qi circulation and harmonize the Stomach. *Huang Lian* (Rhizoma Coptidis) clears interior heat and dries dampness.

VETERINARY MODIFICATIONS

- With Spleen qi deficiency accompanied by coldness and food stagnation, remove *Huang Lian* (Rhizoma Coptidis) and add *Gan Jiang* (Rhizoma Zingiberis).
- With severe damp accumulation, add *Che Qian Zi* (Semen Plantaginis) and *Ze Xie* (Rhizoma Alismatis).
- With nausea and vomiting, add *Ban Xia* (Rhizoma Pinelliae) and *Ding Xiang* (Flos Caryophylli).

CAUTIONS / CONTRAINDICATIONS

Jian Pi Wan is designed to treat food stagnation due to Spleen and Stomach deficiencies. It should not be used to treat food stagnation due to overindulgence in foods, which is an excess condition. Using this formula in an excess condition can potentially aggravate the condition.

SUGGESTED ACUPUNCTURE TREATMENT

1. Points: *Pishu* (BL 20), *Zhangmen* (LR 13), *Weishu* (BL 21), *Zhongwan* (CV 12), *Housanli* (ST 36), *Gongsun* (SP 4), *Yinlingquan* (SP 9), *Neiting* (ST 44), *Shangen* and *Mijiaogan*.

***Jian Pi Wan* (Strengthen the Spleen Pill)**

Diagnosis	Clinical Signs	Treatment	Herbs
Food stagnation and interior heat accumulation due to Spleen and Stomach deficiencies	• Abdominal bloating and borborygmus: food stagnation • Lethargy, poor appetite, decreased food intake, and undigested food in the stools: Spleen and Stomach deficiencies • Loose stools and diarrhea: dampness traveling downward • Greasy tongue coating: dampness • Deficient, weak pulse: deficiency condition	• Strengthens the Spleen and harmonizes the Stomach • Reduces food stagnation and stops diarrhea	• *Ren Shen* (Radix et Rhizoma Ginseng), *Bai Zhu* (Rhizoma Atractylodis Macrocephalae), *Fu Ling* (Poria) and *Gan Cao* (Radix et Rhizoma Glycyrrhizae) tonify qi, strengthen the Spleen and Stomach, dispel dampness, and relieve diarrhea. • *Shan Yao* (Rhizoma Dioscoreae) and *Rou Dou Kou* (Semen Myristicae) strengthen the Spleen and stop diarrhea. • *Shan Zha* (Fructus Crataegi), *Shen Qu* (Massa Fermentata), and *Mai Ya* (Fructus Hordei Germinatus) promote digestion and reduce food stagnation. • *Mu Xiang* (Radix Aucklandiae), *Sha Ren* (Fructus Amomi), and *Chen Pi* (Pericarpium Citri Reticulatae) activate qi and harmonize the Stomach. • *Huang Lian* (Rhizoma Coptidis) clears interior heat and dries dampness.

Jiàn Pí Wán (Strengthen the Spleen Pill)

2. Technique: tonification and/or aquapuncture with vitamin B12.

The objectives are to strengthen the Spleen, harmonize the Stomach, promote digestion, and clear interior heat. *Pishu* (BL 20), the *shu* (transport) point of the Spleen, and *Zhangmen* (LR 13), the *mu* (collecting) point of the Spleen, strengthen the Spleen to promote digestion. *Weishu* (BL 21), the *shu* (transport) point of the Stomach, and *Zhongwan* (CV 12), the *mu* (collecting) point of the Stomach, harmonize the Stomach to remove food stagnation. *Housanli* (ST 36) and *Gongsun* (SP 4) enhance the effects of the above points. *Yinlingquan* (SP 9) dispels dampness and stops diarrhea. Finally, *Neiting* (ST 44) clears heat from the *yangming* channel, which frequently becomes excessive as a result of food stagnation. *Shangen* and *Mijiaogen* are classical points in dogs and horses, respectively, and are very useful in stimulating appetite.

AUTHORS' COMMENTS

Jian Pi Wan literally means "Strengthen the Spleen Pill," because the primary function of this formula is to strengthen the Spleen; and Spleen qi deficiency is often the primary cause of food stagnation. It is a commonly used gastrointestinal formulas in veterinary medicine. It is often prescribed to improve appetite in veterinary patients with deficiency and stagnation from chronic medication, chemotherapy or radiation therapy, chronic illness (cancer, liver or kidney failure), and aging. In contrast to *Bao He Wan* (Preserve Harmony Pill), which treats food stagnation arising from excess, *Jian Pi Wan* is used to treat food stagnation and poor appetite arising from deficiency.

Jian Pi Wan is frequently used to treat cats with inflammatory bowel disease (IBD) characterized by poor appetite, vomiting, and weight loss. It should be given for an appropriate length of time to resolve the disorder. Some cats will require treatment for 4-6 months. A typical dose is 1-2 tea pills or 1 tablet twice daily; most cats will not eat herbs put into their food. In dogs with IBD, it can be used to strengthen the Spleen and act as a preventative measure between acute episodes. It is especially helpful in the treatment of poor appetite due to chemotherapy in cancer patients and for chronic renal failure or cholangiohepatitis in cats. Likewise, *Jian Pi Wan* is very useful in geriatric horses having trouble retaining weight and that are listless and anorexic.

Jian Pi Wan and *Si Jun Zi Tang* (Four-Gentlemen Decoction) both contain *Ren Shen* (Radix et Rhizoma Ginseng), *Bai Zhu* (Rhizoma Atractylodis Macrocephalae), *Fu Ling* (Poria), and *Gan Cao* (Radix et Rhizoma Glycyrrhizae) to tonify qi and strengthen the Spleen. The differences are as follows:

- *Jian Pi Wan* contains large doses of *Bai Zhu* (Rhizoma Atractylodis Macrocephalae) and *Fu Ling* (Poria) to strengthen the Spleen, resolve dampness, and stop diarrhea.
- *Si Jun Zi Tang* contains a larger dose of *Ren Shen* (Radix et Rhizoma Ginseng) to greatly tonify *yuan* (source) *qi*, strengthen the Spleen, and nourish the Stomach.

Section 2

消痞化积剂 — Reducing, Guiding, and Dissolving Formula that Relieves Distention

Zhǐ Shí Xiāo Pǐ Wán

(Immature Bitter Orange Pill to Reduce Focal Distention)

枳實消痞丸

枳实消痞丸

Pinyin Name: *Zhi Shi Xiao Pi Wan*
Literal Name: Immature Bitter Orange Pill to Reduce Focal Distention
Original Source: *Lan Shi Mi Cang* (Secrets from the Orchid Chamber) by Li Gao in 1336

COMPOSITION

Zhi Shi (Fructus Aurantii Immaturus)	15g
Hou Po (Cortex Magnoliae Officinalis), *zhi* (fried with liquid)	12g
Huang Lian (Rhizoma Coptidis)	15g
Ban Xia Qu (Rhizoma Pinelliae Massa Fermentata)	9g
Gan Jiang (Rhizoma Zingiberis)	3g
Ren Shen (Radix et Rhizoma Ginseng)	9g
Bai Zhu (Rhizoma Atractylodis Macrocephalae)	6g
Fu Ling (Poria)	6g
Mai Ya Qu (Fructus Hordei Germinatus Massa Fermentata)	6g
Zhi Gan Cao (Radix et Rhizoma Glycyrrhizae Praeparata cum Melle)	6g

DOSAGE / PREPARATION / ADMINISTRATION

The source text states to grind the ingredients into a fine powder and form into small pills with water. The pills should resemble the size of *Wu Tong Zi* (Semen Firmianae), a small seed approximately 5 mm in diameter. Take 50-70 pills with warm, boiled water between meals. Today, the ingredients are ground into powder and formed into small pills with water. Take 6-9g of pills per dose with warm, boiled water twice daily.

CHINESE THERAPEUTIC ACTIONS

1. Activates qi circulation and reduces fullness and distention
2. Strengthens the Spleen and harmonizes the Stomach

CLINICAL MANIFESTATIONS

Spleen deficiency complicated by qi stagnation and the interlocking of interior heat and cold: food stagnation, epigastric bloating, lack of appetite, lethargy, and irregular bowel movements with mild constipation.

VETERINARY CLINICAL APPLICATIONS

Chronic gastritis, indigestion, bloating, intestinal obstruction, cholelithiasis, and cholecystitis.

EXPLANATION

Zhi Shi Xiao Pi Wan (Immature Bitter Orange Pill to Reduce Focal Distention) treats epigastric bloating complicated with both deficiency and excess conditions. This condition begins with Spleen deficiency and compromised digestive functioning. As the food stagnates, it slowly causes phlegm accumulation, qi stagnation, and interlocking of heat and cold (more heat). Clinical manifestations include food stagnation, epigastric bloating, lethargy, lack of appetite and constipation.

Zhǐ Shí Xiāo Pǐ Wán

(Immature Bitter Orange Pill to Reduce Focal Distention)

***Zhi Shi Xiao Pi Wan* (Immature Bitter Orange Pill to Reduce Focal Distention)**

Diagnosis	Clinical Signs	Treatment	Herbs
Spleen deficiency complicated by qi stagnation and the interlocking of interior heat and cold	• Lack of appetite and lethargy: Spleen deficiency • Food stagnation, epigastric bloating: qi stagnation and phlegm accumulation • Irregular bowel movements: interlocking of heat and cold • Mild constipation: interior heat drying fluids	• Strengthens the Spleen and harmonizes the Stomach • Reduces fullness and distention	• *Zhi Shi* (Fructus Aurantii Immaturus) and *Hou Po* (Cortex Magnoliae Officinalis) activate qi circulation and relieve epigastric fullness and distention. • *Huang Lian* (Rhizoma Coptidis) clears heat and dries dampness. • *Ban Xia Qu* (Rhizoma Pinelliae Massa Fermentata) disperses interior dampness and cold, breaks up clumps, and harmonizes the Stomach. • *Gan Jiang* (Rhizoma Zingiberis) warms the Spleen and dispels cold. • *Ren Shen* (Radix et Rhizoma Ginseng), *Bai Zhu* (Rhizoma Atractylodis Macrocephalae), and *Fu Ling* (Poria) strengthen the Spleen and dry dampness. • *Mai Ya Qu* (Fructus Hordei Germinatus Massa Fermentata) improves digestion and harmonizes the Stomach. • *Zhi Gan Cao* (Radix et Rhizoma Glycyrrhizae Praeparata cum Melle) harmonizes the herbs.

The treatment plan for this syndrome is to activate qi, strengthen the Spleen, and regulate the cold and heat. This formula contains *Zhi Shi* (Fructus Aurantii Immaturus) to break up qi stagnation and reduce epigastric distention. *Hou Po* (Cortex Magnoliae Officinalis) activates qi circulation to relieve epigastric fullness. As a pair, *Zhi Shi* (Fructus Aurantii Immaturus) and *Hou Po* (Cortex Magnoliae Officinalis) have a synergistic effect to regulate qi and relieve both fullness and distention. *Huang Lian* (Rhizoma Coptidis) clears heat and dries dampness. *Ban Xia Qu* (Rhizoma Pinelliae Massa Fermentata) disperses interior dampness and cold, breaks up clumps, and harmonizes the Stomach. A small amount of *Gan Jiang* (Rhizoma Zingiberis) warms the Spleen and dispels cold. *Ren Shen* (Radix et Rhizoma Ginseng), *Bai Zhu* (Rhizoma Atractylodis Macrocephalae), and *Fu Ling* (Poria) strengthen the Spleen and dry dampness. *Mai Ya Qu* (Fructus Hordei Germinatus Massa Fermentata) improves digestion and harmonizes the Stomach. *Zhi Gan Cao* (Radix et Rhizoma Glycyrrhizae Praeparata cum Melle) harmonizes all of the herbs in the formula.

VETERINARY MODIFICATIONS

With epigastric and abdominal pain due to cold, reduce the dose of *Huang Lian* (Rhizoma Coptidis), increase the dose of *Gan Jiang* (Rhizoma Zingiberis), and add *Rou Gui* (Cortex Cinnamomi) and *Gao Liang Jiang* (Rhizoma Alpiniae Officinarum).

CAUTIONS / CONTRAINDICATIONS

Although *Zhi Shi Xiao Pi Wan* has dual effects to purge excess (food stagnation) and tonify deficiency (Spleen deficiency), the main emphasis is to purge excess and clear heat. Therefore, it should be used with caution in patients with severe Spleen deficiency.

PHARMACOLOGICAL EFFECTS

Gastrointestinal: Use of *Zhi Shi Xiao Pi Wan* was associated with stimulating the gastrointestinal tract to increase peristalsis of the intestines and gastric emptying time.[1]

HUMAN CLINICAL STUDIES AND RESEARCH

1. **Chronic gastritis**: One study reported good results using modified *Zhi Shi Xiao Pi Wan* to treat chronic gastritis in 30 patients (22 males and 8 females, between 25-70 years of age, with 1-30 years history of illness). Modifications to the base herbal formula were made as needed. For Liver qi overacting on the Stomach, *Chai Hu* (Radix Bupleuri), *Chen Pi* (Pericarpium Citri Reticulatae), and *Dan Shen* (Radix et Rhizoma Salviae Miltiorrhizae) were added, and *Gan Jiang* (Rhizoma Zingiberis) was removed. For deficiency and cold of the Spleen and Stomach, *Pao*

Zhǐ Shí Xiāo Pǐ Wán

(Immature Bitter Orange Pill to Reduce Focal Distention)

Jiang (Rhizoma Zingiberis Praeparatum) and *Gui Zhi* (Ramulus Cinnamomi) were added, and *Huang Lian* (Rhizoma Coptidis) and *Dan Shen* (Radix et Rhizoma Salviae Miltiorrhizae) were removed. For damp-heat affecting the Spleen and Stomach, *Mu Dan Pi* (Cortex Moutan) and *Zhi Zi* (Fructus Gardeniae) were added. Of 30 patients, the study reported a marked effect in 26 cases, improvement in 3 cases, and no effect in 1 case.[2]

2. **Chronic atrophic gastritis**: One study reported good results using modified *Zhi Shi Xiao Pi Wan* to treat chronic atrophic gastritis in 45 patients. The herbal treatment contained this formula, with modifications based on the condition of the individual patients. For excess heat, the dose of *Huang Lian* (Rhizoma Coptidis) was increased and the dose of *Gan Jiang* (Rhizoma Zingiberis) was reduced. For excess cold, the dose of *Huang Lian* (Rhizoma Coptidis) was decreased and the dose of *Gan Jiang* (Rhizoma Zingiberis) was increased. For frequent belching, *Xuan Fu Hua* (Flos Inulae) was added. The herbs were given three times daily for 1 month per course of treatment, and the patients were monitored for 1 year. Of 45 patients, the study reported significant improvement in 23 cases, improvement in 20 cases, and no effect in 2 cases. The overall effectiveness was 95.6%.[3]
3. **Indigestion**: Use of *Zhi Shi Xiao Pi Wan* was associated with 94.74% effectiveness in treating non-ulcerative indigestion. In addition to the base formula, modifications were made as needed. For Stomach yin deficiency, *Yu Zhu* (Rhizoma Polygonati Odorati) and *Shi Hu* (Caulis Dendrobii) were added, and *Ban Xia* (Rhizoma Pinelliae) and *Sheng Jiang* (Rhizoma Zingiberis Recens) were removed. For constipation, *Da Huang* (Radix et Rhizoma Rhei) and *Gua Lou* (Fructus Trichosanthis) were added. For pain in the upper abdominal area, *Mu Xiang* (Radix Aucklandiae) and *Yan Hu Suo* (Rhizoma Corydalis) were added. For burning sensations in the stomach with acid reflux, *Zuo Jin Wan* (Left Metal Pill) was added. For thick, greasy, white tongue coating, *Dou Kou* (Fructus Amomi Rotundus) was added, and *Bai Zhu* (Rhizoma Atractylodis Macrocephalae) was replaced with *Cang Zhu* (Rhizoma Atractylodis). The herbs were given for 4 weeks per course of treatment. Of 76 patients, the study reported complete recovery in 20 cases, significant improvement in 24 cases, moderate improvement in 28 cases, and no effect in 4 cases.[4]
4. **Intestinal obstruction**: *Zhi Shi Xiao Pi Wan* was used to treat 12 hospitalized patients (between 18-65 years of age) with intestinal obstruction for 1-3 days, associated with inappropriate diet. Modifications to the original formula included substitution of *Ren Shen* (Radix et Rhizoma Ginseng) with *Xi Yang Shen* (Radix Panacis Quinquefolii). Furthermore, *Chuan Lian Zi* (Fructus Toosendan) and *Yan Hu Suo* (Rhizoma Corydalis) were added for severe abdominal pain; *Shen Qu* (Massa Fermentata) and *Shan Zha* (Fructus Crataegi) for severe food stagnation; and *Shi Hu* (Caulis Dendrobii) and *Tian Hua Fen* (Radix Trichosanthis) for severe damage to body fluids. The treatment protocol was to cook the herbs and administer the formula in decoction twice daily. Of 12 patients, 11 had complete recovery, and 1 who did not respond was treated with surgery.[5]
5. **Cholelithiasis and cholecystitis**: Administration of modified *Zhi Shi Xiao Pi Wan* was associated with complete recovery in all 19 patients with cholelithiasis and cholecystitis. Modifications to the base formula included the addition of a larger dose of *Da Huang* (Radix et Rhizoma Rhei) for excess heat; *Chai Hu* (Radix Bupleuri) and *Yu Jin* (Radix Curcumae) for stabbing pain in the hypochondrium; *Zhu Ru* (Caulis Bambusae in Taenia) for nausea and vomiting; *Da Huang* (Radix et Rhizoma Rhei) and *Gua Lou* (Fructus Trichosanthis) for constipation with dry stools; and *Yin Chen* (Herba Artemisiae Scopariae) and *Zhi Zi* (Fructus Gardeniae) for jaundice. Each course of treatment was 5 days.[6]

SUGGESTED ACUPUNCTURE TREATMENT

1. Points: *Neiguan* (PC 6), *Xiawan* (CV 10), *Xuanji* (CV 21), *Shangjuxu* (ST 37), *Tianshu* (ST 25), *Dachangshu* (BL 25), *Housanli* (ST 36), *Pishu* (BL 20), *Yinlingquan* (SP 9), and *Neiting* (ST 44).
2. Technique: even method with moxibustion.

This formula treats a complicated condition, in which there are various problems including Spleen qi deficiency, qi stagnation, and accumulation of interior heat and cold. Therefore, the treatment should focus on strengthening the Spleen, regulating qi, and dispelling interior heat and cold. *Neiguan* (PC 6), *Xiawan* (CV 10) and *Xuanji* (CV 21) regulate qi circulation to relieve abdominal fullness and distention. *Shangjuxu* (ST 37), *Tianshu* (ST 25), *Dachangshu* (BL 25) are the Large Intestine *he* (sea), *mu* (collecting), and *shu* (association) points and promote motility. *Housanli* (ST 36) harmonizes the Stomach to promote digestion. *Pishu* (BL 20) and *Yinlingquan* (SP 9) strengthen the Spleen to dispel dampness. *Neiting* (ST 44) clears heat and dries dampness. Moderate moxibustion may be required to dispel interior cold, but excessive moxibustion should be avoided since this condition already involves interior heat accumulation.

Zhǐ Shí Xiāo Pǐ Wán

(Immature Bitter Orange Pill to Reduce Focal Distention)

AUTHORS' COMMENTS

Jian Pi Wan (Strengthen the Spleen Pill) and *Zhi Shi Xiao Pi Wan* are similar formulas that treat food stagnation and poor digestion, using both tonifying and reducing methods; they treat the combined presentation of both excess and deficiency:

- *Jian Pi Wan* primarily tonifies the Spleen and resolves diarrhea; it secondarily relieves food stagnation.
- *Zhi Shi Xiao Pi Wan* removes stagnation and relieves fullness and distention; it secondarily strengthens the Spleen and Stomach.

Zhi Shi Dao Zhi Wan (Immature Bitter Orange Pill to Guide Out Stagnation) and *Zhi Shi Xiao Pi Wan* (Immature Bitter Orange Pill to Reduce Focal Distention) have similar pinyin names and functions to reduce, guide out and dissolve stagnation and accumulation.

- *Zhi Shi Dao Zhi Wan* is more effective in treating the excess condition of food stagnation and damp-heat accumulation in the Stomach and Intestines.
- *Zhi Shi Xiao Pi Wan* is more suitable for both deficiency and excess conditions characterized by Spleen deficiency, qi stagnation, and the interlocking of interior heat and cold.

References

1. *An Hui Zhong Yi Xue Yuan Xue Bao* (Journal of Anhui University School of Medicine), 1991; 19(3):47.
2. *Zhong Yi Yao Xue Bao* (Report of Chinese Medicine and Herbology), 1991; 3:39.
3. *Shan Xi Zhong Yi* (Shanxi Chinese Medicine), 1997; 7:304.
4. *Si Chuan Zhong Yi* (Sichuan Chinese Medicine), 1998; 7:26.
5. *Zhong Yi Ming Fang Lin Chuang Xin Yong* (Contemporary Clinical Applications of Classic Chinese Formulas), 2001; 502.
6. *Hu Bei Zhong Yi Za Zhi* (Hubei Journal of Chinese Medicine), 1998; 5:38.

Chapter 19 — Summary

— Reducing, Guiding, and Dissolving Formulas

SECTION 1: REDUCING, GUIDING, AND DISSOLVING FORMULAS THAT TREAT FOOD STAGNATION

Name	Similarities	Differences
Bao He Wan (Preserve Harmony Pill)	Promotes digestion, harmonizes the Stomach	Mild to moderate action to treat food stagnation, indigestion and other digestive disorders
Zhi Shi Dao Zhi Wan (Immature Bitter Orange Pill to Guide Out Stagnation)	Reduce and dissolve stagnation, clear damp-heat	Moderate potency, stronger to dispel dampness and treat constipation or diarrhea
Mu Xiang Bing Lang Wan (Aucklandia and Betel Nut Pill)		Strong potency, stronger to activate qi circulation and treat constipation or diarrhea
Jian Pi Wan (Strengthen the Spleen Pill)	Strengthens the Spleen, reduces food stagnation	Strong potency, harmonizes the Stomach, stops diarrhea, and tonifies the Spleen

Bao He Wan (Preserve Harmony Pill) is the principal formula used for any kind of mild to moderate food stagnation, with clinical signs of vomiting, epigastric and abdominal bloating, aversion to food, and belching with a foul smell. It activates digestion and harmonizes the Stomach.

Zhi Shi Dao Zhi Wan (Immature Bitter Orange Pill to Guide Out Stagnation) and ***Mu Xiang Bing Lang Wan*** (Aucklandia and Betel Nut Pill) have similar functions of activating qi circulation and reducing and dissolving stagnation. They are stronger in action than *Bao He Wan* (Preserve Harmony Pill).

- *Zhi Shi Dao Zhi Wan* has a stronger damp-eliminating action. This formula is indicated for patients with stagnation of food and damp-heat in the Stomach and Intestines, causing abdominal pain and diarrhea.
- *Mu Xiang Bing Lang Wan* has a stronger action in breaking up stagnation. It is reserved for more severe forms of stagnation, with both abdominal fullness and pain.

Jian Pi Wan (Strengthen the Spleen Pill) utilizes the tonifying and reducing methods to treat stagnation and accumulation. This formula strengthens the Spleen, harmonizes the Stomach, promotes digestion, and stops diarrhea. It resolves heat and food stagnation with underlying Spleen deficiency. Clinical manifestations include poor appetite, epigastric and abdominal fullness, diarrhea, and a greasy tongue coating.

SECTION 2: REDUCING, GUIDING, AND DISSOLVING FORMULA THAT RELIEVES DISTENTION

Name	Similarities	Differences
Zhi Shi Xiao Pi Wan (Immature Bitter Orange Pill to Reduce Focal Distention)	Reduces, guides, and dissolves accumulation	Relieves epigastric and abdominal bloating, tonifies Spleen

Zhi Shi Xiao Pi Wan (Immature Bitter Orange Pill to Reduce Focal Distention) relieves epigastric and abdominal bloating, strengthens the Spleen, and harmonizes the Stomach. This formula treats Spleen deficiency with interior heat, cold, dampness, and phlegm stagnation. Clinical manifestations include epigastric and abdominal bloating, lack of appetite, lethargy, and mild constipation.

Chapter 20

— Antiparasitic Formulas

驱虫剂

葛洪 Gē Hōng

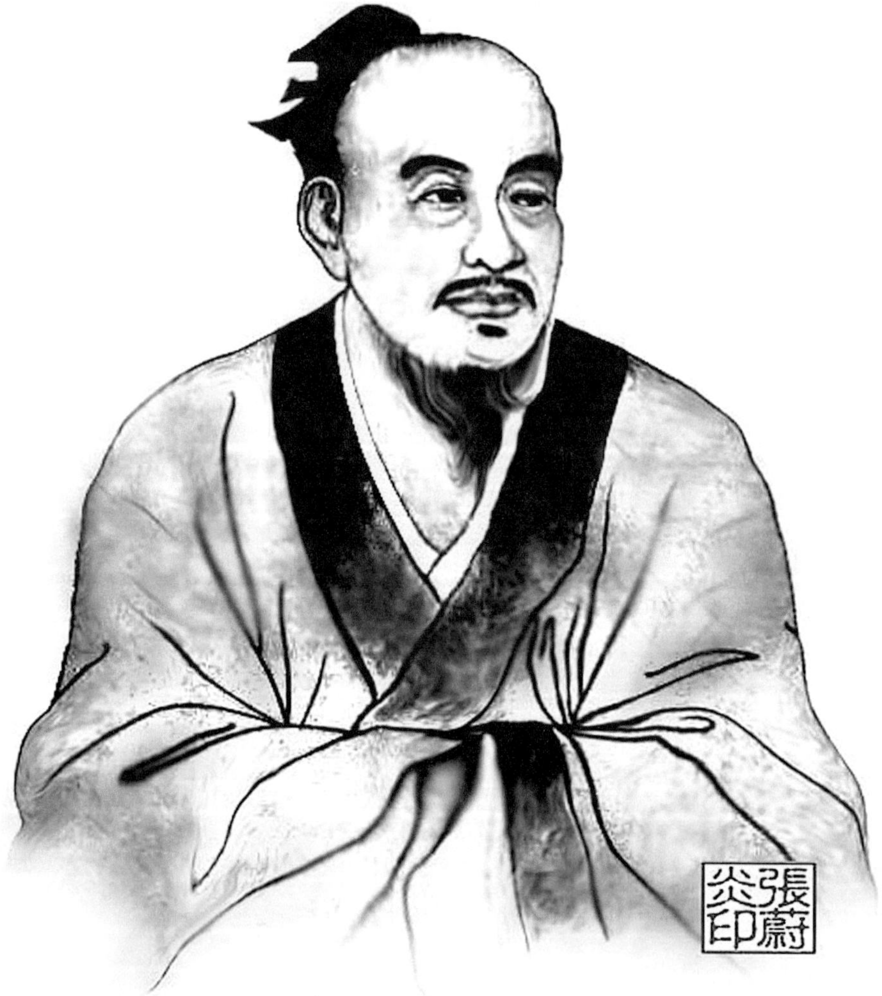

葛洪 Gē Hōng, 284 – 364.

葛洪 Gē Hōng

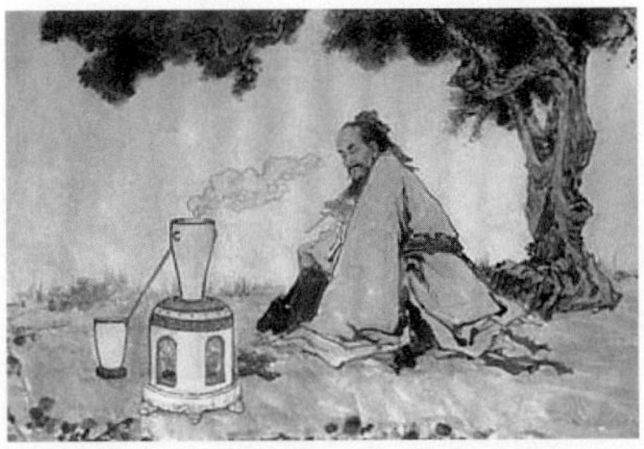

Ge Hong the alchemist

Ge Hong was born in a poor family. When he was thirteen years old, his father died, and his family suffered extreme financial hardship. He began to work to support his family, and during his spare time, he borrowed books and studied diligently. He later became a famed physician and alchemist.

As a physician, he compiled his clinical experiences and published 肘后备急方 *Zhou Hou Bei Ji Fang* (Emergency Formulas to Keep Up One's Sleeve) in 341 CE. This is a valuable text that described details of diseases and their corresponding treatments using herbs that are simple, readily-available, inexpensive, and effective. For example, he is credited as the first person to treat jaundice with *Qing Hao* (Herba Artemisiae Annuae),[1] leg *qi* with milk from cows and sheep,[2] and bites from rabid dogs with the brain marrow from the attacking dog.[3]

As an alchemist, he experimented with various substances to prepare special pills, such as *Xiong Huang* (Realgar), *Liu Huang* (Sulfur), *Dan Fan* (Chalcanthitum), *Xiao Shi* (Niter), *Ci Shi* (Magnetitum), *Zhu Sha* (Cinnabaris), and others. Although many of these substances are no longer used today, he initiated the use of pills and the concept that decoction is not the only dosage form. Ge Hong demonstrated that there are many other viable preparation methods and effective forms of delivery of medicinal substances.

Ge Hong's wife, 鲍姑 Bao Gu, was also a skilled physician. Bao Gu was credited for discovery of moxa and its medicinal properties. Moxa is made by rolling *Ai Ye* (Folium Artemisiae Argyi) into a stick. Since this herb grows all over China, her discovery follows the same principles put forth by her husband, that medicines should be simple, readily-available, inexpensive and effective.

1. Artemisinin from *Qing Hao* (Herba Artemisiae Annuae) is now a standard medication for treating malaria.
2. 脚气 Leg *qi* is a term that describes beriberi, which was treated with beans and milk which contain ample supply of vitamin B_1.
3. The brain marrow of rabid dogs contains antibodies, and has been confirmed to effectively prevent/treat rabies.

Dynasties & Kingdoms	Year
Xia Dynasty 夏	2100-1600 BCE
Shang Dynasty 商	1600-1100 BCE
Zhou Dynasty 周	1100-221 BCE
Qin Dynasty 秦	221-207 BCE
Han Dynasty 漢	206 BCE-220
Three Kingdoms 三國	220-280
Western Jin Dynasty 西晉	**265-316**
Eastern Jin Dynasty 東晉	317-420
Northern and Southern Dynasties 北南朝	420-581
Sui Dynasty 隋	581-618
Tang Dynasty 唐	618-907
Five Dynasties 五代	907-960
Song Dynasty 宋	960-1279
Liao Dynasty 潦	916-1125
Jin Dynasty 金	1115-1234
Yuan Dynasty 元	1271-1368
Ming Dynasty 明	1368-1644
Qing Dynasty 清	1644-1911
Republic of China 中華民國	1912-Present Day
People's Republic of China 中華人民共和國	1949-Present Day

Table of Contents

Chapter 20 — Overview

驱虫剂 — Antiparasitic Formulas

Definition: Antiparasitic formulas consist mainly of antiparasitic herbs that calm, kill and expel various types of parasites from the body. There are many different types of intestinal parasites; each type presents with different clinical manifestations, and each type needs to be treated differently. This chapter emphasizes the treatment of intestinal parasites, such as ascariasis (roundworms), cestodiasis (tapeworms), ancylostomiasis (hookworms), and others.

The common clinical signs of intestinal parasites disorders vary, depending on the type of parasite and the species of the host. The clinical signs can include: weight loss, lethargy, potbellied appearance, intermittent abdominal pain, dry and dull hair coat, diarrhea, and vomiting of clear fluids. If the condition is untreated or treated inappropriately, there may be an inability to grow and thrive, emaciation, enlarged and distended abdomen, and anemia. Conventional de-worming medications are typically used to treat intestinal parasites in domestic animals due to their lack of side effects, rapid onset of action, and efficacy (the complete killing of parasites). Most anti-parasitic herbal formulas contain purgative herbs and substances that can be potentially toxic and are not commonly used in veterinary medicine unless necessary. The primary applications for antiparasitic herbal formulas are in the treatment of resistant, unusual and/or difficult-to-treat parasites (chronic giardiasis, schistosomiasis, echinococcus multilocularis, echinococcus granulosis), and in the treatment of gastrointestinal diseases such as chronic diarrhea, bacterial dysentery, and inflammatory bowel disease.

The mechanisms of antiparasitic formulas are attributed to two main actions: they directly kill the parasites and/or they paralyze the muscles of the parasites, preventing mobility and promoting the parasites' elimination from the gastrointestinal tract. Antiparasitic formulas should be given on an empty stomach for maximum clinical effectiveness.

SUBCATEGORIES OF ACTION

Antiparasitic formulas are usually not divided into subcategories. Clinical signs vary, depending on the type of parasites present. Examples of parasitic infestation, associated clinical signs, and commonly used herbs are as follows:

- Ascariasis (roundworms) is characterized by weight loss despite a good appetite, potbellied appearance, diarrhea, vomiting of worms, worm segments in the stools, and poor growth. Ascariasis may be treated with herbs such as *Shi Jun Zi* (Fructus Quisqualis), *Ku Lian Pi* (Cortex Meliae), *Bing Lang* (Semen Arecae), and *Lei Wan* (Omphalia).
- Cestodiasis (tapeworms) is characterized by stools containing white, rice-like particles (parasite bodies). Cestodiasis may be treated with herbs such as *Bing Lang* (Semen Arecae), *Nan Gua Zi* (Semen Cucurbitae Moschatae), *Fei Zi* (Semen Torreyae), *He Shi* (Fructus Carpesii), and *Wu Yi* (Fructus Ulmi Praeparatus).
- Ancylostomiasis (hookworms) is characterized by pale mucous membranes and a pale tongue, pica, finicky appetite, bloody diarrhea, and lethargy. Ancylostomiasis may be treated with *Ku Lian Pi* (Cortex Meliae), *Fei Zi* (Semen Torreyae), *He Shi* (Fructus Carpesii), *Lei Wan* (Omphalia), and *Mian Ma Guan Zhong* (Rhizoma Dryopteridis Crassirhizomatis).

Chapter 20 — Overview

In addition, antiparasitic herbs and formulas have different characteristics and are used for different general conditions.

- Parasitic infestations characterized by cold should be treated with warm herbs and formulas, such as *Gan Jiang* (Rhizoma Zingiberis) and *Hua Jiao* (Pericarpium Zanthoxyli).
- Parasitic infestations characterized by heat should be treated with the addition of cold herbs and formulas, such as *Hu Huang Lian* (Rhizoma Picrorhizae) and *Huang Bo* (Cortex Phellodendri Chinensis).
- Parasitic infestations characterized by both cold and heat should be treated with two types of herbs: acrid and warm herbs to dispel cold (e.g., *Gan Jiang* [Rhizoma Zingiberis] and *Fu Zi* [Radix Aconiti Lateralis Praeparata]), and bitter and cold herbs to clear heat (e.g., *Huang Lian* [Rhizoma Coptidis] and *Huang Bo* [Cortex Phellodendri Chinensis]). One exemplar formula is *Wu Mei Wan* (Mume Pill).
- Chronic parasitic infestation characterized by malnutrition and Spleen dysfunction should be treated with three types of herbs: herbs that strengthen and harmonize the middle *jiao*, such as *Shen Qu* (Massa Fermentata) and *Mai Ya* (Fructus Hordei Germinatus); herbs that regulate qi and awaken the Stomach, such as *Rou Dou Kou* (Semen Myristicae) and *Mu Xiang* (Radix Aucklandiae); and herbs that clear heat and kill parasites, such as *Huang Lian* (Rhizoma Coptidis) and *Zhu Dan* (Fel Porcus). One representative formula is *Fei Er Wan* (Fat Child Pill).
- Lastly, parasitic infestation characterized by Spleen deficiency should be treated with antiparasitic and tonic herbs, such as *Ren Shen* (Radix et Rhizoma Ginseng), *Fu Ling* (Poria), *Bai Zhu* (Rhizoma Atractylodis Macrocephalae), and *Gan Cao* (Radix et Rhizoma Glycyrrhizae). One exemplar formula is *Bu Dai Wan* (Cloth Sack Pill).

CAUTIONS / CONTRAINDICATIONS

- Fecal examination to verify the type of parasites present is highly recommended before administering a formula to ensure efficacy of the treatment.
- Because these herbs have purging actions, they should be used cautiously or not used at all for weak, pregnant, and/or elderly patients.
- Because some antiparasitic herbs are toxic in nature, they must be dosed properly. Large doses may be associated with adverse effects, but small doses may yield little or no antiparasitic effect.
- These formulas should be taken on an empty stomach. Greasy or oily foods should be avoided when taking these formulas, as digestion and absorption of the formulas could be affected.
- These formulas may cause Spleen and Stomach deficiencies, in which case tonic herbs may be indicated to address the underlying deficiency.

PHARMACOLOGICAL EFFECTS & CLINICAL APPLICATIONS

Antiparasitic formulas are commonly used to treat various types of intestinal parasitic infestations.

- **Parasitic infestations**: The mechanisms of antiparasitic formulas are attributed to two actions: they directly kill the parasites,[1] or they paralyze the muscles of the parasites, inhibit their mobility, and thereby facilitate their elimination from the intestines (parasites with paralyzed muscles cannot physically attach to the intestines of the host and will be expelled).[2,3] Clinical applications of these formulas include ascariasis (roundworms),[4,5] oxyuriasis (pinworms), cestodiasis (tapeworms), ancylostomiasis (hookworms),[6] biliary ascariasis (roundworms),[7] schistosomiasis (trematode worms),[8] and blood flukes.[9] *Wu Mei Wan* (Mume Pill) is one of the most commonly used formulas to treat intestinal parasites.
- **Others**: In addition to treating parasites, certain antiparasitic formulas may also be used to treat other gastrointestinal disorders, such as diarrhea,[10] ulcerative colitis,[11] and irritable bowel syndrome.[12]

Chapter 20 — Overview

References

1. *Zhe Jiang Yi Ke Da Xue Xue Bao* (Journal of Zhejiang Province School of Medicine), 1980; 9(1):1.
2. *Fu Jian Zhong Yi Yao* (Fujian Chinese Medicine and Herbology), 1960; 6:29.
3. *Zhong Cao Yao* (Chinese Herbal Medicine), 1987; 4:28.
4. *Fu Jian Zhong Yi Yao* (Fujian Chinese Medicine and Herbology), 1960; 4:20.
5. *Jiang Su Zhong Yi* (Jiangsu Chinese Medicine), 1959; 9:64.
6. *Zhe Jiang Zhong Yi Za Zhi* (Zhejiang Journal of Chinese Medicine), 1960; 2:65.
7. *Xin Zhong Yi* (New Chinese Medicine), 1995; 1:49.
8. *Zhe Jiang Zhong Yi Za Zhi* (Zhejiang Journal of Chinese Medicine), 1984; 1:15.
9. *Guang Dong Zhong Yi* (Guangdong Chinese Medicine), 1959; 4(7):307.
10. *Jiang Xi Zhong Yi Yao* (Jiangxi Chinese Medicine and Herbology), 1990; 6:45.
11. *Xin Zhong Yi* (New Chinese Medicine), 1981; 6:26.
12. *Gan Su Zhong Yi* (Gansu Chinese Medicine), 1995; 4:24.

Wū Méi Wán (Mume Pill)

烏梅丸
乌梅丸

Pinyin Name: *Wu Mei Wan*
Literal Name: Mume Pill
Alternate Name: Mume Formula
Original Source: *Shang Han Lun* (Discussion of Cold-Induced Disorders) by Zhang Zhong-Jing in the Eastern Han Dynasty

COMPOSITION

Wu Mei (Fructus Mume)	300 pieces or 480g [30g]
Hua Jiao (Pericarpium Zanthoxyli), *chao* (dry-fried) till aromatic	120g [6g]
Xi Xin (Radix et Rhizoma Asari)	180g [3g]
Huang Lian (Rhizoma Coptidis)	480g [6g]
Huang Bo (Cortex Phellodendri Chinensis)	180g [6g]
Gan Jiang (Rhizoma Zingiberis)	300g [9g]
Gui Zhi (Ramulus Cinnamomi)	180g [6g]
Fu Zi (Radix Aconiti Lateralis Praeparata), *pao* (blast-fried)	180g [6g]
Ren Shen (Radix et Rhizoma Ginseng)	180g [6g]
Dang Gui (Radix Angelicae Sinensis)	120g [6g]

DOSAGE / PREPARATION / ADMINISTRATION

The source text states to steep *Wu Mei* (Fructus Mume) in a 50% vinegar solution overnight, then remove the pits and mash the fruits. Dry the mashed fruits under the sun, then mix them with the rest of the ingredients and grind them into powder and form into pills with honey. The pills should resemble the size of *Wu Tong Zi* (Semen Firmianae), a small seed approximately 5 mm in diameter. Take 10 pills [9g] three times daily on an empty stomach with warm, boiled water. Today, this formula may be prepared as a decoction with the doses suggested in brackets. The source text states to avoid cold, raw, or spoiled foods during medication.

CHINESE THERAPEUTIC ACTIONS

1. Warms the internal organs
2. Calms roundworms

CLINICAL MANIFESTATIONS

Ascariasis (roundworms) characterized by heat in the Stomach and cold in the Intestines: weight loss, diarrhea, a potbelly, vomiting of roundworms, abdominal pain, cold paws/extremities and abdominal pain. Also for chronic dysentery and diarrhea.

VETERINARY CLINICAL APPLICATIONS

Ascariasis (roundworms), hookworms, chronic giardia, schistosomiasis, chronic gastritis, bacterial dysentery, chronic dysentery, ulcerative colitis, inflammatory bowel disease and chronic diarrhea.

EXPLANATION

Wu Mei Wan (Mume Pill) treats roundworms characterized by heat in the Stomach and cold in the Intestines. According to traditional Chinese medicine, roundworms prefer warmth and have an aversion to cold. So while they reside in the intestines, they constantly move toward the stomach in search of warmth and food. However, their presence and movement disrupt the normal qi flow in the Stomach and Intestines, causing clinical signs such as abdominal pain, weight loss, diarrhea, a potbelly, and vomiting of roundworms. In cases of severe pain, the flow of yin and yang qi will be disrupted, causing cold paws and extremities.

Treatment of intestinal parasites follows the principle that "sweet taste [of herbs] induces movement [of the parasites], sour taste induces tranquility, acrid taste induces suppression, and bitter taste induces downward movement." *Wu Mei* (Fructus Mume), a sour herb processed with vinegar, calms parasites. *Hua Jiao* (Pericarpium Zanthoxyli) and *Xi Xin* (Radix et Rhizoma Asari) are acrid and warm herbs that warm the interior, dispel cold, and suppress the movement of parasites. *Huang Lian* (Rhizoma Coptidis) and *Huang Bo* (Cortex Phellodendri Chinensis) are bitter and cold herbs that clear heat and drain parasites downward. *Gan Jiang* (Rhizoma Zingiberis), *Gui Zhi* (Ramulus Cinnamomi), and *Fu Zi* (Radix Aconiti Lateralis Praeparata) are acrid and hot herbs that warm the interior and dispel cold. In using herbs that are sour, acrid and bitter, this formula effectively calms the parasites, suppresses their movement, and drains them out of the

Wū Méi Wán (Mume Pill)

***Wu Mei Wan* (Mume Pill)**

Diagnosis	Clinical Signs	Treatment	Herbs
Ascariasis infection characterized by heat and cold	• Weight loss, diarrhea, a potbelly, and vomiting of worms: roundworms • Severe pain and cold limbs: disrupted yin and yang qi circulation	• Warms the internal organs • Calms parasites	• *Wu Mei* (Fructus Mume) calms parasites. • *Hua Jiao* (Pericarpium Zanthoxyli) and *Xi Xin* (Radix et Rhizoma Asari) warm the interior, dispel cold, and suppress the movement of parasites. • *Gan Jiang* (Rhizoma Zingiberis), *Gui Zhi* (Ramulus Cinnamomi), and *Fu Zi* (Radix Aconiti Lateralis Praeparata) warm the interior and dispel cold. • *Huang Lian* (Rhizoma Coptidis) and *Huang Bo* (Cortex Phellodendri Chinensis) clear heat and drain parasites downward. • *Ren Shen* (Radix et Rhizoma Ginseng) and *Dang Gui* (Radix Angelicae Sinensis) tonify qi and blood.

body via defecation. Moreover, it uses both cold herbs to clear heat in the Stomach and hot herbs to dispel cold in the Intestines. Since chronic parasitic infestation often causes generalized weakness and deficiency, this formula contains *Ren Shen* (Radix et Rhizoma Ginseng) and *Dang Gui* (Radix Angelicae Sinensis) to tonify qi and blood.

Interestingly, this formula can treat chronic dysentery and diarrhea with deficiency of *zheng* (upright) *qi*, because such cases are often complicated by the simultaneous presence of cold and heat.

VETERINARY MODIFICATIONS

- To enhance the antiparasitic effect, add *Shi Jun Zi* (Fructus Quisqualis), *Ku Lian Pi* (Cortex Meliae), *Fei Zi* (Semen Torreyae), and *Bing Lang* (Semen Arecae).
- With vomiting, add *Wu Zhu Yu* (Fructus Evodiae) and *Ban Xia* (Rhizoma Pinelliae).
- With severe abdominal pain, add *Mu Xiang* (Radix Aucklandiae) and *Chuan Lian Zi* (Fructus Toosendan).
- With constipation, add *Da Huang* (Radix et Rhizoma Rhei) and *Bing Lang* (Semen Arecae).
- With more heat, remove *Fu Zi* (Radix Aconiti Lateralis Praeparata) and *Gan Jiang* (Rhizoma Zingiberis).
- With more cold, remove *Huang Lian* (Rhizoma Coptidis) and *Huang Bo* (Cortex Phellodendri Chinensis).

CAUTIONS / CONTRAINDICATIONS

- *Wu Mei Wan* may be used to treat chronic dysentery and diarrhea with deficiency of *zheng* (upright) *qi*, if it is characterized by the presence of cold and heat at the same time. Do not use this formula, however, if the dysentery and diarrhea are due to damp-heat.
- This formula should be used with caution during pregnancy.[1]

PHARMACOLOGICAL EFFECTS

1. **Antiparasitic**: *Wu Mei Wan* has been shown to have marked antiparasitic effects against roundworms. The mechanism of this action is attributed to the paralyzing effect of the formula, as the herbs do not actually kill the parasites. It has been suggested that the herbs paralyze the muscles of the parasites, inhibit their mobility, and thereby facilitate the elimination from the intestines.[2,3]
2. **Cholagogic**: *Wu Mei Wan* has been shown to have a stimulating effect on the liver and gallbladder. It increases the production of bile acid by the liver, and stimulates the contraction of the gallbladder.[4,5]
3. **Antibiotic**: Many herbs in *Wu Mei Wan* have shown marked inhibitory effects against various micro-organisms.[6]

HUMAN CLINICAL STUDIES AND RESEARCH

1. **Intestinal ascariasis (roundworms)**: In one study of 8 patients, intestinal obstruction caused by ascariasis was treated effectively using *Wu Mei Wan*. Most patients experienced relief of abdominal pain within 1-2 doses, and complete resolution of the condition in 3 days.[7] Another study of patients also reported marked success expelling roundworms using modified *Wu Mei Wan*, with the addition of *Shi Jun Zi* (Fructus Quisqualis) and *Chuan Lian Zi* (Fructus Toosendan). The treatment protocol was to administer modified *Wu Mei Wan* first to paralyze the roundworms, followed by purgative herbs to expel them with the stools from the intestines.[8]
2. **Biliary ascariasis (roundworms)**: One study of 48 patients reported marked success within 2-13 days using both acupuncture and *Wu Mei Wan* to treat biliary ascariasis.[9] Another study reported good results to relieve pain within 1-3 packs of herbs in 30 of 31 patients using *Wu Mei Wan* plus *Mu Xiang* (Radix Aucklandiae), *Bing Lang* (Semen Arecae) and others.[10] Furthermore, use of modified *Wu*

Mei Wan in 40 patients with biliary ascariasis was associated with a 95% effectiveness. The duration of treatment varied between 2-6 doses.[11] Lastly, one study reported successful treatment of biliary ascariasis in 10 of 11 patients. The herbal treatment was based on *Wu Mei Wan*, with removal of *Huang Bo* (Cortex Phellodendri Chinensis), and the addition of *Wu Zhu Yu* (Fructus Evodiae), *Chuan Lian Zi* (Fructus Toosendan), *Zhi Gan Cao* (Radix et Rhizoma Glycyrrhizae Praeparata cum Melle), and others.[12]

3. **Ascariasis (roundworms) in children**: Complete recovery was reported in 24 patients with intestinal ascariasis when treated with modified *Wu Mei Wan*. Modifications were made based on the presentation of the individuals. For excess heat, *Huang Qin* (Radix Scutellariae) was added, the dose of *Huang Lian* (Rhizoma Coptidis) was increased, and the doses of *Gan Jiang* (Rhizoma Zingiberis) and *Hua Jiao* (Pericarpium Zanthoxyli) were reduced. For excess cold, the doses of *Gan Jiang* (Rhizoma Zingiberis) and *Hua Jiao* (Pericarpium Zanthoxyli) were increased, and the dose of *Huang Lian* (Rhizoma Coptidis) was reduced. For severe abdominal pain, the doses of *Hua Jiao* (Pericarpium Zanthoxyli) and *Gan Cao* (Radix et Rhizoma Glycyrrhizae) were increased, and *Yan Hu Suo* (Rhizoma Corydalis), *Wu Zhu Yu* (Fructus Evodiae), and *Bai Shao* (Radix Paeoniae Alba) were added. For severe nausea and vomiting, the doses of *Wu Mei* (Fructus Mume), *Ban Xia* (Rhizoma Pinelliae), and *Hua Jiao* (Pericarpium Zanthoxyli) were increased, and *Dou Kou* (Fructus Amomi Rotundus) and *Zhu Ru* (Caulis Bambusae in Taenia) were added.[13]
4. **Ancylostomiasis (hookworms)**: One study reported 53.2% effectiveness using *Wu Mei Wan* to treat 60 patients with hookworm infestation.[14]
5. **Schistosomiasis (trematode worms)**: Three hundred and nineteen patients with schistosomiasis were treated with 92.4% effectiveness and 75.9% rate of recovery using *Wu Mei Wan* plus *Da Chai Hu Tang* (Major Bupleurum Decoction) in decoction or pills. The decoction was given once every other day. The pills were made by grinding all the herbs into a fine powder and mixing with honey to make pills. Ten grams of pills were taken per dose, twice daily. The treatment protocol was to use decoctions for acute cases, and pills for chronic cases.[15]
6. **Chronic diarrhea**: Rectal instillation of *Wu Mei Wan* showed 97.8% effectiveness in treating 47 patients with chronic diarrhea of 2-20 years. The treatment protocol was to cook the herbs to yield 200 mL of herbal solution and instill 100 mL of the herbal solution rectally twice daily in the morning and at night.[16]
7. **Bacterial dysentery**: Use of modified *Wu Mei Wan* was associated with complete recovery in 53 of 60 patients with bacterial dysentery. The herbal treatment contained *Wu Mei Wan* plus *Hua Shi* (Talcum) as the base formula. Furthermore, *Gui Zhi* (Ramulus Cinnamomi) and *Xi Xin* (Radix et Rhizoma Asari) were added for aversion to cold; *Ban Xia* (Rhizoma Pinelliae) for nausea and vomiting; *Chi Shao* (Radix Paeoniae Rubra) and *Mu Xiang* (Radix Aucklandiae) for abdominal pain; and *Da Huang* (Radix et Rhizoma Rhei) for rectal tenesmus.[17]
8. **Ulcerative colitis**: According to one study, 25 patients with chronic ulcerative colitis were treated with modified *Wu Mei Wan* with complete recovery in 16 cases, improvement in 7 cases, and no effect in 2 cases.[18]
9. **Irritable bowel syndrome (IBS)**: Use of modified *Wu Mei Wan* was associated with 91% effectiveness in treating IBS in 34 patients (23 males and 11 females). Modifications to *Wu Mei Wan* included the addition of *Ying Su Ke* (Pericarpium Papaveris) and *Yan Hu Suo* (Rhizoma Corydalis) for abdominal pain; dry-fried *Yi Yi Ren* (Semen Coicis) and *Bu Gu Zhi* (Fructus Psoraleae) for diarrhea; *Bai Shao* (Radix Paeoniae Alba) and *Huo Ma Ren* (Fructus Cannabis) for constipation; ginger-processed *Ban Xia* (Rhizoma Pinelliae) and *Zhe Shi* (Haematitum) for nausea and belching. Of 34 patients, the study reported complete recovery in 18 cases, significant improvement in 6 cases, and no response in 3 cases.[19]
10. **Cholecystitis**: One study reported 97.5% effectiveness in treating cholecystitis using modified *Wu Mei Wan*. For acute cholecystitis, *Jin Qian Cao* (Herba Lysimachiae) was added and *Dang Shen* (Radix Codonopsis) was removed from the formula. For chronic illness, *Ji Nei Jin* (Endothelium Corneum Gigeriae Galli) was added. The treatment protocol was to cook the herbs and administer the decoction in two to three equally-divided doses, followed by 10-30 mL of rice vinegar. Of 40 patients, the study reported complete recovery in 12 cases, marked improvement in 15 cases, moderate improvement in 12 cases, and no effect in 1 case.[20]
11. **Cholelithiasis**: Use of modified *Wu Mei Wan* was associated with good result in treating 40 cases of cholelithiasis. In addition to the base formula, *Da Huang* (Radix et Rhizoma Rhei) and *Pu Gong Ying* (Herba Taraxaci) were added for excess heat; larger doses of *Fu Zi* (Radix Aconiti Lateralis Praeparata) and *Gan Jiang* (Rhizoma Zingiberis) were used for excess cold; *Jiang Huang* (Rhizoma Curcumae Longae) and *Chuan Lian Zi* (Fructus Toosendan) for severe hypochondriac pain; *Ban Xia* (Rhizoma Pinelliae) and *Ru Xiang* (Gummi Olibanum) for nausea and vomiting; and *Yin Chen* (Herba Artemisiae Scopariae) and *Yu Jin* (Radix Curcumae) for jaundice. The duration of treatment was 1-3 courses, with 30 days per course. Of 47 patients, the study reported complete resolution in 5 cases, marked improvement in 16 cases, moderate improvement in 20

Wū Méi Wán (Mume Pill)

cases, and no effect in 6 cases. The overall effectiveness was 87.23%.[21]

SUGGESTED ACUPUNCTURE TREATMENT

1. Points: *Baichongwo*, *Juque* (CV 14), *Tianshu* (ST 25), *Zhongwan* (CV 12), *Xiangu* (ST 43), *Housanli* (ST 36), *Sanyinjiao* (SP 6), and *Shenque* (CV 8).
2. Technique: sedation followed by tonification.

Baichongwo is a special point used to treat parasitic infection. *Baichongwo*, literally "hundred insects' nest," is located 1 *cun* above *Xuehai* (SP 10). *Juque* (CV 14) regulates qi circulation and relieves nausea. *Tianshu* (ST 25) and *Zhongwan* (CV 12) restore the normal function of the Intestines to relieve local distention and pain. *Xiangu* (ST 43) clears Stomach heat. *Housanli* (ST 36) and *Sanyinjiao* (SP 6) strengthen the Spleen and Stomach, while tonifying qi and blood. Moxibustion on *Shenque* (CV 8) warms up the interior to dispel cold. Sedation is necessary to eliminate the infestation, while tonification is needed to strengthen the Spleen and tonify qi.

AUTHORS' COMMENTS

Wu Mei Wan is the representative formula for treating ascariasis (roundworms) in Chinese medicine. It can also be used to treat bacterial diarrhea and inflammatory bowel disease, when both conditions involve chronic diarrhea characterized by deficiency and excess with the interlocking of heat (Stomach) and cold (Intestines)."

This formula can also be combined with metronidazole, fenbendazole and/or pyrantel pamoate. Often a combination of conventional antiparasitic drugs and *Wu Mei Wan* can be effective in eliminating chronic giardia infection, when the use of one agent alone is ineffective. The length of treatment is variable and depends on the case.

References

1. *Zhong Yao Ming Fang Yao Li Yu Ying Yong* (Pharmacology and Applications of Famous Herbal Formulas), 1989; 636-637.
2. *Fu Jian Zhong Yi Yao* (Fujian Chinese Medicine and Herbology), 1960; 6:29.
3. *Zhong Cao Yao* (Chinese Herbal Medicine), 1987; 4:28.
4. *Fu Jian Zhong Yi Yao* (Fujian Chinese Medicine and Herbology), 1960; 6:29.
5. *Zhong Cao Yao* (Chinese Herbal Medicine), 1987; 4:28.
6. *Zhong Yi Fang Ji Xian Dai Yan Jiu* (Modern Study of Medical Formulas in Traditional Chinese Medicine), 1997; 1555.
7. *Fu Jian Zhong Yi Yao* (Fujian Chinese Medicine and Herbology), 1960; 4:20.
8. *Jiang Su Zhong Yi* (Jiangsu Chinese Medicine), 1959; 9:64.
9. *Zhong Hua Wai Ke Za Zhi* (Chinese Journal of External Medicine), 1959; 6:547.
10. *Guang Xi Zhong Yi Yao* (Guangxi Chinese Medicine and Herbology), 1981; 3:47.
11. *Shan Xi Zhong Yi* (Shanxi Chinese Medicine), 1985; 1:37.
12. *Xin Zhong Yi* (New Chinese Medicine), 1995; 1:49.
13. *Cheng Du Zhong Yi Xue Yuan Xue Bao* (Journal of Chengdu University of Traditional Chinese Medicine), 1960; 1:45.
14. *Zhe Jiang Zhong Yi Za Zhi* (Zhejiang Journal of Chinese Medicine), 1960; 2:65.
15. *Zhe Jiang Zhong Yi Za Zhi* (Zhejiang Journal of Chinese Medicine), 1984; 1:15.
16. *Jiang Xi Zhong Yi Yao* (Jiangxi Chinese Medicine and Herbology), 1990; 6:45.
17. *Guang Xi Zhong Yi Yao* (Guangxi Chinese Medicine and Herbology), 1981; 3:21.
18. *Xin Zhong Yi* (New Chinese Medicine), 1981; 6:26.
19. *Gan Su Zhong Yi* (Gansu Chinese Medicine), 1995; 4:24.
20. *Shan Xi Zhong Yi* (Shanxi Chinese Medicine), 1993; 7:316.
21. *Zhong Yi Ming Fang Lin Chuang Xin Yong* (Contemporary Clinical Applications of Classic Chinese Formulas), 2001; 153-154.

Féi Ér Wán (Fat Child Pill)

肥兒丸
肥儿丸

Pinyin Name: *Fei Er Wan*
Literal Name: Fat Child Pill
Original Source: *Tai Ping Hui Min He Ji Ju Fang* (Imperial Grace Formulary of the Tai Ping Era) by the Imperial Medical Department in 1078-85

COMPOSITION

Shen Qu (Massa Fermentata), *chao* (dry-fried)	300g
Mai Ya (Fructus Hordei Germinatus), *chao* (dry-fried)	150g
Huang Lian (Rhizoma Coptidis)	300g
Rou Dou Kou (Semen Myristicae), *wei* (roasted)	150g
Mu Xiang (Radix Aucklandiae)	60g
Bing Lang (Semen Arecae), *cuo* (grated) into thin particles and sun-dried	20 pieces [120g]
Shi Jun Zi (Fructus Quisqualis)	150g

DOSAGE / PREPARATION / ADMINISTRATION

The source text states to grind the ingredients into a fine powder and form into small pills using bile from a pig's gallbladder. The pills should resemble *Su Mi* (Semen Setariae) in size. Take 30 pills daily on an empty stomach with warm, boiled water. Adjust the dose according to the age of the patient.

Today, this formula is prepared by grinding the ingredients and sifting the resultant powders together. The mixed powder is then formed into small pills [3g each] using fresh bile from the gallbladder of a pig. Dissolve 1 pill in boiled water and take it on an empty stomach.

CHINESE THERAPEUTIC ACTIONS

1. Kills parasites
2. Reduces accumulation
3. Strengthens the Spleen
4. Clears heat

CLINICAL MANIFESTATIONS

Intestinal parasites and *gan ji* (juvenile malnutrition): abdominal pain, poor digestion, thin or emaciated appearance, lack of appetite, loose stools, enlarged abdomen with swelling and fullness, weak constitution, fatigue, possible nausea and vomiting, dry mouth and thirst, and foul breath. Note: *Gan ji* is defined as infantile malnutrition in humans, but it should be interpreted in veterinary medicine as juvenile malnutrition in animals that fail to thrive.

VETERINARY CLINICAL APPLICATIONS

Parasitic infestation and juvenile malnutrition.

EXPLANATION

Fei Er Wan (Fat Child Pill) treats animals with intestinal parasites with abdominal pain and poor digestion. Chronic parasitic infestation may cause *gan ji* (juvenile malnutrition) characterized by Spleen deficiency and Stomach heat, with clinical signs such as thin or emaciated

***Fei Er Wan* (Fat Child Pill)**

Diagnosis	Clinical Signs	Treatment	Herbs
Intestinal parasites and *gan ji* (juvenile malnutrition)	Abdominal pain, poor digestion, a sallow and yellowish facial complexion, thin or emaciated appearance, enlarged abdomen, fever, foul breath, and loose stools: malnutrition due to parasitic infestation	• Kills parasites • Reduces accumulation • Strengthens the Spleen • Clears heat	• *Shen Qu* (Massa Fermentata) and *Mai Ya* (Fructus Hordei Germinatus) strengthen the Spleen, harmonize the middle *jiao*, and reduce food stagnation. • *Bing Lang* (Semen Arecae) and *Shi Jun Zi* (Fructus Quisqualis) kill and expel parasites. • *Huang Lian* (Rhizoma Coptidis) sedates Stomach heat. • *Rou Dou Kou* (Semen Myristicae) strengthens the Spleen and relieves loose stools. • *Mu Xiang* (Radix Aucklandiae) regulates qi to relieve abdominal pain.

Féi Ér Wán (Fat Child Pill)

appearance, enlarged abdomen, fever, foul breath, and loose stools.

This formula contains *Shen Qu* (Massa Fermentata) and *Mai Ya* (Fructus Hordei Germinatus) to strengthen the Spleen, harmonize the middle *jiao*, and reduce food stagnation. *Huang Lian* (Rhizoma Coptidis) clears Stomach heat. *Rou Dou Kou* (Semen Myristicae), an aromatic herb, strengthens the Spleen and relieves loose stools. *Mu Xiang* (Radix Aucklandiae) regulates qi to relieve abdominal pain. *Bing Lang* (Semen Arecae) and *Shi Jun Zi* (Fructus Quisqualis) kill and expel parasites. Lastly, bile from a pig's gallbladder helps *Huang Lian* (Rhizoma Coptidis) clear heat from the Liver and Stomach.

VETEIRNARY MODIFICATIONS

- With nausea, vomiting, and diarrhea, add *Ban Xia* (Rhizoma Pinelliae) and *Chen Pi* (Pericarpium Citri Reticulatae).
- With weak body constitution accompanied by alternating spells of chills and fever, add *Chai Hu* (Radix Bupleuri) and *Bai Shao* (Radix Paeoniae Alba).
- Without interior heat, remove *Huang Lian* (Rhizoma Coptidis).
- With Spleen and Stomach deficiencies, add *Ren Shen* (Radix et Rhizoma Ginseng) and *Bai Zhu* (Rhizoma Atractylodis Macrocephalae).
- With constipation, add *Da Huang* (Radix et Rhizoma Rhei) and *Zhi Shi* (Fructus Aurantii Immaturus).

CAUTIONS / CONTRAINDICATIONS

- *Fei Er Wan* should ***not*** be used in cases of *gan ji* (juvenile malnutrition) due to Spleen and Stomach deficiencies, as many herbs that expel parasites are rather harsh and may cause more deficiencies.
- Avoid foods that are raw, cold, oily, or greasy while taking this formula.[1]

SUGGESTED ACUPUNCTURE TREATMENT

1. Points: *Baichongwo*, *Pishu* (BL 20), *Housanli* (ST 36), *Tianshu* (ST 25), *Zhongwan* (CV 12), and *Neiting* (ST 44).
2. Technique: tonification and sedation.

The objectives of this treatment are to eliminate intestinal parasites, strengthen the Spleen, and promote digestion. *Baichongwo* is a special point used to treat intestinal parasitic infection. *Baichongwo*, literally "hundred insects' nest," is located 1 *cun* above *Xuehai* (SP 10). *Pishu* (BL 20) and *Housanli* (ST 36) strengthen the Spleen and promote digestion. *Tianshu* (ST 25) and *Zhongwan* (CV 12) regulate qi and relieve abdominal fullness and pain. *Neiting* (ST 44) clears Stomach heat.

AUTHORS' COMMENTS

Fei Er Wan contains herbs that strengthen digestion and kill parasites. Many animals have significant Spleen qi deficiency with endoparasitism, and this formula can be combined with *Si Jun Zi Tang* (Four-Gentlemen Decoction) to improve clinical results. To improve the formula's ability to kill parasites, add *Lu Hui* (Aloe).

Reference

1. *Zhong Yao Ming Fang Yao Li Yu Ying Yong* (Pharmacology and Applications of Famous Herbal Formulas), 1989; 638.

Bù Dài Wán (Cloth Sack Pill)

布袋丸

Pinyin Name: *Bu Dai Wan*
Literal Name: Cloth Sack Pill
Original Source: *Bu Yao Xiu Zhen Xiao Er Fang Lun* (Supplement to the Pocket-Sized Discussion of Formulas for Children)

COMPOSITION

Wu Yi (Fructus Ulmi Praeparatus), *chao* (dry-fried)	60g
Shi Jun Zi (Fructus Quisqualis), *chao* (dry-fried)	60g
Lu Hui (Aloe), *yan* (ground) into thin particles	15g
Ye Ming Sha (Faeces Vespertilionis Murini), *jing* (cleaned)	60g
Ren Shen (Radix et Rhizoma Ginseng)	15g
Bai Zhu (Rhizoma Atractylodis Macrocephalae)	15g
Fu Ling (Poria)	15g
Gan Cao (Radix et Rhizoma Glycyrrhizae)	15g

DOSAGE / PREPARATION / ADMINISTRATION

The source text states to grind the ingredients into a fine powder and form into large pills with water. Each pill should resemble a large bullet and weigh approximately 10g. For administration, place 1 pill in a cheesecloth and cook it with 60g of pork in water until the pork is thoroughly cooked. The pork and the soup are given to children as medication. The pill in the cheesecloth may be used again the next day.

Today, this formula is normally prepared as a powder by proportionally adjusting all of the ingredients and grinding them into powder. Take 3g of powder with pork soup on an empty stomach in the morning, upon awakening.

CHINESE THERAPEUTIC ACTIONS

1. Dispels roundworms and treats *gan ji* (juvenile malnutrition)
2. Tonifies and strengthens the Spleen and Stomach

CLINICAL MANIFESTATIONS

Parasitic infestation with *gan ji* (juvenile malnutrition) in puppies, kittens, and foals: weight loss, exercise intolerance, lethargy, emaciation, a potbelly, dry, lusterless hair, and dull eyes. Note: *Gan ji* is defined as infantile malnutrition in humans, but it should be interpreted in veterinary medicine as juvenile malnutrition in animals that fail to thrive.

VETERINARY CLINICAL APPLICATIONS

Parasitic infestation, malnutrition, and failure to thrive in young animals.

EXPLANATION

Bu Dai Wan (Cloth Sack Pill) treats parasitic infestation in young animals with Spleen deficiency. Chronic infestation of parasites may lead to Spleen and Stomach deficiencies, resulting in weight loss, exercise intolerance, lethargy and emaciation. The potbelly is due to Spleen and Stomach qi deficiencies and stagnation. Because of the decreased absorption of nutrients due to Spleen and Stomach deficiencies, less blood is produced, resulting in dry, lusterless hair and dull eyes.

***Bu Dai Wan* (Cloth Sack Pill)**

Diagnosis	Clinical Signs	Treatment	Herbs
Parasitic infestation and *gan ji* (juvenile malnutrition)	Weight loss, exercise intolerance, lethargy, emaciation, potbelly, dry, lusterless hair, and dull eyes: malnutrition due to parasitic infestation	• Dispels roundworms and treats *gan ji* (juvenile malnutrition) • Tonifies and strengthens the Spleen and Stomach	• *Wu Yi* (Fructus Ulmi Praeparatus) and *Shi Jun Zi* (Fructus Quisqualis) expel roundworms and treat *gan ji* (juvenile malnutrition). • *Lu Hui* (Aloe) expels parasites by purging them out of the body through the bowels. • *Ye Ming Sha* (Faeces Vespertilionis Murini) clears Liver heat and brightens the vision. • *Ren Shen* (Radix et Rhizoma Ginseng), *Bai Zhu* (Rhizoma Atractylodis Macrocephalae), *Fu Ling* (Poria), and *Gan Cao* (Radix et Rhizoma Glycyrrhizae) tonify the Spleen and Stomach.

Bù Dài Wán (Cloth Sack Pill)

Acrid, bitter, and warm, *Wu Yi* (Fructus Ulmi Praeparatus) is combined with sweet and warm *Shi Jun Zi* (Fructus Quisqualis) in this formula to expel roundworms and treat *gan ji* (juvenile malnutrition). Bitter and cold, *Lu Hui* (Aloe) expels the parasites by purging them out of the body through the bowels. *Ye Ming Sha* (Faeces Vespertilionis Murini) clears Liver heat and brightens the vision. Since the root of this syndrome is Spleen and Stomach deficiencies, *Ren Shen* (Radix et Rhizoma Ginseng), *Bai Zhu* (Rhizoma Atractylodis Macrocephalae), *Fu Ling* (Poria), and *Gan Cao* (Radix et Rhizoma Glycyrrhizae) are used to tonify the Spleen and Stomach. Indeed, this formula functions on both tonic and sedative levels to safely and effectively sedates heat and removes parasites without injuring the Spleen and Stomach.

VETERINARY MODIFICATIONS

- With more heat, add *Huang Lian* (Rhizoma Coptidis).
- With food stagnation, add *Shen Qu* (Massa Fermentata) and *Ji Nei Jin* (Endothelium Corneum Gigeriae Galli).

SUGGESTED ACUPUNCTURE TREATMENT

1. Points: *Baichongwo*, *Juque* (CV 14), *Zhongwan* (CV 12), *Tianshu* (ST 25), *Zhangmen* (LR 13), *Qihai* (CV 6), *Shaochong* (HT 9), *Pishu* (BL 20), and *Housanli* (ST 36).
2. Technique: sedation followed by tonification.

This acupuncture treatment is designed to treat parasitic infestation accompanied by Spleen deficiency. *Baichongwo* is a special point used to treat intestinal parasitic infection. *Baichongwo*, literally "hundred insects' nest," is located 1 *cun* above *Xuehai* (SP 10). *Juque* (CV 14), *Zhongwan* (CV 12), and *Tianshu* (ST 25) may regulate qi and remove Stomach and intestinal stagnation. *Zhangmen* (LR 13) and *Qihai* (CV 6) relieve abdominal fullness and distention. *Shaochong* (HT 9) clears Liver heat. Finally, *Pishu* (BL 20) and *Housanli* (ST 36) strengthen the Spleen.

Sedation of the selected points is necessary to eliminate the infestation, and tonification is obligatory to strengthen the Spleen and tonify qi.

AUTHORS' COMMENTS

Bu Dai Wan is a formula that treats chronic parasitic infestation in puppies, kittens, and foals with malnutrition. While the parasite infestation is considered to be an excess condition, the underlying malnutrition represents a deficiency condition. Because of the complexity of this condition, antiparasitic herbs that expel parasites must be used together with tonic herbs to address the underlying deficiencies.

Huà Chóng Wán (Dissolve Parasites Pill)

化蟲丸
化虫丸

Pinyin Name: *Hua Chong Wan*
Literal Name: Dissolve Parasites Pill
Original Source: *Tai Ping Hui Min He Ji Ju Fang* (Imperial Grace Formulary of the Tai Ping Era) by the Imperial Medical Department in 1078-85

COMPOSITION

He Shi (Fructus Carpesii)	1,500g
Ku Lian Pi (Cortex Meliae)	1,500g
Bing Lang (Semen Arecae)	1,500g
Bai Fan (Alumen)	375g
Qian Dan (Minium), *chao* (dry-fried)	1,500g

Note: *Qian Dan* (Minium) is a potentially toxic heavy metal and is rarely used as a medicinal substance today. Its discussion here is included primarily for academic purposes, to reflect the historical use of this substance in its original formulation. Most herbal products today have removed it completely, or replaced it with substitutes with similar functions. For additional information on the toxicity, please refer to *Chinese Medical Herbology and Pharmacology* by John Chen and Tina Chen.

DOSAGE / PREPARATION / ADMINISTRATION

The source text states to grind the ingredients into a fine powder and form into very small pills with flour. The pills should resemble *Huo Ma Ren* (Fructus Cannabis) in size. For infants around one year of age, take 5 pills any time during the day. The pills may be taken with warm rice soup, or warm, boiled water plus 1-2 drops of sesame oil.

CHINESE THERAPEUTIC ACTIONS

Expels and kills various intestinal parasites

CLINICAL MANIFESTATIONS

Intestinal parasites: intermittent, severe pain migrating up and down the abdomen, nausea, and vomiting of clear fluids or parasites.

VETERINARY CLINICAL APPLICATIONS

Ascariasis (roundworms), giardia, coccidia, cestodiasis (tapeworms), cysticercosis and intestinal flukes.

EXPLANATION

Hua Chong Wan (Dissolve Parasites Pill) is designed to treat retention of parasites in the intestines. The intermittent, severe pain migrating up and down the abdomen is due to the upward movement of the parasites. If the parasites affect the Stomach qi flow and cause rising Stomach qi, vomiting of clear fluids or parasites will occur.

This formula contains bitter, acrid, and slightly toxic *He Shi* (Fructus Carpesii) to expel and kill roundworms, pinworms and tapeworms. Bitter, cold, and toxic, *Ku Lian Pi* (Cortex Meliae) relieves abdominal pain and has a strong effect to kill roundworms, hookworms and pinworms. *Bing Lang* (Semen Arecae) activates qi to expel roundworms, tapeworms, hookworms and pinworms from the body. The astringent *Bai Fan* (Alumen) relieves toxicity and calms the parasites. Lastly, the toxic *Qian Dan* (Minium) kills all kinds of parasites.

***Hua Chong Wan* (Dissolve Parasites Pill)**

Diagnosis	Clinical Signs	Treatment	Herbs
Intestinal parasites	• Intermittent, severe pain migrating up and down the abdomen: intestinal parasites • Nausea and vomiting: intestinal parasites affecting Stomach qi circulation	Expels and kills various intestinal parasites	• *He Shi* (Fructus Carpesii), *Ku Lian Pi* (Cortex Meliae), and *Bing Lang* (Semen Arecae) kill and expel various parasites. • *Bai Fan* (Alumen) relieves toxicity and calms the parasites. • *Qian Dan* (Minium) kills all kinds of parasites.

Huà Chóng Wán (Dissolve Parasites Pill)

Today, this formula is used to treat various types of parasitic infections. It can be used as a general formula to clear the intestinal pathways and expel various parasites. However, since the herbs in this formula are strong in nature, caution should be exercised in administering this formula. To prevent possible injury to the qi, it is advisable to use Spleen and Stomach qi-tonifying herbs after administering this formula.

VETERINARY MODIFICATIONS

- With more abdominal pain, add *Zhi Qiao* (Fructus Aurantii) and *Mu Xiang* (Radix Aucklandiae).
- With more heat, add *Huang Lian* (Rhizoma Coptidis) or *Huang Bo* (Cortex Phellodendri Chinensis).
- With intestinal obstruction due to ascariasis (roundworms), add *Hou Po* (Cortex Magnoliae Officinalis), *Zhi Shi* (Fructus Aurantii Immaturus), *Mu Xiang* (Radix Aucklandiae), and *Da Xue Teng* (Caulis Sargentodoxae).

CAUTIONS / CONTRAINDICATIONS

- *Hua Chong Wan* is an extremely potent and slightly toxic formula for the treatment of intestinal parasites. It must be used with caution in juvenile, geriatric and debilitated animals and should not be used in large doses, or for a prolonged period of time. It should be discontinued once the desired effects are achieved. If the parasites are not completely expelled after the first dose, another dose may be given after one week of rest.
- Use of this formula is contraindicated in pregnancy and in patients with loose stools or diarrhea.
- Because this is a potent formula that may injure the body, tonic herbs should be administered after the parasites are cleared to restore the patient's *zheng* (upright) *qi*.

SUGGESTED ACUPUNCTURE TREATMENT

1. Points: *Baichongwo, Tianshu* (ST 25), *Shangjuxu* (ST 37), *Hegu* (LI 4), *Xiawan* (CV 10), and *Liangmen* (ST 21).
2. Technique: sedation.

This is a general treatment for the various types of parasitic infestations in the intestines. *Baichongwo* is a special point used to treat intestinal parasitic infestation. *Baichongwo*, literally "hundred insects' nest," is located 1 *cun* above *Xuehai* (SP 10). *Tianshu* (ST 25), *Shangjuxu* (ST 37), and *Hegu* (LI 4) remove stagnation in the Intestines. *Xiawan* (CV 10) and *Liangmen* (ST 21) are specifically selected to relieve abdominal pain.

AUTHORS' COMMENTS

Hua Chong Wan is a potent antiparasitic formula that may be used to treat various types of intestinal infestation of parasites, including, but not limited to, ascariasis (roundworms), giardia, coccidia, cestodiasis (tapeworms), cysticercosis, and intestinal flukes.

Chapter 20 — Summary

— Antiparasitic Formulas

Name	Similarities	Differences
Wu Mei Wan (Mume Pill)	Expel and/or kill parasites	Tonifies deficiency
Fei Er Wan (Fat Child Pill)		Strengthens the Spleen, clears Stomach heat
Bu Dai Wan (Cloth Sack Pill)		Tonifies Spleen and Stomach deficiencies
Hua Chong Wan (Dissolve Parasites Pill)		Strongly expels and kills intestinal parasites

Wu Mei Wan (Mume Pill) is generally used to treat ascariasis (roundworms) complicated by heat and cold, excess and deficiency. It warms the interior, tonifies the middle *jiao*, dispels cold, and expels the parasites. It is most effective for ascariasis characterized by weight loss, diarrhea, potbelly, and vomiting of roundworms.

Fei Er Wan (Fat Child Pill) and ***Bu Dai Wan*** (Cloth Sack Pill) both treat *gan ji* (juvenile malnutrition) associated with parasitic infestations.

- *Fei Er Wan* clears heat, kills parasites, and strengthens the Spleen to treat *gan ji* (juvenile malnutrition). Clinically, it is used to treat *gan ji* (juvenile malnutrition) characterized by Spleen deficiency and Stomach heat.
- *Bu Dai Wan* expels parasites, strengthens the Spleen, and relieves *gan ji* (juvenile malnutrition). This formula contains more tonic herbs; thus, it is more suitable for *gan ji* (juvenile malnutrition) with Spleen and Stomach deficiencies.

Hua Chong Wan (Dissolve Parasites Pill) can expel and kill intestinal parasites. It has potent antiparasitic effects and may be used to treat a wide variety of parasites, including ascariasis (roundworms), giardia, coccidia, cestodiasis (tapeworms), cysticercosis (bladder worms), and fasciolopsiasis (intestinal flukes).

Chapter 21

— Emetic Formulas

涌吐剂

张从正 Zhāng Cōng-Zhèng

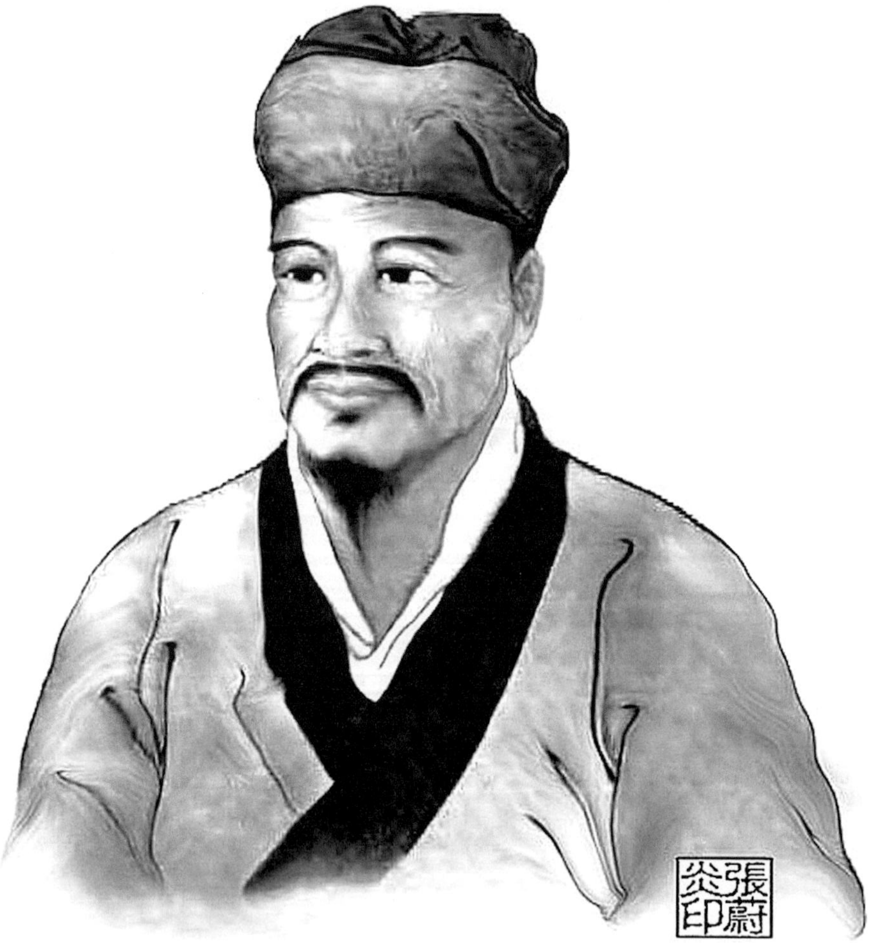

张从正 Zhāng Cōng-Zhèng, also known as
张子和 Zhāng Zǐ-Hé, 1151 – 1231.

张从正 Zhāng Cōng-Zhèng

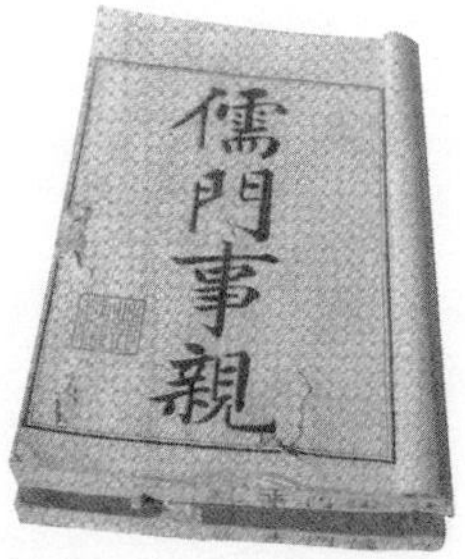

儒门事亲 *Ru Men Shi Qin* (Confucians' Duties to their Parents), published in 1228.

Zhang Cong-Zheng, also known as Zhang Zi-He, is one of the four famous physicians from the period of the Jin and Yuan dynasties. Heavily influenced by Liu Yuan-Su's theories of 火热论 *huo re lun* (discussion of fire and heat), Zhang developed the 攻邪论 *gong xie lun* (discussion on attacking evil). Zhang proposed that all evils are derived from three sources: heaven (wind, cold, summer-heat, dampness, dryness and fire), earth (fog, dew, rain, ice, water and soil) and human (inappropriate diet of excessive sour, bitter, sweet, acrid, salty or bland foods). Correspondingly, all evils can be treated with three methods: *han fa* (sweating) to dispel evil at the exterior, *tu fa* (vomiting) to expel evil from upper body, and *xia fa* (draining downward) to purge evil from the lower body. In contrast to his aggressive treatment methods, Zhang also emphasized the importance of nutrition, and proposed the use of food and herbs to supplement diet and promote longevity. He was the first to establish clear guidelines for nutritional therapy.

Zhang was one of the first to establish the relationship between illnesses and social environment and emotions. Zhang lived and practiced medicine during the end of the Jin dynasty and beginning of the Yuan dynasty, when there was extreme political instability and constant turmoil in the country. Because of this social unrest, people suffered from extreme emotional disturbances, including anger, joy, sadness, fear, worry, and other stressors.

Because of his skills and fame, Zhang was brought to the Imperial Palace as a supreme physician to treat the royal family and court officials. However, he resigned after five years, and opted to live a rambling and leisurely lifestyle that allowed him to read books, write poetry, drink alcohol, and travel around the world. Zhang wrote many works in his lifetime, and is best known for *Ru Men Shi Qin* (Confucians' Duties to their Parents), published in 1228.

Mu Xiang Bing Lang Wan (Aucklandia and Betel Nut Pill) and *Gua Di San* (Melon Pedicle Powder) are two formulas created by Zhang Cong-Zheng that are still in use today.

Dynasties & Kingdoms	Year
Xia Dynasty 夏	2100-1600 BCE
Shang Dynasty 商	1600-1100 BCE
Zhou Dynasty 周	1100-221 BCE
Qin Dynasty 秦	221-207 BCE
Han Dynasty 漢	206 BCE-220
Three Kingdoms 三國	220-280
Western Jin Dynasty 西晉	265-316
Eastern Jin Dynasty 東晉	317-420
Northern and Southern Dynasties 北南朝	420-581
Sui Dynasty 隋	581-618
Tang Dynasty 唐	618-907
Five Dynasties 五代	907-960
Song Dynasty 宋	960-1279
Liao Dynasty 遼	916-1125
Jin Dynasty 金	**1115-1234**
Yuan Dynasty 元	1271-1368
Ming Dynasty 明	1368-1644
Qing Dynasty 清	1644-1911
Republic of China 中華民國	1912-Present Day
People's Republic of China 中華人民共和國	1949-Present Day

Table of Contents

Chapter 21 — Overview

涌吐剂 — Emetic Formulas

Definition: Emetic formulas induce vomiting to treat phlegm stagnation, food accumulation, and the ingestion of poisonous substances. This method of treatment is known as *tu fa* (vomiting), one of the *ba fa* (eight treatment methods) described in the *Huang Di Nei Jing* (Yellow Emperor's Inner Classic) in the first or second century A.D.

These formulas are mainly used to dispel foreign substances from the throat, chest, diaphragm, or epigastrium. Their clinical applications include food stagnation, phlegm stagnation, ingestion of poisonous substances, seizures, *zhong feng* (wind stroke), *bi zheng* (closed disorder) syndrome, *dian kuang* (mania and withdrawal), and *hou bi* (painful obstruction of the throat). Emetic formulas are not typically used in veterinary medicine for the induction of vomiting, as conventional emetic drugs have proven to be more reliable, safe and efficacious. The primary applications of these formulas would be to treat acute poisoning from ingestion of toxic substances and acute food stagnation. Emetic formulas are included here for purposes of discussion and investigation into their potential use.

CAUTIONS / CONTRAINDICATIONS

- Emetic formulas are strong and harsh in nature. Therefore, they should be used with extreme caution in pregnancy, in juvenile, debilitated or geriatric animals, and in cases of blood deficiency, palpitations with shortness of breath, wheezing and dyspnea, and generalized weakness and deficiency. Furthermore, these formulas must be discontinued once the desired effect is achieved.
- The potent and harsh nature of emetic formulas can cause continuous vomiting and injure Stomach qi. For patients that do not cease vomiting after taking the formula, general antidotes such as the fresh juice of *Sheng Jiang* (Rhizoma Zingiberis Recens), cold congee, or cold water should be administered. If these general antidotes do not work, specific antidotes are given. (Specific antidotes vary and are listed in each individual formula monograph.)
- Proper care must be given after emesis to ensure recovery and avoid complications. In order to restore the normal functions of the Spleen and Stomach, animals should consume only congee and other easy-to-digest foods and avoid foods that are greasy, spicy, processed, or hard-to-digest. Also, exposure to wind during and after vomiting should be avoided to prevent the contracting of an exterior condition.
- Accidental poisonings manifest in different clinical signs, depending on the substance ingested. The use of emetic formulas is justified if administered within a short period of time following the ingestion of a poisonous substance, when the injurious matter is still in the stomach and can be ejected by vomiting.
- These formulas should never be used in horses or other species that lack the ability to vomit.
- Emetic formulas should not be used to induce vomiting if corrosive substances have been ingested; this would only cause additional damage to the upper gastrointestinal tract when the corrosive elements are ejected as vomitus.

Chapter 21 — Overview

PHARMACOLOGICAL EFFECTS & CLINICAL APPLICATIONS

Poisoning: The emetic effect of the emetic formulas has been attributed in part to stimulation of the central nervous system and the gastrointestinal tract by herbs such as *Gua Di* (Pedicellus Cucumeris) and *Chang Shan* (Radix Dichroae). Emetic formulas are generally reserved for acute and urgent cases, such as the use of *Gua Di San* (Melon Pedicle Powder) for acute poisoning.[1]

Reference

1. *Zhong Yao Xue* (Chinese Herbology), 1998; 908-909.

Guā Dì Săn (Melon Pedicle Powder)

瓜蒂散

Pinyin Name: *Gua Di San*
Literal Name: Melon Pedicle Powder
Original Source: *Shang Han Lun* (Discussion of Cold-Induced Disorders) by Zhang Zhong-Jing in the Eastern Han Dynasty

COMPOSITION

Gua Di (Pedicellus Cucumeris), *ao* (simmered) until yellow	[1-2g]
Chi Xiao Dou (Semen Phaseoli)	[1-2g]

DOSAGE / PREPARATION / ADMINISTRATION

The source text states to grind equal amounts of the two herbs into a fine powder and sift together. Take 1 spoonful (1-3g) of the powder with a warm, strained decoction made from 6-9g of *Dan Dou Chi* (Semen Sojae Praeparatum). If vomiting is not induced, increase the dose slightly until vomiting is achieved. In addition to using the herbs, vomiting can also be induced physically via the gag reflex. Discontinue the formula when vomiting occurs.

CHINESE THERAPEUTIC ACTIONS

Induces vomiting of phlegm or stagnant food

CLINICAL MANIFESTATIONS

Phlegm or food stagnation in the chest and epigastrium: chest or epigastric distention and hardness causing difficulty in breathing, restlessness, and a slightly superficial pulse.

VETERINARY CLINICAL APPLICATIONS

Acute intoxication, food poisoning, hepatitis, and jaundice.

EXPLANATION

Gua Di San (Melon Pedicle Powder) treats acute and severe phlegm accumulation in the chest, or food stagnation in the epigastrium. The phlegm accumulation and food stagnation may obstruct the proper flow of qi, causing distention and hardness in the chest or epigastrium. Moreover, qi stagnation may lead to the reversed flow of qi, causing difficulty in breathing. Because the stagnation is most severe in the chest region, a slightly superficial pulse may be felt.

This formula uses *Gua Di* (Pedicellus Cucumeris) to induce vomiting of phlegm and stagnant food. *Gua Di* (Pedicellus Cucumeris) also works with *Chi Xiao Dou* (Semen Phaseoli) to expel phlegm and relieve distention and hardness. *Dan Dou Chi* (Semen Sojae Praeparatum) ventilates the Lung, disperses qi stagnation in the chest, and relieves irritability. It also harmonizes the Stomach and regulates the middle *jiao* to prevent the vomiting from damaging the Spleen and Stomach.

CAUTIONS / CONTRAINDICATIONS

- Since *Gua Di* (Pedicellus Cucumeris) is toxic and can easily injure the qi and Stomach, this formula is contraindicated in patients that have Spleen and Stomach deficiencies.
- *Gua Di San* is contraindicated if there is a lack of stagnant phlegm in the chest. Do not use this formula to induce vomiting if the stagnant food has already passed from the stomach to the intestines.
- This formula should only be used in acute and excess conditions. It should be used with extreme caution in geriatric and postpartum patients with blood deficiency, and in those with dizziness and palpitations caused by qi and blood deficiencies.

***Gua Di San* (Melon Pedicle Powder)**

Diagnosis	Clinical Signs	Treatment	Herbs
Phlegm or food stagnation in the chest and epigastrium	• Distention and hardness in the chest or epigastrium: phlegm accumulation and food stagnation • Difficulty in breathing: obstructed qi circulation due to phlegm accumulation and food stagnation	Induces vomiting of phlegm or stagnant food	• *Gua Di* (Pedicellus Cucumeris) induces vomiting of phlegm and stagnant food. • *Chi Xiao Dou* (Semen Phaseoli) expels phlegm and relieves distention and hardness. • *Dan Dou Chi* (Semen Sojae Praeparatum) ventilates the Lung, disperses qi stagnation in the chest, and relieves irritability.

Guā Dì Săn (Melon Pedicle Powder)

- *Gua Di San* must be discontinued when the desired effect is achieved. It must not be used for a prolonged period of time.

HUMAN CLINICAL STUDIES AND RESEARCH

1. **Acute poisoning**: Acute poisoning treated with a modified *Gua Di San* preparation was associated with successful emptying of the stomach in 56 of 58 patients. The overall effectiveness was 96.55%. The average time to empty the stomach of the offending agent was 20.7 minutes. The herbal treatment contained *Gua Di* (Pedicellus Cucumeris), *Sheng Ma* (Rhizoma Cimicifugae), and *Gan Cao* (Radix et Rhizoma Glycyrrhizae). In comparison with other treatment modalities, 58 patients treated with gastric lavage needed an average of 46.4 minutes to empty the stomach, and 56 patients treated with warm water to induce vomiting had only 71.42% effectiveness.[1]
2. **Hepatitis**: Use of *Gua Di San* via intranasal administration has been shown in many studies to effectively treat acute or chronic viral hepatitis.[2] In one study, 153 of 188 patients with acute icteric viral hepatitis showed significant improvement with intranasal administration of 0.1g of *Gua Di San* bilaterally, one time daily, for 3 days per course of treatment.[3]

TOXICOLOGY

Administration of a small dose of *Gua Di San* has not been associated with significant changes to respiration, blood pressure, or heartbeat. However, administration of a large dose has been associated with irregular respiration, decreased blood pressure, reduced heart rate, and eventually, weakened and collapsed respiration.[4] Fatality was reported in one individual eight hours after ingestion of 30g of *Gua Di* (Pedicellus Cucumeris) and 15g of *Chi Xiao Dou* (Semen Phaseoli) on an empty stomach with warm water.[5] Another reported case of fatality involved an individual who ingested *Gua Di San* (actual dose unknown), which subsequently caused gastrointestinal bleeding and eventual fatality on the same day.[6]

TREATMENT OF OVERDOSE

Gua Di San should be used with extreme caution and only when needed. It must be discontinued when the desired effects are achieved. If vomiting persists after the herbs are discontinued, an antidote must be given immediately. Persistent vomiting associated with the use of *Gua Di San* can be relieved with 0.03-0.06 gram of *She Xiang* (Moschus) or 0.3-0.6 gram of *Ding Xiang* (Flos Caryophylli).

SUGGESTED ACUPUNCTURE TREATMENT

1. Points: *Jiuwei* (CV 15) and *Tiantu* (CV 22).
2. Technique: sedation.

The acupuncture treatment here focuses on treating acute and severe stagnation of phlegm or food. *Jiuwei* (CV 15), the *luo* (connecting) point of the *ren* (conception) channel, regulates qi in the Stomach and the chest and eliminates phlegm in the epigastric and thoracic regions. *Tiantu* (CV 22) is a point of intersection between the *yinwei* (linking) and *ren* (conception) channels; it is known for relieving congestion in the chest and esophagus. Sedation of *Tiantu* (CV 22) relieves the feeling of obstruction in the throat.

AUTHORS' COMMENTS

Gua Di San is generally regarded as the standard formula for inducing vomiting. Historically, it has been used to treat severe phlegm accumulation in the chest or food stagnation in the epigastrium. Today, it is also used to treat food poisoning. This formula helps to eliminate offending agents from the stomach and minimizes their further absorption in the digestive tract.

References

1. *Zhong Yi Ming Fang Lin Chuang Xin Yong* (Contemporary Clinical Applications of Classic Chinese Formulas), 2001; 289.
2. *Zhong Yi Ming Fang Lin Chuang Xin Yong* (Contemporary Clinical Applications of Classic Chinese Formulas), 2001; 289.
3. *Ji Lin Zhong Yi Yao* (Jilin Chinese Medicine and Herbology), 1986; 3:12.
4. *Shan Xi Zhong Yi* (Shanxi Chinese Medicine), 1989; 6:39.
5. *Liao Ning Zhong Yi Za Zhi* (Liaoning Journal of Chinese Medicine), 1978; 3:50.
6. *Yao Xue Tong Bao* (Report of Herbology), 1986; 1:42.

Jiù Jí Xī Xián Săn (Urgent Powder to Dilute Saliva)

救急稀涎散

Pinyin Name: *Jiu Ji Xi Xian San*
Literal Name: Urgent Powder to Dilute Saliva
Original Source: *Sheng Ji Zong Lu* (General Collection for Holy Relief) by a staff of court physicians in the Northern Song Dynasty around 1111-1117

COMPOSITION

Zao Jiao (Fructus Gleditsiae)	15g
Bai Fan (Alumen)	30g

DOSAGE / PREPARATION / ADMINISTRATION

The source text states to grind the ingredients into an extremely fine powder. Take 1.5g of the powder with warm water that has been boiled. The dose may be increased (up to 3g) for severe condition. However, avoid overdosing, as it may cause weakness and deficiency.

CHINESE THERAPEUTIC ACTIONS

1. Opens the sensory orifices
2. Dispels phlegm
3. Induces vomiting

CLINICAL MANIFESTATIONS

Zhong feng (wind stroke) and *bi zheng* (closed disorder) syndromes: profuse amount of phlegm and saliva with a rattling sound in the throat, obstruction of qi circulation, decreased muscle tone in the four limbs, altered consciousness or unconsciousness, deviation of the mouth, and a slippery, excess and forceful pulse.

VETERINARY CLINICAL APPLICATIONS

Sudden unconsciousness

EXPLANATION

Jiu Ji Xi Xian San (Urgent Powder to Dilute Saliva) treats animals with *zhong feng* (wind stroke) and *bi zheng* (closed disorder) syndromes characterized by phlegm accumulation. The primary functions of this formula are to dissolve phlegm and open the sensory orifices, and the secondary function is to induce vomiting. As a result of *zhong feng* (wind stroke), phlegm and saliva begin to accumulate in the interior, producing qi stagnation with breathing difficulties, and, in severe cases, *bi zheng* (closed disorder) syndrome with altered consciousness or unconsciousness.

Zao Jiao (Fructus Gleditsiae) opens the orifices by dispelling phlegm, while *Bai Fan* (Alumen) induces vomiting and dissolves phlegm. Once the excessive phlegm and saliva are eliminated, the acute condition of their accumulation will be resolved, hence this formula's name: "Urgent Powder to Dilute Saliva."

CAUTIONS / CONTRAINDICATIONS

Jiu Ji Xi Xian San is designed to treat an urgent situation characterized by acute accumulation of phlegm and saliva. Once this condition is resolved, other herbs and formulas should be used to treat the underlying cause.

SUGGESTED ACUPUNCTURE TREATMENT

1. Points: *Renzhong* (GV 26), *Neiguan* (PC 6), *Laogong* (PC 8), *Fenglong* (ST 40), and *Tiantu* (CV 22).
2. Technique: sedation.

Renzhong (GV 26), *Neiguan* (PC 6), and *Laogong* (PC 8) open the orifices. *Fenglong* (ST 40) and *Tiantu* (CV 22) dissolve phlegm.

***Jiu Ji Xi Xian San* (Urgent Powder to Dilute Saliva)**

Diagnosis	Clinical Signs	Treatment	Herbs
Zhong feng (wind stroke) and *bi zheng* (closed disorder) syndromes	• Profuse amount of phlegm and saliva with a rattling sound in the throat: phlegm obstructing the airways • Altered consciousness or unconsciousness: phlegm obstructing the sensory orifices • Decreased muscle tone in the four limbs and deviation of the mouth: phlegm obstructing the channels and collaterals • Slippery, excess and forceful pulse: phlegm accumulation	• Opens the sensory orifices • Induces vomiting	• *Zao Jiao* (Fructus Gleditsiae) opens the orifices by dispelling phlegm. • *Bai Fan* (Alumen) induces vomiting and dissolves phlegm.

Yán Tāng Tàn Tù Fāng (Salt Decoction to Induce Vomiting)

鹽湯探吐方
盐汤探吐方

Pinyin Name: *Yan Tang Tan Tu Fang*
Literal Name: Salt Decoction to Induce Vomiting
Original Source: *Bei Ji Qian Jin Yao Fang* (Thousands of Golden Prescriptions for Emergencies) by Sun Si-Miao in the Tang Dynasty

COMPOSITION

Shi Yan (Sodium Chloride)

DOSAGE / PREPARATION / ADMINISTRATION

The source text states to dissolve a large amount of *Shi Yan* (Sodium Chloride) in 3 bowls of hot water to make an extremely salty and concentrated solution. Take 1 bowl per dose of the warm solution and repeat with additional doses until all of the stagnant foods are removed via vomiting.

Today, this formula is prepared by dissolving *Shi Yan* (Sodium Chloride) in warm, boiled water until the solution becomes fully saturated. Take 2,000 mL of this preparation per dose to induce vomiting.

CHINESE THERAPEUTIC ACTIONS

Induces vomiting of stagnant food or poisonous substances

CLINICAL MANIFESTATIONS

Food stagnation and sudden turmoil disorder with an inability to vomit or defecate.

VETERINARY CLINICAL APPLICATIONS

Ingestion of poisonous substances

EXPLANATION

Yan Tang Tan Tu Fang (Salt Decoction to Induce Vomiting) treats food stagnation characterized by the patient's inability to vomit. In this syndrome, the patient may have the desire to vomit, but is unable to do so.

This formula uses salt to induce vomiting and relieve stagnation in the body. It is a mild and convenient formula. If the patient does not respond immediately, try administering more salt water.

This formula may also be used for sudden turmoil disorder with severe abdominal pain, in which the patient cannot vomit or defecate. Lastly, it may be used for unconsciousness syndromes that are caused by overeating or Liver qi stagnation.

SUGGESTED ACUPUNCTURE TREATMENT

1. Points: *Neiguan* (PC 6) and *Housanli* (ST 36).
2. Technique: sedation.

Needle *Neiguan* (PC 6) and *Housanli* (ST 36) against the channels with strong manipulation to induce vomiting.

***Yan Tang Tan Tu Fang* (Salt Decoction to Induce Vomiting)**

Diagnosis	Clinical Signs	Treatment	Herbs
Food stagnation	Food stagnation with a desire to vomit	Induces vomiting	*Shi Yan* (Sodium Chloride) induces vomiting and relieves stagnation

Chapter 21 — Summary

— Emetic Formulas

Name	Similarities	Differences
Gua Di San (Melon Pedicle Powder)	Induce vomiting	Strongest emetic effect
Jiu Ji Xi Xian San (Urgent Powder to Dilute Saliva)		Mildest emetic effect
Yan Tang Tan Tu Fang (Salt Decoction to Induce Vomiting)		Moderate and gentle emetic effect

Gua Di San (Melon Pedicle Powder) has the strongest emetic action of these three formulas. It resolves food accumulation in the Stomach and phlegm stagnation in the chest or diaphragm. Clinical manifestations include chest or epigastric fullness and hardness, irritability, and a slightly superficial pulse.

Jiu Ji Xi Xian San (Urgent Powder to Dilute Saliva) has the mildest emetic action of these three formulas. This formula treats *zhong feng* (wind stroke) and *bi zheng* (closed disorder) syndromes with profuse amount of phlegm, obstruction of saliva, and stagnation of qi. Clinical manifestations include decreased muscle tone in the four extremities, altered consciousness or unconsciousness, deviation of the mouth, and a slippery, excess and forceful pulse.

Yan Tang Tan Tu Fang (Salt Decoction to Induce Vomiting) has a gentle and moderate emetic function. It treats the presence of stagnant food or the ingestion of poisonous substances. It is also used for sudden turmoil disorder characterized by the presence of abdominal pain and the inability to vomit or defecate.

Chapter 22

— Formulas that Treat Abscesses and Sores

痈疡剂

龚廷贤 Gŏng Tíng-Xiān

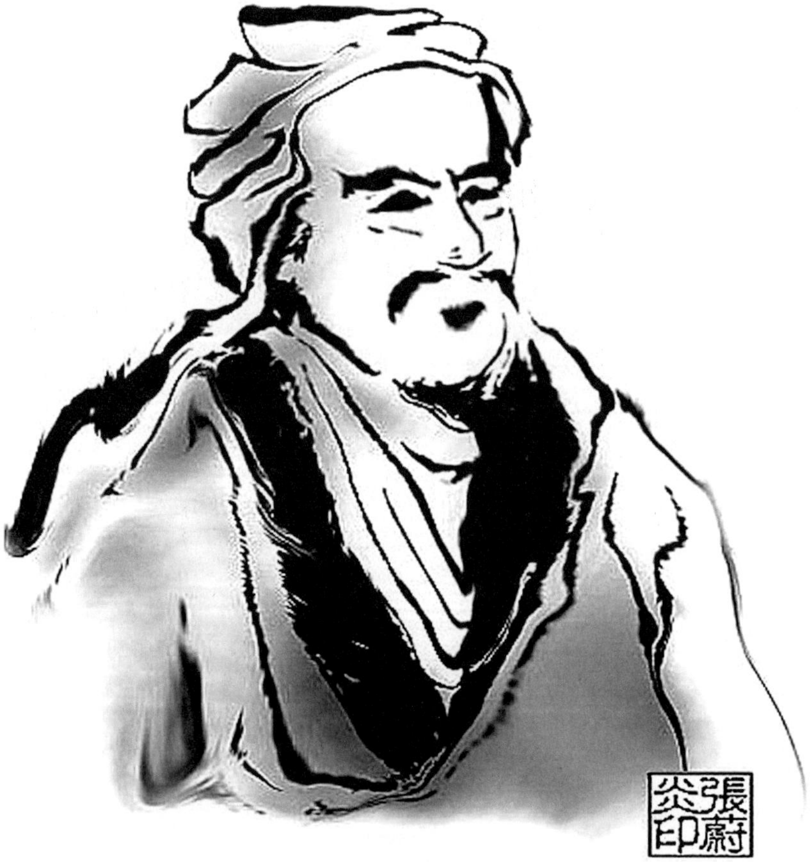

龚廷贤 Gǒng Tíng-Xiān, 1522 – 1619.

龚廷贤 Gǒng Tíng-Xiān

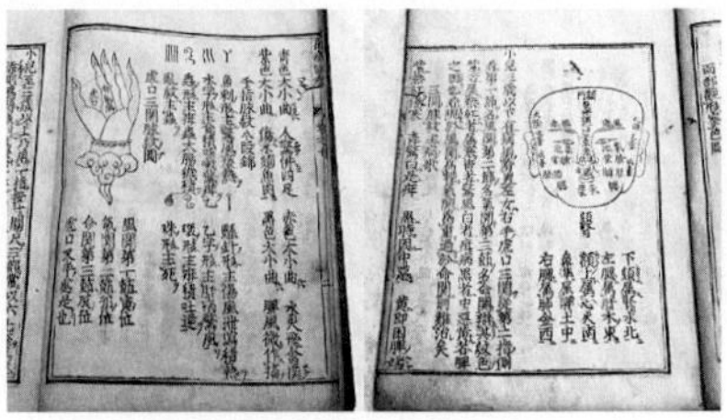

万病回春 *Wan Bing Hui Chun* (Restoration of Health from the Myriad Diseases) in 1587.

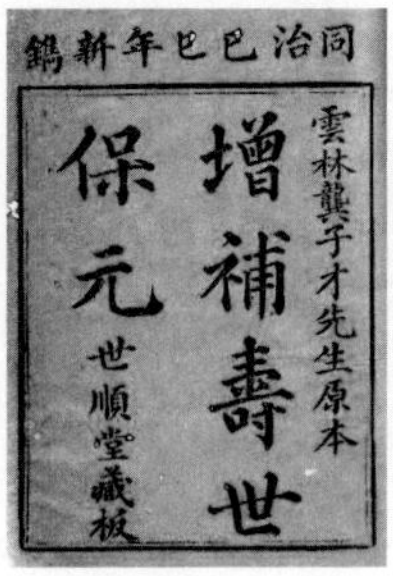

寿世保元 *Shou Shi Bao Yuan* (Achieving Longevity by Guarding the Source) in 1615.

Gong Ting-Xian was one of the most famous physicians of the Ming dynasty in the 16th century. Gong's father was a supreme physician in the Imperial Palace, and subsequently trained him to also become a supreme physician. Gong studied many aspects of medicine, and published many books in his lifetime.

His most famous works include *Wan Bing Hui Chun* (Restoration of Health from the Myriad Diseases) in 1587 and *Shou Shi Bao Yuan* (Achieving Longevity by Guarding the Source) in 1615. The former text totaled 8 volumes, and contained detailed information on differential diagnosis, pathology, treatment, and prevention of, as the name of the text suggests, a myriad of diseases. The latter text contained 10 volumes, and discussed the diagnosis and treatment of internal medicine, external medicine, gynecology, pediatrics and more.

These texts presented many formulas that are commonly prescribed today, such as

- *Jing Jie Lian Qiao Tang* (Schizonepeta and Forsythia Decoction)
- *Shu Gan Tang* (Spread the Liver Decoction)
- *Qing Shang Fang Feng Tang* (Clear the Upper and Guard the Wind Decoction)
- *Wen Qing Yin* (Warming and Clearing Decoction)
- *Fen Xiao Tang* (Separate and Reduce Decoction)
- *Shu Jing Huo Xue Tang* (Relax the Channels and Invigorate the Blood Decoction)
- *Qing Fei Tang* (Clear the Lung Decoction)
- *Qian Jin Nei Tuo San* (Drain-the-Interior Powder Worthy of a Thousand Gold)
- *Shi Liu Wei Liu Qi Yin* (Sixteen-Ingredient Decoction to Flow Qi)
- *San Zhong Kui Jian Tang* (Disperse the Swelling and Break the Hardness Decoction)

Dynasties & Kingdoms	Year
Xia Dynasty 夏	2100-1600 BCE
Shang Dynasty 商	1600-1100 BCE
Zhou Dynasty 周	1100-221 BCE
Qin Dynasty 秦	221-207 BCE
Han Dynasty 漢	206 BCE-220
Three Kingdoms 三國	220-280
Western Jin Dynasty 西晉	265-316
Eastern Jin Dynasty 東晉	317-420
Northern and Southern Dynasties 北南朝	420-581
Sui Dynasty 隋	581-618
Tang Dynasty 唐	618-907
Five Dynasties 五代	907-960
Song Dynasty 宋	960-1279
Liao Dynasty 遼	916-1125
Jin Dynasty 金	1115-1234
Yuan Dynasty 元	1271-1368
Ming Dynasty 明	**1368-1644**
Qing Dynasty 清	1644-1911
Republic of China 中華民國	1912-Present Day
People's Republic of China 中華人民共和國	1949-Present Day

Table of Contents

Chapter 22 — Overview

痈疡剂 — Formulas that Treat Abscesses and Sores

Definition: Formulas that treat abscesses and sores clear heat, eliminate toxins, reduce swellings, drain the interior, discharge pus, promote the generation of new flesh, and astringe ulcerations.

Formulas that treat abscesses and sores have a wide range of clinical applications. They are commonly used to treat both external conditions (including abscesses, sores, cellulitis, boils, multiple abscesses, carbuncles, furuncles, goiter, and malignant and non-malignant tumors) and internal disorders (such as abscesses of the organs). In veterinary medicine, they can be used to treat a wide range of conditions: atopic dermatitis, necrotizing dermatitis, folliculitis, cellulitis, gangrene, vasculitis, mastitis, mammary gland carcinoma, thyroid carcinoma, feline hyperthyroidism, intestinal adenocarcinoma, lymphocytic leukemia, abscesses secondary to bite wounds, osteomyelitis, non-healing wounds and sores, pyoderma, disorders of the lymphatic system, lymphadenitis, lung abscess and intestinal abscess.

Abscesses and sores can either be externally contracted or internally generated. External causes of abscesses and sores include *liu yin* (six exogenous factors), insect or bite wounds, scratch wounds, cuts and burns, and various sport injuries or traumas. Internal causes of abscesses and sores include damages caused by imbalance of *qi qing* (seven emotions), chronic disease (diabetes, Cushing's disease) or an inappropriate diet consisting of too much damp or hot food. These etiological factors can lead to stagnation within the channels and collaterals and disharmony between the qi and blood. If this stagnation is left untreated, heat formation results, and abscesses and sores eventually will form. Other factors, such as cold, dampness, or phlegm, can also stagnate in the muscles, tendons, ligaments, and channels and collaterals to cause either *yin* (deep-rooted) or *yang* (superficial) type of abscesses and sores.

Differential diagnosis of abscesses and sores begins with assessment of whether the condition is externally contracted or internally generated.

- Diagnostic criteria for externally contracted abscesses and sores include differentiation of yin and yang. For example, *yang* (superficial) abscesses and sores are characterized by prominent swelling and inflammation, limited size or surface area with defined borders, redness, and warm, burning sensations in the affected area. On the other hand, *yin* (deep-rooted) abscesses and sores are usually characterized by very slight swelling (almost flat) that may be hard or soft. The affected area is widespread, involves a large surface area, and shows no change in skin color.
- Diagnostic criteria for internally generated abscesses and sores include differentiation of cold or heat, deficiency or excess, and with or without pus. Lung and intestinal abscesses are the most common internal abscess disorders that affect the *zang fu* organs. Pyometra is considered to be an internal abscess of the uterus in Chinese medicine; herbal formulas that treat internal abscesses are not typically used for this condition, as the most common treatment is typically surgical removal of the entire uterus.

External abscesses and sores are treated internally with three main treatment methods: *xiao fa* (reducing method) in the early stage, *tuo fa* (draining method) in the middle stage when there is pus formation, and *bu fa* (tonifying method) in the late stage with ulcerations.

Chapter 22 — Overview

- *Xiao fa* (reducing method) is used in the early stage of abscesses and sores, prior to the formation of pus, to disperse heat and toxins, reduce swelling, and terminate the illness. Specific types of *xiao fa* (reducing method) include the use of herbs that release the exterior, clear heat, warm and unblock, resolve phlegm, move qi, activate blood circulation, and eliminate stagnation.
- *Tuo fa* (draining method) is used in the early to middle stage of abscesses and sores, a stage marked by pus formation with the presence of heat and toxins, or generalized weakness and deficiency with an inability to discharge the pus. *Tuo fa* (draining method) brings the heat and toxins from the deep aspects of the body to the superficial and facilitates the perforation and discharge of pus. However, because this stage is usually characterized by underlying weakness and deficiency, the use of *bu fa* (tonifying method) may be necessary to facilitate the healing process.
- *Bu fa* (tonifying method) is employed in the late stage when the abscesses and sores have perforated and ulcerated, and pus begins to discharge. However, the area of ulceration may not have reduced in size, and the pus may continue to discharge and fails to heal because of underlying deficiencies of qi and blood, Spleen and Stomach, or Liver and Kidney. In these circumstances, *bu fa* (tonifying method) is used to tonify deficiencies, astringe the ulcerations, dry the pus, promote the generation of tissues, and facilitate healing.

Internal abscesses and sores affecting the interior *zang fu* organs should be treated with multiple methods to clear heat, eliminate toxins, and dispel stagnation to reduce swelling. Depending on the individual condition, it may be necessary to add herbs to drain pus and tonify the underlying deficiencies as needed.

SUBCATEGORIES OF ACTION

Formulas that treat abscesses and sores are divided into two subcategories to treat external and internal abscesses and sores.

1. **Formulas that Treat External Abscesses and Sores**

External abscesses and sores can have various presentations and require formulas of corresponding characteristics for treatment. Some formulas emphasize treatment based on differentiation of yin or yang, hot or cold, and excess or deficiency; other formulas focus on the physical location of the abscesses and sores.

- External abscesses and sores characterized by excess, heat, and yang should be treated with formulas that clear heat, eliminate toxins, break the hardness, and reduce the swelling, such as *Xian Fang Huo Ming Yin* (Sublime Formula for Sustaining Life).
- External abscesses and sores characterized by deficiency, cold, and yin should be treated with formulas that tonify, warm and disperse cold, such as *Yang He Tang* (Yang-Heartening Decoction).

Moreover, depending on the nature of the disease (excess or deficiency) and the underlying constitution of the animal, formulas with various functions may be used.

- Exemplar formulas that drain the interior and discharge pus include *Xian Fang Huo Ming Yin* (Sublime Formula for Sustaining Life) and *Wu Wei Xiao Du Yin* (Five-Ingredient Decoction to Eliminate Toxins).
- An exemplar formula that tonifies underlying deficiencies and drains abscesses and sores is *Yang He Tang* (Yang-Heartening Decoction).

Lastly, external abscesses and sores may affect different parts of the body, and thus they require formulas that treat these affected areas. Exemplar formulas in this subcategory include formulas from other chapters that also treat abscesses and sores.

- Formulas that disperse and clear wind-heat are often used to treat abscesses and sores affecting the upper parts of the body (head, face, neck, and shoulders), such as *Niu Bang Jie Ji Tang* (Arctium Decoction to Release the Muscle Layer).

Chapter 22 — Overview

- Formulas that regulate Liver qi circulation, purge fire and eliminate toxins are incorporated to treat abscesses and sores affecting the middle parts of the body (chest, back, and abdomen), such as *Jia Wei Xiao Yao San* (Augmented Rambling Powder) and *Huang Lian Jie Du Tang* (Coptis Decoction to Relieve Toxicity).
- Formulas that clear heat, eliminate toxins, and activate qi and blood circulation in the peripheral channels and collaterals are frequently deployed to treat abscesses and sores affecting the extremities, such as *Si Miao Yong An Tang* (Four-Valiant Decoction for Well-Being).

2. **Formulas that Treat Internal Abscesses and Sores**
Internal abscesses and sores generally affect the lungs and the intestines. Lung abscesses characterized by phlegm, heat, and blood stagnation are treated with formulas, such as *Wei Jing Tang* (Reed Decoction). Intestinal abscesses characterized by damp-heat accumulation and qi and blood stagnation are treated with ormulas, such as *Da Huang Mu Dan Tang* (Rhubarb and Moutan Decoction).

CAUTIONS / CONTRAINDICATIONS

Accurate differential diagnosis and proper selection of treatment methods are essential in obtaining successful results. Incorrect diagnosis or the use of inappropriate treatment methods will delay healing or possibly worsen the condition.

- *Xiao fa* (reducing method) is used in the early stage of abscesses and sores. The use of this strong method is inappropriate in the late stage of abscesses and sores with underlying deficiencies, as it will damage qi and blood and lead to prolonged duration of the illness due to the inability of the ulcerations to heal.
- *Tuo fa* (draining method) is used in the middle stage of abscesses and sores. This method is not recommended if the abscesses and sores are characterized by the presence of excess heat and toxins, which should be treated with herbs that clear heat and eliminate toxins.
- *Bu fa* (tonifying method) is employed in the late stage of abscesses and sores. This method should not be used during the early stage of abscesses and sores, or in cases of accumulation of heat and toxins in the interior, because this method will only contribute to more excess and stagnation.

PHARMACOLOGICAL EFFECTS & CLINICAL APPLICATIONS

Although these formulas are known for treating abscesses and sores, they have a wide variety of pharmacological effects and clinical applications. Formulas that treat external abscesses and sores can treat indications characterized by infections and inflammations that come with abscesses, sores, nodules, and hardness.

- **Dermatological disorders**: These formulas may be used to treat various disorders affecting the skin, such as carbuncles and sores,[1,2] cellulitis,[3] acne vulgaris,[4] gangrene,[5] and erysipelas.[6] Exemplar formulas include *Xian Fang Huo Ming Yin* (Sublime Formula for Sustaining Life), *Si Miao Yong An Tang* (Four-Valiant Decoction for Well-Being), and *Shi Wei Bai Du Tang* (Ten-Ingredient Decoction to Overcome Pathogenic Influences).
- **Blood vessel disorders**: These formulas are effective in treating inflammatory conditions of the blood vessels, such as phlebitis,[7] thrombophlebitis,[8,9,10] thromboangiitis obliterans,[11,12,13] and thrombosis of the iliofemoral vein.[14] Representative formulas include *Xian Fang Huo Ming Yin* (Sublime Formula for Sustaining Life), *Si Miao Yong An Tang* (Four-Valiant Decoction for Well-Being), and *Yang He Tang* (Yang-Heartening Decoction).
- **Breast disorders**: These formulas demonstrate effectiveness in treating various types of breast disorders, such as mastitis,[15,16] breast abscesses,[17] hyperplasia of mammary glands,[18,19] and cystic hyperplasia of the breast.[20] Representative formulas include *Xian Fang Huo Ming Yin* (Sublime Formula for Sustaining Life), *Xiao Luo Wan* (Reduce Scrofula Pill), *Yang He Tang* (Yang-Heartening Decoction), and *Hai Zao Yu Hu Tang* (Sargassum Decoction for the Jade Flask).

Chapter 22 — Overview

- **Throat disorders**: *Xian Fang Huo Ming Yin* (Sublime Formula for Sustaining Life) and *Wu Wei Xiao Du Yin* (Five-Ingredient Decoction to Eliminate Toxins) are two formulas commonly used to treat parotitis, tonsillitis, and peritonsillar abscesses. [21,22,23,24]
- **Others:** Some of these formulas can treat other inflammatory diseases, such as pelvic inflammatory disease,[25,26] appendicular abscess,[27] osteomyelitis,[28,29] and myelitis.[30]

Formulas that treat internal abscesses and sores can also treat various infections and inflammation of the internal organs that give rise to abscesses and sores.

- **Pulmonary disorders**: *Wei Jing Tang* (Reed Decoction) has been shown to effectively treat infection and inflammation of the lungs. The clinical applications of this formula include pulmonary abscesses,[31,32] pneumonia (lobar pneumonia, lobular pneumonia, bronchopneumonia, and mycoplasmal pneumonia),[33] and bronchitis (bronchitis in children, suppurative bronchitis, and chronic bronchitis).[34,35,36]
- **Appendicitis**: These formulas have been used successfully to treat acute appendicitis,[37] chronic appendicitis,[38] ruptured appendicitis with peritonitis,[39] and periappendicular abscess.[40] Two representative formulas are *Da Huang Mu Dan Tang* (Rhubarb and Moutan Decoction) and *Yi Yi Fu Zi Bai Jiang San* (Coicis, Prepared Aconite, and Patrinia Powder).
- **Others**: Formulas that treat internal abscesses and sores have also been shown to treat other diseases characterized by infection and/or inflammation of the internal organs, such as pelvic inflammatory disease, [41,42] acute cholecystitis,[43] ulcerative colitis,[44] chronic prostatitis,[45] and suppurative tonsillitis.[46]

References

1. *He Nan Zhong Yi* (Henan Chinese Medicine), 1988; 5:31.
2. *Hu Bei Zhong Yi Za Zhi* (Hubei Journal of Chinese Medicine), 1988; 6:23.
3. *Liao Ning Zhong Yi Za Zhi* (Liaoning Journal of Chinese Medicine), 1994; 21(5):222.
4. Higaki S, Kitagawa T, Kagoura M, Morohashi M, Yamagishi T. Relationship between Propionibacterium acnes biotypes and Jumi-haidoku-to. Journal of Dermatology. 2000 Oct; 27(10):635-8.
5. *Xin Zhong Yi* (New Chinese Medicine), 1990; 2:27.
6. *Hu Bei Zhong Yi Za Zhi* (Hubei Journal of Chinese Medicine), 1998; 5:32.
7. *Shan Xi Zhong Yi* (Shanxi Chinese Medicine), 1998; 2:74.
8. *Liao Ning Zhong Yi Za Zhi* (Liaoning Journal of Chinese Medicine), 1991; 5:34.
9. *Xin Zhong Yi* (New Chinese Medicine), 1992; 10:24.
10. *Si Chuan Zhong Yi* (Sichuan Chinese Medicine), 1992; 9:37.
11. *Zhong Yi Za Zhi* (Journal of Chinese Medicine), 1980; 1:42.
12. *Tian Jin Yi Yao Za Zhi* (Journal of Tianjin Medicine and Herbology), 1960; 1:1.
13. *Zhe Jiang Zhong Yi Za Zhi* (Zhejiang Journal of Chinese Medicine), 1982; 2:82.
14. *Hei Long Jiang Zhong Yi Yao* (Heilongjiang Chinese Medicine and Herbology), 1997; 3:1.
15. *Nei Meng Gu Zhong Yi Yao* (Traditional Chinese Medicine and Medicinals of Inner Mongolia), 1994; 2:7.
16. *Shi Yong Zhong Yi Yao Za Zhi* (Journal of Practical Chinese Medicine and Medicinals), 1997; 6:13.
17. *Shan Xi Zhong Yi* (Shanxi Chinese Medicine), 1989; 8:366.
18. *Shi Yong Zhong Yi Yao Za Zhi* (Journal of Practical Chinese Medicine and Medicinals), 1998; 11:9.
19. *Shi Yong Zhong Yi Yao Za Zhi* (Journal of Practical Chinese Medicine and Medicinals), 1999; 3:14.
20. *Xin Zhong Yi* (New Chinese Medicine), 1997; 2:18.
21. *Zhong Xi Yi Jie He Za Zhi* (Journal of Integrated Chinese and Western Medicine), 1989; 9(10):612.
22. *He Nan Zhong Yi* (Henan Chinese Medicine), 1995; 5:35.
23. *Shan Dong Zhong Yi Za Zhi* (Shandong Journal of Chinese Medicine), 1992; 11(5):15.
24. *Shang Hai Zhong Yi Yao Za Zhi* (Shanghai Journal of Chinese Medicine and Herbology), 1994; 4:24.
25. *Jiang Su Zhong Yi* (Jiangsu Chinese Medicine), 1996; 6:18.
26. *Fu Jian Yi Yao Za Zhi* (Fujian Journal of Medicine and Herbology), 1994; 4:58.
27. *Zhong Hua Wai Ke Za Zhi* (Chinese Journal of External Medicine), 1960; 2:171.
28. *He Bei Zhong Yi* (Hebei Chinese Medicine), 1989; 3:108.
29. *Jiang Su Zhong Yi* (Jiangsu Chinese Medicine), 1963; 4.
30. *Jiang Xi Zhong Yi Yao* (Jiangxi Chinese Medicine and Herbology), 1997; 5:44.
31. *He Nan Zhong Yi* (Henan Chinese Medicine), 1991; 11(5):24.
32. *Shi Yong Zhong Xi Yi Jie He Za Zhi* (Practical Journal of Integrated Chinese and Western Medicines), 1992; 5(2):83.
33. *Shan Xi Zhong Yi* (Shanxi Chinese Medicine), 1994; 15(8):342.
34. *Shang Hai Zhong Yi Yao Za Zhi* (Shanghai Journal of Chinese Medicine and Herbology), 1983; 10:26.

Chapter 22 — Overview

35. *Shang Hai Zhong Yi Yao Za Zhi* (Shanghai Journal of Chinese Medicine and Herbology), 1959; 2:15.
36. *Jiang Su Zhong Yi* (Jiangsu Chinese Medicine), 1982; 5:14.
37. *Guang Xi Zhong Yi Yao* (Guangxi Chinese Medicine and Herbology), 1986; 3:10.
38. *Tian Jin Yi Yao Za Zhi* (Journal of Tianjin Medicine and Herbology), 1959; 11:411.
39. *Nei Meng Gu Zhong Yi Yao* (Traditional Chinese Medicine and Medicinals of Inner Mongolia), 1993; 2:23.
40. *Yun Nan Zhong Yi Za Zhi* (Yunan Journal of Chinese Medicine), 1995; 2:11.
41. *Guang Xi Zhong Yi Yao* (Guangxi Chinese Medicine and Herbology), 1992; 5:6.
42. *Shan Xi Zhong Yi* (Shanxi Chinese Medicine), 1993; 14(12):533.
43. *Shi Yong Zhong Yi Nei Ke Za Zhi* (Journal of Practical Chinese Internal Medicine), 1992; 3:127.
44. *He Nan Zhong Yi* (Henan Chinese Medicine), 1998; 1:22.
45. *Zhe Jiang Zhong Yi Za Zhi* (Zhejiang Journal of Chinese Medicine), 1993; 8:368.
46. *Liao Ning Zhong Yi Za Zhi* (Liaoning Journal of Chinese Medicine), 1991; 6:36.

Section 1

外痈疡剂 — External Abscesses and Sores

Xiān Fāng Huó Mìng Yǐn (Sublime Formula for Sustaining Life)

仙方活命飲
仙方活命饮

Pinyin Name: *Xian Fang Huo Ming Yin*
Literal Name: Sublime Formula for Sustaining Life
Original Source: *Jiao Zhu Fu Ren Liang Fang* (Revised Fine Formulas for Women) by Bi Li-Zhai in the 16th century

COMPOSITION

Jin Yin Hua (Flos Lonicerae Japonicae)	9g
Fang Feng (Radix Saposhnikoviae)	3g
Bai Zhi (Radix Angelicae Dahuricae)	3g
Dang Gui Wei (Extremitas Radix Angelicae Sinensis)	3g
Chi Shao (Radix Paeoniae Rubra)	3g
Ru Xiang (Gummi Olibanum)	3g
Mo Yao (Myrrha)	3g
Zhe Bei Mu (Bulbus Fritillariae Thunbergii)	3g
Tian Hua Fen (Radix Trichosanthis)	3g
Chuan Shan Jia (Squama Manis), *zhi* (fried with liquid)	3g
Zao Jiao Ci (Spina Gleditsiae), *chao* (dry-fried)	3g
Chen Pi (Pericarpium Citri Reticulatae)	9g
Gan Cao (Radix et Rhizoma Glycyrrhizae)	3g

Note: *Chuan Shan Jia* (Squama Manis) is derived from an endangered animal and is rarely used as a medicinal substance today. Its discussion here is included primarily for academic purposes, to reflect the historical use of this substance in its original formulation. Most herbal products today have removed it completely, or replaced it with substitutes with similar functions.

DOSAGE / PREPARATION / ADMINISTRATION

The source text states to cook the ingredients with 1 large bowl of grain-based liquor and bring it to a boil 5-7 times. Today, it is prepared as a decoction with water or with a 50:50 mixture of water and grain-based liquor.

CHINESE THERAPEUTIC ACTIONS

1. Clears heat and eliminates toxins
2. Reduces swelling and breaks hardness
3. Activates blood circulation and stops pain

CLINICAL MANIFESTATIONS

Early onset of abscesses and sores characterized by accumulation of heat and toxins and stagnation of qi and blood: local redness, swelling and pain with or without fever and trembling, a red tongue, and a rapid, forceful pulse.

VETERINARY CLINICAL APPLICATIONS

Carbuncles (an abscess of the skin that involves hair follicles, sebaceous glands and subcutaneous tissues, made up of multiple furuncles), furuncles (skin boils), vasculitis, mastitis, anal gland abscess, hordeolum (stye), osteomyelitis, and abscesses in rabbits.

EXPLANATION

Xian Fang Huo Ming Yin (Sublime Formula for Sustaining Life) treats early onset of abscesses and sores characterized by accumulation of heat and toxins and stagnation of qi

Xiān Fāng Huó Mìng Yǐn (Sublime Formula for Sustaining Life)

Xian Fang Huo Ming Yin **(Sublime Formula for Sustaining Life)**

Diagnosis	Clinical Signs	Treatment	Herbs
Early onset of abscesses and sores	• Abscesses, sores, local redness and swelling: heat and toxins in the skin and muscles • Local pain: qi and blood stagnation • Fever and trembling: exterior condition • A red tongue: early stage of heat • Rapid, forceful pulse: excess heat condition	• Clears heat and eliminates toxins • Reduces swelling and breaks the hardness • Activates blood circulation and stops pain	• *Jin Yin Hua* (Flos Lonicerae Japonicae) clears heat and eliminates toxins. • *Fang Feng* (Radix Saposhnikoviae) and *Bai Zhi* (Radix Angelicae Dahuricae) disperse and dispel heat toxins. • *Dang Gui Wei* (Extremitas Radix Angelicae Sinensis), *Chi Shao* (Radix Paeoniae Rubra), *Ru Xiang* (Gummi Olibanum), and *Mo Yao* (Myrrha) activate blood circulation and remove blood stagnation. • *Zhe Bei Mu* (Bulbus Fritillariae Thunbergii) and *Tian Hua Fen* (Radix Trichosanthis) resolve phlegm, clear heat, reduce swelling, dispel pus, and break hardness. • *Chuan Shan Jia* (Squama Manis) and *Zao Jiao Ci* (Spina Gleditsiae) drain abscesses and soften nodules. • *Chen Pi* (Pericarpium Citri Reticulatae) regulates the qi flow. • *Gan Cao* (Radix et Rhizoma Glycyrrhizae) clears heat, eliminates toxins, and harmonizes the Stomach.

and blood. It is suitable for early onset of abscesses and sores, in which pus has not yet formed. In this syndrome, heat and toxins in the skin and muscles may cause local redness and swelling, while qi and blood stagnation may cause pain. Since the disease is still located at the exterior, fever and trembling are present. A red tongue with a thin and white or yellow coating indicates that the heat has not yet progressed to the interior organs, while a rapid, forceful pulse suggests excess heat in the body.

Jin Yin Hua (Flos Lonicerae Japonicae) clears heat and eliminates toxins. *Fang Feng* (Radix Saposhnikoviae) and *Bai Zhi* (Radix Angelicae Dahuricae) disperse and dispel heat and toxins from the superficial parts of the body. *Dang Gui Wei* (Extremitas Radix Angelicae Sinensis), *Chi Shao* (Radix Paeoniae Rubra), *Ru Xiang* (Gummi Olibanum), and *Mo Yao* (Myrrha) activate blood circulation and remove blood stagnation to reduce the redness, swelling, and pain. *Zhe Bei Mu* (Bulbus Fritillariae Thunbergii) and *Tian Hua Fen* (Radix Trichosanthis) resolve phlegm, clear heat, reduce swelling, dispel pus, and disperse nodules. *Chuan Shan Jia* (Squama Manis) and *Zao Jiao Ci* (Spina Gleditsiae) open the channels and collaterals to drain the abscesses and soften the nodules. *Chen Pi* (Pericarpium Citri Reticulatae) regulates the qi flow. *Gan Cao* (Radix et Rhizoma Glycyrrhizae) clears heat, eliminates toxins, and harmonizes the Stomach. The use of grain-based liquor helps to activate blood circulation and open the channels and collaterals.

VETERINARY MODIFICATIONS

- For abscesses and sores in the head region, add *Chuan Xiong* (Rhizoma Chuanxiong).
- For abscesses and sores in the chest region, add *Gua Lou* (Fructus Trichosanthis).
- For abscesses and sores in the hypochondriac area, add *Chai Hu* (Radix Bupleuri).
- For abscesses and sores in the waist and back regions, add *Qin Jiao* (Radix Gentianae Macrophyllae).
- For abscesses and sores in the lower extremities, add *Niu Xi* (Radix Achyranthis Bidentatae).
- To enhance the formula's ability to clear heat and eliminate toxins, add one or more of the following: *Zi Hua Di Ding* (Herba Violae), *Pu Gong Ying* (Herba Taraxaci), *Ban Lan Gen* (Radix Isatidis), and/or *Lian Qiao* (Fructus Forsythiae).
- To enhance the formula's ability to eliminate stagnation and soften nodules and hardness, add *Kun Bu* (Thallus Eckloniae), *Tong Cao* (Medulla Tetrapanacis), and *Xia Ku Cao* (Spica Prunellae).
- To improve ability to invigorate blood and resolve stasis, add *Hong Hua* (Flos Carthami) and *Tao Ren* (Semen Persicae).
- With heat in the *xue* (blood) level, add *Di Huang* (Radix Rehmanniae), *Xuan Shen* (Radix Scrophulariae), and *Mu Dan Pi* (Cortex Moutan).
- With qi deficiency, add *Huang Qi* (Radix Astragali) and *Dang Shen* (Radix Codonopsis).

Xiān Fāng Huó Mìng Yǐn (Sublime Formula for Sustaining Life)

CAUTIONS / CONTRAINDICATIONS

- *Xian Fang Huo Ming Yin* should be used with caution in patients with Spleen and Stomach deficiencies, or qi and blood deficiencies. Herbs or formulas that tonify the middle *jiao* should be added as needed.
- This formula is indicated for early stages of abscesses and sores. It is contraindicated for *yin* (deep-rooted) sores, or if the lesions have already ulcerated.

HUMAN CLINICAL STUDIES AND RESEARCH

1. **Abscesses and sores**: One study reported 100% effectiveness using modified *Xian Fang Huo Ming Yin* to treat generalized sores and abscesses.[1] Another study reported 96.3% effectiveness in treating 54 patients with swelling and deep-rooted sores.[2]
2. **Breast abscesses**: Researchers reported complete recovery in 29 of 30 patients with breast abscesses using both oral and topical applications of herbs. Oral formulation was given as a decoction daily, for 7 days per course of treatment, for 1-2 courses total. The formula contained *Jin Yin Hua* (Flos Lonicerae Japonicae) 20g, *Bai Zhi* (Radix Angelicae Dahuricae) 10g, *Dang Gui* (Radix Angelicae Sinensis) 10g, *Chuan Bei Mu* (Bulbus Fritillariae Cirrhosae) 10g, *Fang Feng* (Radix Saposhnikoviae) 10g, *Gan Cao* (Radix et Rhizoma Glycyrrhizae) 10g, *Ru Xiang* (Gummi Olibanum) 6g, *Mo Yao* (Myrrha) 6g, *Zao Jiao Ci* (Spina Gleditsiae) 10g, *Tian Hua Fen* (Radix Trichosanthis) 10g, and *Chen Pi* (Pericarpium Citri Reticulatae) 10g. The treatment protocol was to administer the herbs in decoction with a small amount of grain-based liquor. The topical formulation contained 60g each of *Da Huang* (Radix et Rhizoma Rhei) and *Mang Xiao* (Natrii Sulfas). These two herbs were cooked in 8000 mL of water for 40 minutes, and the decoction was given as a room-temperature herbal wash to the affected area.[3]
3. **Mastitis**: One hundred and eight patients with acute mastitis were treated with modified *Xian Fang Huo Ming Yin*, with complete recovery in 82 cases, marked improvement in 15 cases, slight improvement in 10 cases, and no effect in 1 case. The herbal formula contained *Jin Yin Hua* (Flos Lonicerae Japonicae) 20g, *Fang Feng* (Radix Saposhnikoviae) 10g, *Bai Zhi* (Radix Angelicae Dahuricae) 10g, *Zhe Bei Mu* (Bulbus Fritillariae Thunbergii) 20g, *Tian Hua Fen* (Radix Trichosanthis) 10g, dry-fried *Ru Xiang* (Gummi Olibanum) 10g, dry-fried *Mo Yao* (Myrrha) 10g, vinegar-fried *Chai Hu* (Radix Bupleuri) 20g, vinegar-fried *Xiang Fu* (Rhizoma Cyperi) 12g, *Huang Qin* (Radix Scutellariae) 10g, *Wang Bu Liu Xing* (Semen Vaccariae) 10g, and others as deemed necessary. The treatment protocol was to cook the herbs in water, drink the decoction, and apply the warm herb residue topically to the affected area.[4]
4. **Appendicular abscess**: Use of *Xian Fang Huo Ming Yin* was effective in treating 27 of 30 patients with appendicular abscess. The formula effectively reduced inflammation, relieved pain, and lowered body temperature.[5]
5. **Thrombophlebitis**: Two studies reported good results using modified *Xian Fang Huo Ming Yin* to treat thrombophlebitis. According to the first study, 12 patients were treated with both oral and topical applications of herbs on a daily basis. The herbal formula contained *Jin Yin Hua* (Flos Lonicerae Japonicae) 50g, *Pu Gong Ying* (Herba Taraxaci) 30g, *Lian Qiao* (Fructus Forsythiae) 15g, *Tian Hua Fen* (Radix Trichosanthis) 15g, *Dang Gui* (Radix Angelicae Sinensis) 15g, *Ji Xue Teng* (Caulis Spatholobi) 15g, *Xiang Fu* (Rhizoma Cyperi) 15g, *Chen Pi* (Pericarpium Citri Reticulatae) 15g, *Si Gua Luo* (Retinervus Luffae Fructus) 15g, *Wei Ling Xian* (Radix et Rhizoma Clematidis) 10g, *Fang Feng* (Radix Saposhnikoviae) 10g, *Chuan Shan Jia* (Squama Manis) 10g, *Bai Zhi* (Radix Angelicae Dahuricae) 10g, *Chi Shao* (Radix Paeoniae Rubra) 10g, *Hong Hua* (Flos Carthami) 10g, *Ru Xiang* (Gummi Olibanum) 10g, *Mo Yao* (Myrrha) 10g, *Mu Xiang* (Radix Aucklandiae) 10g, *Cang Zhu* (Rhizoma Atractylodis) 10g, *Huang Bo* (Cortex Phellodendri Chinensis) 10g, *Gan Cao* (Radix et Rhizoma Glycyrrhizae) 10g, *Niu Xi* (Radix Achyranthis Bidentatae) 25g, and 50 mL of grain-based liquor. The treatment protocol was to cook the herbs in water, and drink the decoction. The herb residue was placed inside a cheese cloth which was applied topically to the affected area while warm. Of 12 patients, the study reported complete recovery in 9 cases and marked improvement in 3 cases.[6] In another study, 111 patients with thrombophlebitis were also treated with good results using modified *Xian Fang Huo Ming Yin*. Of 60 patients diagnosed with damp-heat, 49 had complete recovery and 11 had improvement. Of 51 patients diagnosed with blood stagnation, 28 had complete recovery and 20 had improvement.[7]
6. **Anal sinusitis**: One hundred and fifty-six patients with anal sinusitis showed marked improvement using oral and topical application of herbs. The formula for oral ingestion contained *Jin Yin Hua* (Flos Lonicerae Japonicae), *Chen Pi* (Pericarpium Citri Reticulatae), *Gan Cao* (Radix et Rhizoma Glycyrrhizae), *Tian Hua Fen* (Radix Trichosanthis), *Ru Xiang* (Gummi Olibanum), *Mo Yao* (Myrrha), *Dang Gui Wei* (Extremitas Radix Angelicae Sinensis), *Bai Zhi* (Radix Angelicae Dahuricae), *Fang Feng* (Radix Saposhnikoviae), *Chi Shao* (Radix Paeoniae Rubra), *Zao Jiao Ci* (Spina Gleditsiae), processed *Chuan Shan Jia* (Squama Manis), *Da Huang* (Radix et Rhizoma Rhei), and *Huang Bo* (Cortex Phellodendri Chinensis). The herbs used as a topical wash included *Ku Shen* (Radix Sophorae Flavescentis), *Da Huang* (Radix et Rhizoma

Xiān Fāng Huó Mìng Yǐn (Sublime Formula for Sustaining Life)

Rhei), *Mang Xiao* (Natrii Sulfas) and *Huang Bo* (Cortex Phellodendri Chinensis). The duration of treatment was 10-20 days.[8]

7. **Stye**: One study evaluated the use of *Xian Fang Huo Ming Yin* in treating styes in 30 patients (21 males and 9 females, between 8-35 years of age; 24 were affected in one eye, 6 in both eyes). The herbs were administered in decoction daily, with complete recovery in 28 of 30 cases. The duration of treatment was 4-5 days in most patients, and up to 6-7 days in 3 cases. The herbal formula included *Jin Yin Hua* (Flos Lonicerae Japonicae) 25g, *Bai Zhi* (Radix Angelicae Dahuricae) 10g, *Fang Feng* (Radix Saposhnikoviae) 10g, *Dang Gui* (Radix Angelicae Sinensis) 10g, *Chen Pi* (Pericarpium Citri Reticulatae) 10g, *Zhe Bei Mu* (Bulbus Fritillariae Thunbergii) 9g, processed *Chuan Shan Jia* (Squama Manis) 10g, *Chi Shao* (Radix Paeoniae Rubra) 15g, *Tian Hua Fen* (Radix Trichosanthis) 15g, *Zi Hua Di Ding* (Herba Violae) 15g, *Ru Xiang* (Gummi Olibanum) 6g, *Mo Yao* (Myrrha) 6g, and *Gan Cao* (Radix et Rhizoma Glycyrrhizae) 3g. Furthermore, *Pu Gong Ying* (Herba Taraxaci) was added for toxic heat, and *Da Huang* (Radix et Rhizoma Rhei) for constipation. The treatment protocol was to give one pack of herbs in decoction daily.[9]
8. **Pelvic inflammatory disease**: One study reported good results using modified *Xian Fang Huo Ming Yin* to treat pelvic inflammatory disease. The duration of illness varied from 5-22 days among 34 patients (between 21-44 years of age). The herbal formula contained *Chuan Shan Jia* (Squama Manis) 12g, *Tian Hua Fen* (Radix Trichosanthis) 20g, *Gan Cao* (Radix et Rhizoma Glycyrrhizae) 6g, *Ru Xiang* (Gummi Olibanum) 6g, *Mo Yao* (Myrrha) 6g, *Bai Zhi* (Radix Angelicae Dahuricae) 6g, *Chi Shao* (Radix Paeoniae Rubra) 12g, *Zhe Bei Mu* (Bulbus Fritillariae Thunbergii) 12g, *Fang Feng* (Radix Saposhnikoviae) 10g, *Zao Jiao Ci* (Spina Gleditsiae) 12g, *Dang Gui Wei* (Extremitas Radix Angelicae Sinensis) 12g, *Chen Pi* (Pericarpium Citri Reticulatae) 10g, and *Jin Yin Hua* (Flos Lonicerae Japonicae) 30g. *Pu Gong Ying* (Herba Taraxaci), *Gua Lou* (Fructus Trichosanthis), *Huang Bo* (Cortex Phellodendri Chinensis), and *Chi Fu Ling* (Poria Rubra) were added for excess heat; and *Hong Hua* (Flos Carthami), *San Leng* (Rhizoma Sparganii), and *E Zhu* (Rhizoma Curcumae) were added for inflammation and abscesses. The treatment protocol was to cook the herbs in water and drink the decoction in four equally-divided doses daily. In addition, the herb residue was fried with vinegar, placed inside a cheese cloth, and applied topically to the abdominal area for 30 minutes. Of 34 patients, the study reported complete recovery in 15 cases, marked effect in 9 cases, improvement in 8 cases, and no effect in 2 cases. The overall effectiveness was 94.1%.[10]
9. **Cervicitis and vaginitis**: Modified *Xian Fang Huo Ming Yin* was reported to successfully treat 21 patients with cervicitis and 30 patients with vaginitis. In addition to *Xian Fang Huo Ming Yin* as the base formula, *Da Xue Teng* (Caulis Sargentodoxae) and *Bai Jiang Cao* (Herba cum Radice Patriniae) were added for lower abdominal pain; *Tao Ren* (Semen Persicae), *Hong Hua* (Flos Carthami), *San Leng* (Rhizoma Sparganii) and *E Zhu* (Rhizoma Curcumae) were added for lower abdominal hardness and pain that intensify with pressure; and *Gua Lou Zi* (Semen Trichosanthis) and *Dong Gua Zi* (Semen Benincasae) for itching and leukorrhea. Patients were instructed to soak the affected area in an herbal solution made from *Er Cha* (Catechu), *Wu Bei Zi* (Galla Chinensis), *Tong Lu* (Verdigris), *Xiong Huang* (Realgar), *Qing Dai* (Indigo Naturalis), *Bing Pian* (Borneolum Syntheticum), *Hua Jiao* (Pericarpium Zanthoxyli), *She Chuang Zi* (Fructus Cnidii), and *Di Fu Zi* (Fructus Kochiae).
10. **Psoriasis**: Use of *Xian Fang Huo Ming Yin* to treat psoriasis in 25 patients was associated with a 72% rate of recovery and 92% effectiveness. The herbal formula contained *Jin Yin Hua* (Flos Lonicerae Japonicae), *Fang Feng* (Radix Saposhnikoviae), *Bai Zhi* (Radix Angelicae Dahuricae), *Zao Jiao Ci* (Spina Gleditsiae), *Chuan Shan Jia* (Squama Manis), *Tian Hua Fen* (Radix Trichosanthis), *Ru Xiang* (Gummi Olibanum), *Mo Yao* (Myrrha), *Chi Shao* (Radix Paeoniae Rubra), and *Chen Pi* (Pericarpium Citri Reticulatae). The patients were given 6g of pills made from herbal extract, three times daily, for 30 days per course of treatment, for 2 courses total.[11]
11. **Reflux esophagitis**: One study reported complete recovery in 78 of 104 patients with reflux esophagitis who were treated with modified *Xian Fang Huo Ming Yin*. The base formula contained *Jin Yin Hua* (Flos Lonicerae Japonicae) 30g, *Zao Jiao Ci* (Spina Gleditsiae) 30g, *Dang Gui* (Radix Angelicae Sinensis) 12g, *Chen Pi* (Pericarpium Citri Reticulatae) 10g, *Chi Shao* (Radix Paeoniae Rubra) 10g, *Tian Hua Fen* (Radix Trichosanthis) 10g, *Bei Mu* (Bulbus Fritillariae) 6g, processed *Chuan Shan Jia* (Squama Manis) 6g, *Ru Xiang* (Gummi Olibanum) 6g, *Mo Yao* (Myrrha) 6g, and *Gan Cao* (Radix et Rhizoma Glycyrrhizae) 6g. In addition, *Hai Piao Xiao* (Endoconcha Sepiae) 10g and *Wa Leng Zi* (Concha Arcae) 10g were added for acid reflux and belching; *Xian He Cao* (Herba Agrimoniae) 15g and *Ou Jie* (Nodus Nelumbinis Rhizomatis) 10g for bleeding; and *She Gan* (Rhizoma Belamcandae) 10g and *Xuan Shen* (Radix Scrophulariae) 10g for soreness and pain of the throat. The duration of treatment ranged from 1-3 weeks.[12]
12. **Osteoradionecrosis**: Concurrent Western and herbal treatments showed good results in treating 42 patients

with bone necrosis following irradiation. The base formula included *Dang Gui* (Radix Angelicae Sinensis) 12g, *Chuan Shan Jia* (Squama Manis) 12g, *Jin Yin Hua* (Flos Lonicerae Japonicae) 10g, *Tian Hua Fen* (Radix Trichosanthis) 10g, *Bai Zhi* (Radix Angelicae Dahuricae) 10g, *Fang Feng* (Radix Saposhnikoviae) 10g, *Zao Jiao Ci* (Spina Gleditsiae) 10g, *Chen Pi* (Pericarpium Citri Reticulatae) 10g, *Zhe Bei Mu* (Bulbus Fritillariae Thunbergii) 10g, *Ru Xiang* (Gummi Olibanum) 9g, *Mo Yao* (Myrrha) 9g, *Chi Shao* (Radix Paeoniae Rubra) 8g, and *Gan Cao* (Radix et Rhizoma Glycyrrhizae) 8g. Additional modifications were made as deemed necessary. The treatment protocol was to cook the herbs in water, and administer the decoction twice daily in two equally-divided doses before breakfast and at bedtime, for 7 days per course of treatment, for 3-4 courses total. Of 42 patients, the study reported complete recovery in 23 cases, improvement in 14 cases, and no effect in 5 cases.[13] Note: Details of the Western treatment were unavailable at the time of publication.

13. **Osteomyelitis**: Individuals with osteomyelitis were treated with good results using *Xian Fang Huo Ming Yin* and *Yang He Tang* (Yang-Heartening Decoction), plus topical application of other medicine(s). Of 28 patients, the study reported complete recovery in 19 cases after 3-4 months, 4 cases after 5-6 months, and unsatisfactory effect in 5 cases.[14] Note: Details of the medicine(s) used topically were unavailable at the time of publication.
14. **Pneumonia**: Use of modified *Xian Fang Huo Ming Yin* was associated with 87% effectiveness in treating pneumonia in 46 patients (28 males and 18 females, between 18-67 years of age). The herbal formula contained *Jin Yin Hua* (Flos Lonicerae Japonicae) 30g, *Chuan Shan Jia* (Squama Manis) 20g, *Fang Feng* (Radix Saposhnikoviae) 10g, *Bai Zhi* (Radix Angelicae Dahuricae) 12g, *Dang Gui* (Radix Angelicae Sinensis) 10g, *Chen Pi* (Pericarpium Citri Reticulatae) 10g, *Bei Mu* (Bulbus Fritillariae) 10g, *Huang Qin* (Radix Scutellariae) 10g, *Zao Jiao Ci* (Spina Gleditsiae) 20g, *Tian Hua Fen* (Radix Trichosanthis) 15g, *Gan Cao* (Radix et Rhizoma Glycyrrhizae) 5g, *Sang Bai Pi* (Cortex Mori) 12g, and *Jie Geng* (Radix Platycodonis) 12g. *Yu Xing Cao* (Herba Houttuyniae) 30g was added for dark, thick phlegm; and *Gua Lou* (Fructus Trichosanthis) 15g for chest pain. The herbs were given in decoction daily, for 7 days per course of treatment. Of 46 patients, 29 had significant improvement, 11 had moderate improvement, and 6 had no effect.[15]

SUGGESTED ACUPUNCTURE TREATMENT

1. Points: *Quchi* (LI 11), *Hegu* (LI 4), *Zhiyang* (GV 9), *Weizhong* (BL 40), *Xuehai* (SP 10), and *Wenliu* (LI 7).
2. Technique: sedation.

The treatment plan aims to relieve abscesses and sores characterized by heat-toxin accumulation and stagnation of qi and blood. *Quchi* (LI 11), the *he* (uniting) point of the Large Intestine channel, *Hegu* (LI 4), the *yuan* (source) point of the Large Intestine channel, and *Zhiyang* (GV 9) clear heat, sedate fire, and dispel heat toxins. *Weizhong* (BL 40) and *Xuehai* (SP 10) activate the blood and disperse blood stagnation. Finally, *Wenliu* (LI 7) and *Xuehai* (SP 10) dispel heat, regulate the Stomach and Intestines, and reduce swelling.

RELATED FORMULAS

Zhēn Rén Huó Mìng Yǐn

(True Man's Decoction to Revitalize Life)

真人活命飲

真人活命饮

Pinyin Name: *Zhen Ren Huo Ming Yin*

Literal Name: True Man's Decoction to Revitalize Life

Alternate Name: Angelica and Mastic Combination

Original Source: *Yi Fang Ji Jie* (Analytical Collection of Medical Formulas) by Wang Ang in 1682

Bai Zhi (Radix Angelicae Dahuricae)	3g
Zhe Bei Mu (Bulbus Fritillariae Thunbergii)	3g
Fang Feng (Radix Saposhnikoviae)	3g
Dang Gui Wei (Extremitas Radix Angelicae Sinensis)	3g
Gan Cao (Radix et Rhizoma Glycyrrhizae)	3g
Zao Jiao Ci (Spina Gleditsiae), *chao* (dry-fried)	3g
Chuan Shan Jia (Squama Manis), *zhi* (fried with liquid)	3g
Tian Hua Fen (Radix Trichosanthis)	3g
Mo Yao (Myrrha)	3g
Ru Xiang (Gummi Olibanum)	3g
Jin Yin Hua (Flos Lonicerae Japonicae)	9g
Chen Pi (Pericarpium Citri Reticulatae)	9g

Note: *Chuan Shan Jia* (Squama Manis) is derived from an endangered animal and is rarely used as a medicinal substance today. Its discussion here is included primarily for academic purposes, to reflect the historical use of this substance in its original formulation. Most herbal products today have removed it completely, or replaced it with substitutes with similar functions.

Xian Fang Huo Ming Yin and *Zhen Ren Huo Ming Yin* (True Man's Decoction to Revitalize Life) are essentially the same formula, except that *Xian Fang Huo Ming Yin* contains *Chi Shao* (Radix Paeoniae Rubra), while *Zhen Ren Huo Ming Yin* (True Man's Decoction to Revitalize Life) does not.

Xiān Fāng Huó Mìng Yǐn (Sublime Formula for Sustaining Life)

Lián Qiào Bài Dú Sǎn
(Forsythia Powder to Overcome Pathogenic Influences)
連翹敗毒散
连翘败毒散
Pinyin Name: *Lian Qiao Bai Du San*
Literal Name: Forsythia Powder to Overcome Pathogenic Influences
Alternate Names: *Lien Jiao Pai Tu San*, Forsythia Detoxifying Formula
Original Source: *Shang Han Quan Sheng Ji* (All New Collection of Cold-Induced Disorders)

Lian Qiao (Fructus Forsythiae)	[9g]
Zhi Zi (Fructus Gardeniae)	[9g]
Qiang Huo (Rhizoma et Radix Notopterygii)	[8g]
Xuan Shen (Radix Scrophulariae)	[12g]
Bo He (Herba Menthae)	[5g]
Fang Feng (Radix Saposhnikoviae)	[5g]
Chai Hu (Radix Bupleuri)	[6g]
Jie Geng (Radix Platycodonis)	[5g]
Sheng Ma (Rhizoma Cimicifugae)	[5g]
Chuan Xiong (Rhizoma Chuanxiong)	[6g]
Dang Gui (Radix Angelicae Sinensis)	[8g]
Huang Qin (Radix Scutellariae)	[9g]
Bai Shao (Radix Paeoniae Alba)	[10g]
Niu Bang Zi (Fructus Arctii)	[6g]

The source text states to cook the ingredients with *Hong Hua* (Flos Carthami) to make a decoction. However, the doses of the ingredients are unavailable from the source text. Today, the decoction is prepared by using the doses suggested in brackets.

The main actions of *Lian Qiao Bai Du San* (Forsythia Powder to Overcome Pathogenic Influences) are to release wind-heat, clear heat, and eliminate heat and toxins. Clinically, this formula can be used to treat hives, atopic dermatitis with red, itchy skin, strangles in horses and puppies, and abscesses (caseous lymphadenitis) in goats. For the treatment of abscesses in goats, the following herbs should be added to the base formula: to improve the heat-clearing ability, add *Pu Gong Ying* (Herba Taraxaci), *Ban Lan Gen* (Radix Isatidis), and *Jin Yin Hua* (Flos Lonicerae Japonicae); to decrease lymph node swelling, add *Xuan Shen* (Radix Scrophulariae), *Mu Li* (Concha Ostreae), and *Zi Cao* (Radix Arnebiae); for deficiency, add *Huang Qi* (Radix Astragali), *Ren Shen* (Radix et Rhizoma Ginseng), or *Dang Shen* (Radix Codonopsis).

AUTHORS' COMMENTS

In human medicine, *Xian Fang Huo Ming Yin* and *Zhen Ren Huo Ming Yin* (True Man's Decoction to Revitalize Life) are two of the most commonly used formulas for treating all types of abscesses, sores, nodules or swellings that are red, hot, hard, and painful to the touch. The lesions may or may not contain pus. These two formulas can be applied topically to ease pain and swelling in addition to oral administration to maximize clinical effectiveness. In veterinary medicine, *Lian Qiao Bai Du San* (Forsythia Powder to Overcome Pathogenic Influences) is actually used more often than the two formulas mentioned above.

Prostatic abscess in dogs can be effectively treated by using *Xian Fang Huo Ming Yin* in combination with *San Zhong Kui Jian Tang* (Disperse the Swelling and Break the Hardness Decoction) and *Shi Liu Wei Liu Qi Yin* (Sixteen-Ingredient Decoction to Flow Qi). This can be done by combining the prepared formulas together, using extracts in granular or capsule forms.

Xian Fang Huo Ming Yin and *Yang He Tang* (Yang-Heartening Decoction) can be used to treat non-healing fractures with osteomyelitis, in combination with conventional antimicrobials in dogs. It is recommended to add additional herbs to nourish and/or invigorate the blood, such as *Ji Xue Teng* (Caulis Spatholobi), *Dan Shen* (Radix et Rhizoma Salviae Miltiorrhizae), *Tao Ren* (Semen Persicae), or *Ze Lan* (Herba Lycopi). Spleen tonic herbs and/or formulas are typically required, as this formula may require up to six weeks of continuous use for effective results in difficult cases, and most dogs have been on prolonged antibiotic therapy by the time a Chinese medicine practitioner is consulted.

Xian Fang Huo Ming Yin and *Pu Ji Xiao Du Yin* (Universal Benefit Decoction to Eliminate Toxin) both clear heat and eliminate toxins. In severe cases with bacterial resistance, the two formulas can be combined together. Due to the cold and bitter nature of these two formulas, herbs that support the Spleen and Stomach are recommended.

- *Xian Fang Huo Ming Yin*, in addition to clearing heat and eliminating toxins, is better at moving qi and invigorating blood (reducing swelling) to disperse the initial stages of nodules, swellings, carbuncles, and sores; it can be used to treat external and internal abscesses affecting different parts of the body.
- *Pu Ji Xiao Du Yin* focuses on treating toxic heat affecting the upper *jiao*, manifesting in clinical signs such as redness, swelling and pain of the face, difficulty in opening the eyes, sore throat, thirst, and fever. It disperses wind-heat and dispels toxins lodged in the head. Overall, it is stronger at clearing toxic heat than *Xian Fang Huo Ming Yin*.

Xiān Fāng Huó Mìng Yǐn (Sublime Formula for Sustaining Life)

References

1. *He Nan Zhong Yi* (Henan Chinese Medicine), 1988; 5:31.
2. *Hu Bei Zhong Yi Za Zhi* (Hubei Journal of Chinese Medicine), 1988; 6:23.
3. *Shan Xi Zhong Yi* (Shanxi Chinese Medicine), 1989; 8:366.
4. *Nei Meng Gu Zhong Yi Yao* (Traditional Chinese Medicine and Medicinals of Inner Mongolia), 1994; 2:7.
5. *Zhong Hua Wai Ke Za Zhi* (Chinese Journal of External Medicine), 1960; 2:171.
6. *Liao Ning Zhong Yi Za Zhi* (Liaoning Journal of Chinese Medicine), 1991; 5:34.
7. *Xin Zhong Yi* (New Chinese Medicine), 1992; 10:24.
8. *Hu Nan Zhong Yi Xue Yuan Xue Bao* (Journal of Hunan University of Traditional Chinese Medicine), 1994; 2:24.
9. *Hu Bei Zhong Yi Za Zhi* (Hubei Journal of Chinese Medicine), 1989; 4.
10. *Jiang Su Zhong Yi* (Jiangsu Chinese Medicine), 1996; 6:18.
11. *Hu Nan Zhong Yi Xue Yuan Xue Bao* (Journal of Hunan University of Traditional Chinese Medicine), 1998; 3:50.
12. *Zhe Jiang Zhong Yi Za Zhi* (Zhejiang Journal of Chinese Medicine), 1990; 4:155.
13. *Xin Zhong Yi* (New Chinese Medicine), 1999; 10:24.
14. *Xin Zhong Yi* (New Chinese Medicine), 1990; 4:37.
15. *Fu Jian Zhong Yi Yao* (Fujian Chinese Medicine and Herbology), 1997; 4:37.

Jīng Fáng Bài Dú Sǎn

(Schizonepeta and Saposhnikovia Powder to Overcome Pathogenic Influences)

荊防敗毒散

荆防败毒散

Pinyin Name: *Jing Fang Bai Du San*

Literal Name: Schizonepeta and Saposhnikovia Powder to Overcome Pathogenic Influences

Alternate Names: *Ching Fang Pai Tu San*, Schizonepeta and Siler Detoxifying Formula, Schizonepeta and Siler Formula

Original Source: *She Sheng Zhong Miao Fang* (Marvelous Formulas for the Health of Multitudes) by Zhang Shi-Che in 1550

COMPOSITION

Chai Hu (Radix Bupleuri)	4.5g
Qian Hu (Radix Peucedani)	4.5g
Jing Jie (Herba Schizonepetae)	4.5g
Fang Feng (Radix Saposhnikoviae)	4.5g
Qiang Huo (Rhizoma et Radix Notopterygii)	4.5g
Du Huo (Radix Angelicae Pubescentis)	4.5g
Jie Geng (Radix Platycodonis)	4.5g
Chuan Xiong (Rhizoma Chuanxiong)	4.5g
Fu Ling (Poria)	4.5g
Zhi Qiao (Fructus Citri Aurantii)	4.5g
Gan Cao (Radix et Rhizoma Glycyrrhizae)	1.5g [3g]

DOSAGE / PREPARATION / ADMINISTRATION

Prepare the ingredients as a decoction.

CHINESE THERAPEUTIC ACTIONS

1. Releases the exterior and induces diaphoresis
2. Treats skin and external diseases
3. Relieves pain

Jīng Fáng Bài Dú Sǎn

(Schizonepeta and Saposhnikovia Powder to Overcome Pathogenic Influences)

CLINICAL MANIFESTATIONS

Early stage of skin and external diseases: abscesses and sores with redness, swelling and pain, aversion to cold, fever, absence of sweating, no thirst, a red tongue, and a superficial, rapid pulse.

VETERINARY CLINICAL APPLICATIONS

Carbuncles, pustules, boils, urticaria, dermatitis, abscesses, allergic conjunctivitis and scabies.

EXPLANATION

Jing Fang Bai Du San (Schizonepeta and Saposhnikovia Powder to Overcome Pathogenic Influences) primarily treats skin and external disorders, such as abscesses and sores. Local clinical signs include redness, swelling and pain of the affected area, while systemic clinical signs include aversion to cold, fever, absence of sweating, and lack of thirst.

Chai Hu (Radix Bupleuri) and *Qian Hu* (Radix Peucedani) are exterior-releasing herbs that dispel wind and heat. *Jing Jie* (Herba Schizonepetae), *Fang Feng* (Radix Saposhnikoviae), *Qiang Huo* (Rhizoma et Radix Notopterygii), and *Du Huo* (Radix Angelicae Pubescentis) release the exterior, eliminate toxins, and relieve pain. *Jie Geng* (Radix Platycodonis), *Chuan Xiong* (Rhizoma Chuanxiong), and *Fu Ling* (Poria) reduce swelling and inflammation, move the blood, and eliminate pus. *Zhi Qiao* (Fructus Aurantii) regulates qi circulation and removes stagnation. *Gan Cao* (Radix et Rhizoma Glycyrrhizae) harmonizes the herbs.

VETERINARY MODIFICATIONS

- If there is swelling and pain caused by more heat, add *Huang Qin* (Radix Scutellariae) and *Huang Lian* (Rhizoma Coptidis).
- If there is swelling and pain caused by more formation of pus, add *Bai Zhi* (Radix Angelicae Dahuricae) and *Zao Jiao* (Fructus Gleditsiae).
- For acute *bi zheng* (painful obstruction syndrome) caused by wind and dampness, add *Ren Dong Teng* (Caulis Lonicerae Japonicae) and *Sang Zhi* (Ramulus Mori).
- If there is exterior cold and interior heat with a red tongue tip, and a dry mouth, add *Jin Yin Hua* (Flos Lonicerae Japonicae), *Lian Qiao* (Fructus Forsythiae), *Niu Bang Zi* (Fructus Arctii), *Ban Lan Gen* (Radix Isatidis); and remove *Du Huo* (Radix Angelicae Pubescentis) and *Chuan Xiong* (Rhizoma Chuanxiong).

CAUTIONS / CONTRAINDICATIONS

Avoid foods that are raw, cold, oily, or greasy while taking *Jing Fang Bai Du San*.[1]

HUMAN CLINICAL STUDIES AND RESEARCH

High fever: One study reported success in the treatment of high fever in 36 of 45 patients using modified *Jing Fang Bai Du San*. The causes of high fever included postpartum illness, nephritis, respiratory tract infection, and others. The herbal treatment contained *Jing Jie* (Herba Schizonepetae) 30g, *Chai Hu* (Radix Bupleuri) 15g, *Fang Feng* (Radix Saposhnikoviae) 10g, and *Bo He* (Herba Menthae) 10g as the base formula. Modifications varied depending on the causes of fever. For postpartum fever,

***Jing Fang Bai Du San* (Schizonepeta and Saposhnikovia Powder to Overcome Pathogenic Influences)**

Diagnosis	Clinical Signs	Treatment	Herbs
Early stages of skin and external diseases	• Abscesses and sores with redness, swelling and pain: wind, cold and dampness in the muscle layer • Aversion to cold, fever, and absence of sweating: presence of wind at the exterior • Red tongue and a superficial, rapid pulse: exterior condition	• Releases the exterior and induces diaphoresis • Treats skin and external diseases	• *Chai Hu* (Radix Bupleuri) and *Qian Hu* (Radix Peucedani) release wind and heat from the exterior parts of the body. • *Jing Jie* (Herba Schizonepetae), *Fang Feng* (Radix Saposhnikoviae), *Qiang Huo* (Rhizoma et Radix Notopterygii), and *Du Huo* (Radix Angelicae Pubescentis) release the exterior, eliminate toxins, and relieve pain. • *Jie Geng* (Radix Platycodonis), *Chuan Xiong* (Rhizoma Chuanxiong), and *Fu Ling* (Poria) reduce swelling and inflammation, move the blood, and eliminate pus. • *Zhi Qiao* (Fructus Aurantii) regulates qi circulation and removes stagnation. • *Gan Cao* (Radix et Rhizoma Glycyrrhizae) harmonizes the herbs.

Jīng Fáng Bài Dú Sǎn

(Schizonepeta and Saposhnikovia Powder to Overcome Pathogenic Influences)

Dang Shen (Radix Codonopsis) and *Dang Gui* (Radix Angelicae Sinensis) were added. For nephritis and fever, *Jin Qian Cao* (Herba Lysimachiae) and *Qu Mai* (Herba Dianthi) were added. For exterior cold with fever, *Huo Xiang* (Herba Agastaches) and *Hou Po* (Cortex Magnoliae Officinalis) were added. The treatment protocol was to cook the herbs in water and administer the decoction in two equally-divided doses daily.[2]

SUGGESTED ACUPUNCTURE TREATMENT

1. Points: *Fengchi* (GB 20), *Dazhui* (GV 14), *Quchi* (LI 11), *Hegu* (LI 4), *Lingtai* (GV 10), *Shenzhu* (GV 12), and *Weizhong* (BL 40).
2. Technique: even method.

Fengchi (GB 20), *Lingtai* (GV 10), *Shenzhu* (GV 12), and *Dazhui* (GV 14) dispel wind and relieve the exterior. *Quchi* (LI 11) and *Hegu* (LI 4) relieve the exterior and regulate the qi flow of the Lung. *Weizhong* (BL 40) reduces inflammation and eliminates pus and toxins.

RELATED FORMULAS

Jīng Fáng Bài Dú Sǎn (Schizonepeta and Saposhnikovia Powder to Overcome Pathogenic Influences)
荊防敗毒散
荆防败毒散
Pinyin Name: *Jing Fang Bai Du San*
Literal Name: Schizonepeta and Saposhnikovia Powder to Overcome Pathogenic Influences
Original Source: *Qi Xiao Liang Fang* (Fine Formulas with Miraculous Results)

Chai Hu (Radix Bupleuri)	3g
Chuan Xiong (Rhizoma Chuanxiong)	3g
Du Huo (Radix Angelicae Pubescentis)	3g
Fang Feng (Radix Saposhnikoviae)	3g
Fu Ling (Poria)	3g
Jie Geng (Radix Platycodonis)	3g
Jing Jie (Herba Schizonepetae)	3g
Qian Hu (Radix Peucedani)	3g
Qiang Huo (Rhizoma et Radix Notopterygii)	3g
Sheng Jiang (Rhizoma Zingiberis Recens)	3g
Zhi Qiao (Fructus Aurantii)	3g
Gan Cao (Radix et Rhizoma Glycyrrhizae)	1.5g
Bo He (Herba Menthae)	1g

This formula induces sweating, releases the exterior, disperses wind, and dispels dampness. It is used to treat wind, cold and dampness at the exterior, leading to clinical signs such as fever, aversion to cold, neck stiffness, and body aches and pain.

Jīng Fáng Bài Dú Sǎn (Schizonepeta and Saposhnikovia Powder to Overcome Pathogenic Influences)
荊防敗毒散
荆防败毒散
Pinyin Name: *Jing Fang Bai Du San*
Literal Name: Schizonepeta and Saposhnikovia Powder to Overcome Pathogenic Influences
Original Source: *Wan Bing Hui Chun* (Restoration of Health from the Myriad Diseases) by Gong Ting-Xian in 1587

Jing Jie (Herba Schizonepetae)
Fang Feng (Radix Saposhnikoviae)
Qiang Huo (Rhizoma et Radix Notopterygii)
Du Huo (Radix Angelicae Pubescentis)
Chai Hu (Radix Bupleuri)
Qian Hu (Radix Peucedani)
Jie Geng (Radix Platycodonis)
Zhi Qiao (Fructus Aurantii)
Chuan Xiong (Rhizoma Chuanxiong)
Bo He (Herba Menthae)
Jin Yin Hua (Flos Lonicerae Japonicae)
Lian Qiao (Fructus Forsythiae)
Chi Fu Ling (Poria Rubra)

Grind equal proportions of all of the ingredients into powder and prepare as a decoction with *Sheng Jiang* (Rhizoma Zingiberis Recens) and *Bo He* (Herba Menthae).

This formula treats skin and external disorders with suppuration caused by wind-heat and toxins. Suppuration may occur at various parts of the body, including, but not limited to, the skin and glands. The presence of wind is characterized by the exterior clinical sign of aversion to wind and cold; and the presence of heat is characterized by fever. As the disease progresses, suppuration develops as swelling and inflammation at the affected area begin to form and discharge pus. At this time, the treatment must focus on dispelling exterior wind and heat, reducing swelling and inflammation, and eliminating toxins and pus.

Clinical applications of this formula include carbuncles, pustules, boils, urticaria, eczema, dermatitis, abscesses, sores, suppuration, mastitis, proctitis, eye disorders, and scabies.

AUTHORS' COMMENTS

Jing Fang Bai Du San can be used to treat allergic seasonal skin disorders. It is not usually used as a sole formula for this purpose. For allergic dermatitis with skin rashes and

Jīng Fáng Bài Dú Săn

(Schizonepeta and Saposhnikovia Powder to Overcome Pathogenic Influences)

itching, add *Xiao Feng San* (Eliminate Wind Powder) in a 1:1 ratio. If more dampness is present, add *Si Miao San* (Four-Marvel Powder); and if more heat (pyoderma) is present, add *Huang Lian Jie Du Tang* (Coptis Decoction to Relieve Toxicity) or *Yin Qiao San* (Honeysuckle and Forsythia Powder), depending on the clinical signs. This formula is used to treat excess conditions in animals that are otherwise in good condition.

These three "*Jing Fang Bai Du San*" formulas have identical names, but are derived from different sources and have slightly different compositions and applications.

- *Jing Fang Bai Du San* from *She Sheng Zhong Miao Fang* (Marvelous Formulas for the Health of Multitudes) primarily treats early-stage skin and external disorders characterized by wind, cold, and dampness.
- *Jing Fang Bai Du San* from *Qi Xiao Liang Fang* (Fine Formulas with Miraculous Results) also treats early-stage skin and external disorders characterized by wind, cold, and dampness. This formula contains *Sheng Jiang* (Rhizoma Zingiberis Recens) and *Bo He* (Herba Menthae) and is slightly stronger than the previous formula.
- *Jing Fang Bai Du San* from *Wan Bing Hui Chun* (Restoration of Health from the Myriad Diseases) mainly treats skin and external disorders with suppuration, caused by wind, heat, and toxins.

Bai Du San (Overcome Pathogenic Influences Powder) and *Jing Fang Bai Du San* are two very commonly used formulas with similar actions and functions. Both formulas treat external abscesses and sores, but have the following differences:

- *Bai Du San* is more suitable for deficient animals because it contains *Ren Shen* (Radix et Rhizoma Ginseng), which strengthens *yuan* (source) *qi*. In addition, it has only a mild exterior-releasing action, as that is all a weak animal can withstand.
- *Jing Fang Bai Du San* is a potent formula that contains many exterior-releasing herbs, but has no tonic herbs to moderate its exterior-releasing actions. *Jing Fang Bai Du San* is indicated for animals that have no deficiencies.

References

1. *Zhong Yao Ming Fang Yao Li Yu Ying Yong* (Pharmacology and Applications of Famous Herbal Formulas), 1989; 69-70.
2. *Guang Xi Zhong Yi Yao* (Guangxi Chinese Medicine and Herbology), 1989; 4:9.

Wǔ Wèi Xiāo Dú Yǐn

(Five-Ingredient Decoction to Eliminate Toxins)

五味消毒飲
五味消毒饮

Pinyin Name: *Wu Wei Xiao Du Yin*
Literal Name: Five-Ingredient Decoction to Eliminate Toxins
Alternate Name: Dandelion and Wild Chrysanthemum Combination
Original Source: *Yi Zong Jin Jian* (Golden Mirror of the Medical Tradition) by Wu Qian in 1742

COMPOSITION

Jin Yin Hua (Flos Lonicerae Japonicae)	9g [20g]
Zi Hua Di Ding (Herba Violae)	3.6g [15g]
Pu Gong Ying (Herba Taraxaci)	3.6g [15g]
Ye Ju Hua (Flos Chrysanthemi Indici)	3.6g [15g]
Tian Kui Zi (Radix Semiaquilegiae)	3.6g [15g]

DOSAGE / PREPARATION / ADMINISTRATION

The source text states to cook the ingredients with 2 large bowls of water until the liquid is reduced to 80%. Add 0.5 bowl of grain-based liquor and bring it to a boil 2-3 times. Take the hot, strained decoction and cover the body with blankets to promote sweating.

Today, it is prepared as a decoction, with the doses suggested in brackets, and taken with 1-2 spoonfuls of grain-based liquor. The herb residue is crushed into a paste and applied topically to the affected area.

CHINESE THERAPEUTIC ACTIONS

1. Clears heat and eliminates toxins
2. Disperses external carbuncles and furuncles

CLINICAL MANIFESTATIONS

Carbuncles (multiple boils/sores), furuncles (boils), and other types of epithelial inflammations due to accumulation of fire and toxins: local redness, swelling, heat and pain, fever, aversion to cold, carbuncles and furuncles that are hard and deeply rooted, a red tongue, and a rapid pulse.

VETERINARY CLINICAL APPLICATIONS

Generalized infections, cellulitis, febrile disorders, acute pyelonephritis, urinary tract infection, miliary dermatitis, atopic dermatitis, folliculitis, and gingivitis and stomatitis in cats.

EXPLANATION

Wu Wei Xiao Du Yin (Five-Ingredient Decoction to Eliminate Toxins) treats carbuncles, furuncles, and other types of epithelial inflammations characterized by accumulation of fire and toxins. Accumulation of fire and toxins in the interior *zang fu* organs may result in nail-like carbuncles and furuncles that are hard and deeply rooted and are characterized by local redness, swelling, heat, and pain. A red tongue and a rapid pulse suggest that the fire and toxins are located mainly in the interior.

This formula contains *Jin Yin Hua* (Flos Lonicerae Japonicae) to clear heat and eliminate toxins from both the *qi* (energy) and *xue* (blood) levels. *Zi Hua Di Ding* (Herba Violae), *Pu Gong Ying* (Herba Taraxaci), *Ye Ju Hua* (Flos Chrysanthemi Indici), and *Tian Kui Zi* (Radix Semiaquilegiae) clear heat,

***Wu Wei Xiao Du Yin* (Five-Ingredient Decoction to Eliminate Toxins)**

Diagnosis	Clinical Signs	Treatment	Herbs
Carbuncles, furuncles, and other types of epithelial inflammations	• Skin nodules and skin rashes that are deeply rooted: stagnation of fire and toxins • Local redness, swelling, heat, and pain: qi and blood stagnation • Red tongue: heat and toxins • Rapid pulse: heat and toxins	• Clears heat, fire, and toxins • Disperses carbuncles and furuncles	• *Jin Yin Hua* (Flos Lonicerae Japonicae) clears heat and eliminates toxins from both the *qi* (energy) and *xue* (blood) levels. • *Zi Hua Di Ding* (Herba Violae), *Pu Gong Ying* (Herba Taraxaci), *Ye Ju Hua* (Flos Chrysanthemi Indici), and *Tian Kui Zi* (Radix Semiaquilegiae) clear heat, eliminate toxins, cool the blood, disperse nodules, and relieve pain.

Wǔ Wèi Xiāo Dú Yǐn

(Five-Ingredient Decoction to Eliminate Toxins)

eliminate toxins, cool the blood, disperse nodules, and relieve pain. Grain-based liquor helps to activate blood circulation and distribute the herbs to the affected area of the body.

VETERINARY MODIFICATIONS

- With more fire and toxins, add *Lian Qiao* (Fructus Forsythiae), *Ban Zhi Lian* (Herba Scutellariae Barbatae), *Huang Lian* (Rhizoma Coptidis) and increase the dosage of *Zi Hua Di Ding* (Herba Violae).
- With more swelling and inflammation, add *Fang Feng* (Radix Saposhnikoviae) and *Chan Tui* (Periostracum Cicadae).
- With heat in the *xue* (blood) level, add *Chi Shao* (Radix Paeoniae Rubra) and *Mu Dan Pi* (Cortex Moutan).
- For swelling with pus that does not perforate, or sores that have perforated and ulcerated but do not heal, add *Zao Jiao Ci* (Spina Gleditsiae).
- For mastitis with swelling, redness, and pain, add *Gua Lou* (Fructus Trichosanthis), *Bei Mu* (Bulbus Fritillariae), and *Qing Pi* (Pericarpium Citri Reticulatae Viride).
- For infection or inflammation in constitutionally deficient individuals, add *Ren Shen* (Radix et Rhizoma Ginseng) or *Dang Gui Bu Xue Tang* (Tangkuei Decoction to Tonify the Blood).

CAUTIONS / CONTRAINDICATIONS

- *Wu Wei Xiao Du Yin* should be used with caution in patients with Spleen and Stomach deficiencies, or qi and blood deficiencies. This formula is not meant for long-term use unless modified.
- This formula is contraindicated for *yin* (deep-rooted) type of abscesses and sores with underlying deficiencies.

PHARMACOLOGICAL EFFECTS

Antibacterial: According to *in vitro* studies, *Wu Wei Xiao Du Yin* has an inhibitory effect against *Staphylococcus albus, Staphylococcus aureus, alpha-hemolytic streptococcus, beta-hemolytic streptococcus, Salmonella typhi* and *Bacillus proteus*. At high doses, it has an inhibitory effect against *Pseudomonas aeruginosa*. It is ineffective against *E. coli*.[1,2]

HUMAN CLINICAL STUDIES AND RESEARCH

1. **Cellulitis**: Forty-five patients with cellulitis were treated successfully using modified *Wu Wei Xiao Du Yin*. The herbal formula contained *Jin Yin Hua* (Flos Lonicerae Japonicae) 25g, *Ye Ju Hua* (Flos Chrysanthemi Indici) 20g, *Pu Gong Ying* (Herba Taraxaci) 20g, *Zi Hua Di Ding* (Herba Violae) 20g, *Lian Qiao* (Fructus Forsythiae) 25g, *Shi Gao* (Gypsum Fibrosum) 30g, *Bo He* (Herba Menthae) 5g, *Niu Bang Zi* (Fructus Arctii) 15g, *Jiang Can* (Bombyx Batryticatus) 10g, *Mu Dan Pi* (Cortex Moutan) 10g, *Sheng Ma* (Rhizoma Cimicifugae) 10g, and *Zao Jiao Ci* (Spina Gleditsiae) 10g. Furthermore, modifications were made by adding *Da Huang* (Radix et Rhizoma Rhei) 5g and *Xuan Ming Fen* (Natrii Sulfas Exsiccatus) 5g for constipation; *Jing Jie* (Herba Schizonepetae) 15g for aversion to cold; *Gu Sui Bu* (Rhizoma Drynariae) 10g and *Xuan Shen* (Radix Scrophulariae) 10g for chronic illness; and *Ban Lan Gen* (Radix Isatidis) 20g and *Ku Shen* (Radix Sophorae Flavescentis) 15g for severe inflammation. The treatment protocol was to give the herbs in decoction for 6-18 packs of herbs. Of 45 patients, the study reported complete recovery in 30 cases, significant improvement in 10 cases, moderate improvement in 1 case, and no effect in 4 cases. The overall effectiveness was 91.11%.[3]
2. **Shingles**: Administration of 3-6 packs of herbs in decoction was effective in treating all 38 patients with shingles. The herbal treatment contained *Wu Wei Xiao Du Yin* and *Si Wu Tang* (Four-Substance Decoction) as the base formula, with the addition of *Lian Qiao* (Fructus Forsythiae) and *Ban Lan Gen* (Radix Isatidis) for toxic heat; *Long Dan* (Radix et Rhizoma Gentianae) for a bitter taste in the mouth and dysuria; *Da Huang* (Radix et Rhizoma Rhei) for constipation; and *Tu Fu Ling* (Rhizoma Smilacis Glabrae) and a large dose of *Di Huang* (Radix Rehmanniae) for itching and pain.[4]
3. **Febrile disorder**: Use of modified *Wu Wei Xiao Du Yin* was associated with 81.1% effectiveness in treating externally-contracted febrile disorders. In addition to the base formula, modifications were made based on the differential diagnosis of the condition. For exterior wind-heat, *Lian Qiao* (Fructus Forsythiae), *Bo He* (Herba Menthae), and *Lu Gen* (Rhizoma Phragmitis) were added. For exterior wind-cold, *Jing Jie* (Herba Schizonepetae), *Fang Feng* (Radix Saposhnikoviae), and *Qiang Huo* (Rhizoma et Radix Notopterygii) were added. For Lung heat, *Ma Huang* (Herba Ephedrae), *Ku Xing Ren* (Semen Armeniacae Amarum), and *Shi Gao* (Gypsum Fibrosum) were added. For Stomach heat, *Shi Gao* (Gypsum Fibrosum) and *Zhi Mu* (Rhizoma Anemarrhenae) were added. For Gallbladder heat, *Chai Hu* (Radix Bupleuri), *Huang Qin* (Radix Scutellariae), and *Bai Jiang Cao* (Herba cum Radice Patriniae) were added. For Large Intestine heat, *Ge Gen* (Radix Puerariae Lobatae), *Huang Qin* (Radix Scutellariae), and *Huang Lian* (Rhizoma Coptidis) were added. For Urinary Bladder damp-heat, *Mu Tong* (Caulis Akebiae), *Hua Shi* (Talcum), and *Shi Wei* (Folium Pyrrosiae) were added. For constipation, *Da Huang*

Wǔ Wèi Xiāo Dú Yǐn

(Five-Ingredient Decoction to Eliminate Toxins)

(Radix et Rhizoma Rhei) was added. Of 122 patients, the study reported complete recovery in 81 cases, marked improvement in 18 cases, moderate improvement in 16 cases, and no effect in 7 cases.[5]

4. **Viral hepatitis**: Administration of modified *Wu Wei Xiao Du Yin* in decoction daily was effective in treating 248 hepatitis patients (183 hepatitis A cases and 65 hepatitis B). Most patients received 60-100 packs of herbs. However, those with severe conditions required up to 200-300 packs.[6]
5. **Acute cholecystitis**: According to one study, 20 patients with acute cholecystitis were treated with modified *Wu Wei Xiao Du Yin* with 75% effectiveness.[7] Another study reported satisfactory results in all 60 patients (21 males and 39 females) with acute cholecystitis treated with modified *Wu Wei Xiao Du Yin*. The formula was modified by adding *Ze Lan* (Herba Lycopi) and *Fu Ling* (Poria) for dampness; *Dang Gui* (Radix Angelicae Sinensis) and *Tao Ren* (Semen Persicae) for chronic illness; *Da Huang* (Radix et Rhizoma Rhei) and *Po Xiao* (Sal Glauberis) for constipation; *Yan Hu Suo* (Rhizoma Corydalis), *Ru Xiang* (Gummi Olibanum), and *Mo Yao* (Myrrha) for severe pain; *Chen Pi* (Pericarpium Citri Reticulatae) and *Ban Xia* (Rhizoma Pinelliae) for nausea and vomiting; *Yin Chen* (Herba Artemisiae Scopariae) and *Jin Qian Cao* (Herba Lysimachiae) for jaundice; and others as deemed necessary.[8]
6. **Acute pyelonephritis**: Administration of modified *Wu Wei Xiao Du Yin* in decoction daily was associated with 91.4% effectiveness in treating acute pyelonephritis. The duration of treatment ranged from 1-2 courses, with 7 days per course. Of 58 patients with acute pyelonephritis, the study reported complete recovery in 41 cases, improvement in 12 cases, and no effect in 5 cases.[9]
7. **Chronic pyelonephritis**: Administration of modified *Wu Wei Xiao Du Yin* in 13 patients with chronic pyelonephritis was associated with complete recovery in 8 cases, improvement in 3 cases, and no effect in 2 cases.[10]
8. **Glomerulonephritis**: Use of modified *Wu Wei Xiao Du Yin* was associated with marked success in treating glomerulonephritis in children. The herbal treatment contained *Wu Wei Xiao Du Yin* plus *Mu Tong* (Caulis Akebiae) and *Gan Cao* (Radix et Rhizoma Glycyrrhizae) as the base formula. Furthermore, modifications were made as follows: *Ma Huang* (Herba Ephedrae) and *Shi Gao* (Gypsum Fibrosum) for wind and water accumulation; *Wu Ling San* (Five-Ingredient Powder with Poria) for water and damp accumulation; and *Shi Gao* (Gypsum Fibrosum), *Bai Mao Gen* (Rhizoma Imperatae), *Dan Zhu Ye* (Herba Lophatheri), and *Xiao Ji* (Herba Cirsii) for damp-heat accumulation. Of 36 patients, the study reported complete recovery in 30 cases, improvement in 4 cases, and no effect in 2 cases. The overall effectiveness was 94.4%.[11]
9. **Burns**: Fourteen of 15 patients with various degrees of burns were treated successfully with modified *Wu Wei Xiao Du Yin* for prevention and treatment of infection. Depending on the severity of burns and infection, the duration of treatment ranged from 7-21 days. The herbal formula contained *Wu Wei Xiao Du Yin* as the base formula, with the addition of *Dang Shen* (Radix Codonopsis), *Huang Qi* (Radix Astragali), and *Mai Dong* (Radix Ophiopogonis) for qi and yin deficiencies; *Huang Lian Jie Du Tang* (Coptis Decoction to Relieve Toxicity) or *Si Miao San* (Four-Marvel Powder) for fire and toxins; and *Dan Shen* (Radix et Rhizoma Salviae Miltiorrhizae) and *Chi Shao* (Radix Paeoniae Rubra) during the middle stage of recovery.[12]
10. **Myelitis**: Thirteen patients with inflammation of the spinal cord or the bone marrow were treated successfully using both antibiotic drugs and modified *Wu Wei Xiao Du Yin*. Concurrent drug and herb treatment was employed for 3-4 days to control acute infection and inflammation, followed by use of herbs to maintain and consolidate the condition. All 13 patients reported significant improvement or complete recovery within one month. The herbal formula was based on *Wu Wei Xiao Du Yin*, with the removal of *Tian Kui Zi* (Radix Semiaquilegiae), and the addition of processed *Chuan Shan Jia* (Squama Manis) and *Lian Qiao* (Fructus Forsythiae). *Huang Qi* (Radix Astragali) was added for qi deficiency when necessary.[13]
11. **Urinary tract infection**: One study reported 94.6% effectiveness using modified *Wu Wei Xiao Du Yin* to treat 37 children with acute urinary tract infection. In addition to *Wu Wei Xiao Du Yin*, *Chai Hu* (Radix Bupleuri) was added for more heat; *Bai Mao Gen* (Rhizoma Imperatae), *Da Ji* (Herba Cirsii Japonici), and *Xiao Ji* (Herba Cirsii) for hematuria; *Che Qian Zi* (Semen Plantaginis) and *Mu Tong* (Caulis Akebiae) for frequent urination with urgency; and *Huang Qi* (Radix Astragali) for qi deficiency. Of 37 patients, the study reported complete recovery in 26 cases, improvement in 9 cases, and no effect in 2 cases.[14]
12. ***Re lin* (heat dysuria)**: One hundred and fourteen patients out of 128 were successfully treated using modified *Wu Wei Xiao Du Yin*. In addition to the base formula, *Che Qian Zi* (Semen Plantaginis) and *Fu Ling* (Poria) were added for dysuria; *Da Huang* (Radix et Rhizoma Rhei) and *Zhi Shi* (Fructus Aurantii Immaturus) for constipation with a yellow, greasy tongue coating; *Di Huang* (Radix Rehmanniae) and *Bai Mao Gen* (Rhizoma

Wŭ Wèi Xiāo Dú Yĭn

(Five-Ingredient Decoction to Eliminate Toxins)

Imperatae) for damp-heat damaging yin; and *Dang Shen* (Radix Codonopsis) and *Huang Qi* (Radix Astragali) for generalized deficiency.[15]

SUGGESTED ACUPUNCTURE TREATMENT

1. Points: *Lingtai* (GV 10), *Shenzhu* (GV 12), *Hegu* (LI 4), *Weizhong* (BL 40), and *Xuehai* (SP 10).
2. Technique: sedation.

The objectives of this acupuncture treatment are to clear heat, eliminate toxins, and disperse external carbuncles and furuncles. Sedation of *Lingtai* (GV 10) clears heat and fire throughout the body. *Shenzhu* (GV 12) is a special point used to treat various types of epithelial inflammation, such as carbuncles and furuncles. *Hegu* (LI 4) is the *yuan* (source) point of the Large Intestine channel and can sedate heat and eliminate toxins from the *yangming*. Finally, the combination of *Weizhong* (BL 40) and *Xuehai* (SP 10) regulate qi and blood, clear heat from the blood, and reduce swelling and pain.

AUTHORS' COMMENTS

Wu Wei Xiao Du Yin can be used as a base formula for any general infection in veterinary medicine, as it consists of five bitter and cold herbs that clear heat and toxins. The herbs that comprise this formula have been found to have antimicrobial activity and can be used to treat bacterial and viral infections from a conventional medicine perspective. *Wu Wei Xiao Du Yin* was originally used to treat infections affecting the upper *jiao*, as the flower herbs in this formula are light and airy and have a tendency to ascend. This formula is used to treat conditions of excess; it contains no tonic herbs and is quite cold in nature, and so it should not be used in animals with Spleen and Stomach deficiencies without modification, as it will cause vomiting. In modern usage, the applications of this formula have been extended to treat external and internal infections in any region of the body. *Wu Wei Xiao Du Yin* is not typically used alone, but is usually combined with other herbs and conventional antimicrobial drugs (cephalexin, enrofloxacin, ciprofloxacin) to achieve maximum clinical effects.

Wu Wei Xiao Du Yin can be used to treat pyoderma, non-healing wounds, abscess secondary to bite or scratch wounds, and cellulitis. It can also be combined with *Pai Nong San* (Drain the Pus Powder) to help promote the drainage of pus from wounds to accelerate healing. It can be combined with *Tuo Li Xiao Du Yin* (Drain the Interior and Detoxify Decoction) to treat chronic sores, abscesses, and non-healing wounds in weak, geriatric or debilitated animals with underlying qi and blood deficiencies. This formula can be used in the treatment of acute pyelonephritis with edema, dysuria, a red tongue body, and a rapid pulse, or in the treatment of fever that is unresponsive to antibiotics. For these cases, add *Ze Xie* (Rhizoma Alismatis), *Zhi Zi* (Fructus Gardeniae), *Che Qian Zi* (Semen Plantaginis), *Da Huang* (Radix et Rhizoma Rhei), *Dan Shen* (Radix et Rhizoma Salviae Miltiorrhizae), *Lian Qiao* (Fructus Forsythiae), *Huang Bo* (Cortex Phellodendri Chinensis), and *Huang Lian* (Rhizoma Coptidis). For dogs that are deficient, add a small amount of *Bai Zhu* (Rhizoma Atractylodis Macrocephalae), *Huang Qi* (Radix Astragali) and *Dang Shen* (Radix Codonopsis). It can be combined with *Bai Xian Pi* (Cortex Dictamni), *Di Fu Zi* (Fructus Kochiae), *Wu Shao She* (Zaocys) *Zi Cao* (Radix Arnebiae), and *Dan Shen* (Radix et Rhizoma Salviae Miltiorrhizae) to treat damp-heat skin conditions with pruritus.

To improve clinical results in the treatment of perianal dermatitis, this formula can be taken internally, along with the topical application of an herbal wash that contains equal amounts of *Ku Shen* (Radix Sophorae Flavescentis), *Da Huang* (Radix et Rhizoma Rhei), *Huang Bo* (Cortex Phellodendri Chinensis), and *Pu Gong Ying* (Herba Taraxaci).

References

1. *Zhe Jiang Zhong Yi Za Zhi* (Zhejiang Journal of Chinese Medicine), 1978; 1:3.
2. *He Bei Zhong Yi* (Hebei Chinese Medicine), 1980; 2:46.
3. *Liao Ning Zhong Yi Za Zhi* (Liaoning Journal of Chinese Medicine), 1994; 21(5):222.
4. *Yun Nan Zhong Yi Za Zhi* (Yunan Journal of Chinese Medicine), 1994; 3:10.
5. *Hu Bei Zhong Yi Za Zhi* (Hubei Journal of Chinese Medicine), 1989; 4:13.
6. *Shi Zhen Guo Yao Yan Jiu* (Research of Shizhen Herbs), 1994; 1:7.
7. *Hu Bei Zhong Yi Za Zhi* (Hubei Journal of Chinese Medicine), 1989; 4:13.
8. *Shi Zhen Guo Yao Yan Jiu* (Research of Shizhen Herbs), 1993; 2:7.
9. *Shi Yong Zhong Xi Yi Jie He Za Zhi* (Practical Journal of Integrated Chinese and Western Medicines), 1992; 8:466.
10. *Jiang Xi Zhong Yi Yao* (Jiangxi Chinese Medicine and Herbology), 1993; 2:31.
11. *Hu Nan Zhong Yi Za Zhi* (Hunan Journal of Chinese Medicine), 1999; 3:59.
12. *Guang Xi Zhong Yi Yao* (Guangxi Chinese Medicine and Herbology), 1996; 3:24.
13. *Jiang Xi Zhong Yi Yao* (Jiangxi Chinese Medicine and Herbology), 1997; 5:44.
14. *Si Chuan Zhong Yi* (Sichuan Chinese Medicine), 1995; 8:47.
15. *Fu Jian Zhong Yi Yao* (Fujian Chinese Medicine and Herbology), 1996; 2:17.

Sì Miào Yǒng Ān Tāng (Four-Valiant Decoction for Well-Being)

四妙勇安湯
四妙勇安汤

Pinyin Name: *Si Miao Yong An Tang*
Literal Name: Four-Valiant Decoction for Well-Being
Original Source: *Yan Fang Xin Bian* (New Compilation of Time-Tested Formulas) by Bao Xiang-Ao in 1846

COMPOSITION

Jin Yin Hua (Flos Lonicerae Japonicae)	90g [30-90g]
Xuan Shen (Radix Scrophulariae)	90g [30-90g]
Dang Gui (Radix Angelicae Sinensis)	60g [15-30g]
Gan Cao (Radix et Rhizoma Glycyrrhizae)	30g [10-15g]

DOSAGE / PREPARATION / ADMINISTRATION

The source text states to prepare the ingredients as a decoction. The source text specifically emphasizes to use all four herbs in decoction for a total of 10 packs of herbs. Today, this formula may be prepared as a decoction with the doses suggested in brackets.

CHINESE THERAPEUTIC ACTIONS

1. Clears heat and eliminates toxins
2. Activates blood circulation and relieves pain

CLINICAL MANIFESTATIONS

Gangrene: gangrene of the extremities with purulent abscess, dark red discoloration, local inflammation and swelling, possible severe pain, possible fever, thirst, a red tongue body, and a rapid pulse.

VETERINARY CLINICAL APPLICATIONS

Vasculitis, phlebitis, severe necrolytic dermatitis and gangrene.

EXPLANATION

Si Miao Yong An Tang (Four-Valiant Decoction for Well-Being) treats gangrene in the extremities, especially the lower legs, characterized by severe accumulation of heat and toxins. Severe heat and toxin accumulation may injure the body tissues and damage the qi and blood, causing gangrene of the extremities with local inflammation, purulent abscess, dark red discoloration, swelling, and a burning sensation. In acute conditions, there may be severe pain. Fever, thirst, a red tongue, and a rapid pulse suggest interior heat.

This formula contains a large dose of *Jin Yin Hua* (Flos Lonicerae Japonicae) to clear heat and eliminate toxins. *Xuan Shen* (Radix Scrophulariae) purges fire and eliminates toxins. *Dang Gui* (Radix Angelicae Sinensis) activates blood circulation and disperses stagnation. *Gan Cao* (Radix et Rhizoma Glycyrrhizae) assists *Jin Yin Hua* (Flos Lonicerae Japonicae) in clearing heat and eliminating toxins.

VETERINARY MODIFICATIONS

- With more heat and toxins, add *Zi Hua Di Ding* (Herba Violae) and *Lian Qiao* (Fructus Forsythiae), and increase the dosage of *Jin Yin Hua* (Flos Lonicerae Japonicae).
- With severe pain, add *Ru Xiang* (Gummi Olibanum), *Mo Yao* (Myrrha), *Quan Xie* (Scorpio), *Wu Gong* (Scolopendra) and *Bai Shao* (Radix Paeoniae Alba).

Si Miao Yong An Tang **(Four-Valiant Decoction for Well-Being)**

Diagnosis	Clinical Signs	Treatment	Herbs
Gangrene	• Gangrene in the extremities, local inflammation, purulent abscess, dark red discoloration, swelling and a burning sensation: severe heat and toxins damaging the qi and blood • Thirst: heat consuming body fluids • Red tongue and a rapid pulse: interior heat	• Clears heat and eliminates toxins • Activates blood circulation and relieves pain	• *Jin Yin Hua* (Flos Lonicerae Japonicae) clears heat and eliminates toxins. • *Xuan Shen* (Radix Scrophulariae) purges fire and eliminates toxins. • *Dang Gui* (Radix Angelicae Sinensis) activates the blood and disperses stagnation. • *Gan Cao* (Radix et Rhizoma Glycyrrhizae) clears heat, eliminates toxins, and harmonizes all of the herbs.

Sì Miào Yǒng Ān Tāng (Four-Valiant Decoction for Well-Being)

- With more blood stagnation, add *Tao Ren* (Semen Persicae) and *Hong Hua* (Flos Carthami).
- With qi deficiency, add *Huang Qi* (Radix Astragali) and *Dang Shen* (Radix Codonopsis).
- With cold excess and yang deficiency, add *Fu Zi* (Radix Aconiti Lateralis Praeparata), *Gui Zhi* (Ramulus Cinnamomi), and *Lu Jiao Shuang* (Cornu Cervi Degelatinatum).
- With severe swelling and inflammation due to damp-heat, add *Fang Ji* (Radix Stephaniae Tetrandrae), *Huang Bo* (Cortex Phellodendri Chinensis), and *Cang Zhu* (Rhizoma Atractylodis).
- For gangrene in the lower extremities, add *Niu Xi* (Radix Achyranthis Bidentatae) and *Yi Yi Ren* (Semen Coicis).
- For gangrene in the upper extremities, add *Chuan Xiong* (Rhizoma Chuanxiong).
- For gangrene in the trunk of the body, add *Du Zhong* (Cortex Eucommiae).
- For vasculitis, add *Mao Dong Qing* (Radix Ilicis Pubescentis), *Pu Gong Ying* (Herba Taraxaci), *Dan Shen* (Radix et Rhizoma Salviae Miltiorrhizae), *Chi Xiao Dou* (Semen Phaseoli), *Chuan Shan Jia* (Squama Manis), and *Di Long* (Pheretima).

CAUTIONS / CONTRAINDICATIONS

- *Si Miao Yong An Tang* is designed for gangrene characterized by heat and toxins. It is inappropriate for gangrene characterized by cold.
- In severe cases of gangrene in which there is confirmed necrosis of the tissues, the use of this formula is not sufficient. Instead, surgery, or possibly even amputation, is necessary to remove the necrotic tissue.
- The source text states to avoid scratching the affected area while taking this formula.

PHARMACOLOGICAL EFFECTS

1. **Analgesic**: Administration of *Si Miao Yong An Tang* was associated with marked analgesic effects in mice, starting 40 minutes after oral ingestion.[1]
2. **Effect on coagulation**: Administration of *Si Miao Yong An Tang* did not affect coagulation or bleeding time in rabbits and mice.[2]

HUMAN CLINICAL STUDIES AND RESEARCH

1. **Arteriosclerotic gangrene**: One study used modified *Si Miao Yong An Tang* to treat 28 patients with arteriosclerotic gangrene. In addition to the base formula, *Quan Xie* (Scorpio), *Wu Gong* (Scolopendra), and *Bai Shao* (Radix Paeoniae Alba) were added for severe pain; *Pu Gong Ying* (Herba Taraxaci), *Huang Bo* (Cortex Phellodendri Chinensis), and *An Gong Niu Huang Wan* (Calm the Palace Pill with Cattle Gallstone) for heat and toxins; *Dan Shen* (Radix et Rhizoma Salviae Miltiorrhizae), *Tao Ren* (Semen Persicae), and *Hong Hua* (Flos Carthami) for blood stagnation; *Huang Qi* (Radix Astragali), *Bai Zhu* (Rhizoma Atractylodis Macrocephalae), and *Fu Ling* (Poria) for qi deficiency; and *Jue Ming Zi* (Semen Cassiae) for constipation. Of 28 patients, the study reported complete recovery in 19 cases, marked improvement in 3 cases, and no effect in 2 cases.[3]
2. **Thromboangiitis obliterans**: Thirty-three patients (32 males and 1 females) with thromboangiitis obliterans were treated with complete recovery in 16 cases, improvement in 11 cases, and no effect in 6 cases. The herbal formula contained *Si Miao Yong An Tang* plus *Huang Qin* (Radix Scutellariae), *Ban Lan Gen* (Radix Isatidis), and *Chuan Niu Xi* (Radix Cyathulae).[4] Another study reported complete recovery in 28 of 30 patients with thromboangiitis obliterans using *Si Miao Yong An Tang*.[5]
3. **Thrombophlebitis**: Twenty-eight patients with thrombophlebitis were treated with complete recovery in 22 cases, significant effect in 5 cases, and no effect in 1 case. The herbal treatment used *Si Miao Yong An Tang* as the base formula. In addition, depending on the affected area, the following additions were made: *Chuan Xiong* (Rhizoma Chuanxiong) for upper extremities, *Niu Xi* (Radix Achyranthis Bidentatae) for lower extremities, *Du Zhong* (Cortex Eucommiae) for the trunk of the body, and *Chuan Shan Jia* (Squama Manis) for obvious swelling and inflammation.[6]
4. **Phlebitis**: One study reported marked effectiveness using modified *Si Miao Yong An Tang* to treat 32 patients with phlebitis in the lower extremities. Modifications to the base formula included: *Che Qian Zi* (Semen Plantaginis), *Bai Hua She She Cao* (Herba Hedyotis), and *Chuan Niu Xi* (Radix Cyathulae) for early-stage phlebitis; and *Shui Zhi* (Hirudo), *Huang Qi* (Radix Astragali), and *E Zhu* (Rhizoma Curcumae) for late-stage phlebitis. The herbs were cooked in water and the decoction was given orally to the patient. In addition, the herb residue was cooked again in water, and the solution was used as an herbal wash and applied to the affected area. Of 32 patients, the study reported complete recovery in 29 cases and marked improvement in 3 cases.[7]
5. **Thrombosis of iliofemoral vein**: Integrative treatment was found to be effective in 97.2% of patients with iliofemoral vein thrombosis. The herbal treatment contained *Si Miao Yong An Tang*, modified by removing *Gan Cao* (Radix et Rhizoma Glycyrrhizae) and adding *Chuan Xiong* (Rhizoma Chuanxiong), *Da Huang* (Radix et Rhizoma Rhei) and others as needed. In addition, patients also received an intravenous infusion of *Dan Shen* (Radix et Rhizoma Salviae Miltiorrhizae) and oral ingestion of aspirin (300 mg/day for five days, followed by

Sì Miào Yǒng Ān Tāng (Four-Valiant Decoction for Well-Being)

100 mg/day daily). Antibiotic drugs were given if necessary. Of 36 patients, the study reported complete recovery in 28 cases, marked improvement in 7 cases, and no effect in 1 case.[8]

6. **Sciatica**: Use of modified *Si Miao Yong An Tang* in 30 patients with sciatica was associated with complete recovery in 21 cases, marked improvement in 8 cases, and no effect in 1 case. The herbal treatment included *Si Miao Yong An Tang* plus *Wei Ling Xian* (Radix et Rhizoma Clematidis), *Qian Nian Jian* (Rhizoma Homalomenae) and *Chuan Niu Xi* (Radix Cyathulae) as the base formula. Furthermore, modifications to the original formula included the addition of *Huang Bo* (Cortex Phellodendri Chinensis) and *Di Long* (Pheretima) for soreness, heaviness and pain due to damp-heat; *Fu Zi* (Radix Aconiti Lateralis Praeparata) and *Xi Xin* (Radix et Rhizoma Asari) for cold extremities and aversion to cold due to damp-cold; *Du Zhong* (Cortex Eucommiae) and *Sang Ji Sheng* (Herba Taxilli) for low back pain; and *Bai Shao* (Radix Paeoniae Alba), *Yu Zhu* (Rhizoma Polygonati Odorati), and *Shen Jin Cao* (Herba Lycopodii) for muscle spasms, cramps and/or atrophy.[9]

SUGGESTED ACUPUNCTURE TREATMENT

1. Points: *Shenzhu* (GV 12), *Quchi* (LI 11), *Hegu* (LI 4), *Xuehai* (SP 10), *Housanli* (ST 36), *Sanyinjiao* (SP 6), *Jiexi* (ST 41), *Kunlun* (BL 60), *Taixi* (KI 3), and *Shenmai* (BL 62).
2. Technique: sedation.

The four objectives of acupuncture treatment for gangrene include clearing heat, eliminate toxins, activating the blood, and relieving pain. *Shenzhu* (GV 12), *Quchi* (LI 11), and *Hegu* (LI 4) clear heat and eliminate toxins. *Xuehai* (SP 10), *Housanli* (ST 36), and *Sanyinjiao* (SP 6) activate the blood and remove blood stagnation. *Jiexi* (ST 41), *Kunlun* (BL 60), *Shenmai* (BL 62), and *Taixi* (KI 3) regulate qi and open the channels and collaterals.

AUTHORS' COMMENTS

Si Miao Yong An Tang is the representative formula for treating gangrene with underlying yin and blood deficiencies, with such key diagnostic clinical signs as localized inflammation, purulent abscess, dark red discoloration, and swelling.

The original text notes that successful treatment of gangrene requires the use of this formula in large doses for a prolonged duration (at least 10 days). The use of this formula at low doses or for a short period of time will not be effective. This formula is not readily available commercially but can easily be made in-house, as it is composed of only four common herbs. To increase clinical efficacy, it is often combined with herbs that invigorate the blood, such as *Hong Hua* (Flos Carthami), *Tao Ren* (Semen Persicae), *Dan Shen* (Radix et Rhizoma Salviae Miltiorrhizae), and *Ji Xue Teng* (Caulis Spatholobi). It may also be combined with *Pai Nong San* (Drain the Pus Powder) to help drain pus and accelerate healing. Most cases of gangrene in animals occur as a result of injury from neglect, abuse and entrapment. The development of gangrene typically develops secondary to ropes or wires tied around the neck or extremities in domesticated animals. In non-domestic animals (particularly African species), snares are commonly used by poachers, which usually causes the eventual development of gangrene in these animals (gorillas, leopards, antelope, etc). All of these animals may benefit from this formula. Dogs that have vasculitis secondary to snake bite may also be treated with *Si Miao Yong An Tang*.

References

1. *Zhe Jiang Yi Xue* (Zhejiang Journal of Medicine), 1960; 36.
2. *Zhe Jiang Yi Xue* (Zhejiang Journal of Medicine), 1960; 36.
3. *Xin Zhong Yi* (New Chinese Medicine), 1990; 2:27.
4. *Zhong Yi Za Zhi* (Journal of Chinese Medicine), 1980; 1:42.
5. *Tian Jin Yi Yao Za Zhi* (Journal of Tianjin Medicine and Herbology), 1960; 1:1.
6. *Si Chuan Zhong Yi* (Sichuan Chinese Medicine), 1992; 9:37.
7. *Shan Xi Zhong Yi* (Shanxi Chinese Medicine), 1998; 2:74.
8. *Hei Long Jiang Zhong Yi Yao* (Heilongjiang Chinese Medicine and Herbology), 1997; 3:1.
9. *Hu Bei Zhong Yi Za Zhi* (Hubei Journal of Chinese Medicine), 1993; 2:19.

Zǐ Cǎo Gēn Mǔ Lì Tāng (Arnebia and Oyster Shell Decoction)

紫草根牡蠣湯
紫草根牡蛎汤

Pinyin Name: *Zi Cao Gen Mu Li Tang*
Literal Name: Arnebia and Oyster Shell Combination
Alternate Name: *Zi Gen Mu Li Tang*, Lithospermum and Oyster Shell Decoction
Original Source: *Bai Rai Shin Shu* (A New Study of Dermatomycosis and Dermatitis) by Tsursure Katakura

COMPOSITION

Zi Cao (Radix Arnebiae)	3g
Jin Yin Hua (Flos Lonicerae Japonicae)	1.5g
Sheng Ma (Rhizoma Cimicifugae)	2g
Mu Li (Concha Ostreae)	4g
Huang Qi (Radix Astragali)	2g
Dang Gui (Radix Angelicae Sinensis)	5g
Bai Shao (Radix Paeoniae Alba)	3g
Chuan Xiong (Rhizoma Chuanxiong)	3g
Da Huang (Radix et Rhizoma Rhei)	1.5g
Gan Cao (Radix et Rhizoma Glycyrrhizae)	1g

Note: *Zi Cao* (Radix Arnebiae) may be derived from three sources: *Arnebiae euchroma*, *Arnebiae guttata*, and *Lithospermum erythrorhizon*. All three herbs have similar functions and have been used interchangeably in the history of Chinese herbal medicine. However, *Zhong Hua Ren Min Gong He Guo Yao Dian* (Pharmacopoeia of the People's Republic of China) in 2005 identifies the arnebia genus as the official source of *Zi Cao*. Therefore, we have adopted arnebia as the standard nomenclature throughout this text.

DOSAGE / PREPARATION / ADMINISTRATION

The source texts states to cook the herbs in 5 cups of water until the liquid is reduced to 2.5 cups. Take the warm, strained decoction in three equally divided doses daily. Today, the decoction may be prepared using a higher dose of the ingredients (approximately 2-3 times higher).

CHINESE THERAPEUTIC ACTIONS

1. Clears heat and eliminates toxins
2. Reduces swelling and disperses nodules and hardness

CLINICAL MANIFESTATIONS

Malignant abscesses and sores: various types of abscesses, sores, nodules, hardness.

VETERINARY CLINICAL APPLICATIONS

Canine mammary gland adenocarcinoma, mastitis, pyoderma, gangrene.

EXPLANATION

Zi Cao Gen Mu Li Tang (Arnebia and Oyster Shell Decoction) treats various types of dermatological disorders characterized by heat and toxins. It has a broad range of effects and is effective against sores, abscesses, nodules, and hardness.

Zi Cao (Radix Arnebiae) and *Jin Yin Hua* (Flos Lonicerae Japonicae) clear heat and eliminate toxins from the blood. They are also effective in treating various types of chronic and stubborn abscesses and sores due to infection. *Sheng Ma* (Rhizoma Cimicifugae) raises and disperses yang qi while eliminating heat and toxins. *Mu Li* (Concha Ostreae) softens hardness and disperses nodules. *Huang Qi* (Radix Astragali) tonifies qi and promotes healing; it is one of the most important herbs for treating patients with suppurative disorders. *Dang Gui* (Radix Angelicae Sinensis), *Bai Shao* (Radix Paeoniae Alba), and *Chuan Xiong* (Rhizoma Chuanxiong) tonify the blood and strengthen the body. *Da Huang* (Radix et Rhizoma Rhei) drains damp-heat. *Gan Cao* (Radix et Rhizoma Glycyrrhizae) harmonizes all of the herbs in the formula.

Zǐ Cǎo Gēn Mǔ Lì Tāng (Arnebia and Oyster Shell Decoction)

***Zi Cao Gen Mu Li Tang* (Arnebia and Oyster Shell Decoction)**

Diagnosis	Clinical Signs	Treatment	Herbs
Malignant abscesses and sores	Abscesses, sores, nodules and hardness: heat and toxins accumulation	• Clears heat and eliminates toxins • Reduces swelling and disperses nodules and hardness	• *Zi Cao* (Radix Arnebiae) and *Jin Yin Hua* (Flos Lonicerae Japonicae) clear heat and eliminate toxins from the blood. • *Sheng Ma* (Rhizoma Cimicifugae) raises and disperses yang qi while eliminating heat and toxins. • *Mu Li* (Concha Ostreae) softens hardness and disperses nodules. • *Huang Qi* (Radix Astragali) tonifies qi and promotes healing. • *Dang Gui* (Radix Angelicae Sinensis), *Bai Shao* (Radix Paeoniae Alba) and *Chuan Xiong* (Rhizoma Chuanxiong) tonify the blood and strengthen the body. • *Da Huang* (Radix et Rhizoma Rhei) drains damp-heat. • *Gan Cao* (Radix et Rhizoma Glycyrrhizae) harmonizes all of the herbs.

VETERINARY MODIFICATIONS

- With painful bruises and swelling, add *Ru Xiang* (Gummi Olibanum) and *Mo Yao* (Myrrha).
- To clear heat and toxins, add *Lian Qiao* (Fructus Forsythiae) and *Zi Hua Di Ding* (Herba Violae).
- To nourish and move blood and resolve stagnation, add *Dan Shen* (Radix et Rhizoma Salviae Miltiorrhizae) and *Ji Xue Teng* (Caulis Spatholobi).

SUGGESTED ACUPUNCTURE TREATMENT

1. Points: *Xuehai* (SP 10), *Weizhong* (BL 40), *Dazhui* (GV 14), *Shanzhong* (CV 17), *Rugen* (ST 18), *Zigong* (CV 19), *Pishu* (BL 20), *Feishu* (BL 13), *Sanyinjiao* (SP 6), *Tianshu* (ST 25), and *Quchi* (LI 11).
2. Technique: moxibustion, bleeding, and sedation.

Bleed *Weizhong* (BL 40) and sedate *Xuehai* (SP 10) and *Dazhui* (GV 14) to clear heat and eliminate toxins in the blood. Apply moxibustion on *Pishu* (BL 20) and *Feishu* (BL 13) to tonify qi; needle *Sanyinjiao* (SP 6) to tonify blood. Sedate *Tianshu* (ST 25) and *Quchi* (LI 11) to clear heat. If the hardness is in the chest, needle *Shanzhong* (CV 17) and *Rugen* (ST 18); if it is in the genital area, needle *Zigong* (CV 19).

AUTHORS' COMMENTS

Zi Cao Gen Mu Li Tang is effective in treating mammary gland adenocarcinoma in dogs, when combined with the following herbs: *Lian Qiao* (Fructus Forsythiae), *Dan Shen* (Radix et Rhizoma Salviae Miltiorrhizae), *Kun Bu* (Thallus Eckloniae), *Hai Zao* (Sargassum), *Xia Ku Cao* (Spica Prunellae), *Ban Xia* (Rhizoma Pinelliae), *Xiang Fu* (Rhizoma Cyperi), *E Zhu* (Rhizoma Curcumae), *San Leng* (Rhizoma Sparganii), *Bai Hua She She Cao* (Herba Hedyotis), and *Shui Zhi* (Hirudo). Use with caution in animals with deficiency of the middle *jiao*; add herbs or other formulas as needed.

Hăi Zăo Yù Hú Tāng (Sargassum Decoction for the Jade Flask)

海藻玉壺湯
海藻玉壶汤

Pinyin Name: *Hai Zao Yu Hu Tang*
Literal Name: Sargassum Decoction for the Jade Flask
Alternate Name: Sargassum Combination for the Jade Flask
Original Source: *Yi Zong Jin Jian* (Golden Mirror of the Medical Tradition) by Wu Qian in 1742

COMPOSITION

Hai Zao (Sargassum), *xi* (washed)	3g
Kun Bu (Thallus Eckloniae)	3g
Hai Dai (Thallus Laminariae)	1.5g
Zhe Bei Mu (Bulbus Fritillariae Thunbergii)	3g
Ban Xia (Rhizoma Pinelliae), *zhi* (prepared)	3g
Qing Pi (Pericarpium Citri Reticulatae Viride)	3g
Chen Pi (Pericarpium Citri Reticulatae)	3g
Dang Gui (Radix Angelicae Sinensis)	3g
Chuan Xiong (Rhizoma Chuanxiong)	3g
Du Huo (Radix Angelicae Pubescentis)	3g
Lian Qiao (Fructus Forsythiae)	3g
Gan Cao (Radix et Rhizoma Glycyrrhizae)	3g

DOSAGE / PREPARATION / ADMINISTRATION

The source text states to prepare the ingredients as a decoction by cooking the herbs in 2 cups of water until the liquid is reduced down to 80%. Take the decoction before meals if the affected area is in the upper body, and after meals if it is in the lower body.

CHINESE THERAPEUTIC ACTIONS

1. Dissolves phlegm and softens hardness
2. Reduces and disperses goiter and tumor

CLINICAL MANIFESTATIONS

Goiter due to Liver and Spleen disharmony, along with qi and phlegm stagnation: immobile, hard, non-painful goiter in the neck, with no change in skin color and no inflammation.

VETERINARY CLINICAL APPLICATIONS

Goiter, thyroid adenocarcinoma, feline hyperthyroidism, and lymphadenitis.

EXPLANATION

Hai Zao Yu Hu Tang (Sargassum Decoction for the Jade Flask) treats goiter caused by qi and phlegm stagnation, which often arises from the disharmony between the Liver and Spleen. The local qi and phlegm stagnation can then produce blood stagnation. The nodule is usually located in the neck and is immobile, with no color change and no pain; moreover, the nodule does not perforate and is often described as "hard as rock."

This formula uses *Hai Zao* (Sargassum), *Kun Bu* (Thallus Eckloniae), and *Hai Dai* (Thallus Laminariae) to dissolve phlegm and soften nodules. *Zhe Bei Mu* (Bulbus Fritillariae Thunbergii) and *Ban Xia* (Rhizoma Pinelliae) dry dampness and resolve phlegm. *Qing Pi* (Pericarpium Citri Reticulatae Viride) and *Chen Pi* (Pericarpium Citri Reticulatae) regulate qi and spread the Liver. *Dang Gui* (Radix Angelicae Sinensis), *Chuan Xiong* (Rhizoma Chuanxiong), and *Du Huo* (Radix Angelicae Pubescentis) activate blood circulation and disperse the nodule. *Lian Qiao* (Fructus Forsythiae) disperses nodules and reduces swelling. *Gan Cao* (Radix et Rhizoma Glycyrrhizae) harmonizes all of the herbs in the formula.

Hǎi Zǎo Yù Hú Tāng (Sargassum Decoction for the Jade Flask)

***Hai Zao Yu Hu Tang* (Sargassum Decoction for the Jade Flask)**

Diagnosis	Clinical Signs	Treatment	Herbs
Goiter	Hard, immobile goiter in the neck region: Liver and Spleen disharmony, accompanied by qi and phlegm stagnation	• Dissolves phlegm and softens hardness • Reduces and disperses goiter and tumor	• *Hai Zao* (Sargassum), *Kun Bu* (Thallus Eckloniae), and *Hai Dai* (Thallus Laminariae) dissolve phlegm and soften nodules. • *Zhe Bei Mu* (Bulbus Fritillariae Thunbergii) and *Ban Xia* (Rhizoma Pinelliae) dry dampness and resolve phlegm. • *Qing Pi* (Pericarpium Citri Reticulatae Viride) and *Chen Pi* (Pericarpium Citri Reticulatae) regulate qi and smooth the Liver. • *Dang Gui* (Radix Angelicae Sinensis), *Chuan Xiong* (Rhizoma Chuanxiong), and *Du Huo* (Radix Angelicae Pubescentis) activate blood circulation and disperse nodules. • *Lian Qiao* (Fructus Forsythiae) disperses nodules and reduces swelling. • *Gan Cao* (Radix et Rhizoma Glycyrrhizae) harmonizes all of the herbs.

VETERINARY MODIFICATIONS

- For rock-hard nodules, add *San Leng* (Rhizoma Sparganii) and *E Zhu* (Rhizoma Curcumae).
- For nodules associated with Liver qi stagnation, add *Chai Hu* (Radix Bupleuri) and *Xiang Fu* (Rhizoma Cyperi).
- With loose stools due to Spleen deficiency, add *Bai Zhu* (Rhizoma Atractylodis Macrocephalae), *Shan Yao* (Rhizoma Dioscoreae), and *Bai Bian Dou* (Semen Lablab Album).
- With frequent thirst and hunger due to Stomach heat, add *Shi Gao* (Gypsum Fibrosum), *Zhi Mu* (Rhizoma Anemarrhenae), and *Tian Hua Fen* (Radix Trichosanthis).

CAUTIONS / CONTRAINDICATIONS

While taking *Hai Zao Yu Hu Tang*, avoid foods that are sweet, fatty, or heavy in nature.

HUMAN CLINICAL STUDIES AND RESEARCH

Hyperthyroidism: Use of modified *Hai Zao Yu Hu Tang* in 23 patients with hyperthyroidism was associated with 87% effectiveness. The herbal treatment contained *Hai Zao* (Sargassum), *Kun Bu* (Thallus Eckloniae), *Zhe Bei Mu* (Bulbus Fritillariae Thunbergii), *Qing Pi* (Pericarpium Citri Reticulatae Viride), *Chen Pi* (Pericarpium Citri Reticulatae), *Di Huang* (Radix Rehmanniae), *Bai Shao* (Radix Paeoniae Alba), *Tian Dong* (Radix Asparagi), *Xuan Shen* (Radix Scrophulariae), *Xia Ku Cao* (Spica Prunellae), *Huang Qin* (Radix Scutellariae), and *Mu Li* (Concha Ostreae). Clinical results included both subjective and objective improvements, with resolution of clinical signs and normalization of T3 and T4. Of 23 patients, the study reported recovery in 11 cases, improvement in 9 cases, and no effect in 3 cases.[1]

SUGGESTED ACUPUNCTURE TREATMENT

1. Points: *Naohui* (TH 13), *Shaochong* (HT 9), *Xuehai* (SP 10), *Tianding* (LI 17), *Shuitu* (ST 10), and *Hegu* (LI 4).
2. Technique: sedation.

The focus of this treatment is to resolve goiter caused by qi and phlegm stagnation. *Naohui* (TH 13) regulates qi and reduces the nodules, while *Shaochong* (HT 9) regulates Liver qi. *Xuehai* (SP 10) activates the blood. Finally, *Tianding* (LI 17), *Shuitu* (ST 10), and *Hegu* (LI 4) together activate qi, eliminate phlegm stagnation, and reduce lumps and nodules.

AUTHORS' COMMENTS

Hai Zao Yu Hu Tang is one of the most commonly used formulas today for various thyroid disorders with enlargement of the thyroid glands, such as goiter and thyroid tumor. The duration of treatment necessary for improvement ranges from 3-6 months. Should the nodule remain the same size or increase in size, surgery should be considered.

According to *Shi Ba Fan* (Eighteen Incompatibles), *Hai Zao* (Sargassum) and *Gan Cao* (Radix et Rhizoma Glycyrrhizae) are not compatible with each other and should not be used together. However, this formula has been prescribed since 1742, and there has been no reported toxicity or side effects associated with its use. Furthermore, when prescribed, this formula is usually given for approximately 3-6 months. Thus, it is presumed that the use of these two herbs together for the indicated length of time is safe.

Hăi Zăo Yù Hú Tāng (Sargassum Decoction for the Jade Flask)

Hyperthyroidism is the most common endocrine disease of cats. It is typically caused by a benign functional tumor of the thyroid gland, characterized by excess production and secretion of triiodothyronine (T3) and thyroxine (T4), which results in hyper-metabolism. During physical examination, approximately 90% of cats with the disease will have a palpable thyroid mass (goiter). The majority of cats have already been diagnosed with hyperthyroidism by their conventional veterinarian at the time of the initial Chinese veterinary medicine consultation. Chinese medicine is not typically chosen as the primary approach to the treatment of feline hyperthyroidism because conventional therapies are curative. Herbal therapy is slow and prolonged in duration, and cats are difficult to medicate on a long-term basis. However, *Hai Zao Yu Hu Tang* can be used to treat cats with hyperthyroidism that have had adverse reactions to antithyroid drugs, or for those whose overall condition contraindicates nuclear medicine therapy or surgery. This formula is sometimes given prior to nuclear medicine treatment, in addition to other formulas that treat the underlying cause of hyperthyroidism, to strengthen the animal in preparation for the treatment.

Hai Zao Yu Hu Tang must be given for at least 3 months to produce clinically observable results, and like most formulas used to soften hardness and dissolve phlegm, it must be given on a regular basis for optimal results. Other individual herbs that regulate and move qi and blood to promote the resolution of phlegm can be added, such as *Mu Xiang* (Radix Aucklandiae), *Dan Shen* (Radix et Rhizoma Salviae Miltiorrhizae), *Xuan Shen* (Radix Scrophulariae), *Xia Ku Cao* (Spica Prunellae), and *Mu Li* (Concha Ostreae).

There are four formulas that can all be used to treat thyroid enlargement in cats with hyperthyroidism. Their differences are as follows:

- *Hai Zao Yu Hu Tang* (Sargassum Decoction for the Jade Flask) treats thyroid enlargement caused by qi and phlegm stagnation, which often arises from the disharmony between the Liver and Spleen. The local qi and phlegm stagnation can then produce blood stagnation. Nodules and swelling are usually located in the neck and are immobile; they are not painful, do not perforate, and are often described as "hard as rock." This formula must be administered for a minimum of 3-6 months for clinically observable results. These cats will have a red to purple tongue with a greasy coating and a slippery to wiry pulse.
- *Xiao Luo Wan* (Reduce Scrofula Pill) treats thyroid enlargement caused by phlegm and fire. Yin-deficient fire in combination with Liver fire rises to burn and damage the Liver and Gallbladder channels as they travel through the neck, resulting in the formation of lumps and nodules around the ears and the neck. This formula is directed at the branch (enlarged thyroid, lumps and nodules) and not at the root cause of the swellings and is usually modified or combined with another formula to improve clinical efficacy. As a species, cats are very difficult to medicate on a long-term basis. The value of this formula is that it can be added to food, as it only contains three herbs and many cats will eat it without a problem. These cats will have a dry, red tongue with little coating and a thin, wiry, rapid pulse or a thin, slippery pulse.
- *San Zhong Kui Jian Tang* (Disperse the Swelling and Break the Hardness Decoction) treats thyroid enlargement caused by qi and blood stagnation, damp-heat, and phlegm. It treats blood and phlegm accumulation and stagnation in the head and neck, causing nodules, swelling, and hardness in many parts of the body, particularly along the channels of the Liver, Gallbladder, Stomach and *San Jiao* and especially below the ears, under the cheeks/jaw, around the shoulders, and in the axillary region. These accumulations are usually caused by Liver and/or Heart fire flaming upwards to congeal the blood, qi and phlegm and eventually lead to mass formation. This formula is used to treat cats that, in addition to having a thyroid mass, also have other damp-heat conditions that make treatment of their thyroid disease a challenge, such as inflammatory bowel disease, chronic cholangiohepatitis, damp-heat skin (such as military dermatitis), pyelonephritis and diabetes. Unfortunately, many of the cats in this category are weak and debilitated, and this formula is cold and bitter and is best suited for strong animals with excess. Nevertheless, *San Zhong Kui Jian Tang* can still be judiciously used at a low dose, along with Spleen tonic herbs, to initially stabilize cats with multiple damp-heat disorders prior to conventional therapy. Out of the four formulas, *San Zhong Kui Jian Tang* has the greatest ability to treat heat and is not intended for long-term use. These cats will have obvious signs of heat and dampness, feel hot to the touch, can display irritability and aggression, and have a dark red to purple tongue and a rapid, wiry pulse.
- *Shi Liu Wei Liu Qi Yin* (Sixteen-Ingredient Decoction to Flow Qi) treats thyroid enlargement due to long-term qi and blood stagnation (clumping and restraint). It is the most nourishing formula and has very little ability to clear heat. It tonifies and moves qi and blood, expels pus, and disperses swelling. By using herbs that move qi and disperse accumulations, the thyroid mass will dissipate. It can take 3-6 months of treatment before clinical results are seen, and the formula can be used long term. This formula can be used as a adjunct therapy in cats taking oral antithyroid medication (tapazole) to control their hyperthyroidism. It can also be used in cats that are too

Hǎi Zǎo Yù Hú Tāng (Sargassum Decoction for the Jade Flask)

weak and debilitated to take stronger medications and may be combined with *Xiao Luo Wan* (Reduce Scrofula Pill) in these cases. These cats will have a pale pink to light purple tongue and a thin, weak pulse.

References

1. *Nei Meng Gu Zhong Yi Yao* (Traditional Chinese Medicine and Medicinals of Inner Mongolia), 1993; 4:9.

Xiāo Luǒ Wán (Reduce Scrofula Pill)

消瘰丸

Pinyin Name: *Xiao Luo Wan*
Literal Name: Reduce Scrofula Pill
Alternate Name: Scrophularia and Fritillaria Combination
Original Source: *Yi Xue Xin Wu* (Medical Revelations) by Cheng Guo-Peng in 1732

COMPOSITION

Xuan Shen (Radix Scrophulariae), *zheng* (steamed)	120g
Zhe Bei Mu (Bulbus Fritillariae Thunbergii), *zheng* (steamed)	120g
Mu Li (Concha Ostreae), *duan* (calcined) and *yan* (ground) with vinegar	120g

DOSAGE / PREPARATION / ADMINISTRATION

The source text states to first steam *Xuan Shen* (Radix Scrophulariae) and *Zhe Bei Mu* (Bulbus Fritillariae Thunbergii) and calcine and grind *Mu Li* (Concha Ostreae) with vinegar. Then, grind all of the ingredients into powder, mix with honey, and form into pills. Take 9g of pills with boiled water twice daily.

CHINESE THERAPEUTIC ACTIONS

1. Reduces scrofula
2. Nourishes yin
3. Dissolves phlegm and softens hardness

CLINICAL MANIFESTATIONS

Hardness and nodules: hard lumps or nodules anterior or posterior to the ear or in the neck, thyroid gland enlargement (goiter), dry mouth and throat, and a bitter taste in the mouth.

VETERINARY CLINICAL APPLICATIONS

Goiter, feline hyperthyroidism, lymphadenopathy, lymphadenitis and lipomas.

EXPLANATION

Xiao Luo Wan (Reduce Scrofula Pill) treats lumps and nodules around the ears and in the neck. Such nodules

Xiāo Luǒ Wán (Reduce Scrofula Pill)

***Xiao Luo Wan* (Reduce Scrofula Pill)**

Diagnosis	Clinical Signs	Treatment	Herbs
Hardness and nodules	Lumps or nodules around the ears and in the neck	• Reduces scrofula • Nourishes yin • Dissolves phlegm and softens hardness	• *Xuan Shen* (Radix Scrophulariae) nourishes yin and guides fire downward. • *Zhe Bei Mu* (Bulbus Fritillariae Thunbergii) dissolves phlegm and reduces swelling. • *Mu Li* (Concha Ostreae) softens hardness and disperses nodules.

or hardness is often caused by inflammation of the lymph nodes or enlargement of the thyroid gland. Although this formula contains only three herbs, it is very effective. *Xuan Shen* (Radix Scrophulariae) nourishes yin and guides fire downward. *Zhe Bei Mu* (Bulbus Fritillariae Thunbergii) dissolves phlegm and reduces swelling. *Mu Li* (Concha Ostreae) softens hardness and disperses nodules. When combined together, these three herbs treat various hardness and nodules, from early to late stages.

VETERINARY MODIFICATIONS

- With excess phlegm and fire, increase the dose of *Zhe Bei Mu* (Bulbus Fritillariae Thunbergii), and add *Gua Lou* (Fructus Trichosanthis), *Qing Dai* (Indigo Naturalis), and *Ge Qiao* (Concha Meretricis seu Cyclinae).
- With aggression and restlessness, add *Zhi Zi* (Fructus Gardeniae), *Huang Lian* (Rhizoma Coptidis), and *Huang Qin* (Radix Scutellariae).
- With Liver qi stagnation, add *Chai Hu* (Radix Bupleuri), *Xiang Fu* (Rhizoma Cyperi), and *Qing Pi* (Pericarpium Citri Reticulatae Viride).
- With yin-deficient fire, add *Di Gu Pi* (Cortex Lycii), *Mu Dan Pi* (Cortex Moutan), and *Zhi Mu* (Rhizoma Anemarrhenae).

CAUTIONS / CONTRAINDICATIONS

Xiao Luo Wan should be used with caution in patients with Spleen deficiency and loose stools.

HUMAN CLINICAL STUDIES AND RESEARCH

1. **Parotitis**: One study reported improvement in all 406 patients with acute infectious parotitis using oral and topical applications of herbs. *Xiao Luo Wan* was used orally, and *Qing Dai* (Indigo Naturalis) was applied topically to the affected area. Of 290 patients who had unilateral parotitis, the study reported complete recovery in 186 cases, significant recovery in 96 cases, and improvement in 8 cases. Of 116 patients with bilateral parotitis, the study reported complete recovery in 68 cases, significant recovery in 36 cases, and improvement in 12 cases.[1]
2. **Hyperplasia of mammary glands**: One study reported 99.42% effectiveness using *Xiao Luo Wan* plus *Xiao Yao San* (Rambling Powder) to treat 118 patients with unilateral or bilateral hyperplasia of mammary glands. Of 118 patients, the study reported complete recovery in 78 cases, improvement in 34 cases, and no effect in 6 cases.[2]

SUGGESTED ACUPUNCTURE TREATMENT

1. Points: *Tianjing* (TH 10), *Zhaohai* (KI 6), *Lieque* (LU 7), *Fenglong* (ST 40), and local points.
2. Technique: moxibustion.

Tianjing (TH 10) is an effective point for treating pharyngitis and inflammation in the neck. *Zhaohai* (KI 6) and *Lieque* (LU 7) clear heat and benefit the mouth and throat. *Fenglong* (ST 40) resolves phlegm. Local points surrounding swellings may be added, but care should be taken not to insert needles into abscessed glands.

AUTHORS' COMMENTS

Xiao Luo Wan is the representative formula for treating various types of hardness and nodules. Although this formula is literally called "Reduce Scrofula Pill," it may be used for many other types of hardness and nodules.

Xiao Luo Wan has been used to treat lipomas in dogs, in combination with *Shen Ling Bai Zhu San* (Ginseng, Poria, and Atractylodes Macrocephala Powder) and *Zhi Bai Di Huang Wan* (Anemarrhena, Phellodendron, and Rehmannia Pill). It can take 3-6 months to resolve the lipomas. Dietary therapy is essential to nourish yin and body fluids and prevent the formation and continued accumulation of dampness. For swollen, infected, enlarged lymph nodes, it can be combined with *San Zhong Kui Jian Tang* (Disperse the Swelling and Break the Hardness Decoction). For the treatment of feline hyperthyroidism with enlarged thyroid gland, add *Kun Bu* (Thallus Eckloniae), *Hai Zao* (Sargassum), *Xia Ku Cao* (Spica Prunellae), *Chai Hu* (Radix Bupleuri), *Xiang Fu* (Rhizoma Cyperi), and *Bai Shao* (Radix Paeoniae Alba) to help dissolve and soften the thyroid mass and treat the underlying stagnation. Alternatively, add *Jia Wei Xiao Yao San* (Augmented Rambling Powder) to treat the underlying cause of hyperthyroidism, which is typically chronic Liver qi stagnation with the production of heat and fire that eventually damages yin. This combination can be administered 3-6 months prior to conventional therapy with nuclear medicine to strengthen weak and debilitated cats with hyperthyroidism. For the purpose of dissolving nodules, calcined *Mu Li* (Concha Ostreae) should be used instead of the unprocessed form.

References

1. *Zhong Xi Yi Jie He Za Zhi* (Journal of Integrated Chinese and Western Medicine), 1989; 9(10):612.
2. *Shi Yong Zhong Yi Yao Za Zhi* (Journal of Practical Chinese Medicine and Medicinals), 1998; 11:9.

Sàn Zhǒng Kùi Jiān Tāng

(Disperse the Swelling and Break the Hardness Decoction)

散腫潰堅湯

散肿溃坚汤

Pinyin Name: *San Zhong Kui Jian Tang*
Literal Name: Disperse the Swelling and Break the Hardness Decoction
Alternate Names: *San Tsung Kuei Chien Tang*, Forsythia and Laminaria Decoction, Forsythia and Laminaria Combination
Original Source: *Wan Bing Hui Chun* (Restoration of Health from the Myriad Diseases) by Gong Ting-Xian in 1587

COMPOSITION

Hai Zao (Sargassum), *chao* (dry-fried)	15g
Kun Bu (Thallus Eckloniae), *xi* (washed) with cold water	15g
Jie Geng (Radix Platycodonis)	15g
San Leng (Rhizoma Sparganii), *jin* (soaked) in liquor	9g
E Zhu (Rhizoma Curcumae), *jin* (soaked) in liquor	9g
Bai Shao (Radix Paeoniae Alba), *chao* (dry-fried) with liquor	9g
Dang Gui Wei (Extremitas Radix Angelicae Sinensis)	1.5g
Huang Qin (Radix Scutellariae), *chao* (dry-fried) with liquor	9g
Huang Lian (Rhizoma Coptidis)	9g
Long Dan (Radix et Rhizoma Gentianae)	9g
Lian Qiao (Fructus Forsythiae)	9g
Zhi Mu (Rhizoma Anemarrhenae), *jin* (soaked) in liquor	15g
Huang Bo (Cortex Phellodendri Chinensis), *chao* (dry-fried) with liquor	15g
Tian Hua Fen (Radix Trichosanthis)	15g
Chai Hu (Radix Bupleuri)	1.5g
Sheng Ma (Rhizoma Cimicifugae)	1.5g
Ge Gen (Radix Puerariae Lobatae)	9g
Zhi Gan Cao (Radix et Rhizoma Glycyrrhizae Praeparata cum Melle)	15g

Sàn Zhǒng Kùi Jiān Tāng

(Disperse the Swelling and Break the Hardness Decoction)

DOSAGE / PREPARATION / ADMINISTRATION

The source text states to first soak all of the ingredients in water for half a day, then cook until the liquid is reduced by 50%. Take the strained decoction while it is warm.

CHINESE THERAPEUTIC ACTIONS

1. Disperses stagnation and softens hardness
2. Reduces swelling and drains pus

CLINICAL MANIFESTATIONS

Nodules, swelling, and hardness in various parts of the body: suppurative sores, ulcerations, and swellings that remain hard after the discharge of pus and abscess; enlarged thyroid gland.

VETERINARY CLINICAL APPLICATIONS

Cancer, caseous lymphadenitis in the goat, feline hyperthyroidism, thyroid carcinoma, goiter and cellulitis.

EXPLANATION

San Zhong Kui Jian Tang (Disperse the Swelling and Break the Hardness Decoction) treats nodules, swelling, and hardness in various parts of the body, especially below the ears, under the cheeks, around the shoulders, and in the axillary region. It contains many herbs that drain swelling and pus and disperse hardness and stagnation.

Hai Zao (Sargassum), *Kun Bu* (Thallus Eckloniae), and *Jie Geng* (Radix Platycodonis) eliminate phlegm to soften hardness and disperse nodules. *San Leng* (Rhizoma Sparganii) and *E Zhu* (Rhizoma Curcumae) move the blood and eliminate blood stasis to break the hardness. Because these two herbs are rather potent, *Bai Shao* (Radix Paeoniae Alba) and *Dang Gui Wei* (Extremitas Radix Angelicae Sinensis) are added to nourish the blood and moderate their effect. *Huang Qin* (Radix Scutellariae), *Huang Lian* (Rhizoma Coptidis), and *Long Dan* (Radix et Rhizoma Gentianae) clear damp-heat from the upper, middle and lower *jiaos*. *Lian Qiao* (Fructus Forsythiae) clears heat and eliminates toxins. Since these bitter and cold herbs are drying in nature, *Zhi Mu* (Rhizoma Anemarrhenae), *Huang Bo* (Cortex Phellodendri Chinensis), and *Tian Hua Fen* (Radix Trichosanthis) are used to clear deficiency heat and protect yin and fluids. *Chai Hu* (Radix Bupleuri), *Sheng Ma* (Rhizoma Cimicifugae), and *Ge Gen* (Radix Puerariae Lobatae) activate qi circulation

San Zhong Kui Jian Tang **(Disperse the Swelling and Break the Hardness Decoction)**

Diagnosis	Clinical Signs	Treatment	Herbs
Nodules, swelling, and hardness	Nodules, swelling, and hardness with pus and abscess; enlarged thyroid gland	• Disperses stagnation and softens hardness • Reduces swelling and drains pus	• *Hai Zao* (Sargassum), *Kun Bu* (Thallus Eckloniae) and *Jie Geng* (Radix Platycodonis) eliminate phlegm, soften hardness, and disperse nodules. • *San Leng* (Rhizoma Sparganii) and *E Zhu* (Rhizoma Curcumae) move the blood and eliminate blood stasis to break the hardness. • *Bai Shao* (Radix Paeoniae Alba) and *Dang Gui Wei* (Extremitas Radix Angelicae Sinensis) nourish the blood and promote blood circulation. • *Huang Qin* (Radix Scutellariae), *Huang Lian* (Rhizoma Coptidis), and *Long Dan* (Radix et Rhizoma Gentianae) clear damp-heat from the upper, middle and lower *jiaos*. • *Lian Qiao* (Fructus Forsythiae) clears heat and eliminates toxins. • *Zhi Mu* (Rhizoma Anemarrhenae), *Huang Bo* (Cortex Phellodendri Chinensis), and *Tian Hua Fen* (Radix Trichosanthis) clear deficiency heat and protect yin and fluids. • *Chai Hu* (Radix Bupleuri), *Sheng Ma* (Rhizoma Cimicifugae), and *Ge Gen* (Radix Puerariae Lobatae) guide the formula to the upper parts of the body. • *Zhi Gan Cao* (Radix et Rhizoma Glycyrrhizae Praeparata cum Melle) harmonizes all of the herbs.

Sàn Zhǒng Kùi Jiān Tāng

(Disperse the Swelling and Break the Hardness Decoction)

and guide the formula to the upper parts of the body. *Zhi Gan Cao* (Radix et Rhizoma Glycyrrhizae Praeparata cum Melle) harmonizes all of the herbs.

VETERINARY MODIFICATIONS

- For nodules and hardness prior to the formation of pus, add *Jin Yin Hua* (Flos Lonicerae Japonicae) and *Zhi Shi* (Fructus Aurantii Immaturus).
- For nodules and hardness after the formation of pus, add *Huang Qi* (Radix Astragali) and *Bai Zhi* (Radix Angelicae Dahuricae).
- For nodules and hardness with redness, swelling and pain, add *Shi Gao* (Gypsum Fibrosum) and *Zhi Zi* (Fructus Gardeniae).

SUGGESTED ACUPUNCTURE TREATMENT

1. Points: *Tianjing* (TH 10), *Bailao* (extra point), *Quchi* (LI 11), *Zhaohai* (KI 6), *Xuehai* (SP 10), *Geshu* (BL 17), *Sanyinjiao* (SP 6), *Housanli* (ST 36), *Tiantu* (CV 22), and local points.
2. Technique: sedation.

Tianjing (TH 10), *Bailao* (extra point), and local points reduce swelling and soften nodules. *Quchi* (LI 11), *Xuehai* (SP 10), *Zhaohai* (KI 6), *Geshu* (BL 17), *Sanyinjiao* (SP 6), *Housanli* (ST 36), and *Tiantu* (CV 22) clear heat and toxins and regulate qi and blood circulation.

AUTHORS' COMMENTS

San Zhong Kui Jian Tang treats disorders characterized by qi and blood stagnation and damp-heat. It was initially formulated to treat conditions characterized by infection, swelling, and blood and phlegm accumulation and stagnation in the head and neck. Modern application of the formula has been in the treatment of many different types of cancers that include tumors of the head, face, throat and neck. In human medicine, it is currently undergoing intense evaluation for the treatment of breast cancer in women. In veterinary medicine, it has been used to treat thyroid carcinoma, lymphoma, lymphocytic leukemia, mammary adenocarcinoma, liposarcoma, feline hyperthyroidism, and immune-mediated skin disease. It is usually modified, depending on the condition being treated and the constitution of the animal. Goats with caseous lymphadenitis can benefit from this formula, in combination with *Xiao Luo Wan* (Reduce Scrofula Pill). To further reduce swelling and heat, add *Jin Yin Hua* (Flos Lonicerae Japonicae), *Zi Cao* (Radix Arnebiae), and *Mu Dan Pi* (Cortex Moutan).

San Zhong Kui Jian Tang can be used to treat feline hyperthyroidism. It is especially useful for cats with damp-heat affecting the skin or damp-heat in the Intestines, Liver fire, and enlarged thyroid (goiter). It is a strong, cold and bitter formula and should be prescribed with caution in weak cats. A low dose is initially given and then the dose increased over time; herbs should be added as needed to support the middle *jiao*. The primary application is to help resolve damp-heat conditions and reduce thyroid enlargement to stabilize cats prior to nuclear medicine therapy and/or surgery. Once the damp-heat and stagnation (excess) have been resolved another formula is often chosen to continue treatment. *San Zhong Kui Jian Tang* can also be used to treat thyroid adenocarcinoma in dogs; combine it with *Qing Dai* (Indigo Naturalis) and *Dan Shen* (Radix et Rhizoma Salviae Miltiorrhizae) to improve clinical results.

Shí Liù Wèi Liú Qì Yǐn (Sixteen-Ingredient Decoction to Flow Qi)

十六味流氣飲
十六味流气饮

Pinyin Name: *Shi Liu Wei Liu Qi Yin*
Literal Name: Sixteen-Ingredient Decoction to Flow Qi
Alternate Name: Tangkuei Sixteen Herbs Combination
Original Source: *Wan Bing Hui Chun* (Restoration of Health from the Myriad Diseases) by Gong Ting-Xian in 1587

COMPOSITION

Ren Shen (Radix et Rhizoma Ginseng)
Huang Qi (Radix Astragali)
Gan Cao (Radix et Rhizoma Glycyrrhizae)
Dang Gui (Radix Angelicae Sinensis)
Bai Shao (Radix Paeoniae Alba)
Chuan Xiong (Rhizoma Chuanxiong)
Mu Xiang (Radix Aucklandiae)
Bing Lang (Semen Arecae)
Zhi Qiao (Fructus Citri Aurantii)
Hou Po (Cortex Magnoliae Officinalis)
Zi Su Ye (Folium Perillae)
Fang Feng (Radix Saposhnikoviae)
Wu Yao (Radix Linderae)
Bai Zhi (Radix Angelicae Dahuricae)
Gui Zhi (Ramulus Cinnamomi)
Jie Geng (Radix Platycodonis)

DOSAGE / PREPARATION / ADMINISTRATION

The source text states to grate equal proportions of all of the ingredients and prepare as a decoction.

CHINESE THERAPEUTIC ACTIONS

1. Tonifies qi and blood
2. Activates qi and blood circulation
3. Disperses stagnation and drains pus

CLINICAL MANIFESTATIONS

Nodules and hardness due to qi, blood, and phlegm stagnation: nodules and hardness in various parts of the body, such as the neck, mammary glands and abdomen; and goiter.

VETERINARY CLINICAL APPLICATIONS

Malignant and benign mammary gland tumors, intestinal adenocarcinoma, feline hyperthyroidism, and inflammation of the lymph nodes.

EXPLANATION

Shi Liu Wei Liu Qi Yin (Sixteen-Ingredient Decoction to Flow Qi) is one of the best formulas for dispersing nodules and softening hardness. These nodules and lumps may be caused by inflammation of the lymph nodes, goiter, tumor, sores, or abscess of unknown origin.

This formula focuses on treating both the underlying deficiencies (qi and blood) and the stagnations (qi, blood, and phlegm). *Ren Shen* (Radix et Rhizoma Ginseng), *Huang Qi* (Radix Astragali), and *Gan Cao* (Radix et Rhizoma Glycyrrhizae) tonify qi. *Dang Gui* (Radix Angelicae Sinensis), *Bai Shao* (Radix Paeoniae Alba), and *Chuan Xiong* (Rhizoma Chuanxiong) tonify the blood and activate blood circulation. *Mu Xiang* (Radix Aucklandiae), *Bing Lang* (Semen Arecae), *Zhi Qiao* (Fructus Aurantii), *Hou Po* (Cortex Magnoliae Officinalis), *Zi Su Ye* (Folium Perillae), and *Fang Feng* (Radix Saposhnikoviae) regulate the proper flow of qi. *Wu Yao* (Radix Linderae), *Zhi Qiao* (Fructus Aurantii), and *Hou Po* (Cortex Magnoliae Officinalis) break up stubborn qi stagnation. *Bai Zhi* (Radix Angelicae Dahuricae) and *Gui Zhi* (Ramulus Cinnamomi) warm and open the channels and collaterals. *Jie Geng* (Radix Platycodonis) dispels phlegm and drains pus and abscess. Lastly, *Gan Cao* (Radix et Rhizoma Glycyrrhizae) harmonizes all of the herbs in the formula.

Shí Liù Wèi Liú Qì Yǐn (Sixteen-Ingredient Decoction to Flow Qi)

Shi Liu Wei Liu Qi Yin (Sixteen-Ingredient Decoction to Flow Qi)

Diagnosis	Clinical Signs	Treatment	Herbs
Nodules and hardness	Nodules and hardness in various parts of the body: stagnation with underlying deficiency	• Tonifies qi and blood • Activates qi and blood circulation • Disperses stagnation and drains pus	• *Ren Shen* (Radix et Rhizoma Ginseng), *Huang Qi* (Radix Astragali) and *Gan Cao* (Radix et Rhizoma Glycyrrhizae) tonify qi. • *Dang Gui* (Radix Angelicae Sinensis), *Bai Shao* (Radix Paeoniae Alba), and *Chuan Xiong* (Rhizoma Chuanxiong) tonify the blood and activate blood circulation. • *Mu Xiang* (Radix Aucklandiae), *Bing Lang* (Semen Arecae), *Zhi Qiao* (Fructus Aurantii), *Hou Po* (Cortex Magnoliae Officinalis), *Zi Su Ye* (Folium Perillae), and *Fang Feng* (Radix Saposhnikoviae) regulate the proper flow of qi. • *Wu Yao* (Radix Linderae), *Zhi Qiao* (Fructus Aurantii), and *Hou Po* (Cortex Magnoliae Officinalis) break up qi stagnation. • *Bai Zhi* (Radix Angelicae Dahuricae) and *Gui Zhi* (Ramulus Cinnamomi) warm and open the channels and collaterals. • *Jie Geng* (Radix Platycodonis) dispels phlegm and drains pus and abscess. • *Gan Cao* (Radix et Rhizoma Glycyrrhizae) harmonizes all of the herbs.

VETERINARY MODIFICATIONS

- For mammary gland adenocarcinoma, combine with *Wang Bu Liu Xing* (Semen Vaccariae), *Bai Hua She She Cao* (Herba Hedyotis), *Ban Zhi Lian* (Herba Scutellariae Barbatae), *Zao Xiu* (Rhizoma Paridis) and *Dan Shen* (Radix et Rhizoma Salviae Miltiorrhizae).
- For intestinal adenocarcinoma, combine with *San Zhong Kui Jian Tang* (Disperse the Swelling and Break the Hardness Decoction) and add *Qing Dai* (Indigo Naturalis), *Bai Hua She She Cao* (Herba Hedyotis), *Ban Zhi Lian* (Herba Scutellariae Barbatae), *Zao Xiu* (Rhizoma Paridis) and *Dan Shen* (Radix et Rhizoma Salviae Miltiorrhizae).
- For enlarged thyroid gland, add *Xiao Luo Wan* (Reduce Scrofula Pill), *Xia Ku Cao* (Spica Prunellae) and *Dan Shen* (Radix et Rhizoma Salviae Miltiorrhizae).
- For thyroid carcinoma, combine with *San Zhong Kui Jian Tang* (Disperse the Swelling and Break the Hardness Decoction) and add *Qing Dai* (Indigo Naturalis) and *Dan Shen* (Radix et Rhizoma Salviae Miltiorrhizae).

SUGGESTED ACUPUNCTURE TREATMENT

1. Points: *Housanli* (ST 36), *Pishu* (BL 20), *Sanyinjiao* (SP 6), *Geshu* (BL 17), *Shanzhong* (CV 17), *Tianshu* (ST 25), *Qihai* (CV 6), *Hegu* (LI 4), *Taichong* (LR 3), *Tiantu* (CV 22), and local points.
2. Technique: tonification and even method.

Housanli (ST 36) and *Pishu* (BL 20) tonify qi. *Sanyinjiao* (SP 6) and *Geshu* (BL 17) tonify the blood. *Shanzhong* (CV 17), *Tianshu* (ST 25), and *Qihai* (CV 6) regulate qi. *Hegu* (LI 4) and *Taichong* (LR 3) open the channels and collaterals. *Tiantu* (CV 22) dispels phlegm and drains pus. Apply even method on local points to soften nodules and reduce swelling.

AUTHORS' COMMENTS

Shi Liu Wei Liu Qi Yin can be used to treat chronic skin disease, cancer, and thyroid disease due to stagnation of qi and blood. This formula focuses on the nourishment and normalization of the flow of qi and blood to resolve disease and restore homeostasis. It is used to treat chronic conditions and has little ability to clear heat or toxins; modification is necessary if these pathogenic factors are present.

Pái Nóng Sǎn (Drain the Pus Powder)

排膿散
排脓散

Pinyin Name: *Pai Nong San*
Literal Name: Drain the Pus Powder
Alternate Names: *Pai Nung San*, Pus-Expelling Powder, Platycodon and Chih-shih Formula
Original Source: *Jin Gui Yao Lue* (Essentials from the Golden Cabinet) by Zhang Zhong-Jing in the Eastern Han Dynasty

COMPOSITION

Zhi Shi (Fructus Aurantii Immaturus)	16 pieces
Jie Geng (Radix Platycodonis)	1.5g
Bai Shao (Radix Paeoniae Alba)	4.5g

DOSAGE / PREPARATION / ADMINISTRATION

The source text states to grind all of the ingredients into a fine powder. Mix one egg yolk with an equal portion of the herb powder. Take this mixture one time daily with warm water.

CHINESE THERAPEUTIC ACTIONS

1. Dispels pus and eliminates toxins
2. Reduces nodules and disperses stagnation

CLINICAL MANIFESTATIONS

Abscesses and sores: carbuncles, furuncles, sores, cellulitis, boils, and other conditions characterized by the formation of pus, abscess, and discharge.

VETERINARY CLINICAL APPLICATIONS

Carbuncles, furuncles, sores, cellulitis, abscess secondary to bite wounds and cat scratches, lymphadenitis, purulent otitis media, and mastitis.

EXPLANATION

Pai Nong San (Drain the Pus Powder) is designed to treat heat and toxins attacking various parts of the body. While the early stage of heat and toxins involves nodules and hardness, the mid- to late-stages are often characterized by the formation of abscess and the discharge of pus.

This formula contains herbs that dispel pus, eliminate toxins, reduce nodules, and disperse stagnation. *Zhi Shi* (Fructus Aurantii Immaturus), one of the strongest herbs for breaking up stagnant qi and activating qi circulation, reduces the size of the nodules. *Jie Geng* (Radix Platycodonis) is an excellent herb for draining and dispelling pus. Because heat and toxins may consume the blood, *Bai Shao* (Radix Paeoniae Alba) and egg yolk are added to nourish the body.

VETERINARY MODIFICATIONS

- For nodules without ulceration, add *Jin Yin Hua* (Flos Lonicerae Japonicae) and *Lian Qiao* (Fructus Forsythiae).
- For nodules with ulceration, add *Huang Qi* (Radix Astragali) and *Dang Gui* (Radix Angelicae Sinensis).
- With redness, warmth, swelling, and pain, add *Huang Lian* (Rhizoma Coptidis) and *Zhi Zi* (Fructus Gardeniae).
- For sores and cellulitis, add *Tuo Li Xiao Du Yin* (Drain the Interior and Detoxify Decoction).
- To improve ability to drain pus, add *Zao Jiao Ci* (Spina Gleditsiae).
- For the treatment of severe dermatitis, cellulitis or vasculitis, combine with *Si Miao Yong An Tang* (Four-Valiant Decoction for Well-being) and *Dan Shen* (Radix et Rhizoma Salviae Miltiorrhizae).

Pai Nong San (Drain the Pus Powder)

Diagnosis	Clinical Signs	Treatment	Herbs
Abscesses and sores	Nodules and hardness with the formation of abscess and the discharge of pus: heat and toxins attacking the body	• Dispels pus and eliminates toxins • Reduces nodules and disperses stagnation	• *Zhi Shi* (Fructus Aurantii Immaturus) activates qi circulation and breaks up stagnant qi. • *Jie Geng* (Radix Platycodonis) drains and dispels pus. • *Bai Shao* (Radix Paeoniae Alba) and egg yolk tonify the blood and nourish the body.

Pái Nóng Săn (Drain the Pus Powder)

SUGGESTED ACUPUNCTURE TREATMENT

1. Points: *Quchi* (LI 11) and *Qizhuma* (extra point).
2. Technique: moxibustion.

Qizhuma reduces swelling, eliminates toxins, and relieves pain; while *Quchi* (LI 11) disperses nodules and dispels pus. Note: *Qizhuma* is an extra point located 4 *cun* above *Shenmen* (HT 7); it drains pus and eliminates toxins.

Tuō Lǐ Xiāo Dú Yǐn (Drain the Interior and Detoxify Decoction)

托裏消毒飲
托里消毒饮

Pinyin Name: *Tuo Li Xiao Du Yin*
Literal Name: Drain the Interior and Detoxify Decoction
Alternate Names: *Tuo Li Hsiao Tu Yin*, Interior-Drawing and Detoxifying Drink, Gleditsia Combination
Original Source: *Yi Fang Ji Jie* (Analytical Collection of Medical Formulas) by Wang Ang in 1682

COMPOSITION

Ren Shen (Radix et Rhizoma Ginseng)	3g
Bai Zhu (Rhizoma Atractylodis Macrocephalae)	3g
Fu Ling (Poria)	3g
Gan Cao (Radix et Rhizoma Glycyrrhizae)	1.5g
Dang Gui (Radix Angelicae Sinensis)	3g
Bai Shao (Radix Paeoniae Alba)	3g
Chuan Xiong (Rhizoma Chuanxiong)	3g
Huang Qi (Radix Astragali)	3g
Jin Yin Hua (Flos Lonicerae Japonicae)	3g
Jie Geng (Radix Platycodonis)	1.5g
Bai Zhi (Radix Angelicae Dahuricae)	1.5g
Zao Jiao Ci (Spina Gleditsiae)	1.5g

DOSAGE / PREPARATION / ADMINISTRATION

The source text states to cook the ingredients in 2 cups of water until the liquid is reduced to 80%. Take the warm, strained decoction after meals.

CHINESE THERAPEUTIC ACTIONS

1. Tonifies qi and blood
2. Reduces swelling, drains pus, and promotes the generation of new tissues

CLINICAL MANIFESTATIONS

Suppurative disorders in animals with qi and blood deficiencies: nodules and hardness, with or without the discharge of pus and abscess, generalized deficiency, and weakness.

VETERINARY CLINICAL APPLICATIONS

Dermatitis, abscesses, lymphadenitis, otitis media, chronic osteomyelitis, and non-healing sores or wounds in animals with diabetes or undergoing cancer radiation treatments.

Tuō Lǐ Xiāo Dú Yǐn (Drain the Interior and Detoxify Decoction)

EXPLANATION

Tuo Li Xiao Du Yin (Drain the Interior and Detoxify Decoction) treats various types of suppurative disorders with underlying qi and blood deficiencies. It contains herbs to reduce swelling and drain pus to treat abscesses and sores. It also contains herbs to tonify qi, nourish the blood, and promote the generation of new tissues; these actions make it valuable to use in geriatric, weak and debilitated animals.

Ren Shen (Radix et Rhizoma Ginseng), *Bai Zhu* (Rhizoma Atractylodis Macrocephalae), *Fu Ling* (Poria), and *Gan Cao* (Radix et Rhizoma Glycyrrhizae) tonify qi, following the concept of *Si Jun Zi Tang* (Four-Gentlemen Decoction). *Dang Gui* (Radix Angelicae Sinensis), *Bai Shao* (Radix Paeoniae Alba), and *Chuan Xiong* (Rhizoma Chuanxiong) tonify the blood, following the concept of *Si Wu Tang* (Four-Substance Decoction). *Huang Qi* (Radix Astragali), in addition to tonifying qi, can promote the generation of new tissues, thereby facilitating recovery. *Jin Yin Hua* (Flos Lonicerae Japonicae) clears heat, eliminates toxins, and treats all types of suppurative disorders. *Jie Geng* (Radix Platycodonis), *Bai Zhi* (Radix Angelicae Dahuricae), and *Zao Jiao Ci* (Spina Gleditsiae) drain pus and eliminate toxins.

VETERINARY MODIFICATIONS

- For ulcerations with constant discharge of pus, add *Ge Gen* (Radix Puerariae Lobatae) and *Huang Lian* (Rhizoma Coptidis).
- With swelling and pain accompanied by fever, add *Huang Lian Jie Du Tang* (Coptis Decoction to Relieve Toxicity).
- With severe pain, add *Ru Xiang* (Gummi Olibanum) and *Mo Yao* (Myrrha).
- For cellulitis with swelling and pain, add *Pai Nong San* (Drain the Pus Powder).
- For itching, add *Chan Tui* (Periostracum Cicadae) and *Wu Shao She* (Zaocys).
- With toxic heat, combine with *Wu Wei Xiao Du Yin* (Five-Ingredient Decoction to Eliminate Toxins).
- With chronic, severe damp-heat dermatitis with oozing sores and ulcers that won't heal, combine with *Lian Qiao* (Fructus Forsythiae), *Zhi Zi (Fructus Gardeniae)*, *Bai Xian Pi* (Cortex Dictamni), *Di Fu Zi* (Fructus Kochiae), *Tu Fu Ling* (Rhizoma Smilacis Glabrae), *Chi Shao* (Radix Paeoniae Rubra), *Mu Dan Pi* (Cortex Moutan), *Di Huang* (Radix Rehmanniae) and *Dan Shen* (Radix et Rhizoma Salviae Miltiorrhizae).

SUGGESTED ACUPUNCTURE TREATMENT

1. Points: *Sanyinjiao* (SP 6), *Housanli* (ST 36), *Quchi* (LI 11), *Weizhong* (BL 40), *Qiansanli* (LI 10), *Yanglao* (SI 6), *Dingshu* (extra point), and *Qizhuma* (extra point).
2. Technique: moxibustion and even method.

Apply moxibustion on *Housanli* (ST 36) to tonify qi. *Sanyinjiao* (SP 6) tonifies and invigorates blood. *Quchi* (LI 11) and *Weizhong* (BL 40) clear heat and eliminate toxins. Apply moxibustion on *Qiansanli* (LI 10), *Yanglao* (SI 6), *Dingshu*, and *Qizhuma*. Note: *Dingshu* is an extraordinary point located 0.5 *cun* lateral to the *du* (governing) channel, at the same level as the lower border of the spinous process of the tenth thoracic vertebra. *Qizhuma* is an extraordinary point located 4 *cun* above *Shenmen* (HT 7); it drains pus and eliminates toxins.

***Tuo Li Xiao Du Yin* (Drain the Interior and Detoxify Decoction)**

Diagnosis	Clinical Signs	Treatment	Herbs
Suppurative disorders in animals with qi and blood deficiencies	• Nodules and hardness: heat and toxins attacking the body • Discharge of pus and abscess, generalized deficiency and weakness: qi and blood deficiencies	• Strengthens qi and blood • Reduces swelling, drains pus, and promotes the generation of new tissues	• *Ren Shen* (Radix et Rhizoma Ginseng), *Bai Zhu* (Rhizoma Atractylodis Macrocephalae), *Fu Ling* (Poria), and *Gan Cao* (Radix et Rhizoma Glycyrrhizae) tonify qi. • *Dang Gui* (Radix Angelicae Sinensis), *Bai Shao* (Radix Paeoniae Alba), and *Chuan Xiong* (Rhizoma Chuanxiong) tonify the blood. • *Huang Qi* (Radix Astragali) tonifies qi and promotes the generation of new tissues. • *Jin Yin Hua* (Flos Lonicerae Japonicae) clears heat and eliminates toxins. • *Jie Geng* (Radix Platycodonis), *Bai Zhi* (Radix Angelicae Dahuricae), and *Zao Jiao Ci* (Spina Gleditsiae) drain pus and eliminate toxins.

Tuō Lǐ Xiāo Dú Yǐn (Drain the Interior and Detoxify Decoction)

RELATED FORMULA

Tuō Lǐ Xiāo Dú Yǐn
(Drain the Interior and Detoxify Decoction)
托裏消毒飲
托里消毒饮
Pinyin Name: *Tuo Li Xiao Du Yin*
Literal Name: Drain the Interior and Detoxify Decoction
Alternate Names: *Tuo Li Hsiao Tu Yin*, Interior-Drawing and Detoxifying Drink
Original Source: *Wan Bing Hui Chun* (Restoration of Health from the Myriad Diseases) by Gong Ting-Xian in 1587

Huang Qi (Radix Astragali)	6g
Tian Hua Fen (Radix Trichosanthis)	6g
Fang Feng (Radix Saposhnikoviae)	3g
Dang Gui (Radix Angelicae Sinensis)	3g
Chuan Xiong (Rhizoma Chuanxiong)	3g
Bai Zhi (Radix Angelicae Dahuricae)	3g
Jie Geng (Radix Platycodonis)	3g
Hou Po (Cortex Magnoliae Officinalis)	3g
Chuan Shan Jia (Squama Manis)	3g
Zao Jiao (Fructus Gleditsiae)	3g
Jin Yin Hua (Flos Lonicerae Japonicae)	9g
Chen Pi (Pericarpium Citri Reticulatae)	9g

Note: *Chuan Shan Jia* (Squama Manis) is derived from an endangered animal and is rarely used as a medicinal substance today. Its discussion here is included primarily for academic purposes, to reflect the historical use of this substance in its original formulation. Most herbal products today have removed it completely, or replaced it with substitutes with similar functions.

The source text states to cook the ingredients with equal portions of water and grain-based liquor until the liquid is reduced to 70%. Take the warm, strained decoction after meals if the affected area is located on the upper parts of the body, and on an empty stomach before meals if the affected area is located on the lower parts of the body. After the first two decoctions, the remaining decoctions utilize only water to cook the herbs.

This formula tonifies qi and blood, reduces swelling and pus, and promotes the generation of new tissues. Clinically, it treats various abscesses and sores that do not heal after 10-14 days.

The principal and related formulas have the same names, but they are derived from different sources. They have similar functions to treat suppurative disorders in animals with qi and blood deficiencies.

- *Tuo Li Xiao Du Yin,* from *Yi Fang Ji Jie* (Analytical Collection of Medical Formulas) by Wang Ang in 1682, has a stronger effect to tonify qi and blood; thus, it can better address the underlying deficiencies.
- *Tuo Li Xiao Du Yin,* from *Wan Bing Hui Chun* (Restoration of Health from the Myriad Diseases) by Gong Ting-Xian in 1587, has a better function to regulate qi circulation and resolve nodules and hardness.

Yáng Hé Tāng (Yang-Heartening Decoction)

陽和湯

阳和汤

Pinyin Name: *Yang He Tang*
Literal Name: Yang-Heartening Decoction
Original Source: *Wai Ke Zheng Zhi Quan Sheng Ji* (Complete Collection of Patterns and Treatments in External Medicine) by Wang Wei-De in 1740

COMPOSITION

Shu Di Huang (Radix Rehmanniae Praeparata)	30g
Lu Jiao Jiao (Colla Cornus Cervi)	9g
Pao Jiang (Rhizoma Zingiberis Praeparatum), *tan* (charred to ash)	1.5g
Rou Gui (Cortex Cinnamomi), *yan* (ground) into powder	3g
Ma Huang (Herba Ephedrae)	1.5g
Bai Jie Zi (Semen Sinapis)	6g
Gan Cao (Radix et Rhizoma Glycyrrhizae)	3g

DOSAGE / PREPARATION / ADMINISTRATION

The source text states to prepare the ingredients as a decoction.

CHINESE THERAPEUTIC ACTIONS

1. Warms yang and tonifies the blood
2. Disperses cold and eliminates stagnation

CLINICAL MANIFESTATIONS

Yin-type (deep-rooted) sores due to yang deficiency and interior cold stagnation: general swelling, soreness, and pain without local heat on the body and extremities, no change in skin color, no thirst, a pale tongue, and a deep, fine pulse. This formula may be applied for cellulitis, gangrene of the digits, multiple abscesses, and subcutaneous nodules.

VETERINARY CLINICAL APPLICATIONS

Bi zheng (painful obstruction syndrome), back pain, diarrhea, periarthritis of the shoulders, frostbite, osteomyelitis and gangrene.

EXPLANATION

Yang He Tang (Yang-Heartening Decoction) treats *yin*-type (deep-rooted) sores due to yang deficiency and interior cold stagnation. Deficiency of yang may lead to the formation of interior cold, which binds to the bones, muscles, tendons, vessels, or joints. Because of yang deficiency and cold excess, there is an absence of warm or heat sensations. Since the abscesses and sores are located deeper in the tissues, there is no change in skin color. Lastly, *yin*-type (deep-rooted) sores are usually harder to treat since they are anchored deep in the tissues.

***Yang He Tang* (Yang-Heartening Decoction)**

Diagnosis	Clinical Signs	Treatment	Herbs
Yin-type (deep-rooted) sores	• Sores with swelling, soreness, and pain without local heat sensation on the body and extremities, and no change in skin color: stagnation of cold and phlegm with underlying yang and blood deficiencies • Pale tongue and a deep, fine pulse: presence of deficiency and excess conditions	• Warms the yang and tonifies blood • Disperses cold and eliminates stagnation	• *Shu Di Huang* (Radix Rehmanniae Praeparata) warms and nourishes the blood. • *Lu Jiao Jiao* (Colla Cornus Cervi) tonifies *jing* (essence) and strengthens bones and tendons. • *Pao Jiang* (Rhizoma Zingiberis Praeparatum) and *Rou Gui* (Cortex Cinnamomi) warm the body, tonify yang, and disperse cold accumulation. • *Ma Huang* (Herba Ephedrae) opens the skin pores to help disperse the interior cold. • *Bai Jie Zi* (Semen Sinapis) warms the interior and disperses phlegm and cold. • *Gan Cao* (Radix et Rhizoma Glycyrrhizae) eliminates toxins and harmonizes all of the herbs in the formula.

Yáng Hé Tāng (Yang-Heartening Decoction)

This formula contains *Shu Di Huang* (Radix Rehmanniae Praeparata) to warm and nourish the blood. *Lu Jiao Jiao* (Colla Cornus Cervi) tonifies *jing* (essence) and strengthens bones and tendons. *Pao Jiang* (Rhizoma Zingiberis Praeparatum) and *Rou Gui* (Cortex Cinnamomi) warm the body, tonify yang, and disperse cold accumulation. A small amount of *Ma Huang* (Herba Ephedrae) opens the skin pores to help disperse the interior cold through the superficial level. *Bai Jie Zi* (Semen Sinapis) warms the interior and disperses phlegm and cold. It also prevents the warm tonic herbs from creating stagnation in the body. *Gan Cao* (Radix et Rhizoma Glycyrrhizae) eliminates toxins and harmonizes all of the herbs in the formula. Indeed, this formula both tonifies the body and disperses the cold stagnation.

VETERINARY MODIFICATIONS

- With more cold, add *Fu Zi* (Radix Aconiti Lateralis Praeparata).
- With more qi deficiency, add *Dang Shen* (Radix Codonopsis) and *Huang Qi* (Radix Astragali).
- With damp and cold accumulation, add *Xi Xin* (Radix et Rhizoma Asari).

CAUTIONS / CONTRAINDICATIONS

- *Yang He Tang* is contraindicated in the following cases: *yang*-type (shallow-rooted) sores that affect only the superficial parts of the body and are characterized by redness, swelling, burning sensations, and pain; *yin*-type (deep-rooted) sores that have already perforated and ulcerated; and chronic ulceration with heat.
- Once the sores are perforated and ulcerated, *Ma Huang* (Herba Ephedrae) should be removed from this formula to prevent damage to qi and blood.

HUMAN CLINICAL STUDIES AND RESEARCH

1. **Frostbite**: One study reported good results using modified *Yang He Tang* to treat 30 patients with frostbite. In addition to the base formula, modifications were made by adding *Ban Zhi Lian* (Herba Scutellariae Barbatae) for open wounds with discharge, and *Huang Qi* (Radix Astragali) for chronic illness. Most patients recovered within 3-6 packs of herbs, with some needing up to 15 packs.[1]
2. **Thromboangiitis obliterans**: Use of modified *Yang He Tang* in decoction daily was associated with complete recovery in 12 cases and improvement in 8 cases of thromboangiitis obliterans. The herbal treatment contained *Yang He Tang* plus *Dang Gui* (Radix Angelicae Sinensis) and *Dan Shen* (Radix et Rhizoma Salviae Miltiorrhizae). *Jin Yin Hua* (Flos Lonicerae Japonicae) and *Xuan Shen* (Radix Scrophulariae) were added for heat; *Dang Shen* (Radix Codonopsis), *Huang Qi* (Radix Astragali), *Ba Ji Tian* (Radix Morindae Officinalis), and *Yin Yang Huo* (Herba Epimedii) were added for chronic cases.[2]
3. **Peripheral neuritis**: One study reported 90.4% effectiveness using modified *Yang He Tang* to treat 63 patients with peripheral neuritis. The herbal treatment contained *Yang He Tang* plus *Dang Gui* (Radix Angelicae Sinensis) and *Huang Qi* (Radix Astragali) as the base formula. Additional modifications included *Cang Zhu* (Rhizoma Atractylodis) for damp; *Ji Xue Teng* (Caulis Spatholobi) for blood stagnation; *Quan Xie* (Scorpio) and *Wu Gong* (Scolopendra) for wind and phlegm obstructing the channels and collaterals. Of 63 patients, the study reported complete recovery in 43 cases, improvement in 14 cases, and no effect in 6 cases.[3]
4. **Sciatica**: One hundred and sixty-eight patients with sciatica were treated with complete recovery in 130 cases, improvement in 28 cases, and no effect in 10 cases. The herbal treatment contained *Fu Zi* (Radix Aconiti Lateralis Praeparata), *Shu Di Huang* (Radix Rehmanniae Praeparata), *Lu Jiao Jiao* (Colla Cornus Cervi), *Fang Ji* (Radix Stephaniae Tetrandrae), *Xi Xin* (Radix et Rhizoma Asari), *Hong Hua* (Flos Carthami), *Wu Shao She* (Zaocys), and others. The treatment protocol was to cook the herbs in water, and drink the decoction in two equally-divided doses. In addition, the herb residue was placed inside a cloth bag and applied topically to the affected area at bedtime. The duration was 10 days per course of treatment.[4]
5. **Inflammation and pain**: *Yang He Tang* has been shown in many studies to effectively treat inflammation and pain affecting many parts of the body. According to one study, neck pain in 64 patients was treated with 92.2% effectiveness using *Yang He Tang* plus *Gui Zhi* (Ramulus Cinnamomi), *Ge Gen* (Radix Puerariae Lobatae), *Sang Zhi* (Ramulus Mori) and others as needed.[5] According to another study, shoulder pain in 220 patients was treated at 95% effectiveness using *Yang He Tang* plus *Ru Xiang* (Gummi Olibanum), *Mo Yao* (Myrrha), *Bai Shao* (Radix Paeoniae Alba), *Jin Qian Bai Hua She* (Bungarus Parvus), and others.[6] Lastly, 60 patients with chronic lower back pain were treated with good results using modified *Yang He Tang*.[7]
6. **Prolapse of lumbar intervertebral disk**: Use of modified *Yang He Tang* was associated with marked success in treating prolapse of a lumbar intervertebral disk. Of 210 patients, the study reported complete recovery in 148 cases, significant improvement in 28 cases, moderate improvement in 16 cases, and no effect in 18 cases. The overall effectiveness was 91.4%. Most patients responded within 1 month. The herbal formula contained *Yang He Tang* plus *Tu Bie Chong* (Eupolyphaga seu Steleophaga), *Huang Lian* (Rhizoma Coptidis) and *Wu*

Yáng Hé Tāng (Yang-Heartening Decoction)

Gong (Scolopendra) as the base formula. Furthermore, modifications were made by adding processed *Ru Xiang* (Gummi Olibanum), processed *Mo Yao* (Myrrha) and *Di Long* (Pheretima) for severe pain; *Wei Ling Xian* (Radix et Rhizoma Clematidis), *Niu Xi* (Radix Achyranthis Bidentatae), and *Xu Duan* (Radix Dipsaci) for severe lower back pain; *Mu Gua* (Fructus Chaenomelis) and *Du Huo* (Radix Angelicae Pubescentis) for severe leg pain; *Fu Zi* (Radix Aconiti Lateralis Praeparata) for cold; *Cang Zhu* (Rhizoma Atractylodis) and *Fu Ling* (Poria) for dampness; and *Du Zhong* (Cortex Eucommiae) and *Sang Ji Sheng* (Herba Taxilli) for Kidney deficiency.[8]

7. **Osteomyelitis**: Use of *Yang He Tang* has been shown in several studies to effectively treat osteomyelitis. According to one study, use of modified *Yang He Tang* was associated with 95% effectiveness in treating 560 patients with osteomyelitis characterized by yin deficiency and blood stagnation.[9] Another study reported 100% effectiveness using modified *Yang He Tang* to treat osteomyelitis characterized by yang deficiency with cold accumulation.[10] Lastly, suppurative and chronic osteomyelitis have also been treated with good results using this formula.[11,12]
8. **Pain from metastatic carcinoma of bone**: Use of modified *Yang He Tang* was effective in relieving pain associated with metastatic carcinoma of bone. The herbal formula contained *Shu Di Huang* (Radix Rehmanniae Praeparata) 30g, *Rou Gui* (Cortex Cinnamomi) 3g, *Pao Jiang* (Rhizoma Zingiberis Praeparatum) 3g, *Ma Huang* (Herba Ephedrae) 3g, *Lu Jiao Shuang* (Cornu Cervi Degelatinatum) 10g, *Bai Jie Zi* (Semen Sinapis) 6g, *Fu Zi* (Radix Aconiti Lateralis Praeparata) 6g, and *Gan Cao* (Radix et Rhizoma Glycyrrhizae) 5g. The herbs were given in decoction daily, for 1 week per course of treatment.[13]

SUGGESTED ACUPUNCTURE TREATMENT

1. **Points:** *Housanli* (ST 36), *Sanyinjiao* (SP 6), *Xuanzhong* (GB 39), *Shenque* (CV 8), *Zhigou* (TH 6), and *Fenglong* (ST 40).
2. **Technique:** tonification with moxibustion.

The selection of acupuncture points focuses on tonifying yang and blood while eliminating cold stagnation. Clinically, patients may show cellulitis due to yang deficiency and interior cold stagnation. *Housanli* (ST 36) and *Sanyinjiao* (SP 6) nourish *ying* (nutritive) *qi* and blood. *Xuanzhong* (GB 39) also nourishes *ying* (nutritive) *qi*. Moxibustion on *Shenque* (CV 8) tonifies qi and blood. *Zhigou* (TH 6) eliminates cold stagnation, while *Fenglong* (ST 40) dispels phlegm stagnation.

AUTHORS' COMMENTS

Yang He Tang treats *yin*-type (deep-rooted) sores due to yang deficiency and interior cold stagnation. This formula uses a large dose of *Shu Di Huang* (Radix Rehmanniae Praeparata) to tonify yin and nourish the blood. *Ma Huang* (Herba Ephedrae), however, must be used in a small dose (as specified in this formula) to facilitate the ulceration of *yin*-type (deep-rooted) sores. The combination of these two herbs also provides mutual checks and balances. The dispersing nature of *Ma Huang* (Herba Ephedrae) prevents the heavy nature of *Shu Di Huang* (Radix Rehmanniae Praeparata) from creating stagnation; and the heavy nature of *Shu Di Huang* (Radix Rehmanniae Praeparata) prevents the dispersing nature of *Ma Huang* (Herba Ephedrae) from damaging yin and body fluids.

References

1. *Xin Zhong Yi* (New Chinese Medicine), 1989; 3:42.
2. *Zhe Jiang Zhong Yi Za Zhi* (Zhejiang Journal of Chinese Medicine), 1982; 2:82.
3. *Shan Xi Zhong Yi* (Shanxi Chinese Medicine), 1991; 4:160.
4. *Liao Ning Zhong Yi Za Zhi* (Liaoning Journal of Chinese Medicine), 1982; 11:36.
5. *Shan Xi Zhong Yi* (Shanxi Chinese Medicine), 1996; 4:162.
6. *Shan Xi Zhong Yi* (Shanxi Chinese Medicine), 1997; 10:444.
7. *Zhe Jiang Zhong Yi Za Zhi* (Zhejiang Journal of Chinese Medicine), 1998; 4:164.
8. *An Hui Zhong Yi Xue Yuan Xue Bao* (Journal of Anhui University School of Medicine), 1994; 13(1):31.
9. *Bei Jing Zhong Yi Xue Yuan Xue Bao* (Journal of Beijing University School of Medicine), 1991; 14(2):25.
10. *Shan Xi Zhong Yi* (Shanxi Chinese Medicine), 1989; 3:108.
11. *He Bei Zhong Yi* (Hebei Chinese Medicine), 1989; 3:108.
12. *Jiang Su Zhong Yi* (Jiangsu Chinese Medicine), 1963; 4.
13. *Xin Zhong Yi* (New Chinese Medicine), 1994; 26(9):51.

Section 2

内痈疡剂
— Internal Abscesses and Sores

Wěi Jīng Tāng (Reed Decoction)
葦莖湯
苇茎汤

Pinyin Name: *Wei Jing Tang*
Literal Name: Reed Decoction
Original Source: *Bei Ji Qian Jin Yao Fang* (Thousands of Golden Prescriptions for Emergencies) by Sun Si-Miao in the Tang Dynasty

COMPOSITION

Wei Jing (Herba Phragmitis), *qie* (sliced)	2 cups [30g]
Dong Gua Zi (Semen Benincasae)	0.5 cup [24g]
Yi Yi Ren (Semen Coicis)	0.5 cup [30g]
Tao Ren (Semen Persicae)	30 pieces [9g]

DOSAGE / PREPARATION / ADMINISTRATION

The source text states to first cook 2 cups [30g] of *Wei Jing* (Herba Phragmitis) in 20 cups of water until it is reduced to 5 cups. Add the other ingredients and further reduce the decoction from 5 cups to 2 cups. Take 1 cup of decoction per dose to induce vomiting of pus and abscesses.

CHINESE THERAPEUTIC ACTIONS

1. Clears the Lung and dissolves phlegm
2. Dispels stagnation and drains pus

CLINICAL MANIFESTATIONS

Lung abscess: coughing, foul-smelling, yellow sputum with pus and blood, dull pain in the chest; squamous, dry skin; a red tongue and a slippery, rapid pulse.

VETERINARY CLINICAL APPLICATIONS

Pulmonary abscesses, pneumonia, and bronchitis.

EXPLANATION

Wei Jing Tang (Reed Decoction) treats lung abscess with stagnation of heat, toxins, and phlegm. Stagnation in the Lung affects Lung qi circulation, causing coughing and chest pain. Stagnation of heat, toxins, and phlegm also

***Wei Jing Tang* (Reed Decoction)**

Diagnosis	Clinical Signs	Treatment	Herbs
Lung abscess	• Coughing and chest pain: stagnation in the Lung with reversed flow of Lung qi • Foul-smelling, yellow sputum with pus and blood: heat, toxins and phlegm damaging the Lung • Red tongue and a slippery, rapid pulse: heat and phlegm in the interior	• Clears the Lung and dissolves phlegm • Dispels stagnation and drains pus	• *Wei Jing* (Herba Phragmitis) clears the Lung, dispels heat, eliminates phlegm, and drains abscesses. • *Dong Gua Zi* (Semen Benincasae) and *Yi Yi Ren* (Semen Coicis) clear heat, dissolve phlegm, dispel dampness, and drain pus. • *Tao Ren* (Semen Persicae) activates the blood and breaks up blood stagnation.

Wěi Jīng Tāng (Reed Decoction)

damages the Lung, resulting in foul-smelling, yellow sputum with pus and blood. Flaky, dry skin suggests malnourishment of the skin due to lung abscess and obstructed qi and blood circulation.

This formula uses *Wei Jing* (Herba Phragmitis) to clear the Lung and dispel heat. *Dong Gua Zi* (Semen Benincasae) and *Yi Yi Ren* (Semen Coicis) clear heat, dissolve phlegm, dispel dampness, and drain pus. *Tao Ren* (Semen Persicae) activates the blood and breaks up blood stagnation.

VETERINARY MODIFICATIONS

- With cough, sputum, and chest congestion, add *Ting Li Zi* (Semen Descurainiae seu Lepidii).
- With lingering heat accompanied by cough and profuse sputum, add *Si Gua Luo* (Retinervus Luffae Fructus) and *Gua Lou Pi* (Pericarpium Trichosanthis).
- With cough and dyspnea due to pneumonia, combine with *Ma Huang Xing Ren Gan Cao Shi Gao Tang* (Ephedra, Apricot Kernel, Licorice, and Gypsum Decoction).
- For lung abscess that has not yet turned into pus, add *Jin Yin Hua* (Flos Lonicerae Japonicae) and *Yu Xing Cao* (Herba Houttuyniae).
- For lung abscess with a profuse amount of pus, add *Jie Geng* (Radix Platycodonis), *Gan Cao* (Radix et Rhizoma Glycyrrhizae), and *Bei Mu* (Bulbus Fritillariae).
- With heat toxins, add *Jin Yin Hua* (Flos Lonicerae Japonicae), *Lian Qiao* (Fructus Forsythiae), *Yu Xing Cao* (Herba Houttuyniae), *Jie Geng* (Radix Platycodonis) and *Chuan Bei Mu* (Bulbus Fritillariae Cirrhosae); or combine with *Huang Lian Jie Du Tang* (Coptis Decoction to Relieve Toxicity).
- With coughing, add *Pi Pa Ye* (Folium Eriobotryae) and *Gua Lou Pi* (Pericarpium Trichosanthis).

HUMAN CLINICAL STUDIES AND RESEARCH

1. **Pulmonary abscesses**: An integrative treatment using drugs and *Wei Jing Tang* (Reed Decoction) was associated with a marked effect in treating pulmonary abscesses. Of 110 patients, the study reported complete recovery in 68 cases, improvement in 29 cases, and no effect in 13 cases.[1] According to another study, complete recovery was reported in 24 of 26 patients with pulmonary abscesses using *Wei Jing Tang*, *Huang Lian Jie Du Tang* (Coptis Decoction to Relieve Toxicity), and intravenous administration of penicillin.[2]
2. **Pneumonia**: *Wei Jing Tang* has been shown to effectively treat many different types of pneumonia, including but not limited to lobar pneumonia, lobular pneumonia, bronchopneumonia, and mycoplasmal pneumonia.[3]
3. **Bronchitis**: *Wei Jing Tang* has been shown to successfully treat bronchitis in children,[4] suppurative bronchitis,[5] and chronic bronchitis.[6]

SUGGESTED ACUPUNCTURE TREATMENT

1. Points: *Jingqu* (LU 8), *Hegu* (LI 4), *Fenglong* (ST 40), *Xuehai* (SP 10), and *Weizhong* (BL 40).
2. Technique: sedation.

The treatment plan here is to reduce lung abscess and eliminate stagnation of blood, heat, toxins, and phlegm. *Jingqu* (LU 8) and *Hegu* (LI 4) clear Lung heat. *Fenglong* (ST 40) is a special point used to eliminate phlegm and pus stagnation. *Xuehai* (SP 10) and *Weizhong* (BL 40) activate the blood. Overall, through eliminating heat toxins, phlegm, and pus, the lung abscess will gradually subside.

AUTHORS' COMMENTS

Wei Jing Tang treats Lung abscess due to toxic heat obstructing the Lung with stasis of phlegm and blood. It is safe to use at various stages of lung abscess, either before or after the formation of pus. It can be combined with conventional antimicrobial drugs for a synergistic effect. Dogs and cats with the following conditions can benefit from this formula: lung abscess secondary to a foreign body, heartworm disease, lung adenocarcinoma, extension from a liver abscess, penetrating lung trauma (vehicular accident, bite wounds), aspiration pneumonia and abscess, and severe bacterial or fungal pneumonia.

References

1. *He Nan Zhong Yi* (Henan Chinese Medicine), 1991; 11(5):24.
2. *Shi Yong Zhong Xi Yi Jie He Za Zhi* (Practical Journal of Integrated Chinese and Western Medicines), 1992; 5(2):83.
3. *Shan Xi Zhong Yi* (Shanxi Chinese Medicine), 1994; 15(8):342.
4. *Shang Hai Zhong Yi Yao Za Zhi* (Shanghai Journal of Chinese Medicine and Herbology), 1983; 10:26.
5. *Shang Hai Zhong Yi Yao Za Zhi* (Shanghai Journal of Chinese Medicine and Herbology), 1959; 2:15.
6. *Jiang Su Zhong Yi* (Jiangsu Chinese Medicine), 1982; 5:14.

Dà Huáng Mŭ Dān Tāng (Rhubarb and Moutan Decoction)

大黃牡丹湯
大黄牡丹汤

Pinyin Name: *Da Huang Mu Dan Tang*
Literal Name: Rhubarb and Moutan Decoction
Alternate Names: *Ta Huang Mu Tan Pi Tang, Da Huang Mu Dan Pi Tang*, Rhubarb and Moutan Combination
Original Source: *Jin Gui Yao Lue* (Essentials from the Golden Cabinet) by Zhang Zhong-Jing in the Eastern Han Dynasty

COMPOSITION

Da Huang (Radix et Rhizoma Rhei)	12g [18g]
Mang Xiao (Natrii Sulfas)	0.3 cup [9g]
Tao Ren (Semen Persicae)	50 pieces [12g]
Mu Dan Pi (Cortex Moutan)	3g [9g]
Dong Gua Zi (Semen Benincasae)	0.5 cup [30g]

DOSAGE / PREPARATION / ADMINISTRATION

The source text states to cook the ingredients, except *Mang Xiao* (Natrii Sulfas), with 6 cups [1,200 mL] of water until the liquid is reduced to 1 cup [200 mL]. Discard the herb residue, add *Mang Xiao* (Natrii Sulfas) to the strained decoction, bring to a quick boil, and take the decoction immediately. Today, the decoction may be prepared using the doses suggested in brackets.

CHINESE THERAPEUTIC ACTIONS

1. Drains heat and breaks up stagnation
2. Disperses nodules and reduces swellings

CLINICAL MANIFESTATIONS

Early onset of intestinal abscess: swelling and distention of the abdomen, abdominal pain that is worse with palpation, fever, sweating, aversion to cold, a red tongue, and a rapid, slippery to wiry pulse.

VETERINARY CLINICAL APPLICATIONS

Intestinal perforation secondary to foreign body, intestinal volvulus, peritonitis and abscess secondary to intestinal surgery dehiscence.

EXPLANATION

Da Huang Mu Dan Tang (Rhubarb and Moutan Decoction) treats early-stage intestinal abscess caused by accumulation of damp-heat and stagnation of qi and blood in the Intestines. Because stagnation of qi and blood in the Intestines may cause disharmony between the *ying* (nutritive) and *wei* (defensive) levels, fever, sweating, and aversion to cold may occur. The red tongue and the slippery to wiry pulse indicate damp-heat in the interior.

This formula consists of cold downward-draining, damp-heat clearing, and blood-activating herbs. *Da Huang* (Radix et Rhizoma Rhei) quickly purges damp-heat and disperses stagnation. *Mang Xiao* (Natrii Sulfas) softens nodules and reduces swellings. *Tao Ren* (Semen Persicae) and *Mu Dan Pi* (Cortex Moutan) activate blood circulation and cool the blood. *Dong Gua Zi* (Semen Benincasae) clears Intestinal damp-heat and drains pus.

Da Huang Mu Dan Tang **(Rhubarb and Moutan Decoction)**

Diagnosis	Clinical Signs	Treatment	Herbs
Early onset of intestinal abscess	• Swelling and distention of the abdomen, abdominal pain that worsens with palpation: damp-heat accumulation and qi and blood stagnation in the Intestines • Fever, sweating, and aversion to cold: disharmony between the *ying* (nutritive) and *wei* (defensive) levels • Red tongue and a slippery to wiry pulse: damp-heat	• Drains heat and breaks up stagnation • Disperses nodules and reduces swellings	• *Da Huang* (Radix et Rhizoma Rhei) quickly purges damp-heat and disperses stagnation. • *Mang Xiao* (Natrii Sulfas) softens nodules and reduces swellings. • *Tao Ren* (Semen Persicae) and *Mu Dan Pi* (Cortex Moutan) activate blood circulation and cool the blood. • *Dong Gua Zi* (Semen Benincasae) clears Intestinal damp-heat and drains pus.

Dà Huáng Mŭ Dān Tāng (Rhubarb and Moutan Decoction)

VETERINARY MODIFICATIONS

- With severe abdominal pain, add *Chuan Lian Zi* (Fructus Toosendan), *Yan Hu Suo* (Rhizoma Corydalis), *Ru Xiang* (Gummi Olibanum) and *Mo Yao* (Myrrha).
- With abdominal bloating, add *Zhi Shi* (Fructus Aurantii Immaturus), *Hou Po* (Cortex Magnoliae Officinalis), and *Bing Lang* (Semen Arecae).
- With high fever, add *Huang Lian* (Rhizoma Coptidis), *Shi Gao* (Gypsum Fibrosum), *Jin Yin Hua* (Flos Lonicerae Japonicae), *Lian Qiao* (Fructus Forsythiae), *Pu Gong Ying* (Herba Taraxaci), and *Bai Jiang Cao* (Herba cum Radice Patriniae).

CAUTIONS / CONTRAINDICATIONS

- Intestinal abscesses are generally classified as either damp-heat or damp-cold. Animals with intestinal abscesses caused by damp-cold should ***not*** take this formula.
- *Da Huang Mu Dan Tang* is ***not*** suitable for geriatric or weak animals without modification.
- If preparing this formula in decoction, *Da Huang* (Radix et Rhizoma Rhei) does not need to be post-decocted as the emphasis is to clear damp-heat, not to drain or purge downwards. *Mang Xiao* (Natrii Sulfas) should be dissolved in the decoction immediately before serving.

PHARMACOLOGICAL EFFECTS

1. **Antibacterial**: According to *in vitro* studies, *Da Huang Mu Dan Tang* has a potent inhibitory effect against *Staphylococcus* species, and a moderate inhibitory effect against *E. coli*.[1]
2. **Anti-inflammatory**: Both the formula and its ingredients have been shown to reduce inflammation and swelling.[2]
3. **Gastrointestinal**: Administration of *Da Huang Mu Dan Tang* was associated with a stimulatory effect on the gastrointestinal tract; it was shown to increase the intestinal peristalsis and contraction of the appendix.[3,4]
4. **Antioxidant**: One study evaluated several Chinese herbal formulas and found *Da Huang Mu Dan Tang* to have the strongest scavenging activity against three types of free radicals: 1,1-diphenyl-2-picrylhydrazyl (DPPH), superoxide anion radical (O2-.) and hydroxyl radical (OH.). The study suggested that use of *Da Huang Mu Dan Tang* may play a role in treating cerebral ischemia and brain damage, because these disorders are associated with highly reactive oxygen-derived free radicals.[5]

HUMAN CLINICAL STUDIES AND RESEARCH

1. **Acute appendicitis**: Modified *Da Huang Mu Dan Tang* was used with excellent results to treat 224 patients with acute appendicitis. The study included 121 male and 103 female patients, between 7-84 years of age. Out of 224 cases, the study reported complete recovery in 206 cases, and ineffectiveness in 18 cases. The herbal formula was modified as follows: *Chuan Lian Zi* (Fructus Toosendan) and *Chi Shao* (Radix Paeoniae Rubra) were added for stagnation and accumulation; *Jin Yin Hua* (Flos Lonicerae Japonicae) and *Yi Yi Ren* (Semen Coicis) were added for damp-heat; *Huang Lian* (Rhizoma Coptidis) and *Bai Jiang Cao* (Herba cum Radice Patriniae) were added for heat and toxins; *Huang Lian* (Rhizoma Coptidis) and *Hu Zhang* (Rhizoma et Radix Polygoni Cuspidati) for toxic sores; and *Chuan Shan Jia* (Squama Manis) and *Chi Shao* (Radix Paeoniae Rubra) for damp-heat masses.[6]
2. **Ruptured appendicitis with peritonitis**: Modified *Da Huang Mu Dan Tang* and antibiotic drugs were successfully used together to treat 123 patients with ruptured appendicitis and peritonitis. The herbal formula used *Da Huang Mu Dan Tang* plus *Jin Yin Hua* (Flos Lonicerae Japonicae), *Chuan Lian Zi* (Fructus Toosendan), and *Tao Ren* (Semen Persicae) as the base formula, with the addition of *Shi Gao* (Gypsum Fibrosum) and *Tian Hua Fen* (Radix Trichosanthis) for high fever; *Zhu Ru* (Caulis Bambusae in Taenia) and *Lu Gen* (Rhizoma Phragmitis) for nausea and vomiting; *Ru Xiang* (Gummi Olibanum), *Mo Yao* (Myrrha), and *Yan Hu Suo* (Rhizoma Corydalis) for severe pain; and *Bing Pian* (Borneolum Syntheticum) and *Mang Xiao* (Natrii Sulfas) for abscess and swelling in the appendix area. Out of 123 patients, the study reported complete recovery in 75 cases, marked improvement in 44 cases, and no effect in 4 cases.[7]
3. **Acute cholecystitis**: Eighty-eight patients with acute cholecystitis (3 hours to 5 days) were treated with *Da Huang Mu Dan Tang* with good success. Most patients had resolution of clinical signs within 36 hours. Those who did not respond were referred out for emergency treatment. Out of 88 patients, the study reported complete recovery in 57 cases, marked improvement in 22 cases, and no effect in 9 cases.[8]
4. **Chronic prostatitis**: Rectal instillation of modified *Da Huang Mu Dan Tang* was effective in treating patients with chronic prostatitis. In addition to the formula, *Bian Xu* (Herba Polygoni Avicularis) and *Qu Mai* (Herba Dianthi) were added for frequent and painful urination; *Chuan Lian Zi* (Fructus Toosendan) and *Yan Hu Suo* (Rhizoma Corydalis) were added for testicular pain; *Du Zhong* (Cortex Eucommiae) and *Xu Duan* (Radix Dipsaci) were added for lower abdominal pain; *Chuan Shan Jia* (Squama Manis) and *E Zhu* (Rhizoma Curcumae) were added for hardness and nodules of the prostate; and *Pu Gong Ying* (Herba Taraxaci) and *Mo Han Lian* (Herba Ecliptae) were added for presence of white or red blood cells in the seminal fluids. The treatment protocol was to cook the herbs in water, and instill the solution in the rectum one time daily for seven days per course of

Dà Huáng Mŭ Dān Tāng (Rhubarb and Moutan Decoction)

treatment, for a total of 1-8 courses. Out of 60 patients, the study reported complete recovery in 47 cases, and marked improvement in 13 cases.[9]

SUGGESTED ACUPUNCTURE TREATMENT

1. Points: *Shangjuxu* (ST 37), *Tianshu* (ST 25), *Lanwei* (extra point), *Quchi* (LI 11), *Neiting* (ST 44), and *Diji* (SP 8).
2. Technique: sedation.

The treatment plan is to purge heat and reduce swelling. *Shangjuxu* (ST 37), the lower *he* (uniting) point of the Large Intestine and *Tianshu* (ST 25), the *mu* (collecting) point of the Large Intestine, are combined to regulate qi and blood in the Large Intestine. *Lanwei* (an extra point, whose name means "appendix") relieves intestinal abscess and pain. *Quchi* (LI 11) and *Neiting* (ST 44) clear interior heat from the *yangming*. *Diji* (SP 8) relieves abdominal pain.

AUTHORS' COMMENTS

From veterinary medicine perspectives, *Da Huang Mu Dan Tang* could be used in animals to treat internal abscesses that do not respond, or have a poor response, to antibiotic therapy.

References

1. *Zhong Yi Za Zhi* (Journal of Chinese Medicine), 1955, 10:36.
2. *Zhong Yi Fang Ji Xian Dai Yan Jiu* (Modern Study of Medical Formulas in Traditional Chinese Medicine), 1997; 1600.
3. *Shan Dong Yi Xue Yuan Xue Bao* (Journal of Shandong University School of Medicine), 1959; 4:25.
4. *Zhong Yi Fang Ji Xian Dai Yan Jiu* (Modern Study of Medical Formulas in Traditional Chinese Medicine), 1997; 1600.
5. Department of Pharmacy, Tokushima University Hospital, Japan. Studies on attenuation of post-ischemic brain injury by kampo medicines-inhibitory effects of free radical production. I. Yakugaku Zasshi. 1994 Jun; 114(6):388-94.
6. *Guang Xi Zhong Yi Yao* (Guangxi Chinese Medicine and Herbology), 1986; 3:10.
7. *Nei Meng Gu Zhong Yi Yao* (Traditional Chinese Medicine and Medicinals of Inner Mongolia), 1993; 2:23.
8. *Shi Yong Zhong Yi Nei Ke Za Zhi* (Journal of Practical Chinese Internal Medicine), 1992; 3:127.
9. *Zhe Jiang Zhong Yi Za Zhi* (Zhejiang Journal of Chinese Medicine), 1993; 8:368.

Chapter 22 — Summary

— Formulas that Treat Abscesses and Sores

SECTION 1: EXTERNAL ABSCESSES AND SORES

Name	Similarities	Differences
Xian Fang Huo Ming Yin (Sublime Formula for Sustaining Life)	Clear heat, eliminate toxins, release the exterior	Reduces swelling, breaks up hardness, activates blood circulation, stops pain
Jing Fang Bai Du San (Schizonepeta and Saposhnikovia Powder to Overcome Pathogenic Influences)		Strongly releases the exterior, regulates qi and blood circulation
Wu Wei Xiao Du Yin (Five-Ingredient Decoction to Eliminate Toxins)	Clear heat, eliminate toxins	Disperses external carbuncles and furuncles
Si Miao Yong An Tang (Four-Valiant Decoction for Well-Being)		Treats gangrene characterized by heat, fire and toxins
Zi Cao Gen Mu Li Tang (Arnebia and Oyster Shell Decoction)		Treats malignant sores and abscesses
Hai Zao Yu Hu Tang (Sargassum Decoction for the Jade Flask)	Dissolve phlegm, soften hardness, disperse nodules	Treats goiter affecting the neck
Xiao Luo Wan (Reduce Scrofula Pill)		Treats hardness and nodules around the ears and neck
San Zhong Kui Jian Tang (Disperse the Swelling and Break the Hardness Decoction)		Treats hardness and nodules, especially around the ears, cheeks, and shoulders
Shi Liu Wei Liu Qi Yin (Sixteen-Ingredient Decoction to Flow Qi)		Treats hardness and nodules, especially in the neck, mammary glands and abdominal region
Pai Nong San (Drain the Pus Powder)	Tonify deficiencies, drain pus from abscesses and sores	Tonifies the blood
Tuo Li Xiao Du Yin (Drain the Interior and Detoxify Decoction)		Strongly tonifies qi and blood
Yang He Tang (Yang-Heartening Decoction)	Warms yang, dispels cold, treats *yin* (deep-rooted) abscesses and sores	Warms yang, tonifies the blood

Xian Fang Huo Ming Yin (Sublime Formula for Sustaining Life) and ***Jing Fang Bai Du San*** (Schizonepeta and Saposhnikovia Powder to Overcome Pathogenic Influences) have similar functions to release the exterior, clear heat, and eliminate toxins.

- *Xian Fang Huo Ming Yin* treats early onset of abscesses and sores characterized by accumulation of heat and toxins at the exterior with stagnation of qi and blood.
- *Jing Fang Bai Du San* strongly releases the exterior to treat sores and abscesses with exterior clinical signs, such as fever, aversion to cold, and absence of sweating.

Wu Wei Xiao Du Yin (Five-Ingredient Decoction to Eliminate Toxins), ***Si Miao Yong An Tang*** (Four-Valiant Decoction for Well-Being), and ***Zi Cao Gen Mu Li Tang*** (Arnebia and Oyster Shell Decoction) clear heat and eliminate toxins to treat various conditions with abscesses and sores.

- *Wu Wei Xiao Du Yin* treats carbuncles, furuncles, and other types of epithelial inflammation.
- *Si Miao Yong An Tang* treats gangrene of the extremities with local swelling and pus formation.
- *Zi Cao Gen Mu Li Tang* treats malignant abscesses, sores, and ulcers.

Chapter 22 — Summary

Hai Zao Yu Hu Tang (Sargassum Decoction for the Jade Flask), ***Xiao Luo Wan*** (Reduce Scrofula Pill), ***San Zhong Kui Jian Tang*** (Disperse the Swelling and Break the Hardness Decoction), and ***Shi Liu Wei Liu Qi Yin*** (Sixteen-Ingredient Decoction to Flow Qi) have similar functions to dissolve phlegm, soften hardness, and disperse nodules.

- *Hai Zao Yu Hu Tang* treats enlarged thyroid glands in cases of goiter and hyperthyroidism.
- *Xiao Luo Wan* was originally designed to treat scrofula, but may also be used for goiter, thyroiditis, lymphadenitis, parotitis, and hyperplasia of the mammary glands.
- *San Zhong Kui Jian Tang* treats hardness and nodules throughout the body, but is especially effective for areas below the ears and around the shoulders. Clinical applications include cancer, lymphadenitis, hyperthyroidism, goiter, carbuncles, and furuncles.
- *Shi Liu Wei Liu Qi Yin* treats hardness and nodules throughout the body, but is especially effective for regions of the neck, breast and abdomen. Clinical applications include cancer, goiter, and inflammation of the lymph nodes.

Pai Nong San (Drain the Pus Powder) and ***Tuo Li Xiao Du Yin*** (Drain the Interior and Detoxify Decoction) treat mid-to-late stages of abscesses and sores, when affected animals begin to show more underlying deficiencies.

- *Pai Nong San* nourishes the blood, drains pus, and reduces nodules. It is used to treat middle or late stage of abscesses and sores with blood deficiency.
- *Tuo Li Xiao Du Yin* tonifies qi and blood, strengthens the Spleen and Stomach, and drains pus and swellings. It is used to treat late stage of abscesses and sores with severe qi and blood deficiencies.

Yang He Tang (Yang-Heartening Decoction) warms yang, dispels cold, and drains pus from abscesses and sores. It is most effective for *yin*-type (deep-rooted) abscesses and sores with yang deficiency and cold accumulation.

SECTION 2: INTERNAL ABSCESSES AND SORES

Name	Similarities	Differences
Wei Jing Tang (Reed Decoction)	Resolve internal abscesses and sores	Treats lung abscesses
Da Huang Mu Dan Tang (Rhubarb and Moutan Decoction)		Treats intestinal abscesses

Wei Jing Tang (Reed Decoction) clears heat, eliminates toxins, and drains pus. It treats lung abscesses with stagnation of blood, heat, toxins, and phlegm.

Da Huang Mu Dan Tang (Rhubarb and Moutan Decoction) can purge stagnant heat and eliminate toxins. It is excellent for treating early onset of intestinal abscesses.

Part III

— Additional Resources

索引

吴尚先 Wú Shàng-Xían

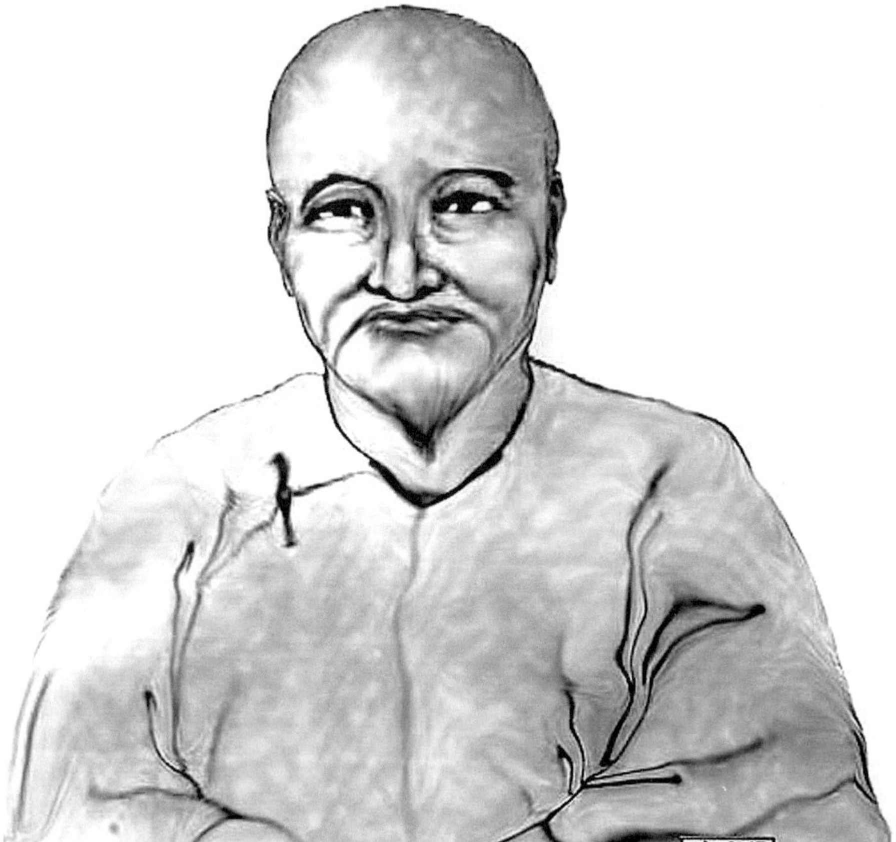

吴尚先 Wú Shàng-Xían, 1806 – 1886.

吴尚先 Wú Shàng-Xian

Wu Shang-Xian specialized in treating both local and systemic disorders via topical applications of herbs. His exploration of topical approaches was motivated by his concern for patients who could not or would not take herbs by oral ingestion, and by his desire to minimize the side effects associated with oral use. In many years of research, Wu explored many different routes of administration, such as oral inhalation, nasal inhalation, topical application, and ophthalmic instillation. He also developed many different dosage forms for medicines, including creams, ointments, plasters, inhalation solutions, and more. Because of his unique treatment methods and uncommon success, he literally treated 4,000 to 5,000 patients per month, and 50,000 to 60,000 patients per year. Wu's style of medicine introduced new options for treatment, and influenced generations of physicians and herbalists, shaping the practice of medicine to this day.

Dynasties & Kingdoms	Year
Xia Dynasty 夏	2100-1600 BCE
Shang Dynasty 商	1600-1100 BCE
Zhou Dynasty 周	1100-221 BCE
Qin Dynasty 秦	221-207 BCE
Han Dynasty 漢	206 BCE-220
Three Kingdoms 三國	220-280
Western Jin Dynasty 西晉	265-316
Eastern Jin Dynasty 東晉	317-420
Northern and Southern Dynasties 北南朝	420-581
Sui Dynasty 隋	581-618
Tang Dynasty 唐	618-907
Five Dynasties 五代	907-960
Song Dynasty 宋	960-1279
Liao Dynasty 遼	916-1125
Jin Dynasty 金	1115-1234
Yuan Dynasty 元	1271-1368
Ming Dynasty 明	1368-1644
Qing Dynasty 清	**1644-1911**
Republic of China 中華民國	1912-Present Day
People's Republic of China 中華人民共和國	1949-Present Day

Table of Contents

Appendix 1

— Formulas Offering Beneficial Effects to Support Pregnancy

Certain formulas have been shown to offer beneficial effects during pregnancy. However, these formulas should be used only under supervision of a qualified healthcare professional, and only when the benefits of using the herbs outweigh the risks.

Symptoms	Formulas
Abdominal pain	• *Dang Gui Shao Yao San* (Tangkuei and Peony Powder) • *Jiao Ai Tang* (Ass-Hide Gelatin and Mugwort Decoction)
Breech presentation of the fetus	• *Ba Zhen Tang* (Eight-Treasure Decoction) with *Huang Qi* (Radix Astragali), *Xu Duan* (Radix Dipsaci) and *Zhi Qiao* (Fructus Aurantii)
Cough	• *Bai He Gu Jin Tang* (Lily Bulb Decoction to Preserve the Metal) • *Liu Jun Zi Tang* (Six-Gentlemen Decoction)
Edema and swelling	• *Wu Ling San* (Five-Ingredient Powder with Poria)
Irritability	• *Qi Ju Di Huang Wan* (Lycium Fruit, Chrysanthemum, and Rehmannia Pill) • *Ba Zhen Tang* (Eight-Treasure Decoction) • *Ban Xia Bai Zhu Tian Ma Tang* (Pinellia, Atractylodes Macrocephala, and Gastrodia Decoction)
Miscarriage, prevention of	• *Bao Chan Wu You Fang* (Preserve Pregnancy and Care-Free Decoction) • *Tai Shan Pan Shi San* (Powder that Gives the Stability of Mount Tai)
Nausea and vomiting	• *Xiang Sha Liu Jun Zi Tang* (Six-Gentlemen Decoction with Aucklandia and Amomum) • *Wen Dan Tang* (Warm the Gallbladder Decoction) • *Ju Pi Zhu Ru Tang* (Tangerine Peel and Bamboo Shaving Decoction)
Restless fetus	• *Bao Chan Wu You Fang* (Preserve Pregnancy and Care-Free Decoction) • *Dang Gui Shao Yao San* (Tangkuei and Peony Powder)
Uterine bleeding	• *Gui Zhi Fu Ling Wan* (Cinnamon Twig and Poria Pill) • *Bao Chan Wu You Fang* (Preserve Pregnancy and Care-Free Decoction)

Appendix 2

— Formulas Offering Beneficial Effects for Post-parturition Care

Certain formulas have been shown to offer beneficial effects for post-parturition care. However, these formulas should be used only under supervision of a qualified healthcare professional, and only when the benefits of using the herbs outweigh the risks.

Symptoms	Formulas
Blood stagnation (retention of lochia)	• *Sheng Hua Tang* (Generation and Transformation Decoction)
Qi and blood deficiencies	• *Ba Zhen Tang* (Eight-Treasure Decoction)
Lactation, insufficient	• *Tong Ru Wan* (Unblock the Breast Pill)
Lactation, excessive	• *Bu Zhong Yi Qi Tang* (Tonify the Middle and Augment the Qi Decoction) with *Qian Shi* (Semen Euryales) and *Wu Wei Zi* (Fructus Schisandrae Chinensis) • *Jia Wei Xiao Yao San* (Augmented Rambling Powder) with *Mu Li* (Concha Ostreae) and *Xia Ku Cao* (Spica Prunellae)
Lactation, termination of	• *Mai Ya* (Fructus Hordei Germinatus) 60g

Appendix 3

— Cautions / Contraindications for the Use of Formulas During Pregnancy

Certain formulas have a recognized potential to endanger or cause harm to a fetus during pregnancy, thus possibly causing birth defects or miscarriages. As a general rule, formulas with potent effects to regulate qi, move blood, or drain downward should be avoided during pregnancy. These formulas are **contraindicated,** or if absolutely necessary, used with **caution** in treatment of pregnant animals. Please note that this is not a comprehensive list - additional information is listed in each formula monograph.

An Gong Niu Huang Wan (Calm the Palace Pill with Cattle Gallstone)

Ba Wei Di Huang Wan (Eight-Ingredient Pill with Rehmannia)

Ba Zheng San (Eight-Herb Powder for Rectification)

Bao He Wan (Preserve Harmony Pill)

Ci Zhu Wan (Magnetite and Cinnabar Pill)

Da Cheng Qi Tang (Major Order the Qi Decoction)

Da Huang Mu Dan Tang (Rhubarb and Moutan Decoction)

Da Huang Zhe Chong Wan (Rhubarb and Eupolyphaga Pill)

Da Jian Zhong Tang (Major Construct the Middle Decoction)

Da Xian Xiong Tang (Major Sinking into the Chest Decoction)

Dang Gui Long Hui Wan (Tangkuei, Gentiana, and Aloe Pill)

Du Huo Ji Sheng Tang (Angelica Pubescens and Taxillus Decoction)

Fang Feng Tong Sheng San (Saposhnikovia Powder that Sagely Unblocks)

Fu Yuan Huo Xue Tang (Revive Health by Invigorating the Blood Decoction)

Fu Zi Li Zhong Wan (Prepared Aconite Pill to Regulate the Middle)

Ge Xia Zhu Yu Tang (Drive Out Blood Stasis Below the Diaphragm Decoction)

Gong Wai Yun Fang (Ectopic Pregnancy Formula)

Gun Tan Wan (Vaporize Phlegm Pill)

Guo Qi Yin (Delayed Menstruation Decoction)

Hei Xi Dan (Lead Special Pill)

Hua Chong Wan (Dissolve Parasites Pill)

Huo Luo Xiao Ling Dan (Fantastically Effective Pill to Invigorate the Collaterals)

Ji Ming San (Powder to Take at Cock's Crow)

Jia Wei Xiao Yao San (Augmented Rambling Powder)

Jin Gui Shen Qi Wan (Kidney Qi Pill from the Golden Cabinet)

Jin Ling Zi San (Melia Toosendan Powder)

Li Zhong Wan (Regulate the Middle Pill)

Liang Ge San (Cool the Diaphragm Powder)

Appendix 3 — Cautions / Contraindications for the Use of Formulas During Pregnancy

Liu Shen Wan (Six-Miracle Pill)
Liu Yi San (Six-to-One Powder)
Ma Huang Fu Zi Xi Xin Tang (Ephedra, Asarum, and Prepared Aconite Decoction)
Ma Zi Ren Wan (Hemp Seed Pill)
Mu Xiang Bing Lang Wan (Aucklandia and Betel Nut Pill)
Ping Wei San (Calm the Stomach Powder)
Qi Li San (Seven-Thousandths of a Tael Powder)
Qian Zheng San (Lead to Symmetry Powder)
Qing Qi Hua Tan Wan (Clear the Qi and Transform Phlegm Pill)
Run Chang Wan (Moisten the Intestines Pill)
San Huang Xie Xin Tang (Three-Yellow Decoction to Sedate the Epigastrium)
San Wu Bei Ji Wan (Three-Substance Pill for Emergencies)
Shao Fu Zhu Yu Tang (Drive Out Blood Stasis in the Lower Abdomen Decoction)
Shen Ling Bai Zhu San (Ginseng, Poria, and Atractylodes Macrocephala Powder)
Shen Tong Zhu Yu Tang (Drive Out Blood Stasis from a Painful Body Decoction)
Sheng Hua Tang (Generation and Transformation Decoction)
Shi Xiao San (Sudden Smile Powder)
Shi Zao Tang (Ten-Jujube Decoction)
Su He Xiang Wan (Liquid Styrax Pill)
Tao He Cheng Qi Tang (Peach Pit Decoction to Order the Qi)
Tao Hong Si Wu Tang (Four-Substance Decoction with Safflower and Peach Pit)
Wu Mei Wan (Mume Pill)
Wu Yao Shun Qi San (Lindera Powder to Smooth the Flow of Qi)
Xi Huang Wan (Cattle Gallstone Pill)
Xiao Huo Luo Dan (Minor Invigorate the Collaterals Special Pill)
Xiao Jin Dan (Minor Gold Special Pill)
Xiao Yao San (Rambling Powder)
Xing Jun San (Troop-Marching Powder)
Xue Fu Zhu Yu Tang (Drive Out Stasis in the Mansion of Blood Decoction)
Yin Chen Hao Tang (Artemisia Scoparia Decoction)
Yu Zhen San (True Jade Powder)
Zhi Bao Dan (Greatest Treasure Special Pill)
Zhi Shi Dao Zhi Wan (Immature Bitter Orange Pill to Guide Out Stagnation)
Zhou Che Wan (Vessel and Vehicle Pill)
Zhu Sha An Shen Wan (Cinnabar Pill to Tranquilize the Spirit)
Zi Jin Ding (Purple Gold Special Pill)
Zi Xue (Purple Snow)
Zuo Jin Wan (Left Metal Pill)

Appendix 4 — Dosing Guidelines

The following table is intended to assist veterinarians in administering proper doses of Chinese herbal formulas. These recommended dosages are a guideline, which is why there is such a wide range of suggestions. Different manufacturers of the same formula may arrive at different strengths so that the practitioner may need to adjust the dose of a given formula and may even require increasing beyond the recommended dose in the table on the following page. Though common sense and a strong knowledge of herbal formulas guided by experience should accompany their use, the vast majority of the formulas in this text have a very wide margin of safety and practitioners should feel comfortable in exploring dose requirements for individual patients. As discussed in the **Dosage** section, modifications may be needed based on the constitution or age of the patient, severity of the condition, and progression of treatment. As with any protocol, patients should be monitored and changes made as necessary. Dosing three times daily is often recommended for best therapeutic effect. Because this schedule can be difficult for many owners, our general recommendations are for twice daily administration. When optimal administration is possible, divide the total daily dose recommended by three. If owners can only dose once daily, use the highest dose listed.

Special Dosing Note: Herbal formula may also be administered via rectal enema. This route of administration may be necessary in emergent cases and for those patients for which oral administration is contraindicated or not possible. Extract granular herb formulas are best suited for rectal use and are easily prepared by mixing with warm water. The dosage required to obtain an effective therapeutic effect is 3-4 times that of the recommended oral dose, and the herbal enema solution retained for a minimum of 5-10 minutes to promote maximum absorption.

Puppies, kittens, foals, and other newborns should be dosed at half of the adult dose.

Appendix 4 — Dosing Guidelines

VETERINARY DOSING GUIDELINES

Animals	Weight	Powder	Extract Granules	Tablets	Pills	Tinctures
Dogs	Up to 15 kg (Up to 25 lbs)	0.5-1.5 g bid	0.5-1 g bid	½ bid	1-3 bid	2-5 drops bid
	15-30 kg (25-50 lbs)	1.5-3 g bid	1-2 g bid	½-1 bid	3-4 bid	5-10 drops bid
	30-45 kg (50-75 lbs)	3-4 g bid	2-3 g bid	1-1½ bid	4-6 bid	10-15 drops bid
	45-60 kg (75-100 lbs)	4-6 g bid	3 g bid	1½-2 bid	6-8 bid	12-20 drops bid
	60-75kg (100-125 lbs)	6-7 g bid	3-4 g bid	2 bid	8-10 bid	15-25 drops bid
Cats	Up to 6 kg (Up to10 lbs)	0.25-0.5 g bid	0.25-0.5 g bid	½ bid	1 bid	1-2 drops bid
	6-9 kg (10-15 lbs)	0.5-1 g bid	0.5 g bid	1 bid	1-2 bid	2 drops bid
	>9 kg (>15 lbs)	1-1.5 g bid	0.5-1 g bid	1 bid	2 bid	2-3 drops bid
Horses*	Minis	5-10 g bid	5-10 g bid	3-5 bid	20 bid	Tinctures in horses are not advised due to volume requirements
	Ponies	10-20 g bid	10-15 g bid	6-8 bid	40-60 bid	
	550-725 kg (900-1200 lbs)	20-30 g bid	15-20 g bid	10 bid	Impractical	
	725-900 kg (1200-1500lbs)	30-40 g bid	20-25 g bid	15 bid	Impractical	

*Ruminants, camelids, and pigs may be dosed like horses, extrapolating for like weights.

Appendix 5

— Weights and Measures: Chinese, British and Metric Systems

CHINESE SYSTEM

1. Measure of Weight

1 *jin* (斤) = 16 *liang* (两)
1 *liang* (两) = 10 *qian* (钱)
1 *qian* (钱) = 10 *fen* (分)
1 *fen* (分) = 10 *li* (厘)

2. Measure of Volume

1 *shi* (石) = 10 *dou* (斗)
1 *dou* (斗) = 10 *sheng* (升)
1 *sheng* (升) = 10 *he* (合)
1 *he* (合) = 10 *shao* (勺)

BRITISH SYSTEM

1. Measure of Weight (Apothecary)

20 grains = 1 scruple
3 scruples (60 grains) = 1 drachm or dram
8 drachms (480 grains) = 1 ounce
12 ounces (5760 grains) = 1 pound

2. Measure of Weight (Avoirdupois)

437½ or 437.5 grains = 1 ounce
16 ounces (7,000 grains) = 1 pound

3. Measure of Volume (Apothecary)

60 minims = 1 fluidrachm or fluidram
8 fluidrachms (480 minims) = 1 fluidounce
16 fluidounces = 1 pint
2 pints (32 fluidounces) = 1 quart
4 quarts (8 pints) = 1 gallon

METRIC SYSTEM

1. Measure of Weight

1 kilogram (kg) = 1,000.000 grams
1 hectogram (hg) = 100.000 grams
1 dekagram (dag) = 10.000 grams
1 gram (g or gm) = 1.000 gram
1 decigram (dg) = 0.100 gram
1 centigram (cg) = 0.010 gram
1 milligram (mg) = 0.001 gram
1 microgram (μg or mcg) = 0.000,001 gram

1 gram (g or gm) = 0.001 kilogram
= 0.010 hectogram
= 0.100 dekagram
= 10 decigrams
= 100 centigrams
= 1,000 milligrams
= 1,000,000 micrograms

2. Measure of Volume

1 kiloliter (kL) = 1,000.000 liters
1 hectoliter (hL) = 100.000 liters
1 dekaliter (daL) = 10.000 liters
1 liter (L) = 1.000 liter
1 deciliter (dL) = 0.100 liter
1 centiliter (cL) = 0.010 liter
1 milliliter (mL) = 0.001 liter
1 microliter (μL) = 0.000,001 liter

1 liter = 0.001 kiloliter
= 0.010 hectoliter
= 0.100 dekaliter
= 10 deciliters
= 100 centiliters
= 1,000 milliliters
= 1,000,000 microliters

Appendix 5 — Weights and Measures: Chinese, British and Metric Systems

METRIC SYSTEM

Multiples and Submultiples		Prefix	Symbols
1,000,000,000,000	(10^{12})	*tera-*	T
1,000,000,000	(10^{9})	*giga-*	G
1,000,000	(10^{6})	*mega-*	M
1,000	(10^{3})	*kilo-*	k
100	(10^{2})	*hecto-*	h
10	(10)	*deka-*	da
0.1	(10^{-1})	*deci-*	d
0.01	(10^{-2})	*centi-*	c
0.001	(10^{-3})	*milli-*	m
0.000,001	(10^{-6})	*micro-*	μ or mc
0.000,000,001	(10^{-9})	*nano-*	n
0.000,000,000,001	(10^{-12})	*pico-*	p
0.000,000,000,000,001	(10^{-15})	*femto-*	f
0.000,000,000,000,000,001	(10^{-18})	*atto-*	a

CONVERSIONS

Weight Conversion
(Chinese Units : Metric : Avoirdupois)

Chinese Units	Grams	Ounces
1 *jin* (斤)	500	17.87
1 *liang* (两)	31.25	1.116875
1 *qian* (钱)	3.125	0.111688
1 *fen* (分)	0.3125	0.011169
1 *li* (厘)	0.03125	0.001117

Volume Conversion
(Chinese Units : Metric : Apothecary)

Chinese Units	Liter	Fluid Ounces
1 *sheng* (升)	1	33.815

Note: Chinese units of weights and measures vary from dynasty to dynasty. Therefore, the conversion of Chinese units to another system is not always simple or straight forward.

Appendix 6

— Convention on International Trade in Endangered Species (CITES)

Trade in herbs and animals listed in Appendix I of Convention on International Trade in Endangered Species (CITES) is strictly prohibited. The discussion of these substances in this text is included only to offer 1) the accurate history of their critically important usage in traditional herbal medicine, and 2) models for appropriate usage of effective substitute substances and alternatives. The information should not be interpreted as condoning illegal use of these endangered species. Additional and updated information may be obtain from www.cites.org.

Endangered Species	Status	Alternatives
Chuan Shan Jia (Squama Manis)	Appendix II	*Wang Bu Liu Xing* (Semen Vaccariae)
Hu Gu (Os Tigris)	Appendix I	*Zhu Gu* (Os Porcus)
She Xiang (Moschus)	Appendix I/II	*Bing Pian* (Borneolum Syntheticum) or *Su He Xiang* (Styrax)
Xi Jiao (Cornu Rhinoceri)	Appendix I	*Shui Niu Jiao* (Cornu Bubali)
Xiong Dan (Fel Ursi)	Appendix I	*Niu Dan* (Fel Bovis)

Appendix 7

— Cross-reference of Single Herb Names

Pinyin Names	Pharmaceutical Names	Chinese Names
A Wei	Resina Ferulae	阿魏
Ai Di Cha	Herba Ardisiae Japonicae	矮地茶
Ai Ye	Folium Artemisiae Argyi	艾叶
Ai Ye Tan	Folium Artemisiae Argyi Carbonisatum	艾叶炭
An Xi Xiang	Benzoinum	安息香
Ba Dou	Fructus Crotonis	巴豆
Ba Dou Shuang	Semen Crotonis Pulveratum	巴豆霜
Ba Ji Tian	Radix Morindae Officinalis	巴戟天
Ba Jiao Feng	Radix Alangii	八角枫
Ba Jiao Hui Xiang	Fructus Anisi Stellati	八角茴香
Ba Li Ma	Fructus Rhododendri	八里麻
Ba Qia	Rhizoma Smilacis Chinae	菝葜
Bai Bian Dou	Semen Lablab Album	白扁豆
Bai Bu	Radix Stemonae	百部
Bai Fan	Alumen	白矾
Bai Fu Ling	Poria Alba	白茯苓
Bai Fu Zi	Rhizoma Typhonii	白附子
Bai Guo	Semen Ginkgo	白果
Bai He	Bulbus Lilii	百合
Bai Hua She She Cao	Herba Hedyotis	白花蛇舌草
Bai Ji	Rhizoma Bletillae	白及
Bai Jiang Cao	Herba cum Radice Patriniae	败酱草
Bai Lian	Radix Ampelopsis	白蔹
Bai Long Chuan Hua Tou	Radix Clerodendron Paniculatum	白龙船花头
Bai Mao Gen	Rhizoma Imperatae	白茅根
Bai Mao Hua	Flos Imperatae	白茅花
Bai Mu Er	Fructificatio Tremellae Fuciformis	白木耳
Bai Mu Tong	Caulis Akebiae Trifoliatae	白木通
Bai Qian	Rhizoma et Radix Cynanchi Stauntonii	白前
Bai Qu Cai	Herba Chelidonii	白屈菜
Bai Shao	Radix Paeoniae Alba	白芍
Bai Tou Weng	Radix Pulsatillae	白头翁
Bai Tou Weng Jing	Caulis Pulsatillae	白头翁茎
Bai Tou Weng Ye	Folium Pulsatillae	白头翁叶
Bai Wei	Radix et Rhizoma Cynanchi Atrati	白薇
Bai Xian Pi	Cortex Dictamni	白鲜皮

Appendix 7 — Cross-reference of Single Herb Names

Pinyin Names	Pharmaceutical Names	Chinese Names
Bai Zhi	Radix Angelicae Dahuricae	白芷
Bai Zhu	Rhizoma Atractylodis Macrocephalae	白术
Bai Zi Ren	Semen Platycladi	柏子仁
Ban Bian Lian	Herba Lobeliae Chinensis	半边莲
Ban Lan Gen	Radix Isatidis	板蓝根
Ban Mao	Mylabris	斑蝥
Ban Xia	Rhizoma Pinelliae	半夏
Ban Xia Qu	Rhizoma Pinelliae Massa Fermentata	半夏曲
Ban Zhi Lian	Herba Scutellariae Barbatae	半枝莲
Bao Ma Zi Pi	Cortex Syringae Amurensis	暴马子皮
Bei Chai Hu	Radix Bupleurum Chinensis	北柴胡
Bei Dou Gen	Rhizoma Menispermi	北豆根
Bei Mu	Bulbus Fritillariae	贝母
Bei Sha Shen	Radix Glehniae	北沙参
Bei Ting Li Zi	Semen Lepidii	北葶苈子
Bi Bo	Fructus Piperis Longi	荜茇
Bi Cheng Qie	Fructus Litseae	荜澄茄
Bi Ma Zi	Semen Ricini	蓖麻子
Bi Zi Cao	Herba Pogonantheri Criniti	笔仔草
Bian Dou Hua	Flos Lablab Album	扁豆花
Bian Dou Yi	Pericarpium Lablab Album	扁豆衣
Bian Xu	Herba Polygoni Avicularis	萹蓄
Bie Jia	Carapax Trionycis	鳖甲
Bie Jia Jiao	Gelatinum Carapax Trionycis	鳖甲胶
Bing Lang	Semen Arecae	槟榔
Bing Pian	Borneolum Syntheticum	冰片
Bo He	Herba Menthae	薄荷
Bo He Nao	Mentholum	薄荷脑
Bo Luo Hui	Herba Macleayae	博落回
Bu Gu Zhi	Fructus Psoraleae	补骨脂
Can Sha	Faeces Bombycis	蚕砂
Cang Er Cao	Herba Xanthii	苍耳草
Cang Er Gen	Radix Xanthii	苍耳根
Cang Er Zi	Fructus Xanthii	苍耳子
Cang Zhu	Rhizoma Atractylodis	苍术
Cao Dou Kou	Semen Alpiniae Katsumadai	草豆蔻
Cao Guo	Fructus Tsaoko	草果
Cao Wu	Radix Aconiti Kusnezoffii	草乌
Cao Wu Ye	Folium Aconiti Kusnezoffii	草乌叶
Ce Bai Ye	Cacumen Platycladi	侧柏叶
Ce Bai Ye Tan	Cacumen Platycladi Carbonisatum	侧柏叶炭

Appendix 7 — Cross-reference of Single Herb Names

Pinyin Names	Pharmaceutical Names	Chinese Names
Cha Chi Huang	Herba Stellariae Aquaticae	茶匙癀
Cha Ye	Folium Camelliae	茶叶
Chai Hu	Radix Bupleuri	柴胡
Chan Su	Venenum Bufonis	蟾酥
Chan Tui	Periostracum Cicadae	蝉蜕
Chang Shan	Radix Dichroae	常山
Chang Zui Lao Guan Cao	Herba Erodii	长嘴老鹳草
Chao Gua Lou Zi	Semen Trichosanthis Tostum	炒瓜蒌子
Che Qian Cao	Herba Plantaginis	车前草
Che Qian Zi	Semen Plantaginis	车前子
Chen Pi	Pericarpium Citri Reticulatae	陈皮
Chen Xiang	Lignum Aquilariae Resinatum	沉香
Chi Fu Ling	Poria Rubra	赤茯苓
Chi Shao	Radix Paeoniae Rubra	赤芍
Chi Shi Zhi	Halloysitum Rubrum	赤石脂
Chi Xiao Dou	Semen Phaseoli	赤小豆
Chong Bai La	Cera Chinensis	虫白蜡
Chong Lou	Rhizoma Paridis	重楼
Chong Wei Zi	Fructus Leonuri	茺蔚子
Chou Wu Tong	Folium Clerodendri Trichotomi	臭梧桐
Chu Chong Ju	Flos Pyrethri	除虫菊
Chu Shi Zi	Fructus Broussonetiae	楮实子
Chuan Bei Mu	Bulbus Fritillariae Cirrhosae	川贝母
Chuan Lian Zi	Fructus Toosendan	川楝子
Chuan Mu Tong	Caulis Clematidis Armandii	川木通
Chuan Mu Xiang	Radix Vladimiriae	川木香
Chuan Niu Xi	Radix Cyathulae	川牛膝
Chuan Shan Jia	Squama Manis	穿山甲
Chuan Shan Long	Rhizoma Dioscoreae Nipponicae	穿山龙
Chuan She Gan	Rhizoma Iridis Tectori	川射干
Chuan Wu	Radix Aconiti	川乌
Chuan Xin Lian	Herba Andrographis	穿心莲
Chuan Xiong	Rhizoma Chuanxiong	川芎
Chui Pen Cao	Herba Sedi	垂盆草
Chun Gen	Radix Ailanthi	椿根
Chun Pi	Cortex Ailanthi	椿皮
Ci Shi	Magnetitum	磁石
Ci Wu Jia	Radix et Rhizoma seu Caulis Acanthopanacis Senticosi	刺五加
Cong	Herba Allii Fistulosi	葱
Cong Bai	Bulbus Allii Fistulosi	葱白
Da Ding Huang	Caulis Euonymi	大疔癀

Appendix 7 — Cross-reference of Single Herb Names

Pinyin Names	Pharmaceutical Names	Chinese Names
Da Dou Huang Juan	Semen Glycines Germinatum	大豆黄卷
Da Feng Zi	Semen Hydnocarpi	大风子
Da Fu Pi	Pericarpium Arecae	大腹皮
Da Huang	Radix et Rhizoma Rhei	大黄
Da Huang Tan	Radix et Rhizoma Rhei Carbonisatus	大黄炭
Da Ji	Radix Euphorbiae seu Knoxiae	大戟
Da Ji	Herba Cirsii Japonici	大蓟
Da Ji Gen	Radix Cirsii Japonici	大蓟根
Da Ji Tan	Herba Cirsii Japonici Carbonisatum	大蓟炭
Da Ji Ye	Folium Cirsii Japonici	大蓟叶
Da Ma Yao	Radix Dolichi	大麻药
Da Qing Ye	Folium Isatidis	大青叶
Da Suan	Bulbus Alli Sativi	大蒜
Da Xiao Ji	Herba Cirsii	大小蓟
Da Xue Teng	Caulis Sargentodoxae	大血藤
Da Ye Ma Dou Ling	Caulis Aristolochiae Kaempferi	大叶马兜铃
Da Zao	Fructus Jujubae	大枣
Dai Mao	Carapax Eretmochelydis Imbricatae	玳瑁
Dan Dou Chi	Semen Sojae Praeparatum	淡豆豉
Dan Fan	Chalcanthite	胆矾
Dan Nan Xing	Arisaema cum Bile	胆南星
Dan Shen	Radix et Rhizoma Salviae Miltiorrhizae	丹参
Dan Zhu Ye	Herba Lophatheri	淡竹叶
Dang Gui	Radix Angelicae Sinensis	当归
Dang Gui Shen	Corpus Radix Angelicae Sinensis	当归身
Dang Gui Tou	Caput Radix Angelicae Sinensis	当归头
Dang Gui Wei	Extremitas Radix Angelicae Sinensis	当归尾
Dang Shen	Radix Codonopsis	党参
Dao Di Wu Gong	Rhizoma Heliminthostachytis	倒地蜈蚣
Dao Diao Jin Zhong	Melothria Maderospatana	倒吊金钟
Dao Dou	Semen Canavaliae	刀豆
Dao Ya	Fructus Oryzae Germinatus	稻芽
Deng Xin Cao	Medulla Junci	灯心草
Deng Zhan Hua	Herba Erigerontis	灯盏花
Di Feng Pi	Cortex Illicii	地枫皮
Di Fu Zi	Fructus Kochiae	地肤子
Di Gu Pi	Cortex Lycii	地骨皮
Di Huang	Radix Rehmanniae	地黄
Di Jin Cao	Herba Euphorbiae Humifusae	地锦草
Di Long	Pheretima	地龙
Di Yu	Radix Sanguisorbae	地榆

Appendix 7 — Cross-reference of Single Herb Names

Pinyin Names	Pharmaceutical Names	Chinese Names
Di Yu Tan	Radix Sanguisorbae Carbonisatum	地榆炭
Dian Qie Cao	Herba Belladonnae	颠茄草
Ding Gong Teng	Caulis Erycibes	丁公藤
Ding Jing Cao	Herba Linderniae	定经草
Ding Shu Xiu	Herba Elephantopus Scaber	丁竖杇
Ding Xiang	Flos Caryophylli	丁香
Ding Xiang Pi	Cortex Caryophylli	丁香皮
Dong Chong Xia Cao	Cordyceps	冬虫夏草
Dong Gua Pi	Exocarpium Benincasae	冬瓜皮
Dong Gua Zi	Semen Benincasae	冬瓜子
Dong Kui Guo	Fructus Malvae	冬葵子
Dong Ling Cao	Herba Rabdosiae	冬凌草
Dong Qing Ye	Folium Ilexis	冬青叶
Dong Yang Shen	Radix et Rhizoma Ginseng Japonica	东洋参
Dou Kou	Fructus Amomi Rotundus	豆蔻
Dou Kou Ke	Pericarpium Amomi Rotundus	豆蔻壳
Du Huo	Radix Angelicae Pubescentis	独活
Du Yi Wei	Herba Lamiophlomis	独一味
Du Zhong	Cortex Eucommiae	杜仲
Du Zhong Ye	Folium Eucommiae	杜仲叶
Duan Ge Qiao	Concha Meretricis seu Cyclinae Calcinata	煅蛤壳
Duan Mu Li	Concha Ostreae Calcinata	煅牡蛎
Duan Shi Gao	Gypsum Fibrosum Praeparatum	煅石膏
Duan Shi Jue Ming	Concha Haliotidis Calcinata	煅石决明
Duan Wa Leng Zi	Concha Arcae Calcinata	煅瓦楞子
Duan Xue Liu	Herba Clinopodii	断血流
Duan Zhen Zhu Mu	Concha Margaritiferae Calcinata	煅珍珠母
Duan Zui Lao Guan Cao	Herba Geranii	短嘴老鹳草
E Bu Shi Cao	Herba Centipedae	鹅不食草
E Jiao	Colla Corii Asini	阿胶
E Zhu	Rhizoma Curcumae	莪术
Er Cha	Catechu	儿茶
Fa Ban Xia	Rhizoma Pinelliae Praeparatum	法半夏
Fan Xie Ye	Folium Sennae	番泻叶
Fang Feng	Radix Saposhnikoviae	防风
Fang Ji	Radix Stephaniae Tetrandrae	防己
Fang Jie Shi	Calcitum	方解石
Fei Zi	Semen Torreyae	榧子
Fen Bi Xie	Rhizoma Dioscoreae Hypoglaucae	粉萆薢
Fen Gen	Radix Puerariae Thomsonii	粉葛
Feng Fang	Nidus Vespae	蜂房

Appendix 7 — Cross-reference of Single Herb Names

Pinyin Names	Pharmaceutical Names	Chinese Names
Feng Jiao	Propolis	峰胶
Feng La	Cera Flava	峰蜡
Feng Mi	Mel	蜂蜜
Feng Wei Cao	Herba Pteris	凤尾草
Feng Xiang Zhi	Resina Liquidambaris	风香脂
Fo Shou	Fructus Citri Sarcodactylis	佛手
Fo Shou Hua	Flos Citri Sarcodactylis	佛手花
Fu Fang Teng	Herba Euonymi	扶芳藤
Fu Hai Shi	Pumice	浮海石
Fu Ling	Poria	茯苓
Fu Ling Pi	Cortex Poria	茯苓皮
Fu Long Gan	Terra Flava Usta	伏龙肝
Fu Pen Zi	Fructus Rubi	覆盆子
Fu Ping	Herba Spirodelae	浮萍
Fu Rong	Radix Hibisci	芙蓉
Fu Rong Ye	Folium Hibisci	芙蓉叶
Fu Shen	Poria Paradicis	茯神
Fu Shou Cao	Herba Adonis	福寿草
Fu Xiao Mai	Fructus Tritici Levis	浮小麦
Fu Zi	Radix Aconiti Lateralis Praeparata	附子
Gan Cao	Radix et Rhizoma Glycyrrhizae	甘草
Gan Jiang	Rhizoma Zingiberis	干姜
Gan Qi	Resina Toxicodendri	干漆
Gan Qing Qing Lan	Herba Dracoephali Tangutici	甘青青兰
Gan Song	Radix et Rhizoma Nardostachydis	甘松
Gan Sui	Radix Kansui	甘遂
Gang Ban Gui	Herba Polygoni Perfoliati	杠板归
Gao Ben	Rhizoma et Radix Ligustici	藁本
Gao Liang Jiang	Rhizoma Alpiniae Officinarum	高良姜
Ge Gen	Radix Puerariae Lobatae	葛根
Ge Hua	Flos Puerariae	葛花
Ge Jie	Gecko	蛤蚧
Ge Qiao	Concha Meretricis seu Cyclinae	蛤壳
Geng Mi	Semen Oryzae	粳米
Geng Tong Cao	Ramulus Aeschynomene Indica	梗通草
Gong Lao Mu	Caulis Mahoniae	功劳木
Gong Lau Ye	Folium Mahoniae	功劳叶
Gou Gu	Os Canitis	狗骨
Gou Gu Ye	Folium Ilicis Cornutae	枸骨叶
Gou Ji	Rhizoma Cibotii	狗脊
Gou Qi Gen	Radix Lycii	枸杞根

Appendix 7 — Cross-reference of Single Herb Names

Pinyin Names	Pharmaceutical Names	Chinese Names
Gou Qi Ye	Folium Lycii	枸杞叶
Gou Qi Zi	Fructus Lycii	枸杞子
Gou Teng	Ramulus Uncariae cum Uncis	钩藤
Gou Wen	Herba Gelsemii Elegantis	钩吻
Gu Jing Cao	Flos Eriocauli	谷精草
Gu Sui Bu	Rhizoma Drynariae	骨碎补
Gu Ya	Fructus Setariae Germinatus	谷芽
Gua Di	Pedicellus Cucumeris	瓜蒂
Gua Lou	Fructus Trichosanthis	瓜蒌
Gua Lou Pi	Pericarpium Trichosanthis	瓜蒌皮
Gua Lou Zi	Semen Trichosanthis	瓜蒌子
Guan Bai Fu	Radix Aconiti Coreani	关白附
Guan Huang Bo	Cortex Phellodendri Amurensis	关黄柏
Guan Mu Tong	Caulis Aristolochiae Manshuriensis	关木通
Guan Ye Jin Si Tao	Herba Hyperici Perforati	贯叶金丝桃
Guang Fang Ji	Radix Aristolochiae Fangchi	广防己
Guang Huo Xiang	Herba Pogostemonis	广藿香
Guang Jin Qian Cao	Herba Desmodii Styracifolii	广金钱草
Guang Zao	Fructus Choerospondiatis	广枣
Gui Ban	Plastrum Testudinis	龟板
Gui Ban Jiao	Gelatinum Plastrum Testudinis	龟板胶
Gui Jia	Carapax et Plastrum Testudinis	龟甲
Gui Jia Jiao	Colla Carapax et Plastrum Testudinis	龟甲胶
Gui Xin	Cortex Rasus Cinnamomi	桂心
Gui Zhen Cao	Herba Bidentis Bipinnatae	鬼针草
Gui Zhi	Ramulus Cinnamomi	桂枝
Hai Dai	Thallus Laminariae	海带
Hai Feng Teng	Caulis Piperis Kadsurae	海风藤
Hai Fu Rong	Herba Limonium Wrightii	海芙蓉
Hai Gou Shen	Testes et Penis Otariae	海狗肾
Hai Jin Sha	Spora Lygodii	海金砂
Hai Long	Syngnathus	海龙
Hai Ma	Hippocampus	海马
Hai Piao Xiao	Endoconcha Sepiae	海螵蛸
Hai Shen	Strichopus Japonicus	海参
Hai Tong Pi	Cortex Erythrinae	海桐皮
Hai Zao	Sargassum	海藻
Han Shui Shi	Mirabilite	寒水石
He Cao Ya	Gemma Agrimoniae	鹤草芽
He Di	Calyx Nelumbinis	荷蒂
He Geng	Caulis Nelumbinis	荷梗

Appendix 7 — Cross-reference of Single Herb Names

Pinyin Names	Pharmaceutical Names	Chinese Names
He Huan Hua	Flos Albiziae	合欢花
He Huan Pi	Cortex Albiziae	合欢皮
He Shi	Fructus Carpesii	鹤虱
He Shou Wu	Radix Polygoni Multiflori	何首乌
He Tao Qiu Pi	Cortex Juglandis	核桃楸皮
He Tao Ren	Semen Juglandis	核桃仁
He Ye	Folium Nelumbinis	荷叶
He Zi	Fructus Chebulae	诃子
Hei Da Zao	Fructus Jujubae Nigrum	黑大枣
Hei Dou	Semen Sojae	黑豆
Hei Xi	Lead	黑锡
Hei Zhi Ma	Semen Sesami Nigrum	黑芝麻
Hei Zhong Cao Zi	Semen Nigellae	黑种草子
Hong Da Ji	Radix Knoxiae	红大戟
Hong Dou Kou	Fructus Galangae	红豆蔻
Hong Fen	Hydrargyri Oxydum Rubrum	红粉
Hong Gu She	Radix Kadsura Japonicae	红骨蛇
Hong Han Lian	Herba Hypericum Ascyron	红旱莲
Hong Hua	Flos Carthami	红花
Hong Jing Tian	Radix et Rhizoma Rhodiolae Crenulatae	红景天
Hong Qi	Radix Hedysari	红芪
Hong Qu	Monascus	红曲
Hong Shen	Radix et Rhizoma Ginseng Rubra	红参
Hong Shi Gao	Gypsum Rubrae	红石膏
Hou Po	Cortex Magnoliae Officinalis	厚朴
Hou Po Hua	Flos Magnoliae Officinalis	厚朴花
Hu Bei Bei Mu	Bulbus Fritillariae Hupehensis	湖北贝母
Hu Gu	Os Tigris	虎骨
Hu Huang Lian	Rhizoma Picrorhizae	胡黄连
Hu Ji Sheng	Herba Visci	槲寄生
Hu Jiao	Fructus Piperis	胡椒
Hu Lu Ba	Semen Trigonellae	胡芦巴
Hu Po	Succinum	琥珀
Hu Yao Huang	Herba Leucas Mollissimae	虎咬癀
Hu Zhang	Rhizoma et Radix Polygoni Cuspidati	虎杖
Hua Jiao	Pericarpium Zanthoxyli	花椒
Hua Ju Hong	Exocarpium Citri Grandis	化橘红
Hua Rui Shi	Ophicalcitum	花蕊石
Hua Shan Shen	Radix Physochlainae	华山参
Hua Shi	Talcum	滑石
Hua Shi Cao	Herba Orthosiphon Aristatus	化石草

Appendix 7 — Cross-reference of Single Herb Names

Pinyin Names	Pharmaceutical Names	Chinese Names
Hua Shi Fen	Pulvis Talci	滑石粉
Huai Hua	Flos Sophorae	槐花
Huai Hua Tan	Flos Sophorae Carbonisatum	槐花炭
Huai Jiao	Fructus Sophorae	槐角
Huai Mi	Flos Sophorae Immaturus	槐米
Huai Tong Ma Dou Ling	Caulis Aristolochiae Moupinensis	淮通马兜铃
Huang Bo	Cortex Phellodendri Chinensis	黄柏
Huang Hua Jia Zhu Tao	Semen Thevetiae	黄花夹竹桃
Huang Jie Zi	Semen Brassicae	黄芥子
Huang Jin	Gold	黄金
Huang Jin Gui	Caulis Vanieriae	黄金桂
Huang Jing	Rhizoma Polygonati	黄精
Huang Jing Zi	Fructus Viticis Negundis	黄荆子
Huang Lian	Rhizoma Coptidis	黄连
Huang Niu Jiao	Cornus Bovis	黄牛角
Huang Qi	Radix Astragali	黄芪
Huang Qin	Radix Scutellariae	黄芩
Huang Shui Qie	Herba Solani	黄水茄
Huang Teng	Caulis Fibraureae	黄藤
Huang Yang Jiao	Cornu Procapra Gutturosa	黄羊角
Huang Yao Zi	Herba Dioscoreae Bulbiferae	黄药子
Huo Ma Ren	Fructus Cannabis	火麻仁
Huo Xiang	Herba Agastaches	藿香
Huo Xiang Ye	Folium Agastaches	藿香叶
Ji Gu Cao	Herba Abri	鸡骨草
Ji Guan Hua	Flos Celosiae Cristatae	鸡冠花
Ji Li	Fructus Tribuli	蒺藜
Ji Nei Jin	Endothelium Corneum Gigeriae Galli	鸡内金
Ji Xiang Teng	Caulis Paederiae	鸡香藤
Ji Xing Zi	Semen Impatientis	急性子
Ji Xue Cao	Herba Centellae	积雪草
Ji Xue Teng	Caulis Spatholobi	鸡血藤
Ji Zi Huang	Galli Vitellus	鸡子黄
Jia Zhu Tao	Folium Cortex et Radix Nerii	夹竹桃
Jian Shen Qu	Massa Fermentata Praeparata	建神曲
Jiang Can	Bombyx Batryticatus	僵蚕
Jiang Huang	Rhizoma Curcumae Longae	姜黄
Jiang Xiang	Lignum Dalbergiae Odoriferae	降香
Jiao Bing Lang	Semen Arecae Praeparata	焦槟榔
Jiao Gu Lan	Rhizoma seu Herba Gynostemmatis	绞股蓝
Jiao Mu	Semen Zanthoxyli Bungeani	椒目

Appendix 7 — Cross-reference of Single Herb Names

Pinyin Names	Pharmaceutical Names	Chinese Names
Jiao Zhi Zi	Fructus Gardeniae Praeparatus	焦栀子
Jie Geng	Radix Platycodonis	桔梗
Jie Lie Xiao Hui Xiang	Herba Hypecoe Leptocarpe	节裂小茴香
Jie Zi	Semen Sinapis	芥子
Jin Bo	Gold foil	金箔
Jin Deng Long	Calyx seu Fructus Physalis	锦灯笼
Jin Fei Cao	Herba Inulae	金沸草
Jin Guo Lan	Radix Tinosporae	金果榄
Jin Meng Shi	Lapis Micae Aureus	金礞石
Jin Qian Bai Hua She	Bungarus Parvus	金钱白花蛇
Jin Qian Cao	Herba Lysimachiae	金钱草
Jin Qiao Mai	Rhizoma Fagopyri Dibotryis	金荞麦
Jin Yin Hua	Flos Lonicerae Japonicae	金银花
Jin Ying Gen	Radix Rosae Laevigatae	金樱根
Jin Ying Zi	Fructus Rosae Laevigatae	金樱子
Jing Da Ji	Radix Euphorbiae Pekinensis	京大戟
Jing Jie	Herba Schizonepetae	荆芥
Jing Jie Sui	Spica Schizonepetae	荆芥穗
Jing Jie Sui Tan	Spica Schizonepetae Carbonisatum	荆芥穗炭
Jing Jie Tan	Herba Schizonepetae Carbonisatum	荆芥炭
Jing Tian San Qi	Herba seu Radix Sedum Aizoom	景天三七
Jiu Cai Zi	Semen Allii Tuberosi	韭菜子
Jiu Ceng Ta	Herba Ocimi Basilici	九层塔
Jiu Jie Chang Pu	Rhizoma Anemones Altaicae	九节菖蒲
Jiu Li Xiang	Folium et Cacumen Murrayae	九里香
Jiu Xiang Chong	Aspongopus	九香虫
Ju He	Semen Citri Reticulatae	橘核
Ju Hong	Exocarpium Citri Rubrum	橘红
Ju Hua	Flos Chrysanthemi	菊花
Ju Ju	Herba et Radix Cichorii	菊苣
Ju Luo	Vascular Citri Reticulatae	橘络
Ju Ye	Folium Citri Reticulatae	橘叶
Ju Ye San Qi	Herba seu Radix Gynura Segetum	菊叶三七
Juan Bai	Herba Selaginellae	卷柏
Jue Ming Zi	Semen Cassiae	决明子
Ku Di Ding	Herba Corydalis Bungeanae	苦地丁
Ku Dou Cao	Herba Sophora Alopecuroidies	苦豆草
Ku Fan	Alumen Exsiccatum	苦矾
Ku Lian Pi	Cortex Meliae	苦楝皮
Ku Lian Zi	Fructus Meliae	苦楝子
Ku Mu	Ramulus et Folium Picrasmae	苦木

Appendix 7 — Cross-reference of Single Herb Names

Pinyin Names	Pharmaceutical Names	Chinese Names
Ku Shen	Radix Sophorae Flavescentis	苦参
Ku Shen Zi	Fructus Sophorae Flavescentis	苦参子
Ku Xing Ren	Semen Armeniacae Amarum	苦杏仁
Ku Xuan Shen	Herba Picriae	苦玄参
Kuan Dong Hua	Flos Farfarae	款冬花
Kun Bu	Thallus Eckloniae	昆布
Lai Fu Zi	Semen Raphani	莱菔子
Lang Du	Radix Euphorbiae Fischerianae	狼毒
Lao Guan Cao	Herba Erodii seu Geranii	老鹳草
Lei Gong Teng	Radix Tripterygii Wilfordii	雷公藤
Lei Wan	Omphalia	雷丸
Li Lu	Radix et Rhizoma Veratri	藜芦
Li Pi	Pericarpium Pyri	梨皮
Li Zhi He	Semen Litchi	荔枝核
Lian Fang	Receptaculum Nelumbinis	莲房
Lian Qian Cao	Herba Glechomae	连钱草
Lian Qiao	Fructus Forsythiae	连翘
Lian Xu	Stamen Nelumbinis	莲须
Lian Zi	Semen Nelumbinis	莲子
Lian Zi Xin	Plumula Nelumbinis	莲子心
Liang Mian Zhen	Radix Zanthoxyli	两面针
Liang Tou Jian	Rhizoma Anemones Raddeanae	两头尖
Liao Da Qing Ye	Folium Polygoni Tinctorii	蓼大青叶
Ling Xiao Hua	Flos Campsis	凌霄花
Ling Yang Jiao	Cornu Saigae Tataricae	羚羊角
Ling Yin Chen	Herba Siphonostegia Chinensis	铃茵陈
Ling Zhi	Ganoderma	灵芝
Liu Huang	Sulfur	硫黄
Liu Ji Nu	Herba Artemisiae Anomalae	刘寄奴
Liu Ye	Folium Salicis Babylonicae	柳叶
Liu Zhi Huang	Herba Solidaginis	柳枝癀
Long Chi	Dens Draconis	龙齿
Long Dan	Radix et Rhizoma Gentianae	龙胆
Long Gu	Os Draconis	龙骨
Long Kui	Herba Solanum Nigrum	龙葵
Long Yan He	Semen Longan	龙眼核
Long Yan Hua	Flos Longan	龙眼花
Long Yan Rou	Arillus Longan	龙眼肉
Lou Lu	Radix Rhapontici	漏芦
Lu Dou	Semen Phaseoli Radiati	绿豆
Lu Dou Yi	Pericarpium Phaseoli Radiati	绿豆衣

Appendix 7 — Cross-reference of Single Herb Names

Pinyin Names	Pharmaceutical Names	Chinese Names
Lu Gan Shi	Galamina	炉甘石
Lu Gen	Rhizoma Phragmitis	芦根
Lu Hui	Aloe	芦荟
Lu Jiao	Cornu Cervi	鹿角
Lu Jiao Jiao	Colla Cornus Cervi	鹿角胶
Lu Jiao Shuang	Cornu Cervi Degelatinatum	鹿角霜
Lu Lu Tong	Fructus Liquidambaris	路路通
Lu Rong	Cornu Cervi Pantotrichum	鹿茸
Lu Song Jiu Mao	Pilus Fructi Malloti	吕宋楸毛
Lu Xian Cao	Herba Pyrolae	鹿衔草
Luo Bu Ma	Herba Apocyni Veneti	罗布麻
Luo Bu Ma Ye	Folium Apocyni Veneti	罗布麻叶
Luo Han Guo	Fructus Momordicae	罗汉果
Luo Han Guo Ye	Folium Momordicae	罗汉果叶
Luo Shi Teng	Caulis Trachelospermi	络石藤
Luo Tuo Peng Zi	Semen Pegani Harmalae	骆驼蓬子
Ma An Teng	Herba Ipomoea Pes-caprae	马鞍藤
Ma Bian Cao	Herba Verbenae	马鞭草
Ma Bo	Lasiosphaera seu Calvatia	马勃
Ma Chi Xian	Herba Portulacae	马齿苋
Ma Dou Ling	Fructus Aristolochiae	马兜铃
Ma Huang	Herba Ephedrae	麻黄
Ma Huang Gen	Radix et Rhizoma Ephedrae	麻黄根
Ma Li Jin	Herba Asclepii	马利筋
Ma Qian Zi	Semen Strychni	马钱子
Ma Qian Zi Fen	Semen Strychni Pulveratum	马钱子粉
Ma Sang	Radix et Folium Coriariae	马桑
Ma Sang Gen	Radix Coriariae	马桑根
Ma Sang Ye	Folium Coriariae	马桑叶
Ma Ti Jin	Herba Dichondrae Repentis	马蹄金
Mai Dong	Radix Ophiopogonis	麦冬
Mai Jiao	Ergota	麦角
Mai Ya	Fructus Hordei Germinatus	麦芽
Mai Ya Qu	Fructus Hordei Germinatus Massa Fermentata	麦芽曲
Man Jing Zi	Fructus Viticis	蔓荆子
Man Shan Hong	Folium Rhododendri Daurici	满山红
Mang Cao	Fructus Illicium Lanceolatum	莽草
Mang Xiao	Natrii Sulfas	芒硝
Mao Dong Qing	Radix Ilicis Pubescentis	毛冬青
Mao Gen	Herba Ranunculi Japonici	毛茛
Mao He Zi	Fructus Terminaliae Billericae	毛诃子

Appendix 7 — Cross-reference of Single Herb Names

Pinyin Names	Pharmaceutical Names	Chinese Names
Mao Zhao Cao	Radix Ranunculi Ternati	猫爪草
Mao Zi Dun Tou	Herba Abutilon Indicum	帽仔盾头
Mei Gui Hua	Flos Rosae Rugosae	玫瑰花
Mei Hua	Flos Mume	梅花
Meng Chong	Tabanus	虻虫
Meng Shi	Lapis Micae seu Chloriti	礞石
Mi Jiao	Cornu Elaphuri	麋角
Mi Meng Hua	Flos Buddlejae	密蒙花
Mi Rong	Cornu Elaphuri Pantotrichum	麋茸
Mi Tuo Seng	Lithargyum	密陀僧
Mian Bi Xie	Rhizoma Dioscoreae Septemlobae	绵萆薢
Mian Hua Zi	Semen Gossypi	棉花子
Mian Ma Guan Zhong	Rhizoma Dryopteridis Crassirhizomatis	绵马贯众
Mian Ma Guan Zhong Tan	Rhizoma Dryopteridis Crassirhizomatis Carbonisatum	绵马贯众炭
Ming Dang Shen	Radix Changii	明党参
Mo Gu Xiao	Caulis Hyptis Capitatae	有骨消
Mo Han Lian	Herba Ecliptae	墨旱莲
Mo Yao	Myrrha	没药
Mu Bie Zi	Semen Momordicae	木鳖子
Mu Dan Pi	Cortex Moutan	牡丹皮
Mu Dan Ye	Folium Moutan	牡丹叶
Mu Ding Xiang	Fructus Caryophylli	母丁香
Mu Fang Ji	Radix Cocculi Trilobi	木防己
Mu Gua	Fructus Chaenomelis	木瓜
Mu Hu Die	Semen Oroxyli	木蝴蝶
Mu Jing Ye	Folium Viticis Negundo	牡荆叶
Mu Li	Concha Ostreae	牡蛎
Mu Ma Dou	Herba Thermopsis Lanceolatae	牧马豆
Mu Tong	Caulis Akebiae	木通
Mu Xiang	Radix Aucklandiae	木香
Mu Zei	Herba Equiseti Hiemalis	木贼
Nan Ban Lan Gen	Rhizoma et Radix Baphicacanthis Cusiae	南板蓝根
Nan Chai Hu	Radix Bupleurum Scorzonerifolfium	南柴胡
Nan Gua Zi	Semen Cucurbitae Moschatae	南瓜子
Nan He Shi	Fructus Carotae	南鹤虱
Nan Sha Shen	Radix Adenophorae	南沙参
Nan Ting Li Zi	Semen Descurainiae	南葶苈子
Nan Wu Wei Zi	Fructus Schisandrae Sphenantherae	南五味子
Nao Yang Hua	Flos Rhododendri Mollis	闹羊花
Niao Bu Su	Ramus Kalopanax Pictus	鸟不宿
Niu Bang Gen	Radix Arctii	牛蒡根

Appendix 7 — Cross-reference of Single Herb Names

Pinyin Names	Pharmaceutical Names	Chinese Names
Niu Bang Zi	Fructus Arctii	牛蒡子
Niu Dan	Fel Bovis	牛胆
Niu Huang	Calculus Bovis	牛黄
Niu Xi	Radix Achyranthis Bidentatae	牛膝
Nu Zhen Zi	Fructus Ligustri Lucidi	女贞子
Nuo Mi	Oryza Glutinosa	糯米
Ou Jie	Nodus Nelumbinis Rhizomatis	藕节
Pang Da Hai	Semen Sterculiae Lychnophorae	胖大海
Pao Jiang	Rhizoma Zingiberis Praeparatum	炮姜
Pao Zai Cao	Herba Physalis Angulatae	炮仔草
Pei Lan	Herba Eupatorii	佩兰
Peng Sha	Borax	硼砂
Pi Pa Ye	Folium Eriobotryae	枇杷叶
Pi Shi	Arsenolite	砒石
Pian Jiang Huang	Rhizoma Wenyujin Concisum	片姜黄
Ping Bei Mu	Bulbus Fritillariae Ussuriensis	平贝母
Po Bu Zi Ye	Folium Cordia Dichotoma	破布子叶
Po Xiao	Sal Glauberis	朴硝
Pu Gong Ying	Herba Taraxaci	蒲公英
Pu Huang	Pollen Typhae	蒲黄
Pu Huang Tan	Pollen Typhae Carbonisatum	蒲黄炭
Pu Tao Zi	Semen Vitis Viniferae	葡萄子
Pu Yin	Radix Wikstroemia Indica	埔银
Qi Dai	Corda Umbilicalis Hominis	脐带
Qi She	Agkistrodon	蕲蛇
Qi Ye Lian	Radix Schefflerae	七叶莲
Qian Cao	Radix et Rhizoma Rubiae	茜草
Qian Cao Tan	Radix et Rhizoma Rubiae Carbonisatus	茜草炭
Qian Ceng Ta	Herba Lycopodii Serrati	千层塔
Qian Dan	Minium	铅丹
Qian Hu	Radix Peucedani	前胡
Qian Jin Zi	Semen Euphorbiae	千金子
Qian Jin Zi Shuang	Semen Euphorbiae Pulveratum	千金子霜
Qian Li Guang	Herba Senecionis Scandens	千里光
Qian Nian Jian	Rhizoma Homalomenae	千年健
Qian Niu Zi	Semen Pharbitidis	牵牛子
Qian Shi	Semen Euryales	芡实
Qiang Huo	Rhizoma et Radix Notopterygii	羌活
Qiao Mai	Semen Fagopyri Esculenti	荞麦
Qin Jiao	Radix Gentianae Macrophyllae	秦艽
Qin Pi	Cortex Fraxini	秦皮

Appendix 7 — Cross-reference of Single Herb Names

Pinyin Names	Pharmaceutical Names	Chinese Names
Qing Dai	Indigo Naturalis	青黛
Qing Fen	Calomelas	轻粉
Qing Feng Teng	Caulis Sinomenii	青风藤
Qing Ge Qiao	Concha Cyclinae	青蛤壳
Qing Guo	Fructus Canarii	青果
Qing Guo Gen	Radix Canarii	青果根
Qing Hao	Herba Artemisiae Annuae	青蒿
Qing Ma Zi	Semen Abutili	苘麻子
Qing Meng Shi	Lapis Chloriti	青礞石
Qing Mu Xiang	Radix Aristolochiae	青木香
Qing Niu Jiao Fen	Cornus Bovis	青牛角粉
Qing Pi	Pericarpium Citri Reticulatae Viride	青皮
Qing Xiang Zi	Semen Celosiae	青葙子
Qing Ye Dan	Herba Swertiae Mileensis	青叶胆
Qu Mai	Herba Dianthi	瞿麦
Quan Shen	Rhizoma Bistortae	拳参
Quan Xie	Scorpio	全蝎
Ren Dong Cao	Herba Lonicerae Japonicae	忍冬草
Ren Dong Teng	Caulis Lonicerae Japonicae	忍冬藤
Ren Gong Niu Huang	Calculus Bovis Artifactus	人工牛黄
Ren Shen	Radix et Rhizoma Ginseng	人参
Ren Shen Ye	Folium Ginseng	人参叶
Ren Zhong Bai	Urinae Hominis Sedimen	人中白
Rou Cong Rong	Herba Cistanches	肉苁蓉
Rou Dou Gen	Radix Myristicae	肉豆根
Rou Dou Kou	Semen Myristicae	肉豆蔻
Rou Gui	Cortex Cinnamomi	肉桂
Ru Xiang	Gummi Olibanum	乳香
Rui Ren	Nux Prinsepiae	蕤仁
San Bai Cao	Herba Saururi	三白草
San Leng	Rhizoma Sparganii	三棱
San Qi	Radix et Rhizoma Notoginseng	三七
San Qi Ye	Folium Notoginseng	三七叶
Sang Bai Pi	Cortex Mori	桑白皮
Sang Ji Sheng	Herba Taxilli	桑寄生
Sang Piao Xiao	Ootheca Mantidis	桑螵蛸
Sang Shen	Fructus Mori	桑椹
Sang Ye	Folium Mori	桑叶
Sang Zhi	Ramulus Mori	桑枝
Sha Ji	Fructus Hippophae	沙棘
Sha Ren	Fructus Amomi	砂仁

Appendix 7 — Cross-reference of Single Herb Names

Pinyin Names	Pharmaceutical Names	Chinese Names
Sha Ren Ke	Pericarpium Amomi	砂仁壳
Sha Shen	Radix Glehniae seu Adenophorae	沙参
Sha Yuan Zi	Semen Astragali Complanati	沙苑子
Shan Ci Gu	Pseudobulbus Cremastrae seu Pleiones	山慈姑
Shan Dou Gen	Radix et Rhizoma Sophorae Tonkinensis	山豆根
Shan Geng Cai	Herba Lobeliae Sessilifoliae	山梗菜
Shan Ma Ti	Radix Rauvolfiae Hainanensis	山马蹄
Shan Mai Dong	Radix Liriopes	山麦冬
Shan Nai	Rhizoma Kaempferiae	山柰
Shan Pu Tao	Radix Vitis Amurensis	山葡萄
Shan Yang Jiao	Cornu Naemorhedis	山羊角
Shan Yao	Rhizoma Dioscoreae	山药
Shan Yin Hua	Flos Lonicerae	山银花
Shan Zha	Fructus Crataegi	山楂
Shan Zha Tan	Fructus Crataegi Carbonisatum	山楂炭
Shan Zha Ye	Folium Crataegi	山楂叶
Shan Zhu Yu	Fructus Corni	山茱萸
Shang Lu	Radix Phytolaccae	商陆
She Chuang Zi	Fructus Cnidii	蛇床子
She Dan	Fel Serpentis	蛇胆
She Gan	Rhizoma Belamcandae	射干
She Tui	Periostracum Serpentis	蛇蜕
She Xiang	Moschus	麝香
Shen Jin Cao	Herba Lycopodii	伸筋草
Shen Qu	Massa Fermentata	神曲
Sheng Fu Zi	Radix Aconiti Lateralis	生附子
Sheng Jiang	Rhizoma Zingiberis Recens	生姜
Sheng Jiang Pi	Pericarpium Zingiberis Recens	生姜皮
Sheng Ma	Rhizoma Cimicifugae	升麻
Sheng Tie Luo	Frusta Ferri	生铁落
Shi Chang Pu	Rhizoma Acori Tatarinowii	石菖蒲
Shi Di	Calyx Kaki	柿蒂
Shi Gao	Gypsum Fibrosum	石膏
Shi Hu	Caulis Dendrobii	石斛
Shi Jue Ming	Concha Haliotidis	石决明
Shi Jun Zi	Fructus Quisqualis	使君子
Shi Lian Zi	Herba Sinocrassulae Indicae	石莲子
Shi Liu Gen Pi	Cortex Radix Granati	石榴根皮
Shi Liu Guo	Fructus Granati	石榴果
Shi Liu Pi	Pericarpium Granati	石榴皮
Shi Liu Pi Tan	Pericarpium Granati Carbonisatum	石榴皮炭

Appendix 7 — Cross-reference of Single Herb Names

Pinyin Names	Pharmaceutical Names	Chinese Names
Shi Luo	Fructus Anethum Graveolens	莳萝
Shi Nan Teng	Ramulus Piper	石南藤
Shi Nan Ye	Folium Photiniae	石南叶
Shi Suan	Bulbus Lycoris	石蒜
Shi Wei	Folium Pyrrosiae	石韦
Shi Xian Tao	Pseudobulbus Pholidotae Chinensis	石仙桃
Shou Wu Teng	Caulis Polygoni Multiflori	首乌藤
Shu Di Huang	Radix Rehmanniae Praeparata	熟地黄
Shu Hua Sha Shen	Radix Adenophorae Remotiflora	疏花沙参
Shu Qi	Folium Dichroae	蜀漆
Shu Wei Huang	Herba Rostellulariae	鼠尾癀
Shuang Liu Huang	Herba Vernoniae Patulae	双柳黄
Shui Ban Xia	Rhizoma Typhonii Flagelliformis	水半夏
Shui Ding Xiang	Herba Ludwigiae Prostratae	水丁香
Shui Fei Ji	Fructus Silybi	水飞蓟
Shui Hong Hua Zi	Fructus Polygoni Orientalis	水红花子
Shui Niu Jiao	Cornu Bubali	水牛角
Shui Yin	Hydrargyrum	水银
Shui Zhi	Hirudo	水蛭
Si Chuan Da Jin Qian Cao	Herba Lysimachia Christinae	四川大金钱草
Si Gua Luo	Retinervus Luffae Fructus	丝瓜络
Song Guo	Fructus Pini	松果
Song Hua Fen	Pollen Pini	松花粉
Song Jie	Lignum Pini Nodi	松节
Song Luo	Herba Usneae	松萝
Song Ye	Folium Pini	松叶
Su He Xiang	Styrax	苏合香
Su Mu	Lignum Sappan	苏木
Suan Zao Ren	Semen Ziziphi Spinosae	酸枣仁
Suo Luo Zi	Semen Aesculi	娑罗子
Suo Yang	Herba Cynomorii	锁阳
Tai Zi Shen	Radix Pseudostellariae	太子参
Tan Xiang	Lignum Santali Albi	檀香
Tao Ren	Semen Persicae	桃仁
Teng Huang	Resina Garciniae	藤黄
Tian Dong	Radix Asparagi	天冬
Tian Hua Fen	Radix Trichosanthis	天花粉
Tian Kui Zi	Radix Semiaquilegiae	天葵子
Tian Ma	Rhizoma Gastrodiae	天麻
Tian Nan Xing	Rhizoma Arisaematis	天南星
Tian Ran Bing Pian	Borneolum	天然冰片

Appendix 7 — Cross-reference of Single Herb Names

Pinyin Names	Pharmaceutical Names	Chinese Names
Tian Shan Xue Lian	Herba Saussureae Involucratae	天山雪莲
Tian Xian Teng	Herba Aristolochiae	天仙藤
Tian Xian Zi	Semen Hyoscyami	天仙子
Tian Zhu Huang	Concretio Silicea Bambusae	天竺黄
Tian Zhu Zi	Fructus Nandinae Domesticae	天竹子
Ting Li Zi	Semen Descurainiae seu Lepidii	葶苈子
Tong Bian	Infantis Urina	童便
Tong Cao	Medulla Tetrapanacis	通草
Tou Gu Cao	Caulis Impatientis	透骨草
Tu Bei Mu	Rhizoma Bolbostematis	土贝母
Tu Bie Chong	Eupolyphaga seu Steleophaga	土鳖虫
Tu Fu Ling	Rhizoma Smilacis Glabrae	土茯苓
Tu Jing Jie	Herba Chenopodii	土荆芥
Tu Jing Pi	Cortex Pseudolaricis	土荆皮
Tu Mu Xiang	Radix Inulae	土木香
Tu Niu Xi	Radix Achyranthis Longifoliae	土牛膝
Tu Rou Gui	Cortex Cinnamomum Burmannium	土肉桂
Tu Si Zi	Semen Cuscutae	菟丝子
Tu Xi Xin	Herba Asari Forbesii	土细辛
Wa Leng Zi	Concha Arcae	瓦楞子
Wa Song	Herba Orostachyis Fimbriati	瓦松
Wan Dian Jin	Radix Ilicis Asprellae	万点金
Wan Nian Qing	Rhizoma et Herba Rohdea	万年青
Wang Bu Liu Xing	Semen Vaccariae	王不留行
Wei Ling Cai	Herba Potentillae Chinensis	委陵菜
Wei Ling Xian	Radix et Rhizoma Clematidis	威灵仙
Wen Ge Qiao	Concha Meretricis	文蛤壳
Wu Bei Zi	Galla Chinensis	五倍子
Wu Gong	Scolopendra	蜈蚣
Wu Jia Pi	Cortex Acanthopanacis	五加皮
Wu Jiu	Cortex Radix Sapii	乌桕
Wu Ling Zhi	Faeces Trogopteri seu Pteromi	五灵脂
Wu Long Cha	Folium Camellia Fermentata	乌龙茶
Wu Mei	Fructus Mume	乌梅
Wu Ming Yi	Pyrolusitum	无名异
Wu Shao She	Zaocys	乌梢蛇
Wu Teng	Ramulus Linderae	乌藤
Wu Tian	Radix et Folium Viticis Quinatae	乌甜
Wu Tong Zi	Semen Firmianae	梧桐子
Wu Wei Zi	Fructus Schisandrae Chinensis	五味子
Wu Yao	Radix Linderae	乌药

Appendix 7 — Cross-reference of Single Herb Names

Pinyin Names	Pharmaceutical Names	Chinese Names
Wu Ye Mu Tong	Caulis Quinata	五叶木通
Wu Yi	Fructus Ulmi Praeparatus	芜荑
Wu Zhu Yu	Fructus Evodiae	吴茱萸
Xi Gua	Fructus Citrulli	西瓜
Xi Gua Cui Pi	Exocarpium Citrulli	西瓜翠皮
Xi Gua Pi	Pericarpium Citrulli	西瓜皮
Xi Gua Shuang	Mirabilitum Praeparatum	西瓜霜
Xi He Liu	Cacumen Tamaricis	西合柳
Xi Hong Hua	Stigma Croci	西红花
Xi Huang	Calculus Bovis	犀黄
Xi Jiao	Cornu Rhinoceri	犀角
Xi Qing Guo	Fructus Chebulae Immaturus	西青果
Xi Shu	Camptotheca	喜树
Xi Xian Cao	Herba Siegesbeckiae	豨莶草
Xi Xin	Radix et Rhizoma Asari	细辛
Xi Yang Shen	Radix Panacis Quinquefolii	西洋参
Xia Ku Cao	Spica Prunellae	夏枯草
Xia Ku Hua	Flos Prunellae	夏枯花
Xia Tian Wu	Rhizoma Corydalis Decumbentis	夏天无
Xian Di Huang	Radix Rehmanniae Recens	鲜地黄
Xian Feng Cao	Herba Bidentis	咸丰草
Xian He Cao	Herba Agrimoniae	仙鹤草
Xian Mao	Rhizoma Curculiginis	仙茅
Xiang Fu	Rhizoma Cyperi	香附
Xiang Jia Pi	Cortex Periplocae	香加皮
Xiang Ru	Herba Moslae	香薷
Xiang Si Cao	Herba Eupatorii Formosani	相思草
Xiang Si Zi	Semen Abrus Precatoris	相思子
Xiang Yuan	Fructus Citri	香橼
Xiao Hui Xiang	Fructus Foeniculi	小茴香
Xiao Ji	Herba Cirsii	小蓟
Xiao Jin Ying	Fructus Rosae Cymosae	小金樱
Xiao Mai	Fructus Tritici	小麦
Xiao Tong Cao	Medulla Stachyuri seu Helwingiae	小通草
Xiao Ye Lian	Fructus Podophylli	小叶莲
Xie Bai	Bulbus Allii Macrostemonis	薤白
Xie Cao	Radix et Rhizoma Valerianae	缬草
Xin Yi	Flos Magnoliae	辛夷
Xing Ren Shu Pi	Cortex Pruni Armeniacae	杏仁树皮
Xiong Dan	Fel Ursi	熊胆
Xiong Huang	Realgar	雄黄

Appendix 7 — Cross-reference of Single Herb Names

Pinyin Names	Pharmaceutical Names	Chinese Names
Xu Chang Qing	Radix et Rhizoma Cynanchi Paniculati	徐长卿
Xu Duan	Radix Dipsaci	续断
Xuan Diao Zi Jing	Ramulus Rubi	悬钓子茎
Xuan Fu Hua	Flos Inulae	旋覆花
Xuan Ming Fen	Natrii Sulfas Exsiccatus	玄明粉
Xuan Shen	Radix Scrophulariae	玄参
Xue Jie	Sanguis Draconis	血竭
Xue Shang Yi Zhi Hao	Radix Aconiti Brachypodi	雪上一枝蒿
Xue Yu Tan	Crinis Carbonisatus	血余炭
Xun Gu Feng	Herba Aristolochiae Mollissimae	寻骨风
Ya Dan Zi	Fructus Bruceae	鸦胆子
Ya Hu Nu	Herba Cissampelotis	亚乎奴
Ya Ma Zi	Semen Lini	亚麻子
Ya She Huang	Herba Lippiae	鸭舌癀
Ya Zhi Cao	Herba Commelinae	鸭跖草
Yan Hu Suo	Rhizoma Corydalis	延胡索
Yang Dan	Fel Capra seu Ovis	羊胆
Yang Jiao Ao	Fructus Strophanthi	羊角拗
Yang Jin Hua	Flos Daturae	洋金花
Yang Qi Shi	Actinolitum	阳起石
Yang Ti	Radix Rumicis Japonici	羊蹄
Ye Ju Hua	Flos Chrysanthemi Indici	野菊花
Ye Ming Sha	Faeces Vespertilionis Murini	夜明砂
Ye Ying Pi	Pericarpium Prunus Pseudocerasus	野樱皮
Yi Bei Mu	Bulbus Fritillariae Pallidiflorae	伊贝母
Yi Mu Cao	Herba Leonuri	益母草
Yi Tang	Maltosum	饴糖
Yi Tiao Gen	Radix Moghaniae	一条根
Yi Wu Gen	Radix Elaeagni	宜梧根
Yi Ye Qiu	Radix Securinegae Suffruticosae	一叶萩
Yi Yi Gen	Radix Coicis	薏苡根
Yi Yi Ren	Semen Coicis	薏苡仁
Yi Zhi	Fructus Alpiniae Oxyphyllae	益智
Yi Zhi Xiang	Herba Vernoniae Cinereae	一枝香
Yin Bo	Silver foil	银箔
Yin Chai Hu	Radix Stellariae	银柴胡
Yin Chen	Herba Artemisiae Scopariae	茵陈
Yin Xing Ye	Folium Ginkgo	银杏叶
Yin Yang Huo	Herba Epimedii	淫羊藿
Yin Yu	Caulis et Folium Skimmiae	茵芋
Ying Su Ke	Pericarpium Papaveris	罂粟壳

Appendix 7 — Cross-reference of Single Herb Names

Pinyin Names	Pharmaceutical Names	Chinese Names
You Chong Zhu	Blattela	油虫珠
Yu Gan Zi	Fructus Phyllanthi	余甘子
Yu Jin	Radix Curcumae	郁金
Yu Li Ren	Semen Pruni	郁李仁
Yu Mi Xu	Stigma Maydis	玉米须
Yu Teng	Radix seu Herba Derridis Trifoliatae	鱼藤
Yu Xing Cao	Herba Houttuyniae	鱼腥草
Yu Yu Liang	Limonitum	禹余粮
Yu Zhi Zi	Fructus Akebiae	预知子
Yu Zhou Lou Lu	Radix Echinopsis	禹州漏芦
Yu Zhu	Rhizoma Polygonati Odorati	玉竹
Yuan Hua	Flos Genkwa	芫花
Yuan Zhi	Radix Polygalae	远志
Yue Ji Hua	Flos Rosae Chinensis	月季花
Yun Zhi	Coriolus	云芝
Zang Chang Pu	Rhizoma Acori Calami	藏菖蒲
Zao Jiao	Fructus Gleditsiae	皂角
Zao Jiao Ci	Spina Gleditsiae	皂角刺
Ze Lan	Herba Lycopi	泽兰
Ze Qi	Herba Euphorbiae Helioscopiae	泽漆
Ze Xie	Rhizoma Alismatis	泽泻
Zhang Mu Xiang	Radix Inulae Racemosae	藏木香
Zhang Nao	Camphora	樟脑
Zhang Ya Cai	Herba Swertae	獐牙菜
Zhao Shan Bai	Folium Rhododendri Micranthi	照山白
Zhe Bei Mu	Bulbus Fritillariae Thunbergii	浙贝母
Zhe Shi	Haematitum	赭石
Zhen Zhu	Margarita	珍珠
Zhen Zhu Mu	Concha Margaritiferae	珍珠母
Zhi Cao Wu	Radix Aconiti Kusnezoffii Praeparata	制草乌
Zhi Chuan Wu	Radix Aconiti Praeparata	制川乌
Zhi Gan Cao	Radix et Rhizoma Glycyrrhizae Praeparata cum Melle	炙甘草
Zhi He Shou Wu	Radix Polygoni Multiflori Praeparata cum Succo Glycines Sojae	炙何首乌
Zhi Hong Qi	Radix Hedysari Praeparata cum Melle	炙红芪
Zhi Huang Qi	Radix Astragali Praeparata cum Melle	炙黄芪
Zhi Ju Zi	Fructus Hoveniae	枳椇子
Zhi Ma Huang	Herba Ephedrae Praeparata	炙麻黄
Zhi Mu	Rhizoma Anemarrhenae	知母
Zhi Qiao	Fructus Aurantii	枳壳
Zhi Qiao Tan	Fructus Aurantii Carbonisatum	枳壳炭

Appendix 7 — Cross-reference of Single Herb Names

Pinyin Names	Pharmaceutical Names	Chinese Names
Zhi Shi	Fructus Aurantii Immaturus	枳实
Zhi Xie Mu Zi	Semen Holarrhena Antidysentericae	止泻木子
Zhi Zi	Fructus Gardeniae	栀子
Zhi Zi Pi	Pericarpium Gardeniae	栀子皮
Zhi Zi Ren	Semen Gardeniae	栀子仁
Zhong Jie Feng	Herba Sarcandrae	肿节风
Zhong Ru Shi	Stalactitum	钟乳石
Zhu Dan	Fel Porcus	猪胆
Zhu Dan Fen	Pulvis Fellis Suis	猪胆粉
Zhu Fan Hua Tou	Rhizoma Mirabilidis	煮饭花头
Zhu Gu	Os Porcus	猪骨
Zhu Jie Shen	Rhizoma Panacis Japonici	竹节参
Zhu Li	Succus Bambusae	竹沥
Zhu Ling	Polyporus	猪苓
Zhu Ru	Caulis Bambusae in Taenia	竹茹
Zhu Sha	Cinnabaris	朱砂
Zhu Sha Gen	Radix Ardisiae Crenatae	朱砂根
Zhu Ya Zao	Fructus Gleditsiae Abnormalis	猪牙皂
Zhu Ye	Herba Phyllostachys	竹叶
Zhu Zi Cao	Herba Euphorbiae Thymifoliae	珠仔草
Zhu Zi Shen	Rhizoma Panacis Majoris	珠子参
Zi Bei Tian Kui	Herba Semiaquilegiae	紫背天葵
Zi Cao	Radix Arnebiae	紫草
Zi He Che	Placenta Hominis	紫河车
Zi Hua Di Ding	Herba Violae	紫花地丁
Zi Jin Pi	Radix Tripterygii Hypoglauci	紫金皮
Zi Ran Tong	Pyritum	自然铜
Zi Shi Ying	Fluoritum	紫石英
Zi Su Geng	Caulis Perillae	紫苏梗
Zi Su Ye	Folium Perillae	紫苏叶
Zi Su Zi	Fructus Perillae	紫苏子
Zi Wan	Radix et Rhizoma Asteris	紫菀
Zi Zhu	Folium Callicarpae	紫珠
Zong Lu	Petiolus Trachycarpi	棕榈
Zong Lu Zi	Fructus Trachycarpi	棕榈子
Zou Ma Tai	Rhizoma Ardisiae	走马胎
Zu Shi Ma	Cortex Daphnes	祖师麻

Appendix 8 — Cross-reference of Herbal Formula Names

Pinyin Names	Literal Names	Chinese Names
Ai Fu Nuan Gong Wan	Mugwort and Cyperus Pill for Warming the Womb	艾附暖宫丸
An Gong Niu Huang Wan	Calm the Palace Pill with Cattle Gallstone	安宫牛黄丸
An Shen Tang	Tranquilize the Spirit Decoction	安神汤
An Zhong San	Calm the Middle Powder	安中散
Ba Wei Dai Xia Fang	Eight-Ingredient Formula for Leukorrhea	八味带下方
Ba Wei Di Huang Wan	Eight-Ingredient Pill with Rehmannia	八味地黄丸
Ba Zhen Tang	Eight-Treasure Decoction	八珍汤
Ba Zheng San	Eight-Herb Powder for Rectification	八正散
Bai Du San	Overcome Pathogenic Influences Powder	败毒散
Bai Du Tang	Overcome Pathogenic Influences Decoction	败毒汤
Bai He Gu Jin Tang	Lily Bulb Decoction to Preserve the Metal	百合固金汤
Bai Hu Jia Cang Zhu Tang	White Tiger plus Atractylodes Decoction	白虎加苍术汤
Bai Hu Jia Gui Zhi Tang	White Tiger plus Cinnamon Twig Decoction	白虎加桂枝汤
Bai Hu Jia Ren Shen Tang	White Tiger plus Ginseng Decoction	白虎加人参汤
Bai Hu Tang	White Tiger Decoction	白虎汤
Bai Mao Gen Tang	Imperata Decoction	白茅根汤
Bai Tong Tang	White Penetrating Decoction	白通汤
Bai Tou Weng Jia Gan Cao E Jiao Tang	Pulsatilla Decoction plus Licorice and Ass-Hide Gelatin	白头翁加甘草阿胶汤
Bai Tou Weng Tang	Pulsatilla Decoction	白头翁汤
Bai Zi Yang Xin Wan	Biota Seed Pill to Nourish the Heart	柏子养心丸
Ban Xia Bai Zhu Tian Ma Tang	Pinellia, Atractylodes Macrocephala, and Gastrodia Decoction	半夏白术天麻汤
Ban Xia Hou Po Tang	Pinellia and Magnolia Bark Decoction	半夏厚朴汤
Ban Xia Xie Xin Tang	Pinellia Decoction to Drain the Epigastrium	半夏泻心汤
Bao Chan Wu You Fang	Preserve Pregnancy and Care-Free Decoction	保产无忧方
Bao He Wan	Preserve Harmony Pill	保和丸
Bao Yuan Tang	Preserve the Basal Decoction	保元汤
Bei Mu Gua Lou San	Fritillaria and Trichosanthes Fruit Powder	贝母瓜蒌散
Bi Xie Fen Qing Yin	Dioscorea Hypoglauca Decoction to Separate the Clear	萆薢分清饮
Bi Yu San	Jasper Powder	碧玉散
Bie Jia Jian Wan	Soft-Shelled Turtle Shell Pill	鳖甲煎丸
Bu Dai Wan	Cloth Sack Pill	布袋丸
Bu Fei E Jiao Tang	Tonify the Lung Decoction with Ass-Hide Gelatin	补肺阿胶汤
Bu Fei Tang	Tonify the Lung Decoction	补肺汤
Bu Gu Wan	Tonify the Bone Pill	补骨丸

Appendix 8 — Cross-reference of Herbal Formula Names

Pinyin Names	Literal Names	Chinese Names
Bu Huan Jin Zheng Qi San	Rectify the Qi Powder Worth More than Gold	不换金正气散
Bu Shen Tang	Tonify the Kidney Decoction	补肾汤
Bu Shen Wan	Tonify the Kidney Pill	补肾丸
Bu Yang Huan Wu Tang	Tonify the Yang to Restore Five Decoction	补阳还五汤
Bu Zhong Yi Qi Tang	Tonify the Middle and Augment the Qi Decoction	补中益气汤
Can Shi Tang	Silkworm Droppings Decoction	蚕矢汤
Cang Er Zi San	Xanthium Powder	苍耳子散
Cang Lin San	Old Rice Granary Powder	仓廪散
Chai Ge Jie Ji Tang	Bupleurum and Kudzu Decoction to Release the Muscle Layer	柴葛解肌汤
Chai Hu An Shen Tang	Bupleurum Decoction to Tranquilize the Spirit	柴胡安神汤
Chai Hu Da Yuan Yin	Bupleurum Decoction to Reach the Membrane Source	柴胡达原饮
Chai Hu Gui Zhi Gan Jiang Tang	Bupleurum, Cinnamon Twig, and Ginger Decoction	柴胡桂枝乾姜汤
Chai Hu Gui Zhi Tang	Bupleurum and Cinnamon Twig Decoction	柴胡桂枝汤
Chai Hu Jia Long Gu Mu Li Tang	Bupleurum plus Dragon Bone and Oyster Shell Decoction	柴胡加龙骨牡蛎汤
Chai Hu Jie Du Tang	Bupleurum Decoction to Relieve Toxicity	柴胡解毒汤
Chai Hu Qing Gan Tang	Bupleurum Decoction to Clear the Liver	柴胡清肝汤
Chai Hu Shu Gan San	Bupleurum Powder to Spread the Liver	柴胡疏肝散
Chai Hu Tang	Bupleurum Decoction	柴胡汤
Chai Hu Xian Xiong Tang	Bupleurum Decoction for Sinking into the Chest	柴胡陷胸汤
Chai Hu Zhi Jie Tang	Bupleurum, Bitter Orange, and Platycodon Decoction	柴胡枳桔汤
Chai Ling Tang	Bupleurum and Poria Decoction	柴苓汤
Chai Ping Tang	Bupleurum and Calm the Stomach Decoction	柴平汤
Chai Xian Tang	Bupleurum Decoction to Raise the Sunken	柴陷汤
Chan Su Wan	Toad Venum Pill	蟾酥丸
Cheng Qi Yang Ying Tang	Order the Qi and Nourish the Nutritive Qi Decoction	承气养营汤
Chi Shi Zhi Yu Yu Liang Tang	Halloysitum and Limonite Decoction	赤石脂禹馀粮汤
Chuan Xiong Cha Tiao San	Ligusticum Chuanxiong Powder to be Taken with Green Tea	川芎茶调散
Ci Zhu Wan	Magnetite and Cinnabar Pill	磁朱丸
Cong Bai Qi Wei Yin	Scallion Decoction with Seven Ingredients	葱白七味饮
Cong Chi Jie Geng Tang	Scallion, Prepared Soybean, and Platycodon Decoction	葱豉桔梗汤
Cong Chi Tang	Scallion and Prepared Soybean Decoction	葱豉汤
Cui Sheng Tang	Birth-Hastening Decoction	催生汤
Da An Wan	Great Tranquility Pill	大安丸
Da Bu Tang	Great Tonifying Decoction	大补汤
Da Bu Yin Wan	Great Tonify the Yin Pill	大补阴丸
Da Chai Hu Tang	Major Bupleurum Decoction	大柴胡汤
Da Cheng Qi Tang	Major Order the Qi Decoction	大承气汤

Appendix 8 — Cross-reference of Herbal Formula Names

Pinyin Names	Literal Names	Chinese Names
Da Ding Feng Zhu	Major Arrest Wind Pearl	大定风珠
Da Fang Feng Tang	Major Saposhnikovia Decoction	大防风汤
Da Huang Fu Zi Tang	Rhubarb and Prepared Aconite Decoction	大黄附子汤
Da Huang Mu Dan Tang	Rhubarb and Moutan Decoction	大黄牡丹汤
Da Huang Zhe Chong Wan	Rhubarb and Eupolyphaga Pill	大黄蟅虫丸
Da Huo Luo Dan	Major Invigorate the Collaterals Special Pill	大活络丹
Da Jian Zhong Tang	Major Construct the Middle Decoction	大建中汤
Da Qiang Huo Tang	Major Notopterygium Decoction	大羌活汤
Da Qin Jiao Tang	Major Gentiana Macrophylla Decoction	大秦艽汤
Da Qing Long Tang	Major Bluegreen Dragon Decoction	大青龙汤
Da Xian Xiong Tang	Major Sinking into the Chest Decoction	大陷胸汤
Da Xian Xiong Wan	Major Sinking into the Chest Pill	大陷胸丸
Da Yuan Yin	Reach the Membrane Source Decoction	达原饮
Dan Shen Yin	Salvia Decoction	丹参饮
Dang Gui Bu Xue Tang	Tangkuei Decoction to Tonify the Blood	当归补血汤
Dang Gui Jian Zhong Tang	Tangkuei Decoction to Construct the Middle	当归建中汤
Dang Gui Liu Huang Tang	Tangkuei and Six-Yellow Decoction	当归六黄汤
Dang Gui Long Hui Wan	Tangkuei, Gentiana, and Aloe Pill	当归龙荟丸
Dang Gui Nian Tong Tang	Tangkuei Decoction to Lift the Pain	当归拈痛汤
Dang Gui San	Tangkuei Powder	当归散
Dang Gui Shao Yao San	Tangkuei and Peony Powder	当归芍药散
Dang Gui Si Ni Jia Wu Zhu Yu Sheng Jiang Tang	Tangkuei Decoction for Frigid Extremities plus Evodia and Fresh Ginger	当归四逆加吴茱萸生姜汤
Dang Gui Si Ni Tang	Tangkuei Decoction for Frigid Extremities	当归四逆汤
Dang Gui Yin Zi	Tangkuei Decoction	当归饮子
Dao Chi San	Guide Out the Red Powder	导赤散
Dao Qi Tang	Conduct the Qi Decoction	导气汤
Dao Shui Fu Ling Tang	Poria Decoction to Drain Water	导水茯苓汤
Dao Tan Tang	Guide Out Phlegm Decoction	导痰汤
Di Huang Yin Zi	Rehmannia Decoction	地黄饮子
Di Tan Tang	Scour Phlegm Decoction	涤痰汤
Ding Chuan Tang	Arrest Wheezing Decoction	定喘汤
Ding Xian Wan	Arrest Seizures Pill	定痫丸
Ding Xiang Shi Di Tang	Clove and Persimmon Calyx Decoction	丁香柿蒂汤
Ding Zhi Wan	Settle the Emotions Pill	定志丸
Du Huo Ji Sheng Tang	Angelica Pubescens and Taxillus Decoction	独活寄生汤
Du Qi Wan	Capital Qi Pill	都气丸
Dun Sou San	Long-Bout Cough Powder	顿嗽散
Duo Ming Wan	Life-Taking Pill	夺命丸
E Jiao Ji Zi Huang Tang	Ass-Hide Gelatin and Egg Yolk Decoction	阿胶鸡子黄汤
Er Chen Tang	Two-Cured Decoction	二陈汤

Appendix 8 — Cross-reference of Herbal Formula Names

Pinyin Names	Literal Names	Chinese Names
Er Long Zuo Ci Wan	Pill for Deafness that Is Kind to the Left [Kidney]	耳聋左慈丸
Er Miao San	Two-Marvel Powder	二妙散
Er Xian Bu Shen Tang	Two-Immortal Decoction to Tonify the Kidney	二仙补肾汤
Er Xian Tang	Two-Immortal Decoction	二仙汤
Er Zhi Wan	Two-Ultimate Pill	二至丸
Er Zhu Tang	Two-Atractylodes Decoction	二术汤
Fa Mu Wan	Quell Wood Pill	伐木丸
Fang Feng Tong Sheng San	Saposhnikovia Powder that Sagely Unblocks	防风通圣散
Fang Ji Fu Ling Tang	Stephania and Poria Decoction	防己茯苓汤
Fang Ji Huang Qi Tang	Stephania and Astragalus Decoction	防己黄芪汤
Fei Er Wan	Fat Child Pill	肥儿丸
Fen Xiao Tang	Separate and Reduce Decoction	分消汤
Fu Fang Ba Zheng San	Revised Eight-Herb Powder	复方八正散
Fu Fang Da Cheng Qi Tang	Revised Major Order the Qi Decoction	复方大承气汤
Fu Ling Tang	Poria Decoction	茯苓汤
Fu Ling Wan	Poria Pill	茯苓丸
Fu Ling Yin	Poria Decoction	茯苓饮
Fu Tu Dan	Poria and Cuscuta Special Pill	茯菟丹
Fu Yuan Huo Xue Tang	Revive Health by Invigorating the Blood Decoction	复元活血汤
Fu Zheng Yi Yan Tang	Support the Upright and Suppress Cancer Decoction	扶正抑癌汤
Fu Zi Li Zhong Wan	Prepared Aconite Pill to Regulate the Middle	附子理中丸
Fu Zi Tang	Prepared Aconite Decoction	附子汤
Gan Cao Gan Jiang Fu Ling Bai Zhu Tang	Licorice, Ginger, Poria and Atractylodes Macrocephala Decoction	甘草乾姜茯苓白术汤
Gan Cao Xie Xin Tang	Licorice Decoction to Drain the Epigastrium	甘草泻心汤
Gan Jiang Ren Shen Ban Xia Wan	Ginger, Ginseng, and Pinellia Pill	乾姜人参半夏丸
Gan Lu Xiao Du Dan	Sweet Dew Special Pill to Eliminate Toxins	甘露消毒丹
Gan Lu Yin	Sweet Dew Decoction	甘露饮
Gan Mai Da Zao Tang	Licorice, Wheat, and Jujube Decoction	甘麦大枣汤
Ge Gen Huang Qin Huang Lian Tang	Kudzu, Coptis, and Scutellaria Decoction	葛根黄芩黄连汤
Ge Gen Huo Xiang Shao Yao Tang	Kudzu, Pogostemon, and Peony Decoction	葛根藿香芍药汤
Ge Gen Tang	Kudzu Decoction	葛根汤
Ge Hua Jie Cheng San	Pueraria Flower Powder for Detoxification and Awakening	葛花解酲散
Ge Xia Zhu Yu Tang	Drive Out Blood Stasis Below the Diaphragm Decoction	膈下逐瘀汤
Gong Wai Yun Fang	Ectopic Pregnancy Formula	宫外孕方
Gou Teng San	Uncaria Powder	钩藤散
Gou Teng Yin	Uncaria Decoction	钩藤饮

Appendix 8 — Cross-reference of Herbal Formula Names

Pinyin Names	Literal Names	Chinese Names
Gu Chong Tang	Stabilize Chong [Thoroughfare Channel] Decoction	固冲汤
Gu Jing Wan	Stabilize the Menses Pill	固经丸
Gua Di San	Melon Pedicle Powder	瓜蒂散
Gua Lou Xie Bai Bai Jiu Tang	Trichosanthes Fruit, Chinese Chive, and Wine Decoction	瓜蒌薤白白酒汤
Gua Lou Xie Bai Ban Xia Tang	Trichosanthes Fruit, Chinese Chive, and Pinellia Decoction	瓜蒌薤白半夏汤
Gua Lou Zhi Shi Tang	Trichosanthes Fruit and Immature Bitter Orange Decoction	瓜蒌枳实汤
Guan Xin Su He Wan	Coronary Styrax Pill	冠心苏合丸
Gui Ling Gan Lu Yin	Cinnamon and Poria Sweet Dew Decoction	桂苓甘露饮
Gui Lu Er Xian Jiao	Tortoise Shell and Deer Antler Syrup	龟鹿二仙胶
Gui Pi An Shen Tang	Restore the Spleen and Tranquilize the Spirit Decoction	归脾安神汤
Gui Pi Tang	Restore the Spleen Decoction	归脾汤
Gui Qi Jian Zhong Tang	Tangkuei and Astragalus Decoction to Construct the Middle	归芪建中汤
Gui Zhi Fu Ling Wan	Cinnamon Twig and Poria Pill	桂枝茯苓丸
Gui Zhi Jia Ge Gen Tang	Cinnamon Twig Decoction plus Kudzu	桂枝加葛根汤
Gui Zhi Jia Hou Po Xing Zi Tang	Cinnamon Twig Decoction plus Magnolia Bark and Apricot Kernel	桂枝加厚朴杏子汤
Gui Zhi Jia Long Gu Mu Li Tang	Cinnamon Twig Decoction plus Dragon Bone and Oyster Shell	桂枝加龙骨牡蛎汤
Gui Zhi Jia Shao Yao Tang	Cinnamon Twig Decoction plus Peony	桂枝加芍药汤
Gui Zhi Ma Huang Ge Ban Tang	Combined Cinnamon Twig and Ephedra Decoction	桂枝麻黄各半汤
Gui Zhi Ren Shen Tang	Cinnamon Twig and Ginseng Decoction	桂枝人参汤
Gui Zhi Shao Yao Zhi Mu Tang	Cinnamon Twig, Peony, and Anemarrhena Decoction	桂枝芍药知母汤
Gui Zhi Tang	Cinnamon Twig Decoction	桂枝汤
Gun Tan Wan	Vaporize Phlegm Pill	滚痰丸
Guo Qi Yin	Delayed Menstruation Decoction	过期饮
Hai Zao Yu Hu Tang	Sargassum Decoction for the Jade Flask	海藻玉壶汤
Hao Qin Qing Dan Tang	Artemisia Annua and Scutellaria Decoction to Clear the Gallbladder	蒿芩清胆汤
He Che Wan Fang	Placenta Pill Formula	河车丸方
Hei Xi Dan	Lead Special Pill	黑锡丹
Hei Xiao Yao San	Black Rambling Powder	黑逍遥散
Hou Po Qi Wu Tang	Seven-Substance Decoction with Magnolia Bark	厚朴七物汤
Hou Po Wen Zhong Tang	Magnolia Bark Decoction for Warming the Middle	厚朴温中汤
Hu Qian Wan	Hidden Tiger Pill	虎潜丸
Hua Ban Tang	Transform Blotches Decoction	化斑汤
Hua Chong Wan	Dissolve Parasites Pill	化虫丸
Hua Gai San	Canopy Powder	华盖散

Appendix 8 — Cross-reference of Herbal Formula Names

Pinyin Names	Literal Names	Chinese Names
Hua Tan Wan	Transform Phlegm Pill	化痰丸
Huai Hua San	Sophora Japonica Flower Powder	槐花散
Huai Jiao Wan	Sophora Japonica Fruit Pill	槐角丸
Huan Shao Dan	Return to Youth Pill	还少丹
Huan Shao Di Huang Wan	Rehmannia Pill to Return to Youth	还少地黄丸
Huang Lian Jie Du Tang	Coptis Decoction to Relieve Toxicity	黄连解毒汤
Huang Lian Shang Qing Wan	Coptis Pill to Clear the Upper	黄连上清丸
Huang Lian Tang	Coptis Decoction	黄连汤
Huang Long Tang	Yellow Dragon Decoction	黄龙汤
Huang Qi Fang Feng Tang	Astragalus Decoction to Guard the Wind	黄芪防风汤
Huang Qi Gui Zhi Wu Wu Tang	Astragalus and Cinnamon Twig Five-Substance Decoction	黄芪桂枝五物汤
Huang Qi Jian Zhong Tang	Astragalus Decoction to Construct the Middle	黄芪建中汤
Huang Qin Hua Shi Tang	Scutellaria and Talcum Decoction	黄芩滑石汤
Huang Qin Tang	Scutellaria Decoction	黄芩汤
Huang Tu Tang	Yellow Earth Decoction	黄土汤
Hui Yang Jiu Ji Tang	Restore and Revive the Yang Decoction	回阳救急汤
Huo Luo Xiao Ling Dan	Fantastically Effective Pill to Invigorate the Collaterals	活络效灵丹
Huo Ming Yin	Revitalize Life Decoction	活命饮
Huo Po Xia Ling Tang	Agastache, Magnolia Bark, Pinellia, and Poria Decoction	藿朴夏苓汤
Huo Ren Cong Chi Tang	Scallion and Prepared Soybean Decoction from the Book to Safeguard Life	活人葱豉汤
Huo Xiang Zheng Qi San	Agastache Powder to Rectify the Qi	藿香正气散
Huo Xue Shun Qi Tang	Invigorate the Blood and Smooth the Qi Decoction	活血顺气汤
Huo Xue Tong Lin Tang	Invigorate the Blood to Unblock Dysuria Decoction	活血通淋汤
Huo Xue Zhi Tong Tang	Invigorate the Blood and Stop Pain Decoction	活血止痛汤
Ji Chuan Jian	Benefit the River [Flow] Decoction	济川煎
Ji Ming San	Powder to Take at Cock's Crow	鸡鸣散
Ji Sheng Shen Qi Wan	Kidney Qi Pill from Formulas that Aid the Living	济生肾气丸
Ji Su San	Peppermint Powder	鸡苏散
Ji Tong Tang	Spine Pain Decoction	脊痛汤
Jia Jian Cheng Qi Tang	Modified Order the Qi Decoction	加减承气汤
Jia Jian Fu Mai Tang	Modified Restore the Pulse Decoction	加减复脉汤
Jia Jian Wei Rui Tang	Modified Polygonatum Odoratum Decoction	加减葳蕤汤
Jia Jian Xiao Qing Long Tang	Modified Minor Bluegreen Dragon Decoction	加减小青龙汤
Jia Wei Ba Zheng San	Augmented Eight Herb Powder for Rectification	加味八正散
Jia Wei Gua Lou Xie Bai Tang	Augmented Trichosanthes Fruit and Chinese Chive Decoction	加味瓜蒌薤白汤
Jia Wei Huo Luo Dan	Augmented Invigorate the Collaterals Special Pill	加味活络丹
Jia Wei Ma Xing Gan Shi Tang	Augmented Ephedra, Apricot Kernel, Licorice, and Gypsum Decoction	加味麻杏甘石汤

Appendix 8 — Cross-reference of Herbal Formula Names

Pinyin Names	Literal Names	Chinese Names
Jia Wei Ping Wei San	Modified Calm the Stomach Powder	加味平胃散
Jia Wei Qian Zheng San	Augmented Lead to Symmetry Powder	加味牵正散
Jia Wei Shao Yao Gan Cao Tang	Augmented Peony and Licorice Decoction	加味芍药甘草汤
Jia Wei Si Wu Tang	Augmented Four-Substance Decoction	加味四物汤
Jia Wei Xiang Su San	Augmented Cyperus and Perilla Leaf Powder	加味香苏散
Jia Wei Xiao Yao San	Augmented Rambling Powder	加味逍遥散
Jia Wei Xin Yi San	Augmented Magnolia Flower Powder	加味辛夷散
Jia Wei You Gui Wan	Augmented Restore the Right [Kidney] Pill	加味右归丸
Jia Wei Zuo Gui Wan	Augmented Restore the Left [Kidney] Pill	加味左归丸
Jian Bi Tang	Remove Painful Obstruction in the Shoulders Decoction	肩痹汤
Jian Ling Tang	Construct Roof Tiles Decoction	建瓴汤
Jian Pi Wan	Strengthen the Spleen Pill	健脾丸
Jiao Ai Tang	Ass-Hide Gelatin and Mugwort Decoction	胶艾汤
Jie Geng Tang	Platycodon Decoction	桔梗汤
Jin Fei Cao San	Inula Powder	金沸草散
Jin Gui Shen Qi Wan	Kidney Qi Pill from the Golden Cabinet	金匮肾气丸
Jin Jian Fei Er Wan	Golden Pill to Construct a Fat Child	金鉴肥儿丸
Jin Ling Zi San	Melia Toosendan Powder	金铃子散
Jin Suo Gu Jing Wan	Metal Lock Pill to Stabilize the Essence	金锁固精丸
Jing Fang Bai Du San	Schizonepeta and Saposhnikovia Powder to Overcome Pathogenic Influences	荆防败毒散
Jing Fang Er Hao	Neck Formula Two	颈方二号
Jing Fang Yi Hao	Neck Formula One	颈方一号
Jing Jie Lian Qiao Tang	Schizonepeta and Forsythia Decoction	荆芥连翘汤
Jiu Ji Xi Xian San	Urgent Powder to Dilute Saliva	救急稀涎散
Jiu Wei Bing Lang Jia Wu Fu Tang	Areca Nine Decoction plus Evodia and Poria	九味槟榔加吴茯汤
Jiu Wei Qiang Huo Tang	Nine-Herb Decoction with Notopterygium	九味羌活汤
Jiu Xian San	Nine-Immortal Powder	九仙散
Ju Ban Zhi Zhu Wan	Tangerine Peel, Pinellia, Immature Bitter Orange, and Atractylodes Macrocephala Pill	橘半枳术丸
Ju Fang Zhi Bao San	Greatest Treasure Powder from the Imperial Grace Formulary	局方至宝散
Ju He Wan	Tangerine Seed Pill	橘核丸
Ju Hua Cha Tiao San	Chrysanthemum Powder to be Taken with Green Tea	菊花茶调散
Ju Pi Zhu Ru Tang	Tangerine Peel and Bamboo Shaving Decoction	橘皮竹茹汤
Ju Yuan Jian	Lift the Source Decoction	举元煎
Juan Bi Tang	Remove Painful Obstruction Decoction	蠲痹汤
Ke Xue Fang	Coughing of Blood Formula	咳血方
Kong Xian Dan	Control Mucus Special Pill	控涎丹
Leng Xiao Wan	Cold Wheezing Pill	冷哮丸

Appendix 8 — Cross-reference of Herbal Formula Names

Pinyin Names	Literal Names	Chinese Names
Li Zhong An Hui Tang	Regulate the Middle and Calm Roundworms Decoction	理中安蛔汤
Li Zhong Hua Tan Wan	Regulate the Middle and Transform Phlegm Pill	理中化痰丸
Li Zhong Wan	Regulate the Middle Pill	理中丸
Lian Mei An Hui Tang	Picrorhiza and Mume Decoction to Calm Roundworms	连梅安蛔汤
Lian Po Yin	Coptis and Magnolia Bark Decoction	连朴饮
Lian Qiao Bai Du San	Forsythia Powder to Overcome Pathogenic Influences	连翘败毒散
Lian Qiao Jie Du Tang	Forsythia Decoction to Relieve Toxicity	连翘解毒汤
Liang Fu Wan	Galangal and Cyperus Pill	良附丸
Liang Ge San	Cool the Diaphragm Powder	凉膈散
Ling Gan Wu Wei Jiang Xin Tang	Poria, Licorice, Schisandra, Ginger, and Asarum Decoction	苓甘五味姜辛汤
Ling Gui Zhu Gan Tang	Poria, Cinnamon Twig, Atractylodes Macrocephala, and Licorice Decoction	苓桂术甘汤
Ling Jiao Gou Teng Tang	Antelope Horn and Uncaria Decoction	羚角钩藤汤
Liu He Tang	Harmonize the Six Decoction	六和汤
Liu Jun Zi Tang	Six-Gentlemen Decoction	六君子汤
Liu Shen Wan	Six-Miracle Pill	六神丸
Liu Wei Di Huang Wan	Six-Ingredient Pill with Rehmannia	六味地黄丸
Liu Wei Gu Jing Wan	Rehmannia Six and Lotus Stamen Pill	六味固精丸
Liu Yi San	Six-to-One Powder	六一散
Long Dan Jiang Ya Pian	Gentiana Pill to Lower [Blood] Pressure	龙胆降压片
Long Dan Jie Du Tang	Gentiana Decoction to Relieve Toxicity	龙胆解毒汤
Long Dan Xie Gan Tang	Gentiana Decoction to Drain the Liver	龙胆泻肝汤
Ma Huang Fu Zi Gan Cao Tang	Ephedra, Prepared Aconite, and Licorice Decoction	麻黄附子甘草汤
Ma Huang Fu Zi Xi Xin Tang	Ephedra, Asarum, and Prepared Aconite Decoction	麻黄附子细辛汤
Ma Huang Jia Zhu Tang	Ephedra Decoction plus Atractylodes	麻黄加术汤
Ma Huang Tang	Ephedra Decoction	麻黄汤
Ma Huang Xing Ren Gan Cao Shi Gao Tang	Ephedra, Apricot Kernel, Licorice, and Gypsum Decoction	麻黄杏仁甘草石膏汤
Ma Xing Yi Gan Tang	Ephedra, Apricot Kernel, Coicis, and Licorice Decoction	麻杏苡甘汤
Ma Zi Ren Wan	Hemp Seed Pill	麻子仁丸
Ma Zi Run Chang Wan	Hemp Seed Pill to Moisten the Intestines	麻子润肠丸
Mai Men Dong Tang	Ophiopogonis Decoction	麦门冬汤
Mai Men Yang Yin Tang	Ophiopogonis Decoction to Nourish the Yin	麦门养阴汤
Mai Wei Di Huang Wan	Ophiopogonis, Schisandra, and Rehmannia Pill	麦味地黄丸
Ming Mu Di Huang Wan	Improve Vision Pill with Rehmannia	明目地黄丸
Mu Fang Ji Tang	Cocculus Decoction	木防己汤
Mu Li San	Oyster Shell Powder	牡蛎散
Mu Xiang Bing Lang Wan	Aucklandia and Betel Nut Pill	木香槟榔丸
Nao Wei Kang Wan	Benefit Brain Atrophy Pill	脑萎康丸

Appendix 8 — Cross-reference of Herbal Formula Names

Pinyin Names	Literal Names	Chinese Names
Nei Bu Huang Qi Tang	Tonify the Interior Decoction with Astragalus	内补黄芪汤
Nian Tong Tang	Lift the Pain Decoction	拈痛汤
Ning Sou Wan	Quiet the Cough Pill	宁嗽丸
Niu Bang Jie Ji Tang	Arctium Decoction to Release the Muscle Layer	牛蒡解肌汤
Niu Huang Qing Xin Wan	Cattle Gallstone Pill to Clear the Heart	牛黄清心丸
Nu Ke Bai Zi Ren Wan	Platycladus Seed Pill for Females	女科柏子仁丸
Nuan Gan Jian	Warm the Liver Decoction	暖肝煎
Pai Nong San	Drain the Pus Powder	排脓散
Ping Wei San	Calm the Stomach Powder	平胃散
Po Bu Zi Ye Tang	Cordia Decoction	破布子叶汤
Pu Ji Xiao Du Yin	Universal Benefit Decoction to Eliminate Toxin	普济消毒饮
Qi Bao Mei Ran Dan	Seven-Treasure Special Pill for Beautiful Whiskers	七宝美髯丹
Qi Ju Di Huang Wan	Lycium Fruit, Chrysanthemum, and Rehmannia Pill	杞菊地黄丸
Qi Li San	Seven-Thousandths of a Tael Powder	七厘散
Qi Pi Wan	Guide the Spleen Pill	启脾丸
Qi Wei Bai Zhu San	Seven-Ingredient Powder with Atractylodes Macrocephala	七味白术散
Qian Jin Nei Tuo San	Drain the Interior Powder Worthy of a Thousand Gold	千金内托散
Qian Zheng San	Lead to Symmetry Powder	牵正散
Qiang Huo Sheng Shi Tang	Notopterygium Decoction to Overcome Dampness	羌活胜湿汤
Qiao He Tang	Forsythia and Mint Decoction	翘荷汤
Qin Jiao Bie Jia San	Gentiana Macrophylla and Soft-Shelled Turtle Shell Powder	秦艽鳖甲散
Qing Bi Tang	Clear the Nose Decoction	清鼻汤
Qing Chang Tang	Clear the Intestines Decoction	清肠汤
Qing Chang Yin	Clear the Intestines Drink	清肠饮
Qing Dai Tang	Clear the Discharge Decoction	清带汤
Qing Fei Tang	Clear the Lung Decoction	清肺汤
Qing Fei Yin	Clear the Lung Drink	清肺饮
Qing Gu San	Cool the Bones Powder	清骨散
Qing Hao Bie Jia Tang	Artemisia Annua and Soft-Shelled Turtle Shell Decoction	青蒿鳖甲汤
Qing Liang Yin	Clearing and Cooling Decoction	清凉饮
Qing Luo Yin	Clear the Collaterals Decoction	清络饮
Qing Pi Yin	Clear the Spleen Decoction	清脾饮
Qing Qi Hua Tan Wan	Clear the Qi and Transform Phlegm Pill	清气化痰丸
Qing Re Jie Du Tang	Clear Heat and Relieve Toxicity Decoction	清热解毒汤
Qing Re Liang Xue Tang	Clear Heat and Cool the Blood Decoction	清热凉血汤
Qing Re Tong Lin Tang	Clear Heat to Unblock Dysuria Decoction	清热通淋汤
Qing Shang Fang Feng Tang	Clear the Upper and Guard the Wind Decoction	清上防风汤
Qing Shu Yi Qi Tang	Clear Summer-Heat and Augment the Qi Decoction	清暑益气汤
Qing Wei San	Clear the Stomach Powder	清胃散

Appendix 8 — Cross-reference of Herbal Formula Names

Pinyin Names	Literal Names	Chinese Names
Qing Wei Tang	Clear the Stomach Decoction	清胃汤
Qing Wen Bai Du Yin	Clear Epidemics and Overcome Pathogenic Influences Decoction	清瘟败毒饮
Qing Xin Li Ge Tang	Clear the Epigastrium and Benefit the Diaphragm Decoction	清心利膈汤
Qing Xin Lian Zi Yin	Lotus Seed Decoction to Clear the Heart	清心莲子饮
Qing Ying Tang	Clear the Nutritive Level Decoction	清营汤
Qing Zao Jiu Fei Tang	Eliminate Dryness and Rescue the Lung Decoction	清燥救肺汤
Qiong Yu Gao	Beautiful Jade Paste	琼玉膏
Qu Feng San	Dispel Wind Powder	祛风散
Qu Mai Zhi Zhu Wan	Medicated Leaven, Barley Sprout, Immature Bitter Orange, and Atractylodes Macrocephala Pill	曲蘖枳术丸
Ren Shen Bai Du San	Ginseng Powder to Overcome Pathogenic Influences	人参败毒散
Ren Shen Chong Cao Tang	Ginseng and Cordyceps Decoction	人参虫草汤
Ren Shen Da Bu Tang	Ginseng Great Tonifying Decoction	人参大补汤
Ren Shen Dang Shao San	Ginseng, Tangkuei, and Peony Powder	人参当芍散
Ren Shen Ge Jie San	Ginseng and Gecko Powder	人参蛤蚧散
Ren Shen Hu Tao Tang	Ginseng and Walnut Decoction	人参胡桃汤
Ren Shen Tang	Ginseng Decoction	人参汤
Ren Shen Xie Fei Tang	Ginseng Decoction to Sedate the Lung	人参泻肺汤
Ren Shen Yang Ying Tang	Ginseng Decoction to Nourish the Nutritive Qi	人参养荣汤
Run Chang Wan	Moisten the Intestines Pill	润肠丸
San Ao Tang	Three-Unbinding Decoction	三拗汤
San Bi Tang	Three-Painful Obstruction Decoction	三痹汤
San Ceng Hui Xiang Wan	Fennel Seed Pill with Three Levels	三层茴香丸
San Huang Shi Gao Tang	Three-Yellow and Gypsum Decoction	三黄石膏汤
San Huang Xie Xin Tang	Three-Yellow Decoction to Sedate the Epigastrium	三黄泻心汤
San Jia An Shen Wan	Three-Shell Pill to Tranquilize the Spirit	三甲安神汤
San Jia Fu Mai Tang	Three-Shell Decoction to Restore the Pulse	三甲复脉汤
San Jian Gao	Three Constructive Paste	三建膏
San Jiao Zhu Yu Tang	Drive Out Blood Stasis in Three *Jiaos* Decoction	三焦逐瘀汤
San Jin Pai Shi Tang	Three Gold Decoction to Expel Stone	三金排石汤
San Miao Wan	Three-Marvel Pill	三妙丸
San Ren Tang	Three-Nut Decoction	三仁汤
San Sheng San	Three-Sage Powder	三圣散
San Wu Bai San	Three-Substance White Powder	三物白散
San Wu Bei Ji Wan	Three-Substance Pill for Emergencies	三物备急丸
San Wu Xiang Ru Yin	Mosla Three Decoction	三物香薷饮
San Zhong Kui Jian Tang	Disperse the Swelling and Break the Hardness Decoction	散肿溃坚汤
San Zi Jiang Qi Tang	Three-Seed Decoction for Directing Qi Downward	三子降气汤
San Zi Yang Qin Tang	Three-Seed Decoction to Nourish One's Parents	三子养亲汤

Appendix 8 — Cross-reference of Herbal Formula Names

Pinyin Names	Literal Names	Chinese Names
Sang Ju Yin	Mulberry Leaf and Chrysanthemum Decoction	桑菊饮
Sang Ma Wan	Mulberry Leaf and Sesame Seed Pill	桑麻丸
Sang Piao Xiao San	Mantis Egg-Case Powder	桑螵蛸散
Sang Xing Tang	Mulberry Leaf and Apricot Kernel Decoction	桑杏汤
Sang Zhi Shi Gao Zhi Mu Tang	Mulberry Twig, Gypsum, and Anemarrhena Decoction	桑枝石膏知母汤
Sha Shen Mai Dong Tang	Glehnia and Ophiopogonis Decoction	沙参麦冬汤
Shan Zha Hua Tan Tang	Crataegus Decoction to Transform Phlegm	山楂化痰汤
Shan Zha Tang	Crataegus Decoction	山楂汤
Shang Zhong Xia Tong Yong Tong Feng Wan	Upper, Middle, and Lower General Use Pill for Wind-Pain	上中下通用痛风丸
Shao Fu Zhu Yu Tang	Drive Out Blood Stasis in the Lower Abdomen Decoction	少腹逐瘀汤
Shao Yao Gan Cao Tang	Peony and Licorice Decoction	芍药甘草汤
Shao Yao Hou Po Tang	Peony and Magnolia Bark Decoction	芍药厚朴汤
Shao Yao Tang	Peony Decoction	芍药汤
Shao Yao Yi Yi Ren Tang	Peony and Coicis Decoction	芍药薏苡仁汤
She Gan Ma Huang Tang	Belamcanda and Ephedra Decoction	射干麻黄汤
Shen Fu Tang	Ginseng and Prepared Aconite Decoction	参附汤
Shen Ling Bai Zhu San	Ginseng, Poria, and Atractylodes Macrocephala Powder	参苓白术散
Shen Ling San	Ginseng and Poria Powder	参苓散
Shen Mi Tang	Mysterious Decoction	神秘汤
Shen Su Yin	Ginseng and Perilla Leaf Decoction	参苏饮
Shen Tong Zhu Yu Tang	Drive Out Blood Stasis from a Painful Body Decoction	身痛逐瘀汤
Shen Xi Dan	Magical Rhinoceros Special Pill	神犀丹
Shen Xiao Tuo Li San	Miraculous Powder for Supporting the Interior	神效托里散
Sheng Hua Tang	Generation and Transformation Decoction	生化汤
Sheng Jiang Xie Xin Tang	Fresh Ginger Decoction to Drain the Epigastrium	生姜泻心汤
Sheng Ma Ge Gen Tang	Cimicifuga and Kudzu Decoction	升麻葛根汤
Sheng Mai San	Generate the Pulse Powder	生脉散
Sheng Tie Luo Yin	Iron Filings Decoction	生铁落饮
Sheng Xian Tang	Raise the Sinking Decoction	升陷汤
Sheng Yang San Huo Tang	Raise the Yang and Disperse the Fire Decoction	升阳散火汤
Sheng Yu Tang	Sage-Like Healing Decoction	圣愈汤
Shi Bu Wan	Ten-Tonic Pill	十补丸
Shi Di Tang	Persimmon Calyx Decoction	柿蒂汤
Shi Gao Tang	Gypsum Decoction	石膏汤
Shi Hu Ye Guang Wan	Dendrobium Pill for Night Vision	石斛夜光丸
Shi Hui San	Ten Partially-Charred Substances Powder	十灰散
Shi Liu Wei Liu Qi Yin	Sixteen-Ingredient Decoction to Flow Qi	十六味流气饮
Shi Pi San	Bolster the Spleen Powder	实脾散
Shi Quan Da Bu Tang	All-Inclusive Great Tonifying Decoction	十全大补汤
Shi Shen Tang	Ten-Immortal Decoction	十神汤

Appendix 8 — Cross-reference of Herbal Formula Names

Pinyin Names	Literal Names	Chinese Names
Shi Wei Bai Du Tang	Ten-Ingredient Decoction to Overcome Pathogenic Influences	十味败毒汤
Shi Wei Di Huang Wan	Ten-Ingredient Pill with Rehmannia	十味地黄丸
Shi Wei Wen Dan Tang	Ten-Ingredient Decoction to Warm the Gallbladder	十味温胆汤
Shi Wei Xiang Ru Yin	Ten-Ingredient Decoction with Mosla	十味香薷饮
Shi Wei Xiao Yao San	Ten-Ingredient Rambling Powder	十味逍遥散
Shi Xiao San	Sudden Smile Powder	失笑散
Shi Zao Tang	Ten-Jujube Decoction	十枣汤
Shou Nian San	Pinch Powder	手拈散
Shou Wu Pian	Polygonum Pill	首乌片
Shu Gan Tang	Spread the Liver Decoction	疏肝汤
Shu Jin Li An San	Relax the Tendons and Instill Peace Powder	疏筋立安散
Shu Jing Huo Xue Tang	Relax the Channels and Invigorate the Blood Decoction	疏经活血汤
Shu Zao Yin Zi	Spread and Unblock Decoction	疏凿饮子
Shuang Jie Tong Sheng San	Double Relieve Powder that Sagely Unblocks	双解通圣散
Shui Lu Er Xian Dan	Water and Earth Two Immortals Special Pill	水陆二仙丹
Si Jun Zi Tang	Four-Gentlemen Decoction	四君子汤
Si Ling San	Four-Ingredient Powder with Poria	四苓散
Si Miao Wan	Four-Marvel Pill	四妙丸
Si Miao Yong An Tang	Four-Valiant Decoction for Well-Being	四妙勇安汤
Si Mo Tang	Four Milled-Herbs Decoction	四磨汤
Si Ni Jia Ren Shen Tang	Frigid Extremities Decoction plus Ginseng	四逆加人参汤
Si Ni San	Frigid Extremities Powder	四逆散
Si Ni Tang	Frigid Extremities Decoction	四逆汤
Si Shen Wan	Four-Miracle Pill	四神丸
Si Sheng Wan	Four-Fresh Pill	四生丸
Si Wu Tang	Four-Substance Decoction	四物汤
Su He Xiang Wan	Liquid Styrax Pill	苏合香丸
Su Zi Jiang Qi Tang	Perilla Fruit Decoction for Directing Qi Downward	苏子降气汤
Suan Zao Ren Tang	Sour Jujube Decoction	酸枣仁汤
Suo Quan Wan	Shut the Sluice Pill	缩泉丸
Tai Shan Pan Shi San	Powder that Gives the Stability of Mount Tai	泰山磐石散
Tao He Cheng Qi Tang	Peach Pit Decoction to Order the Qi	桃核承气汤
Tao Hong Si Wu Tang	Four-Substance Decoction with Safflower and Peach Pit	桃红四物汤
Tao Hua Tang	Peach Blossom Decoction	桃花汤
Tian Ma Gou Teng Yin	Gastrodia and Uncaria Decoction	天麻钩藤饮
Tian Ma Jiang Ya Pian	Gastrodia Pill to Lower [Blood] Pressure	天麻降压片
Tian Tai Wu Yao San	Top-Quality Lindera Powder	天台乌药散
Tian Wang Bu Xin Dan	Emperor of Heaven's Special Pill to Tonify the Heart	天王补心丹
Tiao Jing Er Hao	Regulate Mense Formula Two	调经二号
Tiao Jing San Hao	Regulate Mense Formula Three	调经三号

Appendix 8 — Cross-reference of Herbal Formula Names

Pinyin Names	Literal Names	Chinese Names
Tiao Jing Si Hao	Regulate Mense Formula Four	调经四号
Tiao Jing Yi Hao	Regulate Mense Formula One	调经一号
Tiao Wei Cheng Qi Tang	Regulate the Stomach and Order the Qi Decoction	调胃承气汤
Ting Li Da Zao Xie Fei Tang	Descurainia and Jujube Decoction to Drain the Lung	葶苈大枣泻肺汤
Tong Feng Wan	Wind-Pain Pill	痛风丸
Tong Mai Si Ni Tang	Unblock the Pulse Decoction for Frigid Extremities	通脉四逆汤
Tong Qiao Huo Xue Tang	Unblock the Orifices and Invigorate the Blood Decoction	通窍活血汤
Tong Ru Wan	Unblock the Breast Pill	通乳丸
Tong Xie Yao Fang	Important Formula for Painful Diarrhea	痛泻要方
Tou Nong San	Discharge Pus Powder	透脓散
Tuo Li Tou Nong Tang	Drain the Interior and Discharge Pus Decoction	托里透脓汤
Tuo Li Xiao Du Yin	Drain the Interior and Detoxify Decoction	托里消毒饮
Wan Dai Tang	End Discharge Decoction	完带汤
Wei Jing Tang	Reed Decoction	苇茎汤
Wei Ling Tang	Calm the Stomach and Poria Decoction	胃苓汤
Wei Rui Tang	Polygonatum Odoratum Decoction	葳蕤汤
Wen Dan Tang	Warm the Gallbladder Decoction	温胆汤
Wen Jing Tang	Warm the Channels Decoction	温经汤
Wen Jing Zhi Tong Tang	Warm the Channel and Stop Pain Decoction	温经止痛汤
Wen Pi Tang	Warm the Spleen Decoction	温脾汤
Wen Qing Yin	Warming and Clearing Decoction	温清饮
Wu Hu Zhui Feng San	Five-Tiger Powder to Pursue Wind	五虎追风散
Wu Ji San	Five-Accumulation Powder	五积散
Wu Ji Wan	Wu Ji Pill	戊己丸
Wu Lin San	Five-Ingredient Powder for Painful Urinary Dysfunction	五淋散
Wu Ling San	Five-Ingredient Powder with Poria	五苓散
Wu Mei Wan	Mume Pill	乌梅丸
Wu Mo Yin Zi	Five Milled-Herbs Decoction	五磨饮子
Wu Pi San	Five-Peel Powder	五皮散
Wu Ren Wan	Five-Seed Pill	五仁丸
Wu Shen Tang	Five-Miracle Decoction	五神汤
Wu Wei Xiao Du Yin	Five-Ingredient Decoction to Eliminate Toxins	五味消毒饮
Wu Yao Shun Qi San	Lindera Powder to Smooth the Flow of Qi	乌药顺气散
Wu Zhu Yu Tang	Evodia Decoction	吴茱萸汤
Xi Gan Ming Mu San	Wash the Liver and Brighten the Eyes Powder	洗肝明目散
Xi Huang Wan	Cattle Gallstone Pill	犀黄丸
Xi Jiao Di Huang Tang	Rhinoceros Horn and Rehmannia Decoction	犀角地黄汤
Xi Tong Fang Er Hao	Knee Pain Formula Two	膝痛方二号
Xi Tong Fang Yi Hao	Knee Pain Formula One	膝痛方一号
Xia Yu Xue Tang	Drain Blood Stasis Decoction	下血瘀汤

Appendix 8 — Cross-reference of Herbal Formula Names

Pinyin Names	Literal Names	Chinese Names
Xian Fang Huo Ming Yin	Sublime Formula for Sustaining Life	仙方活命饮
Xiang Fu Wan	Cyperus Pill	香砂丸
Xiang Lian Wan	Aucklandia and Coptis Pill	香连丸
Xiang Ru San	Mosla Powder	香薷散
Xiang Sha Liu Jun Zi Tang	Six-Gentlemen Decoction with Cyperus and Amomum	香砂六君子汤
Xiang Sha Liu Jun Zi Tang	Six-Gentlemen Decoction with Aucklandia and Amomum	香砂六君子汤
Xiang Sha Ping Wei San	Cyperus and Amomum Powder to Calm the Stomach	香砂平胃散
Xiang Sha Yang Wei Tang	Nourish the Stomach Decoction with Aucklandia and Amomum	香砂养胃汤
Xiang Sha Zhi Zhu Wan	Aucklandia, Amomum, Immature Bitter Orange, and Atractylodes Macrocephala Pill	香砂枳术丸
Xiang Sheng Po Di San	Loud Sound Powder for a Broken Flute	响声破笛散
Xiang Su Cong Chi Tang	Cyperus, Perilla Leaf, Scallion, and Prepared Soybean Decoction	香苏葱豉汤
Xiang Su San	Cyperus and Perilla Leaf Powder	香苏散
Xiao Ban Xia Jia Fu Ling Tang	Minor Pinellia and Poria Decoction	小半夏加茯苓汤
Xiao Chai Hu Tang	Minor Bupleurum Decoction	小柴胡汤
Xiao Cheng Qi Tang	Minor Order the Qi Decoction	小承气汤
Xiao Ding Feng Zhu	Minor Arrest Wind Pearl	小定风珠
Xiao Er Hui Chun Dan	Return of Spring Special Pill [Pediatric]	小儿回春丹
Xiao Feng San	Eliminate Wind Powder	消风散
Xiao Huo Luo Dan	Minor Invigorate the Collaterals Special Pill	小活络丹
Xiao Ji Yin Zi	Cirsium Decoction	小蓟饮子
Xiao Jian Zhong Tang	Minor Construct the Middle Decoction	小建中汤
Xiao Jin Dan	Minor Gold Special Pill	小金丹
Xiao Ke Fang	Wasting and Thirsting Formula	消渴方
Xiao Luo Wan	Reduce Scrofula Pill	消瘰丸
Xiao Qing Long Jia Shi Gao Tang	Minor Bluegreen Dragon Decoction plus Gypsum	小青龙加石膏汤
Xiao Qing Long Tang	Minor Bluegreen Dragon Decoction	小青龙汤
Xiao San Tang Er Hao	Dissolve and Disperse Decoction Formula Two	消散汤二号
Xiao San Tang Yi Hao	Dissolve and Disperse Decoction Formula One	消散汤一号
Xiao Xian Xiong Tang	Minor Sinking into the Chest Decoction	小陷胸汤
Xiao Xu Ming Tang	Minor Prolong Life Decoction	小续命汤
Xiao Yao San	Rambling Powder	逍遥散
Xie Bai San	Drain the White Powder	泻白散
Xie Huang San	Drain the Yellow Powder	泻黄散
Xie Qing Wan	Drain the Green Pill	泻青丸
Xin Jia Huang Long Tang	Newly-Augmented Yellow Dragon Decoction	新加黄龙汤
Xin Jia Xiang Ru Yin	Newly-Augmented Mosla Decoction	新加香薷饮

Appendix 8 — Cross-reference of Herbal Formula Names

Pinyin Names	Literal Names	Chinese Names
Xin Yi Qing Fei Yin	Magnolia Decoction to Clear the Lung	辛夷清肺饮
Xin Yi San	Magnolia Flower Powder	辛夷散
Xin Zhi Ju Pi Zhu Ru Tang	Newly-Formulated Tangerine Peel and Bamboo Shaving Decoction	新制橘皮竹茹汤
Xing Jun San	Troop-Marching Powder	行军散
Xing Su San	Apricot Kernel and Perilla Leaf Powder	杏苏散
Xing Su Yin	Apricot Kernel and Perilla Leaf Decoction	杏苏饮
Xing Xiao Wan	Awake and Disperse Pill	醒消丸
Xiong Gui Tiao Xue Yin	Cnidium and Tangkuei Decoction to Regulate Blood	芎归调血饮
Xu Ming Tang	Prolong Life Decoction	续命汤
Xuan Du Fa Biao Tang	Dissipate Toxins and Release the Exterior Decoction	宣毒发表汤
Xuan Fu Dai Zhe Shi Tang	Inula and Hematite Decoction	旋覆代赭石汤
Xue Fu Zhu Yu Tang	Drive Out Stasis in the Mansion of Blood Decoction	血府逐瘀汤
Yan Hu Er Hao	Corydalis Formula Two	延胡二号
Yan Hu Suo San	Corydalis Powder	延胡索散
Yan Hu Yi Hao	Corydalis Formula One	延胡一号
Yan Tang Tan Tu Fang	Salt Decoction to Induce Vomiting	盐汤探吐方
Yang He Tang	Yang-Heartening Decoction	阳和汤
Yang Xin Dan	Nourish the Heart Pill	养心丹
Yang Xin Tang	Nourish the Heart Decoction	养心汤
Yang Yin Qing Fei Tang	Nourish the Yin and Clear the Lung Decoction	养阴清肺汤
Yao Tong Fang Er Hao	Low Back Formula Two	腰痛方二号
Yao Tong Fang Yi Hao	Low Back Formula One	腰痛方一号
Yi Gan San	Restrain the Liver Powder	抑肝散
Yi Gong San	Extraordinary Merit Powder	异功散
Yi Guan Jian	Linking Decoction	一贯煎
Yi Huang Tang	Change the Yellow [Discharge] Decoction	易黄汤
Yi Qi Cong Ming Tang	Augment the Qi and Increase Acuity Decoction	益气聪明汤
Yi Yi Fu Zi Bai Jiang San	Coicis, Prepared Aconite, and Patrinia Powder	薏苡附子败酱散
Yi Yi Ren Tang	Coicis Decoction	薏苡仁汤
Yi Yuan San	Benefit the Basal Powder	益元散
Yi Zi Tang	Yi Word Decoction	乙字汤
Yin Chen Hao Tang	Artemisia Scoparia Decoction	茵陈蒿汤
Yin Chen Pai Shi Tang	Artemisia Scoparia Decoction to Expel Stone	茵陈排石汤
Yin Chen Si Ni Tang	Artemisia Scoparia Decoction for Frigid Extremities	茵陈四逆汤
Yin Chen Wu Ling San	Artemisia Scoparia and Five-Ingredient Powder with Poria	茵陈五苓散
Yin Hua Jie Du Tang	Honeysuckle Decoction to Relieve Toxicity	银花解毒汤
Yin Qiao Jie Du San	Honeysuckle and Forsythia Powder to Relieve Toxicity	银翘解毒散
Yin Qiao San	Honeysuckle and Forsythia Powder	银翘散

Appendix 8 — Cross-reference of Herbal Formula Names

Pinyin Names	Literal Names	Chinese Names
Yin Qiao Tang	Honeysuckle and Forsythia Decoction	银翘汤
You Bi Tang	Benefit the Nose Decoction	优鼻汤
You Gui Wan	Restore the Right [Kidney] Pill	右归丸
You Gui Yin	Restore the Right [Kidney] Decoction	右归饮
Yu Nu Jian	Jade Woman Decoction	玉女煎
Yu Ping Feng San	Jade Windscreen Powder	玉屏风散
Yu Quan Wan	Jade Spring Pill	玉泉丸
Yu Ye Tang	Jade Fluid Decoction	玉液汤
Yu Zhen San	True Jade Powder	玉真散
Yue Bi Jia Zhu Tang	Maidservant from Yue Decoction plus Atractylodes	越婢加术汤
Yue Bi Tang	Maidservant from Yue Decoction	越婢汤
Yue Hua Wan	Moonlight Pill	月华丸
Yue Ju Wan	Escape Restraint Pill	越鞠丸
Zai Zao San	Renewal Powder	再造散
Zeng Ye Cheng Qi Tang	Increase the Fluids and Order the Qi Decoction	增液承气汤
Zeng Ye Tang	Increase the Fluids Decoction	增液汤
Zhe Chong Yin	Break the Conflict Decoction	折冲饮
Zhen Gan Xi Feng Tang	Sedate the Liver and Extinguish Wind Decoction	镇肝熄风汤
Zhen Ling Dan	Rouse the Spirits Special Pill	震灵丹
Zhen Ren Huo Ming Yin	True Man's Decoction to Revitalize Life	真人活命饮
Zhen Ren Yang Zang Tang	True Man's Decoction for Nourishing the Organs	真人养脏汤
Zhen Wu Tang	True Warrior Decoction	真武汤
Zhen Zhong Dan	Pillow Special Pill	枕中丹
Zhen Zhu Mu Wan	Mother of Pearl Pill	珍珠母丸
Zheng Gu Zi Jin Dan	Purple and Gold Pill for Righteous Bones	正骨紫金丹
Zhi Bai Di Huang Wan	Anemarrhena, Phellodendron, and Rehmannia Pill	知柏地黄丸
Zhi Bao Dan	Greatest Treasure Special Pill	至宝丹
Zhi Gan Cao Tang	Honey-Fried Licorice Decoction	炙甘草汤
Zhi Jing San	Stop Spasms Powder	止痉散
Zhi Ke Tang	Stop Coughing Decoction	止咳汤
Zhi Shi Dao Zhi Wan	Immature Bitter Orange Pill to Guide Out Stagnation	枳实导滞丸
Zhi Shi Shao Yao San	Immature Bitter Orange and Peony Powder	枳实芍药散
Zhi Shi Xiao Pi Wan	Immature Bitter Orange Pill to Reduce Focal Distention	枳实消痞丸
Zhi Shi Xie Bai Gui Zhi Tang	Immature Bitter Orange, Chinese Chive, and Cinnamon Twig Decoction	枳实薤白桂枝汤
Zhi Sou San	Stop Coughing Powder	止嗽散
Zhi Suo Er Chen Tang	Two-Cured Decoction with Aurantium and Cardamon	枳缩二陈汤
Zhi Xue Tang	Stop Bleeding Decoction	止血汤
Zhi Zhu Tang	Immature Bitter Orange and Atractylodes Macrocephala Decoction	枳术汤

Appendix 8 — Cross-reference of Herbal Formula Names

Pinyin Names	Literal Names	Chinese Names
Zhi Zhu Wan	Immature Bitter Orange and Atractylodes Macrocephala Pill	枳术丸
Zhi Zhuo Gu Ben Wan	Treat the Turbidity and Guard the Root Pill	治浊固本丸
Zhi Zi Bo Pi Tang	Gardenia and Phellodendron Decoction	栀子柏皮汤
Zhi Zi Chi Tang	Gardenia and Soja Decoction	栀子豉汤
Zhi Zi Jiang Huo Tang	Gardenia Decoction to Descend Fire	栀子降火汤
Zhi Zi Qing Gan Tang	Gardenia Decoction to Clear the Liver	栀子清肝汤
Zhong He Tang	Middle-Heartening Decoction	中和汤
Zhou Che Wan	Vessel and Vehicle Pill	舟车丸
Zhu Ling Tang	Polyporus Decoction	猪苓汤
Zhu Ru Wen Dan Tang	Bamboo Decoction to Warm the Gallbladder	竹茹温胆汤
Zhu Sha An Shen Wan	Cinnabar Pill to Tranquilize the Spirit	朱砂安神丸
Zhu Ye Liu Bang Tang	Lophatherum, Tamarisk and Arctium Decoction	竹叶柳蒡汤
Zhu Ye Shi Gao Tang	Bamboo Leaves and Gypsum Decoction	竹叶石膏汤
Zhu Yu Tang	Drive Out Blood Stasis Decoction	逐瘀汤
Zhuang Jin Tang	Strengthen the Tendon Decoction	壮筋汤
Zi Cao Gen Mu Li Tang	Arnebia and Oyster Shell Decoction	紫草根牡蛎汤
Zi Jin Ding	Purple Gold Special Pill	紫金锭
Zi Shen Ming Mu Tang	Nourish the Kidney to Brighten the Eyes Decoction	滋肾明目汤
Zi Shen Tong Er Tang	Nourish the Kidney to Unblock the Ears Decoction	滋肾通耳汤
Zi Sheng Wan	Nourish Life Pill	资生丸
Zi Wan Tang	Aster Decoction	紫菀汤
Zi Xue	Purple Snow	紫雪
Zi Yin Di Huang Wan	Rehmannia Pill to Nourish Yin	滋阴地黄丸
Zi Yin Jiang Huo Tang	Nourish Yin and Descend the Fire Decoction	滋阴降火汤
Zi Yin Qing Re Tang	Nourish Yin and Clear Heat Decoction	滋阴清热汤
Zuo Gui Wan	Restore the Left [Kidney] Pill	左归丸
Zuo Gui Yin	Restore the Left [Kidney] Decoction	左归饮
Zuo Jin Wan	Left Metal Pill	左金丸

Appendix 9 — Tables of Famous Doctors

Table 1. Famous Doctors – in Chapter Order

Chapters	Names
Part I. Overview	黄帝 Huang Di (Yellow Emperor), dates unknown.
Part II. Formula Monographs	神农 Shen Nong (Divine Husbandman), dates unknown.
1. Exterior-Releasing Formulas	张仲景 Zhang Zhong-Jing, also known as 张机 Zhang Ji, 150-219 CE.
2. Downward Draining Formulas	张景岳 Zhang Jing-Yue, also known as 张介宾 Zhang Jie-Bin, 1563-1640.
3. Harmonizing Formulas	吴有性 Wu You-Xing, also known as 吴又可 Wu You-Ke, 1580's-1660's.
4. Exterior- and Interior-Releasing Formulas	刘完素 Liu Yuan-Su, 1120-1200.
5. Heat-Clearing Formulas	叶桂 Ye Gui, also known as 叶天士 Ye Tian-Shi, 1666-1745.
6. Summer-Heat Dispelling Formulas	吴塘 Wu Tang, also known as 吴鞠通 Wu Ju-Tong, 1758-1836.
7. Interior-Warming Formulas	王叔和 Wang Shu-He, third century.
8. Tonic Formulas	钱乙 Qian Yi, 1032-1113.
9. *Shen*-Calming Formulas	扁鹊 Bian Que, also known as 秦越人 Qin Yue-Ren, 407-310 BCE.
10. Orifice-Opening Formulas	华佗 Hua Tuo, 110-207 CE.
11. Astringent Formulas	傅山 Fu Shan, also known as 傅青主 Fu Qing-Zhu, 1607-1684.
12. Qi-Regulating Formulas	李时珍 Li Shi-Zhen, 1518-1593.
13. Blood-Regulating Formulas	王清任 Wang Qing-Ren, 1768-1831.
14. Wind-Expelling Formulas	王焘 Wang Tao, 670-755.
15. Dryness-Relieving Formulas	陶弘景 Tao Hong-Jing, 456-536.
16. Damp-Dispelling Formulas	王肯堂 Wang Ken-Tang, 1549-1613.
17. Wind-Damp Dispelling Formulas	孙思邈 Sun Si-Miao, 581-682.
18. Phlegm-Dispelling Formulas	朱震亨 Zhu Zhen-Heng, also known as 朱丹溪 Zhu Dan-Xi, 1281-1358.
19. Reducing, Guiding and Dissolving Formulas	李杲 Li Gao, also known as 李东垣 Li Dong-Heng, 1180-1251.
20. Antiparasitic Formulas	葛洪 Ge Hong, 284-364.
21. Emetic Formulas	张从正 Zhang Cong-Zheng, also known as 张子和 Zhang Zi-He, 1151-1231.
22. Formulas that Treat Abscesses and Sores	龚廷贤 Gong Ting-Xian, 1522-1619.
Part III. Additional Resources	吴尚先 Wu Shang-Xian, 1806-1886.

Appendix 9 — Tables of Famous Doctors

Table 2. Famous Doctors – According to Chronology of Chinese Dynasties

Dynasties & Kingdoms		Year	Names
Xia Period 夏		2100-1600 BCE	黄帝 Huang Di (Yellow Emperor), dates unknown. 神农 Shen Nong (Divine Husbandman), dates unknown.
Shang Period 商		1600-1100 BCE	
Zhou Period 周	Western Zhou Period 西周	1100-771 BCE	孙阳 Sun Yang, 680-610 BCE. 扁鹊 Bian Que, also known as 秦越人 Qin Yue-Ren, 407-310 BCE.
	Eastern Period 东周	770-256 BCE	
	Spring and Autumn Period 春秋	770-476 BCE	
	Warring States 战国	475-221 BCE	
Qin Dynasty 秦		221-207 BCE	
Han Dynasty 汉	Western Han 西汉	206 BCE- 24	华佗 Hua Tuo, 110-207 CE. 张仲景 Zhang Zhong-Jing, also known as 张机 Zhang Ji, 150-219 CE.
	Eastern Han 东汉	25-220	
Three Kingdoms 三国	Wei 魏	220-265	王叔和 Wang Shu-He, third century.
	Shu 蜀	221-263	
	Wu 吴	222-280	
Western Jin Dynasty 西晋		265-316	葛洪 Ge Hong, 284-364.
Eastern Jin Dynasty 东晋		317-420	
Northern and Southern Dynasties 北南朝	Southern 南朝	420-589	陶弘景 Tao Hong-Jing, 456-536.
	Northern 北朝	386-581	
Sui Dynasty 隋		581-618	孙思邈 Sun Si-Miao, 581-682.
Tang Dynasty 唐		618-907	王焘 Wang Tao, 670-755.
Five Dynasties 五代	Later Liang 后梁	907-923	
	Later Tang 后唐	923-936	
	Later Jin 后晋	936-947	
	Later Han 后汉	947-950	
	Later Zhou 后周	951-960	
Song Dynasty 宋	Northern Song 北宋	960-1127	
	Southern Song 南宋	1127-1279	

Appendix 9 — Tables of Famous Doctors

Dynasties & Kingdoms	Year	Names
Liao Dynasty 潦	916-1125	钱乙 Qian Yi, 1032-1113.
Jin Dynasty 金	1115-1234	刘完素 Liu Yuan-Su, 1120-1200. 张从正 Zhang Cong-Zheng, also known as 张子和 Zhang Zi-He, 1151-1231. 李杲 Li Gao, also known as 李东垣 Li Dong-Heng, 1180-1251.
Yuan Dynasty 元	1271-1368	朱震亨 Zhu Zhen-Heng, also known as 朱丹溪 Zhu Dan-Xi, 1281-1358.
Ming Dynasty 明	1368-1644	李时珍 Li Shi-Zhen, 1518-1593. 龚廷贤 Gong Ting-Xian, 1522-1619. 王肯堂 Wang Ken-Tang, 1549-1613. 张景岳 Zhang Jing-Yue, also known as 张介宾 Zhang Jie-Bin, 1563-1640. 吴有性 Wu You-Xing, also known as 吴又可 Wu You-Ke, 1580's-1660's. 傅山 Fu Shan, also known as 傅青主 Fu Qing-Zhu, 1607-1684.
Qing Dynasty 清	1644-1911	叶桂 Ye Gui, also known as 叶天士 Ye Tian-Shi, 1666-1745. 吴塘 Wu Tang, also known as 吴鞠通 Wu Ju-Tong, 1758-1836. 王清任 Wang Qing-Ren, 1768-1831. 吴尚先 Wu Shang-Xian, 1806-1886.
Republic of China 中华民国	1911-Present Day	
People's Republic of China 中华人民共和国	1949-Present Day	

Appendix 9 — Tables of Famous Doctors

Table 3. Famous Doctors – in Alphabetical Order

Names	Chapters
扁鹊 Bian Que, also known as 秦越人 Qin Yue-Ren, 407-310 BCE.	9. *Shen*-Calming Formulas
傅山 Fu Shan, also known as 傅青主 Fu Qing-Zhu, 1607-1684.	11. Astringent Formulas
葛洪 Ge Hong, 284-364.	20. Antiparasitic Formulas
龚廷贤 Gong Ting-Xian, 1522-1619.	22. Formulas that Treat Abscesses and Sores
华佗 Hua Tuo, 110-207 CE.	10. Orifice-Opening Formulas
黄帝 Huang Di (Yellow Emperor), dates unknown.	Part I. Overview
李杲 Li Gao, also known as 李东垣 Li Dong-Heng, 1180-1251.	19. Reducing, Guiding and Dissolving Formulas
李时珍 Li Shi-Zhen, 1518-1593.	12. Qi-Regulating Formulas
刘完素 Liu Yuan-Su, 1120-1200.	4. Exterior- and Interior-Releasing Formulas
钱乙 Qian Yi, 1032-1113.	8. Tonic Formulas
神农 Shen Nong (Divine Husbandman), dates unknown.	Part II. Formula Monographs
孙思邈 Sun Si-Miao, 581-682.	17. Wind-Damp Dispelling Formulas
陶弘景 Tao Hong-Jing, 456-536.	15. Dryness-Relieving Formulas
王肯堂 Wang Ken-Tang, 1549-1613.	16. Damp-Dispelling Formulas
王清任 Wang Qing-Ren, 1768-1831.	13. Blood-Regulating Formulas
王叔和 Wang Shu-He, third century.	7. Interior-Warming Formulas
王焘 Wang Tao, 670-755.	14. Wind-Expelling Formulas
吴尚先 Wu Shang-Xian, 1806-1886.	Part III. Additional Resources
吴塘 Wu Tang, also known as 吴鞠通 Wu Ju-Tong, 1758-1836.	6. Summer-Heat Dispelling Formulas
吴有性 Wu You-Xing, also known as 吴又可 Wu You-Ke, 1580's-1660's.	3. Harmonizing Formulas
叶桂 Ye Gui, also known as 叶天士 Ye Tian-Shi, 1666-1745.	5. Heat-Clearing Formulas
张从正 Zhang Cong-Zheng, also known as 张子和 Zhang Zi-He, 1151-1231.	21. Emetic Formulas
张景岳 Zhang Jing-Yue, also known as 张介宾 Zhang Jie-Bin, 1563-1640.	2. Downward Draining Formulas
张仲景 Zhang Zhong-Jing, also known as 张机 Zhang Ji, 150-219 CE.	1. Exterior-Releasing Formulas
朱震亨 Zhu Zhen-Heng, also known as 朱丹溪 Zhu Dan-Xi, 1281-1358.	18. Phlegm-Dispelling Formulas

Bibliography of Historical Texts

Pinyin Names (Translated Names)	**Chinese Names**
Bai Rai Shin Shu (A New Study of Dermatomycosis and Dermatitis) by Tsursure Katakura	
Bai Yi Xuan Fang (Selected Formulas)	百一选方
Bao Ying Cuo Yao (Synopsis of Caring for Infants) by Xue Kai in 1555	保婴撮要
Bei Ji Qian Jin Yao Fang (Thousands of Golden Prescriptions for Emergencies) by Sun Si-Miao in Tang Dynasty	备急千金要方
Ben Cao Bei Yao (Essentials of the Materia Medica) by Wang Ang in 1751	本草备要
Ben Cao Cong Xin (Thoroughly Revised Materia Medica) by Wu Yi-Luo in 1751	本草从新
Ben Cao Fa Hui (Elaboration of the Materia Medica) by Xu Yan-Chun in Ming Dynasty	本草发挥
Ben Cao Gang Mu (Materia Medica) by Li Shi-Zhen in 1578	本草纲目
Ben Cao Gang Mu Shi Yi (Omissions from the Grand Materia Medica) by Zhao Xue-Min in 1765	本草纲目拾遗
Ben Cao Hui Yan (Treasury of Words on the Materia Medica) by Ni Zhu-Mo in 1624	本草汇言
Ben Cao Jing Ji Zhu (Collection of Commentaries on the Classic of the Materia Medica) by Tao Hong-Jing in 480-498 B.C.	本草经集注
Ben Cao Meng Quan (Hidden Aspects of the Materia Medica) by Chen Jia-Mo in 1565	本草蒙荃
Ben Cao Pin Hui Jing Yao (Essentials of Materia Medica) by Liu Wen-Tai in 1505	本草品汇精要
Ben Cao Qiu Zheng (Verification of Materia Medica) by Huang Gong-Xiu in 1769	本草求正
Ben Cao Shi Yi (Omissions from the [Classic of the] Materia Medica) by Chen Cang-Qi in 741 A.D.	本草拾遗
Ben Cao Yan Yi (Extension of the Materia Medica) by Kou Zong-Shi in 1116	本草衍义
Ben Cao Yan Yi Bu Yi (Supplement to the Extension of the Materia Medica) by Zhu Zhen-Heng in 1347	本草衍义补遗
Ben Cao Yuan Shi (Origins of the Materia Medica) by Li Zhong-Li in Ming Dynasty	本草原始
Ben Cao Zai Xin (Renewed Materia Medica)	本草再新
Ben Cao Zheng (Rectification of the Materia Medica)	本草正
Ben Cao Zheng Yi (Truth and False Information of Materia Medica) by Zhang Shan-Lei in 1920	本草正义
Ben Jing (Divine Husbandman's Classic of the Materia Medica) in the second century	本经
Ben Jing Feng Yuan (Journey to the Origin of the Classic of Materia Medica) by Zhang Lu in 1670	本经逢原
Bian Zheng Lun (Records of Differential Diagnosis)	辨证论
Bo Ai Xin Jian (Manual of Universal Lover from the Heart) by Wei Zhi in 1525	博爱心鉴
Bu Yao Xiu Zhen Xiao Er Fang Lun (Supplement to the Pocket-Sized Discussion of Formulas for Children)	补要袖诊小儿方论
Chang Yong Zhong Cao Yao Shou Ce (Handbook of Commonly Used Traditional Chinese Herbs) by Guangzhou People's Liberation Army Medical Brigade	常用中草药手册
Cheng Fang Bian Du (Convenient Reader of Established Formulas) by Zhang Bing-Cheng in 1904	成方便读
Cheng Fang Qie Yong (Practical Formulas) by Wu Yi-Luo in 1761	成方切用
Chong Ding Ji Sheng Fang (Revised Formulas to Aid the Living)	重订济生方
Chong Ding Tong Su Shang Han Lun (Revised Popular Guide to the Discussion of Cold-Induced Disorders) by Yu Gen-Chu in Qing Dynasty	重订通俗伤寒论
Chong Ding Yan Shi Ji Sheng Fang (Revised Formulas to Aid the Living from Yan's Family)	重订严氏济生方
Chong Lou Yu Yao (Jade Key to Many Towers) by Zheng Mei-Run in 1838	重楼玉钥

BIBLIOGRAPHY OF HISTORICAL TEXTS B

Bibliography of Historical Texts

Pinyin Names (Translated Names)	**Chinese Names**
Ci Shi Nan Zhi (Hard-Won Knowledge) by Wang Hao-Gu in 1308	此事难知
Dan Xi Xin Fa (Teachings of [Zhu] Dan-Xi) by Zhu Zhen-Heng in 1481	丹溪心法
Dan Xi Xin Fa Fu Yu (Additions to the Teachings for [Zhu] Dan-Xi) by Fang Guang-Lei in 1536	丹溪心法附余
De Pei Ben Cao (Materia Medica of Combinations)	得配本草
Dong Heng Shi Xiao Fang (Tested and Effective Formulas by Dong Heng) by Dong Heng in 1266	东恒试效方
Dong Tian Ao Zhi (Profound Purpose from the Heavenly Abode) by Chen Shi-Duo in 1694	洞天奥旨
Dong Yi Bao Jian (Precious Mirror of Oriental Medicine) by Xu Sun in 1611	东医宝鉴
Dou Zhen Shi Yi Xin Fa (Teachings of Generations of Physicians about Pox) by Wan Quan in 1568	痘疹世医心法
Fang Ji Xue (Traditional Chinese Medical Formulas) by Shanghai College of Traditional Chinese Medicine in 1975	方剂学
Fu Ke Chan Lun Fang (Discussion of Formulas for Obstetrics and Gynecology)	妇科常论方
Fu Qing Zhu Nu Ke (Women's Diseases According to Fu Qing-Zhu) by Fu Shan in 1827	傅青主女科
Fu Ren Da Quan Liang Fang (Complete Fine Formulas for Women) by Chen Zi-Ming in 1237	妇人大全良方
Fu Ren Liang Fang (Fine Formulas for Women) by Chen Zi-Ming in 1237	妇人良方
Fu Shou Jing Fang (Exquisite Formulas for Fostering Longevity) by Wu Min in 1530	扶寿精防
Gan Zheng Ji Yao (Essential Compilation of Infectious Syndromes) by Yan Hong-Zhi in 1920	感证辑要
Gu Jin Ming Fang (Famous Classic and Contemporary Formulas) by Luo Mei in 1675	古今名方
Gu Jin Yi Jian (Medical Mirror of the Past and Present) by Gong Xin-Zuan in Ming Dynasty	古今医鉴
Gu Jin Yi Tong Da Quan (Comprehensive Collection of Medicine Past and Present) by Xu Chun-Fu in 1556	古今医通大全
Guang Wen Yi Lun (Discussion of Widespread Warm Epidemics) by Dai Tian-Zhang in 1722	广温疫论
Guangxi Zhong Yao Zhi (Guangxi Journal of Chinese Herbal Medicines)	广西中药志
Guizhou Min Jian Yao Wu (Folk Medicina from Guizhou)	贵州民间药物
Hai Jing Ben Cao (Materia Medica from the Ocean)	海经本草
Hai Yao Ben Cao (Materia Medica of Herbs from [Across the] Seas) by Li Xun in 907-960 A.D.	海药本草
Han Shi Yi Tong (Comprehensive Medicine According to Master Han) by Han Mao in 1522	韩氏医通
Hong Shi Ji Yan Fang (Time-Tested Formulas of Hong Family)	洪氏集验方
Huang Di Nei Jing (Yellow Emperor's Inner Classic) in the second century A.D.	黄帝内经
Huang Di Su Wen Xuan Ming Lun Fang (Formulas from the Discussion Illuminating the Yellow Emperor's Basic Questions) by Liu Yuan-Su in 1172	黄帝素问宣明论方
Huo Luan Lun (Discussion of Sudden Turmoil Disorders) by Wan Shi-Xiong in 1862	藿乱论
Ji Sheng Fang (Formulas to Aid the Living) by Yan Yong-He in 1253	济生方
Ji Yin Gang Mu (Materia Medica to Aid Yin) by Wu Zhi-Wang in 1620	济阴纲目
Jia You Ben Cao (Materia Medica of the Jia You Era) by Zhang Yu-Xi and Su Song in 1057-1060	嘉佑本草
Jiang Su Zhi Wu Zhi (Jiangsu Journal of Botany)	江苏植物志
Jiao Zhu Fu Ren Liang Fang (Revised Fine Formulas for Women) by Bi Li-Zhai in 16th century	校注妇人良方
Jin Gui Yao Lue (Essentials from the Golden Cabinet) by Zhang Zhong-Jing in Eastern Han	金匮要略
Jing Shi Zheng Lei Bei Ji Ben Cao (Differentiation and Application of Materia Medica) by Tang Shen-Wei in 1082	经史证类备急本草

Bibliography of Historical Texts

Pinyin Names (Translated Names)	Chinese Names
Jing Xiu Tang Yao Shuo (Herbal Teachings from the Respectfully Decorated Hall) by Qian Shu-Tian	敬修堂药说
Jing Yue Quan Shu (Collected Treatises of [Zhang] Jing Yue) by Zhang Jie-Bin (Zhang Jing-Yue) in 1624	景岳全书
Jiu Huang Ben Cao (Materia Medica to Rescue Emergencies)	救荒本草
Ju Fang (Imperial Formulary) by the Imperial Medical Department in 1078-85	局方
Kai Bao Ben Cao (Materia Medica of the Kai Bao Era) by Ma Zhi in 973-974 A.D.	开宝本草
Lan Shi Mi Cang (Secrets from the Orchid Chamber) by Li Gao in 1336	兰室秘藏
Lan Tai Gui Fan (Guidelines from Lan-Tai) by Xu Da-Chun in 1764	兰台轨范
Lei Bian Zhu Shi Ji Yan Yi Fang (Effective Medical Formulas Arranged by Category by Doctor Zhu) by Zhu Zuo in 1266	类编朱氏集验医方
Lei Gong Pao Zhi Lun (Grandfather Lei's Discussions of Herb Preparation) by Lei Xiao in 470 A.D.	雷公炮制抡
Lei Zheng Huo Ren Shu (Book to Safeguard Life Arranged According to Pattern) by Zhu Gong in 1108	类证活人书
Liang Fang Yi Ye (Small Collection of Fine Formulas) by Xie Yuan-Qing in 1842	良方集腋
Lin Zheng Zhi Nan Yi An (Case Histories from the Compass of Clinical Patterns) by Ye Tian-Shi in 1746	临证指南医案
Ling Nan Cai Yao Lu (Records of Picking Herbs in Guangdong)	岭南采药录
Ling Shu (Magic Pivot) in the second century A.D.	灵枢
Liu Zhou Yi Hua (Medical Dialogues from Liuzhou) by Wei Zhi-Xiu in mid-16th century	柳州医话
Lu Chan Yan Ben Cao (Materia Medica from Steep Mountain-sides)	履巉岩本草
Meika Hosen (A Selection of Famous Physicians' Prescriptions) by Yoshine Hirai	名家方选
Ming Yi Bie Lu (Miscellaneous Records of Famous Physicians) by Tao Hong-Jing in 500 A.D.	名医别录
Ming Yi Za Zhu (Miscellaneous Books of Ming Medicine) by Wang Lun in 1549 A.D.	明医杂著
Ming Yi Zhi Zhang (Displays of Enlightened Physicians) by Huang Fu-Zhong in 16th century	名医指掌
Nanning Shi Yao Wu Zhi (Nanning City Medicines)	南宁市药物志
Nei Jing (Inner Classic) in the second century A.D.	内经
Nei Jing Shi Yi Fang Lun (Enumeration of Formulas Omitted from the Inner Classic) by Luo Long-Ji in Song Dynasty	内经拾遗方论
Nei Ke Zhai Yao (Summary of Internal Medicine) by Wen Sheng in mid-19th century	内科摘要
Nei Wai Shang Bian Huo Lun (Clarifying Doubts about Injury from Internal and External Causes) by Li Gao in 1247	内外伤辨惑论
Pi Wei Lun (Discussion of the Spleen and Stomach) by Li Gao in 1249	脾胃论
Pian Yu Xin Shu (Text from Heart of Jade) by Wu Quan in the mid-16th century	片玉心书
Pin Hui Jing Yao (Essentials of (Herbal) Distinctions)	品汇精要
Pu Ji Ben Shi Fang (Formulas of Universal Benefit from My Practice) by Xu Shu-Wei in 1132	普济本事方
Pu Ji Fang (Formulas of Universal Benefit) by Teng Hong in Ming Dynasty	普济方
Qi Xiao Hai Shang Xian Fang Mi Ben (Secret Text of Extraordinary Effective Beneficial Formulas from Across the Seas)	奇效海上仙方秘本
Qi Xiao Liang Fang (Fine Formulas with Miraculous Results)	奇效良方
Qian Jin Yao Fang (Thousand Ducat Prescriptions) by Sun Si-Miao in 581-685 A.D.	千金要方
Qian Jin Yi Fang (Supplement to the Thousand Ducat Formulas) by Sun Si-Miao in 682 A.D.	千金翼方

Bibliography of Historical Texts

Pinyin Names (Translated Names)	Chinese Names
Qian Tian Jia Fang (Family Formulas of Qian Tian-Jia)	浅田家方
Qing Cao Shi Jie (The World of Herbs) by Zhong Ding-Chuan in 1992	青草世界
Qing Cao Yao Han Shou Jiao Cai (Textbook of Botanical Medicine) by Zhong Ding-Chuan in 1992	青草药函授教材
Quan Guo Zhong Cheng Yao Chu Fang Ji (National Collection of Chinese Herbal Prepared Medicines) in 1949	全国中成药处方剂
Ren Zhai Zhi Zhi (Straight Directions of Benevolent Aid) by Yang Tu-Ying in 1264	仁斋直指
Ri Hua Zi Ben Cao (Materia Medica of Ri Hua-Zi) by Ri Hua-Zi in 713 A.D.	日华子本草
Ri Yong Ben Cao (Household Materia Medica) by Wu Rui in 1330	日用本草
Ru Men Shi Qin (Confucians' Duties to their Parents) by Zhang Cong-Zheng in 1228	儒门事亲
San Yin Ji Yi Bing Zheng Fang Lun (Discussion of Illnesses, Patterns, and Formulas Related to the Unification of the Three Etiologies) by Chen Yan in 1174	三因即一病证方论
Shang Hai Shi Zhong Cheng Yao Zhi Ji Gui Fan (Shanghai Municipal Standards for the Manufacturing of Chinese Prepared Medicines) in 1970	上海市中成药制剂规范
Shang Han Biao Ben Xin Fa Lei Cui (Collection of Methods Related to the Manifestation and Root of Cold-Induced Disorders)	伤寒标本心法类萃
Shang Han Liu Shu (Six Texts on Cold-Induced Disorders) by Tao Hua in 1445	伤寒六书
Shang Han Lun (Discussion of Cold-Induced Disorders) by Zhang Zhong-Jing in Eastern Han	伤寒论
Shang Han Lun Ming Li Lun (Clarification of the Theory of Cold Induced Disorders) by Cheng Wu-Ji in 1156	伤寒论明理论
Shang Han Ming Li Yao Fang Lun (Clarification of the Formulas and Herbs of Cold Induced Disorders) by Cheng Wu-Ji	伤寒明理药方论
Shang Han Quan Sheng Ji (All-New Collection of Cold Induced Disorders)	伤寒全生集
Shang Han Za Bing Lun (Discussion of Cold-Induced Disorders and Miscellaneous Diseases) by Zhang Zhong-Jing in Eastern Han	伤寒杂病论
Shang Han Zhi Ge Fang Lun (Direct Investigations of Formulas for Cold-Induced Disorders) by Liu Yuan-Su in Jin Dynasty	伤寒直格方论
She Sheng Mi Pou (Secrets Investigations into Obtaining Health) by Hong Ji in 1638	摄生秘剖
She Sheng Zhong Miao Fang (Marvelous Formulas for the Health of Multitudes) by Zhang Shi-Che in 1550	摄生众妙方
Shen Nong Ben Cao Jing (Divine Husbandman's Classic of the Materia Medica) in the second century	神农本草经
Shen Nong Ben Cao Jing Shu (Revised Divine Husbandman's Classic of the Materia Medica) by Miao Xi-Yong in 1625	神农本草经书
Shen Shi Yao Han (Scrutiny of the Priceless Jade Case) by Fu Ren-Yu in 1644	审视瑶函
Shen Shi Zun Sheng Shu (Master Shen's Book for Revering Life) by Shen Jin-Ao in 1773	沈氏尊生书
Sheng Ji Jing (Holy Relief Reference) by Zhao Ji in Jin Dynasty	圣济经
Sheng Ji Zong Lu (General Collection for Holy Relief) by a staff of court physicians of Northern Song Dynasty around 1111-1117	圣剂总录
Shi Bing Lun (Discussion of Seasonal Diseases) by Lei Feng in 1882	时病论
Shi Chuan En Jia Chuan Fang (Family Formulas from Shi Chuan-En)	史传恩家传方
Shi Fang Ge Kuo (Collected Songs about Contemporary Formulas) by Chen Nian-Zi in 1801	时方歌括
Shi Liao Ben Cao (Materia Medica of Diet Therapy) by Meng Shan in the seventh century	食疗本草
Shi Wu Ben Cao (Food as Materia Medica) by Lu He-Ming in 701-704 A.D.	食物本草

Bibliography of Historical Texts

Pinyin Names (Translated Names)	**Chinese Names**
Shi Yao Shen Shu (Miraculous Book of Ten Remedies) by Ge Qian-Sun in 1348	十药神书
Shi Yi De Xiao Fang (Effective Formulas from Generations of Physicians) by Wei Yi-Lin in 1345	世医得效方
Shi Yong Tian Ran Yao Wu (Practical Natural Medicine) by Zheng Bing-Chuan in 1997	实用天然药物
Shou Shi Bao Yuan (Achieving Longevity by Guarding the Source) by Gong Ting-Xian in early 17th century	寿世保元
Shu Ben Cao (Materia Medica of Sichuan) by Han Bao-Sheng in 935-960 A.D.	蜀本草
Si He Ting Ji Fang (Collection of Formulas of Si He-Ting)	饲鹤亭集方
Sichuan Zhong Yao Zhi (Sichuan Journal of Chinese Herbal Medicines)	四川中药志
Su Shen Liang Fang (Fine Formulas by Su and Shen) in Song Dynasty	苏沉良方
Su Wen (Basic Questions) in the second century A.D.	素问
Su Wen Bing Ji Qi Yi Bao Ming Ji (Collection of Writings on the Mechanism of Illness, Suitability of Qi, and the Safeguarding of Life as Discussed in the Basic Questions) by Zhang Yuan-Su in 1186	素问病机气宜保命集
Tai Ping Hui Min He Ji Ju Fang (Imperial Grace Formulary of the Tai Ping Era) by the Imperial Medical Department in 1078-85	太平惠民和济局方
Tai Ping Sheng Hui Fang (Holy Grace Formulary of the Tai Ping Era) by Wang Huai-Yin in Song Dynasty	太平圣惠方
Tai Wan Min Jian Yao (Folk Medicine of Taiwan) by Gao Mu-Chun in 1985	台湾民间药
Tai Wan Zhi Wu Yao Cai Zhi (Medicinal Plants of Taiwan)	台湾植物药材志
Tang Ben Cao (Tang Materia Medica) by Su Jing in 659 A.D.	唐本草
Tang Ye Ben Cao (Materia Medica for Decoctions) by Wang Hao-Gu in 1306	汤液本草
Ti Ren Hui Bian (Compilation of Materials of Benevolence for the Body) by Peng Yong-Guang in 1549	体仁汇编
Tong Su Shang Han Lun (Plain Version of Discussion of Cold-Induced Disorders)	通俗伤寒论
Tu Jing Ben Cao (Illustrated Classic of the Materia Medica) by Su Song in 1061	图经本草
Wai Dan Ben Cao (Materia Medica for External Elixirs)	外丹本草
Wai Ke Fa Hui (External Medicine Elaboration) by Xue Yi in 1528	外科发挥
Wai Ke Zheng Zhi Quan Sheng Ji (Complete Collection of Patterns and Treatments in External Medicine) by Wang Wei-De in 1740	外科症治全生集
Wai Ke Zheng Zhi Zhun Sheng (Standards of Patterns and Treatments in External Medicine) by Wang Ken-Tang in Ming Dynasty	外科症治准绳
Wai Ke Zheng Zong (True Lineage of External Medicine) by Chen Shi-Gong in 1617	外科正宗
Wai Tai Mi Yao (Arcane Essentials from the Imperial Library) by Wang Tao in 752 A.D.	外台秘要
Wan Bing Hui Chun (Restoration of Health from the Myriad Diseases) by Gong Ting-Xian in 1587	万病回春
Wei Sheng Bao Jian (Precious Mirror of Health) by Luo Tian-Yi in Yuan Dynasty	卫生宝鉴
Wei Yao Tiao Bian (Cataloged Differentiation of Erroneous Medicines)	伪药条辨
Wen Bing Tiao Bian (Systematic Differentiation of Warm Disease) by Wu Ju-Tong in 1798	温病条辨
Wen Re Jing Wei (Warp and Woof of Warm-Febrile Diseases) by Wang Meng-Ying in 1852	温热经纬
Wen Yi Lun (Discussion of Epidemic Warm Disease) by Wu You-Xing in 1642	温疫论
Wu Pu Ben Cao (Wu Pu's Materia Medica)	吴普本草
Wu Shi Er Bing Fang (Prescriptions for Fifty-Two Kinds of Diseases) in approximately third century B.C.	五十二病方

Bibliography of Historical Texts

Pinyin Names (Translated Names)	**Chinese Names**
Xi Yuan Ji Lu Jiao Yi (Correction and Explanation of the Wrongly Accused)	洗冤集录校译
Xian Dai Shi Yong Zhong Yao (Modern Practical Chinese Medicines)	现代实用中药
Xian Shou Li Shang Xu Duan Mi Fang (Secret Recipes of Treating Wounds and Bone-Setting Taught by Celestials) by Taoist Lin in 846 A.D.	仙授理伤续断秘方
Xian Xing Zhai Yi Xue Guang Bi Ji (Wide-Ranging Medical Notes from the First-Awakened Studio) by Miao Xi-Yong in 1613	先醒斋医学广笔记
Xiao Er Yao Zheng Zhi Jue (Craft of Medicinal Treatment for Childhood Disease Patterns) by Qian Yi in 1119	小儿药症直决
Xin Xiu Ben Cao (Newly Revised Materia Medica) by Su Jing in 657-659 A.D.	新修本草
Xu Ming Yi Lei An (Continuation of Famous Physicians' Cases Organized by Categories) by Wei Zhi-Xiu in 1770	续名医类案
Xuan Ming Lun Fang (Discussion of Dispersing and Brightening Formulas) by Liu Yuan-Su in Jin and Yuan Dynasties	宣明论方
Yan Fang Xin Bian (New Compilation of Time-Tested Formulas) by Bao Xiang-Ao in 1846	验方新编
Yang Ke Xin De Ji (Collection of Personal Expertises Concerning Skin Lesions) by Gao Bing-Jun in 1805	疡科心得集
Yang Shi Jia Zang Fang (Collected Formulas of the Yang Family) by Yang Tan in 1178	杨氏家藏方
Yang Shi Mi Fang (Secret Formulas of Yang Family)	杨氏秘方
Yao Cai Xue (Study of Medicinal Substances)	药材学
Yao Pu (Medicinal Recipes) by Hou Ning-Ji	药谱
Yao Xing Ben Cao (Materia Medica of Medicinal Properties) by Zhen Quan in 600 A.D.	药性本草
Ye Shi Nu Ke (Ye's Women's Diseases)	叶氏女科
Yi Bian (Ordinary Medicine) by Wang San-Cai in 1587	医便
Yi Fang Ji Jie (Analytical Collection of Medical Formulas) by Wang Ang in 1682	医方集解
Yi Fang Kao (Investigation of Medical Formulas) by Wu Kun in 1584	医方考
Yi Fang Xin Jie (New Explanations of Medical Formulas) by Ma You-Du in 1980	医方新解
Yi Guan (Thorough Knowledge of Medicine) by Zhao Xian-Ke in 1617	医贯
Yi Guan Tang (Linking Clinic)	一贯堂
Yi Ji (Levels of Medicine)	医级
Yi Ji Bao Jian (Precious Mirror for Advancement of Medicine) by Dong Xi-Yuan in 1777	医籍宝鉴
Yi Lin Gai Cuo (Corrections of Errors Among Physicians) by Wang Qing-Ren in 1830	医林改错
Yi Lue Liu Shu (Six Texts on the Essentials of Medicine)	医略六书
Yi Men Fa Lu (Precepts for Physicians) by Yu Chang in 1658	医门法律
Yi Xue Fa Ming (Medical Innovations) by Li Gao in Jin Dynasty	医学发明
Yi Xue Qi Yuan (Origins of the Medicine) by Zhang Yuan-Su in Yuan Dynasty	医学启原
Yi Xue Quan Shu (Complete Book of Medicine) by Xu Si-He	医学全书
Yi Xue Ru Men (Introduction to Medicine) by Li Ting in 1575	医学入门
Yi Xue Xin Wu (Medical Revelations) by Cheng Guo-Peng in 1732	医学心悟
Yi Xue Zheng Zhuan (True Lineage of Medicine) by Yu Tian-Min in 1515	医学正传
Yi Xue Zhong Zhong Can Xi Lu (Records of Heart-Felt Experiences in Medicine With Reference to the West) by Zhang Xi-Chun in 1918-34	医学衷中参西录
Yi Yuan (Bases of Medicine) by Shi Shou-Tang in 1861	医原

Bibliography of Historical Texts

Pinyin Names (Translated Names)	**Chinese Names**
Yi Zhen Yi De (Achievements Regarding Epidemic Rashes) by Yu Shi-Yu in 1794	疫疹一得
Yi Zong Jin Jian (Golden Mirror of the Medical Tradition) by Wu Qian in 1742	医宗金鉴
Yin Pian Xin Can (New References of Prepared Medicines)	饮片新参
Yin Shan Zheng Yao (Correct Guide to Eating and Drinking)	饮膳正要
Yong Lei Qian Fang (Everlasting Categorization of Seal Formulas)	永类钤方
Yuan Ji Qi Wei (Explanation of the Subtitles of the Original Mechanism) by Ni Wei-De in 1370	原机启微
Yuan Nan Yang (Asada's Prescriptions) by Sohaku Asada	
Za Bing Yuan Liu Xi Zhu (Wondrous Lantern for Peering into Origin and Development of Miscellaneous Diseases) by Shen Jin-Ao in 1773	杂病源流犀烛
Za Bing Zheng Zhi Xin Yi (New Significance of Patterns and Treatment in Miscellaneous Diseases)	杂病证治新义
Zeng Bu Nei Jing Shi Yi (Supplement to the Formulas Omitted from the Inner Classic)	增补内经拾遗
Zhang San Feng Xian Chuan Fang (Divine Formulas from Zhang Sanfeng)	张三丰仙传方
Zhang Shi Yi Tong (Comprehensive Medicine According to Master Zhang) by Zhang Lu-Xuan in 1695	张氏医通
Zhen Nan Ben Cao (Materia Medica of South Yunnan) by Lan Mao in Qing Dynasty	滇南本草
Zhen Zhu Nang (Pouch of Pearls) by Zhang Yuan-Su in 1186	珍珠囊
Zheng He Sheng Ji Zong Lu (Comprehensive Recording of Sage-Like Benefit from the Zheng He Era) by Sheng Fu in 1122	政和圣济总录
Zheng Lei Ben Cao (Materia Medica Arranged According to Pattern) by Tang Shen-Wei in 1082	证类本草
Zheng Shi Jia Chuan Nu Ke Wan Jin Fang (Zheng's Family Formulas for Women's Disorders)	郑氏家传女科万金方
Zheng Ti Lei Yao (Catalogued Essentials for Correcting the Body) by Bi Li-Zhai (Ji) in 1529	正体类要
Zheng Yin Mai Zhi (Pattern, Cause, Pulse, and Treatment) by Qin Jing-Ming in 1702	证因脉治
Zheng Zhi Zhun Sheng (Standards of Patterns and Treatments) by Wang Ken-Tang in 1602	症治准绳
Zhi Wu Ming Shi Tu Kao (Illustrated Guide for Nomenclature and Identification of Botanical Products)	植物名实图考
Zhong Guo Guo Yao Gu You Cheng Fang Xuan Ji (A Selection of Traditional Prescriptions of Chinese Medicine) by Chinese Herbal Medicine Committee of the Ministry of the Interior in 1967	中国国药故有成方选集
Zhong Guo Yao Dian (Dictionary of Chinese Medicine) in 1977	中国药典
Zhong Guo Yao Yong Zhi Wu Zi (Chinese Journal of Medicinal Botanicals)	中国药用植物志
Zhong Guo Zhi Wu Zi (Chinese Journal of Botany)	中国植物志
Zhong Xi Yi Jie He Zhi Liao Ji Fu Zheng (Combined Chinese and Western Medical Treatment of the Acute Abdomen) by Nankai Hospital of Tianjin in 1973	中西医结合治疗急腹症
Zhong Yao Yao Ming Ci Dian (Dictionary on Nomenclature of Chinese Herbs)	中药药名词典
Zhong Yao Zhi (Journal of Traditional Chinese Herbal Medicines)	中药志
Zhong Yao Zhi Ji Shou Ce (Handbook of Traditional Chinese Medicinal Preparations)	中药制剂手册
Zhong Yi Fu Ke Zhi Liao Xue (Traditional Chinese Medical Treatment of Women's Disorders) by Chengdu College of Traditional Chinese Medicine in 1970	中医妇科治疗学
Zhong Yi Nei Ke Xue (Traditional Chinese Internal Medicine) by Shanghai College of Traditional Chinese Medicine in 1970	中医内科学

Bibliography of Historical Texts

Pinyin Names (Translated Names)	Chinese Names
Zhong Yi Shang Ke Xue (Traditional Chinese Traumatology) in 1949	中医伤科学
Zhong Yi Yan Ke Xue (Traditional Chinese Opthalmology) by Chengdu College of Traditional Chinese Medicine in 1970	中医眼科学
Zhong Zang Jing (Treasury Classic) by Hua Tuo in the Han Dynasty	中藏经
Zhou Hou Bei Ji Fang (Emergency Formulas to Keep Up One's Sleeve) by Ge Hong in 341 A.D.	肘后备急方
Zhou Hou Fang (Formulas to Keep Up One's Sleeve)	肘后方

Bibliography of Contemporary References

Pinyin Names (Translated Names)	Chinese Names
Ai Zheng (Cancer)	癌症
An Hui Yi Xue (Anhui Medicine)	安徽医学
An Hui Zhong Yi Lin Chuang Za Zi (Anhui Journal of Clinical Chinese Medicine)	安徽中医临床杂志
An Hui Zhong Yi Xue Yuan Xue Bao (Journal of Anhui University School of Medicine)	安徽中医学院学报
An Yi Xue Bao (Anyi Medical Journal)	安医学报
Bai Qiu En Yi Ke Da Xue Xue Bao (Journal of Baiqiuen University of Medicine)	白求恩医科大学学报
Bei Jing Yi Ke Da Xue Xue Bao (Journal of Beijing University of Medicine)	北京医科大学学报
Bei Jing Yi Xue (Beijing Medicine)	北京医学
Bei Jing Yi Xue Yuan Xue Bao (Journal of Beijing School of Medicine)	北京医学院学报
Bei Jing Zhong Yi (Beijing Chinese Medicine)	北京中医
Bei Jing Zhong Yi Xue Yuan Xue Bao (Journal of Beijing University School of Medicine)	北京中医学院学报
Bei Jing Zhong Yi Yao Da Xue Xue Bao (Journal of Beijing University of Medicine and Medicinals)	北京中医药大学学报
Bei Jing Zhong Yi Za Zhi (Beijing Journal of Chinese Medicine)	北京中医杂志
Ben Cao Cong Xin (Revised Herbal Materia Medica)	本草从新
Chang Chun Zhong Yi Xue Yuan Xue Bao (Journal of Changchun University of Chinese Medicine)	长春中医学院学报
Chang Yong Zhong Cao Yao Zhong Du Yu Ji Jiu (Poisoning and Treatment of Commonly-Used Chinese Herbs)	常用中草药中毒与急救
Chang Yong Zhong Yao Cheng Fen Yu Yao Li Shou Ce (A Handbook of the Composition and Pharmacology of Common Chinese Drugs)	常用中药成分与药理手册
Chang Yong Zhong Yao De Ying Yong (Application of Commonly-Used Chinese Herbs)	常用中药的应用
Chang Yong Zhong Yao Xian Dai Yan Jiu Yu Lin Chuang (Recent Study & Clinical Application of Common Traditional Chinese Medicine)	常用中药现代研究与临床
Chen Tzu Yen Chiu (Acupuncture Research)	针灸研究
Cheng Du Zhong Yi Xue Yuan Xue Bao (Journal of Chengdu University of Traditional Chinese Medicine)	成都中医学院学报
Chi Jiao Yi Sheng Za Zhi (Journal of Barefoot Doctors)	赤脚医生杂志
Chong Qing Yi Yao (Chongching Medicine and Herbology)	重庆医药
Chong Qing Zhong Yi Yao Za Zi (Chongching Journal of Chinese Medicine and Medicinals)	重庆中医药杂志
Chuan Dong Zhong Yi Za Zhi (Chuandong Journal of Chinese Medicine)	川东中医杂志
Da Zhong Yi Xue (Public Medicine)	大众医学
Dang Dai Ming Yi Lin Zhen Jing Hua Zhong Liu Juan Ji (Essential Clinical Experience of Famous Modern Doctors - Cancer Volume)	当代明医临证精华-肿瘤卷辑
Di Er Jun Yi Da Xue Xue Bao (Journal of Second Military University of Medicine)	第二军医大学学报
Di Yi Jun Yi Da Xue Xue Bao (Journal of First Military University of Medicine)	第一军医大学学报
Dong Bei Zhi Wu Zhi (Northeast Journal of Herbal Medicine)	东北植物志
Dong Jing Yi Shi Xin Zhi (Tokyo Journal of Medicine)	东京医师新知
Dong Wu Xue Za Zhi (Journal of Zoology)	动物学杂志
Fang Ji Xue (Chinese Herbal Formulas)	方剂学
Fang She Yi Xue (Journal of Radiology)	放射医学
Fu Chan Ke Bing Shi Yong Fang (Practical Formulas for Obstetrics and Gynecology Disorders)	妇产科病实用方

Bibliography of Contemporary References

Pinyin Names (Translated Names)	Chinese Names
Fu Chan Ke Qing Bao Zi Liao (Journal of Gynecology)	妇产科情报资料
Fu Jian Jun Qu Wei Sheng Bu (Health Department of Fujian Military)	福建军区卫生部
Fu Jian Min Jian Cao Yao (Local Herbs of the Fujian)	福建民间草药
Fu Jian Sheng Yi Yao Yan Jiu Suo (Fujian Province Institute of Medicine and Herbal Research)	福建省医药研究所
Fu Jian Yi Xue Yuan Xue Bao (Journal of Fujian University of Medicine)	福建医学院学报
Fu Jian Yi Yao Za Zhi (Fujian Journal of Medicine and Herbology)	福建医药杂志
Fu Jian Yi Za Zhi (Fujian Journal of Chinese Medicine)	福建医杂志
Fu Jian Zhong Yi Yao (Fujian Chinese Medicine and Herbology)	福建中医药
Fu Ke Jing Sui (Essence of Obstetrics and Gynecology)	妇科精髓
Fu Ke Lin Chuang Jing Hua (Clinical Pearl of Obstetrics and Gynecology)	妇科临床精华
Fu Zhou Yi Yao (Fuzhou Medicine and Medicinals)	福州医药
Gan Su Zhong Yi (Gansu Chinese Medicine)	甘肃中医
Gan Su Zhong Yi Xue Yuan Xue Bao (Journal of Gansu University of Chinese Medicine)	甘肃中医学院学报
Guang Dong Yi Xue (Guangdong Medicine)	广东医学
Guang Dong Yi Yao Za Zhi (Guangdong Journal of Medicine and Herbology)	广东医药杂志
Guang Dong Zhong Yi (Guangdong Chinese Medicine)	广东中医
Guang Ming Zhong Yi (Guangming Chinese Medicine)	光明中医
Guang Xi Ben Cao (Guangxi Materia Medica)	广西本草
Guang Xi Chi Jiao Yi Sheng (Guangxi Barefoot Doctor)	广西赤脚医生
Guang Xi Wei Sheng (Guangxi Province Public Health)	广西卫生
Guang Xi Yi Xue (Guangxi Medicine)	广西医学
Guang Xi Yi Xue Yuan Xue Bao (Journal of Guangxi University of Medicine)	广西医学院学报
Guang Xi Zhi Wu (Guangxi Plants)	广西植物
Guang Xi Zhi Wu Tu Zhi (Illustrated Guide of Guangxi Plants)	广西植物图志
Guang Xi Zhong Yi Yao (Guangxi Chinese Medicine and Herbology)	广西中医药
Guang Zhou Yi Yao (Guangzhou Medicine and Medicinals)	广州医药
Guang Zhou Zhong Yi Xue Yuan Xue Bao (Journal of Guangzhou University of Chinese Medicine)	广州中医学院学报
Gui Yang Yi Xue Yuan Xue Bao (Journal of Guiyang Medical University)	贵阳医学院学报
Gui Yang Zhong Yi Xue Yuan Xue Bao (Journal of Guiyang Chinese Medical University)	贵阳中医学院学报
Gui Zhou Cao Yao (Guizhou Herbology)	贵州草药
Gui Zhou Yao Xun (Guizhou Journal of Herbology)	贵州药讯
Gui Zhou Yi Yao (Medicine and Medicinals from Guizhou)	贵州医药
Guo Wai Yao Xue Zhi Wu Yao Fen Ce (Foreign Study of Medicine: Herbology)	国外药学植物药分册
Guo Wai Yi Xue (Foreign Medicine)	国外医学
Guo Wai Yi Xue Can Kao Za Zhi (Foreign Journal of Medicine)	国外医学参考杂志
Guo Wai Yi Xue Can Kao Zi Liao (Foreign Reference of Medicine)	国外医学参考资料
Guo Wai Yi Xue Zhong Yi Zhong Yao Fen Ce (Monograph of Chinese Herbology from Foreign Medicine)	国外医学中医中药分册
Guo Wai Yi Yao Zhi Wu Yao Fen Ce (Monograph of Foreign Botanical Medicine)	国外医药植物药分册
Guo Yao De Yao Li Xue (Pharmacology of Chinese Herbs)	国药的药理学

Bibliography of Contemporary References

Pinyin Names (Translated Names)	Chinese Names
Ha Er Bing Yi Ke Da Xue (Haerbing University of Medicine)	哈尔滨医科大学
Ha Er Bing Yi Ke Da Xue Xue Bao (Journal of Haerbing University of Medicine)	哈尔滨医科大学学报
Ha Er Bing Zhong Yi (Haerbing Chinese Medicine)	哈尔滨中医
Ha Yi Da Xue Bao (Journal of Ha Medical University)	哈医大学报
Hai Jun Yi Xue (Navy Medicine)	海军医学
Hai Yang Yao Wu Za Zhi (Journal of Herbs from the Sea)	海洋药物杂志
Hai Yao Ben Cao (Sea of Herbal Pharmacopia)	海药本草
Han Fang Yi Xue (Kampo Medicine)	汉方医学
He Bei Xin Yi Yao (Hebei New Medicine and Herbology)	河北新医药
He Bei Yi Yao (Hebei Medicine and Herbology)	河北医药
He Bei Zhong Yi (Hebei Chinese Medicine)	河北中医
He Bei Zhong Yi Za Zhi (Hebei Journal of Chinese Medicine)	河北中医杂志
He Han Yi Yao Xue Hui Zhi (Hehan Journal of Medicine and Herbology)	和汉医药学会志
He Nan Yi Ke Da Xue Xue Bao (Journal of Henan University School of Medicine)	河南医科大学学报
He Nan Yi Xue Yuan Xue Bao (Journal of Henan University of Medicine)	河南医学院学报
He Nan Yi Yao (Henan Medicine and Herbology)	河南医药
He Nan Zhong Yi (Henan Chinese Medicine)	河南中医
He Nan Zhong Yi Xue Yuan Xue Bao (Journal of University of Henan School of Medicine)	河南中医学院学报
Hei Long Jiang Zhong Yi Yao (Heilongjiang Chinese Medicine and Herbology)	黑龙江中医药
Hu Bei Wei Sheng (Hubei Health)	湖北卫生
Hu Bei Yi Sheng (Hubei Doctor)	湖北医生
Hu Bei Yi Xue Yuan Xue Bao (Journal of Hubei College of Medicine)	湖北医学院学报
Hu Bei Zhong Yi Xue Yuan Xue Bao (Journal of Hubei University of Medicine)	湖北中医学院学报
Hu Bei Zhong Yi Za Zhi (Hubei Journal of Chinese Medicine)	湖北中医杂志
Hu Nan Sheng Jie He Bing Yan Jiu Yuan (Hunan Treatment and Research Center of Tuberculosis)	湖南省结核病研究院
Hu Nan Wei Sheng Fang Yi Tong Xun (Hunan Journal of Preventative Health)	湖南卫生防疫通讯
Hu Nan Yi Cao Gong Ye Yan Jiu (Hunan Research and Industry of Medicine and Medicinals)	湖南医草工业研究
Hu Nan Yi Ke Da Xue Xue Bao (Journal of Hunan University School of Medicine)	湖南医科大学学报
Hu Nan Yi Xue (Hunan Medicine)	湖南医学
Hu Nan Yi Xue Yuan Xue Bao (Medical Journal of Hunan University of Medicine)	湖南医学院学报
Hu Nan Yi Yao Za Zhi (Hunan Journal of Medicine and Herbology)	湖南医药杂志
Hu Nan Zhong Yi (Hunan Journal of Traditional Chinese Medicine)	湖南中医
Hu Nan Zhong Yi Xue Yuan Xue Bao (Journal of Hunan University of Traditional Chinese Medicine)	湖南中医学院学报
Hu Nan Zhong Yi Za Zhi (Hunan Journal of Chinese Medicine)	湖南中医杂志
Hua Xi Kou Qiang Yi Xue Za Zhi (Huaxi Journal of Stomatology)	华西口腔医学杂志
Hua Xi Yao Xue Za Zhi (Huaxi Herbal Journal)	华西药学杂志
Hua Xi Yi Xue Za Zhi (Huaxi Medical Journal)	华西医学杂志
Hua Xue Xue Bao (Journal of Chemistry)	化学学报
Huo Xue Hua Yu Yan Jiu (Research on Blood-Activating and Stasis-Eliminating Herbs)	活血化瘀研究
Ji Lin Wei Sheng (Jilin Public Health)	吉林卫生

Bibliography of Contemporary References

Pinyin Names (Translated Names)	Chinese Names
Ji Lin Yi Sheng (Jilin Doctor)	吉林医生
Ji Lin Yi Xue (Jilin Medicine)	吉林医学
Ji Lin Yi Xue Yuan Xue Bao (Journal of Jilin University of Medicine)	吉林医学院学报
Ji Lin Zhong Yi (Jilin Chinese Medicine)	吉林中医
Ji Lin Zhong Yi Yao (Jilin Chinese Medicine and Herbology)	吉林中医药
Jiang Su Xin Yi Xue Yuan (New Jiangsu University of Medicine)	江苏新医学院
Jiang Su Yi Ke Da Xue Xue Bao (Journal of Jiangsu University of Medicine)	江苏医科大学学报
Jiang Su Yi Xue (Jiangsu Medical Journal)	江苏医学
Jiang Su Yi Yao (Jiangsu Journal of Medicine and Herbology)	江苏医药
Jiang Su Zhong Yi (Jiangsu Chinese Medicine)	江苏中医
Jiang Su Zhong Yi Yao (Jiangsu Medicine and Herbology)	江苏中医药
Jiang Su Zhong Yi Za Zhi (Jiangsu Journal of Chinese Medicine)	江苏中医杂志
Jiang Xi Xin Yi Yao (Jiangxi New Medicine and Herbology)	江西新医药
Jiang Xi Yi Xue Yuan Xue Bao (Medical Journal of Jiangxi University of Medicine)	江西医学院学报
Jiang Xi Yi Yao (Jiangxi Medicine and Herbology)	江西医药
Jiang Xi Yi Yao Za Zhi (Jiangxi Journal of Medicine and Herbology)	江西医药杂志
Jiang Xi Zhong Yi Yao (Jiangxi Chinese Medicine and Herbology)	江西中医药
Jing Xian Dai 25 Wei Zhong Yi Ming Jia Fu Ke Jing Yan (Experiences of 25 Modern Obstetrics and Gynecology Experts)	近现代二十五位中医名家妇科经验
Jin Yi Ke Ji (Jinyi Science and Technology)	锦医科技
Jin Zhou Yi Xue Yuan Xue Bao (Journal of Jinzhou University of Medicine)	锦州医学院学报
Jing Fang Yan Jiu (Research of Experienced Formulas)	经方研究
Jun Shi Yi Xue Jian Xun (Military Medicine Notes)	军事医学简讯
Kang Sheng Su (Antibiotic)	抗生素
Ke Ji Tong Bao (Newspaper of Science and Technology)	科技通报
Ke Ji Tong Xun (Journal of Science and Technology)	科技通讯
Ke Ji Zi Liao (Scientific Techniques and Knowledge)	科技资料
Ke Xue Chu Ban She (Scientific Press)	科学出版社
Ke Xue Tong Bao (Journal of Science)	科学通报
Ke Yan Tong Xun (Journal of Science and Research)	科研通讯
Lan Zhou Yi Xue Yuan Xue Bao (Journal of Lanzhou University of Medicine)	兰州医学院学报
Lao Nian Xue Za Zhi (Journal of Geriatrics)	老年学杂志
Liao Ning Yi Xue (Liaoning Medicine)	辽宁医学
Liao Ning Yi Xue Za Zhi (Liaoning Journal of Medicine)	辽宁医学杂志
Liao Ning Yi Yao (Liaoning Medicine and Herbology)	辽宁医药
Liao Ning Zhong Ji Yi Kan (Liaoning Journal of Medium Medicine)	辽宁中级医刊
Liao Ning Zhong Yi (Liaoning Chinese Medicine)	辽宁中医
Liao Ning Zhong Yi Za Zhi (Liaoning Journal of Chinese Medicine)	辽宁中医杂志
Lin Chuang Gan Dan Bing Za Zhi (Clinical Journal of Hepatic and Gallbladder Diseases)	临床肝胆病杂志
Lin Chuang Pi Fu Ke Za Zhi (Journal of Clinical Dermatology)	临床皮肤科杂志
Lin Chuang Shou Ce You Du Zhong Yao Shi Yong (Clinical Handbook on Applications of Toxic Chinese Herbs)	临床手册有毒中药实用

Bibliography of Contemporary References

Pinyin Names (Translated Names)	Chinese Names
Lin Chuang Yi Shi Zhen Liao Ji Qiao (Clinical Treatment & Techniques)	临床医师诊疗技巧
Lin Chuang Zhong Yao Xue (Clinical Chinese Pharmacology)	临床中药学
Liu Feng Wu Fu Ke Jing Yen (Experience of Obstetrics and Gynecology from Master Liu Feng Wu)	刘奉五妇科经验
Lu Zhou Yi Xue Yuan Xue Bao (Journal of Luzhou Institution of Medicine)	泸州医学院学报
Mei Rong Mei Fa Zhong Yi Gu Fang (Ancient Chinese Formulas for Beautiful Face and Hair)	美容美发中医古方
Mei Rong Yu Wu Guan Bing Wai Zhi Du Te Xin Liao Fa (New Treatments for Cosmetology and the Five Senses)	美容与五官病外之独特新疗法
Meika Hosen (A Selection of Famous Physicians' Prescriptions)	名家方选
Min Guo Yi Xue Za Zhi (Medical Journal of People's Republic of China)	民国医学杂志
Ming Yi Bie Lun (Theories of Famous Doctors)	名医别论
Nan Jing Yi Xue Yuan Xue Bao (Journal of Nanjing University of Medicine)	南京医学院学报
Nan Jing Zhong Yi Xue Yuan Xue Bao (Journal of Nanjing University of Traditional Chinese Medicine)	南京中医学院学报
Nan Jing Zhong Yi Yao Da Xue Xue Bao (Journal of Nanjing University of Traditional Chinese Medicine and Medicinals)	南京中医药大学学报
Nei Ke (Internal Medicine)	内科
Nei Meng Gu Zhong Yi Yao (Traditional Chinese Medicine and Medicinals of Inner Mongolia)	内蒙古中医药
Nei Meng Gu Zhong Yi Za Zi (Inner Mongolia Journal of Traditional Chinese Medicine)	内蒙古中医杂志
Pi Fu Bing Fang Zhi Yan Jiu Tong Xun (Research Journal on Prevention and Treatment of Dermatological Disorders)	皮肤病防治研究通讯
Qing Dao Yi Xue Yuan Bao Dao (Medical Journal of Qingdao Institution)	青岛医学院报导
Qing Dao Yi Xue Yuan Xue Bao (Journal of Qingdao Institution of Medicine)	青岛医学院学报
Qing Hai Yi Yao Za Zhi (Qinghai Journal of Medicine and Herbology)	青海医药杂志
Quan Guo Zhong Yi Er Ke Xue (National Chinese Pediatrics)	全国中医儿科学
Ren Min Jun Yi (Military Reserve Medicine)	人民军医
Ren Min Wei Sheng Chu Ban She (Journal of People's Public Health)	人民卫生出版社
Ri Ben Yao Li Xue Za Zhi (Japanese Journal of Herbology)	日本药理学杂志
Ri Ben Yao Wu Xue Za Zhi (Japanese Journal of Pharmacology)	日本药物学杂志
Shan Dong Ke Xue Ji Shu Chu Ban She (Shandong Science Publication)	山东科学技术出版社
Shan Dong Yi Kan (Shandong Medical Journal)	山东医刊
Shan Dong Yi Ke Da Xue Xue Bao (Journal of Shandong University of Medicine)	山东医科大学学报
Shan Dong Yi Xue Yuan Xue Bao (Journal of Shandong University School of Medicine)	山东医学院学报
Shan Dong Yi Yao (Shandong Medicine and Herbology)	山东医药
Shan Dong Yi Yao Gong Ye (Shandong Pharmaceutical Industry)	山东医药工业
Shan Dong Zhong Cao Yao Shou Ce (Handbook of Shandong Herbs)	山东中草药手册
Shan Dong Zhong Yi Xue Yuan Xue Bao (Journal of Shandong University School of Chinese Medicine)	山东中医学院学报
Shan Dong Zhong Yi Za Zhi (Shandong Journal of Chinese Medicine)	山东中医杂志
Shan Xi Xin Yi Yao (New Medicine and Herbology of Shanxi)	陕西新医药
Shan Xi Xin Zhong Yi (New Shanxi Chinese Medicine)	陕西新中医
Shan Xi Yi Kan (Shanxi Journal of Medicine)	陕西医刊

Bibliography of Contemporary References

Pinyin Names (Translated Names)	Chinese Names
Shan Xi Yi Xue Za Zhi (Shanxi Journal of Medicine)	陕西医学杂志
Shan Xi Yi Yao (Shanxi Medicine and Herbology)	陕西医药
Shan Xi Yi Yao Za Zhi (Shanxi Journal of Medicine and Herbology)	陕西医药杂志
Shan Xi Zhong Yi (Shanxi Chinese Medicine)	陕西中医
Shan Xi Zhong Yi Xue Yuan Xue Bao (Journal of Shanxi University School of Chinese Medicine)	陕西中医学院学报
Shan Xi Zhong Yi Za Zhi (Shanxi Journal Chinese Medicine)	陕西中医杂志
Shang Hai Chi Jiao Yi Sheng Za Zhi (Shanghai Journal of Barefoot Doctors)	上海赤脚医生杂志
Shang Hai Di Er Yi Ke Da Xue Xue Bao (Journal of Second Shanghai University College of Medicine)	上海第二医科大学学报
Shang Hai Di Yi Xue Yuan Xue Bao (Journal of First Shanghai Medical College)	上海第一学院学报
Shang Hai Ke Xue Ji Shu Chu Ban She (Shanghai Science and Technology Publishing Company)	上海科学技术出版社
Shang Hai Ren Min Chu Ban She (People's Press of Shanghai)	上海人民出版社
Shang Hai Yao Wu Shi Yan (Shanghai Research of Medicine)	上海药物实验
Shang Hai Yi Ke Da Xue Xue Bao (Journal of Shanghai University of Medicine)	上海医科大学学报
Shang Hai Yi Xue (Shanghai Medicine)	上海医学
Shang Hai Yi Yao Za Zhi (Shanghai Journal of Medicine and Herbology)	上海医药杂志
Shang Hai Zhong Yi Xue Yuan Xue Bao (Journal of Shanghai University of Chinese Medicine)	上海中医学院学报
Shang Hai Zhong Yi Yao Za Zhi (Shanghai Journal of Chinese Medicine and Herbology)	上海中医药杂志
Shang Hai Zhong Yi Za Zhi (Shanghai Journal of Chinese Medicine)	上海中医杂志
Shen De Yan Jiu (Research of Kidney)	肾的研究
Shen Jing Jing Shen Ji Bing Za Zhi (Journal of Psychiatric Disorders)	神经精神疾病杂志
Shen Nong Ben Cao Jing (Shen Nong Materia Medica)	神农本草经
Shen Yang Yao Xue Yuan Xue Bao (Journal of Shenyang College of Pharmacy)	沈阳药学院学报
Shen Yang Yi Xue Yuan Xue Bao (Journal of Shenyang University of Medicine)	沈阳医学院学报
Sheng Cao Yao Xing Bei Yao (Essentials of Raw Herbal Medicine)	生草药性备要
Sheng Li Xue Bao (Physiology News)	生理学报
Sheng Wu Hua Xue Yu Sheng Wu Wu Li Xue Bao (Journal of Biochemistry and Biophysiology)	生物化学与生物物理学报
Sheng Yao Xue Za Zhi (Journal of Raw Herbology)	生药学杂志
Shi Yong Kou Qiang Yi Xue Za Zhi (Journal of Medical Stomatology)	实用口腔医学杂志
Shi Yong Nei Ke Za Zhi (Practical Journal of Internal Medicine)	实用内科杂志
Shi Yong Yi Xue Za Zhi (Practical Journal of Medicine)	实用医学杂志
Shi Yong Zhong Liu Xue Za Zhi (Practical Journal of Cancer)	实用肿瘤学杂志
Shi Yong Zhong Xi Yi Jie He Fu Ke Xue (Practical Integrated Medicine: Obstetrics and Gynecology)	实用中西医结合妇科学
Shi Yong Zhong Xi Yi Jie He Za Zhi (Practical Journal of Integrated Chinese and Western Medicines)	实用中西医结合杂志
Shi Yong Zhong Xi Yi Jie He Zhen Duan Zhi Liao Xue (Practical Diagnostic and Therapeutics of Integrated Traditional Chinese and Western Medicine)	实用中西医结合诊断治疗学
Shi Yong Zhong Yi Mei Rong Jian Shen 3,000 Fang (3,000 Practical TCM Cosmetology Formulas)	实用中医美容健身3000方

Bibliography of Contemporary References

Pinyin Names (Translated Names)	Chinese Names
Shi Yong Zhong Yi Nei Ke Za Zhi (Journal of Practical Chinese Internal Medicine)	实用中医内科杂志
Shi Yong Zhong Yi Yao Za Zhi (Journal of Practical Chinese Medicine and Medicinals)	实用中医药杂志
Shi Yong Zhong Yi Za Zhi (Journal of Practical Chinese Medicine)	实用中医杂志
Shi Zhen Guo Yao Yan Jiu (Research of Shizhen Herbs)	时珍国药研究
Shi Zhen Guo Yi Guo Yao (Shizhen National Herbs and Medicine)	时珍国医国药
Shou Pi Guo Jia Ji Ming Lao Zhong Yi Xiao Yan Mi Fang Jing Xuan (Experienced Secret Formulas from Nationally Famous TCM Doctors)	首批国家级名老中医效验秘方精选
Si Chuan Sheng Zhong Liu Fang Zhi Zi Liao Xuan Bian (Sichuan Journal of Cancer Prevention and Treatment)	四川省肿瘤防治资料选编
Si Chuan Yi Xue (Sichuan Medicine)	四川医学
Si Chuan Yi Xue Yuan Xue Bao (Journal of Sichuan School of Medicine)	四川医学院学报
Si Chuan Zhong Cao Yao Tong Xun (Sichuan Journal of Chinese Herbology)	四川中草药通讯
Si Chuan Zhong Yi (Sichuan Chinese Medicine)	四川中医
Su Zhou Yi Xue Yuan Xue Bao (Journal of Suzhou University of Medicine)	苏州医学院学报
Tai Wan Yi Xue Hui Za Zhi (Journal of Taiwan Medical Association)	台湾医学会杂志
Tai Wan Zhi Wu Yao Cao (Manual of Vegetable Drugs in Taiwan)	台湾植物药草
Te Chan Ke Xue Shi Yan (Research of Special Scientific Projects)	特产科学实验
Tian Jin Yi Xue Za Zhi (Journal of Tianjin Medicine and Herbology)	天津医学杂志
Tian Jin Yi Yao (Tianjin Medicine and Herbology)	天津医药
Tian Jin Yi Yao Tong Xun (Publication of Tianjin Medicine and Herbology)	天津医药通讯
Tian Jin Yi Yao Za Zhi (Journal of Tianjin Medicine and Herbology)	天津中医药杂志
Tian Jin Zhong Yi (Tianjin Chinese Medicine)	天津中医
Tie Dao Yi Xue (Tiedao Medicine)	铁道医学
Tong Ji Yi Ke Da Xue Xue Bao (Journal of Tongji University of Medicine)	同济医科大学学报
Wu Han Xin Yi Yao (Wuhan New Medicine and Herbology)	武汉新医药
Wu Han Xin Zhong Yi (Wuhan New Chinese Medicine)	武汉新中医
Wu Han Yi Xue Yuan Xue Bao (Journal of Wuhan University School of Medicine)	武汉医学院学报
Wu Han Yi Xue Za Zhi (Wuhan Journal of Medicine)	武汉医学杂志
Wu Shi Er Bing Fang (Fifty-two Disease Patterns & Formulas)	五十二病方
Xi An Yi Ke Da Xue Xue Bao (Journal of Xian University School of Medicine)	西安医科大学学报
Xi An Yi Xue Yuan Xue Bao (Journal of Xian University School of Medicine)	西安医学院学报
Xi Bei Yi Yao Za Zhi (Northwest Journal of Herbal Medicine)	西北医药杂志
Xi Xue Xue Bao (Academic Journal of Medicine)	西学学报
Xi Yao Yan Jiu Tong Xun (Research Journal of Medicine and Herbology)	西药研究通讯
Xian Dai Ben Cao Gang Mu (Contemporary Materia Medica)	现代本草纲目
Xian Dai Shi Yong Yao Xue (Practical Applications of Modern Herbal Medicine)	现代实用药学
Xian Dai Zhong Yao Yao Li Xue (Contemporary Pharmacology of Chinese Herbs)	现代中药药理学
Xiang Cun Yi Xue (Suburban Medicine)	乡村医学
Xiang Gang Zhong Yi Yao Nian Jian (Chinese Medicine and Medicinals of Hong Kong)	香港中医药年鉴
Xin Hua Ben Cao Gang Mu (New Chinese Materia Medica)	新华本草纲目
Xin Jiang Zhong Cao Yao Shou Ce (Xinjiang Handbook of Chinese Herbs)	新疆中草药手册
Xin Jiang Zhong Yi Yao (Xinjiang Chinese Medicine and Herbology)	新疆中医药

Bibliography of Contemporary References

Pinyin Names (Translated Names)	Chinese Names
Xin Yao Yu Lin Chuang (New Medicine and the Clinical Application)	新药与临床
Xin Yi Xue (New Medicine)	新医学
Xin Yi Yao Tong Xun (Journal of New Medicine and Herbology)	新医药通讯
Xin Yi Yao Xue Za Zhi (New Journal of Medicine and Herbology)	新医药学杂志
Xin Zhang Xue Guan Ji Bing (Cardiovascular Diseases)	心脏血管疾病
Xin Zhong Yao Xue (New Chinese Herbal Medicine)	新中药学
Xin Zhong Yi (New Chinese Medicine)	新中医
Xin Zhong Yi Yao (New Chinese Medicine and Medicinals)	新中医药
Yan Ke Tong Xun (Journal of Ophthalmology)	眼科通讯
Yao Jian Gong Zuo Tong Xun (Journal of Herbal Preparations)	药检工作通讯
Yao Li Shi Yan Fang Fa Xue (Research Methodology of Herbal Medicine)	药理实验方法学
Yao Li Xue (Pharmacology)	药理学
Yao Wu Fen Xi Za Zhi (Journal of Herbal Analysis)	药物分析杂志
Yao Xue Qing Bao Tong Xun (Journal of Herbal Information)	药学情报通讯
Yao Xue Tong Bao (Report of Herbology)	药学通报
Yao Xue Xue Bao (Journal of Herbology)	药学学报
Yao Xue Za Zhi (Journal of Medicinals)	药学杂志
Yao Yong Zhi Wu Da Ci Dian (Dictionary of Medicinal Herbs)	药用植物大辞典
Yi Fang Xin Jie (New Explanation for Medical Formulas)	医方新解
Yi Xue Ji Shu Zi Liao (Resource of Medical Techniques)	医学技术资料
Yi Xue Qing Kuang Jiao Liu (Medical Information Exchange)	医学情况交流
Yi Xue Wei Sheng Tong Xun (Journal of Medicine and Sanitation)	医学卫生通讯
Yi Xue Xue Bao (Report of Medicine)	医学学报
Yi Xue Yan Jiu Tong Xun (Report of Medical Studies)	医学研究通讯
Yi Xue Zhong Yang Za Zhi (Central Journal of Medicine)	医学中央杂志
Yi Yao Gong Ye (Pharmaceutical Industry)	医药工业
Yi Yao Ke Ji Za Zhi (Journal of Medical Technology)	医药科技杂志
Yi Yao Wei Sheng (Medicine, Medicinals, and Sanitation)	医药卫生
Yi Yao Xue (Study of Medicine and Medicinals)	医药学
Yi Yao Yan Jiu Tong Xun (Research Journal of Medicine and Medicinals)	医药研究通讯
Yi Yao Za Zhi (Journal of Medicine and Herbology)	医药杂志
Ying Yang Xue Bao (Report of Nutrition)	营养学报
You Du Zhong Yao Jian Bie Pao Zhi Yu Bao Guan (Identification, Preparation and Storage of Toxic Chinese Herbs)	有毒中药鉴别泡制与保管
Yu Bei Yi Xue Zhuan Ke Xue Xiao (Yubei University of Medicine)	预备医学专科学校
Yun Nan Yi Xue Za Zhi (Yunan Journal of Medicine)	云南医学杂志
Yun Nan Yi Yao (Yunan Medicine and Herbology)	云南医药
Yun Nan Zhong Yao Zhi (Yunan Journal of Chinese Herbal Medicine)	云南中药志
Yun Nan Zhong Yi (Yunnan Journal of Traditional Chinese Medicine)	云南中医
Yun Nan Zhong Yi Xue Yuan Xue Bao (Journal of Yunnan University School of Medicine)	云南中医学院学报
Yun Nan Zhong Yi Za Zhi (Yunan Journal of Chinese Medicine)	云南中医杂志
Yun Nan Zhong Yi Zhong Yao Za Zhi (Yunan Journal of Chinese Medicine and Medicinals)	云南中医中药杂志

Bibliography of Contemporary References

Pinyin Names (Translated Names)	**Chinese Names**
Zhe Jiang Min Jian Chang Yong Cao Yao (Commonly Used Herbs in Zhejiang)	浙江民间常用草药
Zhe Jiang Wei Sheng Shi Yan Yuan (Zhejiang Department of Health Research)	浙江卫生实验院
Zhe Jiang Yao Xue (Zhejiang Journal of Chinese Herbology)	浙江药学
Zhe Jiang Yi Ke Da Xue Xue Bao (Journal of Zhejiang Province School of Medicine)	浙江医科大学学报
Zhe Jiang Yi Xue (Zhejiang Journal of Medicine)	浙江医学
Zhe Jiang Zhong Yi Xue Yuan Xue Bao (Journal of Zhejiang University of Chinese Medicine)	浙江中医学院学报
Zhe Jiang Zhong Yi Yao (Zhejiang Chinese Medicine and Herbology)	浙江中医药
Zhe Jiang Zhong Yi Za Zhi (Zhejiang Journal of Chinese Medicine)	浙江中医杂志
Zhi Wu Yao You Xiao Cheng Fen Shou Ce (Manual of Plant Medicinals and Their Active Constituents)	植物药有效成份手册
Zhi Wu Zi Yuan Yu Huan Jing (Source and Environment of Plants)	植物资源与环境
Zhong Cao Tong Xun (Journal of Chinese Herbs)	中草通讯
Zhong Cao Yao (Chinese Herbal Medicine)	中草药
Zhong Cao Yao Cheng Fen Hua Xue (Composition and Chemistry of Chinese Herbs)	中草药成分化学
Zhong Cao Yao Fang Ji De Ying Yong (Applications of Chinese Herbal Formulas)	中草药方剂的应用
Zhong Cao Yao Tong Xun (Journal of Chinese Herbal Medicine)	中草药通讯
Zhong Cao Yao Xue (Study of Chinese Herbal Medicine)	中草药学
Zhong Cao Yao Yao Li Xue (Herbology of Chinese Medicinals)	中草药药理学
Zhong Cheng Yao (Study of Chinese Patent Medicine)	中成药
Zhong Cheng Yao Yan Jiu (Research of Chinese Patent Medicine)	中成药研究
Zhong Guo Bing Li Sheng Li Za Zhi (Chinese Journal of Pathology and Biology)	中国病理生理杂志
Zhong Guo Fang Lao (Chinese Prevention of Tuberculosis)	中国防劳
Zhong Guo Fang Lao Za Zhi (Chinese Journal on Prevention of Tuberculosis)	中国防劳杂志
Zhong Guo Gang Chang Bing Za Zhi (Chinese Journal of Proctology)	中国肛肠病杂志
Zhong Guo Gang Chang Za Zhi (Chinese Journal of Anus and Intestines)	中国肛肠杂志
Zhong Guo Kang Fu Yi Xue Za Zhi (Chinese Journal of Rehabilitation)	中国康复医学杂志
Zhong Guo Mian Yi Xue Za Zhi (Chinese Journal of Immunology)	中国免疫学杂志
Zhong Guo Nong Cun Yi Xue (Chinese Agricultural Medicine)	中国农村医学
Zhong Guo Shen Jing Jing Shen Ke Za Zhi (Chinese Journal of Psychiatric Disorders)	中国神经精神科杂志
Zhong Guo Sheng Li Ke Xue Hui, Di Er Ci Hui (Chinese Convention on Biophysiology, 2nd Annual Convention)	中国生理科学会第二次会
Zhong Guo Shi Yong Nei Ke Za Zhi (Chinese Journal of Practical Internal Medicine)	中国实用内科杂志
Zhong Guo Shou Yi Za Zhi (Chinese Journal of Husbandry)	中国兽医杂志
Zhong Guo Xiang Cun Xin Xi (Suburb Doctors of China)	中国乡村信息
Zhong Guo Yao Chai Xue (Chinese Herbal Botany)	中国药材学
Zhong Guo Yao Ci Dian (Dictionary of Chinese Medicinal Plants)	中国药辞典
Zhong Guo Yao Ke Da Xue Xue Bao (Journal of University of Chinese Herbology)	中国药科大学学报
Zhong Guo Yao Li Tong Xun (Journal of Chinese Herbal Studies)	中国药理通讯
Zhong Guo Yao Li Xue Bao (Chinese Herbal Pharmacology Journal)	中国药理学报
Zhong Guo Yao Li Xue Tong Bao (Journal of Chinese Herbal Pharmacology)	中国药理学通报
Zhong Guo Yao Li Xue Yu Du Li Xue Za Zhi (Journal of Herbology and Toxicology)	中国药理学与毒理学杂志
Zhong Guo Yao Xue Da Ci Dian (Grand Dictionary of Chinese Herbal Medicine)	中国药学大辞典

Bibliography of Contemporary References

Pinyin Names (Translated Names)	Chinese Names
Zhong Guo Yi Ke Da Xue Xue Bao (Journal of University of Chinese Medicine)	中国医科大学学报
Zhong Guo Yi Xue Da Ci Dian (Grand Dictionary of Chinese Medicine)	中国医学大辞典
Zhong Guo Yi Xue Ke Xue Xue Bao (Journal of Chinese Medical Science University)	中国医学科学学报
Zhong Guo Yi Yao Bao (Chinese Journal of Medicine and Medicinals)	中国医药报
Zhong Guo Yi Yao Ke Xue Yuan Lun Wen Zhai Yao (Abstract from Chinese University of Medicine and Science)	中国医药科学院论文摘要
Zhong Guo Yi Yao Xue Bao (Chinese Journal of Medicine and Herbology)	中国医药学报
Zhong Guo Yi Yuan Yao Xue Za Zhi (Chinese Hospital Journal of Herbology)	中国医院药学杂志
Zhong Guo Zhong Xi Yi Jie He Za Zhi (Chinese Journal of Integrative Chinese and Western Medicine)	中国中西医结合杂志
Zhong Guo Zhong Yao Za Zhi (People's Republic of China Journal of Chinese Herbology)	中国中药杂志
Zhong Guo Zhong Yi Yao Xue Bao (Chinese Journal of Chinese Medicine and Herbology)	中国中医药学报
Zhong Hua Bing Li Xue Za Zhi (Chinese Journal of Pathology)	中华病理学杂志
Zhong Hua Er Bi Hou Ke Za Zhi (Chinese Journal of Otolaryngology)	中华耳鼻喉科杂志
Zhong Hua Er Ke Za Zhi (Chinese Journal of Pediatrics)	中华儿科杂志
Zhong Hua Fu Chan Ke Za Zhi (Chinese Journal of Obstetrics and Gynecology)	中华妇产科杂志
Zhong Hua Ji Sheng Chong Chuan Ran Bing Za Zhi (Chinese Journal of Infectious Parasitic Diseases)	中华寄生虫传染病杂志
Zhong Hua Jie He Bing Ke Za Zhi (Chinese Journal of Tuberculosis)	中华结核病科杂志
Zhong Hua Kou Qiang Ke Za Zhi (Chinese Journal of Stomatology)	中华口腔科杂志
Zhong Hua Mi Niao Wai Ke (Chinese Journal of Urology and External Medicine)	中华泌尿外科
Zhong Hua Nei Ke Xue Za Zhi (Journal of Chinese Internal Medicine)	中华内科学杂志
Zhong Hua Nei Ke Za Zhi (Chinese Journal of Internal Medicine)	中华内科杂志
Zhong Hua Pi Fu Ke Xue Za Zhi (Chinese Journal of Dermatology)	中华皮肤科学杂志
Zhong Hua Ren Min Gong He Guo Yao Dian (Chinese Herbal Pharmacopoeia by People's Republic of China)	中华人民共和国药典
Zhong Hua Shen Jing Jing Shen Ke Za Zhi (Chinese Journal of Neurology and Psychiatry)	中华神经精神科杂志
Zhong Hua Wai Ke Za Zhi (Chinese Journal of External Medicine)	中华外科杂志
Zhong Hua Xin Xue Guan Bing Za Zhi (Chinese Journal of Cardiology)	中华心血管病杂志
Zhong Hua Xin Yi Xue Bao (Chinese Journal of New Medicine)	中华新医学报
Zhong Hua Xue Yi Xue Za Zhi (Chinese Journal on Study of Hematology)	中华血液学杂志
Zhong Hua Xue Yi Za Zhi (Chinese Journal of Hematology)	中华血液杂志
Zhong Hua Yan Ke Za Zhi (Chinese Journal of Ophthalmology)	中华眼科杂志
Zhong Hua Yi Liao Za Zhi (Journal of Chinese Therapies)	中华医疗杂志
Zhong Hua Yi Xue Za Zhi (Chinese Journal of Medicine)	中华医学杂志
Zhong Hua Yi Yao Xue Bao (Chinese Journal of Medicinal and Herbology)	中华医药学报
Zhong Hua Yu Fang Yi Xue Za Zhi (Chinese Journal of Preventative Medicine)	中华预防医学杂志
Zhong Hua Zhong Liu Za Zhi (Chinese Journal of Cancer)	中华肿瘤杂志
Zhong Ji Yi Kan (Medium Medical Journal)	中级医刊
Zhong Liu Bian Bing Zhuan Fang Zhi Liao (Differential Diagnosis and Treatment for Cancer)	肿瘤辨病专方治疗
Zhong Liu Yu Fang Yan Jiu (Tumor Prevention and Research)	肿瘤预防研究
Zhong Liu Yu Zhi Tong Xun (Journal of Prevention and Treatment of Cancer)	肿瘤预治通讯

Bibliography of Contemporary References

Pinyin Names (Translated Names)	Chinese Names
Zhong Xi Yi Jie He Fang Zhi Yan Jiu Xue Guan Zhi Liao (Research on Prevention and Treatment of Cardiovascular Disorders Using Integrated Chinese and Western Medicines)	中西医结合防治研究血管治疗
Zhong Xi Yi Jie He Yan Jiu Zi Liao (Research Information on Integration of Chinese and Western Medicine)	中西医结合研究资料
Zhong Xi Yi Jie He Za Zhi (Journal of Integrated Chinese and Western Medicine)	中西医结合杂志
Zhong Xi Yi Yao Za Zhi (Journal of Chinese and Western Medicine)	中西医药杂志
Zhong Yao Bu Liang Fan Ying Yu Zhi Liao (Adverse Reactions and Treatment of Chinese Herbal Medicine)	中药不良反应与治疗
Zhong Yao Cai (Study of Chinese Herbal Material)	中药材
Zhong Yao Cai Ke Ji (Science and Technology of Chinese Herbal Material)	中药材科技
Zhong Yao Ci Hai (Encyclopedia of Chinese Herbs)	中药辞海
Zhong Yao Da Ci Dian (Dictionary of Chinese Herbs)	中药大辞典
Zhong Yao Du Li Xue (Toxicology of Chinese Herbs)	中药毒理学
Zhong Yao Lin Zheng Ying Yong (Clinical Applications of Chinese Herbs)	中药淋症应用
Zhong Yao Tong Bao (Journal of Chinese Herbology)	中药通报
Zhong Yao Xian Dai Yan Jiu Yu Ying Yong (Modern Study of Traditional Chinese Medicine)	中药现代研究与应用
Zhong Yao Xue (Chinese Herbology)	中药学
Zhong Yao Yan Jiu (Research of Chinese Herbology)	中药研究
Zhong Yao Yao Li Du Li Yu Lin Chuang (Pharmacology, Toxicology and Clinical Applications of Chinese Herbs)	中药药理毒理与临床
Zhong Yao Yao Li Xue (Study of Chinese Herbology)	中药药理学
Zhong Yao Yao Li Yu Du Li Za Zhi (Journal of Pharmacology and Toxicology of Chinese Herbs)	中药药理与毒理杂志
Zhong Yao Yao Li Yu Lin Chuang (Pharmacology and Clinical Applications of Chinese Herbs)	中药药理与临床
Zhong Yao Yao Li Yu Ying Yong (Pharmacology and Applications of Chinese Herbs)	中药药理与应用
Zhong Yao Yu Jian Mei (Chinese Herbs and Cosmotology)	中药与健美
Zhong Yao Zhi (Chinese Herbology Journal)	中药志
Zhong Yao Zhong Du Yu Ji Jiu (Poisoning and Treatment of Chinese Herbs)	中药中毒与急救
Zhong Yi Er Ke Za Zhi (Chinese Medical Journal of Pediatrics)	中医儿科杂志
Zhong Yi Fang Ji Da Ci Dian (Grand Dictionary of Chinese Herbal Formulas)	中医方剂大辞典
Zhong Yi Fang Ji De Yao Li Yu Ying Yong (Pharmacology and Applications of Chinese Herbal Formulas)	中医方剂的药理与应用
Zhong Yi Fang Ji Lin Chuan Shou Ce (Clinical Handbook of Chinese Herbal Formulae)	中医方剂临床手册
Zhong Yi Fang Ji Xian Dai Yan Jiu (Modern Study of Medical Formulae in Traditional Chinese Medicine)	中医方剂现代研究
Zhong Yi Fu Ke Xue (Traditional Chinese Medicine of Obstetrics and Gynecology)	中医妇科学
Zhong Yi Han Shou Tong Xun (Reports of Chinese Medicine)	中医函授通讯
Zhong Yi Lin Chuan Fang Ji Xue (Clinical Study of Chinese Herbal Formulas)	中医临床方剂学
Zhong Yi Ming Fang Lin Chuang Xin Yong (Contemporary Clinical Applications of Classic Chinese Formulas)	中医名方临床新用
Zhong Yi Xue (Chinese Herbal Medicine)	中医学
Zhong Yi Yan Jiu Yuan (Research Hospital of Chinese Medicine)	中医研究院

Bibliography of Contemporary References

Pinyin Names (Translated Names)	Chinese Names
Zhong Yi Yao Li (Pharmacology of Chinese Herbs)	中医药理
Zhong Yi Yao Xin Xi (Information on Chinese Medicine and Herbology)	中医药信息
Zhong Yi Yao Xue Bao (Report of Chinese Medicine and Herbology)	中医药学报
Zhong Yi Yao Yan Jiu (Research of Chinese Medicine and Herbology)	中医药研究
Zhong Yi Yao Yan Jiu Can Kao (Research and Discussion of Chinese Medicine and Herbology)	中医药研究参考
Zhong Yi Yao Yan Jiu Zi Liao (Research and Resource of Chinese Medicine and Herbology)	中医药研究资料
Zhong Yi Za Zhi (Journal of Chinese Medicine)	中医杂志
Zhong Yuan Yi Kan (Resource Journal of Chinese Medicine)	中原医刊

Glossary

The first column consists of the terms used in the body of the text. Subsequent columns provide correlation to the Chinese characters, pinyin transliteration, previous translation by Wiseman and Feng, and finally, a definition of the term.

When a Chinese term is important to the understanding of a theoretical or clinical concept, or when it is a term familiar to many students and practitioners of Chinese Herbal Medicine, that term is given in pinyin in the text, with an accompanying translation, if needed. However, for lesser-known terms, English translations have been used in the body of the text, with the glossary provided to assist interested individuals in making connections with the Chinese.

The authors have carefully considered the translation of each term and have offered the clearest and most practical translation they could discover, based on the consideration of both the Chinese terminology and nuances of standard American English usage. In some cases, this differs slightly from translations offered by Wiseman and Feng, which we have included here for purposes of assisting readers already familiar with their work. These small differences in no way diminish our respect for and appreciation of the diligence with which our esteemed colleagues have worked to provide thorough, extensive and effective bridges in understanding via their work.

Terminology	Chinese	Pinyin	Wiseman & Feng	Definition
5 a.m. diarrhea	五更泄	*wu geng xie*	fifth-watch diarrhea	Characterized by early morning (approximately 5 a.m.) diarrhea, this is often caused by Kidney deficiency.
Accumulation	积聚	*ji ju*	accumulation and gathering	An inclusive term describing the accumulation of *ji* (yin substances) and *ju* (yang substances), that may occur in any organ. Clinical presentation differs, depending on the area(s) and organ(s) affected.
Ah shi point	阿是穴	*ah shi xue*	a-shi point	A type of acupuncture point having no fixed location or name, but corresponding to an underlying disorder. Stimulating an *ah shi* point elicits tenderness and pain.
Ao (simmer)	熬	*ao*		A method that slowly cooks the herbs using low heat, extracts active constituents, and removes excess water.
Ba gang bian zheng (eight principle differentiation)	八纲辨证	*ba gang bian zheng*	eight-principle pattern identification	A system of differential diagnosis based on patterns of imbalance or disharmony of the eight factors: exterior and interior location, cold and hot attributes, deficiency and excess states, and yin and yang qualities.
Ba hui (eight meeting) points	八会穴	*ba hui xue*	eight meeting points	A set of eight points corresponding to *zang* (solid organs), *fu* (hollow organs), qi, blood, tendons, vessels, bones and marrows.
Ban (blend)	拌	*ban*		To mix medicinal substances.
Bang (scrape)	镑	*bang*	flaking	A method used to process horn substances to obtain thin flakes. This method increases the surface area and enhances extraction of active ingredients.
Bei (stone-bake)	焙	*bei*	stone-baking	A method to indirectly dry the herbs without changing their color by placing the herbs on a heated stone.
Ben tun (running piglet)	奔豚	*ben tun*	running piglet	A sensation of qi rushing upwards from the lower abdomen to the chest, epigastrium and throat. There will generally be concurrent pain, discomfort, alternation of heat and cold, and palpitations.
Beng lou (flooding and spotting)	崩漏	*beng lou*	flooding and spotting	A condition that includes massive uterine bleeding at irregular intervals and incessant dripping of blood from the uterus.

Glossary

Terminology	Chinese	Pinyin	Wiseman & Feng	Definition
Bi zheng (closed disorder)	闭证	*bi zheng*	block pattern	Characterized by clenched jaws, tight fists, unconsciousness, a warm body and cold extremities; this generally occurs in wind stroke or febrile disorders, with heat attacking the *ying* (nutritive) and *xue* (blood) levels.
Bi zheng (painful obstruction syndrome)	痹证	*bi zheng*	impediment pattern	A pain condition characterized by stagnation and obstruction that may affect any tissue and/or organ.
Big pulse	大脉	*da mai*	big pulse	A broad pulse.
Blood	血	*xue*	blood	The red, viscous fluid in the body that comprises nutrients, body fluids and Kidney *jing* (essence).
Blood deficiency	血虚	*xue xu*	blood vacuity	Pale, lusterless face, pale lips, dizziness, vertigo, palpitations, insomnia, coldness and numbness of the extremities, and a fine, weak pulse illustrate this condition, caused by loss of blood, excessive thinking and worrying, the presence of parasites, or injury to the internal organs.
Blood desiccation	血枯	*xue ku*	blood desiccation	Following profuse loss of blood, a condition characterized by dizziness, a feeling of weightlessness of the extremities, and amenorrhea.
Blood stagnation/stasis	血瘀	*xue yu*	blood stasis	A condition characterized by obstructed blood flow, leading to dark purplish skin color, dried or scaly skin, pain at a fixed location, pain that intensifies with pressure, fullness and distention of the lower abdomen, amenorrhea, black, tarry stools, and a dark purple tongue with black spots. Blood stagnation/stasis may be caused by external injuries, menstrual irregularities, qi stagnation and cold stagnation. Blood stagnation refers to mild to moderate obstruction of blood circulation. Blood stasis refers to moderate to severe obstruction of blood circulation, possibly with clotting.
Bo (open)	擘	*bo*		To open the medicinal substances to allow maximum extraction of active ingredients.
Body fluids	津液	*jin ye*	fluids	An all-inclusive term that describes all the fluids in the body, including tears, saliva, sweat, blood and fluids that lubricate the joints.
Bound pulse	结脉	*jie mai*	bound pulse	A slow pulse with pulses at irregular intervals.
Bowl	盅	*zhong*		A traditional unit of measurement for volume. The exact unit varies depending on the place and time in history.
Breast abscess	乳痈	*ru yong*	mammary welling-abscess	A hard breast abscess accompanied by distention and pain, chills and fever, and obstructed flow of breast milk; this is generally caused by Liver qi stagnation, Stomach fire, or stasis of breast milk.
Bu fa (tonifying)	补法	*bu fa*	supplementation	A method of treatment that nourishes, enriches, supplements, and benefits qi, blood, yin, and yang in the *zang fu* organs.
Chang feng (intestinal wind)	肠风	*chang feng*	intestinal wind	A condition caused by wind attacking the intestines, leading to the presence of bright red blood in the stools.

Glossary

Terminology	Chinese	Pinyin	Wiseman & Feng	Definition
Chao (dry-fry)	炒	*chao*	stir-frying	Parching or tossing medicinal substances in a heated wok. This method increases the warmth of the herb, harmonizes and moderates therapeutic effects, and facilitates extraction of active constituents.
Chao huang (dry-fry to yellow)	炒黄	*chao huang*		Parching or tossing medicinal substances in a heated wok until they become yellow in color.
Chao jiao (dry-fry to burnt)	炒焦	*chao jiao*	scorch-frying	Parching or tossing at high temperature until the medicinal substances are burnt on the outside.
Chao tan (dry-fry to ash)	炒炭	*chao tan*	char-frying	Parching or tossing at high temperature until the medicinal substances turn into ash.
Chen yao (deputy herb)	臣药	*chen yao*	minister	The second of four guiding principles in herbal formulation: *Jun Chen Zuo Shi* (Chief, Deputy, Assistant, Envoy). This herb serves two main functions: 1) to reinforce the effect of *jun yao* (chief herb) to treat the key disease or symptom; and 2) to treat the associated or coexisting diseases or symptoms.
Chi position	尺	*chi*	cubit	The third (most proximal) position on the wrist for pulse diagnosis; it represents Kidney yang (right hand) and Kidney yin (left hand).
Chong (thoroughfare) channel	冲脉	*chong mai*	thoroughfare vessel	One of the eight extraordinary vessels which controls the twelve channels. Also known as the "sea of blood," as it has functions related to blood and gynecology.
Chong fu (take drenched)	冲服	*chong fu*	take drenched	Infusing the medicinal substances into water, decoction or other liquid before ingestion.
Chu (pestle)	杵	*chu*		Using a club-shaped implement to pound or grind medicinal substances in a mortar. This method increases the surface area and enhances extraction of active ingredients.
Clumping	结	*jie*	bind	This describes the formation of a solid mass or masses from one or more substances, such as phlegm, heat or cold.
Cold	寒	*han*	cold	Cold is a yin pathogenic factor that attacks both the outside and inside of the body and is characterized by contraction and stagnation. Clinical presentation of cold includes chills, shivering, aversion to cold, cold extremities, pale face and lips, the presence of undigested food in the stools, and clear urine.
Collapse	厥	*jue*	reversal	A condition of sudden collapse and loss of consciousness that generally can be reversed. The causes of collapse include cold, heat, phlegm and dietary injury, among others.
Controlling sequence	相克	*xiang ke*	restraining	A concept of *wu xing* (five element) theory that describes the orderly sequence in which one element controls the growth of another.
Cui (quench)	淬	*cui*	calcining and quenching	Heating medicinal substances at high temperature until they turn red, followed by dipping them in cold water or vinegar. This method makes the substances brittle to facilitate pulverization.

Glossary

Terminology	Chinese	Pinyin	Wiseman & Feng	Definition
Cun position	寸	*cun*	cun	The first (most distal) position on the wrist for pulse diagnosis; it represents the Lung (right hand) and the Heart (left hand).
Cuo (grate)	锉	*cuo*	grating	To reduce hard medicinal substances into small particles. This method increases the surface area and enhances extraction of active ingredients.
Cup	升	*sheng*		A traditional unit of measurement for both volume (approximately 200 mL) and weight (approximately 18-30g). Today, *sheng* has been standardized to 1,000 mL.
Da tou wen (swollen head epidemic)	大头瘟	*da tou wen*	massive head scourge	An epidemic disease characterized by redness and swelling of the face and sore throat, caused by wind, heat and toxins attacking the face and head.
Dai (girdle) channel	带脉	*dai mai*	girdling vessel	Another of the eight extraordinary vessels, this one serves to bind all of the channels together, and influences lower extremity function.
Damp	湿	*shi*	damp	Damp is a pathogenic factor that occurs mainly in the late summer or in places with high humidity. Dampness is characterized by heaviness and turbidity, which may lead to such symptoms as feeling heaviness in the head and extremities, general fatigue, and fullness in the chest and epigastrium. Dampness is also characterized by increased viscosity of substances and stagnation, such as in cases of abscesses, oozing ulcers, leukorrhea with foul discharge, and arthritis.
Damp rash	湿疹	*shi zhen*		Red eruption of the skin characterized by wind, dampness and heat.
Dao (pound)	捣	*dao*	crushing	To reduce medicinal substances into particles by crushing or grinding. This method increases the surface area and enhances extraction of active ingredients.
De qi (arrival of qi)	的气	*de qi*	obtaining qi	Qi sensation (numbness, pressure, swelling, warmth or other) that follows insertion and manipulation of acupuncture needles.
Debilitation	劳	*lao*	taxation	Generalized weakness resulting from persistent mental and physical wear and tear on the body.
Deep pulse	沉脉	*chen mai*	sunken pulse	A pulse that is distinct at the deep level. It cannot be felt with light pressure of the fingers, but can only be felt with heavy pressure.
Deficiency	虚	*xu*	vacuity	Deficiency refers to a state of insufficiency (such as deficiency of qi, blood, yin or yang), or decreased ability of the organ to carry out its normal physiological functioning (Spleen deficiency, Kidney deficiency, and so on). Deficiency occurs due to congenital deficiency, lack of nourishment, or long-term illness.
Deficient pulse	虚脉	*xu mai*	vacuous pulse	A soggy pulse that is also fine and forceless. It feels soft, weak and forceless, at all three levels.
Dian kuang (mania and withdrawal)	癫狂	*dian kuang*	mania and withdrawal	An inclusive term for various types of mental illness. *Dian* (withdrawal) represents yin disorders: the individual is quiet and socially inactive. *Kuang* (mania) represents yang disorders: the individual is irritable, restless, and physically active.

Glossary

Terminology	Chinese	Pinyin	Wiseman & Feng	Definition
Do not expose to heat	不见火	*bu jian huo*		To avoid direct or indirect contact with fire or high temperature.
Drooling phlegm	痰涎	*tan xian*	phlegm-drool	Characterized by profuse dripping of saliva in children; this is generally caused by wind-heat attacking the Spleen, resulting in its inability to properly process water.
Drum skin pulse	革脉	*ge mai*	drum skin pulse	A pulse that is string-like and empty in the middle.
Drum-like abdominal distention	鼓胀	*gu zhang*	drum distention	Characterized by severe fullness and distention, resulting in the abdomen resembling a drum; this may be caused by emotional constraint, inappropriate diet, excessive use of alcohol, or intestinal parasites.
Dryness	乾	*gan*	dry	Dryness is a pathogenic factor that invades the body in late autumn when there is a lack of moisture in the environment. Dryness consumes yin and body fluids, and may lead to clinical presentations such as dry and chapped skin, dryness of the mouth and throat, thirst, dry cough with little sputum, and so on.
Du (governing) channel	督脉	*du mai*	governing vessel	Confluence of all yang vessels, one of the eight extraordinary vessels, also known as the "sea of yang qi." It influences brain and spinal column functioning.
Duan (calcine)	煅	*duan*	calcination	A preparation method to make medicinal substances crisp and brittle by burning them directly or indirectly in a container. This method is often reserved for minerals or shell-like substances to facilitate pulverization.
Dun (stew)	炖	*dun*	double-boiling	To boil slowly or with simmering heat.
Dysentery	痢疾	*li ji*	dysentery	A disorder characterized by abdominal pain, increased frequency but decreased volume of bowel movements, tenesmus, and the presence of undigested food, mucus, and blood in the stool.
Earth	土	*tu*	earth	Another of the five elements, earth corresponds to ripeness and late summer, to sweet flavors, transformation, and centeredness. The corresponding organ is the Spleen.
Epidemic toxin	疫毒	*yi du*	epidemic toxin	An epidemic pathogenic factor that attacks and affects the entire community, regardless of individual health and constitution.
Epilepsy	痫证	*xian zheng*	epilepsy pattern	Characterized by altered consciousness and muscle convulsions, this disorder occurs frequently in children because they have not yet gained fully-developed defenses against external pathogens. Factors commonly causing seizure include wind, heat, phlegm and inappropriate diet.
Excess	实	*shi*	repletion	Excess refers to the state of surplus or overload that creates a pathologic condition in the body, such as when there is excess heat, formation or accumulation of phlegm, or blood stagnation, among others. Excess conditions occur in the case of invasion of exogenous pathogenic factors or in disharmony of the internal organs.
Excess pulse	实脉	*shi mai*	replete pulse	A broad, large and forceful pulse upon arrival and departure. It feels very forceful at all three levels.

Glossary

Terminology	Chinese	Pinyin	Wiseman & Feng	Definition
Exterior	表	*biao*	exterior	The outside of the body, such as the skin, mouth, nose and nostrils. Pathogenic factors are often said to attack the exterior prior to invading the interior. The clinical presentation of an exterior syndrome includes headache, muscle aches and pain, nasal congestion, coughing and so on.
Exterior and interior	表里	*biao li*	exterior and interior	A term used to indicate differentiation between the exterior and interior parts of the body.
Faint pulse	微脉	*wei mai*	faint pulse	A pulse that is extremely fine, forceless, and indistinct.
Febrile diseases	热病	*re bing*	heat disease	A term that describes all externally-contracted diseases characterized by heat.
Fen sui (pulverize)	粉碎	*fen sui*		To reduce medicinal substances by crushing, beating, or grinding into powder. This method increases the surface area and enhances extraction of active ingredients.
Feng lao bing (wind consumption disease)	风劳病	*feng lao bing*	wind taxation disease	A yin-deficient heat syndrome characterized by tidal fever and steaming bones sensation, caused by maltreatment of an exterior condition leading to formation of heat in the interior damaging yin and blood.
Feng shi (wind-damp)	风湿	*feng shi*	wind-damp	A condition caused by invasion of wind-dampness, leading to pain and limited movements of the joints, muscles and bones.
Feng shui (wind water)	风水	*feng shui*	wind water	A condition caused by invasion of wind to the exterior parts of the body, leading to swelling and water accumulation.
Filth and fetidness	秽	*hui*	foulness	Terms used to describe things that are dirty, foul, or turbid, such as foods or pathogenic factors.
Fine pulse	细脉	*xi mai*	fine pulse	A small and well-defined pulse. It feels narrow, like a fine thread, but is very distinct and clear.
Fire	火	*huo*	fire	Fire is one of the five elements, associated with upward movement of energy, the sparkling flaring of fire, and summer. The corresponding organ is the Heart. In disease terminology, fire is a yang pathogenic factor representing a severe form of heat.
Firm pulse	牢脉	*lao mai*	firm pulse	A pulse that is deep and forceful.
Five elements	五行	*wu xing*	five phases	A theory which evaluates all things according to elements of water, wood, fire, earth and metal. The theory is also used to explain anatomy, physiology, and pathology of the human body, as well as treatment strategies.
Floating edema	浮肿	*fu zhong*	puffy swelling	A symptom characterized by fluid accumulation in superficial parts of the body. This is generally caused by Lung, Spleen or Kidney deficiency, and the consequent inability to properly regulate water metabolism pathways.
Focal distention	痞满	*pi man*	glomus fullness	Fullness, distention and oppression in the chest and abdomen, caused by food retention, phlegm stagnation, and/or damp-heat accumulation.
Fright and palpitations	惊悸	*jing ji*	fright palpitations	A condition of emotional instability and increased sensitivity to stimulus caused by Heart qi deficiency.

Glossary

Terminology	Chinese	Pinyin	Wiseman & Feng	Definition
Frightened wind	惊风	*jing feng*	fright wind	Literally "frightened wind," this describes seizures and convulsions in children. It is most common in children under the age of five, with incidence gradually decreasing with increased age. Clinical presentations include high fever, red eyes, convulsion, opisthotonos, clenched jaws, tight fists, eyes rolled upward, and urinary and bowel incontinence.
Fu (hollow organ)	腑	*fu*	bowel	The hollow organs of the body are the Small Intestine, Large Intestine, Gallbladder, Stomach and Urinary Bladder.
Gallbladder	胆	*dan*	gallbladder	Paired with the Liver, the Gallbladder stores bile and excretes it to the intestines to facilitate digestion.
Gan ji (infantile malnutrition)	疳疾	*gan ji*	gan disease	A disorder characterized by the inability of the Spleen and Stomach to properly transform and transport food. Generally occurring in children under five years of age, *gan ji* is characterized by a sallow facial appearance, weight loss, thin hair, poor appetite, abdominal distention, and irregular bowel movements.
Gao lin (cloudy dysuria)	膏淋	*gao lin*	unctuous strangury	A urinary tract disorder in which the urine has a milky or cloudy appearance, and may be slightly pink (an indication of bleeding). This is caused by damp-heat attacking the Urinary Bladder, leading to the bladder's inability to clear turbid substances.
Generating sequence	相生	*xiang sheng*	engendering	A concept of *wu xing* (five element) theory that describes the orderly sequence in which one element promotes the generation of another.
Gu (food) *qi*	谷气	*gu qi*		Qi that is derived from the ingestion and absorption of food.
Guan position	关	*guan*	bar	The second (middle) position on the wrist for pulse diagnosis represents the Spleen (right hand) and the Liver (left hand).
Half-body perspiration	半身汗	*ban shen han*		Half-body perspiration refers to sweating only on half of the body, such as the left or right side, or upper or lower half. This condition occurs because of obstruction of the channels and collaterals caused by wind-phlegm or wind-dampness. It may also be caused by disharmony of qi and blood, or of *ying* (nutritive) and *wei* (defensive) levels.
Han fa (sweating)	汗法	*han fa*	diaphoresis	A method of treatment that induces a mild sweat by ventilating and dispersing Lung qi, and regulating and harmonizing the *ying* (nutritive) and *wei* (defensive) levels. Sweating is primarily used to expel pathogenic factors at the exterior (skin) level to treat common cold, influenza, the early stage of measles, acute edema (especially above the waist), abscesses and sores with fever and chills, dysentery with exterior signs and symptoms, and many others.
He (uniting) point	合穴	*he xue*	uniting point	Known as "uniting" or "sea" point, this point represents the flow of qi where it is vast and deep, near the elbows or knees.

Glossary

Terminology	Chinese	Pinyin	Wiseman & Feng	Definition
He fa (harmonizing)	和法	*he fa*	harmonization	A method of treatment that regulates and accords complicated patterns of disease that affect multiple parts of the body. Harmonizing is generally used to treat such disorders as *shaoyang* syndrome, *mo yuan* (membrane source) disorders, disharmony of the Liver and Spleen, concurrent presentation of heat in the Stomach and cold in the Intestines, irregularities of qi and blood, and disharmony of the nutritive and defensive levels.
He xi feng (crane's knee wind)	鹤膝风	*he xi feng*	crane's-knee wind	A condition in which the knees are swollen and enlarged, but the muscles above and below the knees are atrophied.
Heart	心	*xin*	heart	The Heart functions to control the blood channels and house the *shen* (spirit). It connects to the Small Intestine and opens to the tongue, and is associated with the fire element.
Heat	热	*re*	heat	Heat is a yang pathogenic factor that attacks both external and internal aspects of the body; it is characterized by the tendency to disperse outwards and to consume yin and fluids. Clinical presentations of heat include a wide variety of signs and symptoms, such as fever, inflammation, infection, bleeding, and others.
Heat in the blood	血热	*xue re*	blood heat	A condition characterized by nosebleeds, coughing of blood, and late-afternoon fever, because of heat affecting the *xue* (blood) level.
Hernial disorder	疝气	*shan qi*	mounting qi	Historically, this term covers a wide variety of disorders related to both internal and external genitalia, in men and women. More recently, it refers specifically to disorders of the male external genitalia (testicles and scrotum).
Hidden pulse	伏脉	*fu mai*	hidden pulse	A pulse that is distinct at the deep level, deeper than the deep pulse.
Hong (bake)	烘	*hong*		A method to directly dry the herbs at low temperature without charring it.
Hou bi (painful obstruction of the throat)	喉痹	*hou bi*	throat impediment	Redness, swelling and pain of the throat caused mainly by wind-cold at the exterior, or Liver or Lung fire in the interior.
Hua (dissolve)	化	*hua*	transform	To cause to pass into solution.
Hui (influential) point	会穴	*hui xue*	meeting point	Referred to as "meeting" or "influential" points, these eight points individually represent one of the following: *zang*, *fu*, qi, blood, tendons, channels, bones or marrow.
Hun (ethereal soul)	魂	*hun*	ethereal soul	Similar to the Western interpretation of "soul" or "spirit," the *hun* functions to maintain mental and psychological health and well-being. It has been said that the Liver stores blood, and blood contains *hun*. Therefore, disorders of the *hun* are often secondary to the inability of the Liver to store blood; or, secondary to deficiency of Liver blood.

Glossary

Terminology	Chinese	Pinyin	Wiseman & Feng	Definition
Insulting sequence	相侮	*xiang wu*	rebellion	A concept of *wu xing* (five element) theory that describes the situation in which an element normally controlled by another reverses the sequence and suppresses or reduces what is normally the controlling element.
Interior	里	*li*	interior	Internal aspects of the body, such as organs, bone marrow, and the *qi* (energy) and *xue* (blood) levels. Pathogenic factors may affect the interior of the body directly or indirectly (via the exterior). Clinical presentation of interior conditions varies significantly, depending on the area and/or organs affected.
Intermittent pulse	代脉	*dai mai*	intermittent pulse	A pulse interspersed with more relatively regular pauses.
Intestinal abscess	肠痈	*chang yong*	intestinal welling-abscess	Intestinal abscesses generally arise from inappropriate diet or emotional disturbances (excessive anger or worry), and are characterized by abdominal pain.
Irritability	烦	*fan*	vexation	A state of impatience, anger, annoyance, and increased sensitivity to stimulus.
Jian (decoct)	煎	*jian*	decoct, brew	To boil medicinal substances in water to extract their active ingredients.
Jie xiong (stagnant chest)	结胸	*jie xiong*	chest bind	A condition caused by stagnation in the chest of pathogenic heat or cold with retention of fluid, phlegm or blood.
Jin (soak)	浸	*jin*	soaking, steeping	To infuse or steep medicinal substances in water or other fluids over a period of time.
Jin (thin body fluid)	津	*jin*	liquid	An inclusive term that describes body fluids of lesser density, such as tears, saliva and sweat.
Jing (clean)	净	*jing*		To remove unwanted or non-medicinal parts from medicinal substances.
Jing (essence)	精	*jing*	essence	The basic substance that makes up the human body and sustains the vital functions of the internal organs. Derived prenatally from one's parents, and postnatally from food, essence is stored in the Kidney.
Jing (river) point	经穴	*jing xue*	river point	Commonly referred to as either "traversing" or "river" points, these points suggest that the flow of qi at the forearms or lower legs has attained a large volume.
Jing (well) point	井穴	*jing xue*	well point	"Well" points represent the beginning of qi circulation within channels, at the most distal parts of the body, where qi flow is still small and shallow.
Jueyin	厥阴	*jue yin*	reverting yin	The last of six stages in the paradigm of yin and yang. This describes the degree of pathology of disease according to the *Shang Han Lun* (Discussion of Cold-Induced Disorders) text. It also identifies the level attributed to the Liver and Pericardium channels that travel throughout the body.
Jun yao (chief herb)	君药	*jun yao*	sovereign	The first of four guiding principles in herbal formulation: *Jun Chen Zuo Shi* (Chief, Deputy, Assistant, Envoy). It is the essential ingredient used at a large dosage to maximize the effect and treat the key disease or symptom.

Glossary

Terminology	Chinese	Pinyin	Wiseman & Feng	Definition
Kidney	肾	*shen*	kidney	The Kidney controls growth, maturation, reproduction and aging. It produces marrow that forms the brain and spinal cord, and it promotes production of bones and blood. Furthermore, it dominates body fluids and receives qi from air via the Lung. Associated with the water element, the Kidney connects with the Urinary Bladder, opens to the ears, and houses the faculty of *zhi* (will power).
Lao lin (fatigue dysuria)	劳淋	*lao lin*	taxation strangury	A urinary tract disorder involving increased frequency of urination, especially with physical stress and exertion. Accompanying symptoms include fatigue, lower back and knee soreness and pain, with dribbling urine, but no pain during urination. This is caused when prolonged exertion leads to Spleen and Kidney exhaustion and inability to control the normal flow of water and urination.
Large Intestine	大肠	*da chang*	large intestine	Connected to the Small Intestine, the Large Intestine absorbs nutrients and water from food.
Large spoon	方寸匕	*fang cun bi*		A large spoon that contains approximately 6-9 grams of powdered herbs.
Leg *qi*	脚气	*jiao qi*	leg qi	A disorder of the leg(s) characterized by numbness, soreness, pain, weakness, possible swelling and cramps, and possible atrophy of leg muscles. Accompanying symptoms may include nausea, vomiting, dyspnea, incoherent speech, and palpitations. Generally caused by wind, damp, and toxins attacking the legs, it overlaps in symptomology with beriberi.
Li feng (dysenteric wind)	痢风	*li feng*		A condition of constitutional weakness and deficiency caused by chronic dysentery, in which wind attacks the legs leading to weakness, pain, paralysis, and inability to walk.
Lin zheng (dysuria syndrome)	淋证	*lin zheng*	strangury pattern	Dysuria syndrome refers to a condition of frequent and painful urination, abdominal pain, and/or pain radiating to the lower back.
Liu jing bian zheng (six stages differentiation)	六经辨证	*liu jing bian zheng*	six-channel pattern identification	A system of differential diagnosis based on identifying patterns of disharmony by relationship to the energetic stages *taiyang, yangming, shaoyang, taiyin, shaoyin,* and *jueyin.*
Liu yin (six exogenous factors)	六淫	*liu yin*	six excesses	The six exogenous climatic conditions that may cause illness when in excess, including wind, cold, summer-heat, dampness, dryness, and fire.
Liver	肝	*gan*	liver	The Liver stores blood, maintains proper flow of qi, and controls tendons. It connects to the Gallbladder, opens to the eyes, and is associated with the wood element.
Long pulse	长脉	*chang mai*	long pulse	A pulse that can be felt beyond the *cun* and *chi* positions.
Loss of qi with hemorrhage	气随血脱	*qi sui xue tuo*	qi deserting with the blood	A dangerous dynamic in which qi is lost because it flows out with the blood in severe bleeding.
Lower *jiao*	下焦	*xia jiao*	lower burner	The lower *jiao* represents the hypogastrium, and includes the functions of the Kidney and the Urinary Bladder.
Lung	肺	*fei*	lung	The Lung controls breathing and the flow of air, regulates water passages, and dominates the skin and hair. It connects with the Large Intestine, opens to the nose, and is associated with the metal element.

Glossary

Terminology	Chinese	Pinyin	Wiseman & Feng	Definition
Lung abscess	肺痈	*fei yong*	pulmonary welling-abscess	A disorder characterized by cough, chest fullness, fever and chills, rapid pulse, dry throat without thirst, foul-smelling sputum, and profuse discharge of sputum. It is generally caused by wind-heat attacking the Lung.
Luo (connecting) point	络穴	*luo xue*	network point	Known as "connecting" or "vessel" points, these points assist communication between the yang external and yin internal channels. Fifteen points in all represent each of the twelve channels and one on each of the front, back and side of the trunk.
Malaria	疟疾	*nue ji*	malaria	An infectious disorder characterized by alternation of chills, fever and perspiration. This disorder occurs most frequently in summer and fall, and is diagnosed as wind, cold, summer-damp, and damp attacking the *ying* (nutritive) and *wei* (defensive) levels.
Mammary aggregation	乳癖	*ru pi*	mammary aggregation	A breast nodule of variable size, slightly mobile, not painful, not of cold or hot origin, does not cause a change in local skin color, nor erupt or cause ulceration. These form primarily because of Liver qi stagnation.
Mammary 'rock'	乳岩	*ru yan*	mammary rock	Single or multiple breast nodules similar in size to jujubes, that do not cause pain, itching, redness or heat sensations, and may continue to grow in size. Most common in women past middle age, this is caused by emotional constraint and obstructed flow of Liver and Spleen qi.
Man (fullness)	满	*man*	fullness	*Man* (fullness) is the feeling of bloating and fullness in the epigastric and abdominal regions.
Metal	金	*jin*	metal	One of the five elements, metal has inward or contracting movement, represents autumn and harvest, and is associated with the Lung.
Middle *jiao*	中焦	*zhong jiao*	middle burner	The middle *jiao* represents the epigastrium, and includes the functions of the Spleen and Stomach.
Ming men (life gate)	命门	*ming men*	life gate	This is key to the overall vitality of the individual. A strong *ming men* (life gate) often indicates that an individual is in great health and will age slowly. A weak *ming men* is often evident in persons who look older than their actual age, and suffer from numerous age-related illnesses.
Moderate pulse	缓脉	*huan mai*	moderate pulse	A slow pulse with approximately three or more beats per respiration.
Mo yuan (membrane source)	膜原	*mo yuan*	membrane source	A term used in *wen bing* (warm disease) to describe a space situated midway between the exterior and the interior of the body where warm disease factors tend to settle.
Mu (collecting) point	募穴	*mu xue*	alarm point	Commonly referred to as "alarm" or "collecting" points, these twelve points individually represent where the qi of a specific internal organ passes on the chest and abdomen.

Glossary

Terminology	Chinese	Pinyin	Wiseman & Feng	Definition
Mumps	痄腮	*zha sai*	mumps	An acute infectious disorder commonly seen in children. Clinical presentations include swelling and pain of the parotid glands, chills and fever, difficulty chewing, and discomfort of the entire body. Most common in winter and spring, it may occur in any season, and is caused by wind-heat (entering the body through the mouth and nose) that becomes blocked in the *shaoyang* channels.
Night perspiration	盗汗	*dao han*	night sweating	Night perspiration refers to sweating that occurs during sleep, and stops when one awakens. It is an indication of yin deficiency.
Over-acting sequence	相乘	*xiang cheng*	overwhelming	A concept of *wu xing* (five element) theory that describes a situation in which a controlling element suppresses or reduces the controlled element instead of controlling its growth or activity.
Pao (blast-fry)	炮	*pao*	blast-drying	To stir fry medicinal substances in an iron wok over intense fire until their surface becomes dark-brown, burnt, or cracked open.
Pericardium	心包	*xin bao*	pericardium	The Pericardium is the external covering of the Heart. It functions as the protective barrier of the Heart against pathological factors, and connects with the *San Jiao*.
Persistent, indeterminate hunger	嘈杂	*cao za*	clamoring stomach	An uncomfortable sensation that mimics pain yet is not painful, that mimics hunger yet the person is not hungry. This condition is usually caused by fire, phlegm accumulation, qi stagnation, or food retention.
Perspiration of the palms and soles	手足心汗	*shou zhu xin han*	sweating in the (heart of the) palms and soles	Profuse perspiration of the hands and feet is an indication of yin deficiency with heat. It is often caused by excessive thinking and worrying that leads to injuries of the Heart and Spleen.
Phlegm	痰	*tan*	phlegm	Phlegm is a by-product formed from water and damp stagnation. The presence of phlegm may obstruct healthy flow and cause illness throughout the body, damaging the Lung, Heart, Stomach, peripheral channels and collaterals, throat and skin.
Pi (distention)	痞	*pi*	glomus	*Pi* (distention) is the feeling of oppression, obstruction, and increased pressure in the chest and epigastric regions.
Pi shui (skin water)	皮水	*pi shui*	skin water	Severe and generalized edema due to Spleen deficiency and damp accumulation, with symptoms such as pitting edema and heaviness and pain of the body and limbs.
Piao (rinse)	漂	*piao*	long rinsing	To steep or soak medicinal substances with frequent change of water to remove dirt, odor or toxicity.
Plum-pit *qi*	梅核气	*mei he qi*	plum-pit qi	The feeling of having a foreign substance, such as a plum pit, obstructing the throat which cannot be expectorated or swallowed.
Po (break open)	破	*po*		To force open.
Po (corporeal soul)	魄	*po*	corporeal soul	A term that refers to basic human instinct and reaction, such as the ability to smell, taste, see, distinguish between cold and hot, and the ability of the newborn to nurse and feed. The main function of *po*, which resides in the Lung, is to maintain physical awareness in order to react and adapt to the external environment.

Glossary

Terminology	Chinese	Pinyin	Wiseman & Feng	Definition
Post-decoct	后下	*hou xia*	add at end	A specific instruction when preparing a decoction, to add specific herbs near the end of the cooking process and then continue cooking the herbs for approximately 5 to 10 additional minutes.
Pre-decoct	先煎	*xian jian*	predecoct	Instruction to cook a certain herb or herbs first (usually for 30 minutes, but this varies) before adding the rest of the herbs to cook a decoction.
Profuse sweating	大汗	*da han*	great sweating	Profuse perspiration often leads to depletion of body fluids. It may occur because of excessive heat or yang collapse.
Qi	气	*qi*	qi	Qi represents the vital energy needed for proper functioning and existence of the organs and the body.
Qi (energy) level	气分	*qi fen*	qi aspect	*Qi* (energy) level refers to the second of four levels of febrile infections. Heat attacking the *qi* level may affect such organs as the Stomach, Lung, Intestines, Gallbladder and Spleen. Clinical presentations will vary depending on the organ(s) affected.
Qi and blood deficiency	气血两虚	*qi xue liang xu*	dual vacuity of qi and blood	Insufficiency of both qi and blood, which influences basic organ functions more strongly than insufficiency of either one alone.
Qi and blood stagnation	气滞血瘀	*qi zhi xue yu*	qi stagnation and blood stasis	Obstructed flow of both qi and blood.
Qi collapse	气陷	*qi xian*	qi fall	Severe insufficiency of qi results in collapse of vital functions.
Qi deficiency	气虚	*qi xu*	qi vacuity	A condition in which insufficient quantity of qi affects body or organ functions.
Qi deficiency bleeding	气虚失血	*qi xu shi xue*	qi vacuity bleeding	Bleeding caused by insufficiency of qi, and its consequent inability to properly guide the flow of blood.
Qi lin (qi dysuria)	气淋	*qi lin*	qi strangury	A urinary tract disorder characterized by obstructed urinary flow, lower abdominal distention and pain, and green-blue tongue color. It is caused by Liver stagnation leading to obstructed flow of qi and urine.
Qi qing (seven emotions)	七情	*qi qing*	seven affects	The seven emotional factors that may cause illness when out of balance, including joy, anger, melancholy, thought (over-thinking), grief, fear and fright.
Qi stagnation	气滞	*qi zhi*	qi stagnation	Obstructed qi flow in internal organs or peripheral channels and collaterals, caused by a variety of factors, including inappropriate diet, emotional disturbance, environmental factors, or external injuries.
Qi xue jin ye bian zheng (qi, blood, and body fluid differentiation)	气血津液辨证	*qi xue jin ye bian zheng*	qi, blood and fluids pattern identification	A system of differential diagnosis based on patterns of disharmony of qi, blood, and body fluids.
Qie (slice)	切	*qie*	cutting	To cut open. This method increases the surface area, creates standard portion weights and sizes, facilitates drying, and prolongs shelf life.
Qing fa (clearing)	清法	*qing fa*	clearing	A method of treatment that clears heat, purges fire and cools the blood to treat diseases characterized by warmth, heat, fire, and toxins.

Glossary

Terminology	Chinese	Pinyin	Wiseman & Feng	Definition
Racing pulse	疾脉	*ji mai*	racing pulse	A fast pulse with seven or more beats per respiration.
Rapid pulse	数脉	*shu mai*	rapid pulse	A fast pulse with six or more beats per respiration.
Re bi (heat painful obstruction)	热痹	*re bi*	heat impediment	One type of *bi zheng* (painful obstruction syndrome) characterized by local redness, swelling, burning sensations and pain. The development of heat is often caused by prolonged obstruction of the channels and collaterals by wind, cold or damp.
Re jue (heat reversal)	热厥	*re jue*	heat reversal	A morbid condition in which excessive pathogenic heat leads to consumption of body fluids which impairs the normal circulation of yang qi and results in cold extremities.
Re lin (heat dysuria)	热淋	*re lin*	heat strangury	A urinary tract disorder characterized by frequent urination, painful and burning sensations upon urination, yellow urine, muscle cramps and pain in the lower abdomen, and a bitter taste in the mouth. This condition is caused by damp-heat attacking the lower *jiao*.
Rebellious qi	气逆	*qi ni*	qi counterflow	Rebellious qi is the flow of qi opposite of its normal or appropriate direction, such as the flow of Lung qi upwards, that leads to coughing.
Ren (conception) channel	任脉	*ren mai*	conception vessel	The confluence of all yin vessels, one of the eight extraordinary vessels. Also known as the "sea of yin qi," it relates to urogenital, gynecological and obstetrical functions.
Restless fetus	胎动不安	*tai dong bu an*	stirring fetus	Constant downward movement of the fetus, abdominal pain, sore back, and perhaps bleeding, are generally caused by qi deficiency, blood deficiency, Kidney deficiency, heat in the blood, or external injuries.
Rock-like breast abscess	乳石痈	*ru shi yong*	rock-like mammary welling-abscess	A rock-hard breast abscess.
Rough pulse	涩脉	*se mai*	rough pulse	A pulse that does not flow smoothly. It feels hesitant, rough and uneven; pulse deficits can often be present with this pulse type
Run (moisten)	润	*run*		To soak the herbs in water to soften the substances prior to slicing, or to ensure complete extraction prior to cooking in decoctions.
San Jiao	三焦	*san jiao*	triple burner	The *San Jiao* is not an anatomical organ, but a generalization of different sections of the body compartment. The *San Jiao* is divided into upper, middle and lower sectors.
San Jiao bian zheng (triple burner differentiation)	三焦辨证	*san jiao bian zheng*	triple burner pattern identification	A system of differential diagnosis based on locating patterns of disharmony in the upper *jiao*, middle *jiao,* or lower *jiao.*
Scallion-stalk pulse	芤脉	*kou mai*	scallion-stalk pulse	A large superficial pulse that feels empty in the middle upon pressure.
Scattered pulse	散脉	*san mai*	scattered pulse	A large superficial pulse without root.
Scoop	合子	*he zi*		A device used to measure herbs, such as *Dan Dou Chi* (Semen Sojae Praeparatum).

Glossary

Terminology	Chinese	Pinyin	Wiseman & Feng	Definition
Seven emotions	七情	*qi qing*	seven affects	Joy, anger, melancholy, thought (over-thinking), grief, fear and fright. An excess of any of the seven emotions may create illness.
Sha zhang (acute filthy disease)	痧胀	*sha zhang*	sand distention	A disease contracted primarily via ingestion of filthy (raw, dirty or unclean) foods, leading to fever, chest oppression, abdominal distention, nausea, vomiting and diarrhea.
Shang han (cold damage)	伤寒	*shang han*	cold damage	A collective term for disorders caused by cold externally-contracted pathogens, diagnosed and treated via *Liu Jing Bian Zheng* (Six Stages Differentiation).
Shang Han Lun (Discussion of Cold-Induced Disorders)	伤寒论	*shang han lun*	on cold damage	A text written by Zhang Zhong-Jing in the Eastern Han dynasty that focuses on diagnosis and treatment of cold-induced disorders. The basic principles of diagnosis and treatment are based on *Liu Jing Bian Zheng* (Six Stages Differentiation).
Shao (burn)	烧	*shao*	burn	To treat the medicinal substances with heat or fire.
Shaoyang	少阳	*shao yang*	lesser yang	Third of six stages in the paradigm of yin and yang. This term identifies the degree of pathology of disease according to the *Shang Han Lun* (Discussion of Cold-Induced Disorders) text. It also describes the level attributed to the Gallbladder and *San Jiao* channels that travel throughout the body.
Shaoyin	少阴	*shao yin*	lesser yin	The fifth of six stages in the paradigm of yin and yang. This term describes the degree of pathology of disease according to the *Shang Han Lun* (Discussion of Cold-Induced Disorders) text. It also identifies the level attributed to the Heart and Kidney channels that travel throughout the body.
Shen (spirit)	神	*shen*	spirit	A term that refers to the entire presentation of the human being, including energy levels, the state of consciousness, and the ability to think and reason. Because it is housed in the Heart, disorders affecting the Heart may also lead to disturbance of the *shen* (spirit).
Shi (hardness)	实	*shi*	repletion	*Shi* (hardness) is the excess condition in which the dry hard stools are interlocked with heat, causing constipation and abdominal pain that intensifies with palpation.
Shi lin (stone dysuria)	石淋	*shi lin*	stone strangury	A urinary tract disorder characterized by lower abdominal tightness and pain, the presence of sandy particles (and possibly blood) in the urine, difficult and painful urination, or sudden termination of the stream of urine. This is caused by damp-heat attacking the lower *jiao*, drying fluids, and leading to the formation of stones.
Shi yao (envoy herb)	使药	*shi yao*	courier	The fourth of four guiding principles in herbal formulation: *Jun Chen Zuo Shi* (Chief, Deputy, Assistant, Envoy). This herb has two main functions: 1) it acts as a channel-guiding herb to direct the formula to the affected channels/areas of the body; and 2) it harmonizes all of the herbs within the formula. *Shi yao* (envoy herb) is usually used only in small doses.

Glossary

Terminology	Chinese	Pinyin	Wiseman & Feng	Definition
Shi-re lin (damp-heat dysuria)	湿热淋	*shi re lin*	damp-heat strangury	A urinary tract disorder characterized by frequent urination, painful and burning sensations upon urination, yellow urine, muscle cramps and pain in the lower abdomen, and a bitter taste in the mouth, all caused by damp heat attacking the lower *jiao*. Other symptoms of damp-heat may include nausea, vomiting, constipation, a yellow, greasy tongue coating, and a slippery, rapid pulse.
Shivering perspiration	战汗	*zhan han*	shivering	Shivering perspiration is a phenomenon that occurs when the body fights against pathogenic factors. The prognosis is good if the patient has a normal temperature after perspiring. The prognosis is poor if the patient becomes fidgety and irritable after perspiring.
Short pulse	短脉	*duan mai*	short pulse	A pulse that can be felt only at *guan* position.
Shu (stream) point	输穴	*shu xue*	stream point	Commonly referred to as "stream" points, these are usually located near the wrists or ankles and suggest that the flow of qi is now of sufficient quantity to carry out these functions.
Shu (transport) point	俞穴	*shu xue*	transport point	Known as "associated points of the back," or "transporting" points, these are twelve points on the upper and lower back where the qi of the internal organs passes. Each represents an organ.
Shui fei (refine with water)	水飞	*shui fei*	water-grinding	A technique to reduce medicinal substances into fine particles by repeatedly grinding them in water.
Skipping pulse	促脉	*cu mai*	skipping pulse	A relatively fast pulse that is broken up by regular pauses.
Slippery pulse	滑脉	*hua mai*	slippery pulse	A pulse that feels smooth and flowing. It feels smooth and rounded and slides away from pressure when pressed.
Slow pulse	迟脉	*chi mai*	slow pulse	A pulse with three or less beats per respiration.
Small Intestine	小肠	*xiao chang*	small intestine	Connecting to the Stomach and Large Intestine, the Small Intestine absorbs nutrients from food.
Small pulse	小脉	*xiao mai*	small pulse	A fine and well-defined pulse. Same as fine pulse.
Small spoon	钱匕	*qian bi*		A small spoon that contains approximately 1.5-1.8 grams of powdered herbs.
Soggy pulse	濡脉	*ru mai*	soggy pulse	A pulse that is fine and floating.
Sores	疮疡	*chuang yang*	sore	An inclusive term for skin lesions, boils, ulcers, carbuncles and furuncles.
Spleen	脾	*pi*	spleen	The Spleen governs the transportation and transformation of food, controls blood, and dominates muscle. It connects with the Stomach, opens to the mouth, and represents the earth element.
Spontaneous sweating	自汗	*zi han*	spontaneous sweating	Spontaneous perspiration, especially after only mild physical activities, is an indication of *wei* (defensive) *qi* deficiency.
Steaming bones sensation	骨蒸	*gu zheng*	steaming bone	A Kidney disorder characterized by heat and steaming sensations originating from the bone marrow. Accompanying symptoms include bodily coldness in the mornings and warm sensations in the evenings, irritability, restlessness, disturbed sleep, red urine, low back pain, cold hands and feet, and warm palms and soles.

Glossary

Terminology	Chinese	Pinyin	Wiseman & Feng	Definition
Stifling sensation	闷	*men*	oppression	An oppressive and congested feeling in the chest that leads to difficulties in breathing deeply.
Stirred pulse	动脉	*dong mai*	stirred pulse	A forceful rapid slippery pulse.
Stomach	胃	*wei*	stomach	Connecting to the mouth through the esophagus, the Stomach receives and decomposes food to facilitate digestion and absorption.
Sudden turmoil	霍乱	*huo luan*	sudden turmoil	An acute disorder characterized by sudden onset of nausea, vomiting, and chest and abdominal pain. Generally occurring in summer and fall, it is usually caused by inappropriate diet, leading to dysfunction of the stomach and intestines.
Summer heat	暑	*shu*	summerheat	Summer heat is a yang pathogenic factor that occurs only in the summer, and is comprised of both heat and damp characteristics, including upward direction and dispersion. Clinical presentations of summer heat include excessive perspiration, thirst, shortness of breath, fatigue, elevated body temperature, heavy sensations in the extremities, poor appetite, and a feeling of congestion in the chest.
Superficial pulse	浮脉	*fu mai*	floating pulse	A pulse that is more pronounced at the superficial level. It can be easily felt with light finger pressure, but is easily obliterated by heavy pressure.
Supreme physician	太医	*tai yi*	supreme physician	Physicians that practice in the Imperial Palace to treat the royalties and their court members.
Surging pulse	洪脉	*hong mai*	surging pulse	A pulse that is broad, large and forceful at all three levels.
Sweaty head	头汗	*tou han*	sweating head	Head perspiration generally arises from heat affecting the upper and middle *jiaos*, possibly accompanied by irritability, thirst, a yellow tongue coating, and a rapid pulse.
Taiyang	太阳	*tai yang*	greater yang	First of six stages in the paradigm of yin and yang, identifying the degree of pathology of disease according to the *Shang Han Lun* (Discussion of Cold-Induced Disorders) text. It also names the level attributed to the Small Intestine and Urinary Bladder channels that travel throughout the body.
Taiyin	太阴	*tai yin*	greater yin	The fourth of six stages in the paradigm of yin and yang. This term describes the degree of pathology of disease according to the *Shang Han Lun* (Discussion of Cold-Induced Disorders) text. It also identifies the level attributed to the Spleen and Lung channels that travel throughout the body.
Tan (char to ash)	炭	*tan*		Charring at high temperature until the medicinal substances turn into ash. This method harmonizes and moderates therapeutic effects, reduces side effects, and potentiates the 'stop bleeding' properties of specific substances.
Tan yin (phlegm retention)	痰饮	*tan yin*	phlegm-rheum	Phlegm retention caused by accumulation of water and dampness, this may occur at various organs and tissues in the body, leading to different illnesses and clinical presentations.
Tight pulse	紧脉	*jin mai*	tight pulse	A pulse that is forceful and string-like.

Glossary

Terminology	Chinese	Pinyin	Wiseman & Feng	Definition
Tong bi (extremely painful obstruction)	痛痹	*tong bi*	painful impediment	One type of *bi zheng* (painful obstruction syndrome) characterized by cold. Similar to cold that is stationary and constricting, *tong bi* is distinguished by severe pain at a fixed location. This type of pain intensifies with exposure to cold, and is relieved by exposure to warmth.
Toxin	毒	*du*	toxin	A toxin is any substance that is potentially harmful to the body. 'Toxin' also describes a pathogenic factor that may cause illness either on the exterior or in the interior of the body. Clinical manifestations of toxicity include pus, abscesses, sores, ulcerations, swelling and inflammation.
Tu fa (vomiting)	吐法	*tu fa*	ejection	A method of treatment that induces emesis to eliminate phlegm, stagnant food, or toxic matters from the throat, chest and diaphragm, or epigastrium. Vomiting induces qi to move upwards and outwards to treat ingestion of poisonous substances, severe cases of food stagnation, sudden turmoil disorder with vomiting and diarrhea, mania and withdrawal caused by phlegm accumulation, and *zhong feng* (wind stroke) with phlegm accumulation.
Tuo zheng (abandoned syndrome)	脱证	*tuo zheng*	desertion pattern	Characterized by profuse sweating, cold extremities, open mouth and closed eyes, and urinary incontinence, this condition occurs when there is severe exhaustion of yin, yang, qi and blood.
Upper *jiao*	上焦	*shang jiao*	upper burner	The upper *jiao* represents the chest, and includes functions of the Heart and the Lung.
Urinary Bladder	膀胱	*pang guang*	bladder	The Urinary Bladder stores and excretes urine.
Uroschesis	癃闭	*long bi*	dribbling urinary block	A disorder in which there is little or no urination, brought about by any of the following: heat in the Urinary Bladder, Kidney yang deficiency, qi deficiency, qi stagnation, or body fluid deficiencies.
Wan bi (stubborn painful obstruction)	顽痹	*wan bi*	insensitive impediment	One type of *bi zheng* (painful obstruction syndrome) that generally occurs after chronic or repetitive injuries to the same areas, causing stiffness, numbness, and lack of mobility.
Warm epidemics	温疫	*wen yi*	warm epidemic	Contagious diseases characterized by heat, with clinical manifestations such as fever, headache, irritability, thirst, vomiting, and with or without sweating.
Water	水	*shui*	water	Water is one of the five elements, associated with winter, with the Kidney, downward movement, and the ability to store or accumulate.
Water and fluid stagnation	水液停滞	*shui ye ting zhi*		Obstructed flow of water and thick fluids in the body.
Weak pulse	弱脉	*ruo mai*	weak pulse	A deep and forceless pulse.
Wei (defensive) level	卫分	*wei fen*	defense aspect	The first of four levels affected by febrile infections. Heat attacking the *wei* (defensive) level is characterized by disorders of the Lung, with such symptoms as fever, headache, dry mouth, thirst, cough, and sore throat, and a red tongue, and superficial, rapid pulse.

Glossary

Terminology	Chinese	Pinyin	Wiseman & Feng	Definition
Wei (defensive) *qi*	卫气	*wei qi*	defense qi	A type of yang qi responsible for warming the exterior, nourishing the skin and muscles, circulating under the skin to prevent invasion by external pathogenic factors, and controlling the skin pores and perspiration. It is generated by the Spleen and Stomach from the essence of food, controlled by the Lung, and resides in the upper *jiao*.
Wei (roast)	煨	*wei*		To cook and parch by wrapping the herbs in wet cloth, paper, or mud, and heating this bundle in hot cinders until the coating has turned black or burned away. This method reduces toxicity or moderates the drastic actions of some herbs.
Wei bi (atrophic painful obstruction)	痿痹	*wei bi*	wilting impediment	One type of *bi zheng* (painful obstruction syndrome) caused by deficiency of the Liver and Kidney, with such presentations as atrophy, weakness and pain of the muscles and bones.
Wei qi ying xue bian zheng (defensive, qi, nutritive, blood differentiation)	卫气营血辨证	*wei qi ying xue bian zheng*	four aspect pattern identification	A system of differential diagnosis based on patterns of disharmony found in the *wei* (defensive) level, *qi* (energy) level, *ying* (nutritive) level or *xue* (blood) level.
Wei zheng (atrophy) syndrome)	痿证	*wei zheng*	wilting pattern	A condition involving decreasing muscle mass and physical strength of the extremities, especially the legs; generally caused by the concurrent presence of excess and deficiency factors.
Wen bing (warm disease)	温病	*wen bing*	warm disease	Acute illnesses caused by externally contracted heat factors: diagnosed and treated based on *Wei Qi Ying Xue Bian Zheng* (Defensive, Qi, Nutritive, Blood Differentiation) and *San Jiao Bian Zheng* (Triple Burner Differentiation).
Wen fa (warming)	温法	*wen fa*	warming	A method of treatment that warms the interior, dispels cold, restores yang, and unblocks channels and collaterals. Warming is usually used to treat the presence of cold affecting the normal functions of *zang fu* organs, or stagnation of cold blocking the channels and collaterals.
Wheezing and dyspnea	哮喘	*xiao chuan*	wheezing and panting	A disorder characterized by wheezing, dyspnea and hurried respiration.
Wind	风	*feng*	wind	Wind is a pathogenic factor that attacks the body through the pores. Wind is a yang pathogenic factor characterized by upward, outward dispersion. Clinical presentation of exterior wind includes headache, nasal obstruction, sore throat, aversion to wind and sweating.
Wind rash	风疹	*feng zhen*	wind papules	An infectious skin disorder commonly seen during winter and spring in children under five years of age. Generally caused by wind-heat attack, it is characterized by itching, rashes and wheals of various sizes.
Wiry pulse	弦脉	*xian mai*	wiry pulse	A pulse that feels like a string of a musical instrument. It has decreased flexibility, feels straight and long, like pressing a violin string.

Glossary

Terminology	Chinese	Pinyin	Wiseman & Feng	Definition
Wood	木	*mu*	wood	One of the five elements, wood represents the expansive energy of Spring, moving outward in all directions, and is associated with the Liver.
Wu shu (five transport) points	五输穴	*wu shu xue*	five transport points	Located below the knees and elbows, these points represent the growth of qi from small to large volume. Their name suggests images of the flow of water. It starts with only a small quantity in a *jing* (well), gushes out into a *ying* (spring), flows from shallow to deep as a *shu* (stream), traverses like a *jing* (river) through the continent, and finally unites with the *he* (sea).
Wu xin re (five-center heat)	五心热	*wu xin re*	vexing heat in the five hearts	A condition characterized by yin-deficient heat in which there is a warm sensation in the middle of the chest, palms and soles.
Xi (cleft) point	郄穴	*xi xue*	cleft point	"Accumulating" or "cleft" points represent the holes or crevices where circulating qi accumulates. There are a total of sixteen such points, one for each of the twelve regular channels, as well as the *yangqiao*, *yinqiao*, *yangwei* and *yinwei* channels.
Xi (wash)	洗	*xi*		To remove unwanted substances or odor with water.
Xia fa (draining downwards)	下法	*xia fa*	precipitation	A method of treatment that cleanses the Stomach and Intestines, induces defecation, and eliminates pathogenic accumulation from the body. This method is generally used to treat stagnant food, dry stools, cold accumulation, hot accumulation, blood stasis, phlegm stagnation, water stagnation, and parasitic infestation.
Xiao fa (reducing)	消法	*xiao fa*	dispersion	A method of treatment that dissolves and disperses hardness and nodules to treat accumulation and stagnation of various substances, such as food, qi, blood, phlegm, water, and parasites. Reducing may be used to treat a wide variety of illness due to various causes.
Xiao ke (wasting and thirsting)	消渴	*xiao ke*	dispersion-thirst	A pathological condition characterized by increased intake of water and food, increased frequency of urination, and decreased body weight.
Xing bi (mobile painful obstruction)	行痹	*xing bi*	moving impediment	One type of *bi zheng* (painful obstruction syndrome) caused by wind attacking the body. Similar to wind that is light and mobile, *xing bi* is characterized by pain in the upper body, specifically pain that travels from one area to another.
Xiong bi (painful obstruction of the chest)	胸痹	*xiong bi*	chest impediment	Characterized by feelings of chest congestion, pain and discomfort, this condition is usually caused by factors such as cold excess, yang deficiency, or phlegm stagnation.
Xuan yin (pleural effusion)	悬饮	*xuan yin*	suspended rheum	Accumulation of *yin* (invisible phlegm) in the chest and hypochondrium causing pain with coughing, breathing, and rotation of the trunk.
Xue (blood) level	血分	*xue fen*	blood aspect	*Xue* (blood) level refers to the fourth level of febrile infections. Heat attacking the *xue* level is characterized by disorders of the Heart and Liver, with such symptoms as high fever, anger, mania, various types of bleeding, delirium, convulsions and clenched jaws.

Glossary

Terminology	Chinese	Pinyin	Wiseman & Feng	Definition
Xue bi (blood painful obstruction)	血痹	*xue bi*	blood impediment	One type of *bi zheng* (painful obstruction syndrome) that is related to blood. Dull pain may be caused by blood deficiency and the inability to nourish the tendons and bones. Sharp pain is often related to blood stagnation blocking the channels and collaterals.
Xue lin (bloody dysuria)	血淋	*xue lin*	blood strangury	A urinary tract disorder characterized by the presence of blood or blood clots in the urine, and burning sensations and pain during urination. Accompanying symptoms may include fatigue, back pain, a pale red tongue, and a fine, rapid pulse. This condition is caused by damp-heat attacking the lower *jiao*, leading to bleeding and obstructed flow of qi and urine.
Ya (press)	轧	*ya*		To push or squeeze into small particles. This method increases the surface area and enhances extraction of active ingredients.
Yan (drown)	淹	*yan*		To soak or steep in water or other liquids.
Yan (grind)	研	*yan*	grinding	To reduce into small particles with a mortar and pestle. This method increases the surface area and enhances extraction of active ingredients.
Yang	阳	*yang*	yang	Yang is the complement to and opposite of yin. Anatomically, it represents the upper, posterior and exterior parts of the body. Physiologically, it represents body functioning, such as the energy level, rate of metabolism, and state of awareness. Pathologically, it represents disharmony or imbalance of body organs.
Yang (melt)	烊	*yang*		To dissolve or disintegrate in water or other liquids.
Yangming	阳明	*yang ming*	yang brightness	Second of the six stages in the paradigm of yin and yang, this term describes the degree of pathology of disease according to the *Shang Han Lun* (Discussion of Cold-Induced Disorders) text. It also identifies the level given the Stomach and Large Intestine channels that travel throughout the body.
Yangqiao (movement) channel	阳跷脉	*yang qiao mai*	yang springing vessel	Of the eight extraordinary vessels, this one pairs with *yinqiao* to maintain proper sleep cycles and control movement and balance.
Yangwei (linking) channel	阳维脉	*yang wei mai*	yang linking vessel	Of the eight extraordinary vessels, this one dominates the exterior in cooperation with *yinwei,* to balance yin and yang in the four extremities.
Ye (thick body fluid)	液	*ye*	humor	An inclusive term that describes body fluids of higher density, such as the fluid that lubricates the joints and moistens the bone marrow.
Yi (intellect)	意	*yi*	intellect	The ability to think, study, memorize, focus, understand, and all other cognitive activities. It resides in the Spleen. Therefore, excessive use of *yi* may consume the Spleen, and deficiency of the Spleen may interfere with the optimal performance of *yi* (intellect).

Glossary

Terminology	Chinese	Pinyin	Wiseman & Feng	Definition
Yin	阴	*yin*	yin	Yin is the complement to and opposite of yang. Anatomically, it represents the lower, anterior and interior parts of the body. Physiologically, it represents the substances of the body, such as blood, sweat, saliva and body fluids. Pathologically, it represents the disharmony or imbalance of body organs.
Yin (invisible phlegm)	饮	*yin*	rheum	*Yin* (invisible phlegm) is the by-product formed from stagnation of water and dampness. *Yin* is the less viscous form of *tan* (phlegm).
Yin shui (yin edema)	阴水	*yin shui*	yin water	A type of edema caused by yang qi deficiency, with generalized deficiency and cold manifestations such as cold hands and feet and loose stools.
Ying (nutritive) level	营分	*ying fen*	construction aspect	The *ying* (nutritive) level refers to the third of four levels of febrile infections. Heat attacking the *ying* level is characterized by disorders of the Heart, with such symptoms as fever, thirst, irritability, delirium, red tongue and fine, rapid pulse.
Ying (nutritive) *qi*	营气	*ying qi*	construction qi	The qi produced by Spleen and Stomach and circulates within blood vessels to nourish the entire body.
Ying (spring) point	荥穴	*ying xue*	spring point	"Gushing" or "spring" points are located in distal parts of the body; their name suggests that qi has begun to flow in larger quantity.
Yinqiao (movement) channel	阴跷脉	*yin qiao mai*	yin springing vessel	Of the eight extraordinary vessels, this one pairs with *yangqiao* to maintain proper sleep cycles and control movement and balance.
Yinwei (linking) channel	阴维脉	*yin wei mai*	yin linking vessel	Another of the eight extraordinary vessels: in cooperation with *yangwei*, this one dominates the interior; to balance yin and yang in the four extremities.
Yuan (source) point	原穴	*yuan xue*	source point	Known as "source" points, these are locations to which the qi of the organs flows and is retained. There are twelve such points, each representing a channel and an organ.
Yuan (source) *qi*	原气	*yuan qi*	source qi	The most basic and most important qi in the body, *yuan* (source) *qi* is derived prenatally from the *jing* (essence) of one's parents, and postnatally from the essence of food. It is distributed throughout the body to maintain health and well-being.
Zang (solid organ)	脏	*zang*	viscus	Solid organs of the body, including the Heart, Lung, Spleen, Liver and Kidney.
Zang du (solid organ toxin)	脏毒	*zang du*	visceral toxin	A condition caused by presence of toxin attacking the solid organ leading to dysentery with presence of dark black blood in the stools.
Zang fu	脏腑	*zang fu*	bowels and viscera	The general term for the five *zang* (solid) and six *fu* (hollow) organs.
Zang fu bian zheng (organ pattern differentiation)	脏腑辨证	*zang fu bian zheng*	organ pattern identification	A system of differential diagnosis based on patterns of disharmony of *zang* (solid) organs and *fu* (hollow) organs.

Glossary

Terminology	Chinese	Pinyin	Wiseman & Feng	Definition
Zang zao (restless organ)	脏躁	*zang zao*	visceral agitation	In middle-aged to geriatric women, this disorder is characterized by symptomology such as emotional instability, mental confusion, crying, episodes of extreme sadness or happiness, and increased sensitivity to stimulus.
Zao (dryness)	燥	zao	dryness	*Zao* (dryness) refers to the dry compacted stool, which feels hard upon abdominal palpation.
Zha (crush)	砸	*zha*		To reduce medicinal substances into particles by pounding. This method increases the surface area and enhances extraction of active ingredients.
Zheng (steam)	蒸	*zheng*	steam	A preparation method to heat the medicinal substances with steam. This method indirectly introduces heat and water to the herbs to alter the therapeutic effect or reduce toxicity.
Zheng (upright) *qi*	正气	*zheng qi*	right qi	A term that summarizes the positive strength generated by healthy functioning of the organs. In comparison to the pathogenic factors, *zheng* (upright) *qi* also represents one's immunity.
Zhi (fry with liquid)	炙	*zhi*	mix-frying	Stir-frying with liquid to improve effectiveness, enhance smell, or reduce side effects. Liquids used for frying include honey, grain-based liquor, vinegar, ginger juice, and salt water.
Zhi (prepared)	制	*zhi*	prepare	To process medicinal substances with different methods.
Zhi (will-power)	志	*zhi*	mind	A term that encompasses will-power and memory. Stored by the Kidney, *zhi* controls drive, determination, motivation, memory and will-power.
Zhong (central) *qi*	中气	*zhong qi*	center qi	The qi of the middle *jiao* represents the healthy functioning of the Spleen and Stomach to transport and transform food and nutrients.
Zhong feng (wind stroke)	中风	*zhong feng*	wind stroke	An acute disorder of semi- or un-consciousness, deviation of the eyes or mouth, hemiparalysis, and difficulty with speech. The cause of the illness is predominantly wind, but this may be accompanied by blood deficiency, phlegm, fire, or other pathogens.
Zhong qi (qi stroke)	中气	*zhong qi*	qi stroke	A condition characterized by stagnated or reversed flow of qi, caused by internal injuries, accumulation of dampness and phlegm, or imbalance of the seven emotions.
Zhou bi (generalized painful obstruction)	周痹	*zhou bi*	generalized impediment	One type of *bi zheng* (painful obstruction syndrome) characterized by generalized pain that also affects the bones and joints.
Zhu (boiling)	煮	*zhu*	boil	Cooking certain medicinal substances in boiling water or another medium to enhance the therapeutic effect or reduce toxicity.
Zhuo bi (fixed painful obstruction)	著痹	*zhuo bi*	fixed impediment	One type of *bi zheng* (painful obstruction syndrome) that often occurs when dampness affects specific, fixed areas. Similar to dampness that is heavy and sinking, *zhuo bi* is characterized by pain and swelling in the lower extremities.

Glossary

Terminology	Chinese	Pinyin	Wiseman & Feng	Definition
Zong (essential) *qi*	宗气	*zong qi*	ancestral qi	*Zong* (essential) *qi* is derived from air taken in by the Lung, and nutrients absorbed by the Spleen and Stomach. It functions to maintain proper ventilation of the Lung and circulation of the Heart.
Zuo yao (assistant herb)	佐药	*zuo yao*	assistant	The third of four guiding principles in herbal formulation: *Jun Chen Zuo Shi* (Chief, Deputy, Assistant, Envoy). This herb has three main functions: 1) it reinforces the effect of *jun yao* (chief herb) or *chen yao* (deputy herb) to treat the disease, or directly treats the secondary symptoms; 2) it counteracts the toxicity or minimizes the drastic effects of the *jun yao* (chief herb) or *chen yao* (deputy herb); and 3) it has an opposite effect as, but works in synergy with, the *jun yao* (chief herb) to treat the most serious and complex disorders.

Index

Words in bold indicate primary formula and chapter names.
Page numbers in **bold** indicate main entries.
Page numbers in ***bold italics*** indicate entries in Appendix or Glossary.

INDEX

Index

Index

Index

Index

Index

Index

Index

Index

Index

Index

Index

Index

Index

Index

INDEX

I

Index

Index

INDEX

Index

Index

Index

Index

Index

Index

Index

Index

Index

INDEX
I

Index

Index

Index

Index

Index

Index

INDEX

Index

Index

Index

Index

Index

Index

Index

Index

Index

Index

Index

Index

Index

Index

Index

Index

Index

Index

Index

Index

Index

Index

Index

Index

Index

Index

Index

Index

Index

Index

Index

Index

Index

Index

Index

Index

About the Authors

John K. Chen, Ph.D., Pharm.D., O.M.D., L.Ac.

Dr. John Chen actively participates in education, research and the frontiers of contemporary application of herbal medicine. In addition to developing professional continuing education seminars and serving as a senior lecturer through the widely-respected Lotus Institute of Integrative Medicine, Dr. Chen speaks at seminars and conferences for universities and local, state, national and international educational and professional organizations. A professor at the University of Southern California School of Pharmacy and numerous colleges/universities of traditional Chinese medicine, Dr. Chen is also a member of the Herbal Medicine Committee for the American Association of Acupuncture and Oriental Medicine (AAAOM) and an herbal consultant for the California State Oriental Medicine Association (CSOMA). A recognized authority on Chinese herbal medicine and western (allopathic) pharmacology, Dr. Chen has written extensively on Oriental medicine and alternative complementary/integrative medicine for professional publications, journals and texts, drawing on his wealth of specialty post-graduate training and experience in mainland China in herbology as applied in internal medicine, and on his doctoral degrees from the University of Southern California (USC) School of Pharmacy and South Baylo University of Oriental Medicine. An editorial board member for the peer-reviewed journal of the American Academy of Medical Acupuncture (AAMA), *Medical Acupuncture*, John Chen was also a board member of the 1999 *Los Angeles Times* Festival Honorary Committee and speaker on Herbal Medicine for the City of Los Angeles First Annual Festival of Health. Appearing in the Discovery Channel 1999 six-hour documentary on alternative and complementary medicine, Dr. Chen served as the expert resource on Traditional Chinese Medicine. He also was a guest speaker on herb-drug interactions in 1998 for the annual USC Bergen Brunswig convention, during which he addressed over 400 pharmacists and medical doctors. Dr. Chen maintains his consulting practice in Southern California.

Tina T. Chen, M.S., L.Ac.

Tina Chen is an active and respected educator in Oriental medicine and Chinese herbal medicine. In addition to lecturing on TCM Gynecology and Cosmetology across North America through the widely-respected Lotus Institute of Integrative Medicine, Ms. Chen is active on the faculty of South Baylo University of Oriental Medicine and has been an active contributor to professional journals and publications. She has served as Southern California Chair of the Education Committee for the California State Oriental Medical Association (CSOMA), and as an examiner for the California State License Exam for acupuncturists, and from 1996-2001 maintained private practice of acupuncture and herbal medicine through Chen's Clinic in La Puente, California. Her teaching and consulting is grounded in extensive post-graduate training in herbal medicine, and TCM gynecology and cosmetology in numerous hospitals in mainland China. This included concentrated training sponsored by the World Health Organization (WHO) in Guang-An-Men Hospital of Traditional Chinese Medicine, Beijing, in the People's Republic of China, specializing in internal medicine, acupuncture and gynecology; also intensive clinical training in internal medicine and gynecology at First Tien-Jin Hospital, People's Republic of China; and at An-Hui Hospital, People's Republic of China, advanced training in internal medicine. Tina Chen's expertise in translation includes serving as translation specialist for the International Association of Integrating East-West Medicine from 1996-2000, the 1996 Third Annual International Acupuncture and Massage Conference sponsored by the Acupuncture and Massage Institute of America, and the California State Association of Oriental Medicine (CSOMA) in 1990. Licensed by the Acupuncture Board in California, Tina Chen also holds certification from the World Health Organization in internal medicine and gynecology. A graduate of South Baylo University of Oriental Medicine, she also earned a B.A. from the University of California at Irvine School of Humanities, in East Asian Language and Literature. She maintains a consulting practice in Southern California.

About the Authors

Signe Beebe, D.V.M.

Dr. Signe Beebe is a graduate of the Purdue University School of Veterinary Medicine, and has practiced integrative medicine since 1995. She is certified in veterinary acupuncture, Chinese herbology, Chinese food therapy and veterinary tui-na by the Chi Institute of Chinese Veterinary Medicine and China National Society of TCVM, and has completed the certificate program in Canine Rehabilitation and Physical Therapy at the University of Tennessee. Dr. Beebe owns the Integrative Veterinary Center in Sacramento, California, where she combines conventional medical therapies with Chinese medicine. Dr. Beebe is an assistant editor and advisory board member of the American Journal of Traditional Chinese Veterinary Medicine (AJTCVM). She is the co-author of "Clinical Handbook of Chinese Veterinary Herbal Medicine", and she regularly lectures at scientific meetings in the US and internationally.

Michael Salewski, D.V.M

Dr. Michael Salewski is a graduate of the Virginia-Maryland Regional College of Veterinary Medicine. He currently practices in Carlton, Oregon at Hindsight Veterinary Care, which treats exclusively using the modalities of TCVM and chiropractic. He co-authored *Clinical Handbook of Chinese Veterinary Herbal Medicine* and is currently working on a book about equine chiropractic care.

Notes

Notes